PEDIATRIC
Ophthalmology and Strabismus

For Elsevier:
Executive Content Strategist: *Russell Gabbedy*
Content Development Specialist: *Poppy Garraway*
Content Coordinator: *Sam Crowe*
Project Manager: *Vinod Kumar*
Design: *Miles Hitchen*
Illustration Manager: *Jennifer Rose*
Illustrator: *Antbits Ltd*
Marketing Manager(s) (UK/USA): *Gaynor Jones/Carla Holloway*

This book is due for return on or before the last date shown below.

PEDIATRIC
Ophthalmology
and Strabismus

FOURTH EDITION

Creig S Hoyt, MD, MA
Emeritus Professor and Chair
University of California
San Francisco, CA, USA

David Taylor, FRCOphth, FRCS, DSc(Med)
Professor Emeritus
Paediatric Ophthalmology
Institute of Child Health
University College London;
Director, Examinations Programme
International Council of Ophthalmology
London, UK

For additional online content visit
expertconsult.com

Edinburgh   London   New York   Oxford   Philadelphia   St Louis   Sydney   Toronto   2013

ELSEVIER
SAUNDERS

© 2013, Elsevier Limited/All rights reserved.

First edition 1990
Second edition 1997
Third edition 2005

The right of Creig S Hoyt and David Taylor to be identified as author of this work has been asserted by him in accordance with the Copyright, Designs and Patents Act 1988.

Notices
Knowledge and best practice in this field are constantly changing. As new research and experience broaden our understanding, changes in research methods, professional practices, or medical treatment may become necessary.

Practitioners and researchers must always rely on their own experience and knowledge in evaluating and using any information, methods, compounds, or experiments described herein. In using such information or methods they should be mindful of their own safety and the safety of others, including parties for whom they have a professional responsibility.

With respect to any drug or pharmaceutical products identified, readers are advised to check the most current information provided (i) on procedures featured or (ii) by the manufacturer of each product to be administered, to verify the recommended dose or formula, the method and duration of administration, and contraindications. It is the responsibility of practitioners, relying on their own experience and knowledge of their patients, to make diagnoses, to determine dosages and the best treatment for each individual patient, and to take all appropriate safety precautions.

To the fullest extent of the law, neither the Publisher nor the authors, contributors, or editors, assume any liability for any injury and/or damage to persons or property as a matter of products liability, negligence or otherwise, or from any use or operation of any methods, products, instructions, or ideas contained in the material herein.

ISBN: 9780702046919
Ebook ISBN: 9781455737819

ELSEVIER your source for books, journals and multimedia in the health sciences
www.elsevierhealth.com

Working together to grow libraries in developing countries
www.elsevier.com | www.bookaid.org | www.sabre.org

ELSEVIER   BOOK AID International   Sabre Foundation

The publisher's policy is to use **paper manufactured from sustainable forests**

Printed in China
Last digit is the print number: 9 8 7 6 5 4 3 2 1

Contents

Contents

Video contents

Foreword

I was lucky in that the first edition of this book was published around the time I started my fellowship training in paediatric ophthalmology. It was then, and remains now, the most comprehensive, well-illustrated and authoritative work on the subject, and was an invaluable aid to a trainee new to the field. This new edition is a masterpiece of concision, and the editors have done a marvellous job in marshalling their international troupe of chapter authors to produce an updated version which stands comparison with any medical textbook. This is, above all, a practical work, designed to communicate relevant information to clinicians struggling with difficult clinical problems affecting children's eyes and vision. My own copy of the first edition is battered with use, and I have no doubt that my copy of this edition will suffer the same fate.

Michael P Clarke MA, MB, B Chir, DO, FRCS, FRCOphth
Head of Department of Ophthalmology
Consultant Ophthalmologist
Eye Department
Royal Victoria Infirmary
Newcastle-upon-Tyne, UK

There is an old African proverb "If you want to go fast, go alone. If you want to go far, go together." An extension of that might read "If you want to go very far, go with an outstanding group of the most accomplished people you can find." This new edition of *Pediatric Ophthalmology and Strabismus* represents the fulfillment of this advice. The two outstanding editors of this masterpiece, David Taylor and Creig Hoyt, have presented us with gifts of wisdom from a cast of over 100 of the most erudite and respected authorities representing all aspects of pediatric ophthalmology and strabismus. The third edition of *Pediatric Ophthalmology and Strabismus* was published seven year ago, and this field has been advancing at a blistering pace. As such, this, the fourth edition is a welcome and needed addition to our libraries and personal bookshelves. In addition to in-depth scholarly chapters on every conceivable aspect of pediatric ophthalmology and strabismus, there is an entire section, containing 34 chapters, that discuss those common practical problems clinicians face every day, for which ready answers are heretofore rarely outlined. In keeping with the explosion in digital technology, this book includes access to videography of many eye movement disorders—a most appropriate addition. This tour-de-force is not only the perfect reference book, but will make for an enjoyable and fulfilling cover-to-cover read.

Burton J Kushner MD
John W. And Helen Doolittle Professor
Department of Ophthalmology and Visual Sciences
University of Wisconsin
Madison, WI, USA

This book on *Pediatric Ophthalmology and Strabismus* is a real treasure, indeed a magnum opus. It is certainly a labour of love for the extremely experienced and seasoned authors, with a wealth of lifetime experience devoted to paediatric eye care. This book is very wide in its scope, yet up-to-date in all aspects.

The book covers basics of pediatric ophthalmology like growth and development, milestones, normative data and epidemiology. It has chapters on the aspects of history taking, examination, genetics and investigations. The book presents the disorders of the eye as a whole and deals with the individual systems involving the pediatric age group quite comprehensively. The aspects of strabismus, ocular motility and amblyopia have received a special attention. A nice innovation is the section on common practical problems in *pediatric ophthalmology and strabismus*, which deals with all the possible complaints that parents come up with. The chapters have been presented very well with a listing of contents, excellent tabulations, extensive photographic illustrations, line diagrams and references.

It must have been a gigantic task to get the contributions of so many authors to make up the 124 chapters and put them together in a lovely wholesome book which is an aesthetic delight. A must read book for all ophthalmologists and residents, more so for those with a special interest in pediatric ophthalmology.

Ashok K Grover MD (AIIMS),
MANMS, FRCS (Glasgow) FIMSA, FICO
Awarded Padma Shri by the President of India
Past President
All India Ophthalmological society
Chairman
Department of Ophthalmology
Sir Ganga Ram Hospital
Chief Executive Officer (CEO)
Vision Eye Centres, Siri Fort Road and Patel Nagar
New Delhi, India

This quality book on *Pediatric Ophthalmology and Strabismus*, now in its fourth edition, deserves to rank among the great textbooks in ophthalmology.

Based on Taylor and Hoyt's third edition of *Pediatric Ophthalmology and Strabismus*, this edition embraces the new knowledge that has emerged in the eight years since their last publication in 2004. It further details the evolving understanding of genetics and embryology in ophthalmology and reviews recent advances in ocular imaging and electrophysiological studies. It draws attention to systemic implications of ocular presentations. The completely revised strabismus section is enhanced with a concise but comprehensive summary of surgical techniques and complications.

Both Professors David Taylor and Creig Hoyt, in addition to their contributions to the practice of pediatric ophthalmology and clinical research, bring a background of neurology and neurophysiology to their role as editors. Their editing, in addition to their personal contributions, does justice to the distinguished contributions of multiple expert authors. The text is enhanced by outstanding clinical photos, illustrations, tables, on-line videos and core references. A constancy of style and presentation adds to the pleasure of study.

This book deserves a place, not only in the medical libraries of universities, but in the hands of ophthalmologists and pediatricians and all those aware that ocular anomalies in childhood can have relevance to adult presentations and disorders.

Frank A Billson
Emeritus Professor
Department of Ophthalmology
University of Sydney
Director
Sight For Life Foundation
Sydney, NSW
Australia

Preface

More than with previous editions of this book we have been questioned, entertained, criticized, but on occasions, encouraged by our friends and colleagues about undertaking this 4th edition. We have heard, "Aren't books dead?," "Why put so much work into a new edition?," "What is wrong with the 3rd edition?," "Who will buy it?," "Medical books become so outdated so quickly, is it really worth it?," "Aren't you guys supposed to be retired?" Except for the last query, we too have seriously pondered all of these issues. We recognize the many challenges to producing a useful, accurate textbook in this period of dramatic innovation but diminishing resources. Nonetheless, we believe that with the combination of concise, up-to-date, and authoritative contributions provided by our expert collaborators and the insight and expertise of our Elsevier editorial team this new edition successfully meets these complex challenges.

While writing this preface we Googled "death of the book" and were informed that there were 272 000 000 matches available after 0.16 seconds of search. Thought-provoking? Without a doubt. Discouraging? Perhaps, but perhaps not. We both still enjoy teaching students and trainees. We admit that we are struck by how ubiquitous computers and tablet devices are in the lecture hall and seminar room. They commonly outnumber print books. Certainly, print books are less frequently purchased by today's physicians-in-training than in our distant era of training. Testimony about this change in reading material was dramatically provided by Amazon who, in April 2011, reported that it sold 105 e-books for every 100 print books. We note that Amazon is not a neutral observer of this phenomenon as it developed and sells one of the major e-platforms and aggressively promotes e-books on its website. In any case, there is evidence to suggest that there is a place for both print and e-book versions of medical textbooks. In a recent assessment of the use of print and electronic medical textbooks Ugaz and Resnick (J Med Libr Assoc 2008; 96: 145–7) concluded:

1. Convenience, remote access, ability to search within the text favored e-books, but
2. For reading large segments of the text the print book was preferred.

Some of you will be reading this in a print version while others will be looking at it on one of the e-platforms on which the text is available. We are extremely grateful that our publishers, Elsevier Ltd, were bold and wise in their suggestion, indeed insistence, that this edition of our book be made available in both print and electronic formats. Moreover, they have committed the resources necessary to make each format available in the highest quality. We believe "the book" is not dead, but it is certainly changing. In partnership with Elsevier we have attempted to change this 4th edition to meet the needs of current and future readers. Other changes include an active website where readers can view and download videos and an extensive photographic library. Throughout the text a video-camera icon can be seen in the margin. In the web version of the text readers can see surgical and clinical videos related to that portion of the text. Readers will also note that only selected references are printed at the end of each chapter in the hard copy. Three or four core references are highlighted for the reader. A complete list of references can be found on the website. The website also provides a means for us to update material in the future as scientific advancements dictate. A traditional textbook this edition is not.

In the 17th century the French satiric moralist, La Bruyere, asserted that, "We came too late to say anything which has not been said already." Surely, he was not speaking of medical knowledge. The short half-life of biomedical information is well recognized if, at times, exaggerated. Most of the chapters for the third edition were written in 2004. Since then there have been significant advances in our understanding of the genetic and molecular biologic mechanisms responsible for childhood retinal and corneal disorders. Although the last decades saw neurophysiology play a central role in major advances in eye care in children, the next decades will surely see genetics at the center of most new advances. Changing details of tumor biology have promoted advancements in the treatment of retinoblastoma, rhabdomyosarcoma, and hemangioma. Careful prospective treatment trials of amblyopia have challenged previous ideas about treatment modalities, duration of treatment and expected outcomes. The expanding epidemic of the multihandicapped blind child in the developed world challenges pediatric ophthalmologists to better understand visual cortex physiology and plasticity in order to provide knowledgeable counsel to parents and teachers. The surgical techniques used to remove cataracts in children are undergoing refinement and improvement; the postoperative optical correction continues to be a challenging obstacle being actively investigated by several authorities in the field. These and many other new and evolving issues in the diagnosis and management of visual disorders in children are discussed in detail in this edition. In the past medicine endorsed blood letting, astrology, and urine charts. Mindful of this, every effort has been made to exclude from this edition not only outdated information but also what might pass for historical curiosities.

A textbook of this breadth cannot be undertaken without a cadre of unique experts who are not only recognized as legitimate authorities in their fields of interest but also are gifted communicators of their expertise. We are fortunate to have engaged 129 coauthors with these skills for this edition. We asked many of them to write a masterful, up-to-date, well-focused, definitive but compressed chapter amplified by new and instructive illustrations. We asked our coauthors to write each chapter from the point of view of not only their knowledge of the field but also their personal experience. C. S. Lewis while Professor of English Literature at Magdalene College, Cambridge said, "We read to know we are not alone." We wanted you, the reader, to know that you are not alone as you seek information in this book. The authors are your consultants who have extensive experience with the problems described in this book.

Our coauthors have not only succeeded in fulfilling their mandate, but have exceeded it by providing some of the most engaging and provocative narratives about childhood visual disorders. We were thrilled to read their manuscripts as they were submitted to us. We learned much from each of the authors and considered it a privilege to be the first to read their treatises. Our debt to these colleagues is profound and enduring. We thank them for their contributions and their willingness to actively assist in the details of the demanding editorial process. We believe the resulting text succeeds in being definitive and comprehensive, but also highly readable. Its detail does not prevent it from being quickly searched for specific information. We resisted the temptation to expand to a multivolume text not only because of the resulting increase in cost, but also in the belief that a single volume text is more versatile and would be used not just in a library or office but also in the clinic and classroom.

Once again, Elsevier has provided us with the expertise and resources necessary to make the process of completing a project of this scope not only manageable but intellectually rewarding. We are especially indebted to Poppy Garraway who was, like a good physician, always affable, available, and extremely able. For several months we contacted her several times daily with a myriad of quandaries and queries. Unfailingly, she responded quickly with sage solutions and reassurances. Vinod Kumar, Project Manager, based in Chennai, answered our numerous questions immediately, charmingly and seemingly oblivious to the numerous time zones that separated us. Russell Gabbedy quietly but efficiently steered the project forward through the labyrinthine structures of a large publishing conglomerate with much more on its corporate plate than disorders of children's eyes. We thank them and all their colleagues.

Despite the peripatetic nature of much of our lives we both spent our more than thirty years as pediatric ophthalmologists in a single institution. The Children's Hospital at Great Ormond Street and the University of California San Francisco provided us with the opportunity to care for children with a wide range of visual problems but also the facilities, staff, and resources to ensure that the care we could provide would be uncompromised. The clinical staff, our professional colleagues, and, most especially, our students supported and stimulated us throughout those three decades. We fear that along the way we have not sufficiently expressed our gratitude to them. As inadequate as it may be, we wish to recognize their essential contributions to this book. Those years of busy clinics and long surgical lists were demanding but never routine, dull, or boring. We feel extremely fortunate to have been able to work in such rewarding environments with so many talented individuals dedicated to the care of the children.

In 1977, one of our mentors, Professor William Hoyt, insisted that we should meet. We did. As a result we have shared a rewarding professional relationship and an even more rich and nuanced personal friendship that has taken us from the deserts of Oman to the jungles of Malaysia. Thank you, Bill! To Anna and Debbie we offer our feeble apologies for missed meals, interrupted conversations, and the endless sound of computer keys at all hours of the day and night.

Creig S Hoyt and David Taylor

List of Contributors

Nisha R Acharya MD, MS
Associate Professor
Department of Ophthalmology
F.I. Proctor Foundation
University of California
San Francisco, CA, USA

James F Acheson MRCP, FRCOphth
Consultant Ophthalmologist
National Hospital for Neurology and Neurosurgery
London, UK

Gillian G W Adams FRCS (Ed), FRCOphth
Consultant Ophthalmic Surgeon
Strabismus, Neuro ophthalmology and Paediatric Services
Moorfields Eye Hospital
London, UK

John R Ainsworth MD, FRCOphth
Paediatric Ophthalmologist,
Retinoblastoma and Paediatric Ophthalmology Service
Birmingham Children's Hospital
Birmingham, UK

Alejandra de Alba Campomanes MD, MPH
Assistant Professor
Department of Ophthalmology and Pediatrics
University of California, San Francisco;
Director
Pediatric Ophthalmology and Adult Strabismus
San Francisco General Hospital
San Francisco, CA, USA

Louise E Allen MBBS, MD, FRCOphth
Consultant Paediatric Ophthalmologist and Associate Lecturer
Addenbrooke's Hospital
Cambridge University Hospital NHS Foundation Trust
Cambridge, UK

Jane Louise Ashworth BMBCh, FRCOphth, PhD
Consultant Paediatric Ophthalmologist
Manchester Royal Eye Hospital
Manchester, UK

Pinar Aydin MD, PhD
Professor of Ophthalmology and Neuro-ophthalmologist
International Council of Ophthalmology, Head of Ethics Committee
Kavaklidere, Ankara, Turkey

Valérie Biousse MD
Cyrus H. Stoner Professor of Ophthalmology
Professor of Ophthalmology and Neurology
Emory University School of Medicine
Altanta, Georgia, USA

Susmito Biswas FRCOphth
Consultant Ophthalmologist and Honorary Clinical Lecturer
Manchester Royal Eye Hospital
Manchester, UK

Graeme C M Black DPhil, FRCOphth
Professor
Honorary Consultant in Genetics and Ophthalmology
Genetic Medicine
University of Manchester;
Central Manchester University Hospitals NHS Foundation Trust
St Mary's Hospital
Manchester, UK

Joanna Black MD FRANZCO
Visiting Medical Specialist
Women's and Children's Hospital
Adelaide, SA, Australia

Thomas M Bosley MD
Professor
Department of Ophthalmology
King Saud University
Riyadh, Saudi Arabia

Richard J C Bowman MA, MD, FRCOphth
Consultant Ophthalmologist
Great Ormond Street Hospital
London, UK

John A Bradbury FRCS, FRCOphth
Consultant Ophthalmologist
Bradford Royal Infirmary
Bradford, UK

Michael C Brodsky MD
Professor of Ophthalmology & Neurology
Mayo Clinic
Rochester, MN, USA

John L Brookes BSc (Hons), MBBS (Lond), FRCOphth
Consultant Ophthalmic Surgeon
Glaucoma Service
Moorfields Eye Hospital
London, UK

Donal Brosnahan MB, BCh, BAO, FRCOphth
Consultant Ophthalmologist
Department of Ophthalmology
Royal Victoria Eye and Ear Hospital
Dublin, Ireland

J Raymond Buncic MD, FRCSC
Professor
Department of Ophthalmology
University Of Toronto
Toronto, Ontario, Canada

Jayne E Camuglia MBBS, BSc
Registrar, Department of Ophthalmology
Royal Children's Hospital
Brisbane, QLD, Australia

Susan M Carden MBBS, FRANZCO, FRACS, PHD
Senior Lecturer
Department of Paediatrics
Royal Children's Hospital
University of Melbourne
Victoria, Australia

Ingele Casteels MD, PhD
Department of Ophthalmology
University Hospitals Leuven
Leuven, Belgium

Kara Cavuoto MD
Clinical Fellow
Pediatric Ophthalmology & Strabismus
Bascom Palmer Eye Institute
University of Miami Miller School of Medicine
Miami, FA, USA

Wilma Y Chang BSc
Research Assistant
Department of Ophthalmology and Visual Sciences
University of British Columbia
Vancouver, BC, Canada

Michael P Clarke MA, MB, BChir, DO, FRCS, FRCOphth
Consultant Paediatric OphthalmologistNewcastle Eye CentreNewcastle
Upon Tyne Hospitals
NHS Foundation TrustReader in Ophthalmology
Newcastle UniversityNewcastle upon Tyne, UK

J Richard O Collin MA, MB, BChir, FRCS, FRCOphth
Consultant Surgeon
Adnexal Service
Moorfields Eye Hospital, and Honorary
Consultant Ophthalmic Surgeon
Great Ormond Street Hospital for Children
London, UK

John Crompton MBBS, FRANZCO, FRACS
Clinical Associate Professor
Head of Eye Department,Institute of Ophthalmology & Visual Science, University of Adelaide/Royal Adelaide
Hospital, Adelaide, SA, Australia

Emmett T Cunningham Jr MD, PhD, MPH
Director
The Uveitis Service
Department of Ophthalmology
California Pacific Medical Center
San Francisco, CA;
Adjunct Clinical Professor of Ophthalmology
Stanford University School of Medicine
Stanford, CA, USA

Kenneth K Dahn BS
Research Assistant
Smith-Kettlewell Eye Research Institute
San Francisco, CA, USA

Susan H Day MD
Chair and Program Director
Department of Ophthalmology
California Pacific Medical Center
San Francisco, CA, USA

Hélène Dollfus MD, PhD
Professor of Medical Genetics
Center for Rare Diseases in Genetic
Ophthalmology (CARGO)
Avenir INSERM Laboratory
University Hospital of Strasbourg
Strasbourg, France

Gordon N Dutton MD, FRCS Ed Hon, FRCOphth
Emeritus Professor of Vision Science
Glasgow Caledonian University
Honorary Senior Research Fellow
University of Glasgow
Glasgow, Scotland

Clive Edelsten MA, MRCP, FRCOphth
Consultant Ophthalmologist
Department of Rheumatology
Great Ormond Street Hospital
London, UK

James Elder MBBS, FRANZCO, FRACS
Consultant Ophthalmologist
The Royal Children's Hospital
Pediatric Ophthalmologist
Royal Women's Hospital;
Associate Professor
Department of Paediatrics
University of Melbourne
Melbourne, VIC, Australia

John S Elston BSc, MD, FRCOphth
Consultant Ophthalmologist in Paediatrics &
Neuro-ophthalmology
John Radcliffe Hospital Oxford
Senior Lecturer
University of Oxford
Oxford, UK

Alistair R Fielder FRCP, FRCS, FRCOphth
Professor Emeritus of Ophthalmology
Department of Optometry & Visual Science
City University
London, UK

David R Fitzpatrick MD
Professor
Medical & Developmental Genetics
MRC Human Genetics Unit
Western General Hospital
Edinburgh, UK

Anne B Fulton MD
Professor
Department of Ophthalmology
Harvard Medical School;
Senior Associate in Ophthalmology
Children's Hospital
Boston, MA, USA

Peter J Francis MD, PhD, FRCOphth
Associate Professor
Casey Eye Institute
Oregon Health and Science University
Portland, OR
USA

Douglas Frederick MD
Professor
Dept of Ophthalmology
Stanford University School of Medicine
Stanford, CA, USA

Charlotte L Funnell MBChB, MRCOphth,
FRCOphth
Consultant Ophthalmologist
Epsom and St Helier University Hospitals
Sutton, UK

Brenda L Gallie MD, FRCSC, OOnt
Professor of Molecular Genetics
Medical Biophysics, and Ophthalmology
University of Toronto;
Director Retinoblastoma Program
Hospital for Sick Children;
Senior Scientist
Ontario Cancer Institute
University Health Network
Toronto, ON, Canada

Megan M Geloneck MD
Resident Physician
Richard S. Ruiz Department of Ophthalmology &
Visual Sciences
The University of Texas at Houston
Houston, TX, USA

Clare E Gilbert MB, ChB, FRCOphth, MD, MSc
Professor of International Eye Health
International Centre for Eye Health
Faculty of Clinical Research
London School of Hygiene & Tropical Medicine
London, UK

Glen A Gole MD, FRANZCO
Professor of Ophthalmology
Discipline of Paediatrics and Child Health
Royal Children's Hospital
University of Queensland
Brisbane, QLD, Australia

William V Good MD
Senior Scientist
Smith Kettlewell Eye Research Institute
San Francisco, CA, USA

Irene Gottlob MD
Professor of Ophthalmology
Ophthalmology Group
University of Leicester
Leicester, UK

Philip G Griffiths FRCS, FRCOphth
Consultant Ophthalmologist, Honorary Clinical
Senior Lecturer
Eye Department, Royal Victoria Infirmary
Newcastle upon Tyne, UK

John R B Grigg MB, BS, FRANZCO, FRACS
Head, Discipline of Ophthalmology
Sydney Medical School;
Save Sight Institute
The University of Sydney;
Consultant Ophthalmologist
Sydney Eye Hospital;
Visiting Medical Officer
Sydney Children's Hospital Network (Randwick
and Westmead)
Sydney, NSW, Australia

Christopher J Hammond MA, MD, MRCP,
FRCOphth
Frost Professor of Ophthalmology and NIHR
Senior Research Fellow
Departments of Ophthalmology and Twin Research
& Genetic Epidemiology
King's College London
St Thomas' Hospital
London, UK

Nancy N Hanna MD
Summa Health System
Akron, OH, USA

Georgina Hall
Genetic Medicine
Central Manchester University Hospitals
NHS Foundation TrustSt Mary's Hospital
London, UK

Ronald M Hansen PhD
Instructor
Harvard Medical School
Research Associate in Ophthalmology
Children's Hospital
Boston, MA, USA

Yoshikazu Hatsukawa MD
Eye Department,
Osaka Medical Centre
Murodo-cho, Izumi, Japan

Hugo W A Henderson BA, MBBS, FRCOphth
Oculoplastic Fellow
Adnexal Service
Moorfields Eye Hospital
London, UK

Richard W Hertle MD, FAAO, FACS, FAAP
Chief of Pediatric Ophthalmology
Director
Children's Vision Center
Akron Children's Hospital
Akron, OH;
Professor
Department of Surgery
College of Medicine
Northeast Ohio Medical College
Rootstown, OH, USA

Göran D Hildebrand BM, BCH, MD, MPhil, DCH, FEBO, FRCS, FRCOphth
Consultant Ophthalmic Surgeon
Royal Berkshire Hospital
Reading
King Edward VII Hospital
Windsor, UK

Melanie Hingorani, MA, MBBS, MD, FRCOphth
Consultant Paediatric Ophthalmologist
Moorfields Eye Hospital
London, UK

Peter Hodgkins BSc (Hons), MBChB, FRCS, FRCOpth
Consultant Ophthalmologist
Southampton University Hospitals NHS Trust
Honorary Clinical Lecturer
Southampton Eye Unit
Southampton, UK

David A Hollander MD, MBA
Assistant Clinical Professor of Ophthalmology
Jules Stein Eye Institute, David Geffen School of Medicine at UCLA
Greater Los Angeles VA Medical Center
Los Angeles, CA, USA

Gerd S Holmström MD, PHD
Professor
Department of Neuroscience/Ophthalmology
Uppsala University
Uppsala, Sweden

Graham E Holder BSc, MSc, PhD
Consultant Electrophysiologist
Director of Electrophysiology
Moorfields Eye Hospital
London, UK

Creig Hoyt MD, MA
Emeritus Professor and Chair
University of California
San Francisco, CA, USA

David G Hunter MD, PhD
Ophthalmologist-in-Chief
Boston Children's Hospital;
Professor of Ophthalmology
Harvard Medical School
Boston, MA, USA

Robyn V Jamieson MBBS(Hons I), PhD, FRACP
Associate Professor
Sydney Medical School
University of Sydney
Sydney, NSW, Australia

James E Jan MD, FRCPCC
Clinical Professor
Senior Research Scientist Emeritus
Department of Pediatrics
Division of Child Neurology
University of British Columbia
Vancouver, BC, Canada

Saurabh Jain MBBS, MS, FRCOphth
Consultant Ophthalmic Surgeon
Department of Ophthalmology
Royal Free London NHS Foundation Trust
London, UK

Hanne Jensen MD, PhD
Associate Professor
Eye Clinic
Kennedy Center
Glostrup, Denmark

Rohit Jolly MBBS, BSc (Hons)
Foundation Year 2 House Officer
Department of Ophthalmology
Royal Free Hospital
London, UK

Robert C Kersten MD
Professor of Clinical Ophthalmology
University of California San Francisco
UCSF Department of Ophthalmology
San Francisco, CA, USA

Phillippe Kestelyn MD, PhD, MPH
Professor in Ophthalmology
Head and Chair Department of Ophthalmology
Ghent University Hospital
Ghent, Belgium

Peng T Khaw PhD, FRCS, FRCP, FRCOphth, FRCPath, FSBiol, FARVO, FMedS
Professor of Glaucoma and Ocular Healing
Director of National Biomedical Research Centre
Moorfields Eye Hospital and UCL Institute of Ophthalmology;
Director of Research and Development
Moorfields Eye Hospital;
Programme Director of Eyes and Vision Theme
UCL Partners Academic Health Science Centre
UCL Institute of Ophthalmology
London, UK

Stephen P Kraft MD, FRCSC
Professor
Department of Ophthalmology and Vision Sciences
Faculty of Medicine
University of Toronto
Toronto, ON, Canada

Burton J Kushner MD
John W. And Helen Doolittle Professor
Department of Ophthalmology and Visual Sciences
University of Wisconsin
Madison, WI, USA

Robert A Kyle MD, MACP
Professor of Medicine,
Laboratory Medicine & Pathology
Mayo Clinic
Rochester, MN, USA

Scott R Lambert MD
R. Howard Dobbs Professor of Ophthalmology
Emory University
Chief of Ophthalmology
Children's Healthcare of Atlanta at Egleston
Atlanta, GA, USA

G Robert LaRoche MD, FRCSC
Professor of Ophthalmology
Department of Ophthalmology and Visual Sciences
Dalhousie University
Halifax, NS, Canada

David Laws FRCS, FRCOphth, DO
Consultant Ophthalmologist
ABM University Health Board
Swansea, UK

Andrew G Lee MD
Professor of Ophthalmology, Neurology, and Neurological Surgery
Weill Cornell Medical College, New York, NY;
Chair Department of Ophthalmology
The Methodist Hospital, Houston, TX;
Clinical Professor
Department of Ophthalmology & Visual Sciences
The University of Texas Medical Branch
Galveston, TX;
Baylor College of Medicine
Houston, TX, USA

Alki Liasis MD
Consultant Electrophysiologist
Clinical and Academic Department of Ophthalmology
Great Ormond Street Hospital
London, UK

Christopher Lloyd MBBS, DO, FRCS, FRCOphth
Consultant Paediatric Ophthalmologist
Manchester Royal Eye Hospital;
Hon. Senior Lecturer
University of Manchester
Manchester, UK

Christopher J Lyons MB, FRCS, FRCOphth, FRCS(C)
Professor
Department of Ophthalmology and
Visual Sciences
University of British Columbia;
Head
Department of Ophthalmology
BC Children's Hospital
Vancouver, BC, Canada

Caroline J MacEwen MD, FRCS, FRCOphth, FFSEM
Professor
Department of Ophthalmology
Ninewells Hospital and University of Dundee
Dundee, UK

D Luisa Mayer PhD
Clinical Assistant Professor
Department of Ophthalmology
Harvard Medical School
Associate Professor
Department of Specialty and Advanced Care
New England College of Optometry
Boston, Massachusetts

Craig A McKeown MD
Professor of Clinical Ophthalmology
Bascom Palmer Eye Institute
University Of Miami Miller School of Medicine
Miami, FL, USA

Stephen D McLeod MD
Professor and Chair
Department of Ophthalmology
University of California San Francisco
San Francisco, CA, USA

Michel Michaelides MBBS, MD, FRCOphth
Consultant Ophthalmic Surgeon and Clinical
Senior Lecturer
Genetics, Medical Retina and Paediatric Services
Moorfields Eye Hospital and UCL Institute of
Ophthalmology
London, UK

Joel M Miller PhD
Principle Investigator and Senior Scientist
Smith-Kettlewell Eye Research Institute
San Francisco, CA, USA

Neil R Miller MD
Professor of Ophthalmology, Neurology and
Neurosurgery
Frank B. Walsh Professor of Neuro-Ophthalmology
Johns Hopkins Medical Institutions
Baltimore, MD, USA

Nor Fadhilah Mohamad MBBS(UM),
MMed(Ophth)(UM),
Honorary Clinical Fellow
Department of Neuro-Ophthalmology
National Hospital for Neurology and Neurosurgery
Richard Desmond Children's Eye Centre
Moorfields Eye Hospital
London, UK

Hans Ulrik Møller PhD
Consultant Pediatric Ophthalmologist
Eye Clinic
Viborg Hospital
Viborg, Denmark

Anthony T Moore MA, FRCS, FRCOphth
Duke Elder Professor of Ophthalmology
Institute of Ophthalmology
University College, London
Honorary Consultant Ophthalmologist
Moorfields Eye Hospital and Hospital for Children
Great Ormond Street
London, UK

Andrew Alan Myles Morris MB, BCh, PhD,
FRCPCH
Consultant in Paediatric Metabolic Medicine
Genetic Medicine
Central Manchester University Hospitals NHS
Foundation Trust
Manchester, UK

Robert Morris MRCP, FRCS, FRCPOphth
Consultant Ophthalmic Surgeon
Southampton Eye Unit
Southampton General Hospital
Southampton, UK

Anne Moskowitz OD, PhD
Research Associate
Department of Ophthalmology
Children's Hospital and Harvard Medical School
Boston, MA, USA

Nancy J Newman MD
LeoDelle Jolley Professor of Ophthalmology,
Professor of Ophthalmology and Neurology,
Instructor in Neurological Surgery
Emory University School of Medicine
Atlanta, Georgia;
Lecturer in Ophthalmology
Harvard Medical School
Boston, MA, USA

Ken K Nischal FRCOphth
Professor of Ophthalmology,
School of Medicine
University of Pittsburgh;
Division Chief
Department of Pediatric Ophthalmology,
Strabismus and Adult Motility
UPMC Eye Center and Children's Hospital of
Pittsburgh
Pittsburgh, PA, USA

Hiroshi Nishikawa MA, MD, FRCS (Plast)
Clinical Lead
Department of Plastic Surgery
Birmingham Children's Hospital
Birmingham, UK

Michael O'Keefe FRCS
Professor of Paediatric Ophthalmology
University College Dublin;
Eye Department
The Children's University Hospital
Dublin, Ireland

Maria Papadopoulos MB, BS, FRACO
Consultant Ophthalmic Surgeon
Glaucoma Service
Moorfields Eye Hospital
London, UK

Manoj V Parulekar MS, FRCS
Consultant Ophthalmologist
Birmingham Children's Hospital
Birmingham, UK

Cameron F Parsa MD
Associate Professor of Ophthalmology
Department of Ophthalmology and Visual Sciences
University of Wisconsin School of Medicine and
Public Health-Madison
Madison, Wisconsin, USA

Carlos E Pavesio FRCOphth
Consultant Ophthalmic Surgeon
Moorfields Eye Hospital
Professorial Unit
City Road
London, UK

Derrick C Pau MD
Clinical Fellow
Department of Ophthalmology
The Methodist Hospital
Houston, TX, USA

Evelyn A Paysse MD
Professor
Departments of Ophthalmology and Pediatrics
Baylor College of Medicine
Houston, TX, USA

Erika Mota Pereira MD
Visiting Assistant Professor of Ophthalmology,
University of Texas Southwestern Medical Center,
Dallas, Texas, USA,
Consultant Pediatric Ophthalmologist
Federal University of Minas Gerais
Belo Horizonte, Minas Gerais, Brazil

Rachel Fiona Pilling MB, ChB, MA, FRCOphth
Consultant Ophthalmologist
Department of Ophthalmology
Bradford Teaching Hospitals
NHS Foundation Trust
West Yorkshire, UK

Venkatesh Prajna MD
Chief Consultant
Cornea & External Eye Diseases
Aravind Eye Hospital & Postgraduate Institute of
Ophthalmology
Madurai, Tamilnadu, India

Frank A Proudlock PhD
Lecturer
Ophthalmology Group
University of Leicester
Robert Kilpatrick Clinical Sciences Building
Leicester Royal Infirmary
Leicester, UK

Anthony Quinn MBChB, FRANZCO, FRCOphth,
DCH
Consultant Ophthalmic Surgeon
Royal Devon & Exeter Hospital
Exeter, UK

Graham E Quinn MD, MSCE
Professor
The Children's Hospital of Philadelphia
University of Pennsylvania School of Medicine
Philadelphia, PA, USA

Jugnoo S Rahi MSc, PhD, MRCPCH, FRCOphth
Professor of Ophthalmic Epidemiology,
Honorary Consultant Ophthalmologist,
Director, Ulverscroft Vision Research Group
Institute of Child Health, UCL and Institute of
Ophthalmology, UCL
Great Ormond Street Hospital NHS Trust
London, UK

Muralidhar Rajamani MD, DNB, MRCO, FRCS
Consultant
Department of Pediatric Ophthalmology and
Strabismus
Aravind Eye Hospital & Postgraduate Institute of
Ophthalmology
Madurai, Tamilnadu, India

M Ashwin Reddy MA, MB, BChir, MD, FRCOphth
Consultant Ophthalmologist
Barts and The London NHS Trust
Moorfields Eye Hospital (Honorary)
Great Ormond St Hospital (Honorary)
London, UK

Michael X Repka MD
Professor of Ophthalmology & Pediatrics
Wilmer Ophthalmological Institute
Johns Hopkins Hospital
Baltimore, MD, USA

Bruce Richard MBBS, MS, FRCS (Plast)
Consultant Plastic Surgeon
Department of Plastic Surgery
Birmingham Children's Hospital
Birmingham UK

Jack Rootman MD, FRCSC
Professor
Department of Ophthalmology and Visual Sciences
Department of Pathology and Laboratory Sciences
University of British Columbia
Vancouver, BC, Canada

Isabelle M Russell-Eggitt MA, MB, BChir, DO, FRCS, FRCOphth
Consultant Paediatric Ophthalmologist
Clinical and Academic Department of Ophthalmology
Great Ormond Street Hospital for Children
London, UK

Tina Rutar MD
Assistant Professor of Ophthalmology and Pediatrics
Department of Ophthalmology
University of California San Francisco
San Francisco, CA, USA

Luis Carlos Ferreira de Sá MD
Consultant Ophthalmologist
University of Sao Paulo
Sao Paulo, Brazil

Reecha Sachdeva MD
Ophthalmology Resident
Cole Eye Institute
Cleveland Clinic
Cleveland, OH, USA

Mandeep Sagoo MB, PhD, MRCOphth
Senior Lecturer in Ophthalmology
UCL Institute of Ophthalmology;
Honorary Consultant Ophthalmic Surgeon
Medical Retina Service
Moorfields Eye Hospital;
Honorary Consultant Ophthalmic Surgeon
St. Bartholomew's and Royal London Hospitals
London, UK

Alison Salt MBBS, MSc, DCH, FRCPCH, FRACP
Consultant Paediatrician
Great Ormond Street Hospital for Children
Foundation Trust Honorary Senior Lecturer
Institute of Child Health, UCL
London, UK

Alvina Pauline D Santiago MD
Clinical Associate Professor
University of the Philippines College of Medicine
Sentro Oftalmologico Jose Rizal
Manila, Philippines

Richard L Scawn FRCOphth
Specialist Registrar
Moorfields Eye Hospital NHS Trust
London, UK

Alan B Scott MD
Senior Scientist
The Smith-Kettlewell Eye Research Institute
San Francisco, CA, USA

Jay Self BM FRCOphth PhD
Research and Clinical Fellow University of Southampton Manchester Royal Eye Hospital Manchester, UK

Panagiotis Sergouniotis MD, PhD
Clinical Research Fellow
UCL Institute of Ophthalmology and Moorfields Eye Hospital
London, UK

Ankoor S Shah MD, PhD
Department of Ophthalmology
Boston Children's Hospital
Instructor of Ophthalmology
Harvard Medical School
Boston, MA, USA

Akbar Shakoor MD
Uveitis fellow
F.I. Proctor Foundation
University of California
San Francisco, CA, USA

Carol L Shields MD
Associate Director
Wills Eye Hospital
Philadelphia, PA, USA
USA

Jerry A Shields MD
Director
Wills Eye Hospital
Philadelphia, PA, USA

Ian Simmons FRCOphth, FRANZCO
Consultant Paediatric Ophthalmologist
Eye Department
Leeds Teaching Hospitals NHS Trust
St James University Hospital
Leeds, UK

John J Sloper MA, DPhil, FRCS, FRCOphth
Consultant
Strabismus and Paediatric Service
Moorfields Eye Hospital
London, UK

Martin P Snead MA, MD, FRCS, FRCOphth
Consultant Vitreoretinal Surgeon
Vitreoretinal Service
Cambridge University NHS Foundation Trust
Cambridge, UK

Carlos R Souza-Dias MD
Titular Professor
Department of Ophthalmology
Faculty of Medical Sciences
Santa Casa de Misericórdia de São Paulo
São Paulo, Brazil

Jane C Sowden PhD
Professor in Developmental Biology and Genetics
UCL Institute of Child Health
University College London
London, UK

Lynne Speedwell FCOptom, MSc (Health Psychol), DCLP, FAAO, FBCLA
Head of Optometry
Great Ormond Street Hospital for Children;
Principal Optometrist
Moorfields Eye Hospital
London, UK

Jay M Stewart MD
Associate Professor of Clinical Ophthalmology
University of California
San Francisco, CA, USA

Yoshiko Sugiyama MD
Department of Ophthalmology
Kanazawa University Hospital
Graduate School of Medical Science
Kanazawa, Ishikawa, Japan

Aileen Sy BA
Medical Student
University of California
San Francisco, CA, USA

Naomi Tan MBChB, BSc(hons)
Ophthalmology Specialist Trainee
London Deanery
London, UK

David Taylor FRCOphth, FRCS, DSc(Med)
Professor Emeritus
Paediatric Ophthalmology
Institute of Child Health
University College London;
Director, Examinations Programme
International Council of Ophthalmology
London, UK

Robert H Taylor FRCOphth, FRCS (Glasg)
Consultant Ophthalmologist
Eye Department
York Hospital
York, UK

Dorothy A Thompson PhD
Consultant Clinical Scientist in Visual Electrophysiology
Clinical and Academic Department of Ophthalmology
Great Ormond Street Hospital for Children NHS Trust
London, UK

Chris Timms DBO (T)
Head Orthoptist
Moorfields Eye Hospital
London, UK

Elias I Traboulsi MD
Director
Head of the Department of Pediatric
Ophthalmology
Center for Genetic Eye Diseases
Cleveland Clinic's Cole Eye Institute;
Professor of Ophthalmology
Director
Ophthalmology Residency Program
Chairman
Department of Graduate Medical Education
Cleveland Clinic Lerner College of Medicine
Case Western Reserve University
Cleveland, Ohio, USA

Stephen John Tuft MD, MChir, FRCOphth
Director
Corneal Service
Moorfields Eye Hospital
London, UK

Lawrence Tychsen MD
Professor
Ophthalmology and Visual Sciences, Pediatrics,
Anatomy and Neurobiology
St. Louis Children's Hospital at Washington
University Medical Center
St. Louis, MO, USA

Jimmy M Uddin MD, BOPSS, FRCOphth
Consultant Ophthalmic Surgeon
Moorfields Eye Hospital
London, UK

Alain Verloes MD, PhD
Head
Clinical Genetics Unit
Hôpital Robert Debre
Paris, France

**Anthony J Vivian BSc, (Hons) MBBS, FRCS,
FRCOphth**
Consultant Ophthalmic Surgeon
Addenbrookes Hospital
Cambridge and West Suffolk Hospital
Bury St Edmunds, Suffolk, UK;
East Anglia Regional Clinical Governance Director
(Ophthalmology) Audit Lead Consultant
Addenbrookes Hospital
Cambridge, UK

Patrick Watts MBBS, MS, FRCS, FRCOphth
Consultant Paediatric Ophthalmologist
University Hospital of Wales
Cardiff, UK

David R Weakley MD
Professor of Ophthalmology and Pediatrics
University of Texas Southwestern Medical Center
Dallas, Texas, USA

David Webb MD, FRCP, FRCPath, MRCPH
Consultant Haematologist
Great Ormond Street Children's Hospital
London, UK

James Edmond Wraith FRCPCH
Professor of Paediatric Inherited Metabolic Disease
Manchester Academic Health Science Centre
Department of Genetic Medicine
St. Mary's Hospital
Manchester, UK

**Patrick Yu-Wai-Man BMedSci, MBBS, PhD,
FRCOphth**
MRC Clinician Scientist,
Mitochondrial Research Group
Institute of Genetic Medicine
Newcastle University;
Academic Clinical Lecturer
Department of Ophthalmology
Royal Victoria Infirmary
Newcastle Upon Tyne, UK
Institute of Child Health, UCL

Epidemiology and the world-wide impact of visual impairment in children

Jugnoo S Rahi • Clare E Gilbert

This chapter aims to familiarize the reader with important issues about epidemiological studies of childhood visual impairment (VI), severe visual impairment (SVI), or blindness (Boxes 1.1 and 1.2), and to synthesize current data to provide a global picture of the frequency, causes, and prevention of VI and blindness in childhood.

Specific issues in the epidemiological study of visual impairment in childhood

- Case definition. A standard definition applicable to all children remains problematic, see below.
- Rarity. Visual impairment and blindness in childhood are uncommon, posing challenges in achieving sufficiently large and representative populations of affected children to allow precise and unbiased study.
- Complex, multidisciplinary management. For a complete picture, information must be sought from the professionals involved in the care of VI or blind children which, in the case of the many children with additional

---

Box 1.1

What is ophthalmic epidemiology?

This science comprises "studies upon people."[1] It has both its origins and its applications in clinical and public health ophthalmology.

Through primary research or by secondary approaches, e.g. systematic literature review and meta-analysis, epidemiology aims to:

- shed light on the causes and natural history of ophthalmic disorders
- enhance the accuracy and efficiency of diagnosis
- improve the effectiveness of treatment and preventive strategies
- provide quantitative information for planning of services

Box 1.2

Epidemiological reasoning

This is based on the following principles:

- The occurrence of disease is not random, rather a balance between causal and protective factors
- Disease causation, modification, and prevention are studied by systematic investigation of populations to gain a more complete view than can be achieved by studying individuals
- The inference that an association between a risk factor and a disease is causal requires:

1. the exclusion of chance, bias, or confounding as alternative explanations for the observed association
2. evidence of a consistent, strong, and biologically plausible association, in temporal sequence, preferably exhibiting a dose–response relationship

---

non-ophthalmic impairments or chronic disorders, adds further layers of complexity.

- Lifecourse approach. A key concept in child health is to understand the biological, environmental, and lifestyle/social influences at all life stages (preconceptional, prenatal, perinatal, and childhood), and how they combine to set and change health trajectories. Lifecourse approaches are increasingly applied to the study of VI and eye disease affecting children or originating in childhood.[2]
- Long-term outcomes. In all pediatric disciplines, developmental issues must be taken into account. Assessment of meaningful outcomes, such as final visual

function or educational placement, requires long-term follow-up.

- Ethics. Issues of proxy consent (by parents) and children's autonomy regarding treatment decisions increasingly impact on participation in ophthalmic epidemiological research.

Framing the question

Clinical or service provision decisions are ideally based on "three-part questions" that incorporate the reference population (e.g. children under 2 years with infantile esotropia), the risk factor or the intervention (e.g. prematurity or strabismus surgery), and the outcomes (e.g. parent-reported improvement in cosmesis and objective improvement in alignment and stereopsis). The focus of the question – be it frequency, causes, or treatment/prevention of disease – determines the study design required to address it, e.g. a descriptive, cross-sectional prevalence survey, or an analytical study (either observational, e.g. case–control or cohort studies, or interventional, e.g. randomized controlled trials).

Who is a visually impaired child?

The affected child, their parents, teacher, social worker, rehabilitation specialist, paediatrician or ophthalmologist are likely to have differing, but equally valid answers to this question. Comparisons within and between countries, and over time, of the frequency, causes, treatment, or prevention of VI require a standard definition. The WHO taxonomy (Table 1.1) is based on the acuity in the better seeing eye measured with optical correction if worn. It has been adopted for epidemiological research, despite the difficulties of measuring visual acuity in very young children and those unable to cooperate with formal testing. Thus, there is a need for a better classification applicable to children of different ages that allows

consideration of other visual parameters (near acuity, visual fields, binocularity, and contrast sensitivity).

Two measures are recognized in clinical practice and research:

1. *Functional vision* assesses the child's ability to undertake tasks of daily living dependent on vision, such as navigating independently.
2. *Vision-related quality of life* elicits the child's and/or parent's view of the gap, caused by the visually impairing disorder and its therapy, between the child's expectations and experiences in terms of his/her physical, emotional/psychological, cognitive, and social functioning.[3] Interest in patient-reported outcomes and experience measures (PROMs and PREMs) coincides with the WHO International Classification of Functioning Disability and Health, a classification and measurement of health, and health-related domains which has underpinned the understanding of disability.[4]

Measuring the frequency and burden of childhood visual impairment

The analogy of running a bath (or filling a water trough) illustrates measures of frequency and burden of disease. The speed at which water runs into the bath equates with *incidence*, i.e. the rate of new occurrence of disease in a given population over a specified time. For example, in the UK the annual incidence of congenital cataract is 2.5 per 10 000 children aged 1 year or less.[5]

The degree to which the bath (or water trough) is full at a particular moment is a balance between how fast water is running in and how much is running out. How full the bath is equates to the *prevalence* of disease, i.e. the proportion of a given population that has the disease or condition of interest at a particular time. This reflects both the incidence of the disease and its duration, i.e. new cases of disease added to the population while others are "lost" from it through death, cure, or migration. For example, the UK prevalence in childhood of amblyopia with an acuity of worse than logMAR 0.3 (6/12, 20/40, 0.5) is about 1%.

The comparison of how a bath is "valued" more broadly, versus a shower or staying unwashed, might equate with measures of utility such as disability-adjusted life years (DALYs) or quality-adjusted life years (QALYs).[6] These incorporate morbidity and mortality into a single measure used to compare states of health within and between countries to identify economic and other priorities in health-care provision. Throughout the world, blindness is categorized in the penultimate class of increasingly severe disability.[6]

Prevalence and incidence data provide complementary information. Incidence identifies and monitors trends which reflect changing exposure to risk factors, or emergence of new exposures and in provision of services and planning research, e.g. estimating likely recruitment time in clinical trials. Prevalence measures the magnitude of the problem in a community at a given time. It helps allocate resources and can be used to evaluate services, if changes in prevalence can be attributed solely to changes in outcome or duration of disease as a result of treatment rather than changes in underlying incidence.

Table 1.1 – World Health Organization classification of levels of visual impairment

Level of visual impairment	Visual acuity in better eye with optical correction (if worn)
Slight, if acuity less than 6/7.5	6/18 or better.
Visual impairment (VI)	Worse than 6/18 up to 6/60
Severe visual impairment (SVI)	Worse than 6/60 up to 3/60 (logMAR 1.1 to 1.3)
Blind (BL)	Worse than 3/60 (worse than logMAR 1.3) to no light perception or Visual field < 10 degrees around central fixation

Note: Adapted with permission from World Health Organization (WHO). International Statistical Classification of Diseases and Health Related Problems. 10th Revision. Geneva, World Health Organisation, 1992.
MAR, minimum angle of resolution.
6/7.5 = logMAR 0.10, 20/25, 0.86/18 = logMAR 0.48, 20/60, 0.33
6/60 = logMAR 1.0, 20/200, 0.10
3/60 = logMAR 1.3, 20/400, 1.31.0

Sources of information on frequency and causes of visual impairment

There are a number of sources of epidemiological information about childhood VI or blindness but, in reality, only a few are available in most countries. This explains the currently incomplete picture of VI (Box 1.3).

1. Population-based prevalence studies. These represent a source of precise, representative estimates of burden (frequency) and causes. However, the few studies of whole populations of children with VI, such as the British national birth cohort studies,[2,7] need to be very large (a study of 100 000 children is required in an industrialized country to identify 100 to 200 children with VI or blindness): costly and difficult!
2. Population-based incidence studies. Studies of incident (newly occurring) VI are even more difficult, explaining their rarity.[11]
3. Special needs/disability registers, surveys, and surveillance. Specific studies and/or surveillance systems[8] or registers of childhood disability can provide information about VI, but it is important to recognize the potential for bias as certain visually impaired children may be over-represented in these sources, e.g. those with multiple impairment.
4. Studies of schools for the visually impaired. In developing countries, studies of children in special education provide information on causes, but these are biased because many blind children (particularly with additional non-ophthalmic impairments) may not have access to special education. With other facility-based studies, e.g. from clinic attendees, the intrepretation of findings and their extrapolation to other populations needs to take these biases into account.
5. Visual impairment registers. These exist in many industrialized countries but, if registration is voluntary and not a prerequisite for accessing special educational or social services, then registers may be incomplete as well as biased, reflecting differences in parental preferences and professionals' practices regarding registration of eligible children.[9]
6. Visual impairment teams. Increasingly children in industrialized settings are evaluated by multidisciplinary teams and if these serve geographically defined populations then useful information can be derived.
7. Disorder-specific ophthalmic surveillance schemes. Research on uncommon ophthalmic conditions in children can be undertaken using population-based surveillance schemes, such as those for congenital anomalies (e.g. for study of anophthalmia or microphthalmia) or adverse drug reactions (e.g. for study of visual loss with vigabatrin), although under-ascertainment can occur. The national active surveillance scheme comprising all senior ophthalmologists in the United Kingdom (the British Ophthalmological Surveillance Unit)[10] studied uncommon disorders, including the first population-based incidence study of SVI and blindness in childhood:[11] an important model for pediatric ophthalmic epidemiological research.
8. Community-based rehabilitation programs. In many developing countries rehabilitation of blind and VI children within the community is being adopted. Where the size of the catchment population is known, it is possible to estimate prevalence and obtain population-based data on causes.[12]
9. Surveillance using key informants. In many developing countries, it may be possible to identify key community and religious leaders, health-care workers, and others who know their communities well and thus can identify children believed to have VI or ocular disorders. This can be combined with the size of the population at risk, to estimate prevalence and population-based data on the causes.[12]

Irrespective of the sources, there is often under-ascertainment, or biased ascertainment. In industrialized countries, families from socially disadvantaged groups or ethnic minorities are less likely to participate in research about health services for visually impaired children,[13] especially in research on rare disorders, when a large and representative sample must be achieved for optimal analysis. Multiple sources gain a more complete and reliable picture of causes and frequency of childhood VI.

Impact of visual impairment

Visual impairment in childhood impacts on all aspects of the child's development and shapes the adult they become, influencing employment, social prospects, and lifelong opportunities[14-16] (see Chapter 59). Although the prevalence and incidence of VI are lower in children than in adults, the years of life lived with VI ("person-years of visual impairment") are considerable. Personal and social costs are important, but difficult to measure (see Box 1.3). The economic costs of childhood VI in terms of loss of economic productivity are considerable: a quarter of the costs of adult blindness in some countries.[17] One estimate of the annual cumulative loss of gross national product attributable to childhood VI was US$ 22 billion.[17]

Visual impairment in the broader context of childhood disability

Multiple impairments

In industrialized countries, at least half of all severely visually impaired and blind children also have motor, sensory, or learning impairments or chronic systemic disorders which confer further disadvantages for them in development, education, and independence.[11,18] It is probably a smaller proportion in developing countries, reflecting the relative importance of conditions such as ophthalmia neonatorum which result in purely ocular disease, and high mortality rates among children who are blind from conditions which are associated with multiple impairment, such as congenital rubella syndrome, cortical blindness following cerebral malaria, meningitis, or cerebral tumors.

For research on etiology and interventions, and for provision of services, there are two populations:

1. Children with isolated VI.
2. Children with VI and other impairments or systemic diseases.

Mortality

Children with visual impairment are more likely to die than other children. In developing countries[19,20] about half of children who become blind die within a few years[19,20] because the causes of their blindness are often associated with high mortality e.g., vitamin A deficiency, measles infection. In the industrialized world, visually impaired children also may have higher mortality rates: in the UK, 10% of VI children die in the year following diagnosis of SVI or blindness.[11]

Prevalence studies of older visually impaired children exclude those who died before school age and underestimate the true frequency thus providing a biased picture.

Groups at high risk of visual impairment

In research and resource allocation VI is just one of many childhood disabilities. Certain children are at increased risk of visual loss: those of low birth weight, the socioeconomically deprived,[11] and those from ethnic minorities.[11] Because these higher risk groups are also less likely to participate in health services research,[14] there is selection bias by sociodemographic factors.

Frequency of childhood visual impairment and blindness

Prevalence

There is an association between prevalence of blindness in children and under-5 mortality rates (U5MRs) for a country, enabling this indicator to be used as a proxy for blindness rates in children.[21] In industrialized countries, where U5MRs are less than 20/1000 live births, the prevalence of blindness is approximately 3–4 per 10 000 children. In countries with U5MRs of >250/1000 live births (e.g. in sub-Saharan Africa), the prevalence of blindness is nearer 12–15 per 10 000 children. This reflects three factors:

1. Exposure to risks and potentially blinding conditions not found in affluent regions (e.g. vitamin A deficiency, cerebral malaria).
2. The occurrence of conditions adequately controlled elsewhere (e.g. measles infection through immunization).
3. Limited access to services and treatments which ameliorate disease progression (e.g. management of retinopathy of prematurity, ROP) or which restore visual function (e.g. high-quality management of cataract).

In 1999, at the launch of VISION 2020, there were an estimated 1.4 million blind children in the world (Table 1.2).[19] This figure was derived using U5MRs for 1994 in each country (i.e. reflecting the midpoint of the 16 years of childhood) and the child population of each country for 1999. The data in

Table 1.2 – Estimates of the prevalence and number of blind children by World Bank region in 1999 and in 2010

World Bank region	Estimates in 1999			Estimates in 2010			Change between 1999 and 2010	
	Child pop. (millions)	Previous estimate	Blind children	Child pop. (millions)	Previous estimate	Blind children	In child population (%)	In estimate of blind children (%)
EME+FSE	248	3.6	90 000	244	2.9	70 000	−1.6	−22.2
LAC	170	5.9	100 000	170	4.2	71 000	−0.2	−29.0
MEC	240	7.9	190 000	241	7.0	168 000	0.4	−11.6
China	340	6.2	210 000	340	3.4	116 000	0.1	−44.8
OAI	260	8.5	220 000	266	5.1	136 000	2.3	−38.2
India	350	7.7	270 000	345	8.1	280 000	−1.6	3.7
SSA	260	12.3	320 000	274	15.3	419 000	5.5	30.9
TOTAL:	1868	7.5	1 400 000	1880	6.7	1 260 000	0.6	−10.0

EME = Established Market Economies; FSE = Former Socialist Economies; LAC = Latin America and Caribbean; OAI = Other Asia and Islands; SSA = sub-Saharan Africa.
Note: Data for countries in EME and FSE regions have been combined as some countries changed their designation between 1999 and 2010.

Table 1.2 are presented by World Bank region, in which countries are grouped by socioeconomic status assessed by a composite of factors, such as maternal education level, which predict general child health and are associated with ophthalmic disease and visual impairment. The figures were revised in 2010 and, because of falling U5MRs, the estimate has fallen by 10% to 1.26 million (see Table 1.2).[20] However, the revised estimates show that the number of blind children in two World Bank regions has not decreased: in India the number of blind children has increased slightly despite a stable child population and in sub-Saharan Africa, where U5MRs are increasing and the child population continues to grow. The greatest change is in China: with a stable child population U5MRs have fallen over recent decades.

The prevalence of VI is not known for many world regions.[20,22] However, severe visual impairment (SVI) and blindness (BL) account for one-third of all levels of visual impairment. In industrialized countries, the combined prevalence of VI, SVI, and BL is about 10 to 22 per 10 000 children aged <16 years, while in some developing countries it is 30 to 40 per 10 000.[20,22]

Incidence

Estimates of the incidence of childhood VI are available for only a few countries (see Box 1.3). Using pooled data from Scandinavian VI registers, the annual incidence of VI, SVI, and BL combined was 0.8 per 10 000 individuals <9 years old in 1993.[23] From a population-based study in the UK, the annual age group-specific incidence was highest in the first year of life at 4.0 per 10 000, the cumulative incidence increasing to 5.3 per 10 000 by 5 years old, and to 5.9 per 10 000 by 16 years old.[11]

"Causes" of visual impairment

Understanding the relative importance of causes of VI, including comparisons between countries and within countries over time, has been enhanced by introduction of a dual taxonomy in which, for each child, the "anatomical site" affected is assigned together with etiological factors categorized according to the timing of their action.[24] This classification started in developing countries, now extended to research in industrialized countries,[11] and is shown in Table 1.3.

Variation by region and over time

Data from a variety of sources, collected or reclassified using this classification system in 1999, are presented in Tables 1.4 and 1.5. Most of the data from developing countries come from examining children in schools for the blind; from industrialized countries, mainly from blind registers. Lesions of the higher visual pathways, in the context of preterm birth, predominate in the wealthiest countries. Acquired conditions of childhood leading to corneal scarring predominate in the poorest countries.

Insufficient data on the causes of blindness in children have been published between 1999 and 2010 to allow re-analysis by region. However, the reduction in mortality and blindness in Asian countries may be attributable to the declining incidence of measles infection and vitamin A deficiency among pre-school-age children. Cataract is now the most important *avoidable* cause of childhood blindness in many regions (Table 1.6).

Table 1.3 – Classification of the causes of childhood visual impairment or blindness, according to the anatomical site(s) affected, and the etiological factors by their timing of action

Anatomical site(s) affected	Etiological factor(s) by timing of action
Whole globe and anterior segment	**Prenatal**
Microphthalmia/anophthalmia	Hereditary
Anterior segment dysgenesis	Autosomal recessive or autosomal
Coloboma – multiple sites	dominant
Others	X-linked
Glaucoma	Chromosomal
Primary	Mitochondrial
Secondary	Hypoxia/ischemia
	Infection
Cornea	Prenatal drug
Sclerocornea	Others
Keratomalacia	Presumed prenatal but factor
Other corneal scar	unknown
Dystrophy	**Perinatal + neonatal**
Lens	Hypoxia/ischemia
Cataract	Infection
Aphakia	Non-accidental injury
Subluxed	Others
	Presumed peri/neonatal but factor
Uvea	unknown
Anidiria	**Childhood**
Uveitis	
Coloboma – single site	Tumor
Retina	Nutritional
	Infection
Retinopathy of prematurity	Hydrocephalus/increased
Retinal and macular dystrophies	intracranial pressure
Albinism	Hypoxia/ischemia
Retinitis/neuroretinitis	Abusive trauma
Retinal detachment	Accidental injury
Retinoblastoma	Specific systemic disorders
Other	Presumed childhood but factor
Optic nerve	unknown
Hypoplasia	**Undetermined timing of insult**
Atrophy – primary or secondary	**and factors unknown**
Neuritis/neuropathy	
Others	
Cerebral/visual pathways	
Neurodegenerative disorders	
Hypoxic/ischemic encephalopathy	
Abusive head trauma	
Infection	
Structural abnormalities	
Tumor	
Other	
Other	
Idiopathic nystagmus	
High refractive error	

Note: Modified with permission from Gilbert C, Foster A, Negrel AD et al. Childhood blindness: a new form for recording causes of visual loss in children. Bull World Health Organ 1993; 71: 485–489.

The causes of visual impairment in children in a country reflect the prevailing balance between the biological, environmental, and social determinants of ophthalmic disorders and the strategies and resources available for their prevention or treatment. Hence the regional variations in the relative

Table 1.4 – Regional variation in the causes of blindness in children: anatomical sites affected (data for 1999)

| | Region | | | | | | | |
| | Wealthiest ◄ | | | | | | ► | Poorest |
Anatomical site affected	EME (% total)	FSE (% total)	LAC (% total)	MEC (% total)	China (% total)	India (% total)	OAI (% total)	SSA (% total)
Globe/ant. seg.	10	12	12	14	26	25	21	9
Glaucoma	1	3	8	5	9	3	6	6
Cornea	1	2	8	8	4	27	21	36
Lens	8	11	7	20	19	11	19	9
Uvea	2	5	2	4	1	5	3	5
Retina	25	44	47	38	25	22	21	20
Optic nerve	25	15	12	8	14	6	7	10
CVP and other	28	8	4	3	2	1	2	5
Total:	100	100	100	100	100	100	100	100

Ant. seg. = anterior segment; CVP = cerebral visual pathways; EME = Established Market Economies; FSE = Former Socialist Economies; LAC = Latin America and Caribbean; OAI = Other Asia and Islands; SSA = sub-Saharan Africa.
Note: Data for countries in EME and FSE regions have been combined as some countries changed their designation between 1999 and 2010.

Table 1.5 – Regional variation in the causes of blindness in children: etiological factors according to timing of action (data for 1999)

| | Region | | | | | | | |
| | Wealthiest ◄ | | | | | | ► | Poorest |
Timing of action	EME (% total)	FSE (% total)	LAC (% total)	MEC (% total)	China (% total)	India (% total)	OAI (% total)	SSA (% total)
Prenatal (definite)								
1. Hereditary	45	18	22	53	31	26	27	20
2. Intrauterine	7	6	8	2	0	2	3	3
Perinatal (definite)	24	28	28	1	2	2	9	6
Childhood (definite)	10	5	10	7	14	28	14	34
Unknown[a]	14	43	32	37	53	42	47	37
Total:	100	100	100	100	100	100	100	100

[a]Availabled data used for this table require classification as "unknown" of those disorders with presumed other "timing of action," e.g. congenital anomalies presumed to be of prenatal origin.
EME = Established Market Economies; FSE = Former Socialist Economies; LAC = Latin America and Caribbean; OAI = Other Asia and Islands; SSA = sub-Saharan Africa.
Note: Data for countries in EME and FSE regions have been combined as some countries changed their designation between 1999 and 2010.

importance of disorders (see Tables 1.4 and 1.5), although data from different sources or that using different case definitions may not be comparable.

The balance between risk factors and treatment or prevention accompanying economic and social development explains the major national trends. For example, in the industrialized world, ophthalmia neonatorum and other causes of corneal scarring have substantially diminished, while cerebral VI, ROP, and the inherited retinal dystrophies have emerged.[19] Congenital cataract remains an important cause of severe visual loss in many developing countries despite the recent marked improvement in visual outcomes in industrialized nations. The most notable recent change has occurred in the "middle income"

countries of Latin America and Eastern Europe where ROP is now the commonest cause of child blindness.[25] This trend is likely to continue in rapidly developing economies in Asia as they expand neonatal care services with increased survival of premature babies.

Other sources of variations in the pattern of causes

The relative importance of disorders will also vary by the level of visual impairment studied. Albinism or congenital cataract are relatively more important if children with all levels of VI

Table 1.6 – Estimates of the number of blind children and the major avoidable causes for a population of 10 million people, by level of economic development

Economic development	Blindness prevalence estimate[a] (/10,000)	Estimates for a total population of 10 million		Major avoidable causes
		Children (N)	Blind children (N)	
High	3–4	2 million	600–800	• Cataract • Glaucoma • Retinopathy of prematurity • Non-accidental injury
Medium	5–7	3 million	1500–2100	• Retinopathy of prematurity • Cataract • Glaucoma
Low	8–11	4 million	3200–4400	• Cataract • Corneal scarring from VADD; ON; measles • Retinopathy of prematurity in urban area • Glaucoma
Very low	12–15	5 million	6000–7500	• Corneal scarring from VADD; ON; measles; HTER • Cataract • Glaucoma

[a]Estimate derived from association with under-5 mortality rates.
HTER = harmful traditional eye remedies; ON = ophthalmia neonatorum; VADD = vitamin A deficiency disorders.

(VI, SVI, or BL) are studied, whereas ROP and cerebral VI are more important if only those with blindness are studied.

Patterns may differ according to whether prevalent cases or incident cases are studied, as survival may be important. Studies restricted to secondary school-age children with established visual loss (prevalent cases) underestimate the number of children with disorders that are also associated with early mortality, e.g. corneal scarring from acute vitamin A deficiency or cerebral visual impairment associated with extremely low birth weight or severe systemic diseases. Such bias may be particularly important in countries with limited access to specialist health care.

None of the data presented in this chapter include children with visual impairment due to undiagnosed or uncorrected refractive error alone. This represents a large population of children – possibly 2 million currently – the majority of whom live in Southeast Asia and have uncorrected myopia (see Box 1.3).

Prevention of visual impairment and blindness in childhood: "VISION 2020"

Children are a priority in "VISION 2020,"[19,21] the global initiative for the elimination of avoidable VI led by the World Health Organization and the International Agency for Prevention of Blindness. As the causes of visual loss vary, country-specific plans and programs are being developed and implemented, based on the priorities for prevention, treatment, and rehabilitation. All programs combine disease control strategies with the development of human resources, technology, and infrastructure. In many countries these programs will interface with existing broader governmental initiatives to improve the health of children or improve services for children with disability.

Reducing blindness due to ROP requires improvement of neonatal services to prevent severe disease from occurring, as well as secondary prevention through screening and early treatment.

Strategies to prevent visual impairment or blindness can be categorized as follows:

1. Primary prevention: to prevent the occurrence of ophthalmic disease. Examples include high-coverage rubella immunization programs, preventing congenital rubella-associated cataract; vitamin A supplementation and measles immunization to prevent corneal scarring; face washing and antibiotic treatment to control trachoma; avoidance of ocular teratogens in pregnancy through public and antenatal health education campaigns; excellent neonatal care to prevent ROP, and preconceptional genetic counseling of families with genetic eye disease.

2. Secondary prevention: to prevent established ophthalmic disease from causing serious visual loss. This includes both screening and surveillance to ensure early detection and prompt referral of children with suspected ophthalmic disease, such as cataract.[26] It incorporates prompt specialist treatment by pediatric ophthalmic professionals of disorders such as ROP, cataract, glaucoma, and amblyopia.

3. Tertiary prevention: to maximize residual visual function and prevent disadvantage due to established visual impairment. This includes interventions aimed at improving visual function even though good vision cannot be achieved, e.g. management of late presenting childhood cataract or optical iridectomy for late presenting central corneal scarring. Tertiary prevention also incorporates assessing and meeting special educational needs, providing low vision aids, mobility

training, and other rehabilitation programs, and providing social support and services to families of children with irreversible visual loss.

The role of ophthalmic professionals in prevention of childhood visual impairment

Ophthalmic professionals have a key role in the implementation of preventive strategies through their ability to:

- Provide specialist pediatric ophthalmic care, combining medical, surgical, and optical management of specific disorders.
- Educate and train non-ophthalmic colleagues, such as pediatricians, family doctors, optometrists or community eye workers, to ensure implementation of programs aimed at early detection and prompt referral of children suspected of having eye diseases, those at high risk for VI, those with major neurodevelopmental disorders, or those with a family history of blinding eye disease.
- Contribute to multidisciplinary VI teams, ideally combining medical, educational, and social service professionals, to ensure comprehensive and coordinated care of all VI children and their families.
- Contribute to assessments of special educational needs and certification of eligibility for special services, in particular notification to VI registers.
- Contribute to monitoring VI in their population.
- To participate in epidemiological research that strengthens the evidence base for practice and policy.

Selected further reading

Rothman KJ, Greenland S, Lash TL, editors. Modern Epidemiology, 3rd ed. Philadelphia: Lippincott Williams & Wilkins; 2008.

Sackett DL, Haynes RB, Guyatt GH, Tugwell P. Clinical Epidemiology, 2nd ed. Boston: Little Brown; 1991.

References

1. Last JM and International Epidemiological Association. A Dictionary of Epidemiology, 2nd ed. New York: Oxford University Press; 1988: xiv, 141.
2. Rahi J, Cumberland PM, Peckham CS. Myopia over the lifecourse: prevalence and early life influences in the 1958 British birth cohort. Ophthalmology 2011; 118: 797–804.
3. Eiser C, Morse R. Quality-of-life measures in chronic diseases of childhood. Health Technol Assess 2001; 5: 1–157.
4. World Health Organization. International Classification of Functioning, Disability and Health (ICF). Geneva: World Health Organization; 2001.
5. Rahi JS, Dezateux C. Measuring and interpreting the incidence of congenital ocular anomalies: lessons from a national study of congenital cataract in the UK. Invest Ophthalmol Vis Sci 2001; 42: 1444–1448.
6. Murray CJ, Lopez AD. Regional patterns of disability-free life expectancy and disability-adjusted life expectancy: global Burden of Disease Study. Lancet 1997; 349: 1347–1352.
7. Pathai S, Cumberland PM, Rahi JS. Prevalence of and early-life influences on childhood strabismus: findings from the Millennium Cohort Study. Arch Pediatr Adolesc Med 2010; 164: 250–257.
8. Mervis CA. Aetiology of childhood vision impairment, metropolitan Atlanta, 1991–93. Paediatr Perinatal Epidemiol 2000; 14: 70–77.
9. Bunce CW, Xing A, Wormald W. Causes of blind and partial sight certifications in England and Wales: April 2007-March 2008. Eye (Lond) 2010; 24: 1692–1699.
10. Foot B, Stanford M, Rahi J. The British Ophthalmological Surveillance Unit: an evaluation of the first 3 years. Eye (Lond) 2003; 17: 9–15.
11. Rahi JS, Cable N. Severe visual impairment and blindness in children in the UK. Lancet 2003; 362: 1359–1365.
12. Muhit MA, Shah S, Gilbert C. The key informant method: a novel means of ascertaining blind children in Bangladesh. Br J Ophthalmol 2007; 91: 995–999.
13. Tadic V, Hamblion EL, Keeley S, et al. "Silent voices" in health services research: ethnicity and socioeconomic variation in participation in studies of quality of life in childhood visual disability. Invest Ophthalmol Vis Sci 2010; 51: 1886–1890.
14. Jan JE, Freeman RD. Who is a visually impaired child? Dev Med Child Neurol 1998; 40: 65–67.
15. Jan JE, Freeman RD, Scott EP. The family of the visually impaired child. In: Jan JE, Scott EP, editors. Visual Impairment in Children and Adolescents. New York: Grune & Stratton; 1977; 159–186.
16. Nixon HL. Mainstreaming and the American Dream: Sociological Perspectives on Coping with Blind and Visually Impaired Children. New York: American Foundation for the Blind; 1991.
17. Shamanna BR, Dandona L, Rao GN. Economic burden of blindness in India. Indian J Ophthalmol 1998; 46: 169–172.
18. Rahi JS, Dezateux C. Epidemiology of visual impairment. In: David TJ, editor. Recent Advances in Paediatrics, 19. London: Churchill Livingstone; 2001: 97–114.
19. Gilbert C, Foster A. Childhood blindness in the context of VISION 2020: the right to sight. Bull World Health Organ 2001; 79: 227–232.
20. Gilbert C, Rahi J. Magnitude and Causes. In: Johnson GJ, et al., editors. Epidemiology of Eye Disease. London and Singapore: Imperial College Press/World Scientific; 2011.
21. World Health Organization. Preventing blindness in children. WHO/PBL/00.77. Geneva: World Health Organization; 2000.
22. Gilbert CE, Anderton L, Dandona L, et al. Prevalence of visual impairment in children: a review of available data. Ophthalmic Epidemiol 1999; 6: 73–82.
23. Rosenberg T, Flage T, Hansen E, et al. Incidence of registered visual impairment in the Nordic child population. Br J Ophthalmol 1996; 80: 49–53.
24. Gilbert C, Steinkuller PG, Du L, et al. Childhood blindness: a new form for recording causes of visual loss in children. Bull World Health Org 1993; 71: 485–489.
25. Gilbert C. Retinopathy of prematurity: a global perspective of the epidemics, population of babies at risk and implications for control. Early Hum Dev 2008; 84: 77–82.
26. Rahi JS, Cumberland PM, Peckham CS. Improving detection of blindness in childhood: the British Childhood Vision Impairment study. Pediatrics 2010; 126: e895–e903.

Clinical embryology and development of the eye

Robyn V Jamieson • John R B Grigg

This chapter deals with the embryology of the eye. We concentrate on organogenesis of the globe and then examine the differentiation of the components of the eye and provide the anatomical substrate for developmental ocular conditions.

The vertebrate eye is formed through coordinated interactions between neuroepithelium, surface ectoderm, and extraocular mesenchyme.[1] The neuroectoderm gives rise to the retina, iris, and optic nerve; the surface ectoderm forms the lens and corneal epithelium; the extraocular mesenchyme comprising mesodermal and neural crest cells gives rise to the corneal stroma, corneal endothelium, extraocular muscles, and fibrous and vascular coats of the eye.[2]

Three main periods can be distinguished in the prenatal development of the eye:

1. *Embryogenesis* includes the establishment of the primary organ rudiments and finishes when the optic groove (optic sulcus), which is considered the anlage of the eye, appears on either side of the midline at the expanded cranial end of the open neural folds around the end of the third gestational week.
2. *Organogenesis* includes the development of the primary organ rudiments and extends to the end of the eighth week.
3. *Differentiation* involves the differentiation of the primitive organs into a fully or partially active organ starting at the beginning of the third month. During this period, the retina, optic nerve, and anterior rim of the optic cup mature and the vitreous, lens, and angle structures develop[3] (Table 2.1, see also Chapter 4 and 6).

Embryogenesis and eye development

Vertebrate early eye formation follows a conserved sequence of events. Soon after gastrulation (formation of the three layers

ectoderm, mesoderm, and endoderm) begins, the eye field is specified in the anterior neural plate. The first morphologic landmarks are bilateral indentations (optic sulci or pits), at approximately 22 days, in the neural folds at the cranial end of the embryo.

Eye organogenesis (4th–8th week gestation human)

Fourth week

In the fourth week, the optic pits deepen and form the optic vesicles (OVs) which are evaginations of the lateral walls of the diencephalon. The OVs are connected to the forebrain by the optic stalk (a short tube that eventually forms the optic nerve) (Fig. 2.1A). Interaction between the OV and surface ectoderm (SE) induces the lens placode, and the wall of the OV in contact with the SE thickens to form the retinal disk. Towards the end of the fourth week invagination begins to transform the OV into the optic cup (OC). Simultaneously, the primordia of the extraocular muscles appear as condensations in the periocular mesenchyme. Disruptions in these early steps lead to severe congenital anomalies, including anophthalmia, microphthalmia, and optic fissure closure defects (coloboma).[5,6]

Fifth week

The process of invagination of the OV to form the OC predominates in the fifth week. Invagination involves the retinal *disk*, lens plate, and the ventrocaudal wall of the OV (Fig. 2.1B). Invagination of the retinal *disk* of the OV leads to formation of the inner layer of the OC which becomes the neural retina, while the external layer of the OC will become the retinal pigment epithelium (RPE) (Fig. 2.1C). The OC is not continuous, and forms a fold inferiorly and ventrally that is continuous with the optic stalk. This fold, called the embryonic (optic) fissure (Fig. 2.3), allows the passage of the hyaloid artery into the OC. The primary vitreous develops around the hyaloid vasculature. The process of invagination also involves the lens placode (plate), which leads to the formation of the lens pit. The lens pit deepens to become the lens vesicle. Further development leads to the lens vesicle

Table 2.1 – Overview of eye development[4]

Gestational age	Developmental milestone
22 days	Optic primordia appears
2nd month	Hyaloid artery fills embryonic fissure Closure of embryonic fissure begins Lid folds appear Neural crest cells (corneal endothelium) migrate centrally; corneal stroma follows Choroidal vasculature starts to develop Axons from ganglion cells migrate to optic nerve
3rd month	Sclera condenses Lid folds meet and fuse
4th month	Retinal vessels grow into nerve fiber layer near optic disc Schlemm's canal appears Glands and cilia develop in lids
5th month	Photoreceptors develop inner segments Lids begin to separate
6th month	Dilator muscle of iris forms
7th month	Central fovea thins Fibrous lamina cribrosa forms Choroidal melanocytes produce pigment
8th month	Iris sphincter develops Chamber angle completes formation Hyaloid vessels regress Retinal vessels reach periphery Myelination of optic nerve fibers is complete to lamina cribrosa Pupillary membrane disappears

separating from the SE.[7] The lens vesicle is large and fills the OC.[8] The SE becomes the corneal epithelium (Fig. 2.1D).[1,3]

Sixth week

In the sixth week the optic fissure closes after the edges of the OC that border the fissure become closely apposed. The pattern of gene expression at those apposed edges must be spatially and temporally appropriate to bring about fusion.[9] The embryonic fissure closure begins in the middle and then extends anteriorly and posteriorly (see Fig. 2.3).

The development of the retina progresses with the RPE forming a single layer of cuboidal cells. A primitive Bruch's membrane arises. The sensory retina thickens due to proliferation of cells in the germinative zone of the inner layer of the OC. At this stage, retinal ganglion cell axons, which form the optic nerve fibers, first enter the optic stalk to exit the primitive eye[4] (Fig. 2.1E). The secondary vitreous, a cellular structure with associated extracellular matrix (ECM), forms and remodels the primary vitreous filling the remaining retrolenticular space.[10]

Seventh week

The main events during the seventh week include the maturation of the RPE, the development of the sensory retina with the formation of outer and inner neuroblastic layers at the posterior pole. Primary lens fibers form to obliterate the cavity in the lens vesicle. The periocular mesenchyme evolves with the formation of the choroidal vasculature posteriorly and the development of the anterior segment (Fig. 2.1F).

The anterior periocular mesenchyme in the mammal has contributions from neural crest and mesodermal cells, whereas in the chick there are only neural crest contributions. The mesenchymal cells migrate forward so that cells of neural crest and mesodermal origin contribute to the corneal stroma, endothelium, and trabecular meshwork: Schlemm's canal (SC) is of mesodermal origin (Fig. 2.2).

Eighth week

In the eighth week, there is marked development of the optic nerve as ganglion cells differentiate; by the end of this week, 2.67 million axons have formed. Optic nerve axons start to make contact with the brain and establish a rudimentary chiasm.[11] The RPE nears maturation with the appearance of melanosomes. Müller cells appear now and extend radial fibers inwards to form the internal limiting membrane and outward toward the future external limiting membrane.

Corneal differentiation includes endothelial cells starting to form Descemet's membrane; the corneal stroma consists of 5–8 rows of cells and the corneal epithelium is evolving to a stratified squamous epithelium.

The lens develops rapidly during this period. The primary lens fibers fill the lens vesicle. The intracellular organelles disappear. The equatorial epithelial cells begin to divide and new cells are pushed posteriorly, then elongate and become the secondary lens fibers. With the formation of the secondary lens fibers, there is development of the lens bow which represents the nuclei of the secondary lens fibers. They form an arc with a forward convexity (Fig. 2.1E). The lens "sutures" develop where the secondary lens fibers meet in a linear pattern at the anterior and posterior poles of the lens. The sutures initially are in a Y shape anteriorly and an inverted Y (ʌ) posteriorly.[7,12]

The four rectus muscles insert into the sphenoid bone and the trochlea develops. The lacrimal glands form from the superotemporal quadrant of the conjunctival sac.

Differentiation and maturation of elements

Cornea

The cornea's main function as a transparent "window" derives from its unique structure and composition permitting the transmission and refraction of light.[13] It consists of three layers: an outer epithelial layer, a middle stromal layer consisting of a collagen-rich ECM interspersed with keratocytes, and an inner endothelial cell layer.

The corneal epithelium develops from SE and its maturation is related to eyelid development. Rudimentary lids fuse 8 weeks after ovulation and do not separate until 26 weeks.[14] Bowman's membrane, which underlies the corneal epithelium, develops from the processes of superficial mesenchymal stromal cells. It first becomes apparent around week 16 and is easily recognizable by the fifth month.[15]

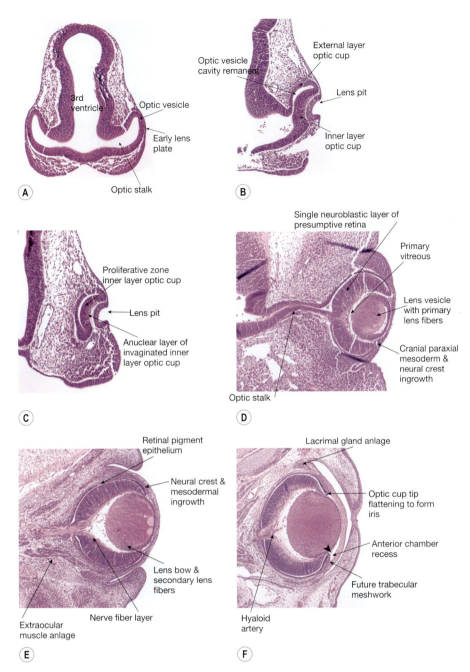

Fig. 2.1 (A) Optic vesicle formation on the lateral wall of the diencephalon. The optic stalk connects the optic vesicle to the forebrain. (9.5 days' gestation (DG) mouse equivalent 26 DG human). (B) Optic vesicle invagination and lens vesicle formation (early 10.5 DG mouse equivalent 28 DG human). (C) Invagination of lens pit and bilayered optic cup forming from invaginated optic vesicle (late day 10.5 DG mouse equivalent 32 DG human). (D) Optic fissure closure, lens vesicle formation and primary vitreous (12.5 DG mouse equivalent 44 DG human). (E) Nerve fiber layer formation, neural crest migration and lens bow formation (14.5 DG mouse equivalent 56–60 DG human). (F) The eye at the end of organogenesis. Cornea, early iris formation, extraocular muscle anlage and lacrimal gland clearly visible. Arrowhead shows pupillary membrane (16.5 DG mouse equivalent >60 days human).

The beginnings of the corneoscleral junction, which will become the limbus, appear at the end of the eighth week. This is marked by a change in stromal appearance at the periphery of the cornea, with cells acquiring a more polymorphic shape and losing regular orientation. By week 11, this junction is well demarcated. In place of the limbal folds identifiable in adult corneas, a ridge-like structure circumscribes and demarcates the developing cornea. This represents the primitive corneal epithelial stem cell niche.[15]

The mature corneal endothelial and stromal layers, the mesenchymal layer of the limbus, and the trabecular meshwork in mammals each consist of two mature cell lineages, one derived from the neural crest and the other from the mesoderm. The mesoderm-derived cells mature to a mix of antigen-presenting cells. These include dendritic cells and macrophages in the limbus and peripheral cornea. Mesenchymal stromal cells of neural crest and mesodermal origin migrate into the space between the corneal epithelium and corneal endothelium and become keratoblasts. The keratoblasts proliferate and synthesize high levels of hyaluronan to form an embryonic corneal stroma ECM. The keratoblasts differentiate into keratocytes which synthesize collagens and keratan sulfate proteoglycans that replace the hyaluronan/water-rich ECM with a densely packed collagen fibril-type ECM.[16] Differentiation of the stroma and endothelium depends on signals from the lens epithelium, although the nature of the responsible molecule(s) is not known.[17]

The corneal stroma, uniquely, has a homogeneous distribution of small diameter 25–30 nm collagen fibrils regularly packed in lamellae. This arrangement minimizes light scattering and permits transparency. The corneal stroma consists primarily of collagen type I, lesser amounts of collagen

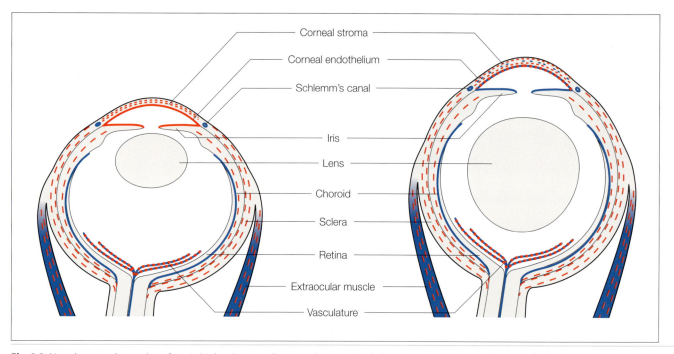

Fig. 2.2 Neural crest and mesoderm fates in bird and mammalian eyes. Cross-sectional diagrams summarizing similarities and differences in contributions of neural crest (red) and mesoderm (blue) to adult chicken and mouse eyes. The major differences occur in the anterior segment. Reproduced with permission Gage PJ et al 2005.[19]

type V, and four proteoglycans, three with keratan sulfate chains, and one with a chondroitin sulfate chain. The core proteins of the proteoglycans and collagen type V regulate the growth of collagen fibrils. The overall sizes of the proteoglycans are small enough to fit in the spaces between the collagen fibrils and regulate their spacing.

Anterior chamber structures

Iris

The most posterior layer of the iris is the pigmented epithelium; anterior to this are the iris muscles and further anteriorly lies the iris stroma. The iris root is attached to the ciliary body (CB) and to the cornea–sclera junction. This region is known as the iridocorneal angle.

The iris arises from the anterior margin of the OC neuroepithelium and the periocular mesenchyme. This includes specification of the peripheral OC to a non-neuronal fate, migration of cells from the surrounding periocular mesenchyme, and formation of the sphincter and dilator smooth muscles from the neuroectoderm.[18] The iris stroma in mice originates from both neural crest and mesoderm.[19,20]

Ciliary body

The ciliary body (CB) shares a common embryonic origin with the iris but develops into a functionally different structure. The CB extends from the iris root anteriorly, to the ora serrata posteriorly, and consists of ciliary muscles (meridional, radial, and circular fibers) and ciliary processes. Each ciliary process (fold) comprises an inner capillary core surrounded by a loose stroma, which is covered by a double-layered secretory epithelium. The outer ciliary epithelium is pigmented, while the inner ciliary epithelium (closest to the lens) is non-pigmented. The undulating ciliary processes provide a large surface area

for secretion of aqueous humor, glycoproteins of the vitreous body, antioxidant enzymes, and neuropeptides.[21] The non-pigmented epithelial cells of the CB are the main source of fibrillin secreted into the zonular fibers connecting the CB to the lens.[22] These zonular fibers and the ciliary muscles mediate lens accommodation. The ciliary muscles also serve in regulating aqueous humor outflow through the trabecular meshwork and uveoscleral outflow pathways.[23]

Trabecular meshwork

Trabecular meshwork formation begins around the fourth month of gestation.[24] The mesenchymal cells of the trabecular meshwork form a wedge-shaped structure between the corneal endothelium and the deeper stroma (Fig. 2.1F). During the fourth to sixth months, there is a 50% increase in cross-sectional area and threefold increase in volume of the trabecular anlage.

Schlemm's canal (SC) forms from a venous plexus anterior to the trabecular anlage which becomes visible in the 16th week of gestation.[25] By 24 weeks, SC is present throughout the entire circumference. By 36 weeks, SC and outer collecting channels are clearly defined and connected by intercanalicular links. The development of this system continues postnatally; an adult-like configuration is achieved by 8 years.[25]

Pupillary membrane

During mammalian lens development, a transient capillary meshwork known as the pupillary membrane (PM) forms in the pupil area. The PM reaches its maximal development by 12–13 weeks' gestation[26] (Figs 2.1F and 2.4). The PM nourishes the anterior surface of the lens and then regresses to clear the optical path. The regression may be due to iris movement leading to altered blood flow in the PM and apoptosis.[27] The regression of the PM occurs in a programmed

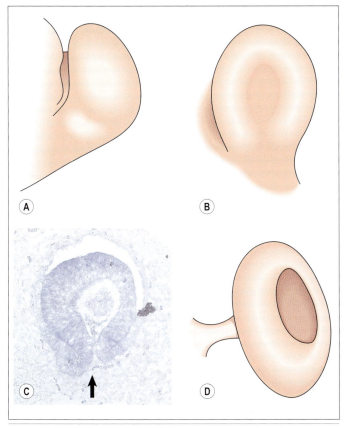

Fig. 2.3 Optic vesicle invagination three dimensional representation (A) Optic vesicle outpouching (9.5 DG mouse 32 DG human), (B) Optic fissure closing (C) Parasaggital section of mouse eye just prior to fissure closure (reproduced from Mihlec et al[50]) (D) Fusion of optic fissure (A, B, D reproduced with permission from Fitzpatrick and van Heyningen)[5].

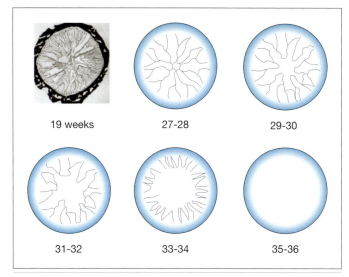

Fig. 2.4 Pupillary membrane regression. The pupillary membrane is fully develped by 13 weeks' gestation. (Top left) Clinical appearance at 19 weeks' gestation (adapted from Zhu et al.[26]). Schematic regression stages (modified from Hittner et al.[28]) at around 29–30 weeks the central quarter of the membrane clears, at 31–32 weeks the central half clears, at 33–34 weeks only a peripheral rim of membrane remains. By 35–36 weeks the membrane has completely regressed.

manner at consistent time points. The stage of regression of the PM is a useful guide to the gestational age of a premature infant. At 27–28 weeks' gestation the PM fully covers the pupil. The central vessels are progressively lost until 35–36 weeks' gestation when the membrane is no longer present[28] (see Fig. 2.4).

Lens

The lens consists of tightly packed fiber cells with a specialized organization. Lens fiber cell terminal differentiation is accompanied by synthesis and short-range ordered packing of crystallin proteins, which provide the transparent and refractive medium through which light passes. The programmed removal of organelles from differentiating lens fiber cells contributes toward lens transparency through formation of an organelle-free zone.[29] At term, the lens is 6 mm in diameter and grows to 9–10 mm in adult life.

Vitreous and hyaloid system

The hyaloid system is well established by 10 weeks' gestation.[26] The tunica vasculosa lentis anastomoses with the annular vessel at the anterior border of the OC and connects to the choroidal vasculature. The hyaloid system has no veins: all

hyaloid vessels are arteries. The venous drainage is via the choroidal veins.[30] The development of the hyaloid vascular system is complete around the fourth month and provides all nutrients to the intraocular components of the developing eye. With the appearance of the developing retinal vasculature at approximately the fifth month of gestation the first signs of hyaloid vessel regression can be detected.[30]

The primary vitreous composed of fibrillar material, mesenchymal cells, and vascular channels forms around the hyaloid vasculature and is gradually remodelled. The secondary vitreous consists principally of a network of type II collagen fibrils. There is gradual remodeling of the vitreous with subsequent condensations of thicker collagen fibers. Blood flow in the hyaloid artery ceases around the seventh month; it is almost completely atrophied by birth.

Retina

The two layers of the OC give rise to the outer retinal pigment epithelium and the inner neural retina (Fig. 2.1C,D). The RPE is required for growth of the eye, and it contributes to control of proper lamination of the neural retina. The basal laminar of the RPE, Bruch's membrane, forms a functional unit with the RPE and choriocapillaris. It is involved in the essential exchange of numerous biomolecules, oxygen, nutrients, and waste products between these tissues.[31]

Differentiation of the neural retina begins at the end of the sixth week. At any location in the retina, there is a fixed birth sequence of retinal cells. Ganglion cells, horizontal cells, and cone photoreceptors are born first, followed by amacrine and bipolar cells, with rod photoreceptors and, last, the Müller cells.[32] At 10–11 weeks' gestation, a region in the outer nuclear layer of the central retina $< 500\ \mu m$ in diameter, about 1500 μm temporal to the optic disc, and comprising only differentiating cone photoreceptors is the first indication of the developing fovea. In primates, it is the initiation point for most developmental events in the retina, including cessation of mitosis, morphologic maturation, apoptosis, opsin expression, and synaptogenesis.[33] Developmental events then radiate from this region across the retina.[33]

The differentiated outer nuclear layer is a single layer of only cones, which will be at the center of the adult fovea. Human rods and cones are arranged in a precise spatial mosaic. L and M cones reach peak spatial density in the center of the fovea, while S cones are absent from the central 100 μm and rods are absent from the central 300 μm of the adult fovea.

In the weeks before birth, photoreceptor morphology becomes more mature across the entire retina. At week 34, cones and rods near the pure cone area of the fovea have outer segments and are forming elongated axons, which terminate in distinct synaptic pedicles in the network of neuronal processes of the outer plexiform layer.[33] While foveal cones are among the first cells in the retina to differentiate, they are the last to attain adult characteristics. In comparison, cones in the periphery are mature in the perinatal human retina.[32]

Genetic ablation of the RPE or disruption of RPE specification genes results in microphthalmia, RPE-to-retina transdifferentiation, and coloboma during murine eye development.[1]

Vascularization of the retina involves proliferation and migration of astrocytes and endothelial cells so that, from 14 to 15 weeks' gestation, the vessels spread outward from the disc and reach the peripheral retina around birth.[34] The stimulus for vascular growth is dependent on the retinal neurons becoming metabolically active, using up oxygen, causing local hypoxia, and causing retinal astrocytes to secrete vascular endothelial growth factor (VEGF), which promotes growth of endothelial cells and formation of retinal blood vessels. When the blood vessels open up and carry oxygenated blood to the area, the hypoxia is relieved, and astrocytic VEGF production decreases to baseline levels. Thus, blood vessel formation is matched to oxygen demand.[35]

The foveal region is never vascularized during normal development, and the foveal avascular zone is fully demarcated by around 28 weeks' gestation in humans.[36] The inhibition of retinal vessels at the fovea is contributed to by expression of a gradient of antiangiogenic or antiproliferative factors such as transforming growth factor-β or fibroblast growth factor-2, centered on the incipient fovea.[34] At the fovea, the retina is adapted morphologically to its blood supply because the development of retinal vessels is inhibited. This is the converse of the rest of the retina and may provide a clue to the susceptibility of the macular to disease.[37]

Optic nerve

The optic nerve develops from the edges of the optic fissure, which can be divided into two adjoining parts: the optic groove, derived from the optic stalk, and the retinal fissure derived from the ventral OV (see Fig. 2.1D). The optic disc forms at the transition between the optic groove and retinal fissure.[38] Axons and hyaloid artery at the developing optic disc become encircled by a ring of compact neuroepithelial cells, characterized by the expression of the paired-boxed transcription factor Pax2.[39] These neuroepithelial cells have a significant role in retinal ganglion cell (RGC) axon guidance. RGC axons initially extend along the vitreous surface of the neural retina and follow a centripetal route towards the center of the retina.

Within the retina, RGC axons grow in close contact with Müller glial cell endfeet and with the vitreous basal lamina, both of which express cell adhesion and ECM molecules.[2,40] The number of RGC axons entering the optic nerve peaks at 3.7 million around 16–17 weeks' gestation. The number of axons then decline, stabilizing at about 1.1 million axons by week 29 of gestation. This figure agrees with an estimate of 1.1–1.3 million optic axons in the human adult.[41] This redundancy contributes to the retinotopic organization being mapped to the cortex via activity-dependent mechanisms.

Extraocular muscles

Craniofacial muscles develop from unsegmented prechordal and paraxial mesoderm. They also receive contributions from the neural crest. The extraocular muscles (EOMs) differ from craniofacial muscles formed in the branchial arches by having different upstream activators of the muscle regulatory transcriptional cassette.[42] EOMs also have unique gene expression profiles including the presence of embryonic and cardiac muscle proteins and higher levels of enzymes, which make the EOMs resistant to many forms of muscular dystrophy.[42]

Lacrimal system

The lacrimal apparatus is divided into secretory and excretory components. The secretory system comprises those structures which contribute to the formation of the tear film, mainly the lacrimal gland. The excretory system, formed by the lacrimal puncta, lacrimal canaliculi, lacrimal sac, and nasolacrimal duct, collects the tear film and drains it into the nasal cavity.[43]

Three stages in lacrimal gland morphogenesis are identified:

1. The presumptive glandular stage at 7–8 weeks' gestation characterized by a thickening of the superior fornix epithelium together with surrounding mesenchymal condensation.
2. The bud stage characterized initially by the appearance of nodular formations in the region of the superior conjunctival fornix and concluding with the appearance of lumina within the epithelial buds.
3. The glandular maturity stage at 9–16 weeks' gestation, when the gland begins to take on the morphology of adulthood.[44]

The excretory lacrimal system begins to develop at 6–7 weeks' gestation when the lacrimal groove is observed between the maxillary and external nasal processes. The lacrimal cord develops at 8 weeks' gestation. By 9–16 weeks, the palpebral orbicular muscle primordium has formed along with the lumen of the excretory lacrimal system and formation of the tendon of the medial palpebral ligament.

Cranial nerves

Twelve pairs of cranial nerves (CN) form during the fifth and sixth weeks of development. They are classified into three groups based on their embryologic origins. The somatic efferent cranial nerves are: oculomotor (CNIII – the majority of the nerve), trochlear (CNIV), abducence (CNVI), and hypoglossal (CNXII). The nerves of the branchial arches include: CN V, VII, IX, and X. The special sensory nerves are: CNI, CNII, and CNVIII.

Within the brain (as opposed to the spinal cord), motor neuron organization is subservient to neuromeric organization. The cranial motor neurons are organized within individual rhombomeres (neuromere of the rhombencephalon) or in adjacent neuromeric pairs. The oculomotor (III) nucleus is located in the posterior midbrain, the trochlear (IV) nucleus in the anterior rhombomere 1 (r1), the trigeminal (V) nucleus in rhombomeres 2 and 3, the abducens (VI) nucleus in rhombomeres 4 and 5, the facial (VII) nucleus in rhombomeres 5 and 6, and the glossopharyngeal (IX) nuclear in rhomobomeres 6 and 7. The midbrain and each hindbrain segment have their own molecular "address" reflected by the expression of a unique combination of transcription factors.[45]

Normal development and function of the efferent cranial nerves is critical for normal development of the extraocular muscles. Stromal cell-derived factor-1 (SDF-1) and hepatocyte growth factor (HGF) play roles in oculomotor and trochlear axon guidance. SDF-1 and HGF are expressed in the mesenchyme around the nerve exit points. SDF-1 and HGF are also expressed around the extraocular muscles and increase the outgrowth of oculomotor/trochlear axons, implicating them in patterning these nerve–muscle projections[46] (see also Chapter 82).

Emmetropization

The human eye is programmed to achieve emmetropia in youth and to maintain emmetropia with advancing years. The visual image is critical in refractive development and the controlling mechanism(s) in emmetropia are largely localized to the retina.[47,48,49]

Embryology resources are well developed online (see http://www.ncl.ac.uk/igm/EADHB/ for detailed images).

References

1. Fuhrmann S. Eye morphogenesis and patterning of the optic vesicle. Curr Top Dev Biol 2010; 93: 61–84.
2. Harada T, Harada C, Parada LF. Molecular regulation of visual system development: more than meets the eye. Genes Dev 2007; 21: 367–78.
3. Barishak Y. Embryology of the Eye and its Adnexa, 2nd ed. Basel: Karger; 2001.
5. Fitzpatrick DR, van Heyningen V. Developmental eye disorders. Curr Opin Genet Dev 2005; 15: 348–53.
7. Lovicu F, McAvoy J, de Iongh R. Understanding the role of growth factors in embryonic development: insights from the lens. R Soc Lond Philos Trans B Biol Sci 2011; 366: 1204–18.
8. Gunhaga L. The lens: a classical model of embryonic induction providing new insights into cell determination in early development. R Soc Lond Philos Trans B Biol Sci 2011; 366: 1193–203.
10. Ponsioen TL, Hooymans JMM, Los LI. Remodelling of the human vitreous and vitreoretinal interface – a dynamic process. Progr Retinal Eye Res 2010; 29: 580–95.
12. Lovicu FJ, Robinson ML, editors. Development of the Ocular Lens. Cambridge, UK: Cambridge University Press; 2004.

13. Quantock AJ, Young RD. Development of the corneal stroma, and the collagen-proteoglycan associations that help define its structure and function. Dev Dynamics 2008; 237: 2607–21.
15. Davies SB, Di Girolamo N. Corneal stem cells and their origins: significance in developmental biology. Stem Cells Dev 2010; 19: 1651–62.
16. Hassell JR, Birk DE. The molecular basis of corneal transparency. Exp Eye Res 2010; 91: 326–35.
18. Davis-Silberman N, Ashery-Padan R. Iris development in vertebrates; genetic and molecular considerations. Brain Res 2008; 1192: 17–28.
19. Gage PJ, Rhoades W, Prucka SK, Hjalt T. Fate maps of neural crest and mesoderm in the mammalian eye. Invest Ophthalmol Vis Sci 2005; 46: 4200–8.
21. Bishop PN, Takanosu M, le Goff M, Mayne R. The role of the posterior ciliary body in the biosynthesis of vitreous humour. Eye 2002; 16: 454–60.
23. Napier HRL, Kidson SH. Molecular events in early development of the ciliary body: a question of folding. Exp Eye Res 2007; 84: 615–25.
25. Ramirez JM, Ramirez AI, Salazar JJ, et al. Schlemm's canal and the collector channels at different developmental stages in the human eye. Cells Tissues Organs 2004; 178: 180–5.
26. Zhu M, Provis JM, Penfold PL. The human hyaloid vasculature: cellular phenotypes and interrelationships. [Research Support, Non-US Gov't]. Exp Eye Res 1999; 68: 553–63.
27. Morizane Y, Mohri S, Kosaka J, et al. Iris movement mediates vascular apoptosis during rat pupillary membrane regression. Am J Physiol Regul Integr Comp Physiol 2006; 290: R819–25.
28. Hittner HM, Hirsch NJ, Rudolph AJ. Assessment of gestational age by examination of the anterior vascular capsule of the lens. J Pediatrics 1977; 91: 455–8.
32. Provis JM, Penfold PL, Cornish EE, et al. Anatomy and development of the macula: specialisation and the vulnerability to macular degeneration. Clin Exp Optom 2005; 88: 269–81.
33. Hendrickson A, Bumsted-O'Brien K, Natoli R, et al. Rod photoreceptor differentiation in fetal and infant human retina. Exp Eye Res 2008; 87: 415–26.
35. Stone J, Itin A, Alon T, et al. Development of the retinal vasculture is mediated by hypoxia-induced vascular endothelial growth factor (VEGF) expression by neuroglia. J Neurosci 1995; 15: 4738–47.
36. Provis JM, Hendrickson AE. The foveal avascular region of developing human retina. Arch Ophthalmol 2008; 126: 507–11.
37. Provis JM. Development of the primate retinal vasculature. Progr Retinal Eye Res 2001; 20: 799–821.
41. Provis JM, van Driel D, Billson FA, Russell P. Human fetal optic nerve: overproduction and elimination of retinal axons during development. J Comp Neurol 1985; 238: 92–100.
43. de la Cuadra-Blanco C, Peces-Pena MD, Janez-Escalada L, Merida-Velasco JR. Morphogenesis of the human excretory lacrimal system. J Anat 2006; 209: 127–35.
44. de la Cuadra-Blanco C, Peces Peña M, Mérida-Velasco J. Morphogenesis of the human lacrimal gland. J Anat 2003; 203: 531–6.
48. Smith EL, 3rd, Huang J, Hung L-F, et al. Hemiretinal form deprivation: evidence for local control of eye growth and refractive development in infant monkeys. Invest Ophthalmol Vis Sci 2009; 50: 5057–69.
50. Mihelec M, Abraham P, Gibson K, et al. Novel SOX2 partner-factor domain mutation in a four generation family. Eur J Hum Gen 2009; 17: 1417–22.

 Access the complete reference list online at

http://www.expertconsult.com

Developmental biology of the eye

David R Fitzpatrick

Introduction

Developmental biology provides an understanding of the mechanisms controlling the four-dimensional changes in shape (morphogenesis), cell type diversity (histogenesis), and functional maturation during embryogenesis and early development. Ocular development is a popular system for developmental biologists since the structure of the eye is similar throughout vertebrate evolution and the molecular basis of development is highly conserved in the well-studied invertebrate animal model, the fruit fly, *Drosophila melanogaster*.

For both ethical and technical reasons, experimental developmental biology is not possible in humans. This limitation is likely to change with the ability to induce trans-differentiation of adult human cells into induced pluripotent stems (**iPS**) cells.[1] An ever-increasing understanding of the genetic basis of human malformations combined with the availability of patient-derived iPS cells predicts that human developmental biology will be an important and rapidly growing field. However, our current knowledge of eye development comes from *Drosophila* and vertebrate models: frogs (*Xenopus laevus*, *Xenopus tropicalis*), fish (zebrafish: *Danio rerio*, medaka: *Oryzias latipes*), chick (*Gallus gallus*), and mouse (*Mus musculus*). Each has strengths and weaknesses. For example, chick embryos have been extensively used for fate mapping (Box 3.1) and tissue recombination experiments, but there are few natural

mutations available for study and genetic manipulation is difficult. In mice, it is possible to inactivate almost any gene in a targeted manner via homologous recombination (see Box 3.1) in embryonic stem cells, but very early development is difficult to visualize since this is a placental mammal. Although exact equivalence of animal model experimental data with orthologous processes in humans is unlikely given the expansion of gene families through evolutionary genome duplication and existence of species-specific phenomena, it is likely that many of the developmental mechanisms will be common and generalizable.

Important concepts and processes in developmental biology

Differentiation

The fertilized egg is a totipotent cell, i.e. one cell can give rise to all embryonic and extra-embryonic tissues. Differentiation is a progressive loss of "stem-ness" associated with increasing functional specialization of the daughter cells. This process ends with terminal differentiation where the cell exits the cell cycle and changes the cellular machinery to fulfill its assigned function. The ancestry of the rod photoreceptor cell would be represented as fertilized egg → blastomere cell → inner cell mass cell → primitive ectodermal cell → neuroectodermal cell → optic field cell → optic vesicle cell → retinal progenitor cell → photoreceptor. This sequence of any developing cell is known as the fate map.

Cell migration

Embryogenesis involves dramatic shape changes over short periods of time. Much of this change is due to differential growth rates within and between tissues. However, there is a subset of cells that shows remarkable migration from their birth place to distant regions of the embryos. The best known of these traveling cells are neural crest cells which form on the lips of the neural fold along the length of the neural tube. The cranial neural crest cells are important in eye development. The molecular basis of the movement of neural crest cells is evolving and many of the master control genes for this process are also important in mediating cancer invasion and metastasis.[2]

Definition of terms

Domain – a specific region or amino acid sequence in a protein with a particular function

Fate mapping – a technique developed by Vogt to trace the specific regions of an early embryo

Gastrulation – process in early embryonic development whereby the single-layered blastula is reorganized into the trilaminar gastrula

Haploinsufficiency – the situation where an individual who is heterozygous for a certain gene mutation is clinically affected because a single copy of the gene is incapable of providing sufficient protein to maintain normal function

Homeobox – a short, usually highly conserved DNA sequence in various genes that encodes a homeodomain

Homeodomain – a domain in a protein that is encoded by a homeobox that recognizes and binds to specific DNA sequences in genes regulated by the homeotic gene

Homologous recombination – a type of genetic recombination in which nucleotide sequences are exchanged between two similar or identical molecules of DNA

Ligand – a signal-triggering molecule that binds to a site on a target protein

Morphogens – secreted proteins that organize surrounding tissues into distinct territories thus governing the pattern of tissue development

Morphogen gradients – morphogens produced from a defined localized source form a concentration gradient as they spread through the tissue. The graded signal acts directly on cells in a concentration-dependent fashion

Nodal proteins – a subset of transforming growth factor-beta (TGFβ) family responsible for mesoderm induction, patterning of the nervous system, and determination of dorsal-ventral axis in embryos

Nodal signaling – a signal transduction pathway involving nodal proteins which are essential in pattern formation and differentiation during embryogenesis

Notch signaling pathway – a cell signaling system important for cell–cell communication and involving gene regulation mechanisms that control multiple cell differentiation during embryonic and adult life

Null mutant – a mutation in a gene that leads to it not being transcribed into RNA and/or translated into a functional protein

Orthologous genes – genes in different species that are similar to each other because they originated by vertical descent from a single gene of the last common ancestor

Paralogue – a pair of genes that derive from the same ancestral gene

Sequence homology – situation where nucleic acid or protein sequences are similar because they have a common evolutionary origin

Signal transduction – process whereby an extracellular signaling molecule activates a membrane receptor that in turn alters intracellular molecules

Transcription – the process of creating a complementary RNA copy of a sequence of DNA. It is the first step leading to gene expression

Programmed cell death

In many developmental tissues a proportion of the constituent cells will be seen to undergo a process where there is nuclear fragmentation leading to death. This process is microscopically and molecularly distinct from senescence and is known as apoptosis or programmed cell death (PCD).[3] The correct functioning of PCD is crucial to the normal development of many organs and appears to prune excess cells.

Signaling

Signaling is one of the most important processes in developmental biology. It involves interaction of a ligand (see Box 3.1) with a receptor, which then effects a change, usually altering protein phosphorylation and/or the transcriptional (see Box 3.1) profile of the receptor-bearing cell. Ligands can be proteins (e.g. Sonic hedgehog) or small molecules (e.g. all-*trans-retinoic acid*). The receptors (e.g. fibroblast growth factor receptors) can be on the cell surface or intracellular (e.g. retinoic acid receptors). The ligand–receptor interaction often leads to a signal transduction (see Box 3.1) cascade (e.g. MAPK pathway). Some ligand–receptor interactions activate several different signal transduction pathways when the most commonly used pathway is known as canonical (e.g. beta catenin activation in Wnt signaling) and the alternative pathways known as non-canonical. There are many different signaling pathways used during eye development (Fig. 3.1).

Morphogen gradients (see Box 3.1) involve a diffusible ligand exerting concentration-dependent differential effects on target tissues. This important concept is summarized in the so-called French flag model (Fig. 3.2).

Transcription factor codes

Transcription factors (TFs) are proteins that reversibly bind – either alone or in combination with other TFs – to specific sequences of DNA called binding sites to exert a *cis*-regulatory effect on one or more genes. The expression of combinations of TF – the TF code – can be used to mark a region of apparently undifferentiated tissue that will become a specific structure. TFs are often used as marker genes to determine tissue fate. An example of this is given in the next section where the TF *RAX* is used to define the eye field.

Specific developmental events in eye development

The eye field and the preplacodal region

Following gastrulation (see Box 3.1), the three germ layers (endoderm, mesoderm, and ectoderm) are established and neural identity begins with formation of the neural plate (Fig. 3.3A,B). The first molecular evidence of eye development is a single "virtual" structure, the eye field, that extends across the midline and is defined by discrete and overlapping expression domains of different TFs – the eye field transcription factors (EFTFs) (see Box 3.1). Rax is the EFTF most commonly used as a marker of the eye field (Fig. 3.3C). Mutations in the human *RAX* gene are a rare cause of human microphthalmia. Homozygous null mutations of *Rax* in mice result in complete

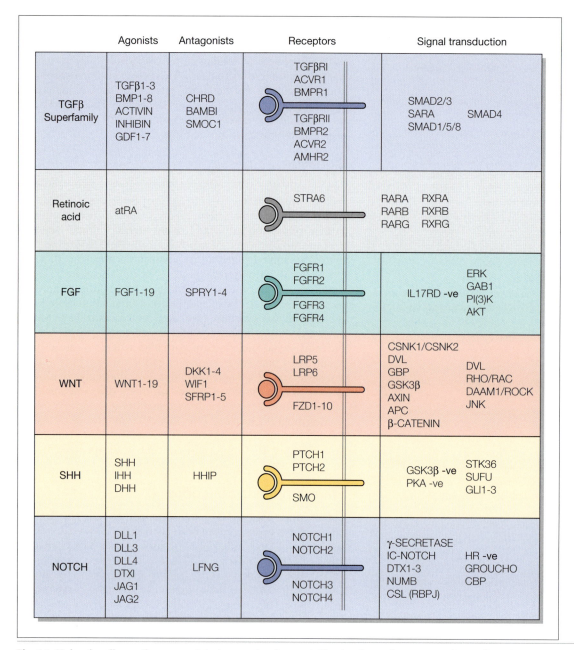

	Agonists	Antagonists	Receptors	Signal transduction	
TGFβ Superfamily	TGFβ1-3 BMP1-8 ACTIVIN INHIBIN GDF1-7	CHRD BAMBI SMOC1	TGFβRI ACVR1 BMPR1 / TGFβRII BMPR2 ACVR2 AMHR2	SMAD2/3 SARA SMAD1/5/8	SMAD4
Retinoic acid	atRA		STRA6	RARA RARB RARG	RXRA RXRB RXRG
FGF	FGF1-19	SPRY1-4	FGFR1 FGFR2 / FGFR3 FGFR4	IL17RD -ve	ERK GAB1 PI(3)K AKT
WNT	WNT1-19	DKK1-4 WIF1 SFRP1-5	LRP5 LRP6 / FZD1-10	CSNK1/CSNK2 DVL GBP GSK3β AXIN APC β-CATENIN	DVL RHO/RAC DAAM1/ROCK JNK
SHH	SHH IHH DHH	HHIP	PTCH1 PTCH2 / SMO	GSK3β -ve PKA -ve	STK36 SUFU GLI1-3
NOTCH	DLL1 DLL3 DLL4 DTXI JAG1 JAG2	LFNG	NOTCH1 NOTCH2 / NOTCH3 NOTCH4	γ-SECRETASE IC-NOTCH DTX1-3 NUMB CSL (RBPJ)	HR -ve GROUCHO CBP

Fig. 3.1 Major signaling pathways used during eye development. The signaling pathways are made up of ligands, antagonists, receptors, and signal transduction effectors. The pathways are named after the ligands, which are either groups of proteins that are related by sequence homology (see Box 3.1) or small molecules. Some receptor–ligand interactions may use more than one signal transduction cascade depending on cell context.

absence of eye structures, due to a failure in formation of the optic sulci that give rise to the optic cups. Other EFTFs include *Otx2*, the earliest molecular delineator of the eye field. Heterozygous loss-of-function mutations in *OTX2* cause severe ocular malformations in humans. The EFTF *Lxh2* has an expression domain within that of *Rax*. Targeted mutations in the mouse *Lhx2* gene cause anophthalmia. As with many EFTFs, LHX2 functions later in eye development. *Hesx1* is not a classical EFTF but loss of *Hesx1* expression in the anterior neural plate of mouse embryos results in anophthalmia and microphthalmia, whereas human mutations are associated with septo-optic dysplasia.

In common with many developmental processes, the eye field is a result of a balance of different signaling activities with competing morphogen gradients originating in neighboring tissues and often having antagonistic functions – some signals promoting formation of the eye field and others inhibitory.[4] Ligands of the Wnt signaling system are secreted from midbrain and paraxial mesoderm regions. A reduction or an increase in Wnt signaling will result in an increase or a decrease in the size of the eye field, respectively. For example, artificially overexpressing an inhibitor of Wnt signaling, *dickkopf1*, in zebrafish causes the eye field to get bigger, whereas homozygous loss-of-function mutations in a different inhibitor of Wnt signaling *axin1* causes reduced eye size.[5] In *Xenopus* embryos Notch signaling also induces the eye field and, of note, hypomorphic mutations of Notch2 in mice causes bilateral microphthalmia. The preplacodal region is a band of ectoderm surrounding the optic field and neural plate which will migrate to form the lens placode.

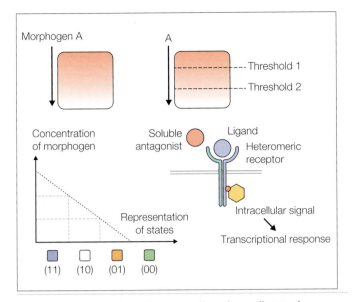

Fig. 3.2 Translation of morphogen gradients into cell state change.
Morphogen gradients are created by diffusible ligands for signaling cascade.
The source of ligand production will represent the peak of the concentration
gradient and factors such as the nature of the extracellular environment and
the catabolism or internalization of the ligand will influence the slope and
extent of the gradient. The signaling gradient is translated into changes in cell
state using a threshold-dependent mechanism. This can be diagrammatically
represented by the "French flag" model in which specific points on the slope
of signaling gradient will result in a change in the differentiated state of a
group of cells that lie between the threshold points. The concept of signal
transduction is represented by the competition between soluble ligands and
antagonists competing for interaction with the receptor complex. If the ligand
binds, it will then trigger the signal transduction to effect the proteomic or
transcriptomic change within the cell.

The eye field must be bisected in the midline in order for
two separate eyes to form: failure results in cyclopia. Nodal
signal from the underlying prechordal plate mesoderm results
in down-regulation of *Pax6* and *Rax* expression in the ventral
midline with the newly separated domains demarcating the
two bilateral optic primordia. Nodal ligands are members of
the TGFβ superfamily of signaling molecules. In zebrafish, the
mutants, *Cyclops*, *oep* (one-eyed pinhead), and *sqt* (squint), all
have cyclopia[6] and failure to form ventral forebrain due to a
loss-of-function mutation in the Nodal pathway. The Nodal
effect is mediated via inductions of *Sonic hedgehog* (*Shh*) expression; both mice and humans with *Shh/SHH* mutations develop
cyclopia and holoprosencephaly (see Chapter 56).

Following splitting of the eye field, the bilateral presumptive
neural retina (PNR) fields are visible as a pair of shallow
grooves (optic sulci) on the anterior neural plate; these will
ultimately form the optic vesicles (OVs). Definition of the
medial and lateral boundaries of the PNR are maintained by
continued Shh signaling from the prechordal mesenchyme
and bone morphogenetic protein (BMP) signaling from the
paraxial mesenchyme, respectively.[7] This process is crucial for
normal eye development since the blind cavefish *Astyanax* is
anophthalmic as the result of an evolutionary mutation producing hyperactivation of the Shh signaling cascade in the
midline.[8,9] This moves the medial boundary of the PNR more
laterally resulting in smaller OVs.

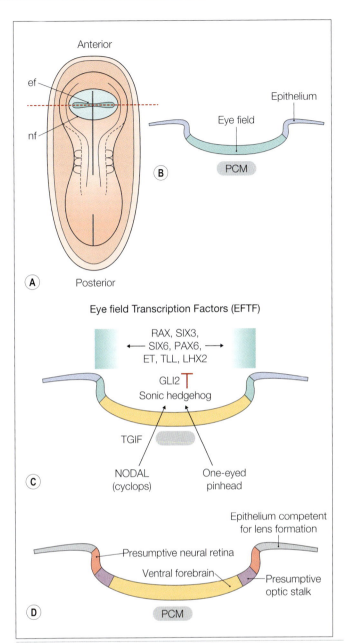

Fig. 3.3 Splitting the eye field. (A) The eye field (ef) is a virtual structure that
forms within the neural field (nf) on the dorsum of the early embryo. (B) A
section through the eye field shows it to be a plate of neuroepithelial cells
spanning the midline and overlying a structure called the precordal
mesenchyme (PCM) which is a rostral continuation of the notocord. Expression
of a group of eye field transcription factors (EFTFs) mark the eye field at this
stage. (C) Sonic hedgehog (SHH) signaling via GLI2 from the PCM acts to inhibit
expression of the EFTF in the midline and split the eye field. (D) SHH also acts to
pattern the now bilateral eye field into the medial presumptive optic stalk
(green) and the more lateral presumptive neural retina (yellow). At this stage
most of the surface ectoderm is competent to produce a lens vesicle.

The optic vesicle and optic stalk

The midline gradient of Shh signaling also differentiates the
optic stalk from optic cup. *Shh* induces expression of the optic
stalk markers, *Pax2*, *Vax1*, and *Vax2*. Overexpression of *Shh* at
this stage results in expanded expression of the ventral marker
Pax2 and the suppression of *Pax6*.[10] Reciprocal transcriptional
repression between *Pax2* and *Pax6* creates a boundary demarcating the future optic stalk region and the PNR,[11] i.e. *Pax2*

expression is a marker of the presumptive optic stalk and *Pax6* the PNR. Human loss-of-function mutations in *Pax2* cause optic nerve coloboma, a failure to complete optic fissure closure. This is presumed to be the result of an expansion of the PAX6 domain into the presumptive optic stalk region at the expense of the *PAX2* domain. Loss-of-function mutations in *Vax2*, or its paralogue (see Box 3.1), *Vax1*, cause optic nerve coloboma in mice, apparently via failure of repression of PAX6 expression.[12] In zebrafish, *Vax1* and *Vax2* genes are expressed in overlapping ventral domains within the developing eyes and their abrogation results in failure of fissure closure and the expansion of neural retina into ventral regions. A further level of control of Vax1/2 function is via the control of the nuclear localization of these proteins through SHH signaling.[13]

Shh, retinoic acid (RA), and BMP4 pattern the developing OV to confer proximoventral and dorsal–distal characteristics on the neuroectoderm. *Bmp4* is expressed in the distal OV and subsequently within dorsal regions of the optic cup. Overexpression of *Bmp4* expands the *Pax6* expression domain thus repressing *Pax2*. Phenotypically, this results in the extension of retinal pigmented epithelium (RPE) into forebrain regions.[10] A similar phenotype is associated with loss of Smoc1, a BMP antagonist, in mice. *SMOC1* mutations in humans result in severe anophthalmia as part of the ophthalmo-acromelic syndrome.[14] Overexpression of another BMP antagonist, Noggin, increases *Pax2* and decreases *Pax6* expression. Treatment of *Xenopus* embryos with RA leads to ventralization of the dorsal OV with expansion of *Vax2* expression domain dorsally.[10] Loss-of-function mutations in RA receptors reduce the size of the ventral retina resulting in failure of the optic fissure to close. Loss of multiple RA receptors results in additional ventral abnormalities, including the absence of ventral iris.[11]

Patterning of neural retina in the optic vesicle

Shh and BMP4 promote dorsal–ventral polarity within the presumptive neural retina (PNR) of the OV (Fig. 3.4). Bmp4 is induced by Lhx2 and in turn induces *Tbx5* expression in the dorsal PNR, while Shh induces *Vax2* expression ventrally. Overexpression of *Bmp4* in *Xenopus* causes expansion of *Tbx5* expression domain ventrally with suppression of *Vax2*. Tbx5 and Vax2 negatively regulate each other in the PNR to impart dorsal and ventral identity. Vsx2 (previously known as *Chx10*), a paired-like homeodomain (see Box 3.1) transcription factor, is expressed in the PNR adjacent to the lens placode in response to inductive fibroblast growth factor (Fgf) signaling from the surface ectoderm. Mutations in *VSX2* lead to microphthalmia in humans and mice. Removal of the lens placode from cultured OV causes abnormal differentiation that can be rescued by exogenous Fgf.

Involvement and development of the RPE

The retinal pigmented epithelium (RPE) develops from dorsal neuroectoderm of the early OV and is required for morphogenesis of the neural retina. Microphthalmia associated transcription factor, *Mitf*, a basic helix-loop-helix leucine zipper

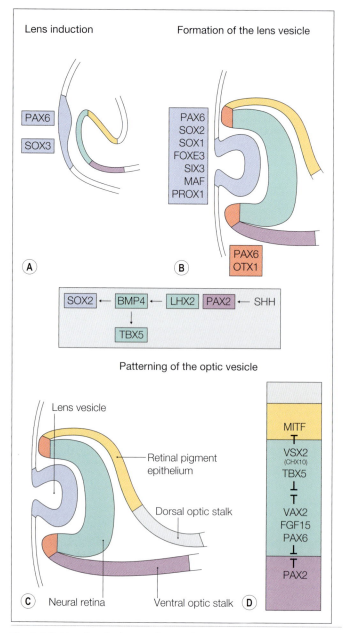

Fig. 3.4 Patterning the lens, retina, and RPE. (A) The formation of the lens requires signaling between the surface ectoderm and the optic vesicle to form the lens placode. The optic stalk is patterned by induction of PAX2 via SHH. LHX2 induces expression of BMP4 in the PNR which in turn induces SOX2 expression in the surface ectoderm; this triggers a cascade of TF expression in the lens placode to induce lens vesicle formation (B, C). BMP4 also induces expression of TBX5. (D) A complex network of transcription factors acts by induction and repression to form the boundaries between the optic stalk and the PNR and the PNR and the RPE.

family gene, is expressed in the future RPE in both mouse and chick. Mutations in *Mitf* cause microphthalmia or anophthalmia in rodents and fish but not humans. *Otx1* and *Otx2* are transcription factors initially expressed throughout the PNR but later mark the presumptive RPE during optic cup formation. Loss-of-function mutations in *Otx* genes in mice result in RPE patterning defects and replacement with ectopic neural retina, while in *Mitf* mutant mice *Otx2* expression is lost. Both proteins co-localize within nuclei of RPE cells and may cooperate to activate other RPE genes. *Mitf* is also a transcriptional target of *Pax6*; both are co-expressed in the presumptive RPE with *Pax6* being restricted to the PNR at later stages.[15]

Lens development

As with many parts of eye development, Pax6 is a key player in lens development. Initially, Pax6 is expressed throughout the head ectoderm but then becomes restricted to the presumptive lens placode as the result of TGFβ signals from the underlying migratory cranial neural crest cells. Pax6 misexpression in *Xenopus* results in ectopic lens formation in developing OVs.[16] Pax6, the Meis family of transcription factors, Bmp7 and Fgf signaling define the regional localization of the placode prior to ectodermal thickening.[17] Both Bmp4-null and Bmp7-null mice do not induce lens development. Disruption of Fgf signaling results in a reduction in placodal Pax6 expression and causes defects in early lens development and lens pit invagination. Co-binding of Sox2 (or Sox1) and Pax6 to enhancers is necessary for early lens crystallin gene expression. The forkhead family gene FoxE3 is a Pax6 target gene, which is expressed in the presumptive lens placode. FoxE3 mutations in humans and mice cause aphakia and microphthalmia. In Mab21l1 mutants, FoxE3 expression is absent in the lens placode yet Pax6 is unaffected, suggesting that activation of Mab21l1 lies between placodal Pax6 and FoxE3 activation.[17] Mab21l1-deficient mice have rudimentary lenses as a result of insufficient invagination of the placode due to insufficient expression of FoxE3 with normal expression of Pax6, Sox2, and Six3. The MAF family of basic leucine zipper transcription factors is also implicated in lens development and is regulated by Pax6.

Once the lens vesicle has separated from the surface ectoderm Prox1 expression is essential for the differentiation and elongation of lens fiber cells with Prox1 mutant lenses failing to polarize and elongate resulting in a hollow lens.[18] Pax6 remains expressed in the lens epithelium until just after the time of vacuole closure, whereas Sox2 is down-regulated soon after vacuole formation. Sox1 is expressed throughout the lens at this time, replacing expression of Sox2 and being present in primary fiber cells. Mutations in mouse Sox1 cause cataracts.

Differentiation of the neural retina

The differentiation of the multipotent retinal progenitors involves the interaction of activating and repressing bHLH transcription factors[19] with each retinal cell type having a unique bHLH factor combinatorial code. Hes1 and Hes5 are both repressive bHLH molecules and double null mutants (see Box 3.1) lack OVs. Retinal ganglion cells (RGCs) are generated from progenitors co-expressing Pax6 and the bHLH activator gene atoh7. Sox2 is expressed widely in neural progenitors. Human heterozygous loss-of-function mutations in Sox2 cause bilateral anophthalmia and severe microphthalmia cases.[20] Hypomorphic mutations in mouse Sox2 result in the loss of RGCs and cause disrupted cell lamination within the neural retina. The decreased levels of Sox2 are associated with reduced Notch1 and Hes-5 expression, while atoh7 and Pax6 are up-regulated. These data are consistent with a key role for Sox2 in the maintenance of retinal neural progenitors.

Shh acts as a retinal precursor cell mitogen increasing neuron cell numbers in culture experiments.[21] The Shh receptor, Patched, is expressed in the neuroblastic layer of the retina in a pattern that follows the wave of differentiating ganglion cells, first observed in the GCL and then later within the INL. The bHLH activators Neurod1 and Neurod4 are expressed in differentiating amacrine cells. In double mutant mice, amacrine cells are completely missing while ganglion and Müller glial cell numbers are increased. Co-expression of Pax6/Neurod1 or Pax6/Neurod1/Neurod4 promotes amacrine cell differentiation, while co-expression of Pax6/Neurod4 results in more horizontal than amacrine cells. Bipolar cells co-express Vsx2/Neurod4/Ascl1 (another bHLH activator). Horizontal cells require co-expression of Pax6/Neurod4/Prox1/Foxn4. Rods and cones require co-expression of Neurod1, Ascl1, Crx, and Otx2. Crx is necessary for normal cone and rod function and is implicated in human photoreceptor degeneration and Leber's congenital amaurosis (LCA; MIM#602225) (see Chapter 44).

Closure of the optic fissure

The optic fissure begins as a deep groove that runs from the ventral rim of the OV continuously along the ventral aspect of the entire outgrowth that provides a channel for hyaloid blood vessels to enter the lentiretinal space (the area between the lens vesicle and the inner wall of the optic cup). Fusion of the fissure begins with apposition of the inferior lips of the ventralmost optic cup and continues anteriorly toward its rim and posteriorly along the optic stalk. Little is known about the genetic factors underlying the fusion event; however, failure of this process results in the commonest major eye malformation, optic fissure closure defects (OFCD, e.g. iris, retina, or optic nerve coloboma). *Pax2* and *Vax2* are expressed in the ventral optic stalk and have both been implicated in OFCD. Patients with Pax2 mutations develop optic nerve coloboma,[22] while both Pax2 and Vax2 knockout mice display colobomata, suggesting that genes expressed in the ventral portion of the OV in the early stages of development may contribute and coordinate the closure of the optic fissure. CHD7 mutations are a common cause of syndromal OFCD as a component of CHARGE syndrome[23] (see Chapter 51). The cause of the vast majority of non-syndromal OFCD cases remains unknown although *PAX6*, *SOX2*, and *SHH* mutations have been reported in a few cases.

Cornea and anterior segment development

The cornea, lens, and anterior segment structures (ciliary body, iris, vitreous, and trabecular meshwork) are formed by contributions from various cell populations from distinct origins in spatially and temporally coordinated interactions. The cornea is derived from both surface ectoderm and neural crest-derived periocular mesenchyme cells. The ectodermal cells secrete a collagen-rich matrix that attracts the surrounding mesenchymal cells to form the stroma of the future corneal epithelium. A second wave of mesenchymal cells forms the corneal endothelium, or posterior stroma. Other neural crest-derived mesenchymal cells line the anterior chamber; iris stroma, and trabecular meshwork. The transcription factor Lmxb1 is required for the normal development of the latter structure.[24] Normal dosage of PAX6 is required for formation of the iris with haploinsufficiency (see Box 3.1) leading to aniridia in humans and mice. PITX2 and FOXC1 are also crucial for normal anterior segment development.[25,26] The pigmented region of iris develops from an outgrowth from the tip of the optic cup margin; the iris muscles form from the outer layer of the optic cup margin. The aqueous humor is secreted into the anterior chamber by the ciliary body epithelium and exits through the trabecular meshwork at the angle of the eye, which has at its anterior the cornea, while the iris is positioned at its posterior. These structures control the flux of aqueous humor in the anterior segment, and maintenance of intraocular pressure is highly important in both the development of the anterior segment and in the adult organ itself.

Summary

Our understanding of the molecular basis of eye development has benefited from an ongoing dialogue between basic developmental biologists and human geneticists, which has successfully elucidated critical patterning and signaling events involved in early development of the lens, retina, and RPE. The emergence of new high-throughput sequencing technologies should increase the pace of discovery dramatically.

References

1. Okita K, Ichisaka T, Yamanaka S. Generation of germline-competent induced pluripotent stem cells. Nature 2007; 448: 313–317.

2. Kuriyama S, Mayor R. Molecular analysis of neural crest migration. Philos Trans R Soc Lond B Biol Sci 2008; 363: 1349–1362.

3. Wyllie AH, Kerr JF, Currie AR. Cell death: the significance of apoptosis. Int Rev Cytol 1980; 68: 251–306.

4. Esteve P, Bovolenta P. Secreted inducers in vertebrate eye development: more functions for old morphogens. Curr Opin Neurobiol 2006; 16: 13–19.

5. de Iongh RU, Abud HE, Hime GR. WNT/Frizzled signaling in eye development and disease. Front Biosci 2006; 11: 2442–2464.

6. Brand M, Heisenberg CP, Warga RM, et al. Mutations affecting development of the midline and general body shape during zebrafish embryogenesis. Development 1996; 123: 129–142.

7. Teraoka ME, Paschaki M, Muta Y, Ladher RK. Rostral paraxial mesoderm regulates refinement of the eye field through the bone morphogenetic protein (BMP) pathway. Dev Biol 2009; 330: 389–398.

8. Pottin K, Hinaux H, Retaux S. Restoring eye size in *Astyanax mexicanus* blind cavefish embryos through modulation of the Shh and Fgf8 forebrain organising centres. Development 2011; 138: 2467–2476.

9. Yamamoto Y, Stock DW, Jeffery WR. Hedgehog signalling controls eye degeneration in blind cavefish. Nature 2004; 431: 844–847.

10. Sasagawa S, Takabatake T, Takabatake Y, et al. Axes establishment during eye morphogenesis in Xenopus by coordinate and antagonistic actions of BMP4, Shh, and RA. Genesis 2002; 33: 86–96.

11. Chow RL, Lang RA. Early eye development in vertebrates. Annu Rev Cell Dev Biol 2001; 17: 255–296.

12. Mui SH, Kim JW, Lemke G, Bertuzzi S. Vax genes ventralize the embryonic eye. Genes Dev 2005; 19: 1249–1259.

13. Kim JW, Lemke G. Hedgehog-regulated localization of Vax2 controls eye development. Genes Dev 2006; 20: 2833–2847.

14. Rainger J, van Beusekom E, Ramsay JK, et al. Loss of the BMP antagonist, SMOC-1, causes ophthalmo-acromelic (Waardenburg anophthalmia) syndrome in humans and mice. PLoS Genet 2011; 7: e1002114.

15. Martinez-Morales JR, Rodrigo I, Bovolenta P. Eye development: a view from the retina pigmented epithelium. Bioessays 2004; 26: 766–777.

16. Zuber ME, Gestri G, Viczian AS, et al. Specification of the vertebrate eye by a network of eye field transcription factors. Development 2003; 130: 5155–5167.

17. Lang RA. Pathways regulating lens induction in the mouse. Int J Dev Biol 2004; 48: 783–791.

18. Wigle JT, Chowdhury K, Gruss P, Oliver G. Prox1 function is crucial for mouse lens-fibre elongation. Nat Genet 1999; 21: 318–322.

19. Hatakeyama J, Kageyama R. Retinal cell fate determination and bHLH factors. Semin Cell Dev Biol 2004; 15: 83–89.

20. Fitzpatrick DR, van Heyningen V. Developmental eye disorders. Curr Opin Genet Dev 2005; 15: 348–353.

21. Wang YP, Dakubo G, Howley P, et al. Development of normal retinal organization depends on Sonic hedgehog signaling from ganglion cells. Nat Neurosci 2002; 5: 831–832.

22. Sanyanusin P, Schimmenti LA, McNoe LA, et al. Mutation of the PAX2 gene in a family with optic nerve colobomas, renal anomalies and vesicoureteral reflux. Nat Genet 1995; 9: 358–364.

23. Chang L, Blain D, Bertuzzi S, Brooks BP. Uveal coloboma: clinical and basic science update. Curr Opin Ophthalmol 2006; 17: 447–470.

24. Liu P, Johnson RL. Lmx1b is required for murine trabecular meshwork formation and for maintenance of corneal transparency. Dev Dyn 2010; 239: 2161–2171.

25. Gage PJ, Zacharias AL. Signaling "cross-talk" is integrated by transcription factors in the development of the anterior segment in the eye. Dev Dyn 2009; 238: 2149–2162.

26. Skarie JM, Link BA. FoxC1 is essential for vascular basement membrane integrity and hyaloid vessel morphogenesis. Invest Ophthalmol Vis Sci 2009; 50: 5026–5034.

Normal and abnormal visual development

Anne B Fulton • Ronald M Hansen • Anne Moskowitz • D Luisa Mayer

Introduction

Development of visual function accompanies development of the eye and brain. The eye grows and the retinal ganglion cell axons find their way out of the eye and, via the optic nerve and neural visual pathways, reach visual cortex targets. As the eye grows, optical properties of the eye change and, normally, emmetropization occurs.[1] Retinal cells move to pave the expanding peripheral retina and to create a fovea that matures to mediate exquisite visual resolution.[2-4] Myelination of the optic nerve fibers continues until approximately age 2 years.[5] Also, after birth, brain myelination continues, brain volume increases, and brain organization matures.[6,7] Concurrently, as the infant develops, visual capabilities increase and become more adult-like.

Diseases of the eye and visual system may decrease visual capabilities, while increases in these capabilities accompany development. Functional deficits may occur even if abnormalities in structure and chemistry are undetectable. In children, sorting out what is due to immaturity versus disease is fundamental. Repeated measures over time help separate effects of development from effects of disease.

Rigorous, non-invasive psychophysical and electrophysiological tests, originally used to study normal visual development in infants, have been modified for clinical application. For measurement of vision, stimuli must be specified in precise physical terms. There must be a reliable relationship of the stimulus to the child's response. Comparison to normal values for age is crucial for valid interpretation of vision test results.

Measurement provides critical information that complements clinical history and observation. Interpretation of the numeric results of an individual patient's vision test includes comparison to normal values for age, such as the mean and prediction interval for normal.[8] Data obtained in serial measurements can be compared to the patient's own prior results to chart the patient's course.

We limit our discussion to those visual functions that are regularly measured clinically, such as visual acuity and visual fields, and those that have been used to investigate strabismus and amblyopia and retinal dystrophies of early onset. The visual functions that are informative in these conditions, in addition to visual acuity and visual fields, are contrast sensitivity, vernier acuity, stereoacuity, and dark adapted visual threshold. For each visual function, we present quantitative information about normal development and comment on the structural and neurophysiological bases for these sensory functions. Some visual functions are mediated by the central retina (grating and letter acuity; contrast sensitivity; vernier acuity; stereoacuity) and others by the peripheral retina (dark adapted, rod mediated visual threshold; visual field). The most commonly measured visual function, visual acuity, evaluates the function of the entire visual pathway. Some visual functions are tested mainly to evaluate the function of the retina (dark adapted visual threshold). Vernier acuity and stereoacuity are non-invasive assessments of processes in the brain. Human retinal and visual development is covered in a more comprehensive fashion elsewhere.[9-11]

Visual acuity

Visual acuity is mediated by the fovea, which projects to a large region of the primary visual cortex. By measuring acuity, the examiner assesses function along the entire visual pathway.

Visual acuity is defined as the finest detail (minimum angle of resolution, MAR) that is detectable.[12-14] Letters of overall size 5 minutes of arc and stroke width 1 minute of arc are designated according to different conventions as 20/20 or 6/6 Snellen, 1.0 decimal, or 0.0 logMAR. 20/200 symbols are 10 times larger. Letter acuity of 20/200 is one of the main criteria for legal blindness in many countries and thus a determinant of eligibility for vision support services where they exist.

In infants and young children who do not read letters or follow instructions for matching, acuity is tested using procedures that keep the child's response under stimulus control during preferential looking (PL), psychophysical (Fig. 4.1) or visual evoked potential (VEP) electrophysiological procedures. The stimuli are repetitive patterns, usually gratings (stripes) specified in minutes of arc (min arc) or cycles per degree (cpd). The development of normal acuity is summarized in Figure 4.2 and Table 4.1. Acuity increases systematically with age (see Fig. 4.2) despite the use of different stimuli (gratings, symbols) and procedures (preferential looking, matching, recognition). At age 2.5 to 3 years developmentally normal children can be tested using symbols and a matching task. Before that age, acuity measurements are accomplished using PL or VEP procedures. For convenience, mean values of normal acuity along with the prediction interval for normal (8) at selected ages are listed in Table 4.1.

During infancy, acuity measured using VEP[15-18] is higher than that obtained using PL.[19,20] In a healthy infant at age 6 months, average PL acuity is 6 min arc and average VEP acuity is approximately 2 min arc.[21,22] The elements of a 20/120 letter subtend 6 min arc, and those of a 20/40 letter subtend 2 min arc. VEP acuity is constrained by processes in the eye, the pathway from the eye to the visual cortex, and the visual cortex.[17] The same processes also constrain PL acuity, but, additionally, PL acuity requires processing in higher neural areas, attention,[23] and eye–head movement. Differences in stimuli, analysis techniques, and response measures also contribute to the VEP–PL difference.

During development, acuity is limited in part by immaturities of the fovea. The fetal fovea becomes identifiable as a ~1665 μm diameter rod free retinal region at about 22 weeks' gestation.[4] By term, the diameter of this immature central retinal region containing exclusively cones has decreased to ~1100 μm; the diameter continues to decrease and reaches the adult diameter (~700 μm) by 15 months.[4] The fovea

continues to mature until approximately age 3 years.[2,24,25] The cones first develop inner segments, which are wider than those in adults, and then outer segments. As the diameter of the rod free zone diminishes, the cone center-to-center spacing decreases, and the inner segments become more slender as the foveal pit develops.[2,26] These features of the foveal cones partially account for low acuity in young infants; there are also post-receptor immaturities which have been documented using the multifocal electroretinogram.[27] Furthermore, immaturities of visual processes in the brain are recognized.[7,28-30]

Assessments of acuity contribute to diagnosis and to assessment of severity and course of disease (Fig. 4.3). PL acuity tests have been used widely for assessment of infant and childhood ophthalmic disorders.[31-35] PL and VEP tests also can measure acuity in patients with cognitive impairment; PL tests have been more widely used. On average, about an octave deficit (a halving of spatial frequency) in acuity was found in patients with cognitive impairment even if the eyes were normal.[36,37]

In diverse ophthalmic disorders the deficit in letter acuity often exceeds that in grating acuity. This was demonstrated in mature subjects with amblyopia who could perform both letter and grating acuity tests. Letter acuity for the amblyopic eye was on average 1.5 times worse than grating acuity.[38] Compared to the simple repetitive pattern of gratings, letters have complex spatial content. For those patients for whom, due to age or ability, grating acuity by PL or VEP provides the feasible test, interpretation of the grating acuity rests on a foundation of knowledge about the relationship of grating and letter acuity in patients. If grating acuities are reported to educators and agencies without explanation, children may be unnecessarily declared ineligible for services.[39,40]

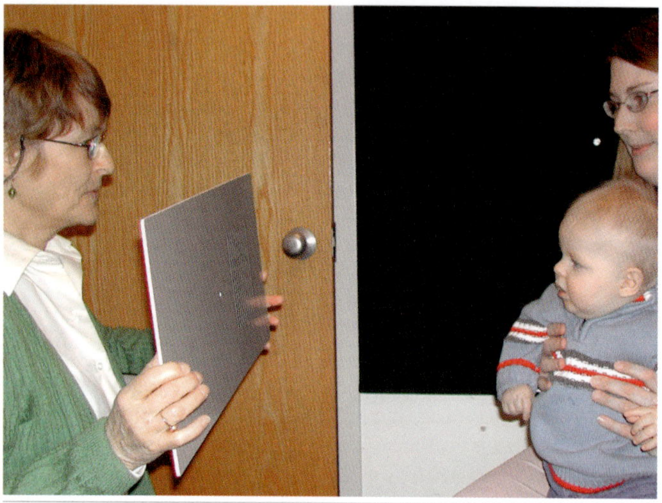

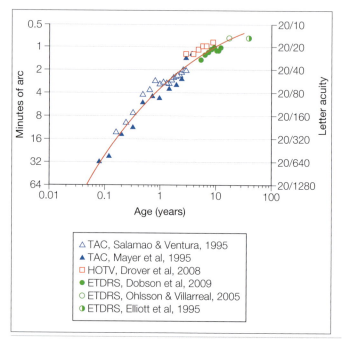

Fig. 4.1 **Preferential looking test of acuity using the Teller Acuity Cards (TAC).** The 10-month-old is seated on his mother's lap. The examiner shows a series of cards with black and white stripes (gratings) on the left (or the right), starting with wide stripes. The examiner, who is unaware of the right-left position of the stripes, must judge the stripe location based on the infant's head and eye movement response.[19] Acuity is taken as the narrowest stripes to which the infant responds.

Fig. 4.2 **Development of acuity in normal subjects.** The mean monocular acuity is shown as a function of age. Grating acuity (triangles) from age 1 month to 4 years was obtained using the Teller Acuity Card (TAC) preferential looking procedure.[19,20] HOTV letters (squares) were used to measure acuity from age 3 to 9 years.[124] ETDRS letters (circles) were used for children from 5 to 12 years,[125] 17- and 18-year-olds,[126] and adults.[127] The smooth curve drawn by eye describes average acuity as a function of age.

Table 4.1 – Acuity Development. Mean visual acuity and 95% prediction interval.

Age	Min arc	Sn VA	95% Prediction limits*		Age	Min arc	Sn VA	95% Prediction limits*	
			Lower	Upper				Lower	Upper
Grating acuity					9		~20/20	~20/41	~20/10
1 month	32.84		65.68	16.42	10		~20/20	~20/39	~20/10
2	15.72		31.45	7.86	11		~20/19	~20/38	~20/9
3	10.63		21.26	5.32	12		~20/18	~20/36	~20/9
4	8.20		16.39	4.10	Adult		~20/15	~20/30	~20/8
5	6.76		13.53	3.38	**Conversion of acuity metrics.**				
6	5.82		11.64	2.91	**Snellen**	**Min arc**	**Cpd**	**Dec VA**	**LogMAR**
7	5.14		10.29	2.57	20/2400	120.00	0.25	0.008	2.08
8	4.64		9.28	2.32	20/1600	80.00	0.38	0.013	1.90
9	4.24		8.49	2.12	20/1200	60.00	0.50	0.017	1.78
10	3.93		7.85	1.96	20/800	40.00	0.75	0.025	1.60
11	3.66		7.33	1.83	20/600	30.00	1.00	0.033	1.48
12	3.45		6.89	1.72	20/400	20.00	1.50	0.050	1.30
15	2.96		5.91	1.48	20/300	15.00	2.00	0.067	1.18
18	2.62		5.25	1.31	**20/200**	**10.00**	**3.00**	**0.100**	**1.00**
21	2.38		4.76	1.19	20/150	7.50	4.00	0.133	0.88
24	2.19		4.39	1.10	20/100	5.00	3.00	0.200	0.70
30	1.93		3.85	0.96	20/80	4.00	7.50	0.250	0.60
36	1.74		3.48	0.87	20/60	6.00	10.00	0.333	0.48
48	1.49		2.99	0.75	20/50	2.50	12.00	0.400	0.40
Symbol acuity					20/40	2.00	15.00	0.500	0.30
3 years		~20/35	~20/70	~20/17	20/30	1.50	20.00	0.667	0.18
4		~20/30	~20/60	~20/15	20/25	1.25	24.00	0.800	0.10
5		~20/27	~20/53	~20/13	**20/20**	**1.00**	**30.00**	**1.000**	**0.00**
6		~20/25	~20/49	~20/12	20/15	0.75	40.00	1.333	−0.12
7		~20/23	~20/46	~20/11	20/10	0.50	60.00	2.000	−0.30
8		~20/22	~20/43	~20/11					

*The prediction interval is the range within which values of 95% of the normal population are expected (8).

Contrast sensitivity

In the real world, objects of widely varying contrast are encountered. Visual acuity is typically tested using high contrast stimuli and, therefore, fails to capture important information about vision. For detection at lower contrast, stimulus elements must be larger than at high contrast (Fig. 4.4). PL[41-44] and VEP[45-47] procedures have been modified to study development of normal contrast sensitivity and clinical conditions. Contrast sensitivity is tested in older children using commercially available charts with gratings or letters.[48,49]

Patients with retinal degenerations or optic nerve demyelination often have low contrast sensitivity. Patients with such disorders may have 20/40, or even 20/20, acuity at high contrast (>95%) and 20/100 acuity at low contrast (10%). On real world tasks, poor contrast sensitivity causes difficulty on everyday vision-mediated tasks even though acuity measured in high contrast conditions may indicate only mild to moderate deficits. This can baffle educators and other caregivers, but may be readily clarified if recognized by the ophthalmologist. Documentation of low contrast sensitivity supports requests for appropriate educational planning.

Vernier acuity and stereoacuity

Vernier acuity and stereoacuity require the processing of visual information in the brain. These functions depend upon integrity of the fovea and optic nerve and complex cortical processing; thus they are higher order visual processes.

Vernier acuity

Vernier acuity is the ability to detect discontinuity in a line.[13,14,50] This is critical to pattern perception. In healthy adults, vernier acuity is approximately an order of magnitude better than letter acuity.[51] Development of normal vernier acuity has been

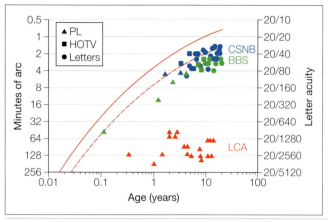

Fig. 4.3 Acuity in patients. Data are from a patient with Bardet-Biedl syndrome (BBS, *BBS7*; green symbols), X-linked congenital stationary night blindness (CSNB, blue symbols), and Leber's congenital amaurosis (LCA, *CRB1*; red symbols). The solid red line, re-plotted from Fig. 4.2, describes average acuity as a function of age and the dashed line the lower 95% prediction limit of normal;[8] see also Table 4.1. Age appropriate tests were used for the patient with BBS and CSNB. In the patients with BBS, acuity remains near the lower limits of normal for age and shows a developmental increase; over the same interval, his dark adapted visual threshold worsened. In the patient with CSNB, visual acuity remained stable as did his dark adapted visual threshold. Acuity in the patient with LCA, who had marked macular atrophy, was measured using the gratings of the preferential looking test. This patient's dark adapted visual threshold worsened significantly during childhood (youngest patient in Fig. 4.6). An octave variability in repeated measures of acuity may be expected in children.

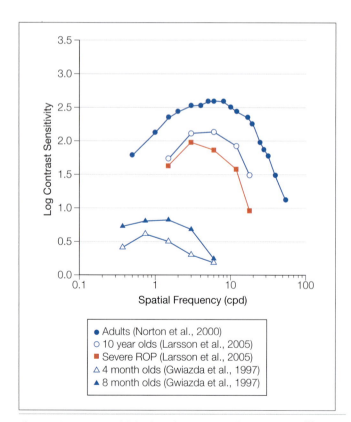

Fig. 4.4 Contrast sensitivity functions. Date are for healthy adult,[128] child,[129] and infant subjects[44] and for pediatric patients with a history of treated retinopathy of prematurity.[129] Data are re-plotted from the cited references. All data were obtained using psychophysical procedures.

studied using PL[52-56] and VEP[57] procedures. Vernier acuity and grating acuity develop at different rates (Fig. 4.5); vernier acuity surpasses grating acuity during infancy[52,54] and childhood.[55,56] Adult levels are reached later for vernier than for grating acuity.[55,57]

Vernier acuity is relatively tolerant to defocus, motion, and, in some conditions, luminance.[58-60] Tests of vernier acuity are, therefore, potentially robust for clinical application. The advantages, however, are offset by susceptibility of vernier acuity to practice effects and attention.[61,62] Although vernier is better than letter acuity in healthy adults (see Fig. 4.5), in amblyopia, deficits in vernier and letter acuity are similar.[38] In children with cerebral visual impairment, deficits in vernier acuity are greater than deficits in grating acuity.[63] The wider use of vernier acuity tests to detect and monitor pediatric ophthalmic disorders warrants consideration.

Stereoacuity

Development of normal stereoacuity has been well studied.[64-68] Infants may demonstrate stereopsis as early as 2 to 3 months, but most show onset at 3 to 5 months of age. The course of stereoacuity development is more rapid than that of grating acuity (see Fig. 4.5). Thresholds are 3 to 5 min arc by age 6 months; in adults, stereoacuity is 1 min arc or better. The onset of infantile esotropia occurs when stereoacuity is normally undergoing rapid development.[69] Stereoacuity tests may detect strabismus and amblyopia,[67,70] and stereoacuity is used to assess outcomes of treatment for esotropia.[71,72]

Dark adapted visual threshold

The ability to detect dim spots of light in the dark develops in early infancy. The test spot must be brighter for detection by a

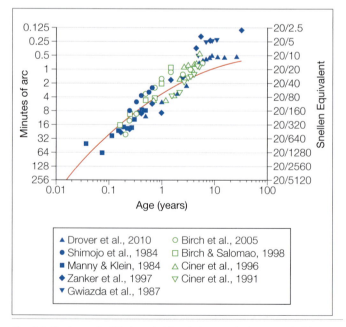

Fig. 4.5 Vernier acuity (filled symbols) and stereoacuity (open symbols) as a function of age in healthy subjects. Data are re-plotted from the cited studies.[52-56,65,67,68,130] The smooth red curve, which shows average acuity as a function of age, is re-plotted from Fig. 4.2.

young infant than by an adult. At age 4 weeks, threshold is on average 1.4 log unit above that in adults.[10,73,74] By age 6 months, the threshold has become equivalent to that in adults.[10]

Threshold is measured following a period of dark adaptation using a modified PL procedure. The stimuli must be carefully specified and controlled.[10] Stimuli are chosen to favor detection by the rod system. Spectral sensitivity functions confirm that dark adapted thresholds are rod mediated in infants as young as age 4 weeks.[73,75,76] The threshold is constrained by catch of photons by rods. By term, the infant's retina has an adult complement of rods. The infant's rod outer segments are shorter and contain less rhodopsin than adults.[77] Therefore, more light must fall on the infant's retina to produce the same response as in an adult.[10,73,77-79] Normally, there is a delay in developmental elongation of the 10° eccentric rod outer segments compared to those in more peripheral (30°) retina; this is accompanied by a delay in development of the 10° eccentric dark adapted threshold. Studies of rod mediated spatial summation show that infants' receptive fields are larger than in the mature retina;[80,81] immaturities of infantile temporal summation are attributed to the rod photoreceptor.[82]

The dark adapted visual threshold mediated by rod photoreceptors in the peripheral retina has been studied in children with retinal disease;[83-86] it can be used to follow retinal disease even when the electroretinogram is markedly attenuated.[86,87] Figure 4.6 shows representative results from patients with Leber's congenital amaurosis (LCA). A 1 log unit worsening of threshold indicates significant progression of disease.[86] Near peripheral (10°) threshold development in infants with a history of retinopathy of prematurity (ROP) is delayed relative to that in term-born infants.[83] The ROP subjects with near peripheral threshold elevation have altered function of the rods in that retinal region.[88] Deficits in peripheral rod thresholds are associated with deficits in post-receptor retinal sensitivity.[89]

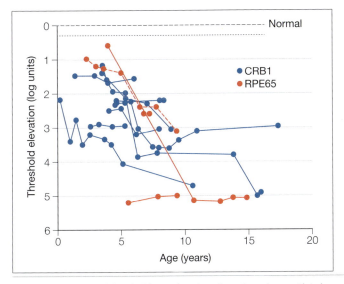

Fig. 4.6 Dark adapted thresholds as a function of age in patients with Leber congenital amaurosis due to changes in *CRB1* or *RPE65* genes. The normal mean threshold is at zero; the dotted line indicates 2 standard deviations below the mean. Shown are thresholds for detecting 10° diameter, 50 ms duration spots presented 20° to the right or left of a small red fixation light.[10] The majority of these patients had worsening thresholds.

Visual fields

The peripheral visual field is assessed in light adapted conditions. Stimuli are presented at selected sites in the periphery. The examiner must provide a procedure by which the patient's response can be reliably related to the stimulus. Adults and older children are capable of communicating their response by buzzer press or similar. Their thresholds for reliable detection of peripheral stimuli can be determined rapidly using automated equipment and standardized statistical procedures. Acceptable reliability indices in automated static perimetry can be obtained in normal 8-year-olds[90,91] and, after a training session, in some children as young as 5 years.[92] Non-automated procedures, such as Goldmann kinetic perimetry, are feasible in children at 4 years, particularly if cast as a computer game.[93] In our opinion, conventional testing should be attempted as young as possible in children at risk of field defects. The youngster's central fixation and subsequent head and eye movement response (orienting response) to the stimulus must be under strict surveillance by the examiner.

Maturation of the peripheral visual field in normal infants and children has been studied. The visual field extent in term-born neonates is significantly smaller than in older children and adults.[94,95] The horizontal extent of the visual field increases monotonically from age 2 months through infancy; by age 1.5 to 4 years, binocular and monocular field extent is 90–95% of that in adults. In children age 4 to 10 years, the visual field extent obtained with arc or hemispheric perimeters approximates that obtained by Goldmann kinetic perimetry.[94,96-103] Maturation of the nasal compared to temporal field may be delayed, although not all studies agree.[94,98,99] Variability in infant and child visual field extent is high; the 95% confidence interval is typically +/− 10 to 15 degrees for monocular field extent.[94,97,98] Attention and visual immaturity limit visual field extent.

Patients with cognitive impairment or neurologic limitations who cannot attend sufficiently for tests using automated or other conventional perimeters are tested using alternative procedures. Some of these procedures were devised to study development of the peripheral visual field in normal infants. Psychophysical schemes similar to those used in PL assessments of visual acuity can impose rigor on visual field testing of pediatric patients.

Confrontation testing is the most commonly used alternative test. The patient must have adequate looking behavior to respond to targets such as toys or lights. The examiner must be alert to the patient's fixation behavior before presentation of the stimulus. The fixation target is typically the examiner's face. The examiner must be alert to the patient's orienting response to the peripheral stimulus. Typically the stimulus is presented starting in the far periphery and is moved slowly toward the center. Each quadrant must be tested. Spurious responses to the examiner's movements confound confrontation testing. To reduce this, a slender wand with lighted tip may be used. Game-like ploys are important for sustaining attention. Standard stimuli and procedures for confrontation testing are not established. The clinician should use the same stimuli and procedure from one test session to the next. The stimuli (in contrast to those used in modern, automated equipment) are well above detection threshold and the sampling of the peripheral visual space is coarse; small scotomata will be missed. Accordingly, these procedures are suitable for defining large, absolute defects such as hemianopia or quadrantanopia produced by retro-chiasmal disease, inferior altitudinal field loss due to white matter injury of prematurity in the parietal-occipital regions of the brain[104] (see Chapter 56), and constriction of the visual field caused by retinal degeneration or drug toxicity.[93,105]

An arc perimeter (Fig. 4.7) or modified hemispheric perimeter provides an advantage over confrontation testing because numeric results are obtained. A map of the patient's responses to stimuli at selected peripheral eccentricities can be specified. Stimuli have included white spheres, LEDs, and other small lights. Responses in each quadrant along the major obliques (45°, 135°, 225°, and 315°) must be measured. Children's visual fields mapped using kinetic arc perimetry have high variability, even when the same stimuli and procedures are used as in some ROP and other studies.[105-107] If monocular visual field testing is not feasible, binocular testing may yield useful information about the child's visual capabilities.

There are a number of matters peculiar to infants' behavior that impact performance of the visual field test. The balance of attention between central and peripheral stimuli influences measured field extent. A too-salient central stimulus may inhibit the infant's ability to disengage and orient toward the peripheral stimulus.[94,108] Ideally, the central stimulus should be similar to the peripheral stimulus in luminance and spatial extent. Spatial extent of the stimulus, rate of central movement, and rate of flicker all have demonstrable effect on field extent in infants.[109-112] Sounds synchronized with presentation of central and peripheral stimuli may enhance attention and orienting in young infants, but not in toddlers.[94] Notably, the parameters that affect infants' fields have little effect on adults' fields.[110,111]

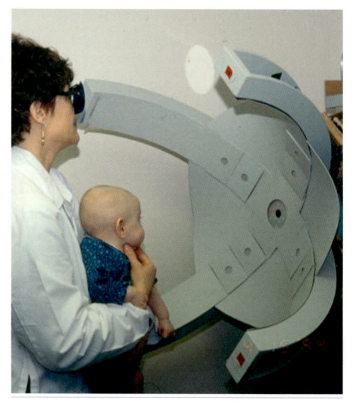

Fig. 4.7 An experimental arc perimeter used to test peripheral field in infants. A healthy infant, age 5 months, is looking at the central fixation display. The infant's orienting eye–head movement response will indicate detection of the peripheral stimulus. The peripheral stimulus is a flickering yellow LED presented along the arcs. The examiner, who is masked to the location of the yellow stimulus by wearing glasses with blue filters, uses a video system (not shown) to monitor the infant's fixation and report responses.[131]

Delayed development of visual responsiveness

The integrated development of structure and function of the eye and the visual pathways enables visual responsiveness at a very young age. A healthy, term-born infant usually starts smiling responsively at 5 weeks and fixes and follows readily by age 2 months. In some infants without conspicuous ophthalmic or medical abnormalities, the visual behavior does not meet normal developmental milestones. The term delayed visual maturation (DVM) has been applied to this problem.[113] DVM may be due more to a delay in development of visual *attention* than to identifiable pathophysiology of the visual system.[114]

Young infants lacking visual responsiveness are taken to the ophthalmologist because of suspected blindness. In some, no ophthalmic or neurologic abnormality is found and, in others, ophthalmic disease will be evident. Additionally, there are those who will be found to have disease of the brain, and still others without any specific clinical abnormalities of the eye or the brain, who will subsequently be diagnosed with a disorder which has associated cognitive impairment or neurodevelopmental disability. The universe of visually unresponsive young infants includes diverse diagnoses. Schemes for categorizing infants with visual delays have sought to organize a mass of information.[115,116] Among those infants in

whom the results of ophthalmic and neurologic examinations are normal, many rapidly develop normal visual responsiveness. A subset of such infants is subsequently found to have cognitive impairment.[116] Hoyt[114] followed, for two decades, patients who in infancy had isolated delays in visual responsiveness. Nearly all developed excellent visual acuity, but more than half manifested neurodevelopmental disorders, usually learning disabilities.[114]

There are several specific ophthalmic conditions that we encounter repeatedly in infants with visual inattention. Optic nerve hypoplasia is a structural abnormality found in some of these infants. Detectable (although sometimes subtle) ophthalmic anomalies occur in the various forms of albinism, perhaps the most common specific diagnosis underlying visual unresponsiveness in infancy.[117]

If another diagnosis cannot be secured, evaluation for severe congenital retinal dystrophy (e.g. LCA) by electroretinographic testing should be done (see Chapter 44). Even if visual inattention is profound in early infancy, patients with severe ocular disorders (including optic nerve hypoplasia and LCA) may show some developmental increments in PL acuity, presumably due to continuing maturation of the regions of the brain subserving vision.[32,118]

Among young, visually inattentive infants, we also find congenital anomalies of retinal function, achromatopsia, and congenital stationary night blindness (see Chapter 44). We narrow the differential diagnosis by electroretinography and then secure the diagnosis by molecular genetic study.

If the eye is not at fault, brain disorders must be considered as the cause of the infant's visual inattention. Structural abnormalities of the brain are found by MRI (see Chapter 56). Still other infants may have seizure activity; in particular, seizure activity in the frontal or parietal lobes is associated with reduced visual responsiveness even in the absence of brain malformation.[114]

Acuity measured by PL or VEP in infants with delayed visual responsiveness is variable, ranging from severely reduced[115] to normal for age.[119] The variability is not surprising given the diverse underlying diagnoses, the multiple components that must mature to produce visual responsiveness, and the fact that approximately half of the brain is dedicated to visual processing.[120] Fantz and co-workers originally considered PL as an assessment of infants' development generally, not only to assess acuity.[121] In our experience, young infants who show little or no visual responsiveness to faces or lights may have measurable PL acuity that is within the range of normal for age. These infants typically proceed to develop good vision. A substantial proportion of them may, however, have neurodevelopmental issues that become apparent later in infancy or childhood.

What underlies the delay in visual responsiveness in infants who clinically have normal eyes? Many answers may eventually be forthcoming. Studies using functional MRI techniques to study mature subjects with achromatopsia or albinism (diagnoses that we find in some infants with delayed visual responsiveness) show anomalous organization of vision-driven activity in the brain.[122,123] These anomalies of the brain's circuitry are too subtle to be detected by routine MRI studies. The processes that govern the turning on of an infant's vision will surely become more completely understood, including the sudden switching on of vision in those with isolated visual delays. We believe that working toward a specific diagnosis is the way to provide the best possible care of these patients.

Finally, we caution that young infants with poor vision often have delays in motor, social, and even language development. In the absence of visual input (such as facial expressions) coordination of social cues and motor development does not occur. This situation may mislead family and physicians. Early, thorough evaluation of the eyes, including electro-diagnostics if indicated, is the ophthalmologist's contribution to minimizing the likelihood of an incorrect diagnosis of global developmental delay in the visually unresponsive infant.

References

3. Packer O, Hendrickson AE, Curcio CA. Development redistribution of photoreceptors across the *Macaca nemestrina* (pigtail macaque) retina. J Comp Neurol 1990; 298: 472–93.
4. Yuodelis C, Hendrickson A. A qualitative and quantitative analysis of the human fovea during development. Vision Res 1986; 26: 847–55.
6. Atkinson J. The Developing Visual Brain. New York, NY: Oxford University Press; 2000.
9. Daw NW. Visual Development, 2nd ed. New York: Springer; 2006.
10. Fulton AB, Hansen RM, Moskowitz A, Akula JD. The neurovascular retina in retinopathy of prematurity. Prog Retin Eye Res 2009; 28: 452–82.
11. Braddick O, Atkinson J. Development of human visual function. Vision Res 2011; 26 [Epub ahead of print].
12. Hamer RD, Mayer DL. The development of spatial vision. In: Albert DM, Jakobiec FA, editors. Principles and Practice of Ophthalmology. Philadelphia: Harcourt Brace Jovanovich, Inc. 1993: 578–608.
17. Fulton AB, Hansen RM, Moskowitz A. Assessment of vision in infants and young children In: Celesia GC, editor. Handbook of Clinical Neurophysiology, Disorders of Visual Processing. Amsterdam: Elsevier; 2005: 218.
18. Birch EE. Assessing infant acuity, fusion, and steropsis with visual evoked potentials. In: Heckenlively JR, Arden JB, editors. Principles and Practice of Clinical Electrophysiology of Vision. Cambridge, MA: MIT Press; 2006: 356.
25. Hendrickson AE. The morphologic development of human and monkey retina. In: Albert DM, Jakobiec FA, editors. Principles and Practice of Ophthalmology: Basic Sciences. Philadelphia: WB Saunders; 1994: 561–77.
27. Hansen RM, Moskowitz A, Fulton AB. Multifocal ERG responses in infants. Invest Ophthalmol Vis Sci 2009; 50: 470–5.
29. Candy TR, Crowell JA, Banks MS. Optical, receptoral, and retinal constraints on foveal and peripheral vision in the human neonate. Vision Res 1998; 38: 3857–70.
33. Lim M, Soul JS, Hansen RM, et al. Development of visual acuity in children with cerebral visual impairment. Arch Ophthalmol 2005; 123: 1215–20.
35. Good WV. Final results of the Early Treatment for Retinopathy of Prematurity (ETROP) randomized trial. Trans Am Ophthalmol Soc 2004; 102: 233–48; discussion 48–50.
38. McKee SP, Levi DM, Movshon JA. The pattern of visual deficits in amblyopia. J Vis 2003; 3: 380–405.
44. Gwiazda J, Bauer J, Thorn F, Held R. Development of spatial contrast sensitivity from infancy to adulthood: psychophysical data. Optom Vis Sci 1997; 74: 785–9.
57. Skoczenski AM, Norcia AM. Development of VEP Vernier acuity and grating acuity in human infants. Invest Ophthalmol Vis Sci 1999; 40: 2411–7.
66. Birch E, Petrig B. FPL and VEP measures of fusion, stereopsis and stereoacuity in normal infants. Vision Res 1996; 36: 1321–7.
73. Hansen RM, Fulton AB. Development of scotopic retinal sensitivity. In: Simons K, editor. Early Visual Development, Normal and Abnormal, Ch. 8. Oxford: Oxford University Press; 1994: 130–42.
74. Hansen RM, Fulton AB. The course of maturation of rod-mediated visual thresholds in infants. Invest Ophthalmol Vis Sci 1999; 40: 1883–6.
77. Fulton AB, Dodge J, Hansen RM, Williams TP. The rhodopsin content of human eyes. Invest Ophthalmol Vis Sci 1999; 40: 1878–83.
78. Fulton AB, Hansen RM. The development of scotopic sensitivity. Invest Ophthalmol Vis Sci 2000; 41: 1588–96.
83. Barnaby AM, Hansen RM, Moskowitz A, Fulton AB. Development of scotopic visual thresholds in retinopathy of prematurity. Invest Ophthalmol Vis Sci 2007; 48: 4854–60.
86. Hansen RM, Eklund SE, Benador IY, et al. Retinal degeneration in children: dark adapted visual threshold and arteriolar diameter. Vision Res 2008; 48: 325–31.
89. Harris ME, Moskowitz A, Fulton AB, Hansen RM. Long-term effects of retinopathy of prematurity (ROP) on rod and rod-driven function. Doc Ophthalmol 2010; 122: 19–27.
93. Mayer DL, Fulton AB. Visual fields. In: Taylor D, Hoyt CS, editors. Pediatric Ophthalmology and Strabismus, 3rd ed. Edinburgh: Elsevier Saunders; 2005: 78–86.
96. Dobson V, Brown AM, Harvey EM, Narter DB. Visual field extent in children 3.5–30 months of age tested with a double-arc LED perimeter. Vision Res 1998; 38: 2743–60.
104. Jacobson L, Flodmark O, Martin L. Visual field defects in prematurely born patients with white matter damage of immaturity: a multiple-case study. Acta Ophthalmol Scand 2006; 84: 357–62.
114. Hoyt CS. Constenbader lecture. Delayed visual maturation: the apparently blind infant. J AAPOS 2004; 8: 215–9.

115. Tresidder J, Fielder AR, Nicholson J. Delayed visual maturation: ophthalmic and neurodevelopmental aspects. Dev Med Child Neurol 1990; 32: 872–81.

120. Van Essen DC. Organization of visual areas in macaque and human cerebral cortex. In: Chalupa LM, Werner JS, editors. The Visual Neurosciences, vol. 1. Cambridge, MA: The MIT Press; 2004: 507–21.

130. Birch EE, Morale SE, Jeffrey BG, et al. Measurement of stereoacuity outcomes at ages 1 to 24 months: Randot Stereocards. J AAPOS 2005; 9: 31–6.

Access the complete reference list online at

http://www.expertconsult.com

Emmetropization, refraction and refractive errors: control of postnatal eye growth, current and developing treatments

Christopher J Hammond

Chapter contents

The eye is one of the first recognizable organs during embryogenesis. Its development depends upon the orderly differentiation and migration of endoderm, mesoderm, neural and surface ectoderm, and neural crest tissue. Knowledge of ocular organogenesis helps to understand diagnosis and treatment of children with congenital ocular anomalies. Ocular anomalies are commonly associated with other structural anomalies, and their recognition can help in the diagnosis of infants with syndromes. Genetic factors control eye development and growth in utero. At birth, development is incomplete: postnatal growth, development, and organization of the eye and the visual pathway to the cortex is important for the normal development of vision.

Refractive error represents a mismatch between the eye's focal length and its axial length. Infant eyes undergo emmetropization whereby the average amount and the variance in the distribution of refractive errors are reduced. The precise mechanisms coordinating the optical and structural development of the eye are not completely understood. Animal experiments suggest that this process is guided by feedback from visual input, which has led to the search for risk factors and ways of stopping excess axial eye growth which is responsible for myopia and its progression.

Refractive error is the most common eye disorder, affecting over a third of adults, and is the cause of a significant burden of visual impairment in the world. The prevalence varies widely among countries; myopia is associated with education, urbanization, and affluence. The prevalence of myopia varies between 7% and 70% depending on the age, occupation, and educational status of those studied.[1] In some East Asian countries, myopia is becoming more common; indeed, it has reached epidemic proportions with over 80% of school leavers and up to 50% of 9-year-olds being myopic.[2] Myopia prevalence is increasing in developed countries with an approximate 1 diopter myopic shift in the US population between 1971 and 1999–2004.[3] The blinding complications of myopia (myopic retinal degeneration, retinal detachment, glaucoma, cataract) occur in highly myopic eyes (pathological myopia). The younger the onset, the faster the rate of progression and the higher the end myopic results. UK data suggests children myopic before the age of 9 years are likely to be at least 6 diopters myopic by adulthood.[4]

Postnatal growth and emmetropization

Refractive error is a mismatch between the optical refractive determinants of the eye (corneal curvature, lens power and location, and axial length). At birth, the eye is rarely emmetropic, and is significantly smaller than the adult eye (Table 5.1); the refractive error of the newborn eye ranges between +2.0 and +4.0 diopters (D) with an almost normal (Gaussian) distribution (Fig. 5.1A).[5] Within 2 years, this variability of

Table 5.1 – Newborn vs. adult ocular parameters

	Newborn	**Adult**
Axial length	16.8 mm	23.0 mm
Mean keratometry	55 D	43 D
Optic nerve length	24 mm	30 mm
Corneal diameter	10 mm	10.6 mm (vertical) × 11.7 mm (horiz.)
Corneal thickness	581 µm	545 µm
Pars plana length	0.5–1.05 mm	3.5–4 mm
Orbital volume	7 cc	30 cc

refractive error decreases and the mean value shifts so that the eye becomes closer to emmetropia. The population distribution becomes more leptokurtotic, which means it is more clustered around the mean value (Fig. 5.1B). This process is called emmetropization and, within populations, it is possible to predict shifts in refractive error so that most of the infants born hyperopic become emmetropic by 6 to 8 years of age. Eye growth is rapid, and reaches 90% of adult proportions by the age of 4. As the cornea flattens, it loses refractive power, which is balanced by increasing axial length. Whether this balance is guided by genetically encoded mechanisms or is affected by environmental influences has been debated for centuries. Most likely both nature and nurture affect the way the eye develops. By adulthood, the distribution of refractive error is similarly leptokurtotic, and there is a left skew in the distribution of the myopic subjects (Fig. 5.1C).[6]

Support for the assertion that eye growth is genetically regulated comes from studies of heritability and epidemiology. Almost all studies of refractive error, and in particular myopia, have shown that the strongest risk factors are having one or two parents who are myopic,[7] and pediatric ophthalmologists recognize the hyperopic/esotropic family attending their practices. While this might be ascribed to families sharing the same environmental risk factors, twin studies control for this shared environment by comparing concordance between monozygotic (identical) and dizygotic (fraternal) twin pairs. Twin studies, across ages and cultures, show a high heritability of refractive error, of the order of 80–90%.[8,9] This is not to say that the environment is not important. Strong temporal trends in myopia prevalence must be due to environmental factors. However, genetic factors appear important in determining where a person lies within the population distribution of a society at a particular time. Recently, genome-wide association studies have reported the association of several genes with refractive error,[10,11] and further genes will be identified. Like many complex traits, myopia susceptibility is conferred by many genes of small effect.

While Kepler suggested a local eye-mediated control of refractive error in the 17th century, myopia studies have been difficult to design, given the need for longitudinal data, and difficulties measuring the amount of close activity in children, and trying to control for factors including lighting, nutritional and other measures. There has been relatively little research into hyperopia, but risk factors for myopia are generally protective for hyperopia and vice versa.

There is a significant association of myopia with near work, educational level of attainment, and IQ.[12] The classic study by Zylbermann et al.[13] showed a significantly higher level of myopia in boys in orthodox schools in Israel, compared to boys in ordinary schools (81% vs. 27%) from the same genetic background. Girls in orthodox schools did not show this increased prevalence. Factors other than simply the amount of reading time, such as reading distance, lighting and a child's ability to concentrate on reading, are difficult to study. A significant amount of myopia is of adult-onset, after the age of 16.[14] This appears to be strongly related to education and the amount of close work. Recent studies have shown a protective effect for outdoor activity. In a comparison between 6-year-olds of East Asian descent in Singapore and Sydney, the hugely increased prevalence in Singapore (30% vs. 3%) was partly ascribed to 3 hours vs. 14 hours outside each week – and this is not just because children were not doing close work.[15] Other

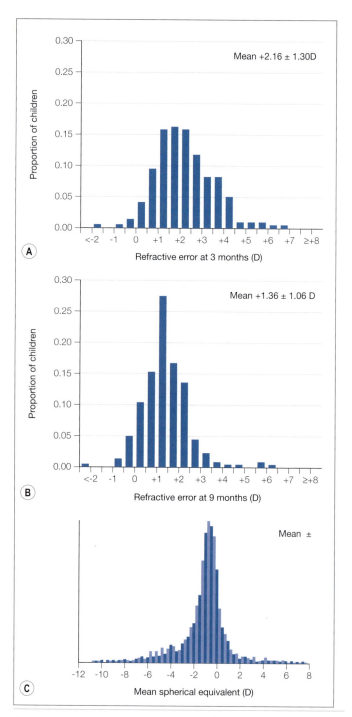

(A)

(B)

(C)

Fig. 5.1 Distribution of refractive error at different ages. (A) At 3 months of age; (B) at 20 months of age (from Mutti et al. Invest Ophthalmol Vis Sci 2005; 46: 3074–80); (C) an adult population distribution (in 1958 British Birth Cohort age 45 years) (from Simpson et al. Invest Ophthalmol Vis Sci 2007; 48: 4421–5).

risk factors for myopia include prematurity, low birth weight for gestational age, gender, greater maternal age, higher paternal occupational social class, and maternal smoking in early pregnancy as well as stature and socioeconomic class in adults.[16]

Animal models of myopia have studied the effect of visual input on the developing eye. Avian models (chicks), primate models (Macaque monkeys), marmosets, or tree shrews are commonly used.[17] These models have shown that when the eye is deprived of formed visual image early in life, axial myopia develops. Both axial myopia and axial hyperopia can be induced with defocusing spectacles or contact lenses placed in front of the eye of young animals; the changes are reversible. Much of the signaling is locally mediated and can occur in the presence of a sectioned optic nerve. Optical defocus leads to biochemical changes, which in turn result in changes in the sclera and choroid of the animals, resulting in axial myopia. Recent studies have cast doubt on the role of the macula, which had been the target of therapies, given the association between close work/accommodation and myopia. The driver of myopia progression may be the peripheral retina.[18]

Treatment of refractive errors

In young children, cycloplegic refraction is essential to establish the true refractive error; glasses should not be prescribed in preschool children without this, given the difficulty of subjective refraction in this age group.

Myopia

At what threshold should myopia be corrected in young children? There is no clear evidence base, but preverbal children have little need for good distance acuity, and preschool children often have a close working distance and no requirement for full distance correction. Guidelines from the American Academy of Ophthalmology's Preferred Practice Pattern[19] and the Pediatric Eye Disease Investigator Group (PEDIG)[20] both set 3 D of myopia as a threshold for correction in young children and the threshold may be even higher in myopic infants. For school-age children, I recommend full correction, but given that myopia is not generally amblyogenic, there is no insistence on a child having to wear their spectacles. Most children with significant myopia and of school age, however, are happy to wear their correction.

Treatments of myopia to prevent or slow progression (which occurs in the vast majority of children), as opposed to correction of the refractive error to enable normal visual acuity, have been based on either the close work theory or animal models of myopia. There are some practitioners who routinely undercorrect myopes, on the grounds that myopic individuals have an accommodation lag. Myopes do not fully accommodate to a near target compared to emmetropes; a slight undercorrection means reduced accommodation need. A randomized controlled trial in Malaysia showed faster progression in the group who were undercorrected by 0.75 D compared to the fully corrected group;[21] the current evidence does not support undercorrection. Soft contact lenses do not reduce or increase myopia progression. An RCT of rigid gas-permeable contact lenses versus spectacles, the CLAMP study, showed a slight reduction in progression over 3 years (1.56 D cf. 2.19 D) but not significant enough to justify the intervention.[22]

There have been several studies attempting to slow progression by reducing accommodation, by comparing single vision spectacles versus progressive add (varifocal) lenses (PAL). Studies in Hong Kong[23] and the United States (COMET study)[24] showed statistically significant slowing of progression using PAL, but only by a clinically insignificant amount of 0.2 D over 2 years (1.28 D vs. 1.48 D in the COMET). To date, trials of

optical manipulation have been disappointing in reducing myopia progression.

Animal models suggested a powerful effect of antimuscarinic agents in stopping eye growth. Atropine has been studied in children. The ATOM study in Singapore randomized 200 children to atropine drops in one eye, and showed a significant reduction in progression (two-thirds of eyes with atropine progressed less than 0.5 D in 2 years, compared to only 16% of untreated eyes).[25] However, after cessation of treatment there was a rapid catch-up in treated eyes. This raises the question whether some of the effect was a deep cycloplegia, and there is the question of how long treatment would be needed. Given the side-effects of photosensitivity and near blur (necessitating reading addition), few ophthalmologists treat myopia progression with atropine. There was hope that pirenzipine, a relatively selective M1 muscarinic inhibitor with fewer cycloplegia/dilation side-effects, would be effective. RCTs in the United States[26] and Singapore[27] showed an approximately halving of progression; however, this drug has never reached the market.

The recent focus on the peripheral retina in development and progression of myopia, and the protective effects of outdoor activity, means new treatments are being developed, including optical devices to cast a relatively myopic image onto the peripheral retina (bifocal contact lenses, or 360° multifocal spectacles), trials of increasing outdoor activity, and tinted lenses to approximate outdoor light frequencies. However, the present evidence basis suggests there is no effective treatment to reduce myopia progression; initial trials of spectacle designs to cast a less hyperopic defocus on peripheral retina have been disappointing. Orthokeratology, a treatment involving overnight rigid contact lens wear to flatten the cornea, is being used increasingly in children. As well as avoiding the need for spectacles, the flattening (which wears off, causing some change in refractive error over the day) may cast a more hyperopic defocus in the periphery and slow progression. There is some risk of corneal infection with these lenses. Trials are awaited. At present it seems sensible to recommend children spend time outdoors each day, not doing close work.

Hyperopia

Spectacle prescription for hyperopia poses challenges, given the fact that it is normal for children to be hyperopic and they have large accommodative reserves. Where visual acuity is reduced for age and a significant hyperopic refractive error is found on cycloplegic retinoscopy, correction is usually required, but this may apply only to those children who are very hyperopic (less than 1% of the population are >4 D). Low levels of hyperopia are not normally associated with reduced vision. Most ophthalmologists will slightly undercorrect the hyperopic child with no strabismus, to mimic "normal" hyperopia in the hope that emmetropization will occur. Yet, the evidence suggests few children with hyperopia more than 4 D will ever emmetropize. Full correction of hyperopic refractive errors measured using cycloplegia is essential in management of strabismus; children with accommodative esotropia should not be undercorrected. In children who are orthotropic the degree of undercorrection varies according to the age of the child and the degree of refractive error. My practice is an undercorrection of 1–2 D in children under the age of 6, and undercorrection of 1 D in children older than 6 years. PEDIG studies have undercorrected (symmetric) hyperopia by 1.5 D.[20]

There is controversy about treatment of asymptomatic hyperopic children. Practice differs between optometrists and ophthalmologists. Many optometrists believe that reading ability is helped by hyperopic spectacles, though a good study from Helveston et al. suggested, in the presence of good distance acuity, there was no relationship between reading ability, school performance, and degree of hyperopia.[28] Hyperopia is the most significant risk factor for esotropia: Atkinson et al. showed children with hyperopia >+3.50 D had a 13 times greater risk of developing strabismus or amblyopia than did children who had no significant hyperopia.[29] Prescribing spectacles for the hyperopia decreased the risk substantially, but the risk for strabismus in these children remained four times greater than in the general population. It seems logical to prescribe for children > 3.5 D, and to consider smaller amounts of hyperopia in children with difficulty reading or with other symptoms. Apart from anisometropia, children will tend to vote with their feet: if the spectacles help, they will wear them. If they perceive no benefit, they won't! Some older children who are 2 D or more hyperopic benefit from a correction when doing close work at school, or for computer use. The American Academy Preferred Practices Patterns recommendations suggest correcting 4.5 D in children aged 3 years and younger, and correcting reduced acuity or strabismus in children 4 years and over.[19]

Astigmatism

Symmetric astigmatism <1.5 D rarely causes loss of visual acuity or amblyopia, particularly meridional astigmatism, and does not require correction in young children. Where there is compound astigmatism and the spherical equivalent falls within the conoid of Sturm onto the retina, the acuity may be surprisingly good. The PEDIG studies have shown that spectacle correction alone brings acuity improvement even in anisometropic children; prescribing astigmatic correction in preschool children may be unnecessary. However, given acuity is usually reduced with astigmatism levels ≥2 D, most ophthalmologists prescribe at this level when it is found. Astigmatism with an oblique axis may reduce vision more, and I prescribe ≥1.5 D for older school-age children. Many research studies have used a prescribing cut-off of >1 D astigmatism; I recommend prescribing on visual acuity and symptoms, given reliable testing at older ages.

Anisometropia

Anisometropia is a strong amblyogenic stimulus (see Chapter 70). Generally, differences of more than 1 D in spherical equivalent and 1.0–1.5 D cylindrical correction are considered significantly amblyogenic warranting correction. Prescribing guidelines suggest full correction of the anisometropia, although hyperopic correction can be symmetrically reduced (in the absence of strabismus), maintaining the anisometropic difference. Age at correction is again controversial. Results are better at younger ages, but many anisometropic children can gain normal acuity even if spectacles are prescribed at relatively older ages – even after 8 years, as demonstrated in the PEDIG studies.[30] The role of refractive surgery in amblyopia is discussed in Chapter 68.

References

1. Saw SM, Katz J, Schein OD, et al. Epidemiology of myopia. Epidemi Rev 1996; 18: 175–87.
2. Morgan I, Rose K. How genetic is school myopia? Prog Retin Eye Res 2005; 24: 1–38.
3. Vitale S, Sperduto RD, Ferris FL, III. Increased prevalence of myopia in the United States between 1971–1972 and 1999–2004. Arch Ophthalmol 2009; 127: 1632–9.
4. Farbrother JE, Kirov G, Owen MJ, Guggenheim JA. Family aggregation of high myopia: estimation of the sibling recurrence risk ratio. Invest Ophthalmol Vis Sci 2004; 45: 2873–8.
5. Mutti DO, Mitchell GL, Jones LA, et al. Axial growth and changes in lenticular and corneal power during emmetropization in infants. Invest Ophthalmol Vis Sci 2005; 46: 3074–80.
6. Simpson CL, Hysi P, Bhattacharya SS, et al. The roles of PAX6 and SOX2 in myopia: lessons from the 1958 British Birth Cohort. Invest Ophthalmol Vis Sci 2007; 48: 4421–5.
7. Mutti DO, Mitchell GL, Moeschberger ML, et al. Parental myopia, near work, school achievement, and children's refractive error. Invest Ophthalmol Vis Sci 2002; 43: 3633–40.
8. Lopes MC, Andrew T, Carbonaro F, et al. Estimating heritability and shared environmental effects for refractive error in twin and family studies. Invest Ophthalmol Vis Sci 2009; 50: 126–31.
9. Dirani M, Chamberlain M, Garoufalis P, et al. Refractive errors in twin studies. Twin Res Hum Genet 2006; 9: 566–72.
10. Hysi PG, Young TL, Mackey DA, et al. A genome-wide association study for myopia and refractive error identifies a susceptibility locus at 15q25. Nat Genet 2010; 42: 902–5.
11. Solouki AM, Verhoeven VJ, van Duijn CM, et al. A genome-wide association study identifies a susceptibility locus for refractive errors and myopia at 15q14. Nat Genet 2010; 42: 897–901.
12. Tay MT, Au Eong KG, Ng CY, Lim MK. Myopia and educational attainment in 421,116 young Singaporean males. Ann Acad Med Singapore 1992; 21: 785–91.
13. Zylbermann R, Landau D, Berson D. The influence of study habits on myopia in Jewish teenagers. J Pediatr Ophthalmol Strabismus 1993; 30: 319–22.
14. Cumberland PM, Peckham CS, Rahi JS. Inferring myopia over the lifecourse from uncorrected distance visual acuity in childhood. Br J Ophthalmol 2007; 91: 151–3.
15. Rose KA, Morgan IG, Smith W, et al. Myopia, lifestyle, and schooling in students of Chinese ethnicity in Singapore and Sydney. Arch Ophthalmol 2008; 126: 527–30.
16. Rahi JS, Cumberland PM, Peckham CS. Myopia over the lifecourse: prevalence and early life influences in the 1958 British birth cohort. Ophthalmology 2011; 118: 797–804.
17. Wallman J, Winawer J. Homeostasis of eye growth and the question of myopia. Neuron 2004; 43: 447–68.
18. Smith EL, III, Ramamirtham R, Qiao-Grider Y, et al. Effects of foveal ablation on emmetropization and form-deprivation myopia. Invest Ophthalmol Vis Sci 2007; 48: 3914–22.
19. American Academy of Ophthalmology. Preferred Practice Pattern: refractive errors and refractive surgery. 2007. http://one.aao.org/CE/PracticeGuidelines/PPP_Content.aspx?cid=e6930284-2c41-48d5-afd2-631dec586286
20. Pediatric Eye Disease Investigator Group. Refractive Error Correction Protocol. 2006. http://pedig.jaeb.org/Studies.aspx?RecID=9
21. Chung K, Mohidin N, O'Leary DJ. Undercorrection of myopia enhances rather than inhibits myopia progression. Vision Res 2002; 42: 2555–9.
22. Walline JJ, Jones LA, Mutti DO, Zadnik K. A randomized trial of the effects of rigid contact lenses on myopia progression. Arch Ophthalmol 2004; 122: 1760–6.
23. Edwards MH, Li RW, Lam CS, et al. The Hong Kong progressive lens myopia control study: study design and main findings. Invest Ophthalmol Vis Sci 2002; 43: 2852–8.
24. Gwiazda J, Hyman L, Hussein M, et al. A randomized clinical trial of progressive addition lenses versus single vision lenses on the progression of myopia in children. Invest Ophthalmol Vis Sci 2003; 44: 1492–500.

25. Chua WH, Balakrishnan V, Chan YH, et al. Atropine for the treatment of childhood myopia. Ophthalmology 2006; 113: 2285–91.

26. Siatkowski RM, Cotter SA, Crockett RS, et al. Two-year multicenter, randomized, double-masked, placebo-controlled, parallel safety and efficacy study of 2% pirenzepine ophthalmic gel in children with myopia. J AAPOS 2008; 12: 332–9.

27. Tan DT, Lam DS, Chua WH, et al. One-year multicenter, double-masked, placebo-controlled, parallel safety and efficacy study of 2% pirenzepine ophthalmic gel in children with myopia. Ophthalmology 2005; 112: 84–91.

28. Helveston EM, Weber JC, Miller K, et al. Visual function and academic performance. Am J Ophthalmol 1985; 99: 346–55.

29. Atkinson J, Braddick O, Robier B, et al. Two infant vision screening programmes: prediction and prevention of strabismus and amblyopia from photo- and videorefractive screening. Eye 1996; 10: 189–98.

30. Cotter SA, Edwards AR, Wallace DK, et al. Treatment of anisometropic amblyopia in children with refractive correction. Ophthalmology 2006; 113: 895–903.

Milestones and normative data

Hans Ulrik Møller

At birth, eye size looks adult-like because the corneal diameter is only 1.7 mm smaller than in an adult, but volume increases threefold and weight doubles on maturity. In the full-term newborn eye volume is 3.25 cm^3 and weight is 3.40 g. The weight increases 40% by the middle of the second year and 70% by the fifth year.

The development of the eye parts is meticulously sequenced, and understanding the milestones of development is needed to assess clinical observations.

Intercanthal distance and palpebra

Abnormalities in the distance between the inner canthi and the outer canthi and the size and shape of the palpebral fissure are important features in craniofacial malformations and fetal alcohol syndrome. A fast non-contact method of measuring facial components is provided in Fig. 6.1A,B.[1]

Palpebral fissure changes in early childhood have been studied by analyzing digital imaging:[2] during the first 3 months of life the upper eyelid is at its lowest position, later rising to its maximum between the age of 3 to 6 months, and then declining until adulthood. The lower eyelid is close to the pupil center at birth, dropping until the age of 18 months

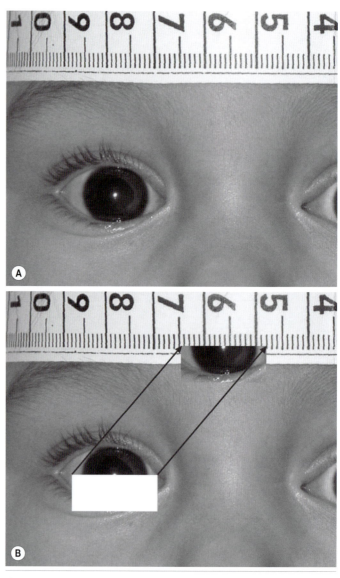

Fig. 6.1 (A) Photograph showing non-contact measurement of corneal diameter in children. Before digital photography of a child's eyes, a paper ruler was taped on the forehead. (B) After uploading the image to a computer, a rectangle is cut using the computer mouse, with the upper line passing through the cornea's widest horizontal diameter. This rectangle then is dragged to the ruler to read the corneal diameter, in this case 12.5 mm. From Lagrèze WA, Zobor G. A method for noncontact measurement of corneal diameter in children. Am J Ophthalmol 2007; 144: 141–2.

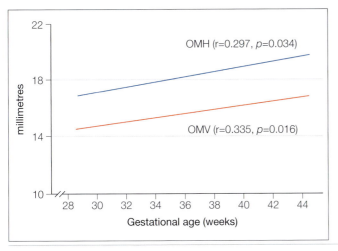

Fig. 6.2 Interocular distance. Linear regression relationship and standard error of the estimate between orbital margin horizontal (OMH) and vertical (OMV) diameters and gestational age. Correlation coefficients with *p* values are indicated. Data from Isenberg et al.[3] With permission from American Academy of Ophthalmology.

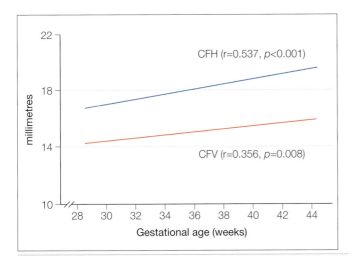

Fig. 6.3 Linear regression relationship and standard error of the estimate between conjunctival fornix horizontal (CFH) and vertical (CFV) diameters and gestational age. Correlation coefficients with *p* values are indicated. Data from Isenberg et al.[3] With permission from American Academy of Ophthalmology.

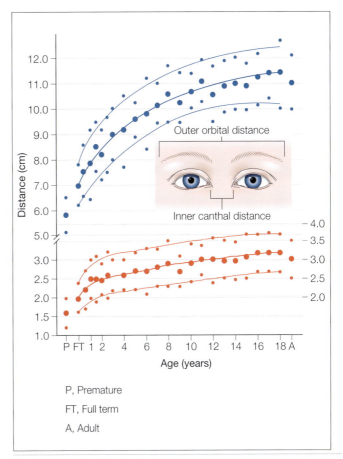

Fig. 6.4 Graphs of inner canthal and outer orbital distances. The large points represent the mean value for each age group, the smaller points represent 2 SD from the mean. The heavy line approximates the 50th percentile, while the shaded area roughly encompasses the range from the 3rd to the 97th percentile. Data from Laestadius et al.[7] With permission from Elsevier.

A universal approach is the canthus index:

$$\text{Canthus index} = \frac{\text{Inner canthus distance} \times 100}{\text{Outer canthus distance}}\%$$

Normals, unrelated to age, lie between 28.4 and 38%.[8] The canthus index of over 1000 children between 6 and 18 years old was determined as follows:[9]

	Boys	Girls
6 years	38.2% (SD 2.1%)	38.3% (SD 1.8%)
16 years	37.1% (SD 2.6%)	36.6% (SD 1.9%)

Tear secretion

Tearing is not a problem when holding open the eyelids on the youngest premature babies. Later, in preterm babies (30–37 weeks after conception) mean basal tear (with topical anesthesia) secretion is 6.2 (±4.5 SD) mm and at term 9.2 (±4.3) mm tested with a Schirmer tear test strip. Mean reflex tear secretion is 7.4 (±4.8) mm in preterm and 13.2 (±6.5) mm in term infants.[10]

when its position stabilizes. A single lower eyelid crease is common at birth, a double crease at the age of 36 months. Figure 6.2 shows the linear relationship between gestational age and orbital margin horizontal (OMH), as well as vertical (OMV) diameters in the unborn child.[3] There is a linear relationship between gestational age and conjunctival fornix horizontal (CFH) and conjunctival fornix vertical (CFV) diameters (Fig. 6.3).[3]

The palpebral fissures are 15±2 mm at 32 weeks of gestation, 17±2 mm at birth, 24±3 mm at 2 years of age, and 27±3 mm at the age of 14.[4,5] Inter-racial differences exist: the palpebral fissure is longer in Black Americans.[6]

Inner canthal distance and outer orbital distance are 16 and 59 mm, respectively, in premature infants; 20±4 and 69±8 mm in newborn babies; 26±6 and 88±10 mm at the age of 3; and 31±5 and 111±12 mm at the age of 14 (Fig. 6.4).[7]

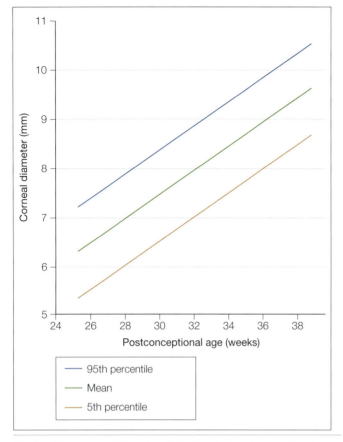

Fig. 6.5 Mean corneal diameter plotted against postconceptional age.
From Tucker SM, Enzenauer RW, Levin AV, et al. Corneal diameter, axial length, and intraocular pressure in premature infants. Ophthalmology 1992; 99: 1296–300.[11] With permission from American Academy of Ophthalmology.

Table 6.1 – Central corneal thickness (CCT) and curvature (R) in newborns and children

Age group	No.	CCT (mm ± SEM)	R (mm ± SEM)
Premature newborns	6	0.545 ± 0.014	6.35 ± 0.09
Mature newborns	19	0.541 ± 0.006	7.11 ± 0.07
Children 2–4 years	10	0.520 ± 0.007	7.73 ± 0.09
Children 5–9 years	15	0.520 ± 0.005	7.81 ± 0.09
Children 10–14 years	11	0.520 ± 0.007	8.01 ± 0.05
Adults (own group and data from literature)		~0.52	~7.8

From Ehlers N, Sørensen T, Bramsen T, et al. Central corneal thickness in newborns and children. Acta Ophthalmol (Copenh) 1976; 54: 285–90. With permission from Blackwell Publishing Ltd.

Table 6.2 – Central and peripheral corneal thickness (mm) in newborn babies

Corneal thickness	Age (hours)		
	0–24	24–48	48–72
Central	0.58	0.56	0.54
Peripheral	0.63	0.63	0.61

From Portellinha W, Belfort R, Jr. Central and peripheral corneal thickness in newborns. Acta Ophthalmol (Copenh) 1991; 69: 247–50. With permission from Blackwell Publishing Ltd.

Cornea

The premature cornea lacks luster and clarity, making some diagnoses difficult. Shallow anterior chambers, miotic pupils, and bluish irides are features of prematurity. The corneal diameter in infants at 25–37 weeks postconceptional age increases by 0.5 mm every 15 days from 6.2 to 9.0 mm (Fig. 6.5).[11,12] The horizontal and vertical diameters of the cornea in full-term boys are 9.8±0.33 mm and 10.4±0.35 mm and in girls 10.1±0.33 mm and 10.7±0.29 mm.[13] Two millimeters of growth in corneal diameter (approximately 20%) occurs in early infancy and early childhood. An adult value of 11.7 mm is reached by 7 years.

Central corneal thickness

Abnormal thickness of the central cornea influences intraocular pressure, but also corneal hysteresis may play a role in children. Central corneal thickness (CCT) in a full-term baby is 0.54 mm greater than in a 1-year-old child. CCTs measured with optical pachymetry and corneal curvature are given for premature and full-term babies in Table 6.1.[14]

CCT in premature infants below 33 weeks gives a mean of 0.656 mm (SD±0.103 mm) 5 days postnatally and 0.566 (SD±0.064) at the age of 110 days.[15] In full-term neonates,[16] CCT is 0.573±0.052 mm (range 0.450–0.691 mm) with a peripheral corneal thickness of 0.650±0.062 mm (range 0.520–0.830 mm). Table 6.2 shows the decrease in thickness during the first few days of life.

Another study[17] confirmed the above data and also measured peripheral corneal thickness: superior corneal thickness was 0.696±0.055 mm, inferior was 0.744±0.062 mm, nasal was 0.742±0.058 mm, and temporal was 0.748±0.055 mm. Adult values are reached at about 3 years of age. There is no significant difference of CCT among racial subgroups.[18]

Keratocyte density is around 60 000 cells per cubic millimeter in infancy with a decline of 0.3% per year through life.

Endothelial cell counts exceed 10 000 cells per square millimeter at 12 weeks of gestation, 50% of this at birth and 4000 cells per square millimeter in childhood.

Pupil size and reaction to light

The pupil, in relative darkness, has a mean diameter of 4.7 mm at 26 weeks postconceptional age. The pupils subsequently become progressively smaller, reaching 3.4 mm at 29 weeks. There is no reaction to light until 30.6 weeks (±1 week) postconceptional age.[19] Figure 6.6 shows the change of pupil diameter in relative darkness (< 10 ft-c) in preterm neonates. The mean pupil size is 3.8 mm (SD ± 0.8 mm) in the newborn period. The incidence of anisocoria of less than 1 mm is 21%; no difference was greater than 1 mm.[20]

The crystalline lens

The lens grows throughout life; information on lens thickness is included in the section "Axial length."

The lens capsule doubles its thickness from birth to old age.

Pars plana and ora serrata

The average pars plana of third trimester fetuses is 1.17 mm in width, which is one-third of that in the adult eye. The distance between the sclerocorneal limbus and the ora serrata is 3.22 mm nasally and 3.33 mm temporally (Table 6.3).[21] Similar figures were obtained from examination of 76 paraffin-embedded normal eyes from 1-week-old to 6-year-old children.[22]

Seventy-six percent of the development of the ciliary body occurs by the age of 24 months. The pars plana, which occupies 75% of the total length of the ciliary body, follows a similar course. The external distance from the limbus to the ora serrata is 0.3–0.4 mm more than the corresponding dimension of the ciliary body in these specimens.

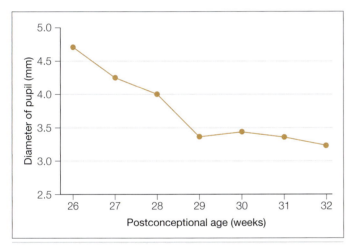

Fig. 6.6 The diameter of the pupil in relative darkness in preterm neonates. With permission from Isenberg SJ, Molarte A, Vazquez M. The fixed and dilated pupils of premature neonates. Am J Ophthalmol 1990; 110: 168–71.

Optic disc parameters

The diagnosis of optic nerve hypoplasia is a subjective one because it is not only optic nerve size that is important. The optic disc dimensions of 66 children of low refraction error aged 2–10 years was studied by fundus photography (Table 6.4A).[23] The vertical disc diameter, the disc area, and the cup-to-disc ratio were significantly larger in Black than in White children. The optic disc dimensions (excluding the meninges), studied at autopsy,[24] produce slightly different results due to fixation shrinkage (13%), but the measurements correlate well with the photographic study (Tables 6.4B and 6.4C). Approximately 50% of optic disc and nerve growth occurs by 20 weeks of gestation and 75% by birth. Ninety-five percent of the growth of the optic disc and nerve occurs before the age of 1 year.

Axial length

In week 9 of fetal life the eye has a sagittal diameter of 1 mm, increasing to a mean of 5.1 mm by the age of 12 weeks.[25]

The total axial length of the premature eye (25–37 weeks postconceptional age) increases linearly from 12.6 to 16.2 mm.[11] Measurements from a later study[26] are given in Table 6.5.

Table 6.3 – Values (mm) of the distance from sclerocorneal limbus to the ora serrata in the nasal, temporal, superior, and inferior meridians (mean ± SD) in fetuses aged 24–40 weeks[20]

Nasal meridian	Temporal meridian	Superior meridian	Inferior meridian
3.22	3.33	3.23	3.27
0.30	0.35	0.36	0.37

From Bonomo PP. Pars plana and ora serrata anatomotopographic study of fetal eyes. Acta Ophthalmol (Copenh) 1989; 67: 145–50. With permission from Blackwell Publishing Ltd.

Table 6.4A – Optic disc parameters in 66 volunteers[23]

No. of volunteers	Race	Sex	Age	Cycloplegic refraction	Vertical disk diameter (mm)	Horizontal disk diameter (mm)	Cup-to-disk ratio	Area (mm²)	Neuroretinal rim area (mm²)
16	Black	Female	7.0	+0.8	2.11	1.84	0.32	3.05	2.57
			2.5	1.4	0.21	0.17	0.21	0.54	0.50
14	Black	Male	7.0	+0.5	2.13	1.85	0.40	3.11	2.46
			2.4	0.7	0.19	0.19	0.20	0.56	0.58
18	White	Female	5.2	+1.0	1.88	1.73	0.10	2.57	2.52
			2.4	1.1	0.20	0.17	0.11	0.49	0.48
18	White	Male	6.1	+0.7	1.94	1.79	0.20	2.74	2.54
			2.2	0.7	0.22	0.22	0.18	0.59	0.58

Values are expressed as means; SDs are listed under the means.
With permission from Mansour AM. Racial variation of the optic disc parameters in children. Ophthalmic Surg 1992; 33: 469–71. © 1992 Slack Inc.

Table 6.4B – Mean vertical and horizontal diameters and area of the optic disc for each age group

| Age | No. of subjects | Mean diameter (mm) (SD) | | Mean area (mm²) (SD) |
		Vertical	Horizontal	
<40 weeks' gestation	20	1.10 (0.21)	0.93 (0.15)	0.82 (0.26)
Term to 6 months	13	1.37 (0.21)	1.13 (0.19)	1.25 (0.40)
6 months to 2 years	12	1.57 (0.15)	1.40 (0.17)	1.73 (0.32)
2–10 years	17	1.64 (0.20)	1.43 (0.19)	1.87 (0.44)
>10 years	31	1.73 (0.23)	1.59 (0.21)	2.19 (0.54)

From Rimmer S, Keating C, Chou T, et al. Growth of the human optic disc and nerve during gestation, childhood, and early adulthood. Am J Ophthalmol 1993; 116: 748–53.

Table 6.4C – Mean vertical and horizontal diameters and area of the optic nerve for each age group

| Age | No. of subjects | Mean diameter (mm) (SD) | | Mean area (mm²) (SD) |
		Vertical	Horizontal	
<40 weeks' gestation	20	1.96 (0.36)	1.79 (0.43)	2.85 (1.16)
Term to 6 months	13	2.38 (0.22)	2.23 (0.30)	4.22 (0.87)
6 months to 2 years	12	2.70 (0.33)	2.55 (0.32)	5.47 (1.26)
2–10 years	17	2.84 (0.39)	2.64 (0.27)	5.95 (1.26)
>10 years	30	3.06 (0.39)	2.85 (0.32)	6.95 (1.62)

From Rimmer S, Keating C, Chou T, et al. Growth of the human optic disc and nerve during gestation, childhood, and early adulthood. Am J Ophthalmol 1993; 116: 748–53, with permission.

Ultrasound measurements of the newborn eye[27] are as follows:

1. Average anterior chamber depth (including the cornea) 2.6 mm (2.4 to 2.9 mm).
2. Average lens thickness 3.6 mm(3.4 to 3.9 mm).
3. Average vitreous length 10.4 mm(8.9 to 11.2 mm).
4. The total length of the newborn eye is 16.6 mm (15.3 to 17.6 mm).

The postnatal growth of the emmetropic eye can be divided into three growth periods:[28]

1. A rapid postnatal phase with an increase in length of 3.7–3.8 mm during the first 18 months.
2. A slower phase from the second to the fifth year of life with an increase in length of 1.1–1.2 mm.

Table 6.5 – Numerical parameters of ocular axial length, and axial growth rate from fetal age 20 weeks to the age of 3 years

Age (weeks)[a]	Axial length (mm)	Growth rate (mm/week)
20	10.08	0.66
30	14.74	0.32
40 (term)	17.02	0.16
50	18.24	0.092
60	18.97	0.059
70	19.48	0.044
80	19.87	0.035
90 (about 1 year)	20.19	0.030
100	20.47	0.026
120	20.93	0.021
140 (about 2 years)	21.31	0.017
170	21.75	0.013
200 (about 3 years)	22.07	0.009

[a]<40 weeks = fetal; >40 weeks = post-term.
From Fledelius HC, Christensen AC. Reappraisal of the human ocular growth curve in fetal life, infancy and early childhood. Br J Ophthalmol 1996; 80: 918–21.

3. A slow juvenile phase, which lasts until the age of 13 years with an increase of 1.3–1.4 mm after which longitudinal growth is minimal.

See Table 6.6 and Fig. 6.7.[28]

Extraocular muscles and sclera

Most of the enlargement of the eye is in the first 6 months of extrauterine life. All diameters increase. The cornea and the iris have about 80% of their adult dimensions at birth. The posterior segment grows more postnatally. Therefore, in squint surgery in the very young child it is more difficult to predict outcomes (Tables 6.7A–6.7C).

The thickness of the sclera in 6-, 9-, and 20-month specimens is 0.45 mm, similar to that in adult eyes.[29]

Children's visual function questionnaire

An instrument to document quality of life is retrievable from http://www.retinafoundation.org/questionnaire.htm, describing data for children up to 7 years of age undergoing different treatment modalities to detect resulting changes in quality of life.[30]

Visual acuity

Postnatal maturation of the visual pathways plays an important role in visual development. At birth, the macula is immature. The fovea reaches histological maturity as late as between

Table 6.6 – Axial length (mm) in male series

Length of axis (mm)	Days	Months		Years													
	1–5	6	9	1–2	2–3	3–4	4–5	5–6	6–7	7–8	8–9	9–10	10–11	11–12	12–13	13–14
No. of eyes	86	2	4	36	118	110	100	64	64	70	100	80	56	52	56	24
Mean	16.78	18.21	19.05	20.61	20.79	21.27	21.68	21.85	21.97	22.09	22.33	22.43	22.50	22.70	22.97	23.15
SD	0.51	—	—	0.47	0.61	0.55	0.58	0.59	0.71	0.62	0.51	0.47	0.47	0.82	0.71	0.38
SE	0.055	—	—	0.078	0.056	0.052	0.058	0.074	0.089	0.074	0.051	0.053	0.063	0.114	0.095	0.078

SD, standard deviation; SE, standard error.
From Larsen JS. The sagittal growth of the eye. I–IV. Acta Ophthalmol (Copenh) 1971; 49: 239–62, 427–40, 441–53, 873–86. With permission from Blackwell Publishing Ltd.

Table 6.7A – Breadth of rectus muscle insertions (mm)

Age	No. of specimens	Superior	Medial	Inferior	Lateral
Neonatal	10	7.5	7.6	6.8	6.9
2–3 months	4	7.3	6.8	6.7	7.0
6 months	4	8.9	9.0	8.3	8.4
9 months	4	8.8	8.7	8.3	8.2
20 months	2	10.2	8.9	9.3	7.8
Adult	5	10.8	10.5	9.8	9.2

With permission from Swan KC, Wilkins JH. Extraocular muscle surgery in early infancy: anatomical factors. J Pediatr Ophthalmol Strabismus 1984; 21: 44–9. © 1984 Slack Inc.

Table 6.7B – Millimeters from clear cornea to rectus muscle insertions

Age	No. of specimens	Superior		Medial		Inferior		Lateral	
		Nasal end	Temporal end	Sup. end	Inf. end	Nasal end	Temporal end	Sup. end	Inf. end
Neonatal	10	6.1	7.6	4.7	5.3	6.0	6.6	6.4	5.8
2 months	3	5.5	5.8	5.2	6.0	5.2	6.2	7.8	5.8
3 months	3	6.9	7.5	5.1	5.8	6.6	7.5	7.5	7.0
6 months	4	7.4	8.3	5.8	6.6	7.2	9.0	7.2	7.1
9 months	4	7.2	9.3	6.2	6.9	7.7	8.8	7.5	7.1
20 months	2	7.1	8.7	7.3	7.6	8.5	9.3	8.5	8.5
Adult	5	7.4	10.0	7.8	7.7	8.0	9.2	8.4	8.5

With permission from Swan KC, Wilkins JH. Extraocular muscle surgery in early infancy: anatomical factors. J Pediatr Ophthalmol Strabismus 1984; 21: 44–9. © 1984 Slack Inc.

Table 6.7C – Distance in millimeters of oblique muscle insertions from clear cornea and optic nerve

Age	No. of specimens	Superior oblique				Inferior oblique			
		To cornea		To optic nerve		To cornea		To optic nerve	
		Ant. edge	Post. edge	Ant. edge	Post. edge	Ant. edge	Post. edge	Ant. edge	Post. edge
Neonatal	8	9.0	11.6	10.6	5.6	10.2	14.8	8.6	2.2
2–3 months	4	10.3	12.8	10.3	5.6	12.1	16.2	8.2	2.3
6–9 months	8	12.3	14.2	12.0	6.4	13.9	18.0	10.8	3.2
20 months	2	14.2	15.3	12.2	7.8	15.5	19.3	11.7	4.6
Adult	3	14.7	17.7	14.6	8.3	16.2	20.5	14.2	6.6

With permission from Swan KC, Wilkins JH. Extraocular muscle surgery in early infancy: anatomical factors. J Pediatr Ophthalmol Strabismus 1984; 21: 44–9. © 1984 Slack Inc.

15 and 45 months of age. Myelination of the optic nerve is not complete until at least the age of 2 years.

"The period between 1 and 3 months is a period of radical changes in visual capabilities and behavior. A rapid rise in acuity, the appearance of the low-frequency cut in contrast sensitivity, the emergence of smooth pursuit eye movements and of symmetrical optokinetic nystagmus, and possibly the establishment of functional binocular vision all occur roughly together."[31]

Lid closure is seen on illumination with a bright light in babies of 25 weeks' gestation. The pupillary reflex to light is seen from weeks 29 to 31. Discriminative visual function and "tracking" eye movements are present by 31–33 weeks' gestational age.[32]

The acuity of the newborn infant is close to 6/240 and, at 7 weeks of age, the infant has eye-to-face contact. Visual acuity rapidly increases to 6/180–6/90 at 2–3 months. At 6 months,

visual acuity is between 6/18 and 6/9. The assessment of visual acuity, however, depends on the testing method. Table 6.8 summarizes pooled information of visual development.

Full accommodative ability is not established until 3–4 months of age. Yet, it does not appear to be a major limiting factor on reported acuity values.

Stereoacuity can be demonstrated by the age of 16 weeks. By 21 weeks infants have a stereoacuity of 1 minute of arc or better.[33] Median Randot stereoacuities are 100 seconds of arc for 3-year-olds, 70 seconds of arc for 4-year-olds, 50 seconds of arc for 5-year-olds, 40 seconds of arc for 6-year-olds and 45 seconds of arc for 7-year-olds.[34]

Results of visuoperceptual testing in a cohort of children aged 4–15 years revealed that visual acuity in the better eye was ≥1.0 (≤0.0 logMAR) in 79% of subjects. None of the children had visual acuity <0.5 (>0.3 logMAR) in the better eye. Amblyopia was found in 0.7% of the subjects. Signs of visuoperceptual problems were reported in 3% of the children.[35]

Nevertheless it is difficult to know precisely at what age adult acuity is normally attained!

Visual field

The visual field of the infant depends on the distance at which the target is presented, whether static or kinetic fields are investigated, how interesting the targets are, and whether a fixation target is present. Between 2 and 4 months the child develops the ability to switch attention to a new object.

The binocular visual field shows little development between birth and 7 weeks. After 2 months there is a rapid expansion of the field until 6–8 months of age. The visual field increases at a slower rate up to 12 months (Fig. 6.8). An asymmetry of 13° or more should be considered pathological.[36,37] Normative data for 4- to 12-year-old children are shown in Table 6.9.[37]

Refraction, corneal curvature, and astigmatism

Most authorities agree that neonatal refractions are distributed in a bell-shaped curve around +2 diopters (D).[38] Later, there is a shift toward emmetropia. In a group of older Swedish children, 68% had no refractive errors, 9% were hyperopic (≥2.0 diopters in spherical equivalent), and 6% were myopic (≥0.5 diopters spherical equivalent).[35] The range of astigmatism is difficult to study due to off-axis retinoscopy errors. One study of non-cycloplegic refractions in children aged 0–6 years revealed a minus cylinder against-the-rule before the age of 4.5 years and a minus cylinder with-the-rule after that age.[39]

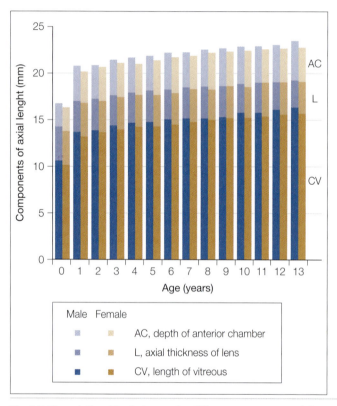

Fig. 6.7 The relationships between the different components of the eye during the growth period. An ultrasound oculometric study. From Larsen JS. The sagittal growth of the eye. I–IV. Acta Ophthalmol (Copenh) 1971; 49: 239–62, 427–40, 441–53, 873–86.[28] With permission from Blackwell Publishing Ltd.

Table 6.8 – Visual acuity according to different methods, given as Snellen equivalents

Technique	Newborn	2 months	4 months	6 months	1 year
Optokinetic nystagmus	20/400	20/400	20/200		20/60
Preferential looking (one study)	20/400	20/200	20/200	20/150	20/50
Preferential looking (other study)	20/800 to 20/1600	20/1200	20/400	20/300	20/100
Visual evoked potential	20/100 to 20/200	20/80	20/80	20/20 to 20/40	20/40

Information pooled from different sources.

Table 6.9 – Mean extent of visual field in degrees (± SEM) in each meridian for five age groups

Age group	ST	IT	IN	SN
Right eye				
4 years	59.2 (2.1)	84.7 (1.6)	51.4 (2.4)	47.8 (1.8)
5 years	63.4 (2.4)	88.1 (1.9)	52.4 (2.6)	51.7 (1.6)
7 years	66.8 (1.5)	86.0 (2.0)	53.6 (2.0)	58.4 (1.3)
10 years	66.9 (2.3)	86.7 (1.7)	57.9 (1.9)	60.2 (1.3)
Adult	72.6 (2.7)	94.9 (1.4)	54.0 (1.7)	60.2 (2.1)
Left eye				
4 years	66.1 (2.6)	83.8 (2.5)	59.2 (2.9)	49.1 (1.7)
5 years	66.7 (2.8)	83.0 (2.3)	54.8 (2.3)	52.4 (1.9)
7 years	73.7 (1.4)	89.4 (1.7)	51.9 (1.5)	55.9 (1.3)
10 years	71.8 (2.5)	86.7 (1.8)	52.9 (2.1)	55.8 (2.5)
Adult	70.7 (2.5)	93.4 (1.7)	52.4 (2.0)	57.7 (2.1)

S, superior; I, inferior; T, temporal; N, nasal.
With permission from Wilson M, Quinn G, Dobson V, Breton M. Normative values for visual fields in 4- to 12-year-old children using kinetic perimetry. J Pediatr Ophthalmol Strabismus 1991; 28: 151–4. © 1991 Slack Inc.

The smaller eyes of premature and full-term babies have a more curved cornea of 6.35 mm in curvature radius in contrast to the adult with 7.8 mm (see Table 6.1).[40] Keratometer measurements in one study in premature infants were 53.1 ± 1.5 diopters, in neonates 48.4 ± 1.7 diopters, at 1 month 45.9 ± 2.3 diopters, and at 36 months 42.9 ± 1.3 diopters. Another study reported 47.59 diopters (SD ± 2.10; range 44.08–50.75 diopters) in the newborn, 45.56 diopters (SD ± 2.70; 40.13–52.75 diopters) in the 12- to 18-month age group and stabilization of the cornea at the age of 54 months with an average of 42.69 diopters (SD ± 1.89; range 40.50–47.50 diopters).[41] Videokeratography reveals that neonates have steep, high astigmatic (generally with-the-rule) corneas at birth that flatten significantly by the age of 6 months. At birth, the central corneal power measured 48.5 diopters and astigmatism measured 6.0 diopters usually with-the-rule with a mean axis of 95 degrees. Neonates delivered vaginally had a greater frequency of with-the-rule astigmatism than those delivered by cesarean section. By 6 months, the mean central corneal power and astigmatism decreased to 43.0 diopters and 2.3, respectively.[42]

There is considerable variation in the nature and severity of refractive errors reported from different areas of the world.

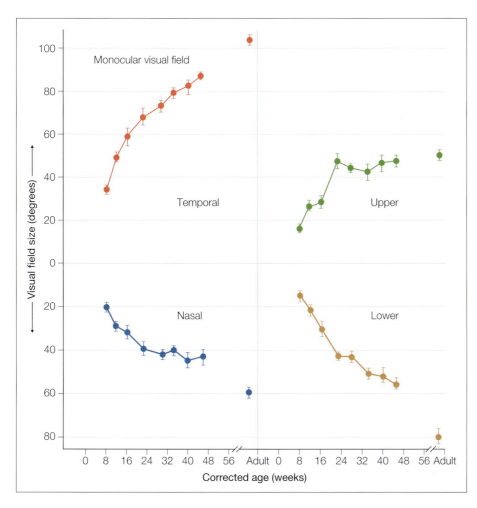

Fig. 6.8 Development of monocular visual field. The horizontal (left) and vertical (right) meridians. Error bars indicate 2 SEM. From Mohn G, van Hof-van Duin J. Development of the binocular and monocular visual fields of human infants during the first year of life. Clin Visual Sci 1986; 1: 51–64, as well as personal communication 1994.

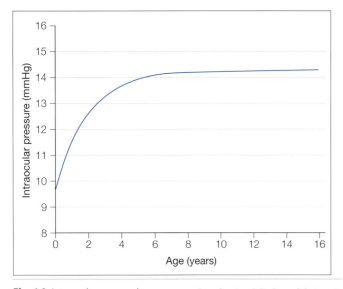

Fig. 6.9 Intraocular pressure by age group. From Pensiero S, Da Pozzo S, Perissutti P, et al. Normal intraocular pressure in children. J Pediatr Ophthalmol Strabismus 1992; 29: 79–84. © 1992 Slack Inc.

Intraocular pressure

An awake measurement of intraocular pressure in children is difficult and a general anesthetic is often required. The anesthetic agents used and the depth of anesthesia may affect the outcome of the measurements. Most studies show the intraocular pressure is lower in children than in adults. Babies who were 3–11 weeks premature had a mean intraocular pressure of 18 mmHg (13–24 mmHg) with a Perkins tonometer and topical anesthesia.[43] Lower values of 11.4 mmHg have been reported in full-term neonates.[44] Somewhat different results were obtained with a hand-held Tonopen. Wth an applanation tonometer, a mean intraocular pressure of 10.3 mmHg was found in 70 premature babies, aged 25–37 weeks.[11]

The intraocular pressure in 460 subjects aged 0–16 years measured with a non-contact Keeler Pulsair tonometer was reported to be 9 mmHg in neonates, increasing to 14 mmHg at the age of 5 years (Fig. 6.9).[45] Averaged Pulsair readings agreed well with Perkins applanation tonometry values in a study of children measured under general anesthesia.[46,47] The new ICare rebound tonometer, in a group of infants, gave a mean intraocular pressure of 11.82±2.67 mmHg with no statistically significant difference between two observers.[47]

Some drugs and procedures affect intraocular pressure under general anesthesia, such as suxamethonium, laryngoscopy, and intubation. Large amounts of some anesthetic agents, such as halothane, reduce intraocular pressure. Dear et al.[48] found that the mean intraocular pressure among 60 infants was 12 mmHg in normal eyes and 22 mmHg in eyes with glaucoma after induction on spontaneous ventilation using nitrous oxide and halothane or isoflurane. Using atracurium and controlled ventilation, there was a slight increase in intraocular pressure. They recommended measuring the intraocular pressure just after induction, before intubation. These recommendations have been endorsed by other studies.[49] Ketamine administration during the first 6 minutes of the procedure[50] is probably the best choice, but there are reservations about using it in infants.

References

2. Paiva RS, Minaire-Filho AM, Cruz AA. Palpebral fissure changes in early childhood. J Pediatr Ophthalmol Strabismus 2001; 38: 219–23.
4. Jones KL, Hanson JW, Smith DW. Palpebral fissure size in newborn infants. J Pediatr 1978; 92: 787.
7. Laestadius ND, Aase JM, Smith DW. Normal inner canthal and outer orbital dimensions. J Pediatr 1969; 74: 465–8.
10. Isenberg SJ, Apt L, McCarty JA, et al. Development of tearing in preterm and term neonates. Arch Ophthalmol 1998; 116: 773–6.
12. al-Umran KU, Pandolfi MF. Corneal diameter in premature infants. Br J Ophthalmol 1992; 76: 292–3.
14. Ehlers N, Sørensen T, Bramsen T, Poulsen EH. Central corneal thickness in newborns and children. Acta Ophthalmol (Copenh) 1976; 54: 285–90.
17. Remon L, Cristobal JA, Castillo J, et al. Central and peripheral corneal thickness in full-term newborns by ultrasonic pachymetry. Invest Ophthalmol Vis Sci 1992; 33: 3080–3.
18. Hussein MAW, Paysse EA, Bell NP, et al. Corneal thickness in children. Am J Ophthalmol 2004; 138: 744–8.
20. Roarty JD, Keltner JL. Normal pupil size and anisocoria in newborn infants. Arch Ophthalmol 1990; 108: 94–5.
23. Mansour AM. Racial variation of the optic disc parameters in children. Ophthalmic Surg 1992; 33: 469–71.
26. Fledelius HC, Christensen AC. Reappraisal of the human ocular growth curve in fetal life, infancy and early childhood. Br J Ophthalmol 1996; 80: 918–21.
30. Birch EE, Cheng CS, Felius J. Validity and reliability of the children's visual function questionnaire (CVFQ). J AAPOS 2007; 11: 473–9.
32. Dubowitz LM, Dubowitz V, Morante A, Verghote M. Visual function in the preterm and full-term newborn infant. Dev Med Child Neurol 1980; 22: 465–75.
33. Held R, Birch E, Gwiazda J. Stereoacuity of human infants. Proc Natl Acad Sci USA 1980; 77: 5572–4.
35. Grönlund MA, Andersson S, Aring E, et al. Ophthalmological findings in a sample of Swedish children aged 4–15years. Acta Ophthalmol Scand 2006; 84: 169–76.
37. Wilson M, Quinn G, Dobson V, Breton M. Normative values for visual fields in 4- to 12-year-old children using kinetic perimetry. J Pediatr Ophthalmol Strabismus 1991; 28: 151–4.
42. Isenberg SJ, Signore M Del, Chen A, et al. Corneal topography of neonates and infants. Arch Ophthalmol 2004; 122: 1767–71.
45. Pensiero S, Da Pozzo S, Perissutti P, et al. Normal intraocular pressure in children. J Pediatr Ophthalmol Strabismus 1992; 29: 79–84.
47. Lundvall A, Svedberg H, Chen E. Application of ICare rebound tonometer in healthy infants. J Glaucoma 2011; 20: 7–9
48. Dear G de L, Hammerton M, Hatch DJ, Taylor D. Anaesthesia and intra-ocular pressure in young children. Anaesthesia 1987; 42: 259–65.
49. Watcha MF, Chu FC, Stevens JL, Forestner JE. Effects of halothane on intraocular pressure in anesthetized children. Anesth Analg 1990; 71: 181–4.

 Access the complete reference list online at http://www.expertconsult.com

Examination, history and special tests in pediatric ophthalmology

G Robert LaRoche

Table 7.1 – The 19 chronologic steps of a pediatric ophthalmology consultation – a progressive level of "intrusiveness" maximizes the cooperation and yield

1	Observe before formal encounter – waiting room, on the way to the examinig room
2	Say "Hi" to child
3	Observe while greeting – body language (body & head), postures, visual behavior
4	Child in the chair alone, on parent's lap, or in parent's arms
5	History – parent, child, family photo album
6	Brückner's
7	None dissociating binocularity tests – two-pencil test (2PT), Lang, Frisby. Head posture
8	VA* – binocular, better eye, worse eye
9	Dynamic retinoscopy
10	Extraocular muscles (EOM) – the frame
**	
11	Pupils, corneal diameter, lids – fixation target, ruler with photo
12	Refined binocularity tests – progressive dissociation
13	Confrontation fields
14	Strabismus assessment
15	Drops
16	Intraocular pressure (IOP)
17	Refraction
18	Fundus
19	Reward

*VA Monocular visual acuity (VA) testing might influence the results of binocularity assessment due to dissociation.
**This line denotes the point from which the examination requires equipment and manipulations near the child's eyes. From here on, the child's cooperation becomes a key issue.

Parents of new pediatric ophthalmology patients often ask: "How on earth are you going to do this?" In fact, the child's problem will be easily assessed with a little play, a few key tricks, and a dose of spontaneity and patience. A speedy uncreative visit will rarely yield a thorough assessment.

Assent and consent

Our ethical responsibilities as caregivers of children are essential. The omniscient doctor used to make all the decisions; now, with patient advocacy and participatory decisions, we have to share more of our responsibility for the good of our young patients and their families. The children also have a right to the truth.[1] In consent, we try to define the limits of our young patients' autonomy: what decisions can a child make on the information we provide? When can they evaluate risks, consequences, and benefits? Should we obtain a child's assent, without coercion, to proceed with an unpleasant examination or treatment in the face of unequivocal parental consent? More on these issues in Chapter 58.

It is all about the child

Personality, timing, and the planned investigations all have their influence on the patient's cooperation (Table 7.1). A crying infant will not yield useful information on its visual potential, but calming feeding – breast or bottle – can lead to a few moments of conclusive observation of a visual response. A worried 3-year-old with juvenile idiopathic arthritis might not volunteer for a slit-lamp examination, but given the chance to first talk about a cherished new pair of sneakers, or be

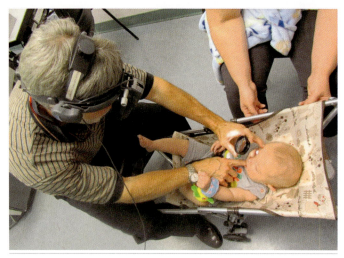

Fig. 7.1 Indirect ophthalmoscopy in infants. An example of unconventional assessment techniques necessary in infants. Here the examination is carried out successfully in the patient's own comfort zone: a stroller and a good suck on the examiner's finger.

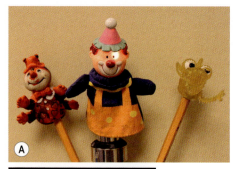

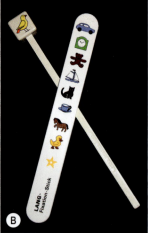

Fig. 7.2 Near fixation targets. (A) Finger puppets. All able to transmit light, giving creative possibilities to enhance their attractiveness. (B) Lang fixation stick and cube. These have become a standard the world around.

shown how to do it by a sibling, may eagerly allow a good view of cells and flare. A shy teenager with papilledema might open up as soon as Mom leaves the room. Mostly, it is all in the act – how you do it!

The equipment

A successful examination room needs toys to satisfy children: small near fixation targets (silent, so not to test hearing) with a few able to transmit an internal light, an audible distant fixating target able to attract attention, and, finally, rewards to give. How many visual targets? "One toy, one gaze, one look" is a good rule (Fig. 7.2). In addition to the usual ophthalmic equipment, a portable slit-lamp and tonometer and appropriate vision charts complete the set. Other special equipment for infant vision, examination of premature newborns, full orthoptic assessment, and electrodiagnostic and imaging investigations are useful in specific circumstances.

History: include the children

Taking a history is crucial. The clues augment elusive clinical signs in a non-cooperative child. Time and opportunism, however, are of the essence. Loquacious parents with genetic disease, a room full of siblings and friends, etc., all distract from the task at hand. While it is tempting to get most of the history from the parents, the child's perspective can be revealing. A parent might provide a very different account of a poorly compliant amblyopic child who has had a great summer at the grandparents' without having to wear that patch! Important details become known only when we gain the confidence of our young patients. Examples include being bullied about wearing spectacles, or emergency room stories about pellet guns changed when only the mother is present. Poor family dynamics, "blame games," avoidance, and miscommunications, socioeconomic and cultural issues can all be barriers. The mother is the usual key to a successful outcome. Her understanding, cooperation, and engagement in the care

process are essential.[2] Finally, pictures can play a big part of the historical record. A few family good photographs can give enough clues to target the examination for a diagnosis of Duane's retraction syndrome, or Brown's syndrome. Retinoblastoma is sometimes detected by images of a white pupil in family photographs.

A no-touch approach at first

With children, simple observation should be the first priority. Simply watch, with a "hands off" approach before intervening. Start with the least intrusive tests. Specialized ancillary tests are usually done after the initial clinical assessment, based on specific diagnostic requirements (Chapters 8 and 9).

Say "Hi"! Break the ice, address the child, be friendly, get down to eye level, and avoid white coats. On the first visit, the ophthalmologist is a stranger and, except for infants, most children are reluctant to open up to strangers. Clothes, shoes or toys, stuffed animals's name – these are all good topics of conversation that create a welcoming atmosphere. Children love play and the examination should be a game as much as possible.

Observe While greeting, observe the head position (incomitant strabismus, nystagmus, or a field defect), evidence of photophobia (corneal disease, retinal dystrophies, glaucoma), body language as evidence of a visual handicap or behavioral peculiarities (extreme hyperactivity, inattention, withdrawal, or violence of the abused child), and the possible clues of

Table 7.2 – Visual developmental milestones relevant to a pediatric ophthalmology examination in young children

Age group	Fine motor-adaptive	Personal/social	Language (receptive and expressive)
0–4 weeks	Visual following from side to midline (90° arc)	Regards human faces with interest	
2 months		Smiles responsively	
3 months	Looks at object placed in hand Looks promptly at objects in midline Follows visually in 180° arc and in circular pattern		
4 months	Reach and grasp begin Looks at objects in hand	Excited when toys presented	
5 months		Distinguishes strangers from family	
6 months		Pushes adult hand away to reject	
8 months		Finger feeds	Responds to name when called (turns)
9 months	Explores pellet with index finger		
10 months		Imitates nursery tricks (modeled), e.g. pat-a-cake Bangs two cubes together in imitation	
12 months		Hands over toy on request with accompanying hand-out gesture	
24 months	Threads shoelace through hole		
48 months	Picks longer of two lines	Buttons up	Points to colors on request (red/blue, yellow/green)

Adapted from Goldbloom R. Pediatric Clinical Skills, 4th ed. Philadelphia: Elsevier; 2011. With permission from Elsevier.

developmental delay, especially associated with abnormal visual functions (Table 7.2).

Head/body posture A visually impaired child often holds the head down even in dimmer lighting while a glaucomatous patient will do so more dramatically in a brighter environment. Photophobia is a presentation that should prompt investigation! Head thrusts or nodding can be of diagnostic help with the abnormal eye movements in ocular motor apraxia (saccadic initiation failure) and spasmus nutans. An abnormal head posture increasing with visual effort is seen with nystagmus or incomitant strabismus. A lot can be quickly learned by simply observing.

Visual behavior The allegedly blind infant who brightens up, follows, and fixes objects when the lights are turned down classically suggests a cone dystrophy. Subtle clues can be useful, like the excess tearing of the symptomatic hyperope, or the close distance fixation in a high myopia. Does the child show random or purposeful conjugate gaze movements? Do the parents report frequent episodes of staring at lights as evidence of very low vision? Is this an hysteric who avoids visual fixation of any object, or is this an autistic child who typically looks preferentially at objects but avoids eye contact? Is there a nystagmus, a null position?

Where to sit for the examination Many young children will be comfortable, quieter, and more cooperative on their parent's lap. A few want to start the visit in their parent's arms away from the usual diagnostic area with its strange machines. Infants can be assessed quite satisfactorily in this manner. Flexibility is essential (Fig. 7.1)!

Parents as a resource Refer to other people in the room to relieve the tension of the child feeling at the center of attention. "Who are these people?" "Is this your sister?" "Is that a real baby in that stroller?" This is also the time for a short history with the guardian on the current problem. Then hear the child's own story: a daily headache becomes a rare occurrence, or vice versa. A complaint of poor vision is really a wish to wear spectacles like the big sister, and so on. Next comes the family history; looking at the family photo album is helpful if they have it. This should not be a protracted affair; things get boring or stressful for a child sitting and waiting for something to happen; further details can be gathered later. Do not just take a history: the first visit is the time to examine both parents.

Do not have too many in the room which may be a source of distraction and noise. The best scenario is to have just the child in the office with a cooperative parent or two. A good friend in the same age group can be calming for a 6- to 10-year-old. Someone might have to hold a non-cooperative child. In decubitus, a preferred position for drop instillation, or sitting and facing the examiner, the parents quickly learn how effective they can be to help and comfort their child (Fig. 7.3).

Targeted examination

Guided by the history and the early clues of observation, the ophthalmologist should first evaluate the most promising components of the examination. As this is a non-systematic approach, a checklist that includes all the possible components

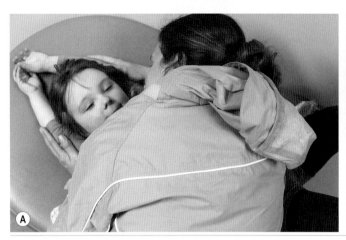 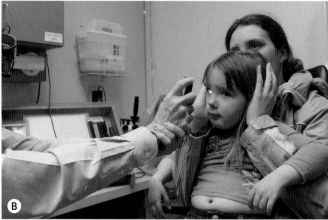

Fig. 7.3 Parent hold. Parents can help physically stabilize their children for crucial parts of the examination. Either in the supine position with the elbows pressed against the head (A) or sitting facing the examiner (B). Both positions involves a close proximity of the parent's soothing voice to help calm the child.

is important. As the visit progresses, the items are checked, and, based on what is needed and what can be achieved, consideration can be given to a second visit, specialized ancillary tests, or an examination under sedation if needed.

Bruckner's test Bruckner's technique is the best way to introduce ophthalmic instruments to a child.[3] A quick look with a direct ophthalmoscope at a distance can detect visually significant opacities, large refractive errors, and some ocular misalignments (see Fig. 7.7). The test includes the brightness of the pupil reflex when the light of a direct ophthalmoscope is aimed at the eyes before dilation in a semi-darkened room. The color and homogeneity as well as the overall symmetry of the findings between the two eyes is observed. The position of the corneal Purkinje images in each eye can detect a gross strabismus. The few seconds required for the Bruckner's test early in the consultation can help answer crucial questions about cataract, corneal scar, congenital pupillary membrane, strabismus, or anisometropia.

Binocularity: first no dissociation, no glasses At around 2 years of age, a child's binocularity can be assessed. Already at age 3 to 4 months, binocularity is established to some degree[4] and infants with early ocular motor difficulties such as Duane's retraction syndrome can adopt a compensatory head posture.

Do not dissociate a child with a potentially binocular condition before properly assessing binocularity. Cooperation will be greatly facilitated by tests that do not involve anything coming near the child's face. The two-pencil test (2PT), the Frisby and the Lang stereotests assess binocularity through the measurement of stereopsis without the interference of dissociating components (Fig. 7.4); they are introduced as a form of play. The 2PT involves a real 3D target to match in real space and tests stereopsis in the order of 2000–3000 seconds of arc.[5] The Frisby stereotest is stationary, but also involves real spatial separation of its targets and is an easy game for toddlers. The Lang stereotest requires haploscopic image dissociation to produce a stereo effect of its targets, but does so without the need for glasses. The Lang's visual targets are very child-friendly, simple, and can measure at least three stereoacuity levels. Children as young as 2 years old will direct their gaze toward the perceived 3D targets. Other more demanding and dissociating tests can be carried out after these.

Vision assessment Measurement of vision of each eye can be "risky" as it involves a degree of intrusiveness that has been avoided in the initial examination. If conducted carefully and cheerfully, it fits well within a play scenario leading to much information. The tests vary with age, but the strategy is the same: binocular vision first, to get a best acuity and establish a "comfort zone" for the child, then the expected better eye, before finally testing the poorer eye. Measuring binocular visual acuity can lead to more information than just vision level: a critical look at the child's behavior can be revealing. An increasing head turn as the child is progressing down a vision chart will confirm the significance of a seemingly mild nystagmus. There may be decreased binocular vision at distance in an intermittently exotropic child trying to control the deviation by accommodative effort.[6] A fast, but accurate session is essential to avoid boredom, loss of concentration, or undue stress. Learning, memorizing, and peeking are all tricks that can fool unsuspicious examiners.

Infants will preferentially look at a normal human face[7] (Fig. 7.5). They will do so while awake, calm, and happy; the best time is halfway through a feed. In this manner, one can confirm the presence of normal visual processing. One can also observe the exaggerated lid opening of a sighted infant when the surrounding lights are dimmed abruptly. We can see the quick re-fixation of a sighted baby toward a preferred visual target, like a face, after having been submitted to a spin that has generated good oculovestibular movements.

To compare the vision of each eye, one can compare behavior when one eye is obstructed compared to the other (Fig. 7.6). A more critical evaluation will assess the *ocular fixation behavior* to a target (CSM fixation: central, in the middle of the pupil; steady, without nystagmus or other eye instability; maintained, even if a monocular short interruption occurs). In these situations, the visual or general behavior of the child is compared as each eye is tested separately after the initial binocular assessment.

Another useful method of comparing one eye to the other is to challenge a maintained fixation with a vertical prism. A 10 to 16 diopter (10–16Δ) prism is used in this way to help visualize any eye re-fixation movement.[8] This simple method is particularly useful in the absence of horizontal strabismus in a child with suspected unequal vision. In esotropic youngsters too young for quantitative measurements, symmetry of

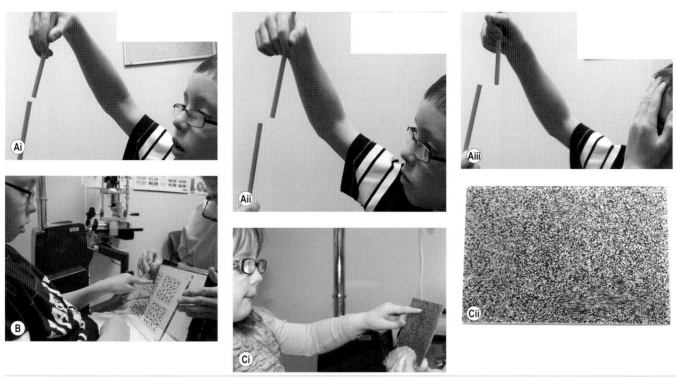

Fig. 7.4 Non-dissociating stereotests. (A) The 2 PT has its limitations because of the many motor components involved, but it provides a real life demonstration of "3-D" vision with straight eyes, as it does here in this esotropic child with high AC/A who shows the advantage of looking through his bifocals. Note to keep the targets at eye level. (B) The Frisby test can give false positive clues of stereopsis if the image plate is rotated on its axis or the patient's head shifts sideways. Easy to administer, it is a good test in the right conditions. (C) The Lang stereotest can be interpreted by watching the patient point or simply gaze at the targets seen only stereoscopically. Here again, however, movements of either the test card or the patient's head can help find monocular clues (apparent increased scrambling of the random dot array in the location of the stereotargets). Note the curvature given to the card by the examiner to make it match the curvature of Panum's area. (D) The popular Titmus is still in use in many clinics and offices. It requires dissociating glasses and uses guiding forms to its stereotargets as opposed to other tests with purely random dot arrays.

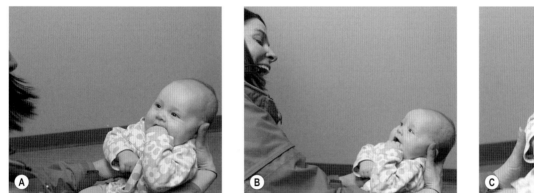

Fig. 7.5 Infant follow face. The examiner holds the infant with good support of the head. The child is happy and relaxed, hence receptive. The face of the examiner is slowly panned across the baby's visual field while observing the child's eyes and head turn in unison with the moving target. The intended movements of the head are easily felt by the supporting hand. The eyes of the examiner's face being of such importance here, it is suggested to remove one's glasses to avoid reflections. A moving but silent mouth with its contrasting contours has been shown to enhance the attractiveness of the target face for infants as young as 3–4 months.

cross fixation or latent nystagmus are both indirect methods of confirming equal vision. On the other hand, sine wave grating tests, including optokinetic nystagmus, visual evoked potentials, and preferential looking cards, estimate vision levels in children. Children prefer to look at simple high contrast gratings but the tests perform poorly in detecting interocular vision differences due to amblyopia and can overestimate the potential recognition vision capacity. Their

usefulness is limited to assessing the progress of deeply amblyopic eyes early in treatment or in handicapped children.[9,10] They are not a necessity for most pediatric ophthalmology practice.

Recognition quantitative visual acuity tests use comparison games and comprise highly standardized logarithmic distribution of visual targets, such as the HOTV (named after the letters used) and LH (after their author, Lea Hyvärinen) tests. They

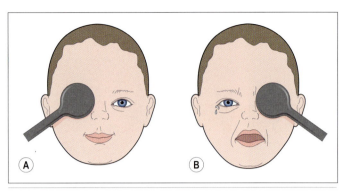

Fig. 7.6 Evaluation of vision in infants. A child with poor vision in one eye (here the right), may not object to having the poorly seeing eye covered (A), but will show displeasure when the good or better eye is covered (B). This can translate in behavioral changes, or active avoidance measures with head movements or pushing of the cover with the hand. (From Goldbloom R. Pediatric Clinical Skills, 4th ed. Philadelphia: Elsevier; 2011. With permission from Elsevier.)

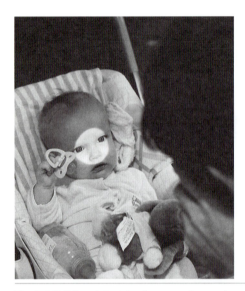

Fig. 7.7 Brückner's test. In all cases, make sure the patient is comfortable, least disturbed, and with his or her own things. Stay at about 0.6 m away with the widest beam of the ophthalmoscope encompassing both pupils. Focus the lense for the working distance and compare both corneal reflection and fundus red reflex for symmetry, homogeneity, and brightness. (From Goldbloom R. Pediatric Clinical Skills, 4th ed. Philadelphia: Elsevier; 2011. With permission from Elsevier.)

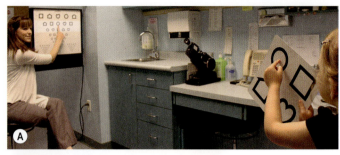

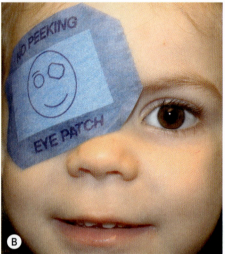

Fig. 7.8 LH logMAR vision chart for children. A well standardized and validated visual acuity (VA) test, the Leah Hivarinnen comparative recognition VA chart has become a gold standard in children of all ages. It can be used in children as young as 36 months. At 41 months, the testability in the general population is good.

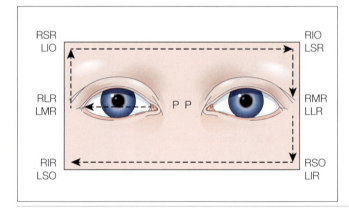

Fig. 7.9 The frame used to evaluate comitance of a strabismus. A slow continuous movement of the dim fixating light along an imaginary frame around the patient's eyes allows the assessment of all 12 extraocular muscles. LIO, left inferior oblique; LIR, left inferior rectus; LLR; left lateral rectus; LMR, left medial rectus; LSO, left superior oblique; LSR, left superior rectus; PP, primary position; RIO, right inferior oblique; RIR, right inferior rectus; RLR, right lateral rectus; RMR, right medial rectus; RSO, right superior oblique; RSR, right superior rectus. (From Goldbloom R. Pediatric Clinical Skills, 4th ed. Philadelphia: Elsevier; 2011. With permission from Elsevier.)

have become standards in visual acuity testing in children too young to complete the ETDRS or other chart (Re:HOTV/LH standards and age) (Fig. 7.8). Most reports show good reliability starting at age 40 months.

Dynamic retinoscopy This technique ensures that a young child is able to accommodate.[11] Its usefulness can be shown in trisomy 21 or cerebral palsy children who show hypoaccommodation. The technique requires only the child's short attention to a visual target placed on the retinoscope while the child's ability to conteract minus lenses is confirmed by retinoscopy.

Version, ductions, null position To evaluate all six extraocular muscles, a quick and dynamic assessment of versions can be carried out by involving the mental representation of a virtual picture frame in front of the patient's face, the corners of which are the targets to reach with a fixation object (Fig. 7.9). The

"frame" is quick and facilitates detection of a muscle dysfunction from any cause. In a cooperative child, monocular testing differentiates version vs. duction deficits.

For infants or less cooperative children, easily evaluating at least four extraocular muscles –hence two cranial nerves – can

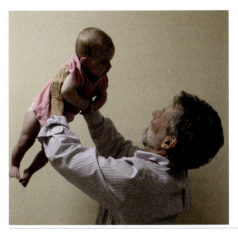

Fig. 7.10 Spin the baby for horizontal extraocular movements. Horizontal strabismus can appear to have limited abduction or adduction in infants. Stimulating an oculocephalic response will elicit full movements by rotating with the child in one's arms while watching the eye movements. Note the forward tilt of 30° to line-up the horizontal semicircular canal with the plane of rotation, enhancing the response. A sighted child will also have the ability to stop a postrotational nystagmus, in contrast to the tonic eye deviation in the direction of the rotation of the blind patient.

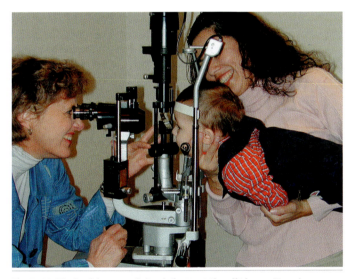

Fig. 7.11 Method for examining infants at the slit-lamp. First, the ophthalmologist sets up the slit-lamp microscope so that it is ready for the most important task (i.e. looking for transillumination using a coaxial beam). While the parent (or clinic assistant) holds the baby with the left arm under his tummy, she places his head on the white strap, continually encouraging him.

be done quickly with minimal equipment in one of two pediatric versions of the doll's head maneuver. Both lateral recti (cranial nerve VI) and medial recti (cranial nerve III, inferior branch) can be tested. For an infant, one needs only a rotating stool; a quick turn in each direction while holding the child up in front of one's eyes, with a slight tilt forward to maximize utricular responses, is all that is needed to confirm full horizontal movements (Fig. 7.10). This will solve the frequent conundrum of a poorly abducting eye in an otherwise normal esotropic infant tested initially with versions. For older children, if no neck anomaly exists, a quick short movement of the head induces the same response and may reveal full eye movement.

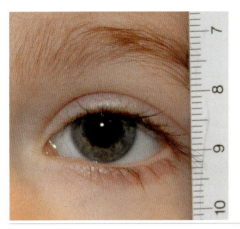

Fig. 7.12 Precise measurements by photograph. A calibrating ruler placed in the same plane as the object of interest of a photograph will provide the accurate reference for the measurement of that object, be it a pupillary or corneal diameter, or an interpalpebral fissure.

Next step: touching and other methods of annoying the child – the second part of the examination

At this point, you must ask yourself if the patient is ready to proceed with the rest of the examination.

Use the company Take advantage of those in the room who came with the child; if they are older or looking more at ease, conduct key tests on them first. That may be a parent but a stuffed animal or doll can also do the trick.

Pupils and corneal diameter he full evaluation of the pupillary responses and measurements of corneal diameters in children is a challenge. Fixation targets are essential for both near and distance: compelling and noisy for distance, and accommodative and interesting for near, all that you can find at hand. Magnification is sometimes useful (surgical 2.5× loupes come in handy) and the ability to easily modify the room lighting while observing the pupils. The pupillary responses to light and dark, not only the diameter measurements but also the dynamic response, give invaluable information. The simple observation of the pupils' behavior while turning the room lights on can be sufficient: normal pupils will constrict, while those of an achromat will dilate initially (paradoxical pupil) (see Chapter 46 and 63); the opposite happens when the lights are turned back on. Finally, a photograph might become the only reliable documentation available to assess corneal diameters or a reported anisocoria. A picture of the child's face with a millimeter ruler in the field (Fig. 7.12) helps measure landmarks.[12]

Lids By the child chewing food or drinking liquid one can witness in infants the lid movements of Marcus Gunn's jaw winking or other misinnervations. Congenital or acquired synkinesis involving the lid can be subtle and cannot be elicited without full and appropriate stimulation of the mastication muscles.

Binocularity If the preliminary testing is not sufficient, more refined binocularity testing can be used at this juncture using the necessary glasses, prisms, and various testing complexities.

51

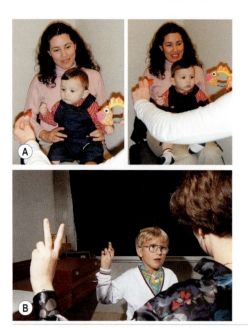

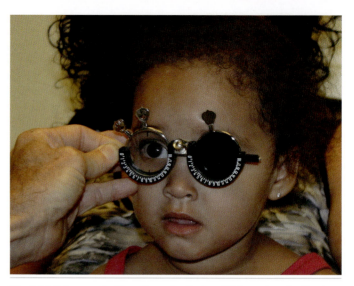

Fig. 7.14 Sciascopy in the axis, and cylinders. While paying attention to one's working distance, any technique that will ensure a cycloplegic refractive sciascopic measurement in the visual axis will ensure precise measurements. When cylinders are involved, an infant trial frame without temple pieces will serve wonders in providing both a good cache as well as helping to find the correct axis.

Fig. 7.13 (A) Assessing the visual field of infants. The tester attracts the baby's attention to a toy (right) while bringing in an object, in this case a dropper bottle, silently from the child's right side to see whether the child's attention is drawn to it – which in this case (left) it is! Although seemingly crude, if defects are detected by these methods, they are likely to be functionally significant in the future. (Photo by Dr Hung Pham.) (B) Demonstration of finger counting technique to assess visual fields in older children. While the tester watches the fixation, the child tells her when the tester's fingers are wiggling or may watch or count the fingers if able to do so.

Confrontation fields A reliable visual field analysis in many young patients is critical. Quantitative results can be obtained on the Goldmann perimeter at around 5 years of age in cooperative children. Automated machines are reliable only later. Therefore, a good confrontation technique is necessary. A fast, fun, and simple field test is essential and no equipment is required except for one's fingers and a bit of patience. In younger children, use moving fingers as targets; in older patients, finger counting is best. In both instances, one's face –or nose for more precision– is the fixation target. With the very little ones, only a binocular testing can be carried out; it might be possible to test an older child with confrontation central field or red saturation assessment similar to adults (Fig. 7.13).

Strabismus assessment In addition to observation of head posture, variable angles, fixation behavior, and cross fixation behavior, prism cover test and alternate cover test as well as sensory testing can be performed to a certain degree in children of all ages. Appropriate accommodative targets are essential for reliable measurements. At least one 6 m target, and ideally a window to the outside world – literally – will be essential for the evaluation of exotropic patients. No one carries out these measurements better then a well trained orthoptist and these professionals excel in the evaluation of children, especially those with strabismus and amblyopia.

Slit-lamp examination The success of an anterior segment examination in a child is largely dependent on their comfort. In stressful emergencies, the challenge can be insurmountable. The short working distance of our instruments is not readily tolerated by many children. 2.5× magnification operating loupes can be useful for surface problems. A Bruckner's test with the direct ophthalmoscope set at +5 D can help for media opacities. The less imposing portable slit-lamp can be of help, while the conventional slit-lamp can be used in cooperative children. Infants can be propped up and restrained by adults for a slit-lamp view (Fig. 7.11).

Refraction Retinoscopy (sciascopy) can measure the true refractive error of an eye only when performed in line with the visual axis, especially when astigmatism is present. Cycloplegic refraction is essential. A non-traumatic, effective technique to instill a cycloplegic drop in children is important. Most cycloplegic drops sting; try them yourself! Cycloplegic refractions are therefore often left to the end of the first visit. Teaching the parents how to instill the cycloplegic at home is worth the extra effort. One drop of most cycloplegic agents is insufficient to achieve good accommodative paralysis in dark-eyed individuals. A solution: pre-treat the corneal epithelium with a topical anesthetic, followed by the instillation of the cycloplegic of choice. Local anesthetics loosen the epithelial tight junctions, enhancing the intracamerular penetration of the cycloplegics. Topical anesthetics are also better tolerated and make the whole episode more acceptable. A higher concentration (e.g. 2% cyclopentolate) may help. Another difficulty with retinoscopy in youngsters is cooperation with refractive trial lenses placed close to their faces. The offering of a +/−0.12 diopter lens to hold on to, or two of them to play percussion, is a trick that has saved this author much time. The precision of the axis measurements of cylinders improves by placing lenses in a trial frame. For younger children, using the frames without the temple pieces greatly helps (Fig. 7.14). With all children who can sit willingly in the examination chair, it is worth trying the phoropter. A good seating position ensures a precise, fast, and reliable refraction. It is a fun experience once it is highlighted how their side of the machine feels like looking through the glasses of a well known mouse cartoon character (Fig. 7.15). A calm environment is essential for refracting

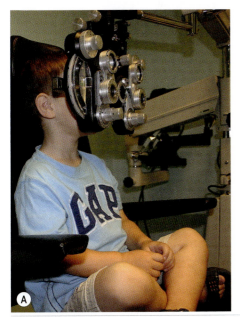
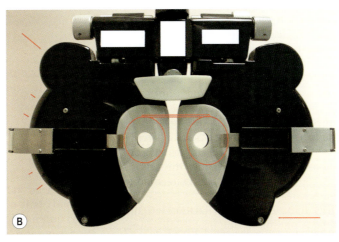

Fig. 7.15 The phoropter and children. (A) As soon as a child can sit, in theory the phoroptor can be used for refractions. A sitting position with good stable posture is essential. (B) On the patient's side, familial features of the famous iconic cartoon mouse become obvious with a little imagination: ears, cheeks, whiskers.

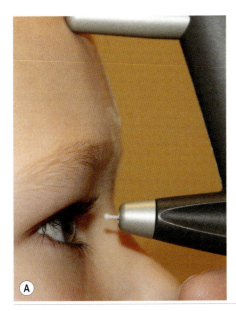
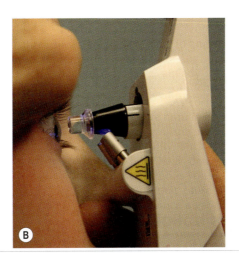
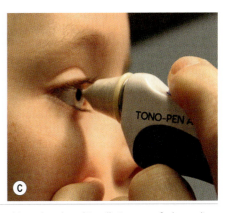

Fig. 7.16 Tonometers in the pediatric age. Note the wide-eyed relaxed-looking child in all these photos. Anything other than this will give you a faulty reading with any instrument.

children and a continuous dialogue between child and refractionist in a quiet and dimmed room will resolve many challenging cases.

Intraocular pressure measurement Seasoned clinicians shine in their ability to "extract" reliable IOP measurements from the least likely candidates. One reliable measurement can make the difference between a discharge or many more visits, including examinations under sedation or anesthesia. Reliability of readings is a major issue, not only because of the variability of thickness of the child's cornea, but also because of the profound effect the examination can have on the measurements obtained. All anesthetics modify the pressure to some extent,

most decreasing it. Any kind of crying, intubation, or forceful lid opening will dramatically raise it. Some instruments are reliable only in a certain range of pressure reading (e.g. tonopen types); others are difficult to use in smaller eyes (e.g. Perkins, Goldmann). All require a relaxed wide-eyed patient. Careful scheduling to take advantage of feeding and nap times is essential (Fig. 7.16).

Fundus examination Most children do not object to the brightness of the indirect ophthalmoscope and will cooperate for a direct ophthalmoscopic examination, as long as an interesting fixation target is made available. The use of fantastical themes to describe what one sees in the fundus is always welcomed and helps allay fears of the unknown. The child's own body parts are perfect visual targets for the peripheral retinal exam. Most know where their left big toe, ear or shoulder is, and will look in the right direction, especially if asked to move those body parts. A 20 D aspheric lense with the indirect ophthalmoscope will facilitate the estimation of vessel caliber, disk size, and macular position. The 28 D is sufficient for an overview of things, but should only be used in conjunction with the 20 D. Children who cooperate well with the slit-lamp examination will allow a good examination with the 78 D or 90 D lenses for a detailed assessment of the posterior pole. These patients will also be cooperative for optical coherence tomography (see Chapter 9). For the others, those who would rather leave the building as soon as they look into the light of the indirect ophthalmoscope, a good restraining technique rarely fails to help obtain a reasonable fundus examination. The level of suspicion will dictate the quality of the examination required and the efforts put into it but, usually, the clinic setting will be satisfactory. The parents are always invited to participate and help. It is better for them to know and understand what is taking place than be alarmed by cries and screams from the other side of a door.

Finally: rewarding success

A good visit cannot end without celebration, rewards, reinforcement, and conditioning. A child who receives positive feedback after showing some good will or after controlling their fears will remember the reward or gift. Stickers are universally welcomed as long as they are current, so keep up with the cultural icons of your young patients. "High fives," hand shakes, and hugs all have their place in the right occasions, as long as the parents are present and comfortable with it. Colorful patches with printed modern designs are welcome as a novelty by many patients with amblyopia. A photo club poster of patching children and a certificate for those who reach their goal are popular in our clinic. Parents should also be rewarded. A progress chart of their child's vision does marvels in celebrating gains as well as reinforcing the need to pick up the efforts when needed. After all is said and done, a smiling child, thankful parents, and a feeling of worth are what constitute our rewards.

References

1. Kenny N, Skinner L. Assessing the appropriate role for children in health decisions. In: Goldbloom RB, editor. Pediatric Clinical Skills, 4th edn. Philadelphia: Elsevier/Saunders; 2011: 307–16.
2. Becker MH, Drachman RH, Kirscht JP. Predicting mother's compliance with pediatric medical regimens. J Pediatr 1972; 81: 843–54.
3. Roe LD, Guyton DL. The light that leaks: Brückner and the red reflex. Surv Ophthalmol 1984; 28: 665–70.
4. Thorn F, Gwiazda J, Cruz AA, et al. The development of eye alignment, convergence and sensory binocularity in young infants. Invest Ophthalmol Vis Sci 1994; 35: 544–53.
5. von Noorden, GK, Campos E. Two-Pencil Test, Binocular Vision and Ocular Motility, 6th ed. St Louis: Elsevier/Mosby; 2002: 304–6.
6. Walsh LA, LaRoche GR, Tremblay F. The use of binocular visual acuity in the assessment of intermittent exotropia. J AAPOS 2000; 4: 154–7.
7. Slater A, Quinn PC. Face recognition in the newborn infant. Inf Child Dev 2001; 10: 21–4.
8. Wright K, Walonker F, Edelman P. 10 diopter fixation test for amblyopia. Arch Ophthalmol 1981; 99: 1242–6.
9. Kushner B, Lucchese NJ, Morton GV. Grading visual acuity with teller cards compared with snellen visual acuity in literate patients. Arch Ophthalmol 1995; 113: 485–93.
10. Drover JR, Wyatt LM, Stager DR, Birch EE. Teller acuity cards are effective in detecting amblyopia. Optom Vis Sci 2009; 86: 755–9.
11. McClelland JF, Saunders KJ. The repeatability and validity of dynamic retinoscopy in assessing the accommodative response. Ophthalmic Physiol Opt 2003; 23: 243–50.
12. Puvanachandra N, Lyons CJ. Rapid measurement of corneal diameter in children: validation of a clinic-based digital photographic technique. J AAPOS 2009; 13: 287–8.

Visual electrophysiology: how it can help you and your patient

Dorothy A Thompson • Alki Liasis

Introduction

Pediatric visual electrophysiology can be a challenge, but provides information about the working of retina and visual pathways that we cannot achieve by other means. This functional assessment helps us with early diagnosis, prognosis, and an objective means of monitoring neurologic and ocular sequelae.

There are international guidelines and standards for performing visual electrophysiologic tests (e.g. ISCEV, the International Society for Clinical Electrophysiology of Vision, available at http://www.iscev.org, or International Federation of Clinical Neurophysiology at http://www.ifcn.info). We apply, and extend, ISCEV adult protocols in able children, i.e. children who can sit still and follow instructions for 30 minutes or more. With younger, or less compliant, children we use adapted protocols that are robust enough to provide comparable information without restraint, sedation, or anesthesia.

As children have short attention spans we may need to use distraction to encourage reproducible results. We need to be flexible and responsive during the test to adapt the protocol, and the order of tests within a protocol. This may be prompted by ongoing analysis and interpretation, or a change in compliance. This enables us to meet the needs of a child in a way they enjoy, yet answer the clinical question in a time efficient way! The overarching aim is to minimize stress and anxiety to child, carer, and staff. This optimizes results and enhances our chance of reliable future monitoring.

The tests

Clinical visual electrophysiologic tests include the electro-oculogram (EOG) and the electroretinogram (ERG), which assess the function of the retinal pigment epithelium (RPE) and retina, and the visual evoked potential (VEP), which assesses the integrity of the postretinal pathways to the striate visual cortex particularly the macular pathways. The retinotopic representation of the macula on the gyri of the occipital lobes is most accessible to surface VEP electrodes.

Behavioral compliance is the limiting factor in pediatric visual electrophysiology testing. To record an EOG the child will have to sit still and make saccades every minute for 15 minutes in the dark then 15 minutes in the light; for the pattern ERG (PERG) or multifocal ERG (mfERG) they need steady fixation with good focus and for an ISCEV ERG they will need to dark adapt for 20 minutes and light adapt for 10 minutes. This may be possible for exceptional youngsters, but it is more likely from ages 5 years upwards. Our adaptive protocol may be applied from birth onwards and aims for a total chair time of 30 minutes during which time pattern VEPs (PVEPs) and flash ERGs are carried out contemporaneously with flash VEPs.

To illustrate this we have applied our GOSH (Great Ormond Street Hospital) protocol to two common questions arising at different ages. The flow chart outlines the diagnostic algorithm and hierarchy of testing (Fig. 8.1). We have added short notes on the technical aspects of the methodology at the end of the chapter. Artefacts can mimic physiologic responses and must be excluded before findings from complementary tests may be interpreted as consistent (see Fig. 8.1).

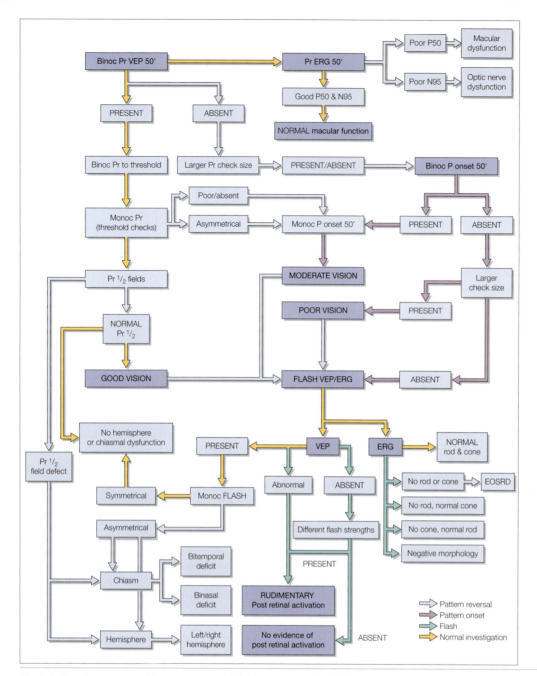

Fig. 8.1 All testing can start with pattern reversal 50′ checks presented to both eyes. Depending upon the response we may proceed to smaller reversing checks and monocular testing, or divert to pattern onset stimulation. After pattern stimulation is completed flash stimulation is used to contemporaneously record ERGs and VEPs. Transoccipital asymmetries are noted throughout and explored in all three stimulus modalities and when possible with half field stimulation. With suspected voluntary defocus the PERG is recorded simultaneously with the pattern reversal VEP. This robust combination strategy can be used to investigate diverse clinical questions as the two examples outline:

1. Babies: unstable eye movements, is this congenital motor nystagmus? Looking for an anterior visual pathway problem:
   Possibilities –
   • Retina: early onset severe retinal dystrophy (EOSRD), cone dysfunction and congenital stationary night blindness (CSNB)
      – need stimuli to separate rod and cone activity and distinguish photoreceptors from inner retina activity (a- and b-wave).
   • Optic nerve: optic nerve hypoplasia
      – need monocular flash and PVEPs to compare interocular amplitudes and latency on the midline electrode.
   • Chiasmal anomaly: albinism (require flash infancy and pattern onset stimulation for older children), chiasmal hypoplasia, glioma
      – need monocular stimulation and a transoccipital array of electrodes to look for transoccipital distribution of VEP.
2. Teenagers: questioning whether there is a functional element to measured subnormal vision:
   • Simultaneous PERG and PVEP
      – control defocus: cycloplegic full correction for viewing distance, observe direction of gaze.

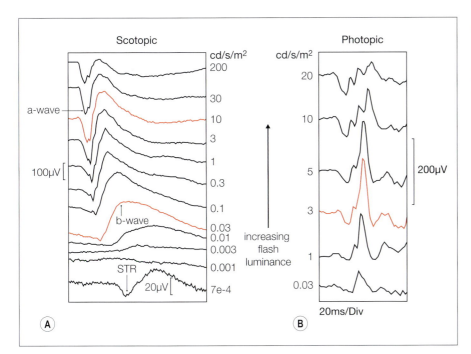

Fig. 8.2 Scotopic (A) and photopic (B) luminance response series. ERGs to ISCEV standard flash strengths are shown in red. (A) from bottom to top shows first the development of the rod driven b-wave and then the a-wave as flash strength increases. (B) shows the photopic hill phenomenon with smaller b-wave amplitude to higher flash strengths.

What do the responses tell us? An aide memoire for a busy clinician

The electro-oculogram

The EOG is used to investigate if a maculopathy is due to retinal pigment epitheliopathy. The standing potential of the eye due to voltage across apical and basal surfaces of the RPE is around 6 millivolts, with maximal positivity detected at the corneal apex. Electrodes placed on the medial and lateral canthi measure a large potential change during a saccade: the electrode closest to the cornea becomes positive relative to the electrode furthest from the cornea. This is the EOG and it is displayed as a voltage/time plot. Eye movements, including nystagmus, can be characterized graphically. The EOG potential increases in light and decreases in the dark.[1] With reproducible eye movements, e.g. saccades of known size, this variation can be measured and expressed as the Arden ratio (light rise/dark trough) and values below 1.6–1.8 are abnormal. The voltage change with light is a consequence of the phagocytosis of outer segment discs and transport of retinal binding proteins at the apical end of the RPE. If the photoreceptors are sick, both the ERG and the EOG are affected. The EOG is diagnostically potent when the Arden ratio is abnormal and the rod ERG is normal as this discriminates a primary retinal condition from an epitheliopathy, e.g. bestrophin mutations (see Chapter 45).[2]

The electroretinogram

The ERG is used to distinguish cone and rod dysfunction and photoreceptor from inner retinal dysfunction. The ERG is measured in microvolts and its size and shape depend upon the relative proportion and extent of rods and cones that are excited and the size of the retinal area stimulated.[3] Rods and cones can be preferentially stimulated by flashes of different colors, strength, and duration presented under different states of dark and light adaptation. The gradual evolution of the ERG waveform with increasing flash strength is shown in Fig. 8.2A scotopically and Fig. 8.2B photopically.

To very dim lights, a small scotopic threshold response (STR) has been described but clinically this is difficult to achieve and is used rarely. As flash strength increases a late (60 ms), round, positive b-wave emerges. This is the rod driven b-wave, which reflects inner retinal activity associated mainly with depolarizing on-bipolar cells. The change of b-wave amplitude with flash strength can be described by a Naka-Rushton function, derived from the Michaelis-Menton equation, but the derived parameters will vary according to the method of curve fitting. In clinical circumstances these need to be interpreted with care.[4]

$$V/V_{max} = Int/Int + K$$

where V = trough-to-peak amplitude of the b-wave, V_{max} = maximum value of trough-to-peak amplitude, Int = flash strength in troland/second, K = semisaturation value, i.e. when Int = K, V is $V_{max}/2$.

As the flash strength further increases an early negative a-wave precedes the b-wave. The a-wave becomes larger and faster with increasing flash strength reflecting photoreceptor hyperpolarization. To the brightest flashes the leading edge of the scotopic a-wave models rod phototransduction.[5]

Measures of a- and b-waves are used most clinically, but other ERG waves can be useful. These include:

1. Oscillatory potentials – a series of wavelets between the a- and b-waves, vulnerable to disturbances of retinal circulation.[6]
2. The photopic negative response – reflecting proximal retinal activity, vulnerable in glaucoma and in potassium channelopathies.[7]
3. The c-wave – related to the EOG, due to a depletion of potassium ions in the space between RPE.

4. The d-wave – an off pathway response. Rods use the on pathway through the inner retina; cones use both on and off pathways. The d-wave is associated with decreases in light under photopic conditions, and is best seen in response to prolonged on–off flashes (on >90 ms). This is an important extra stimulus for investigating "negative," no b-wave ERGs, e.g. subtyping CSNB (see Chapter 44).[8] Usually b- and d-waves are superimposed in the ERGs to short duration (<10 ms) flashes.

Flash ERG amplitudes are proportional to the area of functional retina. When a ganzfeld flash scatters light uniformly over the whole retina the summated ERG can mask a small, localized lesion, e.g. maculopathy. Focal flashes, patterned, and multifocal stimuli avoid intraocular scatter and test localized retinal regions. These require steady fixation.

PERGs are elicited by pattern reversing checks. The waveform is biphasic with positivity at 50 ms and a negativity at 95 ms, termed p50 and n95, respectively. The p50 represents distal retina activity while the n95 characterizes more proximal retina and ganglion cell function.[9] PERGs investigate suspected early maculopathy, but can investigate optic nerve (retinal ganglion cell) dysfunction and distinguish optic nerve from cortical dysfunction. We record PERGs simultaneously with PVEPs using a large (30°) field, and small (15°) fields. The small retinal areas stimulated result in small signal amplitudes (around 0.5–8 μV), with corneal electrodes that allow good focus, and need interrupted signal averaging to avoid blinks and eye movement artefact (Fig. 8.3).

Multifocal stimulation allows focal ERG responses to be recorded simultaneously from many regions of the retina.[10] An array of hexagons are scaled in size with retinal eccentricity to elicit responses of equal size. Each hexagon flashes on and off in an M-sequence. This is a pseudorandom algorithm that guarantees that no stimulus sequence is repeated during an examination. At any one time, on average, half of the hexagons are black and the other half white. The stimulation rate is high, causing a flickering appearance of the screen, but with relatively stable mean luminance. Each element starts the sequence at a different place to every other element. If the difference in starting point in the sequence (the lag) is longer than the response duration, each element generates a response uncorrelated with every other element. Responses unaffected by stimulation of other areas are termed first-order components; second-order components represent temporal interactions between flashes and short lags relative to the duration of the response. It is important to interpret the trace arrays rather than rely on the associated isopotential contour maps which can be misleading. The mfERG waveforms are mathematical constructs not tiny ERGs, and do not directly reflect a- and b-wave sources. mfERGs, like PERGs, are very sensitive to fixation instabilities. Application in children is largely untried.

The visual evoked potential

The VEP is recorded from the occipital region of the scalp. It reflects depolarization of lamina 4c of the striate cortex (area V_1) by the retinogeniculo afferent volley.[11,12] Retinotopic activity from the central 5°, predominantly lower field, dominates the VEP, and PVEPs in children can act as an index of macular pathway function. If the PVEP is abnormal, it is important to rule out primary retinal dysfunction at the macula using PERG, mfERG, and/or fundal imaging. In the presence of known maculopathy or degraded PERG/mfERGs the PVEP waveform may still provide useful information about residual macular and paramacular function. We record PVEPs with both eyes open before monocular testing. We use a transoccipital array of electrodes, large full field (30°) and, where possible, half-field stimulation, to discriminate optic nerve, chiasmal, and hemisphere anomalies (Fig. 8.4).

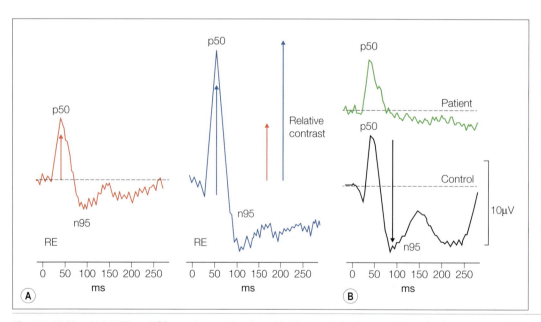

Fig. 8.3 (A) RE and LE PERGs to 50′ from a 3-year-old patient with RE posterior lenticonus. p50 amplitude is proportional to contrast. The RE PERG amplitude reflects the relative contrast loss due to RE cataract. (B) Top trace is RE PERGs to 25′ from 6-year-old patient with kidney failure. Loss of n95 indicates visual loss due to ON compromise not retinal dysfunction. RE, right eye; LE, left eye.

Use of different types of stimulation: pattern reversal, pattern onset, and flash stimulation

Pattern reversal VEPs have a simple triphasic waveform that is maintained across the lifespan with a major positive peak around 100 ms by 7 months of age, called p100 (components are defined by their polarity: p for positive, n negative; the numbers are the latency of the peak after the stimulus). The shape of the full field pattern reversal VEP may become bifid (p-n-p) if a central scotoma reduces the macular contribution, e.g. seen in dominant optic atrophy (see Chapter 52). The bifid waveform is due to enhancement of paramacular contributions n105 and p135. Half-field stimulation can delineate macular and paramacular peaks. We use a wide range of checksizes from 400′ to 6.25′ presented 3/s after 6 weeks of life.

Pattern onset stimulation is attention grabbing, robust to eye movements, and is preferred in nystagmus or to prevent active defocus. Its waveform is complex and three components have spatially separate generator sources: CI, a positivity around 90 ms; CII, negativity at about 110 ms; and CIII, a prominent positivity at around 180–200 ms.[13,14] Different peaks emerge at different ages: the initial positive CI is most prominent in children and depends upon contrast and luminance. CII emerges in later childhood and depends more on contour. These changes mean it can be difficult to use pattern onset VEPs for monitoring longitudinally.[15]

Flash stimulation is robust and can be effective through closed lids. A control ERG recorded at the same time as the VEP can ensure the level of retinal stimulation. We use both flash and pattern stimulation, and often also both pattern reversal and onset stimulation to provide overlapping and complementary evidence of visual pathway function, particularly transoccipital asymmetries.

Flash and pattern reversal VEPs show paradoxical localization. For example, the right half field stimulation of the left hemisphere is detected over the right occipital electrode. This is due to orientation of the cortex activated and is a consequence of our large-field stimulation and a reference electrode placed at the mid-frontal position.[16] Pattern onset VEPs do not show this. The right half field response is detected anatomically appropriately over the left occiput. A comparison of full field pattern onset and reversal VEP transoccipital asymmetries are at times useful to determine if VEP occipital asymmetry is due to pathology, especially in those children with flat or asymmetric skulls who cannot manage half field stimulation.[17]

Visual acuity and the VEP

It is alluring to try to condense PVEPs into a single number descriptor of vision acuity; unfortunately, the relationship is not so simple. In normal children an estimate of visual acuity may be based on the amplitude of PVEPs elicited by patterns of decreasing element size.[18] Threshold VEP acuity is derived from the smallest pattern size to give a response above noise level, or an extrapolation to zero amplitude on a graph of amplitude versus spatial frequency.[19] Although PVEPs show some correlation with behavioral acuity, it is not realistic to expect a direct correlation in a clinical population. For example, as neurons are lost in optic atrophy the PVEPs will become markedly attenuated and degraded, yet if the receptive fields of the few remaining functioning neurons are closely spaced in the central

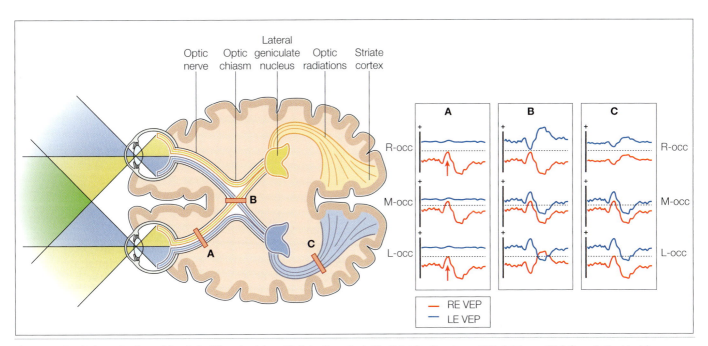

Fig. 8.4 Schematic projection of the right (blue shade) and left (yellow shade) half fields of each eye (RE, right eye; LE, left eye). The black bars superimposed on the pathway represent lesions at (A) left optic nerve, (B) chiasm, and (C) left optic radiations and occipital cortex. The occipital distribution of schematic VEPs caused by these lesions are shown from RE (in red) and LE (in blue) aligned with the electrode sites right (R-occ) and left (L-occ) lateral and the mid-occipital (M-occ) channels. Column a shows a reduced LE VEP and a symmetric distribution of the RE VEP where lateral channel amplitudes are similar (arrowed). Column b shows a crossed asymmetry where the transoccipital distribution of one eye is the mirror image of the other, i.e. the RE VEP is negative (downwards deflection) on the left occiput and the LE VEP is negative over the right occiput. This indicates chiasmal dysfunction. Column c shows each eye has the same, homonymous, distribution reduced over the right occiput. This homonymous distribution or uncrossed asymmetry suggests hemisphere dysfunction. Due to paradoxical lateralization this distribution of flash and pattern reversal VEPs means dysfunction of the right half field representation in the left hemisphere.

field, recognition acuity can be surprisingly good, even with marked optic disc pallor. Estimates of acuity development are higher with VEP techniques in the first 12–18 months of life; after this behavioral estimates exceed VEP acuity.[20] Recognition acuity is an interpretation of high contrast, static images by higher association areas. Discrepancies from a VEP measure of striate cortex activity should not surprise. Nevertheless, PVEPs are a useful index of macular pathway function and provide a qualitative indication of the vision level the retinogeniculate pathway can support. We consider that a pattern reversal VEP to 50' or smaller checks suggests good vision levels, to 100'–200' moderate, and to 400' poor vision levels. If a flash VEP is detected, but no PVEP is recorded, this suggests vision is rudimentary. PVEPs show little intersession variation and are reliable for serial monitoring and are particularly useful for interocular comparisons in infancy.[21]

When the rate of stimulation increases, individual transient PVEP waveforms merge and become sinusoidal. This is a steady state response and is used in sweep VEPs, where many different pattern sizes or contrast levels are swept through rapidly.[22,23] The steady state VEP is analyzed by Fourier techniques into amplitude and phase data. It is possible to determine signal to noise thresholds during acquisition before proceeding to smaller patterns – a step acuity VEP. The sweep technique can provide a number (usually in cpd) to describe acuity or contrast sensitivity quickly, but there is a loss of information about waveform and often transoccipital distribution. These fast rates drive the maturing visual system faster than optimal for highest acuity. As VEP waveforms are such important diagnostic indicators we prefer transient PVEP recording for routine clinical practice (Fig. 8.5).

Technical factors

Visual stimuli include transient flashes of different intensities, durations, temporal rates, colors, patterns, and multifocal mosaics.

Visual stimulators

Flash

Commercial flash stimulators include hand-held strobes, which are advantageous in pediatric testing. They can be manipulated to follow an alert, but restless, child and eye position can be directly observed. Ganzfelds scatter light uniformly over the retina and are available as static domes with chin rests, or smaller hand-held LED versions that are held close to the eye. It is important that these have integral cameras to ensure the eye is open and stimulated properly.

Patterns

Patterned stimuli are computer generated and presented on cathode ray tube (CRT) that are no longer commercially available, liquid crystal diode (LCD), plasma display panels (PDP), or back projection systems. Triggers for response acquisition with CRTs are synchronized with the raster rate generating the image. If running at 50 Hz, there could be a 20 ms difference in latency between a PVEP recorded looking at the top left of the screen compared to the bottom right. LCD screens have an inherent luminance flash artefact generated in the pattern due to timing differences in on and off switching. PDPs avoid both

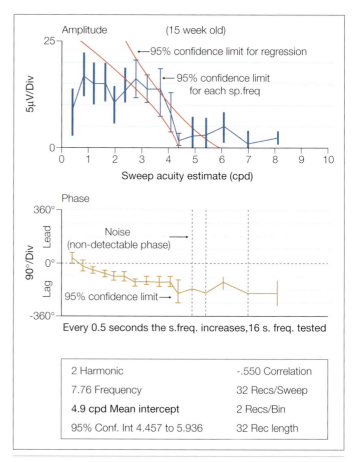

Fig. 8.5 Sweep VEP. Rapid stimulation rates are used to elicit a quasi-sinusoidal VEP characterized by its amplitude and phase. A range of spatial frequencies is presented. There is a trend for VEP amplitude to decrease with increasing spatial frequency. A regression to the baseline or noise level is computed to give an acuity estimate in this case 4.9 cpd.

these issues. We use a large-field PDP with the advantage of the near simultaneous generation of a pattern uniformly over the screen without luminance artefact. Its multisynch capabilities means it allows us to switch quickly between the stimulus and a cartoon DVD during the test to maintain attention whilst a separate audio output keeps soundtrack continuity when patterns are presented.

Field size

Large field sizes (around 30°) are important in pediatric practice, allowing a child some variation of gaze direction whilst still fully stimulating a central, macular, 10° field. Smaller fields are more prone to spurious transoccipital asymmetries when fixation direction varies to the edge of the field.

Check sizes

Patterns prevent light scatter by containing equal numbers of black-and-white elements (usually checks, more rarely gratings) that either counterphase (reverse from black to white) or appear from a background of uniform gray field of equal mean luminance (pattern onset). A wide range of check sizes is important to ensure consistency, provide a broad baseline for monitoring, and intraocular comparison. The diagonal dimension of a single check gives the cycles per degree equivalent.

ERG electrodes

A range of different sized contact lens electrodes are needed for pediatric work, but these are not used often in the UK and Europe because of concerns about cross infection. Disposable corneal electrodes, e.g. DTL, gold foil and HK loop electrodes, are preferred and inferior periorbital skin electrodes are used frequently in younger children. An ERG recorded with a skin electrode is 12–15% of the amplitude of a corneal electrode, but still substantial, i.e. exceeding 10 µV (with corneal electrodes mfERG are measured in nanovolts, PERGs are under 2–5 µV, and adult VEPs ≤5 µV).[24,25] The skin ERG waveform and timings are similar to corneal electrode ERGs. It is important to ensure the cornea is positioned towards the skin electrode, e.g. a child is encouraged to look downwards, or if there is strabismus, or a shallow midface, the skin electrode may be displaced and gaze directed over it. If the child is asleep and eye rolls up, it is possible to record a completely inverted ERG trace.[26]

Refractive error

The PERG is sensitive to 0.5 DS blur, but the pattern reversal VEP is robust to 8 D blur of 60′ checks. These two responses can be recorded together to ensure accurate focus. If there is a doubt about focus, as may occur in patients with suspected functional overlay, then PERGs and PVEPs may be recorded after cycloplegia and correction for stimulator distance, e.g. +1 D added for a viewing distance of 1 m.

Dilation

For our combined protocol we want best focus for pattern reversal VEPs. We do not dilate for the flash ERG protocol which immediately follows the PVEP recording. Pupillary dilation aims to standardize amplitudes, but causes only 12–15% amplitude change.[25,26] Extremes of pupil size or anisocoria are noted, but numerical correction factors for variation in retinal illuminance rarely are applied to clinical ERGs. Recording ERGs to a wide a range of flash strengths ensures this is overcome empirically.

Dark adaptation

It is not practical to have pediatric normative data for abbreviated dark adaptation. Ranges would be required for each 5 minute dark interval for each month of the first year of life. We take the same time point under darkened conditions without long dark adaption and stimulate with dim blue flashes to bias the photoreceptor contribution to be predominantly rod driven. The ERG wave shape provides feedback about the predominant contributing cells as the retina acts like an adaptive photometer.

Maturation

Retinal sensitivity is poor at birth. ISCEV defined flash stimuli include the possibility of non-detectable ERGs in early infancy.[27] In essence, brighter flash stimuli are needed. If anesthesia is used, this can delay the time to peak and diminish the b-wave, particularly.[28] Myelination and synaptogenesis and pruning influence the latency of the pattern reversal VEP, which shortens rapidly to within 10% of adult values in the first 7 months of life. A newborn VEP latency is around 240 ms. It is better to stimulate at 1/second and increase the acquisition time window to 450 ms to ensure capture of responses. After 8 weeks of age, stimulation of 3/second and shortening the time window to 300 ms speeds up data acquisition. There continue to be morphologic changes throughout life and it is important for each laboratory to acquire full normative data sets, sampling frequently in the first 12 months of life.

Summary

Visual EDTs are non-invasive and objective and are ideal tests for children. To get the most information from each child in the least time we combine and adapt stimulation protocols according to individual need. We distract by interleaving cartoon DVDs with patterned stimuli, having continuous sound tracks, music, audio books, noisy toys, and, most importantly, reassure and encourage through personal interaction and play. These are key to attracting attention and gaze direction and a successful recording. We compare responses against age-matched normative data, after artefacts and confounders are excluded. Data obtained from a combined ERG and VEP assessment can localize dysfunction along the visual pathway and provide a qualitative estimate of vision. We provide complementary and supplementary information in many diverse clinical presentations, ranging from an infant who does not fix and follow and has unusual eye movements, to amblyopia not responding to patching, investigation of headaches, and assessment of children who cannot communicate for behavioral assessments.

The prognostic significance of visual EDT results must be weighed in the light of clinical data and with an awareness of maturational changes. Clinical visual EDTs assess the "visual hardware," but do not tell us about the "software." They may suggest the quality of pattern vision which the retinogeniculostriate pathway may support, but clinical EDTs cannot tell how well a child will be able to use the visual data that reaches the striate cortex.

References

1. Arden G, Barrada A, Kelsey JH. New clinical test of retinal function based on the standing potential of the eye. J Physiol 1962; 46: 449–67.
2. Dev Borman A, Davidson AE, O'Sullivan J, et al. Childhood onset autosomal recessive bestrophinopathy. Arch Ophthalmol 2011; 129: 1088–93.
3. Granit R. Sensory Mechanisms of the Retina. London: Oxford University Press; 1947.
4. Evans LS, Peachey NS, Marchese AL. Comparison of three methods of estimating the parameters of the Naka-Rushton equation. Doc Ophthalmol 1993; 84: 19–30.
5. Pugh E, Lamb T. Phototransduction in vertebrate rods and cones: molecular mechanisms of amplification, recovery and light adaptation. In: Stavenga DG, de Grip WJ, Pugh, EN, Jr, editors. Handbook of Biological Physics, vol. 3. Amsterdam: Elsevier; 2000: 183–254.

6. Wachtmeister L. Oscillatory potentials in the retina: what do they reveal? Prog Ret Eye Res 1998; 17: 485–521.

7. Thompson DA, Feather S, Stanescu HC, et al. Altered electroretinograms in patients with KCNJ10 mutations and EAST syndrome. J Physiol 2011; 589: 1681–90.

8. Sieving PA. Photopic ON- and OFF-pathway abnormalities in retinal dystrophies. Trans Am Ophthalmol Soc 1993; 91: 701–73.

9. Holder G. Pattern electroretinography (PERG) and an integrated approach to visual pathway diagnosis. In: Fishman GA, Birch D, Holder GE, et al, editors. Electrophysiologic Testing in Disorders of the Retina, Optic Nerve, and Visual Pathway, 2nd ed. Ophthalmology Monograph 2. San Francisco: Foundation of the American Academy of Ophthalmology; 2001: 197–235.

10. Hood DC, Bach M, Brigell M, et al. ISCEV standard for clinical multifocal electroretinography (mfERG) (2011 edition). Doc Ophthalmol 2012; 124: 1–13.

11. Schroeder CE, Tenke CE, Givre SJ, et al. Striate cortical contribution to the surface recorded pattern reversal VEP in the alert monkey. Vision Res 1991; 31: 1143–57. (Erratum in: Vision Res 1991; 31: 1).

12. Givre SJ, Schroeder CE, Arezzo JC. Contribution of extra striate area V4 to the surface recorded flash VEP in the awake macaque. Vision Res 1994; 34: 415–28.

13. Jeffreys DA, Axford JG. Source localisations of pattern-specific components of human visual evoked potentials I. Component of striate cortical origin. Exp Brain Res 1972; 6: 1–21.

14. Jeffreys DA, Axford JG. Source localisations of pattern-specific components of human visual evoked potentials II. Component of extra-striate cortical origin. Exp Brain Res 1972; 6: 22–40.

15. Shawkat FS, Kriss A. A study of the effects of contrast change on pattern VEPs, and the transition between onset, reversal and offset modes of stimulation. Doc Ophthalmol 2000; 101: 73–89.

16. Barrett G, Blumhardt L, Halliday A, et al. A paradox in the lateralization of the visual evoked response. Nature 1976; 261: 253–5.

17. Mellow TB, Liasis A, Lyons R, Thompson D. When do asymmetrical full-field pattern reversal visual evoked potentials indicate visual pathway dysfunction in children? Doc Ophthalmol 2011; 122: 9–18.

18. Sokol S. Measurement of infant visual acuity from pattern reversal evoked potentials. Vision Res 1978; 18: 33–9.

19. Allen D, Tyler C, Norcia A. Development of grating acuity and contrast sensitivity in the central and peripheral visual field of the human infant. Vision Res 1996; 36: 1945–53.

20. Marg E, Freeman DN, Peltzman P, et al. Visual acuity development in human infants: evoked potential measurements. Invest Ophthalmol Vis Sci 1976; 15: 150–3.

21. Liasis A, Thompson DA, Hayward R, et al. Sustained raised intracranial pressure implicated only by pattern reversal visual evoked potentials after cranial vault expansion surgery. Pediatr Neurosurg 2003; 39: 75–80.

22. Tyler CW, Apkarian P, Levi DM, et al. Rapid assessment of visual function: an electronic sweep technique for the pattern visual evoked potential. Invest Ophthalmol Vis Sci 1979; 18: 703–13.

23. Norcia A, Tyler C, Hamer R, et al. Measurement of spatial contrast sensitivity with the swept contrast VEP. Vision Res 1989; 29; 627–37.

24. Esakowitz L, Kriss A, Shawkat F. A comparison of flash electroretinograms recorded from Burian Allen, JET, C-Glide, gold foil, DTL, and skin electrodes. Eye 1993; 7: 169–71.

25. Bradshaw K, Hansen R, Fulton A. Comparison of ERGs recorded with skin and corneal-contact electrodes in normal children and adults. Doc Ophthalmol 2004; 109: 43–55.

26. Kriss A. Skin ERGs: their effectiveness in paediatric visual assessment, confounding factors, and comparison with ERGs recorded using various types of corneal electrode. Int J Psychophysiol 1994; 16: 137–46. Review.

27. Fulton AB, Hansen RM, Westall CA. Development of ERG responses: the ISCEV rod, maximal and cone responses in normal subjects. Doc Ophthalmol 2003; 107: 235–41.

28. Iohom G, Gardiner C, Whyte A, et al. Abnormalities of contrast sensitivity and electroretinogram following sevoflurane anaesthesia. Eur J Anaesthesiol 2004; 21: 646–52.

Imaging the fundus

Göran D Hildebrand

Von Helmholtz' invention in 1850 of the first clinical direct ophthalmoscope marked the dawn of modern ophthalmology. Direct ophthalmoscopy and later the development of the binocular indirect ophthalmoscope, the slit-lamp, and a range of high-powered aspheric lenses, enabled the imaging of the human fundus, paving the way for the systematic study of intraocular structures and their diseases by direct observation in vivo.[1]

Though ophthalmoscopy remains the initial technique for fundal examination, the ophthalmologist has at his disposal an impressive range of sophisticated imaging techniques which have dramatically increased the ability to investigate the fundus.

Imaging dependent on the state of the media

Confocal scanning laser ophthalmoscopy

In conventional fundus photography, the entire fundus is flooded with a bright flash to visualize its composite structures. In confocal scanning laser ophthalmoscopy (cSLO), a small focused laser point is rapidly swept across the retina pixel by pixel in a raster pattern. Because imaging is confocal, interfering stray light from adjacent structures is minimized, thereby improving contrast. The use of several laser sources permits the imaging of the retina, RPE, and the optic nerve by different wavelengths according to their respective absorption, reflection, and excitation properties (Fig. 9.1). Confocal imaging also enables in-depth structural analysis of the retina and optic nerve, layer by layer, and three-dimensional digital reconstruction, e.g. in the Heidelberg Retina Tomogram (HRT, Heidelberg Engineering, Heidelberg, Germany). The latest SLOs offer not only facilities for digital fluorescein/indocyanine green angiography, but also autofluorescence, red-free and infrared

imaging as well as high-resolution Fourier-domain optical coherence tomography (OCT) all in one machine (Spectralis, Heidelberg Engineering, Heidelberg, Germany).

Autofluorescence

Retinal autofluorescence[2] relies primarily on the content of fluorophores in the lipofuscin granules of RPE cells. Therefore, it serves as a non-invasive indicator of the health of the RPE and outer retina: increased autofluorescence indicates abnormal accumulation of lipofuscin in the post-mitotic RPE cell. It therefore serves as an indicator of RPE *dysfunction* and is seen in a large number of retinal disorders, for instance in Best's and Stargardt's disease. Loss of autofluorescence is an indicator of RPE *atrophy*.

Normally, the optic disc is not autofluorescent due to the absence of RPE cells in the optic disc area. However, focal hyper-autofluorescence is pathgnomonic for superficial optic disc drusen. Because the autofluorescence signal is two orders of magnitude smaller than the fluorescence in fluorescein angiography, autofluorescence scanning needs to be performed before fluorescein is administered for angiography.

Fluorescein and indocyanine green angiography

Digital SLO angiography provides much greater temporal resolution and detail than is possible with conventional serial photography.[3] Unlike in adults, fluorescein (excitation maximum at 490 nm) and indocyanine green (excitation maximum at 805 nm) angiography is uncommonly used in children due to a combination of factors: rarer appropriate pathology and practical concerns of more difficult intravenous access (though oral administration is possible) and administration of intravenous drugs in a child in an eye unit. If angiography in a child is deemed necessary, it must only be carried out with all necessary equipment, drugs, and medical staff trained in pediatric resuscitation available.

Red-free and infrared imaging

Red-free imaging is particularly useful for highlighting vascular structures and nerve fiber layer defects in the inner

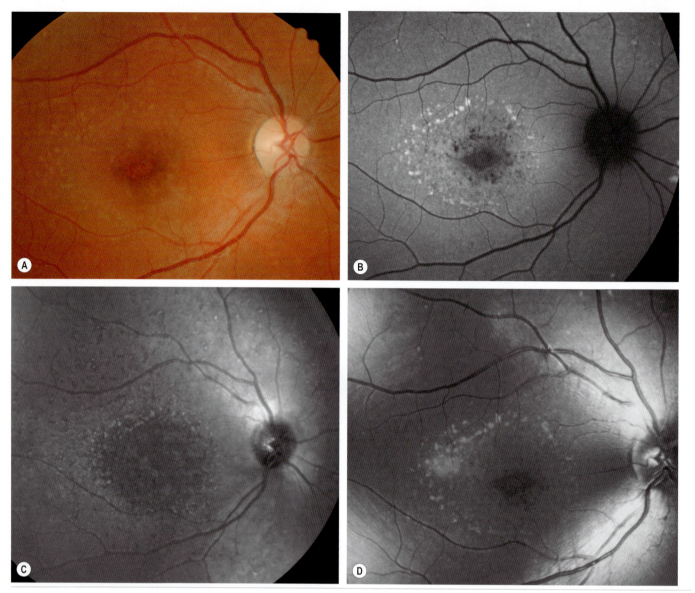

Fig. 9.1 Light of different wavelengths penetrates and is reflected and absorbed differently by different retinal structures. This is why the same fundus, in this case of a patient with Stargardt's disease, reveals different patterns and extent of involvement with conventional color photography (A) and confocal scanning laser autofluorescence (B), infrared (C), and red-free (D) imaging. Spectralis, Heidelberg Engineering, Heidelberg, Germany.

retina. Red-free imaging is available with some scanning laser ophthalmoscopes (see Fig. 9.1) and, of course, by using the green filter on the slit-lamp or direct ophthalmoscope. Infrared imaging has been studied in Stargardt's disease and may play a particular role in visualizing subretinal structures.[4,5]

Wide-field imaging

The RetCam system (Clarity Medical, Pleasanton, California, US) provides wide-field imaging of up to 130° (Fig. 9.2). Because it can be used to visualize and document the posterior and much of the peripheral retina, it is common in screening for retinopathy of prematurity and the documentation of non-accidental injuries in babies. In addition to color images, it can also be used for fluorescein angiography. It requires eye contact.

The Staurenghi 150° contact lens has been used in suitable older patients to obtain high-resolution wide-field cSLO

autofluorescence, infrared, red-free, fluorescein, and indocyanine angiography imaging.

Ultra-wide-field confocal scanning laser

A further technological advance has been the development of ultra-wide-field confocal scanning laser imaging (Optos, Dunfermline, UK). Using an internal parabolic mirror, the scanner can capture up to 200° internal angle (Fig. 9.3), or more than 80% of the entire retina, in a single image through an undilated pupil. This compares very favorably to about 6°, 30° and 45–55° with the direct and indirect ophthalmoscope and a conventional fundus camera, respectively. No eye contact is required and the image is produced in the correct orientation. In addition to color, wide-angle red-free, autofluorescence, and fluorescein angiography, imaging can be carried out by simultaneous laser scanning with blue (488 nm, retina), green

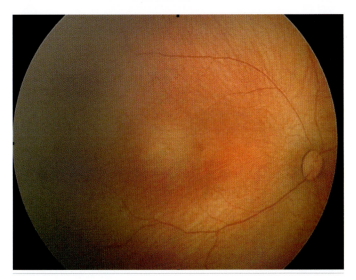

Fig. 9.2 Wide-field RetCam imaging of a normal posterior fundus in a premature baby.

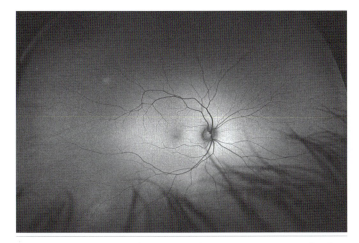

Fig. 9.3 Ultra-wide-field confocal scanning laser imaging (Optos, Dunfermline, UK) captures about 80% of the entire retina in a single view through an undilated pupil, as seen here. In addition to color photography, ultra-wide-angle red-free, autofluorescence (seen here), and fluorescein angiography imaging can be carried out with this instrument. It should find a wider application in pediatric practice.

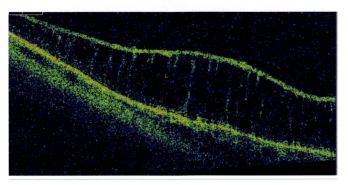

Fig. 9.4 Time domain OCT cross-section demonstrating foveal schisis in a child with X-linked retinoschisis.

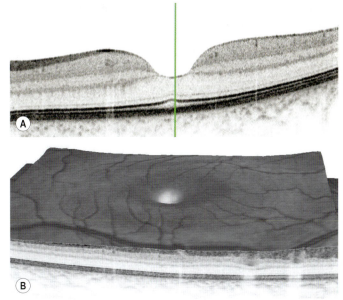

Fig. 9.5 Fourier (Spectral) domain OCT gives the highest available resolution of structural detail of the retina and optic nerve. The degree of cross-sectional histological detail provides an "optical biopsy" in vivo and in real time. The tissue is not removed as in conventional biopsy and, therefore, can be examined repeatedly for monitoring. (A) and (B) show the normal cross-sectional and three-dimensional anatomy of the foveola (foveolar reflex), the foveal clivus, and the perifoveal mound (annular reflex) in a healthy 6-year-old boy. The papillomacular bundle can be clearly seen as an increasingly thick superficial ganglion fiber layer in (A).

(532 nm, from sensory retina to RPE), and red (633 nm, RPE and choroid) wavelengths. The main limitations are cost and the requirement for the child to be able to sit still during the exam in front of the machine and ideally to focus on a target light.

Time and Fourier domain optical coherence tomography: "in vivo histology"

Optical coherence tomography (OCT) has become one of the most important imaging techniques in daily clinical practice. It is non-invasive, fast, safe, and easy to perform, reproducible, and allows cross-sectional and three-dimensional measurements in real time. The resolution is now so good that OCT has been likened to "in vivo histology" and taking an "optical biopsy."

The greater resolution is achieved because OCT is based on light (near infrared, 800–1400 nm), exploiting the differential reflective properties of ocular tissues. The earlier versions used time domain imaging (Fig. 9.4), taking only 512 A-scans in 1.3 second and reconstructing them into two- or three-dimensional images. The introduction of Fourier or Spectral domain OCT (Figs 9.5 and 9.6) now permits up to 400 000 A-scans per second[6] and resolution of up to 3 μm.[7]

Posterior segment OCT provides qualitative and quantitative assessment of the macula/retina (Fig. 9.7), the neurofiber layer, and the optic nerve head. It is increasingly employed in a number of ophthalmic and neurologic conditions.[7-10] OCT has been proposed to have a role in differentiating between optic nerve head drusen and optic disc edema (Figs 9.8 and 9.9)[11] and in monitoring idiopathic intracranial hypertension.[12] Hand-held Fourier domain OCTs have been developed for use in babies and small children.[13] Other applications in children include "shaken baby syndrome",[14] the management of cystoid macular edema in uveitis,[15] and choroidal neovascular membranes.[16]

The Spectralis ophthalmic imaging system combines simultaneous high-resolution confocal scanning laser imaging (infrared, red-free, autofluorescence, fluorescein angiography, and ICG angiography; Fig. 9.10) with high-resolution Spectral domain OCT scanning (Heidelberg Engineering), while eye tracking technology enables the stabilization of the image.

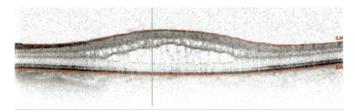

Fig. 9.6 Fourier (Spectral) domain cross-sectional OCT in cystoid macular edema.

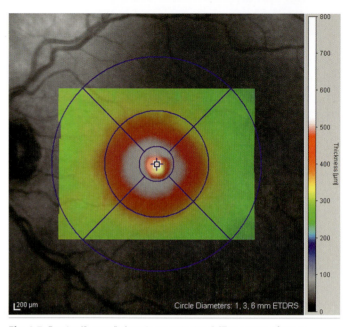

Fig. 9.7 Fourier (Spectral) domain quantitative OCT mapping of tissue thickness in a patient with a macular hole.

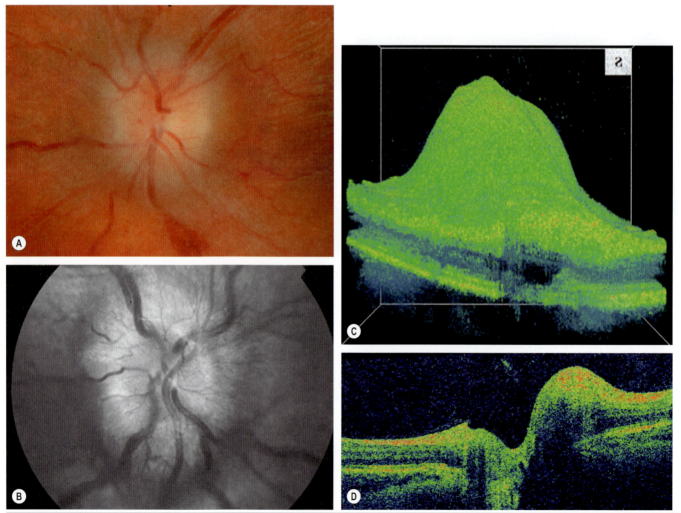

Fig. 9.8 Papilledema in a 14-year-old with hydrocephalus (A, C, and D). Color photography shows a raised optic disc with blurred margins, filling of the cup, hyperemia, telangiectasia, vessel tortuosity and dilation, vessel obscuration by surrounding opaque retinal tissue, disc and retinal hemorrhages. Disc telangiectasia is best seen in red-free images (B, in a different patient). OCT confirms marked swelling of the nerve fiber layer as the cause for the grossly raised optic disc (C and D). The papilledema resolved after emergency ventriculostomy of the third ventricle.

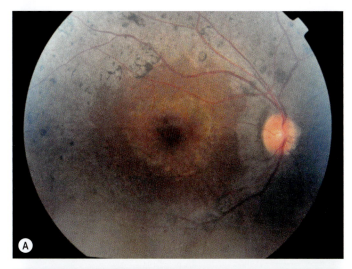

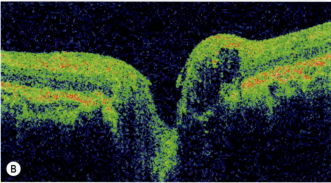

Fig. 9.9 In small children, optic disc drusen tend to be buried and become more superficial and visible with age. Drusen are usually isolated coincidental findings, but may be associated with other findings, such as maculopathy or retinopathy, as in this patient with retinitis pigmentosa (A). Unlike in papilledema (see Fig. 9.8D), the nerve fiber layer is not swollen and either normal (with buried deep drusen early on) or atrophic (with superficial drusen, B).

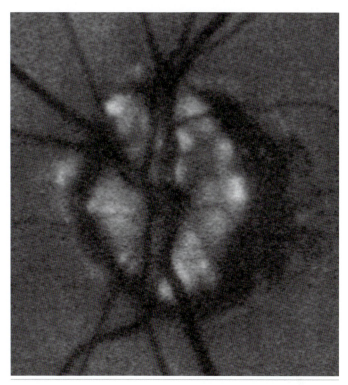

Fig. 9.10 Optic disc drusen can be detected by their autofluorescence as seen here with a confocal scanning laser ophthalmoscope. However, in very small children, the drusen are often too small and too buried to be seen on autofluorescence.

Future OCTs will likely achieve spatial resolution at the cellular level. The combination of ultra-high spatial resolution with other modalities, such as blood flow and spectroscopy, will enable non-invasive high-resolution and depth-resolved functional retinal imaging in vivo.

Imaging independent of the state of the media

Ultrasound, computed tomography, and magnetic resonance imaging

When the media are too opaque to visualize the fundal structures directly (e.g. dense cataract, complete hyphema, vitreous hemorrhage, intraocular tumor) or when structures that are not directly visible by light alone (e.g. deep optic nerve head, optic nerve, orbit and brain) need to be examined, imaging options include ultrasound, computed tomography (CT), and magnetic resonance imaging (MRI), albeit at much lower resolution. Though the resolution of a conventional good quality B-mode ultrasound is only about 150 μm (compared to 3–5 μm in a Fourier domain high-resolution OCT), ultrasound is particularly invaluable in the following situations:

1. Determining the presence of a retinal detachment
2. In looking for optic disc drusen (Figs 9.11 and 9.12)
3. In the further assessment of an intraocular tumor (Fig. 9.13)

Though CT can visualize the calcification in optic disc drusen, CT of the orbit should not generally be carried out for this indication alone, as an ultrasound will provide the same answer with less time, cost, and no radiation to the patient and greater sensitivity. The main indication for CT or MRI is usually to exclude further or associated pathology in the orbit, the optic nerve, or the brain.

Prenatal ultrasound scans can detect eye abnormalities very early in the pregnancy (Fig. 9.14) and can be used to help manage the pregnancy and, if appropriate, to enable early treatment after birth.

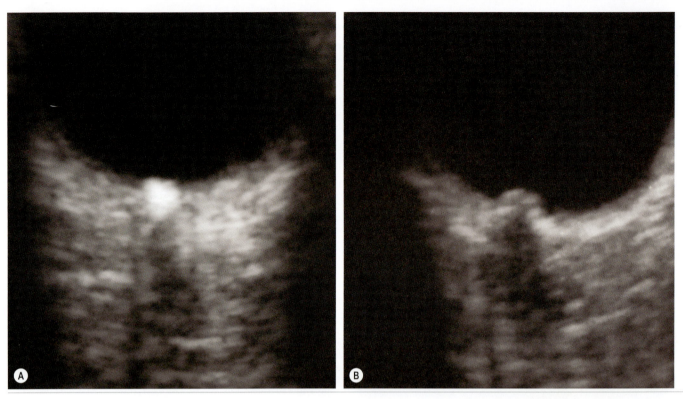

Fig. 9.11 B scan ultrasound is the most sensitive test in detecting drusen even when they are buried. Ultrasound also helps to differentiate between optic disc drusen (A) and optic disc papilledema (B).

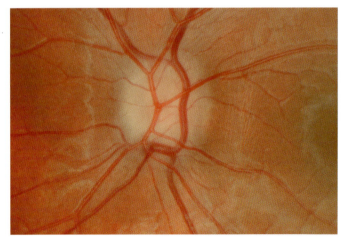

Fig. 9.12 The presence of optic drusen does not exclude the co-presence of intracranial hypertension, as seen here. This 14-year-old obese girl complained of chronic headaches, nausea, intermittent diplopia, and rushing ear sounds. Lumbar puncture confirmed a raised opening pressure with otherwise normal MRI, MRV, and cerebrospinal fluid findings and a diagnosis of idiopathic intracranial hypertension was made. Examination of the optic disc revealed trifurcation of the central retinal artery and an ectopic origin of the central retinal vein from outside the optic disc in both eyes. Ultrasound examination and autofluorescence confirmed the co-presence of optic disc drusen with idiopathic intracranial hypertension.

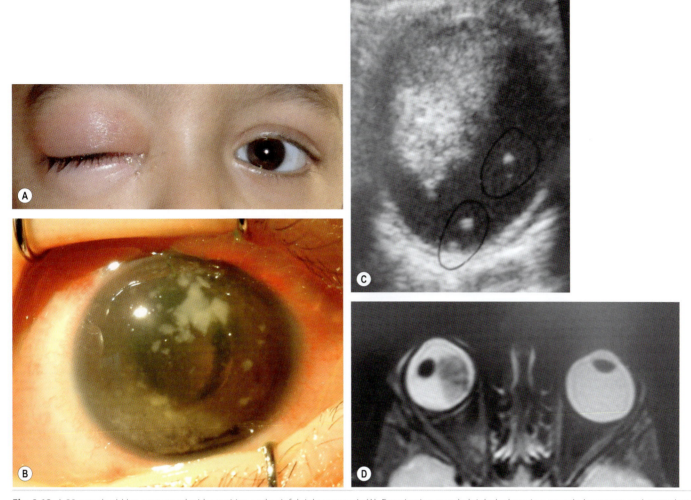

Fig. 9.13 A 20-month-old boy presented with vomiting and painful right proptosis (A). Examination revealed right leukocoria, a pseudo-hypopyon and secondary glaucoma with buphthalmos and an intraocular pressure of 40 mmHg (B). B mode ultrasonongraphy demonstrated a large calcified endophytic mass and widespread vitreous seeding (C). MRI showed secondary displacement of the lens by the advanced retinoblastoma, but no orbital, optic nerve, or intracranial involvement (D). He underwent subsequent enucleation and chemotherapy. Reprinted with permission of Oxford University Press.[17]

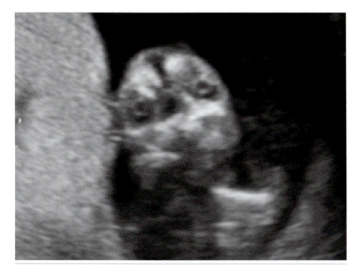

Fig. 9.14 Prenatal ultrasonography of the eyes in a 13-week-old fetus. Courtesy of Prof. Nicolaides, King's College, London.

References

1. Hildebrand GD, Fielder AR. Anatomy and physiology of the retina. In: Reynolds JD, Olitsky SE, editors. Pediatric Retina. Heidelberg: Springer; 2011: 39–65.
2. Holz F, Schmitz-Valckenberg S, Spaids RF, Bird AC, editors. Atlas of Fundus Autofluorescence Imaging. Heidelberg: Springer; 2007.
3. Holz FG, Dithmar S. Fluorescence Angiography in Ophthalmology. Fluorescein Angiography, Indocyanine Green Angiography and Fundus Autofluorescence. Heidelberg: Springer; 2008.
4. Elsner AE, Burns SA, Weiter JJ, Delori FC. Infrared imaging of sub-retinal structures in the human ocular fundus. Vision Res 1996; 36: 191–205.
5. Anastasakis A, Fishman GA, Lindeman M, et al. Infrared scanning laser ophthalmoscope imaging of the macula and its correlation with functional loss and structural changes in patients with Stargardt disease. Retina 2011; 31: 949–58.
6. Potsaid B, Baumann B, Huang D, et al. Ultrahigh speed 1050 nm swept source/Fourier domain OCT retinal and anterior segment imaging at 100,000 to 400,000 axial scans per second. Opt Express 2010; 18: 20029–48.

7. Sakata LM, Deleon-Ortega J, Sakata V, Girkin CA. Optical coherence tomography of the retina and optic nerve: a review. Clin Exp Ophthalmol 2009; 37: 90–9.

8. Subei AM, Eggenberger ER. Optical coherence tomography: another useful tool in a neuro-ophthalmologist's armamentarium. Curr Opin Ophthalmol 2009; 20: 462–6.

9. Mendoza-Santiesteban CE, Gonzalez-Garcia A, Hedges TR 3rd, et al. Optical coherence tomography for neuro-ophthalmologic diagnoses. Semin Ophthalmol 2010; 25: 144–54.

10. Jindahra P, Hedges TR, Mendoza-Santiesteban CE, Plant GT. Optical coherence tomography of the retina: applications in neurology. Curr Opin Neurol 2010 ;23: 16–23.

11. Lee KM, Woo SJ, Hwang JM. Differentiation of optic nerve head drusen and optic disc edema with spectral-domain optical coherence tomography. Ophthalmology 2011; 118: 971–7.

12. Skau M, Sander B, Milea D, Jensen R. Disease activity in idiopathic intracranial hypertension: a 3-month follow-up study. J Neurol 2011; 258: 277–83.

13. Maldonado RS, Izatt JA, Sarin N, et al. Optimizing hand-held spectral domain optical coherence tomography imaging for neonates, infants, and children. Invest Ophthalmol Vis Sci 2010; 51: 2678–85.

14. Sturm V, Landau K, Menke MN. Optical coherence tomography findings in Shaken Baby syndrome. Am J Ophthalmol 2008; 146: 363–8.

15. Skarmoutsos F, Sandhu SS, Voros GM, Shafiq A. The use of optical coherence tomography in the management of cystoid macular edema in pediatric uveitis. J AAPOS 2006; 10: 173–4.

16. Kohly RP, Muni RH, Kertes PJ, Lam WC. Management of pediatric choroidal neovascular membranes with intravitreal anti-VEGF agents: a retrospective consecutive case series. Can J Ophthalmol 2011; 46: 46–50.

17. Hildebrand GD. Examination of the Uncooperative Child. In: Wright KW, Strube YN, editors. Pediatric Ophthalmology and Strabismus, 3rd ed. Oxford: Oxford University Press (in press).

Genetics and pediatric ophthalmology

Graeme C M Black • Georgina Hall

Background

In developed countries, half of the conditions causing childhood blind and partially sighted registration are genetic,[1-3] a figure that is likely to be underestimated. In many developing countries where childhood visual disability is significantly commoner, genetic conditions also represent an important group contributing to childhood blindness.[1,4-6] "Genetic" conditions referred to in this context are monogenic, (Mendelian) conditions. Since many issues regarding diagnosis and counseling apply to the group as a whole, this allows a common approach to clinical management. However, the substantial genetic contribution to common diseases, i.e. the delineation of genetic variants in the complement pathway as contributors to AMD, and normal quantitative traits (corneal thickness, optic nerve size) underlines the observation that molecular genetic discoveries are not limited to Mendelian disease.

The study of inherited ocular disease represents one of the successes of modern molecular genetics, from the description of linkage of xlRP[7] to the identification of the first adRP gene encoding rhodopsin.[8] The Human Genome Project has accelerated the understanding of the molecular basis of human genetic disease. Now, over 200 gene loci and 150 genes have been described underlying human monogenic retinal disorders, implying a level of complexity unsuspected 20 years ago (http://www.sph.uth.tmc.edu/retnet/).

Mendelian inheritance

The human genome is divided among 46 (23 pairs, humans are diploid) physically distinct chromosomes. There are 22 pairs of autosomes plus two sex chromosomes: in the female two X chromosomes, in the male an X and a Y. Human chromosomes vary widely in size and the genes mutated in monogenic ocular disorders are scattered randomly.

Autosomal dominant inheritance (Fig. 10.1)

Autosomal dominant (AD) conditions are caused by mutations in genes on chromosomes 1–22. An affected individual carries one normal and one mutated copy of the gene (i.e. the condition is expressed in the heterozygous state). In most families with AD conditions there are multiple generations with both males and females affected to a similar degree, and male to male transition. Affected individuals have a 1 in 2 chance of passing a mutated gene to each offspring, regardless of sex. The risk to offspring of unaffected individuals is that of the general population, provided that unaffected individuals are certain not to carry the mutated copy of the gene.

Expressivity

Within one family, individuals affected by a single gene disorder carry the same genetic fault. However, the manifestations of that condition may vary widely. The condition or more properly the, mutant allele is said to demonstrate *variable expressivity*. Examples include Marfan's syndrome, neurofibromatosis type I, and oculocutaneous albinism whose ocular and extraocular manifestations vary widely amongst those who carry a mutation. Phenoptypic severity in one individual may have little or no implication for predicting disease severity for siblings or offspring. This leads to uncertainty around interpreting predictive or prenatal genetic testing and means that examining the parents of affected children is *essential* in determining the presence of mild features and predicting dominant (50%) risks for future offspring.

Penetrance

For some AD conditions, the probability of gene carriers developing symptoms is not 100% (i.e. the mutation shows *reduced*

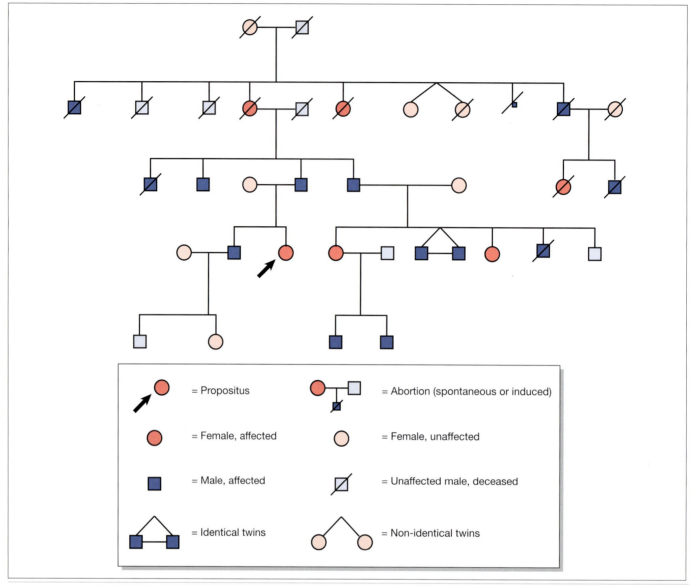

Fig. 10.1 Pedigree construction illustrating autosomal dominant inheritance.

penetrance). Therefore, for many conditions (e.g. forms of AD retinitis pigmentosa (adRP), coloboma, or congenital cataract), gene carriers may not have signs of the condition but have an identical risk for their offspring as those who do. This is another reason for examining the parents of a child with, for example, coloboma or anterior segment dysgenesis. The availability of genetic testing is helpful in providing accurate risks.

New mutations

Dominant conditions may arise *de novo*. In this case, there is no family history and the condition has arisen as the result of a copying error from one parent's DNA. This is seen in many cases of aniridia or retinoblastoma. In such cases, the recurrence risks for future siblings are much lower than 50%. The figure will not be zero due to the risk of *gonadal mosaicism* (i.e. one parent carrying the mutation in a proportion of his/her sperm or eggs).

The exact nature of a *de novo* mutation is difficult to predict – for cases of sporadic aniridia, a deletion can remove other neighboring genes. This is seen in WAGR syndrome where a deletion causes Wilms' tumor, aniridia, genitourinary abnormalities, and intellectual retardation.[9-11] This is termed a *contiguous gene syndrome*. It is for this reason that patients with sporadic aniridia require either renal ultrasound screening or molecular evidence that the Wilms' tumor gene, WT1, is unaffected by the new mutation (Fig. 10.2).

Once a new AD mutation has arisen, an affected individual has a 50% risk for their own offspring. Examples of these conditions include rare forms of Leber's congenital amaurosis (caused by mutations of the *CRX* gene) and retinoblastoma (caused by mutations in the RB1 gene). As RB1 mutation may also show reduced penetrance, the presence of unaffected parents could either mean that an affected child carries a *de novo* mutation or that the parent carries a mutation which exhibits reduced penetrance. Genetic testing may help

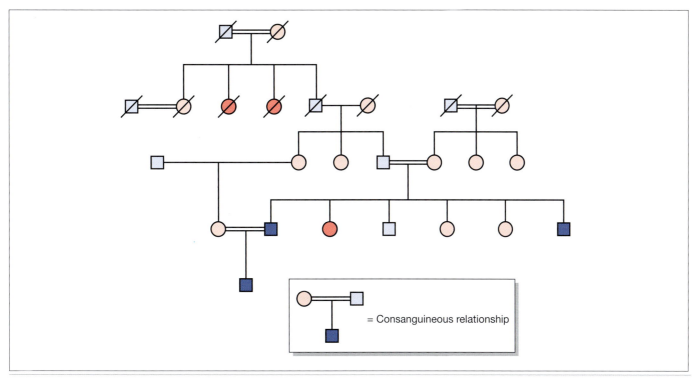

Fig. 10.2 **Pedigree construction illustrating autosomal recessive inheritance in the presence of consanguinity.**

to identify those carrying disease-causing genes and define risks to family members.

Autosomal recessive inheritance (Fig. 10.3)

For autosomal recessive (AR) conditions, affected individuals carry faults on both copies of a given gene (either homozygous where both copies carry the same mutation, or compound heterozygotes where each copy carries a different pathogenic gene fault). Conditions inherited in this fashion include oculocutaneous albinism, autosomal recessive congenital cataract, most forms of Leber's congenital amaurosis, and achromatopsia.

Parents carry one normal and one mutant gene copy but have normal vision as the normal copy is sufficient to produce normal function. For two carrier parents, the risk of having an affected child is $\frac{1}{4}$. Unaffected children have a $\frac{2}{3}$ risk of being carriers.

Recessive conditions can appear as "sporadic" in a family where all parents and siblings are healthy, particularly in smaller families. In the absence of genetic testing, predicting AR inheritance is difficult and may be inferred on the basis of lack of vertical transmission (unaffected parents) and exclusion of X-linked inheritance.

Calculating carrier frequencies in the general population is complex. For inherited eye conditions, where one condition may be caused by many different genes (e.g. retinal dystrophy), accurately predicting the frequency of any one of those genes in a given population is often not possible. For Stargardt's disease with an estimated disease frequency of 1 in 10 000[12] and a carrier frequency of 1 in 50, the risk to the offspring of an affected individual and their children is low (~1% and 0.65%, respectively).

Cousin marriages increase the likelihood that spouses carry an identical gene change. In many ethnic groups, cousin marriages are an important part of family culture. Discussion of the increased risks to future children, if close cousins marry, must be done with sensitivity and appreciation of the cultural issues.

X-linked inheritance (Fig. 10.4)

"Sex linked" conditions are caused by mutations in X chromosome genes. As males have only one X chromosome, such a genetic mutation will be manifest. Heterozygous females will be "carriers" and either unaffected or more mildly affected. The essential features of X-linked inheritance are the presence of affected males (of greater severity than females) and lack of father to son transmission. Females of affected males are obligate carriers. Female carriers have a 50% chance of passing on the mutation, with each son having a 50% chance of being affected, and half their daughters being "carriers." X-linked conditions include Nance-Horan syndrome, Norrie's disease, retinitis pigmentosa (xLRP), congenital stationary night blindness, choroideremia, and retinoschisis.

Female carriers

Classically, it is assumed that X-linked conditions only affect males. This is true for conditions such as retinoschisis and Norrie's disease. However for others, such as X-linked xLRP, there may be phenotypic manifestations seen in heterozygous females, although these may be milder and of later onset than in males. This makes the identification of X-linked pedigrees difficult and places importance on careful history taking. Phenotypic manifestations in females may be highly variable, due to X-inactivation. In a number of X-linked conditions, females

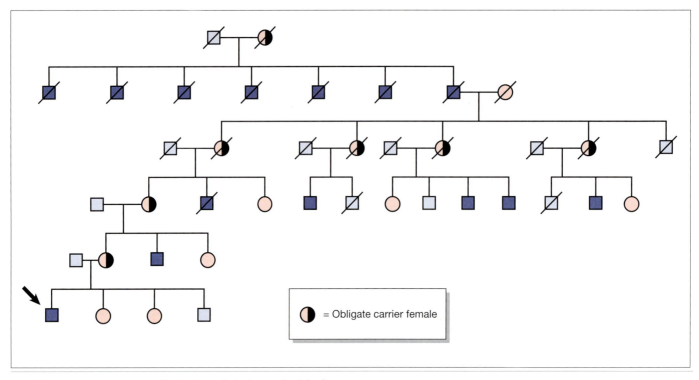

Fig. 10.3 Pedigree construction illustrating x-linked recessive inheritance.

◑ = Obligate carrier female

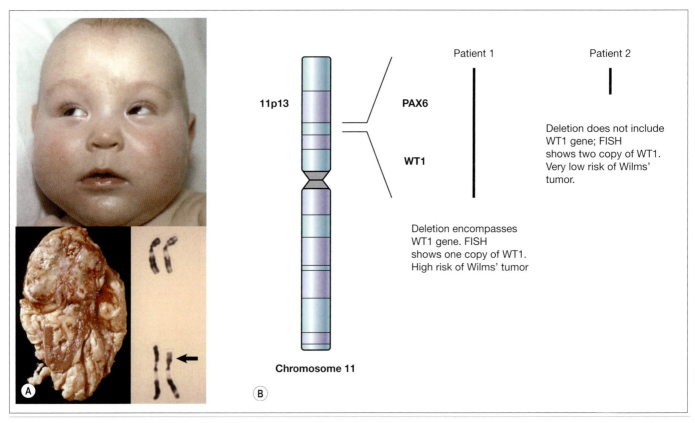

11p13

PAX6

WT1

Chromosome 11

Patient 1

Patient 2

Deletion does not include WT1 gene; FISH shows two copy of WT1. Very low risk of Wilms' tumor.

Deletion encompasses WT1 gene. FISH shows one copy of WT1. High risk of Wilms' tumor

A

B

Fig. 10.4 Aniridia caused by deletion of chromosome 11. (A) A young child presented with delay, genitourinary abnormalities, and aniridia. There was no family history of aniridia. He was found to have a Wilms' tumor in the superior pole of his kidney. Karyotype analysis revealed a cytogenetically visible 11p deletion which encompasses the PAX6 (aniridia) and the WT1 (Wilms' tumor) gene. (B) Patients 1 and 2 are born with sporadic aniridia. Chromosome analysis is normal. Cytogenetic (FISH) analysis shows two copies of the WT1 gene in patient 2 but not patient 1 – patient 1 is at high risk of Wilms' tumor.

may show characteristic ocular signs despite the absence of symptoms (choroideremia, Lowe's syndrome) that can help diagnosis and identification of carriers.

Like dominant inheritance, new mutations in X-linked genes are reported and gonadal mosaicism must be considered in cases of isolated males where the mother has been shown not to be a carrier on a blood sample.

Mitochondrial, or maternal, inheritance

Mitochondria are cellular cytoplasmic organelles. They contain their own small circular genome (16 000–17 000 base pairs of DNA) distinct from the nuclear genome. Mitochondrial DNA (mtDNA) encodes a small number of genes, including important components of the electron-transport chain. mtDNA gene mutations include Leber's hereditary optic neuropathy (LHON) and Kearnes-Sayre syndrome (KSS).

Mitochondria are inherited exclusively from the ovum. For this reason, an mtDNA mutation can only be passed on from mother to child, which is thus *maternally inherited*. LHON is the best known of the maternally inherited ophthalmic genetic conditions. It is atypical because it shows a male bias.

Maternally inherited conditions are highly variable. In many cases where individuals carry mtDNA mutations in all of their cells, as is seen for most patients with LHON, the basis for this variability is poorly understood. However, with

mitochondrial myopathies such as KSS, only a proportion of the mitochondria carry mtDNA mutations, a state termed heteroplasmy. Since each cell has many mitochondria, heteroplasmy (where the ratio of mutant to normal mtDNA may vary between the cells or tissues of a single individual or between different individuals of the same family) can contribute to phenotypic variability. This makes the estimation of prognosis challenging.

Genetic heterogeneity

Similar or identical genetic disorders may be caused by mutations in one of several genes. For example, conditions such as adRP, Usher's syndrome, and Bardet-Biedl syndrome are not single disorders but groups of clinically indistinguishable conditions (Table 10.1).

The concept that defects in more than one gene may cause indistinguishable phenotypic manifestations is termed *genetic or locus heterogeneity*. This has implications for diagnosis, counseling, and genetic testing.

It is commonly recognized that different defects within one gene may cause a wide range of different clinical entities (Table 10.2) which is called *allelic heterogeneity*. This may be caused by different effects of distinct mutations within the same gene

Table 10.1 – Examples of locus heterogeneity amongst inherited ophthalmic conditions

Condition	Inheritance pattern	Locus number	Gene	Chromosomal location
Retinitis pigmentosa	Autosomal dominant	RP18	PRPF3	1q13–q23
		RP4	RHO	3q21–q24
		RP7	PRPH2	6p21.2–cen
		RP9	PAP1	7p13–p15
		RP10	IMPDH1	7q31.3
		RP1	ORP1	8q11–q13
		RP27	NRL	14q11.2
		RP13	PRPF8	17p13.3
		RP17	CA4	17q22
		RP11	PRPF31	19q13.4
		RP30	FSCN2	17q25.3
		RP48	GUCA1B	6p21.1
		RP42	KLHL7	7p15.3
		RP37	N2RE3	15q23
			RDH12	14q24.1
		RP35	SEMA4A	1q22
		RP33	SNRNP200	2q11.2
		RP31	TOPORS	9p21.1
			CRX	19q13.32
Bardet-Biedl syndrome	Autosomal recessive	BBS1		11q13
		BBS2		16q12.2
		BBS3	ARL6	3q11.2
		BBS4		15q24.1
		BBS5	DKFZp7621194	2q31.1
		BBS6	MKKS	20.12.2
		BBS7		4q27
		BBS8	TTC8	14q32.11
		BBS9	PTHB1	7q14.3
		BBS10	C12orf58	12q21.2
		BBS11	TRIM32	9q33.1
		BBS12		4q27

Table 10.2 – Examples of allelic heterogeneity amongst inherited ophthalmic conditions

Chromosomal location	Gene	Condition	Inheritance pattern
5q31	BIGH3	Reis-Bucklers' dystrophy	AD
		Thiel-Behnke dystrophy	AD
		Granular dystrophy	AD
		Avellino dystrophy	AD
		Lattice dystrophy (type I)	AD
Xp11	NDP	Norrie's disease	XL
		Familial exudative vitreoretinopathy	XL
6p21.1-cen	RDS/peripherin	adRP	AD
		Pattern/butterfly macular dystrophy	AD
		Central areolar choroidal dystrophy	AD
3q21–q24	Rhodopsin	adRP	AD
		arRP	AR
		Congenital stationary night-blindness	AD
		Sectoral RP	AD

since the phenotypic outcome of a genetic change is influenced by the mutation, its position/type, and its effect on the encoded protein.

Genetic counseling

Individuals and families request genetic counseling to understand the condition, the risks of becoming affected or of passing it on to children, and the options around genetic testing, reproduction, and management. Genetic counseling aims to help individuals understand information, choose appropriate courses of action, and make the best possible adjustment to a disorder.

Accurate diagnosis is central to effective genetic counseling. Many inherited eye conditions are diagnosed clinically, requiring specialist clinicians and often a multidisciplinary approach including genetic, ophthalmic, and electrophysiology expertise. A detailed family history involving a three-generational pedigree, examination (often multiple family members), as well as a clinical history including systemic features are fundamental to diagnosis. Awareness of both ocular and extraocular manifestations of conditions is critical.

Genetic counseling for inherited eye conditions can present particular challenges. The heterogeneity and overlapping phenotypes makes diagnosis difficult for patients to understand. Many inherited retinal diseases cause progressive deterioration of vision requiring on-going adjustment to loss of

independence. Communication needs of visually impaired individuals means that information has to be provided in suitable formats.

Genetic testing

Molecular testing has become cheaper and more widely available, and is now employed in the clinic. Clinicians need a general understanding of its power and capabilities. It is likely that this will be focused mainly on gene sequencing for inherited ocular single gene disorders. Testing is performed as a means of supplementing detailed clinical examination and investigation. The aim is to clarify diagnosis, for example amongst conditions of extreme genetic heterogeneity that are clinically indistinguishable. In the future, gene-specific therapies (pharmacologic or gene-based) may require genetic diagnosis to direct treatment. While estimation of risk for an individual affected, for example, by a dominantly inherited condition is straightforward, it is more complex for relatives of individuals affected by dominant phenotypes that show reduced penetrance (dominant optic atrophy and AD congenital cataract) or the children of females in a pedigree where males are affected by X-linked retinoschisis.

Molecular testing may be performed on a DNA sample extracted from the peripheral blood or a saliva sample, from a single affected individual (the proband), or from an extended family. Once a pathogenic mutation has been identified, this can be used to screen other family members, born or unborn.

What is a mutation?

Genetic variation is consequent upon the process of DNA mutation. A wide range of mutational mechanisms have been described in human genetic disease and for Mendelian disease. The majority are all-or-none phenomena: affected individuals carry pathogenic genetic changes ("mutations") while unaffected individuals do not. In such cases, affected individuals of a single family carry the identical genetic change and this change is fixed. This sets apart a small group of conditions, such as myotonic dystrophy, which have "dynamic" mutations in which a genetic alteration may vary among different generations of a single family.

Chromosomal alterations

The grossest pathogenic genetic changes are alterations at the level of the chromosome: that is, cytogenetically visible rearrangements such as deletions, inversions, duplications, and translocations. Such "genomic imbalance" is poorly tolerated and only a small fraction of all possible imbalances are ever observed. Such changes include trisomies (e.g. Trisomy 21 or Down's syndrome) and large chromosome deletions (e.g. chromosome 11p deletion associated with WAGR syndrome, see above).

Submicroscopic genomic rearrangements

It is now possible to compare variation in DNA copy number among individuals at a refined level. "Submicroscopic genomic rearrangements" include both losses of genetic material (microdeletions) and gains (microduplications) and are associated with human genetic disease. For example, submicroscopic deletions have been described on the X chromosome in choroideremia, xLRP, and Norrie's disease.

Single gene mutations

Many inherited ocular diseases result from pathogenic changes in a single gene. Single base substitutions, also termed "point mutations," are the best characterized. The Cardiff Human Gene Mutation Database (http://www.biobase-international.com) is an online repository of human genes in which pathogenic mutations are found. Pathogenic point mutations may result in the substitution of one encoded amino acid for another (*missense mutation*). Where this has a deleterious effect on protein function, it may be associated with human disease. A single base alteration that changes a codon normally used to specify an amino acid to a stop codon is termed a *nonsense mutation*. The majority of nonsense mutations cause a reduction in the amount of protein that is produced via the translational machinery.

After transcription the immature mRNA molecule is spliced to form the mature mRNA. Splicing is a complex process requiring the interaction of a large protein complex (the spliceosome) with mRNA molecules. A large number of mutations – in particular those that lie at or close to the junctions between introns and exons – disrupt the splicing process (*splicing mutations*).

Small deletions/insertions, in which up to 20 base pairs of DNA are either deleted or inserted, are another common DNA mutation that cause monogenic human disease. *Insertion/deletion mutations* that are not a multiple of three bases will alter the reading frame of the gene and introduce a premature termination codon. The majority result in an mRNA that is not translated into a polypeptide.

DNA sequencing

For Mendelian disorders, the majority of affected individuals are thought to carry a single pathogenic DNA alteration or mutation. The majority of such variants are in or close to the coding sequences of an increasingly large list of genes.

Conventional DNA sequencing

Until recently, DNA sequencing has been achieved by conventional techniques. In order to do this, short fragments of each gene (perhaps 300–500 base pairs) are amplified using polymerase chain reaction. Consequently, the process of sequencing a small gene is easier and cheaper than a large gene. The study of 10 genes of identical size is 10 times the work of analyzing a single gene. Such work is time-consuming and expensive. There are a number of scenarios in which gene testing is possible to direct clinical management. For xLRP, where the majority of patients have mutations in one of two genes (RP2 and RPGR), a conventional sequencing strategy is straightforward and practical using current technologies. This is true for the stromal corneal dystrophies that are linked to chromosome 5q31 and caused by mutations in the TGFBI gene, where the range of mutations causing granular, lattice type I, and Bowman's layer (Thiel-Behnke and Reis-Buckler) dystrophies is very limited.[13]

Mutation testing can be complicated even when a condition is caused by mutations in a single gene. For example, Cohen's syndrome and Alstrom's syndrome remain difficult to test for as a consequence of the size and complexity of the genes that are mutated in each of these conditions.[14,15] In the case of *ABCA4* (mutated in Stargardt's disease), which encompasses 51 exons and 6000–7000 base pairs of DNA, gene sequencing remains an enormous task. Furthermore, the pick-up rate of mutations, amongst those known to harbor mutations in *ABCA4*, is considerably less than 100%. This means a negative result is of limited value. Finally, for some genes such as *ABCA4*, there is a significant degree of normal variation in both the gene and its encoded protein. The task of defining whether a variation which alters a single amino acid is pathogenic remains onerous.[16]

High-throughput DNA sequencing

For genetically heterogeneous conditions (e.g. congenital cataract, optic neuropathies, arRP, Usher's syndrome) where a large number of genes can be mutated and where no single gene is prevalent, diagnostic strategies based on conventional DNA sequencing are impractical. The design of DNA chips that enable the identification of previously described mutations have had some success (e.g. Leber's congenital amaurosis, Stargardt's disease), but these techniques are heavily biased toward previously studied populations and are of limited success.[17]

Next generation or massively parallel DNA sequencing promises to transform this situation. These developments allow the sequencing of whole human genomes, or offer the capacity to analyze, in each patient, all of the exons of all their genes, or any subset of them. These technologic developments have already proved highly successful at accelerating the process of identifying unknown genes mutated in human diseases.[18] As costs reduce (it is predicted that sequencing of an entire human genome could soon cost as little as $1000), there is a realistic promise that large-scale gene analysis may become a reality. Such developments will create further challenges in how large datasets are stored, since such platforms produce enormous volumes of data. Furthermore, as many of the variants that cause human ocular disease are missense variants, and since a great number of our genes vary in a manner that also cause amino acid substitutions, the challenge will be to select a single pathogenic variant from the large quantity of benign changes that each individual will be found to carry.

Genetic testing: counseling and ethical issues

Genetic testing is increasingly available. Families and clinicians may use genetic testing to confirm the diagnosis and inheritance pattern and, potentially in the future, to increase opportunities to take part in gene-specific treatment trials. Genetic testing can have significant and far-reaching consequences for the individual and their family. Individuals choosing genetic testing may need to think about how they will inform their wider family, the impact on reproductive decisions and other life choices, and additional implications such as health and life insurance. Counseling and informed consent is important when considering a genetic test.

Predictive or presymptomatic testing

In late-onset conditions where the causative gene mutation is known (e.g. *TIMP3* and Sorsby's fundus dystrophy[19]), asymptomatic individuals at 50% risk may choose to have a predictive genetic test to discover if they are carriers. For late-onset genetic conditions, such as Huntington's disease and cancer predisposing syndromes, appropriate counseling protocols, exploring the pros and cons of testing, the impact on the individual and life decisions, the psychosocial support in adapting to the result, and other issues such as insurance are essential.[20,21] The principles are similar with individuals facing untreatable progressive deterioration of their vision affecting life choices, independence, and emotional well-being.

Carrier testing

In recessive and X-linked conditions, where a genetic mutation has been identified in an affected individual, other family members may choose to have carrier testing. In consanguineous families, family members may learn if they are also carrier couples. Women may choose to have carrier testing in X-linked conditions in order to make decisions around reproduction, prenatal testing, or to be more prepared and informed about the risks to future sons. The impact of this information on the couple and the support required after testing should be explored as part of the testing process.

Childhood testing

In childhood-onset conditions where genetic test results impact on clinical management or support parenting/education decisions, testing may be appropriate. However, careful counseling and preparation for parents making these decisions is essential as knowledge around genetic status and risk can have significant impacts upon parenting. For conditions where symptoms may not begin until adulthood, it is generally advised to wait until an individual is old enough to make their own decisions.

Prenatal testing

Where a gene mutation is known in a family, prenatal testing is an option for couples. Chorionic villus sampling (at 11 weeks) and amniocentesis (at 16 weeks) allow accurate genetic diagnosis. As invasive tests, there is a small risk of miscarriage. Consideration needs to be given as to why individuals want a test. Decisions to terminate or continue with an affected pregnancy are individual and influenced by personal experience, coping strategies, and available support. While prenatal genetic testing is uncommon in later onset eye conditions, families with early onset blindness or multiple congenital anomaly syndromes such as Lowe's and Norrie's disease do consider prenatal diagnosis and termination of affected pregnancies. Preimplantation genetic diagnosis involves testing IVF embryos prior to implantation back into the womb. This is becoming available for a number of genetic eye conditions but brings its own ethical and counseling issues.

Clinical examination

A clinical examination may have the same impact as a genetic test. An asymptomatic individual may have subtle ocular changes revealing their genetic status. Therefore, ophthalmologists must be prepared to offer information and counseling before examination for inherited eye conditions so that individuals are aware of and prepared for the implications of abnormal findings.

References

1. Gilbert C, Foster A. Childhood blindness in the context of VISION 2020 – the right to sight. Bull World Health Org 2001; 79: 227–32.
2. Rahi JS, Cable N. British Childhood Visual Impairment Study Group. Severe visual impairment and blindness in children in the UK. Lancet 2003; 362: 1359–65.
3. Alagaratnam J, Sharma TK, Lim CS, Fleck BW. A survey of visual impairment in children attending the Royal Blind School, Edinburgh using the WHO childhood visual impairment database. Eye 2002; 16: 557–61.
4. Dandona R, Dandona L. Childhood blindness in India: a population based perspective. Br J Ophthalmol 2003; 87: 263–5.
5. Reddy SC, Tan BC. Causes of childhood blindness in Malaysia: results from a national study of blind school students. Int Ophthalmol 2001; 24: 53–9.
6. Rogers NK, Gilbert CE, Foster A, et al. Childhood blindness in Uzbekistan. Eye 1999; 13: 65–70.
7. Bhattacharya SS, Wright AF, Clayton JF, et al. Close genetic linkage between X-linked retinitis pigmentosa and a restriction fragment length polymorphism identified by recombinant DNA probe L1.28. Nature 1984; 309: 253–5.
8. Dryja TP, McGee TL, Reichel E, Hahn LB, et al. A point mutation of the rhodopsin gene in one form of retinitis pigmentosa. Nature 1990; 343: 364–6.
9. Andersen SR, Geertinger P, Larsen HW, et al. Aniridia, cataract and gonadoblastoma in a mentally retarded girl with deletion of chromosome II: a clinicopathological case report. Ophthalmologica 1977; 176: 171–7.
10. Crolla JA, van Heyningen V. Frequent chromosome aberrations revealed by molecular cytogenetic studies in patients with aniridia. Am J Hum Genet 2002; 71: 1138–49.
11. Crolla JA, Cawdery JE, Oley CA, et al. A FISH approach to defining the extent and possible clinical significance of deletions at the WAGR locus. J Med Genet. 1997; 34: 207–12.
12. Blacharski PA. Fundus flavimaculatus. In: Newsome DA, editor. Retinal Dystrophies and Degenerations. New York: Raven Press; 1988: 135–59.
13. Munier FL, Frueh BE, Othenin-Girard P, et al. BIGH3 mutation spectrum in corneal dystrophies. Invest Ophthalmol Vis Sci 2002; 43: 949–54.
14. Marshall JD, Hinman EG, Collin GB, et al. Spectrum of ALMS1 variants and evaluation of genotype-phenotype correlations in Alström syndrome. Hum Mutat 2007; 28: 1114–23.
15. Parri V, Katzaki E, Uliana V, et al. High frequency of COH1 intragenic deletions and duplications detected by MLPA in patients with Cohen syndrome. Eur J Hum Genet 2010; 10: 1133–40.
16. Webster AR, Heon E, Lotery AJ, et al. An analysis of allelic variation in the ABCA4 gene. Invest Ophthalmol Vis Sci 2001; 42: 1179–89.
17. Zernant J, Külm M, Dharmaraj S, et al. Genotyping microarray (disease chip) for Leber congenital amaurosis: detection of modifier alleles. Invest Ophthalmol Vis Sci 2005; 46: 3052–9.
18. Züchner S, Dallman J, Wen R, et al. Whole-exome sequencing links a variant in DHDDS to retinitis pigmentosa. Am J Hum Genet 2011; 88: 201–6.
19. Weber BH, Vogt G, Pruett RC, et al. Mutations in the tissue inhibitor of metalloproteinases-3 (TIMP3) in patients with Sorsby's fundus dystrophy. Nat Genet 1994; 8: 352–6.
20. Craufurd D, Donnai D, Kerzin-Storrar L, Osborn M. Testing of children for "adult" genetic diseases. Lancet 1990; 335: 1406.
21. Craufurd D, Tyler A. Predictive testing for Huntington's disease: protocol of the UK Huntington's Prediction Consortium. J Med Genet 1992; 29: 915–8.

Ocular manifestations of intrauterine infections

Akbar Shakoor • Aileen Sy • Nisha Acharya

Maternal infection during pregnancy may have significant consequences to the developing fetus. The "TORCHES" (toxoplasmosis, other agents, rubella, cytomegalovirus, herpes viruses, and syphilis) syndromes are commonly associated with ocular manifestations in the neonate, rarely lymphocytic choriomeningitis and West Nile virus. The infectious agents are transmitted to the fetus through hematogenous spread, through the genitourinary tract or at delivery.

Clinical diagnosis alone is difficult. Chorioretinal scars are common but non-specific. Laboratory testing: cultures, antibody titers and polymerase chain reaction (PCR) aid in confirming the pathogen. Improved screening and prophylaxis of pregnant women at risk may reduce these potentially devastating infections.

Congenital rubella

Rubella is an RNA virus that causes a prodrome of low-grade fever and upper respiratory symptoms prior to a maculopapular rash. Gregg described cataracts, microphthalmos, heart defects, and growth retardation in infants of mothers with rubella early in pregnancy.[1] The congenital rubella syndrome (CRS) now includes most organ systems, commonly with microphthalmia, cataracts, retinopathy, sensorineural hearing loss, various cardiac defects, neurologic abnormalities (microcephaly, mental retardation), bone defects, hepatosplenomegaly, and endocrine abnormalities (diabetes, thyroid disorders).[2-4]

Rubella virus infects the placenta and damages placental endothelial cells which enter the fetal circulation.[5] Infants of mothers infected within the first 16 weeks of gestation suffer the greatest damage. After the first trimester, deafness and retinopathy are the main manifestations.[3,6] The pathogenesis is not well understood.[5] During the first trimester, the fetus relies on maternal IgG, placental transfer of which is inefficient early in gestation.[5] By the second trimester, increased maternal antibody and a developing fetal immune system give greater protection.[5]

Ocular disease affects 78–88% of CRS patients and damages the cornea (keratitis, corneal edema, corneal clouding), iris (hypoplasia, chronic iridocyclitis), lens (cataracts), and retina (pigmentary retinopathy),[4,7,8] causing glaucoma, microphthalmos, optic atrophy, dacryostenosis, nystagmus, strabismus, keratoconus, corneal hydrops, and spontaneous lens resorbtion.[4,7-11]

Pigmentary retinopathy is the commonest ocular finding, affecting up to 60% of CRS patients (Fig. 11.1).[4,7,11] It is characterized by mottled ("salt and pepper") pigmentary changes throughout the fundus, especially in the posterior pole.[11,12] Histopathology shows depigmentation of the retinal pigment epithelium without inflammation.[13] Visual prognosis is good

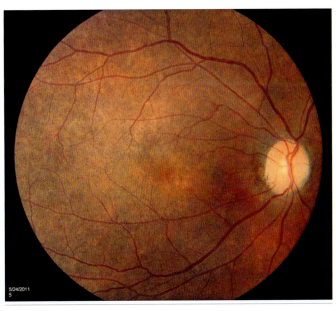

Fig. 11.1 Pigmentary retinopathy in congenital rubella. Courtesy of Emmett Cunningham.

and the electroretinogram is usually normal. Subretinal neo-vascularization, typically occurring after early childhood, may precipitously decrease vision[12] but may carry a relatively good prognosis.

Cataracts affect 27–34% of children with CRS.[4,7] They are characterized by a central opacity surrounded by clear peripheral zone and are usually bilateral.[4,7,13] Rubella virus persists in the lens causing a strong inflammatory reaction after cataract surgery.[11,14]

Glaucoma may be secondary to congenital malformation of the angle or to chronic iridocyclitis or cataracts.[4,7,8,13] Microphthalmos is associated with cataracts, glaucoma, and poor visual acuity.[4,7]

Persistent ocular rubella infection, congenital or acquired, has been associated with Fuchs' heterochromic iridocyclitis (FHI).[15,16] There is a decrease in FHI cases after a rubella vaccination program but the mechanism remains unclear.[17,18]

Diagnosis of rubella infection in the fetus is by enzyme immunoassay for IgG and IgM, culture and PCR of fetal blood, chorionic villous or amniotic fluid.[3] In infants, diagnosis is by rubella-specific IgM, which is 100% detectable in the first 3 months of life but undetectable by 18 months.[3] Diagnosis can also be made by PCR of rubella virus from samples of the lens and saliva.[3,14]

Following the rubella vaccination program in the USA, rubella and CRS rapidly decreased and rubella was no longer endemic in the USA by 2004.[2,19] Worldwide, CRS still affects about 100 000 infants each year, but vaccination programs are increasing.[20] The theoretical risk of malformation means pregnancy is a contraindication to rubella vaccination.[2,3] There have been cases of rubella re-infection in vaccinated women, but the risk of fetal damage is then very low.[2,3]

Toxoplasmosis

Toxoplasma gondii is an obligate intracellular protozoan that causes intracranial calcification and retinochoroiditis.[21] Other manifestations of congenital toxoplasmosis include seizures, hydrocephalus, hepatosplenomegaly, jaundice, anemia, and fever.[22]

Human infection with toxoplasma is caused by ingestion of bradyzoites in raw or undercooked meat, particularly pork and lamb. Infection can also result from ingestion of oocysts in water, soil, or food contaminated by cat feces. Marked regional differences in the prevalence of seropositivity to toxoplasmosis occur due to differing dietary practices and sanitation standards. Serologic evidence for toxoplasma infection exists in up to a third of the world's population[23] and it is responsible for the majority of congenital and acquired infectious uveitis. Whereas the rate of maternal–fetal transmission of toxoplasmosis is fairly high, rapid maternal diagnosis and prenatal treatment with antibiotics can significantly lower the rates of vertical transmission.

The prevalence of toxoplasma seropositivity varies with age. In the USA, antibodies to toxoplasma are present in 5% of children aged 5 or below and in more than 60% of people aged 80 or above. The prevalence of seropositivity in women of child-bearing age is 30%,[13] implying that 70% are at risk for acute infection during pregnancy and vertical transmission of the protozoan. Seropositivity elsewhere may be higher.[24,25] The incidence of congenital toxoplasmosis syndrome is 1–10 per

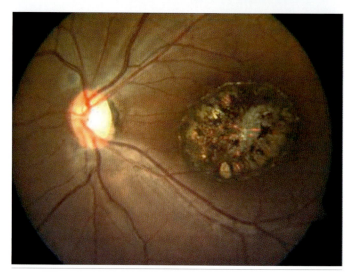

Fig. 11.2 Macular chorioretinal scar due to congenital toxoplasmosis. Courtesy of Dr. Mamta Agarwal.

10 000 live births[23,26] and varies significantly in different geographic regions.

The most recognizable ocular manifestation of congenital toxoplasmosis is the chorioretinal lesion (Fig. 11.2); it is more likely, in congenital disease, to be macular or peripapillary[27] and to be associated with a staphyloma than in acquired disease. Other ocular manifestations include strabismus, microphthalmos, cataract, nystagmus, panuveitis, and optic atrophy.[27]

Maternal toxoplasmosis can be diagnosed by testing serum for antibodies. If both IgG and IgM are negative, infection has not occurred. Positive IgG with a negative IgM is evidence of prior infection.[28] The presence of IgM antibodies with or without positive IgG should initiate further work-up with confirmatory testing including the Sabin-Feldman test, IgG avidity (measures the strength of antigen binding to antibody)[28] and ELISA (enzyme-linked immunosorbent assay) for IgG, IgM, and IgA. High IgG avidity indicates less recent infection.[29] PCR testing of amniotic fluid or fetal blood may be useful.[30] Fetal ultrasonography can detect abnormalities consistent with congenital infection.[31,32]

Serologic evidence of vertical transmission exists in only 10–15% of newborns when maternal toxoplasma infection occurs during the first trimester.[28] Congenital abnormalities in such cases are likely to be more severe. Administration of spiramycin, a macrolide that does not cross the placenta, reduces the sequelae among infected infants though not the rate of maternal–fetal transmission.[33] When maternal toxoplasma infection occurs during the third trimester, fetal transmission is about 75%.[13] Then, maternal treatment with pyrimethamine and sulfadiazine may be administered but, due to concerns about teratogenicity, it is not appropriate during early pregnancy. The macrolide, azithromycin, has been used for the prevention of vertical transmission; at least, it reduces congenital ocular infection in a rodent model.[34] In immunocompromised women, vertical transmission can occur without a recent acute infection.[35] Particular care should be taken in HIV-infected women with a CD4+ count of 200/mm^3 or less: administration of spiramycin for the duration of the pregnancy may then be considered.

Cytomegalovirus

Cytomegalovirus (CMV) is a ubiquitous human pathogen and, like other herpes viruses, can manifest as a primary acquired, latent, and reactivated viral infection. It is the commonest congenital infection in the developed world complicating up to 1% of live births. Ten to fifteen percent of neonates with congenital CMV have clinically apparent disease, 20–30% of which are fatal.[36,37] Complications of symptomatic congenital disease include intrauterine growth retardation, petechial rash, cerebral calcifications, cortical malformations (Fig. 11.3), microcephaly, hepatosplenomegaly, thrombocytopenia, anemia, jaundice, and visual impairment from chorioretinitis. Of the surviving primarily symptomatic neonates, 90% have late manifestations of the infection including delays in psychomotor development, neurologic impairment, hearing loss, and chorioretinitis. In congenitally infected children not symptomatic within the first 30 days of life, milder neurologic sequelae occur in up to 15%.[36,37] Vision loss in congenital CMV infection is secondary to chorioretinopathy, optic neuropathy, and cortical vision loss.[36] In immunocompetent newborns, CMV chorioretinitis, ranging from mild chorioretinal scarring to retinal necrosis, occurs in up to 20% of symptomatic neonates. Commonly, a necrotizing chorioretinitis is seen that resolves to leave scars less densely pigmented than those in congenital toxoplasmosis.[38] Focal vitritis overlying the lesions has been described. Active retinitis is infrequent and is without the hemorrhages seen in CMV retinitis in the immunocompromised child.[36] Asymptomatic children with no retinal lesions may later develop CMV retinitis, so continued monitoring is recommended. Other infrequent ocular complications include keratopathy, cataracts, microphthalmos, and strabismus, which occurs in up to 29%.[36]

Vertical transmission of CMV is usually the result of primary maternal infection though reactivation of latent infection can result in maternal–fetal transmission. The risk of transmission is highest when primary infection occurs during the third trimester,[39,40] but the risk of severe fetal injury is greatest in the first trimester.[41] Primary infection in the first trimester is associated with a lower rate of transmission to the fetus.[39,40]

Serologic screening for primary maternal CMV infection is not routinely conducted due to a lack of effective prenatal treatment or vaccination and because the majority of CMV infections in immunocompetent patients are clinically silent.[42] However, prenatal diagnosis is feasible when seroconversion of maternal IgM antibodies occurs in a previously seronegative woman.[43] If primary maternal infection is diagnosed, fetal infection can be assessed non-invasively by ultrasonography or by CMV isolation in amniotic fluid by PCR or culture. In the neonate, PCR testing and culture of saliva, urine, and dried blood spot specimens can be performed.[42] Isolation of the virus through serologic testing in the first 3 weeks of life is evidence for congenital infection.

Acquired CMV infection is effectively treated with foscarnet, ganciclovir, and its orally absorbed ester, valganciclovir. Unfortunately, prenatal administration of these antiviral agents does not diminish maternal–fetal transmission.[42] Treatment of the congenitally infected infant with ganciclovir decreases the severity of sensorineural hearing loss,[37,44] but has little effect on neurodevelopmental outcomes[37] or visual impairment. Anecdotally, active CMV chorioretinitis in infants can be treated to good effect with intravenous ganciclovir.

Herpes simplex virus

Neonatal herpes simplex virus (HSV) infection affects 1 in 3000 to 20 000 births, with the majority of infections secondary to HSV-2.[45,46] Newborn infection is more likely in mothers with primary HSV infection than recurrent infection.[45] Among mothers with primary HSV infection, HSV infection of the infant occurs in 33–50%.[45] Congenital anomalies occur in 12% of infected infants.[47]

Intrauterine infection (5%)

Intrauterine infection is caused by maternal viremia or by ascending infection from premature rupture of membranes.[45] Infection can lead to hydrops fetalis and fetal death.[49] Surviving infants suffer intrauterine growth retardation, prematurity, and a triad of dermatologic (recurrent, grouped cutaneous vesicles), ocular (chorioretinitis, microphthalmia), and neurologic (microcephaly, intracranial calcifications, encephalitis, psychomotor retardation) abnormalities.[49] Visceral, limb, and bone abnormalities have been reported.[49]

Perinatal infections (85%)

1. Localized disease affecting the skin, eyes, or mouth (SEM). SEM disease has the best prognosis but can disseminate.[46,48]
2. Central nervous system (CNS) disease. This presents at around day 16–19 with seizures, lethargy, fever, tremors, and bulging fontanelles.[48]
3. Disseminated disease affecting multiple organ systems.[48] This can present as sepsis with multiorgan failure (respiratory collapse, liver failure, disseminated intravascular coagulation); mortality is high.[46,48]

Ocular defects occur in 17% of HSV-infected neonates.[50] Ocular pathology in the acute phase of neonatal HSV infection is most commonly blepharoconjunctivitis with vesicles on

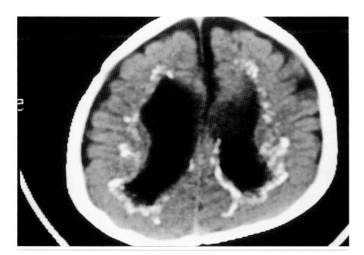

Fig. 11.3 Congenital CMV infection with periventricular calcification, hydrocephalus, and cerebral atrophy shown on this CT scan.

eyelids and keratitis with epithelial dendrites.[50,51] Chorioretinitis is common, with well-demarcated hyperpigmented lesions affecting the peripheral retina, often accompanied by vitritis, and resulting in chorioretinal scars.[50,51] Strabismus and nystagmus are common in children with neurologic disorders.[50,51] Late ocular manifestations include chorioretinal scarring, optic neuritis and atrophy, corneal scarring, and cataracts.[50,51] Rarely, infants develop acute fulminant retinitis.

Postnatal infection (10%)

Recurrence of HSV can result in acute retinal necrosis (ARN). In ARN, one or more foci of retinal necrosis are located in the peripheral retina that spread rapidly and circumferentially, with occlusive vasculopathy, arteriolar involvement, and prominent vitreous and anterior chamber inflammation.[52,53] HSV-2 is the commonest cause of ARN in childhood and such cases are reactivations or recurrences of congenital or neonatal HSV infection.[52-54] PCR of the vitreous or aqueous fluids for varicella zoster virus (VZV) and HSV may help.[52,53]

Diagnosis of neonatal HSV can be made by culture and PCR. Virus culture is usually from samples of skin or mucous lesions or from the conjunctivae, oropharynx, rectum, or urine.[48] PCR can be performed on samples of the nasopharynx, cerebrospinal fluid (CSF), blood, and skin.[55] Diagnosis with PCR is more common than culture in suspected CNS disease as CSF cultures can be negative.[45,55]

Neonatal HSV is treated with intravenous acyclovir 60 mg/kg/day divided every 8 hours for 14 days if limited to skin, eyes, and mouth, and for 21 days if disseminated or in patients with CNS disease.[48] Early initiation of antiviral therapy is important and can lead to improved outcomes.[55] Recurrences are common.[48,56-58] In children, ocular HSV may be treated with oral and/or topical antivirals with topical corticosteroids for immune stromal involvement.[56-58] Prolonged antiviral therapy reduces recurrences, but may cause transient neutropenia.[59]

Syphilis

Congenital syphilis occurs when the fetus is exposed to *Treponema pallidum* in the second and third trimesters. Transmission in the first trimester usually results in fetal death. Maternal–fetal transmission of syphilis occurs in almost all pregnancies complicated by primary untreated maternal infection. Most infants born to mothers with secondary syphilis show signs of congenital syphilis.[60] Latent syphilis can also be transmitted vertically. More than 12 million adult cases and half a million pregnancies are affected worldwide annually.[61,62] After a decrease in acquired syphilis in the 1980s and 1990s, the incidence of infection has increased recently, consequently with an increase in congenital syphilis.[60]

The classic "triad" of congenital syphilis includes interstitial keratitis, nerve deafness, and dental malformations ("Hutchinson's teeth").[63] "Early" manifestations occur in infancy due to active infection including skeletal abnormalities, rhinitis, a maculopapular rash, fissures around the lips, nares and anus, hepatosplenomegaly, anemia, and uveitis. "Late" manifestations are secondary to ongoing inflammatory sequelae of the infection and occur after 2 years of life;[61] they include nerve deafness, bone changes, dental abnormalities, and interstitial keratitis (IK).

Ocular manifestations of congenital syphilis include chorioretinitis, IK, anterior uveitis, iridoschisis, and optic atrophy. Cataracts may be present but are usually a result of anterior segment inflammation from uveitis. Up to 40% of children with untreated congenital syphilis develop IK when 5–20 years of age, bilateral in 80%. It is both an infectious and a hypersensitivity keratitis,[64] which may progress despite adequate intravenous antibiotics and it also requires treatment with topical steroids. Earlier in the disease, IK is associated with anterior uveitis. Deep stromal neovascularization is consistent and secondary glaucoma may occur. Syphilitic chorioretinitis manifests as peripheral areas of pigment mottling.

Pregnant women should be screened for syphilis early in pregnancy and again before delivery.[65] Serologic testing may be divided into treponemal tests such as FTA-ABS, the microhemagglutination assay for *T. pallidum*, and the *Treponema pallidum* particle agglutination assay TP-PA and non-treponemal tests including the Venereal Disease Research Laboratory test (VDRL) and Rapid Plasma Reagin (RPR). A quantitative assay of non-treponemal serology with a titer four times higher than the maternal titer indicates congenital infection. Treponemal tests are almost always positive in infants with congenital syphilis and should be performed with a non-treponemal test to increase specificity. In cases with active cutaneous lesions, dark field microscopy may be employed to isolate treponemes. A lumbar puncture and CSF serology and examination to assess for asymptomatic neurosyphilis should be done in any child with congenital syphilis.[66]

Pregnant women with HIV are at a higher risk of having active syphilis; however, a higher rate of false negatives occurs in these patients.[62] Infants born to HIV positive women should be screened for any clinical manifestations of congenital infection in addition to serologic testing.

Parenteral penicillin G is the treatment for congenital syphilis and 10–14 days of procaine penicillin administered intramuscularly or 10–14 days of intravenous aqueous penicillin is usually adequate. Higher concentrations in the CSF are obtained with intravenous therapy than with intramuscular dosing.[62] Serologic testing should be repeated every 3 months after treatment until serum VDRL or RPR is negative or titers are less than four times their original value. If serum non-treponemal antibody titers remain elevated or begin to rise, CSF analysis should be repeated and parenteral penicillin G repeated.

Varicella zoster virus

Primary infection by varicella zoster virus (VZV) is called varicella, or chickenpox. Intrauterine infection is rare: more than 90% of women of child-bearing age have virus-specific immunity.[67] Infection in the first and second trimesters may lead to congenital varicella syndrome (CVS), while maternal infection near term may result in neonatal disseminated infection.

Manifestations of CVS include dermatomal skin lesions, neurologic defects, ocular manifestations, and limb hypoplasia. Ocular defects include chorioretinitis, cataracts, microphthalmos, optic nerve hypoplasia, and Horner's syndrome (Fig. 11.4). VZV has a high affinity for the nervous system and nearly one-third of affected infants die during the first few months.[67]

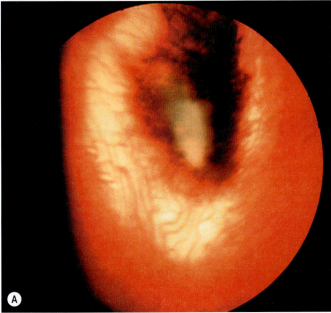
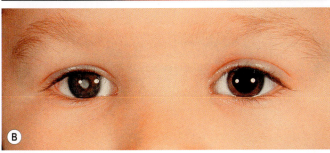
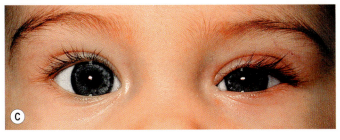

Fig. 11.4 Congenital varicella. (A) Chorioretinal scar in a child with congenital varicella syndrome (B) Congenital varicella with congenital cataract and microphthalmos (C) Congenital varicella with Horner syndrome in the left eye.

Prevention includes vaccination of seronegative women prior to pregnancy and avoidance of exposure to varicella zoster during pregnancy. There are no controlled studies on the utility of antiviral therapy in preventing CVS or that varicella zoster immunoglobulin prevents fetal transmission. Varicella vaccination has reduced congenital and neonatal varicella in Australia following its introduction in 2005 and its use around the world is increasing.[67]

Other intrauterine infections

Lymphocytic choriomeningitis virus is an RNA virus with a rodent reservoir. Transmission to humans may be airborne, from contamination of food by infected mouse urine, feces and saliva, or from bites by infected mice. Transmission to the fetus occurs during maternal viremia. Systemic findings in the neonate include macrocephaly or microcephaly, hydrocephalus, meningitis, hepatosplenomegaly, and neurologic abnormalities such as cerebral palsy, mental retardation, and seizures. The most common ocular manifestation is chorioretinal scarring, most often in the periphery but also occurring in the macula.

West Nile virus is an RNA flavivirus transmitted to humans by mosquito bites. Transmission to babies transplacentally and through breast milk may occur. Most infections are asymptomatic but, rarely, pharyngitis, arthralgia, a skin rash, encephalitis, meningitis, or paralysis occur. Chorioretinal scarring is the most common ocular manifestation and has been reported in congenital infection.

There are no known effective treatments for these conditions.[13]

References

3. Banatvala JE, Brown DW. Rubella. Lancet 2004; 363: 1127–37.
4. Givens KT, Lee DA, Jones T, Ilstrup DM. Congenital rubella syndrome: ophthalmic manifestations and associated systemic disorders. Br J Ophthalmol 1993; 77: 358–63.
7. Khandekar R, Al Awaidy S, Ganesh A, Bawikar S. An epidemiological and clinical study of ocular manifestations of congenital rubella syndrome in Omani children. Arch Ophthalmol 2004; 122: 541–5.
10. Yoser SL, Forster DJ, Rao NA. Systemic viral infections and their retinal and choroidal manifestations. Surv Ophthalmol 1993; 37: 313–52.
11. Mets MB, Chhabra MS. Eye manifestations of intrauterine infections and their impact on childhood blindness. Surv Ophthalmol 2008; 53: 95–111.
13. de Groot-Mijnes JD, de Visser L, Rothova A, et al. Rubella virus is associated with Fuchs heterochromic iridocyclitis. Am J Ophthalmol 2006; 141: 212–4.
14. Quentin CD, Reiber H. Fuchs heterochromic cyclitis: rubella virus antibodies and genome in aqueous humor. Am J Ophthalmol 2004; 138: 46–54.
15. Birnbaum AD, Tessler HH, Schultz KL, et al. Epidemiologic relationship between Fuchs heterochromic iridocyclitis and the United States rubella vaccination program. Am J Ophthalmol 2007; 144: 424–8.
16. Suzuki J, Goto H, Komase K, et al. Rubella virus as a possible etiological agent of Fuchs heterochromic iridocyclitis. Graefes Arch Clin Exp Ophthalmol 2010;248:1487–91.
17. Reef SE, Frey TK, Theall K, et al. The changing epidemiology of rubella in the 1990s: on the verge of elimination and new challenges for control and prevention. JAMA 2002; 287: 464–72.
21. Montoya JG, Liesenfeld O. Toxoplasmosis. Lancet 2004; 363: 1965–76.

Fetal infection occurs by transplacental transmission. CVS may be caused by intrauterine zoster-like VZV reactivations because of the immunologic immaturity of the fetus in the first two trimesters of pregnancy. The criteria to establish a diagnosis of congenital varicella are:

1. Appearance of maternal varicella during pregnancy
2. Presence of congenital skin lesions and/or neurologic defects
3. Eye findings as described above, and limb hypoplasia
4. Proof of intrauterine VZV infection by detection of viral DNA in the infant
5. Presence of specific IgM/persistence of IgG beyond 7 months of age, and/or
6. The appearance of zoster during early infancy.[65]

22. Villena I, Ancelle T, Delmas C, et al. Congenital toxoplasmosis in France in 2007: first results from a national surveillance system. Euro Surveill 2010 Jun 24; 15(25). pii: 19600.

23. Desmonts G, Couvreur J. Congenital toxoplasmosis: a prospective study of 378 pregnancies. N Engl J Med 1974; 290: 1110–6.

25. Delair E, Latkany P, Noble AG, et al. Clinical manifestations of ocular toxoplasmosis. Ocul Immunol Inflamm 2011 Apr; 19: 91–102.

29. Montoya JG, Rosso F. Diagnosis and management of toxoplasmosis. Clin Perinatol 2005; 32: 705–26.

31. Foulon W, Villena I, Stray-Pedersen B, et al. Treatment of toxoplasmosis during pregnancy: a multicenter study of impact on fetal transmission and children's sequelae at age 1 year. Am J Obstet Gynecol 1999; 180: 410–5.

34. Coats DK, Demmler GJ, Paysse EA, et al. Ophthalmologic findings in children with congenital cytomegalovirus infection. J AAPOS 2000; 4: 110–6.

35. Michaels MG, Greenberg DP, Sabo DL, Wald ER. Treatment of children with congenital cytomegalovirus infection with ganciclovir. Pediatr Infect Dis J 2003; 22: 504–9.

41. Yinon Y, Farine D, Yudin MH. Screening, diagnosis, and management of cytomegalovirus infection in pregnancy. Obstet Gynecol Surv 2010 Nov; 65: 736–43.

43. Waggoner-Fountain LA, Grossman LB. Herpes simplex virus. Pediatrics in Review/American Academy of Pediatrics 2004; 25: 86–93.

44. Kimberlin DW, Lin CY, Jacobs RF, et al. Natural history of neonatal herpes simplex virus infections in the acyclovir era. Pediatrics 2001; 108: 223–9.

46. Marquez L, Levy ML, Munoz FM, Palazzi DL. A report of three cases and review of intrauterine herpes simplex virus infection. Pediatri Infec Dis J 2011; 30: 153–7.

51. Van Gelder RN, Willig JL, Holland GN, Kaplan HJ. Herpes simplex virus type 2 as a cause of acute retinal necrosis syndrome in young patients. Ophthalmology 2001; 108: 869–76.

52. Thompson WS, Culbertson WW, Smiddy WE, et al. Acute retinal necrosis caused by reactivation of herpes simplex virus type 2. Am J Ophthalmol 1994; 118: 205–11.

53. Wolfert SI, de Jong EP, Vossen AC, et al. Diagnostic and therapeutic management for suspected neonatal herpes simplex virus infection. J Clin Virol 2011; 51: 8–11.

55. Schwartz GS, Holland EJ. Oral acyclovir for the management of herpes simplex virus keratitis in children. Ophthalmology 2000; 107: 278–82.

58. CDCP. Update on emerging infections: news from the Centers for Disease Control and Prevention. Congenital syphilis – United States 2003–2008. Ann Emerg Med 2010 Sep; 56: 295–6.

60. Woods CR. Syphilis in children: congenital and acquired. Semin Pediatr Infect Dis 2005; 16: 245–57.

65. Sauerbrei A, Wutzler P. The congenital varicella syndrome. J Perinatol 2000; 20: 548–54.

66. Khandaker G, Marshall H, Peadon E, et al. Congenital and neonatal varicella: impact of the national varicella vaccination programme in Australia. Arch Dis Child 2011; 96: 453–6.

Access the complete reference list online at

http://www.expertconsult.com

SECTION 3
Infections, allergic and
external eye disorders

CHAPTER **12**

Neonatal conjunctivitis (ophthalmia neonatorum)

Tina Rutar

Chapter contents

Neonatal conjunctivitis is an inflammation or infection of the conjunctiva occurring within the first month of life. The three categories of neonatal conjunctivitis are chemical, bacterial, and viral. Many forms of neonatal conjunctivitis are self-limited and not vision threatening; others have important systemic associations or can cause blindness.

Conjunctival injection, chemosis, discharge, and eyelid edema can occur with all subtypes of neonatal conjunctivitis. Additional clinical signs, such as laterality, severity of injection and chemosis, character of discharge, presence of conjunctival pseudomembranes, or skin vesicles, can be suggestive of specific etiologies. The clinical history, including maternal prenatal history, can help guide appropriate laboratory testing.

Neonatal conjunctivitis is the most common infection in the first month of life, with an incidence from 1% to 24%.[1]

Prophylaxis

Credé first reported the use of ocular prophylaxis for ophthalmia neonatorum; application of silver nitrate to the eyes of newborns decreased the incidence of ophthalmia neonatorum from 7.8% to 0.17%.[2] Prior to the widespread use of prophylaxis, ophthalmia neonatorum was a common diagnosis in schools for the blind.[2] Corneal scarring, including that caused by ophthalmia neonatorum, remains the leading cause of childhood blindness in Africa.[3]

Types of prophylaxis include: silver nitrate 1%, povidone iodine 2.5%, erythromycin ointment 0.5%, and tetracycline ointment 1%. These agents are administered to the inferior conjunctival fornix of both eyes within 1 hour of an infant's delivery. Silver nitrate is most likely among the prophylactic agents to cause chemical conjunctivitis. Silver nitrate and tetracycline have equal 83–93% efficacy in the prevention of gonococcal ophthalmia neonatorum.[4] In a controlled trial of 3117 Kenyan newborns, povidone iodine 2.5% was more effective than erythromycin or silver nitrate for prophylaxis of infectious conjunctivitis.[5] However, in a randomized controlled trial involving 410 Israeli newborns, povidone iodine was marginally less effective in preventing infectious conjunctivitis and more likely to cause chemical conjunctivitis compared to tetracycline.[6]

In the United States, erythromycin 0.5% is used as the topical prophylactic agent. The other agents are not commercially available there. During an erythromycin shortage in 2009, the Centers for Disease Control recommended topical azithromycin 1% solution, or, if unavailable, topical gentamicin 0.3% or tobramycin 0.3% ointments. Azithromycin is approximately 10 times more costly than povidone iodine prepared by a hospital pharmacy.[7] Topical gentamicin can cause periocular ulcerative dermatitis.[8]

Chemical conjunctivitis

Chemical conjunctivitis develops within 1–2 days after the administration of a topical agent and is bilateral. Gram stain shows leukocytes but no organisms. Withdrawal of the offending agent results in resolution of symptoms within 2 days.

Chlamydial conjunctivitis

The prevalence of *Chlamydia trachomatis* among pregnant women ranges from 2% to 20%; the higher rates are among younger women, and those without prenatal care.[9] The likelihood that an infant born to a mother with untreated *C. trachomatis* infection develops symptomatic conjunctivitis ranges from 20% to 50%.[4,10]

Chlamydial conjunctivitis (Fig. 12.1A) typically develops 5–14 days after delivery. Though more common among infants born vaginally, it can occur after cesarean section delivery.

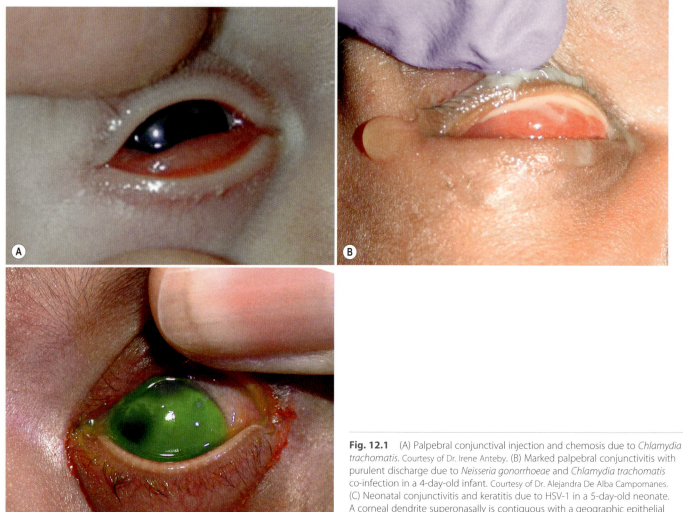

Fig. 12.1 (A) Palpebral conjunctival injection and chemosis due to *Chlamydia trachomatis*. Courtesy of Dr. Irene Anteby. (B) Marked palpebral conjunctivitis with purulent discharge due to *Neisseria gonorrhoeae* and *Chlamydia trachomatis* co-infection in a 4-day-old infant. Courtesy of Dr. Alejandra De Alba Campomanes. (C) Neonatal conjunctivitis and keratitis due to HSV-1 in a 5-day-old neonate. A corneal dendrite superonasally is contiguous with a geographic epithelial defect centrally and temporally. Despite treatment with intravenous acyclovir, the patient developed HSV encephalitis. Courtesy of Dr. John Ross Ainsworth.

The conjunctivitis is unilateral or bilateral, and the discharge is mucopurulent. Pseudomembrane formation can occur. Untreated, the conjunctivitis resolves after weeks to months, but can cause conjunctival and corneal scarring.

The diagnosis is made by isolating *Chlamydia* via culture obtained by scraping the palpebral conjunctiva for epithelial cells. Intracellular inclusions can be demonstrated on Giemsa stain. PCR testing, which is equivalent to culture for detection of *C. trachomatis* in conjunctival specimens, is also available.

Chlamydial conjunctivitis is associated with nasal congestion, otitis media, and pneumonia occurring at 4–12 weeks of life. Chlamydial conjunctivitis is treated with oral erythromycin (50 mg/kg divided into 4 daily doses) for 14 days.[9] Asymptomatic infants born to mothers with untreated *C. trachomatis* infection are not treated prophylactically, in part because erythromycin can cause infantile hypertrophic pyloric stenosis.[11] For infants with conjunctivitis but no sign of pneumonia, systemic erythromycin can be delayed while awaiting confirmatory diagnostic tests for *Chlamydia*. Oral azithromycin (20 mg/kg daily for 3 days) is an alternative treatment, though experience with its use in neonates is limited. The mother and her sexual partners should be treated with a single dose of oral azithromycin (1 g) and be evaluated for other sexually transmitted diseases.

Gonococcal conjunctivitis

The prevalence of gonococcal cervical infection among women in developed countries is typically less than 1%; however, the prevalence in some countries is as high as 22%.[12] Newborns of mothers with gonococcal infection who do not receive prophylaxis have a 30–47% likelihood of developing conjunctivitis after vaginal delivery.[10,12] The gonococcal transmission rate increases to 68% if the mother is also infected with *Chlamydia*.[10] Gonococcal conjunctivitis is also possible among infants born by cesarean section.

Infants typically exhibit symptoms 2–5 days after delivery. The conjunctivitis has an aggressive course, with profuse purulent discharge, and severe conjunctival injection, chemosis, and eyelid edema (Fig. 12.1B). Gonococcus can invade the cornea through intact corneal epithelium. Corneal involvement begins with coarse white peripheral infiltrates. Ulceration can occur by the second week of infection. Corneal scarring due to neovascularization and corneal perforation are significant concerns.[4] One study showed that 4 of 25 patients (16%) with gonococcal conjunctivitis developed corneal involvement.[13]

Infants born to *N. gonorrhoeae* infected mothers, whether or not conjunctivitis develops, should be treated prophylactically with a single dose of IV or IM ceftriaxone (25–50 mg/kg up to 125 mg maximal) or cefotaxime (100 mg/kg IM or IV) if the infant has hyperbilirubinemia.[9] Infants with suspected gonococcal conjunctivitis should undergo Gram stain and culture using modified Thayer-Martin medium prior to receiving antibiotics. Gram negative diplococci on Gram stain have a sensitivity of 86% and specificity of 90% for gonococcal conjunctivitis.[13] Blood and cerebrospinal fluid (CSF) cultures should be obtained to assess for bacteremia and meningitis, and the baby should be monitored clinically for septic arthritis. Because of frequent maternal co-infection with *Chlamydia*, Giemsa stain and chlamydial culture should also be performed. In the presence of systemic infection, the cephalosporin course is extended to 7–14 days. Topical antibiotics are unnecessary; however, frequent saline lavage of the purulent discharge is recommended. The mother and her sexual partners should be treated for gonococcus and presumptively for *Chlamydia*, and they should be evaluated for other sexually transmitted diseases.

Bacterial (not chlamydial or gonococcal) conjunctivitis

Neonatal nasopharyngeal colonization rather than maternal vaginal colonization is implicated in most bacterial conjunctivitides not due to *Chlamydia* or *Gonococcus*.[14] *Staphylococcus aureus, Streptococcus pneumoniae, Streptococcus viridans, Enterococcus* spp., and *Haemophilus* spp. are more commonly isolated from neonates with conjunctivitis compared to controls without.[14,15] Bacterial conjunctivitis has an onset at days 5–14 of life and can be unilateral or bilateral. Bacteria can be cultured on chocolate and blood agar. Some positive cultures represent colonizing rather than disease-causing bacteria. A broad-spectrum topical antibiotic can be used until culture results are available, but many cases resolve without treatment.

Herpetic conjunctivitis

Herpes simplex virus (HSV) can rarely cause neonatal conjunctivitis. Neonates can become infected via vaginal delivery or ascending intrauterine infection if the mother has genital HSV. The risk of infection is far greater if the mother has primary rather than reactivated genital HSV: 25–60% vs. 2%. Neonates can also become infected via direct contact with caregivers who have herpes labialis or herpetic whitlow.[9]

Ophthalmic manifestations of neonatal HSV include eyelid vesicles and erythema, conjunctivitis, keratitis, and anterior uveitis (Fig. 12.1C). The keratitis can involve all layers of the cornea and does not follow the disease patterns seen in adults. Ophthalmic manifestations usually occur 5–14 days after exposure. Neonatal HSV keratoconjunctivitis typically occurs in the setting of systemic disease, which can be disseminated (pneumonitis, hepatitis), meningoencephalitis, or skin/eye/mucous membrane disease. The onset of systemic disease can be delayed, up to 6 weeks of life.

HSV culture (of conjunctiva, corneal epithelium, or skin vesicle scraping), CSF analysis, including HSV PCR (polymerase chain reaction), and liver function tests should be obtained in neonates with suspected HSV keratoconjunctivitis. More rapid diagnostic techniques include direct fluorescent antibody staining or enzyme immunoassay detection of HSV antigens within scrapings. HSV PCR can also be performed on swabs and scrapings. HSV antibody testing is not useful in neonates.

Asymptomatic infants are treated with prophylactic IV acyclovir if they are born to mothers with primary genital HSV at the time of vaginal delivery, or if surface cultures grow HSV. Neonatal HSV infection is treated with IV acyclovir (60 mg/kg per day 3 times daily) for 14 days, or for 21 days in the presence of disseminated or CNS disease.[9] Adjunct therapy with topical trifluorouridine 1%, iododeoxyuridine 0.1%, or vidarabine 3% can be considered. A topical steroid may be added for corneal stromal and endothelial disease, and topical steroid and cycloplegia for uveitis. Babies with neonatal HSV have a high risk of death and are hospitalized for the duration of IV treatment.[9] They are also at high risk of HSV reactivation, and prophylactic acyclovir should be continued for at least six months after hospital discharge.[16]

Neonatal conjunctivitis in hospitalized patients

Hospitalized neonates acquire infection via hospital workers and instrumentation, and via assisted ventilation, which is thought to increase the contact of nasopharyngeal flora with the eye.[16] Additionally, most of these infants are premature or have multiple comorbidities. Coagulase-negative staphylococci, *Staphylococcus aureus* and *Klebsiella* spp. were the most commonly isolated species in a study of 200 neonates in a US intensive care nursery.[17] Methicillin-resistant *Staphylococcus aureus* has caused conjunctivitis outbreaks in neonatal intensive care units;[18] its incidence is increasing.[19]

Laboratory testing

The clinical history guides the appropriate laboratory testing. If multiple infectious causes are in the differential diagnosis, the following tests help narrow the diagnosis:

- Gram stain
- Giemsa stain
- Chlamydial culture or PCR
- Gonococcal culture on Thayer-Martin medium
- Bacterial cultures using blood and chocolate agar
- HSV culture, PCR, direct fluorescent antibody or enzyme immunoassays

Approximately half of clinically evident neonatal conjunctivitides have negative culture results.[14]

References

1. Fransen L, Klauss V. Neonatal ophthalmia in the developing world: epidemiology, etiology, management and control. Int Ophthalmol 1988; 11: 189–96.

2. Forbes GB, Forbes GM. Silver nitrate and the eyes of the newborn: Crede's contribution to preventive medicine. Am J Dis Child 1971; 121: 1–3.

3. Foster A, Sommer A. Childhood blindness from corneal ulceration in Africa: causes, prevention, and treatment. Bull World Health Organ 1986; 64: 619–23.

4. Laga M, Meheus A, Piot P. Epidemiology and control of gonococcal ophthalmia neonatorum. Bull World Health Organ 1989; 67: 471–7.

5. Isenberg SJ, Apt L, Wood M. A controlled trial of povidone-iodine as prophylaxis against ophthalmia neonatorum. N Engl J Med 1995; 332: 562–6.

6. David M, Rumelt S, Weintraub Z. Efficacy comparison between povidone iodine 2.5% and tetracycline 1% in prevention of ophthalmia neonatorum. Ophthalmology

7. Keenan JD, Eckert S, Rutar T. Cost analysis of povidone-iodine for ophthalmia neonatorum prophylaxis. Arch Ophthalmol 2010; 128: 136–7.

8. Binenbaum G, et al. Periocular ulcerative dermatitis associated with gentamicin ointment prophylaxis in newborns. J Pediatr 2010; 156: 320–1.

9. AAP. Red Book: Report of the Committee on Infectious Diseases. Elk Grove Village, IL: American Academy of Pediatrics; 2009.

10. Laga M, et al. Epidemiology of ophthalmia neonatorum in Kenya. Lancet 1986; 2: 1145–9.

11. Rosenman MB, et al. Oral erythromycin prophylaxis vs watchful waiting in caring for newborns exposed to Chlamydia trachomatis. Arch Pediatr Adolesc Med 2003; 157: 565–71.

12. Galega FP, Heymann DL, Nasah BT. Gonococcal ophthalmia neonatorum: the case for prophylaxis in tropical Africa. Bull World Health Organ 1984; 62: 95–8.

13. Fransen L, et al. Ophthalmia neonatorum in Nairobi, Kenya: the roles of Neisseria gonorrhoeae and Chlamydia trachomatis. J Infect Dis 1986; 153: 862–9.

14. Krohn MA, et al. The bacterial etiology of conjunctivitis in early infancy. Eye Prophylaxis Study Group. Am J Epidemiol 1993; 138: 326–32.

15. Sandstrom KI, et al. Microbial causes of neonatal conjunctivitis. J Pediatr 1984; 105: 706–11.

16. Kimberlin DW, Whitley RJ, Wan W, et al. Oral acyclovir suppression and neurodevelopment after neonatal herpes. N Engl J Med 2011; 365: 1284–92.

17. Haas J, et al. Epidemiology and diagnosis of hospital-acquired conjunctivitis among neonatal intensive care unit patients. Pediatr Infect Dis J 2005; 24: 586–9.

18. Cimolai N. Ocular methicillin-resistant Staphylococcus aureus infections in a newborn intensive care cohort. Am J Ophthalmol 2006; 142: 183–4.

19. Lessa FC, et al. Trends in incidence of late-onset methicillin-resistant Staphylococcus aureus infection in neonatal intensive care units: data from the National Nosocomial Infections Surveillance System, 1995–2004. Pediatr Infect Dis J 2009; 28: 577–81.

Preseptal and orbital cellulitis

Jimmy M Uddin • Richard L Scawn

The diagnosis of infective preseptal and orbital cellulitis is clinical. The goal is to prevent rapid deterioration and serious sequelae such as visual loss, cavernous sinus thrombosis, cerebral abscess, osteomyelitis, and septicemia. It must be managed promptly with appropriate antibiotics and medical support within a multidisciplinary team consisting of pediatricians, ophthalmologists, ENT surgeons, nurses, and radiologists. Regular evaluation for progression of signs or deterioration of the clinical picture is essential. Neuroimaging may be necessary to determine the extent of the disease.

Anatomy and terminology

The orbital septum marks the anterior extent of the orbit. It is firmly adherent at the orbital rim with the orbital periosteum as the arcus marginalis; it extends to the upper and lower tarsal plates. Preseptal cellulitis is a descriptive term for patients who present with symptoms and signs of inflammation confined largely to the eyelids: pain, redness, and swelling. The orbital septum acts as a physical barrier to lesions spreading posteriorly to the orbit. Orbital cellulitis involves infection of the postseptal space and usually results from adjacent infected sinuses, commonly the ethmoids. Many vessels and nerves pierce the thin lamina papyracea between the ethmoid sinuses and the orbit: infection easily spreads through these and other naturally occurring perforations, lifting off the loosely attached periosteum within the anterior orbit, resulting in a subperiosteal abscess. An orbital abscess results from an infectious breach of the periosteum or seeding into the orbit. Extension of infection from the ethmoids into the brain may result in meningitis and cerebral abscesses. The presence of decreased, painful eye movements, proptosis, optic neuropathy, or radiological evidence of orbital inflammation or collections signifies orbital cellulitis.

The drainage of the eyelids, sinuses, and orbits is largely by the orbital venous system, which empties into the cavernous sinus via the superior and inferior orbital veins. Since it is devoid of valves, infection may spread in both preseptal and orbital cellulitis, leading to the serious sight- and life-threatening complication of cavernous sinus thrombosis.

Classification

Infective orbital cellulitis and its complications can be classified into five types which are not mutually exclusive and do not necessarily progress in that order[1] (Table 13.1):

Table 13.1 – Classification of orbital cellulitis

Stage	Signs and symptoms	CT findings
Preseptal cellulitis	Eyelid swelling, occasional fever	If performed, sinusitis may be present
Orbital cellulitis	Proptosis, decreased painful eye movements, chemosis	Sinusitis, mild soft tissue changes in the orbit
Subperiosteal abscess	Signs of orbital cellulitis, systemic involvement	Subperiosteal abscess, globe displacement, soft tissue changes in the orbit
Orbital abscess	Signs of orbital cellulitis, systemic involvement, ophthalmoplegia, visual loss	Orbital collection of pus with marked soft tissue changes of the fat and muscles
Intracranial complication	Signs of orbital or rarely preseptal cellulitis, marked proptosis, cranial nerve palsies (III, IV, V, VI)	Intracranial changes: cavernous sinus thrombosis, extradural abscess, meningitis, and osteomyelitis

Modified from Uzcategui N, Warman R, Smith A, et al. Clinical practice guidelines for the management of orbital cellulitis. J Pediatr Ophthalmol Strabismus 1998; 35: 73–9. © 1998 Slack Inc.

1. Preseptal cellulitis
2. Orbital cellulitis
3. Subperiosteal abscess
4. Orbital abscess
5. Cavernous sinus thrombosis

Preseptal cellulitis

Preseptal cellulitis is five times more common than orbital cellulitis, especially in children under the age of 5 years.[2,3] It is often secondary to lid and cutaneous infections – styes, impetigo, erysipelas, herpes simplex, varicella, or dacryocystitis (Figs 13.1, 13.2, and 13.3). It is also associated with upper respiratory tract infections, uncomplicated sinusitis (Fig. 13.4), or lid trauma.

Infective preseptal cellulitis must be distinguished from other causes of lid edema such as adenoviral keratoconjunctivitis, atopic conjunctivitis, or, rarely, Kawasaki's disease.[4] In one series, 16% of children referred with preseptal cellulitis were found to have adenoviral keratoconjunctivitis.[5]

Clinical assessment

History

Children with preseptal cellulitis associated with an upper respiratory tract infection or sinusitis present in the winter months with preceding nasal discharge, cough, fever, localized tenderness, and general malaise, followed by unilateral eyelid swelling. Bilateral involvement is rare. There is history of a localized lid infection or trauma with swelling spreading from an identifiable point.

Examination

The child may be generally unwell and febrile. The cellulitis ranges from a mild localized involvement, with or without an abscess, to generalized tense upper and lower lid edema spreading to the cheek and brow, precluding examination of the eye. Localized causes such as styes, trauma, and dacryocystitis should be evident. There is an absence of proptosis; optic nerve functions and extraocular movements are normal.

It can be difficult to differentiate between preseptal and orbital cellulitis and the diagnosis may change from preseptal to orbital cellulitis if orbital signs become more obvious, clinically or by imaging.[6]

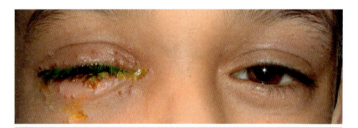

Fig. 13.1 Preseptal cellulitis secondary to eczema herpeticum.

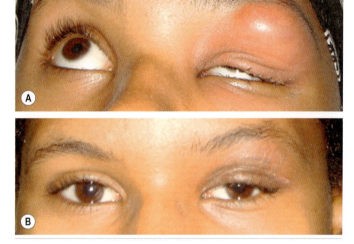

Fig. 13.2 (A) Preseptal cellulitis associated with a lid abscess. Normal eye movements with a white eye (patient looking up). (B) Intravenous antibiotics and surgical drainage resolved her condition.

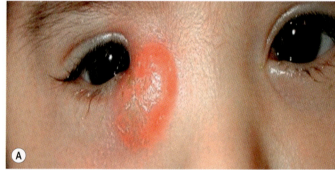

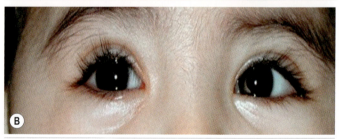

Fig. 13.3 (A) Cellulitis associated with dacryocystitis in a 1-year-old child. (B) Acute infection resolved with antibiotics. Patient subsequently underwent probing to treat the underlying mucocele.

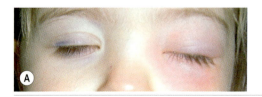
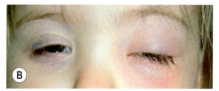
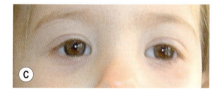

Fig. 13.4 Preseptal/orbital cellulitis treated successfully with intravenous antibiotics. (A) At presentation with swollen lids and possibly mild proptosis. Patient was admitted under pediatricians, ophthalmologist, and ENT. She was treated immediately with intravenous antibiotics. No imaging was performed. (B) Responding to antibiotics within 12 hours. (C) Fully resolved at 4 days.

The clinical picture varies with the organism involved. In staphylococcal infections there is a purulent discharge, while *Haemophilus* infection leads to a non-purulent cellulitis with a characteristic bluish-purple discoloration of the eyelid with irritability, raised temperature, and otitis media (Fig. 13.5). In streptococcal infection there is usually a sharply demarcated red area of induration,[7] heat, and marked tenderness (Fig. 13.6A,B). Preseptal cellulitis may be complicated by meningitis, particularly if the infection is due to *Haemophilus influenzae* type B.[8]

Management

In children who develop preseptal cellulitis following an upper respiratory tract infection, cultures should be taken from the nose, throat, conjunctiva, and any accessible aspirates of the periorbital edema.

Children with mild to moderate preseptal cellulitis can be managed in the same way as uncomplicated sinusitis on an outpatient basis with oral broad spectrum antibiotics or as an inpatient with intravenous antibiotics, if more severe (Table 13.2).[9,10]

Admission, intravenous antibiotics, and close observation may be more appropriate in more severe preseptal cellulitis, young children, the immunocompromised, or those who are systemically unwell.

A CT scan to assess orbital, sinus, and brain involvement is indicated when lid swelling prevents an adequate examination of the globe.[11]

Children with a local cause for the periorbital edema, such as dacryocystitis, need specific treatment for the underlying condition and rarely need further investigation.

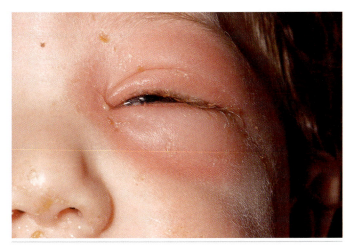

Fig. 13.5 Preseptal cellulitis due to *Haemophilus influenzae* in a 6-month-old infant.

Table 13.2 – Initial antibiotic treatment of preseptal and orbital cellulitis

Preseptal cellulitis	Associated with upper respiratory tract infection Cefuroxime 100–150 mg/kg per day or amoxicillin-clavulanate (augmentin) or ampicillin 50–100 mg/kg per day and chloramphenicol 75–100 mg/kg per day (IV in divided doses)
Orbital cellulitis	Ceftazidime 100–150 mg/kg per day or cefotaxime 100–150 mg/kg per day or oxacillin or nafcillin 150–200 mg/kg per day (in divided doses) Ceftriaxone: 80 mg/kg (max 4 g/day) Flucloxacillin: 50 mg/kg qds IV (max 2 g/dose) Co-Amoxiclav: 30 mg/kg tds (max 1.2 g/dose) Metronidazole: 7.5 mg/kg tds (max 500 mg/dose) Vancomycin should be considered in resistant cases Clindamycin should be added in necrotizing fasciitis

Note: You should consult your own pharmacy for correct doses.
The exact dose will vary with age and severity of infection.
There may be local variations in pathogens and antibiotic resistance.

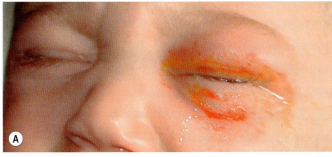
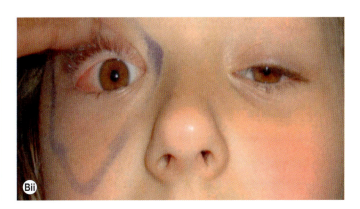

Fig. 13.6 (A) Streptoccocal preseptal cellulitis in a 12-month-old child. (B) It is useful to mark the extent of cellulitis for monitoring purposes. This 10-year-old girl had proptosis and responded to IV antibiotics.

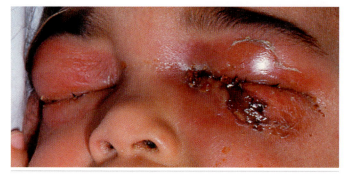

Fig. 13.7 Beta-hemolytic *Streptococcus* may cause necrotizing fasciitis, as shown here. Courtesy of Mr G. Rose.

Lid trauma may result in suppurative cellulitis, when the causative agent is *Staphylococcus aureus* or a beta-hemolytic *Streptococcus*. It is usually sufficient to culture the wound discharge as there is rarely any bacteremia; blood cultures are usually negative.[12] Parenteral antibiotics are administered and tetanus prophylaxis is provided, if appropriate. If the skin has been penetrated by organic material or animal bites, antibiotics should be included coverage for anerobic organisms.

Rarely, beta-hemolytic *Streptococcus* may cause necrotizing fasciitis. It is characterized by a rapidly progressive tense and shiny cellulitis with excessive edema and poorly demarcated borders with a violaceous skin discoloration. Necrosis develops and streptococcal toxic shock syndrome is common (Fig. 13.7). Treatment is with immediate hospitalization with a multidisciplinary team implementing resuscitation and medical support with immediate high-dose intravenous antibiotics including a penicillin or third-generation cephalosporin and clindamycin. Surgical debridement should be considered if there is not a clear response to medical treatment.[13,14]

Orbital cellulitis

Etiology

Infective orbital cellulitis is more frequent in children over 5 years (average age 7 years). In over 90% it is secondary to sinusitis,[12,15] especially of the ethmoid. It is more common in cold weather when the frequency of sinusitis increases. Other less common causes are penetrating orbital trauma, especially when there is a retained foreign body, dental infections,[16] extraocular muscle and retinal surgery,[17] and hematogenous spread during a systemic infectious illness.

Orbital cellulitis is always serious and potentially sight- and life-threatening, giving rise to a variety of systemic and ocular complications (Box 13.1). In the preantibiotic era one-fifth of patients died from septic intracranial complications; one-third of the survivors lost vision in the affected eye.[18] This poor outlook has been dramatically altered by effective antibiotics and the changing spectrum of causative organisms but prompt diagnosis and vigorous treatment are still essential.

History

The usual presentation is with a painful red eye and increasing lid edema in a child who has had a recent upper respiratory tract infection. The child is usually miserable, pyrexial, and unwell.

Box 13.1

Complications of orbital cellulitis

Optic neuritis
Optic atrophy
Exposure keratitis
Central retinal artery occlusion[19]
Retinal and choroidal ischemia[20]
Subperiosteal and orbital abscess[23, 24]
Cavernous sinus thrombosis
Meningitis[12]
Brain abscess
Septicemia[22]

Table 13.3 – The differential diagnosis of inflammatory proptosis

Infection	Orbital cellulitis or cavernous sinus thrombosis
Idiopathic and specific inflammation	Orbital idiopathic inflammation, myositis, sarcoidosis, and Wegener's granulomatosis
Neoplasia	Leukemia, Burkitt's lymphoma, rhabdomyosarcoma, ruptured retinoblastoma, metastatic carcinoma, histiocytosis X (Letterer-Siwe variety), dermoid cyst (rupture and inflammation), and ethmoid osteoma
Trauma	Traumatic hematoma, orbital emphysema, retained foreign body
Systemic	Sickle cell disease (bone infarction) conditions
Endocrine	Dysthyroid exophthalmos (very rare) dysfunction

Modified from Jain A, Rubin PA. Orbital cellulitis in children. Int Ophthalmol Clin 2001; 41: 71–86.

Examination

There are signs of orbital dysfunction, including proptosis, reduced and painful extraocular movements, and optic nerve dysfunction. There may be involvement of cranial nerves III, IV, and VI, especially with superior orbital fissure and cavernous sinus involvement. Visual loss, when it occurs, is usually due to an optic neuropathy but may also be caused by exposure keratitis or a retinal vascular occlusion.[19,20]

The acute, sometimes explosive, onset of pain, fever, and systemic illness helps to differentiate orbital cellulitis from most other causes of inflammatory proptosis which should always be considered when seeing a patient with cellulitis (Table 13.3) (Fig. 13.8A–D).

Orbital cellulitis is partially constrained by the septum at the arcus marginalis; the preseptal soft tissue signs may be less dramatic than those in preseptal cellulitis. Conjunctival chemosis and injection may be subtle or even absent.

Management

Children with orbital cellulitis should be admitted under the care of pediatricians, ophthalmologists, ENT surgeons, and the infectious disease team. Blood cultures, nasal, throat, and conjunctival microbiology swabs may be taken. These are often negative, but a positive result is helpful in planning antibiotic treatment. This should not delay immediate and appropriate intravenous antibiotics and fluid resuscitation where necessary.

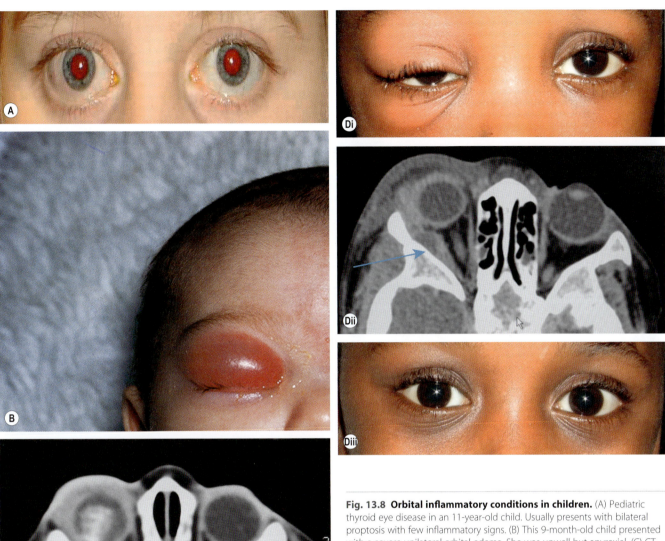

Fig. 13.8 Orbital inflammatory conditions in children. (A) Pediatric thyroid eye disease in an 11-year-old child. Usually presents with bilateral proptosis with few inflammatory signs. (B) This 9-month-old child presented with a severe unilateral orbital edema. She was unwell but apyrexial. (C) CT scan shows bilateral retinoblastoma; large and calcified on the right, small on the left. She was treated with systemic steroids, which abolished the orbital edema, the right eye was enucleated, and the left was given local treatment. She is alive and well 7 years later with a left visual acuity of 6/5. (Di) Orbital cellulitis in a child with sickle cell crisis; (Dii) CT scan shows lateral orbital abscess with possible bone infarction (arrow); (Diii) resolved with antibiotics and fluid management.

The initial treatment of orbital cellulitis in infants should be with a high-dose intravenous third-generation cephalosporin such as cefotaxime, ceftazidime, or ceftriaxone combined with a penicillinase-resistant penicillin. In older children, sinusitis is frequently caused by mixed aerobic and anaerobic organisms; so, clindamycin may be substituted for penicillinase-resistant penicillin. Metronidazole is now being increasingly used in younger children. An alternative regimen is the combination of penicillinase-resistant penicillin with chloramphenicol (see Table 13.2). The initial regime may be modified after culture results. Nasal decongestants such as ephedrine may be helpful in promoting intranasal drainage of infected sinuses. The child should be monitored closely for deterioration of ocular and systemic signs and management modified.

Orbital imaging

Computed tomography (CT) is the investigation of choice. CT is usually readily available. The quick acquisition of images, compared to magnetic resonance imaging (MRI), make it ideal for children in the urgent care setting of orbital cellulitis. CT will define the extent of sinus disease, subperiosteal or orbital abscess, and intracranial involvement. Although a CT scan may detect subperiosteal (Figs 13.9 and 13.10) and orbital abscesses not apparent clinically or on plain films,[11,21] the management of mild and moderate orbital cellulitis without optic nerve compromise or intracranial complications is initially medical. Imaging may be unnecessary unless there is a poor response to intravenous antibiotics, increasing systemic signs, progression of orbital signs, or expectant surgical management. MRI scanning is advantageous in that there is no

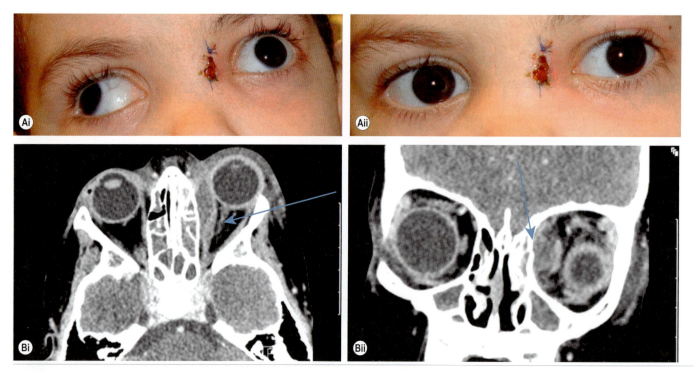

Fig. 13.9 (A) 5-year-old child with a large medial subperiosteal abscess with poor adduction responded poorly to antibiotics and required drainage of the abscess through an external approach. (B) CT scan shows ethmoid sinusitis and lens shape deformity of the subperiosteal abscess (arrows) in the axial and coronal planes.

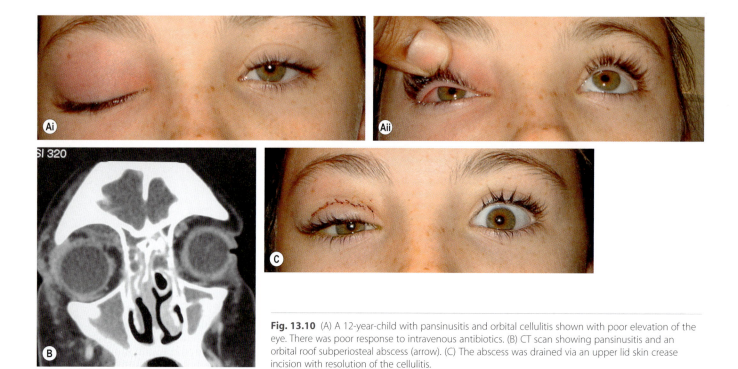

Fig. 13.10 (A) A 12-year-child with pansinusitis and orbital cellulitis shown with poor elevation of the eye. There was poor response to intravenous antibiotics. (B) CT scan showing pansinusitis and an orbital roof subperiosteal abscess (arrow). (C) The abscess was drained via an upper lid skin crease incision with resolution of the cellulitis.

radiation exposure, but the long acquisition time and the need for sedation or anesthesia in children makes it a second line modality. It is more sensitive than CT in detecting intracranial complications such as cavernous sinus thrombosis where a false negative CT is more likely in early disease. MRI may be more sensitive than CT in delineating the extent of fungal sinus disease. The T2 weighted MRI in mycotic infection may appear hypodense due to paramagnetic material produced by the fungi.[22]

Sinus X-rays may be difficult to interpret in small children due to the lack of development of the sinuses and are generally unhelpful.

Microbiology of preseptal and orbital cellulitis

Historically, the most feared pathogen in both preseptal and orbital cellulitis, as well as sinusitis, was *H. influenzae* type B (Hib). Vaccination against Hib was widely available from 1990. In a study of 315 preseptal and orbital cellulitis cases 297 were preseptal and 18 were orbital cellulitis. Before 1990, 12% were found to be Hib-related cellulitis and after 1990, 3.5%. The overall rate of cellulitis also declined by 60% in the 1990s.[3] The dramatic decline of culture-positive infection may be due to higher threshold for admission (managed care), improved general child health, and earlier and more aggressive outpatient use of antibiotics (e.g. oral cephalosporins).

In younger children, the most common pathogens, after the decline in Hib infections, became *Staphylococcus aureus* and *Staphylococcus epidermidis*; *Streptococcus pneumoniae*, *S. pyogenes*, and *S. sanguinis*; and *Moraxella catarrhalis*.[3,6] This mirrors the microbiology of sinusitis. Older children have bacteriologically more complex sinus infections and, therefore, orbital cellulitis.[23] Polymicrobial infections and anaerobic infections are more common in older children.

Methicillin-resistant *S. aureus* (MRSA) orbital cellulitis is a serious concern. The empiric antibiotic choice is changing with the increasing use of vancomycin even in areas with a low prevalence of MRSA. MRSA was reported in as high as 73% of all *S. aureus* orbital cellulitis isolates in one recent US study.[24] However, two other contemporary studies reported 1% of patients or 12% of *S. aureus* isolates to be methicillin resistant.[25,26] The variation highlights the need for obtaining microbiology samples where possible and developing a locally tailored antibiotic policy in conjunction with a microbiologist. Treatment options for MRSA orbital cellulitis include vancomycin or clindamycin.

Fungal infections are rare but should be considered when orbital cellulitis occurs in an immunosuppressed or diabetic child.[27] Those with cystic fibrosis are more likely to be infected with *Pseudomonas aeruginosa* or *S. aureus*.

Subperiosteal and orbital abscess

The incidence of subperiosteal and orbital abscess complicating orbital cellulitis was about 10%,[28] but is now declining. Most have sinus infection. In subperiosteal abscess, a purulent infection within a sinus, usually the ethmoids, breaks through the thin orbital bony wall (lamina papyracea) and lies beneath the loosely adherent periosteum, which is easily lifted off the bone, giving a convex "lens" type of appearance on CT scanning. An orbital abscess occurs either when a subperiosteal abscess breaches the periorbita or when a collection of pus forms within the orbit.

The common causative organism is *Staphylococcus* but *Streptococcus*, *H. influenzae*, and anerobic organisms may also be responsible. It should be suspected whenever there is marked systemic toxicity and orbital signs, or when orbital cellulitis is slow to respond to adequate intravenous antibiotics. The presence of subperiosteal abscess may be indicated by lateral displacement of the globe away from the infected sinus, impaired adduction, and resistance to retropulsion.[29]

All studies have recommended hospitalization for intravenous antibiotic therapy (see Table 13.2) and repeated eye examinations to evaluate progression of infection or involvement of the optic nerve.

CT scanning (Fig. 13.4) at presentation is not always necessary, especially if there is mild orbital cellulitis with clear findings of sinusitis and no optic nerve compromise or intracranial signs but is indicated if the presentation is unusual, severe, in an older child, or there are optic nerve or intracranial signs. If the child does not respond to treatment, it would be advisable to image the sinuses, orbits, and intracranial compartment with a CT scan (Figs 13.11 and 13.12). A contrast-enhanced scan gives additional information in differentiating an abscess, which is amenable to drainage, from a phlegmon (purulent tissue inflammation), which is not.

An orbital abscess should be drained. The management of subperiosteal abscess is more controversial[6] because they may resolve with medical treatment.[6,23,30]

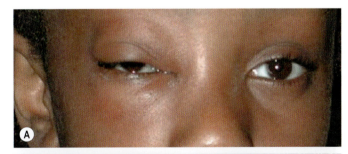

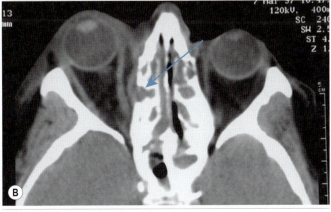

Fig. 13.11 (A) 7-year-old child with right orbital cellulitis, proptosis, white eye, limitation of eye movements, but no optic nerve compromise. (B) CT scan shows ethmoid sinusitis, significant proptosis, and a small medial subperiosteal abscess (arrow). He was successfully treated with antibiotics alone and did not need surgical intervention

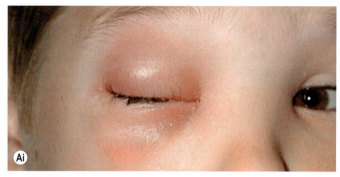

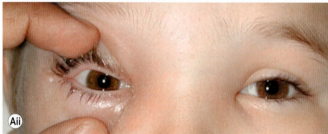

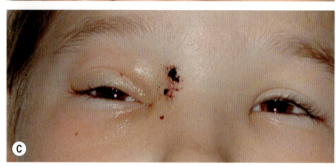

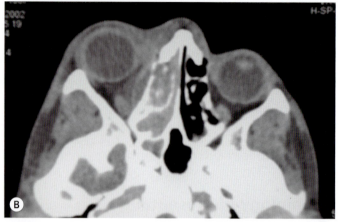

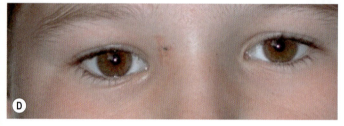

Fig. 13.12 (A) Orbital cellulitis with a white eye. (B) CT scan shows sinusitis and a subperiosteal abscess (arrow). Child deteriorated despite adequate intravenous antibiotics. (C) Drainage of ethmoid sinus and subperiosteal abscess was performed. (D) Patient made a good recovery.

In a review of 37 patients with subperiosteal abscess secondary to sinusitis resolution occurred in 83% of patients under 9 years of age who were treated medically or who had negative cultures on drainage.[31] In contrast, only 25% of those aged between 9 and 14 years cleared without drainage or had negative cultures on drainage. The remaining group, aged 15 years and over, were refractory to medical therapy alone. In a review of the management of subperiosteal abscess the authors found if the abscess was smaller than 10 mm, medical treatment alone was successful in 81% of patients. In contrast, 92% of patients with an abscess larger than 10 mm underwent surgery.[32]

Nine children (2 months to 4 years) with subperiosteal abscesses were managed with a third-generation cephalosporin and vancomycin in the first 24 to 36 hours; only one required surgical drainage, this case being culture-negative. This supports an initial medical management approach for most patients with subperiosteal or orbital abscesses resulting in orbital cellulitis.[6]

Garcia and Harris[23] advocate a non-surgical management of subperiosteal abscess with the presence of four criteria:

1. Age less than 9 years
2. No visual compromise
3. Medial abscess of modest size
4. No intracranial or frontal sinus involvement

In their prospective study of 29 patients fulfilling the above criteria, 27 (93%) were managed successfully with only medical therapy. Only two patients had surgical intervention with successful outcomes.[23]

It seems reasonable to initially treat medically if vision is normal, there is no intracranial extension, the subperiosteal abscess is of moderate size, and the child is under 9 years of age (see Figs 13.11 and 13.12).

Osteomyelitis of the superior maxilla

This rare condition, which usually presents in the first few months of life with fever, general malaise, and marked periorbital edema, may be confused with orbital cellulitis or subperiosteal abscess. The diagnosis should be suspected if there is pus in the nostril and edema of the alveolus and palate on the affected side. An oral fistula may be present. Imaging supports the diagnosis. *Staphylococcus aureus* is the usual infecting organism. Treatment is with high-dose intravenous antibiotics chosen on the basis of culture and sensitivity and surgical drainage of the abscess preferably via the nose.

Cavernous sinus thrombosis

Since the introduction of antibiotics this dreaded complication of orbital cellulitis has become rare. Previously, mortality was almost 100%.[33] In its early stages, cavernous sinus thrombosis may be difficult to distinguish clinically from orbital cellulitis. There is more severe pain, a marked systemic illness, proptosis develops rapidly, and there may be third, fourth, and sixth cranial nerve palsies compared with the mechanical limitation seen in orbital cellulitis.

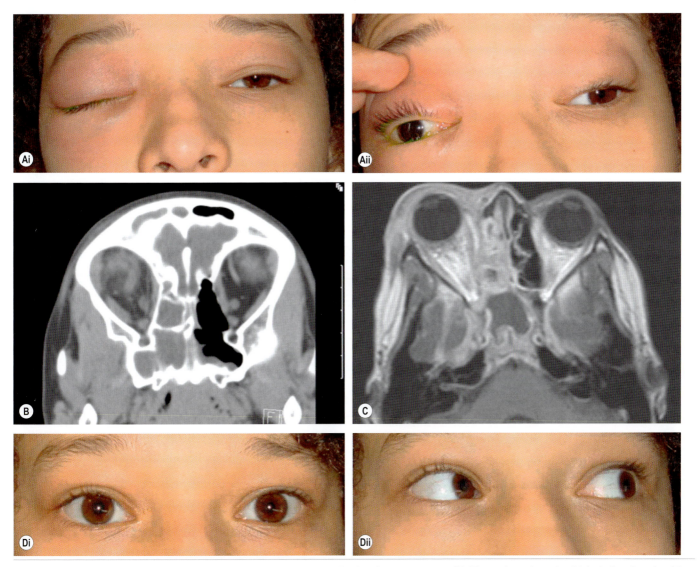

Fig. 13.13 (A) A very unwell 13-year-child with orbital cellulitis, proptosis, and reduced eye movements. (B) CT scan showed pansinusitis including the ethmoids and sphenoid sinus and a dilated cavernous sinus and superior ophthalmic vein (arrows). (C) MRI confirmed a cavernous sinus thrombosis, with flow voids. (D) She made an excellent recovery with antibiotics and anticoagulation.

Hyperalgesia in the distribution of the fifth cranial nerve is common. The presence of retinal venous dilatation and optic disc swelling, especially if bilateral, is very suggestive of cavernous sinus thrombosis. In the later stages, bilateral involvement in cavernous sinus thrombosis makes the clinical distinction from orbital cellulitis easier.

Diagnosis can be supported by CT findings and better confirmed with an MRI scan. Cavernous sinus thrombosis is most frequently associated with *S. aureus* infection[34] (Fig. 13.13).

Management is best undertaken by a pediatric neurologist or neurosurgeon and involves treatment with high-dose intravenous antibiotics. The use of anticoagulants and systemic steroids requires careful consideration.

Fungal orbital cellulitis orbital mucormycosis

Orbital fungal infection should be suspected in any diabetic or immunosuppressed[25] child or one with gastroenteritis and metabolic acidosis[35] who develops a rapidly progressive orbital cellulitis, especially if accompanied by necrosis of the skin or nasal mucosa.

Fungal orbital cellulitis has been described in otherwise healthy children.[36,37] Untreated, it is rapidly fatal.

Colonization of the sinuses by spores followed by direct or hematogenous spread to the orbit occurs, which is heralded by periorbital pain, marked lid edema, conjunctival chemosis, and proptosis. Later, spread to the orbital apex results in third, fourth, and sixth cranial nerve palsies and optic neuropathy. Mucomycosis and aspergillosis have a tendency to invade vessel walls causing thrombosis and subsequent ischemia. Involvement of the facial arteries causes gangrene of the nose, palate, and facial tissues resulting in necrosis. Central retinal artery occlusion and cerebral infarction can result. Once spread to the cavernous sinus and intracranial vessels occurs the prognosis is very poor.

Scrapings from infected tissues should be cultured and Gram and Giemsa stained. Larger tissue biopsies should be fixed in 10% formalin and processed for histologic examination. These

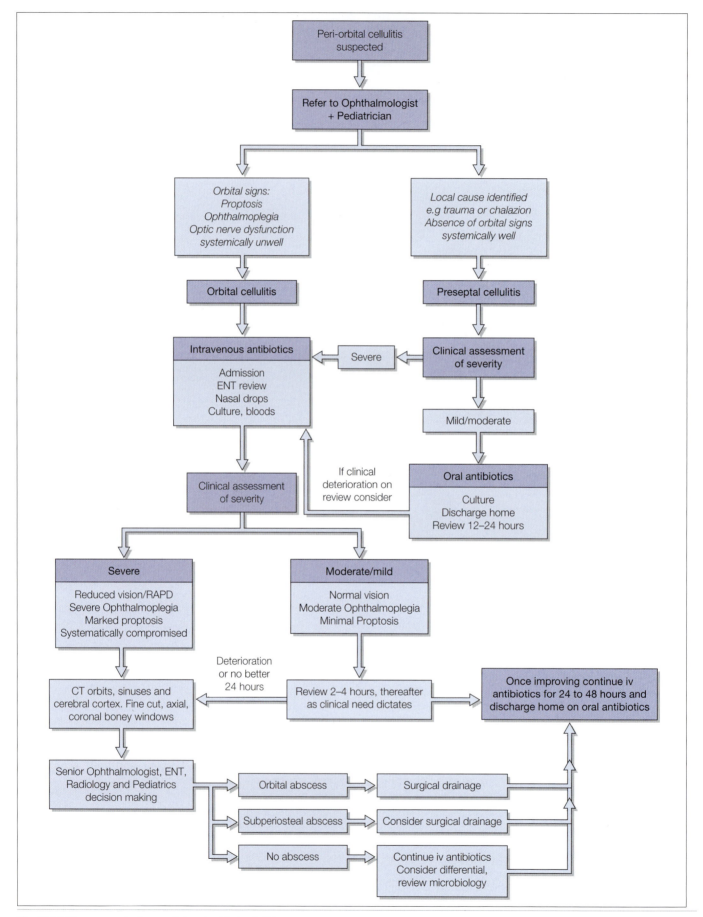

Fig. 13.14 Management of preseptal and orbital cellulitis.

fungi have an affinity for hematoxylin and are, therefore, easily recognized in hematoxylin and eosin sections.

The management consists of specific antifungal therapy, correction of the underlying metabolic or immunologic abnormality and surgical debridement of necrotic tissues. The specific treatment of choice is amphotericin B, which should be given intravenously and may also be used locally to irrigate infected sinuses.[38] It is nephrotoxic so renal function should be carefully monitored.

For further information on the management of preseptal and orbital cellulitis please see Fig. 13.14.

References

1. Chandler JR, Langenbrunner DJ, Stevens ER. The pathogenesis of orbital complications of acute sinusitis. Laryngoscope 1970; 80: 1414–28.
2. Uzcategui N, Warman R, Smith A, Howard CW. Clinical practice guidelines for the management of orbital cellulitis. J Pediatr Ophthalmol Strabismus 1998; 35: 73–9
3. Ambati BK, Ambati J, Azar N, et al. Periorbital and orbital cellulitis before and after the advent of Haemophilus influenzae type B vaccination. Ophthalmology 2000; 107: 1450–3.
4. Sheard RM, Pandey KR, Barnes ND, Vivian AJ. Kawasaki disease presenting as orbital cellulitis. J Pediatr Ophthalmol Strabismus 2000; 37: 123–5.
5. Ruttum MS, Ogawa G. Adenovirus conjunctivitis mimics preseptal and orbital cellulitis in young children. Pediatr Infect Dis J 1996; 15: 266–7.
6. Starkey CR, Steele RW. Medical management of orbital cellulitis. Pediatr Infect Dis J 2001; 20: 1002–5.
7. Jones DB. Discussion on paper by Weiss et al. Bacterial periorbital cellulitis and orbital cellulitis in childhood. Ophthalmology 1983; 90: 201–3.
8. Ciarallo LR, Rowe PC. Lumbar puncture in children with periorbital and orbital cellulitis. J Pediatr 1993; 122: 355–9.
9. Durand M. Intravenous antibiotics in sinusitis. Otolaryngol Head Neck Surg 1999; 7: 7.
10. Healy GB. Comment on: "Chandler et al. The pathogenesis of orbital complications in acute sinusitis. Laryngoscope 1970; 80: 1414–28." Laryngoscope 1997; 107: 441–6.
11. Goldberg F, Berne AS, Oski FA. Differentiation of orbital cellulitis from preseptal cellulitis by computed tomography. Paediatrics 1978; 62: 1000–5.
12. Weiss A, Friendly D, Eglin K, et al. Bacterial periorbital and orbital cellulitis in childhood. Ophthalmology 1983; 90: 195–203.
13. Rose GE, Howard DJ, Watts MR. Periorbital necrotising fasciitis. Eye 1991; 5: 736–40.
14. Stevens DL. Streptococcal toxic shock syndrome associated with necrotizing fasciitis. Annu Rev Med 2000; 51: 271–88.
15. Watters E, Wallar PH, Hiles DA, Michaels RH. Acute orbital cellulitis. Arch Ophthalmol 1976; 94: 785–8.
16. Flood TP, Braude LS, Jampol LM, Herzog S. Computed tomography in the management of orbital infections associated with dental disease. Br J Ophthalmol 1982; 66: 269–74.
17. von Noorden GK. Orbital cellulitis following extraocular muscle surgery. Am J Ophthalmol 1972; 74: 627–9.
18. Duke-Elder S. Acute orbital inflammations. In: Duke-Elder S, editor. The Ocular Adnexa. London: Henry Kimpton; 1952: 5427–48. (System of Ophthalmology, Vol. 5.)
19. Jarrett WH, Gutman FA. Ocular complications of infection in the paranasal sinuses. Arch Ophthalmol 1969; 81: 683–8.
20. Sherry T. Acute infarction of the choroid and retina. Br J Ophthalmol 1973; 57: 133–7.
21. Rudloe TF, Harper MB, Prabhu SP, et al. Acute periorbital infections: who needs emergency imaging? Pediatrics 2010; 125: e719–26.
22. Eustis HS, Mafee MF, Walton C, Mondonca J. MR imaging and CT of orbital infections and complications in acute rhinosinusitis. Radiol Clin North Am 1998; 36: 1165–83.
23. Garcia GH, Harris GJ. Criteria for nonsurgical management of subperiosteal abscess of the orbit. Ophthalmology 2000; 107: 1454–58
24. Jain A, Rubin PA. Orbital cellulitis in children. Int Ophthalmol Clin 2001; 41: 71–86.
25. Seltz LB, Smith J, Durairaj VD, et al. Microbiology and antibiotic management of orbital cellulitis. Pediatrics 2011; 127: e566–72.
26. McKinley SH, Yen MT, Miller AM, Yen KG. Microbiology of pediatric orbital cellulitis. Am J Ophthalmol 2007; 144: 497–501.
27. Schwartz JN, Donnelly EH, Klintworth GK. Ocular and orbital phycomycosis. Surv Ophthalmol 1977; 22: 3–28.
28. Hornblass A, Herschorn BJ, Stern K, Grimes C. Orbital abscess. Surv Ophthalmol 1984; 29: 169–78.
29. Harris GJ. Subperiosteal abscess of the orbit. Arch Ophthalmol 1983; 101: 751–7.
30. Rubin SE, Zito J. Orbital sub-periosteal abscess responding to medical therapy. J Pediatr Ophthalmol Strabismus 1994; 31: 325–6.
31. Harris GJ. Subperiosteal abscess of the orbit. Ophthalmology 1994; 101: 585–95.
32. Ryan JT, Preciado DA, Bauman N, et al. Management of pediatric orbital cellulitis in patients with radiographic findings of subperiosteal abscess. Otolaryngol Head Neck Surg 2009; 140: 907–11
33. Grove WE. Septic and aseptic types of thrombosis of the cavernous sinus. Arch Otolaryngol 1936; 24: 29–50.
34. Southwick FS, Richardson EP, Swartz MN. Septic thrombosis of the dural sinuses. Medicine 1986; 65: 82–106.
35. Hale LM. Orbito-cerebral phycomycosis. Arch Ophthalmol 1971; 86: 39–43.
36. Blodi FC, Hannah FT, Wadsworth JA. Lethal orbitocerebral phycomycosis in otherwise healthy children. Am J Ophthalmol 1969; 67: 698–705.
37. Whitehurst FO, Listen TE. Orbital aspergillosis: report of a case in a child. J Pediatr Ophthalmol 1981; 18: 50–4.
38. Lee EJ, Lee MY, Hung YC, Wang LC. Orbital rhinocerebral mucormycosis associated with diabetic ketoacidosis: report of survival of a 10-year-old boy. J Formos Med Assoc 1998; 97: 720–3.

Endophthalmitis

Donal Brosnahan

Infectious endophthalmitis occurs when bacteria, fungi, parasites, or viruses enter the eye following a breach of the outer wall of the eye (exogenous endophthalmitis), or when microorganisms enter the eye from a source elsewhere in the body (endogenous endophthalmitis). Exogenous endophthalmitis most frequently arises following surgery but may be a consequence of trauma. Endogenous endophthalmitis usually results from hematogenous spread of infection. Exogenous endophthalmitis may be sub-classified into acute and chronic. The classification of endophthalmitis is important as each type has a characteristic clinical setting, differing spectrum of microorganisms, and varying visual prognosis.

Clinical presentation

The presentation of bacterial endophthalmitis depends on the route of infection and the virulence of the microorganism. Acute postoperative endophthalmitis typically presents 1–3 days after surgery with pain and decreased vision. There is often lid swelling, conjunctival injection, corneal edema, and chemosis. Intraocular findings include uveitis, hypopyon, vitreous cells, and occasionally sheathing of blood vessels. In children, presentation and treatment are often delayed particularly following trauma where occult penetration may go undetected.

Infection with less virulent organisms may result in chronic or late onset endophthalmitis, which may run an indolent course with exacerbations and remissions. Intraocular inflammation is less severe, but hypopyon and vitreous activity may be present. The presence of creamy white plaques on the posterior capsule following cataract surgery is suggestive of *Propionibacterium* infection. In endophthalmitis following penetrating injury there may be a persistent severe uveitis and

vitreous haze with infiltration of the wound edges. Retinal periphlebitis may be an early sign of bacterial endophthalmitis. Endophthalmitis should be suspected after intraocular surgery or traumatic perforation whenever the inflammation is greater than expected. Serial and frequent examinations may be necessary. The main differential diagnoses are fungal endophthalmitis and severe uveitis. Rarely, retinoblastoma or metastatic tumor may present with uveitis and hypopyon.

Exogenous bacterial endophthalmitis

Cataract surgery

Exogenous endophthalmitis in adults occurs most frequently following intraocular surgery (70–80%). Cataract extraction has a reported incidence of postoperative endophthalmitis of 0.1–0.38%[1] (Fig. 14.1). Good et al. reported an incidence of 0.45% in a retrospective review of 641 cases of cataract extraction in children.[2] Wheeler et al. reported an incidence of 0.07% in children undergoing cataract and glaucoma surgery.[3]

Endophthalmitis following cataract surgery in adults is associated with rupture of the posterior capsule. Surgery for congenital cataract, whether lensectomy or lens aspiration, usually involves breach of the posterior capsule. Therefore, one might expect a higher incidence of postoperative endophthalmitis

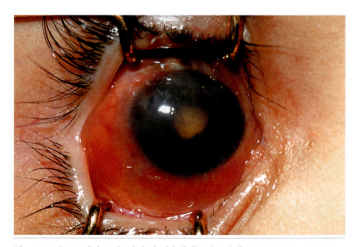

Fig. 14.1 Bacterial endophthalmitis following infant cataract surgery and intraocular lens implantation.

similar to that reported in intracapsular cataract, posterior capsular tear, and anterior vitrectomy.

Toxic anterior segment syndrome (TASS) may be difficult to distinguish from infective endophthalmitis. TASS is a sterile inflammatory response usually occurring in the first 48 hours following cataract surgery. If doubt exists as to whether the patient has endophthalmitis or TASS, vitreous biopsy and intravitreal antibiotics are warranted.

The Endophthalmitis Vitrectomy Study (EVS) studied 420 cases of infectious endophthalmitis presenting within 6 weeks of cataract extraction or secondary intraocular lens implantation.[4] Positive culture was obtained from 69.3% of intraocular specimens. Gram-positive bacteria were isolated in 94.2% of cases and Gram-negative bacteria in 6.5% of isolates. *Staphylococcus epidermidis*, normal skin flora, was by far the most common gram-positive isolate (70%), followed by *Staphylococcus aureus* (9.9%), *Streptococcus* spp. (2.2%), and *Propionibacterium acnes*. *Proteus* and *Pseudomonas* were the most common Gram-negative organisms. *Haemophilus influenzae* has also been identified in other series.[5] Weinstein's study of children with endophthalmitis reported similar results, 75% of culture positive cases being caused by Gram-positive organisms.[6] *Staphylococcus epidermidis*, *Streptococcus pneumoniae*, and *Staphylococcus aureus* have been identified as the most frequent infecting agents in children following cataract extraction.

Trauma

Trauma is a significant cause of exogenous endophthalmitis in children. Endophthalmitis following penetrating injury accounted for 44% of cases in a 10-year review of pediatric endophthalmitis.[7] The incidence of endophthalmitis after penetrating injury ranges from 4% to 20% and is particularly high when injury occurs in a rural setting.[8] Eight-five percent of patients in the Endophthalmitis Vitrectomy Study (EVS) achieved final visual acuity of 20/400 or better while only 22–42% achieved this level of acuity following post-traumatic endophthalmitis.[4,9]

Poor visual outcome results from delayed diagnosis and treatment. Damage to ocular structures and retained intraocular foreign body also are contributory factors to poor visual outcome. In adults with post-traumatic endophthalmitis, *Staphylococcus epidermidis* and *Bacillus* spp. are the most frequent pathogens. In a review of post-traumatic endophthalmitis in children *Streptococcal* spp. were isolated in 25.9%, *Staphylococcus* in 18.5%, and *Bacillus* spp. in 22% of cases.

Glaucoma filtration surgery

Infection associated with filtration surgery is often subclassified into blebitis, defined as mucopurulent material in and around the bleb associated with anterior segment activity but without hypopyon. If a hypopyon is present, or there is evidence of vitreous activity, a diagnosis of endophthalmitis is made. Endophthalmitis may occur soon after surgery, but is frequently reported many years after surgery. Antimetabolites such as 5-fluorouracil (5-FU) and mitomycin C are used to augment filtration surgery in childhood glaucoma. While improving the success rate of filtration surgery they increase the risk of postoperative endophthalmitis. When intraoperative 5-FU is used, the reported incidence of endophthalmitis is 1–5.7%. The incidence of endophthalmitis is 0.3–4.9% when mitomycin C is applied.[10]

Implantation of glaucoma drainage devices is associated with increased rates of endophthalmitis. A review of 542 eyes with Ahmed valve insertion noted an endophthalmitis rate significantly higher in children. The incidence in adults was 1.7%, compared to 4.4% in children.[11] Endophthalmitis is often associated with conjunctival erosion and tube exposure; inferior placement of bleb or drainage device is also associated with higher rates of infection. When endophthalmitis is related to glaucoma surgery, the spectrum of microorganisms differs from that in cataract surgery in that streptococcal species predominate. *Haemophilus influenzae* is also isolated more frequently than *Staphylococcus epidermidis*. This difference may reflect the fact that endophthalmitis is often of late onset with invasion of microorganisms through thin walled or leaking blebs.[12] Jampel et al. found increased incidence of endophthalmitis associated with full thickness filtration procedures, inferior placed blebs, bleb leakage, and the use of mitomycin.[13] If endophthalmitis develops in the early postoperative period, *Staphylococcus epidermidis* is more frequently cultured.

Strabismus surgery

Endophthalmitis following strabismus surgery is rare, with an incidence of 1:3500 to 1:185000.[14] Scleral perforation is thought to be a prerequisite for the development of endophthalmitis following strabismus surgery. Spatulated needles have greatly reduced the frequency of scleral perforation during strabismus surgery. Needles and sutures are frequently contaminated despite the use of preoperative povidone-iodine. Carothers et al. noted 19% of needles and 24% of sutures were culture positive in patients undergoing strabismus surgery.[15] When scleral perforation has been noted, a dilated fundal examination is indicated and laser photocoagulation or cryotherapy to any retinal lesions should be considered. Many surgeons would ask the help of a retinal surgeon in this (see Chapter 86). Periocular and systemic antibiotics may reduce the risk of endophthalmitis following perforation.

Streptococcus pneumoniae, *Staphylococcus aureus*, *Haemophilus influenzae*, and *Staphylococcus epidermidis* have been isolated in cases of endophthalmitis associated with strabismus surgery. It appears that infection with more virulent organisms is more frequent than infection following cataract surgery. Visual prognosis is poor as a consequence of delayed diagnosis and the virulence of the infecting organisms.

Intravitreal injection

Anti-vascular endothelial growth factor (anti-VEGF) is an effective treatment for some forms of retinopathy of prematurity. Anti-VEGF is delivered by intravitreal injection; in adults endophthalmitis rates range from 0.019% to 0.07% when it is used to treat age-related macular degeneration.[16] Exogenous endophthalmitis may also arise secondary to suppurative keratitis associated with exposure or trauma (Fig. 14.2).

Prevention

The patient is the most common source of postoperative infection. Children with extraocular infection, blepharitis, conjunctivitis, or with impaired nasolacrimal drainage should have surgery deferred until these are remedied. Surgery should

Box 14.1

Initial antibiotic treatment of bacterial endophthalmitis

Intravitreal antibiotics

Vancomycin 1 mg in 0.1 ml of normal saline

and ceftazidime 2.25 mg in 0.1 ml of normal saline

or Amikacin 0.4 mg in 0.1 ml of normal saline and

ceftazidime 2 mg in 0.1 ml of normal saline

Systemic antibiotics

Vancomycin 44 mg/kg per day

and ceftazidime 100–150 mg/kg per day

or Ciprofloxacin 5–10 mg/kg per day

Topical antibiotics

Vancomycin 50 mg/ml hourly

and ceftazidime 50 mg/ml hourly

or Gentamicin 14 mg/ml hourly

Box 14.2

Risk factors for endogenous endophthalmitis in children

Bacterial

Immunosuppression

Bacterial endocarditis

Meningococcal infection

Gastrointestinal sepsis

Fungal

Prematurity

Parenteral nutrition

Immunosuppression

Broad-spectrum antibiotics

Retinopathy of prematurity

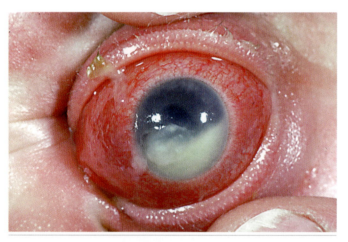

Fig. 14.2 Endophthalmitis with hypopyon following exposure keratitis in an infant with Crouzon's disease.

also be deferred in the presence of upper respiratory tract infection.

Preoperative application of aqueous povidone-iodine 5% solution to the conjunctival sac decreases bacterial counts and probably reduces the incidence of endophthalmitis; however, it must be applied at least 3 minutes prior to surgery. In cases of penetrating injury, povidone-iodine should not be applied.

A prospective study by the European Society of Cataract and Refractive Surgeons demonstrated a fivefold decrease in the incidence of postoperative endophthalmitis in patients undergoing phacoemulsification surgery when intracameral cefuroxime (1 mg in 0.1 ml) was given at the end of surgery.[17] It is likely that intracameral cefuroxime results in reduced infection rates in pediatric cataract surgery. Antibiotics in irrigating solutions during cataract surgery do not decrease the incidence of endophthalmitis. Many surgeons inject antibiotics subconjunctivally when performing intraocular surgery; its effectiveness is unproven. There may be a beneficial effect from administering intravitreal antibiotics after repair of penetrating injuries where there is a known higher rate of endophthalmitis.

Management

If endophthalmitis is suspected, it is essential to proceed rapidly and obtain aqueous and vitreous samples before starting antibiotic treatment. General anesthesia will be required to allow thorough examination, collection of specimens, and delivery of intravitreal antibiotics. The microbiologist should be informed to ensure that appropriate culture media are available in the operating room and also to perform Gram and Giemsa stains. Specimens should be sent immediately to the laboratory. Aqueous and vitreous specimens are plated on appropriate agar to facilitate culture of the potential pathogens, e.g. blood agar, chocolate agar, and Sabouraud's dextrose agar. Specimens should be placed on glass slides for Gram and Giemsa stains. Culture for up to 2 weeks is required to allow growth of anaerobes such as *Propionibacterium spp.* and fungal species. *Propionibacterium acnes* may be sequestered in folds of the posterior capsule and, if suspected, removal of capsular remnants for culture may be helpful in confirming the diagnosis.

Polymerase chain reaction (PCR) is a highly sensitive and specific test, which can be employed to rapidly identify bacteria, fungi, and viruses resulting in early diagnosis and appropriate antibiotic therapy. It is particularly helpful in culture-negative cases or when the patient has been commenced on antimicrobial therapy before samples are obtained. Care must be taken to minimize the risk of contamination of the specimen with environmental organisms, which may cause a false positive PCR result. Positive PCR results with a negative culture must be interpreted with caution; always consider whether the PCR result is a recognized ocular pathogen and also consider the clinical context.

Vitreous samples are preferably obtained using a mechanical cutter: 0.2 ml is removed for culture and staining. Care must be taken in infants as the pars plana is poorly developed. Therefore, sclerotomies should be anteriorly placed. If an intraocular lens has not been inserted, an anterior approach is possible.

Once vitreous sampling has been completed, antibiotics are injected into the vitreous cavity: vancomycin, 1 mg in 0.1 ml of normal saline, and ceftazidime, 2 mg in 0.1 ml of normal saline. Vancomycin is effective against Gram-positive bacteria and ceftazidime against Gram-negative organisms.

Dexamethasone, 0.4 mg in 0.1 ml, may also be given intravitreally to reduce the inflammatory response. Antibiotics are delivered with a 30-gauge needle using separate syringes for each antibiotic. Most antibiotic has left the eye by 48 hours and consideration should be given to repeating the injections after this period.

The EVS did not show any additional benefit from using systemic antibiotics to supplement intravitreal therapy. In the EVS, systemic treatment consisted of amikacin and ceftazidime; however, this may be suboptimal as vancomycin is more effective against Gram-positive cocci. Systemic antimicrobial therapy is indicated in cases of endogenous endophthalmitis secondary to blood stream infection or infection at a distant focus.

Subconjunctival antibiotics do not penetrate the vitreous cavity well and have limited use. Topical antibiotics may be used to supplement intravitreal injection if there is superficial infection or suppurative keratitis (vancomycin 50 mg/ml and ceftazidime 50 mg/ml or amikacin 25 mg/ml). Treatment regimens need to take into account the clinical setting and the likely infecting microorganisms. Antibiotic therapy should be reviewed in the light of clinical response and culture results.

Consult with your vitreoretinal colleagues for consideration of early virectomy. The management of endophthalmitis following cataract has been greatly influenced by the EVS. The key findings of this study were:

1. Immediate vitrectomy is not indicated if the visual acuity is better than light perception.
2. If visual acuity is light perception only then there is a significant benefit from vitrectomy.
3. There is no additional therapeutic benefit from the use of systemic antibiotics.

Vitrectomy decreases the bacterial load and removes toxins and inflammatory mediators from the eye. Removal of opaque vitreous will hasten visual rehabilitation. It may be very difficult in some children to establish a reliable visual acuity. It should be noted that in this study the systemic antibiotics used differed from those given intravitreally and would not therefore have helped to maintain intraocular antibiotic levels. The role of vitrectomy in endophthalmitis associated with strabismus or glaucoma surgery has not been established. However, the same general principles apply.

Endogenous bacterial endophthalmitis

Endogenous or metastatic bacterial endophthalmitis results from hematogenous spread from a distant focus such as bacterial endocarditis, meningitis, abdominal sepsis, or otitis media. Two to eight percent of all bacterial endophthalmitis cases are endogenous and are frequently bilateral (14–50%).[18] Although symptoms and signs are similar to exogenous endophthalmitis, the clinical setting is different. Systemic symptoms may predominate. Initially, ophthalmological features may be mild and the diagnosis delayed. The presence of red eye in a patient with sepsis should prompt early and full ophthalmological examination.

Endogenous endophthalmitis most frequently results from Gram-positive organisms such as *Staphylococcus aureus*, *Streptococcus pneumoniae*, and *Listeria monocytogenes*. Gram-negative infection results from *Neisseria meningitides*,

Haemophilus influenzae, *Klebsiella* spp. and *Escherichia coli*. Gram-positive organisms predominate in North America and Europe with Gram-negative organisms more frequently isolated in Asia.[19] *Klebsiella* species predominate in East Asia, often associated with cholangiohepatitis and liver abscess. Premature infants are more likely to develop endophthalmitis secondary to *Pseudomonas aeruginosa* and *Streptococcus pneumoniae*. These infants are immunocompromised and often dependent on ventilators and humidifiers, which may be a source of nosocomial infection.

Once the diagnosis is suspected, systemic antimicrobial therapy should be commenced. If an infective agent has not been identified from blood culture, aqueous and vitreous specimens should be obtained and intravitreal antibiotics administered covering both Gram-positive and Gram-negative organisms. Blood cultures are positive in up to 72% of cases and are useful in guiding initial antibiotic therapy. If the child presents to the ophthalmologist, urgent assessment by a pediatrician or infectious diseases specialist is indicated. The role of vitrectomy is not established; no prospective studies have been undertaken.

Exogenous fungal endophthalmitis

Exogenous fungal endophthalmitis may complicate penetrating eye injury especially when it occurs in a rural setting and in the presence of retained organic foreign body or fungal keratitis. Presentation may not be until weeks or months after injury. Progressive uveitis, hypopyon, vitritis, and vitreous abscess following penetrating injury should give rise to suspicion of fungal endophthalmitis. Aqueous and vitreous samples should be obtained promptly. Giemsa stain may identify hyphae confirming the diagnosis and facilitating early treatment with intravitreal amphotericin B. Vitrectomy should be considered if there is significant vitreous involvement.

Endogenous fungal endophthalmitis

Endogenous fungal endophthalmitis is usually associated with candida septicemia. Risk factors include immunosuppression, intravenous feeding, and prematurity. *Candida albicans* is the organism most commonly identified in endogenous fungal endophthalmitis although *Aspergillus fumigatus* and *Histoplasma capsulatum*, *Coccidioides immitis*, *Blastomyces dermatiditis*, *Cryptococcus neoformans*, and *Sporotrichum schenckii* have all been implicated.

Neonatal endophthalmitis is almost always endogenous and results from systemic candidiasis. In neonates, candidemia is associated with central venous catheters, parenteral nutrition and the use of broad-spectrum antibiotics. A recent review of the incidence of neonatal endogenous endophthalmitis in the United States demonstrated a significant reduction in the incidence (8.71 cases per 100 000 live births in 1998 and 4.14 cases per 100 000 live births in 2006).[20] This decrease may result from improved care and earlier treatment of neonates with candidemia. Candidemia, retinopathy of prematurity and low birth weight were significant risk factors in the development of endophthalmitis in this study. The presence of retinopathy of prematurity was associated with a twofold increase in the rate of endophthalmitis.

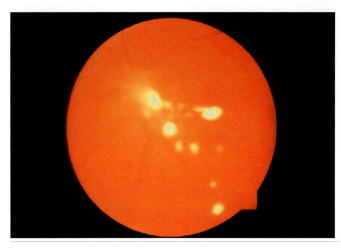

Fig. 14.3 Endogenous *Candida* endophthalmitis in an immunosuppressed child. Note characteristic "string of pearls" appearance of vitreous infiltrates.

Ocular involvement may take the form of chorioretinitis where pale creamy white lesions are noted in the choroid with a predilection for the posterior pole. These lesions may extend into the vitreous to form "puff balls" which, when multiple, have a "string of pearls" appearance (Fig. 14.3). There may be areas of retinal hemorrhage with white centers similar to Roth's spots. Vitreous inflammation is variable. The anterior segments may be involved and secondary cataract has been reported. Early diagnosis and systemic treatment will prevent the progression of chorioretinal lesions to diffuse endophthalmitis. *Aspergillus* endophthalmitis is typically more severe with large confluent areas of chorioretinitis.

Clinical features may suggest the diagnosis; however, blood and urine cultures are useful in diagnosis. If there are positive cultures from blood or urine, it is not necessary to perform vitreous sampling. Giemsa stain and Sabouraud's media are used to identify and culture fungi. PCR is also employed and can rapidly identify fungi from intraocular samples.

In endophthalmitis associated with candidemia, systemic administration of fluocytosine is indicated. Fluocytosine has superior ocular penetration to amphotericin B and is less toxic. If a species other than *Candida* is suspected or confirmed, amphotericin B is more appropriate as it is active against a broader range of fungi. Amphotericin B has significant systemic side effects including nephrotoxicity, neutropenia, and hypokalemia. The use of the liposomal version of amphotericin B (L-AMB) is less toxic than the deoxycholate forms. If there is only chorioretinal involvement without significant vitreous involvement, systemic treatment may suffice. In the presence of vitreous involvement, intravitreal amphotericin B (5 μg in 0.1 ml of normal saline) may be given as an adjunct to systemic therapy. The use of intravitreal steroid remains controversial.

References

1. Desai P, Minassenian DC, Reidy A. National cataract survey 1997–8: a report of the results of the clinical outcomes. Br J Ophthalmol 1999; 83: 1336–40.
2. Good WV, Hing S, Irvine AR, et al. Postoperative endophthalmitis in children following cataract surgery. J Pediatr Ophthalmol Strabismus 1990; 27: 283–5.
3. Wheeler DT, Stager DR, Weakley DR. Endophthalmitis following pediatric intraocular surgery for congenital cataract and congenital glaucoma. J Pediatr Ophthalmol Strabismus 1992; 29: 139–41.
4. Endophthalmitis Vitrectomy Study Group. Results of the Endophthalmitis Vitrectomy Study. Arch Ophthalmol 1995; 113: 1479–96.
5. Doft BH. The endophthalmitis vitrectomy study. Arch Ophthalmol 1991; 109: 487–8.
6. Weinstein GS, Mondino BJ, Weinberg RJ, et al. Endophthalmitis in a pediatric population. Ann Ophthalmol 1979; 11: 935–43.
7. Thordsen JE, Harris L, Hubbard GB 3rd. Pediatric endophthalmitis: a 10-year consecutive series. Retina 2009; 29: 127–36.
8. Verbraeken H, Rysselaere M. Post-traumatic endophthalmitis. Eur J Ophthalmol 1994; 4: 1–5.
9. Sternberg P Jr, Martin DF. Management of endophthalmitis in the post-endophthalmitis vitrectomy study era. Arch Ophthalmol 2001; 119: 754–5.
10. Ang GS, Varga Z, Shaarway T. Postoperative infection in penetrating versus non-pentrating glaucoma surgery. Br J Ophthalmol 2010; 94: 1571–6.
11. Al-Torbak AA, Al-Shahwan S, Al-Jadaan l, et al. Endophthalmitis associated with Ahmed glaucoma valve implant. Br J Ophthalmol 2005; 89: 454–8.
12. Lehmann OJ, Bunce A, Matheson MM, et al. Risk factors for the development of post-trabeculectomy endophthalmitis. Br J Ophthalmol 2000; 84: 1349–53.
13. Jampel HD, Quigley HA, Kerrigan-Baumrind LA, et al. Glaucoma Surgical Outcome Study Group: risk factors for late-onset infection following glaucoma filtration surgery. Arch Ophthalmol 2001; 119: 1001–8.
14. Recchia FM, Baumal CR, Sivalingam A, et al. Endophthalmitis after pediatric strabismus surgery. Arch Ophthalmol 2000; 118: 939–44.
15. Carothers TS, Coats DK, McCreery KM, et al. Quantification of incidental needle and suture contamination during strabismus surgery. Binoc Vis Strabismus Q 2003; 18: 75–9.
16. Sampat KM, Garg SJ. Complications of intravitreal injections. Curr Opin Ophthalmol 2010; 21: 178–83.
17. ESCRS Endophthalmitis Study Group. Prophylaxis of postoperative endophthalmitis following cataract surgery: results of the ESCRS multicentre study and identification of risk factors. JCRS 2007; 29: 20–6.
18. Okada AA, Johnson RP, Liles WC, et al. Endogenous bacterial endophthalmitis: report of a ten year retrospective study. Ophthalmology 1994; 101: 832–8.
19. Wong JS, Chan TK, Lee HM, et al. Endogenous bacterial endophthalmitis: an East Asia experience and a reappraisal of a severe ocular affliction. Ophthalmology 2000; 107: 1483–91.
20. Moshfeghi AA, Charalel RA, Hernandez-Boussard T, et al. Declining incidence of neonatal endophthalmitis in the United States. Am J Ophthalmol 2011; 151: 59–65.

External eye disease and the oculocutaneous disorders

Stephen J Tuft

This chapter focuses on the most common external eye conditions in children, especially conjunctivitis, blepharokeratoconjunctivitis, and allergic eye disease (Fig. 15.1).

Blepharokeratoconjunctivitis

Blepharitis is common in all age groups: it is a disorder of the lid margins with or without obvious inflammation. Lid disease can involve the anterior lid margin (lash follicles) or posterior lid margin (meibomian glands).[1] Corneal disease occurs with both. The clinical features include:

- Conjunctivitis
- Styes and meibomian cysts
- Keratitis
- Dermatologic disease

In children, dermatologic associations (rosacea and acne vulgaris) are less common,[2] but corneal disease is more likely to progress to significant vision loss without obvious surface inflammation, termed blepharokeratoconjunctivitis (BKC)[3] (Table 15.1).

Keratitis is unusual in **acute** blepharitis, commonly caused by styes from infected lash follicles (hordoleum), impetigo, herpes simplex infection, or meibomian cysts.

Pathogenesis of blepharokeratoconjunctivitis

BKC is a delayed hypersensitivity response to bacterial antigens released into the tear film. The release of breakdown products of meibomian gland lipid into the tear film may cause

Table 15.1 – Features of pediatric blepharokeratoconjunctivitis

Associated skin disease	Acne rosacea Acne vulgaris Atopic dermatitis Less common than in adults		
Symptoms[a]	Photophobia Pain Eye rubbing Redness Watering Discharge Blur (older children)		
Signs[b]	Lids[c] Inspissated meibomian ducts Crusting Collarettes Notching of lid margins Meibomian cysts Styes	Conjunctiva[c] Bulbar hyperemia Tarsal papillary hyperplasia Tarsal follicles Lipid crystals Phlyctenules	Cornea Punctate epitheliopathy Marginal keratitis Phlyctenules Axial supepithelial scar Thinning Sectorial vascularization

[a]Some patients may be asymptomatic.
[b]Signs may be very asymmetric or even unilateral.
[c]Lid and conjunctival change can be minimal even with corneal disease.

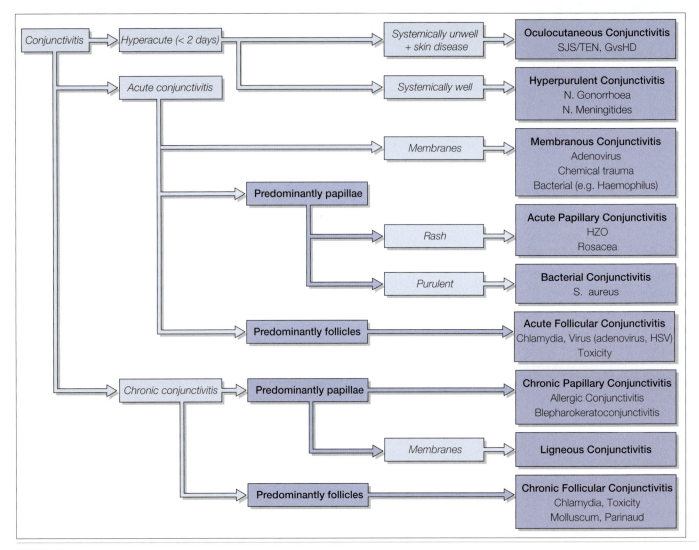

Fig. 15.1 Algorithm for assessment of conjunctivitis.

inflammation. An unstable tear film amplifies the effect through surface drying. An immunologic mechanism is supported by the observation that rabbits immunized with *Staphylococcus aureus* or with the bacterial cell wall component ribitol teichoic acid develop ulcerative keratitis, phlyctenules, and marginal corneal ulcers.[4,5] Posterior lid margin disease is not the result of infection. Clinically, there is keratinization of the ductules of the meibomian glands and meibomian gland "drop out."[6]

The symptoms of early cases of BKC are chronically uncomfortable red eyes (Fig. 15.2). The disease can be very asymmetric or unilateral, with photophobia if there is keratitis (Table 15.1). Photophobia can limit activity. There may be eye rubbing and crusting in the morning, but discharge is not a major feature. The disease can remain asymptomatic until reduced vision or a corneal opacity alerts the patient or parents.

The signs of anterior blepharitis include scales and collarettes at the bases of the lashes (Fig. 15.3). The appearance of the posterior lid margin can be surprisingly normal, or there may be inspissation of the meibomian gland openings with expression of white sebum following gentle lid pressure. In more active disease there is a mixed papillary and follicular change especially in the upper and lower tarsal conjunctiva

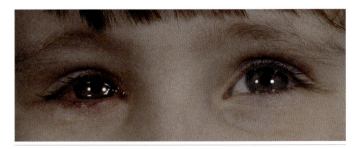

Fig. 15.2 Red and watery right eye of child with blepharokeratoconjunctivitis. There is anterior blepharitis and a reactive ptosis.

(Fig. 15.4) with limbitis and conjunctival or corneal phlyctenules (Figs 15.5 and 15.6). A phlyctenule (or phlycten) is a small white collection of polymorphs and leukocytes with an overlying epithelial defect. Conjunctival crystals are not always present but are a specific sign for this condition (Fig. 15.7).[7] The corneal signs range from a mild inferior punctate keratopathy to diffuse corneal stain with fluorescein

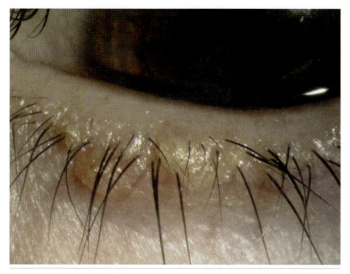

Fig. 15.3 **Crusting at the base of the lashes in anterior blepharitis.**

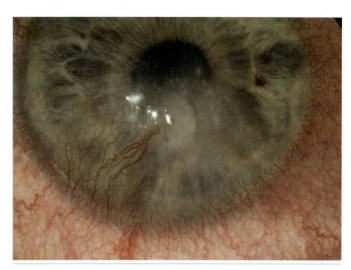

Fig. 15.6 **A recurrent corneal phlyctenule.** There is scar, thinning, and vascularization of the cornea that reduce vision.

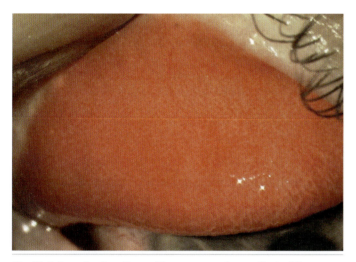

Fig. 15.4 **A predominantly papillary response in a patient with very active blepharokeratoconjunctivitis.**

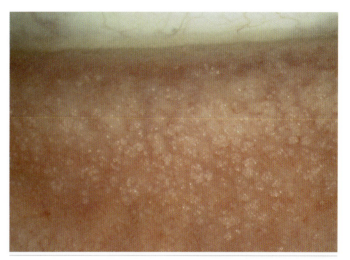

Fig. 15.7 **Numerous subconjunctival crystalline deposits in blepharokeratoconjunctivitis.**

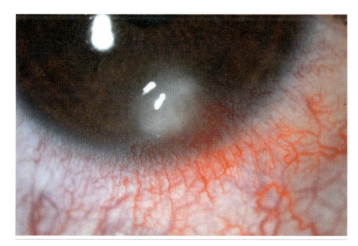

Fig. 15.5 **Acute phlyctenule at the limbus.** The lesion is raised with an epithelial defect. There is early corneal vascularization.

(Fig. 15.8). More severe corneal changes include peripheral corneal thinning and vascularization at the site of previous phlyctenules (Fig. 15.9). Vision loss may be severe and insidious. It is reversible if it is the result of epitheliopathy, but permanent if it is from central extension of peripheral corneal disease or diffuse central stromal scar. Some patients have corneal changes compatible with BKC but with minimal or absent lid and conjunctival change.

Treatment of blepharokeratoconjunctivitis

- Treat acute infection or styes with a warm compress and a short course of topical antibiotic (Table 15.2).
- Meibomian cysts tend to resolve spontaneously but they should be incised if they do not resolve after 3 months, or if they affect vision by altering lid position. A course of oral antibiotic (e.g. doxycycline) should be considered for recurrent cysts.
- For chronic disease, a daily warm compress followed by lid cleaning with a cotton bud moistened in boiled water

followed by topical antibiotic ointment. This can take 4–6 weeks to work.

- Topical corticosteroid is the basis of treatment for most cases of BKC with conjunctival phlyctenules or significant corneal disease. For example, fluoromethalone 0.1% four times a day, reducing to once daily after 4 weeks.

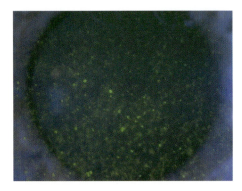

Fig. 15.8 Punctate epithelial erosion and microcysts secondary to blepharitis. Stained with fluorescein.

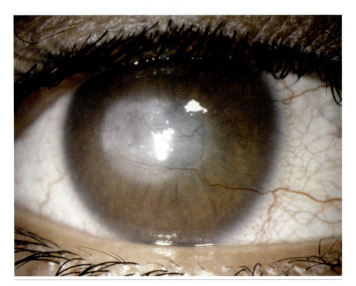

Fig. 15.9 Dense axial cornea scar associated with blepharokerato-conjunctivitis. The patient was relatively asymptomatic until a corneal opacity was noted.

Long-term treatment (i.e. for years) with low-dose steroid may be required.

- Treat visually significant keratitis with long-term (8–12 weeks) low-dose oral antibiotic (Table 15.2).[8] Corneal phlyctenules can rarely lead to perforation of the cornea and loss of vision due to scarring. They should be treated with intensive topical corticosteroids and topical antibiotics if there is an epithelial defect. Systemic antibiotics reduce the frequency and severity of relapses of phlyctenular disease.
- The effect of manual expression of the meibomian gland secretions is debated and it is difficult to perform without sedation in young children.
- Dietary supplement with oral flaxseed oil has been recommended.[9]
- Rarely, for inexorable corneal opacification, systemic immunosuppression (e.g. with mycophenolate) is required.
- Secondary microbial keratitis can occur; it should be treated immediately.
- An axial corneal opacity or irregular astigmatism may cause amblyopia. Visual correction may be possible in older children using a rigid contact lens.

The great majority of cases of phlyctenular disease in developed countries are associated with staphylococcal lid margin disease, but phlyctenules are associated with tuberculosis, and very rarely with helminthiasis, leishmaniasis, and candidiasis.[10] In areas where tuberculosis is common, a child with a phlyctenule should be screened for tuberculosis.

Other uncommon causes of chronic blepharokeratoconjunctivitis

Lesions of discoid lupus erythematosus at the lash margin may mimic chronic blepharitis. These may respond to topical treatment with steroid but systemic therapy (e.g. hydroxychloroquine) is usually required.[11] Lash infestation by crab lice (*Phthirus pubis*) can cause low-grade irritation and conjunctivitis (Fig. 15.10). Removal of the eggs (nits) and lice at the slit-lamp followed by application of white soft paraffin eye ointment to the lid margin twice daily for 10 days to smother the lice is effective. An alternative is pilocarpine 4% gel, which is toxic to adult lice. Insecticides (e.g. permethrin 1%, malathion 1%) are not licensed for ocular use; they are used

Table 15.2 – Antibiotic treatment for blepharokeratoconjunctivitis

Indication + common pathogens	First line treatment	Alternatives
Posterior blepharitis Affect meibomian glands and gland orifices • *Staphylococcus aureus* • *Staphylococcus epidermidis*	Oc Chloramphenicol 1% Applied after eye lid hygiene and at night	Oc Polyfax (polymyxin B sulphate 10 000 units, bacitracin zinc 500 units/g) Oc Fusidic acid Azithromycin gel
	po Erythromycin 125 mg bd Until clinical improvement noted (usually 2 to 4 weeks)	po Doxycycline 50–100 mg od For children >12 years of age
Anterior blepharitis Seborrheic blepharitis of the lashes • *Staphylococcus aureus*	Oc Chloramphenicol 1% after eye lid hygiene at night	Oc Polyfax (polymyxin B sulphate 10 000 units, bacitracin zinc 500 units/g) bd Oc Fusidic acid every night

Doxycycline should not be used in children under 12 years and patients should be warned about skin sensitivity to sunlight and gastrointestinal side-effects.

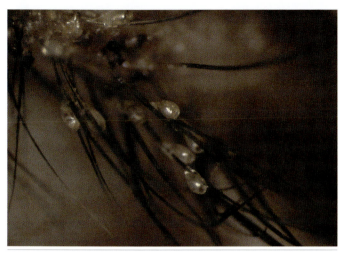

Fig. 15.10 *Phthirus pubis* **infestation of the lashes.** Adults can be seen superiorly at the bases of the lashes with eggs (nits) adherent to the shaft of the lashes.

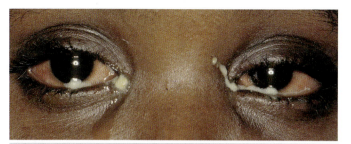

Fig. 15.11 **Acute bacterial conjunctivitis.** Bilateral purulent discharge is an index of bacterial infection.

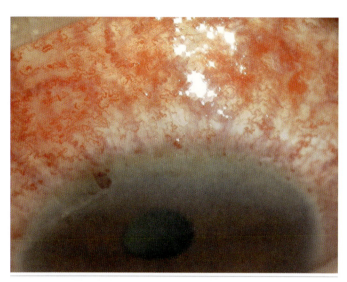

Fig. 15.12 *Neisseria gonorrhoeae* **conjunctivitis.** There is intense congestion of the vessels with petechial hemorrhages. There may be a hyperpurulent discharge and a tendency for corneal thinning at the superior limbus.

in shampoos but they cause irritation. Decontamination of bed wear is essential. A pediatrician should be involved and screening for sexually transmitted infection such as chlamydia may be indicated.

Conjunctivitis

The causes of conjunctivitis are outlined in Fig. 15.1. Cultures are only necessary when there is:

1. Photophobia
2. Loss of vision
3. Hyperacute conjunctivitis, or
4. Chronic conjunctivitis (symptoms >2 weeks).

Ophthalmia neonatorum (infection before 28 days) is discussed in Chapter 12.

Acute conjunctivitis

Acute bacterial conjunctivitis is common in young children. It is bilateral in 70% of cases with a mucopurulent discharge, diffuse bulbar redness, and papillary hypertrophy of the upper tarsal plate conjunctiva. *Haemphilus influenzae*, *Streptococcus pneumoniae*, *Moraxella catarrhalis*, and *Staphylococcus aureus* are the most common pathogens.[12-14] One-quarter of children with conjunctivitis have a symptomatic otitis media,[15,16] which usually spontaneously resolves.[17] Viruses (adenovirus, picornovirus, herpes virus) are isolated in 6% of cases,[14] and preauricular adenopathy is one of the few characteristic features of viral infection. Chemical irritation, BKC, and allergic conjunctivitis should be considered as alternative causes. Herpes simplex virus (HSV) rarely causes follicular conjunctivitis, just 5% of cases in one Japanese study.[18]

Acute infective conjunctivitis is typically self-limiting and resolves spontaneously over 2 weeks (65% in 2–5 days) (Fig. 15.11). Sight threatening complications are uncommon. Management for most cases is irrigation with boiled water and the removal of secretions on the lid with a moist cotton pad. Antibiotics are unnecessary for the majority of cases although, if used within 5 days of onset of symptoms, they accelerate the resolution of symptoms and bacterial clearance.[19,20] Complications of untreated disease are unusual. There is no evidence to support the superiority of any particular antibiotic. It is not necessary to exclude children from school unless there is an epidemic.

Hyperpurulent conjunctivitis

Hyperpurulent conjunctivitis requires urgent attention: it may be associated with severe corneal and systemic disease. Patients are typically febrile with a rapid onset of periocular swelling, mucopurulent discharge, pain, hemorrhagic conjunctivitis and chemosis with possible preauricular lymphadenopathy. Swelling and photophobia may make examination difficult. It is important to exclude infection with *Neisseria gonorrhoeae* and *N. meningitidis*, although *Staphylococcus*, *Streptococcus*, *Haemophilus*, and *Pseudomonas* spp. may rarely cause a similar picture (Figs 15.12 and 15.13). *Neisseria gonorrhoeae* conjunctivitis is not always sexually acquired, although this possibility should be excluded. Infection has occurred with the use of traditional medicines containing infected urine.[21,22] *Neisseria gonorrhoeae* causes a rapidly progressive ulcerative keratitis with a characteristic superior corneal gutter that can rapidly perforate. *Neisseria meningitidis* conjunctivitis is usually acquired by airborne spread within schools. Although less severe, in 15% it causes epithelial breakdown and ulcerative keratitis.[23] Metastatic spread of *N. menigitidis* to the eye can occur as a terminal event following septicemia.

Membranous conjunctivitis

Differentiating membranous and pseudomembranous conjunctivitis is not useful. Any severe conjunctivitis (infectious, chemical, immune) can lead to membrane formation with corneal infiltrates and epithelial sloughing. Resolution may be accompanied by conjunctival scarring with symblepharon and secondary entropion or trichiasis. Potential causes include:

- Adenovirus and HSV
- *Neisseria* spp.
- Stevens-Johnson syndrome, toxic epidermal necrolysis
- *Corynebacterium diphtheriae* (rare in developed countries)

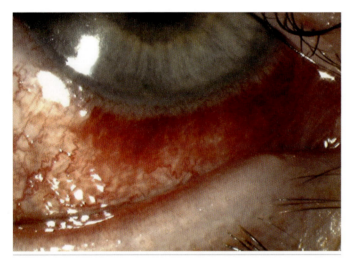

Fig. 15.13 Primary *N. meningitidis* conjunctivitis in a child.
Subconjunctival hemorrhages and epithelial defects are a common feature.

- *Streptococcus pyogenes, Haemophilus influenza, Staphylococcus aureus*
- Accidental injury (chemical) or artefacta

Diagnosis and investigation of conjunctivitis

Conjunctivitis is a clinical diagnosis. Investigation is only indicated for persistent conjunctivitis or hyperpurulent conjunctivitis. Samples should include an urgent Gram stain and culture on blood agar. Polymerase chain reaction (PCR) should exclude *Neisseria* spp., chlamydia, adenovirus, and HSV. Treatment guidelines are presented in Table 15.3.

Systemic treatment for microbial conjunctivitis

Systemic treatment is required for patients with hyperpurulent conjunctivitis, if there is evidence of generalized infection, and immunosuppressed patients. These patients should be admitted until the diagnosis and management have been confirmed. Consultation with an infectious diseases specialist should be made. Patients with otitis media and hyperpurulent conjunctivitis may harbor identical strains of *Haemophilus influenzae* in both sites; systemic therapy is indicated.[24]

Acute follicular conjunctivitis

Acute follicular/mixed conjunctivitis is characteristic of infection by viral or chlamydial organisms. Viral infectious keratoconjunctivitis
This is an important cause of ocular morbidity and visual loss worldwide. Herpes simplex virus (HSV), varicella-zoster virus (VZV), adenovirus, and enterovirus are common causes.

Adenoviral keratoconjunctivitis

In many parts of the world adenoviral keratoconjunctivitis is the most common viral infection of the ocular surface, causing community or clinic-based epidemics. The cause depends on

Table 15.3 – Antibiotic treatment for conjunctivitis

Indication + common pathogens	First line treatment	Alternative
Acute conjunctivitis[a] • *Haemophilus influenzae* • *Moraxella catarrhalis* • *Streptococcus pneumoniae* • *Staphylococcus aureus*	Observation, or G Chloramphenicol 0.5% qds for 7–10 days	A fluoroquinolone, e.g. G Levofloxacin 0.5% qds for 7 days (prescribe if Gram-negative infection suspected)
Hyperacute bacterial conjunctivitis • *Neisseria gonorrhoeae* • *Neisseria meningitidis* Note Seek opinion from genitourinary and infectious diseases specialist	IM Ceftriaxone once daily for 3 days G Cefuroxime (PF) 5% hourly for 24 hours, then six times a day until resolved	IM Spectinomycin once daily for 3 days G Ceftazidime (PF) 5% or a fluoroquinolone hourly for 24 hours, then six times a day until resolved
Chlamydia conjunctivitis • *Chlamydia trachomatis* Note Seek genitourinary opinion Treat sexual partners of parents/carers if necessary	Oc Erythromycin 0.5% tds until review by genitourinary specialist PO Azithromycin 1 g STAT (for children who weigh ≥45 kg)	PO Doxycycline 100 mg bd or 200 mg daily for 7 days for children over 12 years of age

[a]Acute conjunctivitis has a 65% chance of resolving without treatment within 2–5 days.

the route of referral. A British study of children seen in primary care with acute infective conjunctivitis found that 8% of cases were due to adenovirus infection.[14] An American study of adults and children seen in an ophthalmic emergency room found that 62% of cases of acute infective conjunctivitis were due to adenovirus.[25] The clinical signs of the ocular pathogenic strains (serotypes 8, 19, and 37) are indistinguishable, but viral serotyping is routine in some countries (e.g. Japan). This permits epidemiologic tracking of outbreaks. Classification of disease subtypes (pharyngoconjunctival fever, epidemic keratoconjunctivitis) related to specific serotypes is of limited value.

Adenovirus infection causes acute lid swelling, follicular conjunctivitis, petechial hemorrhages, conjunctival membranes, and preauricular lymphadenopathy (Fig. 15.14). There may be an upper respiratory tract infection, vomiting and abdominal pain, urethritis, and cervicitis. Corneal epithelial sloughing and anterior uveitis can occur. Usually, a focal epithelial keratitis develops in 3 to 5 days, followed after 2 weeks by the development of immune mediated focal subepithelial infiltrates (Fig. 15.15). After 3 weeks, the epithelial changes subside, leaving subepithelial scarring and irregular astigmatism that often resolves over 6 months but which may be permanent. Subconjunctival scarring is common but not progressive or clinically significant. Diagnosis can be confirmed by PCR.[26] Because there may be 4–10 days of virus shedding before clinical disease is apparent, and because adenovirus can survive on dry surfaces, spread of infection between patients and clinicians is common.
There are no controlled trials showing a benefit of topical steroid or antiviral therapy for adenoviral keratoconjunctivitis. Treatment is based on symptomatic relief such as cold compress.[27,28] Topical corticosteroid should be restricted to cases with visual reduction secondary to keratitis[29] or if there is a membranous conjunctivitis or uveitis, but this may lengthen the period of virus shedding. Topical steroid is safe and unlikely to precipitate herpetic epithelial disease even if there is HSV conjunctivitis.[18] Topical non-steroidal agents, interferon, and antivirals (acyclovir, trifluorothymidine) have no effect and should not be used (Table 15.4). The lack of effective treatment

has led to strict protocols to limit nosocomial virus spread.[30] Patients with an acute conjunctivitis should be seen promptly in a separate area of the clinic where they cannot mix with other patients; equipment should be decontaminated after use.

Herpes simplex blepharoconjunctivitis

Herpes simplex conjunctivitis or blepharoconjunctivitis (Fig. 15.16) is less common than bacterial conjunctivitis in children. It is not known if it is a primary infection or recurrent disease following asymptomatic primary infection. It is often unilateral, follicular, and associated with preauricular lymphadenopathy. Blepharoconjunctivitis can be severe if there is coexisting atopic dermatitis (eczema herpeticum). There may be a diffuse punctate keratitis or a dendritic ulcer, with multiple dendrites or geographic lesions in the presence of atopic dermatitis or vernal keratoconjunctivitis. It is often self-limiting but healing is accelerated by treatment with an antiviral such as acyclovir ointment or trifluorothymidine drops five times a day for 1 week. Oral acyclovir is effective, especially for eczema herpeticum.

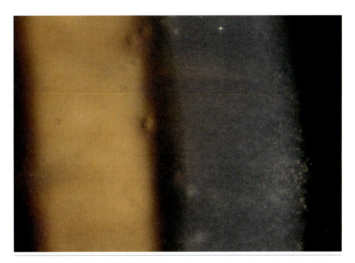

Fig. 15.15 Raised epithelial lesions of acute adenovirus keratitis. After a week the lesions flatten with the onset of anterior stromal scarring and irregular astigmatism.

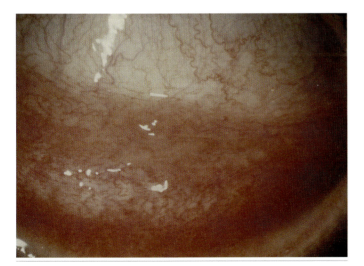

Fig. 15.14 Conjunctival follicular response in acute adenovirus infection. A papillary change may predominate over the upper tarsal conjunctiva.

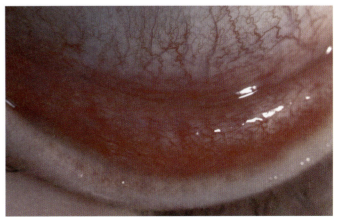

Fig. 15.16 A mild follicular conjunctivitis associated with herpes simplex infection. Confirmed by PCR.

Table 15.4 – Treatment options for viral conjunctivitis

Indication + common pathogens	First line treatment	Alternative
Viral conjunctivitis • Herpes simplex virus Usually subsides without treatment within 4–7 days unless complications occur	Acyclovir eye ointment 3% 5× daily for 7 days (or continue for at least 3 days after complete healing) or Oral acyclovir 200 mg 5× daily for 5 days	Trifluorothymidine eye drops 1% (Pres/PF) 5× daily for 7 days
Viral conjunctivitis • Varicella (herpes) zoster virus Notes: Exclude HIV/immunosuppression	Oral acyclovir 800 mg 5× daily for 7 days	
Viral conjunctivitis • Adenovirus • Enterovirus Notes: Highly contagious. Self-limited, with improvement of symptoms and signs within 5–14 days	Nil	

- For adenovirus infection instruct patient to avoid sharing personal items (towels, sheets, pillows, etc.), use meticulous hand washing, and avoid close personal contact for approximately 2 weeks.
- There is no effective treatment for adenovirus infection; however, artificial tears, topical antihistamines, or cold compresses may be used to mitigate symptoms.
- Dose reduction required when using oral antivirals in renally impaired patients.

Acute hemorrhagic conjunctivitis

Large outbreaks of acute hemorrhagic conjunctivitis caused by enterovirus 70 or coxsackievirus A24 occurred in central Africa and Asia in the 1980s.[31] It has a rapid onset and resolution with characteristic petechial subconjunctival hemorrhages, without permanent corneal change. Direct inoculation and the use of traditional eye medicines, rather than the fecal–oral route, spreads the infection. Confirmation of infection is by PCR. There is no effective treatment; management relies on infection control. The outcome is usually benign, although a polio-like paralysis (radiculomyelitis) develops in one in 10 000 enterovirus 70 patients.[32]

Chlamydia conjunctivitis

Outside the neonatal period, infection with *Chlamydia trachomatis* serotypes D–K is usually sexually acquired. There is a mixed follicular and papillary conjunctivitis with mucopurulent discharge and preauricular lymphadenopathy. The follicles may be prominent in the lower tarsal and bulbar conjunctiva. These should be distinguished from normal childhood follicles in the fornix and at the superior border of the tarsal plate. The superior cornea can show a superficial punctate keratitis followed by subepithelial opacities and peripheral vessels. Diagnosis is by conjunctival smears submitted for PCR or nucleic acid amplification tests. Treatment is with a single dose of azithromycin or a course of erythromycin or doxycycline. Children should be investigated for other sexually transmitted diseases (e.g. *N. gonorrheae)*, and assessed for potential sexual abuse.

Trachoma

This is an important cause of external eye disease and the leading infectious cause of blindness. Repeated infection with serotypes A–C of *Chlamydia trachomatis* can cause conjunctivitis in children that progresses to scarring and blindness as adults. Without reinfection, it is a self-limiting disease. In 2002, at least 1.3 million people were blind from trachoma.

Currently, 40 million people have active disease in the 50 countries where it is endemic, principally in poor rural communities in sub-Saharan Africa.[33] It has disappeared from most developed countries. Transmission is by direct contact with eye or nasal secretions, eye-seeking flies, or by aerosol.

In some endemic areas, 80% of children have active disease and scarring disease can be seen in late childhood. Active disease in children is usually characterized by a mixed follicular and papillary response best seen over the everted upper tarsal plate, often accompanied by a severe inflammatory response that obscures the underlying vessels over the tarsal plate, and a superior pannus.[34] Resolved follicles at the superior limbus leave depressions (Herbert's pits) that are pathognomonic of previous infection. Corneal blindness is the result of trichiasis, dry eye, secondary infection, and vascularization.

Control of the disease is by implementation of the SAFE strategy:

S = Surgery for trichiasis
A = mass distribution of Antibiotics
F = Facial cleanliness
E = Environmental improvement

Treatment of acute conjunctivitis is with a single dose of oral azithromycin (20 mg kg body weight), or 6 weeks of 1% tetracycline ointment.[35] Topical azithromycin is an alternative. Mass treatment is recommended when the prevalence of active infection is >5%.[33] Clinical signs may persist for months after active infection has been eliminated. If there is trichiasis, lash epilation and lid taping are short-term options prior to lid eversion surgery.[36]

Chronic follicular conjunctivitis

This should be distinguished from the appearance of the normal conjunctiva in children, who may have prominent follicles in the fornix but without subconjunctival infiltration that obscures the vertical pattern of tarsal conjunctival vessels. Chronic reinfection with *Chlamydia trachomatis* is a cause of chronic follicular conjunctivitis along with other rare chlamydial infections (feline pneumonitis, psittacosis, and lymphogranuloma venereum). Chronic canaliculitis and secondary conjunctivitis caused by *Actinomyces* spp. is rare in children. Hypersensitivity to medications (preservatives, especially in ocular hypotensives) can produce a follicular response. Other potential causes are described below.

Molluscum contagiosum

Molluscum contagiosum is a double stranded DNA poxvirus. Transmission is by direct contact or autoinoculation to the eye. Molluscum lesions are umbilicated; when on the lid or close to the lash line they can easily be missed (Fig. 15.17). In this location they can cause a chronic follicular conjunctivitis, usually unilateral with a peak incidence at ages 2 to 4 years. Multiple lesions can develop in patients with atopy and in the immunosuppressed. Treatment is by expression or curettage of the core of the lesion, facilitated by making a small incision in the inner margin of the lesion with the tip of a needle – cautery or cryotherapy may cause depigmentation of the lid margin and loss of lashes; resolution is then rapid. Chronic cases can develop a punctate keratopathy with secondary peripheral vascularization.

Parinaud's oculoglandular syndrome

This rare condition causes a unilateral granulomatous conjunctivitis with surrounding follicles, often associated with fever and ipsilateral regional lymphadenopathy.[37] It is a variant of cat-scratch disease, which is usually caused by a Gram negative bacterium, *Bartonella henselae*, following a scratch from a cat or inoculation of contaminated cat-flea feces into the conjunctiva. The diagnosis is confirmed by a rising IgG serology, indirect fluorescent antibody for *Bartonella* spp., or PCR from affected tissue. There is a tendency to resolution but treatment is with oral azithromycin, doxycycline, or ciprofloxacin. Other rarer causative agents are tularemia (*Francisella tularensis*), sporotrichosis, tuberculosis, and chlamydia.

Ophthalmia nodosa

This is a granulomatous reaction of the conjunctiva or cornea to implanted plant or insect hairs. There is rapid onset of irritation, photophobia, and chemosis after exposure. Migration of barbed hairs into the tissue is aggravated by eye rubbing. Intraocular penetration of the hairs can occur, with symptoms of chronic keratoconjunctivitis, uveitis, vitritis or chorioretinitis.[38] Caterpillar hairs (setae) were the first reported causative agent but hairs from pet tarantulas (e.g. Chilean rose tarantula – *Grammostola rosea*) are now more common. Tarantulas release a cloud of hairs as a defensive ploy when threatened. Protruding hairs can be removed, but physical removal of buried hairs is usually impossible. Mild topical steroid is effective to control inflammation. Conjunctival granulomas can be excised (Fig. 15.18).[39]

Conjunctival folliculosis

Folliculosis is a marked follicular response without other signs of ocular inflammation mostly seen in adolescents and young adults. There may be only mild discomfort; the follicles may have been noted coincidentally. The follicles may be present on the tarsal, forniceal, and bulbar conjunctiva (Fig. 15.19).

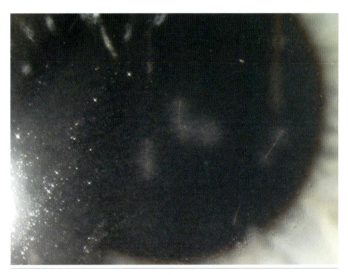

Fig. 15.18 Tarantula hairs embedded in the cornea. There was an associated mild conjunctivitis.

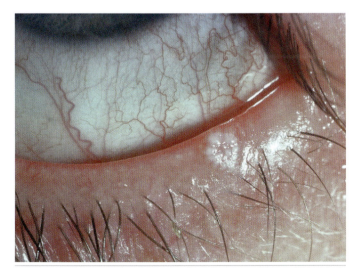

Fig. 15.17 An umbilicated lesion of molluscum contagiosum on the lid margin. There may be an associated follicular conjunctivitis and corneal vascularization in neglected cases.

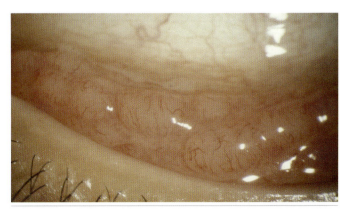

Fig. 15.19 Numerous large follicles in the inferior fornix (folliculosis). The patient was asymptomatic.

Treatment or investigation is not usually required. A trial of topical steroid or oral doxycycline is appropriate but spontaneous resolution occurs: it may take years.

Chronic papillary conjunctivitis

Vernal keratoconjunctivitis

Vernal keratoconjunctivitis (VKC) is an atopic disease in which an allergic response is mounted to common environmental allergens, dust or pollen. The mild ocular allergic diseases are seasonal and perennial allergic conjunctivitis. VKC has an early onset with a high expectation for eventual resolution, and atopic keratoconjunctivitis that is unremitting, typically developing in older patients with severe atopic dermatitis (eczema).

Clinical features

VKC usually develops in the first decade of life (82% by age 10 years with a mean age of 7 years). In 95% of cases there is remission by the late teens.[40,41] In Africa, India, and the Middle East it is a substantial public health problem, accounting for 3% of eye clinic patients, and 10% of outpatient attendances.[42] It affects 3–10% of children in Africa and the Middle East.[43,44] The prevalence in Western Europe is less than 0.03%.[43] VKC is more common in males although the gender difference is less marked in the tropics.[45] In temperate regions, 45% to 75% of patients have a history of asthma or eczema; in tropical regions this is lower (0–40%). There is a family history of atopy in 50% of patients, although the expression (eczema, asthma, or allergic rhinitis) may vary in different family members. Limbal VKC is more frequent in patients of African or Asian descent; this racial predisposition persists after migration to temperate regions.[46]

Symptoms of VKC consist of itch, photophobia, discomfort, blepharospasm, blurred vision, and mucous discharge. The disease can be markedly asymmetric. The skin of the lids may be eczematous with excoriation at the canthi and a reactive ptosis (Fig. 15.20). Papillary hypertrophy and cellular infiltration over the upper tarsal plates obscures the pattern of underlying vessels. Giant papillae (>1 mm diameter) give a cobblestone appearance and, in active disease, mucus accumulates between the papillae (Fig. 15.21). Papillae can form at the limbus appearing as gelatinous or vascular mounds with white Horner-Trantas dots (aggregates of degenerated eosinophils and epithelial cells) on the apices (Fig. 15.22). Reticular scarring can develop over the upper tarsal plate, rarely of

clinical significance.[47] VKC is classified as palpebral, limbal, or combined disease according to the distribution of the giant papillae. Palpebral or combined limbal and palpebral diseases behave similarly, whereas purely limbal disease, which is the more common form in tropical regions, is a more benign variant in temperate regions.[48]

Corneal changes

In mild disease there may be punctate epithelial erosions on the superior and central cornea. If there is active palpebral disease, mucus may be deposited on the superior corneal epithelium (Fig. 15.23), which can stimulate the formation of superficial corneal neovascularization. If there is severe palpebral disease, this may progress to corneal epithelial necrosis (macroerosion) caused by the toxic agents (e.g. eosinophilic major basic protein) released from the epithelium of the upper tarsal conjunctiva (Fig. 15.24).[49] An epithelial erosion may heal completely with early intensive treatment, but in neglected cases mucus and calcium deposition on Bowman's layer can prevent re-epithelialization and a vernal plaque (shield ulcer) develops (Fig. 15.25). These plaques rarely vascularize, but

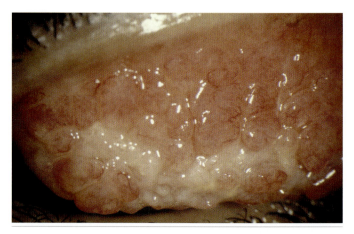

Fig. 15.21 Active palpebral vernal keratoconjunctivitis. There are giant papillae with adherent mucus.

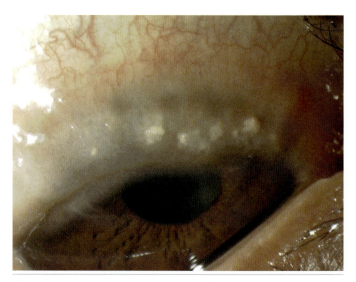

Fig. 15.22 Limbal vernal keratoconjunctivitis. White Trantas' dots have formed on the apices of the limbal papillae. There is a secondary pseudogerontoxon centrally.

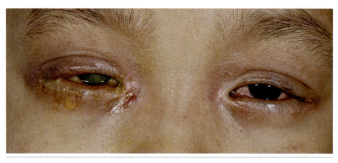

Fig. 15.20 Severe signs in a 6-year-old child with vernal keratoconjunctivitis. The lids are thickened with loss of lashes. There is also an abrasion on the side of the nose from eye rubbing. A right corneal plaque has developed.

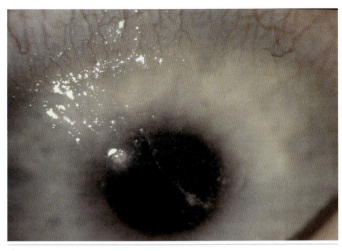

Fig. 15.23 Mucus adherent to the superior corneal epithelium in a case with palpebral vernal keratoconjunctivitis.

they cause intense discomfort. Because there is a risk of secondary infection, including crystalline keratopathy, a prophylactic antibiotic should be prescribed (Fig. 15.26). Although visual loss from limbal disease is uncommon an arcuate infiltrate can develop adjacent to limbal papillae (pseudogerontoxon), and there may be cystic degeneration of the conjunctiva in previously affected areas. In tropical regions, untreated limbal VKC is an important cause of visual loss.

Associated disease

Patients with VKC may have other conditions that affect their vision:

1. Herpes simplex keratitis.
2. Keratoconus in up to 26% of patients.
3. A characteristic anterior capsular cataract in 8%.[50]
4. Complications of unsupervised steroid treatment in up to 20%.[51]

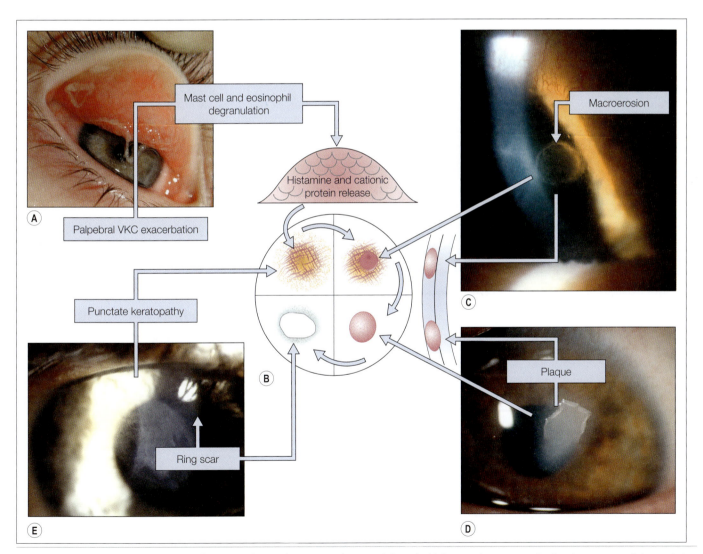

Fig. 15.24 The pathogenesis of vernal plaque. (A) The tarsal conjunctiva becomes inflamed with increased mucous production due to mast cell degranulation and histamine release. Eosinophil degranulation releases cationic proteins that are epitheliotoxic resulting in (B) associated corneal punctate keratopathy with adherent mucous. (C) If the inflammation continues a confluent area of epithelium breaks down to form a macroerosion. (D) Epithelial and eosinophilic debris are deposited on Bowman's membrane in the base of the macroerosion to form a vernal plaque. (E) Whether this is removed with lamellar dissection or epithelializes a ring scar results. The diagram illustrates the corneal staining pattern with Rose Bengal. (Figure D reproduced with permission from Bruns T, Breathnach S, et al. The Skin and Eyes. In: Rook's Textbook of Dermatology, 7th ed. London: Blackwell Publishing Ltd; 2004)

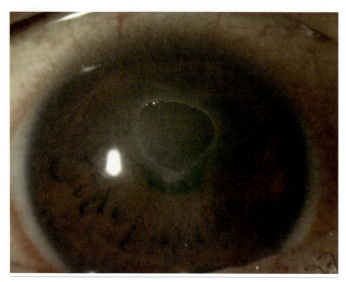

Fig. 15.25 Large corneal plaque in a case with palpebral vernal keratoconjunctivitis. The base of the defect is calcified.

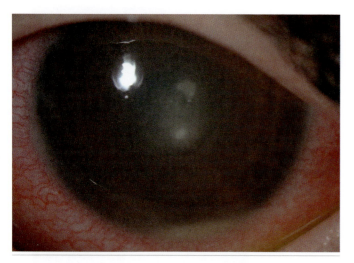

Fig. 15.26 Secondary bacterial infection of a vernal plaque. Prophylactic antibiotic should be used until a plaque has healed.

The risk of visual loss is greatest in tropical regions, varying between 0% and 10%.

The higher rate of visual loss in tropical areas is related to poor access to treatment and coexistent disease such as trachoma and bacterial conjunctivitis. In developed countries, minor visual loss from corneal scar occurs in about 6% of patients;[52] 25% of patients with VKC in Western Europe develop corneal complications.[43]

Disease mechanisms

In atopy a subpopulation of T lymphocytes (Th2) is abnormally expanded; these cells drive the disease process via the type I (IgE-mediated) immediate hypersensitivity response. Th2 cells generate cytokines and interleukins (IL-3, IL-4, and IL-13) that promote the synthesis of IgE by B cells.[53,54] When an allergen comes into contact with conjunctival mast cells coated with IgE antibodies specific to that allergen, the mast cell degranulates and releases histamine and other cytokines that recruit other inflammatory cells such as eosinophils, which in turn attract more inflammatory cells.[55] Additional inflammatory mediators are released into the tissue and tears.[56]

Tarsal and limbal papillae consist of a central vascular core of mononuclear cells surrounded by edematous connective tissue infiltrated with plasma cells, mast cells, activated eosinophils, and lymphocytes.[57] Squamous metaplasia of the overlying epithelium may also contain mast cells but a reduced number of goblet cells. Scar tissue (collagen type III) forms in the core of the papillae.

Mechanical irritation can precipitate a clinical picture similar to VKC: "contact lens associated giant papillary conjunctivitis (GPC)." The role of secondary irritation (diesel particles, infection, or smoke) amplifying the symptoms of VKC has not been fully explored. The genetic basis for VKC is not fully determined. An altered epithelial and mucosal barrier function is important, allowing environmental allergens access to the immune system. Mutations in the filaggrin gene, a protein that controls keratin aggregation, may be significant.[58]

The diagnosis of VKC is based on characteristic clinical signs. Investigations to support the diagnosis are not widely available. The following may be helpful:

- Total serum IgE and tear IgE are usually elevated, but these measurements are non-specifically elevated if there is atopic dermatitis.
- Measurement of local IgE production by radio-allergosorbent test confirms allergic conjunctivitis but is only available in some specialist departments.[41,59]
- A cytology specimen, taken by swabbing the conjunctiva with a nylon brush, will contain eosinophils and MC_T mast cells (tryptase positive, chymase negative) if there is severe allergic eye disease.[60]
- "Allergy testing" is not indicated in the majority of patients. In temperate regions epidermal or conjunctival challenge testing shows that at least 50% of patients are sensitive to house dust mite allergen, pollens, and animal dander.[41,59] Testing for local environmental allergens (pollens, house dust mite, etc.) can support an atopic basis for the disease, but patients may react to several allergens with no indication as to which is causing the allergic conjunctivitis. Conversely, allergen-specific conjunctival provocation may reveal sensitivity to allergens that do not provoke a response by skin testing. In the same individual the allergens provoking asthma and allergic conjunctivitis may be different. Advice should be sought from a clinical allergist if the disease is refractory.

Management

There is the potential to retain good vision in the majority of cases of VKC, and iatrogenic disease must be avoided. The presence of papillae is not a good indicator of activity. This is best reflected by the presence of mucus between the papillae, Trantas dots, mucus adherent to the corneal epithelium, as well as corneal epithelial breakdown, vascularization, and ulceration. A grading system for severity of disease based on the size of superior tarsal papillae and associated scarring, the presence of limbal papillae, the extent of encroachment of the papillae onto the peripheral cornea, and secondary corneal changes has been proposed.[61] Medical management is proportional to symptoms and signs; intensive topical corticosteroid is reserved for crises (Fig. 15.27).[61] The following should be considered:

- Allergen avoidance by eliminating feather pillows, carpets, pets. Allergens are often locally distributed, but

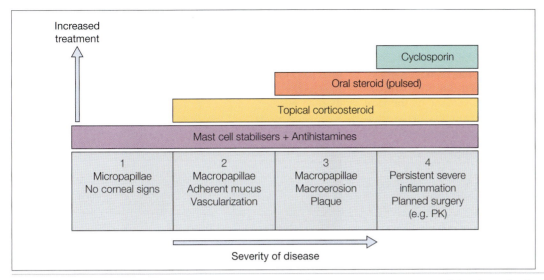

Fig. 15.27 The stepladder of treatment for severe allergic eye disease. With increasing severity of clinical signs (grades 1–4) treatment is added to control the disease. PK, penetrating keratoplasty.

geographic treatment by relocation may not be practical. The patient's school may need to be informed that VKC is not an infection. School staff may need to administer treatment during the school day.

- An oral antihistamine can help sleep and reduce nocturnal eye rubbing.
- Topical medications are effective, but no one agent is superior.[62] For mild disease, topical histamine (H_1) antagonists (levocobastine 0.05%, emedastine 0.05%) produce rapid symptomatic relief. Topical cromones (sodium cromoglycate 2–4%, nedocromil sodium 2%) and other mast cell stabilizers (lodoxamide 0.1%) prevent mast cell degranulation. Dual action agents active against H_1 receptors and mast cell degranulation (e.g. olopatadine 0.1%) have been introduced. All are safe for long-term maintenance therapy, reducing the number and severity of exacerbations and the need for supplementary topical corticosteroid.
- Topical acetylcysteine 5–10% reduces mucus adherence to the cornea during exacerbations.
- The role of topical non-steroidal agents (diclofenac 0.1%, ketorolac 0.5%), a potentially safe option, needs better evaluation.
- Topical corticosteroid is very effective, but patients should be carefully monitored for side-effects (glaucoma, cataract, and ocular herpetic infection). Synthetic steroids (fluoromethalone, loteprednol, rimexolone) may reduce the risk of glaucoma and cataract. Steroid ointment, such as betamethasone, may be useful at night to reduce treatment frequency.
- Steroid injected into the supratarsal space after lid eversion (0.5–1.0 ml of either dexamethasone (4 mg/ml) or triamcinolone (40 mg/ml)) is reserved for severe disease not responding to topical treatment, or given following surgery for a vernal plaque.
- Cyclosporin A (0.05% to 2%) is safe in children.[63] It is an alternative to topical corticosteroid, but probably less well tolerated, less effective, and more expensive.[64] The

safety of topical antimetabolites such as mitomycin 0.01% needs to be confirmed.[65]

- Systemic immunosuppression with corticosteroids, cyclosporin A, tacrolimus, or azathioprine is reserved for severe unremitting disease with corneal complications. Leukotriene receptor antagonists (e.g. montelukast) appear to only be effective if there is associated atopic asthma.[66] Molecular antagonists of IgE (e.g. omalizumab) and immunoglobulin are very expensive and have not yet been fully evaluated.
- Surgical excision or cryotherapy of papillae produces only temporary remission. Application of mitomycin 0.02% after excision may reduce the rate of recurrence.[67] Cryotherapy at the limbus risks causing limbal stem cell failure.
- Treatment of vernal plaque is by superficial keratectomy after the local allergic disease has been medically controlled. The epithelium should be reflected to show the full extent of the plaque and the plaque debrided or "peeled" from the surface. A minimum depth of tissue should be removed. There is no advantage in using laser phototherapeutic keratectomy. An amniotic membrane graft may rarely be required for a large persistent epithelial defect. A bandage contact lens is not an alternative to effective medical management. It increases the risk of secondary infection.

For severe unremitting disease, a short period of supervised treatment in hospital may be required.

Treatment for GPC includes replacing scratched contact lenses or prostheses, optimizing their fit to reduce conjunctival trauma, and the use of a rigorous hygiene and protein removing tablets 1–2 times weekly. Topical corticosteroids can be used freely in blind eyes with prostheses.

Oculocutaneous conjunctivitis

Autoimmune blistering skin diseases caused by production of autoantibodies directed against various specific epitopes in the adhesion structures of the skin and mucous membrane are rare in children. The most frequent pediatric immunobullous disease is linear IgA disease; pemphigoid, dermatitis herpetiformis and pemphigus are less common. Identification of the autoantigens involved has improved diagnosis.

Erythema multiforme minor causes a self-limiting papillary conjunctivitis with relatively minor involvement of the skin and mucosa. It is a reaction to HSV infection. Erythema multiforme major is now more commonly referred to as Stevens-Johnson syndrome/toxic epidermal necrolysis.

Stevens-Johnson syndrome and toxic epidermal necrolysis

Stevens-Johnson syndrome (SJS) and the more severe variant, toxic epidermal necrolysis (TEN), are a spectrum of disease with potentially devastating ocular consequences. SJS is defined as having <10% body surface area skin involvement and TEN as >30% affected. There is a characteristic prodrome of fever, malaise, and upper respiratory infection.[68] The typical erythematous macules and target lesions can progress to vesicular lesions and skin necrosis. In severe disease even slight rubbing leads to exfoliation of the outer epidermis (Nikolsky's sign). Any mucosal surface can be affected; lesions are most common on the lips and oral mucosa. The mortality rate of SJS is 1–5%, and of TEN is 25–35%; this can rise to 90% if large areas of epidermis are involved. More than 50% of patients surviving TEN suffer long-term sequelae.[69,70] The annual incidence in all ages is approximately 1.9 per 10^6 in Europe, lower in some ethnic groups. The incidence in HIV positive patients is much higher. Eighty percent of patients hospitalized for treatment of SJS/TEN will develop eye disease, and 35% continue with chronic disease.[71] It is the eye disease that causes the most profound long-term morbidity because it can progress over years after the acute episode has resolved.

The most commonly associated trigger factors for these diseases are HSV infection, mycoplasma pneumonia, and exposure to drugs. Sulfonamides, phenobarbital, carbamazepine, and lamotrigine are strongly associated with a risk of SJS or TEN in children, with lesser associations with valproic acid, non-steroidal anti-inflammatory drugs, and paracetamol.[72] In some cases no precipitating factor is identified.

The mechanism of disease involves Fas-Fas ligand interaction and cytotoxic T-lymphocyte activation that results in keratinocyte apoptosis, which is the basis of the skin and mucosal lesions.[73,74] Histologically, there is lymphocyte aggregation at the dermal/epidermal interface and a perivasculitis.

Acute ocular complications usually occur concurrently with the skin disease but may precede it by several days.[75] The early signs include conjunctivitis with a mucous discharge, conjunctival membranes, and sloughing of the conjunctival epithelium (Figs 15.28 and 15.29). Conjunctival ulceration over the tarsal plates is common but may be difficult to confirm due to lid swelling. Corneal epithelial defects may progress to corneal ulceration with the potential for microbial superinfection (Fig. 15.30). Progressive sight threatening corneal complications can result from conjunctival scarring involving the lid margin, tarsus, and loss of the fornix. Late complications may result from damage to the limbal epithelial stem cells and from chronic inflammation or infection causing corneal opacity and neovascularization (Figs 15.31–15.34).

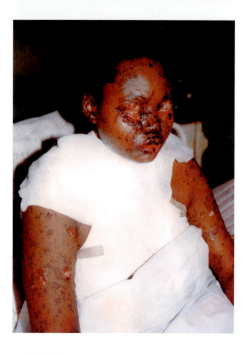

Fig. 15.28 Skin and lid lesions in acute Stevens-Johnson syndrome.

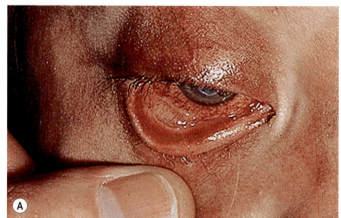

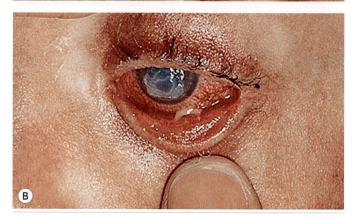

Fig. 15.29 Conjunctival inflammation and necrosis in acute Stevens-Johnson syndrome. There is an associated keratitis (A) and a full thickness loss of conjunctival epithelium (B).

Management of SJS/TEN

Supportive management in the acute phase of the disease is essential. Patients are critically ill and require transfer to a regional burns unit or intensive care department for skin care and medical support. Identification and removal of the

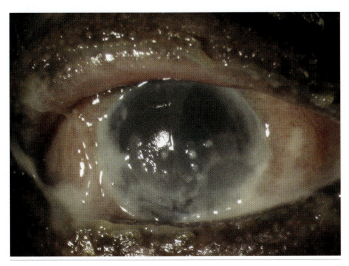

Fig. 15.30 Eye 3 weeks after onset of Stevens-Johnson syndrome. There is a subtotal epithelial defect over the cornea and conjunctiva with excessive mucus accumulation.

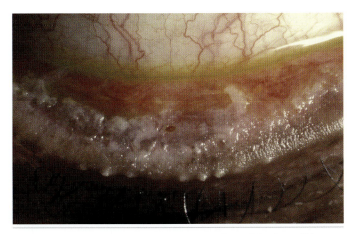

Fig. 15.31 Keratinization of the posterior surface of the lower lid margin in Stevens-Johnson syndrome. Keratinization is an important risk for microbial keratitis and vascularization.

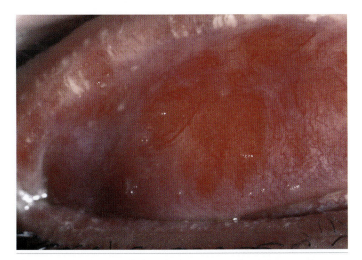

Fig. 15.32 The characteristic reticular pattern of scarring over the upper tarsal plate that is a consequence of acute Stevens-Johnson syndrome. The meibomian gland orifices open onto the posterior lid margin.

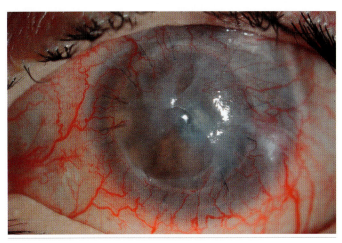

Fig. 15.33 Persistent epithelial defect and melting in a graft required to treat a perforated cornea in late stage Stevens-Johnson syndrome.

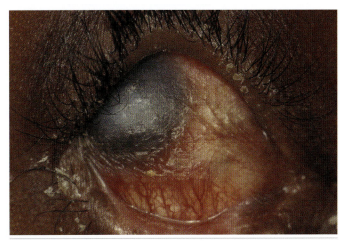

Fig. 15.34 A dry keratinized ocular surface in end stage ocular disease following Stevens-Johnson syndrome.

inciting agent is important. There is some evidence that systemic corticosteroids or intravenous immunoglobulin (IVIG) improve the prognosis of SJS compared to supportive care alone, while IVIG or other agents such as tumor necrosis factor alpha inhibitors (e.g. infliximab) and oral cyclosporin improve the prognosis of TEN.[69] However, this is controversial.[76] Early treatment with pulsed intravenous methylprednisolone may improve the final visual outcome.[77]

There is no standardized treatment for the prevention of ocular complications. There is some correlation between early signs of ocular involvement and the final visual outcome.[78] The use of topical corticosteroid or an amniotic membrane onlay to preserve vision and prevent scarring may be beneficial.[79] Periodic lysis of conjunctival adhesions with a glass rod, removal of membranes, or insertion of a symblepharon ring may be helpful although there is no proof of benefit. Lid taping or lubricant ointment must be used if the patient is anesthetized to prevent exposure keratitis. Topical corticosteroid[75] or cyclosporin may help reduce severe conjunctival inflammation, but they should be used cautiously when there is a corneal epithelial defect because bacterial superinfection of an epithelial defect can progress rapidly. An amniotic membrane sutured to cover the entire ocular surface from lid margin to lid margin as a temporary biologic bandage may limit symblepharon formation and prevent limbal stem cell failure if performed within 2 weeks of onset of symptoms.[80,81] Episodes of conjunctival inflammation may persist after the systemic disease has resolved or recur much later (recurrent SJS) in a clinical pattern similar to ocular mucous membrane pemphigoid. These recurrences do not occur in non-ocular tissues; their pathogenesis is obscure.[82]

In the chronic phase of the disease (>1 month from onset) treatment focuses on management of chronic ocular surface disease by eliminating or minimizing toxicity from topical treatments and to introduce immunosuppressive therapy if there is recurrent inflammation or progressive cicatrization. Successful management depends on the identification of the contributing components of the ocular surface disease, which must all be managed for successful control of the diseases (see below). Severe conjunctival inflammation leads to the following sequence of events (Table 15.5):

- Loss of goblet cells and the accessory conjunctival lacrimal glands.
- Loss of the posterior lid margin with migration of the openings of the meibomian glands onto the posterior lid surface with meibomian gland dysfunction. Metaplasia of the meibomian gland duct epithelium is accompanied by abnormal lashes that grow from the gland opening (distichiasis). Keratinization extending onto the posterior lid margin is a particular risk for progressive corneal vascularization and opacification.
- An unstable tear film and a secondary punctate keratopathy causes chronic discomfort, photophobia, and reduced vision. Keratinization of the corneal surface results in severe discomfort and loss of vision.
- Conjunctival inflammation leads to a coarse reticular pattern of scarring over the upper tarsal plate. Conjunctival scarring can lead to lid shortening and entropion, resulting in corneal abrasion from trichiasis. Incomplete lid closure (lagophthalmos) is common.
- Trichiasis, dry eye disease, exposure, and poor surface healing mean that any abrasion can lead to a persistent corneal epithelial defect. This may progress rapidly to corneal stromal melt and perforation, particularly if there is microbial infection.

- Acute severe inflammation or chronic ocular surface disease may lead to ocular surface failure from loss of corneal epithelial stem cells.

Graft-versus-host disease

Hemopoietic allogeneic stem cell transplantation (allo-SCT) is used to treat a number of malignant and non-malignant hematologic disorders and some inherited diseases. The main complication of allo-SCT, developing in 40% of patients after an HLA-matched graft, is acute (<3 months after graft) systemic graft-versus-host disease (GvHD). A proportion progress to chronic disease.[83] The mechanism is the recognition by donor cytotoxic T lymphocytes of host alloantigens on antigen presenting cells. GvHD affects the gastrointestinal tract, liver, skin, and lungs.[83] Ten percent of patients develop conjunctival involvement during acute GvHD, with hyperemia and edema, the formation of conjunctival membranes, subconjunctival hemorrhage, and corneal epithelial breakdown. Ocular involvement in acute disease is an index of subsequent mortality.[84-86] In chronic GvHD ocular complications occur in up to 90% of patients, especially if there is skin or mouth involvement, with conjunctival fibrosis involving the ductules of the lacrimal gland.[84-88] Corneal disease and chronic uveitis are the primary causes of visual loss. The principal ocular complication is dry eye disease, developing in 40–60% of patients, with a poor tear film, punctate erosions, and filamentary keratitis. There may be necrosis of the lid margins with secondary keratinization of the posterior lid margin and conjunctiva, trichiasis, entropion, and auto-occlusion of the punctae.[87] GvHD is a potentially blinding disease. In one study, severe ocular complications (bacterial keratitis or corneal perforation) occurred in 13% of 620 patients who had received bone marrow transplantation or allo-SCT (Fig. 15.35).[89] The incidence of severe ocular complications may be reduced by planned ophthalmic review and early treatment.[88] Patients are at risk during the required bone marrow suppression before an allo-SCT of corneal involvement from herpes virus infections (simplex, zoster, Epstein-Barr).

Table 15.5 – Ocular effects of chronic ocular surface disease

Ocular effects	Symptoms and signs
Loss of goblet cells	Poor tear film
Loss of lacrimal gland	Dry eye disease
Meibomian gland drop out	Punctate corneal epithelial stain
Posterior lid margin loss	Persistent epithelial defect
Posterior migration of meibomian gland orifices	Vascularization
Keratinization, particularly of the posterior lid margin	Scar
	Visual loss
Conjunctival scarring and symblepharon	
Entropion	
Trichiasis	
Exposure	
Ocular surface stem cell failure	

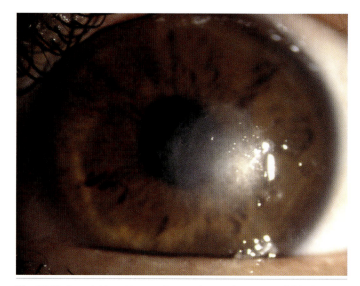

Fig. 15.35 Bacterial keratitis complicating dry eye disease in a child who developed graft-versus-host disease following bone marrow transplantation.

Initial management is intensive preservative-free lubricants (e.g. hyaluronic acid). A hematologist should supervise the management of systemic GvHD with treatment with systemic corticosteroid, cyclosporin A, or mycophenolate. Additional management options for chronic ocular surface disease are described below.

Inherited abnormalities of the epidermal microfilament assembly structure can cause severe corneal and ocular surface disease. Epidermolysis bullosa is described in Chapter 33.[90] Laryngo-onychocutaneous syndrome (LOGIC or Shabbir's syndrome) falls within this group of diseases. It is an autosomal recessive condition described in consanguineous Punjabi Muslim families that comprises skin, laryngeal, and ocular mucous membrane sloughing and granulation tissue. It is evident in the first year of life and is relentlessly progressive (Fig. 15.36). The conjunctival changes are resistant to treatment, although fornix reconstruction using amniotic membrane may be partly effective. The gene lies on chromosome 18q11.2, a region that includes the LAMA3 gene that encodes the laminin subunit alpha-3. Loss-of-function mutations of this gene cause the lethal skin disorder Herlitz' type junctional epidermolysis bullosa.[91] Similarly, Meesmann's epithelial corneal dystrophy is an autosomal dominant epithelial dystrophy that is the result of mutations of the KT3 or KT12 genes, part of the microfilament system (see Chapter 34). Patients may develop photophobia and blepharospasm within the first months of life, and there is a risk of amblyopia.

Corneal limbus stem cell failure (ocular surface failure)

Corneal epithelial stem cells are located in the basal layer of the epithelium at the limbus. Epithelial stem cell deficiency can result from chemical or thermal injury, or develop after acquired inflammation in conditions such as SJS of VKC. Congenital causes include aniridia, ectodermal dysplasia, in which there is an absence of the meibomian gland orifices, and the autoimmune polyendocrinopathies (Fig. 15.37).[92] The final common pathway of disease is conjunctivalization of the surface of the cornea in which the epithelial layer contains goblet cells and the epithelial cells themselves express an altered cytokeratin profile (CK19) that is characteristic of conjunctiva (Fig. 15.38).[93-95] There is often poor vision from vascularization and scarring. The eye is uncomfortable due to an unstable epithelial surface. In bilateral disease there is often a severe reduction in quality of life.[96-98]

Ocular surface failure is a difficult management problem. For unilateral disease (e.g. burns) a corneal epithelial phenotype can be restored by direct transfer of limbal tissue from the unaffected eye.[99] In bilateral disease a living related donor (parent, sibling) may contribute tissue, or a cadaveric donor can be used combined with systemic immunosuppression. An oversized or eccentric keratoplasty that includes part of the limbus can also be used if there is associated corneal stromal opacity. In adults, a successful outcome at 3 years following an autograft has been reported in 74–100% of cases;[99-102] in childhood the outcome is not clear. The results using unrelated donor tissue are worse (21–54%).[103-105] Laboratory-based techniques of cultured limbal epithelial transplantation have also been developed.[106] The cells are obtained from a biopsy of limbal tissue or oral mucosa. There is an attempt to increase

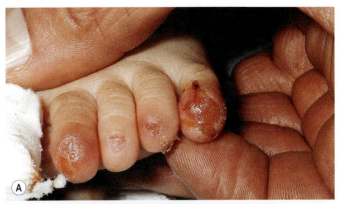

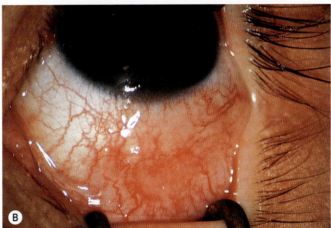

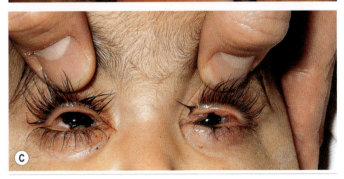

Fig. 15.36 Laryngo-onycho-cutaneous (Shabbir or LOGIC) syndrome. This syndrome comprises laryngeal, nail bed (A), oral, and esophageal lesions. In (B) a conjunctival granuloma with a necrotic slough can be seen, and in (C) there is bilateral conjunctival and nasal mucosal and skin involvement.

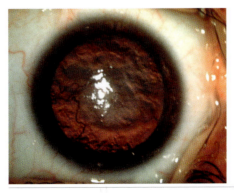

Fig. 15.37 Corneal vascularization and scarring in a child with autoimmune polyendocrinopathy. The mechanism is thought to be corneal limbus stem cell failure.

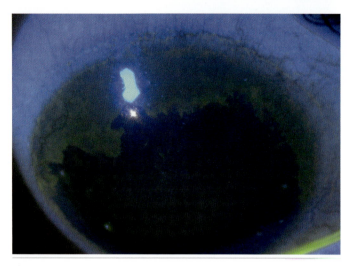

Fig. 15.38 Peripheral conjunctivalization of the cornea in a child with aniridia as shown by late stain with fluorescein. With time the abnormal epithelium may advance to cover the whole cornea.

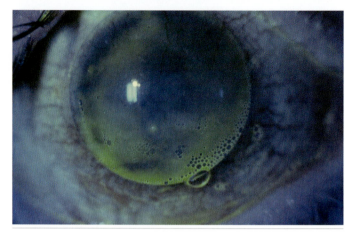

Fig. 15.39 A limbal-fit rigid contact lens used to improve vision following corneal scarring from Stevens-Johnson syndrome.

the proportion of highly proliferative cells (stem cells) in the sample, or direct outgrowth of epithelial cells from the biopsy is encouraged. A sheet of cultured epithelial cells rich in stem cells or transient amplifying cells attached to a carrier such as amniotic membrane is transplanted onto the prepared surface of the recipient cornea.[107] Laboratory-based methods are difficult and expensive. They are currently only available in a small number of specialist centers.

Management of severe ocular surface disease

The following options apply to the management of severe ocular surface disease whatever the cause:

- Dry eye disease: use non-preserved lubricants with an ointment (e.g. white soft paraffin) at bedtime. Hyaluronic acid drops 0.1% to 0.4% have a long surface residence time. Autologous serum drops are effective in adults but of limited utility in small children. Temporary punctual occlusion with silicone plugs or permanent punctal occlusion with diathermy conserves tears.
- Chronic surface inflammation: topical corticosteroid (e.g. prednisolone 0.5%) or preservative-free synthetic steroid. Calcineurin antagonists (cyclosporin 0.05% to 2%, or tacrolimus 0.03%, if available). Filamentary keratitis: mucolytic drops – acetylcysteine 5–10%.
- Toxicity: eliminate preservatives in drops. Use preservative-free medications, especially benzalkonium chloride, and aminoglycoside antibiotics. Recovery from the effects of toxicity may take several weeks.
- Trichiasis: epilate lashes in the short term. Electrolysis for occasional lashes, cryotherapy for groups of misdirected lashes, and surgery for entropion.
- Blepharitis: lid hygiene, topical antibiotic ointment, and oral erythromycin or doxycycline.
- Keratinization: topical retinoic acid 0.05% is effective in 30% of patients but only available from specialized manufacturing pharmacies.
- Persistent corneal epithelial defect: treat exposure, infection, and trichiasis if present. Try intensive preservative-free lubricants, then therapeutic lenses (e.g.

silicone hydrogel, or rigid corneal lens, or scleral lenses in very dry eyes) (Fig. 15.39). If this is unsuccessful, close the eye with a temporary botulinum toxin tarsorrhaphy or a lid suture. Alternatively, an amniotic membrane onlay graft with a temporary tarsorrhaphy.

- Corneal perforation: temporize with therapeutic contact lenses and/or corneal glue. If a keratoplasty is necessary, perform a lamellar rather than a penetrating procedure.
- Disease unresponsive to topical therapy (intense conjunctival inflammation, secondary corneal disease, progressive conjunctival scarring): systemic immunosuppressives may be required. Azathioprine and cyclosporin can be used separately or combined. A short course of high-dose oral prednisolone (1 mg/kg) can be used for rapid control until other agents are effective.
- Secondary corneal neovascularization: isolated vessels can be occluded by fine needle diathermy. Topical steroid or subconjunctival bevacizumab are options for more diffuse vascularization.
- Management of end stage bilateral corneal opacity due to scarring, neovascularization, and keratinization can be formidable, especially with severe dry eye disease. The results of ocular surface reconstruction by limbal allograft are poor in the presence of dry eye.[105] A Boston keratoprosthesis if the eye is moist or osteo-odontokeratoprosthesis for cases with severe dry eye may be considered.[108] A conjunctival flap may be more appropriate if the eye is uncomfortable and there is no visual potential.

Toxic and hypersensitivity keratoconjunctivitis

In children who require long-term topical medication for glaucoma, allergic conjunctivitis, or recurrent herpes simplex keratitis, toxicity should be considered as a cause for conjunctival hyperemia, follicular and papillary conjunctival reactions, or delayed epithelial healing (Fig. 15.40). Secondary conjunctival scarring (pseudopemphigoid) and punctal stenosis can occur. There may be redness and an eczematous change of the periorbital skin. The most common sensitizing agents are atropine, pilocarpine, guanethidine, epinephrine, antivirals, benzalkonium chloride (as a preservative), and aminoglycosides.

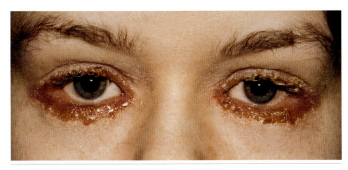

Fig. 15.40 Severe contact dermatitis following topical application of a cromoglycate for allergic eye disease.

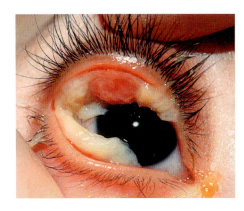

Fig. 15.41 Ligneous conjunctivitis showing typical membranes. The central area of thickened hyperemic conjunctiva on the upper tarsus is the appearance that is sometimes seen in chronic cases which may no longer have membranes.

Treatment is elimination of the causative agent and a short course of topical steroid if there is severe inflammation.[109]

Corneal or conjunctival artefacta

Conjunctivitis artefacta is uncommon in children. Self-medication (e.g. topical anesthetic abuse) or self-harm are common causes in adults and may be seen in older children. Non-accidental injury from parents or carers should be considered (see Chapter 67). Suggestive features of artefacta are signs that do not fit established patterns of disease, such as epithelial defects extending onto the conjunctiva, unilateral disease, involvement of only a defined region of the ocular surface, and failure to improve on therapy. It is often very difficult to be certain of the diagnosis. "Mucous fishing" in allergic conjunctivitis, corneal anesthesia, and molluscum should be excluded. There should be a frank discussion with the child and parents of the possibility that this may be the diagnosis, and involvement of a pediatrician and social services if necessary.[110]

Ligneous conjunctivitis

Ligneous conjunctivitis is the most common manifestation of type I plasminogen deficiency (hypoplasminogenemia). There is an inability to break down fibrin clots due to an absence of plasmin; wound healing is arrested at the stage of granulation tissue formation.[111-113] It is usually seen in infants and young children of all ethnic groups, with a slight female preponderance. Untreated the disease can persist for decades. It is usually an autosomal recessive disorder with a homozygous or compound heterozygous defect in the plasminogen gene (chromosome 6q26).[114] Typically, it involves the upper tarsal conjunctiva although the bulbar and lower tarsal conjunctiva may be involved (Fig. 15.41). Lesions have a yellow–white or red appearance and a woody texture. The disease may be precipitated by infection, trauma, or surgery. Fifty percent of cases are bilateral. Secondary corneal involvement occurs in 30% of cases with associated loss of vision. Lesions of extraocular mucosal sites are less common but include the gingiva, ear, respiratory tract, female genitourinary tract, skin, and renal collecting system. Several children with ligneous conjunctivitis have developed hydrocephalus.[113]

Management should involve a hematologist. There will be early recurrence if surgical excision is performed without appropriate ancillary treatment. Conservative therapy should be considered in patients who are asymptomatic without corneal involvement. Before the demonstration of the role of plasminogen, a success of 75% was achieved with excision with meticulous hemostasis, and immediate hourly application of topical heparin and steroid continued until inflammation had subsided. Multiple treatments are sometimes required.[115] Systemic or topical plasminogen concentrates are now the treatment of choice;[116] systemic treatment is preferred as this is a multisystem disorder. Unfortunately, plasminogen concentrate is currently not available commercially for either systemic or local treatment. Topical plasmin is ineffective; it is rapidly broken down in the tear film.[117]

Keratoconjunctivitis is one of the ocular manifestations of biotinidase deficiency, a condition treated with oral biotin (vitamin B$_7$) supplements. If untreated, children may have seizures, hypotonia, alopecia, seborrhoic dermatitis, and optic atrophy.[118]

Keratitis

Corneal infection is rare in the normal eye because of the protective effects of corneal sensation and the blink reflex, as well as the presence of innate antimicrobial agents (e.g. defensins) in the tear film and ocular surface. Keratitis can occur if any of these are compromised. Visual rehabilitation and prevention of amblyopia are particular concerns in younger children with corneal inflammation.

Microbial keratitis

The main risk factors for microbial infection in children are trauma, ocular surface disease (VKC, trichiasis, BKC, congenital corneal anesthesia, exposure from orbital tumor, dry eye disease, and exposure from other causes such as icthyosis), systemic disease (systemic immunodeficiency, SJS/TEN, vitamin A deficiency and measles), and prior corneal surgery.[119-124] Orthokeratology (correction of refractive error by moulding the cornea with a soft contact lens) in adolescents is a particular risk reported mostly from Asian countries.[125] The relative contribution of these risk factors varies with age, gender, and geographic location. In children up to 3 years of age, systemic illness and congenital external ocular disease are the main risk factors. In developing countries, protein-energy malnutrition and vitamin A deficiency is a significant risk factor under 5 years.[126] In adolescents, contact lens wear is an important cause of microbial keratitis in the developed world.[120,121,123,124] Boys have a higher rate of microbial keratitis than girls, possibly because of higher rates of trauma (Figs 15.42 and 15.43).

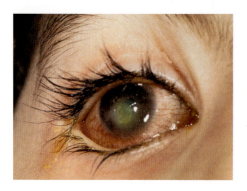

Fig. 15.42 Bacterial keratitis that developed following corneal exposure in a child with Möbius syndrome.

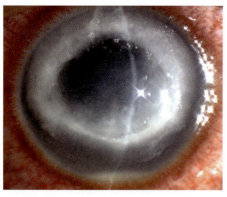

Fig. 15.43 Severe corneal ulceration secondary to *Pseudomonas aeruginosa* in an adolescent wearing a soft contact lens for myopia. There is extensive corneal melting and an hypopyon.

Table 15.6 – Distinguishing features of suppurative keratitis and sterile keratitis

Presumed microbial	Presumed sterile
Central lesions	Peripheral lesions
Lesions >1 mm diameter	Lesions <1 mm in diameter, or >1 mm diameter at the limbus
Epithelial defect	Intact epithelium (early) or small epithelial defect
Severe, progressive pain	
Severe corneal suppuration with lysis	Mild, non-progressive pain
Uveitis	Mild corneal suppuration
	No uveitis

The organisms responsible vary. All centers report high rates of coagulase-negative *Staphylococcus*, *Staphylococcus aureus*, and *Streptococcus* spp. in younger children. *Pseudomonas* infection is more common in older children and is associated with contact lens wear. Fungus infection accounts for 10–18% of cases and filamentary fungal infections (*Fusarium*, *Aspergillus*) are common following trauma in subtropical and tropical environments,[127] with yeast (*Candida* spp.) a particular risk factor in debilitated children. Polymicrobial infections are also common.

Immune (sterile) keratitis can occur. It results from immune mediated inflammation. Immune infiltrates tend to be small and peripheral on the cornea without a large epithelial defect. They respond rapidly to topical antibiotic and low-dose topical corticosteroid. If the diagnosis is in doubt, they should be managed as infectious keratitis (Table 15.6).

Initial examination

This should record:

- Dimensions of the lesion. The maximum length and width of the epithelial defect and infiltrate, and distance from limbus.

Table 15.7 – Investigations for suspected microbial keratitis

Organism	Histology	Culture
Common bacterial isolates	Gram stain	Blood agar Nutrient broth
Facultative bacterial isolates		
• *Mycobacteria* spp.	Ziehl-Neelson	Lowenstein-Jensen
• *Nocardia* spp.	Gram stain	
Anaerobes	Gram stain	Thioglycolate broth
Acanthamoeba	Immunofluorescence Calcofluor white	Non-nutrient agar seeded with killed *Escherichia coli*
Fungi	Silver stain Calcofluor white	Sabouraud's agar Blood agar
Microsporidium	Gram stain Periodic acid-Schiff	No growth in vitro

- Stromal thinning expressed as a percentage of normal corneal thickness.
- Anterior chamber activity including presence of fibrin, cells, and flare.
- The presence and height of a hypopyon.
- Evidence of perforation.
- Remediable risk factors for infection such as trichiasis or exposure.

Investigation

Children with suspected microbial infection should be treated immediately with an appropriate broad-spectrum antibiotic. Diagnostic tests are not essential and may require sedation of the patient. Obtaining a sample for culture and sensitivity testing provides epidemiologic data and guidance for alternative treatment if there is failure to respond or deterioration on treatment. Culture is essential if:

- The clinical diagnosis is uncertain.
- There is a failure to respond to empiric first line treatment.
- An unusual pathogen is suspected (e.g. fungus, amoeba, microsporidium).

Minimum investigation should include a slide for microscopy and Gram stain with material inoculated on blood agar plates (Table 15.7). Most fungi will grow on blood agar. Non-nutrient agar and Sabaraud's agar should be included if acanthamoeba or fungi are suspected. Samples should be inoculated directly onto the media and not placed in transport media. Samples are taken as a mini biopsy with a 21 G hypodermic needle from the edges of the lesion. Growth of most pathogens can be expected after 48 hours. Cultures for fungi and acanthamoeba should be incubated for up to 7 days. Sensitivity testing is normally reported for bacteria and fungi, but not acanthamoeba. Histologic examination should include immunohistochemistry for acanthamoeba cysts and trophozoites and a silver stain for fungal hyphae. Confocal microscopy can confirm the presence of fungi and acanthamoeba cysts; this procedure may be possible in older children.[128]

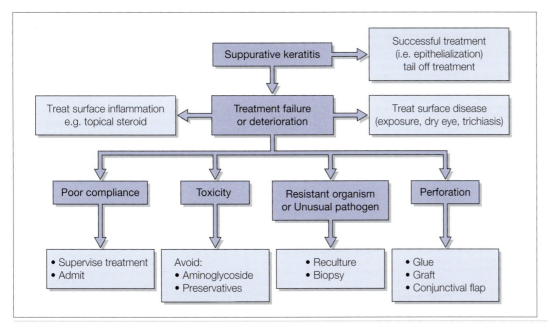

Fig. 15.44 Algorithm for evaluating response to treatment of suppurative keratitis.

Treatment

The goals of treatment are sterilization of the cornea and healing. Sterilization may be rapid; it precedes epithelial healing and resolution of inflammation.[129]

Choice of initial antibiotics

This depends on local epidemiologic data on the common corneal pathogens and their antimicrobial susceptibilities (Table 15.8). In temperate climates, bacterial isolates account for over 90% of the infections. In tropical climates, 50% may be fungal infection. Polymicrobial infection is present in 5–10% of cases. The choice of topical antibiotics for bacterial keratitis is outlined in Table 15.8 but selections should be modified if regionally appropriate. The first line option is fluoroquinolone monotherapy or a combination of a fortified aminoglycoside and fortified cephalosporin (neither are commercially available). In adults these alternatives are comparable in effect.[130,131] Although aminoglycoside and fluoroquinolone resistance is a problem in some parts of the USA and India, it is not currently in the UK. Because fluoroquinolones may not adequately treat streptococcal species, it is prudent to use a combination of a fluoroquinolone and a fortified cephalosporin because streptococcal infection is common in young children.[132]

Sterilization phase

Treatment with hourly drops is given initially: 48 hours duration gives a wide margin of safety. Admission is preferable unless good compliance is guaranteed. Topical treatment is reduced to 4 times daily until healing has occurred (i.e. re-epithelialization of the cornea). Fungal and amoebic infections require prolonged treatment to ensure sterilization. Systemic antimicrobials are only necessary for ulcers adjacent to the limbus to prevent scleral spread, or if there is actual or incipient corneal perforation. Adjunctive therapies may include cycloplegia, analgesics, and hypotensive agents for secondary glaucoma. A subconjunctival injection of a broad-spectrum antibiotic can be given if an examination under anesthesia has been necessary or if there is poor compliance, but it does not achieve higher corneal concentrations than topical treatment.

Once treatment has been started there can be an initial increase in inflammatory signs due to endotoxin release. Definite evidence of progression after 48 hours (increased stromal thinning, or a clear expansion of the ulcer) implies the patient is insensitive to treatment or there is poor compliance. Patients should be admitted if necessary and the microbiology results reviewed. A change to an alternative therapy is not indicated at this stage unless there is antimicrobial resistance to the primary therapy. Complications are common in children. Even with early recognition and appropriate management surgery rates range from 6% to 28%.[119-123] If there is threatened or actual perforation, application of cyanoacrylate glue may stabilize the situation. Urgent lamellar or penetrating keratoplasty (PK) may be required although there is a high risk of graft failure and amblyopia. A conjunctival flap may be more appropriate for large perforations in infants. If there is deterioration or indolent inflammation after 1 week, repeat culture for fastidious organisms or a biopsy are indicated.

The healing phase

Even after sterilization of the corneal ulcer, healing may be delayed by persistent inflammation, toxicity to treatment, or failure to treat the precipitating causes (e.g. exposure, dry eye disease) (Fig. 15.44). Non-preserved medications should be used if possible and ocular surface disease should be treated.

Use of topical corticosteroids

Topical corticosteroids reduce inflammation that may be delaying healing. However, they must be introduced cautiously because they potentiate the growth of fungi and herpes simplex infection. In adults, there is no clear benefit for the use of corticosteroids as adjunctive therapy in the management of microbial keratitis.[133,134] Healing without topical steroid will occur but is slower than when steroid is used. In patients with a PK in whom fungal infection is excluded topical

Table 15.8 – Treatment options for microbial keratitis

Common pathogens	First line treatment	Alternatives
• *Staphylococcus aureus* • *Streptococcus pneumoniae* • *Pseudomonas aeruginosa* • *Serratia marcescens*	Fluoroquinolone, e.g. G Levofloxacin 0.5% hourly (day and night) for 2 days then hourly (day) for 3 days then qds until resolution	G Cefuroxime 5% hourly then taper according to severity until resolution plus G Gentamicin 1.5% hourly then taper The following antibiotics can be used if available according to sensitivity results: G Penicillin 0.3% G Amikacin 2.5% G Ceftazidime 5% G Vancomycin 5%
Mycobacterium keratitis • *M. chelonae* • *M. fortuitum* • *M. flavescens*	G Amikacin 2.5% hourly plus G Levofloxacin 0.5% hourly	G Clarithromycin 1% hourly plus PO Moxifloxacin
Fungal keratitis • *Candida* spp. • *Aspergillus* spp. • *Fusarium* spp.	G Econazole 1% (arachis oil) hourly then taper frequency until resolution (active against *Candida* spp. and some *Aspergillus* spp.) or G Voriconazole 1% (active against *Candida* spp., *Aspergillus* spp. and *Fusarium* spp.) or G Amphotericin 0.15% (active against *Candida* spp. and *Aspergillus* spp.)	G Miconazole 1% (arachis oil) (active against *Candida* spp. and some *Aspergillus* spp.) G Chlorhexidine 0.2%
	For lesions that potentially extend into the anterior chamber or into the sclera – add systemic therapy PO Fluconazole bd (active against *Candida*) or PO Itraconazole bd (active against *Aspergillus*)	PO Voriconazole (active against *Fusarium* spp., *Aspergillus* spp., and fluconazole resistant *Candida* spp.) Intralesional voriconazole 50 μg in 0.1 ml repeat weekly as needed (reconstituted from a 200 mg IV vial)
• *Acanthamoeba* spp. Recommended regimen: Hourly day and night for 48 hours then Hourly by day for 72 hours then every 2 hours for 3–4 weeks then tailored to each individual case No clinical evidence to suggest that dual therapy is more effective than monotherapy with polyhexamethylene biguanide alone	G Polyhexamethylene biguanide 0.02% or G Chlorhexidine digluconate 0.02% plus G Propamidine isethionate (Brolene) or G Hexamidine diisethionate (Desomedine)	If unresponsive to both combinations of first line therapy consider G Polyhexamethylene biguanide 0.06% G Chlorhexidine 0.2%

corticosteroid therapy should be introduced at the outset of infection to protect against allograft rejection. Topical cyclosporin may be an option to control inflammation in cases where fungal infection is suspected; this does not potentiate fungal growth.

Progressive or indolent microbial keratitis

Progressive microbial keratitis after 5 days of intensive broad-spectrum topical antibiotic treatment is an indication for re-culture using specialist media (Table 15.7) or corneal biopsy, with debridement of the ulcer to enhance antimicrobial penetration. Stopping treatment for 24 hours prior to re-culture may increase the chance of recovering a pathogen, but there is a risk that an infection can advance rapidly during this time. When a biopsy is performed, half should be sent for histology, the other half pulverized and cultured. A microbiologist should be consulted regarding optimum media for isolation, which would normally include a modified Ziehl-Neelsen plate. Slow growing pathogens can take 3 weeks to grow in culture and the laboratory should be asked to perform extended incubation. A trial of therapy directed at the organism most likely to be causing the infection on clinical and epidemiologic grounds can be started while waiting for the pathology results.

Fungal keratitis is characterized by a white stromal infiltrate with feathery borders, satellite lesions, hypopyon, and endothelial plaque formation. Treatment is dependent on local epidemiologic data. Suggested antifungal therapies are shown in Table 15.8.[135] In the USA and some other countries commercially available natamycin 5% is the drug of choice for filamentary fungal infection, with amphotericin B used for *Candida* spp. Oral treatment is recommended for deep stromal filamentary fungal infection because of risk of hyphal growth through Descemet's layer into the anterior chamber.[136] Subconjunctival, intrastromal, or intracameral injection of amphotericin are additional treatment options to achieve therapeutic levels of drug. Early excisional keratoplasty may be required to control progressive filamentary fungal infections.

Acanthamoeba infection in children is rare but may be associated with contact lens wear or trauma. Delay in diagnosis can seriously affect outcome.[119,137] Treatment options are presented in Table 15.8. While epithelial disease is relatively easy to eliminate, stromal infection can require months of treatment before the acanthamoeba cysts are killed. More detailed management options are presented elsewhere.[137]

Microsporidium keratitis is an emerging cause of corneal infection in some regions. Large series from Singapore and Southern India report infections in immunocompetent patients related to soil contamination, trauma, and contact lens wear. The most common appearance is a coarse punctate epitheliopathy. Diagnosis is confirmed by histologic examination of an epithelial biopsy. Although topical fluoroquinolones have been recommended,[138] the disease is self-limiting with a good visual outcome.[139] *Microsporidium* stromal disease is extremely rare and difficult to eradicate. Excisional keratoplasty is often required. Treatment options for stromal disease include topical Fumadil-B 0.3% (active drug fumagillin) and oral albendazole.

Herpes simplex virus keratitis

Herpes simplex virus (HSV) is the most common infectious cause of corneal blindness in developed countries. It is also an important cause of visual loss in developing countries, particularly in association with endemic measles. It is less common in children than adults.

Primary infection with HSV may be subclinical and remote from the site of recurrent disease. Acute conjunctivitis may represent primary infection. After infection the virus is carried to the sensory ganglion where a latent infection is established. Stimuli such as fever, hormonal change, ultraviolet radiation, trauma, and trigeminal nerve injury may then reactivate HSV, which is transported in axons to the ocular surface causing recurrent disease. The virus may maintain latency within the cornea and HSV can be spread by corneal transplantation.[140] The HSV1 strain is usually responsible for ocular or labial disease; HSV2 causes urogenital infection and is associated with herpetic ophthalmia neonatorum. HSV1 and HSV2 reside equally in almost all ganglia; local factors favor HSV1 reactivation from the trigeminal ganglion.[141] Transmission of HSV is facilitated in conditions of crowding and poor hygiene. Malnutrition, measles, and malaria may suppress cell-mediated immunity and be associated with severe unilateral and bilateral HSV infection.[142]

Because primary HSV infections may be asymptomatic in two-thirds of cases, clinical surveys underestimate the incidence and prevalence.[14] Serology is used to define the prevalence of prior infection, and this reflects latency. Age, geographic location and socioeconomic status affect the prevalence. Using PCR the detection of HSV in the trigeminal ganglion suggests a prevalence of 18.2% by 20 years of age, but crowding may be a risk factor for early exposure and in Africa 70–80% have HSV1 antibodies by adolescence. 10 million people worldwide may have herpetic eye disease.[143]

There are different patterns of HSV keratitis. The clinical picture may vary over time and multiple features may be present in the same cornea:

- Epithelial lesions (dendritic ulcer, geographic ulcer). This is the result of virus replication and is the most common presentation of recurrent ocular HSV (Fig. 15.45). A geographic ulcer is nominally >1 mm diameter and associated with concurrent topical corticosteroid treatment or allergic eye disease.

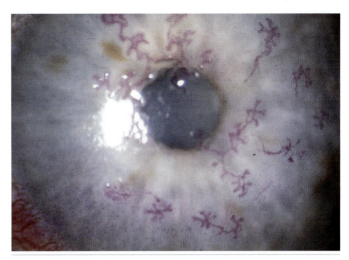
Fig. 15.45 Multiple dendrites from herpes simplex infection complicating vernal keratoconjunctivitis.

- Neurotrophic keratitis (metaherpetic ulceration, persistent epithelial defect) is secondary to corneal anesthesia or toxicity.
- Necrotizing keratitis (immune keratitis). Active stromal infection with an inflammatory response causing stromal melting.
- Endothelialitis (disciform keratitis). The primary target of viral replication is the corneal endothelium, which is damaged, with secondary edema of the overlying stroma.[144,145]

Viral antigen is detectable in stromal disease but replication is an important component. Lymphocytes (Th1) are essential for stromal inflammation; Langerhans antigen presenting cells participate in the immune response. Polymorphonuclear neutrophils are critical for viral clearance but also mediate tissue destruction.

Following a first episode of keratitis the rate for recurrence of ocular HSV increases from 20% at 2 years postinfection, to 40% at 5 years, and 70% at 7 years. After the first episode of corneal involvement 32–40% of the patients experience a recurrent herpetic ulcer: 25% experience disciform keratitis or stromal keratouveitis, 5% experience ocular hypertension, and 6% develop scarring sufficient to decrease visual acuity.[146] Bilateral disease occurs in 12% of patients, especially in atopes (who are at risk of eczema herpeticum) and the immunosuppressed. HSV is more severe in children than in adults, especially if they are immunosuppressed, in whom viral shedding and recurrences are more common. Recurrent disease is associated with visual loss, but with prompt treatment the visual consequences can be minimized; 90–94% of patients maintain vision of >6/12 but 3% are 6/36 or worse.[146] HSV keratitis accounts for 3–10% of all PKs performed in the UK and the USA.[147]

Management

Summary guidelines are:

- Epithelial HSV disease (dendritic ulcer, geographic ulcer) is the result of viral replication, and is treated with a topical antiviral agent (Table 15.9). Oral antiviral and topical corticosteroid is not required.

Table 15.9 – Treatment options for viral keratitis

Pathogen	First line treatment	Alternative
Viral keratitis • *Herpes simplex virus (HSV)*	Oc acyclovir 3% 5× daily For prophylaxis of stromal keratitis and keratouveitis PO acyclovir 400 mg bd under specialist supervision (modify dose according to age)	G Trifluridine 1% 5× daily

- Stromal disease is treated with steroid to reduce destructive inflammation, but covered with an antiviral agent to prevent enhanced viral replication (dendritic keratitis). Both treatments are gradually reduced as the inflammation subsides. A topical non-steroidal anti-inflammatory agent or topical cyclosporin are alternatives to steroid but less effective.
- Latent virus cannot be eliminated, but viral resistance is not usually a problem except in the immunosuppressed because each reactivation occurs with naive virus.

The antiviral agents used to treat HSV disease are purine or pyrimidine analogs that are incorporated to form abnormal viral DNA (Table 15.9). Topical trifluorothymidine (F_3T, trifluridine) and acycloguanosine (acyclovir) have low toxicity and achieve virucidal concentrations in the stroma and anterior chamber, effectively covering adjunctive steroid treatment. Acyclovir has the advantage that it can be used systemically. Both F_3T and acyclovir are active against HSV1 and HSV2. Other topical agents, such as ganciclovir and foscarnet, are equivalent to F_3T or acyclovir in treating dendritic or geographic ulcers.[148] Topical interferon may have a small additional effect when used in conjunction with a topical antiviral, but it is expensive and not generally available. Oral acyclovir did not hasten healing of epithelial disease when used in combination with topical treatment. Debriding infected corneal epithelium is effective, but adjunctive virucidal agents are needed to avert an early recurrence of epithelial keratitis. The sample obtained from epithelial debridement can be sent for PCR confirmation of HSV infection.

The Herpes Eye Disease Study Group treatment guidelines are as follows:

- For stromal disease (e.g. disciform keratitis), topical steroid (1% prednisolone phosphate four times daily), in conjunction with topical antiviral cover, reduces recovery time by 68% with no increased risk of recurrence at 6 months.[149]
- There is no additional effect of oral acyclovir over topical steroid and F_3T when treating stromal keratitis.[150]
- After epithelial HSV a 3-week course of oral acyclovir (400 mg 5 times a day) does not prevent stromal disease in the subsequent year.[151]
- Prophylactic treatment with acyclovir (400 mg bd) reduces epithelial recurrences and stromal recurrences in patients with prior stromal disease by about 50% over 12 months.[152] Prophylactic treatment is usually restricted to patients with bilateral disease, prior HSV keratitis in atopes, or the immunosuppressed, especially following corneal surgery.

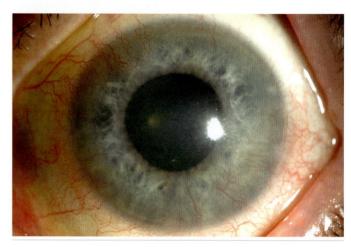

Fig. 15.46 **Peripheral corneal vascularization and opacity following herpes zoster ophthalmicus.**

- Oral acyclovir (400 mg bd for 6 months) reduces the risk of HSV recurrence after PK.[153]

Herpes zoster ophthalmicus

The varicella virus can become latent in sensory ganglia in up to 100% of cases. The diagnosis of herpes zoster ophthalmicus (HZO) is usually clinical, with a painful rash over the upper lid and forehead with a particular risk of corneal involvement if the side of the nose is involved (Hutchinson's sign). However, the rash may be minimal and PCR testing can be used to confirm a primary infection. There is a gradual increase in exposure to VZV with age; in developed countries antibodies to VZV are present in 99% of the population by the age of 40 years.[154-156] The incidence in children <18 years is less than 1.5 : 1000 individuals. HZO is normally associated with reducing antibodies to VZV and it is, therefore, uncommon in children unless they are immunosuppressed (e.g. chemotherapy or radiotherapy). Immunosuppression can trigger a reactivation of vesicular rash. 9–16% of patients have trigeminal involvement (HZO), of whom 50–72% have ocular involvement, and 20% have corneal involvement. It is not known how vaccination for VZV (against chickenpox) will affect the incidence and severity of HZO.[157]

Corneal involvement during the early stages of herpes zoster ophthalmicus can present as a dendritic or stromal keratitis (Fig. 15.46), occasionally associated with uveitis, glaucoma, progressive outer retinal necrosis, and scleritis. The epithelial disease of acute HZO is the result of mucus accumulation on the epithelial surface rather than viral replication, but coinfection with HSV is possible. The use of topical antiviral at this stage is a wise precaution. Recurrent corneal inflammatory disease after 2–3 months does not reflect viral replication and a topical antiviral is not normally prescribed.

Oral antivirals reduce the severity of acute HZO and the frequency of late onset inflammatory corneal disease by 50%, but have no proven effect on reducing late complications such as neurotrophic keratitis or postherpetic neuralgia.[158,159] Oral acyclovir is generally prescribed for 5 days within 72 hours of the onset of rash. Valacyclovir and famcyclovir are not approved for pediatric use.[160,161] Topical acyclovir is not recommended to treat the rash of zoster. Management of neurotrophic keratitis is with topical lubricants or corneal protection (e.g. tarsorrhaphy).

Interstitial keratitis

Interstitial keratitis (IK) is an immune mediated, non-ulcerative inflammation of the corneal stroma (Fig. 15.47). The epithelium and endothelium are unaffected. In a minority of cases, it is associated with potentially severe systemic disease that requires medical management. HSV is the most common cause, but there are numerous other causes, although the majority are rare.[162] IK may be unilateral or bilateral, diffuse, sectorial, peripheral, focal, and may affect any layer of the stroma. There may be vascularization or an associated uveitis.

Symptoms include photophobia and discomfort, although some cases may be asymptomatic and first noted by the parents. There is corneal opacity often with perilimbal injection. Untreated the inflammation can lead to secondary neovascularization, with residual ghost vessels when the acute phase settles. It is the result of a hypersensitivity response to antigens, or antigen bearing cells, in the corneal stroma. Treatment with topical steroids is effective unless there is associated secondary scarring or lipid keratopathy, which will be permanent. If HSV is a potential diagnosis, treatment should be topical or oral acyclovir.

The principal causes are viral, bacterial, and protozoal. Particularly if the IK is inactive, the majority of cases have no identifiable cause (i.e. idiopathic).[163]

- Herpes simplex stromal keratitis is the most common cause for active IK in developed countries, accounting for over 70% of cases.
- Herpes zoster stromal keratitis is the second most common cause, presenting as either a focal anterior stromal keratitis or a late diffuse keratitis associated with scarring, vascularization, and lipid deposition.
- Epstein-Barr virus and mumps virus can cause multifocal discrete anterior stromal opacities that develop several days or weeks after systemic disease. It may respond to topical steroid. Systemic antiviral therapy is not required.
- Congenital syphilis (acquired infection with the spirochete *Treponema pallidum)* is rare in children, although it was once synonymous with IK and is still a major cause of IK worldwide. Screening during pregnancy and treatment with antibiotics has dramatically reduced the incidence.[164] The features are diffuse corneal edema that is bilateral in 80% of cases followed by circumferential intense deep vascularization (salmon patch). Secondary degenerative changes progress into adulthood.

The associated signs of congenital syphilis are nerve deafness, abnormal teeth, and characteristic changes of the nose and face. Diagnosis is confirmed by serologic testing. Systemic treatment is essential, but the corneal changes are helped by topical steroid.

- Tuberculosis is most frequently associated with granulomatous uveitis, but IK may be associated with sectorial sclerokeratitis.
- Leprosy is uncommon in children. The stromal infiltration of leprosy is a bilateral superotemporal wedge of infiltration followed by vascularization. Secondary corneal anesthesia and lagophthalmos due to involvement of the Vth and VIIth cranial nerves is more common in adults.[165]
- Lyme disease is caused by tick-transmitted infection with a number of different species of the spirochete *Borrelia*. There is a history of travel to endemic areas in North America and Eurasia and preceding flu-like symptoms of skin lesions (bull's eye rash, erythema migrans), CNS, heart and joint involvement. The commonest ocular feature (10% of cases) is a mild transient conjunctivitis and periorbital edema, with corneal changes (3% of cases) a late feature, with nummular opacities that may vascularize in untreated disease.[166,167] Optic neuritis, intermediate uveitis, retinal vasculitis and cranial nerve palsies may occur. Diagnosis is confirmed by an ELISA (enzyme-linked immunosorbent assay) or PCR of serum, and systemic treatment with amoxicillin or doxycycline is required, although the corneal changes respond to topical steroid.
- Onchocerciasis (river blindness) is a regionally important cause of corneal opacity that is becoming less common with eradication programs. It is caused by infection by the parasitic helminth *Onchocerca volvulus* that is transmitted by Similium blackflies in endemic areas. Inflammation is stimulated by microfilaria that have migrated from the conjunctiva into the cornea where they have died.[168] In children a pattern of superficial punctate lesions (snowflake keratitis) due to inflammation stimulated by dead parasites in the cornea is seen. In adults, this may progress to sclerosing keratitis that spreads centrally from the limbus in the interpalpebral zone accompanied by deep vascularization. Vision may be lost as a result of retinitis or secondary glaucoma. Treatment is with oral ivermectin, usually given as part of a community-based eradication program. Leishmaniasis and trypanosomiasis are protozoal infections that can cause IK.

Cogan's syndrome is a rare autoimmune disease that can occur in children although the mean age of onset is in the 30s. There is inflammation directed against an antigen found in the cornea and inner ear, with an associated vasculitis. Onset of eye discomfort, redness, and photophobia may be preceded by an upper respiratory tract infection in half of cases. The early corneal changes are bilateral peripheral focal posterior stromal opacities with subepithelial infiltrates, with mild secondary vascularization. There may be a gradual onset of symptoms of nausea, vertigo, and tinnitus similar to Ménière's disease. Atypical Cogan's syndrome may have conjunctivitis, subconjunctival hemorrhage, episcleritis, uveitis, and retinal vasculitis. Atypical features should alert the clinician to the possibility

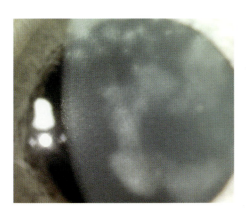

Fig. 15.47 Interstitial keratitis following herpes simplex infection.

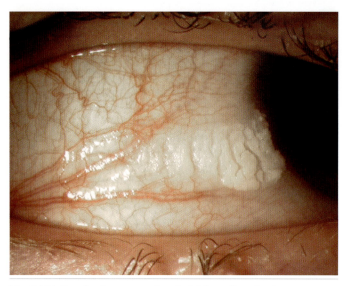

Fig. 15.48 Keratin plaque associated with hereditary benign intraepithelial dyskeratosis.

of alternative diagnoses, such as juvenile arthritis, ulcerative keratitis, etc. There are no specific laboratory abnormalities. The importance of recognizing this condition is the association with deafness and vestibular symptoms. Urgent treatment with high doses of oral corticosteroid is required to prevent rapid progression of auditory loss, although this develops in 50% of cases despite treatment. Late onset aortitis can occur.[169]

Thygeson's superficial punctate keratitis

This can occur in young children. There may be photophobia, discomfort, and blurred vision. Coarse elevated epithelial lesions with minimal stromal reaction and an absence of vascularization is pathognomonic. Blepharokeratoconjunctivitis should be excluded. Initial treatment is with topical lubricants. Topical steroid is effective but may prolong the course of the disease. Topical cyclosporin is also effective. A therapeutic contact lens may be an option in older children.

Ichthyosis

These skin disorders can affect the external eye in varying degrees. There may only be lid margin inflammation producing superficial corneal opacity (e.g. X-linked ichthyosis), or severe corneal exposure and infection (e.g. lamellar ichthyosis).

Hereditary benign intraepithelial dyskeratosis

Hereditary benign intraepithelial dyskeratosis is an autosomal dominant disorder characterized by elevated epithelial plaques on the ocular and oral mucous membranes (Fig. 15.48). It occurs primarily, but not exclusively, in individuals of American Indian heritage. It is the result of a duplication in chromosome 4 (4q35).[170] There is photophobia and blepharospasm with secondary corneal scarring and vascularization. Vitamin A deficiency should be excluded as a cause of conjunctival keratinization. Topical lubricants provide symptomatic relief.

References

3. Viswalingam M, Rauz S, Morlet N, Dart JK. Blepharo-keratoconjunctivitis in children: diagnosis and treatment. Br J Ophthalmol 2005; 89: 400–3.

9. Jones SM, Weinstein JM, Cumberland P, et al. Visual outcome and corneal changes in children with chronic blepharo-keratoconjunctivitis. Ophthalmology 2007; 114: 2271–80.

14. Rose PW, Harnden A, Brueggemann AB, et al. Chloramphenicol treatment for acute infective conjunctivitis in children in primary care: a randomised double-blind placebo-controlled trial. Lancet 2005; 366: 37–43.

20. Sheikh A, Hurwitz B. Antibiotics versus placebo for acute bacterial conjunctivitis. Cochrane Database Syst Rev 2006: CD001211.

27. Ward JB, Siojo LG, Waller SG. A prospective, masked clinical trial of trifluridine, dexamethasone, and artificial tears in the treatment of epidemic keratoconjunctivitis. Cornea 1993; 12: 216–21.

30. Dart JK, El-Amir AN, Maddison T, et al. Identification and control of nosocomial adenovirus keratoconjunctivitis in an ophthalmic department. Br J Ophthalmol 2009; 93: 18–20.

33. Hu VH, Harding-Esch EM, Burton MJ, et al. Epidemiology and control of trachoma: systematic review. Trop Med Int Health 2010; 15: 673–91.

43. Bremond-Gignac D, Donadieu J, Leonardi A, et al. Prevalence of vernal keratoconjunctivitis: a rare disease? Br J Ophthalmol 2008; 92: 1097–102.

47. Kumar S. Vernal keratoconjunctivitis: a major review. Acta Ophthalmol 2009; 87: 133–47.

56. Leonardi A, Sathe S, Bortolotti M, et al. Cytokines, matrix metalloproteases, angiogenic and growth factors in tears of normal subjects and vernal keratoconjunctivitis patients. Allergy 2009; 64: 710–17.

62. Mantelli F, Santos MS, Petitti T, et al. Systematic review and meta-analysis of randomised clinical trials on topical treatments for vernal keratoconjunctivitis. Br J Ophthalmol 2007; 91: 1656–61.

63. Pucci N, Caputo R, Mori F, et al. Long-term safety and efficacy of topical cyclosporine in 156 children with vernal keratoconjunctivitis. Int J Immunopathol Pharmacol 2010; 23: 865–71.

68. Letko E, Papaliodis DN, Papaliodis GN, et al. Stevens-Johnson syndrome and toxic epidermal necrolysis: a review of the literature. Ann Allergy Asthma Immunol 2005; 94: 419–36.

75. Sotozono C, Ueta M, Koizumi N, et al. Diagnosis and treatment of Stevens-Johnson syndrome and toxic epidermal necrolysis with ocular complications. Ophthalmology 2009; 116: 685–90.

81. Shay E, Kheirkhah A, Liang L, et al. Amniotic membrane transplantation as a new therapy for the acute ocular manifestations of Stevens-Johnson syndrome and toxic epidermal necrolysis. Surv Ophthalmol 2009; 54: 686–96.

85. Riemens A, te Boome L, Imhof S, et al. Current insights into ocular graft-versus-host disease. Curr Opin Ophthalmol 2010; 21: 485–94.

97. Kolli S, Ahmad S, Lako M, Figueiredo F. Successful clinical implementation of corneal epithelial stem cell therapy for treatment of unilateral limbal stem cell deficiency. Stem Cells 2010; 28: 597–610.

101. Santos MS, Gomes JA, Hofling-Lima AL, et al. Survival analysis of conjunctival limbal grafts and amniotic membrane transplantation in eyes with total limbal stem cell deficiency. Am J Ophthalmol 2005; 140: 223–30.

107. Shortt AJ, Tuft SJ, Daniels JT. Ex vivo cultured limbal epithelial transplantation. A clinical perspective. Ocular Surface 2010; 8: 80–90.

109. Dart J. Corneal toxicity: the epithelium and stroma in iatrogenic and factitious disease. Eye 2003; 1: 886–92.

113. Schuster V, Seregard S. Ligneous conjunctivitis. Surv Ophthalmol 2003; 48: 369–88.

124. Wong VW, Lai TY, Chi SC, Lam DC. Pediatric ocular surface infections: a 5-year review of demographics, clinical features, risk factors, microbiological results, and treatment. Cornea 2011; 30: 995–1002.

126. Jhanji V, Naithani P, Lamoureux E, et al. Immunization and nutritional profile of cases with atraumatic microbial keratitis in preschool age group. Am J Ophthalmol 2011; 151: 1035–40.

132. Kaye S, Tuft S, Neal T, et al. Bacterial susceptibility to topical antimicrobials and clinical outcome in bacterial keratitis. Invest Ophthamol Vis Sci 2010; 51: 362–8.

136. Galarreta DJ, Tuft SJ, Ramsay A, Dart JK. Fungal keratitis in London: microbiological and clinical evaluation. Cornea 2007; 26: 1082–6.

137. Dart JK, Saw VP, Kilvington S. Acanthamoeba keratitis: diagnosis and treatment update 2009. Am J Ophthalmol 2009; 148: 487–99 e482.

145. Chong EM, Wilhelmus KR, Matoba AY, et al. Herpes simplex virus keratitis in children. Am J Ophthalmol 2004; 138: 474–5.

155. Liesegang TJ. Herpes zoster ophthalmicus natural history, risk factors, clinical presentation, and morbidity. Ophthalmology 2008; 115: S3–12.

162. Knox CM, Holsclaw DS. Interstitial keratitis. Int Ophthalmol Clin 1998; 38: 183–95.

167. Huppertz HI, Munchmeier D, Lieb W. Ocular manifestations in children and adolescents with Lyme arthritis. Br J Ophthalmol 1999; 83: 1149–52.

 Access the complete reference list online at
http://www.expertconsult.com

Ocular manifestations of HIV/AIDS in children

Emmett T Cunningham Jr. • Philippe Kestelyn • Carlos E Pavesio

Chapter contents

HIV/AIDS-related illnesses are among the leading causes of morbidity and mortality worldwide.[1] Each day, over 7000 persons become infected with HIV and 5000 persons die from complications related to their infection. Roughly 2.5 million children 15 years of age or less currently have HIV/AIDS. This number increased by approximately 370000 in 2009, representing over 1000 newly infected children per day. Ocular complications occur in 70% or more of adults and up to 50% of children with HIV/AIDS if not treated with antiretroviral therapy.[1,2]

The introduction of multidrug combination therapy changed the face of HIV/AIDS-related eye disease. Termed *H*ighly *A*ctive *A*nti*R*etroviral *T*herapy (HAART), this regimen uses a combination of potent antiretrovirals to inhibit replication of HIV. Patients on HAART experience a dramatic improvement in helper CD4+ T cell populations and a marked decline in viral titers, resulting in fewer opportunistic infections, reduced morbidity and mortality, and improved quality of life. Despite the decline in the incidence of ocular complications in patients taking HAART, they continue to occur and remain an important cause of disability in HIV-infected patients. This is particularly true in the developing world, where access to HAART varies considerably from country to country.[2]

HIV/AIDS: global and regional epidemiology

The 2010 report from The Joint United Nations Program on HIV/AIDS (UNAIDS) and the World Health Organization (WHO) on the global HIV/AIDS epidemic estimated that 33.3 million (31.4–35.3 million) people were living with HIV in 2009, 90% of whom were unaware of their infection.

Roughly 15.9 million (14.8–17.2 million) were women and 2.5 million (1.6–3.4 million) were children under 15 years of age (Table 16.1). The prevalence of HIV infection in children varies, with over 90% of all children with HIV/AIDS living in Africa (Fig. 16.1). It has been estimated that 16.6 million (14.4–18.8 million) children under the age of 18 have lost one or both parents to HIV/AIDS, and of the 1.8 million (1.6–2.1 million) people who died of HIV/AIDS-related illnesses in 2009, 260 000 (150 000–360 000) were children under 15 years of age.[1]

Transmission of HIV in children

While high-risk behaviors such as injection drug use, unprotected commercial sex, and unprotected sex between men contributes to HIV transmission, most HIV infections in adults occur during unprotected heterosexual intercourse.[2] Most HIV-positive children acquired their infection in utero, at delivery, or while breast feeding – so-called <u>M</u>other <u>T</u>o <u>C</u>hild

Table 16.1 – Global summary of HIV/AIDS as of 2009

Number of people living with HIV/AIDS in 2009	
Total	33.3 million (31.4–35.3 million)
Adults	30.8 million (29.2–32.6 million)
Women	15.9 million (14.8–17.2 million)
Children under 15 years of age	2.5 million (1.6–3.4 million)
Number of people newly infected with HIV in 2009	
Total	2.6 million (2.3–2.8 million)
Adults	2.2 million (2.0–2.4 million)
Children under 15 years of age	370 000 (230 000–510 000)
Number of HIV/AIDS-related deaths in 2009	
Total	1.8 million (1.6–2.1 million)
Adults	1.6 million (1.4–1.8 million)
Children under 15 years of age	260 000 (150 000–360 000)

The numbers in parentheses represent confidence intervals based on the best available information.
From UNAIDS, Report on the global AIDS epidemic, 2010. http://www.unaids.org/globalreport/Global_report.htm.

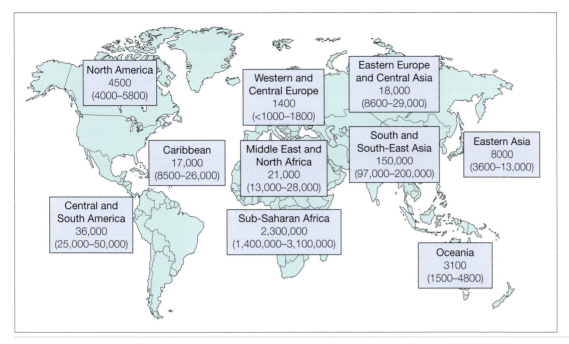

Fig. 16.1 2009 number of children less than 15 years of age with HIV/AIDS by region. Roughly 90% of the 2.5 million children estimated to be infected by HIV live in Africa. Modified from UNAIDS, Report on the global AIDS epidemic, 2010. http://www.unaids.org/globalreport/Global_report.htm.

Transmission (MTCT). Prior to the advent of obstetric and antiretroviral interventions, up to 40% of infants born to infected mothers contracted HIV infection. This included 20% to 25% of infections that occurred in utero, 35% to 50% that occurred during delivery, and 25% to 35% who were HIV negative at birth, and within the first 6 weeks of delivery, but who became infected later, presumably as a result of transmission through breast milk.[3] These rates have since declined dramatically in North America, Western Europe, and other resource-rich regions, where current total perinatal transmission rates vary from 1% to 3%. The incidence of MTCT in many resource-poor regions remains high due to the high prevalence of HIV in women of child-bearing age, a lack of access to antiretroviral prophylaxis, and few feasible alternatives to breastfeeding. Sub-Saharan Africa has the highest burden of HIV disease overall, accounting for 80% to 90% of perinatal infections and children infected by HIV.[1]

Diagnosis of HIV/AIDS in children

The Centers for Disease Control and Prevention (CDC) case definition[4] of HIV infection among children aged less than 18 months recognizes four categories:

1. Definitely HIV-infected
2. Presumptively HIV-infected
3. Presumptively uninfected with HIV
4. Definitively uninfected with HIV.

The presence of maternal antibodies can make diagnostic laboratory testing for HIV infection among children aged less than 18 months unreliable; these children with perinatal HIV exposure who develop an AIDS-defining illness (Box 16.1) are considered presumptively HIV-infected.

A child aged less than 18 months is categorized as definitively HIV-infected if born to an HIV-infected mother and

testing of the infant (excluding cord blood testing) shows a positive result on two separate specimens from one or more of the following HIV virologic (non-antibody) tests:

- HIV nucleic acid (DNA or RNA) detection
- HIV p24 antigen test, including neutralization assay, for a child aged less than or equal to 1 month
- HIV isolation (viral culture)

A child aged less than 18 months born to an HIV-infected mother is categorized as definitively uninfected with HIV if:

1. The criteria for definitive HIV infection are not met, and
2. At least two negative HIV DNA or RNA virologic tests from separate specimens are obtained.

The CDC laboratory criteria for reportable HIV infection among persons aged 18 months to less than 13 years exclude confirmation of HIV infection through the diagnosis of AIDS-defining conditions alone. Laboratory confirmation of HIV infection is required for all reported cases of HIV infection among children in this age group.

Children aged 18 months to less than 13 years are categorized as having AIDS if the criteria for HIV infection are met and at least one of the AIDS-defining conditions has been documented (see Box 16.1). Once HIV infection has been established, early initiation of both HAART and *Pneumocystis jirovecii* pneumonia prophylaxis, followed by scheduled administration of routine vaccinations for infants is recommended.[5]

In 2007, the World Health Organization (WHO) revised the HIV infection and AIDS clinical staging system and the clinical and surveillance case definitions.[6] They recommended reporting cases of HIV infection as HIV infection or advanced HIV disease (AHD), which includes AIDS. All cases of HIV infection, AHD, and AIDS require a confirmed diagnosis of HIV infection based on laboratory testing. The revised WHO surveillance case definitions include the following four stages:

Box 16.1

AIDS-defining conditions for children less than 13 years of age, adolescents, and adults

- Bacterial infections, multiple or recurrent[a]
- Candidiasis of bronchi, trachea, or lungs
- Candidiasis of esophagus[b]
- Cervical cancer, invasive[c]
- Coccidioidomycosis, disseminated or extrapulmonary
- Cryptococcosis, extrapulmonary
- Cryptosporidiosis, chronic intestinal (greater than 1 month's duration)
- Cytomegalovirus disease (other than liver, spleen, or nodes), onset at age >1 month
- Cytomegalovirus retinitis (with loss of vision)[b]
- Encephalopathy, HIV related
- Herpes simplex: chronic ulcers (greater than 1 month's duration) or bronchitis, pneumonitis, or esophagitis (onset at age greater than 1 month)
- Histoplasmosis, disseminated or extrapulmonary
- Isosporiasis, chronic intestinal (greater than 1 month's duration)
- Kaposi's sarcoma[b]

- Lymphoid interstitial pneumonia or pulmonary lymphoid hyperplasia complex[a,b]
- Lymphoma, Burkitt's (or equivalent term)
- Lymphoma, immunoblastic (or equivalent term)
- Lymphoma, primary, of brain
- *Mycobacterium avium* complex or *Mycobacterium kansasii*, disseminated or extrapulmonary[b]
- *Mycobacterium tuberculosis* of any site, pulmonary,[b,c] disseminated,[b] or extrapulmonary[b]
- *Mycobacterium*, other species or unidentified species, disseminated[b] or extrapulmonary[b]
- *Pneumocystis jirovecii* pneumonia[b]
- Pneumonia, recurrent[b,c]
- Progressive multifocal leukoencephalopathy
- *Salmonella* septicemia, recurrent
- Toxoplasmosis of brain, onset at age less than 1 month[b]
- Wasting syndrome attributed to HIV

[a]Only among children aged less than 13 years. (CDC. 1994 Revised classification system for human immunodeficiency virus infection in children less than 13 years of age. MMWR 1994; 43[No. RR-12].)
[b]Condition that might be diagnosed presumptively.
[c]Only among adults and adolescents aged ≥13 years. (CDC. 1993 Revised classification system for HIV infection and expanded surveillance case definition for AIDS among adolescents and adults. MMWR 1992; 41[No. RR-17].)
For surveillance purposes patients are categorized as having AIDS only if the criteria for HIV infection are met. Adapted from Schneider E, Whitmore S, Glynn KM, et al. Centers for Disease Control and Prevention (CDC). Revised surveillance case definitions for HIV infection among adults, adolescents, and children aged <18 months and for HIV infection and AIDS among children aged 18 months to <13 years – United States, 2008. MMWR Recomm Rep. 2008; 57(RR-10): 1–12.

Table 16.2 – WHO classification of HIV-associated immunodeficiency using CD4+ T cell counts and percentages

Classification of HIV associated immunodeficiency	Age-related CD4+ T cell values			
	≤11 months (CD4%)	12–35 months (CD4%)	36–59 months (CD4%)	≥5 years (cells/mm³ or CD4%)
Not significant	>35%	>30%	>25%	>500 cells/mm³
Mild	30–35%	25–30%	20–25%	350–499 cells/mm³
Advanced	25–29%	20–24%	15–19%	200–349 cells/mm³
Severe	<25%	<20%	<15%	<200 cells/mm³ or <15%

asymptomatic HIV infection, or stage 1; mildly symptomatic HIV infection, or stage 2; AHD, or stage 3; and AIDS, or stage 4.[6,7] An HIV-positive child's level of immunosuppression may be staged using circulating CD4+ T cell levels. Whereas absolute CD4+ T cell counts are typically used in adults, absolute counts normally decline dramatically over the first 5 years of life; so, for young children CD4+ T cell percentages provide best estimates of disease severity. The WHO classification of HIV-associated immunodeficiency in young children is shown in Table 16.2. A similar system recommended by the CDC grades the immune status of HIV-infected children using either CD4+ T cell counts or percentages as stage 1, 2, 3 (Table 16.3).[8] In comparison, adults with an absolute CD4+ T cell count less than 200 cells/mm³ are characterized as having AIDS; those with a count less than 100 cells/mm³ are considered profoundly immunosuppressed and at greatest risk of developing one or more ocular complications, including cytomegalovirus (CMV) and other necrotizing herpetic retinitis.[8]

Ocular manifestations of HIV/AIDS in children

Literature on the ocular manifestation of HIV/AIDS in children is limited (Table 16.4),[8-17] but suggests that ocular aspects of HIV infection differ between children and adults in several important respects. First, ocular complications of HIV/AIDS are less common in children than in adults. This is particularly true for CMV retinitis (Fig. 16.2) and HIV retinopathy (cotton-wool spots), which occur in fewer than 5% of untreated HIV-positive children, compared to 30% or more of untreated

Table 16.3 – Surveillance case definition for HIV infection among adults and adolescents (aged ≥13 years) – United States, 2008

Stage	Laboratory evidence[a]	Clinical evidence
Stage 1	Laboratory confirmation of HIV infection *and* CD4+ T-lymphocyte count of ≥500 cells/μl *or* CD4+ T-lymphocyte percentage of ≥29	None required (but no AIDS-defining condition)
Stage 2	Laboratory confirmation of HIV infection *and* CD4+ T-lymphocyte count of 200–499 cells/μl *or* CD4+ T-lymphocyte percentage of 14–28	None required (but no AIDS-defining condition)
Stage 3 (AIDS)	Laboratory confirmation of HIV infection *and* CD4+ T-lymphocyte count of <200 cells/μl *or* CD4+ T-lymphocyte percentage of <14[b]	*Or* documentation of an AIDS-defining condition (with laboratory confirmation of HIV infection)[b]
Stage unknown[c]	Laboratory confirmation of HIV infection *and* no information on CD4+ T-lymphocyte count or percentage	*And* no information on presence of AIDS-defining conditions

[a]The CD4+ T-lymphocyte percentage is the percentage of total lymphocytes. If the CD4+ T-lymphocyte count and percentage do not correspond to the same HIV infection stage, select the more severe stage.

[b]Documentation of an AIDS-defining condition (Appendix A) supersedes a CD4+ T-lymphocyte count of ≥200 cells/μL and a CD4+ T-lymphocyte percentage of total lymphocytes of ≥14. Definitive diagnostic methods of these are in the 1993 revised HIV classification system and the expanded AIDS case definition (CDC. 1993 Revised classification system for HIV infection and expanded surveillance case definition of AIDS among adolescents and adults. MMWR 1992;41 (No. RR-17) and from the National Notifiable Diseases Surveillance System (available at http://www.cdc.gov/epo/dphsi/casedet/case_definitions.htm).

[c]Although cases with no information on CD4+ T-lymphocyte count or percentage or on the presence of AIDS-defining conditions can be classified as stage unknown, every effort should be made to report CD4+ T-lymphocyte counts or percentages and the presence of AIDS-defining conditions at the time of diagnosis. Additional CD4+ T-lymphocyte counts or percentages and any identified AIDS-defining conditions can be reported as recommended. (Council of State and Territorial Epidemiologists. Laboratory reporting of clinical test results indicative of HIV infection: new standards for a new era of surveillance and prevention [Position Statement 04-ID-07]; 2004. Available at http://www.cste.org/ps/2004pdf/04-ID-07-final.pdf.)

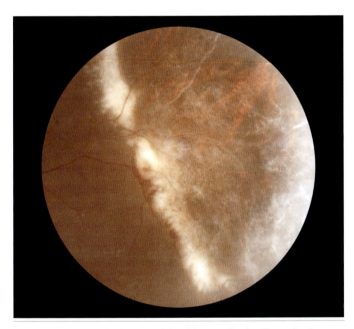

Fig. 16.2 Cytomegalovirus retinitis with an active leading edge in a child with AIDS from Rwanda.

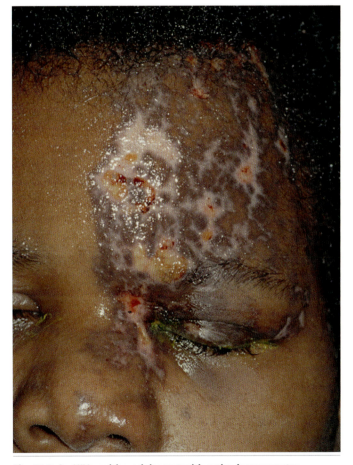

Fig. 16.3 An HIV-positive adolescent with active herpes zoster ophthalmicus.

adults.[8] Herpes zoster ophthalmicus (HZO; Fig. 16.3) appears to be less common in HIV-infected children as compared to adults,[18] although zoster dermatitis has been reported as an early complication of immune reconstitution in children receiving HAART.[19,20] Second, a distinctive retinal vasculitis[21] (Fig. 16.4), not commonly recognized in adults, is seen in about 3% of HIV-infected children in the USA[10] and France,[11] and from 30% to 40% of HIV-positive children in Africa.[14,15] Vascular inflammation is typically bilateral and peripheral with periphlebitis occurring three times more often than periarteritis. This peripheral retinal vasculitis may be associated with a generalized lymphadenopathy, including salivary

Table 16.4 – Prevalence of ocular complications in clinic-based pediatric cohorts

Study	Location	Sample size	Male:Female	Age range (months)	Average age (months)	Number (%) with eye involvement	Peripheral retinal vasculitis – number (%)	Cytomegalovirus retinitis – number (%)	HIV retinopathy (cotton-wool spots) number (%)	Chorioretinitis – number (%)	Herpes zoster ophthalmicus – number (%)	Other – number (%)
Almeida et al., 2007[17]	Brazil	111	0.63:1	5–153	26.4	19 (17.1%)	0 (0)	1 (0.9%)	0 (0%)	2 (1.8%)	1 (0.9%)	Blepharitis – 6 (5.4%); allergic conjunctivitis – 4 (3.6%); dry eye – 2 (1.8%)
Esposito et al., 2006[16]	Italy	117	1.09:1	1–268	196	9 (8.1%)	0 (0%)	8 (6.8%)	0 (0%)	1 (0.9%)	0 (0%)	
Ikoona et al., 2003[15]	Uganda	158	0.82 – 1	6–183	42	55 (34.8%)	49 (31.0%)	6 (3.8%)	0 (0%)		3 (1.9%)	Molluscum contagiosum – 16 (10.1%); conjunctival xerosis – 14 (8.9%); keratitis – 11(7.0%); optic atrophy – 5 (3.2%)
Kestelyn et al., 2000[14]	Rwanda	162	1.25:1	2–168	30	88 (54.3%)	63 (38.9%)	3 (1.9%)	4 (2.5%)	8 (4.9%)	2 (1.2%)	Conjunctival xerosis – 2(1.2%); subconjunctival hemorrhage – 2 (1.2%); conjunctival telangiectasis – 1 (0.6%); palpebral abscesses – 1 (0.6%)
Padhani et al., 2000[13]	Tanzania	62	1.06:1	18–168	44.5	24 (38.7%)	2 (3.2%)	0 (0%)	0 (0%)	0 (0%)	0 (0%)	Conjunctival xerosis – 15 (24.2%); phlyctenules – 3 (4.8%); macular edema – 8 (12.9%); retinal hemorrhages – 2 (3.2%); optic atrophy – 1 (1.6%); retinal NV – 1 (1.6%)
Hammond et al., 1997[12]	UK	98	NR	8–122	NR	5 (5.1%)	0 (0%)	3 (3.1%)	0 (0%)	0 (0%)	0 (0%)	Progressive outer retinal necrosis – 1 (1.05%); allergic conjunctivitis – 1 (1.0%)
Girard et al., 1997[11]	France	33	1.09:1	20–192	57	7 (21.2%)	1 (3.0%)	0 (0%)	0 (0%)	1 (3.0%)	1 (3.0%)	Bacterial conjunctivitis – 3 (9.1%); conjunctivitis associated with febrile rash – 3 (9.1%); retinal vascular tortuosity – 2 (6.1%); disc swelling – 2 (6.1%); molluscum contagiosum – 1 (3.0%); herpetic keratitis 1 (3.0%); chalazion 1 (3.0%); small, punctate, white retinal lesions 1 (3.0%)
de Smet et al., 1992[10]	USA	160	NR	NR	73	29 (18.1%)	5 (3.1%)	10 (6.3%)	4 (2.5%)	1 (0.6%)	0 (0%)	Heterotrophia – 10 (6.3%); 2,3'-dideoxyinosine retinal toxicity – 15 (9.4%)
Dennehy et al., 1989[9]	USA	40	1.11 – 1	1–68	23	8 (20%)	0 (0%)	2 (5.0%)	3 (7.5%)	0 (0%)	0 (0%)	Retinal hemorrhages – 2 (5%); molluscum contagiosum – 2 (5%); preseptal cellulitis – 1 (2.5%)

NR = not reported.

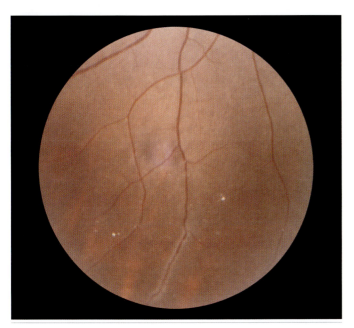

Fig. 16.4 An HIV-positive child from Africa with peripheral retinal vasculitis and several nearby superficial, small, punctate, white retinal lesions.

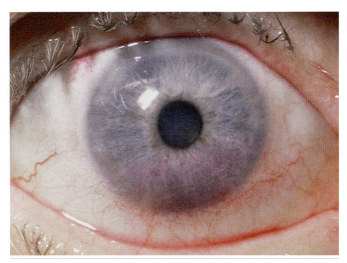

Fig. 16.5 An HIV-positive patient with keratoconjunctivitis sicca and prominent Rose Bengal staining of the inferior conjunctiva and cornea.

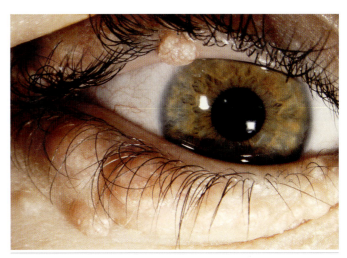

Fig. 16.6 An HIV-positive adolescent with hemophilia and both upper and lower lid molluscum contagiosum lesions.

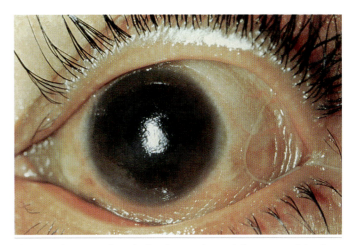

Fig. 16.7 Severe conjunctival and corneal xerosis in a young Asian boy. A prominent mucus strand is evident near the lateral canthus. *Courtesy of Dr. Alfred Sommer.*

and lacrimal gland involvement, and Lymphocytic Interstitial Pneumonia (LIP), suggesting that these children might have the same immunopathological response occurring at different body sites. Prior to the introduction of HAART, HIV-positive children with LIP had a relatively good survival as compared to overall cohorts of HIV-infected children. LIP with salivary and lacrimal gland involvement in HIV-positive children may be analogous to Diffuse Infiltrative Lymphocytosis Syndrome (DILS) in adults – an HIV-associated disorder characterized by chronic circulating and visceral CD8+ T cell infiltration, including involvement of the lung and salivary and lacrimal glands.[14]

Orbital and adnexal complications of HIV/AIDS occur in adults, and include orbital cellulitis and tumors, most notably lymphoma and Kaposi's sarcoma.[8] Orbital and adnexal involvement in HIV-positive infants and children is less common, although a single HIV-infected child with preseptal cellulitis was reported[9] (Table 16.4). A "fetal AIDS syndrome" consisting of downward obliquity of the eyes, prominent palpebral fissures, hypertelorism, and blue sclerae has been described.[22]

Prior to the introduction of HAART, up to 20% of HIV/AIDS adults had anterior segment complications, most notably conjunctival telangiectasis, keratoconjunctivitis sicca (Fig. 16.5), infectious keratitis, and molluscum contagiosum (Fig. 16.6).[8] Similar complications occur in children (see Table 16.4). Almeida et al.[17] observed dry eye in 2 of 111 HIV-infected children in Brazil. Conjunctival xerosis (Fig. 16.7), presumably due to the combined effects of malnutrition, vitamin A deficiency, and HIV-related malabsorption and diarrhea, has been noted in Africa[13-15] in 1.2%[14] to 24.2%[13] of pediatric HIV/AIDS patients. Zaborowski et al.[23] described seven black African boys from South Africa with HIV-associated arthritis and bilateral intraocular inflammation, including three with anterior uveitis and four with intermediate uveitis. Five of 10 affected eyes had cataract and two had cystoid macular edema. Although the intraocular inflammation resembled juvenile idiopathic arthritis associated uveitis, being insidious and asymptomatic in onset and bilateral and non-granulomatous in character, patients with HIV-associated arthritis and uveitis are different. They all were male, antinuclear antibody negative, and six of the seven had polyarticular joint involvement. Isolated cases of bacterial conjunctivitis, allergic conjunctivitis, otherwise unspecified keratitis and conjunctivitis, conjunctival telangiectasis, subconjunctival hemorrhage, and blepharitis have also been noted in HIV-infected children (see Table 16.2). The relationship of these findings to the child's underlying HIV infection has yet to be established.

In addition to isolated cases of CMV retinitis, HIV retinopathy, and the distinctive peripheral retinal vasculitis, posterior segment complications in children with HIV/AIDS include isolated cases of increased retinal vascular tortuosity, disc swelling, macular edema, toxoplasmic retinochoroiditis, non-CMV herpetic retinitis,[24] small punctate white retinal lesions (see Fig. 16.4), chorioretinitis of undetermined cause, and dideoxyinosine toxicity (see Table 16.4). Some of these findings may have been unrelated to the HIV status of the children.

Children infected by HIV are at increased risk of neurodevelopmental delay and increased incidence of neuro-ophthalmic complications. De Smet et al.[10] found heterotropia in 6.3% of their cohort. Isolated cases of optic atrophy of undetermined cause have been noted in children with HIV/AIDS.[13,15]

Ophthalmic screening and monitoring of HIV-infected children

Recommendations for ophthalmic screening and monitoring of HIV-infected children are not available. However, we recommend that all infants of HIV-positive mothers be screened for ocular complications shortly following birth and then every 2 to 3 months until their HIV status is known. Once HIV positivity is established, screening of children without ocular complications should be determined by overall level of immunosuppression (see Table 16.2). In the absence of ocular signs or symptoms, we recommend that children with severe immunosuppression receive a dilated eye examination every 2 to 3 months, that those with advanced immunosuppression be examined every 6 months, and that those with mild or no immunosuppression be seen annually. Once one or more ocular complications of HIV/AIDS have been identified, follow-up varies and depends upon the treatment status of the complication(s), as well as the age and immune status of the child.

References

1. UNAIDS. Report on the global AIDS epidemic, 2010. http://www.unaids.org/globalreport/Global_report.htm.
2. London NJ, Shukla D, Heiden D, et al. HIV/AIDS in the developing world. Int Ophthalmol Clin 2010; 50: 201–18.
3. Fowler MG, Gable AR, Lampe MA, et al. Perinatal HIV and its prevention: progress toward an HIV-free generation. Clin Perinatol 2010; 37: 699–719.
4. Schneider E, Whitmore S, Glynn KM, et al. Centers for Disease Control and Prevention (CDC). Revised surveillance case definitions for HIV infection among adults, adolescents, and children aged <18 months and for HIV infection and AIDS among children aged 18 months to <13 years – United States, 2008. MMWR Recomm Rep 2008; 57(RR-10): 1–12.
5. Camacho-Gonzalez AF, Ross AC, Chakraborty R. The clinical care of the HIV-1-infected infant. Clin Perinatol 2010; 37: 873–85.
6. World Health Organization (WHO). WHO case definitions of HIV for surveillance and revised clinical staging and immunological classification of HIV-related disease in adults and children. Geneva, Switzerland: WHO Press; 2007. Available at http://www.who.int/hiv/pub/guidelines/hivstaging/en/index.html.
7. WHO. Management of HIV Infection and Antiretroviral Therapy in Infants and Children. A Clinical Manual. WHO Technical Publication No. 51; 2006.
8. Cunningham ET Jr, Belfort R Jr. HIV/AIDS and the Eye: A Global Perspective. San Francisco: American Academy of Ophthalmology, 2002: Ophthalmology Monographs; Volume 15.
9. Dennehy PJ, Warman R, Flynn JT, et al. Ocular manifestations in pediatric patients with acquired immunodeficiency syndrome. Arch Ophthalmol 1989; 107: 978–82.
10. de Smet MD, Butler KM, Rubin BK, et al. The ocular complications of HIV in the pediatric population. In: Dernouchamps JP, Verougstraete C, Caspers-Velu L, Tassignon MJ, editors. Proceedings of the Third International Symposium on Uveitis. Recent Advances in Uveitis, 1992: 315–9.
11. Girard B, Prevost-Moravia G, Courpotin C, Lasfargues G. Ocular manifestations in a pediatric HIV positive population. J Fr Ophthalmol 1997; 20: 49–60.
12. Hammond CJ, Evans JA, Shah SM, et al. The spectrum of eye disease in children with AIDS due to vertically transmitted HIV disease: clinical findings, virology and recommendations for surveillance. Graefe's Arch Clin Exp Ophthalmol 1997; 235: 125–9.
13. Padhani DH, Manji KP, Mtanda AT. Ocular manifestations in children with HIV infection in Dar es Salaam, Tanzania. J Trop Pediatr 2000; 46: 145–8.
14. Kestelyn P, Lepage P, Karita E, Van de Perre P. Ocular manifestations of infection with the human immunodeficiency virus in an Af pediatric population. Ocul Immunol Infect 2000; 8: 263–73.
15. Ikoona E, Kalyesubula I, Kawuma M. Ocular manifestations in paediatric HIV/AIDS patients in Mulago Hospital, Uganda. Afr Health Sci 2003; 3: 83–6.
16. Esposito S, Porta A, Bojanin J, et al. Effect of highly active antiretroviral therapy (HAART) on the natural history of ocular manifestations in HIV-infected children. Eye 2006; 20: 595–7.
17. Almeida FPP, Paula JS, Martins MC, et al. Ocular manifestations in pediatric patients with HIV infection in the post-HAART era in southern Brazil. Eye 2007; 21: 1017–18.
18. Pandey N, Chandrakar AK, Adile SL, et al. Human immunodeficiency virus infection in a child presenting as herpes zoster ophthalmicus. J Indian Med Assoc 2007; 105: 216–17.
19. Tangsinmankong N, Kamchaisatian W, Lujan-Zilbermann J, et al. Varicella zoster as a manifestation of immune restoration disease in HIV-infected children. J Allergy Clin Immunol 2004; 113: 742–6.
20. Wang ME, Castillo ME, Montano SM, Zunt JR. Immune reconstitution inflammatory syndrome in human immunodeficiency virus-infected children in Peru. Pediatr Infect Dis J 2009; 28: 900–3.
21. Kestelyn P, Lepage P, Van de Perre P. Perivasculitis of the retinal vessels as an important sign in children with the AIDS-related complex. Am J Ophthalmol 1985; 100: 614–15.
22. Marion RW, Wiznia AA, Hutcheon G, Rubinstein A. Fetal AIDS syndrome score. Correlation between severity of dysmorphism and age at diagnosis of immunodeficiency. AJDC 1987; 141: 429–31.
23. Zaborowski AG, Parbhoo D, Chinniah K, Visser L. Uveitis in children with human immunodeficiency virus-associated arthritis. J AAPOS 2008; 12: 608–10.
24. Purdy KW, Heckenlively JR, Church JA, Keller MA. Progressive outer retinal necrosis caused by varicella-zoster virus in children with acquired immunodeficiency syndrome. Pediatr Infect Dis J 2003; 22: 384–6.

Disorders of the eye as a whole

Reecha Sachdeva · Elias I Traboulsi

The ophthalmologist needs to make an exact diagnosis in patients with eyes that are smaller than normal, or with malformations affecting anterior or posterior structures. A precise diagnosis allows good counseling of patients and families and an educated guess at visual outcomes and screening for possible future complications. Conditions that are associated with a small ocular size include microphthalmos and anophthalmos, nanophthalmos, persistent hyperplastic primary vitreous, and some cases of aniridia and Peters' anomaly.

Anophthalmos and microphthalmos

Anophthalmos and microphthalmos are rare, with an incidence of between 2 and 19 per 100 000 live births, respectively.[1-3] They are often associated with systemic malformations. Although reported risk factors include maternal age over 40 years, multiple births, low birth weight, and low gestational age, there is no unifying causation, and clustering of cases, which might suggest an environmental cause, probably does not occur.[1,2,4,5]

Anophthalmos

Anophthalmos is when the eye is non-existent (Fig. 17.1) or, more commonly, when it is not visible and a tiny cystic remnant of the eye is identified on pathology. The term, "clinical anophthalmos," emphasizes that there is a spectrum in which anophthalmos merges with microphthalmos. True anophthalmos is sometimes associated with absence of the optic nerve and chiasm, as in some patients with *SOX2* mutations.[6]

Secondary abnormalities of the orbit occur, with orbital growth universally retarded to some extent. Extraocular muscles may be absent and the optic foramen size is often decreased. The conjunctival sac may be small. Although the absence of a developing eye does not affect the initial development of a bony orbit,[7] the growth of the orbit is highly influenced by the presence or absence of an eye. The mean axial length of the human full-term neonatal and adult eyes are approximately 17 and 23.8 mm, respectively,[8] with the normal neonatal eye measuring 70% of the adult size.[9] Orbital volume increases dramatically during the first 3 years of life, especially in the first year.

While orbital volume cannot be assessed using plain radiographs, the horizontal and vertical sizes of the orbital openings from the orbital rim can be measured and are reduced in adults with congenital anophthalmos, or in those enucleated within the first year of life. This retardation of orbital growth is halved when an orbital implant is used, and the severity of the overall reduction in volume diminishes if the insult occurs at a later date. Orbital growth appears to be complete by the age of 15 years; subsequent enucleation will not result in appreciable size difference.[10]

Anophthalmos is a complete failure of budding of the optic vesicle or early arrest of its development. Consecutive or degenerative anophthalmos is when an optic vesicle formed, but subsequently degenerated. The presence of optic nerves, chiasm, or tract with anophthalmos may indicate this pathogenesis.

Many causes for anophthalmos have been proposed; these merge with the causes of microphthalmos (see next section).

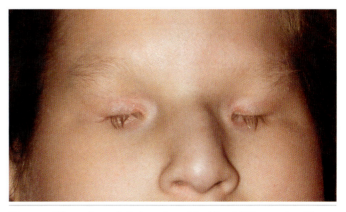

Fig. 17.1 Bilateral anophthalmos in a girl with a *SOX2* mutation. There was absence of all visual pathways.

Bilaterality and increased severity imply an early teratogenic or genetic developmental event.[11] In isolated cases, inheritance may be autosomal dominant[12] or autosomal recessive.[13] In families with clear Mendelian inheritance, ocular pathology may be asymmetric or even unilateral. Mutations in *SOX2* are one of the more common causes of anophthalmos.[14]

Microphthalmos

The volume of a microphthalmic eye is reduced. Often, clinical suspicion arises from a corneal diameter less than 10 mm in adults. Although microphthalmos is usually associated with a small cornea, there may be microphthalmos with a normal cornea, and microcornea without microphthalmos.[15,16] Ultrasonographic determination of an axial length less than 21 mm in an adult or 19 mm in a 1-year-old child substantiates a diagnosis of microphthalmos.[17] This represents a reduction of 2 standard deviations or more below normal.

Bilateral microphthalmos[18] occurs in approximately 10% of blind children.[19] The effect of microphthalmos on vision depends on whether it is bilateral, the severity of the microphthalmos, and associated ocular malformations – specifically, the degree of retinal maldevelopment, horizontal corneal diameter, and the presence or absence of cataract and coloboma.[20]

Microphthalmos may be simple (without other ocular defects) or complex (associated with anterior segment malformations, cataracts, retinal or vitreous disease, or more complex malformations).[17,21] It can be further divided into colobomatous (Fig. 17.2) and non-colobomatous on the basis of associated uveal abnormalities.[15,22] The association between eye growth and closure of the fetal fissure is important since closure of the cleft is completed early in development.[23]

Microphthalmos represents a non-specific growth failure of the eye in response to prenatal insults and genetic defects. Inadequate postnatal growth, secondary to decreased size of the optic cup, altered vitreous composition, and low intraocular pressure, may play a role in the pathogenesis of simple microphthalmos.[21] Posterior segment abnormalities and complex microphthalmos may be secondary to inadequate production of secondary vitreous.[17] Microphthalmos can be classified according to mode of inheritance, environmental causes, chromosomal aberration, as well as syndromic associations that have additional systemic abnormalities. (For a complete search of inherited conditions associated with microphthalmos and anophthalmos, see http://www.ncbi.nlm.nih.gov/omim.)[7,15]

Idiopathic isolated microphthalmos

Vision is variably affected, depending on the degree to which the eye is microphthalmic as well as associated high errors of refraction and consequent amblyopia.

Inherited isolated microphthalmos

Although most cases are sporadic,[24,25] some are autosomal dominant.[26] Some families (Fig. 17.3) have dominant inheritance of colobomatous microphthalmos, with variable expression with extreme microphthalmos at one end of the spectrum and coloboma at the other. A high rate of consanguinity suggests an autosomal recessive inheritance in some cases.[13,27] X-linked recessive inheritance occurs, sometimes with mental retardation.[28]

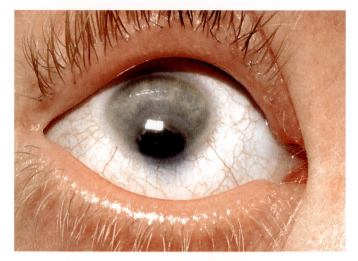

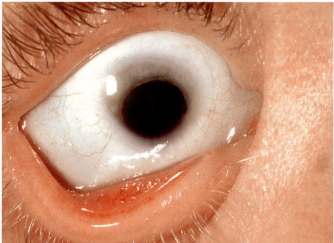

Fig. 17.2 Colobomatous microphthalmos. Both eyes are generally small with an inferior coloboma in the fundus. Although vision was limited to an acuity of 2/60 in each eye, the patient had a useful field and navigated without problems.

Microphthalmos with orbital cyst

This form of microphthalmos presents with a bulge behind the lower lid from birth (Fig. 17.4A). It is secondary to failure of optic fissure closure and the protrusion of a cyst from the coloboma. It has been confused with a congenital cystic eye,[29] but the two are different. In the latter, the eye is replaced by a cystic structure and there is no lens or other normal eye structures. In microphthalmos with cyst, the small eye often cannot be seen and a neoplasm may be suspected. The cyst usually communicates with the eye.[30-32] Presentation may be as an orbital mass distending the lids and hiding the eye, or as proptosis in which a microphthalmic eye is visible. Ultrasonography and CT or MRI scanning aid in diagnosis (Fig. 17.4B).[31] Most cases of microphthalmos with cyst are sporadic; familial cases have been reported, with presumed autosomal recessive inheritance.[30,33,34]

Management is initially conservative, especially for small cysts. Large cysts may be managed with repeated aspiration or by surgical removal.[31,35-37] If the cyst is not growing rapidly, it may be left in place until some orbital growth is achieved. Because of the communication of the cyst with the eye, removal

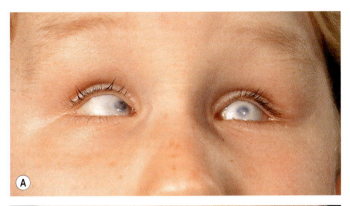

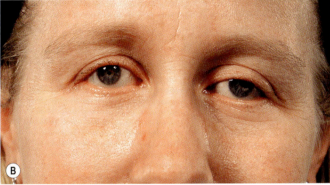

Fig. 17.3 (A) Bilateral marked non-colobomatous microphthalmos. (B) Mother of the child in (A) showing bilateral non-colobomatous microphthalmos.

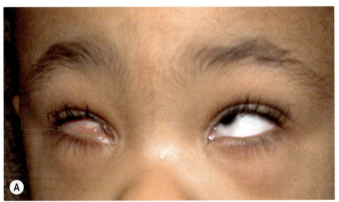

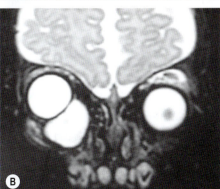

Fig. 17.4 (A) Bulge in right lower lid is due to pressure from cyst behind it. Ipsilateral eye is microphthalmic and has a coloboma. (B) MRI of same patient shows small eye with attached cyst.

of the cyst may deflate the microphthalmic eye necessitating its removal.

Microphthalmos with cryptophthalmos

Cryptophthalmos implies a varying degree of skin covering the eyeball, with variable cutaneous adhesions to the cornea.[38] It is usually bilateral with a variable degree of severity. Unilateral cases have been described.

Francois described three subgroups of cryptophthalmos:[39]

1. Complete cryptophthalmos (Fig. 17.5): the lids are replaced by a layer of skin without lashes or glands that is fused with the microphthalmic eye without a conjunctival sac. Normal electrophysiological responses have been recorded.[40]
2. Incomplete cryptophthalmos (Fig. 17.6): the lids are colobomatous (often medially) or rudimentary and there is a small conjunctival sac. The exposed cornea is often opaque.
3. An abortive form: the upper lid is partly fused with the upper cornea and conjunctiva and may be colobomatous.[38] The globe is often small.

A fourth autosomal dominant type exists in which the upper lid is very tall and fused with the lower one at the margins. There is a normal complement of lashes. A dimple in the upper lid indicates where it is attached to the underlying eyeball.[41]

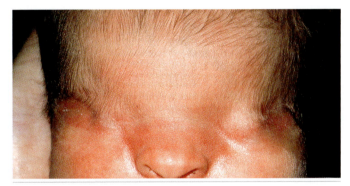

Fig. 17.5 Complete cryptophthalmos. Note the characteristic continuation of the forehead skin onto the cheek. There is an abnormal hairline extending to the brow.

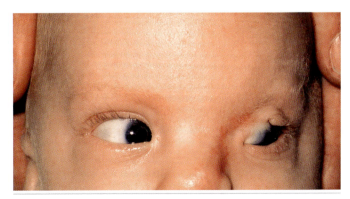

Fig. 17.6 Partial cryptophthalmos of the left eye. The eye is small and the cornea is opaque. There is a colobomatous upper lid and a characteristic "lick" of hair from the temple to the brow with a unilateral nose abnormality.

The systemic associations with cryptophthalmos and microphthalmos include nose deformities, cleft lip and palate, syndactyly, abnormal genitalia, renal agenesis, mental retardation, and many others.[38,42,43]

Microphthalmos with ocular and systemic malformations

Other eye malformations and systemic abnormalities are frequent in microphthalmos. Numerous syndromes associated with microphthalmos have been reported (http://www.ncbi.nlm.nih.gov/omim).[44]

Microphthalmos with ocular abnormalities

Microphthalmos is a non-specific response to a wide variety of influences. It occurs with many severe eye diseases, including anterior segment malformations such as Peters' anomaly or cataracts, especially in the context of a chromosomal abnormality,[45] persistent hyperplastic primary vitreous (PHPV),[46] and multisystem syndromes such as the oculodentodigital syndrome.[47] Microphthalmos may be secondary to severe, widespread intraocular disease including retinopathy of prematurity, retinal dysplasia, retinal folds,[48] retinal degeneration and glaucoma. A three-generation family has been described with aniridia, anophthalmos, and microcephaly.[49] Coloboma is the most common associated ocular malformation with microphthalmos and is found in many microphthalmos syndromes.[50,51]

Microphthalmos with systemic malformations

Up to 50% of patients with anophthalmos and microphthalmos have associated systemic abnormalities.[9,52] Many patients with microphthalmos-associated syndromes, especially chromosomal disorders, are mentally retarded[28,53,54] or have cleft palate with and without macrosomia.[55]

The most common syndromic cause of colobomatous microphthalmos is the CHARGE syndrome (Coloboma, Heart abnormalities, Atresia of the choanae, Retardation of growth and development, Genitourinary abnormalities, and Ear/hearing abnormalities).[50] Patients can have cranial nerve abnormalities such as facial nerve palsy, craniofacial clefting, dysphagia/esophageal abnormalities, duplication of the thumb, and congenital brain abnormalities, particularly of the forebrain.[56,57] Although most cases are sporadic, autosomal dominant transmission has been reported.[58] Mutations in the *CHD7* gene are responsible for 60% of CHARGE cases, with possible genotype–phenotype correlation.[59,60] *CHD7* encodes a putative chromodomain protein widely expressed in the neuroectoderm and in neural crest cells during human development.[61] Mutation in the *SEMA3E* gene can result in CHARGE syndrome.[62]

The Temple-al-Gazali syndrome (Fig. 17.7) also referred to as X-linked dominant microphthalmos with linear skin defects (MLS) syndrome or the microphthalmos, dermal aplasia, and sclerocornea (MIDAS) syndrome results from a deletion of Xp22.2-pter.[63,64] Patients have linear, irregular areas of skin aplasia especially of the head and neck, microphthalmos with variable sclerocornea, and, sometimes, abnormal intelligence.[65-67] The condition is lethal in XY males.

Fryns "anophthalmos plus" syndrome is microphthalmos or anophthalmos, cleft lip or palate, and sacral neural tube defect.[68] The branchio-oculofacial syndrome combines a broad nose with large lateral pillars, branchial sinuses, and orbital

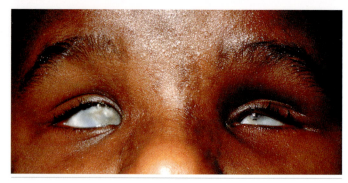

Fig. 17.7 Microphthalmos, dermal aplasia, and sclerocornea (MIDAS or Temple-al-Gazali) syndrome showing extreme microphthalmos and characteristic skin lesions.

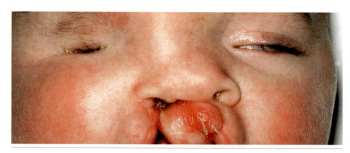

Fig. 17.8 Right clinical anophthalmos, left microphthalmos in a child with bilateral cleft lip and palate associated with fronto-facio-nasal dysplasia.

cysts.[69,70] Other microphthalmos syndromes with facial defects include fronto-facio-nasal dysplasia (Fig. 17.8),[71] and the cerebro-oculo-nasal syndrome in which there is an asociation of anophthalmos/microphthalmos, abnormal nares, and central nervous system anomalies.[72]

In Delleman's syndrome there is an association of skin tags, punched-out lesions of the skin on the ears and elsewhere, mental retardation, hydrocephalus, brain malformations, and orbital cysts.[73,74]

Microphthalmos has been described in patients with growth retardation, microcephaly, brachycephaly, oligophrenia syndrome (GOMBO syndrome).[75]

The eyes can be quite small in some patients with the oculo-dento-digital syndrome, characterized by bilateral digital anomalies (Fig. 17.9) with cutaneous syndactyly of fingers and camptodactyly,[47,76] thin nose with hypoplastic alae nasi and small nares, partial dental agenesis, enamel hypoplasia, and glaucoma.[77,78]

Patients with the less common recessive variety are more likely to have microphthalmos.[79] The syndrome results from mutations in Connexin 43. Iris cysts and anomalous retinal development may occur.[80]

Waardenburg's recessive anophthalmos syndrome includes microphthalmos with syndactyly, oligodactyly, and other limb defects and mental retardation.[81]

Patients with the X-linked recessive Lenz' microphthalmos syndrome have microphthalmos with mental retardation, malformed ears, and skeletal anomalies.[51,82,83] The gene maps to Xq27-q28 but has not been identified yet.

The autosomal recessive Warburg's MICRO syndrome comprises microphakia, microphthalmos, characteristic

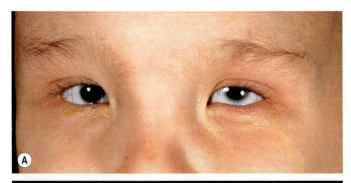

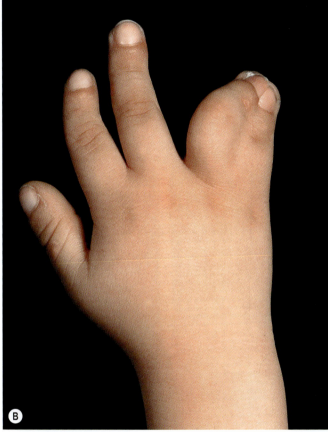

Fig. 17.9 (A) Bilateral microphthalmos, thin nose, and epicanthic folds in a patient with the oculo-dento-digital syndrome. (B) Cutaneous syndactyly of fingers and camptodactyly in the oculo-dento-digital syndrome.

lens opacity, atonic pupils, cortical visual impairment, microcephaly, developmental delay by 6 months of age, and microgenitalia in males.[84,85] It can be caused by mutations in the gene encoding the catalytic subunit of the RAB3 GTPase-activating protein complex (RAB3GAP).[86]

Gene mutations associated with anophthalmos and microphthalmos

A large number of chromosomal deletions, duplications, and translocations have been linked to anophthalmos and microphthalmos, often in association with well-delineated syndromic conditions.[87] A number of genes have been identified as causes of anophthalmos and microphthalmos.

SOX2

The *SOX2* gene located at 3q26.3-27 is a major causative gene of microphthalmos and anophthalmos with an autosomal-dominant inheritance pattern. De novo heterozygous loss-of-function point mutations account for 10–20% of bilateral anophthalmos and severe microphthalmos.[14] It is expressed at critical stages of eye development[88] and mutations have been associated with sclerocornea, cataract, persistent hyperplastic primary vitreous, optic disc dysplasia, mental retardation, neurologic abnormalities,[6] facial dysmorphism, failure to thrive and anomalies of the gastrointestinal, pituitary gland, and genital systems.

PAX6

Mutations in this gene on chromosome 11p13 generally cause aniridia, but may rarely cause autosomal-dominant panocular malformations, microphthalmos, and anophthalmos.[3,89] *PAX6* and *SOX2* interact and play a regulatory role in lens induction in several animal models.[90]

PAX2

Mutations in *PAX2* are found in cases of the renal-coloboma syndrome (ocular colobomas, vesicoureteral reflux, and kidney anomalies).[91] The eyes are sometimes small (see Chapter 51).

CHX10

Human *CHX10* is expressed in progenitor cells of the developing neuroretina and in the inner nuclear layer of the mature retina. The human microphthalmos locus was mapped on chromosome 14q24.3; *CHX10* mutations were identified in non-syndromic autosomal recessive microphthalmos, cataracts, and severe abnormalities of the iris.[92]

FOXE3

Mutations in this gene on chromosome 1p32 have been associated with microphthalmos and lens agenesis.[93] The locus had been previously linked to congenital primary aphakia.

OTX2

This gene located at 14q22-23, is a bicoid-type homeodomain transcription factor expressed in the neuroretina and brain. Heterozygous loss-of-function mutations account for 2% of anophthalmos and severe microphthalmos.[88]

BMP4

This gene, also at 14q22-23, is a candidate gene for anophthalmos. As a member of the transforming growth factor-β1 superfamily of secretory signaling molecules, it is important in optic vesicle formation, lens induction, and anterior and posterior segment development.[88]

Additional mutations associated with microphthalmos and anophthalmos have been identified in *RX*,[94,95] *BCOR*,[96] and *STRA6*, among others.[97] Several loci for dominant, recessive, and X-linked inherited microphthalmos have been identified (http://www.ncbi.nlm.nih.gov/omim).

While cluster studies have failed to identify causal links between environmental factors and microphthalmos/anophthalmos,[5] prenatal infection with rubella, toxoplasmosis, varicella, cytomegalovirus, parvovirus B19, influenza, and coxsackie A9 have been implicated.[2,9,98,99] Maternal vitamin A toxicity,[100] hyperthermia,[101] X-ray exposure, and prenatal drug exposure (thalidomide, warfarin, alcohol, the fungicide benomyl) have been postulated as potential non-infectious etiologies.[8]

Other disorders of the eye as a whole

Nanophthalmos

Nanophthalmos (Fig. 17.10) is a rare condition characterized by eyes whose axial length is less than 20 mm in adults. There is high hypermetropia, a weak but thick sclera with abnormal collagen,[102] a tendency toward angle closure glaucoma in young patients,[103] and uveal effusion. Some cases are autosomal recessive. Sundin and associates found a frameshift mutation in the original recessive nanophthalmos kindred and four independent mutations in the *MFRP* gene on 11q23.3.[104,105] There is an increased fibronectin level in nanophthalmic sclera and cells: it is a compound involved with cellular adhesion and healing.[106] Nanophthalmos may result from an abnormality in composition of sclera that prevents its normal expansion as the eye grows.

Any surgery, but especially intraocular surgery and even laser trabeculoplasty,[107-110] may be complicated by severe uveal

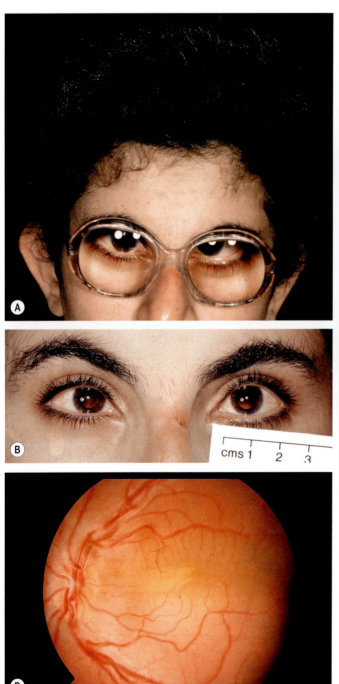

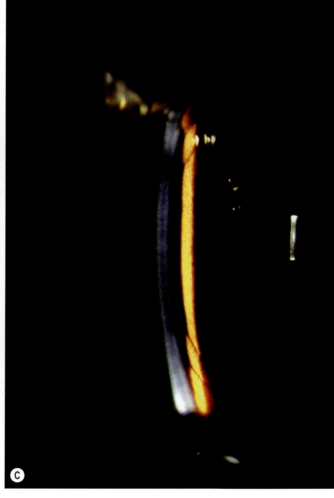

Fig. 17.10 (A) Patient with nanophthalmos wearing high hypermetropic glasses. The phakic correction was +10.00 D right, +11.00 left. (B) Patient with nanophthalmos with small eyes and abnormal red reflex with coaxial illumination. (C) Shallow anterior chamber in patient with nanophthalmos. The eyes are prone to angle closure glaucoma. (D) Retinal appearance in a patient with nanophthalmos showing a crowded optic disc and prominent yellow foveal pigment with a fold between the fovea and the macula. Nanophthalmic eyes are very prone to choroidal effusions spontaneously or in response to intraocular surgery.

effusion. Vortex vein decompression may reduce the incidence of uveal effusion.[107]

Cyclopia and synophthalmos

Complete (cyclopia) or partial (synophthalmos) fusion of the two eyes is very rare. The brain fails to develop two hemispheres and the orbit has gross deformities.[111-113] They are rarely compatible with life. The brain is almost always malformed; the telencephalon fails to divide and a large dorsal cyst develops. The orbit is markedly affected as a consequence of the abnormal development of midline mesodermal structures. The normal nasal cavity is replaced by the "pseudo-orbit."[114] The eyes are more commonly partly fused with one optic nerve and no chiasm. Other intraocular abnormalities such as persistent hyperplastic primary vitreous, cataract, coloboma, and microcornea may exist.[115]

Chromosomal aberrations are common.[116] Familial occurrences and association with consanguineous marriages have also been noted.[117] Other etiologic considerations include maternal health and toxic factors.[118]

Clinical evaluation and management of anophthalmos and microphthalmos

The ophthalmologist faced with a new patient with microphthalmos must address several questions:

1. Is this an isolated ocular problem or are there associated systemic malformations?
2. What is the level of vision?
3. What is the refractive error? Is amblyopia present?
4. Are colobomas present? Do they involve the fovea?
5. Are there other ocular malformations?
6. Is there evidence of congenital infection, chromosomal abnormality, or environmental factors?
7. Is this genetically determined and heritable with recurrence risks in siblings?
8. Are there life-threatening associations (cardiac, brain, or renal defects) or factors that may alter parental expectations (mental retardation or deafness)?

Following family and medical history, physical examination, review of systems, appropriate chromosomal testing, and molecular genetic testing are ordered. Neuro- and orbital imaging and possibly renal ultrasonography and audiological assessment may be needed.

Clinical diagnosis of anophthalmos may be difficult. To differentiate between anophthalmos and extreme microphthalmos, the examiner can touch the lids to feel for any globe movements from residual extraocular muscle function. Diagnosis may be aided by corneal diameter measurements. Bulging of the lower lid may be observed in patients with microphthalmos with cyst. Unilateral anophthalmos is often associated with anomalies of the other eye. Detailed examination of both eyes is crucial.[119] Eye examination of both parents and any siblings needs to be undertaken. Small visually insignificant colobomas in otherwise normal eyes indicate carrier state of the mutation.

Vision should be assessed and may require electrodiagnostic testing in infants (see Chapter 8). Visual evoked potential may demonstrate reduced, but useful, function in patients with clinical anophthalmos. The evaluation of visual potential is imperative; it may guide the approach to socket expansion if indicated. Ophthalmologists should withhold prognostication of visual potential based on degree of microphthalmos and ocular malformation. Patients with very small eyes and even large colobomas may have preserved vision.

Neuroimaging or ultrasound may demonstrate extremely microphthalmic eyes, but histological sectioning is needed to determine the presence of neural ectoderm-derived cells (in microphthalmos) or their absence (in anophthalmos). Ultrasound is useful to determine a decreased axial length in microphthalmic eyes. MRI is important as many conditions associated with microphthalmos and anophthalmos affect brain development.[120]

Ophthalmic intervention may be limited to glasses to offset amblyogenic refractive errors, helping the ocularist in management and fitting of cosmetic shells or contact lenses in non-seeing eyes, and diagnosing and treating glaucoma and cataracts. Microphthalmic eyes with corneal opacities may rarely require corneal grafting, but such interventions should be weighed against the risk of making the situation worse by precipitating glaucoma or more corneal opacification with graft failure. In patients with unilateral microphthalmos and poor vision, protective glasses should be prescribed.

Underdevelopment of the bony orbit, eyelids, and fornices leads to the inability to retain a prosthesis later in life. Mild microphthalmos may be managed with enlarging conformers, which should be translucent if there is vision. While anophthalmos is initially managed similarly with a conformer in the first several weeks of life, serial static implants or expandable implants may be used after 6 months of age to increase orbital volume. Complications of orbital implants include wound dehiscence, extrusion, or inadequate stimulation of bony growth.[8] Hydrophylic expanders held in place by tarsorrhaphy may allow growth of the bony orbit.[9] Controversially, some advocate early removal of a non-seeing microphthalmic eye with replacement of tissue by dermis fat graft or ball implant. In cases of microphthalmos with cyst, surgical intervention may be delayed as orbital growth is more likely if the eye and cyst are left in place.[9]

Proper referral to multidisciplinary teams is optimal. Because midline neurologic and pituitary abnormalities are common, referral to neurology and endocrinology may be indicated. In cases of bilateral anophthalmos or severe microphthalmos with no light perception, melatonin may establish regular nocturnal sleep patterns (see Chapter 121).[9] If no syndromic findings are identified initially, evaluation may be repeated at 3–5 years. Many syndromes may not fully manifest until later in childhood. Referral to a low vision specialist, occupational therapist, and other agencies may be indicated.

The benefits of genetic evaluation are threefold. In cases of severe vision loss, identification of a potential cause may ease the guilt felt by some parents. Known syndromic findings of mutations of certain genes or chromosomal rearrangements may drive multidisciplinary approach and screening. Genetic counseling may aid in risk assessment for future siblings of the affected child. However, given the number of genes identified with a link to anophthalmos and microphthalmos, genetic counseling may be difficult. Even when a causal mutation is identified, gonadal mosaicism and variable penetrance may make recurrence risk prediction difficult.[8,88] For example, there

145

have been observations of normal parents of affected children carrying loss of function *SOX2* and *OTX2* mutations.[8] Given systemic comorbidities identified with many mutations, the patient's siblings may be tested for genetic abnormalities. With unbalanced chromosomal translocation, with parents having rearrangements, the risk to siblings is higher and genetic testing should be recommended.

Prenatal diagnosis can be made by ultrasound early in the second trimester.[121] Transvaginal ultrasound may identify anophthalmos and microphthalmos. Cytogenetic studies may be conducted on amniotic fluid samples at 14 weeks' gestation, or on chorionic villus samples at 10–12 weeks' gestation. These may be useful when an anomaly is identified on ultrasonography, to identify gene mutations associated with neurologic anomalies and other systemic findings.

References

1. Shaw GM, Carmichael SL, Yang W, et al. Epidemiologic characteristics of anophthalmia and bilateral microphthalmia among 2.5 million births in California, 1989–1997. Am J Med Genet A 2005; 137: 36–40.

3. Morrison D, FitzPatrick D, Hanson I, et al. National study of microphthalmia, anophthalmia, and coloboma (MAC) in Scotland: investigation of genetic aetiology. J Med Genet 2002; 39: 16–22.

9. Ragge NK, Subak-Sharpe ID, Collin JR. A practical guide to the management of anophthalmia and microphthalmia. Eye (Lond) 2007; 21: 1290–300.

14. Fantes J, Ragge NK, Lynch SA, et al. Mutations in SOX2 cause anophthalmia. Nat Genet 2003; 33: 461–3.

20. Elder MJ. Aetiology of severe visual impairment and blindness in microphthalmos. Br J Ophthalmol 1994; 78: 332–4.

29. Hayashi N, Repka MX, Ueno H, et al. Congenital cystic eye: report of two cases and review of the literature. Surv Ophthalmol 1999; 44: 173–9.

35. Raynor M, Hodgkins P. Microphthalmos with cyst: preservation of the eye by repeated aspiration. J Pediatr Ophthalmol Strabismus 2001; 38: 245–6.

36. McLean CJ, Ragge NK, Jones RB, Collin JR. The management of orbital cysts associated with congenital microphthalmos and anophthalmos. Br J Ophthalmol 2003; 87: 860–3.

44. Baraitser MW, R, Russel-Eggitt I, et al. GENEEYE. Bushey: London Medical Databases; 2003.

52. Maumenee I, Mitchell T. Colobomatous malformations of the eye. Trans Am Ophthalmol Soc 1990.

57. Blake KD, Hartshorne TS, Lawand C, et al. Cranial nerve manifestations in CHARGE syndrome. Am J Med Genet A 2008; 146A: 585–92.

59. Lalani SR, Safiullah AM, Fernbach SD, et al. Spectrum of CHD7 mutations in 110 individuals with CHARGE syndrome and genotype-phenotype correlation. Am J Hum Genet 2006; 78: 303–14.

66. McLeod SD, Sugar J, Elejalde BR, et al. Gazali-Temple syndrome. Arch Ophthalmol 1994; 112: 851–2.

68. Makhoul IR, Soudack M, Kochavi O, et al. Anophthalmia-plus syndrome: a clinical report and review of the literature. Am J Med Genet A 2007; 143: 64–8.

83. Ng D, Hadley DW, Tifft CJ, Biesecker LG. Genetic heterogeneity of syndromic X-linked recessive microphthalmia-anophthalmia: is Lenz microphthalmia a single disorder? Am J Med Genet 2002; 110: 308–14.

84. Warburg M, Sjo O, Fledelius HC, Pedersen SA. Autosomal recessive microcephaly, microcornea, congenital cataract, mental retardation, optic atrophy, and hypogenitalism. Micro syndrome. Am J Dis Child 1993; 147: 1309–12.

86. Aligianis IA, Johnson CA, Gissen P, et al. Mutations of the catalytic subunit of RAB3GAP cause Warburg Micro syndrome. Nat Genet 2005; 37: 221–3.

91. Cunliffe HE, McNoe LA, Ward TA, et al. The prevalence of PAX2 mutations in patients with isolated colobomas or colobomas associated with urogenital anomalies. J Med Genet 1998; 35: 806–12.

95. London NJS, Kessler P, Williams B, et al. Sequence alterations in RX in patients with microphthalmia, anophthalmia, and/or coloboma. Mol Vis 2009; 15: 162–7.

100. Ozeki H, Shirai S. Developmental eye abnormalities in mouse fetuses induced by retinoic acid. Jpn J Ophthalmol 1998; 42: 162–7.

101. Milunsky A, Ulcickas M, Rothman KJ, et al. Maternal heat exposure and neural tube defects. JAMA 1992; 268: 882–5.

104. Sundin OH, Leppert GS, Silva ED, et al. Extreme hyperopia is the result of null mutations in MFRP, which encodes a Frizzled-related protein. Proc Natl Acad Sci USA 2005; 102: 9553–8.

105. Sundin OH, Dharmaraj S, Bhutto IA, et al. Developmental basis of nanophthalmos: MFRP is required for both prenatal ocular growth and postnatal emmetropization. Ophthalmic Genet 2008; 29: 1–9.

113. Situ D, Reifel CW, Smith R, et al. Investigation of a cyclopic, human, term fetus by use of magnetic resonance imaging (MRI). J Anat 2002; 200: 431–8.

119. O'Keefe M, Webb M, Pashby RC, Wagman RD. Clinical anophthalmos. Br J Ophthalmol 1987; 71: 635–8.

120. Mathers PH, Grinberg A, Mahon KA, Jamrich M. The Rx homeobox gene is essential for vertebrate eye development. Nature 1997; 387: 603–7.

Access the complete reference list online at
http://www.expertconsult.com

Developmental anomalies of the lids

Hélène Dollfus • Alain Verloes

Major developmental anomalies create significant medical problems.[1] They often require specific surgical or medical management. Minor anomalies are features that vary from those commonly seen in the normal population; they do not cause increased morbidity. Major anomalies are not a variation of the normal spectrum. Developmental anomalies of the eyelids can belong to both categories. They can be isolated or observed in a syndromic context.

Single developmental anomalies are divided into four categories:[2]

1. A deformation is caused by an abnormal external force (usually, but not always) before birth, that results in an abnormal growth or formation of a body part.
2. A disruption occurs when a normally growing region is disrupted by some process, such as anoxic necrosis. Usually, disruptions and deformations are isolated and not associated with multiple congenital anomalies.
3. A malformation is an abnormal development of a body part due to an underlying genetic, epigenetic, or environmental or stochastic factor that alters normal development.
4. A dysplasia is an alteration of an intrinsic cellular architecture that can appear, or evolve with time (by opposition to a malformation). Malformation and dysplasia are not mutually exclusive: a malformation can be underlined by a tissue dysplasia.

When several developmental anomalies are present, three situations are defined:

1. An association is a group of anomalies that occur more frequently together than expected by chance, but which do not have a unified underlying etiology. Many associations described in the literature are syndromes (such as the CHARGE "association").
2. A sequence is a group of anomalies that stem from a single major anomaly that alters the development of other surrounding or related tissues or structures. The term "field defect" describes malformations of distinct anatomic structures located in a particular region of the body.
3. A syndrome is a well-characterized constellation of major and minor anomalies that occur together in a predictable fashion, presumably due to a unique underlying etiology that may be monogenic, chromosomal, mitochondrial, or teratogenic in origin. A syndrome is clinically defined, and several distinct etiologies may be causative (e.g. Bardet-Biedl syndrome can be caused by more than 16 different gene defects).

Normal development and anatomy of the eyelids

Embryology of the eyelids

Development of the eyelids is characterized by three main stages:

1. Initial development
2. Fusion
3. Final reopening.

Initial development

During the first month of embryonic development, the optic vesicle is covered by a thin layer of surface ectoderm. During the second month, active cellular proliferation of the adjacent mesoderm results in the formation of a circular fold of mesoderm lined by ectoderm. This fold constitutes the rudiments of the eyelid, which gradually elongates over the eye. The mesodermal portion of the upper lid arises from the frontal nasal process, the lower lid from the maxillary process. The covering layer of ectoderm becomes skin on the outside, conjunctiva on the inside. Tarsal plate, connective, and muscles of the eyelids are derived from the mesodermal core.

Fusion

Fusion of the eyelids by an epithelial seal begins at the two extremities at 8 weeks and is soon complete, covering the corneal epithelium. The eyelids remain adherent to each other until the end of the fifth to the seventh month.

Final reopening

Separation begins from the nasal side, and is usually completed during the sixth or seventh month of development. Very rarely, this process is incomplete at birth in a full-term infant (Fig. 18.1).[3] The specialized structures in the lids develop between 8 weeks and 7 months. By term, the lid is fully developed.

Morphology and anatomy of the eyelids

The eyelids have several characteristic horizontal and vertical folds.

The most conspicuous is a well-demarcated horizontal skin crease 3–4 mm above the upper lid margin, which flattens out on depression and becomes deeply recessed when the upper lid is elevated. It divides each lid into an orbital and tarsal portion. The orbital portion lies between the margin of the orbit and the crease; the tarsal portion lies in direct relationship to the globe. A tarsal plate composed of dense connective tissue is found in both the upper and lower eyelids. The upper lid tarsal plate has a marginal length of 29 mm and is 10–12 mm wide. The lower lid tarsal plate is 4 mm wide.

The palpebral fissure is the entrance into the conjunctival sac bounded by the margins of the eyelids; it forms an asymmetrical ellipse that undergoes complex changes during infancy.[4] After birth, the upper lid has its lowest position with the lower eyelid margin close to the pupil center. Between ages 3 and 6 months, the position of the upper lid reaches its maximum. The distance between the pupil center and the lower eyelid margin increases linearly until age 18 months.[4] By adulthood, the upper eyelid covers the upper 1–2 mm of the cornea, the lower lid lies slightly below its inferior margin.[5] Palpebral fissures have a slight outer-upward inclination as the

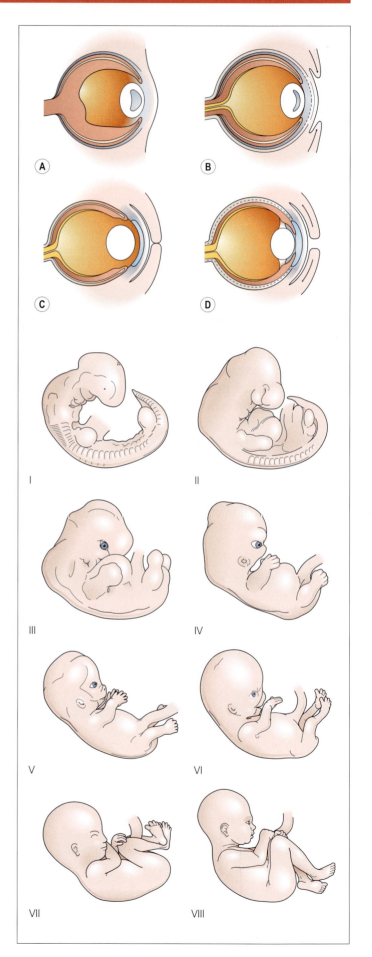

Fig. 18.1 Development of the eyelids. Schematic representation of the eyelids and the development of the embryo and the fetus (after 2 months). (A–D) Main stages of the development of the eyelids. (A) Before 6 weeks: optic vesicle covered with surface ectoderm. (B) Between 6 and 8 weeks: superior and inferior folds elongated over the eye. (C) Soon after 8 weeks of development: fusion of the superior and inferior folds of the eyelids until the seventh month. (D) From the seventh month to birth; the eyelids are open. (I–VIII) Main stages of development of a human being with regard to eyelid development. (I) Embryo aged 31–35 days (no eyelids). (II) Embryo aged 6 weeks (the eyelids start to appear). (III) Embryo aged 7 weeks. (IV, V) Embryo during the 8th week. (VI) Embryo aged 9 weeks (the eyelids have started to fuse). (VII) Fetus aged 4 months (eyelids are fused). (VIII) Fetus close to birth (eyelid can open).

outer canthus is positioned 1 or 2 mm higher than the inner canthus. The normal orientation of the eyelids varies depending on ethnic origin. Palpebral fissure length increases during normal development.[6]

The principal muscle involved in opening the upper lid and in maintaining normal lid position is the levator palpebrae superioris. Müller's muscle and the frontalis muscle play accessory roles.

The levator palpebrae superioris arises as a short tendon blended with the origin of the superior rectus from the undersurface of the lesser wing of the sphenoid bone. The levator palpebrae superioris is innervated by branches from the superior division of the oculomotor nerve.

Müller's muscle is a thin band of smooth muscle fibers 10 mm in width that arise on the inferior surface of the levator palpebrae superioris. It courses anteriorly, between the levator aponeurosis and the conjunctiva of the upper eyelid to insert into the superior margin of the tarsus. Branches of the sympathetic nerve innervate Müller's muscle. The eyelid is indirectly elevated by attachment of the frontalis muscle into the superior orbital portions of the orbicularis oculi muscle. The frontalis muscle is innervated by the temporal branch of the facial nerve.

Clinical evaluation of the eyelids

Dysmorphology is the study of abnormal development. Guidelines were proposed by an international group for most dysmorphologic terms.[7-10]

The clinical assessment of craniofacial features, including eyelid malformations, is based on the overall subjective qualitative clinical evaluation and on objective quantitative measurements. Qualitative anomalies are easy to define as present or absent. The frequency of a feature in the general population defined as a "variant" (present in more than 1% of people)

must be distinguished from an "anomaly." A number of anomalies useful in dysmorphology are quantitative. An objective definition of an abnormal phenotype requires knowledge of the normal variation of the trait (usually defined as ±2 SD (standard deviation) for any measurement) in a population. Some anomalies are subjective (e.g. "a coarse face").

Morphologic measurements can be easily performed with a transparent ruler. The measurements are compared to a normal database.[5]

Clinical landmarks

Many lid anomalies are correlated with an abnormal orbital structure. Hypertelorism and hypotelorism, for instance, influence the appearance of the eyelids. The normal distance between the orbits varies during embryogenesis and after birth in accordance with craniofacial development.

The embryonic separation of the globes (the angle between the optic nerves at the chiasm of the fetus) progresses from a 180° angle between the ocular axes in the first weeks of development to 70° at birth, 68° in adulthood [11,12] (Fig. 18.2A). The interorbital distance (the shortest distance between the inner walls of the orbits) increases with age[13] (Fig. 18.2B). The most accurate interorbital measurements are obtained from X-rays (Waters half-axial projection, or posteroanterior cephalograms) or computed tomograms.[14]

Clinical evaluation of the interocular distances is based on the measurement of the following lid-based landmarks:[15-19]

- Interpupillary distance
- Inner intercanthal distance
- Outer intercanthal distances
- Horizontal palpebral length.

An approximate "rule of thumb" is that the inner intercanthal distance should be equivalent to the palpebral length (Fig. 18.3).

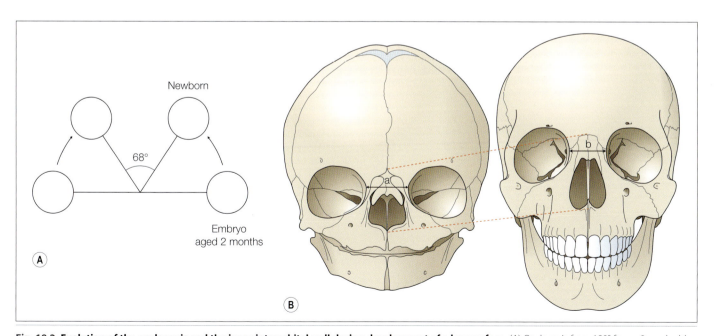

Fig. 18.2 Evolution of the ocular axis and the inner interorbital wall during development of a human face. (A) Ocular axis from 180° for an 8-week-old embryo to 68° for a newborn (adapted from Zimmermann et al.[8]). (B) Evolution of the bony orbit: a face from a newborn compared to an adult.

There are tables presenting the change in interocular distances according to age. The clinical method for assessing interocular distance is based on a biometric study that includes measurements of the inner intercanthal distance, the outer intercanthal distance, and the interpupillary distance in Caucasians from birth to 14 years. The normal intercanthal distance is 20 ± 2 mm (1 SD) at birth, increasing to 26 ± 1.5 mm by 2 years of age. The normal interpupillary distance is 39 ± 3 mm at birth, increasing to 48 ± 2 mm by 2 years of age.[4]

Ethnic variations of orbital features are important; comparison of newborns from England and Africa showed that the Caucasian and the African newborns had the same inner canthal distance, whereas the outer canthal distance and palpebral fissure length were significantly smaller in Caucasian newborns than in African newborns.[20]

Normal growth curves for many physical parameters have been compiled by Hall et al.[21]

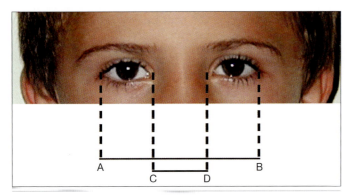

Fig. 18.3 Normal interocular distances. "The rule of the thumb" in a 5-year-old child: inner intercanthal distance is equivalent to palpebral length (AB = BC = CD).

Eyelid developmental anomalies

Developmental anomalies of the eyelids include variable eyelid malformations. Systematic clinical eyelid evaluation is based on:

1. Distances between the eyelids
2. General morphology of the eyelids
3. Palpebral fissures and slanting
4. Position of the eyelid, and
5. Evaluation of the eyebrows and eyelashes.

Developmental anomalies of the periorbital region

Abnormal distances between the eyelids and orbits

Conditions with abnormal distances between the eyelid landmarks are defined in Table 18.1 and schematically presented in Fig. 18.4.

Appreciation of the interocular distance is biased by the shape of the nasal bridge between the glabella and the inferior boundary of the nasal bone on a vertical axis, and between the inner canthi on a horizontal axis. Excessive interocular distance can be falsely suggested by a flat nasal bridge; prominent nasal bridges can give a false appearance of hypotelorism.

Hypertelorism

Hypertelorism corresponds to an interpupillary distance of more than 2 SD above the mean. It results from excessive distance between the medial wall or bony orbits. Hypertelorism occurs in more than 550 disorders (Figs 18.5 and 18.6) and is often subjectively appreciated and confused with telecanthus. Three pathogenic mechanisms have been suggested:[13]

Table 18.1 – Conditions with abnormal spacing of the orbits and eyelids

Condition	Definition	Comments
Hypertelorism	Increased distance of the inner and outer intercanthal distances	1. Not only the increased inner intercanthal distance (a common mistake) 2. Exclude erroneous hypertelorism (misleading adjacent structures) in cases of: Flat nasal bridge Epicanthic folds Exotropia Widely spaced eyebrows Narrow palpebral fissures Isolated dystopia canthorum
Hypotelorism	Reduced distance between the medial walls of the orbits with reduced inner and outer intercanthal distances	Exclude illusory hypotelorism in cases of: Esotropia Closely spaced eyebrows
Telecanthus	Increased distance between the inner canthi Primary telecanthus: increased distance between the inner canthi (normally spaced outer canthi and normal interpupillary measurement) Secondary telecanthus: increased inner canthi distance (associated with ocular hypertelorism)	Often mistaken as hypertelorism
Dystopia canthorum	Similar to secondary telecanthus (telecanthus) together with lateral displacement of the lacrimal puncta	Clinical tip: an imaginary vertical line passing through the lacrimal punctum cuts the cornea

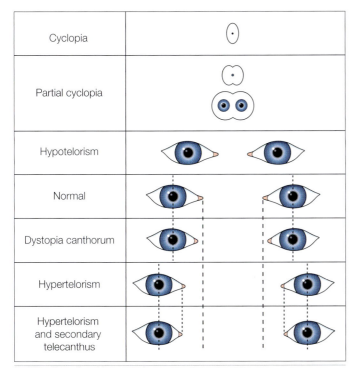

Cyclopia	
Partial cyclopia	
Hypotelorism	
Normal	
Dystopia canthorum	
Hypertelorism	
Hypertelorism and secondary telecanthus	

Fig. 18.4 The spectrum of abnormal distances between the eyes from cyclopia to hypertelorism.

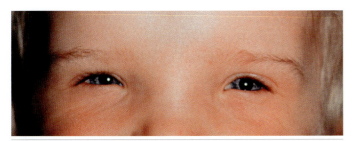

Fig. 18.5 Hypertelorism in Optiz' syndrome (esophageal abnormalities, hypospadias, and other midline defects). (Image courtesy of Clinique Ophthalmologique des Hôpitaux Universitaires de Strasbourg.)

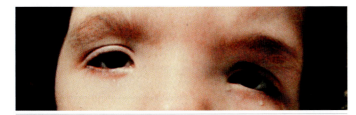

Fig. 18.6 Hypertelorism in Coffin-Lowry syndrome (a mental retardation syndrome).

1. The early ossification of the lesser wings of the sphenoid, fixing the orbits in fetal position
2. The failure of development of the nasal capsule, allowing the primitive brain vesicle to protrude into the space normally occupied by the capsule, resulting in morphokinetic arrest in the position of the eyes as in frontal encephalocele (see Chapter 56)[22]
3. A disturbance in the development of the skull base as in craniosynostosis syndromes (i.e. Crouzon's or Apert's syndromes) or in midfacial malformations such as frontonasal dysplasia.

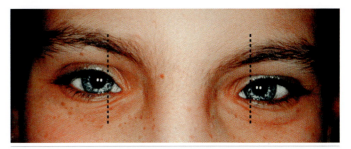

Fig. 18.7 Telecanthus and dystopia canthorum. A teenager with Waardenburg's syndrome. Note that an imaginary vertical line at the level of the puncta cuts the cornea.

The widow's peak (frontal hairline with bilateral arcs to a low point in the midline of the forehead) is a consequence of ocular hypertelorism: the two fields of hair suppression are further apart than usual with the fields failing to overlap sufficiently high on the forehead. Widow's peak is common in disorders with major hypertelorism, such as Opitz G/BBG syndrome (OMIM#145410).

Telecanthus and dystopia canthorum

Telecanthus is defined as a distance between the inner canthi more than 2 SD above the mean for age, sex, and ethnicity. It is common and often associated with hypertelorism. Dystopia canthorum is a specific feature of Waardenburg's syndrome (WS) type 1[23] (Fig. 18.7), where telecanthus results from abnormal outward displacement of the inner canthi relative to the ocular globe. This condition is an autosomal dominant syndrome with variable expressivity, characterized by:

1. Dystopia canthorum with a broad nasal root
2. Poliosis and a white forelock
3. Heterochromia irides, and
4. Sensorineural hearing loss.[24]

WS type 2 differs from WS type 1 by the absence of dystopia canthorum. Type 3 is the homozygous state of type 1 with limb anomalies; type 4, a genetically heterogeneous, autosomal dominant or autosomal recessive disorder, is associated with Hirschsprung's disease.[25]

Hypotelorism

Hypotelorism is an interpupillary distance more than 2 SD below the mean. Hypotelorism occurs in more than 60 syndromes (Fig. 18.8). It can result from premature closure of the metopic sutures resulting in vertical frontal ridge, up-slanted palpebral fissures and hypotelorism.[26]

Hypotelorism can also result from insufficient development of the brain hemispheres, as in holoprosencephaly. Holoprosencephaly is a rare brain anomaly, frequently associated with facial anomalies (see Chapter 56).[27,28] It results from an early abnormal formation of the telencephalic vesicles: they remain partially or totally fused. Holoprosencephaly usually leads to underdevelopment of middle facial structures. Severity of midfacial anomalies usually correlates with the severity of the underlying brain malformation,[29,30] forming a spectrum that goes from:

- A single median orbit with fused eye globes (cyclopia with or without synophthalmia), to
- Nasal and premaxillary agenesis, to

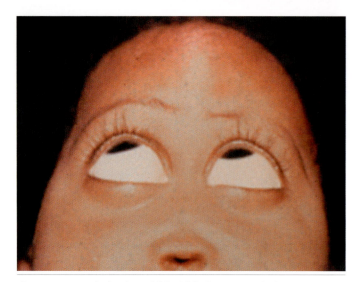

Fig. 18.8 Hypotelorism in a child with holoprosencephaly. (Courtesy of Pr Sylvie Odent.)

- A single central maxillary incisor with hypotelorism (see Table 18.1).

Holoprosencephaly may be due to environmental/maternal factors (such as maternal diabetes), chromosomal abnormalities (trisomy 13, 18q deletion), or single gene defects[31] (Table 18.2).

Abnormal aspect of the inner canthus

Epicanthus palpebralis

Epicanthus palpebralis (or epicanthal fold) is a vertical cutaneous fold arising from the nasal root and directed toward the internal part of the upper lids (Fig. 18.9). It can be subdivided into the areas where they occur such as preseptal, pretarsal, or orbital. The fold may cover the inner canthus. It is normal in fetuses of all ethnic origins and common in young children with a flat nasal bridge. Epicanthus palpebralis is a normal feature in many populations, mostly Asians. It is common in syndromes where the nasal bridge is flat, such as trisomy 21. Epicanthus often vanishes with age.

Epicanthus inversus

Epicanthus inversus is a fold of skin starting at the medial aspect of the lower lid and arching upward to cover the medial canthus (see blepharophimosis; Chapter 19). It is the hallmark of the blepharophimosis–ptosis–epicanthus inversus syndrome (BPES).

Major malformations of the eyelids

Ablepharon

Ablepharon is the absence of lids. It occurs in several settings:

1. Neu-Laxova syndrome – with intrauterine growth retardation, syndactyly, swollen "collodion" skin, microcephaly, and severe developmental brain defects.[32]

2. Autosomal dominant ablepharon-macrostomia syndrome – absent or rudimentary eyelids,[33] a hypoplastic nose, ambiguous genitalia, absent zygoma, and macrostomia with possible familial recurrence[34] (Fig. 18.10).

3. Say-Barber syndrome[35] – hypertrichosis of the back, macrostomia, microblepharon, ectropion, and sometimes ablepharon. It could be allelic to ablepharon-macrostomia syndrome.

Cryptophthalmos (see Chapter 17)

Cryptophthalmos is rare: there is failure of development of the eyelid folds with continuity of the skin from the forehead to the cheek.[36,37] In complete cryptophthalmos, the epithelium that is normally differentiated into cornea and conjunctiva becomes part of the skin that passes continuously from the forehead to the cheek. The eyebrow is usually absent and the globes are microphthalmic. In the incomplete form, a rudimentary lid and conjunctival sac is present. Abortive cryptophthalmos presents with a normal lower lid and an absent or abnormal upper lid, the forehead skin passing directly to and fusing with the superior cornea (Fig. 18.11).

Cryptophthalmos may be an isolated finding or present as part of Fraser's syndrome.[36] Fraser's syndrome is a rare autosomal recessive syndrome with cryptophthalmos, hypoplasia of the genitalia, laryngeal stenosis, and renal hypoplasia or agenesis.

Ankyloblepharon

Ankyloblepharon is partial or complete adhesion of the ciliary margins of the superior and inferior eyelids. Ankyloblepharon filiforme ad natum is usually a sporadic isolated malformation in which the upper and lower lids are joined by tags (easily cured by a simple surgical procedure)[38] (Fig. 18.12). Ankyloblepharon may be inherited as an autosomal dominant trait. It may occur in association with ectodermal defects and cleft lip and/or palate in Hay-Wells syndrome,[39] an allelic variant of the ectodactyly– ectodermal dysplasia–cleft lip palate (EEC) syndrome (see Chapter 28). Ankyloblepharon may occur in trisomy 18.[40]

Clefting or notching of the eyelids ("coloboma")

Notches or clefts of the eyelid have been described as eyelid colobomas, but there is no embryologic relation with defects due to malclosure of the embryologic fissure. They are usually triangular with the base at the lid margin. The size varies from a discrete notch to a major defect with exposure keratopathy requiring surgery.[41]

Eyelid colobomas may occur in all areas of the eyelids but are most common in the nasal half of the upper lid. More than one lid may be involved; there may be multiple colobomas in the same lid. The eye may be normal or have abnormalities such as corneal opacities, and iris and retinal colobomas extending to microphthalmos and anophthalmos. There may be associated bands limiting ocular motility; strabismus is common.[42] The cause of eyelid colobomas remains uncertain. They may be equivalent to facial clefts, but intrauterine factors may play a major role.[43] Amniotic bands may cause mechanical disruptive clefting of the eyelids in the amniotic deformity, adhesions, mutilations (ADAM) syndrome.[44]

Table 18.2 – Gene identification in syndromes with developmental eyelid anomalies cited in this chapter (updated August 2011)

Name of syndrome	Inheritance patten	Type of eyelid anomaly	Gene name (reference)	Extraocular manifestation
Alopecia universalis	AD	Absent eyebrows and eyelashes	*HR* (human homolog of mouse hairless gene)[99]	Absent hair on all the body
Apert's syndrome		Hypertelorism Protrusion of the eyes Asymmetry of orbits Strabismus	*FGFR2* (fibroblast growth factor receptor 2)[100]	Craniosynostosis Complete syndactyly
BPES type I and type II	AD	Blepharophimosis Ptosis Epicanthus inversus	*FOXL2* (Forkhead box L 2)[101,102]	Ovarian failure in type II
Coffin-Lowry syndrome		Hypertelorism Down-slanting palpebral fissures	*RPS6KA3*[103]	X-linked mental retardation syndrome
Cohen's syndrome	AR	Wavy eyelid Retinal dystrophy	*COH1*[104]	Microcephaly, mental retardation, intermittent neutropenia, truncular obesity
Cornelia de Lange syndrome	AD, XLD (*SMC1A* gene)	Thin, penciled eyebrows Thick eyebrows Synophris	*NIPBL*[105] *SMC1A*[106]	Typical facies, limb reduction defects, pre- and postnatal growth retardation, mental retardation
Crouzon's syndrome	AD	Hypertelorism Protrusion of the eyes Asymmetry of orbits	*FGFR2*[107] *FGFR3*	Craniosynostosis Mild digital anomalies
Ectodermal dysplasia anhydrotic (EDA)	XL	Absent or sparse eyebrows and eyelashes	*EDA1*[108]	Abnormal sweating, peg- or cone-shaped teeth, oligodontia
Fraser's syndrome		Cryptophthalmos	*FRAS*[109] *FREM2*[110]	Renal agenesis or hypoplasia, laryngeal stenosis, syndactyly, genital anomalies
Hay-Wells (EEC syndrome type 3)	AD	Sparse eyebrows and eyelashes	P63[111,112]	Ectrodactyly–ectodermal dysplasia–clefting syndrome
Holoprosencephaly	AD, AR, chromosomal, environmental	Cyclopia or more or less severe secondary hypotelorism	*SHH* (sonic hedgehog)[113] *SIX3*[114] *TGIF*[115] *ZIC2*[116] *PTCH1*[117] *GLI2*[118]	Malformation of the brain induces craniofacial anomaly
Kabuki syndrome	AD	Long palpebral fissures	*MLL2*[119]	Typical dysmorphism, hypotonia, mental retardation
Lymphedema-distichiasis syndrome	AD	Distichiasis Ptosis	*FOXC2*[120,121]	Lymphedema Diabetes mellitus
Noonan's syndrome	AD	Ptosis	*PTPN11*[122] *SOS1 RAF1 KRAS NRAS*[123] *SHOC2*[124]	Pulmonary artery stenosis, cardiomyopathy, short stature, webbing of the neck, pectus excavatum, cryptorchidism
Opitz BBBG syndrome	XL	Hypertelorism Widow's peak	MID1[125]	Laryngeal cleft, hypospadias (X linked)
Rubinstein-Taybi syndrome	AD	Heavy high-arched eyebrows Down-slanting palpebral fissures Ptosis	*CREBBP*[126] *EP300*[127]	Broad thumbs and toes, characteristic facies, mental retardation
Saethre-Chotzen syndrome	AD	Ptosis	*TWIST*[128,129]	Variable, asymmetric craniosynostosis
Setleis' syndrome (focal facial dermal dysplasia)	AR	Absent eyelashes Multiple rows of eyelashes Upslanting eyebrows	*TWIST2*[130]	Bilateral temporal skin defects resembling forceps marks
Treacher-Collins syndrome	AD	Down-slanting palpebral fissures Occasional colobomas of eyelids	*TCOF1*[131]	First branchial arch syndrome
Waardenburg's syndrome types I and III	AD (type III: AR)	Telecanthus Dystopia canthorum Iris heterochromia	*PAX3* (Paired-box 3)[132]	Variable deafness White forelock Type II is the homozygous form (with severe limb anomalies)
Waardenburg's syndrome type II	AD	Iris heterochromia	*MITF*[133] *SNAI2*[134]	Similar to type I, but without telecanthus
Waardenburg's syndrome type IV (or Shah-Waardenburg syndrome)	AD, AR	Iris heterochromia	*EDNRB EDN3 SOX10*[135]	Similar to type II, with Hirschsprung's disease

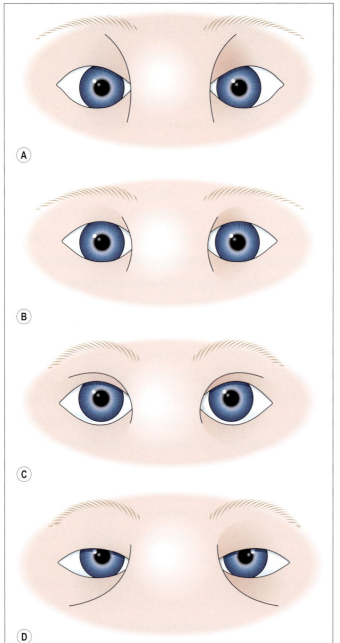

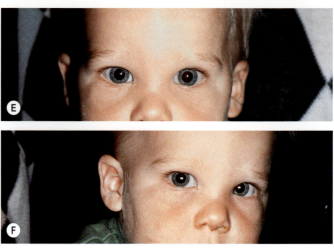

Fig. 18.9 Epicanthus. (A) Superciliaris; (B) palpebralis (most frequent); (C) tarsalis ("Asian epicanthus"); (D) inversus (blepharophimosis–ptosis–epicanthus inversus syndrome). (E) Epicanthus in the straight-ahead position. This child can be seen to have a broad base to his nose and mild epicanthus. In the straight-ahead position his eyes appear straight. (F) On looking right the adducting eye appears to be convergent, giving rise to a pseudosquint.

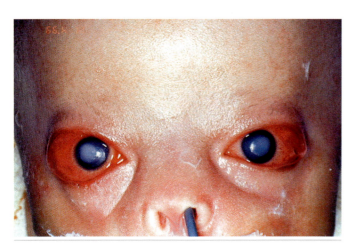

Fig. 18.10 Bilateral ablepharon. Ablepharon-macrostomia syndrome. (Image courtesy of Dr A. A. Cruz.)

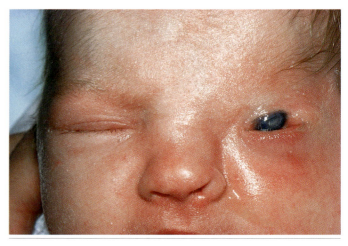

Fig. 18.11 Cryptophthalmos. Unilateral partial abortive cryptophthalmos (symblepharon): the upper lid is fused to the eye.

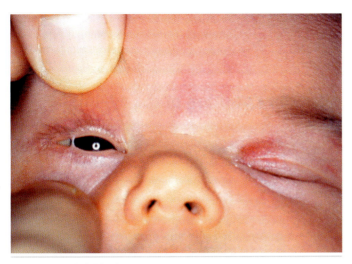

Fig. 18.12 **Ankyloblepharon.** (Image courtesy of Dr A. A. Cruz.)

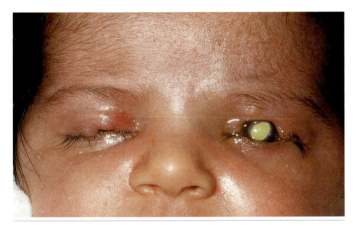

Fig. 18.13 **Coloboma of the eyelid.** Bilateral lid colobomas in a patient with Goldenhar's syndrome. Since birth this child has corneal exposure on the left from a large lid coloboma that has given rise to drying of the cornea, corneal ulceration, and ultimately scarring.

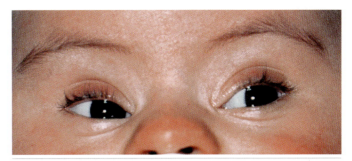

Fig. 18.14 **Up-slanting palpebral fissures in a child with trisomy 21.** (Image courtesy of Clinique Ophthalmologique des Hôpitaux Universitaires de Strasbourg.)

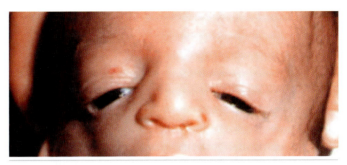

Fig. 18.15 **Down-slanting palpebral fissures in a child with Treacher-Collins syndrome.**

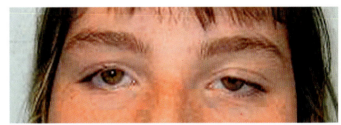

Fig. 18.16 **"Wavy palpebral" fissures in Cohen's syndrome** (associated with retinal dystrophy). (Image courtesy of Dr Y. Alembik.)

Coloboma of the upper lid can occur in the oculo-auriculo-vertebral dysplasia syndrome (Goldenhar's syndrome), which has no clear genetic basis (Fig. 18.13). Coloboma of the lower lid is a common feature of the autosomal dominant Treacher-Collins syndrome.[45,46]

Abnormal palpebral fissures

Orientation of the palpebral fissures

The slant, or inclination, of the palpebral fissure is the angle formed by the line that connects the lateral canthus and the medial canthus of each eye, and horizontal. The normal palpebral slant is slightly up. Palpebral fissures are described as up-slanted when the outer canthus is positioned higher than usual, down-slanted when the outer canthus is lower than usual.

Up-slanted palpebral fissures may be associated with microcephaly. In trisomy 21, up-slanting of the palpebral fissures is the most common ocular and facial feature[47,48] (Fig. 18.14).

Hypoplastic malar bones often result in down-slanted palpebral fissures. It is a characteristic finding in first or second branchial arch malformations such as the Treacher-Collins syndrome characterized by a narrow face with hypoplasia of supraorbital rims, zygomas, and hypoplastic ear (Fig. 18.15).

The palpebral fissure may have a "wave shape" in Cohen's syndrome defined by a specific facial appearance, developmental delay, and retinal degeneration[49] (see Chapter 45) (Fig. 18.16).

Long palpebral fissures

Palpebral fissures are long when the distance between the medial and lateral canthi is more than 2 SD above the mean for age.

Euryblepharon is generalized enlargement of the palpebral aperture, usually greatest laterally.[50] There is localized outward and downward displacement of the lateral canthus, with a downward displacement of the lower lid. This may superficially mimic the appearance of congenital ectropion (the eversion of the whole lower lid defines congenital ectropion). It may occur as an isolated anomaly, may be inherited as an autosomal dominant trait, or may be associated with trisomy 21[51] or with craniofacial dysostosis. Euryblepharon is characteristic of the Kabuki syndrome: postnatal growth retardation, mental retardation, and a facial appearance suggesting the make-up of the actors of a traditional Japanese theater[52,53] (Fig. 18.17).

Short palpebral fissures

Palpebral fissures are short when the distance between the medial and lateral canthi is more than 2 SD below the mean for age.

A moderate reduction of the palpebral length may be the consequence of excessive curvature of the palpebral rim ("almond-shaped fissures") and can be found in trisomy 21.

Blepharophimosis is a reduction in the maximum vertical distance between the upper and lower eyelids combined with short palpebral fissures. Blepharophimosis can be isolated or part of various syndromes. It should not be confused with ptosis (in which palpebral fissures are not shortened).[54]

The fetal alcohol syndrome associates growth retardation, microcephaly, and cognitive impairment. It is one of the most common causes of blepharophimosis.[55]

The blepharophimosis–ptosis–epicanthus inversus syndrome (BPES) is an autosomal dominant condition with marked blepharophimosis, ptosis and hypoplasia of the tarsal plates, and epicanthus inversus (Fig. 18.18). Two clinical types of BPES have been defined:[56]

1. BPES type I: transmission through males only and menstrual irregularity and infertility due to ovarian failure in the affected females.
2. BPES type II: no associated infertility[56] and transmission is through both sexes. Early milestones may be delayed because of hypotonia and backward head tilt.

Ohdo's syndrome is usually sporadic and defined by blepharophimosis, ptosis, dental hypoplasia, partial deafness, and mental retardation.[57] Ptosis and/or blepharophimosis are also observed in chromosomal syndromes. Blepharophimosis with ptosis is, for instance, a hallmark of chromosome 3p deletion.[58]

Abnormal position of the eyelids

Ectropion

Congenital ectropion is an outward rotation of the eyelid margin, frequently associated with overexposure of the palpebral and scleral conjunctiva and cornea. It may occur in the upper or lower lids, rarely as an isolated anomaly. Associations of congenital or acquired ectropion include blepharophimosis syndrome, trisomy 21,[59] mandibulofacial or other facial dysostoses, skin disorders, i.e. lamellar ichthyosis[60] or microphthalmos, buphthalmos, and orbital cysts.

Congenital skin disorders may lead to congenital ectropion in congenital cutis laxa with looseness of the lid or the harlequin ichthyotic babies with cicatricial ectropion (Fig. 18.19).

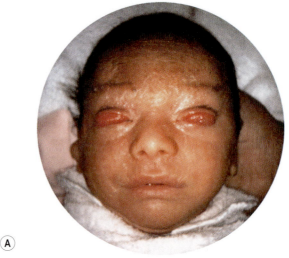

(A)

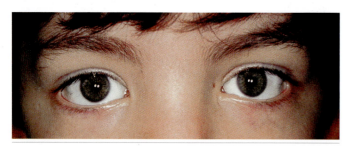

Fig. 18.17 Euryblepharon in Kabuki syndrome.

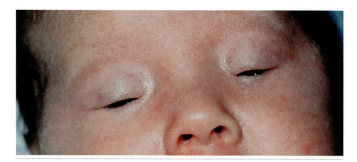

Fig. 18.18 Blepharophimosis–ptosis–epicanthus inversus syndrome in a 2-month-old child.

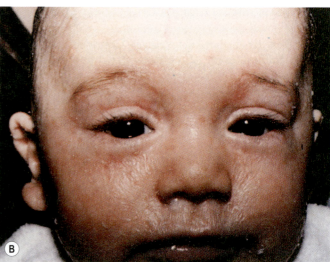

(B)

Fig. 18.19 Ectropion. (A) Bilateral ectropion in a patient with severe congenital ichthyosis. (B) Same patient after bilateral lid suture. (Dr Geoffrey Hipwell's patient.)

Therapy is initially conservative using lubrication. Surgical intervention is indicated for exposure keratitis or cosmesis.

Eversion

Congenital eversion of the lids is an acute ectropion. It can occur intermittently in neonates when the child cries. It is caused by spasm of the orbicularis muscle and usually resolves spontaneously. If it becomes established, the conjunctiva becomes chemotic and may obscure the globe. This condition may be associated with trisomy 21, African origin, and difficult deliveries. It should be treated initially by pressure patching or repositioning of the lids and taping and in second intention with surgery[61] (Fig. 18.20).

Epitarsus

Primary epitarsus is an apron-like fold of conjunctiva attached to the inner surface of the upper lid. It occurs secondary to conjunctivitis and amniotic bands or as a congenital anomaly.[62]

Epiblepharon

Epiblepharon is a condition with a redundant skinfold across either the upper or lower eyelid, which forces the lashes against the cornea. There is a familial tendency. It occurs more frequently in chubby-cheeked and Asian infants.[63] Epiblepharon usually resolves within the first 2 years of life as a result of differential growth of the facial bones; occasionally, surgery to remove a strip of skin and fat from the lid margin is necessary. It is seldom associated with keratitis (Fig. 18.21).

Entropion

Congenital entropion is an inward turning of the lid margin with malposition of the tarsal plate. It usually involves the lower lid, although involvement of the upper lid occurs. Congenital entropion must be distinguished from epiblepharon, where a skinfold causes a secondary turning of the lower lid eyelashes. Entropion may be secondary to microphthalmos and enophthalmos, resulting from lack of support of the posterior border of the eyelid.

The etiology of primary congenital entropion is controversial: hypertrophy of the marginal portion of the orbicularis muscle and disinsertion of the lower lid retractors may be responsible factors.[64-66]

Protection of the cornea is paramount. Congenital entropion, as opposed to congenital epiblepharon, requires prompt surgical intervention to prevent corneal scarring and infection[67] (Fig. 18.22). Surgical procedures involve myocutaneous resection and plication or reattachment of the lower lid retractors to the inferior tarsal border. A trial of simpler treatment may be worthwhile.

Lagophthalmos

Lagophthalmos is the inability to totally close the eyelids. Typically, lagophthalmos is noted during sleep. It may be an isolated finding or part of a syndrome. Lagophthalmos can be associated with ectropion.

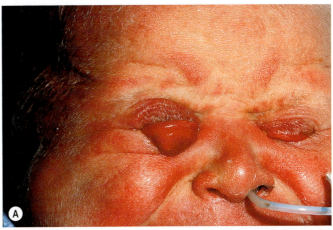

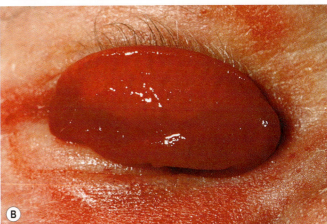

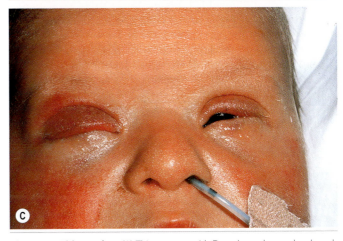

Fig. 18.20 Lid eversion. (A) This neonate with Down's syndrome developed lid eversion when crying that rapidly became permanently present. The birth history was unremarkable. (B) The lid eversion was maintained by the very marked chemosis. (C) After taping the lids for 4 days the swelling resolved, leaving bruising, indicating that hemorrhaging may play a causative role.

Lid retraction in infancy

Occasionally, infants present with a history of one or both eyelids appearing to be retracted. Upper lid retraction exists when the resting position of the lid is above the superior limbus. For lower lid retraction the affected lower lid rests below the inferior limbus. There is often significant asymmetry between the two sides. There are several conditions that can give rise to this appearance:

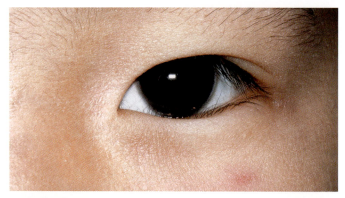

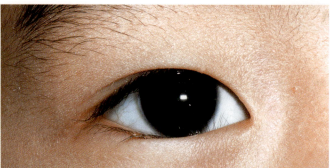

Fig. 18.21 Epiblepharon. In this child the lower lid lashes have turned in from birth, but the cornea has remained undamaged. Spontaneous improvement usually occurs.

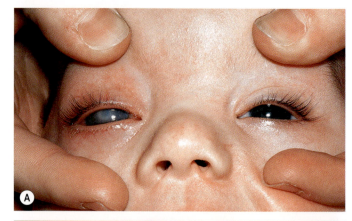

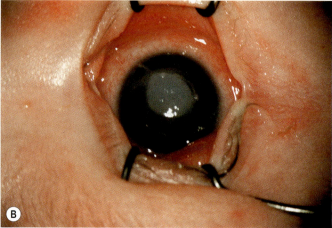

Fig. 18.22 Congenital entropion. (A) Shortly after birth this child's eye was found to be swollen. During examination under anesthetic right upper lid entropion was found. (B) A corneal abrasion caused by the entropion.

1. Physiologic, in the newborn.
2. Congenital idiopathic lid retraction.[68] There are patients in whom one eyelid, usually the upper, is retracted. Several anatomical variants may be responsible for this: an increase in the number and size of the levator muscle fibers or a thickened or shortened levator aponeurosis or orbital septum. No definite etiology has been established.
3. A false appearance of lid retraction may be given by ipsilateral proptosis, contralateral ptosis (when the child is trying to elevate the ptotic lid), inferior rectus fibrosis, double elevator palsy, Brown's syndrome, or orbital pathology, which restrict upward movement of the eye.
4. Bilateral lid elevation with an upgaze palsy is the classic "setting sun" sign in hydrocephalus and dorsal midbrain disease.
5. Lid retraction, unilateral or bilateral, may occur with the Marcus Gunn jaw-winking phenomenon. Sometimes there is no ptosis – the lid just elevates.
6. Neonatal Graves' disease.[69]
7. A sequel to third nerve palsy with aberrant regeneration.[70]
8. Myasthenic patients may have transient lid retraction, a "twitch," after looking down for a period.
9. Lid lag is a defective relaxation of the lids that occurs in hyperthyroidism, myopathic disease, a congenitally short levator tendon,[71] or occasionally myasthenia gravis.
10. Seventh nerve palsy.
11. Levator fibrosis.[72]
12. Vertical nystagmus.

Treatment depends upon the etiology. For primary congenital eyelid retraction, initial management should consist of observation and lubrication. Indications for surgical intervention include corneal exposure and cosmesis.

Ptosis (see Chapter 19)

Ptosis is usually classified as congenital or acquired. A simple congenital dystrophy or dysgenesis of the levator muscle must be distinguished from other causes of ptosis. If the levator is dystrophic, it will not relax properly: there will be lid lag on downgaze. If the levator muscle is not dystrophic, the ptotic eyelid will remain ptotic in all positions of gaze.

The following classification emphasizes this differentiation.

Classification

Congenital ptosis

Simple congenital ptosis is the most common ptosis in childhood (Figs 18.23 to 18.26). It is due to a dystrophy or dysgenesis of the levator palpebrae superioris muscle. Lid lag on downgaze and the extent of the skin crease are usually related to the levator function. In view of the close embryologic development of the levator and superior rectus muscles, it is not surprising that ptosis may be associated with a superior rectus weakness. There is no well-defined pattern of heredity. It is not

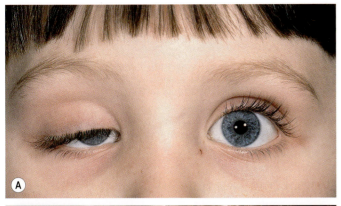

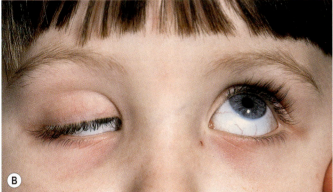

Fig. 18.23 Congenital ptosis. (A) Simple unilateral congenital ptosis. (B) With mildly defective superior rectus action on the right.

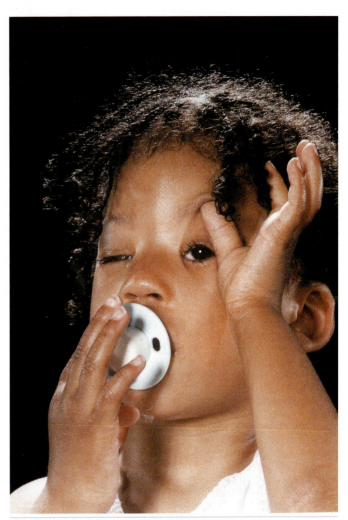

Fig. 18.25 Congenital ptosis. This girl with bilateral ptosis adapts to the condition by lifting her lid any time she wants to see more clearly.

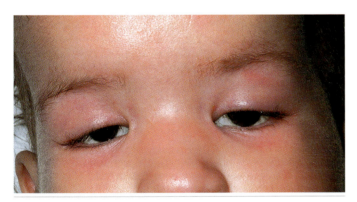

Fig. 18.24 Congenital ptosis. Bilateral severe simple congenital ptosis.

known why an isolated unilateral dystrophy of the levator muscle should be relatively common.

Aponeurotic defects may occur anywhere in the aponeurosis. They are associated with good levator function and no lid lag on downgaze. The most common sites are at the origin or insertion of the aponeurosis. If a defect occurs at the origin and the terminal aponeurosis is normal, there will be ptosis with good levator function and a normal skin crease. If the defect occurs at the insertion of the aponeurosis, as commonly occurs with trauma, the ptosis will be associated with a high skin crease.

Neurogenic defects

A third nerve palsy may be either congenital or acquired (see Chapter 83). There is ptosis and the eye is abducted by the lateral rectus and intorted by the superior oblique muscle.

There may be associated neurologic defects.[72] The pupil is usually, but not always, large with loss of accommodation. Recognition of the complete form is easy, but in partial form the diagnosis may be missed and investigation delayed.

Aberrant third nerve regeneration may occur after a congenital or acquired oculomotor palsy.

Marcus Gunn jaw-winking syndrome is due to an abnormal synkinesis between the levator and, usually, the lateral pterygoid muscle. The affected eyelid is usually ptotic but elevates when the jaw is opened and deviated to the contralateral side (Figs 18.27 and 18.28). A medial pterygoid synkinesis in which the affected eyelid elevates when the jaw is clenched or protruded is less common. Voluntary levator excursion is always decreased. Frequently, there is a weakness of the superior rectus muscle. The condition is usually congenital, sporadic, and unilateral, but acquired and familial cases may occur.

For Horner's syndrome see Chapter 63.

Myogenic ptosis

Progressive external ophthalmoplegia may present in childhood with ptosis, which may initially be unilateral but becomes bilateral (see Chapter 83). There is an associated slowly progressive palsy of all the extraocular muscles, which usually

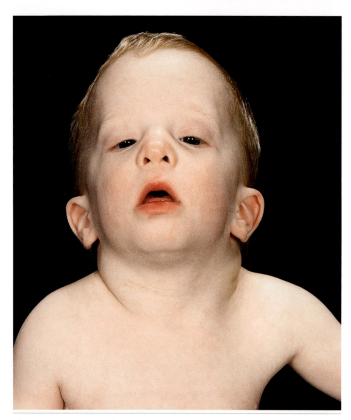

Fig. 18.26 Congenital ptosis. Bilateral congenital ptosis with abnormal head posture. The abnormal head posture is an adaptive mechanism to allow binocular vision.

limits elevation first but progresses until the eyes are practically immobile (Fig. 18.29). The pupil and accommodation are not involved. It may occur sporadically, but it is commonly an autosomal dominant trait.

Histology, electron microscopy, and electromyography suggest that it is a muscular dystrophy. Characteristic ragged red fibers may be seen on muscle biopsy stained with a modified trichrome method. It is probably a generalized mitochondrial abnormality and may progress to involve the orbicularis, facial, pharyngeal, and skeletal muscles, especially of the neck and shoulders. A pigmentary retinopathy and cardiomyopathy may occur. There is an increased anesthetic risk of malignant hyperthermia.

Myasthenia gravis is a chronic disease characterized by an abnormal fatigability of striated muscles (see Chapter 83). It may be confined to a single group of muscles or become generalized. Ten percent of cases occur in children before puberty; it may occur transiently in newborns of myasthenic mothers. There is a familial incidence, but there is no clear hereditary pattern. Many cases are associated with hyperplasia of the thymus or a thymoma. The cause is an autoimmune defect in the acetylcholine mechanism at the neuromuscular junction. Ptosis is usually worse at the end of the day and is often the presenting symptom. Diplopia commonly occurs; the child may present with an unusual squint. The orbicularis oculi is usually also weak.

Easy fatigability causes an increase in the ptosis after repeated up- and downgaze. The abnormality of neuromuscular control may be demonstrated by an overshoot of the eyelid on upgaze.

It is diagnosed:

1. Clinically
2. By antibody studies:
   a. By finding raised levels of anticholinesterase receptor antibody, and
   b. By finding raised levels of IgG antibodies against the muscle-specific kinase
3. By single-fiber electromyography; probably the most sensitive test is looking for "jitter" on the EMG of an affected muscle or, if the eye muscles only are affected, another muscle, and
4. By the pharmacologic test.

In an adult-sized child, 2 mg of Tensilon (edrophonium chloride) is given intravenously as a test dose followed by 8 mg given rapidly. This may produce quick relief of the ptosis.

Unless pre- and post-test parameters (such as a Hess chart or orthoptic measurements) are measured the test is often equivocal except in cases clinically obvious, and this limits the value of the test, which is used less frequently than previously. If the child is less than 10 kg in weight, the dose is reduced or prostigmin (neostigmine) can be given by intramuscular injection 20 minutes after an intramuscular injection of atropine. The test carries a significant risk and must only be carried out in circumstances where resuscitation facilities are immediately available, appropriate to the age of the child.

Pseudoptosis

Pseudoptosis is when the eyelid margin is at the normal level but the eyelid appears ptotic. If the eye is hypotropic, there may be such an apparent ptosis, which disappears when the eye takes up fixation. In enophthalmos, the apparent ptosis can be corrected by restoring the orbital volume. Excess skin from a resolving hemangioma may overhang the lid margin and be another cause of pseudoptosis.

Syndromes with ptosis

Several genetic disorders are associated with ptosis:

1. Noonan syndrome: small stature, a webbed neck, and pulmonary stenosis.
2. Saethre-Chotzen syndrome: an autosomal dominant craniosynostosis syndrome with syndactyly[73] (Fig. 18.30).

Eyebrows and eyelashes

Anomalies of the dermatologic component of the eyelids are also important as isolated or syndromic features.

Prominent eyebrows and/or eyelashes

Prominent eyelashes with highly arched heavy eyebrows associated with down-slanting palpebral fissures and/or ptosis are found in the Rubinstein-Taybi syndrome, a mental retardation syndrome associated with broad thumbs and toes.[74]

Heavy and thick eyebrows occur in metabolic disorders (see Chapter 62), such as the mucopolysaccharidoses, mucolipidoses, and fucosidosis, usually associated with a coarse face (Fig. 18.31).

Distichiasis

Distichiasis is a congenital abnormality with partial or complete accessory rows of eyelashes exiting from the posterior lid

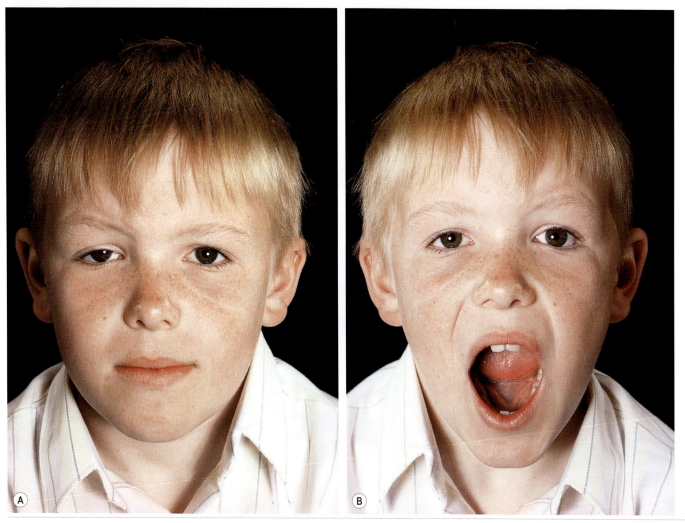

Fig. 18.27 Marcus Gunn ptosis. (A) Right ptosis. (B) With jaw open the right upper lid rises.

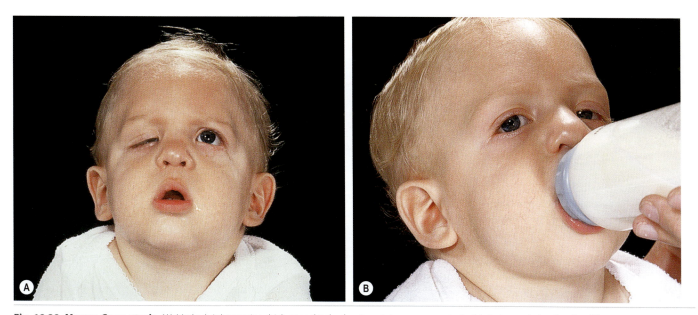

Fig. 18.28 Marcus Gunn ptosis. (A) Marked right ptosis, which completely elevates on jaw movements; in this instance during feeding (B).

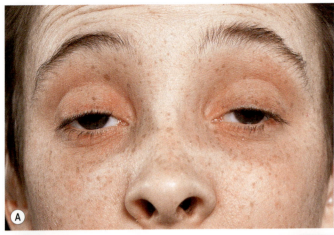

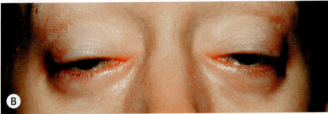

Fig. 18.29 Ptosis in chronic external ophthalmoplegia in a mitochondrial disorder.

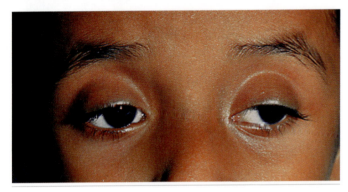

Fig. 18.30 Ptosis in Saenthre-Chotzen syndrome.

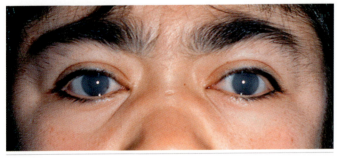

Fig. 18.31 Heavy eyebrows and coarse facies in mucopolysaccharidosis. (Image courtesy of Clinique Ophthalmologique des Hôpitaux Universitaires de Strasbourg.)

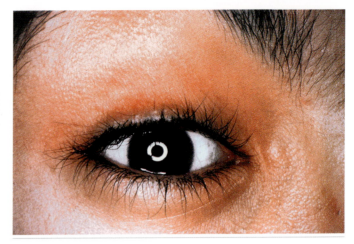

Fig. 18.32 Distichiasis.

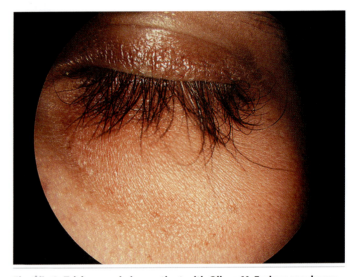

Fig. 18.33 Trichomegaly in a patient with Oliver-McFarlane syndrome. (Image courtesy of Dr L. Santos.)

margin at or near the meibomian gland orifices[75] (Fig. 18.32). It may occur as an isolated anomaly, or be inherited as an autosomal dominant trait. In the autosomal dominant distichiasis-lymphedema syndrome, it is associated with chronic lymphedema of the lower extremities[76,77] possibly associated with a webbed neck, cardiac defects, vertebral anomalies, extradural spinal cysts, and bifid uvula.[78]

In the Setleis syndrome,[79] there are bilateral temporal skin defects resembling forceps marks, absent lashes, or distichiasis, with a coarse facial appearance.[80]

Trichomegaly

Trichomegaly is excessive growth of eyelashes. Trichomegaly can be familial or acquired with human immunodeficiency virus infection or some medical drugs such as interferon alpha treatment.[81] This feature combined with mental retardation and retinal dystrophy is characteristic of Oliver-McFarlane syndrome[82] (Fig. 18.33) (see Chapter 45).

Synophrys

Synophrys is when eyebrows extend to the midline; it is common in naturally hairy persons.

Cornelia de Lange syndrome is the association of mental retardation, growth retardation, limb reduction defect, flared nostrils, and hirsutism with characteristic synophrys and long eyelashes[83,84] (Fig. 18.34).

Synophrys can occur in Waardenburg's syndrome.

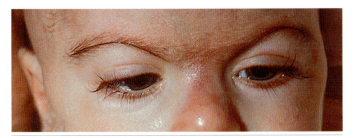

Fig. 18.34 Synophrys in Cornelia de Lange syndrome.

An autosomal recessive condition with a cone–rod dystrophy, hairy face and eyebrows, synophrys, coarse scalp hair, and distichiasis has been described.[85]

Sparse or absent eyebrows and/or eyelashes

Sparse or absent eyebrows and/or eyelashes occurs as an isolated condition or associated with other features. It occurs in many syndromes:

1. Alopecia universalis congenita (generalized atrichia): autosomal recessive condition with absent scalp, pubic, and axillary hair as well as absent eyebrows and eyelashes from birth.[86]
2. GAPO syndrome: growth retardation, alopecia, pseudoanodontia, optic atrophy, glaucoma, and sparse or absent eyebrows and eyelashes.[87,88]
3. Ectodermal dysplasia: a clinical and genetic heterogeneous group of congenital disorders with abnormal development of one or several ectoderm-derived tissues. Sparse eyebrows and eyelashes are classical features.[89]
4. EEC syndrome: an autosomal dominant syndrome with highly variable expression characterized by sparse or absent hair, sparse eyebrows and eyelashes, brittle nails, teeth anomalies, and split hands or ectodactyly.[90,91] The lacrimal duct system is defective in more then 90% (see Chapter 21).
5. Ectodermal dysplasia anhydrotic (EDA): an X-linked condition. The affected males have hypotrichosis, abnormal teeth, and absent sweat glands[92] (Fig. 18.35).

Familial conditions with hypotrichosis/alopecia and retinal degeneration,[93] as well as a syndrome associating alopecia and cataract,[94] have been reported.

Patches of hypotrichosis/alopecia at the level of the eyebrow can be observed in the progressive facial hemiatrophy syndrome or Parry-Romberg syndrome with an "en coup de sabre" appearance and ipsilateral neurologic and eye features such as enophthalmos and retinal telangiectasias[95] (Fig. 18.36).

Trichotillomania is a chronic psychiatric condition defined by uncontrollable hair pulling, the eyelashes being the most commonly affected[96] (Fig. 18.37).

White brows or lashes

White eyelashes and eyebrows occur in oculocutaneous albinism. The lashes and eyebrows are white as is the hair and the skin.

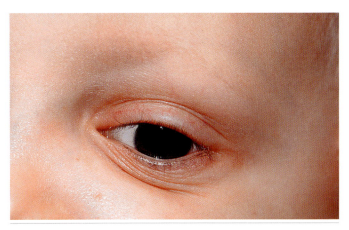

Fig. 18.35 Sparse eyebrows in anhidrotic ectodermal hypoplasia. (Image courtesy of Clinique Ophthalmologique des Hôpitaux Universitaires de Strasbourg.)

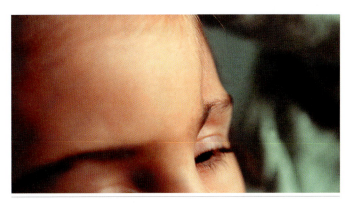

Fig. 18.36 "En coup de sabre" appearance of the eyebrow in Parry-Romberg syndrome.

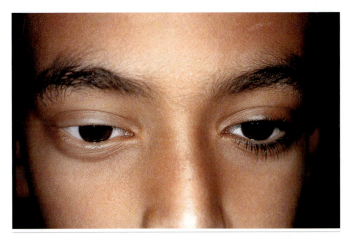

Fig. 18.37 Trichotillomania. The lashes have been plucked. A few remaining broken lashes can be seen in the upper lid.

Poliosis is defined as white brows or lashes in an otherwise normally pigmented individual. Poliosis occurs in Waardenburg's syndrome (Fig. 18.38) and Parry-Romberg syndrome. It is also a feature of the acquired Vogt-Koyangi- Harada syndrome.

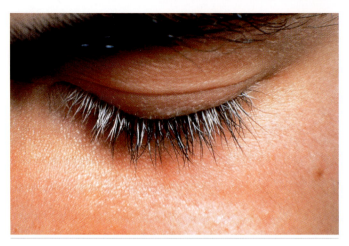

Fig. 18.38 Poliosis in a patient with Waardenburg's syndrome. The poliosis can be clearly seen against the normally dark lashes.

Dysmorphology databases and genes involved in syndromes with eyelid anomalies

Databases in dysmorphology and genetics are based on morphologic analysis of the patient guiding the clinician by submitting a list of possibly corresponding syndromes.[97,98] The clinical observation of the face remains essential. Severe or discrete anomalies may be important in diagnosis. The analysis of these features, with the aid of databases, helps the clinician diagnostically and guides molecular investigations.

Table 18.2 summarizes the genes identified in syndromes with developmental anomalies of the eyelids.

References

1. Jones KL. Smith's Recognizable Patterns of Human Malformation, 5th ed. Philadelphia: Saunders; 1997.
7. Hennekam RC, Cormier-Daire V, Hall JG, et al. Elements of morphology: standard terminology for the nose and philtrum. Am J Med Genet A 2009; 149: 61–76.
8. Allanson JE, Cunniff C, Hoyme HE, et al. Elements of morphology: standard terminology for the head and face. Am J Med Genet A 2009; 149: 6–28.
9. Carey JC, Cohen MM Jr, Curry CJ, et al. Elements of morphology: standard terminology for the lips, mouth, and oral region. Am J Med Genet A 2009; 149: 77–92.
10. Hall BD, Graham JM Jr, Cassidy SB, Opitz JM. Elements of morphology: standard terminology for the periorbital region. Am J Med Genet A 2009; 149: 29–39.
11. Fries PD, Katowitz JA. Congenital craniofacial anomalies of ophthalmic importance. Surv Ophthalmol 1990; 35: 87–119.
21. Hall JG, Allanson JE, Gripp KW, Slavotinek AM. Handbook of Physical Measurement, 2nd ed. Oxford: Oxford University Press; 2007.
24. Read AP, Newton VE. Waardenburg syndrome. J Med Genet 1997; 34: 656–65.
30. Kjaer I, Keeling JW, Graem N. The midline craniofacial skeleton in holoprosencephalic fetuses. J Med Genet 1991; 28: 846–55.
31. Wallis D, Muenke M. Mutations in holoprosencephaly. Hum Mutat 2000; 16: 99–108.
34. Ferraz VEF, Melo DG, Hansing SE, et al. Ablepharon-macrostomia syndrome: first report of familial occurrence. Am J Med Genet 2000; 94: 281–3.
41. Seah LL, Choo CT, Fong KS. Congenital upper lid colobomas. Ophthal Plast Reconstr Surg 2002; 18: 190–5.
46. Hertle RW, Ziylan S, Katowitz JA. Ophthalmic features and visual prognosis in the Treacher–Collins syndrome. Br J Ophthalmol 1993; 77: 642–5.
49. Chandler KE, Kidd A, Al-Gazali L, et al. Diagnostic criteria, clinical characteristics and natural history of Cohen syndrome. J Med Genet 2003; 40: 233–41.
55. Stromland K. Ocular involvement in the fetal alcohol syndrome. Surv Ophthalmol 1987; 31: 277–84.
56. Zlotogora J, Sagi M, Cohen T. The blepharophimosis, ptosis, and epicanthus inversus syndrome: delineation of two types. Am J Hum Genet 1983; 35: 1020–7.
70. Stout AU, Borchert M. Etiology of eyelid retraction in children. J Pediatr Ophthalmol Strabismus 1993; 30: 96–9.
82. Oliver GL, McFarlane DC. Congenital trichomegaly with associated pigmentary degeneration of the retina, dwarfism and mental retardation. Arch Ophthalmol 1965; 74: 169–71.
83. Levin AV, Seidman DJ, Nelson LB, et al. Ophthalmic findings in Cornelia de Lange syndrome. J Pediatr Ophthalmol Strabismus 1990; 27: 94–102.
88. Ilker SS, Ozturk F, Kurt E, et al. Ophthalmic findings in GAPO syndrome. Jpn J Ophthalmol 1999; 43: 48–52.
89. McNab AA, Potts MJ, Welham RA. The EEC syndrome and its ocular manifestations. Br J Ophthalmol 1989; 73: 261–4.
102. De Baere E, Dixon MJ, Small KW, et al. Spectrum of FOXL2 gene mutations in blepharophimosis-ptosis-epicanthus inversus (BPES) families demonstrates a genotype-phenotype correlation. Hum Mol Genet 2001; 10: 1591–600.
105. Krantz ID, McCallum J, DeScipio C, et al. Cornelia de Lange syndrome is caused by mutations in NIPBL, the human homolog of Drosophila melanogaster Nipped-B. Nat Genet 2004; 36: 631–5.
107. Reardon W, Winter RM, Rutland P, et al. Mutations in the fibroblast growth factor receptor 2 gene cause Crouzon syndrome. Nat Genet 1994; 8: 98–103.
110. Jadeja S, Smyth I, Pitera JE, et al. Identification of a new gene mutated in Fraser syndrome and mouse myelencephalic blebs. Nat Genet 2005; 37: 520–5.
112. McGrath JA, Duijf PH, Doetsch V, et al. Hay–Wells syndrome is caused by heterozygous missense mutations in the SAM domain of p63. Hum Mol Genet 2001; 10: 221–9.
113. Roessler E, Belloni E, Gaudenz K, et al. Mutations in the human Sonic Hedgehog gene cause holoproencephaly. Nat Genet 1996; 14: 357–60.
119. Ng SB, Bigham AW, Buckingham KJ, et al. Exome sequencing identifies MLL2 mutations as a cause of Kabuki syndrome. Nat Genet 2010; 42: 790–3.
123. Tartaglia M, Zampino G, Gelb BD. Noonan syndrome: clinical aspects and molecular pathogenesis. Mol Syndromol 2010; 1: 2–26.
135. Pingault V, Ente D, Dastot-Le Moal F, et al. Review and update of mutations causing Waardenburg syndrome. Hum Mutat 2010; 31: 1–16.

Access the complete reference list online at

http://www.expertconsult.com

Lids: Congenital and acquired abnormalities – practical management

Robert C Kersten • Hugo W A Henderson • J Richard O Collin

This chapter concentrates on the practical management of congenital and acquired eyelid lesions. The main indications for eyelid surgery in children are to optimize the potential for useful vision in severe congenital malformations, to prevent amblyopia, to control exposure and breakdown of the ocular surface, and to improve cosmesis. These aims are aligned as reconstructive lid surgery usually results in both improved function and cosmesis.

Complex cases require a careful treatment plan. However, flexibility is often required in oculoplastic surgery, and the surgeon often enters the operating room with the realization that plans may need to be modified.

Management of congenital lid conditions

Lid coloboma

The treatment of lid coloboma is directed toward treating sight-threatening corneal exposure, preventing amblyopia and improving cosmesis. Occasionally, underlying abnormalities which limit ocular motility may need to be addressed.

The coloboma is described in terms of its position using the Tessier classification, and in terms of its extent.[1] An examination is carried out to exclude associated ocular and systemic abnormalities. Initial management aims to protect the ocular surface with lubrication and occlusive dressing taking care not to induce amblyopia with them. A forced duction test is performed on all children with an eyelid coloboma for underlying

adhesions[2] which need early treatment. This should be carried out early and it usually requires an examination under anesthesia. A small coloboma can be closed under the same anesthetic. If a more complicated repair is required, timing depends on the underlying ocular surface protection but delaying repair allows growth of soft tissues increasing options for advancement and closure. If corneal exposure cannot be controlled, the eyelid reconstruction is urgent. A defect less than 25% of the lid length can be repaired by excision of the coloboma margins and direct closure. For defects of 25–50% of lid length, a lateral canthotomy and cantholysis allows the wound edges to come together. For defects of 50% or more, tissue will need to be added from elsewhere. In the lower eyelid, the posterior lamellar can be reconstructed using tarsoconjunctival grafts from the upper lid, together with advancement myocutaneous eyelid flaps or skin grafts. Eyelid sharing procedures are better for older children or eyes in which there is no visual potential, due to the risk of occlusion amblyopia. They may be necessary in cases of uncontrolled exposure; in these circumstances the flap should be divided after 2 weeks, and followed with aggressive occlusion therapy.

The coloboma in Treacher-Collins syndrome (see Chapter 18) is a pseudocoloboma in which there is a defect of subcutaneous tissue rather than a true eyelid discontinuity. The syndrome is variably severe, including an abortive form. Severe cases may require craniofacial surgery prior to eyelid surgery in order to re-establish malar support. In less severe cases, the lids can be built with oculoplastic surgery alone. In mild cases, the lateral canthus can be repositioned with a lateral canthoplasty, but extensive undermining and repositioning of the periocular soft tissues is necessary to maintain the new canthal position. In moderate cases, with absence of vertical and horizontal eyelid soft tissue, the lid can be reconstructed with the use of hard palate mucous membrane grafts or ear cartilage to support the lid. The lateral canthus can be secured with wire fixation to bore holes in the lateral orbital rim. Moderately severe cases may require transposition flaps from the upper to lower lids with a lateral canthal strip.

Cryptophthalmos

Cryptophthalmos is a rare condition in which the upper eyelid and eyebrow fail to develop and the cutaneous epithelium is continuous with conjunctiva at the superior fornix. There is usually severe dysgenesis of the anterior segment as well. The condition can be complete, incomplete, or partial (congenital symblepharon) (see Chapter 18).

In complete cryptophthalmos there is no real chance of gaining vision even with reconstructive surgery. In incomplete cryptophthalmos there may be some chance of achieving useful vision or reasonable cosmesis, but this is unusual: then the same concerns pertain as in eyelid colobomas. The urgency of surgery depends on whether the condition is unilateral or bilateral, the presence of visual potential, and the degree of corneal exposure. If the condition is unilateral, no visual potential exists, and exposure is controlled, surgery should be delayed to allow for the relaxation of tissues, which occurs as the infant matures.[3]

Surgery reconstitutes the components of the anterior and posterior lamellae. Pedicle rotation flaps from the cheek or brow, eyelid sharing, full-thickness skin grafts, and mucous membrane grafts are used. The success of complex lid reconstruction is limited by defective tear production, a lack of healthy conjunctiva and underlying ocular defects associated with the condition, such as corneal and anterior segment dysgenesis. The surgeon must be prepared to perform a corneal graft when reconstruction is undertaken as the lids and cornea are fused in a continuous tissue plane and there is a danger of perforation.

Ablepharon

Complete failure of eyelid development is rare (see Chapter 18). Urgent treatment is required to protect the ocular surface followed by early lid reconstruction. The results depend on the severity of the lid changes and the integrity of the underlying structures. Treatment of true ablepharon has poor results; however, treatment of milder cases (microblepharon), by vertical stretching of the lid and anchoring at the lateral orbital rim, is more successful. Although the eyelid may open minimally initially due to "bow-stringing" of the tight eyelid, this improves significantly within 6–8 weeks of surgery.

Ankyloblepharon

In ankyloblepharon (see Chapter 18) the eyelid margins are partially or completely fused together with a reduction in the palpebral aperture. Ankyloblepharon filiforme adnatum is a similar condition in which one or more skin tags join the two lids and there is usually a normal horizontal palpebral aperture: it is treated by division of the tag or tags.

Ankyloblepharon must be differentiated from blepharophimosis in which the palpebral aperture is reduced and there is telecanthus, but the eyelid margins are normal. Recognition of ankyloblepharon necessitates systemic examination to detect associated abnormalities. The lids are opened along the line of fusion with sharp scissors or a scalpel. A thin strip of skin and orbicularis is excised and the bare lid margin allowed to conjunctivalize. The lid structure and tarsus are usually otherwise normal.

Euryblepharon

Euryblepharon (see Chapter 18) is congenital primary enlargement of the palpebral aperture, usually greatest laterally. There is a localized outward and downward displacement of the lateral canthus and downward displacement of the lower lid.

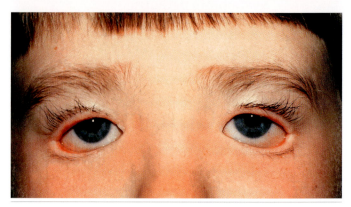

Fig. 19.1 **Bilateral ectropion due to shortage of the anterior lamella in a patient with euryblepharon and blepharophimosis.**

Mild cases may require no treatment or simple lubrication. If there is a danger of corneal exposure, the lateral canthus may be tightened and positioned more superiorly and posteriorly. Wide undermining and repositioning of the soft tissues is necessary or the tissues tend to migrate to their original location. If the eyelid is short vertically, skin grafts and/or posterior lamellar grafts with overlying soft tissue advancement may be required. Free grafts usually result in suboptimal cosmesis in young children.

Ectropion

The initial treatment of ectropion in childhood is conservative, using lubrication to prevent exposure keratitis. Surgery is aimed at treating the underlying cause: shortage of skin or increased lid laxity (paralytic ectropion is discussed later) and is usually delayed until the child is older and has more soft tissue with which to work. Ectropion associated with a shortage of skin occurs in congenital conditions such as Down's syndrome, blepharophimosis (Fig. 19.1), and acquired conditions such as ichthyosis, dermatomyositis, and trauma. A localized scar can be lengthened with a Z-plasty, and a generalized shortage of skin corrected with a skin flap or graft. Increased lid laxity causing ectropion is found in congenital conditions such as megaloblepharon and euryblepharon and can occur after trauma. It is treated with lid-shortening procedures.[4]

Eversion

Treatment of congenital eversion (see Chapter 18) is aimed at repositioning the everted eyelids so that the underlying soft tissue swelling and chemosis can resolve. Once this has occurred, the eyelids remain in proper position. Repositioning the eyelids and pressure patching or taping for 5–7 days is usually sufficient. More severe cases can be treated by intermarginal sutures.

Epiblepharon

Epiblepharon is a horizontal fold of skin across the upper or lower eyelid that may push the lashes against the cornea (see Chapter 18). The lid margin remains in a normal position. Epiblepharon usually resolves by 5–6 years of age as the facial bones grow. It is usually asymptomatic and is seldom associated with keratitis (Fig. 19.2). Surgical intervention is reserved

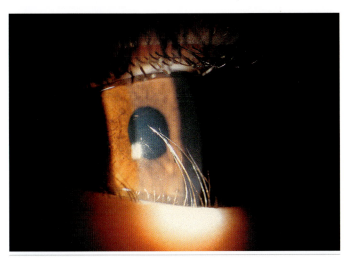

Fig. 19.2 Epiblepharon. In this child the lower lid lashes have turned in from birth, but the cornea has remained undamaged. Spontaneous improvement usually occurs.

for those patients in whom it causes corneal compromise despite conservative treatment (i.e. lubrication) or it persists into adolescence. Quickert sutures can be used in milder cases, or excision of an ellipse of skin and orbicularis muscle with tarsal fixation is used in more severe cases.[5,6]

Entropion

In congenital entropion (see Chapter 18), the eyelid margin is inverted (Figs 19.3 and 19.4). This often requires prompt surgical intervention to prevent corneal infection and scarring. It should be distinguished from epiblepharon, where a skin fold causes a secondary turning of the lower lid lashes. Surgery is directed toward re-everting and stabilizing the eyelid with excision of skin and orbicularis, reattachment of the lower eyelid retractors to the inferior border of the tarsus, and then re-fixating the skin edges to the inferior tarsal border.

Tarsal kink/upper lid entropion

Congenital upper lid entropion is rare but often associated with a horizontal kinking of the tarsus. As with lower lid entropion, there is a risk of corneal scarring and infection. It can be corrected by incising the tarsus along the kink, and then repositioning the anterior lamella of the eyelid (Fig. 19.5).

Distichiasis

Distichiasis is a developmental abnormality in which a second row of cilia emerges from the meibomian gland orifices posterior to the normal eyelashes. The abnormal lashes may be asymptomatic or cause superficial corneal problems. If the patients are symptomatic or show significant corneal staining, treatment is indicated. Electrolysis is the treatment of choice for a single or very few lashes, and can be combined with a posterior cutdown in which a short vertical incision is made through the tarsal plate to expose the lash root, which can be treated with electrolysis under direct vision. For larger numbers of lashes, electrolysis is not effective, takes a long time, and produces tarsal scarring. Cryotherapy is then preferable with a double freeze–thaw cycle for 20 seconds. In the upper lid, a gray line split between the anterior and posterior lamellae

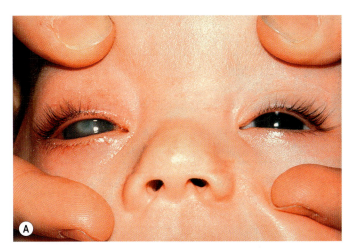

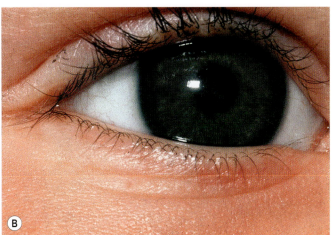

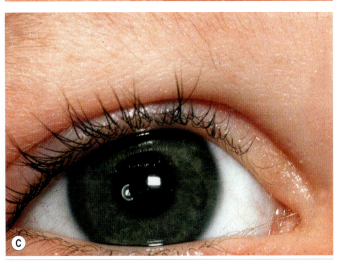

Fig. 19.3 Congenital entropion. (A) Shortly after birth this child's eye was found to be swollen. During examination under anesthetic right upper lid entropion was found with a corneal abrasion caused by the entropion. (B) After taping the lids, the entropion resolved, and (C) ultimately there was only minimal subepithelial opacity.

allows cryotherapy to be applied directly to the tarsus, avoiding damage to the normal lash roots and, in dark-skinned patients, discoloration of the skin. The posterior lamella is then advanced, leaving the raw surface of the tarsal plate to granulate. This prevents contraction of the tarsal plate leading to entropion.

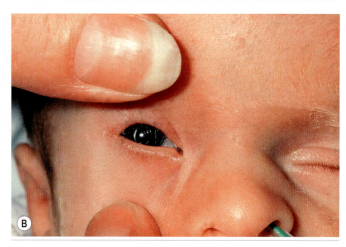

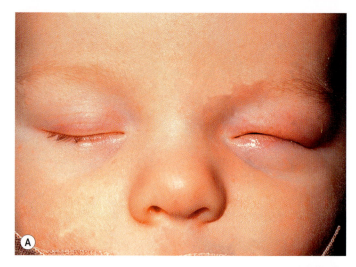

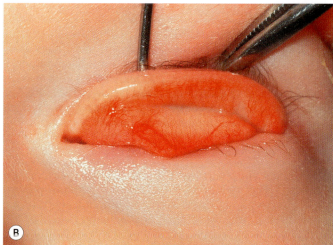

Fig. 19.4 Congenital entropion. (A) This child presented with irritability and an abnormality of the right lids, which were slightly swollen. (B) Same child with the lid everted, showing the lashes inturned and abrading the cornea without damage at this stage. It was treated with simple lid suture and resolved without complication.

Fig. 19.5 Horizontal tarsal kink. (A) This child presented with a swollen and sore left eye with blepharospasm. (B) On eversion of the lid the horizontal kink in the tarsus can be seen. It runs the whole length of the tarsal plate, which is bent to 90°. It was treated by forced eversion using a strabismus hook to straighten the tarsus by force while the margin of the lid was held. This was followed by a week of lid suture, and the condition resolved following that treatment but there was severe corneal scarring and the eye was blind.

Epicanthal folds

Epicanthal folds are folds of skin which extend from the upper eyelid toward the medial canthus. The fundamental difference between epicanthal folds and epiblepharon is that epicanthal folds are caused by a relative shortage of skin where the soft tissue is stretched tautly between the medial eyelid and the medial canthus instead of following the contour of the nasal angle. Epicanthal folds only require urgent treatment if they cause trichiasis or obstruct vision. They are largely an esthetic issue and become less prominent with development of the bridge of the nose and stretching of the overlying skin. As the folds represent lines of skin shortage, they can be broken up and lengthened with various different flaps. A simple epicanthic fold can be treated with a Z-plasty. Two separate Z-plasties can be used when a fold affects both the upper and lower lids. A mild epicanthic fold associated with telecanthus can be treated with a Y–V plasty and shortening of the underlying medial canthal tendon. If there is a marked epicanthic fold associated with telecanthus, a double Z-plasty can be combined with a Y–V plasty.[7,8]

Telecanthus

Telecanthus is an increased width between the medial canthi, with a normal interpupillary distance. If there is an overgrowth of bone with an increase in the interorbital width the condition is referred to as hypertelorism. Telecanthus can usually be improved by shortening the medial canthal tendons without involving a significant reduction in bone.[9] Mild cases can be treated by medial canthal plication with a non-absorbable or wire suture combined with a Y–V plasty. More severe cases may require transnasal wiring combined with a Y–V plasty. Posterior placement of the wire is necessary for a good cosmetic result. The thickness of the anterior lacrimal crest and medial orbital wall bone can be reduced with a burr at the same procedure. If a transnasal wire is required, it is essential to have preoperative radiologic evidence of the height of the cribriform plate to avoid damage to the intracranial structures. The correction of hypertelorism requires craniofacial surgery to mobilize the orbital rims and reduce the intervening ethmoid bones.

Blepharophimosis

"Blepharophimosis" means small eyelids. In the blepharophimosis syndrome, the horizontal palpebral aperture is reduced and this is associated with epicanthus inversus, ptosis, and telecanthus (see Chapter 18).

Treatment is directed toward promoting visual development and improving cosmesis. Patients should be refracted and amblyopia and strabismus are common.[10] Resting lid position determines the urgency of ptosis correction. If a marked ptosis contributes to amblyopia, either by obstructing the visual axis, or by inducing astigmatism, ptosis surgery is urgent.

The treatment of blepharophimosis syndrome is staged. Hypertelorism, epicanthus inversus, and telecanthus can be repaired at one sitting. Various techniques have been described to rearrange the medial canthal tissues, but a simple Y to V advancement with medial canthal tendon plication, or, in the case of more severe telecanthus, transnasal wiring, is most effective. In addition, the epicanthal folds generally improve with development of the mid-face. Ptosis surgery is done as a second procedure because correcting the telecanthus may worsen the ptosis. Moreover, levator function is usually very poor; thus, if there is no risk of amblyopia, ptosis surgery can be delayed until the child is sufficiently developed to carry out a brow suspension with autologous fascia lata or temporalis fascia (Fig. 19.6).

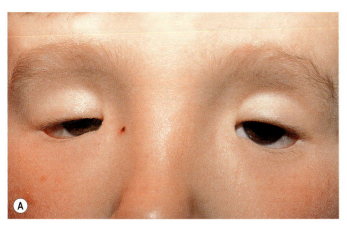

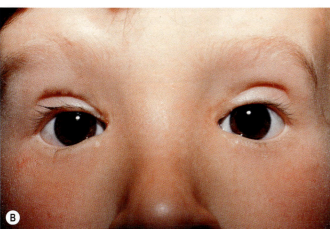

Fig. 19.6 Blepharophimosis. (A) This patient has blepharophimosis syndrome with blepharophimosis, ptosis, and telecanthus. (B) The same child after Y–V canthoplasties followed by brow suspensions with autogenous fascia lata.

Management of congenital and acquired ptosis

Congenital ptosis is usually associated with a dysgenesis of the levator muscle. There is a direct relationship between the levator muscle function, i.e. the excursion of the upper lid between full upgaze and downgaze, and the number of healthy striated muscle fibers. This is the main factor influencing the choice of ptosis surgery. Causes of acquired ptosis include aponeurotic defects, third nerve palsies and associated syndromes, Horner's syndrome, ocular myopathies, and myasthenia. These will influence the choice of surgery by affecting Bell's phenomenon, levator function, the variability of ptosis, etc.

History and examination

Chapter 18 reviews the various causes of congenital vs. acquired ptosis. A careful history to confirm the congenital or acquired nature of the condition and associated phenomenon is important. With congenital ptosis the parents may report that the condition seemed to improve initially after birth and then plateaued after a few months.

A full eye examination should be performed, with attention to the position of the lid on downgaze, levator excursion from down- to upgaze, extraocular motility, facial or eyelid dysmorphism or mass, aberrant movements of the lid associated with extraocular excursions or jaw movement, pupillary size and reactivity, and variability in eyelid height. Best corrected visual acuity, fixation preference, and retinoscopy or subjective refraction should be performed to rule out associated amblyopia. Further investigations may be indicated, for instance with third nerve palsies or congenital Horner's syndrome.[11]

The degree of ptosis should be assessed by comparing the vertical interpalpebral aperture measurements on both sides and assessing the height of the lid above the corneal reflex from a spot source of light (margin-reflex distance.) This obviates inaccuracies from malposition of the lower eyelid. The levator function should be measured by pressing over the brow to prevent any frontalis action and then measuring the excursion of the lid between full up- and downgaze, if the child is old enough to cooperate. The position of the skin crease on both sides and the presence or absence of Bell's phenomenon should be noted as well as orbicularis strength.

Treatment

This depends on the diagnosis and physical findings. Surgical correction is urgent only if there is a risk of amblyopia because the eyelid is inducing asymmetric astigmatism or occluding the visual axis. Even in the setting of severe unilateral ptosis, a chin-up head position is often adopted to maintain binocular fusion. Hence ptosis surgery often may be delayed until the child is old enough for an accurate assessment of levator function, but regular examinations to monitor amblyopia are mandatory. Underlying strabismus should be corrected before undertaking ptosis repair as eyelid height may be affected by strabismus surgery.

With congenital ptosis the levator function and degree of ptosis govern the choice of operation. In mild congenital ptosis, if there is about 2 mm of ptosis with good levator function of 10 mm or more, a Fasanella Servat procedure or müllerectomy predictably elevates the eyelid.

In moderate congenital ptosis with levator function between 5 and 10 mm, a graded levator resection, depending on the amount of levator function and degree of ptosis (Fig. 19.7) is attempted. Either an anterior or a posterior approach to the levator can give satisfactory results. The posterior approach has the advantage that the resected levator muscle is held by pull-out sutures that are tied in the skin crease. If an overcorrection occurs, these can be removed in the early postoperative period and the eyelid lowered. The anterior approach is suitable for a maximum levator resection; it allows wider exposure of the levator muscle and the creation of an enhanced lid fold by directly fixating skin to the underlying distal edge of the cut levator muscle. The disadvantage of a large levator resection is that it increases lagophthalmos and lid lag on downgaze.

In severe congenital ptosis with less than 5 mm of levator function, a frontalis sling is usually necessary. The success of this procedure relies on the intrinsic reflex recruitment of the ipsilateral frontalis muscle. Internal attachment between the frontalis and the eyelid is carried out so that frontalis elevation results in a more efficient eyelid elevation. If it is necessary to elevate an eyelid urgently to prevent amblyopia, this can be done with a unilateral procedure using a non-autogenous material. Many materials have been utilized, but non-autogenous materials carry risk of infection, extrusion, migration due to "cheese-wiring," or degradation with breakage or loss of strength. Of the various options, a 1 mm silicone rod or extruded polytetrafluoroethylene suture offers the best long-term stability. If there is no concern about amblyopia, it is better to wait until the child's leg is large enough to harvest autogenous fascia lata (usually 3 to 4 years) to use as the sling material. A pentagonal sling with opening of the eyelid crease and direct suturing the sling material to tarsal plate allows for

excellent symmetry of eyelid creases. Intraoperative adjustment of lid height and contour can be effected depending on placement of the fixation sutures on the tarsal plate. Controversy exists as to whether unilateral ptosis with poor levator function should be treated with a unilateral sling or if better symmetry can be achieved by excising the normal levator muscle and lifting both eyelids symmetrically with a bilateral brow suspension (Figs 19.8 and 19.9). Excellent symmetry in primary position can usually be obtained with unilateral surgery but asymmetric lid lag will be visible in downgaze. Bilateral surgery, however, places the "normal" eye at risk of exposure.

A frontalis sling is usually ineffective if there is amblyopia as there will be no stimulus for recruitment of the frontalis to clear the visual axis if there is no drive to obtain binocular vision. In this case, a maximal levator resection may be performed. The levator muscle is dissected free of it attachments, including Whitnall's ligament, and the muscle maximally resected (up to 30 mm) and re-sutured to the tarsal plate through an anterior approach. The goal is to leave the eyelid margin at the level of the superior limbus. This approach may lead to lagophthalmos and exposure keratopathy but most young patients will tolerate this with the aid of initial aggressive corneal lubrication. Lagophthalmos usually improves over time, but a severely dystrophic levator muscle is heavily infiltrated with fatty tissue and tends to stretch with recurrence of ptosis over time.

Specific conditions

In the blepharophimosis syndrome levator function is usually poor and bilateral autogenous fascia lata brow suspensions are required. If the levator function is good, bilateral levator resections can be performed. The epicanthus inversus is usually best treated with a medial canthoplasty about 6 months before the lids are lifted.

In Marcus Gunn syndrome, if the jaw-winking element is unobtrusive, the ptosis alone can be corrected based on the levator function. If the jaw-winking is severe, it can be abolished or diminished by transecting the levator muscle and attaching it to periorbita behind the supraorbital rim. The ptosis must then be corrected with a brow suspension procedure. Some cases may become less marked with time. It may be justifiable to delay surgery until the child is old enough to determine the ultimate degree of jaw-wink.

With third nerve lesions the eye should be straightened first with strabismus surgery. Correction of the ptosis depends on the levator function. If Bell's phenomenon is defective, there is a risk of exposure keratitis; ptosis surgery should be more conservative. Congenital third nerve lesions may often display aberrant innervation with cross-signaling between the medial rectus and levator palpebrae superioris (see Chapter 83). In this case, extirpation of the levator and frontalis sling surgery is required. A similar approach is used if there is cyclic third nerve dysfunction.

Horner's syndrome usually does well with a Fasanella Servat or müllerectomy procedure.

Patients with myasthenia gravis should first be managed medically. If ptosis persists, silicone rod frontalis sling allows elevation of the eyelid and postoperative adjustment of eyelid height, if necessary. The two ends of the rod are attached to each other by placing them through a Watzke sleeve; the ends are left long with about a centimeter of excess rod on either

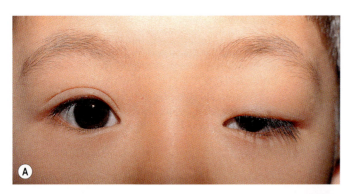

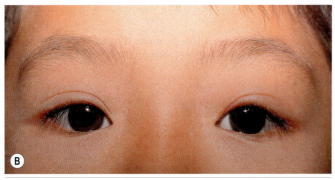

Fig. 19.7 (A) Unilateral simple congenital ptosis. (B) The same child after levator resection.

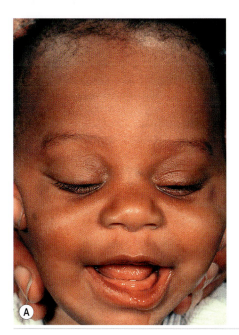
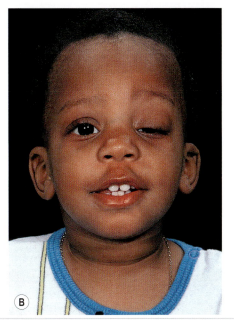
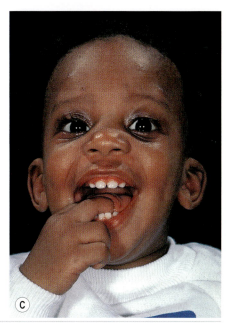

Fig. 19.8 (A) Right ptosis in a 6-month-old baby. It can be seen that there is no lid crease on the right while it is present on the left. The child is looking down during this photograph and the normally ptotic lid is slightly higher than the normal lid, suggesting a dystrophic ptosis. (B) Same child at 2 years of age preoperatively. (C) Same child postoperatively. A bilateral levator sling procedure has been carried out.

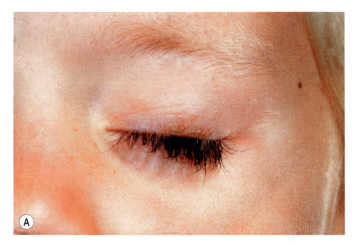

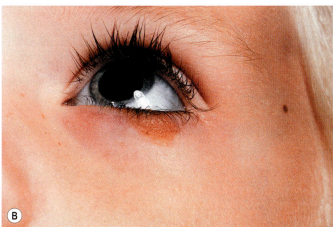

Fig. 19.9 Divided nevus.

side. This allows reopening of the eyebrow incision over the sleeve and loosening of the sling.

Aponeurotic defects occurring congenitally, traumatically, or secondary to blepharochalasis syndrome should be repaired by advancing the levator aponeurosis. This is best done under local anesthesia when the child is older so that intraoperative adjustment of eyelid height and contour can be performed.

In the congenital cranial dysinnervation disorders (see Chapter 82), a brow suspension with careful postoperative management to prevent exposure may give good results.

Lid retraction in infancy

Lid retraction in infancy can be caused by various conditions (see Chapter 18). Major lid retraction with corneal exposure requires urgent treatment with lubrication and early surgery to protect the cornea. Cases of mild lid retraction may benefit from cosmetic surgery that may be delayed into early childhood.

The upper lid can be lowered and the lower lid elevated by recessing the lid retractors provided there is no shortage of skin or conjunctiva. Upper lid retractor recessions through a posterior approach can be used to release Müller's muscle and aponeurosis and correct up to 2 mm of lid retraction. However, posterior approach upper lid retractor recessions inevitably cause a raised skin crease. This does not matter in mild or bilateral cases, but is important in severe unilateral cases. In these, the retractors should be lengthened via an anterior approach levator recession or Z-myotomy or a spacer graft and the skin crease reformed at the desired level. Lower lid retraction may be corrected by retractor recession, usually in combination with a spacer graft.[12]

Seventh nerve palsy

In the newborn the incidence of facial palsy is 0.2%. Birth trauma is the cause of 78% of facial paralysis in this group, and can be caused by forceps delivery, pressure from the maternal sacrum, pressure from the fetal shoulder, or intracranial hemorrhage. Nearly 90% of newborn facial palsies completely recover without treatment, usually by 5 months of age.[13] In infancy or childhood, acquired facial palsy is most often associated with otitis media and mastoiditis.

Bell's palsy is less common in children than in adults. It is manifest as a sudden onset of paralysis of all five divisions of the facial nerve without signs of ear or cerebellopontine angle disease. It is bilateral in 0.3% to 2% of cases, and recurrent in 9% of cases.

In bilateral palsies the resultant disability is dramatically more severe, and can be associated with severe feeding problems. In the newborn it may be associated with Möbius syndrome (see Chapter 82). In childhood, the most common cause in endemic areas is Lyme disease, followed by otitis media and idiopathic.[14]

Although facial nerve palsy in children has a good prognosis, it may be the initial manifestation of a life-threatening disorder such as an intracranial neoplasm or vascular malformation. If there are other neurologic findings, imaging studies are indicated. Progression of facial nerve palsy is usually due to a tumor; in 20% of patients with recurrent facial weakness a tumor is eventually discovered.

The main problems caused by a seventh nerve palsy are corneal exposure, paralytic ectropion, epiphora, and poor cosmesis.[15]

Corneal exposure

Corneal exposure does not usually result from poor lid closure alone as Bell's phenomenon is good in infants; there are usually additional risk factors. These include inadequate Bell's phenomenon, reduction in corneal sensation, lower lid ectropion, treatment on a ventilator, prematurity, or reduction in tear production if the lesion is proximal to the geniculate ganglion. A reduction in corneal sensation is more common after surgical treatment of intracranial tumors although it may be present in Möbius syndrome.

Initial treatment is with lubricants, taping at night, and occasionally occlusive dressings may be required. The lubricants can be stopped for 2 to 3 hours a day, or the other eye patched in order to avoid amblyopia. Occasionally, a temporary lateral tarsorrhaphy may be required to protect the cornea. If there is continued corneal exposure after 6 months, or earlier if there is no chance of recovery, the palpebral aperture can be reduced permanently. The vertical palpebral aperture can be reduced by raising the lower lid with a lateral tarsorrhaphy and medial canthoplasty, by lowering the upper lid with a müllerectomy, or recession of Müller's muscle and the levator muscle, or with a full-thickness blepharotomy. Lid closure can be improved mechanically with upper lid gold weights or springs.

Paralytic ectropion

Paralytic ectropion can be treated by a medial canthoplasty. If required, this can be combined with lateral canthal tightening.

Epiphora (see Chapter 21)

Epiphora is due to the loss of the lacrimal pump mechanism and is exacerbated by lower lid ectropion. Persistent watering after 6 months may be improved by correction of any ectropion with a lateral canthal tightening and medial canthoplasty.

Watering may also occur due to "crocodile tears" in which tearing is associated with salivation due to aberrant innervation of the lacrimal gland by parasympathetic fibers intended for the salivary glands. Crocodile tears may be improved by injections of 2.5 units of botulinum toxin into the palpebral lobe of the lacrimal gland, but this requires a general anesthetic in a child. Severe epiphora of any cause may require a Lester Jones tube: this is difficult to manage in a small child.

Cosmesis

Surgery to raise the brow, reduce the palpebral aperture, and correct ectropion may help. Lower facial paralysis tends to cause progressive facial asymmetry; facial slings or nerve grafting may help restore facial tone and position.

Lid tumors

Nevi

Surgery for nevi is indicated if there is concern for the development of malignant potential, amblyopia due to lid malposition, and cosmesis.

Large, or giant, congenital nevi are associated with a risk of malignant transformation. The risk is related to increasing size of the lesion and may occur in up to 20% of very large congenital hairy nevi. The incidence of malignant transformation in small and medium congenital nevi is controversial, but probably is negligible. Divided nevi ("kissing nevi") are a form of congenital melanocytic nevus that involves the upper and lower lids (Fig. 19.9). Malignant transformation has not been reported in congenital nevi limited to the eyelids. Peak onset of malignant transformation occurs by 2–3 years of age. The lesions are difficult to treat due to their size. Surgery may require numerous stages, with skin grafts and flaps, and the use of tissue expanders. The multiple procedures may result in marked scarring. Dermabrasion, within the first few months and preferably weeks of life, may reduce the chance of malignant transformation, improve cosmesis, and reduce the extent of further surgery.[16]

Acquired nevi are rarely a concern in children, but these lesions are monitored.

Molluscum contagiosum

Molluscum contagiosum are viral lesions which frequently occur on the eyelids (Fig. 19.10). They may rarely obtain large size; "kissing" lesions may occur on the upper and lower lids (Fig. 19.11). They are often associated with a follicular conjunctivitis (Fig. 19.12), which does not resolve until the lesions near the eyelid are eradicated (see Chapter 15). Treatment modalities include curettage and diathermy of the core of the lesion, cryotherapy, and chemical ablatives.

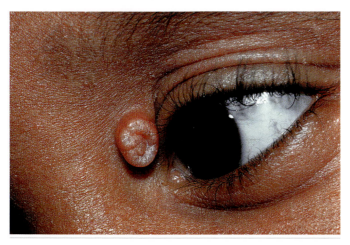

Fig. 19.10 Large molluscum contagiosum lesion. (Dr Susan Day's patient.)

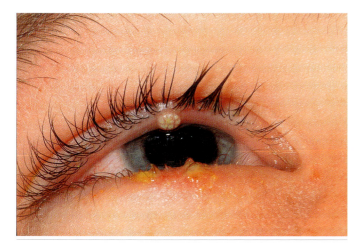

Fig. 19.11 Molluscum contagiosum showing multiple lesions and a follicular conjunctivitis.

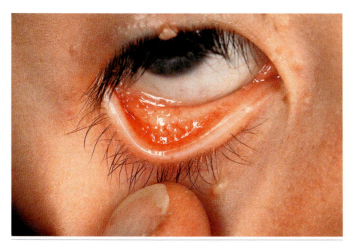

Fig. 19.12 Molluscum contagiosum showing "kiss" lesions on upper and lower lids.

Juvenile xanthogranuloma (see Chapter 27)

Juvenile xanthogranuloma (see Chapter 27) is a benign disease characterized by the development of small yellowish rubbery cutaneous lesions, including eyelid lesions, measuring 1 to 10 mm, in the first 1 to 9 months of life, associated with ocular xanthogranuloma lesions, particularly in the iris; spontaneous hyphema and glaucoma may result.

Complex choristoma

These are rare lid tumors that consist of variable combinations of ectopic tissues (see Chapter 29). They resemble other choristomas such as dermoids and lipodermoids. When acinar elements compose the majority of the tissue, they may have a fleshy appearance or resemble an ectopic lacrimal gland. Mild growth may occur during puberty, but malignant transformation is very rare. They can involve the underlying tissue. Conjunctival lesions may involve tissues deep in the globe; therefore, excision is performed with caution.

Pilomatrixoma (calcifying epithelioma of Malherbe)

A small hard nodule in the eyebrow is likely to be a pilomatrixoma. The overlying skin is intact and may have a pink to purple discoloration. It may be mistaken for a chalazion or dermoid. Treatment is excision.

Lid hamartoma

Lid hamartomas include infantile hemangiomas (see Chapter 20), plexiform neurofibromas (see Chapter 65), lymphangiomas (venolymphatic malformations) (see Chapter 20), and congenital nevi.

Indications for surgery for plexiform neurofibroma and lymphangioma include mechanical ptosis, occlusion amblyopia, astigmatic anisometropic amblyopia, and cosmetic deformity. Surgery for both these lesions is challenging. The lesions may be extensive, involving the lids, orbits, and surrounding facial tissues. Due to their infiltrative nature there may be an increase in growth around puberty. Treatment should be planned in conjunction with allied surgical specialties. In general, less surgical intervention is better than more. Repeated procedures may be necessary over the lifetime of the patient.

Meibomian gland diseases

Chalazia (meibomian cysts)

A chalazion is a lipogranulomatous inflammatory reaction of the meibomian gland that results from obstruction of the gland duct and is usually located in the mid-portion of the tarsus. It may occur on the lid margin if the opening of the duct is involved. A secondary bacterial infection of the surrounding tissue may develop with swelling of the entire lid. Chalazia may cause pressure on the globe and induce astigmatism. Most chalazia ultimately resolve spontaneously; this may be hastened by frequent application of warm compresses. These can be made using a cup of uncooked rice placed in a thin sock and heated for one minute in the microwave oven. If the chalazion is inflamed or secondarily infected, treatment with oral azithromycin (once a week for 3 weeks) is often helpful. There is little role for topical antibiotic drops or ointment since these do not penetrate the tarsal plate. Incision of the posterior tarsal wall of the lesion and curettage is sometimes necessary. This is avoided whenever possible in young children since it requires general anesthesia. Chronic meibomitis and blepharitis may predispose to recurrent chalazia, and can be treated by lid cleaning and antibiotic/hydrocortisone ointment and oral azithromycin (see Chapter 15).

Other diseases of the meibomian glands include the following:

1. Absent or deficient glands: primary congenital ectodermal dysplasia or ichthyosis, or secondary to lid disease.
2. Replacement: primary distichiasis, or secondary distichiasis due to metaplasia.
3. Meibomian seborrhea: associated with seborrheic dermatitis and acne rosacea. The meibum is greasy and solidified.
4. Meibomitis: often occurs with blepharitis. The orifices are red and swollen and sometimes there is soreness with associated lid edema. Treatment is similar to blepharitis.

Acute blepharitis (see Chapter 15)

Acute blepharitis presents with ulceration of the lid margins and is usually caused by *Staphylococcus aureus*, other organisms, and viruses, including *Moraxella* spp., herpes simplex, and various fungi in immunosuppressed patients (Fig. 19.13). Staphylococcal and *Moraxella* blepharitis usually respond well to antibiotic cream and lid hygiene.

Chronic blepharitis (see Chapter 15)

Chronic blepharitis is much more common than the acute form. It presents as irritable, red, and scaly eyelids that are sometimes edematous (Fig. 19.14). The anterior lid margin is usually most affected, but occasionally the posterior lid margin is more red and swollen when the meibomian glands are affected (chronic meibomitis). Chronic infection with *S. aureus*, *Propionibacterium acnes*, or coagulase-negative staphylococcal species may play a role.[17]

Most of the cases of chronic blepharitis have a seborrheic element with greasy, scaly lids associated in some cases with seborrheic dermatitis of the scalp (dandruff), or elsewhere.

Treatment is by regular lid cleaning, with particular attention to the lid margins. Expression of meibomian secretion by firm pressure may help the symptoms of burning and irritation. A 3-week course of oral azithromycin is indicated. Recurrent or severe cases, associated with keratoconjunctivitis, may be treated by a short course of steroid–antibiotic combination ointment.

Lid lice (see Chapter 15)

Lid lice are usually pubic lice rather than head lice because their body shape is more suited to the wider spacing of the lashes. They may be found on slit-lamp examination of the bases of the lashes; their eggs ("nits") may be found attached to the lashes. The pubic hair must be treated with a topical anti-lice shampoo. The lice and nits can be manually removed from the eyelashes and topical non-medicated ointment applied to the lashes three times a day will often asphyxiate remaining lice. Topical physostigmine or pilogel can be applied.

Trichiasis

Trichiasis is an acquired condition of the eyelash roots in which the cilia are misdirected posteriorly causing corneal and conjunctival irritation. In the large majority of cases, it is caused by subtle cicatricial entropion, as evidenced by the anterior migration of the mucocutaneous junction relative to its normal location at the posterior lid margin. The more common causes of trichiasis include chronic blepharitis, Stevens-Johnson syndrome, burns, trachoma, and pemphigus (usually in adults).

The treatment of trichiasis depends on the number of abnormal lashes. One or a few lashes can be treated with electrolysis or surgery to excise the lash roots or resect the affected portion of the eyelid margin. More numerous lashes are best treated with cryotherapy, but all the lashes in the treated area are liable to be destroyed and it may cause depigmentation. In heavily pigmented patients cryotherapy can be combined with a lid-splitting technique as described above for distichiasis.

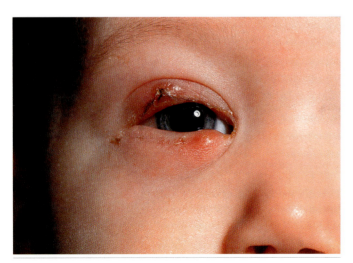

Fig. 19.13 Acute blepharitis with lid ulceration and stye formation.

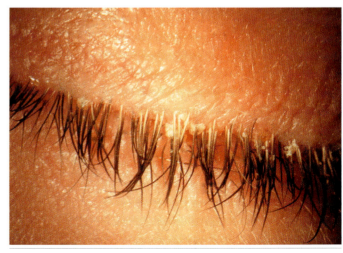

Fig. 19.14 Chronic blepharitis associated with chronic *Staphylococcus* infection.

Socket management

Contracted socket

Early socket growth is rapid (see Chapter 6). At 3 months, the face is only 40% of its adult size; by 5½ years it is 80% of its adult size. The presence of an eye is necessary for normal orbital growth. The loss of an eye, microphthalmia, or anophthalmia all result in abnormal orbital growth, but lack of a normal globe during development in utero leads to much more severe socket hypoplasia than loss of an eye after birth. The aims of socket management in infants are to increase the size of the bony orbit, conjunctival space, and palpebral length, and to promote the normal development of the lid margins and lashes.

Treatment must be started early to avoid a poor esthetic result. If the patient has an orbital cyst associated with microphthalmos or anophthalmos, this may be left to aid socket expansion (see Chapter 17).[18] The socket can be expanded using increasing sizes of orbital conformer. Expandable conformers that do not require serial changes and can be increased in size by injecting saline through a port have become available. These can be placed in the intraconal space and connected to a remote injection port under the skin (e.g. over the ear) or in the conjunctival sac with an anterior port directly accessible through the palpebral fissure.

An alternative is the self-inflating hydrogel expander. This is made of a modified copolymer of methylmethacrylate and vinylpyrrolidone, similar to contact lens material but with more capacity for swelling. It swells 10–12 times in volume, taking about 2 to 6 weeks to expand to its full size in the orbit.

Orbital volume replacement

Sometimes orbital expansion results in an increase in the anteroposterior dimension of the socket without increasing the palpebral fissure length and forniceal depth. The resultant conformer is round and deep and will not promote an increase in vertical and horizontal lid length, and will be difficult to retain. An orbital implant can be inserted, and a thinner conformer used to improve the fornices. Alternatively, if hydrogel expanders are used, a lens-shaped expander can be used to expand the conjunctival space followed by a spherical expander for the orbit.

The lateral fornix is often difficult to enlarge. It may need to be constructed surgically with a mucous membrane graft in order to retain a prosthesis.

Orbital implants available include porous implants of hydroxyapatite and polypropylene, non-porous implants made from silicone and acrylic, and dermis fat grafts. The porous implants have the advantage that they may become integrated into the socket and are less likely to extrude. However, their more abrasive surface may increase the erosion of the overlying conjunctiva and Tenon's capsule resulting in increased likelihood of exposure. There may be the option of pegging the porous implant to improve motility later. However, integration into the socket tissues makes these implants more difficult to remove when an implant may need to be replaced for a larger size. No study has supported the concept that porous implants give better motility unless they are pegged. Since pegging is rarely done due to a 30–40% incidence of

complications, silicone or acrylic implants are generally preferred. Dermis fat grafts have several advantages.[19] In adults, they tend to atrophy, but in children they grow as the child grows and help with socket expansion. They may grow such that they require debulking.[20] The conjunctiva can be attached to the edge of the graft, allowing the conjunctival epithelium to grow over the surface of the graft and increase the size of the conjunctival sac. If further volume augmentation is required, an orbital implant can be placed posterior to the graft.[21] The main disadvantage is donor site morbidity, although this is seldom a problem.

If treatment has failed to achieve adequate orbital expansion, resulting in marked facial asymmetry, craniofacial surgery may be required to augment or repair the orbit. Vascularized flaps to increase soft tissue may be used: for example, in cases of tissue atrophy secondary to radiotherapy.

Discharging sockets

Socket discharge is a common problem in patients with a prosthesis. The common causes are:[22]

1. Prosthesis: poor fit, mechanical irritation, hypersensitive reaction, and poor prosthetic hygiene.
2. Orbital implant: extrusion of implant, conjunctival inclusion cyst, and granuloma formation.
3. Lid: poor closure and infected focus.
4. Socket lining: contracture resulting in a mixture of skin and mucous membrane.
5. Lacrimal system: defective tear production or drainage and dacryocistitis.

Management is to treat the underlying cause.

Lid and adnexal trauma
(see Chapter 66)

Etiology

The majority of pediatric lid and adnexal injuries are accidental in nature, most commonly occurring during domestic activity, play time, or sporting activity.[23,24] Injuries from dog bites are frequent. Accidental penetration by common objects such as pencils or toys occurs frequently when a child carrying one of these stumbles and falls. Lid injuries include contusions, crush injuries, abrasions, lacerations, puncture wounds, and burns. These frequently occur in combination.

Immediate management

A history is taken, noting the time of the injury, nature of any projectile (was it sharp or blunt, metallic or vegetable), the speed of the projectile (was it thrown or shot), height of a fall and the type of surface the child landed on, any loss of consciousness, and any witnesses.

The assessment of the patient starts by examining and treating the patient for all injuries. Any necessary basic life support is given, and a full systemic examination may be required, including a neurologic examination if there is any suspicion of intracranial injury. It is not uncommon for long narrow objects such as pencils to penetrate the intracranial cavity via the orbit when a child carrying them stumbles and falls. A full ocular examination is performed. Visual function is assessed;

if possible the visual acuity is taken. In a young child one evaluates fixation and checks the patient's tolerance of occlusion of the uninjured eye. Check the pupil responses for a relative afferent defect.

The injury is assessed by looking for any damage not readily visible. A small penetrating lid laceration may have extensive underlying damage, including intracranial injury, orbital fractures, optic neuropathy, and injury to the globe. Avulsion injuries of the upper or lower eyelid (e.g. dog bites) are usually accompanied by canalicular injury as this is the weakest part of the eyelid and often the first area to tear. The patient is examined for any evidence of a retained foreign body, missing tissue, and damage to the lacrimal system. The presence of levator function should be noted in upper lid lacerations. If a large hematoma is present, there should be a greater suspicion of damage to the orbit and globe. CT scans are used to look for retained foreign bodies and fractures; MRI scans can be useful to look for a retained organic foreign body and more fully assess intracranial injury. Photographs are taken of any injury for future reference. A tetanus toxoid booster is given as appropriate.

The results of eyelid surgery are not prejudiced by waiting for up to 48 or 72 hours if this allows more time and better facilities to be available.[25] However, upon initial exam the wound should be cleansed and irrigated copiously to prevent infection, subsequent tattooing, or retained foreign bodies. It is examined carefully and the tissues repositioned as accurately as possible. The skin can be closed with absorbable sutures, avoiding a further anesthetic for suture removal. Tissue should not be excised or discarded as the eyelid region has an excellent blood supply; any pedicle should be preserved. It is not usually necessary to cut or "freshen" the wound. In contaminated wounds such as animal bites, prophylactic intravenous antibiotics are given within 1 hour followed by a 1-week course of oral antibiotics.

After initial repair, major revision should be delayed for 6 to 9 months. One then repairs secondary defects such as lid retraction or ptosis unless the patient develops symptoms of corneal exposure that cannot be controlled with simple lubrication or is at risk of developing amblyopia.[25]

Lid margin defects require careful approximation of the lash line and gray line to avoid lid notch, rotation of the lid, and lash abnormalities. The gray line and lash line sutures can be buried to avoid later removal.

Traumatic ptosis

Traumatic ptosis can be caused by:

1. Direct injury or stretching of the aponeurosis or levator muscle.
2. Loss of orbital contents or phthisical eye, lowering the fulcrum of the levator complex.
3. Injury to the superior division of the third nerve or sympathetic nerve supply.
4. Mechanical restriction due to conjunctival, lid, or deep orbital scarring.

Most levator defects should be sutured at the time of the primary repair; however, minor defects can be left as they are likely to heal spontaneously and excessive surgery may lead to lid retraction. Residual ptosis may be repaired at a later date, usually after 6 months or after any improvement has ceased.

Early intervention is indicated if there is any risk of amblyopia. A temporary frontalis sling using removable material such as a Prolene or Supramid suture or a silicone rod may be required. Secondary repair is via an anterior approach. Excision of the scar tissue may leave a gap in the levator complex, requiring a spacer. A dermis fat graft can be used to prevent the reformation of dense adhesions. Treatment of ptosis due to nerve injury is described earlier in this chapter.

Lacrimal drainage injuries

It was formerly believed that the lower canaliculus played a greater role in tear drainage than the upper system. Therefore, some authors recommended that only inferior canalicular lacerations be repaired. Studies of lacrimal scintigraphy after occlusion of either upper or lower punctum have concluded that both play an equal role in tear drainage; injury to either one deserves surgical repair. Although many patients will be asymptomatic as long one of their two canaliculi remains functioning, at least 10% of patients will have epiphora if one punctum is occluded. This increases to more than 50% when subject to globe irritation by exposure to the elements.

The canaliculi should be repaired by suturing the two ends of a canaliculus over an indwelling silicone stent which is usually left in place for three or more months. The white color of the canalicular epithelium can usually be seen with loupe magnification, although the aid of an operating microscope may be required. Injection of fluorescein stained viscoelastic via the opposite punctum (or directly into the sac in cases of upper and lower canalicular damage) may help to identify the canaliculus. Use of a pigtail probe passed through the intact punctum in an attempt to find the lacerated cut end is controversial; it may damage healthy tissue (especially the older hooked instruments). With the use of an operating microscope, good hemostasis, and a thorough knowledge of the anatomy, this is seldom required.

If the canaliculi are to be anastomosed, they are intubated with a self-retaining monocanalicular stent, or with bicanalicular stents. The peri-canalicular soft tissues are closed with 7-0 vicryl sutures. Care is taken to repair the posterior limb of the medial canthal tendon, which is immediately posterior to the medial canaliculus. This maintains the lid in apposition to the globe. In repairing the canaliculus the sutures should be passed into the tissues immediately around the canaliculus and not through its epithelium.[26]

Common canalicular injury is repaired, or opened into the lacrimal sac, the canaliculi intubated and a dacryocystorhinostomy performed.

Canalicular damage near the punctum can be treated by a retrograde dacryocystorhinostomy with marsupialization of the canaliculus into the conjunctival sac. Blockage near the lacrimal sac can be re-treated by excision of the scar and connection of the patent canaliculus to the sac. In either case, at least 8 mm of one canaliculus is necessary for success.

Medial canthal tendon injuries

The anterior limb of the medial canthal tendon seldom needs repair; however, if the posterior limb is damaged and only the anterior limb is repaired, the lid will be anteropositioned. The method of repair of the posterior limb depends on the posterior fixation point available. If the lacrimal drainage system is intact and there is a firm and reasonably positioned medial wall fixation point, the posterior limb and eyelid tissues can be directly attached to the medial orbital wall. If the lacrimal sac must be opened for dacryocystorhinostomy and the tissues behind the lacrimal sac are adequate, a non-absorbable suture can be passed behind the opened lacrimal sac and used to reattach the medial canthus and eyelid tissues medially and posterior to the posterior lacrimal fascia. If there is no adequate ipsilateral fixation point, a "T-shaped" mini-plate can be attached to the anterior lacrimal crest and the tendon sutured to one of its posterior fixation points or a transnasal wire can be used to reposition the medial canthus posteriorly.

Burns

In the acute stage, burns are treated with heavy lubrication or occlusive therapy to protect the cornea. To avoid amblyopia in the young child, the eye may be left for 2 to 3 hours a day without lubrication or the other eye can be patched. In severe cases of exposure, a conjunctival flap may be required to protect the cornea in the chronic stage. Cicatricial contracture of the eyelids is a frequent problem and tarsorrhaphies, lid-sharing procedures, split-thickness skin grafting, and Frost sutures may be necessary to protect the ocular surface. Re-operation is often required due to progressive wound contracture which may continue for months. After 30 days, the lids are reconstructed. Split skin grafts may be required; lid-sharing procedures are avoided where possible to avoid the risk of amblyopia.

References

1. Tessier P, Rouigier J, Wolfe SA. Plastic Surgery of the Orbit and Eyelids. New York: Masson; 1981.
2. Seah LL, Choo CT, Fong KS. Congenital upper lid colobomas: management and visual outcome. Ophthalmic Plast Reconstr Surg 2002; 18: 190–5.
3. Stewart J, Sarada D, Seiff S. Aminotic membrane graft in the surgical management of cryptophthalmos. Ophthalmic Plast Reconstr Surg 2002; 18: 378–80.
4. Morris RJ, Collin JRO. Functional lid surgery in Down's syndrome. Br J Ophthalmol 1986; 73: 494–7.
5. Sundar G, Young SM, Tara S, et al. Epiblepharon in East Asian patients: the Singapore experience. Ophthalmology 2010; 117: 184–9.
6. O'Donnell BA, Collin JRO. Congenital lower eyelid deformity with trichiasis, epiblepharon and entropion. Aust NZ J Ophthalmol 1994; 22: 33–7.
7. Sin-Daw L. Correction of epicanthal fold using the VM-plasty. Br J Plast Surg 2000; 53: 95–9.
8. Takashi F, Motomu M, Katsuki K, Kenichi N. Modified split V-W plasty for entropion with an epicanthal fold in Asian eyelids. Plast Reconstr Surg 2006; 118: 635–42.
9. Lee V, Konrad H, Bunce C, et al. Aetiology and surgical treatment of childhood blepharoptosis. Br J Ophthalmol 2002; 86: 1282–6.
10. Dawson ELM, Hardy TG, Collin JRO, Lee JP. The incidence of strabismus and refractive error in patients with blepharophimosis, ptosis and epicanthus inversus (BPES). Strabismus 2003; 11: 173–7.
11. Finsterer J. Ptosis: causes, presentation and management. Aesthet Plast Surg 2003; 27: 193–204.
12. Collin JRO, Castronovo S, Allen L. Congenital eyelid retraction. Br J Ophthalmol 1990; 9: 542–4.
13. Toelle SP, Boltshauser E. Long-term outcome in children with congenital unilateral facial nerve palsy. Neuropediatrics 2001; 32: 130–5.
14. Cook SP, MacCartney KK, Rose CD, et al. Lyme disease and seventh nerve paralysis in children. Ann J Otolaryngol 1997; 18: 320–3.
15. Lorch M, Teach S. Facial nerve paralysis: etiology and approach to diagnosis and management. Pediatr Emerg Care 2010; 26: 763–9.
16. Reynolds N, Kenealy J, Mercer N. Carbon dioxide laser dermabrasion for giant melanocytic nevi. Plast Reconstr Surg 2003; 111: 2209–14.
17. McCulley JP. Eyelid disorders: the meibomian glands, blepharitis, and contact lenses. Eye Cont Lens Sci Clin Pract 2003; 29: 93–5.
18. McLean CJ, Ragge NK, Jones RB, et al. The management of orbital cysts associated with congenital microphthalmos and anophthalmos. Br J Ophthalmol 2003; 87: 860–3.
19. Mitchell KT, Hollstein DA, White WL, O'Hara MA. The autogenous dermis-fat orbital implant in children. J AAPOS 2001; 5: 367–9.
20. Heher K, Katowitz J, Low J. Unilateral dermis-fat implantation in the pediatric orbit. Ophthalmic Plast Reconstr Surg 1998; 14:81–7.
21. Kazin M, Katowitz J, Fallon M, et al. Evaluation of a collagen/hydroxyapatite implant for orbital reconstruction surgery. Ophthalmic Plast Reconstr Surg 1992; 8: 94–108
22. Custer PL, Kennedy RH, Woog JJ, et al. Orbital implants in enucleation surgery: a report by the American Academy of Ophthalmology. Ophthalmology 2003; 110: 2054–61.
23. Savar A, Kirsvrot J, Rubin P. Canalicular involvement in dog bite related eyelid lacerations. Ophthamic Plastic Reconstr Surg 2008; 24: 296–8.
24. Jordan DR, Ziai S, Gilberg SM, Mawn LA. Pathogenesis of canalicular lacerations. Ophthalmic Plastic Reconstr Surg 2008; 24: 394–8.
25. Chang E, Rubin PA. Management of complex eyelid lacerations. Int Ophthalmol Clin 2002; 42: 187–201.
26. Kersten RC, Kulwin DR. One-stitch canalicular repair: a simplified approach for repair of canalicular laceration. Ophthalmology 1997; 104: 785–9.

Part 2
Lids, brows and oculoplastics

Lid and orbital infantile peri-ocular hemangiomas (capillary hemangiomas) and other vascular disease

Christopher J Lyons • Doug Frederick

Vascular lesions of the orbit include tumors such as capillary and cavernous hemangiomas and hemangiopericytomas together with malformations such as venous-lymphatic malformations (lymphangiomas), orbital varices, and arteriovenous malformations. Infantile peri-ocular hemangiomas (capillary hemangiomas), common benign vascular tumors, are characterized by rapid growth during the first year of life and show regression over the next several years[1,2] Cavernous hemangiomas and hemangiopericytomas are predominantly seen in adults, but may rarely cause proptosis in childhood. Venous-lymphatic malformations (lymphangiomas) are vascular malformations that infrequently present in early childhood and are complicated by bouts of hemorrhage and rapidly progressive enlargement. Varices and arteriovenous malformations primarily present in the second and third decades.

Tumors

Infantile peri-ocular hemangioma (capillary hemangioma)

Infantile peri-ocular hemangioma (capillary hemangioma), a hamartoma, is the most common childhood orbital tumor. It occurs more frequently in females than males in a ratio of $3:2$[3] with no inheritance pattern. Its incidence is increased by prematurity.[4] It is distinguished from other orbital vascular lesions by spontaneous regression. Numerous techniques are available to manage this potentially disfiguring disorder which affects vision: there is no "one size fits all" approach for this unpredictable tumor; patients whose lesion resolves rapidly with treatment could have done so without treatment. We are fearful of uncontrolled growth, as seen in Fig. 20.1. Treatment of periocular hemangiomas is a team effort involving

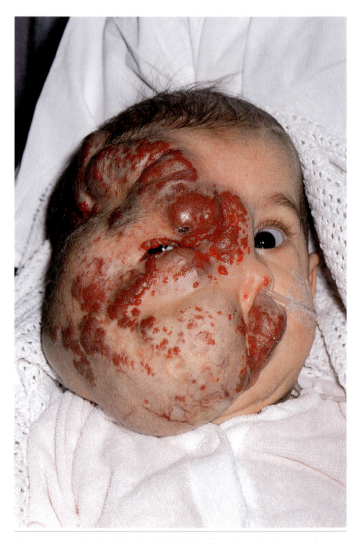

Fig. 20.1 Massive facial and orbital infantile peri-ocular hemangioma (capillary hemangioma).

pediatricians, dermatologists, and ophthalmologists. Decisions to treat using propranolol, systemic or intralesional steroids, or surgery are based on the position of the lesion, the presence of amblyopia, rapidity of growth, and discussion of risk/benefits with informed parents. Children must be followed closely, watching for rebound growth and checking for amblyopia.

Its histopathology varies with its clinical phase; in its early proliferative phase, it consists mostly of numerous dividing endothelial cells; vascular spaces are rare and small. It is rich in mast cells, whose function is not clear. There may be numerous mitotic figures which could lead to an incorrect diagnosis of malignancy in rapidly enlarging lesions. The characterization of poorly differentiated lesions may be helped by reticulin stains or by the identification of factor VIII, which is produced by the endothelial cells, using peroxidase or fluorescein antibody techniques.[3] In more mature tumors, vascular spaces are larger, with fewer flattened endothelial cells. The tumor is not encapsulated and tends to infiltrate surrounding structures. In the involutional phase, the endothelial cells are replaced by adipocytes and there is deposition of fibrous tissue.

The natural history of infantile peri-ocular hemangioma (capillary hemangioma), rapid enlargement followed by spontaneous involution, is unique for vascular tumors. Their vascular endothelium expresses placenta-associated antigens,[5] not expressed by other vascular tumors or normal skin, which has led to speculation that infantile hemangiomas develop either because of angioblasts abnormally differentiating toward placental vascular phenotypes or as the result of placental cell embolization of fetal tissues.[5] The presence of maternal–fetal microchimerism for infants with solitary hemangiomas was supported by a subsequent molecular genetic study.[6] Recently, the potential role for hypoxia in hemangioma development has been stressed.[7]

Clinical features

One-third of infantile peri-ocular hemangiomas (capillary hemangiomas) (Fig. 20.2) are present at birth; all have appeared by the age of 6 months. The appearance of the tumor may be preceded by a faint cutaneous flush. Usually, rapid growth lasting 3 to 6 months is followed by a period of stabilization and then regression (Fig. 20.3). Margileth and Museles[1] found that 30% of 336 hemangiomas had regressed by the age of 3 years, 60% by 4 years, and 76% by 7 years.

Infantile peri-ocular hemangiomas (capillary hemangiomas) are most commonly in the upper lid or orbit (Fig. 20.3).

Their appearance varies according to the depth of involvement (Fig. 20.3A); superficial cutaneous lesions have a red lobulated appearance, giving rise to the name "strawberry" nevus (see Fig. 20.8A). These superficial lesions consist initially of a confluence of telangiectasias that progress to raised, nodular lesions. They may enlarge and become blueish in color with crying. Subcutaneous hemangiomas are often blueish in color. Lesions situated deep to the orbital septum may present with proptosis without cutaneous discoloration. Occasionally, the

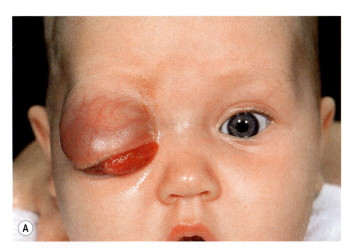

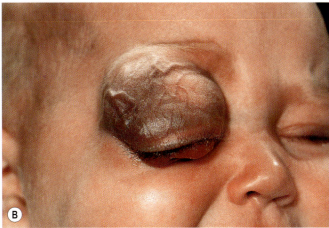

Fig. 20.2 (A) Infantile peri-ocular hemangioma (capillary hemangioma) of the anterior orbit and lid. (B) Same patient when crying showing engorgement and mild increase in size.

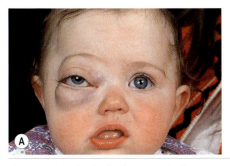 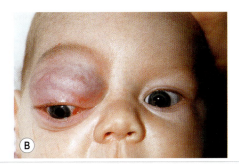 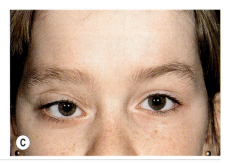

Fig. 20.3 (A) Orbital infantile peri-ocular hemangioma (capillary hemangioma). The mother of this child was accused of having injured her child. (B) Orbital infantile peri-ocular hemangioma (capillary hemangioma) in a child aged 2 months. (C) Same patient as (B) aged 9 years after some spontaneous resolution and surgery. Surgery is usually not necessary and best avoided in most instances.

proptosis is severe enough to cause corneal exposure. One-third of hemangiomas involve several levels of depth. A deeply situated lesion causing only proptosis with no cutaneous signs may present a diagnostic dilemma. A helpful diagnostic sign is the increase in proptosis with crying (Fig. 20.2). In 30% of patients, "strawberry" nevi are found at other cutaneous sites.[2] Occasionally, enormous growth occurs obliterating facial structures (Fig. 20.1).

Amblyopia is common with orbital infantile peri-ocular hemangioma (capillary hemangioma), with a prevalence between 43% and 60%.[2,8] Rarely, this results from occlusion of the visual axis by a bulky tumor. More often it results from distortion of the globe by tumor causing corneal astigmatism. The axis of the corrective plus cylinder is directed toward the tumor. This may persist after the hemangioma has regressed but usually resolves, at least partially, particularly if the hemangioma resolves or is treated early.[9,10] Prolonged occlusion can result in ipsilateral myopia and the resultant anisometropia may be another amblyogenic factor. Secondary strabismus is common as a result of the interruption of binocularity or displacement of the globe by the tumor.

Systemic complications of infantile peri-ocular hemangiomas (capillary hemangiomas) are rare:[3]

1. Kasabach-Merritt syndrome: a potentially life-threatening coagulopathy resulting from consumption of fibrinogen and platelet entrapment within a large vascular hemangioma. It usually responds to platelet replacement and corticosteroids.
2. PHACE(S) syndrome (**p**osterior fossa abnormalities, **h**emangioma, **a**rterial lesions, **c**ardiac abnormalities, **e**ye and **s**ternal abnormalities) with serious cardiovascular and neurologic complications and frequent ocular involvement including amblyopia, strabismus, anterior polar cataract, ptosis, and optic neuropathy.[11] A careful ocular, cardiac, and neurologic examination is necessary for patients with extensive facial infantile peri-ocular hemangiomas (capillary hemangiomas).

Investigation

In the majority of children presenting with proptosis, lid involvement or other cutaneous hemangiomas suggest the diagnosis.

Doppler ultrasound may help to secure the diagnosis.[12] The extent of the lesion can be assessed by computed tomography (CT) scanning. A soft tissue density mass is seen to infiltrate the orbit, with smooth or nodular margins, often crossing boundaries between compartments such as the muscle cone or orbital septum. Bony erosion may be seen. Enhancement is variable, according to the vascularity of the lesion and its stage of development. T2-weighted magnetic resonance imaging (MRI) is useful to delineate the tumor since the lesion is hyperintense due to its intrinsic blood flow (Fig. 20.4). T1-weighted gadolinium-enhanced views with fat suppression to improve contrast give the best assessment of the anatomic relationships of the tumor. Obtaining an magnetic resonance angiogram and venogram (MRA and MRV) at the time of the MRI may rule out other vascular anomalies that can mimic hemangiomas. Lesions confined to the posterior orbit, especially during a period of growth, may occasionally be mistaken for a malignant tumor such as rhabdomyosarcoma; biopsy may be indicated.

Management

Management should be conservative, with treatment of significant refractive error and amblyopia while awaiting spontaneous regression (Fig. 20.5). The appearance of superficial pale stellate areas of scarring ("Herald spots") on a "strawberry" lesion is a useful early indicator of spontaneous regression. Amblyopia therapy should be accompanied by spectacle correction of the astigmatic error of the affected eye with appropriate glasses (Fig. 20.6).

Active treatment to reduce the size of the tumor is only indicated if there is occlusion of the visual axis or if a posterior lesion results in progressive proptosis with optic nerve compression, corneal exposure, and significant or progressive amblyopia. Methods of treatment include topical or systemic beta-blockers,[15-17] local or systemic steroids,[10,13,14] surgical excision,[18] radiotherapy, laser,[19] and injection of sclerosing agents.

A dramatic reduction was noted in the size of infantile peri-ocular hemangiomas (capillary hemangiomas) in children treated with propranolol (Fig. 20.7) for cardiac disorders.[20] At doses of 1–3 mg/kg/day, a response may be seen within a few days. Subsequent studies have shown a response rate of up to 90%; side-effects such as hypotension, bronchospasm, bradycardia, heart block, and hypoglycemia can be avoided with careful monitoring.[15,16] This observation has revolutionized the treatment of hemangiomas; beta-blockers are now the first choice for most ophthalmologists. Topical timolol 0.5% also has been reported to be effective, and with far fewer side-effects than with systemic beta-blockers is appealing.[17] Randomized trials comparing systemic and topical propranolol to corticosteroids are ongoing.

Nowadays steroids are considered a useful but 'second line' alternative to beta-blockers. Kushner[21] reported good results with injection of local steroid into the hemangioma. The steroid should be injected slowly throughout the tumor while the needle is withdrawn to reduce the risk of central retinal artery embolization,[22] a rare complication. Tumor regression should be noted within 2–4 weeks, and further injections may be necessary (Fig. 20.8). Other complications include local fat atrophy, skin hypopigmentation, eyelid necrosis, and periorbital calcification. While systemic side-effects are less common with intralesional rather than systemic steroids, care must be taken to make certain that adrenal insufficiency does not occur during concurrent illness, trauma, or surgical stress.[3,13] Ultrasound guidance may be helpful for posteriorly situated lesions.[23] The whitish skin discoloration that is sometimes noted from superficial accumulation of depot steroid after injection is usually transient. The risk of dissemination of vaccines should lead to discussion with the pediatrician of infants about to have systemic or intralesional steroid treatment.

Systemic steroids (1.5–5.0 mg/kg/day) may be preferable for very extensive or posteriorly situated lesions (Fig. 20.9). The exact dose is undetermined. However, the response of over 90% for doses greater than 3 mg/kg/day falls to less than 70% for doses of 2 mg/kg/day and less.[13] The side-effects of growth retardation, gastrointestinal bleeding, behavior changes, and adrenal suppression may make this therapy less desirable. A rebound increase in size has been noted after discontinuation of oral steroid.

Sight-threatening lesions which have failed to respond to steroids or beta-blockers may be amenable to treatment with

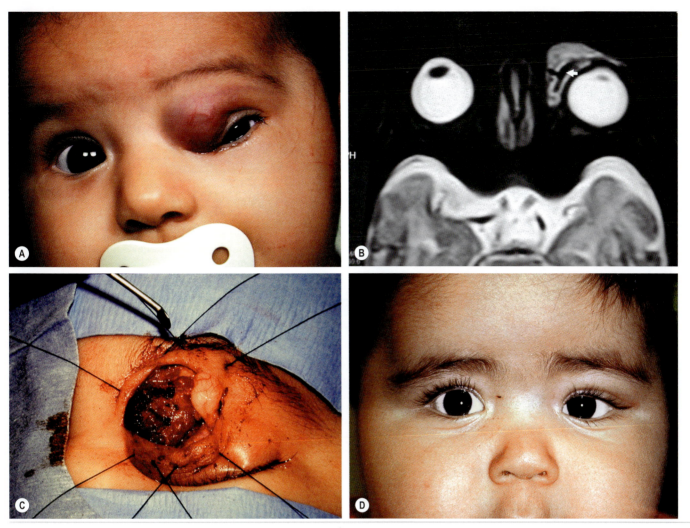

Fig. 20.4 (A) This 2.5-month-old child presented with a large subcutaneous infantile peri-ocular hemangioma (capillary hemangioma) that was unresponsive to steroids and inducing significant astigmatism. (B) T2-weighted MRI demonstrated a relatively well-defined anterior orbital mass with a large central flow void (arrow). (C) Operative photo of the same lesion during excision. (D) After surgery, she had minimal ptosis, and her astigmatism regressed. (Patient of the University of British Columbia. (A) and (B) reproduced with permission from Rootman J. Diseases of the Orbit: A Multidisciplinary Approach. 2nd ed. Philadelphia: Lippincott Williams and Wilkins; 2002: 542.)

interferon alpha 2a,[24,25] although the response to this treatment may be slow and the side-effects uncertain in infants. Other immunomodulators, vincristine and cyclophosphamide, have been used to treat hemangiomas (primarily visceral). Their use in treating infantile orbital infantile peri-ocular hemangiomas (capillary hemangiomas) seems limited.

The carbon dioxide, argon, yttrium–aluminum–garnet (YAG), and dye lasers have been used to treat hemangiomas. Their use is limited by scarring, although the dye laser tuned to 577 or 585 nm with a 10 ms pulse duration may allow selective thermal damage of capillary tissue with minimal scarring and accelerated regression.[19,26] However, pulse dye lasers were designed to treat the thin-walled ectatic vessels of port wine stains not the small-caliber capillaries with great cellularity in infantile peri-ocular hemangiomas (capillary hemangiomas).[27] Radiotherapy and sclerosing agents should no longer be used.

Previously, surgical excision was deferred until the lesion stopped regressing, often after 6 or 7 years of age when any residual cosmetic defect was corrected.[28] However, well-defined lesions causing significant amblyopia through obstruction or astigmatism can safely be removed surgically. The technique requires meticulous hemostasis, but the tumor is readily removed microsurgically after failure to respond to treatment with steroids or beta-blockers, or as a primary treatment[18] (Fig. 20.10).

Hemangiopericytoma

This rare tumor, which ranges from benign to malignant, is derived from the pericyte. It is usually seen in adults but has been reported in early infancy.[29] Its behavior is unpredictable; the usual presentation is with gradually increasing proptosis and mass effect related to a tumor which is usually superiorly placed. On CT scan, it is well-circumscribed showing marked, homogeneous contrast enhancement. There is a pronounced, early blush on angiography. It is usually a locally invasive tumor which recurs locally unless completely excised within its pseudocapsule. This is technically challenging as the tumor is very friable. Ten to 15% develop distant metastasis. Occasionally, these tumors behave very aggressively. In these cases, exenteration may be necessary.[6]

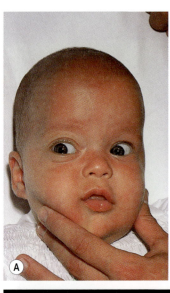
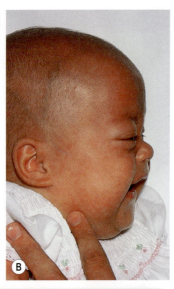

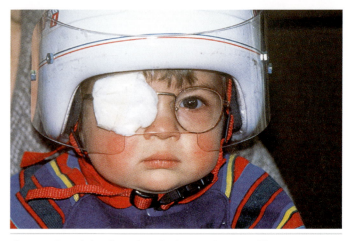

Fig. 20.6 Deep infantile peri-ocular hemangioma (capillary hemangioma) in a 6-month-old boy. A faint blueish tinge is evident in the left lower lid. There is a +4.0 diopter induced cylinder. Occlusion is vital in virtually every case and, in this child, his inventive parents have devised a novel method of preventing him from removing the patch. Eighteen months later the lesion had resolved, as had the cylinder. (Patient of the University of British Columbia.)

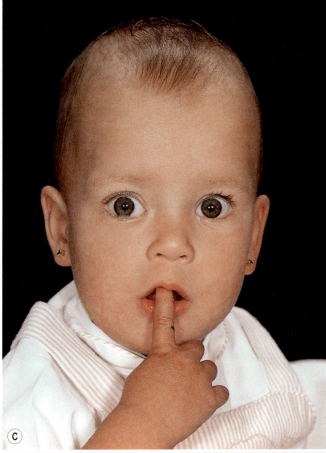

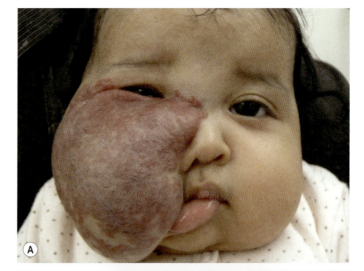

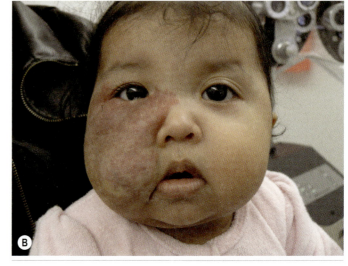

Fig. 20.5 (A,B) Right orbital infantile peri-ocular hemangioma (capillary hemangioma) in a child aged 5 months. (C) Complete resolution without treatment.

Fig. 20.7 (A) A large segmental infantile peri-ocular hemangioma (capillary hemangioma) in a 4-month-old old girl causing inverse ptosis and astigmatism. The hemangioma had grown rapidly in the first month of life and was unresponsive to oral and intralesional steroid treatment. A systemic work up for PHACE syndrome was negative. (B) After 2 months of oral propranolol treatment, the size and thickness of the lesion has decreased and the visual axis cleared. (Courtesy of Tina Rutar.)

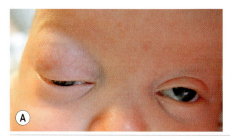
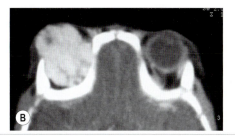
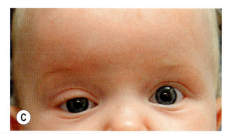

Fig. 20.8 This infant was born at 27 weeks' gestation. Right upper lid swelling was noted at age 6 weeks, and she was seen in our clinic at 16 weeks of age (A). (B) CT scan confirmed infantile peri-ocular hemangioma (capillary hemangioma) showing a poorly defined, enhancing lesion in the superior orbit. An intralesional injection of 40 mg triamcinolone and 20 mg methylprednisolone was given at this time. Repeat injection was planned for 8 weeks later but was deferred due to her clinical improvement. Part-time occlusion of the left eye was used. (C) Three months later, she was equally visually attentive with each eye. No further treatment is planned. (Patient of the University of British Columbia.)

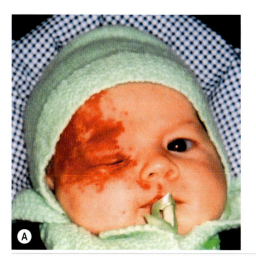
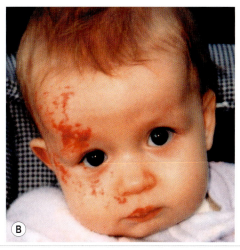
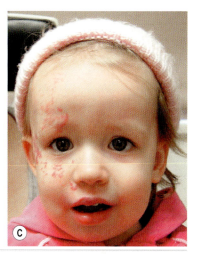

Fig. 20.9 (A) This 6-week-old infant was noted to have right upper lid swelling and discoloration from the second week of life, increasing on crying. There is complete closure of the right eye. Oral steroids were started at 6 weeks of age at 5 mg/kg/day, tapering to nothing over 6 months. (B) By 9 months of age, her Cushingoid features have resolved; the infantile peri-ocular hemangioma (capillary hemangioma) no longer obstructs the right visual axis. (C) At 11 months, the cutaneous changes have largely disappeared. There is no amblyopia. (Patient of the University of British Columbia.)

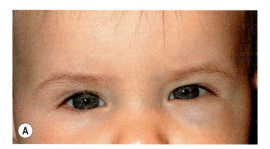
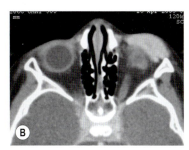

Fig. 20.10 (A) Clinical photograph of an 8-month-old child who presented with a progressive mass of the lower lid, causing astigmatism (+2.50 cylinder at 90°) and upward displacement of the left globe. (B) Contrast-enhanced CT scan demonstrates a relatively well-defined anterior orbital mass involving the left lid and inferior orbit. (C) Intraoperative photo of the same patient at the time of excision of the infantile peri-ocular hemangioma (capillary hemangioma). (D) One month after surgery, his astigmatism resolved. Patient of the University of British Columbia.

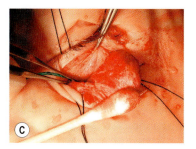
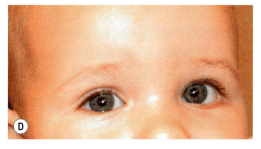

Vascular malformations

Vascular malformations of the orbit are derived from venous (varices and venous-lymphatic malformations (lymphangiomas)) and arterial (arteriovenous malformations) vascular anlagen and constitute an important cause of orbital tumors in childhood. They are best understood in the context of their hemodynamics and can be divided into three types:[30,31]

- Type 1 (no flow) lesions have little connection to the vascular system and include venous-lymphatic malformations (lymphangiomas), or combined venous lymphatic malformations.
- Type 2 (venous flow) lesions are either distensible, with a direct and significant communication to the venous system, or non-distensible, with minimal communication with the venous system. Both types 1 and 2 can be combined, with features both of distensibility and non-distensible hemodynamics.
- Type 3 (arterial flow) lesions include arteriovenous malformations that are characterized by an antegrade high flow through the lesion to the venous system.

Venous-lymphatic malformations (lymphangiomas)

These vascular anomalies usually arise in childhood and are often difficult to manage. They may enlarge gradually, but their expansion can be sudden, from hemorrhage into the lesion. Unlike infantile peri-ocular hemangiomas (capillary hemangiomas), they do not undergo spontaneous regression. Deeply situated lesions are difficult to excise; their margins are poorly defined and they arborize widely throughout the orbit.

Venous-lymphatic malformations (lymphangiomas) accounted for a small proportion of orbital tumors.[32] In one-third of cases, it is apparent at birth or within the first weeks of life[33] and over three-quarters of patients present in the first decade. A female preponderance (ratio 2–3:1) has been reported.[33]

Their occurrence within the orbit is puzzling in view of the absence of lymphatic drainage from the retroseptal tissues. It has been suggested that venous-lymphatic malformations (lymphangiomas) arise from primitive vascular elements within the orbit.[34] However, ultrastructural analysis and immunochemistry have identified lymphatic endothelium in orbital venous-lymphatic malformation (lymphangioma).[35] They do not appear to grow by cellular proliferation; the full extent of the malformation is present at birth, insinuating itself within the normal orbital tissues. Since the vascular channels have characteristics of both lymphatic and venous vessels, the histologic differentiation of venous-lymphatic malformations (lymphangiomas) from orbital varices has been a source of debate.[36-38] Hemodynamically, venous-lymphatic malformations (lymphangiomas) and varices are part of a continuum of venous-derived lesions, differentiated according to the presence or lack of connection to the venous system. Whereas varices are connected and therefore expand with Valsalva maneuver or supine posture, venous-lymphatic malformations (lymphangiomas) are isolated and do not. Lesions may be mixed with both venous and lymphatic components represented within a single mass. The extremes of the spectrum can be differentiated histopathologically; the venous-lymphatic malformations (lymphangiomatous) element has distinctive electron microscopic features.[39] The pathogenesis of these lesions relates to the lack of blood flow and the tendency for sludging, neovascularization, and hemorrhage with recurrent inflammatory episodes and the formation of isolated "chocolate cysts".[31]

Histopathologically, they consist of diaphanous, serous fluid-filled channels lined by endothelium. These have characteristics of true lymphatic channels as well as areas of dysplastic channels. Lymphoid follicles are often present in the stromal components.

The clinical features of venous-lymphatic malformations (lymphangiomas) vary with the extent and depth of orbital involvement.

Superficial

Isolated superficial involvement is comparatively rare and consists of multiple conjunctival cysts filled with clear or xanthochromic fluid, or a subcutaneous blueish cystic swelling of the eyelid. The latter may transilluminate and present with an abrupt localized change in color due to hemorrhage into a pre-existing lesion.[40] Superficial venous-lymphatic malformations (lymphangiomas) are easily accessible and, if unsightly, may be excised with good results.

Deep

The hallmark of deeply situated orbital venous-lymphatic malformations (lymphangiomas) is proptosis (Figs 20.11 and 20.12). Deep venous-lymphatic malformations (lymphangiomas) may present with gradually increasing proptosis with or without ptosis. In contrast to infantile peri-ocular hemangiomas (capillary hemangiomas), the proptosis is variable. An increase with upper respiratory tract infections and other generalized inflammatory states has been ascribed to lymphoid activity within the lesion.

The most typical presentation, however, is with sudden proptosis resulting from hemorrhage into a hitherto unsuspected lesion. The differential diagnoses include other causes of rapidly increasing proptosis such as rhabdomyosarcoma (see Chapter 24), neuroblastoma (see Chapter 26), etc. Examination of the nasal and palatal mucosa may be helpful if it reveals mixed clear fluid and blood-filled blebs of widespread venous-lymphatic malformation (lymphangioma) (Fig. 20.13). Optic nerve compression may occur with rapidly expanding blood-filled "chocolate cyst"[41] (see Fig. 20.11) with decreased visual acuity and disc swelling. It is an indication for urgent orbital intervention to decompress or excise the lesion.

Combined lesions (lymphohemangiomas)

These usually present in infancy, gradually enlarging over many years. Long-standing lesions may be associated with orbital enlargement. The presence of tell-tale conjunctival and lid changes is helpful in making the diagnosis of venous-lymphatic malformation (lymphangioma) (see Fig. 20.13). Hemorrhage into superficial lesions may result in the striking appearance of blood menisci within the conjunctival cysts (Fig. 20.14). These may be accompanied by recurrent subconjunctival hemorrhage and lid ecchymosis. Deep hemorrhage results in proptosis, commonly associated with compressive optic neuropathy. Combined lesions may be large enough to simultaneously involve every orbital space producing gross proptosis and facial deformity, some from extension through the

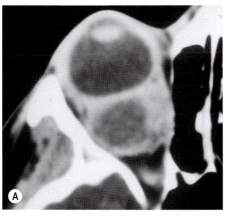

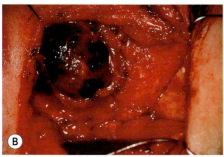

Fig. 20.11 Previously asymptomatic 8-year-old presenting with sudden onset axial proptosis overnight, decreased vision, afferent pupillary defect, and optic disc swelling. (A) CT shows a cystic mass indenting the globe posteriorly. (B) At surgery, the chocolate cyst was identified and decompressed. (Patient of the University of British Columbia.)

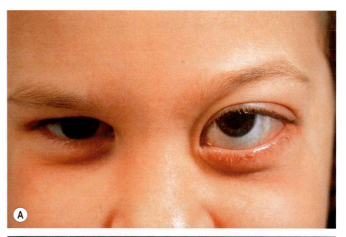

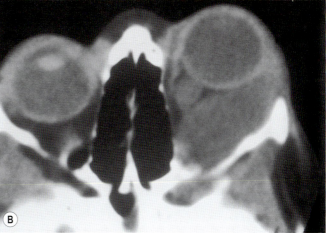

Fig. 20.12 Orbital venous-lymphatic malformation (lymphangioma). (A) Sudden onset of proptosis in the left eye of a previously asymptomatic 5-year-old child. (B) CT scan shows diffuse soft tissue density lesion arborizing through the retrobulbar tissues. (Patient of the University of British Columbia.)

superior orbital fissure, and non-contiguous intracranial vascular abnormalities occur.[42] Since the latter are at risk of bleeding, brain imaging is indicated in patients with orbital venous-lymphatic malformation (lymphangioma).

Investigation

CT scanning shows a soft tissue density mass with poorly defined margins and inhomogeneous enhancement after injection of contrast medium. Bony destruction is absent but large lesions can result in smooth enlargement of the orbit (see Fig. 20.12B). The presence of a cystic component helps differentiate venous-lymphatic malformations (lymphangiomas) from infantile peri-ocular hemangiomas (capillary hemangiomas). Since hemoglobin has paramagnetic qualities changing as blood denatures, blood-containing "chocolate cysts" are well visualized by MRI scanning[43] (Fig. 20.15). The age of intralesional hemorrhages can be assessed since oxyhemoglobin in fresh hemorrhage is hypointense on T1- and T2-weighted images, gradually becoming hyperintense as it is converted to methemoglobin. Later, degradation to ferritin and hemosiderin once again produces a hypointense image. Intravenous contrast in the case of CT scan or gadolinium in MRI is helpful in imaging the most active component of the lesion which should be removed if surgery is contemplated. A review of brain images is indicated for non-contiguous intracranial vascular anomalies.[42]

Management

A conservative approach should preferably be adopted; complete excision is difficult in all but the most superficial lesions

and hemorrhagic cysts tend to shrink with time. Surgery can precipitate further hemorrhage. Bed rest alone or with cold compresses can result in a good outcome even in cases with marked acute proptosis.[44]

Surgery is indicated if there is optic nerve dysfunction, corneal exposure, pain and nausea from raised orbital pressure, or the risk of amblyopia from astigmatism or strabismus. It is possible to temporize by aspirating the cyst contents through a needle under ultrasound guidance. Poor results and frequent morbidity have been reported from attempts at subtotal excision. We feel that surgery, when indicated, should excise as much of the venous-lymphatic malformation (lymphangioma) as is safe, particularly removing the active tissue as well as draining blood cysts with release of their contents. Unlike dermoid or sebaceous cysts, excision of the whole cyst wall is not necessary to avoid recurrence. The carbon dioxide laser may be useful in reducing hemorrhagic complications associated with subtotal excision surgery.[45] Systemic steroids[46] or intralesional OK-432 (group A *Streptococcus pyogenes* of human origin)[47] may reduce the size of these tumors.

Congenital orbital varices

Varices are of high- and low flow-types. Low-flow varices are clinically similar to venous-lymphatic malformations

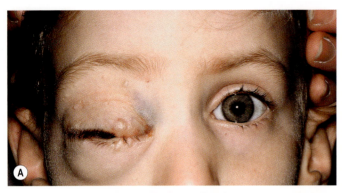

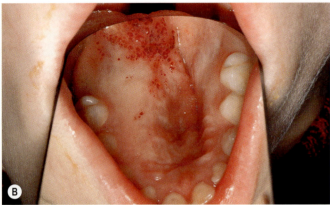

Fig. 20.13 (A) This 4-year-old boy was born after a 32-week gestation. Right proptosis developed by 4 weeks and was progressive despite orbital surgery, until the age of 3 years. It has been static since then. The diagnosis was a venous-lymphatic malformation (lymphangioma). (B) Same patient showing clear and blood-filled cystic lesions on the palate.

(lymphangiomas), with a tendency for sudden, often recurrent hemorrhage,[48] whilst high-flow varices expand with increased jugular venous pressure and rarely bleed.[31]

Distensible orbital varices expand only slowly during childhood and rarely give rise to visual problems. There is often a subconjunctival component (see Fig. 20.14). They often present in adolescence with discomfort on bending over and slow development of enophthalmos and deepening superior sulcus due to fat atrophy and enlargement of the orbit, which may be seen on plain X-rays, along with phleboliths. The main indications for surgical excision are removal of the superficial component for cosmetic reasons or removal of deeper lesions for grave, persistent pain. A combined neuroradiologic method with gluing followed by excision may be worthwhile in cases that demonstrate isolation from the venous system and do not share out-flow with critical orbital structures.[49] Detachable coil embolization may be considered before proceeding with surgery.[50] Some orbital varices may be associated with intracranial varicosities (Fig. 20.16).

Arteriovenous malformations

Arteriovenous malformations are characterized by the development of pulsating exophthalmos with episodes of hemorrhage, thrombosis, or extended, tortuous and engorged vessels secondary to arterialization of out-flow venous channels. They may have an audible bruit and can cause pain when engorged by Valsalva maneuver. Typically, they present in late adolescence or early adult life.

On imaging, arteriovenous malformations are characterized by irregular, rapidly enhancing masses. Doppler studies and CT or MR angiography demonstrate high-flow characteristics. With selective angiography, the lesions consist of engorged proximal arterial supply, a tangled malformation, and a distal venous out-flow (Fig. 20.17).

Arteriovenous malformations can largely be observed. The indications for intervention include recurrent hemorrhage or

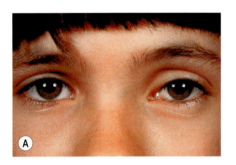

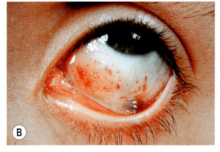

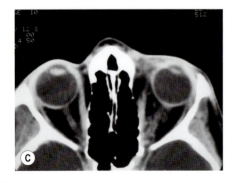

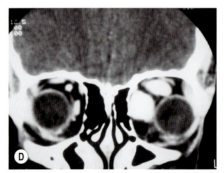

Fig. 20.14 (A) This 12-year-old child presented with an epibulbar lesion on the left side associated with fullness of the upper and lower lids and slight ptosis. (B) The epibulbar surface demonstrates a gelatinous-appearing lesion medially containing many clear fluid-filled cysts along with focal blood cysts, many of which appear to have menisci. In addition in the inferolateral fornix, there appears to be a dark varix. The conjunctival lesion was proven on biopsy to be consistent with a venous-lymphatic malformation (lymphangioma) histologically and by electron microscopy. It was noted also that the superior sulcus appeared somewhat deepened on the left.
(C) Post-contrast CT scan in the axial view shows an irregular lesion occupying the anteromedial orbit around and behind the caruncle. On direct coronal view (D), there is evidence of a posterior orbital varix that appeared with increased venous pressure. This lesion represents a combined venous-lymphatic malformation (lymphangioma) and varix. (Patient of the University of British Columbia.)

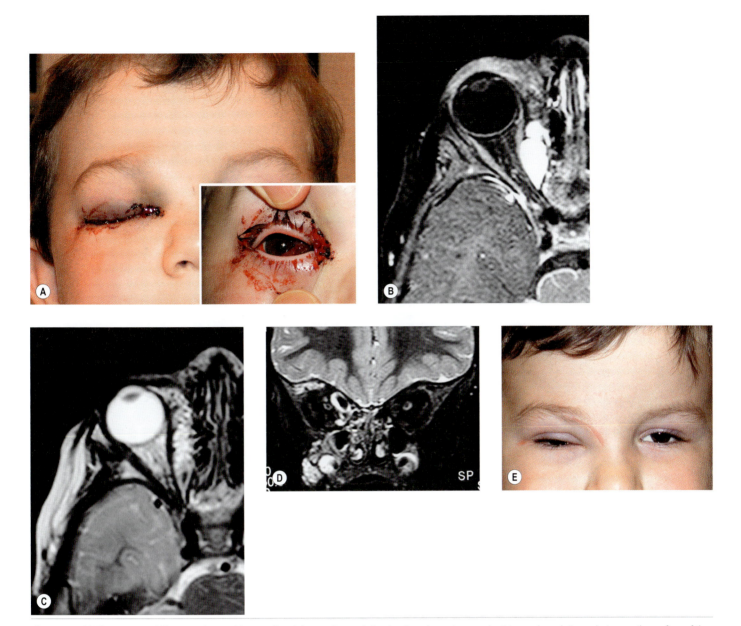

Fig. 20.15 (A) This 2.5-year-old boy was born with a swollen right eye. At age 1, he developed spontaneous bruising and a gelatinous lesion on the surface of the right globe, treated at the time with steroids with improvement. He continued, however, to have constant bleeding from the epibulbar surface, progressive lid closure, and swelling. (B–D) MRI scans demonstrate an extraconal medial lesion that involves the lid and forehead and extends to the apex of the right orbit. Posteriorly, note the cystic components consistent with venous-lymphatic malformation (lymphangioma). The patient underwent excision of his venous-lymphatic malformation (lymphangioma). (E) He did well postoperatively (seen here at 1 month following surgery) with a residual ptosis and persistent lid involvement, which will require future surgery. (Patient of the University of British Columbia. (B–D) with permission from Rootman J. Vascular malformations of the orbit: hemodynamic concepts. Orbit 2003; 22: 103–20.)

persistent pain. The malformations can be removed using selective gluing or embolization of in-flow vessels followed by excision.[51]

Sturge–Weber syndrome (see Chapters 37 and 65)

The port wine stain in Sturge-Weber syndrome can be confused with infantile peri-ocular hemangioma (capillary hemangioma) in their early stage. Infantile peri-ocular hemangiomas (capillary hemangiomas) grow in thickness and breadth within the first few weeks of life; the vascular lesion of Sturge-Weber syndrome remains unchanged. In addition to the triad of glaucoma, port wine stain, and cerebral vascular malformation it can be associated with choroidal hemangioma leading to serous retinal detachment. Orbital involvement is rare[52] with ipsilateral naevus flammeus and orbital vascular malformation causing proptosis without intracranial involvement.

Early results of the use of pulsed dye lasers for naevus flammeus have been encouraging. Treatment with pulse dye laser in the first few years of life can prevent thickening of the skin lesion and results in lightening of the color. Regular intraocular pressure monitoring is indicated.

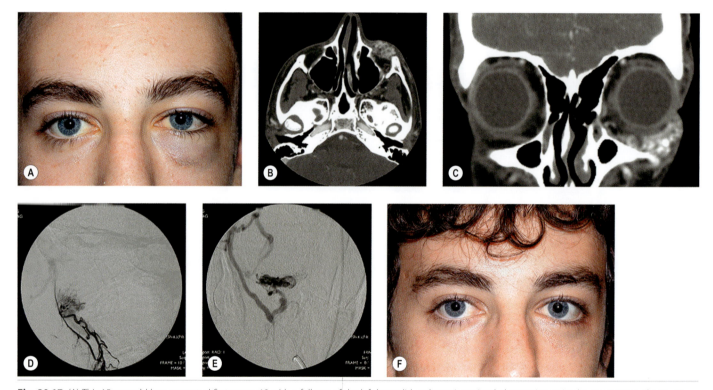

Fig. 20.16 (A) Subconjunctival varicosities in a patient with an orbital and intracranial hemangioma. (B) Contrast-enhanced CT scans showing the intracranial lesion (same patient).

Fig. 20.17 (A) This 15-year-old boy presented first at age 12 with a fullness of the left lower lid and transient visual obscuration episodes on exertion, due to an arteriovenous malformation. He was observed for 2.5 years, during which time the lesion progressed, and it was decided to intervene. He underwent combined embolization and excision of his mass. (B, C) CT angiograms demonstrate the tangle of the arteriovenous malformation in the left inferior orbit and lid. (D) Selective external carotid angiogram shows the external maxillary supply, while the anterior-posterior venous phase angiogram (E) reveals the venous out-flow to the facial and superior ophthalmic veins with facial compression. (F) Photograph of the patient 4 months after his surgery shows his post-operative result. (Patient of the University of British Columbia.)

Rare vascular lesions of the orbit

Klippel-Trenaunay-Weber syndrome
(see Chapter 65)

This syndrome comprises multiple cutaneous nevi associated with various angiomas of one or more limbs, which may show hypertrophy of the soft tissues. Orbital varix is a rare finding.[53]

Blue rubber bleb nevus syndrome

This rare syndrome usually presents in childhood. It consists of multiple blueish cutaneous vascular anomalies associated with angiomas of the gastrointestinal tract, lung, heart, and central nervous system.[54] The cutaneous lesions are soft, rubbery, and compressible. Most cases are sporadic but autosomal dominant inheritance has been reported. Conjunctival, iris, and retinal angiomas may occur and orbital venous malformation.[55]

References

3. Haik BG, Karcioglu ZA, Gordon RA, et al. Capillary hemangioma (infantile periocular hemangioma). Surv Ophthalmol 1994; 38: 399–426.

4. Praveen V, Vidavalur R, Rosencrantz TS, Hussain N. Infantile hemangiomas and retinopathy of prematurity: possible association. Pediatrics 2009; 123: e484–9.

5. North PE, Waner M, Mizeracki A, et al. A unique microvascular phenotype shared by juvenile hemangiomas and human placenta. Arch Dermatol 2001; 137: 559–70.

6. Pittman KM, Losken HW, Kleinman ME, et al. No evidence of maternal-fetal microchimerism in infantile hemangioma: a molecular genetic investigation. J Invest Dermatol 2006; 126: 2533–8.

7. Colonna V, Resta L, Napoli A, Bonifazi E. Placental anomalies in children with infantile hemangioma: clinical and histological observations. Br J Dermatol 2010; 162: 208–9.

10. Weiss AH, Kelly JP. Reappraisal of astigmatism induced by periocular capillary hemangioma and treatment with intralesional corticosteroid injection. Ophthalmology 2008; 115: 390–7.

11. Kroneberg A, Biel F, Ceisler E, et al. Ocular and systemic manifestations of PHACES (Posterior fossa malformations, Hemangiomas, Arterial anomalies, Cardiac defects and coarctation of the Aorta, Eye abnormalities and Sternal abnormalities or ventral developmental defects. J AAPOS 2005; 9: 169–73.

13. Bennett ML, Fleischer AB, Chamlin SL, Frieden IJ. Oral corticosteroid use is effective for cutaneous hemangiomas: an evidence-based evaluation. Arch Dermatol 2001; 137: 1208–13.

14. Nguyen J, Fay A. Pharmacologic therapy for periocular infantile hemangiomas: a review of the literature. Semin Ophthalmol 2009; 24: 178–84.

15. Missoi TG, Lueder GT, Gilbertson K, Bayliss SJ. Oral propranolol for treatment of periocular infantile hemangiomas. Arch Ophthalmol 2011; 129: 899–903.

16. Al Dhaybi R, Superstein R, Millet A. Treatment of periocular infantile hemangiomas with propranolol: case series of 18 children. Ophthalmology 2011; 118: 1184–8.

17. Pope E, Chakkittankandiyil A. Topical timolol gel for infantile hemangiomas. A pilot study. Arch Dermatol 2010; 146; 564–5.

18. Levi M, Schwartz S, Blei J, et al. Surgical treatment of capillary hemangiomas causing amblyopia. J AAPOS 2007; 11: 230–4.

19. Hunzeker CM, Geronemus RG. Treatmernt of superficial hemangiomas of the eyelid using the 595-nm pulsed dye laser. Dermatol Surg 2010; 36: 576–81.

20. Leaute-Labreze C, de la Roque ED, Hubiche T, et al. Propranolol for severe hemangiomas of infancy. N Engl J Med 2008; 358: 2649–51.

24. Ezekowitz RA, Mulliken JB, Folkman J. Interferon alpha-2a therapy for life-threatening hemangiomas of infancy. N Engl J Med 1992; 326: 1456–63.

25. Fledelius HC, Illum N, Jensen H, et al. Interferon-alfa treatment of facial infantile haemangiomas: with emphasis on the sight-threatening varieties. A clinical series. Acta Ophthalmol Scand 2001; 79: 370–3.

27. Frieden I. Early laser treatment of periorbital infantile hemangiomas may work, but is it really the best treatment option? Dermatol Surg 2010; 36: 598–601.

29. Bailey PV, Weber TR, Tracy TF, et al. Congenital hemangiopericytoma: an unusual vascular neoplasm of infancy. Surgery 1993; 114: 936–41.

31. Rootman J. Vascular malformations of the orbit: hemodynamic concepts. Orbit 2003; 22: 103–20.

35. Curlsen C, Schlotzer-Schrehardt U, Breiteneder-Geleff S, Holbach LM. Orbital lymphangioma with positive immunochemistry of lymphatic endothelial markers (vascular endothelium growth factor receptor 3 and podoplanin). Graefes's Arch Clin Exp Ophthalmol 2001; 239: 628–32.

36. Garrity JA. Orbital venous anomalies: a long-standing dilemma [editorial]. Ophthalmology 1997; 104: 903–4.

41. Kazim M, Kennerdell JS, Rothfus W, et al. Orbital lymphangioma: correlation of magnetic resonance images and intraoperative findings. Ophthalmology 1992; 99: 1588–94.

42. Katz SE, Rootman J, Vangveeravong S, et al. Combined venous lymphatic malformations of the orbit (so-called lymphangiomas): association with noncontiguous intracranial vascular anomalies. Ophthalmology 1998; 105: 176–84.

45. Kennerdell JS, Maroon JC, Garrity JA, et al. Surgical management of orbital lymphangioma with the carbon dioxide laser. Am J Ophthalmol 1986; 102: 308–14.

47. Suzuki Y, Obana A, Gohto Y, et al. Management of orbital lymphangioma using intralesional injection of OK-432. Br J Ophthalmol 2000; 84: 614–17.

49. Lacey B, Rootman J, Marotta TR. Distensible venous malformations of the orbit: clinical and hemodynamic features and a new technique of management. Ophthalmology 1999; 106: 1197–209.

51. Warrier S, Prabhakaran VC, Valenzuela A, et al. Orbital arteriovenous malformations. Arch Ophthalmol 2008; 126: 1669–75.

54. Fishman SJ, Smithers CJ, Folkman J, et al. Blue rubber bleb nevus syndrome. Ann Surg 2005; 241: 523–8.

55. McCannel CA, Hoenig J, Umlas J, et al. Orbital lesions in the blue rubber bleb nevus syndrome. Ophthalmology 1996; 103: 933–6.

 Access the complete reference list online at
http://www.expertconsult.com

The lacrimal system

Caroline J MacEwen

Introduction

The lacrimal system consists of a secretory portion and a drainage system. The secretory portion is the lacrimal and accessory lacrimal glands. With the meibomian glands and the goblet cells, they secrete the components of the tear film. The tear film has three layers: the inner mucin layer secreted by the conjunctival goblet cells, the intermediate aqueous layer secreted by the lacrimal and accessory lacrimal glands, and the outer, oily layer secreted by the meibomian glands. The accessory lacrimal glands produce basal tear secretion; the lacrimal gland is responsible for reflex tearing in response to noxious or emotional stimuli.

The drainage system consists of the lacrimal puncta, canaliculi, lacrimal sac, and the nasolacrimal duct. This active system pumps tears from the conjunctival sac into the inferior meatus of the nose.

Tears flow along the lid margins and conjunctival fornices. They are spread across the surface of the eye by blinking. Tears protect the eye by surface lubrication, provision of oxygen and antibacterial substances such as IgA, IgG, and lysozyme, and mechanical removal of irritating substances and cellular debris.

Lacrimal problems in children usually relate to underproduction of tears, causing dry eyes, which is rare but potentially sight-threatening, or reduced drainage of tears, which is much more common but less serious (Box 21.1).

Lacrimal gland

Embryology

The lacrimal gland develops from ectoderm that is supported by mesodermal connective tissue. It continues to grow 3–4 years after birth. Basal tearing is present in infants from birth,

---

Box 21.1

Causes of watery eyes in children

Excess tear production (lacrimation)
Allergic rhinitis
Upper respiratory tract infection
Epiblepharon
Subtarsal foreign body
Iritis
Corneal abrasion/ulceration
Conjunctivitis
Glaucoma

Drainage failure (epiphora)
Congenital nasolacrimal duct obstruction
Skeletal and sinus abnormalities
Lid malposition
Punctal malposition
Punctal occlusion
Anomalous drainage system

---

and reflex tearing begins at any time from birth to several months of age.[1]

Anatomy

The lacrimal gland is an exocrine gland in the anterior aspect of the supratemporal orbit within the bony lacrimal fossa. The majority of the gland lies within this fossa, but the lateral horn of the levator palpebrae superioris separates this orbital part from the palpebral lobe, which extends anteriorly into the supratemporal conjunctival cul-de-sac. The ducts of the gland pass through the palpebral lobe and open on to the conjunctiva in the superior fornix. The lacrimal gland is innervated via the facial (afferent) and trigeminal (efferent) nerves. The accessory glands of Kraus and Wolfring sit in the superior conjunctival fornix.

Congenital abnormalities

Congenital absence is rare, usually occurring in conditions with reduced conjunctiva: anophthalmos, cryptophthalmos, and the lacrimo-auriculo-dento-digital (LADD) syndrome. Anomalous lacrimal ductules that secrete tears on to the skin rather than the conjunctival sac may be found near the lacrimal gland, around the lateral canthus, or in the preauricular region. These are rare but may require dissection and excision.[2]

The embryology of the lacrimal gland is closely linked to that of the conjunctival epithelium. This explains the common supratemporal position of dermoid cysts, near the lacrimal gland.

Other congenital anomalies include orbital ectopic lacrimal gland tissue. A drainage system may not be present in such cases and an enlarging orbital mass may develop. Neoplasms can occur with such ectopic tissue.

Crocodile tears (see Chapter 100) occur from congenital aberrant innervation between the fifth and seventh cranial nerves causing tearing with chewing or sucking.[3]

Dry eyes in children

Congenital causes

Congenital alacrima is rare. It may be due to absence of the lacrimal gland or to it being ectopic in the orbit. Alacrima may be associated with systemic conditions such as the Riley-Day syndrome (familial dysautonomia), anhydrotic ectodermal dysplasia, and Allgrove's syndrome (familial alacrima, achalasia of the cardia, and adrenal deficiency) (see Chapter 98).

Acquired causes

Acquired tear deficiency may be due to pathology of the lacrimal gland, causing failure of tear production, or to conjunctival damage (see Chapter 31), leading to ductule obliteration. The lacrimal gland may be damaged by Epstein-Barr infection, as the result of HIV infection, or in patients with bone marrow transplantation (often associated with graft-versus-host disease). The conjunctiva may be affected by injury (burns), infection, the sequelae of trachoma, Stevens-Johnson syndrome, or toxic epidermal necrolysis.

Sjögren's syndrome is rare in children. It can be a primary autoimmune event or associated with rheumatoid arthritis or systemic lupus erythematosus. Children with Sjögren's syndrome often have lacrimal gland enlargement. They may have recurrent parotid gland swelling and salivary gland involvement. Sjögren's syndrome should be considered in any child with recurrent parotiditis, keratoconjunctivitis sicca, and early tooth decay due to xerostomia.[4]

Chronic blepharitis is uncommon. It usually presents with recurrent chalazia, although the lids may appear normal. The associated poor quality tear film causes patches of dryness and may lead to peripheral corneal vascularization and scarring which can be sight-threatening.

Isotretinoin treatment for acne is a cause of dry eyes in adolescence. This is usually reversible at cessation of the drug.

Children with dry eyes present with irritable, uncomfortable, gritty, red eyes. A reduced tear meniscus is evident with punctate keratopathy, particularly affecting the interpalpebral zone. Staining occurs with fluorescein and Rose Bengal dyes. Severe keratopathy due to concomitant corneal hypoesthesia can be a problem in the Riley-Day syndrome.

Treatment of dry eyes involves copious use of artificial tears and temporary or permanent punctal occlusion in severe cases. Immunomodulation may have a role to play in secondary lacrimal gland failure including that due to infections. Blepharitis should be treated with lid hygiene, lubricants, and systemic antibiotics such as erythromycin or azithromycin. Oral tetracyclines should be avoided in children prior to their second dentition.

Dacryoadenitis

Dacryoadenitis is usually associated with viral infection, mumps, infectious mononucleosis, herpes zoster, tuberculosis, brucella, histoplasmosis, or gonococcal infection. Lacrimal gland swelling may rarely be a sign of childhood Sjögren's disease.

A primary clinical feature of dacryoadenitis is the "S sign" in which there is drooping of the lateral aspect of the upper lid. In acute inflammatory cases, the overlying skin is inflamed. Neuroimaging confirms enlargement and helps rule out other orbital masses. In the long term, dacryoadenitis may damage the lacrimal gland and cause reduced tear secretion.

Dacryoadenitis must be differentiated from a lacrimal gland infarct, which occurs in children with a sickle cell crisis. The onset is rapid, like acute dacryoadenitis.

Treatment of acute dacryocystitis is aimed at the underlying cause.

Lacrimal tumors (see Chapter 26)

Lacrimal tumors are very rare in children. Pseudotumor causing painful swelling may affect the lacrimal gland.[5] Malignant epithelial tumors, including mixed cell adenocystic and other carcinomas, have been recorded in childhood.[6]

Lacrimal gland enlargement is also found in conditions such as sarcoidosis or leukemia. Prolapse of the lacrimal gland, which is commonly bilateral, may present as a subconjunctival mass in the upper outer fornix. This may occur with craniofacial anomalies (see Chapter 28) due to reduced orbital volume and increased orbital pressure.

The lacrimal drainage system

Embryology

The lacrimal outflow system develops between the maxilla and the lateral nasal process from surface ectoderm. By the end of the first trimester this tissue begins to canalize. The puncta usually open with the eyelids during the sixth month of gestation. The nasolacrimal duct opens into the inferior meatus of the nose just before or after term birth. There may be a failure of this canalization process at any part of the system, but this is most frequent at the lower end.[7]

Anatomy

Understanding the lacrimal outflow system is important for the pediatric ophthalmologist, especially for performing probing.

The puncta should be in contact with the globe at the medial aspect of the upper and lower lids. The proximal part of the canaliculus, the ampulla, is a slightly dilated vertical portion 1 mm in length in the young child. The canaliculus then turns 90° to run medially in a horizontal direction. The upper and lower canaliculi join to form the common canaliculus that enters the lateral wall of the lacrimal sac. Rosenmüller's valve prevents reflux of tears from the sac into the canaliculus. The lacrimal sac sits in the bony lacrimal fossa, separated from the middle meatus of the nose by the maxilla and lacrimal bone. The lacrimal sac extends superiorly under the medial canthal ligament to form its fundus. The nasolacrimal duct exits from the lower end of the sac and passes in a downward, lateral, and slightly posterior direction. This duct is surrounded by bone in its upper part but becomes membranous inferiorly. The nasolacrimal duct opens into the medial wall of the inferior meatus of the nose via the valve of Hasner. This ostium is found under the inferior turbinate of the nose, approximately 1 cm directly behind the entrance of the nose in the baby.

Physiology

Tears are actively pumped through the outflow system. During blinking, when the lids close, the canaliculi are shortened and narrowed by contraction of the pretarsal orbicularis muscles. Simultaneously the same muscles pull the lateral sac wall, creating negative pressure inside the sac, sucking fluid into the expanded sac. Further lid closure causes contraction of the orbicularis oculi muscle, which squeezes the tears from the sac into the nasolacrimal duct. At the end of each blink, the sac is empty. As the lids open, the canaliculi and the sac elastically expand. This causes a vacuum within the system into which tears enter via the puncta, and the cycle begins again.

Congenital abnormalities

Common abnormalities, include narrowing (stenosis), blockage (atresia), complete absence (agenesis), or duplication (accessory channels) of any part of the system. A membranous obstruction at the distal end of the nasolacrimal duct is the commonest abnormality, causing congenital nasolacrimal duct obstruction.[7] Obstruction at other sites is rare, but more relevant in older children.

Children with craniofacial abnormalities (see Chapter 28), particularly clefting syndromes, have complex anomalies of the lacrimal outflow system that may involve large areas being either blocked or absent.

Congenital dacryocystocele

A dacryocystocele is a congenital swelling located at the medial canthus due to trapped fluid inside the lacrimal sac and nasolacrimal duct.[8] The fluid is unable to escape from either the upper or lower end of the drainage system as both are blocked. This presents as a tense, blue, non-pulsatile swelling below the medial canthus. It is evident at, or shortly after, birth (Fig. 21.1A). The inferior end of the dacryocystocele projects into the nose (Fig. 21.1B) and in some cases may be responsible for breathing difficulties.[9] If respiratory compromise occurs, urgent treatment is required.

Congenital dacryocystocele must be differentiated from a meningoencephalocele, a meningocele, a mid-line nasal dermoid cyst (see Chapter 29), or a capillary hemangioma (see Chapter 20). An MRI scan is helpful in identifying the dilated sac and nasolacrimal duct and excluding other pathology. Routine imaging is unnecessary; the diagnosis is usually made clinically.

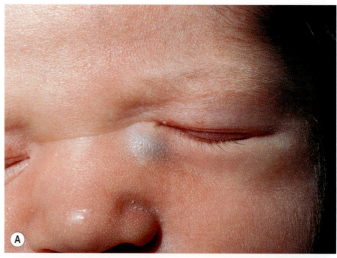

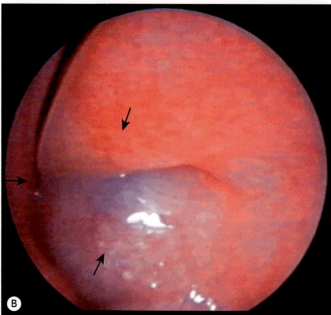

Fig. 21.1 Congenital dacryocystocele. (A) A bluish swelling is seen below the medial canthal tendon. It can present as nasal obstruction. (B) Dacryocystocele viewed from inside the nose, demonstrating the dilated nasolacrimal duct protruding into the nasal cavity, which may cause respiratory distress (left nostril).

Treatment of a dacryocystocele involves observation during the first 2 weeks of life, during which time most spontaneously improve. If it has not settled by this stage, if acute dacryocystitis (Fig. 21.2) or respiratory difficulties develop, then endoscopic drainage of the dacryocystocele into the nose is indicated and the nasal mucosa over the dacryocystocele excised. If acute dacryocystitis has intervened, intravenous antibiotics should be given prior to surgery.

Congenital nasolacrimal duct obstruction

Congenital nasolacrimal duct obstruction represents a delay in maturation of the lacrimal system where it enters the nose, resulting in a persistent membranous obstruction at the valve of Hasner. The diagnosis is made on a history of a watery eye that has been present from the first few weeks of birth. This is

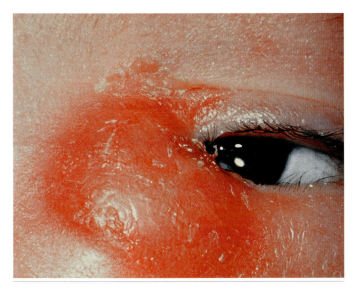

Fig. 21.2 Acute dacryocystitis in a baby with a congenital dacryocystocele. A dacryocystocele is not normally inflamed.

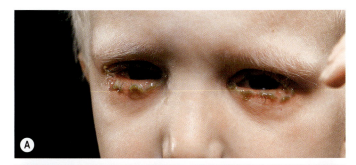

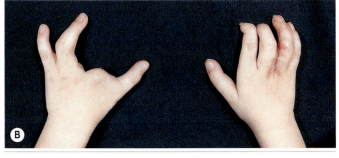

Fig. 21.3 (A) The ectrodactyly, ectodermal dysplasia, clefting (EEC) syndrome is associated with nasolacrimal duct obstruction and (B) "lobster claw" deformity of the hands.

usually unilateral but may be bilateral. If so, it is commonly asymmetrical. Some children develop a mucopurulent discharge that may be constant or intermittent. The eye remains "white" without evidence of active infection, although conjunctivitis may complicate the condition. The child is well with no evidence of irritation or photophobia. The skin around the eye may become red and excoriated. Although usually an isolated abnormality, congenital nasolacrimal duct obstruction may be more frequent in certain conditions, such as EEC syndrome (ectrodactyly, ectodermal dysplasia, clefting; Fig. 21.3) branchio-oculo facial syndrome, craniometaphyseal or craniodiaphysial dysplasia, Down's syndrome, LADD syndrome, and the CHARGE association (Table 21.1).

There is an increased tear meniscus and there may be stickiness or crusting on the lashes. A mucocele may develop. The contents can be expressed into the conjunctival sac.

A fluorescein disappearance test should be performed on children with epiphora. It provides evidence of lacrimal outflow obstruction.[10] Fluorescein 1% is instilled into each lower conjunctival fornix and cobalt blue light from the slit-lamp illuminates the eyes. The tear meniscus is evaluated at 2 and 5 minutes (and at 10 minutes in equivocal cases). Normally, the fluorescein disappears by 5 minutes (graded 0 or 1), but remains present in children with obstruction. This test illustrates clearly the nature of the problem (Fig. 21.4).

Natural history

Congenital nasolacrimal duct obstruction is evident in up to 20% of infants, of which the vast majority become symptomatic during the first month. The natural history is spontaneous resolution with maturation.[11-13] Spontaneous resolution is rapid[11-13] (Fig. 21.5) during the first year of life and continues, at a reduced rate, beyond this into childhood.[14,15]

Conservative treatment

Because of the high rate of spontaneous resolution, observation is recommended until the child is at least 1 year old and even older. Parental education should provide reassurance and information about the etiology and natural history.

Cleansing the lids and lashes with cooled boiled water gently expressing the contents of the lacrimal sac proximally into the conjunctival sac[16] maintains flow in the system and prevents stagnation, reducing any sticky discharge. Massage of the sac may also increase hydrostatic pressure within the lacrimal system. This increases resolution by rupturing the membranous obstruction.[17,18] Parents find this difficult and need clear instructions: press on the sac below the medial canthus with the little finger 2–3 times per day if possible. Vaseline (or liquid paraffin) should be applied to the periocular skin to protect and treat any areas of redness or broken skin.

Antibiotics are not required and should be avoided unless there is evidence of conjunctivitis. Swabs for bacterial growth should only be performed under these conditions as "pathogenic" bacteria are frequently commensals in the conjunctival sacs of normal infants and do not require antibiotic treatment in white watering eyes.[19]

Syringing and probing

If epiphora persists, syringing and probing the lacrimal drainage system is the treatment of choice. The optimum time to intervene remains controversial. In the past, probing was advocated at presentation or after a short period of conservative treatment.[20,21] However, this has become less favored due to better understanding of the natural history of the condition. It has been shown that the earlier probing is performed, the greater is the success rate.[22,23] However, the higher failure rate in older children is probably unrelated to the age of the child, but is due to a process of natural selection.[24-29] As children grow older, more complex and severe obstructions become common because cases of simple membranous obstruction spontaneously resolve. This reduces the success rate of probing in older children and increases the requirement for more extensive surgery.[14] Observation is as effective as probing in

Table 21.1 – Systemic associations of nasolacrimal duct obstruction in children

Syndrome	Genetics	Other eye findings	Systemic findings
Down's syndrome See Chapters 36, 38	Trisomy 21, mosaic or translocation	Up-slanting palpebral fissures, strabismus amblyopia, cataract, blepharitis	Short stature, hypotonia, simian crease, mental retardation, flat nose, small mouth and ears
EEC See Chapters 15, 18, 44 See Fig. 21.3	AD	Photophobia, absent eye lashes	Ectrodactlyly, hypoplasia or aplasia of middle digits, ectodermal dysplasia (absent sweat glands, hair, eyelashes, and brows), clefts (palate/lip)
Branchio-oculo-facial	AD; mutations in TFAP2A gene	Hypertelorism, microphthalmos, cataract, coloboma	Post-auricular branchial cleft defects, cleft lip/palate, low-set ears, malformed nose, hemangiomas of chest and neck
Craniometaphyseal dysplasia	AD/AR; mutations in ANK membrane protein gene	Optic atrophy	Hyperostosis of cranial bones, splayed metaphyses, palsies cranial nerve VII and VIII, delayed teething
Craniodiaphyseal dysplasia	AR/AD	Optic atrophy, strabismus, hypertelorism, exophthalmos	Generalized hyperostosis and sclerosis, growth retardation, parasnasal bossing, deafness, cylindrical long bones
LADD (lacrimo-auriculo-dento-digital)	AD Loss of FGF signaling	Ptosis, keratitis sicca	Hypoplasia, aplasia, or atresia of lacrimal and salivary glands, abnormalities of forearms and fingers, ear anomalies
CHARGE See Chapter 51	AD/sporadic mutations in CHD7	Coloboma	Coloboma, heart defects, atresia choanae, retardation of growth and development, genitourinary problems, ear abnormalities/deafness
Goldenhar's See Chapters 18, 28, 31, 82	Usually sporadic	Lid coloboma, epibulbar/limbal dermoid, Duane syndrome	Macrostoma, hemifacial microsomia, atresia ear canal, ear deformity, misshapen tongue, hemivertebrae, preauricular tags

AD, autosomal dominant; AR, autosomal recessive; FGF, fibroblast growth factor.
Further information: http://www.orpha.net; http://rarediseases.info.nih.gov.

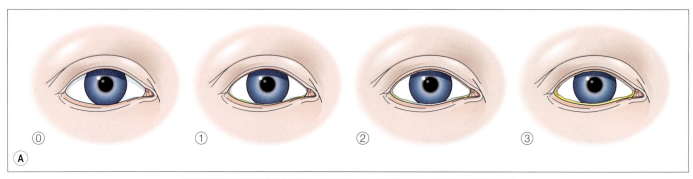

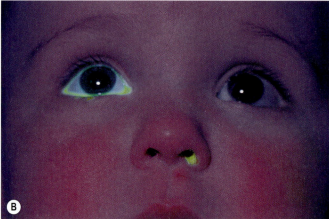

Fig. 21.4 The fluorescein disappearance test. (A) Grading the test is usually performed at 5 or 10 minutes.[24] (B) This child has evidence of delayed fluorescein disappearance test from the right eye, and a patent left system is confirmed by the presence of fluorescein in the nostril.

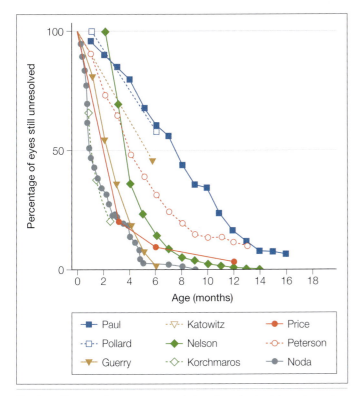

Fig. 21.5 The rate of spontaneous resolution of nasolacrimal duct obstruction expressed as a percentage of those still unresolved at a given age in months.

children up to the age of 2, but probing provides a more rapid result if performed around 12 months of age.[14]

The decision to probe is based on the natural history, severity, and informed parental request. Probing under 12 months of age is generally not recommended, and there is no evidence that it is detrimental to wait until 2 years of age[14,24-28] and probably later if desired.

"Office probing," carried out on awake, restrained babies, which is favored in the USA, is less popular elsewhere because it must be performed no later than 4–6 months of age. This is a stage when at least 50% of those undergoing probing would not require intervention if left until 1 year of age. In addition, iatrogenic damage to the friable nasolacrimal duct, with possible false passage formation may result.

Probing should be carried out in a pediatric environment with the child anesthetized. Probing is diagnostic, as well as therapeutic. In the small number of cases that remain symptomatic the cause of failure can be identified and a management plan formed. This can only be achieved under general anesthesia using a laryngeal mask following full nasal preparation. Probing should be carried out in a step-wise fashion, identifying the patency or obstruction of each area between the puncta and end of the nasolacrimal duct. Probing is a blind procedure and depends on awareness of resistance to the probe as it passes through the system. The use of a nasal endoscope permits direct visualization of the lower end of the nasolacrimal duct which assists in the diagnosis and management.[28]

Each punctum is dilated using a Nettleship dilator. This is introduced in a vertical direction for approximately 1 mm and then rotated through 90° medially to run horizontally parallel to the lid margin to dilate the proximal canaliculus. This is easier if the lid is held taut by pulling the eyelid laterally to straighten out the canaliculus. The lacrimal system should be syringed with fluorescein-stained saline using a disposable cannula. Syringing takes place via each punctum and any areas of resistance or any regurgitation of fluid or mucus are noted. The inside of the nose should be inspected with an endoscope or fluorescein retrieved via a nasal or pharyngeal aspirate. The passage of fluorescein and the amount of resistance are important factors in deciding the site and nature of any abnormality of the lacrimal outflow system.

The following features of syringing are useful in identifying the nature of the obstruction:

- Stenosis at the valve of Hasner, or a narrow inferior meatus caused by a tight inferior turbinate: difficulty in injecting the fluid, regurgitation of clear fluid via the other punctum and fluorescein is identified in the nose.
- Atresia at the lower end of the nasolacrimal duct: resistance to flow of fluid, regurgitation of mucus via the other punctum, and no fluorescein is retrieved from the nose.
- Agenesis (rare): severe resistance to flow, clear fluid regurgitation, no fluorescein in nose.
- Physiologic/functional blockage: free and easy flow of fluorescein into the nose in symptomatic children, indicating a normal anatomic pathway.

If a nasal endoscope is used, it should be introduced into the inferior meatus after infracture of the inferior turbinate. This maneuver is often therapeutic as it opens up a narrow inferior meatus and may stretch a stenotic ostium.[30] The fluorescein-stained fluid should be syringed through the system and observed through the endoscope.

- Atresia is identified as ballooning of the submucosa with no passage of fluorescein.
- Stenosis appears as a poor flow through the narrow valve (Fig. 21.6A).
- A clear free flow indicates either that the infracture has been effective or that the patient has "functional" epiphora.

The system should then be probed via the upper canaliculus using the smallest probe available (usually a Bowman's size 0000). The probe is passed in the same manner as the dilator until it reaches a hard stop that indicates the medial wall of the sac. The probe is withdrawn slightly and rotated 90° so that its tip is pointing downward. It is then advanced gently downward but also slightly posteriorly and laterally to follow the path of the nasolacrimal duct. During passage of the probe the operator should note the level of any resistance. If the probe perforates a persistent membrane at the valve of Hasner, this may be felt as it enters the inferior meatus.

If being performed with endonasal control, in a successful procedure, the probe will be observed entering the inferior meatus through the valve of Hasner (Fig. 21.6B).

Unsuccessful probings are observed when the probe:

- fails to perforate the atretic mucosa (Fig. 21.6C) or
- creates a false passage by missing the valve of Hasner, and either carries on in a submucosal plane to the floor of the nose or enters the meatus through a false and usually ineffective passage.

In the first instance, a cut down onto the probe may be required; in the other it may be possible to steer the probe

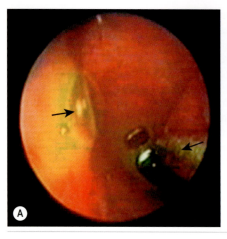 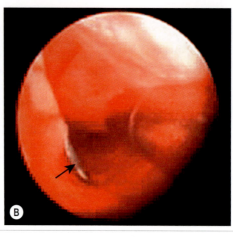 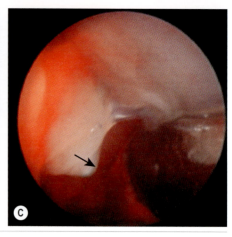

Fig. 21.6 (A) Stenotic flow through the valve of Hasner – right nostril. (B) Probe entering the inferior meatus via the valve of Hasner – right nostril. (C) Probe distending, but not perforating, the mucosa in a case of atresia of the lower end of the nasolacrimal duct – right nostril. (Courtesy of Paul White.)

under direct visualization toward and through the stenotic or atretic valve of Hasner. If the perforation is inadequate and felt to be tight, the probe size should be increased to a maximum size 1. Larger probes should be avoided as they may induce canalicular damage. To confirm patency the syringing should be repeated with fluorescein-stained saline.

Postoperatively a steroid/antibiotic combination should be instilled for 2 weeks. Improvement is usually noted within a few days of the probing. If there has been no improvement by 1 month, it is unlikely that the treatment has been successful.

What to do if probing fails

If probing fails, it is important to identify the reason for failure. Failure is generally due to one of three causes:

1. Failure to create an anatomically patent passage:
    a. a tight inferior meatus due to a large inferior turbinate
    b. failure to perforate the mucosa with the probe
    c. submucosal passage of the probe
    d. false passage formation, or
    e. inadequate size of the perforation.
2. Physiologic (functional) epiphora. Functional epiphora is persistent watering despite a clear, patent, free-flowing syringing, observed endoscopically in the inferior meatus and no resistance felt on probing. All other causes of lacrimation or epiphora must be eliminated. The fluorescein disappearance test demonstrates delay. The cause is probably physiologic pump failure. Such children may have an upper respiratory cause, such as large adenoids. A history regarding nasal symptoms should be taken.
3. Complex abnormalities of the outflow system. Abnormalities of the canaliculi or the proximal nasolacrimal duct become commoner in older children. These abnormalities may be complex, especially in children with abnormal facial skeletons.[31]

A major advantage of endoscopic probing is that these common causes of failure can be identified and treated at the first probing, improving the success rate.[32]

If endoscopic probing was not performed on the first occasion, then this approach is useful in re-probings. It will identify the most frequent causes of failure and permit appropriate treatment.[32] If the initial procedure was an endoscopic procedure, subsequent treatment is dependent on the original findings. Another option is intubation of the system with silicone tubes.[33] However, intubation carries risk of damage to the canaliculi. It may be unnecessary (e.g. in functional cases), and is no more effective than endoscopic probing in repeat cases.[34]

Intubation

Indications for silicone tubes include upper nasolacrimal duct obstruction and canalicular stenosis.[33] Intubation can be employed to treat "failed probings",[35] but the etiology of the failure should be clarified prior to intubation.

Intubation should take place under general anesthetic after the nose has been prepared with decongestant. Nasal endoscopic guidance is used to view the inferior meatus. Tubes come with a metal introducer. Each end is placed through the system via canaliculi, into the sac, and down the nasolacrimal duct into the inferior meatus. They should be retrieved under direct visualization. Ritleng tubes – silicone tubes, inserted via hollow probes which are placed in the lacrimal system – are easier to insert, less traumatic, and more likely to be successful, especially in the hands of a novice.[36] Postoperative treatment consists of a topical antibiotic and steroid preparation into the conjunctival sac.

Possible complications of intubation include cheese-wiring through the canaliculi, dislocation superiorly or inferiorly, infection, and scarring of the drainage system.[37]

The optimum time to leave tubes in place is not known, but 3–6 months is usually recommended.[37] Tubes should be removed under general anesthetic via the nose to prevent aspiration of the tube. This system is then irrigated to remove debris and to confirm patency.

Balloon catheter dilatation of the lacrimal system is an alternative to intubation in patients with failed probing.[38] This has a high success rate similar to that of intubation,[39] but is significantly more expensive. It has been suggested that balloons have a role in the primary treatment of CNLDO, but the results are no better than "blind" probing.[40] The role of balloon dacryoplasty in the management of congenital nasolacrimal duct obstruction still needs to be fully evaluated.

Dacryocystorhinostomy

Children rarely require a dacryocystorhinostomy (DCR), but indications include persistent epiphora despite probing and intubation, complex congenital abnormalities of the lacrimal outflow apparatus (particularly involving the upper nasolacrimal duct), and acquired disease usually caused by infection or trauma.[41] External and endoscopic routes are possible. Excellent success rates, comparable to those of adult DCR, have been reported.[42,43]

Congenital fistulae of the lacrimal outflow system

Fistulae of the lacrimal system in which tracts open onto the skin directly from the puncta, canaliculi, lacrimal sac, or nasolacrimal duct are rare. They may appear as double puncta, or appear in the region of the medial canthus (Fig. 21.7). They are usually non-functioning and should be left untreated unless they allow flow of tears onto the face or result in epiphora (rare). Treatment involves excision of the fistula after ensuring that the remaining outflow system is patent.

Punctal and canalicular abnormalities

Failure of the proximal end of the lacrimal drainage system to canalize may result in punctal stenosis or atresia. This is often asymptomatic especially if only one punctum is abnormal. Narrow puncta should be dilated. Membranous obstruction should be pierced with a needle and dilated. These cases do well, but are often associated with distal abnormalities and a syringing should always be performed.

Abnormalities proximal to the sac result in surprisingly few symptoms. Agenesis should be suspected if the papilla is not readily obvious.[44] If only one punctum is missing, syringing via the other one detects the extent of the damage. Surgery to construct these areas is specialized. Retrograde probing from an external DCR incision may be attempted through the sac; otherwise, a Jones tube is required. This type of surgery may be left until the child is in their teens.

Acquired conditions of the lacrimal drainage apparatus

Canaliculitis

Canaliculitis in children is uncommon but may be due to bacterial or primary herpes simplex infection. Management involves obtaining viral and bacterial cultures and treatment with antibiotics or antiviral agents depending on the clinical and laboratory findings. Probing in the active phase should be avoided.

Acute dacryocystitis

Acute dacryocystitis may accompany non-patent nasolacrimal systems or may occur as a primary event. This is particularly common in infants with dacryocystocele.[45] Treatment comprises prompt intervention with intravenous antibiotics as retrobulbar abscesses may occur. Cultures should be taken of any pus or discharge that can be expressed through the punctum. Probing should not be performed as damage to the congested

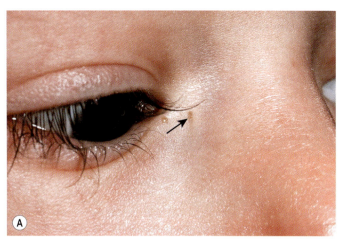

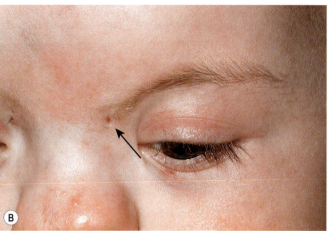

Fig. 21.7 Congenital fistula of the nasolacrimal system. A fistula can be seen as a tiny mark (A) below or (B) above the medial canthus.

epithelium may cause false passage and lead to orbital cellulitis and fistula formation.[46] Skin incisions should not be made during the acute phase as an external fistula may occur. If a mass remains after resolution, evacuation can be performed through the skin with a needle through the lower pole of the sac, although the pus may be inspissated or loculated. Once the infection has resolved, probing should be performed if epiphoria persists.

Acquired nasolacrimal duct obstruction

Acquired nasolacrimal duct obstruction may be caused by diseases of the nose or paranasal sinuses, especially chronic allergic rhinitis or persistent upper respiratory tract infections with enlarged adenoidal lymphoid tissue. These are commoner in older children and adolescents.[47] Rarely, acquired obstruction may herald a more sinister cause such as fibrous dysplasia, cranial metaphysial or cranial diaphysial dysplasia, or tumor formation (see Chapter 25). Treatment should be aimed at the underlying cause.

References

1. Sevel D. Development and congenital abnormalities of the nasolacrimal apparatus. J Pediatr Ophthalmol Strabismus 1981; 18: 13–9.

5. Chavis RM, Garner A, Wright JE. Inflammatory orbital pseudotumour: a clinicopathologic study. Arch Ophthalmol 1978; 96: 1817–22.

9. Edmond JC, Keech RV. Congenital nasolacrimal sac mucocoele associated with respiratory distress. J Pediatr Ophthalmol Strabismus 1991; 28: 287–9.

10. MacEwen CJ, Young JD. The fluorescein disappearance test (FDT): an evaluation of its use in infants. J Pediatr Ophthalmol Strabismus 1991; 28: 302–5.

11. Petersen RA, Robb RM. The natural course of congenital obstruction of the nasolacrimal duct. J Pediatr Ophthalmol Strabismus 1978; 15: 246–50.

13. MacEwen CJ, Young JD. Epiphora during the first year of life. Eye 1991; 5: 596–600.

19. MacEwen CJ, Phillips MG, Young JD. Value of bacterial culturing in the course of congenital nasolacrimal duct (NLD) obstruction. J Pediatr Ophthalmol Strabismus 1994; 31: 246–50.

21. Baker JD. Treatment of congenital nasolacrimal duct obstruction. J Pediatr Ophthalmol Strabismus 1985; 22: 34–6.

22. Katowitz JA, Welsh MG. Timing of initial probing and irrigation in congenital nasolacrimal duct obstruction. Ophthalmology 1987; 94: 698–705.

23. Mannor GE, Rose GE, Frimpong-Ansah K, Ezra E. Factors affecting the success of nasolacrimal duct probing for congenital nasolacrimal duct obstruction. Am J Ophthalmol 1999; 127: 616–7.

25. el-Mansoury J, Calhoun JH, Nelson LB, Harley RD. Results of late probing for congenital nasolacrimal obstruction. Ophthalmology 1986; 93: 1052–4.

26. Nelson LB, Calhoun JH, Menduke H. Medical management of congenital nasolacrimal duct obstruction. Pediatrics 1985; 76: 172–5.

27. Kashkouli MB, Kassaee A, Tabatabaee Z. Initial nasolacrimal duct probing in children under age 5: cure rate and factors affecting success. J AAPOS 2002; 6: 360–3.

28. Wallace J, Cox A, White P, MacEwen CJ. Endoscopic assisted probing for congenital naso-lacrimal duct obstruction. Eye 2006;20:998–1003.

32. MacEwen CJ, Young JD, Barras CW, et al. Value of nasal endoscopy and probing in the diagnosis and management of children with congenital epiphora. Br J Ophthalmol 2001; 85: 314–8.

35. Aggarwal RK, Misson GP, Donaldson I, Willshaw HE. The role of nasolacrimal intubation in the management of childhood epiphora. Eye 1993; 7: 760–2.

36. Pe MR, Langford JD, Lindberg JV, et al. Ritleng intubation for treatment of congenital naso lacrimal duct obstruction. Arch Ophthalmol 1998;116:387–91

37. Welsh MG, Katowitz JA. Timing of Silastic tubing removal after intubation for congenital nasolacrimal duct obstruction. Ophthal Plast Reconstr Surg 1989; 5: 43–8.

38. Becker BB, Berry FD. Balloon catheter dilatation in pediatric patients. Ophthalmic Surg 1991; 22: 750–2.

39. Repka M, Chandler D, Holmes J, et al. Balloon catheter dilation and naso lacrimal intubation for treatment of naso lacrimal duct obstruction after failed probing. Arch Ophthalmol 2009; 127: 633–9

40. Goldich Y, Barkana Y, Zadok D, et al. Balloon catheter dilatation versus probing as primary treatment for congenital dacryostenosis. Br J Ophthalmol 2011; 95: 634–6

41. Billson FA, Taylor HR, Hoyt CS. Trauma to the lacrimal system in children. Am J Ophthalmol 1978; 86: 828–33.

42. Kominek P, Cervenka S. Pediatric endonasal dacryocystorhinostomy: a report of 34 patients. Laryngoscope 2005; 115: 1800–03.

43. Hakin KN, Sullivan TJ, Sharma A, Welham RA. Paediatric dacryocystorhinostomy. Aust NZ J Ophthalmol 1994; 22: 231–5.

44. Lyons CJ, Rosser PM, Welham RA. The management of punctal agenesis. Ophthalmology 1993; 100: 1851–5.

45. Pollard ZF. Treatment of acute dacryocystitis in neonates. J Pediatr Ophthalmol Strabismus 1991; 28: 341–3.

46. Weiss GH, Leib ML. Congenital dacryocystitis and retrobulbar abscess. J Pediatr Ophthalmol Strabismus 1993; 30: 271–2.

47. Sturrock SM, MacEwen CJ, Young JD. Long term results after probing for congenital naso-lacrimal duct obstruction. Br J Ophthalmol 1994; 31: 362–7

Access the complete reference list online at
http://www.expertconsult.com

The management of orbital disease in children

Christopher J Lyons · Wilma Y Chang · Jack Rootman

Chapter contents

Orbital abnormalities in childhood may be congenital or acquired. Congenital abnormalities related to a developmental problem can be confined to the orbit or be part of a more widespread craniofacial malformation. For instance, proptosis may be related to a shallow or small orbit, or the relationship between the orbits may be disturbed: in hypertelorism the orbits are widely separated; in hypotelorism, they are set close together. An orbital wall defect may allow prolapse of intracranial tissue with pulsating exophthalmos or enophthalmos. The orbits develop throughout childhood and congenital absence of the globe, enucleation, or radiotherapy results in failure of normal orbital growth.

Children with acquired orbital disorders most commonly present with signs and symptoms of a mass leading to proptosis or non-axial displacement, soft tissue signs, and/or a palpable orbital mass. Other presentations include reduced vision, restriction of ocular movements, pain and inflammation. Occasionally, a child may present with enophthalmos following orbital trauma.

The relative frequency of the conditions causing proptosis in childhood varies considerably [1-8] depending, in part, on the source of the material. Series from eye hospitals[3] are different from those from neurosurgical[2] or pediatric units.[6] Geographic factors vary: the major causes of proptosis in African children[4] are different from those seen in Europe and North America. Series that rely solely on tissues specimens[1,5,7,8] reflect the incidence of lesions that are excised surgically and exclude the many conditions that can be diagnosed and treated without biopsy or surgery, such as infantile periocular hemangioma, or those in which biopsy may be more conveniently obtained at another site of involvement, such as neuroblastoma or histiocytosis. In that sense, they are not helpful in formulating the differential diagnosis of an individual child with proptosis.

Orbital disease and age

Within the childhood years, defined here as ages up to and including 16 years, important trends in the incidence of the causative disorders at different times of life can help the diagnostic process.

We have reviewed the clinical data of 326 children seen by the orbital service in Vancouver, Canada since 1976 (Table 22.1). This period includes the introduction of the computed tomography (CT) scan, a watershed in the non-invasive investigation of orbital disease. Neoplasia and structural abnormalities (including cysts) account for the great majority of children presenting with orbital disease (Fig. 22.1). This is quite different from adults, in which over 60% of presentations are due to inflammatory causes: structural abnormalities account for less than 15% of cases. However, the distribution of orbital disease in children aged over 11 years is similar to the adult pattern (Fig. 22.2).

Fortunately, only a small proportion of the neoplasia can be considered malignant, which concurs with published series.[6,7,9] Under 2 years of age, the major causes of proptosis are infantile hemangiomas and venous lymphatic malformations (lymphangioma), inclusion and dermoid cysts, and other structural abnormalities. Figure 22.3, which shows the distribution of the major diagnostic groups by age at presentation, indicates that while some lesions are distributed evenly throughout childhood (venous lymphatic malformation, varices, and arteriovenous malformations), others tend to occur within a specific age range. Seven patients with rhabdomyosarcoma were seen, whose ages ranged from 2 to 11 years. The seven patients with Langerhans cell histiocytosis ranged in age from 3 to 9 years. Infantile hemangioma was overwhelmingly more common in early infancy. Inflammatory conditions were increasingly frequent after the age of 5 years, especially orbital cellulitis, non-specific orbital inflammatory syndromes (6 years and over), and thyroid orbitopathy (11 years and over). It is noteworthy that there were two cases of

Table 22.1 – Orbital disease in children: multiseries data comparison

	Rootman[15]		Bullock et al.[10]		Crawford[6]		All series	
	No.	% of series	No.	% of series	No.	% of series	No.	% of all series
Neoplasia								
Optic nerve glioma	17	5.2	5	3.6	17	3.0	39	3.8
Meningioma	2	0.6	2	1.4			4	0.4
Other neurogenic tumor	6	1.8					1	0.1
PNS tumors	19	5.8	9	6.4	14	2.5	42	4.1
Lymphocytic	1	0.3	1	0.7	3	0.5	5	0.5
Other lymphocytic	3	0.9	4	2.9	20	3.6	27	2.6
Histiocytic	7	2.1	1	0.7	20	3.6	28	2.7
Vascular	36	11.0	14	13.6	14	2.5	64	6.2
Secondary/metastatic	5	1.5	4	2.9	21	3.8	30	2.9
Mesenchymal								
Rhabdomyosarcoma	7	2.1	3	2.1	11	2.0	21	2.0
Fibrous	1	0.3	3	2.1	1	0.2	5	0.5
Histiocytic	2	0.6	2	1.4			4	0.4
Bone	3	0.9					3	0.3
Neoplasia	6	1.8	2	1.4	5	0.9	13	1.3
Other	2	0.6	1	0.7			3	0.3
Unknown neoplasia			1	0.7	3	0.5	4	0.4
Lacrimal	2	0.6					2	0.2
Teratoma					1	0.2	1	0.1
Structural								
Cystic	60	18.4	59	42.1	6	1.1	122	11.9
Bone anomalies	9	2.8			50	8.9	59	5.8
Ectopia	13	4.0	11	7.9			24	2.3
Other	3	0.9			2	0.4	4	0.4
Inflammatory								
Infectious diseases	21	6.4			232	41.5	253	24.7
NSOIS	14	4.3	6	4.3	5	0.9	25	2.4
Other – inflammatory	10	3.1	3	2.1			13	1.3
Thyroid orbitopathy	27	8.3			107	19.1	134	13.1
Vascular	46	14.1	9	2.9	14	2.5	69	6.7
Atrophy/degeneration	2	0.6					2	0.2
Unknown	2	0.6			13	2.3	15	1.5
Total	326		140		559		1025	

NSOIS, non-specific orbital inflammatory syndrome; PNS, peripheral nerve sheath.

lacrimal gland carcinoma and four of Wegener's granulomatosis in this series, a reminder that, although rare, these potentially lethal conditions do occur in children.

Clinical assessment

When assessing a child with orbital disease, a history, examination, and differential diagnosis in the context of the child's age are essential before investigations can be planned.

History

The age of onset, laterality (unilateral or bilateral), and the tempo of onset are important clues to the diagnosis. The duration may be difficult to determine accurately and a review of old photographs may be helpful, but proptosis alone is frequently not obvious on photos.

Bilateral proptosis in early infancy is often due to orbital shallowing in craniofacial malformations. This can occasionally be unilateral, as in plagiocephaly. Usually, however, unilateral proptosis is due to the globe being displaced forward by a mass within the orbit.

Some masses such as optic nerve glioma or dermoid cyst grow slowly. Rapidly increasing proptosis suggests a metastatic deposit or rapidly growing tumor such as rhabdomyosarcoma. Rapid tumor growth may be associated with necrosis and hemorrhage resulting in periorbital ecchymosis. The presence of bilateral ecchymosis is suggestive of metastatic neuroblastoma.

A catastrophic onset (within hours) implies a bleed within an (often unsuspected) pre-existing lesion such as a venous lymphatic malformation (lymphangioma). Occasionally, the onset of orbital cellulitis may be very sudden. It is usually accompanied by pain, local inflammation, and limitation of ocular motility in a child who is generally ill and febrile. The presence of clinically detectable orbital and periorbital inflammatory symptoms and signs in childhood is overwhelmingly associated with infection or non-specific orbital inflammatory

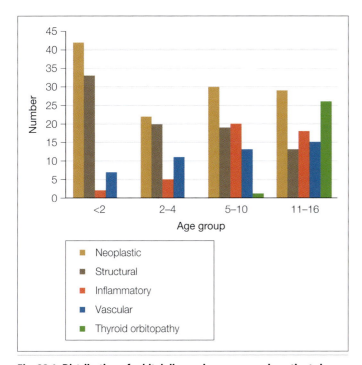

Fig. 22.1 **Distribution of orbital disease by age group in patients less than 17 years of age.**

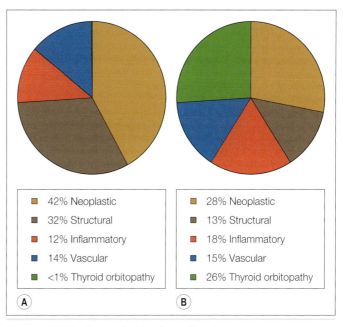

Fig. 22.2 (A) Distribution of orbital disease in patients less than 11 years of age. (B) Distribution of orbital disease in patients 11–17 years.

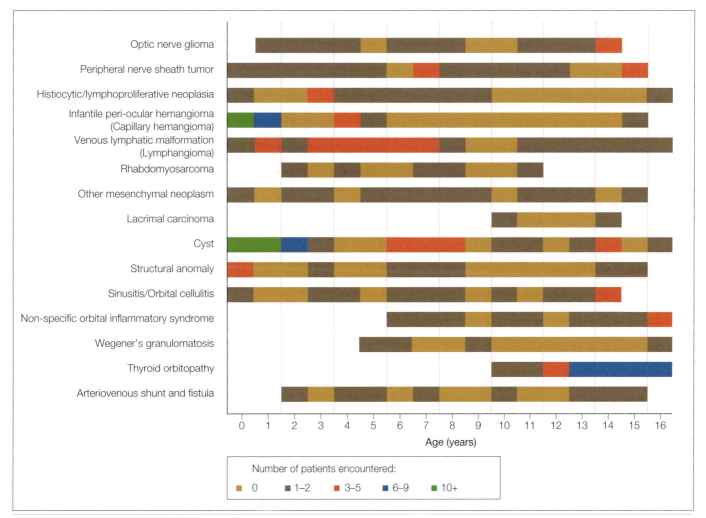

Fig. 22.3 **Age distribution of common orbital diseases.**

disease. Although inflammation is part of the classical description of rhabdomyosarcoma, it is not typical and was absent in all six patients in our series, all of whom did have rapid onset.

Most round-cell tumors in childhood, including rhabdomyosarcoma, granulocytic sarcoma (chloroma) and Ewing's sarcoma, present as a mass developing over weeks in a subacute manner. Neuroblastoma can present with onset of proptosis over days.

An increase in proptosis with crying or straining is suggestive of infantile periocular hemangioma, varices, or absence of the sphenoid wing (as in neurofibromatosis type 1, NF1). This sign is useful in the neonate, where crying almost invariably accompanies a thorough eye examination. When very obvious, its presence helps to exclude malignancy as a cause of the proptosis.

Pulsating exophthalmos may be associated with congenital defects of the orbital wall (as seen in NF1) or encephalocele. Occasionally, large periocular infantile peri-ocular hemangiomas (capillary hemangiomas) pulsate due to their rich arterial blood supply, as may high-flow arteriovenous malformations, though the latter are rare in childhood and more common in adolescence or young adulthood.

Skin discoloration may offer a clue to the underlying etiology. Red is suggestive of the arterial supply of infantile periocular hemangioma which, when superficial to the septum, almost invariably involves the overlying skin. When deep, these may have a blueish or purple hue. Lesions derived from venous anlagen, varices, or venous lymphatic malformations (lymphangiomas) appear blue or purple, as do some cystic lesions, lacrimal, or conjunctival cysts. Some cystic lesions, for instance the cysts associated with colobomatous microphthalmos, are blueish but transilluminate to a focal light. The brownish cutaneous discoloration of hemosiderin is usually caused by previous bleeds into a vascular lymphatic malformation (lymphangioma) or, rarely, by neuroblastoma. Both of these may present with spontaneous ecchymosis.

Examination

Children with proptosis must have a visual assessment. In infants, this may be limited to observing fixation; resentment to cover of the contralateral eye suggests poor vision. The 10-prism diopter base down test may be useful if poor vision is suspected in an orthotropic child. A cover test should be performed and ocular ductions and versions assessed. Limitation of ductions may be due to mechanical restriction by tumor, muscle infiltration, inflammation, edema, or entrapment. Third, fourth, and sixth cranial nerve function should be tested, as well as sensory testing in the Vi and Vii distribution if possible. Occasionally, as in an older child with a blow-out fracture, a forced duction test may be useful to detect muscle restriction.

The site of an orbital mass may be indicated by the direction in which the eye is displaced. A posterior or intraconal tumor results in axial proptosis; an extraconal tumor may displace the eye vertically or laterally. For example, in fibrous dysplasia of the orbit, which most commonly affects the frontal bone, the globe is usually displaced downwards and forwards. Orbital cellulitis secondary to ethmoidal sinus infection usually displaces the globe laterally. Although the globe is displaced away from most mass lesions, it can be displaced toward them, as in the case of cicatrizing lesions within the orbit (Table 22.2).

Enophthalmos

Enophthalmos, recession of the eyeball in the orbit, may occur in the following cases:

1. Following radiotherapy (Fig. 22.4).
2. Sphenoid wing dysplasia and other bone dysplasias.
3. Parry-Romberg syndrome or morphoea (Fig. 22.5).
4. Developmental tumors (Fig. 22.6).
5. Orbital floor blow-out fracture.

Table 22.2 – Causes of mass effect in children (excluding thyroid orbitopathy)

	All years			0–2 years			3–10 years			11–16 years		
	No.	% series	% cohort	No.	% series	% cohort	No.	% series	% cohort	No.	% series	% cohort
Optic nerve gliomas	8	2.5	3.9	1	0.3	1.2	3	0.9	3.7	4	1.2	10.5
Peripheral nerve sheath tumors	8	2.5	3.9	2	0.6	2.4	4	1.2	4.9	2	0.6	5.3
Lymphoproliferative	8	2.5	3.9	1	0.3	1.2	6	1.8	7.3	1	0.3	2.6
Infantile peri-ocular hemangiomas (capillary hemangiomas)	30	9.2	14.8	22	6.8	26.5	5	1.5	6.1	1	0.3	2.6
Bone/mesenchymal tumors	15	4.6	7.4	3	0.9	3.6	8	2.5	9.8	4	1.2	10.5
Congenital cysts and dermolipomas	62	19.1	30.5	37	11.4	44.6	17	5.2	20.7	8	2.5	21.1
Sinusitis/Orbital cellulitis	9	2.8	4.4	0	0.0	0.0	8	2.5	9.8	1	0.3	2.6
Venous lymphatic malformations (lymphangiomas)	26	8.0	12.8	6	1.8	7.2	14	4.3	17.1	7	2.2	18.4
All causes of mass effect	203	62.5		83	25.5		82	25.2		38	11.7	

Number of patients in series with non-thyroid orbital disease, n = 325.

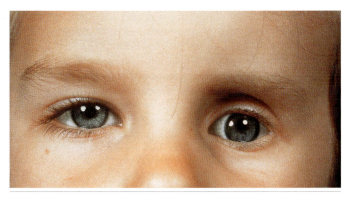

Fig. 22.4 Left enophthalmos following radiotherapy for retinoblastoma. (Patient of the University of British Columbia.)

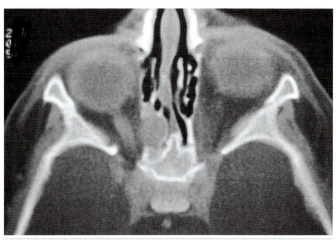

Fig. 22.6 Acquired enophthalmos caused by an astroglial tumor involving the paranasal sinuses.

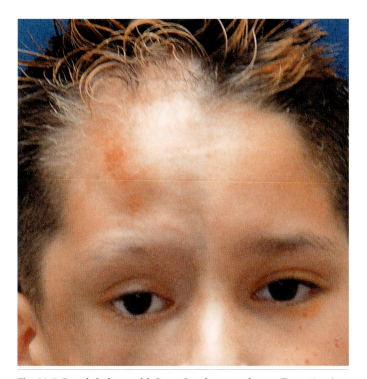

Fig. 22.5 Enophthalmos with Parry-Romberg syndrome. The patient has a chronic right-sided uveitis, atrophy of the subcutaneous tissues, pigmentary changes, and hair loss on the affected side. (Patient of the University of British Columbia.)

Globe position should be recorded using an exophthalmometer and a transparent ruler is used to measure the amount of vertical and horizontal displacement. It is difficult to measure proptosis accurately in infants, but careful observation from above or below often helps to highlight its presence.

Eyelid position should be recorded; retraction or lag may suggest thyroid orbitopathy, but may also be indicative of tethering by tumors such as Langerhans cell histiocytosis.

Slit-lamp examination may show dilated dysmorphic venous channels in the conjunctiva of patients with varices. Venous lymphatic malformation (lymphangioma) may be associated with visible conjunctival lymphangiectasis or cysts, which occasionally contain a meniscus of blood. Lisch nodules on the iris are diagnostic signs of NF1, increasing in number with age and which may suggest plexiform neurofibroma or

sphenoid wing dysplasia with encephalocele as causes of proptosis or a good prognosis for optic nerve glioma but a poorer systemic prognosis from other central nervous system tumors. Juvenile cataract is a marker for NF2 so it suggests meningioma or schwannoma as a cause of orbital mass.

The presence of an afferent pupillary defect suggests optic neuropathy, which may be due to intrinsic disease, as in glioma, or to extrinsic compression, as in fibrous dysplasia involving the optic canal (rare). Field testing might reveal the central scotoma of optic neuropathy. In older children, color vision can be assessed using subjective red desaturation or an Ishihara chart to confirm the presence of an optic neuropathy.

Cycloplegic refraction is important to detect astigmatism due to distortion of the globe by an orbital mass. Retrobulbar lesions tend to result in a hyperopic shift; lesions at or anterior to the equator produce astigmatism. These are important causes of amblyopia.[10] Occasionally, axial myopia may mimic proptosis, particularly when unilateral. Long-term occlusion of an eye, as in uncorrected unilateral ptosis due to infantile periocular hemangioma (capillary hemangioma), results in ipsilateral axial myopia.

Optic disk swelling or atrophy can appear in patients with optic nerve compression or glioma. If the mass is close behind the globe, choroidal folds may be present. Optico-ciliary shunt vessels, classically associated with meningioma, are much more frequently seen in optic nerve glioma in children because they are much more common.

Palpation of the orbit reveals the consistency of a localized mass. Infantile peri-ocular hemangiomas (capillary hemangiomas) feel firm and spongy; their contents cannot be expelled by applied pressure, whereas orbital varices are easily drained of blood, even with gentle pressure. Dermoids should be examined for mobility or fixation and the presence of posterior margin or a tail extending into the orbit or temporalis fossa. A posterior extension or extension through the lateral wall of the orbit is more likely to be present in dermoids that are situated inside the orbital rim than in those directly overlying the rim.

Although the orbit does not have true lymphatics, the preauricular and submandibular lymph nodes should be palpated to exclude enlargement from metastasis, as in rhabdomyosarcoma involving the eyelids, or infection, as in orbital cellulitis.

The evaluation of children with orbital disease should include systemic examination; this may give useful clues to the diagnosis. Café-au-lait spots suggest neurofibromatosis, and skin pigmentation may be seen in fibrous dysplasia. Characteristic skin lesions may also be present in Langerhans cell histiocytosis and juvenile xanthogranuloma. Infantile peri-ocular hemangioma (capillary hemangioma) of the orbit is often associated with cutaneous infantile peri-ocular hemangiomas (capillary hemangiomas) elsewhere. In suspected metastatic disease there may be other involved sites such as an abdominal mass in neuroblastoma or skin, scalp or bony lesions in Langerhans cell histiocytosis. Thyroid orbitopathy may be accompanied by systemic signs or history of hyperthyroidism suggestive of this diagnosis.

Opinions from other specialists, particularly general pediatricians and ENT surgeons, may help to determine the cause of proptosis in a child.

Investigations

Investigating children with proptosis should be guided by the history and clinical findings and tailored to each patient. In some instances, such as craniofacial malformations, the abnormalities fit a clear pattern and further investigations are not warranted although referral to genetics would be appropriate. In others, further tests will be necessary to confirm the suspected diagnosis or to assess the degree of orbital involvement. When other systems are involved, such as extension of tumor into the brain or sinuses or systemic involvement in malignancy, investigation of the child should be planned with the other specialists who may become involved in the child's care.

Radiology

Plain X-rays

Although CT scan is the initial radiologic investigation in most patients with orbital disease, plain X-rays may still be useful in certain circumstances. These include the assessment of orbital bony trauma, localization of a radio-opaque orbital foreign body, and assessment of systemic disease (such as absence of the sphenoid wing in neurofibromatosis).

Sinus X-rays in suspected sinus disease with orbital cellulitis should be interpreted with care, since sinus anatomy is variable under the age of 10 years. Although the finding of bony distortion on the affected side suggests a long-standing or slow-growing process in adults, this sign is unreliable in children, where it may be seen with rapidly enlarging lesions.

The merits of plain X-rays are the ubiquity of the equipment, low cost, and the fact that sedation is rarely required. Although the dose of radiation delivered in a CT scan of the orbit is higher than that used in a plain X-ray, the diagnostic yield is much greater.[11]

Computed tomography and magnetic resonance imaging

Diagnostic imaging of orbital structures was revolutionized by CT. Optimal imaging requires 0.75 to 2 mm slice thickness and both direct coronal and axial images, tailored to the clinical need.[12] Thin slices are indicated for optic nerve and foreign body imaging. High resolution axial images can be reformatted to coronal images without obtaining fresh coronal views. CT provides information about intracranial as well as orbital structures.[12] It yields more information on the presence of calcification and on bony detail; soft tissue and "bone window" settings can be specifically requested.[13] CT can also be used when a ferromagnetic foreign body is suspected. The differential diagnostic yield is increased by the use of contrast agents which enhance vascular lesions, inflammations, and some malignancies.

Sedation is usually necessary under the age of 3–4 years, though the speed of data acquisition has increased significantly. Data capture for orbital CT scan with a 16-slice scanner takes under 10 seconds. The relatively high dose of radiation makes CT useful for initial diagnosis but undesirable for regular follow-up, especially for patients with tumor suppressor gene mutations (retinoblastoma, neurofibromatosis, and rhabdomyosarcoma).

Magnetic resonance imaging (MRI) provides higher resolution of soft tissue without exposure to ionizing radiation.[12] This is important if repeat imaging is necessary, for example a child with NF1 and optic nerve glioma who is being followed regularly. Any plane can be chosen at the time of the examination. Orbital views may be obtained with a 0.5–3.0 tesla field, and surface coils should be used to increase the surface-to-noise ratio. Contrast enhancement can be obtained for similar indications to those outlined above for CT, using gadolinium which results in T1 shortening. Because fat has a bright signal on T1-weighted images, fat saturation techniques must be used to maximize the effect of contrast enhancement in the orbit. This is essential to examine the optic nerve which would otherwise be swamped by the bright fat signal, potentially obscuring an important finding such as optic nerve sheath meningioma, which would be more obvious with CT.

Multiple image sequences can provide characteristic signal patterns, such as the fluid/fluid levels typical of low- or no-flow vascular malformations and aneurysmal bone cysts. Identification and dating of blood within hemorrhagic lesions such as venous lymphatic malformations (lymphangiomas), presence or absence of flow within mass lesions, and contrast enhancement of the optic nerve in optic neuritis are further strengths of this technique.

Disadvantages include the time taken to image an orbit, 20–30 minutes, compared with CT which takes seconds; CT can be used without sedation for much younger patients who can lie still for 2 or 3 minutes. Conversely, most patients under the age of 6 years require sedation or anesthesia (often using only IV propofol as opposed to intubation or laryngeal mask) for MRI because of the noise and duration of the procedure. Other drawbacks include a contraindication for patients with ferromagnetic foreign bodies. A more specific problem of MRI for orbital work is its relative inability to image bone and calcification clearly,[13] which may be important when differentiating glioma from meningioma in the orbit.

Surgery

The surgical approach to the child's orbit differs markedly from that taken in adult orbital disease. This is due to the relative shallowness of the orbit in childhood. Lateral orbitotomy, with lateral orbital wall removal, is unnecessary in most cases since lesions can usually be reached via the anterior approach.

References

1. Porterfield JF. Orbital tumors in children: a report on 214 cases. Int Ophthalmol Clin 1962; 2: 319–26.

2. MacCarty CS, Brown DN. Orbital tumors in children. Clin Neurosurg 1982; 11: 76–84.

3. Youseffi B. Orbital tumors in children: a clinical study of 62 cases. J Pediatr Ophthalmol Strabismus 1969; 6: 177–81.

4. Templeton AC. Orbital tumours in African children. Br J Ophthalmol 1971; 55: 254–61.

5. Eldrup-Jorgensen P, Fledelius H. Orbital tumours in infancy: an analysis of Danish cases from 1943–1962. Acta Ophthalmol 1975; 53: 887–93.

6. Crawford JS. Diseases of the orbit. In: Crawford JS, Morin JD, editors. The Eye in Childhood. New York: Grune and Stratton; 1983: 361–94.

7. Shields JA, Bakewell B, Augsburger JJ, et al. Space occupying orbital masses in children: a review of 250 consecutive biopsies. Ophthalmology 1986; 93: 379–84.

8. Kodsi SR, Shetlar DJ, Campbell RJ, et al. A review of 340 orbital tumors in children during a 60-year period. Am J Ophthalmol 1994; 117: 177–82.

9. Bullock JD, Goldberg SH, Rakes SM. Orbital tumors in children. Ophthal Plast Reconstr Surg 1989; 5: 13–16.

10. Bogan S, Simon JW, Krohel GB, et al. Astigmatism associated with adnexal masses in infancy. Arch Ophthalmol 1987; 105: 1368–70.

11. Weiss RA, Haik BG, Smith ME. Introduction to diagnostic imaging techniques in ophthalmology. Int Ophthalmol Clin 1986; 26: 1–24.

12. Mafee MF, Mafee RF, Malik M, et al. Medical imaging in pediatric ophthalmology. Pediatr Clin N Am 2003; 50: 259–86.

13. Mafee MF. The orbit proper. In: Som PM, Bergeron RT, editors. Head and Neck Imaging, 2nd ed. St. Louis: Mosby; 1991: 747–813.

14. Moseley IF, Sanders MD. Computerized Tomography in Neuro-ophthalmology. London: Chapman and Hall; 1982.

15. Rootman J. Diseases of the Orbit: A Multidisciplinary Approach, 2nd ed. Philadephia: Lippincott Williams and Wilkins; 2003.

Neurogenic tumors

Cameron F Parsa

Optic nerve tumors

Optic glioma

Juvenile gliomas (World Health Organization Grade I pilocytic astrocytomas) consist of a surplus of the astrocytic glial cells supporting axons. They are the most frequent intracranial tumor to affect the visual pathways in children. They may occur anywhere in the brain, however, and are present in approximately 25% of young children with neurofibromatosis type 1 (NF1),[1] itself the most commonly identified pathogenetic mutation in the general population with an incidence of approximately 1/3000. Most of these lesions are detectable by magnetic resonance imaging (MRI) in infancy, but only a fraction ever cause clinical symptoms. A roughly equivalent number of patients also present clinically with juvenile optic gliomas, but do *not* have NF1. Recent evidence reaffirms earlier notions that these tumors represent glial cell hamartomas.[2,3] Grade II and higher malignant gliomas of the anterior visual pathway that behave more aggressively, including glioblastoma multiforme, are recognized in adults[4,5] and may occasionally occur in children;[6–9] their diagnosis and treatment, altogether different, is not addressed here.

Visual pathway gliomas

Gliomas may arise anywhere along the visual pathways. Multifocality is common, and an initial optic nerve presentation later followed by chiasmal involvement should not be assumed to necessarily represent invasion.[10] Multifocal growth, as well as regression, may occur contemporaneously or at different times with either or both optic nerves affected, sparing chiasm, or vice versa (Fig. 23.1).[11] Hence surgical resection of a distal optic nerve tumor may not necessarily prevent later growth more proximally.[10,12] Patients with optic gliomas should

be examined for signs of neurofibromatosis in the eye (in particular melanocytic iris hamartomas termed Sakurai-Lisch nodules), orbit (neurofibromas, sphenoid bone defects), and skin (multiple café-au-lait spots, neurofibromas). Family members should also be examined.

Though some have believed that gliomas occurring in the presence of NF1 have a better visual prognosis compared to those occurring sporadically, such impressions are due to selection biases; since most NF1-associated gliomas are detected by surveillance MRI scans ordered for asymptomatic NF1 patients, many clinically insignificant tumors are thus detected. Individuals without NF1, on the other hand, present to the physician only when they have large, symptomatic masses. Overall survival for those with NF1-associated gliomas, moreover, is worse, since these patients have an underlying mutation in the NF1 tumor suppressor gene, they tend to develop, for reasons not well understood,[13] other, non-neural crest derived, tumors, particularly soft-tissue sarcomas,[14,15] and myelogenous disorders.

Presentation

The age of presentation ranges from birth to between 4 and 12 years generally; the vast majority have presented by 20 years of age.[16] Gliomas involving the intraorbital portion of the nerve may present with axial proptosis[12] (Fig. 23.2). For reasons yet unclear, the enlarged intraorbital portion of the tumor has a predisposition to kink and deflect downward, thus producing an upward rotation of the posterior aspect of the globe (Fig. 23.3A,B): this can produce a nearly pathognomonic feature of mild proptosis in a child with hypotropia or limitation of elevation.[12] Older patients may verbalize visual loss with color vision and field defects.

Chiasmal gliomas may present slightly later with bilateral visual loss, although they may also be discovered during investigation of hydrocephalus, disconjugate nystagmus (see Fig. 23.1), endocrine dysfunction,[2] or in a hitherto asymptomatic patient via neuroimaging studies (Fig. 23.4).[17] The presenting history is usually of slowly deteriorating vision, though in rare cases sudden visual loss can result from hemorrhage within the tumor.[18,19]

Gliomas affecting the chiasm and the nerves asymmetrically may cause a dissociated nystagmus mimicking spasmus nutans.[20] In children, asymmetric nystagmus, particularly in the presence of optic atrophy, poor feeding, or hydrocephalus,

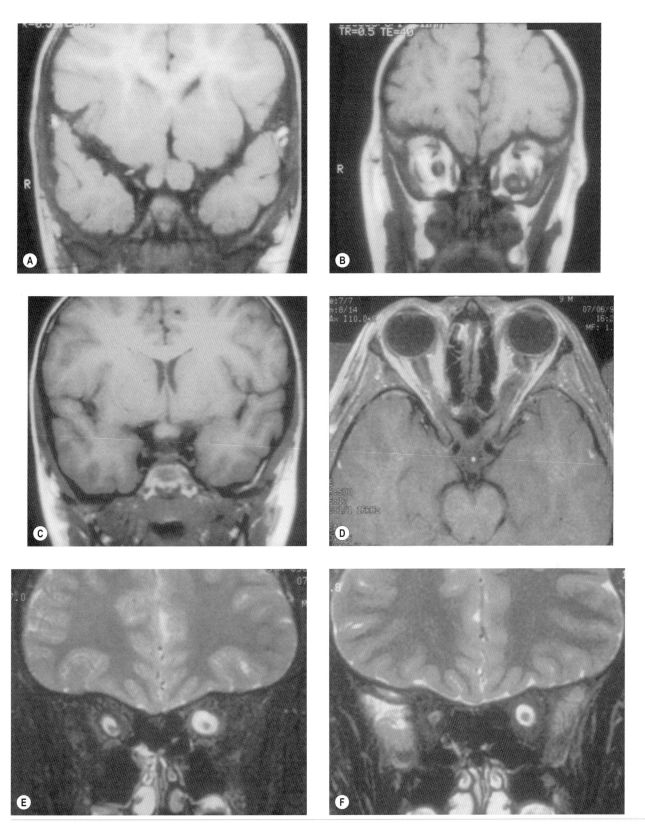

Fig. 23.1 Multifocality of tumoral growth and regression. (A) MRI in a 5-month-old boy with nystagmus and head nodding reveals enlargement of the chiasm, more prominent on the left. (B) Concomitant, bilateral, optic nerve enlargement is also present, more pronounced on the left. A prominent rim of low-signal intensity surrounds a central core of higher signal intensity, greater on the left, the so-called pseudo-CSF sign. (C) MRI 5 years later shows marked spontaneous reduction in the size of the chiasmal portion of the tumor, with the left side now smaller than the right. While the nystagmus had resolved, optic nerve involvement remained unchanged and visual acuity was 20/20 OD and 20/400 OS. (D) MRI after contrast 3 years later shows the chiasm to now be essentially normal in size and signal intensity. (D,E) Both optic nerves, however, still remain unchanged in size, displaying prominent tubular enlargement with downward kinking. Trace optic disk atrophy was present in the right eye with normal acuity, visual field and color vision, but marked disk atrophy was present in the left eye, with acuity decreased now to counting fingers at two feet despite spontaneous shrinkage and normalization in size of the chiasmal portion of the tumor. (F) MRI another 3 years later showed marked reduction bilaterally of the orbital perineural arachnoidal hyperplasia, with no further changes in vision. The "pseudo-CSF" sign seen here notwithstanding, a genetics evaluation of the boy and his family failed to detect any other evidence for NF1. (Patient of the University of California San Francisco Medical Center.)

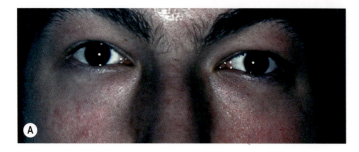

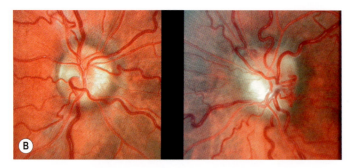

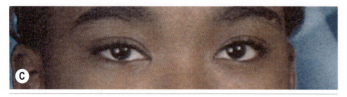

Fig 23.2 15 year old boy with proptosis in the left eye; left eye with optic disc pallor, swelling and optocilliary shunt vessels. Note the right eye has optic atrophy.

is suggestive of chiasmal glioma with or without posterior extension into the optic tracts (see Fig. 23.1).

Involvement of the hypothalamus, whether primary or secondary, can produce various endocrine abnormalities. Precocious puberty is often present in children with chiasmal glioma.[17] Reduced growth and sexual maturation, diabetes insipidus, and obesity may also occur. In infancy, there may be extreme wasting, reduced development, and often the vertical or asymmetric rotary nystagmus mimicking spasmus nutans, an association known as Russell diencephalic syndrome.[6,21]

Optic disk pallor may be noted if there is poor vision. Optociliary shunt vessels are present only if the tumor is in proximity to the globe with swelling of the optic disk compressing the central retinal vein. However, many of these overgrowths of glial cells which are intrinsic to the visual pathway do not significantly affect vision and remain clinically silent (see Fig. 23.4). Visual acuity does not correlate to tumor size or growth; vision can remain unaffected by large uniform tumor involvement along much of the visual pathway, or be extremely compromised by a small irregular growth, or regression, distorting axons focally.[22] Hence, findings from visual evoked potential testing are generally not of use. In the absence of visual symptoms, visual pathway gliomas are rarely identified by fundus examination alone.

Radiographic features

Since the hamartomatous overgrowth of the astrocytic glial cells is intrinsic to the visual pathways, the usual contours of involved structures are preserved. As a result, the radiographic appearances are generally so characteristic that biopsy is not needed to make a diagnosis. Biopsy, moreover, carries a risk of ocular or visual morbidity and is frequently misleading in optic nerve glioma since there may be reactive changes in the surrounding arachnoid similar to, and misinterpreted as, nerve sheath meningioma.[23,24]

MRI (Figs 23.1, 23.4, and 23.5) is thus the modality of choice for evaluation and follow-up. MRI reveals a smooth fusiform optic nerve enlargement with variable gadolinium contrast enhancement. Due to the soft nature of the tumor and its elongation,[25] the optic nerve is commonly kinked in the immediate retrobulbar zone (Figs 23.1, 23.3, and 23.5), a finding which helps to differentiate glioma from the rarer, but stiffer, extrinsic and generally more damaging childhood optic nerve sheath meningioma.[26] Intraorbital optic nerve gliomas found in NF1 also often possess a characteristic feature: a superimposed reactive arachnoid proliferation tied to mucinous accumulation in the perineural subarachnoid space (Fig. 23.6).[10,23] T2-weighted images of NF1 optic nerve gliomas thus much more commonly show an area of high signal intensity (corresponding to the mucinous/high water content element), the so-called "pseudo-CSF" sign, surrounding a central core of lower signal intensity (the intraneural tumor) (see Figs 23.1 and 23.3).[25,27,28] Chiasmal gliomas are noted as an enlarged suprasellar mass with recognizable contours preserved, that may be accompanied by a diagnostic contiguous enlargement of the optic nerve or tract. The adjacent hypothalamus may also be involved.

Computed tomography (CT) scanning reveals a similar smooth fusiform optic nerve enlargement with variable contrast enhancement, but minor degrees of enlargement are relatively difficult to detect. Calcification rarely and only minimally occurs in glioma, whereas it is a common feature of meningioma. When an intracanalicular glioma is present, there is only smooth enlargement of the optic canal, whereas with meningiomas, there can be reactive infiltrative changes in adjacent bone.

Biological behavior and management

By definition, grade I pilocytic gliomas possess only rare, if any, mitotic figures and the majority of tumors demonstrate overall stability[2,14,29] with only limited growth potential during development. Unlike higher grade gliomas, they do not show p53 mutations.[30] They grow mainly by accumulation of mucosubstance, often with cystic enlargement and hydration.[10,29] A few, however, may also show enlargement of the solid tumor component.[31] On the other hand, spontaneous regression may also occur,[11] and once a tumor is discovered, it is as likely to shrink given enough time, as it is to grow initially.[11,32-36] Although as many as 25% of children with NF1 have gliomas,[1,17] such incidences have not been noted in adults with NF1, and virtually no new cases present in adults with, or without, NF1. Misleading terminology is sometimes used to describe mostly adult and grade II and higher gliomas as "pilocytic-like," "atypical pilocytic," or "pilocytic with anaplastic features."[3,8] However, spontaneous anaplastic degeneration of grade I pilocytic astrocytomas does not occur. Reports purporting to show such changes have described only transformations iatrogenic in origin, secondary to the late effects of radiation.[3] Gliomas also do not metastasize in the usual sense; during infancy, rarely, "drop metastases", often asymptomatic in nature, may occur to the leptomeninges via the cerebrospinal fluid (CSF)

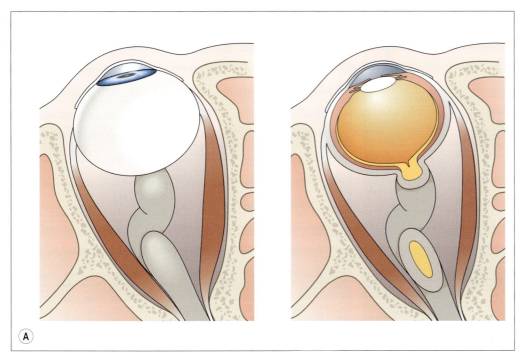

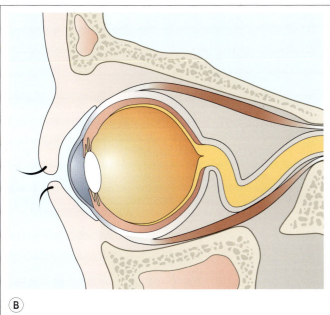

Fig. 23.3A,B Optic nerve kinking. The tubular thickening and elongation of the optic nerve that occurs with glial growth causes the nerve, for reasons not yet entirely clear, to generally kink downward within the orbit, causing the posterior aspect of a slightly proptotic globe to rotate upward. Thus, the clinical presentation of a slightly proptotic, hypotropic eye in a child is nearly pathognomonic for optic nerve glioma. The kinking, which can appear as a nerve discontinuity on axial MRI sections, also serves as a diagnostic aid. The drawings also depict perineural arachnoidal gliomatosis often seen in neurofibromatosis 1. (Reproduced with permission from Imes RK, Hoyt WF. Magnetic resonance imaging signs of optic nerve glioma in neurofibromatosis 1. Am J Ophthalmol 1991; 111: 729–34.)

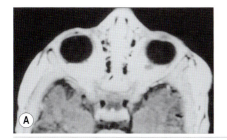
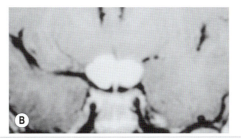
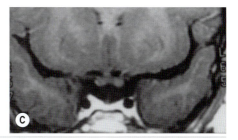

Fig. 23.4 Postnatal tumoral growth and regression. (A) MRI first revealed a normal chiasm and optic pathways in this 3-month-old boy with normal vision, but with multiple café-au-lait spots. (B) Two years later, however, MRI revealed the growth of a large enhancing mass respecting chiasmal contours. Bilateral optic nerve involvement was also noted extending beyond the orbital apex on separate images. Visual acuity, nonetheless, was 20/20 OU with no relative afferent pupillary defect despite trace optic disk atrophy noted in the left eye. (C) Another 2 years later, MRI demonstrated a markedly decreased tumor size, with essentially no enhancement. Visual acuity remained 20/20 OU, while the boy stayed healthy and quite bright. (Patient of the University of California San Francisco Medical Center.)

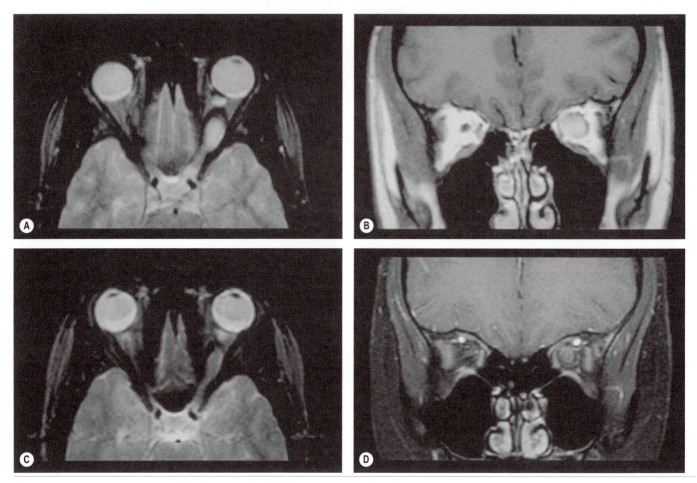

Fig. 23.5 Spontaneous regression of optic nerve glioma in the 14-year-old girl depicted in Figure 23.2. (A) MRI shows a fusiform enlargement of the left optic nerve, hyperintense and homogeneous in signal intensity from the globe up to the chiasm with intervening kink downward creating an apparent discontinuity. The left globe is proptotic and there is widening of the left neural foramen. (B) MRI reveals marked enlargement of the left intraorbital optic nerve, with prominent and homogeneous signal enhancement. (C) MRI 1 year later shows shrinkage of the optic nerve tumor along its entire course, with decrease in signal intensity. The left globe is no longer proptotic. (D) MRI shows clear reduction in optic nerve diameter, with only trace signal enhancement centrally. This girl had been scheduled to receive radiation therapy, but 1 week before this was to be initiated, she reported improved vision. Her planned radiation therapy sessions were cancelled while her vision improved from counting fingers at 4 feet, to 20/15 over the course of the year. Had the patient's radiation therapy been scheduled a week earlier, her improvement would have erroneously been attributed to the treatment. (Patient of the Johns Hopkins Hospital). Anecdotal observations of tumor shrinkage noted following radiation or chemotherapy, particularly when noted long after termination of therapy, are likely due to the phenomenon of spontaneous regression.

passageways after surgical manipulations during ventricular shunt placement, or less commonly, after hemorrhagic cystic degeneration and rupture,[37-40] much as occurs with such lesions noted intraocularly.[41] Given these characteristics, these tumors fulfill the criteria for, and are best described as, glial hamartomas.[2,3,42-45]

Growth of gliomas is a function of both cellular proliferative *and* apoptotic activity; both may be high, or both low, reflecting a steady-state function within a tumor that demonstrates clinical stability.[30,46] For these reasons, histopathologic examinations assessing proliferative activity alone,[8,9,47,48] without also acertaining the rate of apoptosis, cannot provide information of prognostic utility.[11,43] Inherently limited biopsy sampling sizes for tumors that are known to be heterogeneous both in their composition and in their growth patterns and phases, further limits the prognostic potential for such approaches.

Since mitoses are very rare, if at all present, no clinically significant benefit should be expected from antimitotic ionizing radiation beyond that expected from background spontaneous regression in the natural evolution of these tumors.

Due to the severe adverse effects, moreover, of radiation on incompletely myelinated and still developing brain – including severe mental and growth retardation, psychiatric problems, vascular occlusions, and the induction of second tumors – attempts at treatment via ionizing radiation are now contraindicated in children.[29,32,33,49,50] For similar reasons, antimitotic chemotherapy also offers no benefits. In previous studies reporting minor treatment effects, investigators failed to stratify results for those with "low-grade gliomas" into those with grade I pilocytic gliomas versus those with grade II fibrillary astrocytomas. As with initial reports ascribing benefits to radiation therapy, these studies also do not take into account the acknowledged fact of spontaneous regression[11,42,51] and often include instances of tumor regression long after the cessation of therapy as a treatment effect.[52] Loss of vision, moreover, is used in many treatment protocols as a measure to initiate chemotherapy. Declining acuity, however, does not correlate with tumor enlargement[22,29] and can also result from the spontaneous regression of tumors distorting nerve axons. Subsequent immediate radiographic evidence demonstrating tumor

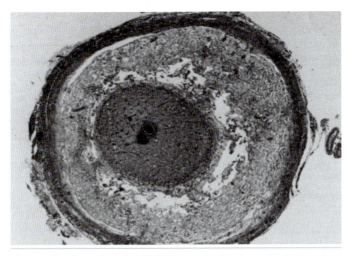

Fig. 23.6 Perineural arachnoidal gliomatosis. The hyperplastic pia and subarachnoid tissues form a dense mass which can mimic meningioma around the atrophic optic nerve. The nerve's peripheral border is arachnoid proper, which shows no reaction of its own. An explanation for this phenomenon may be high protein content serum containing growth factors exuded into the subarachnoid space, providing a nutrient medium for the connective tissue cells. (From Lindenberg R, Walsh FB, Sacks JG. Neuropathology of Vision: An Atlas. Philadelphia: Lea and Febiger; 1973: 77.) Such overgrowth would be more prominent whenever there is an innate tendency for overgrowth of neural tissue or sheaths, such as when there is a mutation in the NF1 tumor suppressor gene. The high water content of this tissue creates the so-called "pseudo-CSF" sign noted on T2-weighted MRI which, in turn, is often considered a radiologic indicator for NF1-associated optic nerve gliomas, though not specifically so. (From Lindenberg R, Walsh FB, Sacks JG. Neuropathology of Vision: An Atlas. Philadelphia: Lea and Febiger; 1973: 130–2.)

size reduction then is erroneously attributed to an effect of treatment.[22] More recent surveys and other studies, some of them specifically addressing in part some of these concerns, have confirmed the lack of beneficial treatment effects in the face of demonstrated toxicities.[35,36,53]

Optic nerve gliomas situated anterior to the chiasm may appear as threatening to involve this structure (see Fig. 23.5). Despite radiologic appearances, convincing evidence is lacking to show such evolution often occurs or that surgical excision of such tumors[24] will prevent anticipated contralateral eye involvement; one may be witnessing instead multicentric nests of cells within different phases of growth (Fig. 23.1) rather than a true progression and invasion of cells moving forward.[10] Resection of the intracranial portion of an optic nerve near the chiasm, furthermore, can endanger chiasmal blood supply, with spreading necrosis. Surgical decompression of an expanded nerve sheath, however, with aspiration of perineural mucoid contents can be considered if visual obscurations are due to mucoid accumulation and hydration. If disfiguring proptosis is present and there is evidence of steady tumoral enlargement on sequential MRI scans, with total absence of the intraocular nerve fiber layer, it is certainly reasonable to surgically remove the intraorbital portion of the nerve, preserving posterior ciliary blood supply and globe for cosmetic purposes.[2,54-56]

With a lack of beneficial radiative or antimitotic chemotherapeutic effects, and with limited indications for surgical intervention of visual pathway gliomas, the emphasis of management must therefore be conservative. A reasonable approach is to follow clinical symptomatology, addressing secondary issues as they may arise, i.e. placing a shunt to deal with an obstructive

hydrocephalus, addressing endocrine abnormalities associated with hypothalmic/chiasmal gliomas, or instituting penalization therapy if a strabismus is present. In rare settings where exophytic growth is noted, when draining symptomatic cysts or mucinoid accumulations may be possible, or whenever there is no hope for visual recovery due to total absence of intraocular nerve fiber layer, excisional surgery can be considered. A comprehensive discussion should take place with the family to ensure their understanding of the lack of efficacy of antimitotic regimens and of the not-inconsequential adverse effects they induce. It follows that frequent neuroimaging in those known to harbor a tumor may not be warranted. Use of the more precise term "hamartoma," rather than the broader designation of "tumor," which is psychologically more threatening and evocative of neoplasms, can be helpful.[42,43] In children who also have NF1, pointing out the melanocytic hamartoma Sakurai-Lisch nodules that grow postnatally on the irides can serve as a helpful educational analogy. More often than not, parents are relieved to hear that their child may not need as many repeated examinations, including MRI scans under sedation, and that they need not agree to some recommendations for current antimitotic treatments that, even by reports of their proponents, provide mediocre results with non-negligible adverse effects, in order to be considered responsible parents. Despite the relatively decreased cavitary space available for the expansion of intracranial masses, until efficacious treatment modalities become available, glial hamartomas which occur either intracranially or intraorbitally should be approached in much the same conservative way that ophthalmologists have to date managed those that occur intraocularly.[2,42,43]

Screening for visual pathway gliomas

Routine neuroimaging is no longer suggested in asymptomatic patients suspected of having NF1 to detect asymptomatic glioma. While this may help to secure the diagnosis of NF1, it does little to assist in patient management.[57]

Meningiomas

Based on autopsy studies, as many as 2–3% of the general population eventually harbors an incidental meningioma. However, meningiomas are very rare in childhood, and only slightly more common in the teenage years. An extrinsic tumor of the neural covering, meningioma results from proliferation of meningothelial cap cells of the arachnoid villi and may arise particularly in association with NF2 (as many as 25% to 40% of children with meningiomas have NF2, which may be diagnosed only later). With respect to the visual system, they may occur within the sheath of the optic nerve, or from the dura of the sphenoid bone, for example, affecting the sphenoid wing and/or parasellar region. Optic nerve sheath tumors, particularly when intracanalicular, present with early visual loss and relatively little mass effect.

Optic nerve sheath meningiomas

In general, they are the second most common optic nerve tumor after gliomas, and the most common tumor of the optic nerve sheath. Unlike the well-described female predilection in adults, a gender difference is not noted in children. This should perhaps not be surprising, given the frequent presence of estrogen and progesterone receptors on these tumors and the diminished gender-differentiated serum levels of estrogen and progesterone prior to puberty. Growth may be faster during infancy (likely a result of other hormonal influences), whereas those who present in the second decade have a clinical course that approaches that of adults with slowly progressive visual loss and mild proptosis.[58] The histologic subtypes do not appear to differ in childhood meningiomas,[59] but their tendency to grow through the dura makes extraocular muscle involvement relatively frequent[56] while intermittent strabismus or diplopia can also otherwise occur as a result of splinting of the optic nerve by the relatively rigid tumor. Circumferential expansion of the tumor around the nerve generally results in a compressive optic neuropathy, though the tumor may sometimes also invade the nerve directly along its pial septae. Duction-induced obscurations may occur at first, followed by visual loss as the tumor enlarges, with progressive constriction of the visual field. An afferent pupillary defect, as well as disk edema or pallor and prominent optociliary shunt vessels, may be present. Although the latter may also occur with optic nerve gliomas, since development of these collateral channels depends on persistent, unyielding compression of the central retinal vein, in general, prominent optociliary vessels associated with disk atrophy are more suggestive of a meningioma in proximity to the optic globe (sometimes referred to, in this setting, as Hoyt-Spencer vessels).[60]

Investigation

MRI with fat suppression and gadolinium contrast will nearly always reveal the tumor and is the modality of choice for defining its extent.[61] MRI will demonstrate an intracanalicular and intracranial involvement more clearly than CT scan. For tumors that extend close to, but not up to the globe, a perioptic "cyst" is often noted.[62,63] This represents a distal expansion of the uninvolved and softer dural sheath, secondary to perineural CSF accumulated, as noted by the author, during normal diurnal intracranial pressure spikes, including those normally induced by changes in position and during Valsalva maneuvers. When cerebrospinal pressure decreases following a spike, the tighter and less elastic encapsulated sheath involved by tumor collapses first, reducing the perineural space and limiting fluid egress, much like a ball-valve mechanism. The distally expanded dural sheath reservoir created, the so-called "cyst," contains CSF reflective of the highest diurnal intracranial pressure, rather than its average. If this compartment retains a pressure higher than the average intraocular pressure, papilledema will develop despite the absence of elevated pressures measured in the physiologic CSF cisterns. When a tumor involves dura closer to the globe, cystic dural expansion may no longer be evident, though the same mechanism, with similar pressure differentials, may still be at play.

Although routine MRI of the intraorbital portion of the optic nerve may not reveal the classical findings of "tram-line" calcification that could be evident on a CT scan, calcification is only present in 50% at the time of diagnosis (Figs. 23.7).[26] Since meningiomas may be quite vascular, enhancement with intravenous contrast and tumor blush on angiography are common features of diagnosis, unlike glioma where they are rare.[6] Furthermore, there may be straightening of the nerve due to tumoral stiffness rather than kinking, a feature common to gliomas. Some investigators have drawn attention to the radiologic similarity of the perineural variant

of non-specific orbital inflammation (such as sarcoid disease) and optic nerve sheath meningioma.[64]

The best diagnostic modality for bony change is CT scan, which may demonstrate the irregular hyperostosis underlying the tumor as it infiltrates the Haversian canal system, inciting hyperostosis and bone proliferation. This can be very useful to detect pneumosinus dilatans, considered pathognomonic for meningiomas located in the intracanalicular area and which themselves may not always be directly visible by either CT or MRI.

Biopsy is not very helpful in differentiating meningioma from glioma, due to the presence of reactive meningeal hyperplasia in the latter, which appears similar to meningioma.[12,23] It should, however, be possible to distinguish these two entities on clinical and radiologic grounds alone.[26,65]

Treatment

The tumor may progress very slowly or even remain stable in size for an extended period of time; since there is no metastatic potential, it is reasonable to observe the tumor to establish the pattern of growth in individual cases and, in children, to allow for further brain myelination and maturation prior to any invasive treatment. Left alone in the long term, however, optic nerve sheath meningiomas almost always result in complete visual loss in the affected eye, and the clinical course is faster in children.[26]

Limited indications exist for surgery. Unless the bulk of the tumor is exophytic outside the dura and away from the nerve, surgical excision invariably leads to blindness due to concomitant disruption and removal of the intricate and delicate arachnoidal and pial vessels which feed the optic nerve as well as the tumor (Fig. 23.8). In special instances, particularly when there have been obscurations on eye movements, fenestration of the nerve sheath along with decompression of a perioptic cyst, *but without removal of the tumor*, may improve vision, though the effect may be relatively short-lasting.[62,63] Nonetheless, surgical excision is the procedure of choice for those with already blind (absent intraocular nerve fiber layer) and disfiguring proptotic eyes, to remove the intraorbital portion of the tumor, leaving the globe and ciliary blood supply intact.[55,56] Recurrences following surgery, many years later, may nonetheless occur with cavernous sinus extensions.

Fortunately, over the past several decades, hyperfractionated confocal stereotactic radiotherapy has proven to be an effective and lasting treatment modality in adults. While it was initially believed that ionizing radiation would prove ineffective against such slow-growing tumors with uncommon mitoses, empiric treatment has proven otherwise.[66,67] Because of the exquisite monitoring of optic nerve function that is possible via visual perimetry, experience with highly focussed ionizing beams to the orbit, minimizing damage to the ocular and brain structures, has conclusively demonstrated the surprising efficacy of this treatment modality, despite the paucity of correlative post-treatment tumor changes visible radiographically. Since no improvement has been noted with equivalent antimitotic chemotherapy,[58] it is presumably the effects of radiation on the tumor vasculature which effectuates this beneficial response. This response, which may be noted just days after treatment, argues strongly for a decompressive effect via vascular deturgescence.[65,68,69] The optimal radiation dose for this modality, however, has not yet been determined in adults, and data is even more limited in children; total doses initially selected

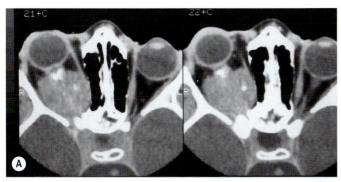

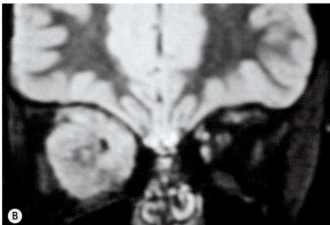

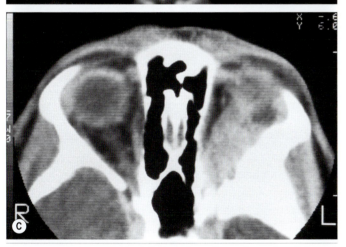

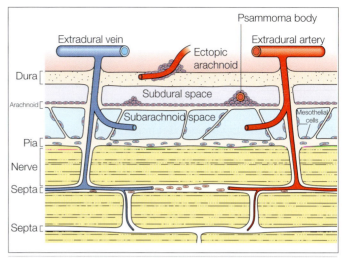

Fig. 23.8 Vascular anatomy of the optic nerve and meninges. Diagram showing the relationship of meninges and small blood vessels to optic nerve fiber bundles and septa. Dural bridges carrying blood vessels connect with the septal system after crossing arachnoid and meningeal spaces. The capillaries of the nerve fiber bundles stay within the septa. Blood supply and drainage take place via extradural vessels. Ectopic arachnoid is not an unusual finding. (From Lindenberg R, Walsh FB, Sacks JG. Neuropatholology of Vision: An Atlas. Philadelphia: Lea and Febiger; 1973: 77.) Although an increase in collateral blood supply from the central retinal artery can allow for the sacrifice of compromised septal vessels when there is slow tumoral growth in the distal portion of the nerve, surgical removal of the meningeal coverings, particularly in areas where no tumor has been present, or more proximally, where no central retinal vessel exists to supply collateral blood flow, will inevitably disrupt functional feeding vessels to the nerve and cause immediate injury.

Fig. 23.7 Orbital meningiomas. (A) Optic nerve meningioma in a 5-year-old boy. CT scan showing some "tram-track" calcification around the distal portion of the optic nerve and orbital expansion on the right. (B) MRI of same patient showing the clear differentiation between the peripheral tumor and the axial optic nerve though calcium is not demonstrated. (C) Sphenoid wing meningioma in a 9-year-old boy: CT scan showing marked hyperostosis on the left. Mild lid swelling and proptosis were also present.

ranged from 54 to 60 Gy, the maximal dose tolerable before significant radiation-induced optic neuropathy or retinopathy occurs. However, a comparison of the radiosurgical series of basal meningiomas over the years shows a trend toward lower treatment doses associated with unchanged excellent tumor control rates, but reduced incidence of radiation-induced adverse side-effects.[70] For optic nerve sheath meningiomas, however, hypofractioned "Gamma knife" delivery should currently be avoided; while the smaller single doses provided (initially 16 Gy, now down to doses of 10–12 Gy) have been as effective for basal meningiomas[70] as the much higher total doses administered over the course of weeks with hyperfractionated therapy (45–54 Gy), a large single dose radiation exposure can cause significant toxicity to sensitive structures such as the optic nerve. Since improvement in visual fields can also be recorded long before hyperfractionated treatment is completed,[71] it seems most logical, particularly for children whose immature brains are far more prone to adverse effects of radiation, to administer such therapy, if considered absolutely necessary, only gradually until an anticipated improvement in visual function is attained, rather than treating empirically with near-maximally tolerated doses. Such improvement can be monitored via visual perimetry if the child is old enough, or alternatively, via visual evoked potentials and other means. Should neuroimaging ever demonstrate recurrent growth, additional cumulative doses of radiation may then be considered. A decline in vision following initial improvement, however, should not necessarily be equated with recurrent tumoral growth.[72] Though a delayed decline in vision can be a result of radiation neuropathy, when other signs for this do not exist, some individuals may respond to optic nerve sheath fenestration.[72] It seems plausible that in such instances the ball-valve mechanism for perineural CSF flow described above may be occurring within a compartment enclosed by the more rigid tumoral nerve sheath that will not show expansion on MRI, and at a distance more removed from the globe where congestion of axoplasmic flow can not be visualized ophthalmoscopically as disk edema.

One should also recall that the risk of radiation-induced malignancy includes a dose-dependent inducement of delayed secondary meningiomas. However, even these tumors are sensitive to radiation therapy so this possibility alone should not dissuade clinicians from potentially sight-preserving treatment.[73] Given the lack of other demonstrated effective treatment modalities,[74] we recommend the use of hyperfractionated conformal stereotactic radiation therapy in older children, titrated, however, only to monitored levels of anticipated visual recovery, rather than to maximally tolerated doses, in order to minimize the very serious potential side-effects on developing brain. In younger children, observation and surgical tactics such as nerve sheath fenestration to delay eventual radiative therapy until brain myelination is complete may be advisable.

Extraoptic intracranial involvement in young patients – sites of ophthalmic relevance are the sphenoid wing (see Fig. 23.7C), suprasellar area, and olfactory groove – should prompt either very close observation or total excision of the lesion. The ophthalmic features reflect the position of the tumor, since those situated medially present with visual loss, cranial nerve palsies, and signs and symptoms of venous obstruction at the orbital apex, while those arising laterally cause mass effect and swelling in the temporalis fossa. Very rarely, meningiomas can arise at extradural sites in children.[75] If total excision is not possible, continued monitoring and observation are warranted until the child may be old enough to receive low-dose adjuvant radiation to preserve visual function and arrest tumor progression, thereby minimizing severe secondary cognitive effects that can otherwise result. Again, it is recommended that any such radiative therapy be minimized by titrating to anticipated recovery of visual potential, rather than by providing the high empiric doses thus far given to adults, which have been based on maximally tolerable tissue dosages. To strike the right balance in determining treatment protocols, with or without radiation, and maximize visual potential while minimizing risks and side-effects, a careful, customized approach to each pediatric patient is necessary.

Rare optic nerve tumors in childhood

Leukemic infiltration of the optic nerve traditionally has a grave systemic prognosis, although with combined radiotherapy and chemotherapy the prognosis is greatly improved when the infiltration is prelaminar and the optic disk has a fluffy appearance with edema and hemorrhage without marked visual loss. Retrolaminar involvement may result in moderate disk swelling but profound visual loss and constitutes an ophthalmic emergency.[76-78] Disk swelling may be present either due to direct infiltration of the nerve, or to elevated intracranial pressure, or both.

Tumors of the optic disk such as melanocytoma, angiomatous malformations, or glial hamartoma (as seen in tuberous sclerosis, or in isolation) may involve the very anterior parts of the optic nerve. Bilateral optic disk gliomas are rare, but they are a sign of NF2.[79] Ganglioma, ganglioglioma,[80] inflammatory lesions, aneurysms, histiocytosis, sarcomas, and other rare entities have also been described.[81,82] Medulloepithelioma is a tumor that arises from the medullary epithelium of the optic vesicle and is much more commonly found in the ciliary body. It can affect the optic nerve head and may extend into the substance of the optic nerve. Both benign and malignant forms have been described. Margo and Kincaid[83] found a vascular

malformation in the retrolaminar portion of two eyes removed for suspicion of retinoblastoma; one eye had a neuroblastic tumor and the other a form of retinal dysplasia.

The importance of many of these rare optic nerve tumors is in the differential diagnosis of the much more common optic nerve glioma, for which biopsy is rarely performed.

Schwannoma

Schwannomas (formerly known as neurilemmomas or neurinomas) are well-circumscribed benign, encapsulated, ovoid, peripheral nerve slow-growing tumors that arise almost exclusively from the Schwann cells of peripheral nerve sheath (Fig. 23.9). They are rare in childhood, generally noted in young to middle-aged patients. Like all tumors involving

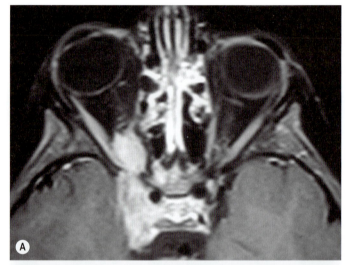

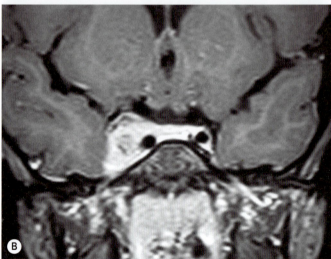

Fig. 23.9 Schwannoma. (A,B) These MRI scans demonstrate a lesion of the gasserian ganglion in a child with NF1 that presented at 19 months of age with right exotropia and a partially dilated right pupil. He had reduced vision due to amblyopia. These images showing heterogeneous tumor signal, corresponding to Antoni A and Antoni B histologic cellular patterns, support a diagnosis of schwannoma versus neurofibroma. The boy developed a ptosis as part of his third nerve palsy, and he was observed and followed clinically and with imaging without progression for 4 years. (Patient of the University of British Columbia.)

neural coverings, they are more common in NF2, but they are also somewhat common in NF1. Unlike neurofibromas, which also arise from Schwann cells and are more common in children with NF1, schwannomas have specific Antoni A areas (frequent nuclear palisading arrangements in a compact and solid structure) and Antoni B areas (a looser and more vascular myxomatous structure), with the latter imparting a heterogeneous signal on MRI which can mimic cavernoma. The sensory nerves are much more frequently affected and thus schwannomas most commonly present in the superior orbit, with a corresponding facial hypesthesia that may help in clinical diagnosis (pain is rare unless the tumor is large). Schwannomas of the ocular motor nerves, particularly the third nerve, are well recognized, however.

Orbital schwannoma generally presents with painless, insidious proptosis. Diplopia may result from third nerve involvement or compression by a tumor in the trigeminal ganglion (see Fig. 23.9). Schwannoma may also occur in the eyelid.[84] Progression tends to be slow and sometimes intermittent over a period of years. Since the tumor is derived from the Schwann cells and is thus typically located along the periphery of the nerve, the mass can be stripped away with meticulous dissection of the tumor and minimal damage to the nerve, though the looser Antoni B areas create a more friable structure making excision somewhat more fragmented.[85] With total excision, recurrence is rare.[56,84,85,86] Spontaneous regression[85] may also be more frequent than previously appreciated, as has recently been noted for vestibular schwannomas.[87] Radiation and chemotherapy are not indicated. Transformation into a malignant Schwann cell tumor is exceedingly rare in adults with many of these apparently trauma or surgically induced. For practical purposes, malignant transformation does not occur in childhood.

References

2. Hoyt WF, Baghdassarian SA. Optic glioma of childhood: natural history and rationale for conservative management. Br J Ophthalmol 1969; 53: 793–8.

3. Parsa CF, Givrad S. Juvenile pilocytic astrocytomas do not undergo spontaneous malignant transformation: grounds for designation as hamartomas. Br J Ophthalmol 2008; 92(1): 40–6.

8. Rodriguez FJ, Scheithauer BW, Burger PC, et al. Anaplasia in pilocytic astrocytoma predicts aggressive behavior. Am J Surg Pathol 2010;43(2):147–60.

10. Anderson DR, Spencer WH. Ultra structural and histochemical observations of optic nerve gliomas. Arch Ophthalmol 1970; 83: 324–35.

11. Parsa CF, Hoyt CS, Lesser RL, et al. Spontaneous regression of optic gliomas: thirteen cases documented by serial neuroimaging. Arch Ophthalmol 2001; 119: 516–29.

12. Wright JE, McDonald WI, Call NB. Management of optic nerve gliomas. Br J Ophthalmol 1980; 64: 545–52.

14. Imes RK, Hoyt WF. Childhood chiasmal gliomas: update on the fate of patients in the 1969 San Francisco study. Br J Ophthalmol 1986; 70: 179–82.

22. Parsa CF. Why visual function does not correlate with glioma size or growth. Arch Ophthalmol 2012; 130: 521–2.

23. Lindenberg R, Walsh FB, Sacks JG. Neuropathology of Vision: An Atlas. Philadelphia: Lea and Febiger; 1973: 130–2.

24. Wright JE, McNab AA, McDonald WI. Optic nerve glioma and the management of optic nerve tumours in the young. Br J Ophthalmol 1989; 73: 967–74.

29. Glaser JS, Hoyt WF, Corbett J. Visual morbidity with chiasmal glioma: long-term studies of visual fields in untreated and irradiated cases. Arch Ophthalmol 1971; 85: 3–12.

32. Smoots DW, Geyer JR, Lieberman DM, Berger MS. Predicting disease progression in childhood cerebellar astrocytoma. Childs Nerv Syst 1998; 14: 636–48.

33. Due-Tønnessen BJ, Helseth E, Scheie D, et al. Long-term outcome after resection of benign cerebellar astrocytomas in children and young adults (0–19 years): report of 110 consecutive cases. Pediatr Neurosurg 2002; 37: 71–80.

34. Palma L, Celli P, Mariottini A. Long-term follow-up of childhood cerebellar astrocytomas after incomplete resection with particular reference to arrested growth of spontaneous tumour regression. Acta Neurochir (Wien) 2004; 146: 581–88.

35. Dalla Via P, Opocher E, Pinello ML, et al. Visual outcome of a cohort of children with neurofibromatosis type 1 and optic pathway glioma followed by a pediatric neuro-oncology program. Neuro-Oncology 2007; 9(4): 430–7.

36. Moreno L, Bautista F, Ashley S, Duncan C, Zacharoulis S. Does chemotherapy affect the visual outcome in children with optic path glioma? A systematic review of the evidence. Eur J Cancer 2010; 46: 2253–9.

42. Parsa CF, Givrad S. Pilocytic astrocytomas as hamartomas: implications for treatment. Br J Ophthalmol 2008; 92(1): 3–6.

43. Parsa CF. Why optic gliomas should be called hamartomas. Ophthal Plast Reconstr Surg 2010; 26(6): 497.

49. Packer RJ, Savino PJ, Bilaniuk LT, et al. Chiasmatic gliomas of childhood: a reappraisal of natural history and effectiveness of cranial irradiation. Childs Brain 1983; 10: 393–403.

51. Schmandt SM, Packer RJ, Vezina LG, Jane J. Spontaneous regression of low-grade astrocytomas in childhood. Pediatr Neurosurg 2000; 32(3): 132–6.

52. Packer RJ, Sutton LN, Bilaniuk LT, et al. Treatment of chiasmatic/hypothalamic gliomas of childhood with chemotherapy: an update. Ann Neurol 1988; 23(1): 79–85.

57. Listernick R, Ferner RE, Liu GT, Gutmann DH. Optic pathway gliomas in neurofibromatosis 1: Controversies and recommendations. Ann Neurol 2007; 61: 189–98.

58. Traunecker H, Mallucci C, Grundy R, et al. Children's cancer and leukaemia group (CCLG): guidelines for the management of intracranial meningioma in children and young people. Br J Neurosurg 2008; 22(1): 13–25 [Commentary by Paul Eldridge p. 24–25].

59. Lee HBH, Garrity JA, Cameron JD, et al. Primary optic nerve sheath meningioma in children. Surv Ophthalmol 2008; 53(6): 543–58.

66. Wilson CB. Meningiomas: genetics, malignancy, and the role of radiation in induction and treatment. The Richard C. Schneider Lecture. J Neurosurg 1994; 81(5): 666–75.

67. Turbin RE, Thompson CR, Kennerdell JS, et al. A long-term visual outcome comparison in patients with optic nerve sheath meningioma managed with observation, surgery, radiotherapy, or surgery and radiotherapy. Ophthalmology 2002; 109(5): 890–9; discussion 899–900.

68. de Alba Campomanes AG, Larson DA, Horton JC. Immediate shrinkage of optociliary shunt vessels after fractionated external beam radiation for meningioma of the optic nerve sheath. AJNR 2008; 29: 1360.

72. Turbin RE, Wladis EJ, Frohman LP, et al. Role for surgery as adjuvant therapy in optic nerve sheath meningioma. Ophthal Plast Reconstr Surg 2006; 22(4): 278–82.

85. Gündüz K, Shields CL, Günalp I, et al. Orbital schwannoma: correlation of magnetic resonance imaging and pathologic findings. Graefes Arch Clin Exp Ophthalmol 2003; 241(7): 593–7.

87. Von Eckardstein KL, Beatty CW, Driscoll CLW, Link MJ. Spontaneous regression of vestibular schwannomas after resection of contralateral tumor in neurofibromatosis type 2. Report of 2 cases. J Neurosurg 2010; 112(1): 158–62.

Access the complete reference list online at
http://www.expertconsult.com

Orbital rhabdomyosarcoma

Jerry A Shields • Carol L Shields

Chapter contents

General considerations

Rhabdomyosarcoma (RMS) is a tumor of the orbit that has received considerable attention in the literature.[1-43] Historically, most children died from this neoplasm, but recent advances in diagnosis and treatment have led to marked improvement in prognosis.[2,3,13,28-33] The ocular region, particularly the orbital soft tissues, represents a major anatomic location for RMS. Orbital RMS is one of the few life-threatening diseases seen initially by the ophthalmologist. Prompt diagnosis and treatment can save the life of the patient. Therefore, eye care physicians should be aware of this tumor, recognize its clinical features, and refer the patient for prompt treatment. In rare instances, RMS has been known to arise in the eyelid, conjunctiva, and even the iris.[1] It can also occur in the orbit as a metastatic tumor from a distant location and can extend secondarily in the orbit from a primary neoplasm in the paranasal sinuses.[2,20] This chapter reviews primary orbital RMS, with emphasis on changing concepts in the diagnosis and management.

RMS is the most common primary orbital malignancy of childhood.[2] In our clinical series of 1264 patients, the 35 cases of orbital RMS accounted for 97% of myogenic tumors and 3% of all orbital lesions.[4] Orbital RMS generally occurs in the first two decades of life with a mean age at diagnosis of 8 years.[1,2] The tumor can originate primarily in the orbit or it can arise in the sinuses or nasal cavity and secondarily extend into the orbit.[2] Orbital RMS has been observed many years after orbital irradiation for retinoblastoma.[11]

Clinical features

Examples of clinical features, imaging studies, and pathology are shown in Figs 24.1 and 24.2 and are discussed in more detail subsequently.

Patients with orbital RMS generally present with proptosis (80–100%), globe displacement (80%), blepharoptosis (30–50%), conjunctival and eyelid swelling (60%), palpable mass (25%), and pain (10%).[1-3] Blepharoptosis is often the first sign in a patient with a superior orbital tumor (Fig. 24.1A). Slightly more advanced cases show downward and lateral displacement of the globe due to the usual superior or superonasal location of the mass in 70% (Fig. 24.1B).

Ophthalmoscopy can occasionally reveal choroidal folds, retinal venous tortuosity, and optic disc edema. Pain occurs in 10% of cases; it usually occurs in more advanced cases. Visual impairment in usually minimal until the tumor becomes advanced. A firm mass is palpable in subcutaneous tissues in about 25% of cases and a fleshy conjunctival component is sometimes visible. RMS in the orbit anteriorly and nasally may produce nasolacrimal duct obstruction, leading to a delay in diagnosis.[2]

Proptosis secondary to orbital RMS can develop more rapidly in newborns and infants. In older children and adults, it tends to have a slower course and rarely attains a large size. In regions where medical care is not readily available, RMS can attain immense proportions and destroy the eye.[2,3]

Diagnostic approaches

Any child in the first two decades of life who presents with symptoms and signs of an orbital mass should be considered to have RMS until proven otherwise. The child should have a detailed history, office examination, and imaging studies, particularly computed tomography (CT) or magnetic resonance imaging (MRI).

Computed tomography

CT is important in the assessment of children with suspected RMS, particularly for the detection of bony involvement by the tumor. With CT, the tumor appears in the early stages as a well-circumscribed, homogeneous, round to ovoid mass that

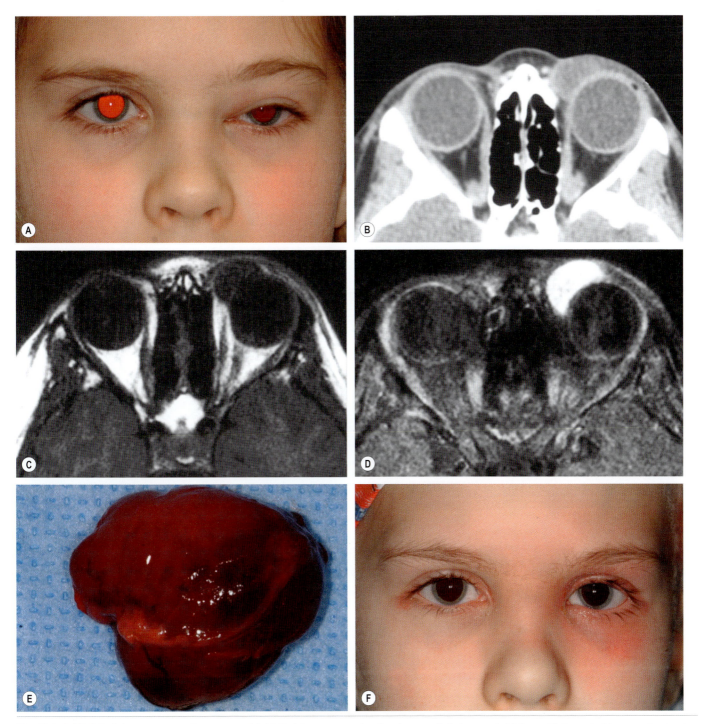

Fig. 24.1 Orbital rhabdomyosarcoma in a young girl. (A) Facial appearance showing downward displacement of left eye. (B) Computed tomography showing solid mass in orbit superonasally (C) MRI in T1-weighted image without enhancement depicting circumscribed orbital mass. (D) MRI in T1-weighted image with enhancement showing enhancement of the malignancy as well as the normal enhancement of extraocular muscles and lacrimal gland. (E) Intact tumor after surgical excision. (F) Slight erythema of periocular skin following irradiation.

is isodense to muscle (Fig. 24.1B). It is usually extraconal in location and is most often found in the superonasal aspect of the orbit. It is usually confined to the orbital soft tissues and does not arise from the extraocular muscles or bone, although it can cause displacement of the rectus muscles. The smaller tumors tend not to invade bone, but larger ones can occasionally erode bone and extend to the sinuses or nasopharynx.

Orbital RMS shows moderate to marked enhancement with contrast agents.[1,2]

Magnetic resonance imaging

MRI, which detects the extent of soft tissue involvement, is a valuable method for diagnosis and surgical planning

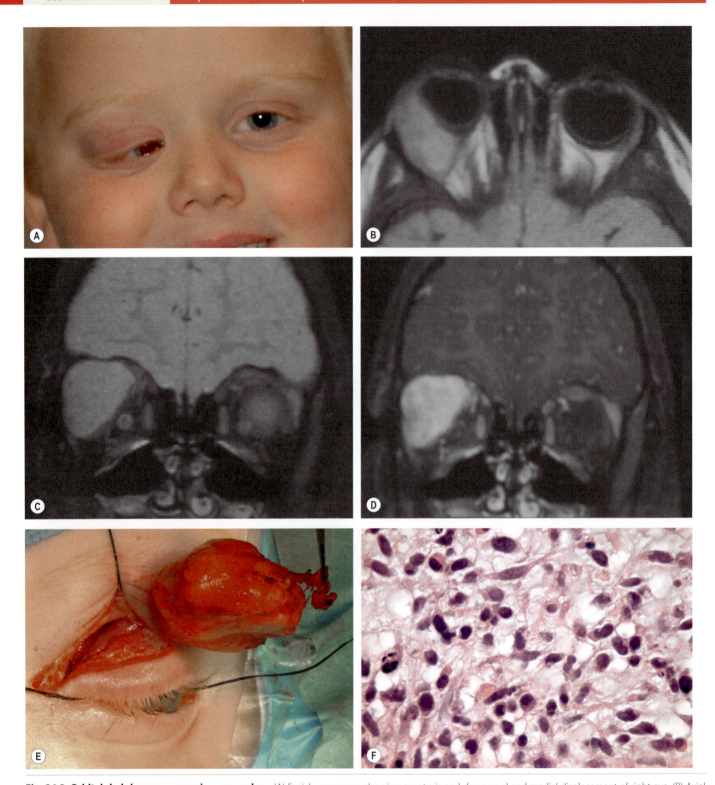

Fig. 24.2 Orbital rhabdomyosarcoma in a young boy. (A) Facial appearance showing proptosis and downward and medial displacement of right eye. (B) Axial MRI showing superotemporal mass. (C) Coronal MRI showing superotemporal mass. (D) Coronal MRI after gadolinium enhancement showing bright enhancement of the vascular malignancy. (E) Tumor removed intact by superolateral orbitotomy. (F) Histopathology showing malignant elongated strap cells and round cells.

for RMS (Figs 24.1C,D and 24.2B–D). With T1-weighted imaging, the tumor appears in the early stages as a round to ovoid mass usually located in the orbital soft tissue superonasally. It has a hypointense signal with respect to orbital fat, but is isointense with respect to extraocular muscles. It generally shows moderate to marked enhancement with gadolinium and is best delineated with fat suppression techniques. On T2-weighted imaging, it is hyperintense to extraocular muscles and orbital fat. It is usually non-cystic, but rare cavitary RMS may resemble a cystic lesion.[14,21]

Biopsy

A biopsy is necessary in cases of suspected RMS in order to establish the diagnosis before initiation of therapy. Based on the findings of clinical examination and imaging studies, the clinician must decide whether to perform an excisional or incisional biopsy.

The question sometimes arises as to whether fine needle aspiration biopsy (FNAB) should be used to establish the diagnosis of orbital RMS. Although there are indications for FNAB of orbital tumors, particularly in the diagnosis of lymphoma and orbital metastasis, we believe that there is no role for FNAB in the primary diagnosis of RMS. The scanty tissue obtained by FNAB is often insufficient for the cytopathologist to establish a diagnosis and the spindle shaped cells are difficult to differentiate from other spindle cell tumors. Furthermore, FNAB could liberate viable tumor cells into the adjacent soft tissues. The best management is generally to remove as much of the tumor as possible; this cannot be achieved with FNAB. Therefore, FNAB should rarely, if ever, be used to make the primary diagnosis of RMS.

Pathology

Orbital RMS probably arises from primitive pleuripotential mesenchymal cells with a propensity to differentiate toward skeletal muscle.[1,2,25] Several histopathologic variations of RMS occur in the orbit. The embryonal type is most common; the alveolar type is the most malignant.[1,2,25] Embryonal RMS is characterized histopathologically by spindle to round cells that show features characteristic of skeletal muscle in various stages of embryogenesis. The predominant cell is an elongated spindle cell that can assume a variety of arrangements and degrees of differentiation (Fig. 24.2F). Generally, the cytoplasm is highly eosinophilic and cross striations can sometimes be identified on routine histopathologic sections or with special stains. The alveolar type appears as loosely arranged, malignant cells with septae that are reminiscent of the pulmonary alveoli. The botryoid type may be a variant of the embryonal type that assumes a papillary configuration.[25]

Immunohistochemical studies provide great assistance in the diagnosis of RMS and in its differentiation from other spindle cell tumors.[1,2] Immunohistochemical studies have become the main approach to establishing the diagnosis. Immunohistochemical markers include antibodies against desmin, muscle-specific actin, and myoglobin that typically show positive reaction to RMS but negative reaction to other round or spindle cell tumors.

With the recent refinements in immunohistochemistry electron microscopy is almost never used in the diagnosis of orbital RMS.

Management

Historical aspects

Until the 1960s, orbital exenteration was the treatment of choice for orbital RMS.[34,35] Most authorities believed that complete surgical removal of the tumor would offer the patient the best chance of survival. However, the mortality rate for patients with orbital RMA continued to be greater than 70% in the early 1970s.[12,34,35] Subsequently, there have been major advances in diagnosis and treatment of orbital RMS. Education of physicians, better access to early medical care, and CT and MRI have advanced early diagnosis of this tumor, allowing prompt management using combined surgery, chemotherapy, and irradiation. Improved survival has resulted from this more conservative approach, with greater than 90% survival in recent years.[28-33] Much of the current information on diagnosis and treatment of RMS has been obtained through collaborative endeavors, mainly through the Intergroup Rhabdomyosarcoma Study Group (IRSG).

Intergroup Rhabdomyosarcoma Study Group

In 1972, IRSG was established to increase knowledge and to improve therapeutic results for RMS. Although these studies have usually been of RMS from all locations, some data pertains specifically to orbital RMS.[36-43]

A staging classification of RMS, employed by the IRSG, is used for RMS:

Group I: localized disease, completely resected.
Group II: microscopic disease remaining after biopsy.
Group III: gross residual disease remaining after biopsy.
Group IV: distant metastasis present at onset.

This classification can assist in selecting treatment and in predicting prognosis; it can be applied to cases of orbital RMS.[2]

Based on information from the IRSG, the management of orbital RMS should include any combination of surgery, irradiation, and chemotherapy.

Surgery

The final diagnosis of orbital RMS should be made on the basis of histopathologic findings following surgery, usually by excisional or incisional biopsy. The excised tissue should be submitted immediately for histopathology. There is usually no need for frozen sections except when the surgeon is uncertain whether representative tumor tissue is biopsied: these sections are not definitive. It may be difficult to differentiate RMS from other neoplasms and inflammatory processes by frozen section examination alone. Processing for light microscopy and immunohistochemical studies should be expedited so that a diagnosis is finalized within 24 to 48 hours.

Several approaches to surgery have been advocated, including orbital exenteration, excisional biopsy, and incisional biopsy. Orbital exenteration is rarely used today as a primary treatment. The ophthalmic surgeon should decide on the approach to biopsy and preferably do a complete excisional biopsy (Figs 24.1E,F 24.2E) to confirm the diagnosis. Prompt referral of the patient to a facility where further management will be a collaborative decision by the ophthalmologists, pathologists, pediatric oncologists and radiation oncologists, preferably under the guidelines of ISRG, is recommended.

Chemotherapy

Chemotherapy is generally the first line of ancillary treatment for children with orbital RMS. Vincristine and actinomycin D are generally employed in appropriate doses, since tumors in the orbit have a favorable outcome with these agents.[13,28-33]

Irradiation

The poor prognosis for patients with orbital RMS following orbital exenteration prompted the use of orbital irradiation (later combined with chemotherapy) for selected patients. The use of radiation is controversial and generally depends on the staging of the disease. Radiation currently employed for orbital RMS (4000 to 5000 cGy) can be associated with ocular complications.[2,3] New techniques, including proton therapy and cyberknife irradiation for orbital RMS, may reduce secondary complications. Details of radiation therapy for RMS are reviewed elsewhere.[31-33,39-45]

Irradiation is often necessary following orbital exenteration for tumor recurrence after standard irradiation and chemotherapy have failed to control the tumor.

Prognosis

Orbital RMS can be highly aggressive locally and can invade the brain and adjacent tissues and metastasize to lung, lymph nodes, and other distant sites. However, using modern therapeutic regimens the survival has improved dramatically. Today, survival is greater than 95% for orbital RMS.[3,4] Factors responsible for the better prognosis for RMS in the orbital region include the more favorable anatomic location, the earlier stage of the disease at the time of diagnosis, more favorable tumor morphology, and, perhaps, patient age.

Summary

RMS, the most common primary orbital malignancy of childhood, requires prompt diagnosis and treatment. It usually occurs in the first two decades of life, when the patient develops rapidly progressive proptosis and displacement of the eye. The tumor can arise primarily in the orbit or it can arise in the sinuses or nasal cavity and secondarily extend to involve the orbit.

Orbital RMS arises from primitive pleuripotential mesenchymal cells with a propensity to differentiate toward skeletal muscle. Several histopathologic variations of RMS occur in the orbit. The embryonal type is most common whereas the alveolar type is the most malignant.

Ophthalmologists should be aware of the clinical features of orbital RMS and order prompt imaging studies to determine the extent of the disease. A carefully planned biopsy should be performed and, if the diagnosis is confirmed, the child should be referred to pediatric oncologists for management. Patients are staged and managed according to the IRSG or similar protocol. The ophthalmologist has an important role in the initial diagnosis and subsequent follow-up of affected patients.

References

1. Shields JA, Shields CL. Myogenic tumors. In: Shields JA, Shields CL, editors. Atlas of Eyelid, Conjunctival and Orbital Tumors, 2nd ed. Philadelphia: Lippincott Williams and Wilkins; 2008: 599–613.
2. Shields JA, Shields CL. Rhabdomyosarcoma: review for the ophthalmologist. The 2001 Henry Dubins Lecture. Surv Ophthalmol 2003; 48: 39–57.
3. Shields CL, Shields JA, Honavar SG, Demirci H. Clinical spectrum of primary ophthalmic rhabdomyosarcoma. Ophthalmology 2001; 108: 2284–92.
4. Shields JA, Shields CL, Scartozzi R. Survey of 1264 patients with orbital tumors and simulating lesions: The 2002 Montgomery Lecture, Part 1. Ophthalmology 2004; 111: 997–1008.
6. Shields JA, Bakewell B, Augsburger JJ, et al. Space-occupying orbital masses in children: a review of 250 consecutive biopsies. Ophthalmology 1986; 93: 379–84.
7. Seregard S. Management of alveolar rhabdomyosarcoma of the orbit. Acta Ophthalmol Scand 2002; 80: 660–4.
9. Wharam M, Beltangady M, Hays D, et al. Localized orbital rhabdomyosarcoma: an interim report of the intergroup rhabdomyosarcoma study committee. Ophthalmology 1987; 94: 251–4.
11. Wilson MC, Shields JA, Shields CL, Litzky L. Orbital rhabdomyosarcoma fifty seven years after radiotherapy for retinoblastoma. Orbit 1996; 15: 97–100.
13. Raney RB, Anderson JR, Kollath J, et al. Late effects of therapy in 94 patients with localized rhabdomyosarcoma of the orbit: Report from the Intergroup Rhabdomyosarcoma Study (IRS)-III, 1984–1991. Med Pediatr Oncol 2000; 34: 413–20.
15. Cescon M, Grazi GL, Assietti R, et al. Embryonal rhabdomyosarcoma of the orbit in a liver transplant recipient. Transpl Int 2003; 16: 437–40.
16. Jung A, Bechtold S, Pfluger T, et al. Orbital rhabdomyosarcoma in Noonan syndrome. J Pediatr Hematol Oncol 2003; 25: 330–2.
17. Lumbroso L, Sigal-Zafrani B, Jouffroy T, et al. Late malignant melanoma after treatment of rhabdomyosarcoma of the orbit during childhood. Arch Ophthalmol 2002; 120: 1087–90.
18. Othmane IS, Shields CL, Shields JA, et al. Primary orbital rhabdomyosarcoma in an adult. Orbit 1999; 18: 183–9.
19. Spahn B, Nenadov-Beck M. Orbital rhabdomyosarcoma: clinicopathologic correlation, management and follow-up in two newborns. A preliminary report. Orbit 2001; 20: 149–56.
20. Amato MM, Esmaeli B, Shore JW. Orbital rhabdomyosarcoma metastatic to the contralateral orbit: a case report. Ophthalmology 2002; 109: 753–6.
21. Fetkenhour DR, Shields CL, Chao AN, et al. Orbital cavitary rhabdomyosarcoma masquerading as lymphangioma. Arch Ophthalmol 2001; 119: 1208–10.
24. Marr BP, Shields CL, Shields JA, Eagle RC Jr. Conjunctival cat-scratch disease simulating rhabdomyosarcoma. J Pediatr Ophthalmol Strabismus 2003; 40: 302–4.
28. Raney B, Walterhouse DO, Meza JL, et al. Results of the Intergroup Rhabdomyosarcoma Study Group D9602 protocol, using vincristine and dactinomycin with or without cyclophosphamide and radiation therapy, for newly diagnosed patients with low-risk embryonal rhabdomyosarcoma: a report from the Soft Tissue Sarcoma Committee of the Children's Oncology Group. J Clin Oncol 2011; 29: 1312–8.
29. Raney B, Stoner J, Anderson J, et al. Soft-Tissue Sarcoma Committee of the Children's Oncology Group. Impact of tumor viability at second-look procedures performed before completing treatment of the Intergroup Rhabdomyosarcoma Study Group protocol IRS-IV, 1991-1997: A report from the Children's Oncology Group. J Pediatr Surg 2010; 45: 2160–8.
30. McDonald MW, Esiashvili N, George BA, et al. Intensity-modulated radiotherapy with use of cone-down boost for pediatric head and neck rhabdomyosarcoma. Int J Radiat Oncol Biol Phys 2008; 72: 884–91.
31. Luu QC, Lasky JL, Moore TB, et al. Treatment of embryonal rhabdomyosarcoma of the sinus and orbit with chemotherapy, radiation, and endoscopic surgery. J Pediatr Surg 2006; 41: e15–7.
32. Wolden SL, Wexler LH, Kraus DH, et al. Intensity-modulated radiotherapy for head and neck rhabdomyosarcoma. Int J Radiat Oncol Biol Phys 2005; 61: 1432–8.
33. Sagerman RH, Cassady JR, Tretter P. Radiation therapy for rhabdomyosarcoma of the orbit. Trans Am Acad Ophthalmol Otolaryngol 1968; 72: 849–53.
36. Crist WM, Anderson JR, Meza JL, et al. Intergroup rhabdomyosarcoma study. IV: Results for patients with nonmetastatic disease. J Clin Oncol 2001; 19: 3091–102.
37. Crist WM, Gehan EA, Ragab AH, et al. Third Intergroup Rhabdomyosarcoma Study. J Clin Oncol 1995; 13: 610–30.

38. Mannor G, Rose GE, Plowman PN, et al. Multidisciplinary management of refractory orbital rhabdomyosarcoma. Ophthalmology 1997; 104: 1198–201.

39. Maurer HM, Gehan EA, Beltangady M, et al. The Intergroup Rhabdomyosarcoma Study II. Cancer 1993; 71: 1904–192.

40. Wharam MD, Hanfelt JJ, Tefft MC, et al. Radiation therapy for rhabdomyosarcoma: Local failure risk for clinical group III patients on Intergroup Rhabdomyosarcoma Study II. Int J Radiat Oncol Biol Phys 1997; 38: 797–804.

41. Wharam M, Beltangady M, Hays D, et al. Localized orbital rhabdomyosarcoma: an interim report of the Intergroup Rhabdomyosarcoma Study Committee. Ophthalmology 1987; 94: 251–4.

42. Baker KS, Anderson JR, Link MP, et al. Benefit of intensified therapy for patients with local or regional embryonal rhabdomyosarcoma: Results from the Intergroup Rhabdomyosarcoma Study IV. J Clin Oncol 2000; 18: 2427–34.

43. Rousseau P, Flamant F, Quintana E, et al. Primary chemotherapy in rhabdomyosarcomas and other malignant mesenchymal tumors of the orbit: Results of the International Society of Pediatric Oncology MMT 84 Study. J Clin Oncol 1994; 12: 516–21.

Access the complete reference list online at
http://www.expertconsult.com

Other mesenchymal abnormalities

Christopher J Lyons • Jack Rootman

Rhabdomyosarcoma is discussed in Chapter 24. Every mesenchymal component of the orbit can give rise to sarcomatous tumors, but these are exceedingly rare and will not be discussed. Nevertheless, they are part of the differential diagnosis of rhabdomyosarcoma.

Dysplasias

Fibrous dysplasia of the orbit

Fibrous dysplasia (FD) is rare, characterized by the replacement of normal bone by a cellular fibrous stroma containing islands of immature bone and osteoid which does not remodel along lines of stress into lamellar bone. It has been reported in infancy[1] but usually presents in childhood; its onset is insidious and it may remain asymptomatic until adulthood. Progression usually slows in the second or third decade, when "bone maturity" is reached, though growth may continue into the fourth decade in some cases. It is important to distinguish it from meningioma[2] and osteosarcoma.

FD may be confined to a single site (monostotic form) or, more rarely, involve multiple bony sites (polyostotic form). Polyostotic FD, which co-exists with cutaneous pigmentation and endocrine abnormalities, is the McCune-Albright syndrome.[3] FD is a non-inheritable disorder caused by mis-sense mutations occurring post-zygotically. These result in failure of mesenchymal precursor cells to differentiate normally into osteoblasts resulting in extensive proliferation of fibrous tissue from abnormally differentiated osteoblast precursors. The GSα mutation can be tested for in peripheral blood.[4]

Clinical features

Three-quarters of patients with orbital FD have the monostotic form affecting several contiguous bones but the disease usually remains unilateral. The craniofacial area is affected in 20% of patients, with a predilection for the frontal, sphenoid, and ethmoid bones. Typically, there is a painless, firm, bony swelling with contour distortion; in the orbit, there is an accompanying mass effect. The clinical presentation depends on the predominant wall involved, most commonly the roof, resulting in proptosis and downward displacement of the globe and orbit.[5,6] The lacrimal fossa may be affected, mimicking a lacrimal gland tumor.[7] Maxillary disease (Fig. 25.1) displaces the eye upwards, with persistent epiphora if the nasolacrimal duct is affected.[8] Sphenoid involvement results in optic nerve compression[5,6] from narrowing of the optic canal (Fig 25.2) or by an associated sphenoid sinus mucocoele.[9] Rarely, involvement of the sella turcica may result in chiasmal compression.[10] Other uncommon neuro-ophthalmic complications include cranial nerve palsies,[11] trigeminal neuralgia, raised intracranial pressure, and papilledema.[11,12] Extensive craniofacial involvement can result in severe cosmetic deformity. Pain may occur, either localized or as a diffuse ipsilateral headache. Visual loss is not uncommon.[5,13] Malignant transformation to osteosarcoma, fibrosarcoma, chondrosarcoma, and giant cell sarcoma occurs in 0.5% of cases increasing to 15% with prior radiotherapy.[13] The accompanying signs are rapid progression, worsening pain, and infiltration of surrounding structures.

The main radiographic feature of FD is expansion of bone. The lesions may be sclerotic, with a dense ground-glass homogeneity, lytic, with increased lucency, or show a mixed picture with alternating areas of lucency and increased density. Most orbital cases are easily diagnosed since they are sclerotic.[5] The main radiologic differential diagnosis includes histiocytosis-X, hyperostotic meningioma, Paget's disease (both rare in children), and some bone tumors. On magnetic resonance imaging (MRI) there is a correlation between T1 and T2 signal intensity and clinical and pathologic activity of the lesion.[14] Occasionally, large cystic lesions form in the orbital wall.[5] These may contain blood (Fig. 25.3) and necrotic debris and can be mistaken for aneurysmal bone cysts.[13] Involvement of

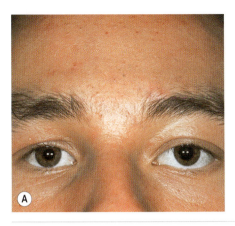
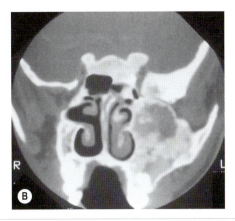
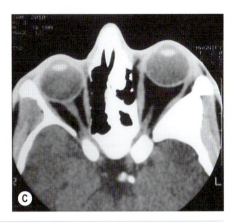

Fig. 25.1 (A) This 16-year-old presented with a history of progressive facial distortion and decreasing vision in the left eye to 20/40. Compressive optic neuropathy was diagnosed secondary to fibrous dysplasia. (B) CT scan of the same case showing cystic fibrous dysplasia involving the orbital apex. (C) Axial CT scan shows optic canal involvement. This was surgically decompressed. (Patient of the University of British Columbia.)

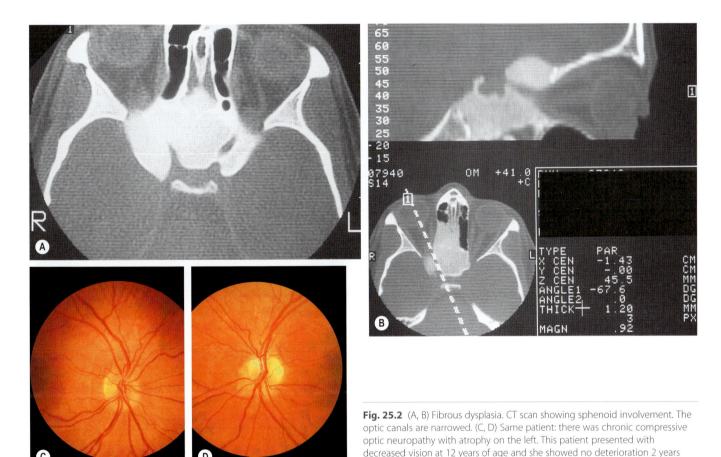

Fig. 25.2 (A, B) Fibrous dysplasia. CT scan showing sphenoid involvement. The optic canals are narrowed. (C, D) Same patient: there was chronic compressive optic neuropathy with atrophy on the left. This patient presented with decreased vision at 12 years of age and she showed no deterioration 2 years later with minimal residual signs or symptoms; she was not treated.

a neighboring sinus may mimic mucocele.[13,15] Computed tomography (CT) scanning with the possible addition of MRI is the best modality to evaluate the extent of cranial and orbital involvement. The optic canal and chiasm should be assessed for signs of compression.

Management

FD is usually benign and self-limiting. However, the final extent and time of arrest of the lesion are unpredictable. Treatment aims to prevent complications, especially optic nerve compression, and improve cosmesis while waiting for spontaneous arrest.

When there is little doubt about the diagnosis, initial observation and repeat radiologic assessment is best. If the lesion in the orbital wall is lytic or cystic, biopsy is usually necessary to confirm the diagnosis. Outside the orbit, the risk of malignant change after radiotherapy is high[16] and is not used.

Surgery is indicated for cosmetic disfigurement, intractable pain, or optic nerve compression. Since dysplastic bone can be vascular, preoperative blood cross-matching is advisable.

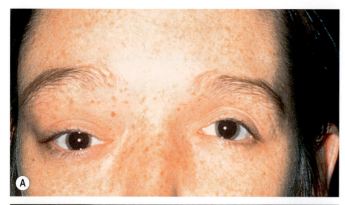

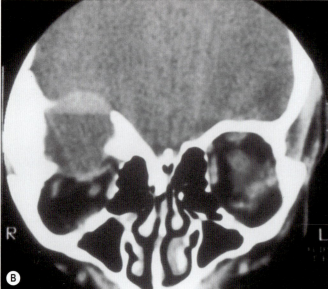

Fig. 25.3 (A) This 22-year-old developed sudden proptosis of the right eye after a history of slowly progressive facial asymmetry from early childhood. (B) CT scan showed the fluid level of a hemorrhage within the cystic dysplastic bone. The diagnosis was fibrous dysplasia. (Patient of the University of British Columbia.)

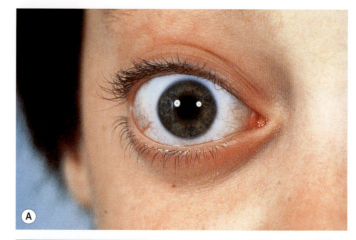

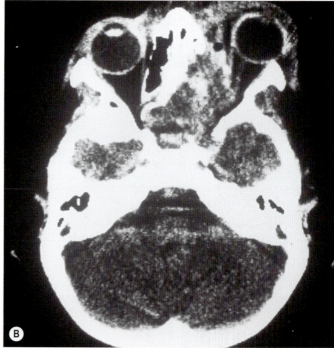

Fig. 25.4 This 10-year-old had a 1-month history of progressive proptosis of the right eye and lateral displacement of the globe. There was gradual loss of vision. Reparative granuloma was diagnosed by intranasal biopsy and the patient underwent lateral rhinotomy and excision of lesion via the ethmoid and maxillary sinuses. (Patient of the University of British Columbia.)

Resection of dysplastic bone around the optic canal can reverse visual loss of early compressive optic neuropathy.[9,13] Steroids may also be useful.[17] When decompressing the optic nerve, rongeurs rather than high speed drills (heat producing) should be used to protect the nerve. Surgery traditionally consisted of de-bulking the lesion. However, the margins of the affected bone are difficult to define clinically and recurrence was common.[6] In the last 20 years, there has been a shift toward more radical excision of all diseased bone and immediate facial and orbital reconstruction using bone grafts[5,18] by combined ophthalmology/craniofacial teams. Whilst some groups report no visual function deterioration following early optic canal decompression, there have been reports of blindness complicating prophylactic nerve decompression.[19] Visual loss is not usually the result of progressive optic canal stenosis but from the rapid expansion of cystic components, FD mucoceles, or hemorrhage.[20] Prophylactic optic canal decompression is not indicated and a conservative approach is warranted, reserving optic canal decompression for patients with progressive or sudden deterioration of visual function.[21]

Bone tumors

Reparative granuloma

Reparative granuloma and aneurysmal bone cyst are parts of a spectrum of reactive giant cell lesions; it may be difficult to differentiate them histologically.

Reparative granulomas (also known as giant cell granulomas) are rare. They affect patients in the first and second decades of life and occur in the mandible, maxilla, and phalanges.[13] The lesion may spread to the maxilla, ethmoid,[22] and sphenoid bones, involving the orbit (Fig. 25.4) and causing proptosis.[23,24] The presentation may be catastrophic if intralesional hemorrhage occurs.[13] Histopathologically, there is a spindle cell stroma with profuse hemorrhagic and hemosiderin content. Osteoblastic giant cells are present within the stroma and new bone may be laid down at the edge of the lesion.

The course is usually benign. Treatment is by surgical curettage; healing occurs by new bone formation. Curettage may need to be repeated or the bony margins resected if the lesion recurs. Radiotherapy is rarely necessary.[23]

Aneurysmal bone cyst

This uncommon lesion usually affects the metaphysis of long bones or the spine, often preceded by trivial trauma. The skull is affected in less than 1% of cases; about one-quarter of these affect the orbit.[25] It is a benign lesion which can usually be differentiated from reparative granuloma by the presence of large blood-filled channels lined by multinucleate giant cells and fibroblasts. However, they can be solid, making this differentiation difficult. The two may coexist.[26]

Aneurysmal bone cysts of the orbit (Fig. 25.5) have been periodically reviewed.[27,28] Most present in the second decade; there is a 5:3 female:male ratio. The history is usually shorter than 3 months with presentations including proptosis, diplopia, ophthalmoplegia,[29] ptosis, headache, visual deterioration due to optic nerve compression, nasal congestion,[25] epistaxis,[30] and epiphora.[31] Most cases involve the orbital roof and result in gradually increasing unilateral proptosis and downward displacement of the globe.[32] The medial and lateral orbital walls can also be involved. Like reparative granulomas, intralesional

hemorrhage may occur, leading to a sudden presentation with signs related to mass effect, occasionally mimicking orbital malignancy in early childhood.[33] Large cysts with intracranial extension may give rise to raised intracranial pressure, papilledema,[34] and optic nerve compression.[13]

Radiologically, irregular expansion with destruction of bone is seen on CT scan, with a thin shell of bone outlining the limits of the lesion. There may be patchy enhancement of the mass or its rim. Hemorrhage and multiple fluid–fluid levels[28] may be evident on MRI or ultrasound.

The treatment of choice is surgical excision or curettage with frozen section[13] and grafting with autogenous bone chips. Repair of the orbital wall with a plate,[28] or craniofacial reconstruction may be indicated at the time of surgery.[27,35] The prognosis is good despite a recurrence rate as high as 66%,[36] usually within 2 years of treatment. Cryotherapy and irradiation have also been used though the latter carries a later risk of osteosarcoma.

Neoplasias

Juvenile ossifying fibroma of the orbit

This rare disorder arises in the bony wall of the orbit, presenting with slowly progressive proptosis. It is similar to, but distinct from, FD.[13]

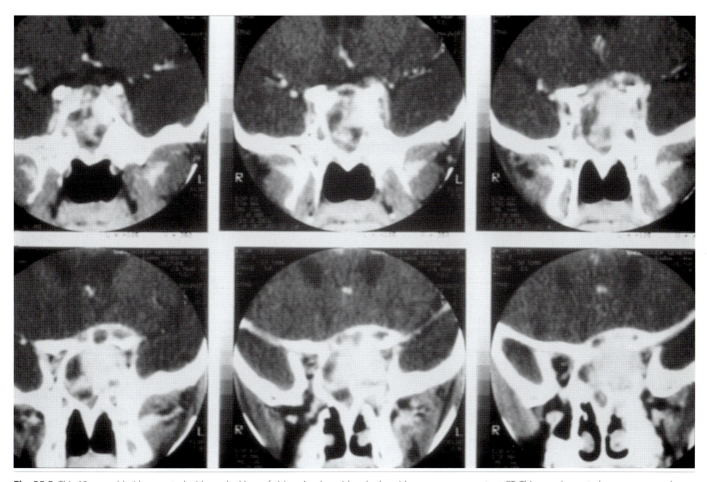

Fig. 25.5 This 12-year-old girl presented with gradual loss of vision. A sphenoid and ethmoid mass was apparent on CT. This was shown to be an aneurysmal bone cyst by intranasal biopsy and she underwent cranio-orbitotomy. (Patient of the University of British Columbia.)

It usually presents with slowly progressive painless globe displacement in adolescence or early adulthood: younger cases have been reported. The orbital roof (Fig. 25.6) or ethmoid bone are the most common sites;[37,38] rarely, maxillary involvement may cause upward displacement of the globe.[39] There may be massive enlargement with considerable morbidity and disfigurement.[38] Diplopia may occur, and posterior tumors may cause apical crowding. Occasionally, inflammation is a feature.[40]

CT scan, which is preferable to MRI,[41] shows a homogeneous central zone with a sclerotic margin expanding a single bone. The lesion is usually clearly demarcated but may grow to involve surrounding bones, sometimes crossing the midline to the other orbit.

Histopathologically, the predominant feature is a central whorled, cellular, vascular stroma surrounded by varying amounts of bone. The more aggressive psammomatoid variant contains islands of lamellar bone or 'ossicles' surrounded by a rim of osteoid and osteoblasts resembling the psammoma bodies of meningioma. The tumors enlarge insidiously; surgery

becomes necessary for most cases. The treatment of choice is complete excision since recurrence is common especially in the presence of residual tumor and with psammomatoid histopathology[38] when regular follow-up is indicated by a multidisciplinary team.[42] Extragnathic cementomas are tumors which behave in a similar fashion.

Other mesenchymal tumors

Osteoblastoma

This benign tumor rarely involves the orbit[43] but can originate from the orbital roof and ethmoid sinuses. It presents with mass effect and globe displacement.[43] Radiologically, osteoblastomas are well circumscribed and may have a lucent center with foci of calcification. The treatment of choice is surgical, either with curettage or more radical excision and reconstruction; both of these may be associated with profuse bleeding due to the vascularity of the tumor. Histologically, it may be difficult to differentiate these from osteoid osteomas.[44] Osteoblastomas tend to be larger, more vascular, and have potential for progressive growth and recurrence. The prognosis is reasonably good but in the spine and long bones they have a 10–15% recurrence rate after curettage.[45] Since sarcomatous transformation has been reported in the skull,[46] complete excision is indicated, preferably by a multidisciplinary team.

Postirradiation osteosarcoma of the orbit (see Chapter 42)

Survivors of familial retinoblastoma are at greater risk of developing a second tumor,[47,48] even in the absence of radiotherapy, due to their genetic predisposition. Recently, retinoblastoma treatment regimes use less radiotherapy for this reason. Most of these tumors are osteosarcomas,[48] which may occur within the field of radiation or at a distant site. Of 693 patients with bilateral retinoblastoma 89 developed second tumors;[48] 58 occurred within the radiation field and 31 outside. The latent period from completion of radiotherapy to development of the second tumor ranged from 10 months to 23 years (mean 10.4 years). The prognosis of osteosarcoma of the orbit is extremely poor; most patients die within a year of diagnosis.

Infantile cortical hyperostosis (Caffey's disease)

This uncommon disorder of unknown etiology affects infants in the first few months of life. It is characterized by sudden onset of fever, irritability, and soft tissue swelling. The soft tissue over the involved bone is swollen and tender. Plain X-rays show subperiosteal new bone formation and cortical thickening. There is usually leukocytosis and raised erythrocyte sedimentation rate. The mandible is the most common bone to be involved, in which case the infants have a characteristic facial appearance with swollen cheeks. It is generally self-limiting and the radiologic appearance reverts to normal within a few months. Involvement of the facial and skull bones may lead to periorbital edema and even proptosis.[49,50] The management is conservative: initially, observation and follow-up radiologic examination of the involved bones. Systemic steroids may be used for persistent disease, or to hasten remission if there is gross swelling.

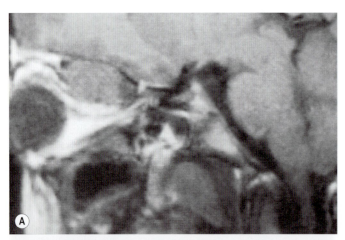

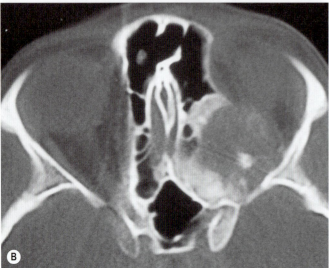

Fig. 25.6 (A) Ossifying fibroma. This 7-year-old child presented with progressive proptosis of the right eye and downward displacement of the globe. The MRI scan shows a mass in the orbital roof displacing the levator–superior rectus complex, the globe and the optic nerve downwards. (B) Same patient. CT scan showing the sclerotic margin of the fibroma.

Osteopetrosis

This rare disorder is due to defective bone resorption by osteoclasts resulting in increased bony thickness and density. There is increased fragility of long bones, narrowing of the marrow cavity and of the bony foramina of the skull (Fig. 25.7). Most patients presenting in childhood have autosomal recessive osteopetrosis which presents in infancy with a very severe "malignant" form, soon fatal if untreated, or a less aggressive form appearing in the first decade.

The malignant form presents in infancy with failure to thrive, anemia, and thrombocytopenia; extramedullary hematopoiesis results in hepatosplenomegaly and lymphadenopathy. It is a cause of neonatal hypocalcemia, causing seizures, due to unopposed osteoblastic function.[51] Bony involvement may result in small orbits with proptosis,[52] narrowing of the cranial foramina, temporal bossing, and nasolacrimal duct obstruction.[53] Optic atrophy follows narrowing of the optic canal and optic nerve compression.[54,55] Compression of other cranial nerves results in facial palsy and deafness.

The bone density on X-ray is uniform without corticomedullary demarcation (see Fig. 25.7). There is broadening of the metaphyses and pathologic fractures are common.

Visual function needs to be monitored with electrophysiology in affected infants.[56,57] Vision may be preserved or improved by early decompression of the optic canal,[58,59] but the procedure is difficult due to the great density of the bone. There is a subgroup of patients with infantile malignant osteopetrosis in whom visual loss results from a rod–cone dystrophy;[56,57,60,61] they may have evidence of widespread neuronal degeneration. A macular chorioretinal abnormality has also been reported.[61] Ocular involvement by age 2 months occurred in half of 33 patients with autosomal recessive osteopetrosis;[62] three had retinal degeneration. Thus, in evaluating a child with osteopetrosis with visual loss, an ERG should always precede optic nerve decompression. Depending on the underlying mutation and severity of the disease, treatment with bone marrow or hematopoietic stem cell transplantation is the best option.[63]

Autosomal dominant osteopetrosis may be discovered in adulthood: it has no ophthalmic complications and a normal life expectancy but numerous orthopedic problems.

Other bone dysplasias

These include craniometaphyseal dysplasia, cranioepiphyseal dysplasia, X-linked hypophosphatemic rickets (Fig. 25.8) and many others which may be characterized by bone thickening, foraminal occlusion, and orbital narrowing.

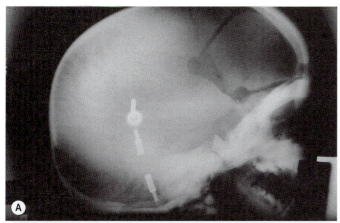
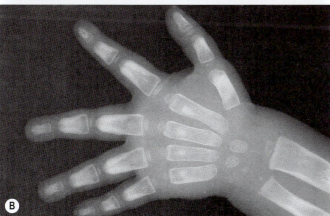

Fig. 25.7 (A) Osteopetrosis. This infant had a bilateral compressive optic neuropathy which failed to respond to optic nerve decompression. He also has a shunt in situ. Bone marrow transplantation has been successful in some cases. (B) X-ray of the hands showing increased density of distal ends of the phalanges (same patient).

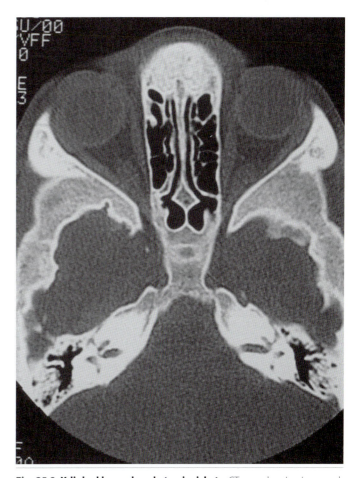

Fig. 25.8 X-linked hypophosphatemic rickets. CT scan showing increased bone density, especially of the cortical bone. There was chronic optic nerve compression which did not deteriorate over a 10-year period while it was monitored by measuring acuity, color vision, pupil reactions, visual fields, and VEPs.

References

1. Joseph E, Kachhara R, Bhattacharya RN, et al. Fibrous dysplasia of the orbit in an infant. Pediatr Neurosurg 2000; 32: 205–8.

3. Albright F, Butler AM, Hampton AO, Smith P. Syndrome characterized by osteitis fibrosa disseminata, areas of pigmentation and endocrine dysfunction with precocious puberty in females. N Engl J Med 1937; 216: 727–46.

4. Garcia RA, Inwards CY, Unni KK. Benign bone tumors: recent developments. Semin Diagn Pathol 2011; 28: 73–85.

5. Moore AT, Buncic JR, Munro IR. Fibrous dysplasia of the orbit in childhood. Ophthalmology 1985; 92: 12–20.

8. Moore RT. Fibrous dysplasia of the orbit. Surv Ophthalmol 1969; 13: 321–34.

13. Rootman J. Diseases of the Orbit: A Multidisciplinary Approach, 2nd ed. Philadelphia: Lippincott Williams & Wilkins; 2002.

15. Char D, Barakos JA, Cobbs CS, Shiel MJ. Fibrous dysplasia. Orbit 2010; 29: 216–18.

19. Edelstein C, Goldberg RA, Rubino G. Unilateral blindness after ipsilateral prophylactic transcranial optic canal decompression for fibrous dysplasia. Am J Ophthalmol 1998; 126: 469–71.

20. Michael CB, Lee AG, Patrinely JR, et al. Visual loss associated with fibrous dysplasia of the anterior skull base: case report and review of the literature. J Neurosurg 2000; 92: 350–4.

24. Hoopes PC, Anderson RL, Blodi FC. Giant cell (reparative) granuloma of the orbit. Ophthalmology 1981; 88: 1361–6.

25. Hunter JV, Yokoyama C, Moseley IF, Wright JE. Aneurysmal bone cyst of the sphenoid with orbital involvement. Br J Ophthalmol 1990; 74: 505–8.

28. Menon J, Brosnahan DM, Jellinek DA. Aneurysmal bone cyst of the orbit: a case report and review of literature. Eye 1999; 13: 764–8.

29. Alkhani A. Left eye proptosis in an 11 year-old child. Can J Neurol Sci 2008; 35: 91–3.

31. Ozdamar Y, Acaroglu G, Kazanci B, et al. Aneurysmal bone cyst of the ethhmoid presenting with proptosis and epiphora. Orbit 2010; 29: 149–51.

36. Biesecker JL, Marcove RC, Huvos AG, Mike V. Aneurysmal bone cysts: a clinicopathologic study of 66 cases. Cancer 1970; 26: 615–25.

37. Blodi FC. Pathology of orbital bones: The XXXII Edward Jackson memorial lecture. Am J Ophthalmol 1976; 81: 1–26.

39. Shields JA, Peyster RG, Handler SD, et al. Massive juvenile ossifying fibroma of maxillary sinus with orbital involvement. Br J Ophthalmol 1985; 69: 392–5.

40. Cruz AA, Alencar VM, Figueiredo AR, et al. Ossifying fibroma: a rare cause of orbital inflammation. Ophthal Plast Reconstr Surg 2008; 24(2): 107–12.

44. McHugh JB, Mukherji SK, Lucas DR. Sino-orbital osteoma: a clinicopathologic study of 45 surgically treated cases with emphasis on tumors with osteoblastoma-like features. Arch Pathol Lab Med 2009; 133: 1587–93.

48. Abramson DH, Ellsworth RM, Kitchin FD, Tung G. Second nonocular tumors in retinoblastoma survivors: are they radiation-induced? Ophthalmology 1984; 91: 1351–5.

51. Chen CJ, Lee MY, Hsu ML, et al. Malignant infantile osteopetrosis initially presenting with neonatal hypocalcemia: case report. Ann Hemat 2003; 82: 64–7.

56. Thompson DA, Kriss A, Taylor D, et al. Early VEP and ERG evidence of visual dysfunction in autosomal recessive osteopetrosis. Neuropediatrics 1998; 29: 137–44.

57. Hoyt CS, Billson FA. Visual loss in osteopetrosis. Am J Dis Child 1979; 133: 955–8.

59. Haines SJ, Erickson DL, Wirts JD. Optic nerve decompression for osteopetrosis in early childhood. Neurosurgery 1988; 23: 407–50.

63. Steward CG. Hematopoietic stem cell transplantation for osteopetrosis. Pediatr Clin N Am 2010; 57: 171–80.

Access the complete reference list online at

http://www.expertconsult.com

Metastatic, secondary and lacrimal gland tumors

Christopher J Lyons • Jack Rootman

Neuroblastoma and Ewing's sarcoma account for most childhood orbital metastatic disease.[1] Wilms' tumor, testicular embryonal sarcoma, ovarian sarcoma, and renal embryonal sarcoma occasionally metastasize to the orbit.[2]

It is important to differentiate between blood-borne deposits of a malignant tumor (metastatic disease) and extension of a tumor into the orbital tissues from an adjacent structure (secondary disease). Retinoblastoma and rhabdomyosarcoma are the most important sources of secondary orbital disease in children (see Chapters 24 and 42).

Metastatic disease

Neuroblastoma

Neuroblastoma is the most common extracranial solid tumor of childhood accounting for 9% of all childhood cancers and is the third leading cause of cancer-related death in children. Its incidence peaks in infancy with a median age at diagnosis of 17 months. It arises from postganglionic sympathetic neuroblasts. Most primary tumors involve the adrenal medulla but they can occur anywhere within the sympathetic nervous system in paraspinal ganglia, neck, or pelvis. This is the most common source of orbital metastasis in children, accounting for 41 of 46 cases of orbital metastatic disease reported by Albert et al;[1] but it is a rare cause of orbital disease representing only 1.5% of 214 orbital tumors reported by Porterfield[3] and 3% of 307 childhood orbital tumors quoted by Nicholson and Green.[2]

Genetics

Only 1–2% of cases have a family history; the underlying genetic mutation has been determined for most of these pedigrees, helping to understand sporadic neuroblastoma. It arises from the interaction of multiple common predisposing genomic variations. The genetic characteristics of each tumor have important prognostic significance; high levels of MYCN (N-myc) proto-oncogene amplification are found in approximately 20% of primary tumors and are associated with a worse outcome for each tumor stage.[4-7]

Hyperdiploidy of tumor cell DNA content confers an improved prognosis for infants under 1 year of age at diagnosis. Conversely, segmental chromosomal alterations are associated with more aggressive disease.[8] Many genetic abnormalities have been identified in primary neuroblastoma tumors but their independent prognostic significance remains unclear. The most frequent somatically acquired copy number abnormality is allelic gain of distal chromosome 17q, identified in over 50% of primary tumors. An unbalanced gain is associated with more aggressive disease and decreased survival. Cellular genomic aberrations are a better prognostic predictor of the tumor's biological behavior than clinical factors such as age and stage at diagnosis. This is important for treatment planning since it is not uncommon for these tumors to regress spontaneously (stage 4S), even if already disseminated to the liver, skin, and bone marrow. If identified early, these infants can be spared the harmful adverse effects of chemotherapy since their survival rate exceeds 95%.[9] In contrast, children with high risk neuroblastoma are often resistant to multimodality treatment and have a 5-year survival rate of 40%.

Clinical presentation

Most cases occur by 3 years[10] and 90% are diagnosed by age 5, the range being from birth to the late teens. The adrenals are the primary site in 51% of cases, but the tumor can arise in the cervical sympathetic chain, mediastinum, or pelvis.[11] Primary orbital neuroblastoma occurs mostly in adults.[12,13] Neuroblastoma is more common in patients with neurofibromatosis type 1 (NF1).

The clinical features vary according to the different sites of origin, tendency for multiple metastases, features related to its hormone secretion, and any paraneoplastic syndrome. Pain, fever, and weight loss are common symptoms; cerebellar encephalopathy (ataxia, myoclonic jerks, opsoclonus of unknown cause), diarrhea (from tumor vasoactive peptide production), Horner's syndrome (sympathetic chain involvement), and hypertension with flushing episodes (catecholamine production) are classic signs of neuroblastoma.

The diagnosis is often not made until the patient has widespread metastases;[14] 40% have metastases at presentation, a proportion which rises to 55% in patients over the age of 1

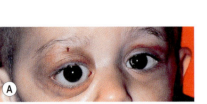
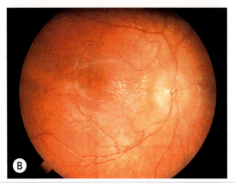
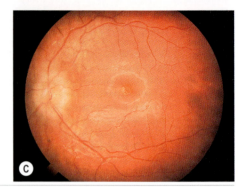

Fig. 26.1 Neuroblastoma. (A) This child presented with bilateral orbital bruising and right proptosis. (Patient of Dr. S. Day.) (B,C) This patient had widespread orbital and cranial bone involvement with raised intracranial pressure and papilledema.

year. Surprisingly, about 10% of tumors and their metastases (stages 1 to 4s) undergo spontaneous regression, something which occurs 100 times more commonly than for any other cancer.[15] This fact underlies the cautious treatment approach outlined below.

Tumor histology ranges from undifferentiated (neuroblastoma) to mature ganglion cells (ganglioneuroblastoma or ganglioneuroma). The histopathological characteristics such as the amount of stroma, degree of differentiation and number of mitotic figures, reflected in the Shimada classification, do have some prognostic value.

Ninety percent of patients have abnormally high levels of vanillylmandelic acid (VMA) in their urine due to catecholamine secretion. The urinary VMA concentration can be useful for diagnosis and to monitor treatment.

Ophthalmic and orbital features

The presence of neuroblastoma in the mediastinum or cervical sympathetic chain may first manifest with Horner's syndrome. This was the underlying diagnosis in two of 10 children with Horner's syndrome reviewed by Woodruff et al.[16] Gibbs et al.[17] described congenital Horner's syndrome in an infant with non-cervical neuroblastoma, suggesting that the two conditions might indicate a widespread dysgenesis of the sympathetic nervous system. Tonic pupils have been reported as a paraneoplastic effect of adrenal neuroblastoma.[18] Iris[19] and choroidal[20] metastases from abdominal neuroblastoma have been described. The presence of opsoclonus (see Chapter 90), a striking large amplitude erratic ocular flutter also known as "dancing eyes syndrome," with or without ataxia and myoclonus, suggests occult localized neuroblastoma.[14] The primary tumor in these cases is in the chest or abdomen and not the brain. It is usually associated with a good prognosis, possibly because only single copies of the N-myc oncogene are present within the tumor cells.[21] Opsoclonus can also be present with multiple N-myc copies, signaling a poor outcome.[22]

Presentation

In 93% of the 46 cases reported by Albert et al.,[1] the primary tumor had been diagnosed prior to presentation with orbital signs. Ninety percent of the 60 patients with orbital metastases reviewed by Musarella et al.[14] had a primary abdominal tumor. Orbital metastases commonly present with sudden onset and rapid progression of proptosis (Fig. 26.1), unilateral or bilateral. Ecchymosis (Fig. 26.2) is present in 25% of cases.[14,23,24] The lesion is usually in the superolateral orbit and zygoma but

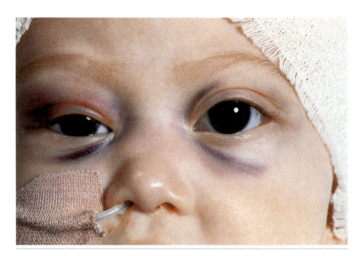

Fig. 26.2 Periorbital ecchymoses in a patient with orbital neuroblastoma.

may occur anywhere within the orbit. Bony lesions give rise to swelling of overlying tissues so periorbital swelling and ptosis may be present. This presentation may be confused with orbital cellulitis or other rapidly progressive orbital tumors such as rhabdomyosarcoma, Ewing's sarcoma, medulloblastoma, Wilms' tumor, and acute lymphoblastic leukemia.[25] A bleed into a pre-existing but clinically unsuspected venous lymphatic malformation (lymphangioma) may also present with sudden onset of proptosis and ecchymosis. The ecchymosis can lead to suspicion of child abuse and diagnostic delay.[26]

Treatment

The main prognostic (risk) factors are the age at diagnosis, stage of disease (Table 26.1), MYCN status, Shimada histology, and ploidy for infants. Survival rates for low risk groups are 90–100%, whilst those for high risk groups range from 20% to 60%.

Low risk neuroblastoma (stages 1 and 2) is treated surgically. The cure rate is greater than 90% for stage 2 neuroblastomas with no further treatment even if small amounts of tumor remain after surgery.[27] Chemotherapy or radiation can cure local recurrence. Stage 4s has a favorable prognosis; the survival rate is almost 100% with observation and supportive care only.[28] Treatment for intermediate risk neuroblastoma includes surgery and chemotherapy with agents including carboplatin, cyclophosphamide, cisplatin, etoposide, and doxorubicin over several months. Radiotherapy is used for incomplete response

Table 26.1 – International neuroblastoma staging system (INSS)

Stage	Description
1	Tumor confined to organ or origin
2	Tumor extends beyond organ of origin but not beyond midline
2a	No lymph node involvement
3	Tumor extends beyond midline with or without bilateral lymph node involvement
4	Tumor disseminated to distant sites
4s	Children younger than 1 year of age with dissemination to liver, skin, or bone marrow without bone involvement and a primary tumor that would otherwise be stage 1 or 2

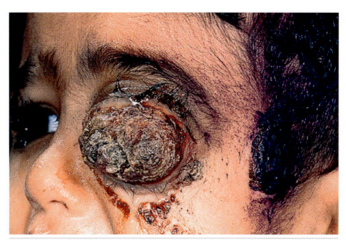

Fig. 26.3 Retinoblastoma. This child with extensive orbital involvement with lymphatic spread (note the pre-auricular gland involvement) is a common presentation in developing countries.

to chemotherapy. Children with stage 3 and infants with stage 4 under 1 year of age and otherwise favorable features have an excellent prognosis of more than 90% survival with moderate treatment. It is important to obtain sufficient material for histopathological and genetic study to determine these patients' moderate risk and spare them the high doses necessary for higher risk groups. High risk patients receive induction chemotherapy followed by high dose chemotherapy and bone marrow transplantation with additional cis-retinoic acid treatment.[29]

Ewing's sarcoma

Ewing's sarcoma is highly malignant and an important cause of mortality and morbidity. This group of neuroectoderm-derived neoplasms includes Ewing's sarcoma, Askin's tumor (in the chest wall), and peripheral primitive neuroectodermal tumors.[30]

The usual age of onset is 10–25 years, especially the first half of the second decade. It is very rare in African and Chinese people. Four percent of primary tumors are in the head and neck, usually the maxilla or mandible, but sometimes the orbital roof.[31] Spread from contiguous structures such as the sinuses may occur. There is a marked tendency to spread to adjacent soft tissues, other bones, and the lungs.[32] Immunohistochemical characteristics help to differentiate Ewing's from other small round cell tumors such as rhabdomyosarcoma, neuroblastoma, and lymphoma. Ewing's sarcomas are often S-100, neuron-specific enolase and surface glycoprotein MIC-2 positive and negative for muscle markers such as desmin or actin. A reciprocal translocation, $t(11:22)(q24;q12)$ is present in 83% of tumors.[33] There is a cytogenetic rearrangement on the long arm of chromosome 22 fusing the EWS gene (whose function is unknown) and members of the ETS family of transcription factors (FLI-1, ERG). This causes deregulation of other genes within the cell and development of the malignant phenotype.[34] In undifferentiated tumors, the diagnosis may be secured by cytogenetic analysis for the translocation or PCR (polymerase chain reaction) for chimeric fusion gene products EWS/FLII or EWS/ERG.

There are numerous reports of primary Ewing's sarcoma involving the orbit, arising from the ethmoid and sphenoid sinuses, roof of the orbit, lesser wing of the sphenoid, and temporal bone. A short history is typical, featuring swelling, globe displacement, strabismus with diplopia and duction limitation, headache, visual loss, pain, and localized bony tenderness.[1,35,36]

On computed tomography (CT) scan, there is a "moth-eaten" unevenly enhancing appearance of the involved bone, associated with a soft tissue mass. The differential diagnosis includes neuroblastoma, rhabdomyosarcoma (if extraskeletal), Langerhans' cell histiocytosis, and osteomyelitis.

In apparently primary orbital tumors, the patient should be evaluated for metastatic disease with a chest CT, radionuclide scan, bone marrow aspirate, and tissue biopsies. Adequate amounts of fresh tissue should be obtained for histopathologic and cytogenetic studies. Treatment of the primary tumor is with multiagent chemotherapy to shrink the tumor before surgical excision. Vincristine, doxorubicin, and cyclophosphamide are the main treatments with, in addition, ifosfamide and etoposide. Although these tumors are radiosensitive and local control may be achieved by radiotherapy, surgery is preferable due to the risk of late radiotherapy complications including osteosarcoma. Histologically clear margins are essential. The prognosis for metastatic disease remains poor; only one-third survive in the long-term. Since there is an appreciable risk of late recurrence or development of a second malignancy, such as osteogenic sarcoma, prolonged follow-up is indicated.

Secondary disease

Retinoblastoma (see Chapter 42)

Retinoblastoma confined within the eye poses little threat to life and is curable.[32,37] The prognosis is greatly worsened by extension into the orbit (Fig. 26.3) or central nervous system or by metastatic disease. The consequences of trans-scleral spread to the orbit and extension into the optic nerve are considered in Chapter 42.

Malignant melanoma

Intraocular melanoma very rarely occurs in infancy and childhood; secondary orbital melanoma is exceedingly rare. Occasionally, orbital malignant melanoma occurs in the neonatal period with extensive involvement of orbital and other facial tissues at presentation.

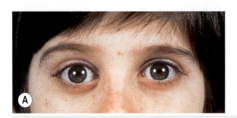
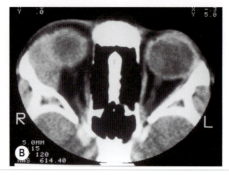
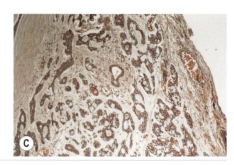

Fig. 26.4 (A) This 10-year-old boy presented with a 1-year history of gradual right orbital enlargement and upper lid swelling. There was no pain or sensory loss. (B) CT scan showed a lacrimal gland mass excavating the frontal bone, without erosion. Even rapidly growing lesions may cause excavation in childhood. (C) It was an adenoid cystic carcinoma of the lacrimal gland. The patient was alive and well 23 years later. (Patient of the University of British Columbia.)

Lacrimal gland tumors

The most common cause of a lacrimal gland fossa mass in childhood is dermoid cyst, since these lesions tend to occur in the upper outer quadrant of the orbit.[2] Inflammatory lesions, including non-specific lacrimal inflammation, Wegener's granulomatosis, sclerosing inflammation, and angiolymphoid hyperplasia are unusual and cystic lesions in this age group include dermoid cysts and lacrimal cysts. Adenoid cystic carcinoma and granulocytic sarcoma (chloroma) are rare but do occur in childhood.

Primary epithelial tumors of the lacrimal gland are rare in young children (Fig. 26.4), more frequent over the age of 10 years. Benign mixed tumor of the lacrimal gland is unusual:[3] cure is effected by complete removal of the tumor, with recurrence if excision is incomplete. They are slowly progressive; the certainty of diagnosis is increased by CT scanning prior to removal.[38]

A few cases of adenoid cystic carcinoma have been reported in children.[3,39,40] They tend to develop rapidly. Alternatively, a pre-existing lesion can present acutely with symptoms which may include pain and paraesthesia due to perineural invasion which often extends microscopically beyond the tumor mass, which is, in part, responsible for the poor prognosis and recurrence after excision.

Radiologically, bone erosion is highly suggestive of malignancy. However, it is important to note that absence of erosion does not exclude malignancy; since bony remodeling occurs rapidly in childhood, localized bony expansion may still be seen with rapidly growing masses such as adenoid cystic carcinoma[41] whereas in adults, this sign would indicate a slow-growing mass such as pleomorphic adenoma.

These tumors may be difficult to distinguish clinically from other lacrimal lesions such as low grade infections, non-specific inflammation,[42] or leukemic deposits[43] and biopsy may be required for confirmation.

Adenoid cystic carcinoma is invasive and carries a poor prognosis despite surgery, radiotherapy, and chemotherapy.[44]

References

1. Albert DM, Rubenstein RA, Scheie HG. Tumor metastasis to the eye. II. Clinical study in infants and children. Am J Ophthalmol 1967; 63: 727–32.

2. Nicholson DH, Green WR. Pediatric Ocular Tumors. New York: Masson; 1981.

3. Porterfield JF. Orbital tumors in children: a report on 214 cases. Int Ophthalmol Clin 1962; 2: 319–26.

5. Deyell RJ, Attyeh EF. Advances in the understanding of constitutional and somatic genomic alterations in neuroblastoma. Cancer Genet 2011; 204: 113–21.

6. Abramson DH, Andracchi S. Orbital granuloma formation after enucleation for intraocular retinoblastoma. Am J Ophthalmol 1997; 123: 567–9.

8. Janoueix-Lerosey I, Schleiermacher G, Michels E, et al. Overall genomic pattern is a predictor of outcome in neuroblastoma. J Clin Oncol 2009; 27: 1026–33.

9. De Bernardi B, Gerrard M, Boni L, et al. Excellent outcome with reduced treatment for infants with disseminated neuroblastoma without MYCN gene amplification. J Clin Oncol 2009; 27: 1034–40.

10. Davis S, Rogers MAM, Pendergrass TW. The evidence and epidemiologic characteristics of neuroblastoma in the United States. Am J Epidemiol 1987; 126: 1063–74.

11. Gross RE, Farber S, Martin LW. Neuroblastoma sympatheticum: a study and report of 217 cases. Pediatrics 1959; 23: 1179–91.

12. Bullock JD, Goldberg SH, Rakes SM, et al. Primary orbital neuroblastoma. Arch Ophthalmol 1989; 107: 1031–3.

13. Jakobiec FA, Klepach GL, Crissman JD, Spoor TC. Primary differentiated neuroblastoma of the orbit. Ophthalmology 1987; 94: 255–66.

14. Musarella MA, Chan HSL, DeBoer G, Gallie BL. Ocular involvement in neuroblastoma: prognostic implications. Ophthalmology 1984; 91: 936–40.

15. Pritchard J, Hickman JA. Why does stage 4s neuroblastoma regress spontaneously? Lancet 1994; 345: 992–3.

16. Woodruff G, Buncic JR, Morin JD. Horner's syndrome in children. J Pediatr Ophthalmol Strabismus 1988; 25: 40–4.

17. Gibbs J, Appleton RE, Martin J, Findlay G. Congenital Horner's syndrome associated with non-cervical neuroblastoma. Dev Med Child Neurol 1992; 34: 642–4.

21. Cohn SL, Salwen H, Herst CV, et al. Single copies of the N-myc oncogene in neuroblastomas from children presenting with the syndrome of opsoclonus-myoclonus. Cancer 1988; 62: 723–6.

22. Hiyama E, Yokoyama T, Ichikawa T, et al. Poor outcome in patients with advanced stage neuroblastoma and coincident opsomyoclonus syndrome. Cancer 1994; 74: 1821–6.

23. Alfano JE. Ophthalmological aspects of neuroblastomatosis: a study of 53 verified cases. Trans Am Acad Ophthalmol Otolaryngol 1968; 72: 830–48.

26. Timmerman R. Images in clinical medicine: raccoon eyes and neuroblastoma. N Engl J Med 2003; 349: E4.

27. Perez CA, Matthay KK, Atkinson JB, et al. Biologic variables in the outcome of stages I and II neuroblastoma treated with surgery as primary therapy: a children's cancer group study. J Clin Oncol 2000; 18: 18–26.

28. Nickerson HJ, Matthay KK, Seeger RC, et al. Favorable biology and outcome of stage IV-S neuroblastoma with supportive care or

minimal therapy: a children's cancer group study. J Clin Oncol 2000; 18: 477–86.

29. Matthay KK, Villablanca JG, Seeger RC, et al. Treatment of high-risk neuroblastoma with intensive chemotherapy, radiotherapy, autologous bone marrow transplantation, and 13-cis-retinoic acid. Children's Cancer Group. N Engl J Med 1999; 341: 1165–73.

31. Alvarez-Berdecia A, Schut L, Bruce DA. Localized primary intracranial Ewing's sarcoma of the orbital roof. Case report. J Neurosurg 1979; 50: 811–13.

32. Jakobiec FA, Jones IS. Metastatic and secondary tumors. In: Duane TD, editor. Clinical Ophthalmology. Hagerstown: Harper and Row; 1983.

34. Shing DC, McMullan DJ, Roberts P, et al. FUS/ERG gene fusions in Ewing's tumors. Cancer Res 2003; 63: 4568–76.

35. Dutton JJ, Rose JG, Jr, DeBacker CM, Gayre G. Orbital Ewing's sarcoma of the orbit. Ophthal Plast Reconstr Surg 2000; 16: 292–300.

36. Bajaj MS, Pushker N, Sen S, et al. Primary Ewing's sarcoma of the orbit: a rare presentation. J Pediatr Ophthalmol Strabismus 2003; 40: 101–4.

40. Shields JA, Bakewell B, Augsburger JJ, et al. Space occupying orbital masses in children: a review of 250 consecutive biopsies. Ophthalmology 1986; 93: 379–84.

41. Rootman J. Diseases of the Orbit: A Multidisciplinary Approach, 2nd ed. Philadelphia: Lippincott Williams & Wilkins; 2002.

43. Kincaid MC, Green WR. Ocular and orbital involvement in leukemia. Surv Ophthalmol 1983; 27: 211–32.

44. Krohel GB, Stewart WB, Chavis RM. Orbital Disease: A Practical Approach. New York: Grune & Stratton; 1981.

Access the complete reference list online at
http://www.expertconsult.com

Part 3
Orbit and lacrimal

Histiocytic, hematopoietic and lymphoproliferative disorders

Christopher J Lyons • Jack Rootman

"Histiocytosis" describes an abnormal proliferation of cells derived from the monocyte-phagocyte system. It is divided into two main groups:

1. Langerhans' cell histiocytosis (LCH, histiocytosis X): abnormal histiocytes are derived from dendritic (granular) Langerhans' cells, involved in antigen presentation.[1,2] These cells have characteristic inclusions visible on electron microscopy.
2. Non-Langerhans' cell histiocytosis results from proliferation of another class of dendritic histiocytes, the dermal dendrocytes, lacking inclusion granules. These are responsible for juvenile xanthogranuloma.

The macrophage system, a third type of histiocytic cell, gives rise, through a polyclonal proliferation, to sinus histiocytosis, also known as Rosai-Dorfman disease.[3] These three histiocytic disorders will be discussed in this chapter.

Langerhans' cell histiocytosis (histiocytosis X)

Langerhans' cell histiocytosis (LCH) is predominantly a childhood disorder with a peak incidence from 1 to 3 years of age and an annual incidence of 4–5 per million.[4] Boys are more frequently affected, though female patients may be younger, with more widespread disease.[5] Langerhans' cells are dendritic histiocytes with minimal phagocytic capacity, involved in immune surveillance. Normally situated at the junction of dermis and epidermis, they migrate to regional lymph nodes after antigen encounter, where they participate in antigen presentation.[6]

LCH lesions are destructive and space-occupying producing a clinical picture which varies with the site and the tissue involved. In children, the disease most commonly affects bones, especially those involved in hematopoiesis, and skin. Lesions may occur in the other organs containing histiocytes and macrophages such as the spleen, liver, lymph nodes, and lung. Data from the early 1990s suggested a monoclonal neoplastic origin to this disorder[6] but further investigation has not shown consistent genomic aberrations.[7] The exact etiology of this disorder remains obscure. Langerhans' cells in the skin multiply from single progenitor cells in embryonic development. LCH cells may react to the local cellular environment including T cells and cytokines in an abnormal manner.[8] The result is highly variable, possibly depending on cell mutations, interaction with immune surveillance and the site of origin of the affected cell.

Alfred Hand[9] first reported polyuria, exophthalmia and skull destruction in a 3-year-old. Subsequently, conditions describing the spectrum of histiocytic disease were given eponymous names; eventually, three different clinical disorders were described:

1. Eosinophilic granuloma, typically affects children aged 4–7 years. The lesions are confined to bone.
2. Hand-Schuller-Christian disease affects younger patients and is more widespread and aggressive with multifocal lesions at the skull base causing the triad of diabetes insipidus (from infiltration of the hypothalamus and/or posterior pituitary), exophthalmos, and bony defects of the skull.
3. Letterer-Siwe disease – often affects children under 2 years of age causing multisystem involvement including cutaneous, lymph node, visceral, ocular, and orbital disease. This is the most aggressive end of the LCH spectrum, and is frequently fatal.

Since there is significant clinical overlap and identical histopathology in all three groups, Lichtenstein[10] called the whole group "histiocytosis X" to emphasize the common cell of origin and the unknown etiology. The term "Langerhans' cell histiocytosis" replaced histiocytosis X in 1987, differentiating conditions in which the abnormal histiocytes are derived from the Langerhans' cell from the other histiocytic disorders. LCH has been subdivided clinically into:

1. Single system disease, which may be limited to a single site (unifocal, usually corresponding to eosinophilic granuloma), or involve multiple sites (multifocal, corresponding to Hand-Schuller-Christian disease)
2. Multisystem disease (systemic, previously known as Letterer-Siwe disease).

Ophthalmic involvement

The most common ophthalmic presentation of LCH is orbital involvement (Fig. 27.1),[5,11] but disease of the globe and brain may also lead to ophthalmic consultation. Intraocular lesions, with infiltration of the uveal tract, are seen most frequently in infants with disseminated LCH.[12] Intracranial involvement may cause visual field defects due to infiltration of the optic nerves, chiasm, or tracts. Cranial neuropathy[13] and raised intracranial pressure are occasional presentations.

Orbital involvement

The orbit is involved in 20% of cases of LCH,[11] usually with the localized form of the disease (eosinophilic granuloma); it is rare in patients whose disease is limited to soft tissue, suggesting that the lesion usually arises in the bone.[11] They are usually situated superotemporally, with a predilection for the frontal and parietal bones and the greater wing of the

sphenoid.[14,15] Radiologically, the lesions are lytic, with a soft tissue component causing expansion of the surrounding tissues (Figs 27.1 to 27.4). Occasionally, lytic bony lesions may be seen radiologically in the absence of any clinical signs.

Clinical features

The usual presentation is with unilateral or bilateral proptosis.[5] Rarely, the proptosis may be extreme causing luxation of the globe.[16] Less commonly, the presentation is with isolated orbital involvement in a previously healthy child, in which case the disease is usually unilateral. Initially, the course may be evanescent and relapsing. An isolated lesion of the superior orbital wall may present with unilateral ptosis or inferonasal globe displacement. The lesions, if superficial, are generally soft to palpation. Optic nerve compression and cranial nerve palsies are rare, but may be seen with extensive orbital involvement.[11] Skin tethering (Fig. 27.5), erythema, and erosion may occur (see Fig. 27.5). Visual loss may be caused by optic nerve compression,[11] optic atrophy due to chronically raised intracranial pressure,[11] chiasmal disease, or intraocular infiltration.[12,17,18] Chronic disseminated LCH (Hand-Schuller-Christian disease) may present with polyuria and polydipsia, and can be associated with growth, thyroid, and gonadotrophic hormone deficiencies.

Investigation

In most children with orbital disease, plain X-rays (Fig. 27.6) will demonstrate a lytic bone lesion. Computed tomography

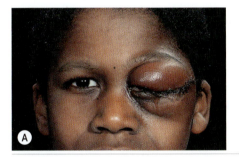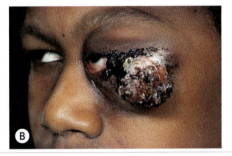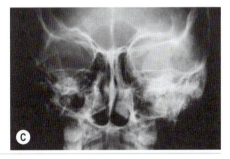

Fig. 27.1 (A) LCH involving the left orbit. (B) The vision is unaffected but progression leads to surface ulceration. (C) Skull X ray shows extensive bony hypertrophy around a chronic lesion. The patient responded to limited excision, curettage and local steroid injection.

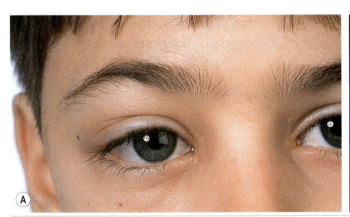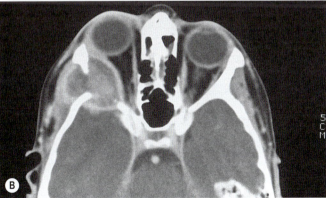

Fig. 27.2 (A) This 9-year-old boy presented with swelling and erythema of the right upper lid of 2 weeks duration. There was 4 mm proptosis. The CT scan (B) showed a mass which had eroded the posterolateral wall of the orbit, into the temporalis fossa. Fine needle biopsy was consistent with LCH. The lesion was excised surgically and irrigated locally with corticosteroid. There was a good response to a tapering course of systemic prednisolone. (Patient of the University of British Columbia.)

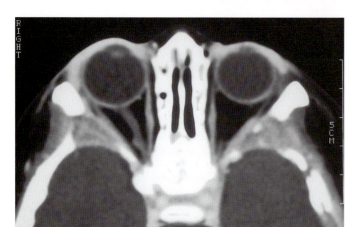

Fig. 27.3 LCH with extensive orbital involvement with bony erosion on CT scan.

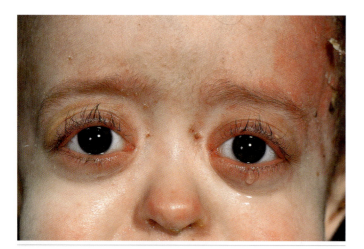

Fig. 27.4 Patient with bilateral LCH, proptosis, and obstructed nasolacrimal duct.

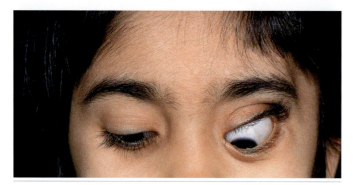

Fig. 27.5 Skin and lid tethering with orbital LCH.

(CT) scan demonstrates an enhancing mass often with a low density center; together with magnetic resonance imaging (MRI) this will delineate the extent of intraorbital bone or intracranial involvement (Fig. 27.7). On MRI, bony lesions are typically hypointense on T1-weighted images with intermediate to high signal intensity on T2-weighted images. Most lesions show moderate to intense contrast enhancement. MRI is preferable for evaluation of intracranial extension.[18] Orbital lesions usually remain extraconal but may spread into the muscle cone.

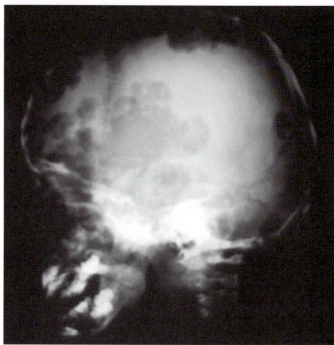

Fig. 27.6 Disseminated Langerhans' cell histiocytosis with punched-out skull lesion.

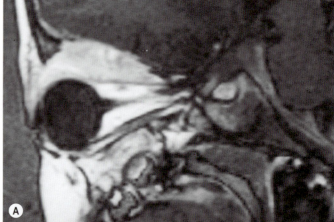

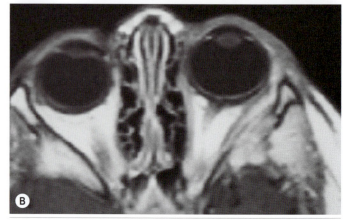

Fig. 27.7 (A, B) LCH showing extensive involvement of the left orbital bones.

The diagnosis is confirmed by histologic examination of involved tissue. In children with multisystem disease, an accessible site such as skin or a peripheral bone should be biopsied; in cases with solitary orbital involvement, orbital biopsy is necessary. Fine needle aspiration may be useful in these circumstances.[19] Children who present to the ophthalmologist should be referred to a pediatric oncologist to determine if there is any systemic involvement. Further investigations may include chest X-ray, skeletal survey, lung and liver function tests, and specific gravity of early morning urine.

Histopathology reveals granulomatous infiltration consisting of histiocytes and multinucleated lipid-laden giant cells, eosinophils (particularly numerous in single site bone-based lesions or "eosinophilic granulomas"), lymphocytes, plasma cells. and neutrophils. Electron microscopy demonstrates typical Langerhans' granules, also known as Birbeck or racket bodies, in about 50% of cases,[20] indicating that the proliferating histiocytes are derivatives of the Langerhans' cells, part of the mononuclear–phagocyte system.[21] Immunohistochemical techniques may be helpful to secure the diagnosis.[2]

Management and prognosis

Close dialogue between the treating ophthalmologist and oncologist in the management of LCH with orbital involvement is essential.[22] Advice from other specialists such as ENT and orthopedic surgery may be needed.

The management of orbital lesions depends on whether there is single system or multisystem disease.[23] Conservative management with careful observation may be justified in patients with single site orbital involvement, where complete spontaneous resolution after incisional biopsy[24] or even fine needle aspiration has been reported. Usually, patients with a single orbital lesion are treated by biopsy and curettage resulting in resolution.[11] Intralesional steroids may be used to hasten remission[11] or reduce pain. If there is marked proptosis or optic nerve compression, a short course of systemic steroids or radiotherapy may be used to induce remission. A radiation dose of 500–600 cGy is usually sufficient. The total dose should not exceed 1000 cGy because of the risk of radiation-induced malignancies in later life. Cosmetically disfiguring lesions of the orbital wall may be removed surgically with curettage. Orbital bone involvement frequently results in arrested growth of the walls with shallowing. This is not related to the use of radiotherapy (Fig. 27.8).

In patients with generalized LCH, orbital involvement will generally respond to systemic chemotherapy. Local radiotherapy may be used in addition if there is progressive proptosis or optic nerve compression.

Children with single system disease, for example of the bone, have a good prognosis.[25,26] The prognosis is poor in multisystem or visceral disease, especially if there is infiltration and failure of key organs such as the bone marrow, liver, and lungs, which may be fatal.[7] Children under the age of 2 years have a mortality rate of 55–60%; death is rare after the age of 3 years. Although some authors have stressed age as the most important prognostic factor, it is really the tendency of infants to develop multisystem disease rather than their age which dictates the poorer prognosis of children aged 2 years and under.[23,27] Response to the initial treatment of multisystem LCH is a good predictor of eventual outcome.[23,28]

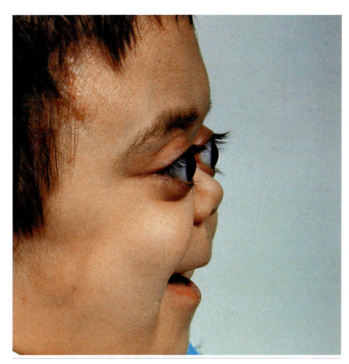

Fig. 27.8 This patient has shallow orbits and exophthalmos due to the arrest of bony development following treatment for orbital Langerhans' cell histiocytosis. (Patient of the University of British Columbia). (With permission from Rootman J. Diseases of the Orbit: A Multidisciplinary Approach, 2nd ed. Philadelphia: Lippincott Williams and Wilkins; 2002: 411.)

Non-Langerhans' cell histiocytosis

Juvenile xanthogranuloma

Juvenile xanthogranuloma (JXG) is a disorder of unknown etiology in which there is abnormal proliferation of non-Langerhans' histiocytes. These, like Langerhans' histiocytes, are probably a group of dendritic cells.[29] It is characteristically a benign skin disorder of infants and young children which tends to undergo spontaneous regression. It is more common in children with neurofibromatosis type 1 (NF1) and can be the first sign of this disorder.[30,31] The simultaneous presence of JXG and NF1 raises the risk of developing juvenile myelomonocytic leukemia 20–30 times,[32] yet screening for leukemia in this group remains controversial.[33] The skin lesions are occasionally accompanied by ocular involvement but ocular involvement can occur without cutaneous lesions. Visceral and bony involvement occurs less commonly than in LCH.[34]

Histopathology

The JXG lesion consists of a mixture of lymphocytes, plasma cells, histiocytes, giant cells, and occasional eosinophils. The distinctive histologic feature is the presence of Touton giant cells, in which a central ring of nuclei encloses an area of eosinophilic cytoplasm surrounded by a foamy cytoplasm (Fig. 27.9). An important electron microscopic feature is the absence of Langerhans' (Birbeck) granules in the histiocytes, distinguishing these lesions from LCH. Immunohistochemistry of JXG is positive for vimentin, CD68, and factor XIIIa immunostains and negative for S100 protein, helping to differentiate this condition from other histiocytic proliferations.[29]

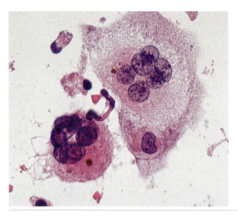

Fig. 27.9 Juvenile xanthogranuloma. Touton giant cell.

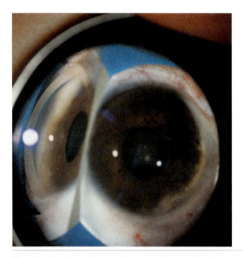

Fig. 27.10 Juvenile xanthogranuloma. Gonioscopy view showing the angle filled with yellowish xanthogranuloma material. It can also be seen in the bottom right of the picture directly.

Ocular involvement

JXG predominantly occurs in infancy and early childhood; in Zimmerman's series[34] 85% of patients with ocular involvement were less than 1 year old, 64% less than 8 months. It occurs in neonates.[35] Patients with ocular disease may occasionally present in adult life.[36] Most have unilateral disease although a few cases with bilateral involvement have been reported.[37] Cutaneous lesions are benign and often self-limited whilst ocular involvement can result in glaucoma and visual loss from optic nerve damage or amblyopia; however, since only 3 or 4 patients of every 1000 with cutaneous JXG develop ocular complications, routine eye screening of all patients is not justified. It could be limited to children with cutaneous involvement under 2 years of age, whose risk of ocular involvement is highest.[38]

The iris is infiltrated in the majority of cases,[34,39] the ciliary body,[34,39] or rarely the choroid and retina[39,40] may also be affected. Rarely, juvenile xanthogranuloma can masquerade as uveitis in childhood in the absence of skin lesions.[39,41]

Typically, a localized or diffuse yellow or fluffy-white iris lesion is evident in one eye of an infant (Fig. 27.10), often accompanied by hyphema (Fig. 27.11). Glaucoma, with corneal edema, photophobia, ocular enlargement, and circum-corneal flush are usually present. There may be uveitis and a

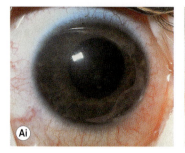
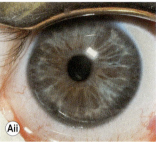
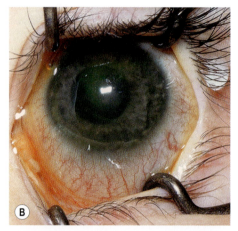
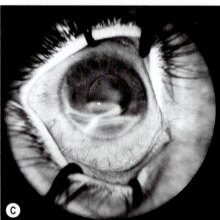
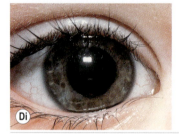
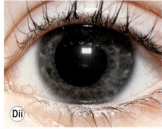

Fig. 27.11 (A–C) Presumed juvenile xanthogranuloma. The patient had presented because of recurrent left hyphema resulting in glaucoma. There was iris vascularization with profuse fluorescein leakage but no frank mass formation. (D) One year later. After 350 cGy radiotherapy there was a very marked improvement and after a period of occlusion of the right eye the acuity was 6/6. No recurrence occurred over 9 years.

xanthochromic flare. In some cases, iris heterochromia is the only presenting sign.

Although typically yellow or creamy-white, the iris lesion may occasionally be very vascular and can be mistaken for a hemangioma. The differential diagnosis of spontaneous hyphema in childhood includes:

1. Trauma (unrecognized or with abuse) (see Chapters 66 and 67)
2. Tumor (retinoblastoma see Chapter 42), dictyoma, LCH, leukemia, neuroblastoma)
3. Rubeosis (secondary to retinopathy of prematurity (see Chapter 43), retinal dysplasia, persistent hyperplastic primary vitreous (see Chapter 41))
4. Iris arteriovenous malformation

Management

If cutaneous lesions are present with an iris lesion, a diagnosis of JXG is best confirmed by skin biopsy. In cases without cutaneous involvement, examination of aqueous from a paracentesis may show typical histiocytes. Diagnostic iris biopsy should be avoided if possible because of the risk of hemorrhage.

Several different treatments have been advocated for uveal lesions, including topical and systemic steroids,[42] radiotherapy, and surgical excision. Medical treatment is preferable because of the risk of extensive hemorrhage following excision. We suggest a short course of topical,[43] subconjunctival,[44] and/or systemic steroids[45] to induce remission, adding a topical beta-blocker or carbonic anhydrase inhibitor if the intraocular pressure is raised. In cases which are unresponsive to steroid, radiotherapy (at a dose not exceeding 500 cGy) may be required.[46]

Optic nerve and retinal involvement

Wertz et al.[40] reported a 20-month-old infant with iris heterochromia in the absence of skin lesions. Hemorrhagic infarction of the retina was accompanied by rubeosis. Histologic examination of the enucleated eye revealed massive infiltration of the optic nerve, disc, retina, and choroid with histiocytes. Touton giant cells, diagnostic of JXG, were present.

Epibulbar lesions

Conjunctival (Fig. 27.12), episcleral, and corneal involvement in JXG are uncommon, presenting as a limbal nodule whose color may be yellow, orange, or pink.[47,48] This may grow over as well as around the cornea, and may accompany intraocular involvement.[49] It may also appear as a yellowish or yellowish-pinkish subconjunctival mass which could be mistaken for subconjunctival lymphoma.[34] Frequently, the lesions gradually regress in which case they may be observed. Enlarging lesions may be treated in the same way as uveal lesions, with topical or systemic steroids or even radiotherapy. Bleeding is occasionally troublesome if the lesion is excised;[50] recurrence is a possibility.

Involvement of the ocular adnexae

Initially, the typical skin lesions (Fig. 27.13) are tense yellow to reddish-brown papules. Later, these become softer and orange or yellow–brown in color. Since they have a predilection for the face, neck, and trunk, it is not surprising that they

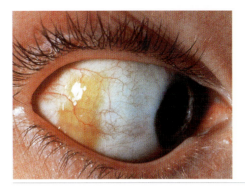

Fig. 27.12 A slowly enlarging yellowish lesion was noticed in the conjunctiva of this 15-year-old boy. Histology showed Touton giant cells, characteristic of juvenile xanthogranuloma. (Patient of the University of British Columbia.)

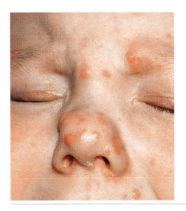

Fig. 27.13 Juvenile xanthogranuloma with skin lesions. Both eyes were glaucomatous (see Chapter 37).

are common on the eyelids. Occasionally, a single lid lesion is the only manifestation of JXG and biopsy may be necessary to make a diagnosis.[51] The nodules usually regress spontaneously within a year but occasionally persist for several years.

Orbital involvement in JXG is uncommon,[34,52,53] but it may cause unilateral proptosis in infancy. Most cases present within the first 6 months of life, often in the absence of cutaneous findings. JXG has been described arising in the lacrimal fossa as a mass causing nasolacrimal duct obstruction in a 2-year-old.[54] The extraocular muscles may be infiltrated, resulting in restrictive strabismus.[34] In contrast to LCH, bony destruction is unusual but may occur.[55] Intracranial involvement is well documented, with a clinical course ranging from spontaneous regression to fatal progression.[53,56,57] If there are no other systemic features, it may be difficult to differentiate between JXG and histiocytosis X clinically, but light and electron microscopy are diagnostic. The lungs, liver, spleen, gastrointestinal tract, and pericardium may be affected.[58] Freyer et al.[57] have reviewed systemic involvement in JXR and stress that, unlike its cutaneous form, significant complications may arise from this disease.

As JXG has a tendency to undergo spontaneous remission, patients with orbital involvement should initially be observed. Patients with progressive proptosis or marked restriction of ocular motility should be given a short course of systemic steroid.[55] If there is no response, low-dose radiotherapy (500 cGy) should be given. The visual and systemic prognosis is usually excellent.

Sinus histiocytosis with massive lymphadenopathy (Rosai-Dorfman disease)

Rosai and Dorfman first used the name "sinus histiocytosis with massive lymphadenopathy" in 1969. Known since then as sinus histiocytosis or Rosai-Dorfman disease, this idiopathic disorder mainly affects children and young adults. In a series of 113 patients[59] the average age was 8.6 years. It is more common in males. The cause is unknown. Massive painless cervical lymphadenopathy is present in the vast majority of patients, often with enlargement of other lymph node groups. Forty-three percent of patients have involvement of extranodal sites;[59] 8.5% of patients with sinus histiocytosis have orbital or eyelid involvement.[60] The upper respiratory tract, salivary gland, skin, testes, and bone can also be affected. The lymphadenopathy is accompanied by fever, neutrophil leukocytosis, polyclonal hypergammaglobulinemia, and a raised erythrocyte sedimentation rate.[61] The signs and symptoms may persist for months or years before recovery.[62]

Patients with ophthalmic involvement usually present with unilateral or bilateral proptosis. In the orbit, soft tissue involvement sparing the bones is most typical (84.6%), followed by eyelid involvement (45.4%),[59,63,64] which may affect all four eyelids.[65] One or both lacrimal glands may also be affected.[66] The tumor mass usually remains extraconal; optic nerve compression is rare but there may be a duction deficit.[61] Less commonly, there is an epibulbar mass without proptosis.[64] Progressive proptosis may lead to corneal exposure, ulceration, and even endophthalmitis.[59,63] Rarely, there may be intraocular lesions with infiltration of the uvea by histiocytes.[59] Relapsing uveitis is an occasional feature which may precede the lymphadenopathy by years.[67] The lack of bony and visceral involvement helps to differentiate it from LCH.

Histopathologic examination of orbital biopsy specimens shows a dense cellular infiltrate of histiocytes, lymphocytes, and plasma cells surrounded by connective tissue. The histopathologic hallmark is lymphophagocytosis in which viable lymphocytes are located in well-defined cytoplasmic vacuoles of intact histiocytes. Electron microscopy fails to demonstrate the typical Birbeck inclusion granules of Langerhans' cells, differentiating this condition from LCH, though, like Langerhans'

cells, the cells are S100-positive and may express CD1a antigen.[3] Malignant lymphoma is an important differential diagnosis.

There is no agreement regarding the treatment of this disorder; high-dose systemic steroids, systemic chemotherapeutic agents such as vinblastine and methotrexate, and radiotherapy[68] have all been used without consistent success. The management of orbital involvement should include frequent assessment of vision and the maintenance of adequate corneal care. Progressive proptosis causing exposure keratitis may require orbital decompression.[59,63] The orbital disease tends to be chronic with occasional recurrences, but the systemic prognosis is good; there was one death in Foucar et al.'s series[59] which may have been related to complications from systemic chemotherapy. Involvement of kidneys, lungs, liver, or associated immunologic disease may be poor prognostic features.[60]

Leukemia (see Chapter 64)

The eye, like the brain, is a relative "pharmacologic sanctuary" in the treatment of leukemia so it is not surprising that recurrent disease frequently manifests within the eye or central nervous system. Orbital involvement may be the first manifestation or part of disseminated leukemia.

Leukemia accounted for 11% of the 27 cases of unilateral proptosis in children reported by Oakhill et al.[69] It was second only to rhabdomyosarcoma (see Chapter 24) in frequency of childhood malignant orbital disease in Porterfield's[70] series. The orbit is more commonly involved in acute than chronic leukemia and, in children, by myeloblastic than lymphoblastic tumors. Ridgway et al.[71] examined 657 children with acute leukemia and found orbital involvement, clinically, in 1%. Yet, Kincaid and Green[72] found postmortem evidence of orbital involvement in 10% of 384 patients.

The clinical features of orbital leukemic involvement include proptosis, lid edema, chemosis, and pain. Both orbits are involved in 2% of patients with orbital leukemia. Proptosis may be due to a mass of leukemic cells or to orbital hemorrhage, which may also appear subconjunctivally and cause eyelid discoloration (Fig. 27.14).[73] Other diseases which may present with rapidly increasing proptosis, chemosis, and hemorrhage must be considered. These include rhabdomyosarcoma, neuroblastoma, Ewing's sarcoma, and orbital

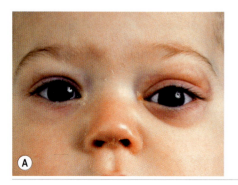
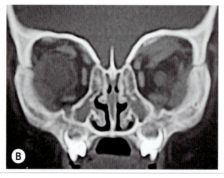
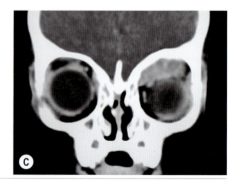

Fig. 27.14 (A) This 10-month-old boy presented with a 3-week history of cough, irritability, and puffy eyes. X-rays showed pneumonia, and complete blood count revealed pancytopenia. He had bilateral lid masses with downward displacement of the left globe and blue-yellow discoloration of the lid. (B,C) CT scan demonstrates a left irregular orbital mass superiorly and inferolaterally, extending to the apex where the bone was irregular. Biopsy demonstrated chloroma, and cytogenetics confirmed a diagnosis of AML M5 with marrow involvement.

cellulitis.[72] Leukemia may present with intraocular involvement in childhood, with conjunctival injection, hypopyon, and glaucoma.[74]

Orbital leukemic deposits are often associated with meningeal involvement[71] and are part of terminal disease,[70,71] although in some cases orbital signs may be the presenting feature of leukemia (chloroma) and biopsy provides the diagnosis. The lacrimal gland[75] or, more rarely, the extraocular muscles[72] may be infiltrated and contiguous sinus disease is a common postmortem finding. The orbit is occasionally the site of opportunistic infection by bacteria or fungi in immunosuppressed leukemic children. Iatrogenic complications include ptosis and extraocular muscle palsy from the use of cytotoxic agents such as vincristine.[76]

Leukemic deposits consist of cells derived from lymphoblasts or myeloblasts. A localized form of acute myeloblastic leukemia has a predilection for the bones of the skull and particularly the orbit where it presents as a rapidly expanding tumor. This was initially called "chloroma," a reference to its greenish color from the pigmented enzyme myeloperoxidase. The term "granulocytic sarcoma," or sometimes myeloid sarcoma, is now used. It is more common in boys; children from Asia, Africa, and Latin America are more likely to be affected.[77] The peak prevalence of orbital granulocytic sarcoma is at age 7–8 years.[78] Granulocytic sarcoma may appear at any time in the course of myeloblastic leukemia. It is not uncommon for this orbital presentation to precede the hematologic diagnosis in which case the diagnosis can be challenging.[79] This was reported in 29 of 33 cases (88%) in Zimmerman's large study of orbital granulocytic sarcoma.[75] In the majority of cases, hematologic changes appear within 2 months. Histologically, it is a poorly differentiated high grade malignancy which should be distinguished from the other round cell tumors of childhood. Its main diagnostic differential, large B-cell lymphoma, is very much rarer in children. The diagnosis of orbital granulocytic sarcoma is based on clinical presentation and biopsy. An elevated white cell count in the peripheral blood with increased peripheral and medullary blasts, as well as the presence of an Auer rod pathognomonic of AML are helpful confirmatory findings. The Leder stain identifying cells with esterase activity (positive in approximately three-quarters of cases) as well as immunohistochemical stains help to secure this diagnosis.

Orbital leukemia is treated by systemic chemotherapy with or without local irradiation. The dose and effect of the latter are not clearly defined.

The prognosis of orbital granulocytic sarcoma is related to the nature of the underlying hematologic malignancy; extramedullary involvement may adversely impact the outcome of the leukemia: Byrd et al. found that half their leukemic patients with granulocytic sarcoma achieved complete remission as compared to 92% without.[80]

Lymphoma

Knowles et al.[81] stated that they had never seen orbital lymphoma as part of systemic nodal disease in children, attesting to the rarity of this disorder in childhood. However, the incidence of lymphoma is increasing in the general population for reasons which are not understood.[82] There are individual case reports of orbital involvement by B, T, and null cell lymphomas[83-85] and the orbit is a site for post-transplantation lymphoproliferative disorders,[86] but the only lymphoma with a predilection for the child, and in particular the head and neck region, is Burkitt's lymphoma.

This high grade undifferentiated lymphocytic tumor most commonly affects children in tropical Africa but occurs sporadically worldwide. The Epstein-Barr virus acts as an oncogene in patients who have been immunologically stimulated by chronic exposure to malaria organisms.[87] The tumor affects males more commonly than females (2 : 1 ratio), with a median age of 7 years at presentation. In 60% of African cases, there is a maxillary tumor causing massive proptosis, but this may only appear late in the disease, since only 13% of patients present with exophthalmos. Non-African cases tend to present later (median age 11 years) with a greater propensity for abdominal involvement, although the head and neck region can be involved.[88,89] Burkitt's lymphoma may also present with cranial nerve palsies or papilledema from central nervous system involvement. Younger patients and those with localized disease have a better prognosis. The tumor responds to chemotherapy with prolonged remission; some patients show immunologic self-cure.[90]

References

2. Pinkus GS, Lones MA, Matsumura F, et al. Langerhans cell histiocytosis immunohistochemical expression of fascin, a dendritic cell marker. Am J Clin Pathol 2002; 118: 335–43.

3. Favara BE, Feller AC, Pauli M, et al. Contemporary classification of histiocytic disorders. The WHO Committee on Histiocytic/ Reticulum Cell Proliferations. Reclassification Working Group of the Histiocyte Society. Med Pediatr Oncol 1997; 29: 157–66.

7. Abla O, Egeler RM, Weitzman S. Langerhans cell histiocytosis: current concepts and treatments. Cancer Treat Res 2010; 36: 354–9.

8. Filipovich A, McClain K, Grom A. Histiocytic disorders: recent insights into pathophysiology and practical guidelines. Biol Blood Marrow Transplant 2010; 16: S82–9.

10. Lichtenstein L. Histiocytosis X: integration of eosinophilic granuloma of bone, Letterer-Siwe disease, and Schuller-Christian disease as related manifestations of a single nosologic entity. AMA Arch Pathol 1953; 56: 84–102.

11. Moore AT, Pritchard J, Taylor DS. Histiocytosis X: an ophthalmological review. Br J Ophthalmol 1985; 69: 7–14.

12. Boztug K, Frimpong-Ansali K, Nanduri VR, Lawson J. Intraocular Langerhans cell histiocytosis in a neonate resulting in bilateral loss of vision. Pediatr Blood Cancer 2006; 47: 633–5.

15. Rootman J. Diseases of the Orbit: A Multidisciplinary Approach, 2nd ed. Philadelphia: Lippincott Williams & Wilkins; 2002.

22. Harris GJ. Langerhans cell histiocytosis of the orbit: a need for interdisciplinary dialogue. Am J Ophthalmol 2006; 141: 374–8.

23. Allen CE, McClain KL. Langerhans histiocytosis: a review of past, current and future therapies. Drugs Today (Barc) 2007; 43: 627–43.

24. Rajendram R, Rose G, Luthert P, et al. Biopsy-confirmed spontaneous resolution of orbital Langerhans cell histiocytosis. Orbit 2005; 24: 39–41.

27. Nezelof C, Barbey S. Histiocytosis: nosology and pathobiology. Pediatr Pathol 1985; 3: 1–41.

29. Dehner LP. Juvenile xanthogranulomas in the first two decades of life: a clinicopathologic study of 174 cases with cutaneous and extracutaneous manifestations. Am J Surg Pathol 2003; 27: 579–93.

31. Raygada M, Arthur DC, Wayne AS, et al. Juvenile xanthogranuloma in a child with previously unsuspected neurofibromatosis type 1 and juvenile myelomonocytic leukemia. Pediatr Blood Cancer 2010; 54: 173–5.

33. De Keyser C, Maudgal P, Legius E, et al. Juvenile xanthogranuloma of the corneoscleral limbus: report of two cases. Ophthal Genet 2011; 32: 54–6.

34. Zimmerman LE. Ocular lesions of juvenile xanthogranuloma: nevoxanthoedothelioma. Am J Ophthalmol 1965; 60: 1011–35.

41. Zamir E, Wang RC, Krishnakumar S, et al. Juvenile xanthogranuloma masquerading as pediatric chronic uveitis: a clinicopathologic study. Surv Ophthalmol 2001; 46: 164–71.

48. Chaudhry IA, Al-Jishi Z, Shamsi FA, Riley F. Juvenile xanthogranuloma of the corneoscleral limbus: case report and review of the literature. Surv Ophthalmol 2004; 49: 608–14.

51. Kuruvilla R, Escaravage GK, Finn AJ, Dutton JJ. Infiltrative subcutaneous juvenile xanthogranuloma of the eyelid in a neonate. Ophthal Plast Reconstr Surg 2009; 25: 330–2.

52. Shields CL, Shields JA, Buchanon HW. Solitary orbital involvement with juvenile xanthogranuloma. Arch Ophthalmol 1990; 108: 1587–9.

59. Foucar E, Rosai J, Dorfman RF. The ophthalmologic manifestations of sinus histiocytosis with massive lymphadenopathy. Am J Ophthalmol 1979; 87: 354–67.

60. Foucar E, Rosai J, Dorfman R. Sinus histiocytosis with massive lymphadenopathy (Rosai-Dorfman disease): review of the entity. Semin Diagn Pathol 1990; 7: 19–73.

62. Rosai J, Dorfman RF. Sinus histiocytosis with massive lymphadenopathy: a pseudolymphomatous benign disorder. Analysis of 34 cases. Cancer 1972; 30: 1174–88.

66. Prabhakaran VC, Bhatnagar A, Sandilla J. Orbital and adnexal Rosai Dorfaman disease. Orbit 2008; 27: 356–62.

70. Porterfield JF. Orbital tumors in children: a report on 214 cases. Int Ophthalmol Clin 1962; 2: 319–26.

77. Stockl FA, Dolmetsch AM, Saornil A, et al. Orbital granulocytic sarcoma. Br J Ophthalmol 1997; 81: 1084–8.

78. Chung EM, Murphey MD, Specht CS, et al. From the archives of the AFIP. Pediatric orbit tumors and tumorlike lesions: osseous lesions of the orbit. Radiographics 2008; 28: 1193–213.

82. Margo CE, Mulla ZD. Malignant tumors of the orbit: analysis of the Florida cancer registry. Ophthalmology 1998; 105: 185–90.

86. Douglas RS, Goldstein SM, Katowitz JA, et al. Orbital presentation of posttransplantation lymphoproliferative disorder: a small case series. Ophthalmology 2002; 109: 2351–5.

 Access the complete reference list online at

http://www.expertconsult.com

Part 3
Orbit and lacrimal

Craniofacial abnormalities

John Crompton • Joanna Black

Introduction

This chapter discusses two main groups of disorders:

1. Craniosynostoses, in which premature closure of sutures causes an abnormally shaped skull, e.g. Crouzon's and Apert's syndromes.
2. The clefting syndromes, in which there is a failure of apposition or fusion of fetal tissues. These include the mandibulofacial dysostoses, e.g. Treacher-Collins and Goldenhar's syndromes.

In addition, frontoethmoidal meningoencephaloceles, midline facial clefts, and amniotic bands are discussed.

Craniosynostosis

Craniosynostosis is premature fusion of one or more cranial vault sutures with resultant skull deformity. It occurs in approximately 1 in 2500 births and may be primary or secondary. Thirty percent of cases are syndromic, usually with multiple suture involvement and associated primary malformations in the face, trunk, or extremities. Syndromic craniosynostosis patients present with significant cosmetic challenges and face complex neurologic, ophthalmologic, and airway difficulties. Non-syndromic ("simple") craniosynostosis may have neurologic or ophthalmologic complications. Some cases of simple craniosynostosis represent the mild end of a spectrum of syndromic disease.[1]

Pathophysiology

Pathogenesis and genetics[1]

The most common craniosynostosis syndromes are autosomal dominant. New mutations are of paternal origin; their risk of occurrence increases with increasing paternal age. Mutations of seven genes are associated with the condition. These belong to four functional groups:

1. Tyrosine-kinase receptors: FGFR1, FGFR2, and FGFR3
2. DNA regulatory molecules
3. TWIST1 and MSX2, ligand receptors
4. EFNB1 and EFNB2 and intracellular cell membrane protein trafficking: RAB23.

Five of these mutations are involved in cell proliferation and ossification and belong to a common molecular pathway. Gain-of-function mutations represent the main molecular mechanism causing the disorders, but loss-of-function may lead to the phenotype. These seven genes account for 30% of syndromic cases. The genetic etiology of non-syndromic craniosynostosis is poorly understood; familial occurrence and associated gene changes within fused sutures are the same for both syndromic and non-syndromic cases.[2] The reader is referred to genetic databases such as the Online Mendelian Inheritance in Man (OMIM) Database (http://www.ncbi.nlm.nih.gov/entrez). Environmental factors have also been implicated in the etiology of craniosynostosis, including maternal smoking and altitude and intrauterine head constraint.[3] Craniosynostosis may occur secondary to various conditions, including shunted hydrocephalus, metabolic disorders such as hyperthyroidism and rickets, and hematologic disorders such as thalassemia and sickle cell anemia.[3]

Effects on the skull

Cranial sutures are fibrous joints providing a malleable quality to the head, allowing vaginal birth and growth of the brain during early development. Premature skull suture fusion results in restricted cranial growth perpendicular to the fused suture and compensatory growth at the remaining open sutures (Fig. 28.1). The principal clinical manifestations have been given Greek or Latin descriptors; identification of the involved suture has found more favor recently. Trigonocephaly ("triangular head") is metopic suture synostosis, scaphocephaly

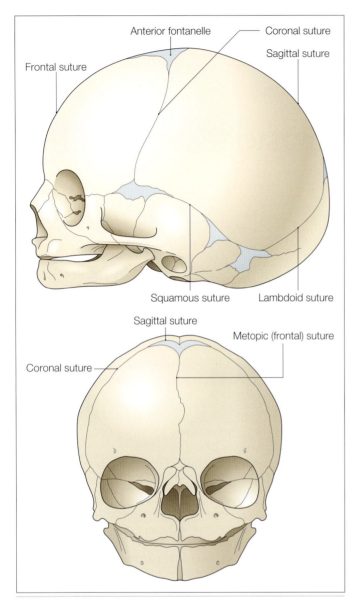

Fig. 28.1 The cranial sutures and fontanelles in an infant skull.

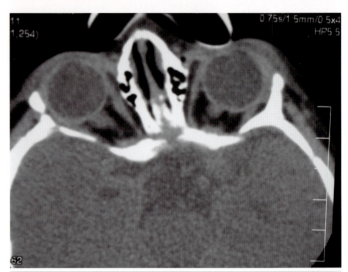

Fig. 28.2 Saethre-Chotzen syndrome. Axial CT of a patient with Saethre-Chotzen syndrome demonstrating shortened orbits and proptosis.

("boat shaped head") is sagittal suture synostosis, plagiocephaly ("twisted head") is either unilateral coronal or unilateral lambdoid suture synostosis, and brachycephaly ("short head") is bilateral coronal suture synostosis (Table 28.1). Multiple suture involvement results in more complex head morphologies such as tryphyllocephaly (Kleeblatschadel, clover leaf, or trilobed skull) or oxycephaly ("towering head"). Premature synostosis also occurs in the cranial base and facial skeleton. Cranial base underdevelopment compounds primary mid-facial hypoplasia through its indirect effects on mid-facial growth. The resulting abnormalities of palate, dentition, airway, and hearing may be severe.

Effects on intracranial pressure, the brain, and optic nerve

Brain development is intimately tied to growth of the skull; children with craniosynostosis may have developmental delay.[4,5] Reported incidences vary widely. Increased intracranial pressure (ICP) may occur in 75% of syndromic patients and

20% of single suture craniosynostosis patients. In syndromic patients four dynamic factors may contribute to raised ICP: restricted skull volume ("craniostenosis"), intracranial venous hypertension, hydrocephalus, and sleep apnea caused by facial deformity.[6] Due to its slowly progressive nature, the majority of patients have no warning symptoms. Radiologic findings are not necessarily related to intracranial pressure recordings and optic nerve swelling is frequently absent. FGFR gene products are found in the optic nerve sheath and, when these are mutated, its failure to dilate may be due to abnormal fibrous tissue in the optic nerve sheath or lamina cribrosa.[7] This increased resistance and the limited autoregulatory capacity within the sheath increases the susceptibility of the optic nerve to decreased cerebral perfusion pressure due to raised ICP, venous hypertension, and obstructive sleep apnea-related CO_2 retention.[8] Sleepapnea-related hypoxia may also contribute to brain and optic nerve damage.

Effects on the orbit

In syndromic craniosynostosis mid-facial hypoplasia and underdevelopment of the skull base lead to shallowing of the orbits, retrusion of the orbital rims, and proptosis (Fig. 28.2). Vision threatening corneal exposure or globe prolapse may occur. Keratinocyte growth factor receptor is a splice variant of FGFR2 and corneal epithelial healing may be abnormal with some FGFR mutations. Lowering of the cribriform plate and anterior cranial fossa floor with overgrowth of the ethmoid complex results in failure of anterior rotation of the orbital axes in fetal life (see Chapter 2), creating divergent orbital axes and hypertelorism (see Chapter 22). This divergence may be greater in the frontal than maxillary planes, resulting in ex-cyclorotation of the orbits (Fig. 28.3). The external manifestation of this is the anti-mongoloid palpebral fissure. Premature closure of the metopic suture may result in hypotelorism. These changes in orbital axis and angulation increase the likelihood of strabismus, which is seen in up to 90% of patients. FGFR2 is expressed in the extraocular muscles (EOMs); this may explain some of the EOM abnormalities, including bifid, hypoplastic or absent muscles, microscopic abnormalities, and a gristly, inelastic feel.[7] FGFR2 is also expressed in the

Table 28.1 – Simple craniosynostosis

Suture involved	Features
Metopic	Ridging of metopic suture Depressed superolateral orbital rims Narrowed intercanthal distance
Unilateral coronal	Ipsilateral forehead and frontoparietal flattening Contralateral frontoparietal bulging Ipsilateral anterior displacement of the zygoma and ear Deviation of nose to contralateral side Shortened orbital roof and superior oblique imbalance
Sagittal	Biparietal narrowing Frontal bossing Ridging of the sagittal suture
Unilateral lambdoid	Ipsilateral occipital flattening Ipsilateral frontal bossing

embryonic rat lens and cornea. This may account for the high incidence of refractive error in these patients.

Management

Diagnosis[2]

Simple craniosynostoses are summarized in Table 28.1 and the most common craniosynostosis syndromes are described in Table 28.2. Syndromic craniosynostosis presents little challenge to detection and may be diagnosed in utero (Fig. 28.4). There are a number of differential diagnoses to consider with simple synostoses. History and examination will usually resolve any uncertainty. Attention should be paid to:

1. The angle of the palpebral fissure
2. The position of the ear

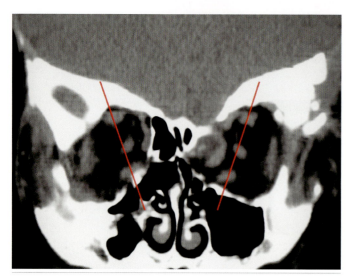

Fig. 28.3 Crouzon's syndrome. Coronal CT in a patient with Crouzon's syndrome demonstrating ex-cyclorotation of the orbits and their contents. A line drawn between the centers of the superior and inferior rectus muscles emphasizes the angle.

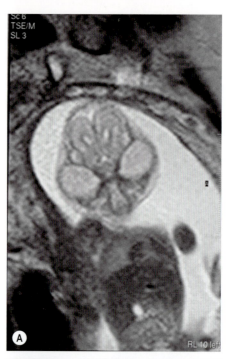

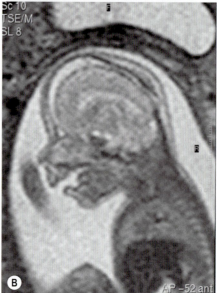

Fig. 28.4 Antenatal ultrasound images of a fetus with Pfeiffer's syndrome.

3. Any twisting of the nasal tip
4. A "bird's eye view" of the head.

The sutures may be palpated for abnormal ridging or immobility. Deformational plagiocephaly, a common condition since the introduction of the "back to sleep" intervention to reduce the risk of sudden infant death syndrome, may be confused with lambdoid synostosis, which is very rare. Deformational plagiocephaly is characterized by a history of development of the head shape in the first few months of life in association with persistent positioning on one side, torticollis, or an inactive or developmentally delayed infant. The resultant occipitoparietal flattening may be differentiated from unilateral lambdoid synostosis by a parallelogram shaped head seen from above and anterior displacement of the ipsilateral ear. Unilateral lambdoid synostosis results in a trapezoidal shaped head from above and the ear is posteriorly displaced (Figs 28.5 and 28.6). The relatively large head and poor neck muscle tone of the premature baby results in a laterally turned head and may result in a long narrow head. The distinction from sagittal synostosis can be made by the mobile sagittal suture and correction of the head shape at 3 months of age as head control increases. Metopic synostosis may present some diagnostic difficulty; it is a spectrum of disease: at one end is the development of a metopic ridge in the first year of life, which usually requires no treatment. This may be differentiated from premature closure of the metopic suture seen in primary microcephaly by normal head circumference. At the other end of the spectrum is classic trigonocephaly characterized by metopic ridging in association with supraorbital recession and hypotelorism (see Chapter 22).

Craniosynostosis is very complex. Decisions about timing and indications for surgery are made with input from specialists from craniofacial, neurosurgical, ENT, dental, orthodontic, anesthetic, psychologic, audiology, speech therapy, nursing, and ophthalmologic services, forming a craniofacial team. Patients require care from birth until their growth is complete at maturity. Treatment options are exclusively surgical with a broad range of available surgical techniques. A primary procedure is typically performed in the first 6 months of life, to allow safe growth of a rapidly expanding brain. Removal of the affected suture by strip craniectomy has largely been replaced by more extensive remodeling procedures and expansion of the cranial cavity, most commonly by fronto-orbital advancement. The growing brain may then exert pressure on the released calvaria and dura, allowing for good correction of the cerebrocranial disproportion and deformity. Bone growth is also good and minimizes the risk of bone defects. From this age until the age of 10, craniosynostosis should be managed expectantly with careful monitoring for evidence of raised intracranial pressure, corneal exposure, and airway problems. Some cases may require further cranial expansion surgery or mid-facial distraction; expectation would be for recurrence where surgery has been performed at a young age. Surgery in the second decade of life is directed at reducing residual deformity. Best results are achieved the closer to completion

Table 28.2 – The most common craniosynostosis syndromes

Syndrome	Clinical features
Apert's 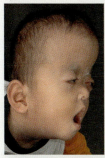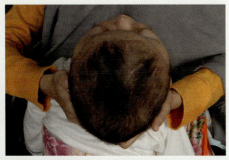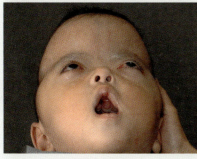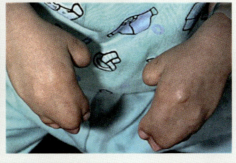	Genetics: AD, FGFR2 CS: bicoronal (antenatal), lambdoid, brachycephaly, cranial base (late childhood) CNS (common): megalencephaly, anomalies septum pellucidum, low IQ, hydrocephalus Face: cleft palate, dental crowding, malocclusion Other: syndactyly (universal), cervical spine fusions, tracheal cartilaginous fusions
Crouzon's 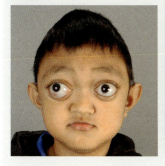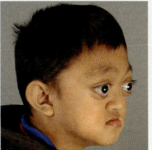	Genetics: AD, variable expressivity, FGFR2, FGFR3 CS (usually in infancy): bicoronal +/− sagittal or lambdoid, cranial base. Head shape variable (scaphocephaly, trigonocephaly, trilobed) CNS (common): Chiari malformation, jugular foramen stenosis, hydrocephalus Face: exorbitism, mid-facial hypoplasia, beaked nose, narrow palate, dental crowding, malocclusion Other: cervical vertebral fusion, tracheal cartilaginous fusions, conductive hearing loss
Pfeiffer's 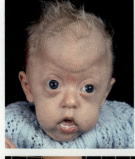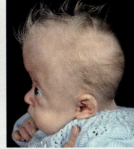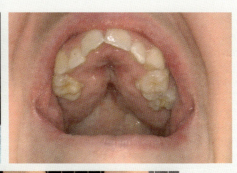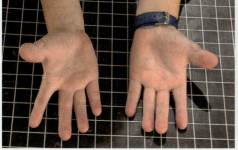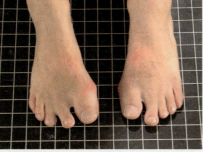	Genetics: AD, incomplete penetrance, FGFR1, FGFR2, FGFR3 Type 1: coronal +/− sagittal CS, normal IQ and life expectancy Type 2: cloverleaf skull, low IQ, synostosis of elbow and forearm Type 3: simple CS, short cranial base, synostosis of elbow and forearm Face: exorbitism, ptosis, ocular anterior segment dysgenesis, mid-facial hypoplasia, malocclusion Other (all 3 types): low set ears, ear tags, broad thumbs and great toes, brachydactyly, syndactyly, cervical vertebral fusions, tracheal cartilaginous fusions, cardiovascular, gastrointestinal, urogenital anomalies

Continued

Table 28.2 – The most common craniosynostosis syndromes **Continued**

Syndrome	Clinical features
Muenke's	Genetics: AD, FGFR3, variable expressivity CS: coronal Other: low IQ, midfacial hypoplasia, ptosis, hand anomalies
Saethre-Chotzen	Genetics: AD, TWIST (one case of FGFR2) CS (not universal): coronal, metopic, lambdoid. Often asymmetric Other: ptosis, high forehead, low hairline, maxillary hypoplasia, narrow or cleft palate, broad great toes, brachydactyly, partial cutaneous syndactyly
Antley-Bixler	Genetics: AR, FGFR2 (one case of FGFR1) CS: coronal, lambdoid Other: severe mid-facial hypoplasia, stenosis or atresia of choanae, low set protruding ears

of growth the procedure is performed. Complications include blood loss, bone defects, scalp scarring, and, most commonly, incomplete correction of the deformity. Residual deformity is particularly common in unilateral or asymmetric synostosis. Whilst fever is common in any surgery penetrating the dura, infection is very rare in procedures not entering the nasopharynx. Despite extensive subperiorbital dissection in fronto-orbital advancement surgery, ophthalmic complications are rare. The effects on ocular alignment are discussed below. Genetic studies have provided potential targets for pharmacologic or genetic modalities of treatment. The development of such non-surgical treatment options may complement or replace current invasive techniques.[9]

Ophthalmic management in craniosynostosis

The ophthalmologist should manage craniosynostosis patients in conjunction with a multidisciplinary specialized craniofacial unit. Examination may be limited by developmental and

speech delay, breathing difficulties, and exposure keratopathy related photophobia. Ophthalmic genotype–phenotype correlations have been reported amongst syndromic craniosynostosis.[10,11] The visual complications amongst non-syndromic craniosynostosis will vary with diagnosis.[12,13] However, similar ophthalmic complications may be seen in patients with any diagnosis.

Vision loss

The most important roles of the ophthalmologist are to ensure adequate protection of exposed corneas, monitor for raised intracranial pressure, and detect and treat vision loss. Syndromic craniosynostosis patients have a visual acuity of 6/12 or worse in at least one eye in 65% of cases; in 40% of cases in the better eye.[14,15] Vision loss is rare in simple metopic and sagittal suture synostosis but is frequent in unilateral coronal synostosis. The majority of non-syndromic and nearly half of syndromic vision loss is due to treatable causes: astigmatism, anisometropia, and amblyopia.[15-17] Astigmatism may be severe,

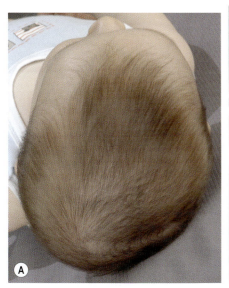

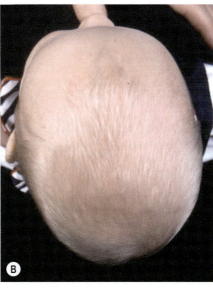

Fig. 28.5 Bird's eye views demonstrating the trapezoidal head malformation seen in lambdoid suture synostosis and parallelogram head malformation seen in deformational plagiocephaly.

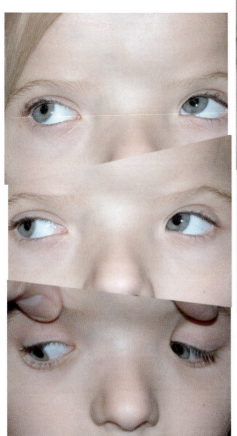

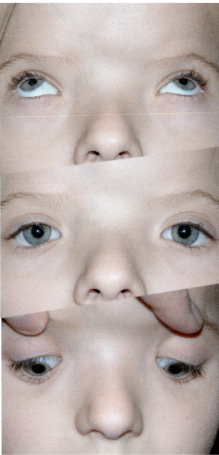

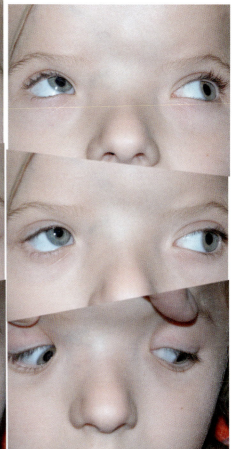

Fig. 28.6 Patient with deformational plagiocephaly demonstrating occipitoparietal flattening and anterior displacement of the ear.

secondary to the shape of the orbits, ptosis, and corneal scarring. Spectacles may need to be customized to allow comfort and acceptance of wear. Atropine penalization may be preferable to occlusion therapy for amblyopia when there is significant proptosis of the globe. Exposure keratopathy due to a shortened orbit is common in syndromic craniosynostosis and causes discomfort, photophobia, examination difficulties, infection, vision loss, and scarring. The cornea should be protected with lubricants; tarsorrhaphy may be necessary, especially in cases of spontaneous globe prolapse or during periods of significant perioperative chemosis and swelling. Tarsorrhaphy, however, may result in lid margin changes, which will undermine ocular surface health in the long term. The definitive treatment is midfacial or frontofacial advancement; the need may necessitate highlighting with the craniofacial team. Distraction devices are the method of choice for this in younger patients; in older patients surgery may be considered.

The optic nerve is susceptible to damage in craniosynostosis and optic neuropathy may manifest as visual acuity or field loss. Photophobia may make assessment of the optic nerve difficult. Papilledema is frequently absent despite raised ICP. Serial pattern reversal visual evoked potentials (VEPs) are a sensitive and reversible marker of visual pathway dysfunction in raised intracranial pressure due to craniosynostosis.[18,19] Since radiology is also unreliable in detecting raised ICP in craniosynostosis, prolonged invasive ICP monitoring is often required to select patients needing early cranial vault expansion surgery. VEP monitoring provides a valuable non-invasive alternative.[19]

Anterior segment dysgenesis has been reported in Pfeiffer's syndrome.[20] Findings include prominent Schwalbe's lines, corectopia, and Peters' anomaly. It is prudent to monitor Pfeiffer's syndrome patients for glaucoma.

Strabismus

Strabismus is reported in as many as 90% of craniosynostosis patients; exotropia is more frequent than esotropia. Dissociated eye movements, most commonly overelevation in adduction and V-pattern, occurs in as many as 44% (Fig. 28.7). Theories as to the cause include desagittalization of the obliques due to divergent orbital axes, increased contact of the inferior oblique and globe due to short orbits, and ex-cyclorotated orbits and EOMs.[21] Ex-cyclorotation of all the EOMs will create an abnormal abducting force in elevation from the superior rectus muscles and an abnormal adducting force in depression from the inferior rectus muscles, resulting in a V pattern. The medial rectus muscles will have an abnormal elevating force in adduction and lateral rectus muscles an abnormal depressing force in abduction, mimicking inferior oblique overaction. Craniosynostosis patients have an abnormally high incidence of absent EOMs: superior oblique and superior rectus are the most commonly affected. Strabismus may be multifactorial in some patients.

Success may be limited in strabismus surgery in craniosynostosis patients; however, a patient's condition is rarely worsened and a measured degree of optimism may be held. The timing of surgery takes into account any prior or planned craniofacial reconstruction. Routine fronto-orbital advancement has little effect on strabismus but surgery to correct hypertelorism often results in an eso-shift. Craniofacial surgery may involve extensive subperiosteal orbital dissection and may result in subconjunctival fibrosis, making surgery more difficult. For these reasons, strabismus surgery should usually be deferred for some postoperative time.[22] Some surgeons advocate early surgery when craniofacial reconstruction has been deferred beyond the first year of life, to establish binocularity. However, the likelihood of a second, postreconstruction procedure must be considered. Perfect alignment may be very difficult to achieve and a binocular patient may face a higher risk of postoperative diplopia.

In V patterns and overelevation in adduction the surgeon should have a high index of suspicion of ex-cyclorotation or muscle anomaly. Other indicators of ex-cyclorotation include ex-cyclorotation of the fundus and torsional movements with vertical OKN stimulation. Preoperative imaging may be useful. The EOMs are most easily identified on coronal CT or MRI immediately posterior to the globe (see Fig. 28.3). Whilst MRI is the "gold standard" imaging technique, 3-D ultrasound imaging is a safe and accurate alternative. Due to short reconstruction times, it may be performed at the time of surgery. It is less accurate at determining extraocular muscle position.[23] If imaging is not possible, surgical alternatives should be planned prior to operation. Some advocate exploration of all six EOMs. Where muscles are absent the risk of anterior segment ischemia needs to be kept in mind.

Horizontal deviations in primary gaze may be treated by standard recession and/or resection surgery; transposition of the rectus muscles may improve the dissociated movements. Coats et al. reported on 14 operated craniosynostosis patients with V pattern with severe oblique dysfunction.[24] Only inferior oblique (IO) myectomy or denervation and extirpation were consistently effective at treating IO overaction; only IO denervation and extirpation improved the superior oblique (SO) underaction. Isolated IO anteriorization and infraplacement of the medial rectus muscles were ineffective. The antielevation syndrome seen after temporal spreading of the insertion in IO anteriorization could worsen the IO overaction of the opposite, adducting eye. Hussein et al. reported nine cases of absent superior oblique tendon confirmed by the exaggerated traction test, seven of which had craniosynostosis.[25] They reported good reduction in IO overaction and divergence in upgaze with IO nasal and anterior transposition. The best responses were seen in those with unilateral absent SO. Good correction of hypotropia due to imaging-confirmed superior rectus muscle absence can be obtained with a Foster modification of the Knapp procedure.[22] The surgery in one case induced a horizontal deviation.

Clefting syndromes

The second major group of craniofacial abnormalities are the clefting syndromes and results from defective apposition or failure of fusion of neighboring structures during embryonic development. Tessier[26] introduced a descriptive classification, numbering them from 0 to 14 in clockwise rotation around

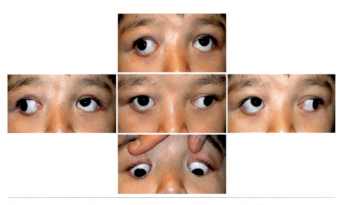

Fig. 28.7 Crouzon's syndrome. Images of a patient with Crouzon's syndrome demonstrating a V pattern and updrift in adduction.

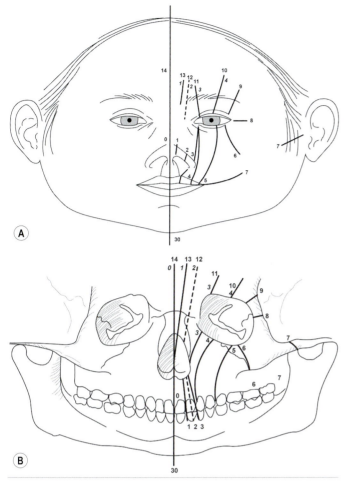

Fig. 28.8 Tessier classification of craniofacial clefts. (A) Soft tissue. (B) Skeletal. (Modified from David DJ, Moore MH, Cooter RD. Tessier clefts revisited with a third dimension. Cleft Palate J 1989; 26: 163–84.)

the orbit (Fig. 28.8). Clefts of midline structures of the nose and forehead are numbered 0 and 1 below the level of the medial canthus and 13 and 14 above. Nasolacrimal and medial canthal clefts are numbered 2, 3 and 4 below and 10, 11 and 12 above and so on. Cleft number 30 is of the mandibular symphysis. Clefts resulting from failure of embryonic closure of the nasolacrimal furrow or from amniotic bands are simply numbered according to their location relative to the eye.

Tessier's system encompasses the eponymously named syndromes of the face including Treacher-Collins and Goldenhar's, as well as craniofacial microsomia, formerly grouped together as mandibulofacial dysostoses, that are primarily due to retarded differentiation of the first branchial arch mesoderm.

Van der Muelen et al.[27] have developed a different classification replacing "cleft" with "dysplasia" and basing it on the embryology of the brain, face, and cranium. This classification explains deformities ranging from anencephaly to lymphangioma by facial clefting and craniosynostosis. However, this system competes with the more simplistic topographic classification of Tessier which we use in this chapter.

The following figures are examples of the individual numbered clefts (with the cleft highlighted on the 3D CT scan)

– some have combinations of clefts, as shown in Figs 28.9 to 28.14).

Cleft number	Common ocular problem
3 & 11	epibulbar dermoid
4 & 10	iris coloboma
5 & 9	microphthalmos
9, 10, 11	upper lid cleft
3, 4, 5, 6	lower lid cleft

Types of lacrimal problems: the puncta may be displaced laterally or be absent and the canaliculi may be disrupted or elongated; the lacrimal sac and/or nasolacrimal duct may be absent, and there may be bony defects of the lacrimal fossa.

Treacher-Collins syndrome

Although this syndrome (TCS) was first described by Berry, Treacher-Collins emphasized the malar deformity; it was expanded by Franceschetti and Zwahlen. The incidence is 1 : 50 000 live births;[28] the mode of inheritance is autosomal dominant with complete penetrance but variable expressivity of a gene on the long arm of chromosome 5 (5q32–33.3).[29] Various gene deletions encoding RNA polymerases 1 and 111 have been identified, confirming the heterogeneity of TCS thus supporting the hypothesis that TCS is a ribosomopathy.[30]

General findings

- Complete form of TCS involves Tessier's clefts 6, 7, and 8 (Fig. 28.14).
- Characteristic facies include hypoplasia of malar and zygomatic bones with deficient inferolateral orbital angles (Fig. 28.15).
- Bird- or fish-like profile results from absence of the nasofrontal angle.
- Lower jaw is hypoplastic with abnormal dentition.
- Respiratory problems result from choanal atresia and mandibular retrusion.
- Malformations of the external ear are common.
- Deafness (50% of cases) results from ossicular chain or inner ear malformations. EARLY AUDIOLOGIC ASSESSMENT ESSENTIAL.
- Accessory auricular appendages and blind fistulae occur between the angle of the mouth and ear.

Ocular findings

- Antimongoloid slant of palpebral fissure.
- Coloboma of lateral one third of lower lid (common) or pseudo-coloboma with hypoplastic cilia, subcutaneous tissues, and muscle; absent lashes on the medial one-third of lower lids (common).
- Canthal dystopia.
- Nasolacrimal obstruction.
- Limbal or orbital dermoids (common), high astigmatism in severely affected cases.
- Severe risk of cognitive deprivation due to astigmatism plus deafness.
- Difficult to fit spectacles in presence of hearing aids and external ear abnormalities.

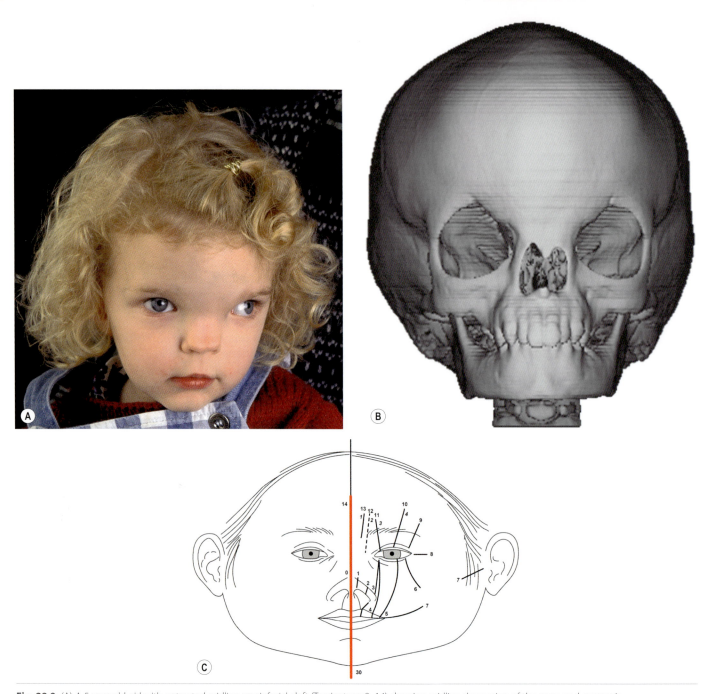

Fig. 28.9 (A) A 5-year-old girl with untreated midline craniofacial cleft (Tessier type 0–14) showing midline depression of the nose, and exotropia. (B) CT reconstruction shows widely displaced orbits and widened nasoethmoid region. (C) Cleft marked in red.

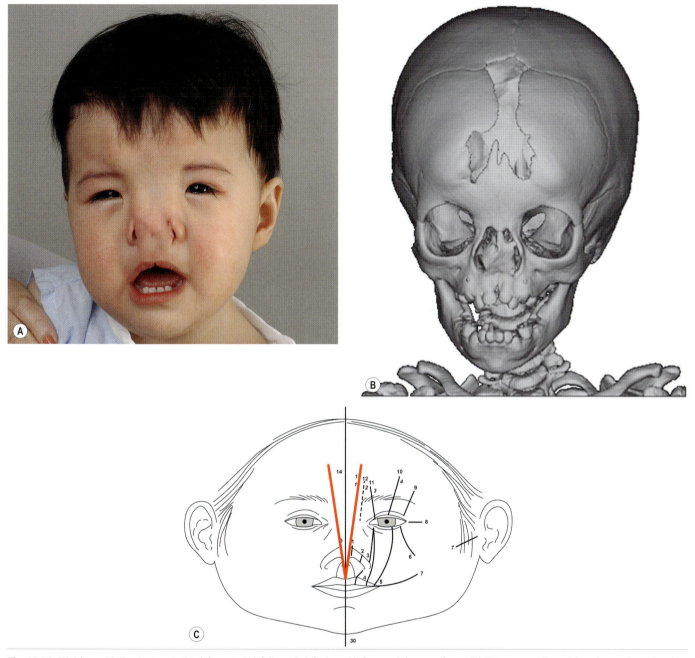

Fig. 28.10 (A) A boy with Tessier type 1–13 cleft: central cleft lip and cleft alae with flattened dorsum of nose. (B) CT reconstruction: widened nasoethmoid region. (C) Clefts marked in red.

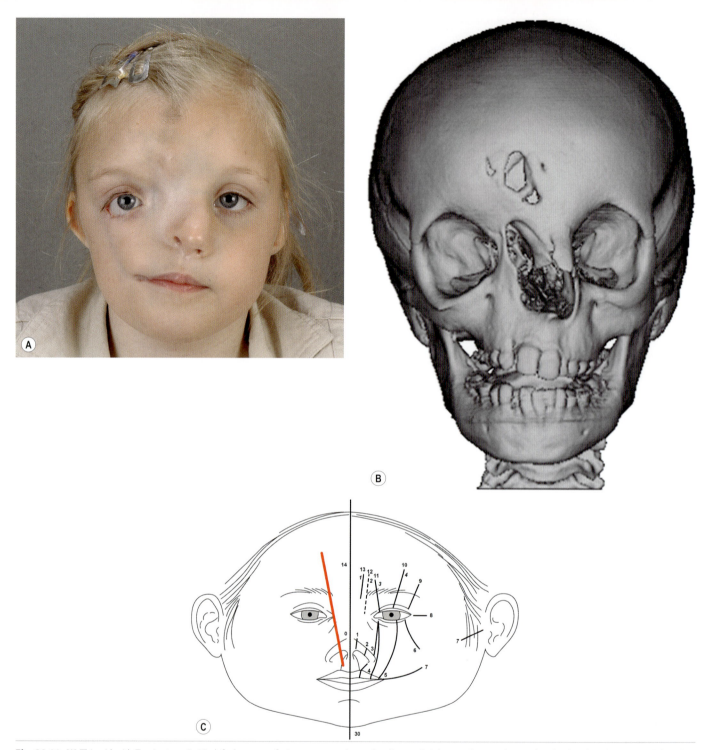

Fig. 28.11 (A) This girl with Tessier type 2–12 cleft shows a soft tissue groove above the distorted right nostril extending up her forehead and a type 5 cleft with vertical soft tissue deficiency between the lateral portion of the lip and the right lower eyelid cleft. (B) CT reconstruction: 2–12 cleft through ethmoids to frontal bone displacing the orbit laterally; 5: abnormal inferolateral orbital rim. (C) Only the 2–12 cleft is shown in red whilst her right 5 cleft corresponds to that shown in black on the left.

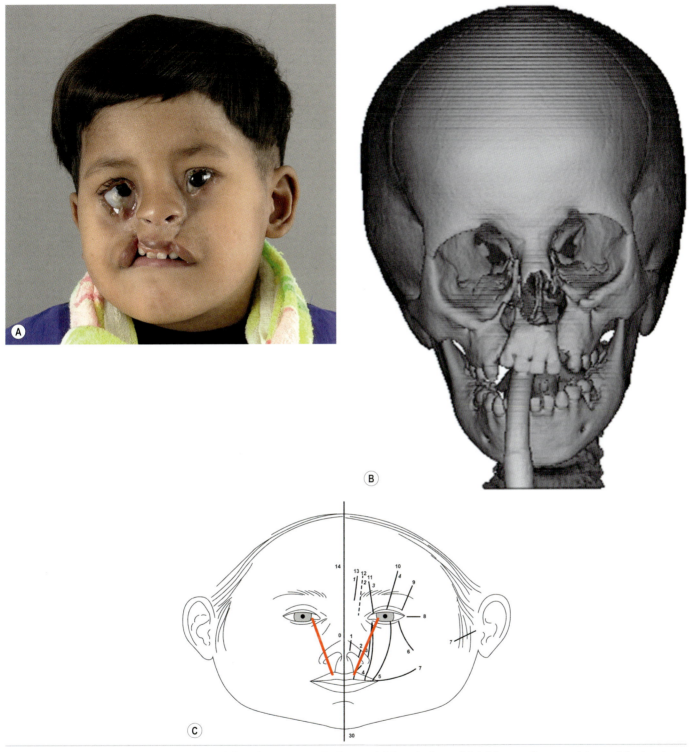

Fig. 28.12 (A) This boy has bilateral Tessier type 4 clefts with severe vertical soft tissue deficiency in the medial cleft lip extending toward the medially placed clefts in the lower and upper eyelids together with marked right orbital dystopia. (B) CT reconstruction shows bilateral clefts of anterior maxillae into orbital rims and the right orbital dystopia. (C) The number 4 clefts are shown in red.

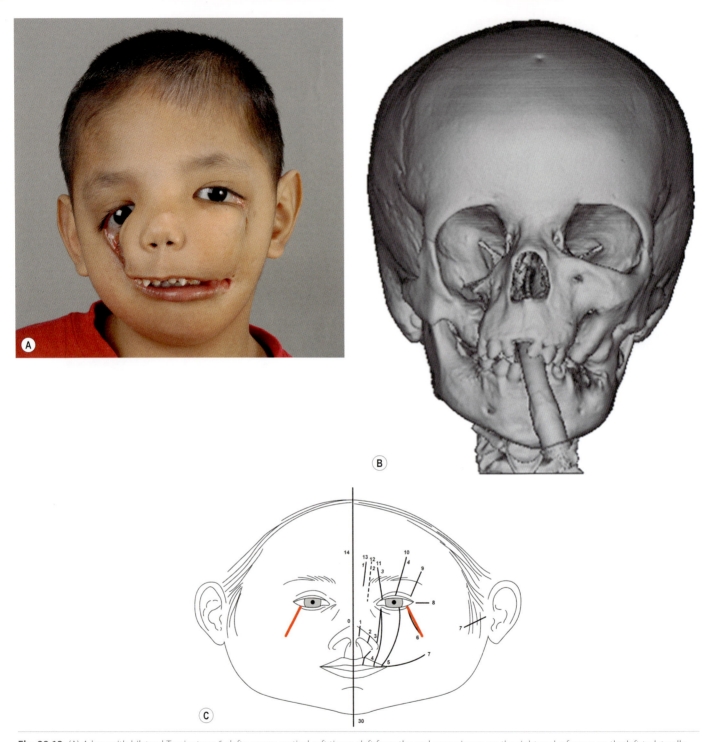

Fig. 28.13 (A) A boy with bilateral Tessier type 6 clefts: severe vertical soft tissue cleft from the oral commissure on the right and a furrow on the left to laterally placed lower eyelid clefts. There is antimongoloid obliquity of the palpebral fissures, some ectropion, and marked right orbital dystopia. (B) CT reconstruction: cleft in region of the right zygomaticomaxillary suture with hypoplasia of the maxilla and orbital rim. (C) Both number 6 clefts shown in red.

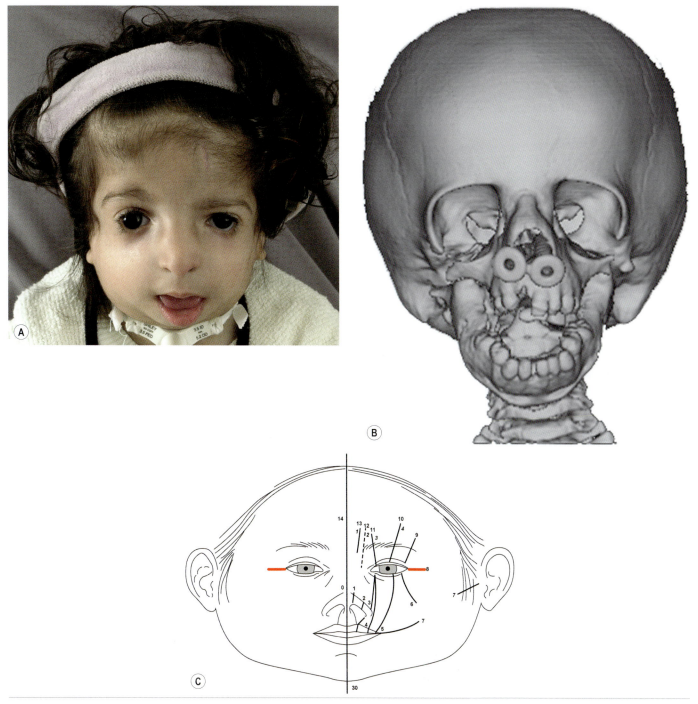

Fig. 28.14 (A) This girl has severe Treacher-Collins syndrome and Tessier cleft type 8 with choanal atresia and mandibular retrusion (hence the tracheostomy), lower eyelid pseudocolobomata and external ear abnormalities. (B) CT reconstruction: deficient lateral orbital wall, rim and floor with hypoplastic malar and zygomatic bones bilaterally. (C) Type 8 clefts shown in red.

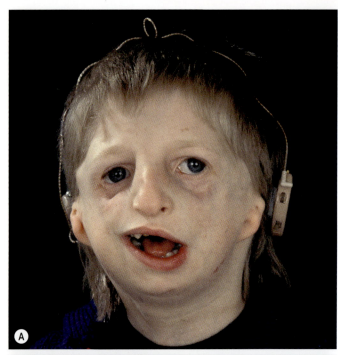

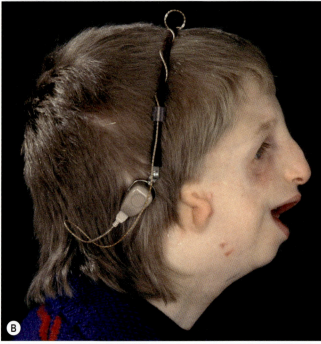

Fig. 28.15 (A) A boy with Treacher-Collins syndrome with mid-face hypoplasia, antimongoloid slant of palpebral fissures, pseudo-coloboma of lateral one third of lower lid, nasolacrimal obstruction, deafness, and external ear abnormalities. (B) Typical "fish-like" profile (absent nasofrontal angle), hypoplastic lower jaw, mouth breathing due to nasal airway obstruction.

Management protocol[31]

1. Birth–2 years: airways and feeding problems, hearing problems.
2. 2–12 years: speech therapy and education, removal of limbal dermoid, oculoplastic repair of lid coloboma, and facial reconstruction with bone or vascular bone flaps.
3. 13–18 years: orthognathic surgery, final facial revision.

4. The abnormal anatomy causes airway management difficulties necessitating anesthetic expertise.

Goldenhar's syndrome

Goldenhar described a syndrome of epibulbar dermoids, preauricular appendages, and mandibular hypoplasia (or hemifacial microsomia) which was expanded by Gorlin et al.[28] to the "oculoauriculovertebral spectrum." Most cases are sporadic but familial cases have been associated with a deletion on the long arm of chromosome 22 (22q11.2).[32]

Expression is variable, ranging from a few preauricular appendages only to bilateral clefting extending from the angles of the mouth to the tragus as well as of the palate and from either side of the frontonasal process to the medial canthi.

General findings

- Facial abnormalities may be bilateral but are usually more severe on one side (Fig. 28.16).
- Preauricular appendages – usually anterior to the tragus +/– fistula to ear.
- Facial asymmetry.
- Bilateral clefting from angle of mouth to tragus and of palate and either side of frontonasal process to medial canthi.
- The "expanded Goldenhar complex" includes vertebral, cardiac, renal, pulmonary, and central nervous system abnormalities (including severe hydrocephalus and mental retardation).

Ocular findings

- Dermolipoma: usually yellowish, subconjunctival, superotemporal orbit. Rarely enlarges – can often be left alone (Fig. 28.17A).
- Epibulbar dermoid: unilateral 50%, bilateral 25%, usually inferotemporal limbus but can occur anywhere on the globe or within orbit. White but often infiltrate of lipid at leading edge in cornea (Fig. 28.17B). May have irritating hairs (Fig. 28.17C). Can increase in size and cause astigmatism and amblyopia.
- Coloboma of iris: cosmetic defect +/– glare problems. May need cosmetic contact lens with painted iris.
- Microphthalmos – common.
- Ocular motility disturbance – common. Duane's syndrome/esotropia/exotropia found in about 25%.[28]
- Ptosis.
- Nasolacrimal duct obstruction and fistula.
- Coloboma of mid third of upper lid in 20%, often with ipsilateral epibulbar lesion.

Goldenhar's syndrome shares a number of features with Treacher-Collin syndrome; a combination of both has been reported.

Frontoethmoidal meningoencephalocele

These are subclassified as to their location: nasofrontal, nasoethmoidal and naso-orbital; their exit hole from the

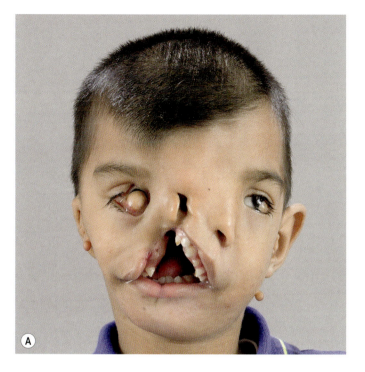

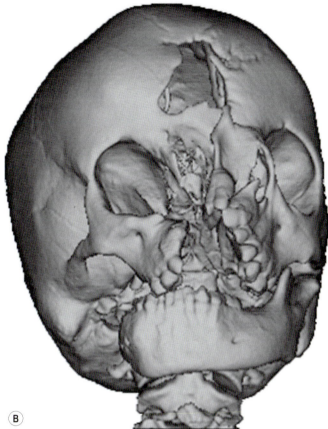

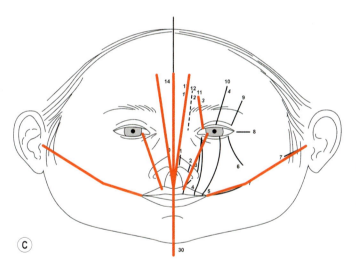

Fig. 28.16 (A) This highly intelligent boy has all the elements of Goldenhar's syndrome combined with complex, multiple midline clefts (Tessier types 30, 0–14, 1–13, 3, 7) with a coloboma of the middle third of the right upper lid with bilateral inferotemporal epibulbar dermoids impairing vision and preauricular appendages. The right lower lid coloboma was part of his maxillary cleft. (B) CT reconstruction shows the frontal defect, the gross orbital dystopia, the maxillary cleft, and the absence of the right mandible and temporomandibular joint. (C) His multiple clefts are shown in red.

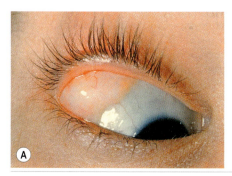

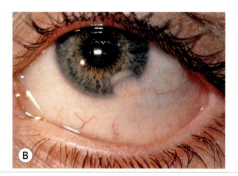

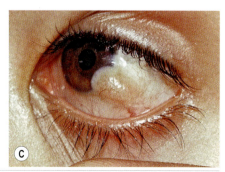

Fig. 28.17 (A) Yellowish subconjunctival dermolipoma in the superotemporal orbit. (B) Epibulbar dermoid at inferotemporal limbus with leading edge lipid infiltrate in cornea. (C) This epibulbar dermoid had irritating hairs growing from it.

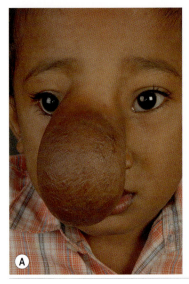
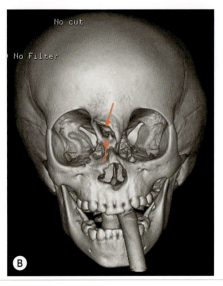
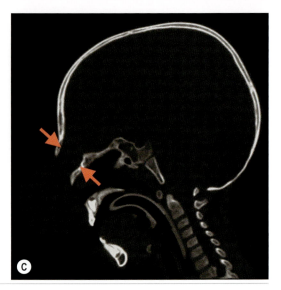

Fig. 28.18 (A) This boy from South-East Asia has a very large nasoethmoidal variety of frontoethmoidal meningoencephalocele causing an exotropia and typical elongation of the face. (B) CT reconstruction with arrows indicating the bony cranial base defect. (C) This sagittal CT scan shows the dysfunctional brain tissue extruding through the region of the foramen cecum (arrowed).

anterior cranial fossa being the foramen cecum. The extruding intracranial contents covered in meninges distort the developing face producing telecanthus, orbital dystopia, elongation of the face, and dental malocclusion (Fig. 28.18).

The clinical presentation depends on the location and extent of the lesion and can vary between a small soft cystic swelling over the bridge of the nose, depressing the nasal structures, to nasal obstruction causing difficulty with breathing and eating. Hypertelorism occurs particularly if there is associated facial clefting producing a midline defect. Ocular problems include strabismus and amblyopia and nasolacrimal drainage problems.

Frontoethmoidal encephaloceles are more frequent in South-East Asia (1:5000 live births), Africa, Malaysia, and Russia.

Management

Hydrocephalus, when present, must be dealt with first then excision of the cele, watertight closure of the dural defect, followed by reconstruction of the skull defect. Early removal of the meningoencephalocele by the craniofacial route allows re-establishment of normal facial growth.[33] The prognosis depends on the presence of additional congenital anomalies.[34] Post craniofacial surgical problems include hydrocephalus, rhinorrhea, secondary encephalocele (if raised ICP and inadequate reconstruction of the frontal bone). We have found that postoperative strabismus nearly always resolves, as does epiphora, which surprises as the lacrimal drainage system is rather tortuous having been stretched considerably by the developing cele.

Midline facial cleft

These may include cleft lip and palate, midline bifid nose, and midline encephalocele plus other intracranial abnormalities.

Such subtle signs as a small notch in the upper lip or in the middle of the nose should alert the clinician to an underlying defect (Fig. 28.19).

Six patients in one series[35] all had midline cleft lip and palate, hypertelorism, absent corpus callosum, and sphenoethmoidal (basal) encephalocele, and five of the six had pituitary deficiency. Two had unilateral and one had bilateral peripapillary staphyloma. Two had bilateral optic disk hypoplasia whilst another had a staphyloma in one eye and a morning glory disk anomaly (MGDA) in the other. A MGDA or optic disk hypoplasia should trigger neuroradiologic investigation to rule out these midline brain defects.

Amniotic bands

These occur when bands of amnion encircle parts of the developing fetus, restricting local growth such as ring constriction of fingers. When the head is affected, the resulting clefts do not follow usual developmental patterns. However, major craniofacial malformations may occur (Fig. 28.20). This sporadic condition affects both sexes equally.[36]

The most common ocular malformations are congenital corneal leukomata or acquired corneal opacities secondary to exposure and eyelid colobomas. The eyelid defects appear to be extensions of facial clefts and are often located adjacent to the corneal opacities. Other associations are microphthalmos, strabismus, hypertelorism, and rarely coloboma of iris and retina.

Craniofacial surgery

The use of nylon skulls,[37] created from 3D CT scans of the patient, allows realistic planning and rehearsal of complex staged reconstructions (Fig. 28.21).

Whilst bone grafting and craniofacial osteotomies correct the underlying skeletal abnormalities, the ultimate success of

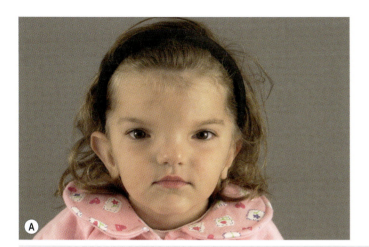

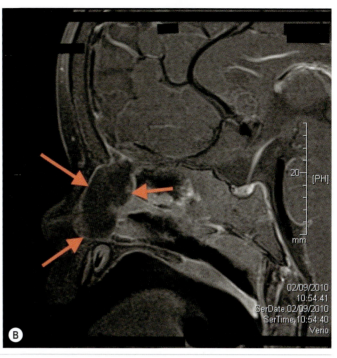

Fig. 28.19 (A) This little girl has subtle external signs of her midline cleft and basal encephalocele: midline nasal furrow and hypertelorism. (B) This other girl's sagittal MRI scan shows a midline basal encephalocele (arrows). She presented with noisy breathing and examination showed cerebrospinal fluid rhinorrhea and a whitish mass up her nostril.

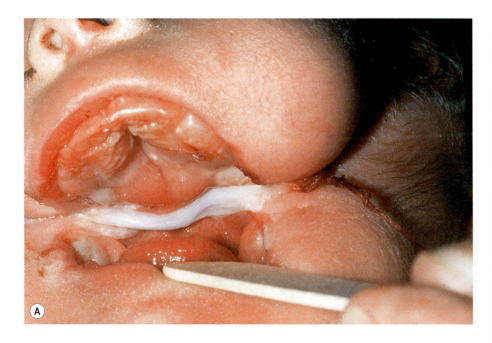

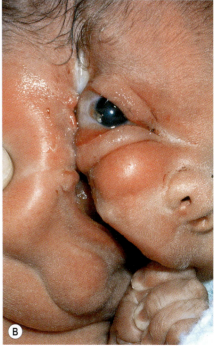

Fig. 28.20 Amniotic bands. (A) A white band can be seen traversing the palate, ending as a cord. (B) The cord cleaves the right maxilla and orbit.

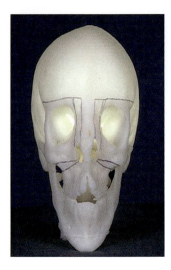

Fig. 28.21 This nylon model constructed from a three-dimensional CT scan of a patient with a midline cleft shows not only the deformity but how the model can be used for surgical planning and rehearsal.

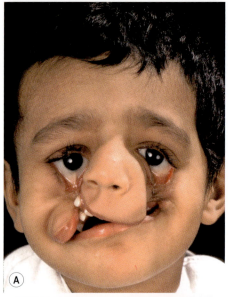

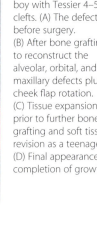

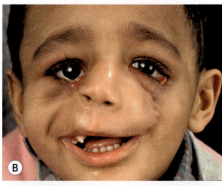

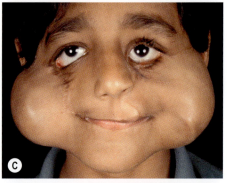

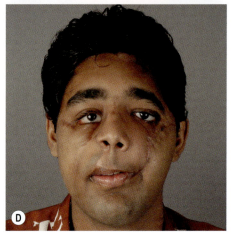

Fig. 28.22 This sequence shows stages in the management of this boy with Tessier 4–5 clefts. (A) The defect before surgery. (B) After bone grafting to reconstruct the alveolar, orbital, and maxillary defects plus cheek flap rotation. (C) Tissue expansion prior to further bone grafting and soft tissue revision as a teenager. (D) Final appearance at completion of growth.

these reconstructions is limited by the deficiency of skin and soft tissue. Craniofacial tissue expansion (Fig. 28.22) prior to the primary correction or the secondary surgery allows tension free closure and improved aesthetic results by using neighboring tissues of the correct color and texture. Surgical protocols have been developed for the various conditions but these often need to be individualized.

The ophthalmologist needs to be aware of the various complications of this specialized surgery.[38]

Neurosurgical complications

- Dural damage, more common in surgical correction of craniosynostosis, leading to cerebrospinal fluid (CSF) leak with potential for infection and rarely a growing fracture.
- Persisting CSF fistula especially with hypertelorism or frontoethmoidal encephalocele correction.
- Intracranial hematoma especially from vascular lesions found in midline clefts.
- Acute hydrocephalus especially after correction of frontoethmoidal meningoencephaloceles.
- Cerebral ischemia can lead to gliosis and epilepsy.

Aspects of ocular complications prior to, during, and after craniofacial surgery include:

- Adequate corneal protection to prevent drying, ulceration, and scarring with long term measures required if poor lid function.
- Monitoring visual acuity and its correction to prevent amblyopia.
- Correction of strabismus.
- Canthal and lid position must be optimized prior to lacrimal surgery.

Diplopia can complicate malposition of the whole orbit, malposition of the globe within the orbit, or from injury to the EOMs. However, in the grosser orbital deformities, binocular vision is rarely present and central suppression prevents diplopia. There is often pre-existing alternating strabismus. Binocularity, when present, will be retained postoperatively provided the optic axes remain parallel. About 10% require squint surgery.

Dystopia can be minimized by the craniofacial surgeon preserving a frontal bar of bone as a reference point for orbital repositioning. Following orbital repositioning, for example for hypertelorism, sixth cranial nerve palsies are common but transient: 90% recover in 6 to 12 months in our experience.

Canthal dystopia is a frequent problem medially with clefts with a medial lid coloboma or deficient canthal ligament. Wedge excision, lower lid advancement, Z-plasties, or other flaps may be needed.

Epiphora is common and probably due to crumpling of the canaliculi. The drainage system is often not present or functional in Tessier no. 3 clefts and in frontoethmoidal meningoencephaloceles. If dacryocystorhinostomy is indicated, it may not be possible to fashion usual nasolacrimal flaps and so out-fracturing techniques from sac to nasal cavity with dilators (e.g. Hegar's cervical) followed by packing with cellulose sponge is often required. Use of Lester Jones or other tubes may not be practical as they require careful follow-up care.

Enophthalmos is common after correction of naso-orbital frontoethmoidal meningoencephalocele. It is difficult to correct even with extensive bone grafting.

A "tight orbit" or "orbital compartment syndrome" is a dreaded complication due to marked edema or hemorrhage causing optic nerve or retinal ischemia or infarction. Pupillary responses and visual acuity must be closely monitored. In such an event, the appropriate orbital decompressive technique will be dictated by the previous operative procedure.

Pressure on the globe or optic nerve by a malpositioned bone graft can occur but direct trauma to those structures is very rare.

We are aware of only two cases of postoperative blindness from 9170 individual non-trauma craniofacial patients treated to date by our clinic.

Infection rarely occurs but is always a risk, especially as the nasal sinuses are opened, of necessity, in craniofacial procedures. Appropriate aseptic techniques and postoperative antibiotic regimes must be followed.

The ophthalmologist as an important member of the craniofacial team

These developmental conditions obviously involve more than just the eye and adnexae and hence ideally the ophthalmologist is a member of a craniofacial surgical team taking a coordinated role in the assessment, planning, surgical correction, and rehabilitation of the patient.

The ophthalmologist must accurately record the preoperative state including visual acuity, presence or otherwise of binocular vision, strabismus and ptosis. The team planning meeting coordinates the sequence of management and surgical steps required by the many surgical specialties involved. Postoperatively the role is reassessment and management of any surgical complications followed by visual rehabilitation. The whole process usually extends over many years – at least until after visual system maturation and often well after cessation of craniofacial growth.

Sadly, patients with craniofacial defects are often shunned or ridiculed by members of society. The ophthalmologist may improve their visual function and cosmesis and is richly rewarded when the patient is enabled to take their rightful place in society.

Acknowledgment

Signed parental consent for publication of all the clinical photographs is held by the Australian Cranio-Facial Unit, Adelaide, South Australia.

References

1. Passos-Bueno MR, Serti Eacute AE, Jehee FS, et al. Genetics of craniosynostosis: genes, syndromes, mutations and genotype-phenotype correlations. Front Oral Biol 2008; 12: 107–43.
2. Komotar RJ, Zacharia BE, Ellis JA, et al. Pitfalls for the pediatrician: positional molding or craniosynostosis? Pediatr Ann 2006; 35: 365–75.
3. Rice DP. Clinical features of syndromic craniosynostosis. Front Oral Biol 2008; 12: 91–106.
4. Raybaud C, Di Rocco C. Brain malformation in syndromic craniosynostoses, a primary disorder of white matter: a review. Childs Nerv Syst 2007; 23: 1379–88.
5. Kapp-Simon KA, Speltz ML, Cunningham ML, et al. Neurodevelopment of children with single suture craniosynostosis: a review. Childs Nerv Syst 2007; 23:269–81.
6. Tamburrini G, Caldarelli M, Massimi L, et al. Intracranial pressure monitoring in children with single suture and complex craniosynostosis: a review. Childs Nerv Syst 2005; 21: 913–21.
7. Khan SH, Britto JA, Evans RD, Nischal KK. Expression of FGFR-2 and FGFR-3 in the normal human fetal orbit. Br J Ophthalmol 2005; 89: 1643–5.
8. Hayward R. Venous hypertension and craniosynostosis. Childs Nerv Syst 2005; 21: 880–8.
9. Melville H, Wang Y, Taub PJ, Jabs EW. Genetic basis of potential therapeutic strategies for craniosynostosis. Am J Med Genet A 2010; 152A: 3007–15.
10. Jadico SK, Huebner A, McDonald-McGinn DM, et al. Ocular phenotype correlations in patients with TWIST versus FGFR3 genetic mutations. J AAPOS 2006; 10: 435–44.
11. Khong JJ, Anderson PJ, Hammerton M, et al. Differential effects of FGFR2 mutation in ophthalmic findings in Apert syndrome. J Craniofac Surg 2007; 18: 39–42.
12. Gupta PC, Foster J, Crowe S, et al. Ophthalmologic findings in patients with nonsyndromic plagiocephaly. J Craniofac Surg 2003; 14: 529–32.
13. Denis D, Genitori L, Bardot J, et al. Ocular findings in trigonocephaly. Graefes Arch Clin Exp Ophthalmol 1994;232:728–33.
14. Khan SH, Nischal KK, Dean F, et al. Visual outcomes and amblyogenic risk factors in craniosynostotic syndromes: a review of 141 cases. Br J Ophthalmol 2003; 87: 999–1003.
15. Tay T, Martin F, Rowe N, et al. Prevalence and causes of visual impairment in craniosynostotic syndromes. Clin Exp Ophthalmol 2006; 34: 434–40.
16. Baranello G, Vasco G, Ricci D, Mercuri E. Visual function in nonsyndromic craniosynostosis: past, present, and future. Childs Nerv Syst 2007; 23: 1461–5.
17. Levy RL, Rogers GF, Mulliken JB, et al. Astigmatism in unilateral coronal synostosis: incidence and laterality. J AAPOS 2007; 11: 367–72.
18. Thompson DA, Liasis A, Hardy S, et al. Prevalence of abnormal pattern reversal visual evoked potentials in craniosynostosis. Plast Reconstr Surg 2006;118:184–92.
19. Liasis A, Nischal KK, Walters B, et al. Monitoring visual function in children with syndromic craniosynostosis: a comparison of 3 methods. Arch Ophthalmol 2006;124:1119–26.
20. Hammerton MA. The ophthalmic features of Pfeiffer syndrome. In: Marchac D, editor. Craniofacial Surgery, Proceedings of the Sixth International Congress of The International Society of Craniofacial Surgery, Saint Tropez (French Riviera); 1995: 157–9.
21. Ron Y, Dagi LR. The etiology of V pattern strabismus in patients with craniosynostosis. Int Ophthalmol Clin 2008; 48: 215–23.

22. Rattigan S, Nischal KK. Foster-type modification of the Knapp procedure for anomalous superior rectus muscles in syndromic craniosynostoses. J AAPOS 2003; 7: 279–82.

23. Somani S, Mackeen LD, Morad Y, et al Assessment of extraocular muscles position and anatomy by 3-dimensional ultrasonography: a trial in craniosynostosis patients. J AAPOS 2003; 7: 54–9.

24. Hussein MA, Stager DR Sr, Beauchamp GR, et al. Anterior and nasal transposition of the inferior oblique muscles in patients with missing superior oblique tendons. J AAPOS 2007; 11: 29–33.

25. Coats DK, Paysse EA, Stager DR. Surgical management of V-pattern strabismus and oblique dysfunction in craniofacial dysostosis. J AAPOS 2000; 4: 338–42.

26. Tessier P. Anatomical classification of facial, craniofacial and laterofacial clefts. J Maxillofac Surg 1976; 4: 69–92.

27. Van der Muelen JC, Mazzola B, StrickerM, et al. Classification of craniofacial malformation. In: Stricker M, van der Muelen JC, Raphael B, et al., editors. Craniofacial Malformation. Edinburgh: Churchill Livingstone; 1990: 149–309.

28. Gorlin RJ, Cohen MM, Hennekam RC. Syndromes of the Head and Neck. New York: Oxford University Press; 2001.

29. Dixon MJ, Dixon J, Houseal T, et al. Narrowing the position of the Treacher Collins syndrome locus to a small interval between three microsatellite markers at 5q32–33.1. Am J Hum Genet 1993; 52: 907–14.

30. Dauwerse JG, Dixon J, Seland S, et al. Mutations in genes encoding subunits of RNA polymerases 1 and 111 cause Treacher Collins syndrome. Nat Genet 2011; 43:20–2.

31. Thompson JT, Anderson PJ, David DJ. Treacher Collins syndrome: protocol management from birth to maturity. J Craniofac Surg 2009; 20:2028–35.

32. Balci S, Enzic O. Goldenhar syndrome phenotype and 22q11 deletion. Am J Med Genet A 2011; 155A(2): 458.

33. David DJ, Sheffield L, Simpson DA, White J. Fronto-ethmoidal meningoencephaloceles: morphology and treatment. B J Plast Surg 1984;37: 271–84.

34. Hoving EW. Nasal encephaloceles. Childs Nerv Syst 2000; 16: 702–6.

35. Hodgkins P, Lees M, Lawson J, et al. Optic disc anomalies and frontonasal dysplasia. Br J Ophthalmol 1998; 82:290–3.

36. Fries PD, Katowitz JA. Congenital craniofacial anomalies of ophthalmic importance. Surv Ophthalmol 1990; 35: 87–119.

37. Abbott JR, Netherway DJ, Wingate PG, et al. Computer generated mandibular model: surgical role. Aust Dent J 1998; 43: 373–6.

38. David DJ. Reconstruction: facial clefts. In: Mathes SJ, editor. Plastic Surgery, Vol 4: Pediatric Plastic Surgery. Philadelphia: Elsevier; 2006: 381–46.

Cystic lesions and ectopias

Christopher J Lyons • Jack Rootman

Cystic lesions

Cystic lesions of the orbit in childhood include dermoid cysts, microphthalmos with cyst, lacrimal ductal cyst, congenital cystic eyeball, encephalocele, sinus mucocele, and teratoma. In some parts of the world parasitic cysts involving organisms such as *Echinococcus* and *Schistosoma* are common; these are rare in Europe and North America.[1] Hemorrhage within orbital venous lymphatic malformations (lymphangiomas) may give rise to "chocolate" cysts. Cystic lesions of the orbital bones may be seen in fibrous dysplasia, ossifying fibroma, and aneurysmal bone cyst. Cystic orbital lesions were reviewed by Lessner et al.[2]

Lacrimal ductal cyst

Lacrimal ductal cysts are rare in childhood but an important part of the differential diagnosis of an orbital mass in the lacrimal gland region. Bullock et al.[3] suggested that lacrimal cysts should be classified by their site of origin: palpebral lobe (simple dacryops), orbital lobe, accessory glands, or ectopic lacrimal gland. Clinically, they may be confused with superficial conjunctival dermoid (though these are more commonly medial) or inclusion cysts as well as parasitic cysts.

Lacrimal ductal cysts most commonly arise from the palpebral lobe in adults but they may occur in teenagers, sometimes with a history of trauma or inflammation. A smooth, transilluminating mass slowly enlarges in the lateral aspect of the upper lid (Fig. 29.1) and may be evident on lid eversion as a blueish cyst. Rarely, they enlarge with crying and can be tender or painful, occasionally resolving spontaneously as the cyst decompresses with a gush of tears. If the patient is symptomatic, surgical excision of the intact cyst is curative. Marsupialization of larger cysts may be necessary.

Cysts in the orbital lobe are rare; they usually present in infancy or early childhood as a tense mass in the lacrimal fossa. They are larger than their palpebral counterparts. They may enlarge, sometimes suddenly due to inflammation or

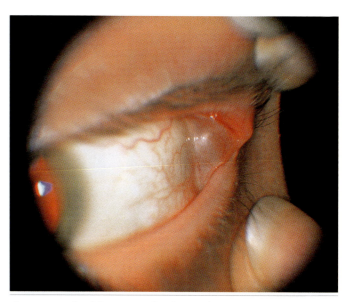

Fig. 29.1 Lacrimal ductal cyst showing as a transilluminating mass in the lateral fornix revealed by pulling the lid away from the globe. (Patient of the University of British Columbia.)

hemorrhage causing proptosis with inferonasal displacement of the globe or even globe subluxation.[4] Deep extension into the posterior orbit may be seen on computed tomography (CT) scan. Excision of the intact cyst is desirable, with lateral orbitotomy if there is posterior extension. Histologically, ductal cysts of the palpebral lobe are lined by an outer layer of myoepithelium and inner layer of cuboidal cells, unlike congenital orbital lobe cysts whose epithelial lining is cuboidal.

Cysts of the accessory glands of Krause and Wolfring may occur, resulting in swelling in the conjunctival fornix. These can be excised via the conjunctiva.

Lacrimal tissue may occasionally occur ectopically within the eye and orbit with an associated cystic component (see below).

Dermoid cyst

Dermoid cysts of the orbit and periorbital region are common in childhood, accounting for 3–9% of orbital masses.[5,6] They are developmental choristomas which arise from ectodermal

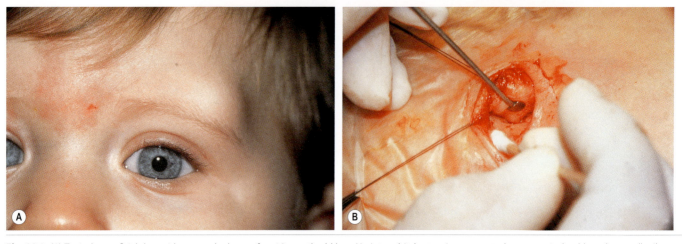

Fig. 29.2 (A) Typical superficial dermoid cyst on the brow of an 18-month-old boy. No intraorbital extension was noted preoperatively, although a small tail was seen to insert into bone at the time of surgery (B). This was divided and cauterized. The cyst was intact. (Patient of the University of British Columbia.)

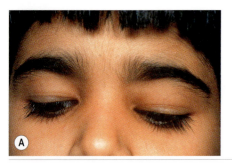
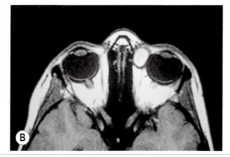
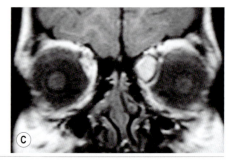

Fig. 29.3 (A) This 10-year-old boy had a gradually enlarging mass in his left upper lid for several years. (B) T1-weighted MRI shows that this is situated anteriorly and its contents are isodense with orbital fat. (C) On coronal view, the mass is seen indenting the globe. It was excised completely and found to be a dermoid cyst. (Patient of the University of British Columbia.)

rests trapped at suture lines or within mesenchyme during orbital development.

The cysts are lined by keratinized stratified squamous epithelium: hair follicles and sebaceous glands are found in their wall. Cyst leakage or rupture may give rise to chronic low-grade granulomas.

Dermoids may be superficial or deep.[7] Conjunctival dermoids are variants, occurring posterior to the septum in the orbit. Most childhood dermoids are superficial.

Superficial dermoids

These often present in infancy as a rounded mass, typically at the superotemporal (Fig. 29.2) margin of the orbit.[8] One-quarter arise in the medial orbit[8,9] (Fig. 29.3); these may be lined by stratified squamous epithelium.[9] They are painless, non-tender, firm, non-fluctuant, and often immobile, fixed to the underlying bone. Since they are usually situated outside the orbit, they cause no displacement of the globe. The orbital rim is palpable behind their posterior edge. Unsuspected deep extension into the temporalis fossa, posterior orbit, or even intracranial space occasionally occurs in apparently superficial dermoid cysts. These "dumbbell" dermoids may present with the typical signs of superficial dermoid, but extend into the temporalis fossa in an hour-glass configuration (Fig. 29.4) and may be associated with temporalis swelling in 1.5–34% of such cases.[10,11] Very rarely, proptosis with or without visual impairment triggered by mastication (masticatory oscillopsia) can result from pressure on a communicating cyst by

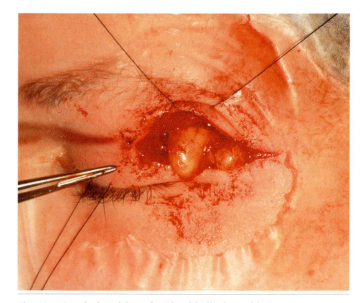

Fig. 29.4 Surgical excision of a "dumbbell" dermoid. The intervening bone has been removed. (Patient of the University of British Columbia.)

temporalis contraction with chewing.[12] Presentation with orbital cellulitis related to a discharging sinus tract arising from an orbital dermoid has been reported.[13] Simultaneous orbital and temporalis fossa dermoid cysts without communication have been described.[14]

The radiologic appearance of a dermoid cyst is characteristic: on CT scan, the best modality to highlight bony features, a rounded discrete mass is associated with thinning and smooth erosion of the underlying bone. The contents are often of heterogeneous density on CT and magnetic resonance imaging (MRI). Fat lucency was noted in 71% of 70 patients,[10] its presence within the cyst is considered diagnostic.[15]

Preoperative assessment of any dermoid cyst is essential to rule out deep extension. If the cyst is small, mobile, and easily palpable for its entire extent, imaging may not be necessary; large cysts with ill-defined, deep margins are best assessed with a CT scan or MRI using 2 mm slices through the lesion, preferably with coronal cuts.

Excision of superficial dermoid cysts is relatively simple. We prefer to do this by the age of 5 years to avoid accidental rupture or inflammatory episodes related to spontaneous leakage.[16] The incision may be situated directly over the lesion above, below, or through the eyebrow. A skin-crease approach[11,17] or endoscopic removal[18] leaves a less conspicuous postoperative scar. Although excision of the intact cyst is desirable, intraoperative rupture is not disastrous if the contents and the entire cyst wall are carefully removed. Decompression of the cyst may be helpful to expose the underlying bone. Failure to excise the cyst wall completely, or residual cyst contents, can elicit a chronic inflammatory reaction with sinus formation and persistent discharge. Cyst rupture with dramatic inflammatory signs were present in only four of 17 patients with ruptured cysts:[19] a low-grade lipogranulomatous response was more common.

A neurosurgical approach with craniectomy may be necessary for safe and complete excision of a dumbbell dermoid extending intracranially.[20]

Deep dermoids

These present in adolescence and adulthood with gradual enlargement and displacement of orbital contents; they can present similarly in infancy.[21] Typically, only their smooth and rounded anterior margin can be palpated although they may extend to the orbital apex.[22] The lesion may not be palpable at all (Fig. 29.5).[23] Proptosis and/or globe displacement are predominant features but ocular motility,[8,24] visual disturbances, and pain may occur. Dermoid cysts may be within[24,25] or attached to the lateral rectus muscle.[26]

The CT findings of deep dermoids are similar to those of superficial dermoids except for the frequent presence of irregular orbital wall defects as well as sclerosis, irregular scalloping, or notching of the underlying bone. The walls of large dermoid cysts may demonstrate irregular "egg-shell" calcification.

The management of deep dermoids can be difficult[22,27,28] since total surgical excision is necessary to prevent complications. Preoperative clinical and radiologic assessment is essential to plan the appropriate surgical approach, which may involve combined anterior and lateral orbitotomies or focal marginotomies.[22] Although it was felt that this surgery was best delayed until bone growth had ceased,[28] such delay may not be necessary to safeguard facial bony growth.

Conjunctival dermoids

One-half of these arise in the medial orbit in relation to the caruncle, usually in teenagers and adults.[22] They are not attached to the orbital bones, and are lined by typical conjunctival epithelium with goblet cells and adnexal structures with

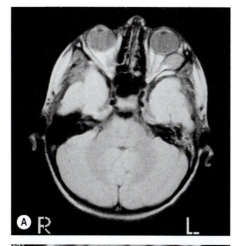

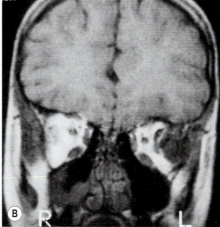

Fig. 29.5 (A) Orbital dermoid. (B) MRI scan showing lateral retro-ocular lesion on the left side.

mucinous or mixed content in the cyst. They are managed by complete excision.

Orbital encephalocele (see Chapter 56)

These rare abnormalities may be congenital or acquired. Congenital lesions arise from a presumed defective separation of neuroectoderm from surface ectoderm, resulting in a bony dehiscence with a "cystic" herniation of dura into the orbit, either alone (meningocele) or with brain tissue (meningoencephalocele). They may be associated with an optic disc anomaly;[29] basal encephalocele should always be excluded in a child with a morning glory disc, especially if there is a midline facial anomaly such as hypertelorism, notched or cleft lip or palate[30] (see Chapter 51). Significant cerebral vascular anomalies may be evident.[31] Orbital encephaloceles may be acquired as a result of head injury and orbital fracture, with herniation of the dura with or without brain through the bony defect.[32,33] Congenital orbital encephaloceles may be anterior or posterior.[34] Anterior lesions herniate through single or multiple defects[35] in the region of the sutures dividing the frontal, ethmoid, lacrimal, and maxillary bones. They usually present as a congenital cystic swelling of the medial orbit extending onto the face, accompanied by telecanthus and, frequently, epiphora. They may present in infancy and early childhood with gradually increasing forward and lateral globe displacement. The medial canthal tendon is usually displaced in an inferolateral direction. Atypical presentations occur, such as the 10 mm blueish cystic mass in the superonasal fornix of a 1-month-old patient which was found to be a meningoencephalocele.[36]

Classically, the cyst increases in size on straining or crying.[4,37] It may be fluctuant, pulsatile, reducible with gentle pressure, and it may transilluminate. Anterior encephaloceles are important in the differential diagnosis of any medial canthal swelling, having been mistaken for sinus mucoceles, dermoid cysts, or nasolacrimal duct mucoceles.[38] A bony defect with intracranial communication is evident on CT scan. Three-dimensional CT reconstruction may be helpful in planning surgery,[39] which is usually performed by neurosurgical and/or maxillofacial teams. Posterior encephaloceles herniate into the orbit via the optic foramen, orbital fissures, or a bony defect. They present with slowly progressive, sometimes pulsatile, proptosis. Occasionally, posterior encephaloceles present later.

Typically, the eye is displaced forwards and downwards[4] and the proptosis increases on straining or crying. Plain X-rays demonstrate enlarged foramina or a bony defect of the posterior orbit. CT scan demonstrates the size and contents of the cyst. Posterior encephaloceles are particularly associated with the sphenoid wing dysplasia of neurofibromatosis type 1 (NF1); they can also be associated with enophthalmos.

Sinus mucocele

The paranasal sinuses are of clinical relevance to childhood orbital disease and it is important to be familiar with their development. All the sinuses are present at birth in a rudimentary form, except the frontal sinus which first appears at the age of 2 years. There are two spurts of enlargement: at the age of 6 or 7 years, coinciding with the eruption of the second dentition, and again at puberty.[40] Since the frontal sinus is the source of most mucoceles, this disorder is rare in childhood. Ethmoidal sinus mucoceles, however, may present in early life,[41] particularly with cystic fibrosis.

A mucocele is a cystic expansion of a paranasal sinus, resulting from obstruction of its ostium. The normal mucous secretions of the respiratory epithelial lining accumulate within the sinus, leading to a gradual expansion with loss of its bony structure. With further expansion, the cystic mass transgresses the orbital wall and displaces the orbital contents. It may also erode into the intracranial space.[42] Eventually, the cyst contents consist of viscous material which may be white, yellow, or brown and enclosed by a fibrous capsule.

Most mucoceles arise anteriorly, affecting frontal or anterior ethmoid sinuses. The usual presentation is with gradually increasing proptosis (Fig. 29.6) with inferolateral or lateral displacement of the globe, appearing clinically as hypertelorism. A firm cystic non-compressible, non-inflammatory swelling may be palpable in the medial orbit. Its extension above the medial canthal tendon should differentiate it from a mucocele of the lacrimal sac. The absence of pulsatility, expansion with straining, and bony skull defect differentiate it from an encephalocele. Sphenoid sinus mucoceles are rare in childhood but sudden blindness from optic nerve compression by a sphenoid sinus mucocele has been reported.[43]

Plain X-rays show a markedly enlarged sinus on the affected side. On CT scan, a smooth-walled cystic lesion, often with egg-shell calcification of the margins arises from the affected

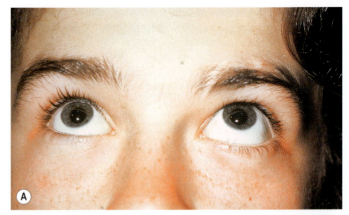

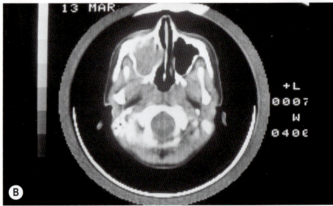

Fig. 29.6 (A) Post-traumatic mucocele. At the age of 9 years, this patient sustained an orbital blow-out fracture which was repaired using a silastic sheet. He is seen here at the age of 14 years; there is proptosis and upward displacement of the globe. (B) CT scanning showed the silastic implant had caused maxillary sinus obstruction and secondary mucocele. The implant was removed and the sinus opened surgically to allow drainage into the nose. (Patient of the University of British Columbia.)

sinus. In childhood, this is most commonly the ethmoid, and there is expansion into the medial orbit with thinning of the wall and destruction of the internal septa.

Since incomplete excision of the cyst wall is frequently followed by recurrence, the cyst walls should be completely removed or the cyst marsupialized to the nasal cavity to prevent recurrence and to re-establish sinus drainage. Excision or drainage of the mucocele is usually performed endoscopically by an ENT surgeon.[44] The transcaruncular approach has been recommended for the management of fronto-ethmoidal mucoceles.[45] After medial incisions are used, careful repositioning of the trochlea is advised to avoid postoperative superior oblique underaction.[46] Other cystic lesions arising in the sinuses, including dentigerous cysts, may also cause proptosis.

Congenital cystic eyeball (anophthalmos with cyst) (see Chapter 17)

True anophthalmia is very rare. More commonly, complete or partial failure of invagination of the optic vesicle before the 7 mm stage results in a "congenital cystic eye" or "anophthalmos with cyst."[47] No recognizable globe is present within the orbit. The congenital cystic "eye" is lined by neuroglial tissue without any normal ocular structures such as lens, ciliary body, or retina. The wall of the cyst is fibrous connective tissue with attached extraocular muscles. The absence of surface ectoderm-derived ocular structures is a common feature which may help with correct diagnosis. Congenital cystic eyeball is rare compared to microphthalmos with cyst, caused by a later defect in embryogenesis.[48]

It presents at birth as a large cystic swelling within the orbit. In contrast to microphthalmos with cyst, the cystic eyeball is usually centrally placed or distends the upper lid;[47,49] the cyst may occasionally be inferior.[48] The fellow eye is usually normal, but contralateral microphthalmos with cyst,[50] persistent hyperplastic primary vitreous, or bilateral congenital cystic eyes have been reported.[48]

The histology is similar to the cystic portion of anophthalmos with cyst: multiple cavities filled with proliferating glial tissue.[48,49] These cystic orbital lesions, occurring in neonates, should be distinguished from teratomas.

Microphthalmos with cyst

Incomplete closure of the fetal fissure between the 7 and 14 mm stage of embryonic development may result in a variety of colobomatous defects of the eye.[51] Eyes with severe colobomas are often microphthalmic and proliferation of neuroectoderm at the lips of the persistent fetal fissure may result in the formation of an orbital cyst which communicates with the eye. The size of the cyst varies enormously.

Several genetic mutations are known to cause anophthalmia and microphthalmia (see Chapter 17). Their association with systemic abnormalities makes their identification particularly important. Many are autosomal dominantly inherited so future siblings are at risk. SOX2,[52] OTX2, PAX2, and PAX6 as well as CHD7 (CHARGE syndrome) are the most frequently implicated mutations; involvement of a geneticist is advisable. Ragge et al. reviewed the diagnosis and multidisciplinary management of anophthalmia and microphthalmia.[53]

Clinical presentation

The manifestations are variable, ranging from an apparently normal eye with a clinically unapparent cyst, an obvious cyst in association with a deformed eye, to an invisible eye displaced by a cyst occupying the whole orbit. Typically, a blueish cystic transilluminating lesion (Fig. 29.7) bulges inferiorly into the lower fornix and lid, displacing a microphthalmic or rudimentary eye under the upper lid.[54] Rarely, the cyst may be present in the upper lid and the eye is displaced downwards.[55] Occasionally, the eye cannot be identified clinically,[54] even under anesthesia. Bilateral involvement is not uncommon. The cyst communicates with the eye via a variably narrow stalk. The microphthalmic eye usually has extremely poor vision and an associated optic nerve and retinal coloboma. The eye, though often very small, usually achieves differentiation with cornea, iris, ciliary body, and lens choroid and retina. The

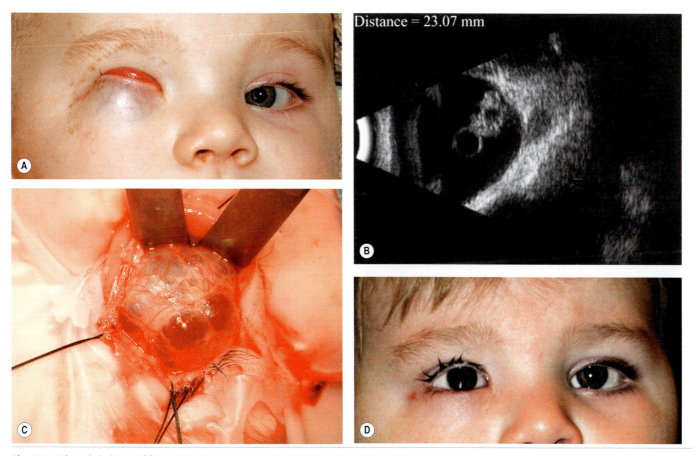

Fig. 29.7 Microphthalmos with cyst. This boy was born with a blueish swelling of the left lower lid which gradually enlarged. At 6 months (A), a large cyst fills the right orbit and distorts the lower lid, leading to conjunctival prolapse and exposure. (B) Imaging showed an expanded orbit with a multilocular cyst and a possible residual eye superior and posterior to the cyst. (C) The mass was excised along with the microphthalmic eye. (D) Postoperative result with prosthesis. (Patient of the University of British Columbia.)

other eye may be normal or may also have an optic nerve or retinal coloboma.[54,56] The extent of the cystic component is best delineated by CT scan, although B-scan ultrasound can also be useful. Small asymptomatic cysts may be found incidentally on CT scan (Fig. 29.8). The glial nature of the cyst lining can be demonstrated by immunohistochemistry.[57]

Management

Most cases require no immediate surgical intervention[56] since the cyst contributes to socket expansion.[50,53] Cyst enlargement resulting in an unsightly appearance can be managed by aspiration; repeated aspiration may be necessary and after multiple aspirations surgery may be indicated. Although it may be difficult to excise the cyst without sacrificing the globe, this can be achieved in patients with mild microphthalmos, with a satisfactory cosmetic outcome.[58]

The presence of an eye is important in inducing normal bony orbital growth. A congenitally anophthalmic socket will have delayed orbital growth and conjunctival contraction of the fornices, which may prevent satisfactory prosthetic fitting. Early orbital volume replacement with an appropriate implant and/or prosthesis is advocated if the globe is small or absent. Various types of conformers and socket expanders can be used

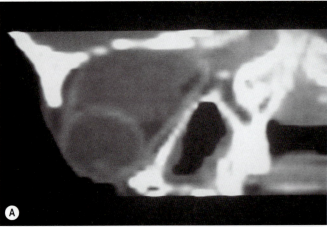

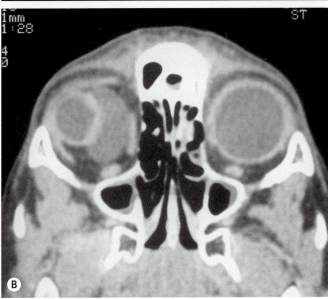

Fig. 29.8 CT scans showing the superior and medial orbital cyst.

to maintain the conjunctival fornices, palpebral fissures, and, perhaps, promote orbital growth.[53]

Early enucleation produces a bony volume reduction; good cosmetic results may be achieved with the use of a large orbital implant at the time of enucleation.[59]

Surprising evidence came from CT three-dimensional reconstruction and volumetric analysis on a small group of patients enucleated in childhood or adult life, with or without orbital implants. There was a bony orbital volume reduction of up to 15%, less than previously thought, and clinically imperceptible. No facial asymmetry was apparent whether or not an orbital implant was used at the time of enucleation in early childhood (0.4–8.0 years), with a follow-up ranging from 25 to 52 years.[60]

Orbital teratoma

Teratomas are tumors that arise from pluripotent embryonic stem cells and consist of elements derived from more than one germ cell layer. Although classically all three layers are represented, only mesoderm is invariable; ectodermal or endodermal elements can be absent. Such tumors should be called "teratoid." The extent of the tumor can be limited to the orbit (primary orbital teratoma) or it may involve the intracranial compartment, cavernous sinus,[61] nose, and sinuses. Occasionally, a much larger primary intracranial tumor invades the orbit secondarily. This usually manifests prenatally as polyhydramnios and is rarely compatible with life.

The usual presentation of a primary orbital teratoma is with unilateral, often massive, proptosis in a newborn child.[62] Teratomas are more common in females by a ratio of 2:1. The globe is often of normal size or slightly small (Fig. 29.9) but it is surrounded by intensely chemotic conjunctiva. It is displaced by a large cystic mass which is often fluctuant and transilluminates but may appear solid. The mass is often intraconal, giving rise to axial displacement with indentation by the four recti. Superior or inferior teratomas can occur. Typically, there is rapid growth after birth as secretions from the epithelial elements of the tumor accumulate within its cystic spaces. Exposure keratopathy, ulceration, and even perforation can complicate the resultant lagophthalmos. The tumor may stretch and adhere to the optic nerve, with optic atrophy. Occasionally, teratomas grow very slowly.[63]

On ultrasound, the tumor is of heterogeneous density and may contain foci of calcification which, along with orbital

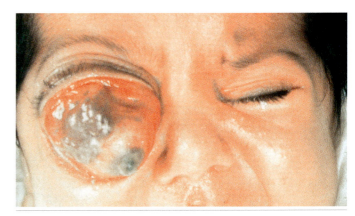

Fig. 29.9 Orbital teratoma.

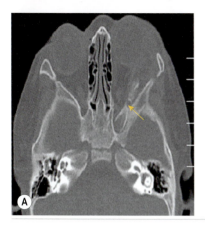
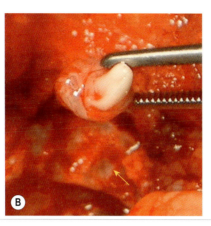
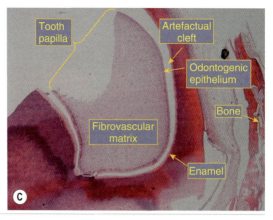

Fig. 29.10 (A) MRI of orbits of a 3-year-old child with slowly progressive proptosis. The arrow shows an area of mixed density in the lateral part of the left orbit. (B) At surgery, three teeth embedded in a bony matrix were found. (C) Histopathology confirmed a fully formed tooth.

enlargement, are evident on plain X-rays. CT and MRI delineate the lesion, define any intracranial extension, and highlight variable density with cystic elements, fat, and, occasionally, teeth (Fig. 29.10).

The treatment of choice is early surgical excision, with preservation of the globe if possible.[62-64] Intraoperative aspiration of fluid from the cystic mass may facilitate tumor removal. With intracranial involvement, a combined orbitotomy and craniotomy is necessary to remove the tumor. Total excision can be difficult. Vision may be preserved in the affected eye.[65] They are rare but the long-term outlook probably mostly depends on the histologic differentiation and the extent of the tumor; respiratory obstruction carries a poor prognosis.[66] Residual tumor can give rise to late recurrence and malignant change;[67] the latter is rare in the orbit.[68]

Parasitic cysts

Echinococcosis (hydatid cyst)

The tapeworm *Echinococcus* is an intestinal parasite of dogs and foxes. Sheep, cattle, or rodents may ingest contaminated feces and become hosts, and dogs become infected by eating their carcasses. Humans ingest ova in contaminated meat, berries, unclean vegetables, or feces from poor hand hygiene. The ova hatch in the intestine, and larvae migrate throughout the body, settling in various organs to form slowly enlarging, fluid-filled cysts full of larvae. Due to the distribution of blood from the portal tract, there is a predilection for the right lobe of the liver. Approximately 1% of infestations involve the orbit,[69] especially the superior and posterior orbit.

Most sheep- and cattle-rearing areas of the world have a high prevalence. Clinically, orbital echinococcosis presents with insidious signs of mass effect, which may be accompanied by chemosis, diplopia, restricted ocular motility, visual loss, and optic atrophy. Rupture of the cyst can result in an acute inflammatory episode.

The diagnosis of orbital echinococcosis is made by ultrasonography, CT (Fig. 29.11), or MRI scanning, which show a cystic mass whose wall is occasionally calcified and contains fluid which is isodense with vitreous. Other confirmatory findings include eosinophilia on a blood film, and positive enzyme-linked immunosorbent assay (ELISA) for echinococcal antibodies; this has over 90% sensitivity and specificity for *Echinococcus*.

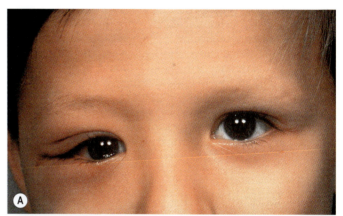
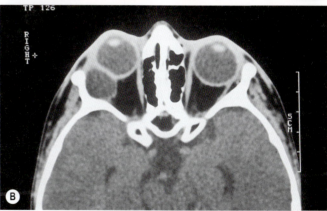

Fig. 29.11 (A) This 9-year-old refugee, who lived in unsanitary conditions, presented with a 6-month history of increasing right upper lid swelling. He has 4 mm of right proptosis, downward displacement of the globe, and lateral ptosis. (B) On CT scan a cystic lesion is found situated posterolaterally to the globe; this was an echinococcal cyst which was excised intact. (Patient of the University of British Columbia.)

Systemic treatment with albendazole is effective and a suitable alternative to surgery in uncomplicated cases.[70] Orbital cysts may be excised intact via a direct or lateral orbitotomy. Intraoperative rupture should be avoided, although technically difficult,[71] since it may be complicated by inflammation and implantation of daughter cysts. Cyst aspiration followed by irrigation with hypertonic saline may destroy daughter cysts.[72]

Hydatid cyst surgery should be accompanied by treatment with albendazole.

Other parasitic infestations of the orbit include cysticercosis and trichinosis, both acquired from pork.

Ectopias

Dermolipoma

These congenital lesions arise as a result of sequestration of skin within the conjunctiva at the time of embryonic development of the eyelids. They are superficial and rarely cystic yet are frequently misdiagnosed as cystic orbital dermoids. They may occur alone or as part of Goldenhar's syndrome spectrum, with lid coloboma, pre-auricular skin tags, hemifacial microsomia, and palatal and hearing abnormalities. They are situated laterally on the bulbar surface, are pink and skin-like due to keratinization (Fig. 29.12), and may have surface hairs which can cause irritation. Rarely, they may contain bony tissue.[73] Frequently, their superior and posterior extensions are close to the lacrimal ducts and levator muscle.[74] Surgery, in response to symptoms of irritation, should be conservative, performed with the microscope and limited to excision of the hair-bearing surface tissues or the interpalpebral lesion,[69,75] identifying and preserving the lacrimal ducts and avoiding the lateral rectus and levator muscles. Attempts at complete excision of dermolipoma with orbital dissection are risky and may cause dry eye, restrictive symblepharon, strabismus, and ptosis.[73,76]

Ectopic lacrimal gland

Lacrimal gland tissue may occasionally occur at ectopic sites within the orbit. Most commonly, it is found in the eyelid or conjunctiva, but it may occur on the cornea or even the iris and choroid.[77] Green and Zimmerman[78] reported eight cases; more have been added to the literature, often in children or teenagers. The ectopic tissue may be situated intra- or extraconally. Typically, the patients present with proptosis; double vision is a common symptom due to muscle restriction from the inflammatory response which the ectopic tissue often incites. The differential diagnosis includes true orbital neoplasms. Investigation, including CT scan, often shows a cystic component.[79] The treatment of choice is surgical excision. If this is incomplete, proptosis may recur.[78] The aberrant tissue may give rise to tumors such as pleomorphic adenoma or adenocarcinoma.[78]

Conjunctival and inclusion cyst

Conjunctival tissue may be sequestered as a primary embryologic malformation[80] or as a result of trauma or surgery.[81] This may occur anywhere on the conjunctiva and may be seen as a blister-like conjunctival swelling, filled with clear fluid. Occasionally, a posterior extension is present, with mass effect. Recurrence is common if the cyst is punctured and complete excision of the wall is indicated for a cure (Fig. 29.13). Histologically, this is conjunctival epithelium. Inclusion cysts may occur on the skin of the eyelids after trauma or surgery.

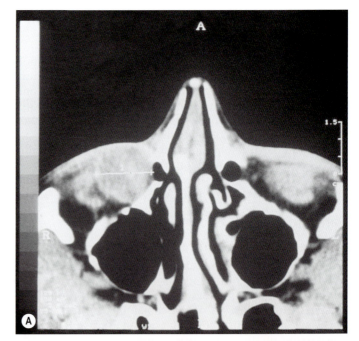

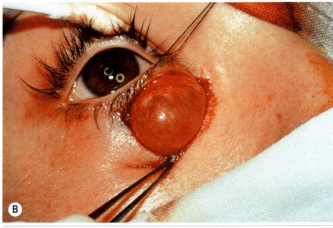

Fig. 29.13 (A) This child had a lower lid swelling, found to be cystic on CT scanning. A conjunctival cyst was excised via a skin incision (B). Differential diagnoses included conjunctival dermoid, ductal cyst, venous lymphatic malformation (lymphangioma) and respiratory cyst. (Dr. Alan McNab's patient.)

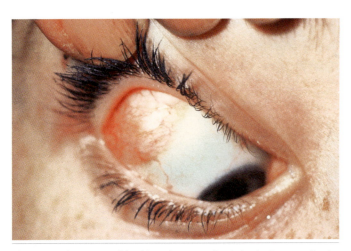

Fig. 29.12 This 16-year-old girl has a long-standing lesion in the upper fornix of the right eye which is consistent with a dermolipoma.

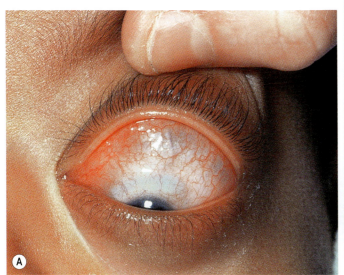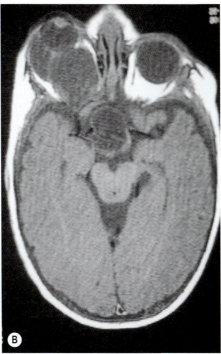

Fig. 29.14 (A) This 1-year-old child had a congenital proptosis with a cystic lesion seen almost surrounding the eye. (B) MRI scanning showed the cystic lesion was contiguous with a cyst in the suprasellar cystern. En bloc excision revealed an ectopic neural cystic hamartoma.

Other cystic lesions

A variety of other very rare, developmental cysts of neural origin may occur (Fig. 29.14).

References

2. Lessner AM, Antle CM, Rootman J, et al. Cystic lesions of the orbit and radiolucent defects of bone. In: Margo CE, Hamed LM, Mames RN, editors. Diagnostic Problems in Clinical Ophthalmology. Philadelphia: WB Saunders; 1994: 87–98.

3. Bullock JD, Fleishman JA, Rosset JS. Lacrimal ductal cysts. Ophthalmology 1986; 93: 1355–60.

9. Shields JA, Kaden IH, Eagle RC, Jr, Shields CL. Orbital dermoid cysts: clinicopathologic correlations, classification, and management. The 1997 Josephine E. Schueler Lecture. Ophthal Plast Reconstr Surg 1997; 13: 265–76.

10. Sathananthan N, Moseley IF, Rose GE, Wright JE. The frequency and clinical significance of bone involvement in outer canthus dermoid cysts. Br J Ophthalmol 1993; 77: 789–94.

15. Nugent RA, Lapointe JS, Rootman J, et al. Orbital dermoids: features on CT. Radiology 1987; 165: 475–8.

16. Abou-Rayyah Y, Rose GE, Konrad H, et al. Clinical, radiological and pathological examination of periocular dermoid cysts: evidence of inflammation from an early age. Eye 2002; 16: 507–12.

19. Satorre J, Antle CM, O'Sullivan R, et al. Orbital lesions with granulomatous inflammation. Can J Ophthalmol 1991; 26: 174–95.

20. Nevrekar D, Abdu E, Selden NR. Craniectomy for a bilobed dermoid cyst in the temporalis fossa and greater wing of the sphenoid bone. Pediatr Neurosurg 2009; 45: 46–8.

22. Sherman RP, Rootman J, Lapointe JS. Orbital dermoids: clinical presentation and management. Br J Ophthalmol 1984; 68: 642–52.

29. Pollock JA, Newton TH, Hoyt WF. Trans-sphenoidal and transethmoidal encephaloceles. Radiology 1968; 90: 442–53.

31. Lenhart PD, Lambert SR, Newman NJ, et al. Intracranial abnormalities with morning glory disk anomaly. Am J Ophthalmol 2006; 142: 644–50.

33. Kumar R, Verma A, Sharma K, et al. Post-traumatic pseudomeningocele of the orbit in a young child. J Pediatr Ophthalmol Strabismus 2003; 40: 110–2.

35. Boonvisut S, Ladpli S, Sujatanond M, et al. Morphologic study of 120 skull base defects in frontoethmoidal encephalomeningoceles. Plast Reconstr Surg 1998; 101: 1784–95.

41. Alberti PW, Marshall HF, Munro-Black JI. Frontal ethmoidal mucocoele as a cause of unilateral proptosis. Br J Ophthalmol 1968; 52: 833–8.

43. Casteels I, De Loof E, Brock P, et al. Sudden blindness in a child: presenting symptom of a sphenoid sinus mucocoele. Br J Ophthalmol 1992; 76: 502–4.

44. Conboy PJ, Jones NS. The place of endoscopic sinus surgery in the treatment of paranasal sinus mucocoeles. Clin Otolaryngol 2003; 28: 207–10.

48. Hayashi N, Repka MX, Ueno H, et al. Congenital cystic eye: report of two cases and review of the literature. Surv Ophthalmol 1999; 44: 173–9.

50. McLean CJ, Ragge NK, Jones RB, Collin JR. The management of orbital cysts associated with congenital microphthalmos and anophthalmos. Br J Ophthalmol 2003; 87: 860–3.

51. Pagon RA. Ocular coloboma. Surv Ophthalmol 1981; 25: 223–36.

53. Ragge N, Subak-Sharpe ID, Collin JRO. A practical guide to the management of anophthalmia and microphthalmia. Eye 2007; 21: 1290–300.

58. Polito E, Leccisotti A. Colobomatous ocular cyst excision with globe preservation. Ophthal Plast Reconstr Surg 1995; 11: 288–92.

60. Hintschich C, Zonneveld F, Baldeschi L, et al. Bony orbital development after early enucleation in humans. Br J Ophthalmol 2001; 85: 205–8.

61. Tobias S, Valarezo J, Meir K, Umansky F. Giant cavernous sinus teratoma. A clinical example of a rare entity: case report. Neurosurgery 2001; 48: 1367–70.

62. Hoyt WF, Joe S. Congenital teratoid cyst. Arch Ophthalmol 1962; 68: 197–201.

65. Morris DS, Fayers T, Dolman PJ. Orbital teratoma: case report and management review. J AAPOS 2009; 13: 605–7.

69. Rootman J. Diseases of the Orbit: A Multidisciplinary Approach, 2nd ed. Philadelphia: Lippincott Williams & Wilkins; 2002.

72. Benazzou S, Arkha Y, Derraz S, et al. Orbital hydatid cyst: review of 10 cases. J Craniomaxillofac Surg 2010; 38: 274–8.

75. McNab AA, Wright JE, Caswell AG. Clinical features and surgical management of dermolipomas. Aust N Z J Ophthalmol 1990; 18: 159–62.

78. Green WR, Zimmerman LE. Ectopic lacrimal gland tissue: report of eight cases with orbital involvement. Arch Ophthalmol 1967; 78: 318–27.

81. Song JS, Finger PT, Kurli M, et al. Giant secondary conjunctival inclusion cysts: a late complication of strabismus surgery. Ophthalmology 2006; 113: 1045–9.

Access the complete reference list online at
http://www.expertconsult.com

Inflammatory disorders

Christopher J Lyons • Jack Rootman

Chapter contents

Inflammatory orbital disorders become more common in the second decade of life, when causes of orbital disease increasingly resemble those found in adulthood.

The principal inflammations can be divided into non-specific orbital inflammatory syndromes (NSOIS) (also known as idiopathic orbital inflammation,[1] and previously known as "inflammatory pseudotumor") and specific causes such as sarcoidosis and Wegener's granulomatosis, both of which are rare but potentially life-threatening. The incidence of thyroid orbitopathy increases in the teenage years, and this is discussed briefly.

Infective orbital cellulitis in early childhood is most commonly related to dacryocystitis or trauma. Over the age of 6 years, and particularly in the second decade, the fully-formed sinuses become the most common source of orbital cellulitis (see Chapter 13).

Non-specific orbital inflammatory syndromes (pseudotumors)

Definition

The child's orbit is occasionally the site of acute or subacute inflammation of unknown cause.[2,3] This entity was previously known as "orbital inflammatory pseudotumor,"[4] a term which, with the advent of CT and MRI and pathologic studies, has been abandoned. Instead, the site of inflammation is identified,[5,6] including anterior, diffuse, apical, myositic, and lacrimal types. Children tend to develop the anterior and diffuse types, but myositis and lacrimal inflammation may occur. Apical involvement is rare. Non-specific sclerosing inflammation of the orbit is very rare in childhood.

These syndromes present acutely or subacutely with inflammatory signs. Although apparently idiopathic, they have many features of an orbital immune reaction.[7] Histologically, there is an influx of lymphocytes, plasma cells, sparse neutrophils, and macrophages. Inflammatory mediators cause edema, vascular dilatation and pain without systemic malaise. In contrast, chronic inflammations and granulomatous diseases cause mass effect as their predominant feature without clinical features of acute inflammation. The common CT profile of acute or subacute NSOIS is a poorly defined margin to the inflammatory focus, as well as contrast enhancement.[8,9] With MRI, T2-weighted sequences with fat suppression and gadolinium can highlight areas of fluid accumulation indicative of inflammatory foci.

Anterior idiopathic orbital inflammation: acute and subacute

This is the most common type of NSOIS in childhood. The inflammatory process is centered on the anterior orbit and adjacent globe (Fig. 30.1). Pain, proptosis, lid swelling, conjunctival injection, and decreased vision are the main presenting features,

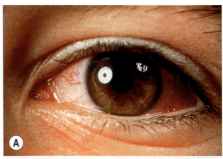
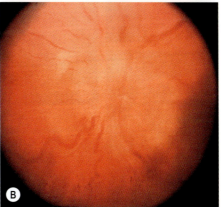

Fig. 30.1 Anterior NSOIS in a 6-year-old boy who presented with a red eye (A), pain on eye movement and decreased vision of 3 days duration. Fundoscopy (B) shows choroidal swelling and papillitis. (Patient from the University of British Columbia.)

with an onset over days or occasionally weeks. Children are more likely to have an associated anterior and posterior uveitis, which can potentially lead to misdiagnosis and erroneous treatment with topical steroid.[3,10,11] The disc may be swollen.[3,12] Systemically, the erythrocyte sedimentation rate may be raised, and there is often cerebrospinal fluid pleocytosis.[12] Disturbances in thyroid function tests and hypothyroidism have also been reported in association with NSOIS.[13,14] CT scans show diffuse anterior orbital inflammation centered on the globe, producing scleral and choroidal thickening with or without serous retinal detachment. The junction of the globe and optic nerve is characteristically obscured on CT scan with inflammatory changes extending along the nerve sheath. On ultrasound, there is a uniform-density infiltrate corresponding to sclerotenonitis, with accentuation of the sub-Tenon's space and doubling of the optic nerve shadow producing a T-shaped shadow (or T-sign) (Fig. 30.2).

Diffuse idiopathic orbital inflammation: acute and subacute

This is clinically similar to the anterior form, although the symptoms and clinical signs are more severe (Fig. 30.3). The eye movements are more restricted and the visual acuity is worse due to serous retinal detachment and/or optic neuropathy. Inflammatory soft tissue changes permeate the whole orbit on CT scan, with a white-out appearance whose density is proportional to the severity of the clinical signs, and which resolves as the condition settles. Again, the T-sign is evident on ultrasonography.

Anterior and diffuse non-specific orbital inflammatory syndromes: differential diagnoses and management

The differential diagnoses include infection such as orbital cellulitis, scleritis, sudden enlargement of a pre-existing lesion such as a ruptured dermoid, hemorrhage into a venous-lymphatic malformation (lymphangioma) or malignancy which, in childhood, may be rhabdomyosarcoma, neuroblastoma, Ewing's sarcoma, or leukemic infiltration. Anterior and diffuse NSOIS are also part of the differential diagnoses of uveitis and serous retinal detachment in childhood. Biopsy of involved orbital tissues should be considered in all but the most typical cases.

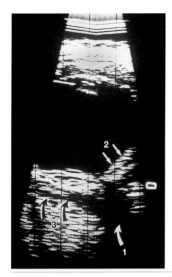

Fig. 30.2 Ultrasound scan of anterior NSOIS showing the T-sign. There is doubling of the optic nerve shadow (1), shallow retinal detachment (2) and accentuation of Tenon's space (3). (Patient from the University of British Columbia.)

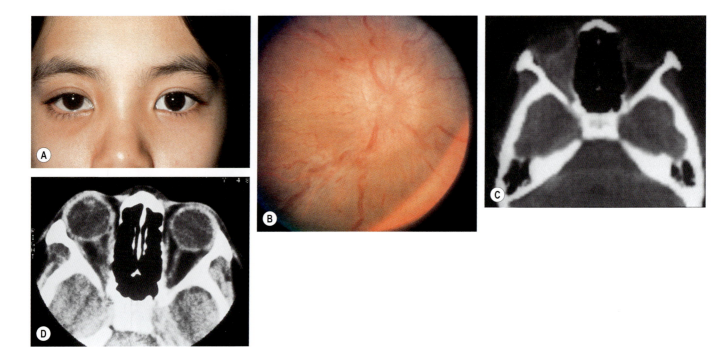

Fig. 30.3 Diffuse NSOIS in a 12-year-old girl who presented with a retrobulbar ache, associated with ptosis (A), and pain on eye movement. There was right-sided uveitis with marked disc swelling (B). On CT scanning (C), there was a "white-out" appearance of the right orbit (similar patient) which resolved after treatment with systemic steroids (D). (Same patient from the University of British Columbia.)

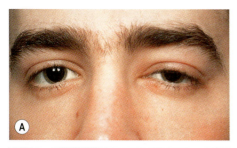

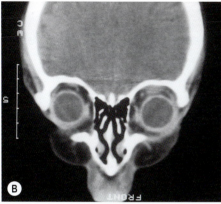

Fig. 30.4 Left superior rectus myositis in a 16-year-old boy. Ptosis (A) and pain limitation of upgaze with diplopia were the presenting signs; this was due to left superior rectus myositis shown as a thickened muscle complex on CT scan (B). (Patient from the University of British Columbia.)

Treatment with non-steroidal anti-inflammatory drugs such as flurbiprofen is tried first. Systemic steroids may be used in addition, or as an alternative in doses for prednisolone of 1–1.5 mg/kg per day. There is usually rapid improvement in symptoms, especially pain, as well as clinical signs. Progress can be monitored by resolution of the clinical, CT, and ultrasound features. This disease may have a recalcitrant course, with frequent recurrences and steroid dependence. High-dose steroid is re-started for recurrence and tapered as quickly as clinical progress will allow, usually over a few weeks. Failure to respond suggests the need for biopsy and the renewed search for a specific etiology. Low-dose radiotherapy has been advocated for biopsy-proven cases that do not respond to steroids. Combined steroids and immunosuppressives may be necessary.

Idiopathic orbital myositis: acute and subacute

This is characterized by proptosis, pain and limitation of eye movement with diplopia, ptosis, lid edema, and conjunctival chemosis. Strabismus is often present with duction limitation in the direction of action of the involved muscle(s).[15] Spasm of the affected muscle also causes restriction of the ipsilateral antagonist with a positive forced duction test. Globe retraction and narrowing of the lid fissure similar to Duane's syndrome is a frequent finding.[16,17]

CT scan shows diffuse muscle enlargement with irregular margins (Fig. 30.4). The muscle enlargement frequently involves the tendon,[18] in contradistinction to thyroid orbitopathy where, typically, the tendon is spared. The superior rectus–levator complex or medial rectus are the most common muscles to be involved, but any muscle can be affected, including the obliques.[19] More than one muscle may simultaneously be involved and bilateral disease may occur.

The cause of orbital myositis is unknown but a number of associations have been reported, including upper respiratory tract infection,[20] Lyme disease,[21] Whipple's disease,[22] and other autoimmune diseases.[23]

The differential diagnoses include thyroid orbitopathy, which differs from idiopathic orbital myositis in that a preceding or concurrent history of thyroid disorder is common, pain is absent, the inferior recti tend to be the first muscles involved (although any muscle may be involved), and sparing of the tendon is apparent on CT scan. In some cases, differentiating between these two conditions can be very difficult[24] and misdiagnosis is not uncommon.[3] Early orbital cellulitis, orbital metastasis, and trichinosis are other differential diagnoses.

Non-steroidal anti-inflammatory treatment has been advocated,[25] but the rapid and dramatic response to steroids is almost diagnostic. We recommend an initial dose of prednisolone of 0.5–1 mg/kg per day, tapering to nothing over 2–4 weeks. Delay in diagnosis and initiation of therapy is associated with recurrence and incomplete resolution of signs.

Idiopathic lacrimal inflammation: acute and subacute

Pain, tenderness, and swelling over the lateral aspect of the upper lid are typical presenting features of this disorder.[26] The lid may have an S-shaped configuration with ptosis which is more marked laterally than medially. The globe is often slightly displaced downward and medially. Slit-lamp examination shows superotemporal conjunctival chemosis and pouting of the excretory lacrimal duct orifices. There is no uveitis. On CT scans, the inflammation is centered on the lacrimal gland, often extending diffusely into the lateral orbit and involving the adjacent globe. The differential diagnoses include bacterial and viral dacryoadenitis, the latter often occurring in association with childhood infections such as mumps or mononucleosis. In this situation, the child is likely to be ill, and generalized lymphadenopathy or salivary gland enlargement may be noted, along with lymphocytosis. Inflammation related to leakage from a dermoid cyst and neoplasia including chloroma (granulocytic sarcoma) are other rare possibilities. Lacrimal gland involvement in orbital sarcoid tends to be chronic, presenting with signs and symptoms of dry eyes, and is rare in childhood.

Acute or subacute lacrimal gland swellings in childhood do not need biopsy if they are related to an obvious viral illness such as mumps or if there are other findings suggestive of mononucleosis. Atypical lesions in patients whose signs and symptoms fail to respond to treatment should have an early biopsy.

Idiopathic lacrimal inflammation is treated with moderate-dose systemic steroids, tapering with resolution of symptoms and signs.

Specific causes of orbital inflammation

The most common cause of orbital inflammation in childhood is infective orbital cellulitis (see Chapter 13). Other childhood orbital inflammatory diseases are comparatively rare, called "specific" since they have a defined clinical, radiologic, biochemical, and histopathologic spectrum, though their underlying cause has not been clearly determined.

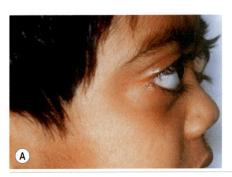
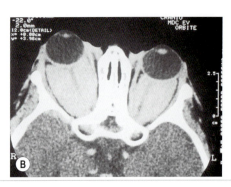
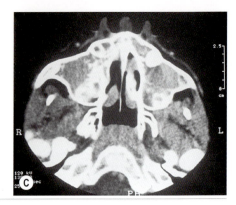

Fig. 30.5 A 7-year-old boy presented with a 3-month history of progressive bilateral proptosis (A). He has positive ANCA titers. CT (B,C) shows widespread involvement of the orbital soft tissues and maxillary sinuses. (Patient from the University of British Columbia.)

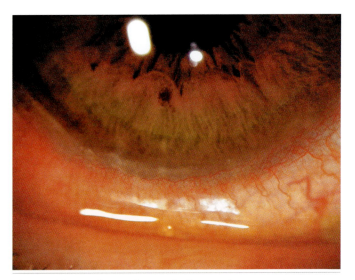

Fig. 30.6 Wegener's granulomatosis. Photograph or cornea demonstrates marginal infiltration with a clear zone between the infiltrate and limbus, a feature characteristic of the disease. (Patient from the University of British Columbia.)

Wegener's granulomatosis

This is a necrotizing granulomatous vasculitis which has a predilection for the airways and the kidneys. The limited form of the disease in which the kidneys are spared has a better prognosis and is more commonly associated with orbital disease.[27] Both forms have the same incidence of ocular and orbital involvement, ranging in different studies from 28% to 45%.[25] Before the introduction of cyclophosphamide, over 90% of affected patients died within 2 years.[28] Although this is not a common disease of childhood, it does occur under the age of 18. Its rarity in childhood commonly leads to a delay in diagnosis.[3]

Clinical features

The onset of orbital Wegener's granulomatosis is often preceded by a history of subacute or chronic low grade disease, with sudden aggravation leading to presentation. The main features are proptosis, which is frequently bilateral, with ocular and facial pain which may be severe. An orbital mass usually develops (Fig. 30.5), displacing the globe, even in patients who initially present with scleritis. The latter is typically nodular and necrotizing, accompanied by characteristic marginal corneal infiltration, which can progress to ulceration. Decreased vision is common and can be related to optic neuropathy.

We have seen five children or adolescents with Wegener's granulomatosis affecting the orbit; lacrimal gland involvement with lid swelling and brawny discoloration occurred in two of these. The orbital disease was bilateral in two patients; midline disease and lacrimal gland involvement was present in the others. All our patients had ENT symptoms in the 3 months prior to presentation, including nasal blockage, discharge or bleeds, pain over the paranasal or mastoid sinuses, and hearing loss or tinnitus. Levi et al[29] recently reviewed ocular involvement as the presenting feature of Wegener's granulomatosis in children.

CT scans show an orbital mass with infiltrative margins obscuring fat and adjacent muscles. Midline bony erosion and sinus involvement may be evident. Histologic changes include areas of fat disruption and focal necrosis with lipid-laden macrophages, giant cells, and evidence of acute inflammatory cells. Vasculitis is often difficult to find in these specimens.[27,30] Fibrosis is common. Stains for fungi and mycobacteria should be performed to exclude them as causes.

Septra (Septrin), an antibiotic combination of trimethoprim and sulphamethoxazole, is a first-line treatment for this condition. Azathioprine is a second-line drug. Cyclophosphamide is effective in Wegener's granulomatosis[31] but is reserved, due to its oncogenic potential, for children who have not responded to the above or who present with severe disease. Antineutrophil cytoplasmic antibodies (cANCA) are specific markers for Wegener's if there is a "cytoplasmic" staining pattern. Their plasma level correlates with disease activity. Failure of these to return to normal after clinical improvement with treatment indicates a high risk of relapse.[32]

Wegener's granulomatosis is rare but occurs in childhood and clinicians should remain alert for this potentially lethal disorder especially in patients with bilateral orbital involvement, particularly with scleritis accompanied by characteristic marginal corneal infiltration (Fig. 30.6). Respiratory tract or sinus (including the mastoid sinuses) involvement further supports this diagnosis.

Sarcoidosis

This chronic granulomatous inflammatory disease of unknown cause is more commonly seen in the orbit as a cause of dacryoadenitis in females aged 30 years and over. Nevertheless, children are occasionally affected; several hundred cases have

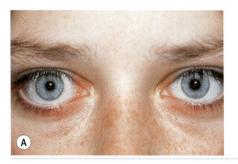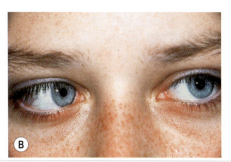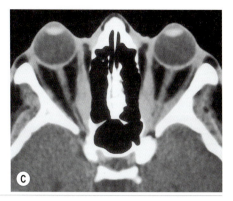

Fig. 30.7 This girl had a 6-year history of double vision at the extremes of gaze. Her past medical history included autoimmune hepatitis and hyperthyroidism, treated with radioiodine. There is lid retraction (A), lid lag, and restriction of abduction with esotropia in lateral gaze (B). Bilateral medial rectus enlargement involving the muscle belly but sparing the tendons is evident on CT scanning (C). (Patient from the University of British Columbia.)

been documented in children under the age of 15 years; the incidence of the disease rapidly increases in the late teens, peaking in the third decade. The risk is increased 3–10 times in African-Americans versus Caucasians, with a slight female preponderance. Age defines to some extent the pattern of systemic involvement: children aged 5 years or less develop uveitis, arthropathy, and skin rash; those aged 8 to 15 have lung involvement with ocular, skin, and spleen involvement in approximately one-third.[33]

Anterior uveitis, which may be chronic and granulomatous or acute, is the commonest finding at presentation, affecting one-quarter to one-half of patients. The eyelid, conjunctiva, sclera, episclera, and lacrimal glands may be involved. Orbital infiltration causing unilateral proptosis has been reported in a 5-year-old child with arthritis.[34] Cornblath et al.[35] reported a 15-year-old boy with pain, diplopia, and ophthalmoplegia from generalized involvement of the extraocular muscles. There was diffuse enlargement of all the muscles on CT, suggesting orbital myositis or thyroid orbitopathy. Unlike the latter,[36] the muscle insertions were enlarged on CT scan.

Thyroid orbitopathy

Approximately 2.5% of all cases of Graves' disease occur in children,[37] and about half of these develop ophthalmic signs.[38,39] In the series from Toronto,[40] it was the second most common cause of proptosis in children (orbital cellulitis was first). Neonatal thyroid orbitopathy is well recognized, affecting the infant of a hyperthyroid mother. It is otherwise rare before puberty; the age of onset is generally from 12 years onwards. It is more prevalent in girls, with a 6 : 1 gender ratio.[41] There is commonly a family or past history of hyperthyroidism. Associations with other autoimmune disorders, diabetes,[41] and Down's syndrome have been reported.

The orbital involvement is mild, often limited to lid edema or retraction. There may be proptosis, sometimes asymmetric, which occasionally warrants orbital decompression.[42]

A few patients develop severe thyroid orbitopathy with marked restriction of ductions[42] (Fig. 30.7A,B) and proptosis with inflammatory signs. The severity of the orbitopathy tends to increase with age.[39] Optic neuropathy and sight-threatening corneal problems have not been described in children. Orbital imaging may show enlarged muscles (Fig. 30.7C) with characteristic sparing of the tendons.

References

1. Harris GJ. Idiopathic orbital inflammation: a pathogenetic construct and treatment strategy. The 2005 ASOPRS Foundation Lecture. Ophthal Plast Reconstr Surg 2006; 11: 79–86.
2. Mottow LS, Jakobiec FA. Idiopathic inflammatory orbital pseudotumor in childhood. I. Clinical characteristics. Arch Ophthalmol 1978; 96: 1410–7.
3. Rootman J. Diseases of the Orbit: A Multidisciplinary Approach, 2nd ed. Philadelphia: Lippincott Williams & Wilkins; 2002.
4. Blodi FC, Gass DJM. Inflammatory pseudotumour of the orbit. Br J Ophthalmol 1968; 2: 79–93.
5. Rootman J, Nugent RA. The classification and management of acute orbital pseudotumours. Ophthalmology 1982; 89: 1040–8.
6. Rootman J. Why pseudotumour is no longer a useful concept [editorial]. Br J Ophthalmol 1998; 82: 339–40.
7. Kennerdell JS, Dresner SC. The non-specific orbital inflammatory syndromes. Surv Ophthalmol 1984; 29: 93–103.
8. Moseley IF, Sanders MD. Computerized Tomography in Neuro-Ophthalmology. London: Chapman and Hall; 1982.
9. Atlas SW, Grossman RI, Savino PJ, et al. Surface coil MRI of orbital pseudotumor. Am J Roentgenol 1987; 148: 803–8.
10. Bloom JN, Graviss ER, Byrne BJ. Orbital pseudotumor in the differential diagnosis of pediatric uveitis. J Pediatr Ophthalmol Strabismus 1992; 29: 59–63.
11. Hertle RW, Granet DB, Goyal AK, Schaffer DB. Orbital pseudotumor in the differential diagnosis of pediatric uveitis [letter]. J Pediatr Ophthalmol Strabismus 1993; 30: 61.
12. Mottow-Lippa L, Jakobiec FA, Smith M. Idiopathic inflammatory orbital pseudotumor in childhood. II. Results of diagnostic tests and biopsies. Ophthalmology 1981; 88: 565–74.
13. Atabay C, Tyutyunikov A, Scalise D, et al. Serum antibodies reactive with eye muscle membrane antigens are detected in patients with non-specific orbital inflammation. Ophthalmology 1995; 102: 145–53.
14. Uddin JM, Rennie CA, Moore AT. Bilateral non-specific orbital inflammation (orbital "pseudotumour"), posterior scleritis, and anterior uveitis associated with hypothyroidism in a child. Br J Ophthalmol 2002; 86: 936.
15. Pollard ZF. Acute rectus muscle palsy in children as a result of orbital myositis. J Pediatr 1996; 128: 230–3.
16. Timms C, Russell-Eggitt IM, Taylor DSI. Simulated (pseudo-) Duane's syndrome secondary to orbital myositis. Binoc Vis Strabismus Q 1989; 4: 109–12.
17. Moorman CM, Elston JS. Acute orbital myositis. Eye 1995; 9: 96–101.
18. Trokel SL, Hilal SK. Recognition and differential diagnosis of enlarged extraocular muscles in computed tomography. Am J Ophthalmol 1979; 87: 503–12.

19. Wan WL, Cano MR, Green RL. Orbital myositis involving the oblique muscles. An echographic study. Ophthalmology 1988; 95: 1522–8.

20. Purcell JJ, Jr, Taulhee WA. Orbital myositis after upper respiratory tract infection. Arch Ophthalmol 1981; 99: 437–8.

21. Seidenberg KB, Leib ML. Orbital myositis with Lyme disease. Am J Ophthalmol 1990; 109: 13–6.

22. Orssaud C, Poisson M, Gardeur D. Myosite orbitaire, recidive d'une maladie de Whipple. J Fr Ophtalmol 1992; 15: 205–8.

23. Weinstein GS, Dresner SC, Slamovits TL, Kennerdell JS. Acute and subacute orbital myositis. Am J Ophthalmol 1983; 96: 209–17.

24. Jellinek EH. The orbital pseudotumor syndrome and its differentiation from endocrine exophthalmos. Brain 1969; 92: 35–58.

25. Robin JB, Schanzlin DJ, Meisler DM, et al. Ocular involvement in the respiratory vasculitides. Surv Ophthalmol 1985; 30: 127–40.

26. Belanger C, Zhang KS, Reddy AK, et al. Inflammatory disorders of the orbit in childhood: a case series. Am J Ophthalmol 2010; 150: 460–3.

27. Perry SR, Rootman J, White VA. The clinical and pathologic constellation of Wegener's granulomatosis of the orbit. Ophthalmology 1997; 104: 683–94.

28. Hollander D, Manning RT. The use of alkylating agents in the treatment of Wegener's granulomatosis. Ann Intern Med 1967; 67: 393–8.

29. Levi M, Kodsi SR, Rubin SE, et al. Ocular involvement as the initial manifestation of Wegener's granulomatosis. J AAPOS 2008; 12: 94–6.

30. Satorre J, Antle CM, O'Sullivan R, et al. Orbital lesions with granulomatous inflammation. Can J Ophthalmol 1991; 26: 174–95.

31. Fauci AS, Haynes BF, Katz P, Wolff SM. Wegener's granulomatosis: prospective clinical and therapeutic experience with 85 patients for 21 years. Ann Intern Med 1983; 98: 76–85.

32. Power WJ, Rodriguez A, Neves RA, et al. Disease relapse in patients with ocular manifestations of Wegener's granulomatosis. Ophthalmology 1995; 102: 154–60.

33. Hoover DL, Khan JA, Giangiacomo J. Pediatric ocular sarcoidosis. Surv Ophthalmol 1986; 30: 215–28.

34. Khan JA, Hoover DL, Giangiacomo J, Singsen BH. Orbital and childhood sarcoidosis. J Pediatr Ophthalmol Strabismus 1986; 23: 190–4.

35. Cornblath WT, Elner V, Rolfe M. Extraocular muscle involvement in sarcoidosis. Ophthalmology 1993; 100: 501–5.

36. Trokel SL, Jakobiec FA. Correlation of CT scanning and pathologic features of ophthalmic Graves' disease. Ophthalmology 1981; 88: 553–64.

37. Bram I. Exophthalmic goiter in children: comments based upon 128 cases in patients of 12 and under. Arch Pediatr 1937; 54: 419–24.

38. Young LA. Dysthyroid ophthalmopathy in children. J Pediatr Ophthalmol Strabismus 1979; 16: 105–7.

39. Uretsky SH, Kennerdell JS, Gutai JP. Graves' ophthalmopathy in childhood and adolescence. Arch Ophthalmol 1980; 98: 1963–4.

40. Crawford JS. Diseases of the orbit. In: Crawford JS, Morin JD, editors. The Eye in Childhood. New York: Grune and Stratton; 1983: 361–94.

41. Hayles AB, Kennedy RL, Beahrs OH, Wollner LB. Exophthalmic goiter in children. J Clin Endocrinol Metab 1959; 19: 138–51.

42. Liu GT, Heher KL, Katowitz JA, et al. Prominent proptosis in childhood thyroid eye disease. Ophthalmology 1996; 103: 779–84.

Conjunctiva and subconjunctival tissue

Venkatesh Prajna • Muralidhar Rajamani

Anatomy

The conjunctiva is a thin, translucent, vascular mucous membrane that lines the inner surface of the eyelids and the anterior surface of the eyeball as far as the limbus. This tissue is arranged in a sac-like fashion and is composed of a palpebral region (covering the inner aspects of the lids), a bulbar region (covering the surface of the sclera), a forniceal region, and a medial semilunar fold.

While the palpebral conjunctiva shares its blood supply with the eyelids, the bulbar component is supplied by the anterior ciliary arteries. The nerve supply to the conjunctiva is through the lacrimal, supraorbital, supratrochlear, and infraorbital branches of the ophthalmic division of the trigeminal nerve.

The conjunctival epithelium varies from 2 to 5 cells in thickness and is continuous with the corneal epithelium at the limbus and with the skin at the margin of the lids. While the bulbar conjunctiva is lined by a stratified non-keratinized squamous epithelium, the forniceal and tarsal regions are lined by columnar and cuboidal types, respectively. A key constituent of the cellular architecture is the presence of goblet cells, which accounts for 10% of the basal cells of the conjunctival epithelium. These cells are more prevalent in the medial forniceal and palpebral regions, and play a vital part in secreting the mucin component of the tear film. There is an increase in the number of these cells during chronic inflammation of conjunctiva, while conditions like pemphigoid and vitamin A deficiency causes a decrease. Other cell types which nestle within the epithelial layers include melanocytes, Langerhans' cells, and intraepithelial lymphocytes.

Beneath the epithelium lies a loose structure called the substantia propria. This structure contains different cell types which mediate immune responses (mast cells, plasma cells, eosinophils, and lymphocytes) interspersed in a vascular network. This arrangement of immune cells, commonly referred to as conjunctiva-associated lymphoid tissue, existing in a vascular environment, is continuously exposed to potential external infective agents and allergens thus serving as a perfect setting for inflammation to set in.

Beneath the conjunctiva lies a fibroelastic tissue, Tenon's capsule, which surrounds the eye ball from the corneoscleral junction to the optic nerve. Tenon's capsule is thicker in children and contains more fibroblasts. Hence surgeries like trabeculectomy performed in children, especially without adjuvant procedures like intraoperative use of antimetabolites, may fail due to the aggressive healing response induced by these fibroblasts.[1]

Conjunctiva in systemic disease

A careful flashlight examination of the conjunctiva in a brightly lit environment often provides comprehensive information about a potential underlying systemic disorder. Information about color, lustre, abnormalities in vascularization, and pigmentation help to suspect an underlying ocular or a systemic cause. A slit-lamp evaluation can then be carried out to focus on the specific area of the pathology.

Vitamin A deficiency

This systemic condition affects organs throughout the body. The ocular manifestation is termed xerophthalmia and affected individuals present with night blindness, conjunctival xerosis, Bitot's spots, corneal xerosis, keratomalacia, and the "xerophthalmic" fundus.

In this condition, the conjunctival epithelium is transformed from the normal columnar to the stratified squamous type. There is an associated loss of goblet cells, formation of a granular cell layer, and keratinization of the surface. The conjunctiva loses its normal lustre and is altered into a dry or unwettable one (Fig. 31.1). It is almost always bilateral. A classic ocular sign is Bitot's spots, which is a superficial, scaly, gray area on the interpalpebral region of the bulbar conjunctiva (Fig. 31.2). *Corynebacterium xerosis* can colonize these spots, and produce a foamy appearance because of the gas-forming nature of these organisms. If untreated, the condition involves the cornea, causing corneal xerosis and finally corneal melting, or keratomalacia.

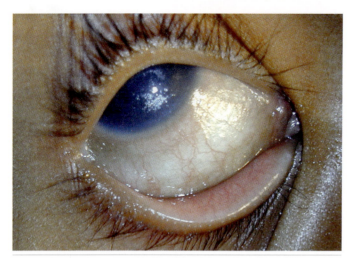

Fig. 31.1 Xerophthalmia. Dry, lustureless, inferior bulbar conjunctiva showing a wrinkled appearance. Associated corneal xerosis is also seen. (Courtesy of Dr. P. Vijayalakshmi, MS.)

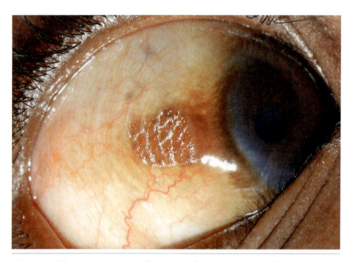

Fig. 31.2 Bitot's spot. A superficial, scaly, foamy Bitot's spot of the bulbar conjunctiva.

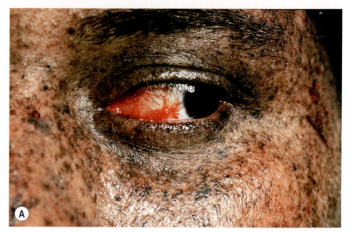

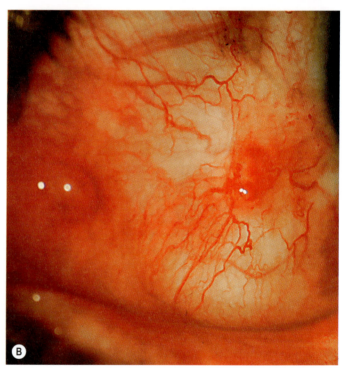

Fig. 31.3 Xeroderma pigmentosa. (A) The widespread skin pigmentation can be seen in this girl of Indian origin. (B) The conjunctiva was affected by multifocal recurrent squamous cell carcinomas.

The diagnosis of xerophthalmia is often clinical and does not require any additional investigations. In doubtful cases, impression cytology of the superficial layers of the conjunctival epithelium may be helpful to show the loss of goblet cells and keratinization of epithelial cells. Oral administration of vitamin A is preferred because it is safe, cost-effective, and highly effective. In affected children above 12 months of age, retinol palmitate (110 mg) or retinol acetate (200 000 IU) are given orally immediately and the dose is repeated the following day. An additional dose should be given 2 weeks later to boost liver resources. Children between 6 and 11 months should receive only half the above-mentioned dose, and children less than 6 months one-quarter of the dose.

Parenteral administration is indicated in those children with conditions such as persistent vomiting, severe stomatitis, and attendant difficulty in deglutition, severe diarrhea with malabsorption, and septic shock. Such children can be treated with intramuscular injection of 55 mg of water-miscible retinol palmitate (100 000 IU), which replaces the first oral dose. This is repeated the next day. Children of less than 1 year are treated with vitamin A in half the prescribed dosage. After the acute phase is over, dietary supplements with provitamin A-rich foods, should be provided.[2]

Xeroderma pigmentosa

This condition is inherited as an autosomal recessive disorder. Symptoms appear in early childhood. Affected individuals present with extreme photophobia, photosensitivity, and typical dark pigmentary changes in the skin. They are at an increased risk for malignant lesions in sun-exposed mucocutaneous and ocular structures (Fig. 31.3A). There is an impaired ability to repair ultraviolet light-induced DNA damage, which results in accumulation of the damaged DNA. This accumulation of abnormal DNA leads to chromosomal mutation and cell death and is thought to be responsible for neoplasms in these individuals.

Conjunctival involvement occurs mostly in the interpalpebral area in the form of xerosis, telangiectasia, chronic conjunctival congestion, pigmentation, pinguecula, and pterygium. Ocular surface neoplasms such as squamous cell carcinoma, basal cell carcinoma, and malignant melanoma may occur, with a predilection for the limbal area (Fig. 31.3B). Corneal changes include exposure keratitis, band-shaped nodular keratopathy, scarring, ulceration, vascularization, and perforation. The posterior segment is usually spared. Elevated symptomatic conjunctival nodules and suspected neoplasms may require repeated excisions; otherwise the treatment is symptomatic.

Sturge-Weber syndrome

This is a congenital disorder with a classical triad of cutaneous facial angioma, leptomeningeal angioma, and ocular involvement (see Chapter 65). The facial angioma typically occurs in the distribution of the ophthalmic division of the trigeminal nerve. Dilated episcleral and conjunctival vessels with aneurysm formation in the limbal area are commonly seen. Glaucoma is a frequent accompaniment (see Chapter 37), especially in patients with severe conjunctival involvement.[3]

Icthyosis

Ichthyosis is a heterogeneous family of at least 28 genetic skin disorders. Most pedigrees are either autosomal dominant or X-linked in their inheritance pattern. A rare autosomal recessive form, lamellar icthyosis, occurs. In all these conditions, dry scaly lesions are present predominantly over the upper half of the body, mainly around the neck, mouth, and trunk. The conjunctiva may become inflamed primarily or secondarily due to lid anomalies like ectropion.[4] A papillary reaction may develop (Fig. 31.4). The treatment is to provide adequate lubrication and to correct the lid abnormalities, if present.

Anemia

Conjunctival pallor is a sensitive and commonly used sign to detect anemia in children. This examination should preferably be done in broad daylight and correlated with the other systemic indicators. An important causative factor, especially in underdeveloped economies, is systemic helminthiasis. Conjunctival pallor can be masked by conjunctival inflammation, notably trachoma.

Leukemias

Involvement of the conjunctiva is not a common feature of leukemia. It occurs in approximately 4% of all patients with this disease. However, it may be the initial sign of the disease or of a relapse. Herein lies the importance of early recognition. The affected individuals present initially with congestion of the bulbar (particularly the perilimbal area) or the palpebral conjunctiva. In some instances, the conjunctiva may be erythematous and chemotic. The lesions are firm and non-tender and often associated with subconjunctival hemorrhage.

Histopathologically, the cells infiltrate all layers of the substantia propria. The infiltration may be diffuse or patchy and typically localize around the blood vessels. The conjunctival lesions usually respond rapidly to systemic chemotherapy.

Measles keratoconjunctivitis

Measles typically produces a bilateral keratoconjunctivitis. The characteristic Koplik's spots may be seen in the conjunctiva. The plica semilunaris may be swollen. Epithelial keratitis may supervene early in children and late in adults. The signs usually resolve without sequelae in the immunocompetent and well-nourished. Treatment is symptomatic and topical anti-inflammatory therapy may provide relief. In children with protein/energy malnutrition, this disease can be particularly devastating. Vitamin A deficiency is also present and may present with rapid keratomalacia. Secondary bacterial infection is common in immunodeficient individuals.

Alkaptonuria

This is a rare autosomal recessive disorder in which an affected individual's urine turns a dark brown-blackish color when exposed to air. It is linked to chromosome 3q21-q24, caused by a deficiency of homogentisic 1,2-dioxygenase.[5] This deficiency results in accumulation of homogentisic acid, which gets deposited in various tissues and organs. Systemic features include pigmentation over the face and nails, calcific and atherosclerotic heart disease, and arthritis. Ocular manifestations include a brown to black pigmentation of the nasal and temporal sclera especially in the area of the horizontal rectus muscle insertions. Pigmentation of the cornea has been reported.

Ataxia telangiectasia (Louis-Bar syndrome)

The condition is a rare autosomal recessive disorder characterized by early onset cerebellar ataxia, oculocutaneous telangiectasia, ocular motor apraxia (saccadic initiation failure), dysarthria, and immunodeficiency. Of these, ataxia is the first sign and is progressive. Chromosomal fragility and increasing susceptibility to ionizing radiation result in a predilection to malignant disorders such as lymphomas and leukemias. Affected individuals tend to have high levels of alpha-fetoprotein in their blood.

The most characteristic ocular involvement is the appearance of a conjunctival telangiectasia that appears around the

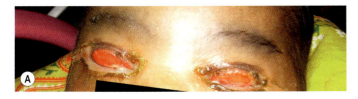

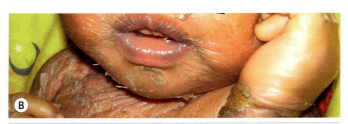

Fig. 31.4 Icthyosis. (A) There is keratinization of the upper palpebral conjunctiva secondary to ectropion of the upper lids. (B) The classical "stretched out" skin lesions are seen predominantly around the mouth and neck.

first decade of life. This lesion is usually seen in the interpalpebral bulbar conjunctiva, but may extend to the fornices. It is caused by ultraviolet damage and can be prevented or minimized by early and consistent use of 100% UV filter lenses. Other associated disorders include hypometric saccades, horizontal ocular motor apraxia, deficient accommodative ability, strabismus, and nystagmus.[6]

Fabry's disease

This X-linked disease is a disorder of lysosomal storage caused by a deficiency of alpha-galactosidase A which degrades glycosphingolipid components of the plasma membranes. This deficiency results in accumulation of glycosphingolipids, especially globotriaosylceramide.[7] Conjunctival vascular tortuosity, telangiectasia and cornea verticellata are common manifestations (see Chapter 62).

Osler-Weber-Rendu syndrome

This is a rare autosomal dominant disorder of blood vessels that can cause excessive bleeding. It is characterized by vascular dilatations in a variety of organ systems. Systemic features include epistaxis, dyspnea on exertion, gastrointestinal bleeding, hemoptysis, and hematuria. The classical ocular abnormality detected is conjunctival telangiectasia.[8] It may present with bloody tears or frank external hemorrhage. Retinal telangiectasia and arteriovenous malformations have been reported. These vessels are stable and can be distinguished from neovascular bundles by the absence of leakage on fundus fluorescein angiography.

Sickle cell disease

The conjunctival signs in this condition are fairly specific. Comma-shaped capillary and venular microaneurysms, which disappear under the heat of the examining lamp, are noted in the inferotemporal quadrant of an otherwise pale conjunctiva. These aneurysms reappear after application of a mild vasoconstrictor. These vascular anomalies are exaggerated during sickling crises.

Conjunctival tumors

Hamartomas

Hamartomas are congenital overgrowths of a normal tissue at their naturally occurring site. Hemangiomas are the most common hamartomatous lesion. They are of two types: capillary and cavernous. The capillary type is more common and can be either an isolated conjunctival lesion or part of a lesion involving the orbit and lids as well. These lesions are detected shortly after birth as elevated, soft nodules (Fig. 31.5) and usually grow and become prominent in the first year of life after which a process of involution occurs.[9] No active intervention is necessary in the vast majority of these cases.

Rarely, the lids, periorbital tissue, conjunctiva, and deeper orbital tissues may also be involved. Extensive angiomatous lesions may preclude visualization of the cornea. Lid involvement causes ptosis. A deeper orbital involvement may cause proptosis which increases with the Valsalva maneuver. Astigmatism can be present if the tumors press on the globe.

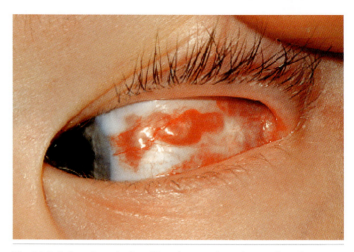

Fig. 31.5 Subconjunctival capillary hemangioma in an otherwise normal child. Although it had regressed spontaneously from being quite large at birth, it was prone to repeated subconjunctival hemorrhages. On this occasion the hemorrhage is contained within the subconjunctival tissue but can be seen to be spreading anteriorly.

Amblyopia may develop because of anisometropia or, rarely, stimulus deprivation. Optic nerve compression, strabismus, and exposure keratitis may be associated with some cases.

Intralesional or systemic steroids or propranolol (see Chapter 20) are used when necessary (almost always) for an orbital component; the response rate is 30–60%. Systemic interferon alpha-2a, previously reserved for life-threatening hemangiomas,[9] is no longer used due to its side effects.

Cavernous hemangioma is a much rarer and larger lesion than the capillary type. It has a higher propensity to involve deeper structures. This tumor does not regress spontaneously and the management is by surgical excision.

Choristomas

Choristomas are congenital tumors comprising a proliferation of normal cells in an abnormal location. Dermoids and lipodermoids are the most common choristomas that present in the conjunctiva. Dermoids are firm lesions with a predilection for the limbus. The surface can either be smooth, dome-shaped, or keratinized with hair formation (Fig. 31.6). A dermoid contains all the tissues of the skin including the dermal adnexal structes such as sebaceous glands and hair. They can present either as an isolated lesion or as a part of Goldenhar's syndrome (oculoauriculovertebral dysplasia), in which the structures that are derived from the first branchial arch are also affected.

Dermoids have a tendency to grow during puberty. They are usually asymptomatic, but large dermoids can cause irritation, cosmetic disfigurement, or significant astigmatism. In these situations, surgical excision can be considered. As these tumors have a tendency to invade deeper structures, donor corneal or scleral tissue should be available at the time of surgery.[10]

Lipodermoids are softer, yellow-colored lesions often occurring at the lateral canthal region. In most instances, the posterior extension cannot be demarcated clearly. Dermal adnexal structures are not seen histopathologically. They seldom require any treatment. Surgery, if required, should be performed with extreme caution to avoid damage to other structures, especially the lacrimal gland, and because extensive excision predisposes to symblepharon.

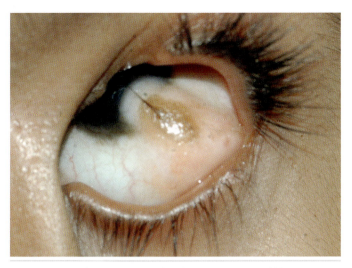

Fig. 31.6 Dermoid. A temporal limbal dermoid in a 5-year-old boy causing significant astigmatism. Hair growth is seen on the surface.

Epithelial tumors

Squamous papillomas present as fleshy and often multiple pedunculated tumors in children. They have a vascular stalk surrounded by acanthotic epithelium and are seen in the caruncle, fornix, and eyelid margin. They are caused by the human papilloma virus type 6. Viral shedding can cause large, confluent areas of ocular surface involvement. The surface of a papilloma flows out like branches of a tree with small vascular fronds on the surface. Topical mitomycin (0.02%) is useful in reducing the size of the tumor. It is applied twice a day for 15 days. Depending on the response, a second or third cycle can be repeated, with a drug-free interval of 15 days. Topical interferon therapy also seems to have some benefit. If the lesion does not respond to these medications, excision followed by cryotherapy can be performed.

Keratoacanthomas are tumors characterized by pseudoepitheliomatous hyperplasia with a central keratin plug. This tumor presents as a painless, firm, grayish-white keratotic nodule which grows rapidly over a period of 3–4 weeks. This benign tumor is often confused with squamous cell carcinoma. Treatment is by complete surgical excision with application of cryotherapy to the base.

Lymphangiectasia

This condition is characterized by dilated lymphatic channels and may be diffuse or localized. The lesion usually occurs in the interpalpebral space and may accumulate blood episodically because of communication with a vein. This can cause surrounding conjunctival edema and a subconjunctival hemorrhage. Small lesions can be observed, but larger lesions require excision.

Lymphangiomas

These tumors are rare and are hamartomatous proliferations lined by endothelium. There is no known hereditary or systemic association. Clinically, in the conjunctiva, they present as clear vessels with variably sized clear fluid-filled cysts either alone or interspersed amongst blood-filled hemangioma vessels. They may increase in size on Valsalva maneuver. Hemorrhage into an orbital lymphangioma can produce rapidly increasing proptosis and present as an ophthalmic emergency (see Chapter 20): the presence of subconjunctival and buccal lymphangioma tissue may be a useful clinical sign of the underlying cause.

Rhabdomyosarcoma

This is the most common malignant orbital tumor in children (see Chapter 24). Conjunctiva is the source of the primary tumor in around 12% of patients with orbital rhabdomyosarcoma.[11] The superior and superonasal areas are commonly involved. They present as light brown colored elevated lesions and may be confused for focal areas of inflammation, papillomas, capillary hemangiomas, or conjunctival cysts. Lack of response to medical management and rapid progression is a characteristic feature which should alert the clinician. Histopathologically, it comprises loosely coherent spindle cells in a myxoid stroma. MRI is needed to reveal orbital extension. Treatment is by radiotherapy and adjuvant chemotherapy.

Neurofibromas and neurilemmomas

These tumors arise from the Schwann cells which lie within the nerve. While neurilemmomas are discrete masses, neurofibromas may present as irregular tortuous lesions that may be local or diffuse. Localized symptomatic neurofibromas can be excised and the diffuse tumors can be managed by periodic partial excision.

Juvenile xanthogranuloma

Juvenile xanthogranuloma is an idiopathic cutaneous eruption of childhood in which conjunctival involvement is very rare (see Chapter 27). Most reported conjunctival cases have been in adults without skin lesions. They present as solitary, elevated conjunctival lesions near the corneoscleral limbus. They are usually round or yellow/flesh-colored masses. Histopathological examination reveals lipid histiocytes, chronic inflammatory cells and the characteristic Touton giant cell. Most conjunctival lesions have been excised in order to establish the diagnosis. However, they may spontaneously involute or respond to topical steroids

Pigmented lesions of the conjunctiva

Pigmentation of the conjunctiva is a common occurrence. The lesions are mostly benign in nature, but rarely can assume a malignant potential. A documented progression of these lesions is a clear indication for surgical removal.

Conjunctival nevus

This is one of the commonest pigmented lesions of the eye. Small, circumscribed lesions have little malignant potential and need not be surgically excised (Fig. 31.7A). However, nevi that show progression, or show features suggestive of feeder vessel vascularization, should be excised (Fig. 31.7B). Nevi can be either junctional, compound, or subepithelial in type. In junctional nevi, the melanocytes are restricted to the basilar epithelium. Compound nevi extend into the substantia propria, but maintain an intraepithelial component. They may develop cystic areas because of entrapment of goblet cells. The

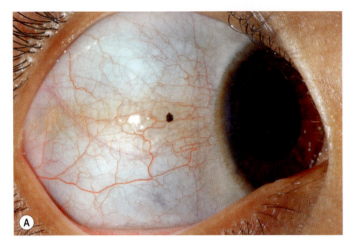

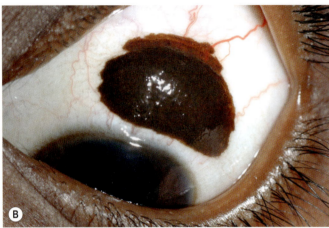

Fig. 31.7 Conjunctival nevus. (A) Small circumscribed pigmentation of the conjunctiva which does not require active surgical intervention. (B) An aggressive looking nevus with suspicious feeder vessels in the superior aspect. This lesion warrants surgical excision and regular follow-up.

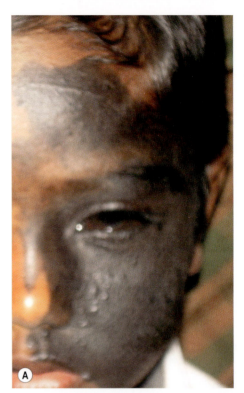

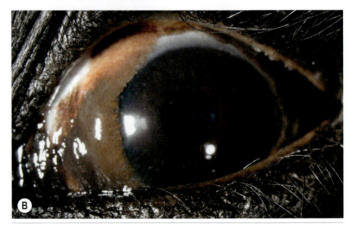

Fig. 31.8 Giant melanocytic nevus. (A) Affecting the left half of the face along with pigmentation of the left eye. (B) A close-up view of the left eye showing dense pigmentation of the conjunctiva more on the nasal half. The surrounding skin of the eyelids also shows dark pigmentary changes.

subepithelial type eventually loses its connection with the basilar epithelium and is confined within the substantia propria.

Melanocytic nevus

This is a rare form of congenital nevus that involves the eyelid skin, conjunctiva, and the face (Fig. 31.8). The surface is jet black, hairy, and often nodular. It carries a high risk of malignant transformation, which is estimated to be as high as 45%. Radical excision and reconstructive surgery is the usual treatment

Nevus of Ota

In this condition, conjunctival or scleral pigmentation (slate-gray or bluish in color) is associated with pigmentation of the periocular tissue as well as the face. The nevi are present at birth. Patients with this condition are at increased risk for developing a uveal melanoma or glaucoma.[12]

Malignant melanoma

This condition is rare in children. Conditions such as dysplastic nevus syndrome, xeroderma pigmentosa, and neurofibromatosis put children at increased risk of developing a malignant melanoma. It is characterized by a rapid growth of pigmented lesions of the conjunctiva, and feeder vessels may be seen.

Involvement of Tenon's capsule and the sclera may restrict the mobility of the tumor over the ocular surface. In suspected cases it is important to check the preauricular and submandibular node for enlargement.

Miscellaneous disorders of conjunctiva

Pyogenic granuloma

An aberrant healing response following trauma or surgery for strabismus can result in an exaggerated fibrovascular response, erroneously referred to as pyogenic granuloma. However, this condition is neither an infection nor a typical granulomatous reaction, but a granulation tissue formation. Rapid growth may simulate a malignancy. A history of preceding trauma or

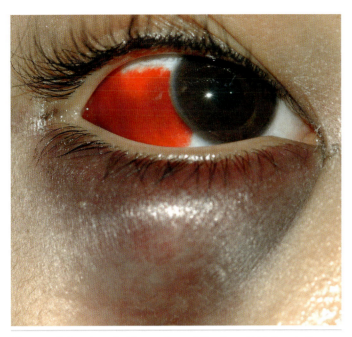

Fig. 31.9 Subconjunctival hemorrhage following a fist injury to the eye. An associated ecchymosis of the lower lid is also seen.

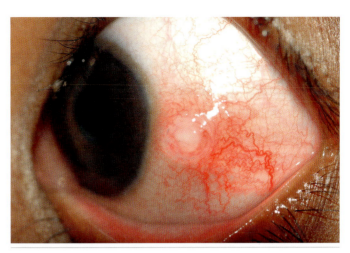

Fig. 31.10 An elevated nodular lesion seen in a 7-year-old girl on anti-tuberculous treatment.

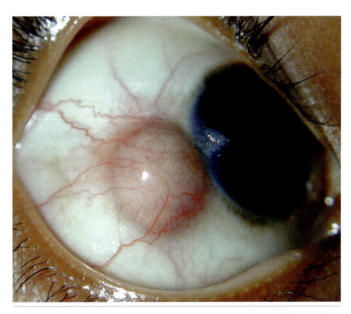

Fig. 31.11 River water granuloma. Well-circumscribed smooth elevated nodular lesion seen in the bulbar conjunctiva. (Courtesy of Dr. Rathinam, DNB.)

surgery helps in making the diagnosis. The condition may resolve spontaneously, but usually some form of treatment is required. A short course of topical steroids may be given, but excision biopsy is the treatment of choice.

Subconjunctival hemorrhage

A subconjunctival hemorrhage often occurs after a seemingly trivial blunt trauma (Fig. 31.9). It can also be seen in conditions which cause a rise in central venous pressure such as a seizure, violent coughing, or sudden straining. It may present in a dramatic manner and may cause considerable consternation. It usually resolves spontaneously within 2 weeks and does not require any treatment. Subconjunctival hemorrhages are also seen in conditions such as leukemia and as a sequelae to some forms of conjunctivitis. In cases of suspected head injury, the presence of a subconjunctival hemorrhage with a poorly defined posterior margin is a matter of grave concern and has to be investigated radiologically.

Conjunctival granulomas

The presence of a variety of lymphoid cells in the substantia propria serves as a perfect setting for the development of inflammatory granulomas following some systemic and local disorders. The common systemic diseases that can cause conjunctival granulomas include sarcoidois, tuberculosis, Parinaud's oculoglandular syndrome, Wegener's granulomatosis, trematode-induced granulomas, and rhinosporidiosis.

Sarcoid nodules manifest as small light brown colored nodules in the conjunctiva[13] and show aggregates of epithelioid histiocytes on histopathological evaluation.

Tuberculosis of the conjunctiva may cause granulomas, tarsal necrosis, conjunctival masses, and small miliary palpebral conjunctival ulcers. Phlyctenular conjunctival response can also be seen in some cases (Fig. 31.10). Coexisting anterior segment involvement may be present.

Trematodes are known to cause conjunctival granulomas.[14] They are acquired by children while swimming in fresh water ponds infested by these trematodes. The granuloma is usually seen as a smooth, enlarged nodular lesion in the bulbar conjunctiva (Fig. 31.11). Coexistent anterior chamber granuloma and corneal inflammation may be seen in some cases. A specific inflammatory reaction known as Splendore-Hoeppli phenomenon has been described with helminthic infections, though the helminths themselves have rarely been isolated. The reaction comprises a central deposit of granular, acellular eosinophilic material surrounded by eosinophils, epithelioid cells, histiocytes, and lymphocytes. Small granulomas may be treated with topical corticosteroids. Large lesions and those that fail conservative management should undergo an excisional biopsy.

Rhinosporidiosis may present as pedunculated granulomas, often seen in the palpebral conjunctiva[15] (Fig. 31.12). The surface is granular and on careful examination reveals pearly

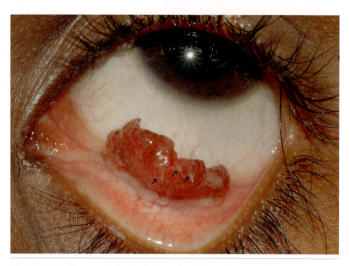

Fig. 31.12 Rhinosporidiosis. Pedunculated irregular granuloma seen in the inferior palpebral conjunctiva. Note the white spherules over the surface of the granuloma. (Courtesy of Dr. Usha Kim, DNB.)

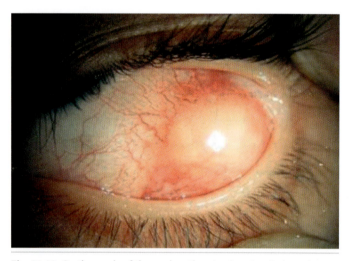

Fig. 31.13 Cysticercosis of the conjunctiva. A subconjunctival translucent cyst in the bulbar conjunctiva caused by cysticercosis.

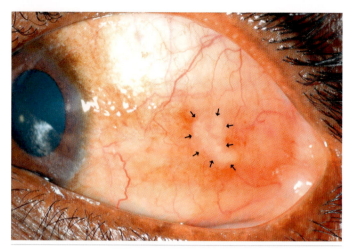

Fig. 31.14 Subconjunctival worm. The contour of this worm, identified later as *Filaria*, is clearly seen.

white studded spores, which have a tendency to bleed on touch. Treatment is by complete excision followed by cryotherapy. This lesion has an extraordinary tendency to bleed during surgery.

Ophthalmia nodosa is a granulomatous nodular conjunctivitis caused by irritation of the eye due to retained capillary hairs of caterpillars, spiders, or bees. Children presenting with this condition often give a history of a fall. Small nodules may be seen in the conjunctiva along with patterned corneal abrasions. These corneal abrasions are due to the hairs embedded in the upper tarsus and their sharp ends rubbing the cornea.

Parasitic infestation of the conjunctiva

This condition is common in endemic areas and usually presents in the cyst form. The common parasitic cysts are cysticercus and hydatid. They may present with inflammation. These parasitic cysts have to be removed in toto along with cryotherapy of the base. Cysticercosis is caused by the larval form of *Taenia solium* known as cysticercosis cellulosae. The cysts are usually subconjunctival in location with a thin

translucent wall (Fig. 31.13). Adjacent orbital structures and muscles may be involved. A chalky white area representing the scolex may be seen which clinches the diagnosis.[16] Spontaneous expulsion of these cysts has been reported. A complete ophthalmic and systemic evaluation is needed to look for other involved areas. Treatment is by mechanical removal with supplementation of systemic antihelminthic treatment. Exuberant inflammatory responses may need a course of systemic steroid therapy.

Ophthalmomyiasis

This term refers to the infestation of the eye by the larval forms of the order Diptera. Implicated species include *Oestrus ovis* (transmitted from sheep and goats by gravid adult flies), *Dermatolabia hominis* (transmitted from cattle and fowl by mosquitoes), *Cuterebra*, *Hipoderma bovi*, *Chrysomyia*, and *Cordylobia*.[17] Conjunctival involvement causes irritation, foreign body sensation, redness, and chemosis. There may be pseudomembrane formation with petechial hemorrhages. Patients may experience perception of movements and slit-lamp examination shows the larvae. The aim of the treatment is to extract the worm mechanically. The worm may be caught with a forceps or pulled out with a suture passed through the larva.

Occasionally, adult worms can be seen presenting in the subconjunctival space with the patient complaining of irritation and foreign body sensation. A slit-lamp evaluation will reveal the contours of the worm (Fig. 31.14). The treatment is by mechanical removal of the worm using a forceps (Video 31.1). In some instances, the worm is entrapped beneath the conjunctiva in close proximity to the extraocular muscles. In these situations, care should be taken to isolate the muscle and extract the worm without injuring the muscle (Video 31.2).

Conjunctival trauma and foreign bodies

The conjunctiva is a common site for foreign bodies, most commonly upper tarsal. An examination after lid eversion is mandatory for any history of trauma and suspicion of foreign body. Various foreign bodies that have been described include insect wings, beetles, cilia, caterpillar hair, seed husk, pieces of wood, twigs (Fig. 31.15), and natural and synthetic fibers. Any foreign body lodged in the conjunctiva evokes an acute

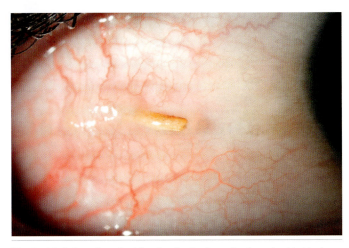

Fig. 31.15 Subconjunctival foreign body. A small twig embedded in the conjunctiva and required mechanical removal.

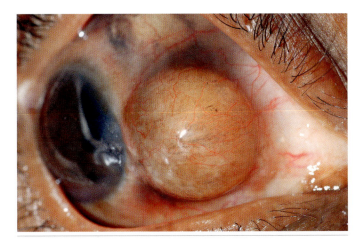

Fig. 31.16 Phacocele. A traumatically anteriorly dislocated lens mimicking a subconjunctival cyst.

inflammatory reaction with a copious outpouring of tears. However, if the foreign body has a large surface area, it may become embedded resulting in a chronic inflammatory response. This causes a granuloma containing epithelioid and foreign body giant cells. The symptoms rapidly abate after the removal of the foreign body. Very rarely, blunt injuries in the eye, especially in older children and young adults, can cause the lens to dislocate anteriorly into the subconjunctival space and may present as a cystic lesion beneath the conjunctiva. This condition, which may mimic a subconjunctival cyst, is referred to as a phacocele (Fig. 31.16), which may also be a presenting sign of Ehlers-Danlos syndrome type 6.

Symblepharon

In this condition, there is an adhesion between the bulbar and palpebral conjunctiva. It commonly occurs in association with congenital lid coloboma. Other causes include a chronic dry eye, chemical burns, and Stevens-Johnson syndrome where the goblet cells are destroyed. Localized symblepharon, without compromise to the visual apparatus, need not be treated. Surgical release and forniceal reconstruction using amniotic membrane or mucous membrane grafts is indicated in severe cases.

References

1. Reynolds JD, Olitsky SE. Pediatric glaucoma. In: Wright KW, Spiegel PH, editors. Pediatric Ophthalmology and Strabismus. New York: Springer; 2002: 483–98.
2. WHO. Vitamin A deficiency and its consequences (accessed Jun 9 2011). Available from: http://www.who.int/nutrition/publications/micronutrients/vitamin_a_deficieny/9241544783/en/index.html.
3. Sullivan TJ, Clarke MP, Morin JD. The ocular manifestations of the Sturge-Weber syndrome. J Pediatr Ophthalmol Strabismus 1992; 29: 349–56.
4. Cruz AA, Menezes FA, Chaves R, et al. Eyelid abnormalities in lamellar ichthyoses. Ophthalmology 2000; 107: 1895–8.
5. Sharma V, Chong YY, Kosmin A. Alkaptonuria presenting with conjunctival lesion. Compr Ther 2007; 33: 71–2.
6. Farr AK, Shalev B, Crawford TO, et al. Ocular manifestations of ataxia-telangiectasia. Am J Ophthalmol 2002; 134: 891–6.
7. Mastropasqua L, Nubile M, Lanzini M, et al. Corneal and conjunctival manifestations in Fabry disease: in vivo confocal microscopy study. Am J Ophthalmol 2006; 141: 709–18.
8. Brant AM, Schachat AP, White RI. Ocular manifestations in hereditary hemorrhagic telangiectasia (Rendu-Osler-Weber disease). Am J Ophthalmol 1989; 107: 642–6.
9. Haik BG, Karcioglu ZA, Gordon RA, Pechous BP. Capillary hemangioma (infantile periocular hemangioma). Surv Ophthalmol 1994; 38: 399–426.
10. Shen YD, Chen WL, Wang IJ, et al. Full-thickness central corneal grafts in lamellar keratoscleroplasty to treat limbal dermoids. Ophthalmology 2005; 112: 1955.
11. Shields CL, Shields JA, Honavar SG, Demirci H. Primary ophthalmic rhabdomyosarcoma in 33 patients. Trans Am Ophthalmol Soc 2001; 99: 133–42; discussion 142–3.
12. Sinha S, Cohen PJ, Schwartz RA. Nevus of Ota in children. Cutis 2008; 82: 25–9.
13. Obenauf CD, Shaw HE, Sydnor CF, Klintworth GK. Sarcoidosis and its ophthalmic manifestations. Am J Ophthalmol 1978; 86: 648–55.
14. Rathinam S, Fritsche TR, Srinivasan M, et al. An outbreak of trematode-induced granulomas of the conjunctiva. Ophthalmology 2001; 108: 1223–9
15. Reidy JJ, Sudesh S, Klafter AB, Olivia C. Infection of the conjunctiva by *Rhinosporidium seeberi*. Surv Ophthalmol 1997; 41: 409–13.
16. Nath K, Gogi R, Zaidi N, Johri A. Cystic lesions of conjunctiva (a clinicopathological study). Indian J Ophthalmol 1983; 31: 1–4.
17. Khurana S, Biswal M, Bhatti HS, et al. Ophthalmomyiasis: three cases from North India. Indian J Med Microbiol 2010; 28: 257–61.

Anterior segment: developmental anomalies

Ken K Nischal • Jane C Sowden

The anterior segment of the eye is an intricate arrangement of interacting tissues essential for vision. The cornea, iris, and the anterior epithelium of the lens form the boundaries of the anterior chamber. Schwalbe's line, the trabecular meshwork, and the scleral spur lie in the anterior chamber angle at the junction of the peripheral cornea and the root of the iris. Aqueous produced by the ciliary body flows into the anterior chamber through the pupil and leaves the eye through the trabecular meshwork into Schlemm's canal and the venous circulation.[1]

Embryology of the anterior segment

Neural crest cells are critical for the development of the anterior segment. They originate at the edge of the neural fold. During neurulation, as the neural tube closes, the neural crest cells undergo an epithelial to mesenchymal transition and migrate away ventrally on either side of the neural tube. The different migratory pathways of the neural crest cells give rise to a wide variety of cell types including a contribution to the developing eye.

In addition to the large contribution from neural crest-derived mesenchymal cells (Table 32.1) to tissues of the anterior segment, the neurectoderm of the optic cup and the surface ectoderm also give rise to anterior segment components. The peripheral edge of the optic cup forms the posterior iris epithelium and the ciliary body epithelium. The surface ectoderm gives rise to the corneal epithelium after the separation of the lens vesicle. Please see Fig. 32.1 for a brief reminder of embryologic development of the eye.

Control of development: responsible genes

Gene mutations causing anterior segment developmental anomalies

Several disease causing genes have been identified (Table 32.2) and animal models have illuminated the essential role of these

Table 32.1 – Origin of tissue of the anterior segment and sites of expression of important genes[4-6]

Embryonic tissue contributing to the anterior segment	Gene expression in early embryonic tissue	Anterior segment tissues (other ocular tissues)	Gene expression in developing angle tissues
Neural crest-derived periocular mesenchymal tissue	Pitx2 Foxc1 Lmx1b	Corneal endothelium Corneal stroma Anterior iris stroma Angle structures: Trabecular meshwork Ciliary muscle (Extraocular muscles) (Sclera) (Choroid)	Foxc1, Pitx2 Foxc1, Pitx2 Foxc1, Pax6 (Pitx2) (Foxc1)
Neurectoderm of the optic cup	Pax6	Pigmented iris epithelium Ciliary epithelium (Retina)	Pax6 Pax6 (Pax6)
Surface ectoderm	Pax6	Lens Corneal epithelium	Pax6, Foxe3, Maf Pax6, Pitx2

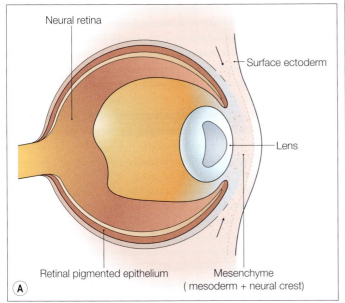

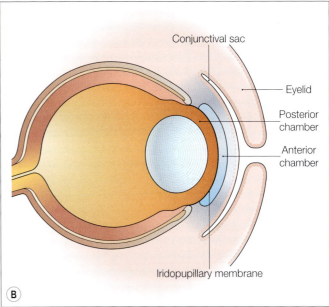

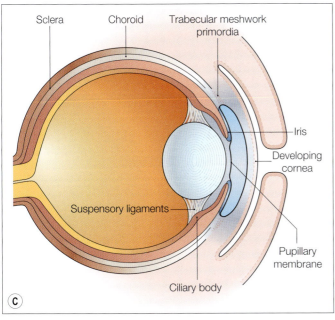

Fig. 32.1 Early development of the anterior segment. (A) By five weeks of development in the human embryo, the lens vesicle has separated from the surface ectoderm and neural crest cells are migrating around the optic cup and between the surface ectoderm and the developing lens. (B) During the seventh week, the mesenchymal layer gives rise to the corneal stroma, bounded by an endothelium, and the anterior iris stroma. This process of differentiation occurs simultaneously with a separation of the two layers to form the anterior chamber between the developing cornea and the iris. (C) A sheet of mesenchyme bridging the future pupil remains until the seventh month of gestation. The edges of the optic cup form the posterior iris epithelium and the ciliary body epithelium.[2,3]

genes in the normal molecular and cellular processes underlying the development of the anterior segment.

Transcription factors and anterior segment development

The majority of genes proven to play critical roles in anterior segment developmental anomalies (ASDAs) all encode transcription factors (Table 32.2), which act by regulating the transcription of other genes, which are their downstream target genes. They coordinate programs of growth and differentiation by either enhancing or repressing the expression of their target genes. Each transcription factor has a different type of DNA-binding domain for the purpose of interacting with the regulatory DNA sequence of its target genes. These DNA-binding domains are highly conserved throughout the animal kingdom, and this is partly why animal models have proved to be so

useful for understanding the function of human genes. *PAX6* and *PITX2* encode proteins containing a paired-type and bicoid-type homeodomain, respectively, whereas FOXC1 encodes a fork-head domain containing protein. These genes are closely related to genes called paired, bicoid, and forkhead, first shown to be essential for development and patterning the body of *Drosophila melanogaster*, an invaluable model system for the discovery of many genes important for human development and disease.

Gene expression in the developing anterior segment: sites of gene action

The sites of gene expression during development of the anterior segment pinpoint their site of action (Fig. 32.1 and Table 32.1). Knowledge of sites of gene expression derives mainly from study of the mouse as a model for mammalian

Table 32.2 – Genes essential for the normal development of the anterior segment and whose mutation causes ASDAs

Human gene	Type	Chromosome location	Human disease	OMIM number
CYP1B1	Enzyme	2p22	Congenital glaucoma	601771
EYA1	Transcription factor	8q13	Branchiootorenal dysplasia ASDA	601653
FOXC1	Transcription factor	6p25	ASDA (iridogoniodysgenesis anomaly, iris hypoplasia, Axenfeld-Rieger anomaly, Axenfeld-Rieger syndrome) Congenital glaucoma	601090
FOXE3	Transcription factor	1p23	ASDA and cataracts Peters' anomaly	601094
LMX1B	Transcription factor	9q34	Nail-patella syndrome	602575
MAF	Transcription factor	16q23	ASDA and cataracts	177075
PAX6	Transcription factor	11p13	Aniridia Peters' anomaly Cataracts ASDA Keratitis Optic nerve hypoplasia and glaucoma Foveal hypoplasia	106210
PITX2	Transcription factor	4q25	ASDA (Axenfeld-Rieger syndrome, iris hypoplasia, iridogoniodysgenesis) Glaucoma	601542
PITX3	Transcription factor	10q25	ASDA and cataracts	602669
LTBP2	Latent TGFβ-binding protein 2	14q24.3	Megalocornea, microspherophakia, congenital glaucoma	602091
COL4A1	Collagen	TYPE IV, ALPHA-1	13q34 Axenfeld-Rieger	120130
B3GALTL	UDP-GAL:BETA-GlcNAc BETA-1,3-GALACTOSYLTRANSFERASE-LIKE	13q12.3	Peters-plus syndrome	610308
KERA	Keratan sulfate proteoglycan	12q21.33	Corneal plana	603228
PXDN	Extracellular matrix-associated protein, peroxidasin	2q25.3	ASDA cataracts microcornea	605158
SLC4A11	SODIUM BORATE COTRANSPORTER	20p13-p12	Corneal dystrophy, Fuchs endothelial, 4,	610206
JAG1	Ligand of the Notch Receptor	20p12	Alagille syndrome with posterior embryotoxon, iris hypoplasia, small corneal diameter, iridocorneal synechiae, and corectopia	601920
LAMB2	Extracellular matrix protein, laminin	3p21	Pierson syndrome with microcoria or ASDA	15032
BMP4	Regulatory molecule	14q22-q23	ASDA with or without anophthalmia/ microphthalmia	112262

development combined with limited expression data from human studies and other animal model or experimental systems. This information helps understand the origin of the abnormalities observed in patients with gene mutations.

The patterns of expression of genes whose mutation causes ASDAs can be considered as three types:

1. Those expressed within migrating periocular neural crest cells (*Foxc1*, *Pitx2*, *Lmx1b*)
2. Those expressed only within the developing lens (*Foxe3*, *Maf*)
3. Those with a more panocular expression including the lens, of which *Pax6* is the only example.

Pax6 is expressed from the earliest stages of eye development and has earned the title of an eye master control gene. *Pax6* expression continues throughout eye development in cells deriving from the neurectoderm of the optic cup and from the anterior surface ectoderm. *Pax6* is expressed in the developing lens, inner and pigmented layers of the iris and ciliary body, the corneal epithelium, and the developing retina. Significantly it is also expressed later in the mesenchymally derived developing trabecular meshwork.

In contrast to the widespread expression of *Pax6*, *Foxc1* and *Pitx2* have a more restricted expression within the developing eye. Both genes are expressed within the mesenchyme around the developing optic cup (the periocular mesenchyme) including the prospective cornea. Their expression is down-regulated as the mesenchyme differentiates, with expression persisting in structures of the developing angle. *Foxc1* and *Pitx2* are both expressed in the forming iris, but not within the neurectoderm of the optic cup or in the lens vesicle.

Understanding gene function through study of animal models

Each human gene whose mutation causes ASDA has a highly related and equivalent gene (an orthologous gene) in the mouse genome. Mice lacking functional copies of these genes show anterior segment abnormalities similar to clinical conditions. The phenotypes of mice heterozygous for a mutation and carrying only one functional gene copy provide models of dominantly inherited clinical conditions. Information from homozygous mouse mutations, although rare in patients, is useful for defining the essential role of key genes. Differences in the genetic regulation of human and mouse eye development exist but the mouse is the best available model and is proving particularly valuable for understanding ASDAs and glaucoma.

Foxc1 and *Pitx2* are essential for corneal development

Developmental arrest and abnormal retention and contraction of the embryonic endothelial layer on portions of the iris and anterior chamber angle have been proposed as the cause of the iris changes, tissue strands, and the abnormalities of Schwalbe's line found in ASDAs.[9]

Heterozygous mutation of the *Foxc1* gene in mice causes ocular abnormalities with marked variable expressivity, which are very similar to patient conditions and the widely variable ocular defects sometimes seen within families sharing the same mutation.[10,11] Ocular defects in the heterozygotes are progressive with a gradual worsening of the corectopia and with the peripheral iridocorneal adhesions becoming more evident over time. Some juvenile mice showed mild corneal opacity progressing to a high incidence of corneal opacification, with neovascularization and cataracts, in older animals.

Studies with mice have also demonstrated that the genetic background influences the penetrance of ocular defects in heterozygotes and is likely to cause some of the variation seen between families carrying the same mutations. However, as a high level of variability is often seen in genetically identical mice, the variation must to a large extent stem from developmental events and may reflect stochastic events relating to levels of key molecules at critical moments of development.

The asymmetric phenotypes often observed between eyes in the same patient also likely reflect such stochastic events.

Mice that are homozygous for mutation of *Foxc1* (called the congenital hydrocephalus, ch, or Mf1 gene-targeted mouse) show a more severe dysgenesis of the anterior segment.[4,12] Histologic analysis shows that the cornea fails to separate from the lens, resulting in the complete absence of an anterior chamber. The outer corneal epithelium is thicker than normal and the stroma is disorganized. There is no differentiation of the inner corneal endothelial layer, and there is a failure to form tight occluding junctions between these posterior endothelial cells necessary for normal physiologic barrier function. Descemet's membrane, the basal lamina secreted by the corneal endothelium, is thus absent. Hypoplasia of the iris stromal mesenchyme and the pigmented layer accompanies the corneal abnormalities, and the eye is typically microphthalmic. The phenotype of these mice suggests that *Foxc1* is essential for conversion of mesenchymal neural crest cells to an endothelium phenotype.

The phenotype of the mice homozygous for *Foxc1* mutation is strikingly similar to that of mice carrying homozygous mutation of another gene implicated in human ASDAs, the *Pitx2* gene. Mice homozygous for mutation of *Pitx2* have displaced, irregular pupils, and this condition is also present in some heterozygotes. In homozygotes, the anterior chamber and the corneal endothelium are absent, and the corneal epithelium is thickened (hypercellular) with undifferentiated mesenchymal cells lying between this epithelium and the optic cup.[13] *Pitx2* appears essential for differentiation of both the mesenchymal and epithelial components of the cornea, tissues derived from the cranial neural crest-derived periocular mesenchyme and the surface ectoderm, respectively. *Pitx2* expression, but not Foxc1 expression, has been reported in the corneal ectoderm (derived from the surface ectoderm).[5] Lack of *Pitx2* in mice also causes failure of extraocular muscle development, reduced eye size (microphthalmia), and delay in optic fissure closure (optic nerve coloboma). These conditions have not been observed in patients with PITX2 mutation.

Mice that lack *Pitx2* also have abnormalities in multiple organs that are essential sites of *Pitx2* gene activity. These include roles for *Pitx2* in left–right asymmetry involved in cardiac positioning and lung asymmetry and pituitary, craniofacial, and tooth development. Only eye and tooth abnormalities are apparent in heterozygote animals,[14] and these are consistent with the dental abnormalities found in patients with PITX2 mutation. Knowledge of other organs critically affected by lack of *Pitx2* is useful for understanding other systemic features often identified in patients with anterior segment dysgenesis. Recently it has been shown that complex severe ASDA phenotypes may be due to digenic inheritance of PITX2 and FOXC1 in humans.[15]

Pax6 and other genes expressed in the developing lens cause ASDAs

It is now well established that mutation or deletion of the PAX6 gene and/or chromosomal rearrangements involving the PAX6 gene on 11p13 underlies most cases of aniridia.[6,16] PAX6 is also more widely implicated in anterior segment malformations. Mice with heterozygous mutations of the *Pax6* gene help in understanding the role of *Pax6* in ASDA as their phenotype resembles the patient conditions associated with

PAX6 mutation. Heterozygous Pax6 (small eye (Sey)) mice have a reduced eye size (microphthalmia) and a wide spectrum of anterior eye defects including iris hypoplasia, iridocorneal adhesions and corneal opacification, incomplete separation of the lens from the cornea (keratolenticular adhesion), vascularized cornea, and cataracts.[17,18]

Peters' anomaly (see later), characterized by keratolenticular and/or iridocorneal adhesion, is a genetically heterogeneous condition. A proportion of cases of Peters' anomaly have PAX6 mutations, and the phenotype of the Sey heterozygous mice resembles that of Peters' anomaly.[19] FOXE3 mutation has been associated with Peters' anomaly, and mice heterozygous for Foxe3 mutation also have central corneal opacity and keratolenticular adhesion similar to that in Peters' anomaly.[20]

The lens plays an essential role in the induction of anterior segment differentiation.[21,22] Analysis of heterozygous Pax6 eyes indicates that haploinsufficiency of Pax6 causes primary defects in the lens and that these underlie secondary complex defects of the anterior segment iris and cornea. Pax6 is highly expressed in anterior lens epithelium and may act indirectly on neural crest-derived mesenchymal cells of the developing anterior segment by regulating the production of lens-derived signaling molecules. Two other genes are implicated in causing ASDA by affecting the inductive properties of the lens. MAF and FOXE3 mutation both cause ASDA with cataracts. In the mouse the Maf and the Foxe3 genes are both primarily expressed in the developing lens and not within the neural crest-derived mesenchymal cells of the developing anterior segment. Recent work has shown that homozygous mutations in FOXE3 result in primary congenital aphakia.[23]

Considering the different roles of the genes implicated in ASDAs suggests a model in which Pax6, Maf, and Foxe3 are involved in the production of secreted signaling factors from the lens important for organizing the anterior segment development. Pitx2, Foxc1, and Lmx1b are essential for the differentiation of the neural crest-derived mesenchymal tissue, which happens in response to factors secreted by the lens. Without these mesenchymally expressed genes the separation between the cornea and the lens to form the anterior chamber, as well as differentiation of the angle drainage structures, does not take place or is incomplete, depending on the gene dosage.

Insights into the etiology of developmental glaucoma from mouse models of ASDA

The relationships between gene mutations, structural abnormalities of the angle, and the high incidence of glaucoma in ASDAs are not well understood. Histology of the anterior chamber angle from patients has shown failure of the intertrabecular spaces and Schlemm's canal to develop. Analysis of mouse models of the human conditions is now conclusively demonstrating that single-gene mutations cause abnormalities in the trabecular meshwork tissue, which obstruct aqueous flow.

In Foxc1 homozygous mice, histologic analysis of the iridocorneal angle identified abnormalities, including small or absent Schlemm's canal, hypoplastic or absent trabecular meshwork, and hypoplastic ciliary body with short and thin ciliary processes.[10] The development of the chamber angle has also been studied in Pax6 heterozygotes. Mesenchymal cells at the angle that normally express Pax6 and differentiate into trabecular meshwork cells next to Schlemm's canal remain undifferentiated, demonstrating that Pax6 is directly required for differentiation of the angle.[18]

In addition to the ASDAs, which have overt abnormalities in the anterior segment associated with glaucoma, new understanding is being gained of primary congenital glaucoma and the genetic pathways that underlie these related disease etiologies. Mice lacking Cyp1b1 have developmental focal abnormalities of the angle similar to those reported in patients with primary congenital glaucoma and CYP1B1 mutation. These defects were small or absent Schlemm's canal, basal lamina (resembling Descemet's membrane) extending from the cornea over the trabecular meshwork, and attachments of the iris to the trabecular meshwork and peripheral cornea (synechiae).

Clinical conditions due to anterior segment developmental anomalies

ASDAs may be considered in terms of their embryologic origin. Therefore they may be:

- Of neural crest cell origin
- Of ectodermal origin
- Of global origin.

Anterior segment developmental anomalies of neural crest cell origin

Posterior embryotoxon

This prominent, anteriorly displaced Schwalbe's line, seen in 8–15% of the normal population appears as a whitish, irregular ridge up to several millimeters from the limbus and is often incomplete. It may be inherited in an autosomal dominant fashion. In isolation, it is not associated with an increased risk of glaucoma.

Ocular associations may include iris adhesions with or without iris changes such as hypoplasia, pseudopolycoria, and/or corectopia, in which case it forms part of the spectrum of the Axenfeld-Rieger anomaly (Fig. 32.2).

The main systemic association is in a jaundiced neonate, in which case its presence may be suggestive of the autosomal dominant condition Alagille syndrome (arteriohepatic dysplasia)[24-26] which is characterized by intrahepatic cholestasis, peripheral pulmonary artery stenosis, peculiar facies, and butterfly vertebral arch defects. Posterior embryotoxon is seen in 90% of all cases and 77% of cases also have iris strands.[24,25]

Since isolated posterior embryotoxon is not associated with glaucoma there is no need for regular review unless other members of the family have features of Axenfeld-Rieger Anomaly/syndrome.

Axenfeld-Rieger syndrome (ARS) has ocular and non-ocular features. The ocular features consist of posterior embryotoxon with iris strands attached, some of which may be very broad and thick and others thread-like. Historically if these were the only findings the term Axenfeld anomaly was used. If in addition iris defects are present then historically this was termed Rieger anomaly. Axenfeld-Rieger anomaly encompasses both now. Iris findings range from stromal hypoplasia, pseudopolycoria, corectopia (pupil displaced toward a thick peripheral iris strand) (Fig. 32.3), and ectropion uveae. The anterior chamber angle is usually open though there may be a high insertion of the iris into the posterior portion of the

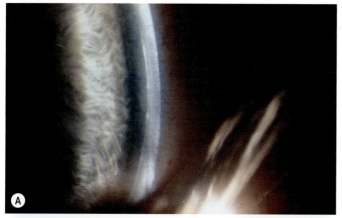

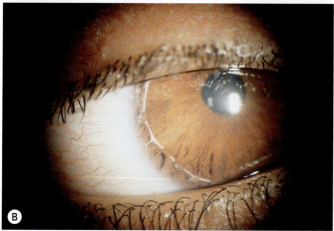

Fig. 32.2 Posterior embryotoxon. (A) Posterior embryotoxon with no associated ocular anomalies is a common but subtle anomaly seen on slit-lamp examination. (B) Marked posterior embryotoxon with iris strands attached (Axenfeld-Rieger anomaly).

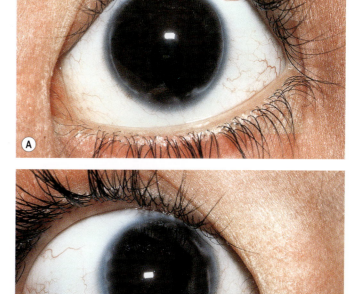

Fig. 32.3 Axenfeld-Rieger anomaly. There is iris hypoplasia, posterior embryotoxon, pseudopolycoria (A), and corectopia with the pupil drawn peripherally.

trabecular meshwork.[9,27,28,33] Occasionally the pupil corectopia is severe enough to warrant surgical pupilloplasty. The pupil may still progress over years to become even more eccentric in placement despite surgery.

Angle and iris changes are usually stable. Glaucoma develops in 50–60% of patients with ARS, usually manifesting itself in childhood or young adulthood. Incomplete development of the trabecular meshwork and Schlemm's canal is thought to occur again due to development arrest occurring during the third trimester, causing obstruction to aqueous outflow and hence glaucoma.[9,28]

Other less frequently occurring ocular features include strabismus, cataracts, limbal dermoids, retinal detachment, macular degeneration, chorioretinal colobomas, and choroidal and optic nerve head hypoplasia.

Familial glaucoma iridogoniodysplasia has been described in one pedigree and entails marked iris hypoplasia, iridocorneal angle anomalies, and, frequently, glaucoma.[29]

IGDA has been described as iridocorneal angle anomalies, iris stromal hypoplasia, and glaucoma in 50% of cases.[30]

IGDS is a rare condition in which iris hypoplasia and iridocorneal angle anomalies are associated with non-ocular features such as jaw and dental abnormalities.[31]

The characteristic non-ocular features of ARS are maxillary hypoplasia, mild prognathism, hypodontia (decreased but

evenly spaced teeth), anodontia/oligodontia (focal absence of teeth), microdontia (reduction in crown size), cone-shaped teeth (Fig. 32.4), and excess periumbilical skin (Fig. 32.5) with or without hernia. Hypertelorism, telecanthus, and a broad flat nose have also been described.[32] Other systemic features that have been reported include growth hormone deficiency and short stature, heart defects, middle ear deafness, mental deficiency, cerebellar anomalies (*FOXC1* mutations), oculocutaneous albinism, hypospadias, abnormal ears, and, in one pedigree, myotonic dystrophy and Peters' anomaly.[9,34]

Management depends on the presenting complication of the structural anomalies. Occasionally there is severe pupillary stenosis for which a large pupilloplasty is required which may be complicated by lens damage and/or late contraction. Severe corectopia without severe stenosis can be adequately treated with occlusion therapy of the less affected eye.

Medical therapy should be used for glaucoma prior to surgical intervention with the exception of infantile cases where goniotomy/trabeculotomy is first choice of treatment. Miotics should be used with caution, since they may cause trabecular meshwork collapse, with a reduction in aqueous outflow.

Trabeculectomy with antimetabolite augmentation appears to be the procedure of choice for most patients with glaucoma secondary to ARS, especially in older children (Fig. 32.6). The

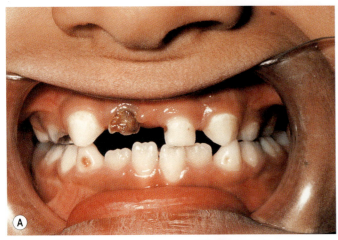

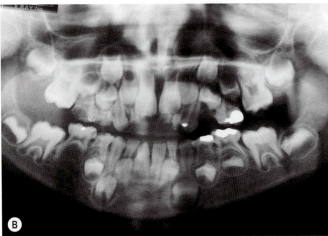

Fig. 32.4 Axenfeld-Rieger syndrome. (A) Widely spaced, some conical, teeth; partial anodontia and caries. (B) Dental X-ray of a patient with ARS.

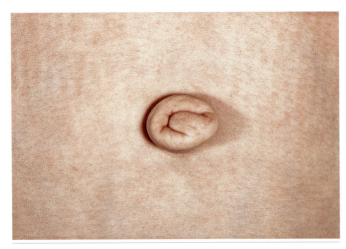

Fig. 32.5 Axenfeld-Rieger syndrome. Excess periumbilical skin in ARS.

use of cycloablation should be considered in cases where, because of cooperation of the child, a drainage procedure would be unsuitable. Draining procedures other than trabeculectomy include the use of drainage tubes with or without antimetabolite augmentation.[35-38]

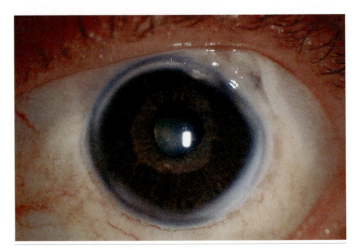

Fig. 32.6 Axenfeld-Rieger syndrome. Trabeculectomy bleb in a child with ARS. There is iris hypoplasia.

Congenital iris ectropion

This is a rare usually unilateral condition in which there is a congenital, non-progressive, non-tractional hyperplasia of the posterior pigment iris epithelium onto the anterior surface of the iris (ectropion). The child is often thought to have mydriasis and anisocoria because of the dark nature of the posterior pigment epithelium. The ectropion may be circumferential (Fig. 32.7) or sectorial. Other ocular features include iris stromal hypoplasia, a high iris insertion into the trabeculum with goniodysgenesis, and secondary glaucoma.

The clinical features are thought to result from an arrest in development with abnormal retention of primordial endothelium, which explains the central iris and angle changes. Although the affected pupil reacts to light and accommodation it may not do so at the same speed as the unaffected eye.[7,39,40] Glaucoma occurs in the majority of these patients usually between early childhood and puberty.

Systemic associations that should be excluded include neurofibromatosis I and Prader-Willi syndrome.

Management of the glaucoma can be difficult with medical therapy often being unsuccessful and augmented trabeculectomy is often the surgical operation of choice.[7,39,40]

Congenital hereditary endothelial dystrophy

Please see Chapter 34.

Posterior polymorphous dystrophy

Please see Chapter 34.

Primary congenital glaucoma

Please see Chapter 37.

ICE syndromes

The iridocorneal endothelial (ICE) syndromes, thought to be due to a primary neural crest cell abnormality, include progressive essential iris atrophy, Chandler syndrome, and the iris-nevus syndrome (also known as Cogan-Reese syndrome).[41-43]

These rare syndromes are even rarer in children. They are unilateral with females affected more than males and are almost exclusively found in white people. However, specular microscopy almost always reveals mild corneal and iris abnormalities in the "unaffected" eye.[44]

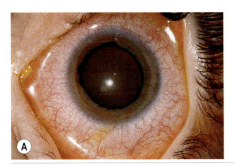
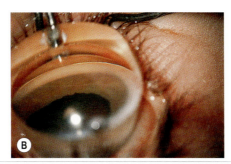
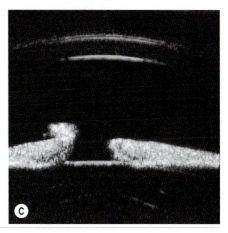

Fig. 32.7 Congenital ectropion uveae. (A) Ectropion uveae, shown as a wide, irregular, dark brown margin to the pupil in a child with glaucoma. (B) Gonioscopic view showing high iris insertion. (C) High-frequency ultrasound image of a child with congenital iris ectropion. Note the frill of posterior pigment epithelium displaced anteriorly.

Specular microscopy studies[45] of early cases of ICE syndrome suggest that a subpopulation of corneal endothelial cells are congenitally abnormal and subsequently migrate/proliferate at a slow rate, resulting in a delayed onset of symptoms or diagnosis. These cells may migrate over the angle and onto the iris to cause different signs such as glaucoma and peripheral anterior synechiae. Descriptions of the trabecular meshwork in a 16-year-old with ICE syndrome show collapsed trabecular beams and decreased intertrabecular spaces.[46]

Progressive iris atrophy shows corectopia, iris ectropion, and pseudopolycoria. Peripheral anterior synechiae often form and gradually become very broad based. Iris holes and thinning occur due to contraction of the membrane formed by the migrating cells. The cornea can appear normal in this condition or have an appearance at the endothelial level similar to that of Fuchs' dystrophy. Glaucoma is not uncommon in this condition and may develop before extensive iris changes. Chandler syndrome is usually associated with corneal edema due to corneal endothelial changes, but iris changes, if present, are much milder than those seen in progressive essential iris atrophy, with glaucoma if present also being more easily controlled medically. Iris-nevus syndrome consists of iris changes either of a nodular type or a flattish pigmented type. These lesions may be associated with varying degrees of iris atrophy and/or corneal endothelial changes.[41-43]

Older patients present with visual disturbance, whereas younger ones usually present due to the finding of pupil disturbance, pseudopolycoria, or pigmentary change of the iris.

Management is purely of any glaucoma that may occur in the first instance. Children are unlikely to require corneal grafting but may do so in their adult lives.[47] Glaucoma management should be attempted initially with aqueous production-suppressing topical treatment but filtering surgery may be needed. Usually antimetabolite augmented trabeculectomy is favored, whereas some authors also advocate the use of drainage tubes.

Anterior segment developmental anomalies of ectodermal origin

The two main conditions in this category are limbal and corneal dermoids, which may be associated with Goldenhar

syndrome with up to 30% of patients being affected[48-50] (see Chapter 29 and Figs 29.2 to 29.4, Figs 32.8 and 32.9).

Anterior segment developmental anomalies of a global origin

The anomalies in this category include megalocornea, microcornea, aniridia, autosomal dominant keratitis, Peters' anomaly, cornea plana, sclerocornea, microphthalmos, and anophthalmos. Of these, microphthalmos and anophthalmos will be discussed in Chapter 24.

Congenital megalocornea

This rare, usually bilateral, condition, thought to be due to defective optic cup growth, results in the cornea growing larger in an attempt to close the gap. Usually inherited as an X-linked recessive trait, mapping to Xq21.3–q22, 90% of patients are males. Female carriers may have slightly enlarged corneal diameters. The remaining cases are autosomal dominant or occasionally autosomal recessive. It is defined as a nonprogressive, enlarged cornea with a horizontal diameter of more than 13 mm, without glaucoma (Fig. 32.10). Myopia is the most common refractive disorder associated with this condition, often accompanied by with-the-rule astigmatism. Associated ocular features include Krukenberg's spindle, increased pigmentation in the trabecular meshwork, iris stromal hypoplasia with iris transillumination, cataracts, ectopia lentis, mosaic corneal dystrophy, and later onset glaucoma. This can be difficult to assess because the cornea is usually thinner than it should be centrally, which can result in artificially lower intraocular pressure measurements using applanation tonometry. Reported associations include Alport's syndrome, craniosynostosis, dwarfism, Down's syndrome, facial hemiatrophy, Marfan's syndrome, mucolipidosis type II, Frank-Ter Haar syndrome (OMIM 249420), megalocornea-mental retardation syndrome.[51-55]

Management consists of careful observation for complications such as cataract formation, dislocated lens, and glaucoma. The iris transillumination can result in difficulty in bright light (usually outdoors), and some patients benefit from tints in their spectacles. Lagophthalmos can be a problem due to improper closure of the eyelids at night, and a lubricating

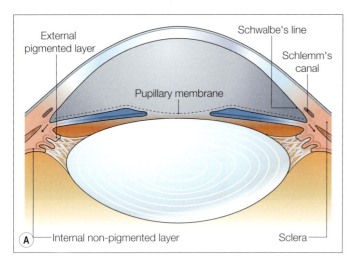

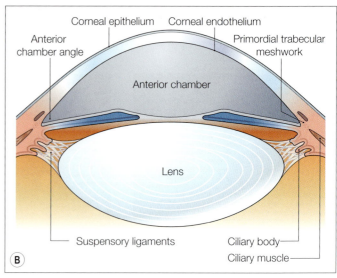

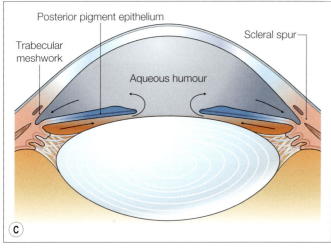

Fig. 32.8 Maturation of the angle of the anterior segment. (A) By 5 months the iris insertion is anterior to the trabecular meshwork primordia. (B) Realignment of the iris insertion gradually uncovers the developing trabecular meshwork. (C) At birth the iris insertion has reached the level of the scleral spur uncovering the angle.[7-9]

eye ointment may be used nightly to prevent exposure problems. Contact lenses can be considered for children with high astigmatism.

Microcornea

This is an uncommon condition defined as any cornea less than 10 mm in horizontal diameter. It may be the result of overgrowth of the tips of the optic cup and may be inherited in an autosomal dominant or recessive manner. If it is an isolated finding with the rest of the eye normal, it is called microcornea, whereas if the anterior segment and the rest of the eye is small, the term is microphthalmos.

Microcornea may be unilateral or bilateral and is usually associated with hypermetropia. Associated ocular findings may include iris colobomas, corectopia, cataracts, microphakia, persistent hyperplastic primary vitreous, retinopathy of prematurity, angle closure glaucoma, infantile glaucoma, and chronic open-angle glaucoma (occurring in up to 20% of patients later in life) (Fig. 32.11).

Systemic associations include Ehlers-Danlos syndrome, Marfan's syndrome, Rieger's syndrome, Norrie syndrome, Trisomy 21, rubella, Turner's syndrome, Waardenburg's syndrome, Weil-Marchesani syndrome, Warburg's microsyndrome, cataract-microcornea syndrome, and acrorenoocular syndrome and microsyndrome.[56-59]

Visual acuity may be normal if it is an isolated finding and if any refractive error is corrected early to avoid amblyopia. The prevalence of congenital corneal opacity (CCO), including Peters' anomaly, "sclerocornea," Congenital hereditary endothelial dystrophy (CHED), and posterior polymorphous dystrophy is approximately 3/100 000.[70]

By making use of ultrasonography, notably ultrasound biomicroscopy (UBM) to help visualize the structures of the anterior segment and prove or disprove the presence of adhesions, improved classification of these conditions can be achieved. In the literature the term sclerocornea and Peters' anomaly has often been used to describe congenital corneal opacification, where the status of anterior segment structures is not known.

It is the opinion of these authors that CCOs are best classified to the subcategories of Peters' anomaly (PA), sclerocornea with cornea plana (S-CNA), and total "sclerocornea" (total opacification of the cornea: S-CCO) based on the clinical features. Then investigations into the causes of such congenital anomalies may follow a logical approach (see Box 32.1).

Peters' anomaly

The designation Peters' anomaly describes iridocorneal or keratolenticular adhesion resulting in central or eccentric, localized, or total corneal opacification (Fig. 32.2). The

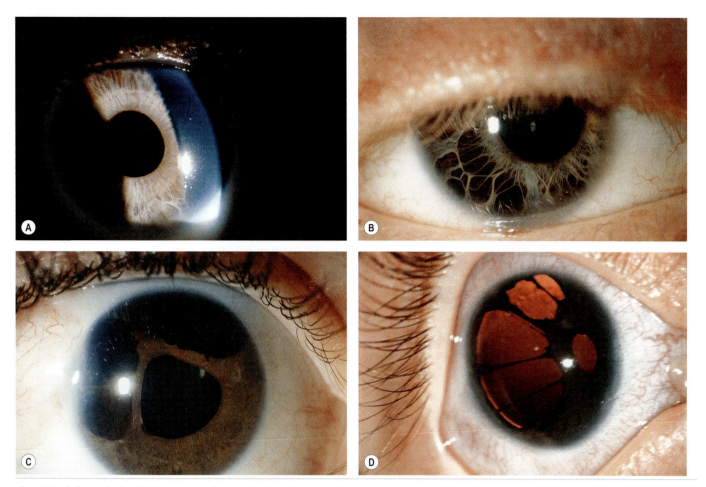

Fig. 32.9 Iris hypoplasia. (A) Iris hypoplasia showing the loss of stroma giving rise to prominence of the sphincter muscle. (B) Marked stromal hypoplasia revealing the posterior pigmented epithelium. (C) Marked stromal hypoplasia giving rise to pseudopolycoria in Axenfeld-Rieger anomaly (ARA). (D) Pseudopolycoria in ARA seen in retroillumination.

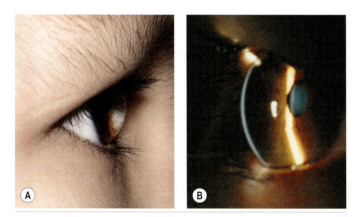

Fig. 32.10 Congenital megalocornea. The horizontal corneal diameter is 13.5 mm, and the anterior chamber is deep as seen in (B). In (A) it is possible to see into the iridocorneal angle without a gonioscope.

pathogenesis of Peters' anomaly is controversial. None of the theories adequately explains all the clinical and histopathologic findings in all forms of Peters' anomaly. Peters' anomaly should be regarded as a heterogeneous group of congenital anomalies with a similar clinical appearance, corneal opacification, resulting from several pathogenic mechanisms including genetic and/or environmental.

It is likely that in those cases where a genetic basis is responsible, accompanying ocular conditions may point to the likely mutation; e.g. aniridia and Peters' anomaly is likely to be due to a *PAX6* mutation whereas Axenfeld-Rieger anomaly/syndrome with Peters' anomaly is likely to be due to *PITX2* mutations.[35,71,72]

Most cases are sporadic, but autosomal recessive and dominant inheritance have been reported.

Peters' anomaly is defined as a congenital central corneal opacity with corresponding defects in the posterior corneal stroma, Descemet's membrane, and endothelium. Eighty percent of cases are bilateral. Glaucoma is present in 50% to 70% of cases.

Peters' anomaly has been often classified into three groups:

1. Posterior corneal defect with leukoma alone (Fig. 32.12)
2. Posterior corneal defect with leukoma and adherent iris strands (Fig. 32.13)
3. Posterior corneal defect with leukoma, adherent iris strands, and keratolenticular contact or cataract (Fig. 32.14).

Posterior corneal defect with leukoma alone is the simplest form of Peters' anomaly and the least documented in the literature. The iris and lens are normal, but a defect in the posterior cornea has produced an overlying opacity, which varies from a mild haze to an elevated vascularized

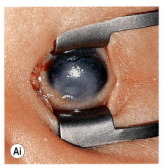
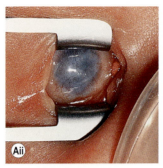

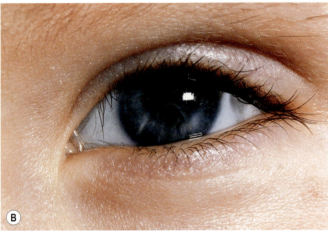

Fig. 32.11 Microcornea. (A) Microcornea in a child with ASDA.
(B) Microcornea with iris and pupil anomalies.

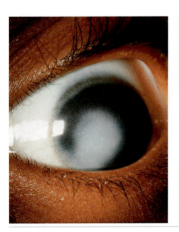
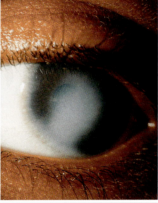

Fig. 32.12 Bilateral Peters' anomaly with eccentric opacification.
Anterior segment imaging will determine whether the cause is iridocorneal
adhesions and/or keratolenticular adhesion.

lesion, and may decrease in the first few years of life. Occasionally the defect is so severe as to cause relative clearing centrally with opacification in the mid-periphery of the cornea (Fig. 32.15). The peripheral cornea is usually clear, allowing visualization of the lens–cornea adhesion with a gonioscope (Fig. 32.16), although scleralization of the limbus is common.[66,67,73-75]

In a recent publication we showed mutations in CYP1B1 associated with congenital corneal opacification and suggest that the original description of von Hippel's ulcer could be explained by such a *CYP1B1* "cytopathy";[77] besides glaucoma no additional ocular sign is seen.

If there are iridocorneal adhesions these usually arise from the collarette and vary from fine strands to broad bands. Keratolenticular adhesions may occur and can be described as one of the following types:

1. The lens may be adherent to the corneal stroma with absence of Descemet's membrane and lens capsule.
2. The lens may be located in a forward position, but only opposed and not adherent to the posterior surface of the cornea.
3. The lens may be in place but with a portion of the anterior capsule and lens cortex in contact with or imbedded in the posterior corneal surface.

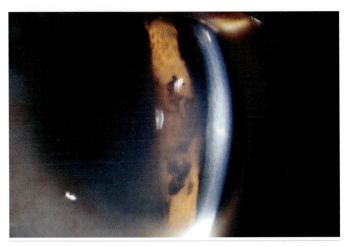

Fig. 32.13 Peters anomaly. Congenital leukoma, which has cleared to reveal iris strands to the posterior surface of the cornea.

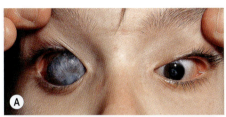

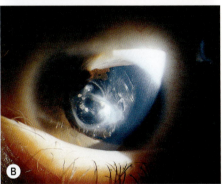

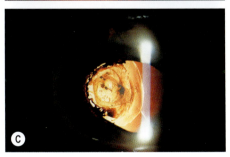

Fig. 32.14 Peters' anomaly. (A) Severe bilateral Peters' anomaly with glaucoma of the right eye. (B) The left eye has iridocorneal and keratolenticular adhesions and iris hypoplasia. The eye is slightly small. (C) The left eye in retroillumination.

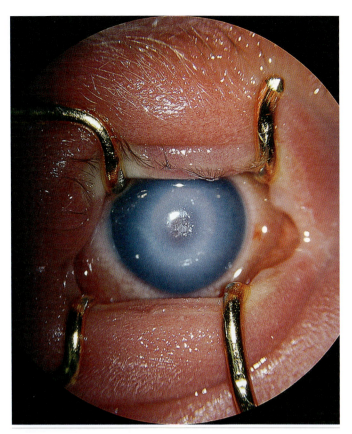

Fig. 32.15 A variant of Peters' anomaly. The posterior corneal defect is so great so as to give relatively clear appearance centrally.

Systemic associations include craniofacial anomalies, congenital heart disease, pulmonary hypoplasia, syndactyly, ear anomalies, genitourinary disorders, central nervous system abnormalities, dwarfism, fetal alcohol syndrome, and chromosomal abnormalities. Peters'-plus syndrome[83] is a rare autosomal recessive disorder comprising short-limb dwarfism, smooth philtrum with thin upper lip, hearing loss, cleft lip/palate, brachymorphism, with short hands and tapering brachydactyly, mental retardation, and bilateral Peters' anomaly. It is associated with mutations in the B3GALTL gene.[78-83]

Histologically findings may vary but include diffuse thickening of Bowman's layer, mild atrophic changes in the overlying epithelium, normal anterior stroma, compressed posterior stromal lamellae partially replaced by fibrous tissue, and a broad central defect of Descemet's membrane and endothelium. The periphery of the cornea usually has an intact Descemet's membrane and endothelium. The anterior chamber is usually deep, except in areas of iridocorneal or keratolenticular adhesions. In other cases absence of Bowman's layer with anterior stromal edema and posterior corneal defect has been described.[69,84]

Management of congenital corneal opacification is quite difficult, and, despite early diagnosis and prompt medical treatment or surgery, many of these cases have a poor outcome. Early penetrating keratoplasty, within the first 3 months, offers the infant the best hope for good vision. Suture removal after 4 to 6 weeks, followed by contact lens fitting and treatment of any amblyopia, is only successful if all involved are committed and motivated. If the reader keeps in mind that the goal of

4. The lens is in place but has a cone-shaped pyramidal cataract axially aligned with a posterior corneal defect.
5. The lens may be in place but has an axial anterior polar or nuclear cataract.

Associated ocular features include Axenfeld-Rieger syndrome or aniridia, microphthalmia, persistent hyperplastic primary vitreous (PHPV), and retinal dysplasia.[30]

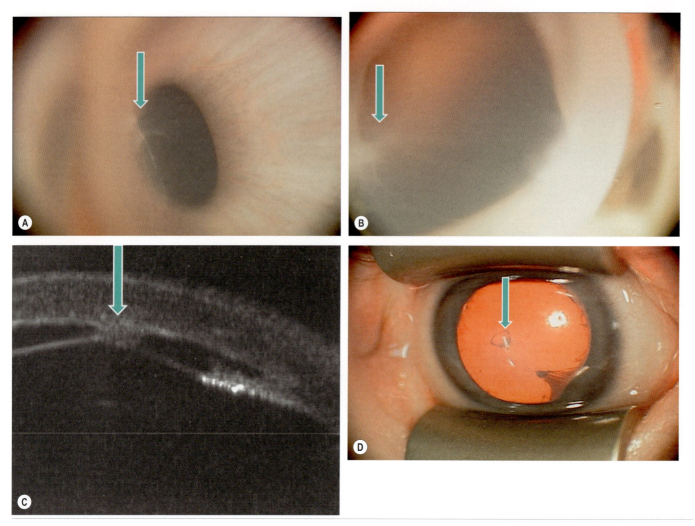

Fig. 32.16 Keratolenticular adhesion (arrow) seen with ultrasound biomicroscopy and clinically. This is a very mild Peters' anomaly.

treatment is to achieve developmental vision at the very least then this allows a better way to counsel parents. Graft rejection is a real issue however, evidence for the use of artifical corneas such as the Boston K-pro in infants is probably not robust yet.[85] However the use of the Boston K-pro in children who have undergone previous corneal grafts which have eventually rejected should be considered. Alternatives to allograft penetrating keratoplasty include broad iridectomies and autorotational keratoplasty.[86,87]

Sclerocornea

In this uncommon, non-inflammatory, non-progressive condition there is extension of opaque scleral tissue and fine vascular conjunctival and episcleral tissue into the peripheral cornea, obscuring the limbus. It is bilateral in 90% of cases. Visual acuity is reduced only if the central cornea is involved. Sclerocornea may be autosomal dominant or recessive (more severe) with 50% of cases being sporadic.

The word "sclerocornea" has caused much confusion;[60] wherever possible the term "sclerocornea" should be assigned to one of the CCO subcategories of sclerocornea with cornea plana (S-CAN; see below) which describes peripheral scleralization with cornea plana, or total "sclerocornea" (total congenital opacification of the cornea: S-CCO), in cases in which

all of the cornea is opaque and resembles the sclera, having first excluded Peters' anomaly using anterior segment imaging. A clinical phenotype of "sclerocornea" may in fact be due to keratolenticular adhesion, which is Peters' anomaly.

This also explains the similarity of some histologic descriptions to Peters' anomaly.[64-67]

Management of sclerocornea consists of surveillance for glaucoma or cataract. In bilateral cases with central involvement, penetrating keratoplasty may be performed but postoperative glaucoma is a major problem. Preoperative assessment with high-frequency ultrasound is advisable to assess the presence of iridocorneal and keratolenticular adhesions.[68,69]

Cornea plana

Cornea plana may be due to an arrest in development at the 4-month fetal stage, which results in a bilateral or unilateral flattening of the corneal curvature with a curvature of less than 43 D (Fig. 32.17). The cornea may be clear or associated with sclerocornea. There is usually hypermetropia and microcornea may also be seen. The recessive and dominant forms share clinical signs such as reduced corneal curvature, indistinct limbus, and arcus lipoides at an early age. The two forms are distinguished by a central, round, and opaque thickening, approximately 5 mm in width, only seen in recessive cases.[61]

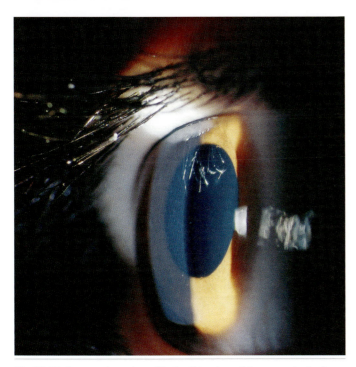

Fig. 32.17 Cornea plana. In profile, the flat nature of the cornea is clearly seen.

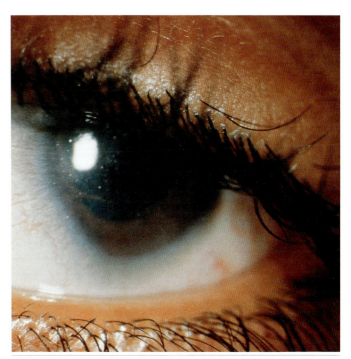

Fig. 32.18 Sclerocornea with cornea plana (S-CNA[60]). There is peripheral scleralization, most likely CNA2.

Autosomal recessive cornea plana (CNA2) may be caused by mutations in the *KERA* gene (12q22), which encodes for keratocan. Keratocan, lumican, and mimecan are keratan sulfate proteoglycans, which are important to the transparency of the cornea.[62]

Sclerocornea with cornea plana (S-CNA) is characterized by peripheral corneal scleralization but a view of the eye through the center of the cornea is possible, and there is always accompanying cornea plana (Figs 32.18 and 32.19).

Associated ocular findings include sclerocornea, infantile glaucoma, angle closure glaucoma and chronic open-angle glaucoma, retinal aplasia, anterior synechiae, aniridia, congenital cataracts, ectopia lentis, choroidal and iris coloboma (Fig. 32.20), blue sclera, pseudoptosis, and microphthalmos. Systemic associations include osteogenesis imperfecta and epidermolysis bullosa.[63]

Management consists of cycloplegic refraction and correction of any refractive error and surveillance for glaucoma.

Autosomal dominant keratitis

This rare recurrent stromal keratitis and corneal vascularization has been shown to be due to mutations in *PAX6*, which are also known to cause aniridia.

The child usually presents with an irritated red eye and is photophobic. It may be associated with foveal hypoplasia. Being autosomal dominant, there is variable expressivity and penetrance within the same pedigree with the mildest phenotype resulting in a 1 or 2 mm circumferential band of corneal opacification and vascularization contiguous with the limbus.[88-90]

Management is difficult and examination under anesthesia may be needed to clinch the diagnosis. Lubrication with artificial tears and ointments is essential. The role of limbal stem cell transplantation is unclear in this condition but early

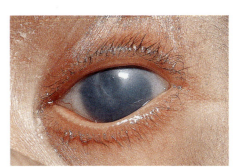

Fig. 32.19 Total congenital corneal opacification (S-CCO[60]) with diffuse non-inflammatory opacity of the cornea. The cause can only be determined by anterior segment imaging.

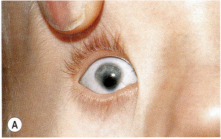

Fig. 32.20 Cornea plana associated with coloboma.

303

recurrence after penetrating keratoplasty has been noted. It is thought that this condition may be a variant of aniridia. If this is so, limbal stem cell transplantation might be a viable option.[89]

Aniridia

Aniridia has a prevalence of 1 in 50 000.[79] Mutations in *PAX6* are responsible for human aniridia,[78] which is a panocular, bilateral disorder with absence of much (Figs 32.21 to 32.23) or most of the iris tissue, although iris hypoplasia may also be seen. Foveal and optic nerve hypoplasia are variably present (Fig. 32.24), resulting in a congenital nystagmus and leading to reduced visual acuity to 6/30 or worse.

Associated ocular features include anterior polar cataracts, often with attached persistent papillary membrane strands, cortical cataract (Fig. 32.25), glaucoma, and corneal opacification, all of which often develop later in childhood (Fig. 32.26). Glaucoma occurs in up to half of all cases and a recent study suggested that, up to the age of 40 years, 15% of patients are diagnosed with glaucoma per age decade.[91]

Corneal opacification occurs secondary to limbal stem cell deficiency in aniridia (Fig. 32.12). Lens subluxation

(Fig. 32.26) can also be associated with aniridia, often with glaucoma.[79,92]

The typical presentation is a baby with nystagmus who has the appearance of absent irides or dilated unresponsive pupils. Photophobia may be present.

Variable expressivity complicates the diagnosis of aniridia. So-called "aniridia with preserved ocular function" has been described as type II aniridia (still linked to 11p13).[95] Visual acuity is more normal, nystagmus is usually not present, and the incidence of cataracts, glaucoma, and corneal opacification is less.

Aniridia can be sporadic or familial. The familial form is autosomal dominant with complete penetrance, but variable expressivity. Two-thirds of all aniridia children have affected parents. It is said that sporadic aniridia is associated with Wilms' tumor in up to one-third of cases.[93]

The Wilms' tumor gene WT1 locus lies close to the *PAX6* gene locus on 11p13. A chromosomal deletion involving both loci results in the association of Wilms' tumor with aniridia.

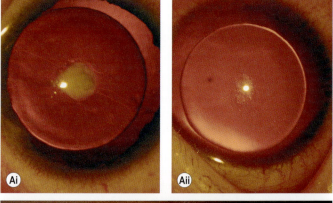

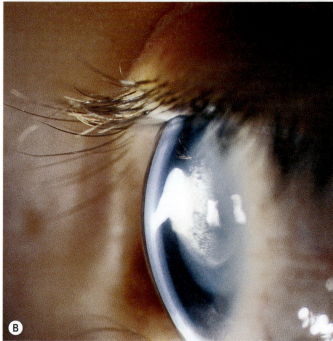

Fig. 32.21 Aniridia. A high-frequency ultrasound of an adolescent with aniridia. Note the iris stump (I), ciliary processes (CP), cornea (C), sclera (S), and lens (L).

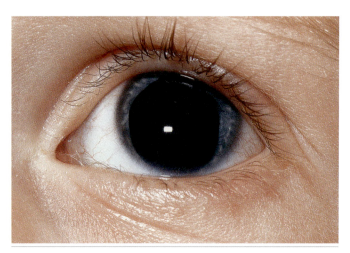

Fig. 32.22 Partial aniridia in a member of an autosomal dominant pedigree.

Fig. 32.23 Aniridia. (A) Aniridia with anterior polar cataract. (B) Aniridia with anterior extension of an anterior polar cataract with attachment to the cornea.

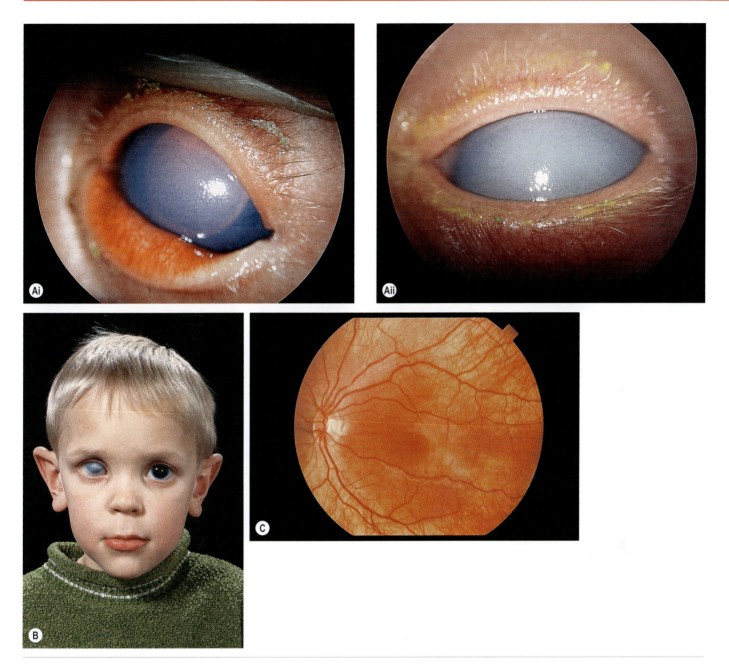

Fig. 32.24 Aniridia. (A) Bilateral severe congenital glaucoma in aniridia. (B) Same patient after multiple surgery showing uncontrolled glaucoma in the right eye and controlled glaucoma in the left. (C) Left fundus of the same patient showing mild foveal hypoplasia. The acuity was 6/18.

In Denmark,[93] patients with sporadic aniridia have a relative risk of 67 (confidence interval: 8.1–241) of developing Wilms' tumor. None of the patients with smaller chromosomal deletions or intragenic mutations were found to develop Wilms' tumor. Familial aniridia patients are said not to be at risk for Wilms' tumor; however, one case has been reported in a child with familial aniridia, but this probably represents a familial 11p13 deletion.[94]

When associated with aniridia, Wilms' tumor is diagnosed before the age of 5 in 80% of cases. The median age at diagnosis is 3 years.

Sporadic aniridia has also been associated with genitourinary abnormalities and mental retardation (AGR triad), a constellation that has been linked with a deletion of the short arm

of chromosome 11 (11p-). Some but not all of these patients get Wilms' tumor (WAGR association). Aniridia can also rarely be associated with ataxia and mental retardation (Gillespie syndrome). Multisystem syndromes and chromosomal abnormalities such as ring chromosome 6 can also include aniridia.[16,96] Ocular associations of aniridia include Peters' anomaly, microcornea, and ectopia lentis.

Management includes genetic analysis to exclude chromosomal deletion. Until the result is known, all children with sporadic aniridia should have repeated abdominal ultrasonographic and clinical examinations. One protocol advised that the child be seen every 3 months until the age of 5, every 6 months until the age of 10, and once a year until the age of 16. However, the examinations are best continued until

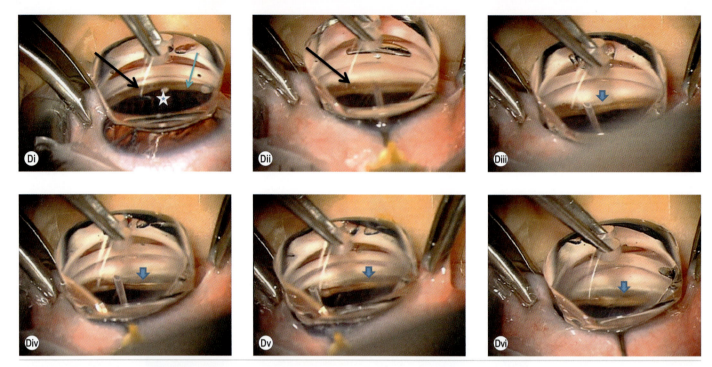

Fig. 32.24 Continued (D) Another case of aniridia: child undergoing goniotomy. The star shows the ciliary processes. There is iris root remnant (child is NOT dilated), and the angle is anomalous. The arrow indicates the developing cleft during successful goniotomy.

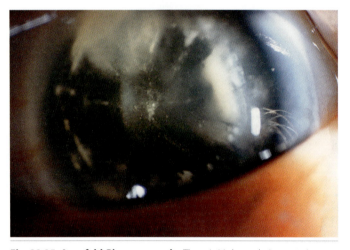

Fig. 32.25 Axenfeld-Rieger anomaly. There is iris hypoplasia, posterior embryotoxon, pseudopolycoria (top of picture), and corectopia with the pupil drawn peripherally.

chromosomal and then intragenic mutational analyses have confirmed a PAX6 mutation only. If chromosomal deletion is found then 3-monthly scans should be performed and the child transferred to the care of a nephrologist.

Management of the ocular condition consists of conservative measures such as correction of any refractive errors with filter lenses to reduce glare, and surveillance for onset of glaucoma. These patients often suffer from chronic angle closure glaucoma, which usually develops later and is difficult to treat. For this reason[97] prophylactic goniotomy in cases of aniridia is sometimes advocated. Cyclodiode laser, drainage tubes, and trabeculectomy with antimetabolite (usually mitomycin) have all been advocated for treatment of established glaucoma uncontrolled by topical medication alone. Usually corneal opacification occurs in adulthood but may occur in children. This may necessitate limbal stem cell transplant and corneal graft.[98]

Penetrating keratoplasty for anterior segment developmental anomalies

Infant penetrating keratoplasty has historically been thought to be a thankless endeavor with poor results.[99,100] However, 35% graft survival at 7 years post graft has been reported in cases of Peters' anomaly,[101] and good visual results have been reported following early penetrating keratoplasty (PKP).[102-104]

Crucial to penetrating keratoplasty in children is the acknowledgment that pediatric ocular tissue behaves differently from that of the adult. The age at which the child's eye becomes more like that of an adult is controversial, but experience suggests that a child over the age of 10 years will have ocular tissue that behaves almost like that of an adult.

High-frequency ultrasound is a well-established tool for the examination of the anterior segment, especially in eyes with corneal opacity.[105-107] It is one of the most challenging conditions to treat surgically,[106] but the use of high-frequency ultrasound evaluation helps determine a more appropriate entry into the anterior chamber.

All cases require a Flieringa ring because the sclera is much less rigid than that of an adult (Fig. 32.27). This is sutured using 8/0 nylon in four quadrants, and the suture is left long so as to stabilize the eye with the long suture ends using Steri-Strips. A pediatric radial corneal marker is used to mark the cornea and allow centration, which aids placement of the trephine. A small paracentesis is made and the anterior chamber hyperinflated with viscoelastic, usually Healon GV.

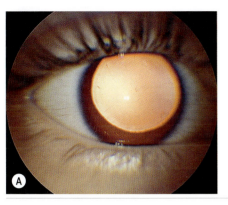 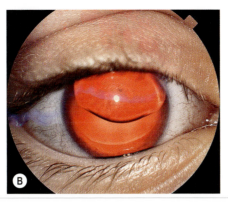 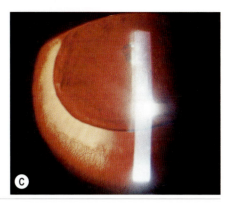

Fig. 32.26 Aniridia. (A) Aniridia with lens subluxation in 1979. (B) Same patient in 1985, showing progressive subluxation. (C) In 1995 there is further subluxation and corneal vascularization.

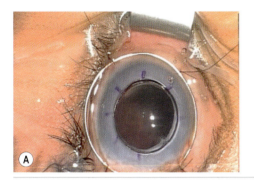 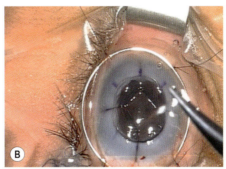 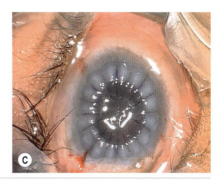

Fig. 32.27 Penetrating keratoplasty in a child with ASDA. Note the flieringa ring and the use of 16 interrupted 10/0 nylon sutures.

Prior to trephination of the host, mannitol is infused according to the weight and age of the child to reduce the intraocular pressure and reduce the risk of expulsive hemorrhage.

A manual trephine is used and, if keratolenticular adhesions or extensive iridocorneal adhesions are present, the anterior chamber is not entered with the trephine. Vacuum trephines such as the Barron-Hessburg are usually not manufactured to a small enough diameter.

The host button is fashioned after initial trephination with a 15° disposable blade so as to avoid excessive damage to the iris and/or lens. In cases of keratolenticular adhesion the lens may be carefully peeled off the cornea but this usually results in cataract formation within a few weeks of the graft. Therefore there is an argument for lens aspiration with sparing of the posterior capsule; this needs surgical capsulectomy through a pars plicata approach usually within a few weeks also, but at least the donor cornea is a little more protected from trauma since the capsulectomy occurs a little deeper in the eye away from the corneal endothelium. All cases of Peters' anomaly or sclerocornea have an iridectomy in four quadrants to try and reduce the incidence of glaucoma. The donor corneal button is oversized by 1 mm in all these cases also to increase the anterior chamber depth There is evidence that this improves outcome.[108] Grafts are sutured using at least 16 10/0 nylon interrupted sutures.

All cases receive subconjunctival antibiotic and steroid injection at the end of the procedure. Intracameral dexamethasone is not routinely used by these authors.

The commonest causes of congenital corneal opacification include "sclerocornea" and Peters' anomaly, both of which are probably part and parcel of the same spectrum of an ASDA. UBM imaging is more reliable in making a definitive diagnosis than just clinical examination alone in such cases.[19] Assessment of presence or absence of the lens, the iris, keratolenticular adhesions, and iridocorneal adhesions all help with surgical planning and also with assessment of surgical prognosis. A classification of congenital corneal opacification has been suggested which can help guide the reader in assessing prognosis[109] (Box 32.1).

The presence or absence of glaucoma must be assessed. If glaucoma is present preoperatively, this again is a poor prognosticator. In these circumstances and if the corneal opacification is bilateral, laser cycloablation (usually cyclodiode laser) is used under UBM guidance to treat the inferior half of the eye. This allows control of the glaucoma with appropriate topical medication, and penetrating keratoplasty can then be performed with the clear understanding that drainage will probably be needed to be placed at a later stage to control the glaucoma. Simultaneous PKP and drainage tube placement in infant eyes is not a route favored by these author.

The tissue reactivity in infants is such that intensive topical steroid/antibiotic preparations are a necessity to prevent fibrin formation, synechiae, and rejection. These are applied half-hourly for the first 24 hours with cycloplegic drops three times daily and antibiotic/steroid ointment at night to allow the infant to sleep. The intensity of drops is tailed off over 2

307

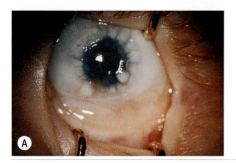
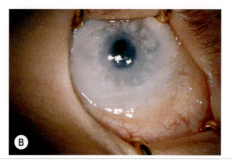
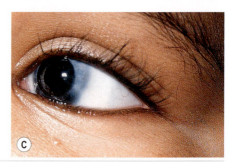

Fig. 32.28 Infant keratoplasty. (A) There is mucous plug formation around loose sutures only 4 weeks post PKP for this case of complete sclerocornea. (B) The same case as in (A) 4 months later. There is peripheral opacification and scarring encroaching on the visual axis. (C) Two years post PKP for Peters' anomaly. The child remains on ciclosporin nightly. (Not the same case as that shown in A and B.)

months, and cycloplegia may continue for the same period. Infants are reviewed twice weekly for the first 6 weeks because the slightest hint of a loose suture or suture vascularization necessitates removal of the offending suture under anesthesia within 24 hours (Fig. 32.28). Failure to do so results in rapid epithelial rejection. In any case, all sutures are removed in infants at the latest by 6 weeks postoperatively.

After 2 weeks, topical ciclosporin A (CsA) eye drops (2% in corn oil) are used twice daily indefinitely to prevent rejection of the corneal graft. There is evidence that topical CsA reaches adequate levels for immunosuppression within the cornea but not necessarily within the eye, and that the combined use of CsA and steroid drops reduces the rate of rejection in high-risk corneal grafts compared to topical steroids only.

In 1977 Waring and Laibson[100] stated "We do not recommend PK in patients with unilateral, congenital corneal opacities. However, those with bilateral cloudy corneas should have an attempt at keratoplasty as early in life as possible." These authors agree with this statement almost in its entirety; the only point of contention is that in some cases the so-called "normal" eye is not normal, only less affected. In these cases the parents should be given the option of keratoplasty with the clear understanding that the prognosis for vision is poor due to the physiologic phenomenon of amblyopia on top of the risks of rejection, infection, and glaucoma.

There is no doubt that if it is understood that the aim of surgery is to give functional vision and not perfect vision and that a partially clear graft that allows delivery of functional vision is still a successful outcome, then infant PKP can be very rewarding for the patient and the surgeon[99-117] (see Figs 32.27 and 32.28).

References

3. O'Rahilly R. The prenatal development of the human eye. Exp Eye Res 1975; 21: 93–112.

6. van Heyningen V, Williamson KA. PAX6 in sensory development. Hum Mol Genet 2002; 11: 1161–67.

15. Kelberman D, Islam L, Holder SE, et al. Digenic inheritance of mutations in FOXC1 and PITX2: correlating transcription factor function and Axenfeld-Rieger disease severity. Hum Mutat 2011; 32(10): 1144–53.

16. Crolla JA, van Heyningen V. Frequent chromosome aberrations revealed by molecular cytogenetic studies in patients with aniridia. Am J Hum Genet 2002; 71: 1138–49.

18. Baulmann, DC, Ohlmann A, Flugel-Koch C, et al. Pax6 heterozygous eyes show defects in chamber angle differentiation that are associated with a wide spectrum of other anterior eye segment abnormalities. Mech Dev 2002; 118: 3–17.

19. Hanson IM, Fletcher JM, Jordan T, et al. Mutations at the PAX6 locus are found in heterogeneous anterior segment malformations including Peters anomaly. Nat Genet 1994; 6: 168–73.

20. Ormestad M, Blixt A, Churchill A, et al. Foxe3 haploinsufficiency in mice: a model for Peters anomaly. Invest Ophthalmol Vis Sci 2002; 43: 1350–7.

21. Beebe DC, Coats JM. The lens organizes the anterior segment: specification of neural crest cell differentiation in the avian eye. Dev Biol 2000; 220: 424–31.

26. Hingorani M, Nischal KK, Davies A, et al. Ocular abnormalities in Alagille syndrome. Ophthalmology 1999; 106: 330–7.

27. Heon E, Sheth BP, Kalenak JW, et al. Linkage of autosomal dominant iris hypoplasia to the region of the Rieger syndrome locus (4q25). Hum Mol Genet 1995; 4: 1435–9.

34. Doward W, Perveen R, Lloyd IC, et al. A mutation in the RIEG1 gene associated with Peters anomaly. Genet 1999; 36: 152–5.

48. Baum JL, Feingold M. Ocular aspects of Goldenhar's syndrome. Am J Ophthalmol 1953; 75: 250.

49. Shields JA, Laibson PR, Augsburger JJ, et al. Central corneal dermoid: a clinicopathologic correlation and review of the literature. Can J Ophthalmol 1986; 21: 23–6.

54. Roche O, Dureau P, Uteza Y, et al. [Congenital megalocornea.] J Fr Ophtalmol 2002; 25: 312–8.

58. Ainsworth JR, Morton JE, Good P, et al. Micro syndrome in Muslim Pakistan children. Ophthalmology 2001; 108: 491–7.

67. Townsend WM, Font RL, Zimmerman LE. Congenital corneal leukomas 2: Histopathologic findings in 19 eyes with central defect in Descemet's membrane. Am J Ophthalmol 1974; 77: 192–206.

69. Nischal KK, Naor J, Jay V, et al. Clinicopathological correlation of congenital corneal opacification using ultrasound biomicroscopy. Br J Ophthalmol 2002; 86: 62–9.

70. Bermejo E, Martinez-Frias ML. Congenital eye malformations: clinical epidemiological analysis of 1,124,654 consecutive births in Spain. Am J Med Genet 1998; 75: 497–504.

74. Waring GO, Rodrigues MM, Laibson PR. Anterior chamber cleavage syndrome: a stepladder classification. Surv Ophthalmol 1975; 20: 3–27.

77. Kelberman D, Islam L, Jacques TS, et al. CYP1B1-related anterior segment developmental anomalies novel mutations for infantile glaucoma and Von Hippel's ulcer revisited. Ophthalmology 2011; 118(9): 1865–73

78. Prosser J, van Heyningen V. PAX6 mutations reviewed. Hum Mutat 1998; 11: 93–108.

82. Lesnik Oberstein SA, Kriek M, White SJ, et al. Peters Plus Syndrome is caused by mutations in B3GALTL, a putative glycosyltransferase. Am J Hum Genet 2006; 79(3): 562–6

87. Haumann GO, Volcker HE, Gackle D. Ipsilateral rotational autokeratoplasty. Klin Monatsbl Augenheilkd 1977; 170: 488–93.

92. Traboulsi EI. Ocular malformations and developmental genes. J AAPOS 1998; 2: 317–23.

93. Gronskov K, Olsen JH, Sand A, et al. Population-based risk estimates of Wilms tumor in sporadic aniridia: a comprehensive mutation screening procedure of PAX6 identifies 80% of mutations in aniridia. Hum Genet 2001; 109: 11–8.

97. Chen TC, Walton DS. Goniosurgery for prevention of aniridic glaucoma. Arch Ophthalmol 1999; 117: 1144–8.

102. Yang LL, Lambert SR, Lynn MJ, et al. Long-term results of corneal graft survival in infants and children with Peters anomaly. Ophthalmology 1999; 106: 833–48.

109. Nischal KK. Congenital corneal opacities: a surgical approach to nomenclature and classification. Eye (Lond) 2007; 21(10): 1326–37.

110. Dana MR, Moyes AL, Games JA, et al. The indications for and outcome in pediatric keratoplasty: a multicenter study. Ophthalmology 1995; 102: 1129–38.

115. Cowden JW. Penetrating keratoplasty in infants and children. Ophthalmology 1990; 97: 324–9.

Access the complete reference list online at
http://www.expertconsult.com

Part 4
External disease and anterior segment

Corneal abnormalities in childhood

Stephen D McLeod

The broad spectrum of disorders that affect the clarity and optical regularity of the cornea are represented in children but developmental and genetic anomalies comprise a larger proportion than in adults. However, many degenerative and dystrophic conditions may not be apparent until adolescence and beyond.

Corneal abnormalities, particularly if monocular or asymmetrical, have the potential to be amblyogenic; in management we should consider not only restoration of optical clarity, but the role that amblyopia might play.

The white cornea at birth poses an important differential diagnosis. The first consideration is congenital glaucoma (see Chapter 37). Intraocular pressure is elevated and the corneal diameter is large. Ruptures in Descemet's membrane may be present. The optic nerves show increasing cupping, often

reversible with intraocular pressure control. Urgent intervention is usually indicated.

Forceps injury is another cause of corneal clouding apparent at birth. Forceps marks may be visible on the lids or cheek. A linear, usually vertical, rupture of Descemet's membrane is present causing corneal edema which always resolves leaving astigmatism. Late corneal decompensation is possible. Metabolic disorders that may cause congenital corneal clouding such as the mucopolysaccharidoses are discussed in Chapter 62; congenital hereditary endothelial and stromal dystrophies are discussed in Chapter 34.

Developmental defects

Embryologic errors

Anterior segment dysgenesis (Chapter 32)

Anterior segment dysgenesis is a spectrum of congenital anterior segment disorders that result from abnormal migration of the waves of neural crest that, from the sixth week of gestation, invade the primary mesenchyme behind the surface ectoderm, giving rise to the corneal endothelium, corneal stroma, angle, and the iris stroma.[1] Thus, anterior segment dysgenesis frequently leads to glaucoma and corneal opacification.

The anterior segment dysgeneses[2-8] have been linked to abnormalities in homeotic genes that control migration and differentiation of neural crest; these include mutations in the PAX6, PITX2, and FOXC1 genes.[2,3,4]

Penetrating keratoplasty for unilateral cases is of limited benefit since the risk of graft failure and amblyopia is high, but may be considered more readily in bilateral cases. Sometimes, penetrating keratoplasty is performed on the eye with more severe opacification, while observing the less affected eye for spontaneous clearing. The success of penetrating keratoplasty in this age group and for this condition is limited; satisfactory visual results are seen in less than 50% of cases due to graft failure, amblyopia, or glaucoma.[9]

Genetic syndromes

Trisomy 18 and trisomy 8 mosaic

Corneal opacification at birth has been observed in some cases of trisomy 18. Corneal abnormalities include stromal

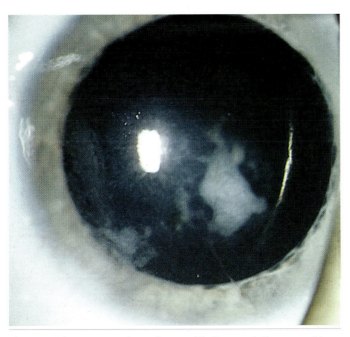

Fig. 33.1 Trisomy 8 mosaic syndrome with characteristic geographic corneal opacity.

hypercellularity, and absence of Bowman's and Descemet's layers. Eyelid abnormalities can lead to ocular surface disease.

Dense corneal opacity has been reported in trisomy 8 mosaic, described as richly vascularized fibrous tissue localized to the superficial layers of the cornea.[10] Spontaneous resolution of this opacity has been observed, but other ophthalmic hallmarks of the disorder including diffuse retinal pigment abnormalities, attenuated ERG, Duane's syndrome, and macular hypoplasia persist (Fig. 33.1).

Ectodermal dysplasia

Ectodermal dysplasia is a rare (1 : 100 000 live births), usually X-linked or autosomal recessive, condition with abnormal eccrine glands, wispy or absent hair, and abnormal teeth or nails. Numerous syndromes make up the ectodermal dysplasia group; the two main groups are the hidrotic and the anhidrotic (or hypohidrotic) forms. Ocular involvement is usually limited to anhidrotic forms.[11]

Ocular abnormalities include blepharitis, conjunctivitis, corneal scarring, pannus, photophobia, decreased tear production, and entropion with trichiasis[12,13] (Fig. 33.2). Meibomian and lacrimal abnormalities may lead to ocular surface disease resulting in keratopathy, infection, and scarring[14] (Fig. 33.3). However, recurrent erosions, pannus, and opacification occur with normal tear film measures; this suggests that the primary pathology may sometimes be limbal stem cell insufficiency. Thus, conjunctival limbal allograft has been suggested for corneal opacification associated with pannus.[15]

Corneal opacities associated with dermatologic conditions

Ichthyosis

The ichthyosiform dermatoses are a group of disorders characterized by scaling. "Harlequin baby" and "collodion baby" are

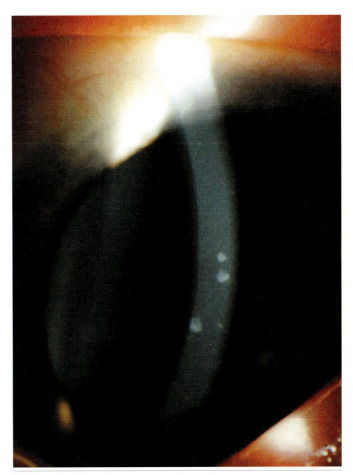

Fig. 33.2 Ectodermal dysplasia with small superficial corneal opacities.

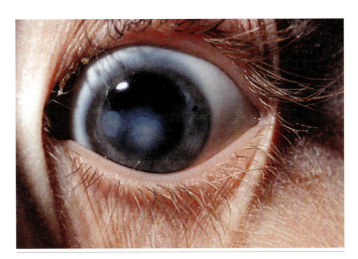

Fig. 33.3 Ectodermal dysplasia with an axial keratopathy. The acuity was 6/24.

extreme congenital forms that may have congenital ectropion.[16] They frequently succumb to skin infections in the neonatal period. Ichthyosis vulgaris is the most common form, inherited as an autosomal dominant trait, with scaling of the extensor surfaces and back. No eye problems occur.

X-linked ichthyosis is congenital and occurs in 1 in 6000 males.[17] Afflicted individuals suffer scaling of the scalp, face and neck, abdomen, and limbs; palms and soles are spared.

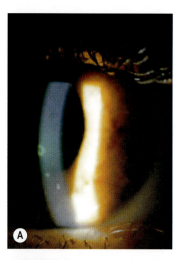

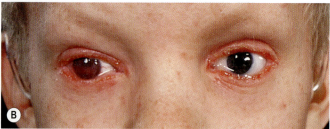

Fig. 33.4 (A) Ichthyosis with fluorescein-staining superficial corneal lesions. (B) KID syndrome with deafness (the patient is using hearing aids) and severe bilateral keratopathy. The left eye has been enucleated.

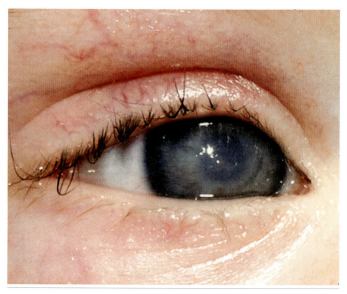

Fig. 33.5 **Epidermolysis bullosa.** Although many cases of epidermolysis bullosa do not have corneal changes, some, like this patient, develop acute epithelial erosions as a result of minor trauma, which if repeated result in permanent corneal opacity and vascularization.

Corneal nerves may be thickened and band keratopathy occurs as an isolated abnormality.[18] Superficial corneal lesions, which stain with fluorescein (Fig. 33.4A), occur; they are usually transient but recur and eventually cause superficial scarring. The scarring and superficial lesions may be caused by eyelid abnormalities, or may occur independently.

Small posterior corneal opacities are located in deep corneal stroma or Descemet's membrane and are not visually significant.[18]

Lamellar ichthyosis and ichthyosis linearis circumflexa are severe autosomal recessive disorders giving rise to ectropion and keratoconjunctivitis mainly due to exposure.[19] This can be so severe as to lead to corneal scarring, infection, and perforation.[20] Epidermolytic hyperkeratosis and erythrokeratoderma variabilis are two autosomal dominant varieties. Ichthyosis occurs in the Sjögren-Larsson syndrome, Netherton's syndrome (ichthyosis, sparse hair, eyebrows, and eyelashes, and atopic diathesis), Refsum's disease, chondrodysplasia punctata, IBIDS syndrome (ichthyosis, brittle hair, impaired intelligence, decreased fertility, and short stature), and the KID syndrome of ichthyosis, deafness, and keratitis[21] (Fig. 33.4B). The keratitis of KID syndrome is attributed to ocular surface drying due to obstruction of the lacrimal gland ductules by shed hyperkeratinized corneal epithelial cells or alternatively to limbal stem cell deficiency.[22] Treatment with lubrication, topical corticosteroids, and antibiotics have been advocated with variable success.

Autoimmune blistering diseases

These disorders are developed from the inflammatory reaction of autoantibodies against specific immunoreactants in the skin and mucous membranes. Ocular involvement includes the skin, conjunctiva, and cornea. Corneal opacity results from ocular surface damage due to dry eye – a result of conjunctivitis, scarring of the lacrimal ductules, and loss of goblet cells – exposure due to cicatricial lid change, trichiasis, and infection.[23]

Specific types of autoimmune blistering diseases in childhood include linear IgA bullous disease and, rarely, mucous membrane pemphigoid.

Erythema multiforme, Stevens-Johnson syndrome, and toxic epidermal necrolysis

Erythema multiforme, Stevens-Johnson syndrome, and toxic epidermal necrolysis (see Chapter 15) are self-limited eruptions of the skin and mucous membranes that are due to a hypersensitivity reaction to environmental factors including drugs and infections.[24] Since the long-term ocular surface compromise and corneal scarring are considered to be a consequence of the severity of the acute event, initial management is directed toward attenuating local inflammation. Amniotic membrane to the eyelid margins, palpebral conjunctiva, bulbar conjunctiva, and cornea is sometimes successsful.[25]

Epidermolysis bullosa

Epidermolysis bullosa is an autosomal recessive disorder caused by mutations in the collagen VII gene that compromises synthesis of collagen VII and anchorage fibrils. This results in generalized blistering of the skin and mucous membranes, beginning in childhood. Ocular complications include eyelid blisters, ectropion, symblepharon formation, tear film abnormalities, goblet cell loss, squamous metaplasia, reduced corneal sensation, recurrent corneal erosions (Fig. 33.5), ulceration, limbal stem cell deficiency, corneal pannus, and scarring. Treatment is challenging with some success using amniotic membrane transplantation and autologous transplantation of cultivated limbal epithelial cells on amniotic membrane.[26,27]

Reiter's syndrome

Reiter's syndrome (reactive arthritis) characterized by inflammatory arthritis of large joints, urethritis, and ocular inflammation is commonly associated with conjunctivitis and iridocyclitis. Mainly peripheral anterior stromal keratitis, epithelial erosions, and more diffuse subepithelial and anterior stromal infiltrates associated with fine conjunctival papillae occur. These lesions resolve with topical corticosteroids.[28]

Vitamin A deficiency and measles (see Chapter 31)

In patients with long-term vitamin A deficiency, the ocular surface can become involved with conjunctival and corneal xerosis, keratinization, severe punctate keratitis, vascularization, and edema. When vitamin A deficiency is accompanied by malnourishment and protein deficiency, keratomalacia, an acute liquefactive necrosis of the cornea can occur (Fig. 33.6), especially when associated with measles infection, herpes

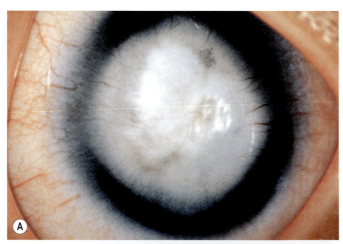

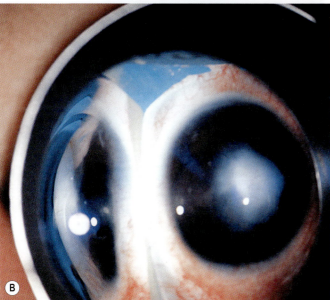

Fig. 33.6 (A) Keratomalacia showing the large axial scar. (B) Gonioscopic view showing the iris attached to the posterior surface of the cornea – leukoma adherens.

simplex, or the use of traditional eye medicines.[29] When diagnosed early, some of these problems are reversible with vitamin A replacement. It may be prevented by diet, vitamin A replacement, and measles vaccination.[30] Higher doses of vitamin A are necessary when the child has worm infestation or diarrhea.[31] Bitot's spot is a triangular foamy-appearing lesion of keratinized tissue that occurs over the conjunctiva in vitamin A deficiency; its presence on the temporal side of the eye suggests active deficiency.[32] Vitamin A deficiency also causes night-blindness.

Infectious keratitis (see Chapter 15)

Infectious keratitis is one of the most vision-threatening consequences of trauma, trachoma, and vitamin A deficiency and related ocular surface disease. It becomes the common denominator leading to blindness associated with numerous ocular and systemic conditions. Traumatic corneal injury is a leading predisposing factor,[33,34,35,36] but the nature of the trauma and the microbiology of subsequent infection varies based on geography. Recently, corneal trauma due to contact lens wear including orthokeratology has emerged as a distinct risk in regions such as Asia with a high prevalence of pediatric contact lens wear.[37-39]

Infections following traumatic injury are most commonly caused by bacteria, but a relatively high rate of fungal infection occurs in areas where filamentous fungal corneal infection is more common, such as South India and China.[33,36] Whether the leading risk factor is traumatic injury or contact lens wear, the most common organisms include both Gram-positive species (staphylococcal and streptococcal species)[33,34,35,37] and Gram-negative species.[36,38]

Infectious keratitis associated with orthokeratology carries an elevated risk for infection with destructive organisms such as *Acanthamoeba*.[39] Aggressive topical treatment with the appropriate antimicrobial agent offers the best chance of a good optical outcome, but amblyopia due to residual corneal scarring and irregular astigmatism after this unilateral condition can have a significant impact on vision.

Herpetic keratitis (see Chapter 15)

Herpetic keratitis is important in the differential diagnosis of corneal epithelial, stromal, or endothelial disease in childhood. Few case series have been reported. Herpetic keratitis in children may differ from that in adults:[40]

1. A higher incidence of bilateral disease (in older individuals this is more commonly associated with atopy).
2. A more intense inflammatory response.
3. A propensity toward stromal scarring.
4. Isolated epithelial keratitis, combined epithelial and stromal keratitis, and keratouveitis. Stromal keratitis is most commonly accompanied by epithelial disease.

An increased risk of recurrence should be considered, but while acyclovir is helpful in the acute phase of all forms of disease, and for prophylaxis in adults the role of prophylactic acyclovir in children has not been addressed prospectively.

Inflammatory keratitis: chronic blepharokeratoconjunctivitis
(see Chapter 15)

Blepharokeratoconjunctivitis is eyelid margin disease with secondary conjunctival and corneal involvement characterized by inflamed eyelids, anterior lid margin telangiectasia, scaling at the base of the cilia, and chronic papillary conjunctivitis. Corneal findings include punctate epitheliopathy, marginal infiltrates, pannus formation, neovascularization, stromal scarring, and lipid keratopathy.[41,42,43]

It is recognized in childhood, but standard treatment regimens that include daily lid hygiene, topical broad spectrum antibiotics, systemic antibiotics, and topical corticosteroids must be modified for children. Systemic antibiotics should be restricted to those appropriate for children such as azithromycin. Care must be taken to manage the potential for intraocular pressure elevation that accompanies chronic topical corticosteroid use, particularly since blepharokeratoconjunctivitis in childhood follows a chronic relapsing course. Amblyopia should be considered in patients with axial stromal scarring.[44]

Interstitial keratitis

Interstitial keratitis describes stromal inflammation, characterized by white cell infiltration and edema that can be followed by neovascularization in prenatal syphilis, mumps, herpes simplex, herpes zoster, varicella vaccination, Epstein-Barr virus infection, leprosy, onchocerciasis, and tuberculosis.[45]

Congenital syphilitic keratitis is typically a bilateral interstitial keratitis that appears between 5 and 15 years of age, and is characterized by a period of intense photophobia, anterior uveitis, and active, deep stromal infiltration and neovascularization followed by regression and resolution over the course of many months to years leaving typical "ghost vessels."[46] The pathogenesis is not well defined.[47] An antigen–antibody complex may be responsible because very few or no spirochetes have been identified in eyes with active keratitis, inflammation does not respond to penicillin and improves with corticosteroids, and antibodies against treponemal antigens have been identified in the cornea.[48]

Cogan's syndrome

Cogan's syndrome consists of interstitial keratitis and audiovestibular disease.[49] Commonly a disease of adulthood, Cogan's syndrome has been recognized in children.[50] The keratitis is usually bilateral, peripheral subepithelial stromal inflammation that can progress to nummular lesions. Deep stromal keratitis can lead to deep stromal neovascularization. The eighth nerve impairment may precede or follow corneal involvement. An association with polyarteritis nodosa and other systemic associations has been described.[51] The cause is unknown although immunologic factors,[52] viral agents,[53] and vasculitis[54] have been implicated. In atypical disease, uveitis replaces corneal inflammation,[55] but the anterior segment inflammation responds well to topical corticosteroids. Although sometimes reversible, hearing loss[56] is more

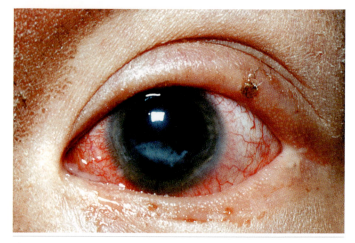

Fig. 33.7 Keratitis. Keratitis resulting from a combination of exposure, drying, and the direct effects of irradiation for orbital rhabdomyosarcoma.

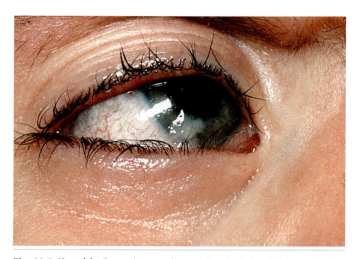

Fig. 33.8 Keratitis. Dry and exposed eye giving rise to keratitis in a patient with seventh nerve palsy associated with the CHARGE association.

commonly persistent; cochlear implants may provide successful rehabilitation.[57]

Corneal trauma

Exposure keratitis

Exposure keratitis is damage to the ocular surface resulting from inadequate lid protection and failure to maintain adequate lubrication and protection of the corneal epithelium. This results in epitheliopathy, subepithelial and anterior stromal scarring, and, later, corneal neovascularization (Fig. 33.7). In severe cases, often associated with infection, persistent epithelial defect, stromal thinning, and corneal perforation can occur.

Eyelid defects (colobomas, etc.) may cause exposure keratitis.[58] Exophthalmos from orbit disease or craniofacial abnormalities (see Chapter 28) can result in poor lid closure, as can seventh nerve palsies (Fig. 33.8). Fifth cranial nerve palsies also result in neurotrophic epitheliopathy; combined fifth and seventh cranial nerve palsies present the greatest therapeutic challenge. Immediate management requires protection of the eye with ointment and lubrication, but surgical intervention, usually tarsorrhaphy, to establish better eyelid protection of the ocular surface may be required.

Corneal anesthesia and hypoesthesia

Defective corneal sensation may give rise to a chronic, recurrent, and severe keratitis. Although termed neurotropic, the main etiologic factors are drying, reduced blinking, and repeated trivial trauma. Defective corneal sensation may arise from any cause of fifth nerve damage. It occurs with trauma, herpes zoster ophthalmicus, developmental or acquired brain stem lesions, and tumors, in particular cerebellopontine angle or pontine tumors. It may occur with herpes simplex keratitis.[59] Corneal hypoesthesia occurs in leprosy, Goldenhar's syndrome,[60] and other oculofacial syndromes.[61] It has been reported in a family of Navajo Indians with an acromutilating neuropathy.[62] It can be found in a subclinical form in Adie's pupil,[63] and is characteristic in the Riley-Day syndrome (Fig. 33.9). It occurs in the MURCS association – Mullerian duct aplasia/hypoplasia, renal agenesis or ectopy, and cervicothoracic somite dysplasia.[64]

Corneal anesthesia may be unilateral,[65] familial,[66] and occasionally associated with fifth nerve motor involvement.[67] A proportion of these children have other neurologic disorders. An element of self-mutilation may be present, which can be difficult to treat – elbow splinting being the most satisfactory method.[68] Children with neurotrophic keratitis (Fig. 33.10) are rarely diagnosed when they are first examined. It is the recurrent nature of the disease and their relative lack of symptoms in spite of evident corneal trauma that draws attention to the

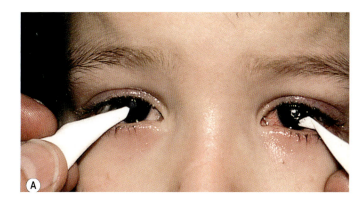

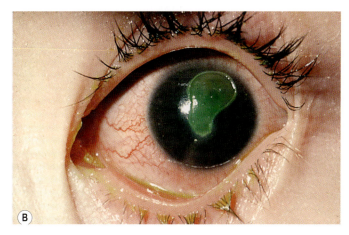

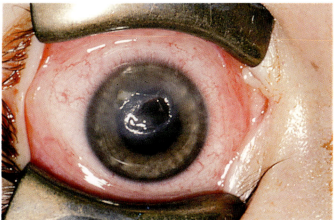

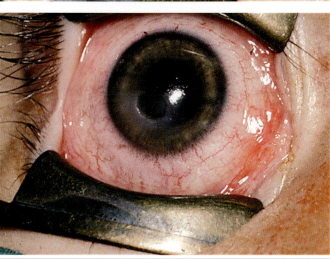

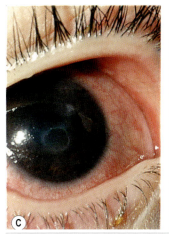
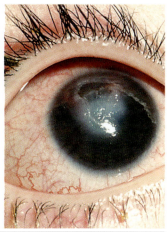

Fig. 33.9 Riley-Day syndrome. This child had a combination of anesthetic corneas and dry eyes that had been treated for several months by topical wetting agents without success. He responded well to a bilateral tarsorrhaphy and lubricant ointment. Later, punctal occlusion allowed enough wetting of his eyes to allow the tarsorrhaphies to be undone.

Fig. 33.10 Neurotrophic keratitis. (A) Profound corneal anesthesia that allows the eye to be touched and for keratitis to occur without pain. There are faint scars on the nose and forehead from painless recurrent trauma. (B) In this child acute episodes of erosion due to direct trauma resulted in corneal scarring. (C) Repeated corneal ulceration and keratitis gave rise to bilateral scarring.

corneal sensory deficit. The presence of scars on the forehead may suggest trigeminal anesthesia. However, in almost any severe keratitis, corneal sensation may be reduced. The corneal anesthesia should be profound to assure the diagnosis. Since the child is usually insensitive to any corneal stimulus, care must be taken during assessment of corneal sensitivity to avoid causing an abrasion.

Cases with lagophthalmos or defective tears are much more severe. This combination is seen in the Riley-Day syndrome, leprosy, and some brain stem lesions. Treatment in small children is very difficult but becomes easier with age; it requires dedicated parents to avoid progressive corneal trauma and blindness. There are a variety of regimes, but the following have been successful in most cases.

Treatment in infancy

Acute epithelial defects are treated with frequent antibiotic drops (without preservative) and ointment with temporary taping of the eye. Frequent use of lubricant drops in mild cases is sufficient, but once a persistent epithelial defect or a pattern of repeated epithelial breakdown is established, the exposed area of the cornea should be reduced. Taping or gluing the lids or using protective bubble shields or spectacles are helpful temporary measures, but an early tarsorrhaphy is the most effective measure. An outer half or third tarsorrhaphy is used, but it is easier to undo than to increase the procedure. Simple lubricating ointment (containing no antibiotic or preservative) is used at night, or day and night in severe cases. This can blur vision and may cause amblyopia in young children, and this should be considered in establishing the schedule of application. Arm-splinting may be necessary to prevent disruption of the ocular surface protection.

Treatment in childhood

Children can be treated with simple ointment in the acute phase but more severe, persistent cases may require tarsorrhaphy. This should be considered before stromal scarring results from epithelial compromise.

Accidental and non-accidental injury

Accidental corneal injury is a leading cause of microbial keratitis and corneal scarring. A spectrum of corneal injuries can occur in child abuse.[69] The presence of lid ecchymoses accompanying corneal injury should arouse suspicion of abuse. A careful history and physical examination should be conducted, searching for other unexplained injuries.

Forceps injuries (Fig. 33.11) cause ruptures of Descemet's membrane usually in a vertical direction which are associated with high astigmatism in the axis of the ruptures, myopia, and amblyopia.[70] Chemical injuries, sometimes repeated, may be due to non-accidental injury[71] (Fig. 33.12).

Hyphema and blood staining

Blood staining of the cornea is a potentially visually significant complication of hyphema following ocular trauma. The incidence ranges from 2% to 11% for subtotal hyphema, to 100% in one study of total hyphema.[72] The severity of hyphema (total versus subtotal) duration, degree of elevation of intraocular pressure, the integrity of the corneal endothelium, and the occurrence of secondary hemorrhages are the factors associated with staining. Patients with sickle cell trait or disease are

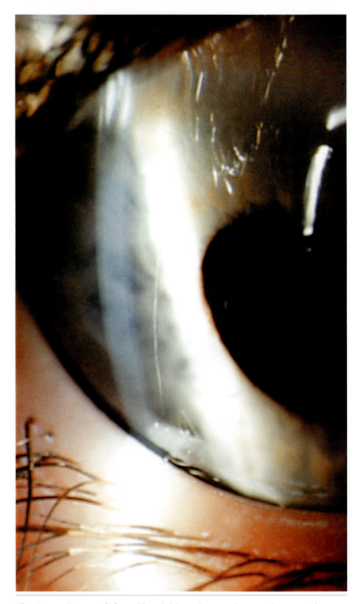

Fig. 33.11 Forceps injury. This child was born with an opalescent right cornea in a normal-sized eye. After a few months the cornea cleared, revealing vertical breaks in Descemet's membrane. The other eye was normal.

particularly susceptible to increases of intraocular pressure that can exacerbate corneal blood staining.[73] Corneal blood staining is of particular concern in infants and children since it can lead to deprivation amblyopia.

The management of traumatic hyphema is controversial. A prospective study of traumatic hyphema suggested that the risk of corneal blood staining in hyphemas that are initially total, do not resolve below 50% at 6 days, and maintain a pressure of greater than 25 mmHg can be reduced by anterior chamber washout.[74] Other elements of care, particularly those directed toward the prevention of rebleed are unresolved. General recommendations include the use of a cycloplegic agent to relieve photophobia and to prevent seclusion pupillae, and bed rest or moderate ambulation with the head elevated to allow settling of the blood. Patients should be examined daily in order to monitor rebleeding, intraocular pressure, the appearance of synechia, and corneal blood staining.

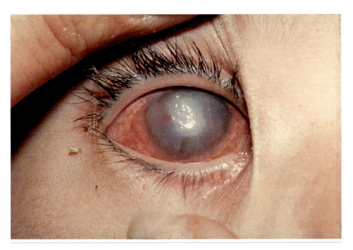

Fig. 33.12 Presumed non-accidental chemical injury to the cornea. This child suddenly developed a profoundly severe keratitis in one eye on the day that his mother's boyfriend left home.

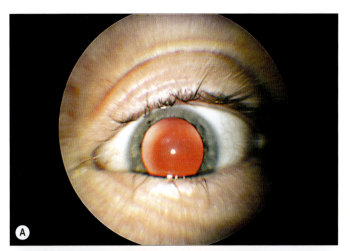

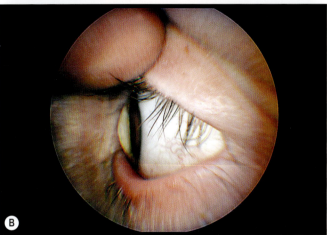

Fig. 33.13 Keratoconus. (A) The retinoscopy reflex in keratoconus is abnormal with no clear end point. (B) Side view showing the conical corneal and the outward bowing of the lower lid (Munson's sign).

The effectiveness of corticosteroids administered either topically or systemically is unclear. Aminocaproic acid and tranexamic acid may reduce secondary hemorrhage risk, although the former is accompanied by gastrointestinal upset and hypotension, and is associated with a slower rate of hyphema clearance.[73] Therefore, pending more robust studies, their use might be limited to cases at higher risk for complications such as patients with sickle cell trait or disease.[73]

Keratoconus (see Chapter 34)

Keratoconus is characterized by bilateral, progressive, noninflammatory central thinning of the cornea. It occurs with a frequency of 1:2000 in the general population.[75] It is frequently familial, with variable expression.[76] Although several loci have been mapped, no mutations in any genes have been identified.[77]

Keratoconus is associated with conditions associated with eye rubbing[78] including atopy, floppy lids, Down's syndrome, retinal dystrophies, and congenital cone/rod dystrophy.[75] Keratoconus may occur in patients with posterior polymorphous dystrophy.[79]

First symptoms are usually of visual impairment. Corneal thinning and apical protrusion that is asymmetric with inferior displacement leads to increasing irregular astigmatism (Fig. 33.13). Rigid contact lens use becomes necessary to compensate for the high degree of corneal irregularity and optical distortion.

Descemet's membrane may rupture leading to acute ingress of aqueous and massive corneal edema or "acute hydrops" (Fig. 33.14). The symptoms of hydrops are blurred vision and hyperemia. It resolves spontaneously over several months, leaving corneal scarring; in some cases, a reduction in apical steepening compared to the pre-hydrops topography develops as the edema clears. Rarely, neovascularization occurs following acute hydrops that increases the risk of rejection in subsequent corneal grafting. Treatment is usually conservative but corticosteroids should be considered for neovascularization.[80] Intracameral injection of long-acting gas, e.g. perfluoropropane, has been used for more rapid resolution of edema.[81]

Most cases of keratoconus can be managed conservatively, with spectacles, toric soft contact lenses, and where irregular astigmatism limits vision, rigid gas-permeable contact lenses.[75] The role of collagen cross-linking to stabilize the cornea and slow progression is under investigation; its role in children is unclear. When the corneal topography precludes a stable contact lens fit, corneal scarring limits vision, or the child develops intolerance to a rigid gas-permeable lens, corneal transplant should be considered. This, however, is uncommon in children. To preserve native endothelium, particularly in younger, higher rejection risk individuals, deep/lamellar keratoplasty has gained in popularity and acceptance. It is technically challenging particularly with stromal thinning, and risks post-graft astigmatism requiring rigid contact lens fitting.

Keratoglobus and blue sclerae

In keratoconus, the stromal thinning occurs in the center of the cornea; in keratoglobus, the thinning is more extensive: the cornea takes on a globular, rather than a conical, appearance best seen in profile. Keratoglobus may be associated with Ehlers-Danlos type VI, brittle cornea syndrome,[82] and the

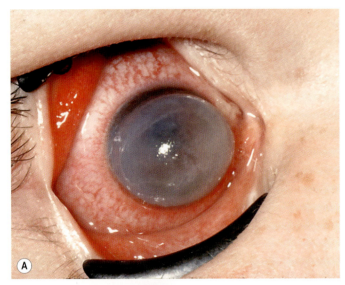

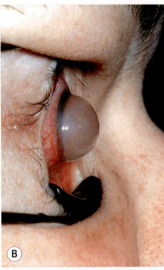

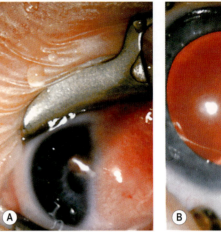

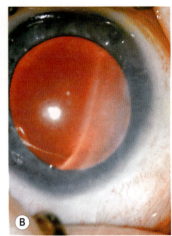

Fig. 33.15 (A) Limbal dermoid that covered half of the cornea and extended posteriorly in the fornix. (B) Same patient, 1 year following lamellar keratectomy carried out at 2 months of age. Although the cosmetic appearance was satisfactory and remained so for 5 years after this photograph the eye was deeply amblyopic due to high astigmatism and the corneal opacity.

Fig. 33.14 (A) Acute hydrops in a child with Down's syndrome and keratoconus. (B) Same patient. Side view showing extreme keratoglobus. After using elbow restraints to stop her rubbing her eyes, bilateral tarsorrhaphies, and padding of the eye, the keratoglobus resolved and became asymptomatic but vision was reduced by axial scarring.

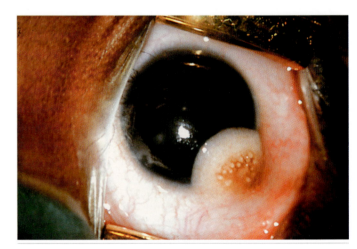

Fig. 33.16 Hairy limbal dermoid.

autosomal recessive syndrome of blue sclerae, joint hyperextensibility, deafness, and mottled teeth.[83]

The characteristic blue discoloration is probably related to thinning of the sclera. Blue sclera is seen in Ehler-Danlos syndrome, cornea plana, peripheral sclerocornea, and microcornea[83,84] and is a consistent finding in osteogenesis imperfecta. Osteogenesis imperfecta is associated with brittle bones and a conductive hearing loss. Six types of osteogenesis imperfecta have been described; four of these are autosomal dominantly inherited and two are recessive. Autosomal recessive osteogenesis imperfecta is characterized by early infant death or severe growth retardation. Infants with osteogenesis imperfecta may have retinal hemorrhages; the mechanism by which they occur is obscure but it is important to remember in suspected non-accidental injury cases. Rarely, blue sclera occurs in the Hallermann-Streiff syndrome and Marfan's syndrome and in association with brittle corneas[85] or ectodermal dysplasia.[86] In infancy many normal children have blue-tinged sclerae as do some older myopic children.

Dermoids

Choristomas are benign congenital overgrowths of normal tissue in an abnormal location; in the eye they consist of a combination of ectodermal elements including keratinized epithelium, hair, and sebaceous glands, and mesodermal elements including fibrous tissue, fat, and blood vessels[87] (Figs 33.15–33.17). Single-tissue choristomas contain ectopic tissues of mesodermal or ectodermal origin,[88] while complex choristomas contain two or more tissues of mesenchymal or ectodermal origin. They may be multiple. Most are sporadic and unilateral.

Corneal dermoids (or lipodermoids) are characteristically a solid mass of dermis-like and pilosebaceous material covered with keratinized, often hairy, squamous epithelium. They are usually at the inferotemporal corneoscleral junction but they

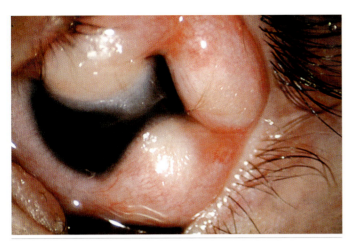

Fig. 33.17 Multiple corneal dermoids in a patient with Goldenhar's syndrome.

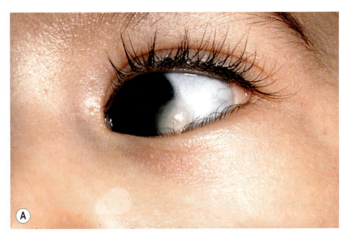

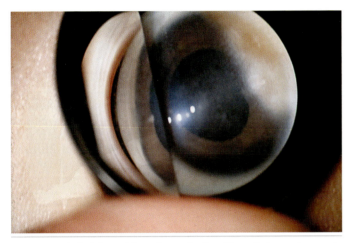

Fig. 33.18 Limbal dermoid: gonioscopic view. Through the gonioscope it can just be seen that the dermoid involves the inner part of the cornea, indicating that caution should be taken during surgery. A full-thickness corneal graft may be the only way to treat this sort of problem and may not be indicated unless the cosmetic appearance is extreme.

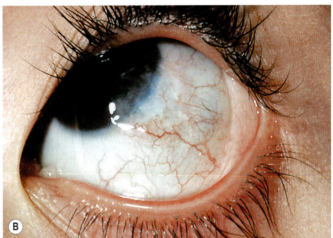

Fig. 33.19 Limbal dermoid. (A) The indication for surgery was the cosmetic appearance. It can be seen that the dermoid is raised and pale colored. (B) Same case as in (a) after lamellar keratectomy. Although there is still some residual corneal opacity the lesion is now flat and cosmetically acceptable.

may be much more widespread and overlie a microphthalmic or staphylomatous eye.[89] Dermoids can involve the entire thickness of the cornea and sclera[90] and can affect vision by occlusion or by distorting the cornea, producing astigmatism and amblyopia.

Dermolipomas are similar to dermoids but have a large amount of fat and few or no pilosebaceous glands. Some are inherited in an autosomal dominant fashion, occasionally X-linked recessive.[91] Dermoids and dermolipomas occur in Goldenhar's syndrome,[92] encephalocraniocutaneous lipomatosis,[93] congenital generalized fibromatosis,[94] and the linear nevus sebaceous syndrome.[95] The gene for one syndrome that segregates as an X-linked trait and is characterized as bilateral, central dermoid tumors sparing the peripheral and deep cornea has been localized to X924-qter.

Treatment is usually necessary on cosmetic grounds but must be preceded by an ocular examination including gonioscopy (Fig. 33.18) and/or high-resolution biomicroscopy to assess the extent of the mass.[96] The lesion can be simply resected to level plane with surrounding tissue, or lamellar keratectomy with the placement of a donor corneal lamellar graft to augment corneal and scleral integrity can be performed[97] (Fig. 33.19). Enucleation is rarely considered for widespread dermoids, but when necessary should be delayed to allow for orbital growth.

Amniotic bands

Amniotic bands may be associated with congenital corneal leukomas or with exposure keratitis from lid defects.[98] The leukoma might be associated with derangement of the anterior segment including absence of the iris and lens, and replacement of the normal corneal tissue with ectodermal and mesodermal derivatives. Displaced amniotic band may prevent the normal induction of the surface ectoderm by the optic vesicle to produce the lens placode, as well as inhibiting the normal invasion of neural crest to produce iris, angle, and corneal structures.[99]

Corneal crystals

Corneal crystals occur in a number of conditions; some have important systemic associations.

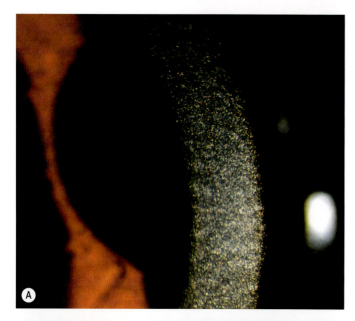

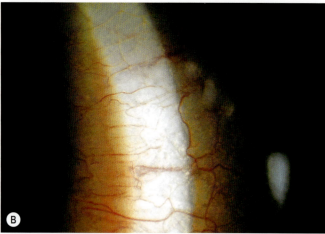

Fig. 33.20 Cystinosis. (A) Corneal crystals can be seen by slit-lamp microscopy. The children are often blonde, fair-skinned, and very photophobic. (B) Crystal deposition occurs in many tissues throughout the body, including the conjunctiva, which can be seen here on slit-lamp biomicroscopy.

Cystinosis (see Chapter 62)

Cystinosis is a rare autosomal recessive lysosomal storage disease with intracellular accumulation of cystine in tissues including the kidneys, bone marrow, pancreas, muscles, brain, and eye.[100] A mutation occurs in the gene CTNS encoding cystinosin on chromosome 17, an integral membrane protein that transports cystine out of the lysosome. Cystinosis is divided into ocular cystinosis with isolated corneal crystal deposition (Fig 33.20) but no systemic findings, and nephropathic cystinosis that appears earlier in life (classic infantile versus juvenile onset or adolescent) and is accompanied by renal tubular Fanconi's syndrome. The more common and severe infantile phenotype presents with growth retardation and renal problems between 6 and 12 months of age, while the intermediate form shows later onset but similar symptoms.[100] The corneal crystals are numerous needle-shaped, highly refractile crystals, initially concentrated in the anterior periphery, but with spread to involve all layers of the cornea

including the endothelium. The crystal deposits of earlier cases are easily identified at the slit-lamp; the increased density in older patients imparts a haze to the cornea that is visible to the naked eye.

The corneal crystals are frequently associated with photophobia of varying severity, sometimes debilitating. They do not usually reduce acuity. Other corneal findings in long-standing cases include superficial punctate keratopathy, recurrent erosions, filamentary keratitis, and band keratopathy.

Oral cystine-depleting agents such as cysteamine, if started early, can preserve renal function and improve growth rates,[101] and have little effect on corneal crystal accumulation.[102] Topical cysteamine is effective in alleviating many ocular symptoms of cystinosis including photophobia, blepharospasm, and eye pain, and promotes dissolution of crystals even in long-standing patients.[100]

Schnyder's corneal dystrophy

Schnyder's corneal dystrophy is a rare, autosomal dominant dystrophy with progressive bilateral corneal opacification caused by the accumulation of cholesterol and lipid in the corneal stroma.[103] The culpable gene is UBIAD1, which is involved in cholesterol metabolism. Only half of patients with this disorder demonstrate corneal crystals on slit-lamp examination.[104] Younger patients have central corneal involvement, and later may develop arcus-like opacity, that ultimately converges centrally creating a diffuse, pan-stromal haze. This can lead to glare and decreased function particularly in daylight; penetrating keratoplasty may be indicated.[103]

Bietti's crystalline dystrophy

Bietti's crystalline dystrophy is a rare, autosomal recessive dystrophy characterized by marginal crystalline deposits in the cornea as well as yellow tinted retinal crystals, tapetoretinal degeneration, and choroidal sclerosis.[105] Decreased visual acuity, night-blindness, and visual field constriction can become apparent as early as the second decade. The responsible gene has been localized on chromosome 4q35, and is thought to represent a disorder of fatty acid and corticosteroid metabolism.[106]

Other causes of corneal crystals include brown-colored uric acid deposits, multiple myeloma, corneal injury with the Dieffenbachia plant due to release of the calcium oxalate present in the sap,[107] and tyrosinemia type II (Fig. 33.21) in which bilateral keratitis is associated with palmar and plantar ulcers and developmental delay. It is treatable with a low tyrosine and phenylalanine diet.

Band keratopathy

Band keratopathy in children is most often the result of ocular inflammation or systemic disease, e.g. juvenile idiopathic arthritis (see Chapter 39). The band (Fig. 33.22) occurs in the interpalpebral region, usually with a clear region between the band and the limbus. Calcium salts precipitate in the basement membrane of the corneal epithelium, Bowman's membrane, and the superficial corneal stroma. The deposits of calcium take on a "Swiss-cheese" appearance. Corneal calcium

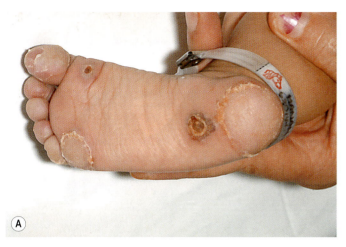

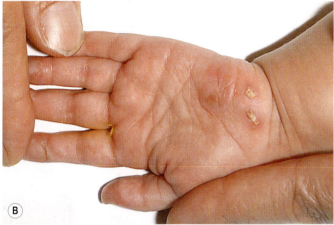

Fig. 33.21 Tyrosinemia type II. (A) Skin lesions on pressure points of the sole. (B) Skin lesions on the pressure points of the palms.

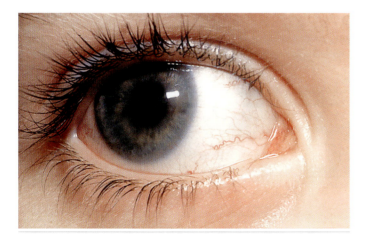

Fig. 33.22 Band keratopathy in a patient with juvenile idiopathic arthritis (see Chapter 39).

deposits can also take the form of corneal calcific degeneration that accompanies advanced anterior segment and globe degeneration in phthisis bulbi, necrotic intraocular neoplasm, extensive trauma, or severe dry eye as in graft-versus-host disease or rheumatoid arthritis. It may involve all corneal layers.[108]

Any condition causing systemic hypercalcemia can cause band keratopathy: e.g. sarcoidosis, parathyroid disease, and multiple myeloma. Chronic ocular inflammation also causes

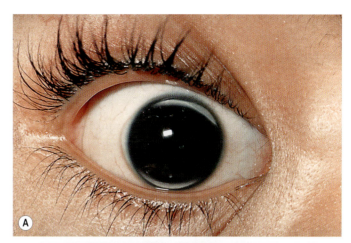

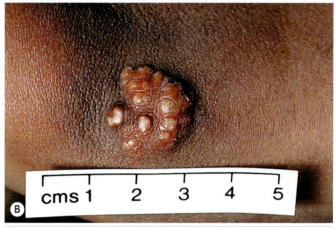

Fig. 33.23 (A) Corneal arcus in a patient with hyperlipidemia. (B) Skin xanthoma in hypercholesterolemia.

band keratopathy. Prolonged corneal edema and glaucoma rarely lead to band formation.

Corneal arcus

Arcus lipoides is due to a deposition of a variety of phospholipids, low-density lipoproteins, and triglycerides in the stroma of the peripheral cornea (Fig. 33.23). Unlike xanthomas, corneal arcus is not invariably associated with hyperlipidemia, but when corneal arcus appears in youth it suggests raised plasma low-density lipoproteins. Arcus is not correlated with plasma high-density lipoprotein or very-low-density lipoprotein. Arcus appears in youth in familial hypercholesterolemia (Fredrickson's type II) and in familial hyperlipoproteinemia (type III).

Corneal nerves

Corneal nerves are visible in the periphery of the normal cornea but may be more visible under certain conditions, including the following:[109]

1. Fuchs' corneal dystrophy
2. Keratoconus
3. Buphthalmos
4. Leprosy
5. Refsum's disease

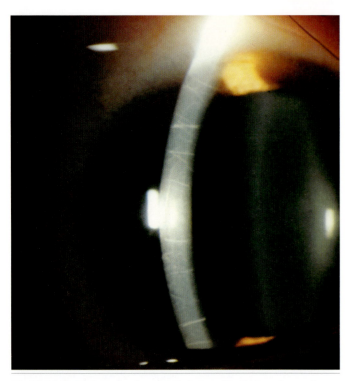

Fig. 33.24 Multiple endocrine neoplasia type IIb. Thickened corneal nerves can be seen crossing even the axial area of the cornea.

6. Ichthyosis
7. Multiple endocrine neoplasia (MEN) type IIb (Fig. 33.24)
8. Neurofibromatosis – rare, may have MENIIb[112]

Multiple endocrine neoplasia

In MEN type IIb, patients show a "marfanoid" habitus, full and fleshy lips, and nodular neuromas on the tip and edges of the tongue and on the margins of the eyelids.[110] Pes cavus, constipation, and peroneal muscular atrophy are due to neuroma formation.[111] It is autosomal dominantly inherited. Prominent corneal nerves within an otherwise normal cornea and nodular subconjunctival tumors are important diagnostic features (Fig. 33.24).[110] Because of a very high incidence of thyroid medullary carcinoma in MEN type IIb, prophylactic thyroidectomy may be recommended in childhood. Pheochromocytoma also occurs. Enlarged corneal nerves may occur in MEN type IIa.[112]

References

1. Harissi-Dagher M, Colby K. Anterior segment dysgenesis: Peters' anomaly and sclerocornea. Int Ophthalmol Clin 2008; 48: 35–42.
4. Iseru SU, Osbourne RJ, Farrall M, et al. Seeing clearly: the dominant and recessive nature of FOXE3 in eye developmental anomalies. Hum Mutat 2009; 10: 1378–86.
6. Bhandari R, Ferri S, Whittaker B, et al. Peters anomaly: review of the literature. Cornea 2011; 30: 939–44.
9. Dana MR, Moyes AL, Gomes JA, et al. The indications for and outcome in pediatric keratoplasty: a multicenter study. Ophthalmology 1995; 102: 1129–38.
15. Daya SM, Ilari FA. Living related conjunctival limbal allograft for the treatment of stem cell deficiency. Ophthalmology 2001; 108: 126–33.
21. Derse M, Wannke E, Payer H. Successful topical cyclosporine A in the therapy of progressive vascularising keratitis in keratitis-ichthyosis-deafness (KID) syndrome. Klin Monatsbl Augenhilkd 2002; 219: 383–6.
23. Laforest C, Huilgol SC, Casson R, et al. Autoimmune bullous diseases: ocular manifestations and management. Drugs 2005; 65: 1767–79.
25. Gregory DG. Treatment of acute Stevens-Johnson syndrome and toxic epidermal necrolysis using amniotic membrane: a review of 10 consecutive cases. Ophthalmology 2011; 118: 908–14.
29. Foster A, Sommer A. Corneal ulceration, measles and childhood blindness in Tanzania. Br J Ophthalmol 1987; 71: 331–43.
37. Wong VW, Lai TY, Chi SC, Lam DS. Pediatric ocular surface infections: a 5-year review of demographics, clinical features, risk factors, microbiological results, and treatment. Cornea 2011; 30: 995–1002.
39. Watt KG, Swarbrick HA. Trends in microbial keratitis associated with orthokeratology. Eye Contact Lens 2007; 33: 373–7.
41. Viswalingam M, Rauz S, Morlet N, Dart JK. Blepharokeratoconjunctivitis in children: diagnosis and treatment. Br J Ophthalmol 2005; 89: 400–3.
50. Gluth MB, Baratz KH, Matteson EL, Driscoll CL. Cogan syndrome: a retrospective review of 60 patients throughout a half century. Mayo Clin Proc 2006; 81: 483–8.
58. Grover AK, Chaudhuri Z, Malik S, et al. Congenital eyelid colobomas in 51 patients. J Pediatr Ophthalmol Strabismus 2009; 46: 151–9.
64. Esakowitz L, Yates JR. Congenital corneal anaesthesia and the MURCS association: a case report. Br J Ophthalmol 1988; 72: 236–9.
68. Trope GE, Jay JL, Dudgeon J, Woodruff G. Self-inflicted corneal injuries in children with congenital anaesthesia. Br J Ophthalmol 1985; 69: 551–4.
73. Gharaibeh A, Savage HI, Scherer RW, et al. Medical interventions for traumatic hyphema. Cochrane Database Syst Rev 2011; 19: CD005431.
76. Karimian F, Aramesh S, Rabei HM, et al. Topographic evaluation of relatives of patients with keratoconus. Cornea 2008; 27: 874–8.
80. Rowson, N, Dart J, Buckley R. Corneal neovascularisation in acute hydrops. Eye 1992; 6: 404–6.
82. Al-Hussain H, Zeisberger SM, Huber PR, et al. Brittle cornea syndrome and its delineation from the kyphoscoliotic type of Ehlers-Danlos syndrome (EDS VI): report on 23 patients and review of the literature. Am J Med Genet A 2004; 124A: 28–34.
85. Zlotogora J, BenEzra D, Cohen T, Cohen E. Syndrome of brittle cornea, blue sclera and joint hyperextensibility. Am J Med Genet 1990; 36: 269–72.
88. Mansour AM, Barber JC, Reinecke RD, Wang FM. Ocular choristomas. Surv Ophthalmol 1989; 33: 339–58.
93. Kodsi SR, Bloom KE, Egbert JE, et al. Ocular and systemic manifestations of encephalocraniocutaneous lipomatosis. Am J Ophthalmol 1994; 118: 77–82.
97. Watts P, Michaeli-Cohen A, Abdoleil M. Outcome of lamellar keratoplasty for limbal dermoids in children. J AAPOS 2002; 6: 209–15.
99. Datta H, Datta S. Anterior segment dysgenesis and absent lens caused by amniotic bands. Clin Dysmorphol 2003; 12: 69–71.
100. Tsilou E, Zhou M, Gahl W, et al. Ophthalmic manifestations and histopathology of infantile nephropathic cystinosis: report of a case and review of the literature. Surv Ophthalmol 2007; 52: 97–105.
101. Gahl WA, Reed GF, Thoene JG, et al. Cysteamine therapy for children with nephropathic cystinosis. N Engl J Med 1987; 316: 971–7.
103. Weiss JS. Schnyder corneal dystrophy. Curr Opin Ophthalmol 2009; 20: 292–8.
106. Lee J, Jiao X, Hejtmancik JF, et al. The metabolism of fatty acids in human Bietti crystalline dystrophy. Invest Ophthalmol Vis Sci 2001; 42: 1707–14.

 Access the complete reference list online at http://www.expertconsult.com

CHAPTER **34**

Corneal dystrophies

Hans Ulrik Møller

Corneal dystrophies are rare Mendelian inherited conditions which exhibit bilateral and usually symmetrical corneal changes.

Nomenclature has been difficult because of controversies about the phenotype definitions. Many authors published different phenotypes under the same headings.

In this chapter, I will focus on a few classic dystrophies, highlighting the clinical presentation in children and emphasizing the differences from the adult. Slit-lamp pictures of the often very subtle changes of corneal dystrophies in children are difficult to take. The clinical pictures in this chapter look almost alike. However, when examining children for a corneal dystrophy, do not look for the well-known adult slit-lamp appearance. You need to look for subtle opacities, similar to the adult clinical picture, but the final diagnosis is made after examining the whole family. Most of the dystrophies are progressive, and the figures illustrate how different the clinical picture may be in youngsters.

Definition

The term dystrophy is from the Greek words *dys* (wrong or difficult) and *trophe* (nourishment). There is no universally accepted definition of the term dystrophy. The word was first used 150 years ago for a group of entities clearly not of traumatic or infectious origin. They were believed to be due to poor nerve supply or nourishment. Most later proved to be genetic in origin, but the word stuck to this group of inherited diseases.

Inherited opacification of the cornea in systemic conditions such as cystinosis are not included here.

Degenerations are secondary, non-genetic processes resulting from aging or previous corneal inflammation.

Classification

Recently an international group of cornea specialists proposed a new classification of 25 entities considered to be

Box 34.1

The International Committee for Classification of Corneal Dystrophies (IC3D): the four levels of corneal dystrophies

Category 1. A well-defined corneal dystrophy in which the gene has been mapped and identified and specific mutations are known

Category 2. A well-defined corneal dystrophy that has been mapped to one or more specific chromosomal loci, but the gene(s) remains to be identified

Category 3. A well-defined clinical corneal dystrophy in which the disorder has not yet been mapped to a chromosomal locus

Category 4. This category is reserved for a suspected new, or previously documented, corneal dystrophy, although the evidence for it being a distinct entity is not yet convincing

The category of a specific corneal dystrophy can be expected to change over time as knowledge advances. Eventually, all valid corneal dystrophies should attain category 1

The classification comprising an extensive description of each condition, clinical pictures, key references, and a few words on onset in childhood can be retrieved at http://www.corneasociety.org/ic3d.

dystrophies.[1] The committee developed a series of descriptive categories as shown in Box 34.1.

Mutation rate

The prevalence and clinical significance of the conditions vary. The founder effect (i.e., an increase in the number of cases of a certain genetic trait due to the introduction of a new mutation in an isolated population) has, in some countries, given rise to publication of large pedigrees of conditions that may be almost non-existent elsewhere.

As the mutation rates for many of the corneal dystrophies are low, it is important to be cautious when diagnosing apparently sporadic cases. A family history *and examination* of family members are mandatory.

Dystrophies related to mutations in the TGFBI gene

New genetic information describes the different allelic mutations within the TGFBI (transforming growth factor-beta induced) gene on chromosome 5q31. They account for many of the classic corneal dystrophies, which are allelic variations of dominant entities of the same gene. Thus, genetic knowledge is bringing order to this field of ophthalmology. Although naming the diseases according to mutation number has not gained universal recognition, most ophthalmologists rely on a genetic analysis to distinguish between the rarer varieties.

Granular dystrophies

Granular corneal dystrophy, type 1 (a category 1 dystrophy)

Granular corneal dystrophy, type 1 is distinguished by discrete granular-appearing corneal opacities in an otherwise clear cornea. This type has several hundred granules in one cornea (mutation R555W).

The opacities are white in direct illumination, and transparent, like a crack in glass, by retro-illumination. At about 5 years of age, these may be brownish and superficial to Bowman's membrane and present in a verticillata configuration (Fig. 34.1A). The granules increase in number and size and progress into the stroma during late childhood while visual deterioration is moderate. There is always a 2 mm clear limbal zone. Unlike most dominant disorders, the expressivity is constant in all generations.

Granular corneal dystrophy, type 2 (a category 1 dystrophy)

Granular corneal dystrophy, type 2 (mutation R124H) is probably the most frequent worldwide; I have seen such patients in six countries. In the past, this has been incorrectly called Avellino dystrophy. Clinically and on electron microscopy, this mutation looks like a mixture of granular and lattice dystrophies with fewer, often larger later in life, elements in the cornea. Vision is affected only if the granules are in the optic axis. It rarely is possible to diagnose until the late teens. Thus a parent carrying this mutation may need genetic analysis to know whether the children inherited the trait (Fig. 34.1B). A so-called superficial, unusual variety (Fig. 34.1C) with a very severe clinical outcome in young children has been described. They have an almost white central cornea before the age of 10 years. These patients are homozygous for this dominant gene.

Lattice corneal dystrophy (a category 1 dystrophy)

Lattice dystrophy (type I, mutation R124C) is also an autosomal dominant condition of the TGFBI gene. Several subtypes have been described; they should be distinguished by genetic analysis. Deposition of amyloid is its hallmark, recognized by three distinct slit-lamp observations:

1. Tiny non-refractile, whitish spots, round or ovoid (Fig. 34.2A).
2. A diffuse axial, anterior stromal haze.
3. White, anterior, stromal dots as well as, in older patients, filamentary lines that are refractile on indirect illumination (Fig. 34.2B).

The deposition may be symmetrical or asymmetrical. The intervening stroma becomes increasingly hazy as time goes by, resulting in glare and worsening of vision. The appearance of the lattice lines gives rise to the name of the condition, but will only become evident in adulthood. Many patients have recurrent erosions.

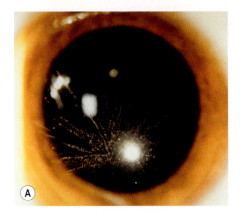

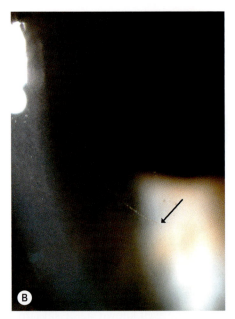

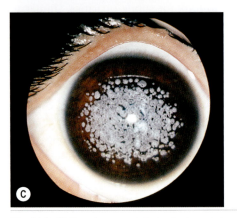

Fig. 34.1 (A) Granular corneal dystrophy, type 1 showing a verticillata-like configuration of the corneal opacities. (B) Granular corneal dystrophy, type 2. A few of these discrete opacities may be all that is visible in a young child. (C) A 7-year-old homozygous patient; granular corneal dystrophy, type 2.

Reis-Bücklers and Thiele-Behnke corneal dystrophies (category 1 dystrophies)

Mutations in that same gene also give rise to Reis-Bücklers corneal dystrophy (mutation R124L) and Thiel-Behnke corneal dystrophy (mutation R555Q and maybe others on

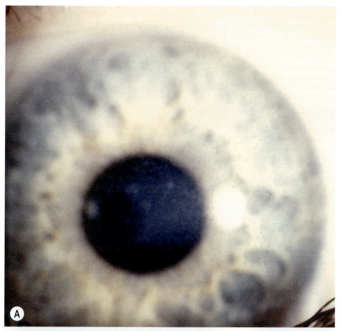

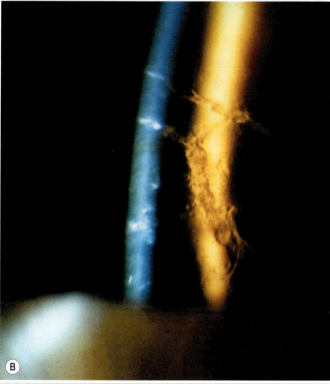

Fig. 34.2 (A) Lattice corneal dystrophy. Early changes showing non-refractile round spots just visible in the pupil. (Courtesy of Mr. A E A Ridgway.) (B) Later changes showing filamentary lines.

chromosome 10q24 – a category 2 variety). Both have early onset recurrent erosions. Reis-Bücklers has confluent irregular subepithelial opacities showing rod-shaped bodies on electron microscopy, as does granular corneal dystrophy. Thiel-Behnke corneal dystrophy has a honeycomb look in the slit-lamp and curly fibers on electron microscopy. Both have subtle superficial opacifications at presentation that progress to give visual problems.

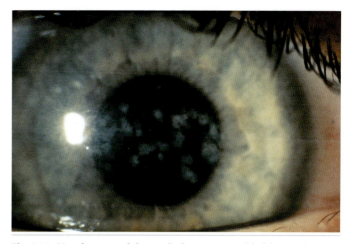

Fig. 34.3 Macular corneal dystrophy in a 13-year-old girl. Typical macular opacities. What cannot be seen in the picture is the opaque ground substance between opacities and the thin cornea.

Dystrophy due to mutations in other genes

Macular corneal dystrophy (a category 1 dystrophy)

Not many ophthalmologists will diagnose macular dystrophy in a very young child; the first findings are very subtle, and hard to diagnose as macular dystrophy, especially if the patient is the first affected in the family. As it is inherited as an autosomal recessive trait, consanguinity is frequent. They comprise nebulous, whitish opacities in the center of the cornea (Fig. 34.3). The cornea is very thin, which is a diagnostic clue. However, over the years it increases in thickness and the corneal stroma becomes increasingly hazy between the opacities with an irregular surface. Deposits of glycosaminoglycan cause the opacifications. The high prevalence of macular dystrophy in Iceland is an example of the founder effect. Macular dystrophy has been linked to chromosome 16; several mutations exist in the CHST6 gene. Progressive visual deterioration is symmetrical and inevitably serious in the second or third decade.

Posterior polymorphous corneal dystrophy (some subtypes are a category 1, some a category 2 dystrophy)

This is also an autosomal dominant dystrophy which may be seen in the very young. It is often asymmetrical and progression, if it occurs, is slow. Thus the corneas in affected children and adults appear similar. Slit-lamp examination shows small, round, discrete, transparent, vesicular lesions (Fig. 34.4) surrounded by a ring of opacity deep in the cornea at the level of Descemet's membrane; geographical and band varieties exist. Do note the words *posterior* and *polymorphous* in the name of the disease; the deep involvement is in contrast to most other corneal dystrophies. The opacities are best seen on retro-illumination.

Posterior polymorphous dystrophy has been linked to chromosome 20q11 (unknown gene) and 1p34–p32.2 in the COL8A gene and 10p11.2 ZEB1 gene.

The symptoms are often mild and vision usually unaffected.

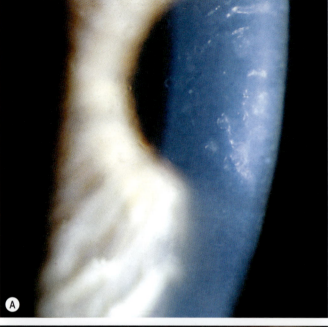

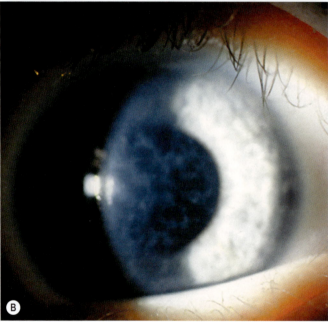

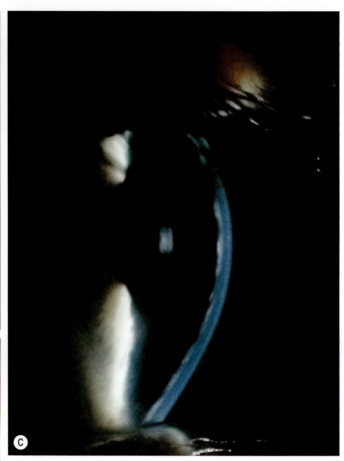

Fig. 34.4 Posterior polymorphous corneal dystrophy. (A) Deep transparent vesicular lesions. (B) Direct illumination showing geographical opacities. (C) Posterior polymorphous corneal dystrophy. Slit-lamp picture showing deep posterior stromal-endothelial ring-like opacities.

Meesmann's corneal dystrophy (a category 1 dystrophy)

This condition has a variable expression. It may be asymptomatic or present in early childhood with ocular irritation and photophobia due to recurrent erosions and a mild blurring of vision. Scarring may later cause changes in the slit-lamp appearance. The typical patient has a huge number of tiny epithelial vesicles (Fig. 34.5). In the young child, small areas may be spared.

Treatment with soft contact lenses may be useful. Corneal abrasion or excimer laser treatment for a decrease in visual acuity caused by basement membrane changes is soon followed by recurrence. Vision is rarely severely affected in children.

Mutations in two loci, 12q13 and 17q12, of the KRT3/ KRT12 gene have been reported.

Schnyder's corneal dystrophy (a category 1 dystrophy)

This autosomal dominant corneal dystrophy can be diagnosed in children but may have a variable expression. The central anterior cornea has a slowly progressing, disc-like central opacification with or without polychromatic crystals (Fig. 34.6). It may be visible in the first decade. In their twenties, patients develop arcus lipoides and a diffuse stromal haze. Vision is variably affected, as some patients have no central crystals. The crystals contain cholesterol and other lipids. The affected gene, UBIAD1, is localized on 1-p36.

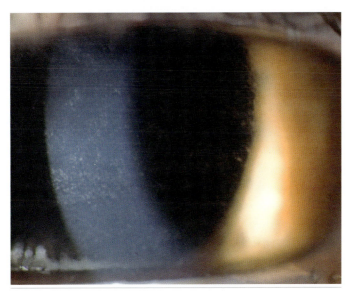

Fig. 34.5 Meesmann's corneal dystrophy showing multiple epithelial vesicles. (Courtesy of K K Nischal.)

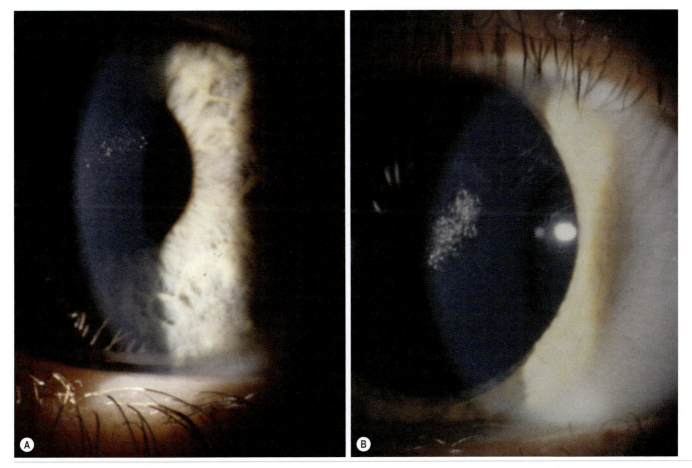

Fig. 34.6 Schnyder's corneal dystrophy. Very discrete subepithelial crystals in a 4-year-old (A) and a 10-year-old patient (B) without any arcus. (Dr. Weiss' patients.)

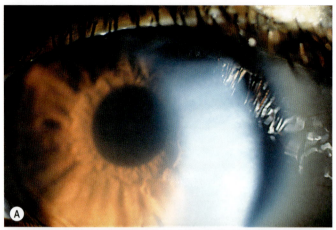

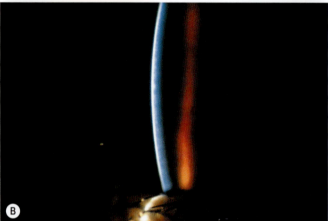

Fig. 34.7 Congenital hereditary endothelial dystrophy. (A) Opaque cornea. (B) Opaque and thickened cornea on slit-lamp illumination.

Congenital hereditary endothelial dystrophy (the autosomal dominant variety is a category 2 dystrophy; the autosomal recessive variety is a category 1 dystrophy)

This important but rare congenital corneal disease was described by Maumenee, a name still used as an eponym, although often it is called by the acronym CHED. Autosomal dominant as well as recessive inheritance patterns exist. The recessive form (chromosome 20p13, SLC4A11 gene) is the more severe and usually presents at birth with diffuse avascular haziness, ground-glass, bluish-white opacity of the cornea (Fig. 34.7) and nystagmus. The dominant form (chromosome 20p11.2–q11.2) develops during the first or second year of life and progresses slowly. This may be a variety of posterior polymorphous corneal dystrophy.

The cornea is thicker than normal. Outcome varies.

Congenital hereditary endothelial dystrophy patients may be observed rather than operated on in early life. A pressure lowering treatment may improve clarity. If grafting is necessary, it carries a good prognosis. Differentiation from congenital glaucoma is important, but often difficult.

Reference

1. Weiss JS, Møller HU, Lisch W, et al. IC3D classification of the corneal dystrophies. Cornea 2008; Suppl 2: 1–42.

The lens

Jay Self • Christopher Lloyd

Anatomy

The crystalline lens, like the cornea, has two principal optical properties: transparency and refractive power. Its structure reflects this. It is a transparent, biconvex, avascular mass of uniquely differentiated epithelial cells. It lies immediately posterior to the iris and is held in position behind the pupil by zonular fibers from the ciliary body.

The lens has an equatorial diameter of 6.5 mm at birth and a maximum anteroposterior thickness of 3.5 mm at the poles. It is completely enveloped by a collagenous capsule, the basement membrane of the cuboidal epithelial cells which lie beneath it in a single layer. The cuboidal cells at the equatorial region of the lens develop throughout life to form spindle-shaped secondary lens fibers. This addition of fibers at the equatorial region slowly changes the morphology of the lens from an almost spherical fetal shape to an elliptical biconvex shape in childhood and early adulthood. The embryonic and fetal nuclei are present at birth. The fetal nucleus is demarcated from the embryonic nucleus by Y-shaped upright sutures anteriorly and inverted Y-shaped sutures posteriorly. Successive nuclear zones are laid down during development. Lens fibers developing after birth contribute to the adult nucleus. Thus, the lens nucleus is made up of densely compacted lens fibers (epithelial cells which have lost their nuclei) with the more peripheral lens cortex less densely packed. Further lens growth mostly affects anteroposterior depth; by early adulthood the lens has a stable equatorial diameter of approximately 9 mm and an anteroposterior depth of 5 mm.

Embryology

The lens develops as a thickening of the surface ectoderm overlying the optic vesicle. This "lens placoid" appears on day 26–27 in the human embryo. In the chick, a tight extracellular matrix-mediated adhesion occurs between the optic vesicle and the surface ectoderm.[1] The mitotically active surface ectoderm is fixed in place, resulting in cell crowding, elongation, and thickening of the placoid. Adhesion of the optic vesicle to the lens placoid ensures eventual alignment of the lens and retina in the visual axis. However, there is no direct cellular contact between the basement membranes of the optic vesicle and surface ectoderm.[2] The lens placoid then invaginates to form the lens pit. This becomes the lens vesicle. Lens vesicle detachment is the initial event leading to formation of the anterior segment of the eye (day 33). It is accompanied by migration of epithelial cells via a keratolenticular stalk, cellular necrosis, and basement membrane breakdown.[3] Disruption to this process by exogenous or endogenous factors can result in anterior segment developmental abnormalities (see Chapter 32). The detached lens vesicle is lined by a single layer of columnar epithelial cells surrounded by a basal lamina, the future lens capsule. Primary lens fiber formation occurs in the epithelial cells lining the posterior surface of the lens vesicle. This is promoted by the adjacent retinal primordium.[4] The lens is thus dependent upon the retinal primordium for cytodifferentiation. The primary lens fibers fill the lumen of the lens vesicle. Elongation of lens cells adjacent to the retina forms the embryonal lens nucleus. The anterior lens cells nearest the corneal primordium remain a cuboidal monolayer and become the lens epithelium. This remains mitotically active for life, providing future lens fiber cells. Epithelial cells differentiate into secondary lens fibers at the lens equator (lens bow). These fibers elongate both anteriorly and posteriorly and insert over the primary lens fibers. They are thickest at the equator. This produces preferential growth of the equatorial diameter of the fetal lens. Secondary lens fibers meet anteriorly and posteriorly at the Y sutures.

Zonular fibers are derived from the non-pigmented ciliary epithelium during the fifth month of gestation. The glycoprotein fibrillin is the main component of the ciliary zonules. There are two isoforms, fibrillin-1 and fibrillin-2. Fibrillin-1 polymers form, without any significant elastin, a structural scaffold of extensible microfibrils. These are arranged in parallel bundles to form the zonular fibers. Disorders affecting the structure or function of these fibrillin-rich microfibrils result in zonular dysfunction, in particular ectopia lentis.[5] Fibrillin-1 gene (FBN1) mutations cause Marfan's syndrome (MFS) possibly some forms of Weill-Marchesani syndrome (WMS) and various other type-1 fibrillinopathy phenotypes in which ectopia lentis is common. Conversely, fibrillin-2 gene (FBN2) mutations can cause Beals' syndrome which is phenotypically similar to MFS but is rarely associated with ectopia lentis (see below).

The tunica vasculosa lentis (TVL) is a vascular network derived from the hyaloid artery posteriorly and a parallel radial palisade of anastomoses with the annular blood vessel laterally. It envelops the developing lens and nourishes it at a time when aqueous production and formation of the anterior chamber have not yet begun. This intraocular network of vessels begins development in the first month of gestation, is maximal in the second to third month, and begins to regress by the fourth month. It has largely disappeared by birth.[6] Persistent TVL is commonly seen in premature neonates and failure of regression of the TVL and hyaloid arteries can cause a range of developmental anomalies collectively termed persistent fetal vasculature (PFV).

Developmental abnormalities of the lens

Anomalous lens development produces a wide range of abnormalities including complete absence of the lens (primary aphakia) and anomalies of lens size, shape, position, and transparency.

Congenital aphakia results from failure of induction of embryonic surface ectoderm to form a lens placoid and lens vesicle and is invariably associated with significant anterior and posterior segment developmental abnormalities and poor visual function. Primary congenital aphakia can result from a variety of teratogenic events (e.g. congenital rubella) in the first 4 weeks of embryogenesis and usually results in microphthalmos, severe anterior segment developmental abnormalities,

and posterior segment colobomata.[7] Secondary congenital aphakia occurs as a result of spontaneous absorption or expulsion of the developing lens. It is associated with less severe ocular anomalies such as PFV.

Microspherophakia is a developmental anomaly with a spherically shaped lens of reduced size and diameter (Fig. 35.1). It may result from abnormal or arrested development of secondary lens fibers. It can occur as an isolated autosomal recessive congenital disorder with mutations in the LTBP2 gene identified in one pedigree[8] or as part of a hereditary systemic disorder, the most common of which are, autosomal dominant and recessive forms of WMS. It is often accompanied by ectopia lentis (Fig. 35.2).

Duplication of the lens is a very rare anomaly associated with corneal metaplasia, uveal coloboma, and cornea plana.[11] It is presumed that metaplastic changes in the surface ectoderm prevent normal lens placoid formation and thus lead to multiple lens vesicles.

Lens coloboma (Fig. 35.3) occurs in areas where there is a failure of zonular development. Lens indentations or scalloped defects in the lens edge demarcate areas of absent zonules.

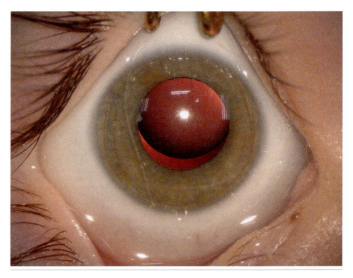

Fig. 35.2 Weill-Marchesani syndrome (WMS). Microspherophakia and upward lens subluxation.

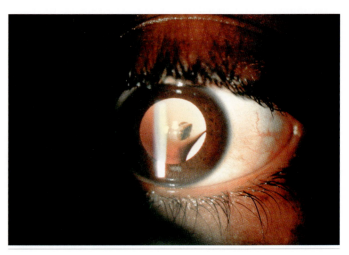

Fig. 35.3 Lens coloboma. Note small cataract adjacent to the coloboma. (Patient of Dr S. Day.)

Fig. 35.1 Weill-Marchesani syndrome (WMS). Microspherophakia with anterior dislocation.

They may occur unilaterally as an isolated anomaly or bilaterally as part of a uveoretinal coloboma phenotype. Lens colobomas may be seen secondary to zonular damage by the congenital ciliary body tumor medulloepithelioma.[9] A localized opacity is often found in the region of the lens coloboma; this is particularly true where it is associated with a ciliary body medulloepithelioma. Most lens colobomas occur inferiorly or inferotemporally.

Lenticonus (Figs 35.4–35.6) and lentiglobus are developmental malformations of the anterior or posterior lens surfaces. Lenticonus is a conical defect and lentiglobus a spherical defect. Posterior surface abnormalities are more common than anterior surface anomalies. Both are usually axial. The resulting refractive error through the central lens is often much more myopic and astigmatic than through the peripheral lens. Lentiglobus is more common than lenticonus and usually unilateral.[10] Lentiglobus is a progressive, well-circumscribed globular bulging of the posterior capsule of the lens. Most cases (95%) are unilateral and there is little evidence that unilateral lentiglobus is a familial condition. In contrast, bilateral posterior lentiglobus is more likely to be inherited as an X-linked or an autosomal dominant trait.[11] It usually presents as the only ocular anomaly; however, it has rarely been associated with microcornea, Duane's syndrome, and anterior lenticonus. Associated cataract is thought to be caused by mechanical stretching of lens fibers. Lenticonus is more common than previously thought.[12] It may be familial with autosomal dominant or X-linked recessive inheritance (Figs 35.4 and 35.5). It may also be seen with Down's syndrome or in the presence of a persistent hyaloid artery remnant (Fig. 35.6).

Anterior lenticonus occurs secondary to an abnormally thin anterior capsule centrally. Approximately 90% of bilateral

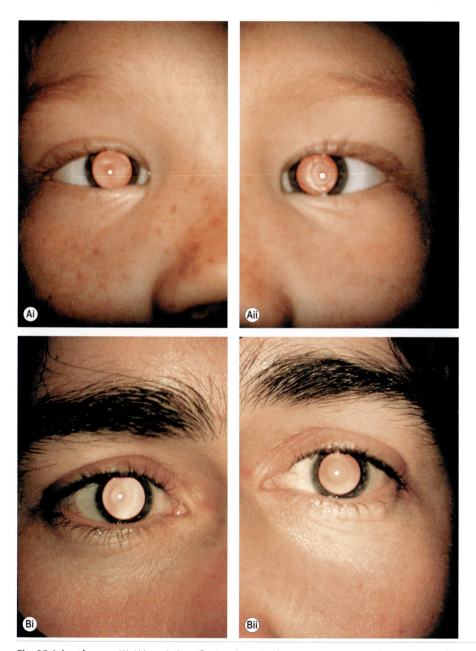

Fig. 35.4 Lenticonus. (A) Although the reflex is a dynamic phenomenon seen on retinoscopy, it can be seen here as a static change in the homogeneity of the red reflex. (B) Mother of patient in (A). Posterior lenticonus is more frequent in boys and may be X-linked.

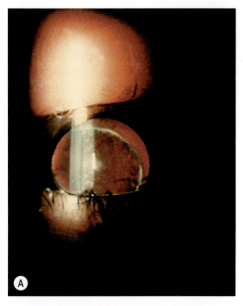

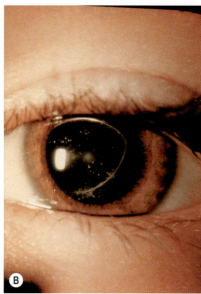

Fig. 35.5 (A) Lenticonus with posterior extension and cataract formation occurring in a healthy girl. (B) Operative photograph with retroillumination on the left showing the defect in the posterior capsule (same patient).

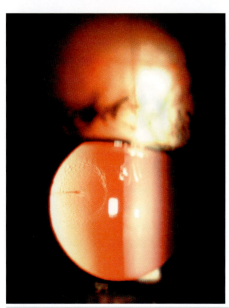

Fig. 35.6 Lenticonic area on the posterior surface of the lens associated with a hyaloid remnant. The presence of the persistent hyaloid remnant suggested that it was important in the pathogenesis.

cases are seen in association with Alport's syndrome, which is a rare basement membrane disorder caused by anomalous type 4 collagen and is characterized by progressive hereditary nephritis, sensorineural hearing loss, and ocular abnormalities. Inheritance is often X-linked (85%), although it can be autosomal recessive (10%) or autosomal dominant (5%). Mutations have been identified in COL4A1-6 genes on three different chromosomes. Males with the X-linked form are usually severely affected but females tend to have a mild form, often with only microscopic hematuria and normal renal function. The ocular abnormalities in the X-linked form are characteristically a dot-and-fleck retinopathy (85%), anterior lenticonus (25%), and rarely a posterior polymorphous corneal dystrophy. Additional ocular abnormalities are not uncommon, including cataracts, posterior lenticonus, and retinal detachment.

Persistence of components of the fetal lens vasculature system, persistent hyperplastic primary vitreous (PHPV), or PFV can lead to persistent pupillary membranes, epicapsular stars, iridohyaloid blood vessels, persistence of the posterior fetal fibrovascular sheath (most commonly called anterior PHPV), and Mittendorff dots (see Chapter 36).

Ectopia lentis

Ectopia lentis or lens dislocation is most commonly due to disorders that disrupt the fibrillin-rich microfibrils of the ciliary zonule affecting its structure and function. Displacement of the lens can range from subtle subluxation to total dislocation due to breakage of most or all of the zonular attachments. Ectopia lentis usually results in reduced visual acuity due to induced refractive error. The most common causes of ectopia lentis include MFS and related type-1 fibrillinopathies, trauma, homocystinuria, and WMS. In addition to the refractive effects, subluxation or luxation can lead to glaucoma.

Marfan's syndrome and the type-1 fibrillinopathies

The fibrillin-1 gene (FBN1) resides on chromosome 15 and the FBN1 protein is a major constituent of microfibrils and the lens zonules. Mutations in FBN1 result in the connective tissue disorder Marfan's syndrome (MFS) as well as a group of related clinical phenotypes collectively termed the type-1 fibrillinopathies.[13] These range from the severe neonatal MFS (usually fatal by age 2) to "simple" ectopia lentis, which is not associated with systemic disease. Autosomal dominant WMS has been described due to a FBN1 mutation in one pedigree. Over 2230 mainly unique mutations have been identified in the FBN1 gene. With the exception of a clustering of FBN1 mutations associated with neonatal MFS no clear genotype–phenotype correlation exists. There is also significant intrafamilial variability between individuals with identical mutations in FBN1. MFS has an incidence of approximately 1 in 10 000 births and is an autosomal dominant disorder. Diagnosis is made using

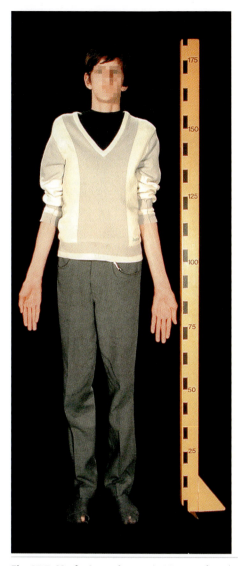

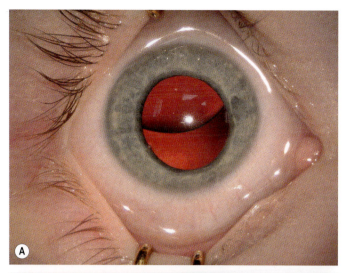

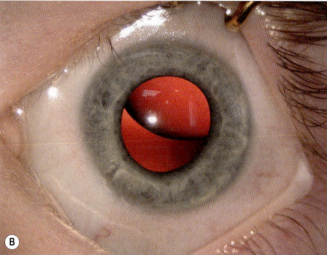

Fig. 35.9 Marfan's syndrome. Upward lens subluxation in the right (A) and left (B) eyes of the same child.

Fig. 35.7 Marfan's syndrome. At 15 years of age he is 1.75 m in height. He has very long limbs, arachnodactyly, and pectus excavatum.

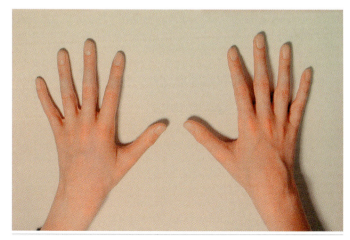

Fig. 35.8 Marfan's syndrome. Arachnodactyly.

the Ghent criteria which incorporate major clinical findings with family history and the results of molecular studies. Associated skeletal abnormalities include tall stature (Fig. 35.7), arachnodactyly (Fig. 35.8), chest wall deformities, and scoliosis. The typical cardiac abnormalities are dilation of the aortic root, mitral valve prolapse, and aortic aneurysm. Ocular findings include ectopia lentis in 60%, axial myopia, corneal flattening, cataract, hypoplasia of the ciliary muscle and iris, open angle glaucoma, and strabismus. Lenses in MFS can sublux in any direction but most commonly displace upward (Fig. 35.9). Zonular fibers in ectopia lentis are fewer in number, thin, stretched, and irregular in diameter.[5] They are also inelastic and more easily broken than normal fibers. The insertion and ultrastructure of zonular fibers attached to the lens capsule in MFS is also abnormal. Reduced synthesis of fibrillin-1 combined with proteolytic degradation of microfibrils accounts for the variable and occasionally progressive nature of some of the clinical manifestations of MFS.[5]

Early lens subluxation can be seen as a flattening or scalloped notching of one lens sector. Zonular fibers typically elongate (Fig. 35.10) and accommodation may be affected. Progression of subluxation is relatively unusual[14] and in

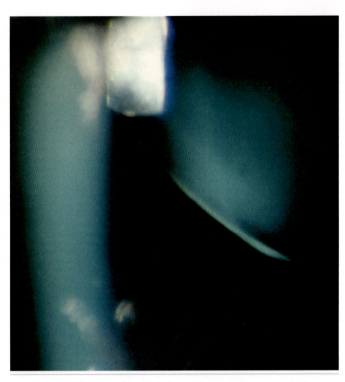

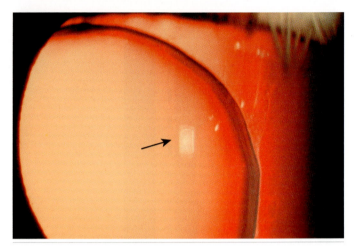

Fig. 35.11 Homocystinuria. Inferiorly dislocated lens with broken, short, and curly zonules. In homocystinuria, the zonules tend to break in their central portion and curl up adjacent to the lens (arrow).

Fig. 35.10 Marfan's syndrome. Dislocated lens with intact stretched zonules. The shadow on the left is the slit beam (out of focus) passing through the cornea.

our experience rarely requires surgical intervention after the age of 10.

Mutations in the *TGFβR2* and *TGFβR1* genes have also been described in MFS and a new group of MFS-related connective tissue disorders: the TGF-β signalopathies.

Homocystinuria

Most homocystine, an intermediate compound of methionine degradation, is remethylated to methionine. It is not ordinarily detectable in plasma or urine. The accumulation of homocysteine and its metabolites (homocystinemia or homocystinuria) is caused by disruption of any of the three interrelated pathways of methionine metabolism:

Type 1: deficiency in the enzyme cystathionine beta-synthase (CBS)
Type 2: defective methylcobalamin synthesis
Type 3: abnormality in the enzyme methylene tetrahydrofolate reductase.

Homocysteinemia is a milder clinical entity than homocystinuria and describes raised plasma levels of homocysteine and is associated with cardiovascular disease and stroke. It may occur in the absence of homocysteinuria and can be caused by genetic predisposition or from a genetic predisposition worsened by comorbid conditions and/or nutritional and environmental factors.

Type 1 homocystinuria is the most prevalent inborn error of methionine metabolism and is an autosomal recessive condition. It occurs in 1 in 300 000 to 1 in 500 000 live births. It is more common in Ireland where there is an incidence of 1 in 52 000. The gene for cystathionine beta-synthetase (CBS) lies on chromosome 21q22.3. Affected individuals are normal

at birth but during early childhood may show neurodevelopmental delay and failure to thrive. Ectopia lentis occurs later along with osteoporosis, fits, psychiatric disorders, and thromboembolic phenomena. However, diagnostic delay is common. Untreated, 90% of individuals develop progressive ectopia lentis.[15] Slit-lamp examination of individuals with ectopia lentis reveals broken and matted zonular fibers (Fig. 35.11). The lens typically subluxates inferiorly or anteriorly and may cause pupil block glaucoma (Fig. 35.12). Patients with homocystinuria are usually tall with elongated limbs and arachnodactyly. They have fair complexions, blue irides, and a malar flush (Fig. 35.13). Kyphoscoliosis, pectus excavatum, high arched palate, and generalized osteoporosis are also common. Other ophthalmic features include progressive myopia (often seen prior to the onset of ectopia lentis), iridodonesis, cataract, iris atrophy, retinal detachment, central retinal artery occlusion, optic atrophy, anterior staphylomas, and corneal opacities.[16] To screen for this disorder, the cyanide nitroprusside test is used, but methionine loading tests and direct measures of urinary and blood methionine are more precise. Early diagnosis and medical treatment significantly improve outcome. Forty percent of individuals respond to high doses of vitamin B6, and for non-responders, dietary restriction of methionine and cysteine supplementation can prevent lens luxation and learning disability.[17] Anesthesia can be complicated by thromboembolic events, and precautions should include optimal biochemical control and preoperative aspirin, intravenous hydration, and compressive stockings. Lens dislocation into the anterior chamber is the most common indication for surgery followed by pupil block glaucoma.[16]

Weill-Marchesani syndrome

Weill-Marchesani syndrome (WMS) is a rare systemic connective tissue disorder. Affected individuals exhibit microspherophakia, ectopia lentis, lenticular myopia, and glaucoma in association with short stature, brachydactyly, and joint stiffness. The lens commonly dislocates into the anterior chamber, causing pupil block glaucoma. Presenile vitreous liquefaction is also reported.[18] It is usually an autosomal recessive disorder which may be caused by mutations in the ADAMTS10 gene on chromosome 19.[19] Autosomal dominant WMS has been

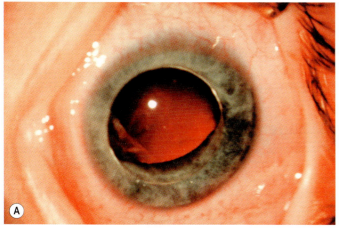

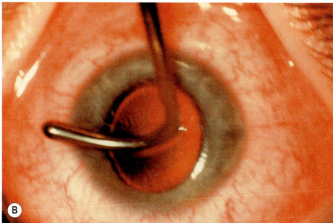

Fig. 35.12 **Homocystinuria.** (A) Anterior/inferior dislocation of the lens, which is jammed in the pupil. (B) Homocystinuria with anterior dislocation and glaucoma. The lens is being repositioned under local anesthetic with a strabismus hook.

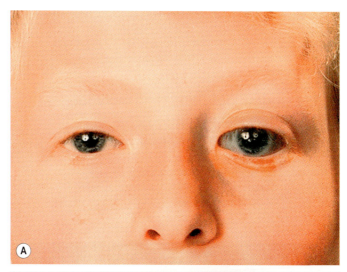

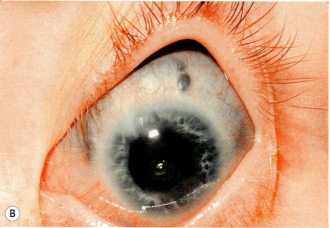

Fig. 35.13 **Homocystinuria.** (A) Fair-haired boy with chronic glaucoma following unreported anterior dislocation of the lens. (B) Despite his age the left eye had become buphthalmic.

described in a pedigree with a mutation in the FBN1 gene (which more commonly causes MFS). A WMS-like syndrome has been described in association with a mutation in the ADAMTS17 gene on chromosome 15.[20] ADAMTS10 and ADAMTS17 belong to a family of proteins called the ADAMTS proteases. A related family of proteins, the ADAMTS-like proteins, includes the ADAMTSL4 protein, the gene for which has been found to be mutated in some pedigrees with isolated autosomal recessive ectopia lentis and ectopia lentis et pupillae (ELeP). These proteins are known to interact with ECM proteins (including fibrillin) and have a role in TGF-β signaling.

Ectopia lentis et pupillae

Ectopia lentis et pupillae (ELeP) is a rare condition that usually exhibits an autosomal recessive inheritance pattern, although a dominant pedigree has been described.[21] It is closely related to autosomal recessive ectopia lentis; both phenotypes have been described in the same pedigree. Lenticular and pupillary ectopia occur in opposite directions, resulting in an oval- or slit-shaped pupil. Poor pupillary dilatation, axial myopia, glaucoma, megalocornea, and iris transillumination defects are also described. Membrane formation on the posterior aspect of the iris has been observed both in histologic sections and on ultrasound biomicroscopy and suggests that the pathogenesis of this condition may be mechanical tethering of the pupil

by a membranous structure with coexistent zonular disruption.[22] Mutations in the ADAMTSL4 gene have been identified in some pedigrees with ELeP and some with autosomal recessive ectopia lentis.

Aniridia (see Chapter 32) and congenital glaucoma (see Chapter 37)

Aniridia is rarely complicated by ectopia lentis. This may be secondary to associated advanced infantile glaucoma and buphthalmos. Surgical removal of the cataracts often found in such individuals may compromise the subsequent success of glaucoma procedures. Sturge-Weber syndrome may also cause secondary ectopia lentis by the same mechanism.

Megalocornea

Ectopia lentis (often inferior) in association with megalocornea (in the absence of raised intraocular pressure) has been described. Cataract may coexist.[23]

Ehlers-Danlos syndrome

Ectopia lentis may rarely occur in association with high myopia in Ehlers-Danlos syndrome.

Trauma

Trauma to the eye may result in zonular damage and ectopia lentis.[24] Rarely this may occur as a result of non-accidental injury.

Sulfite oxidase deficiency and molybdenum cofactor deficiency

These related disorders are rare autosomal recessive inborn errors of sulfite metabolism. Both cause a loss of function of sulfite oxidase leading to CNS toxicity by unknown mechanisms. The diagnosis is suggested in neonates by the association of seizures, abnormal tone, severe neurodevelopmental delay, and ectopia lentis. Affected children usually die in early childhood.[25]

Xanthine oxidase deficiency

This is a very rare cause of ectopia lentis. It is associated with low serum uric acid levels.

Management of ectopia lentis

The ophthalmologist's primary aims for eyes affected by ectopia lentis are restoration of visual function, avoidance of or treatment of amblyopia and the appropriate management

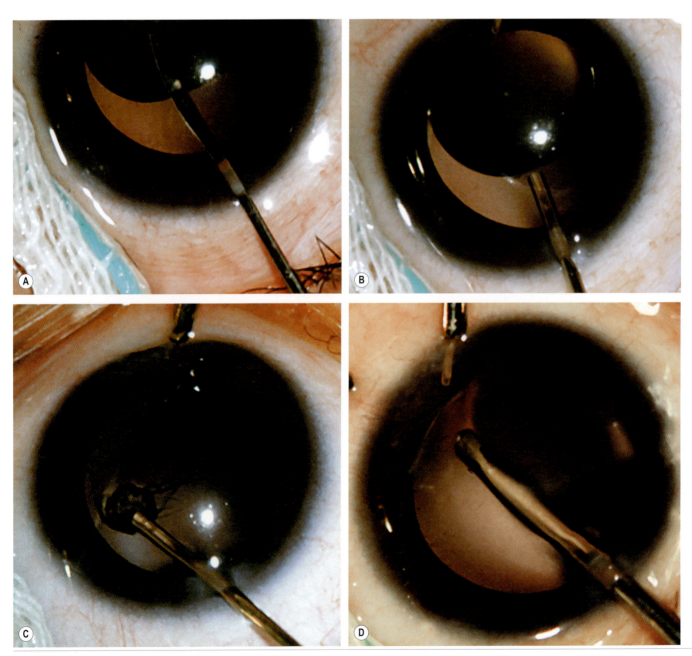

Fig. 35.14 Marfan's syndrome. Lens surgery. (A) The anterior chamber is maintained by a small cannula (not visible on this photograph) and a sharp knife is being used to penetrate the lens capsule. (B) A simple aspiration cannula is inserted into the lens through the capsular incision. (C) All of the lens material is aspirated. (D) A vitrectomy machine is used to clear the remains of the capsule.

of any complications such as glaucoma. Correction of acquired myopia/astigmatism with simple optical measures is all that is required for many children. Spectacles can provide satisfactory optical correction particularly where there is a relatively symmetrical refractive error. However, where there is asymmetrical (or unilateral) ectopia lentis, the use of a contact lens may be necessary to avoid aniseikonia. If the crystalline lens is extensively subluxed, correction of the refractive error of the aphakic zone of the pupil can be be tried. Coexistent pharmacologic pupillary dilatation can aid acceptance of this.

Bilateral ametropic amblyopia has been reported in up to 50% of individuals with ectopia lentis despite good conservative management.[26] This was found to be particularly evident where the lens edge was adjacent to the center of the pupil but where the visual axis was still primarily phakic. Axial high myopia is common in such cases and is possibly secondary to amblyopia.[27] It is postulated that early lens surgery may avoid induced myopia and the subsequent increased risk of retinal detachment. Thus, surgical removal of the lens is indicated in individuals with poor visual acuity due to the pupil being bisected by the lens edge. It is also indicated in those individuals with anterior dislocation of the lens or persistent uveitis due to friction of the displaced lens on the iris. Posteriorly dislocated lenses may be managed conservatively but should be monitored. Signs of glaucoma, uveitis, or retinal degenerative changes are indications for vitreo-lensectomy. The lens is most likely to dislocate anteriorly in homocystinuria. Lens repositioning can often be carried out after pupillary dilatation by using direct mechanical pressure on the cornea with a squint hook. The pupil is then miosed (see Fig. 35.12B).

Microsurgical techniques yield very good results following either limbal or pars plana approach lensectomy for ectopia lentis.[27,28] If the limbal technique is adopted, the vitreous cutter should be introduced into the area of greatest subluxation (Fig. 35.14). Aspiration of the lens material from within the capsular bag prior to completing the capsulectomy ensures lens material is not displaced into the vitreous cavity. Retinal detachment, a frequent problem prior to lensectomy procedures using vitreous cutting instruments, is now a rare complication.[29] Contact lens or spectacle correction of subsequent aphakia is effective and relatively straightforward. In one large study the best-corrected visual acuity of approximately 90% of eyes with ectopia lentis was improved by 2 Snellen lines or more following lensectomy.[29]

YAG laser zonulysis is an alternative technique for moving a lens edge out of the pupillary axis[30] and allows subsequent aphakic correction. Damage to the lens may occur during this procedure, necessitating subsequent lensectomy. This technique is not frequently employed.

The use of IOLs for treatment of aphakia following lensectomy for ectopia lentis remains controversial. Techniques include sclerally sutured IOLs, iris claw lenses, iris fixated lenses, and "in the bag" surgery utilizing capsular anchoring devices or sutured CTRs.[31-34] Reported complications include corneal endothelial cell loss (an average of 14% in the early postoperative period in one study), suture breakage, and/or lens decentration (33% within a few years follow-up in one study) and visual axis opacification requiring surgery for "in the bag" techniques (70% of cases in some studies). Most techniques utilizing IOLs have relatively few long-term results and tend to describe non-inferiority to aphakia corrected with contact lenses rather than superior visual outcomes.

Given the abnormal zonule (and most often other ocular tissues) in children with ectopia lentis, the lack of long-term results and the reported complications with IOLs, the gold standard for refractive correction of those undergoing lensectomy for ectopia lentis remains contact lenses or spectacles.

Visual improvement occurs in nearly all cases, but it may be delayed (often reflecting long-established ametropic amblyopia).[35]

References

1. Hendrix RW, Zwaan J. Changes in the glycoprotein concentration of the extracellular matrix between lens and optic vesicle associated with early lens differentiation. Differentiation 1974; 2: 357–62.

2. Hunt HH. A study of the fine structure of the optic vesicle and lens placode of the chick embryo during induction. Dev Biol 1961; 3: 175–209.

3. Garcia-Porrero JA, Colvee E, Ojeda JL. The mechanisms of cell death and phagocytosis in the early chick lens morphogenesis: a scanning electron microscopy and cytochemical approach. Anat Rec 1984; 208: 123–36.

4. Coulombre JL, Coulombre AJ. Lens development. IV. Size, shape, and orientation. Invest Ophthalmol 1969; 8: 251–7.

5. Ashworth JL, Kielty CM, McLeod D. Fibrillin and the eye. Br J Ophthalmol 2000; 84: 1312–7.

6. Goldberg MF. Persistent fetal vasculature (PFV): an integrated interpretation of signs and symptoms associated with persistent hyperplastic primary vitreous (PHPV). LIV Edward Jackson Memorial Lecture. Am J Ophthalmol 1997; 124: 587–626.

7. Johnson BL, Cheng KP. Congenital aphakia: a clinicopathologic report of three cases. J Pediatr Ophthalmol Strabismus 1997; 34: 35–9.

8. Kumar A, Duvvari MR, Prabhakaran VC, et al. A homozygous mutation in LTBP2 causes isolated microspherophakia. Hum Genet 2010; 128: 365–71.

9. Singh A, Singh AD, Shields CL, Shields JA. Iris neovascularization in children as a manifestation of underlying medulloepithelioma. J Pediatr Ophthalmol Strabismus 2001; 38: 224–8.

10. Crouch ER, Jr, Parks MM. Management of posterior lenticonus complicated by unilateral cataract. Am J Ophthalmol 1978; 85: 503–8.

11. Gibbs ML, Jacobs M, Wilkie AO, Taylor D. Posterior lenticonus: clinical patterns and genetics. J Pediatr Ophthalmol Strabismus 1993; 30: 171–5.

12. Russell-Eggitt IM. Non-syndromic posterior lenticonus a cause of childhood cataract: evidence for X-linked inheritance. Eye (Lond) 2000; 14: 861–3.

13. Fuchs J. Marfan syndrome and other systemic disorders with congenital ectopia lentis: a Danish national survey. Acta Paediatr 1997; 86: 947–52.

14. Maumenee IH. The eye in the Marfan syndrome. Trans Am Ophthalmol Soc 1981; 79: 684–733.

15. Cross HE, Jensen AD. Ocular manifestations in the Marfan syndrome and homocystinuria. Am J Ophthalmol 1973; 75: 405–20.

16. Harrison DA, Mullaney PB, Mesfer SA, et al. Management of ophthalmic complications of homocystinuria. Ophthalmology 1998; 105: 1886–90.

17. Yap S, Rushe H, Howard PM, Naughten ER. The intellectual abilities of early-treated individuals with pyridoxine-nonresponsive homocystinuria due to cystathionine beta-synthase deficiency. J Inherit Metab Dis 2001; 24: 437–47.

18. Evereklioglu C, Hepsen IF, Er H. Weill-Marchesani syndrome in three generations. Eye (Lond) 1999; 13: 773–7.

19. Dagoneau N, Benoist-Lasselin C, Huber C, et al. ADAMTS10 mutations in autosomal recessive Weill-Marchesani syndrome. Am J Hum Genet 2004; 75: 801–6.

20. Morales J, Al-Sharif L, Khalil DS, et al. Homozygous mutations in ADAMTS10 and ADAMTS17 cause lenticular myopia, ectopia lentis, glaucoma, spherophakia, and short stature. Am J Hum Genet 2009; 85: 558–68.

21. Cruysberg JR, Pinckers A. Ectopia lentis et pupillae syndrome in three generations. Br J Ophthalmol 1995; 79: 135–8.

22. Byles DB, Nischal KK, Cheng H. Ectopia lentis et pupillae: a hypothesis revisited. Ophthalmology 1998; 105: 1331–6.

23. Saatci AO, Soylev M, Kavukcu S, et al.. Bilateral megalocornea with unilateral lens subluxation. Ophthal Genet 1997; 18: 35–8.

24. Jarrett WH, II. Dislocation of the lens: a study of 166 hospitalized cases. Arch Ophthalmol 1967; 78: 289–96.

25. Edwards MC, Johnson JL, Marriage B, et al. Isolated sulfite oxidase deficiency: review of two cases in one family. Ophthalmology. 1999; 106: 1957–61.

26. Romano PE, Kerr NC, Hope GM. Bilateral ametropic functional amblyopia in genetic ectopia lentis: its relation to the amount of subluxation, an indicator for early surgical management. Binocul Vis Strabismus Q 2002; 17: 235–41.

27. Salehpour O, Lavy T, Leonard J, Taylor D. The surgical management of nontraumatic ectopic lenses. J Pediatr Ophthalmol Strabismus 1996; 33: 8–13.

28. Reese PD, Weingeist TA. Pars plana management of ectopia lentis in children. Arch Ophthalmol 1987; 105: 1202–4.

29. Halpert M, BenEzra D. Surgery of the hereditary subluxated lens in children. Ophthalmology 1996; 103: 681–6.

30. Tchah HW, Larson RS, Nichols BD, Lindstrom RL. Neodymium:YAG laser zonulysis for treatment of lens subluxation. Ophthalmology 1989; 96: 230–4; discussion 5.

31. Konradsen T, Kugelberg M, Zetterstrom C. Visual outcomes and complications in surgery for ectopia lentis in children. J Cataract Refract Surg 2007; 33: 819–24.

32. Cleary C, Lanigan B, O'Keeffe M. Artisan iris-claw lenses for the correction of aphakia in children following lensectomy for ectopia lentis. Br J Ophthalmol 2011; doi:10.1136.

33. Dureau P, de Laage de Meux P, Edelson C, Caputo G. Iris fixation of foldable intraocular lenses for ectopia lentis in children. J Cataract Refract Surg 2006; 32: 1109–14.

34. Assia EI, Ton Y, Michaeli A. Capsule anchor to manage subluxated lenses: initial clinical experience. J Cataract Refract Surg 2009; 35: 1372–9.

35. Speedwell L, Russell-Eggitt I. Improvement in visual acuity in children with ectopia lentis. J Pediatr Ophthalmol Strabismus 1995; 32: 94–7.

Childhood cataracts

Scott R Lambert

Chapter contents

Incidence

Cataracts, which are opacities of the crystalline lens, are an important problem in children worldwide. The incidence varies, but in the UK the adjusted cumulative incidence at age 1 year is 2.49/10 000, increasing to 3.46/10 000 by age 15 years.[1] Bilateral cataracts are more common than unilateral.

Detection

Because of visual deprivation with both unilateral and bilateral cataracts, successful management requires early detection and referral for treatment. The red reflex should be assessed by direct ophthalmoscopy in the newborn nursery and at each well-child check-up. If an abnormality is detected, referral should be made to an ophthalmologist. Pupillary dilation may be necessary to detect some incomplete cataracts.

Children with visually significant unilateral cataracts often present with strabismus and dense amblyopia. However, visual behavior will usually be unaffected by a *unilateral* cataract, and for this reason the parents may not be aware of it. In contrast, dense *bilateral* cataracts are usually associated with impaired visual behavior. If nystagmus develops, visual prognosis is worse, although it may be reversed by prompt treatment.[2]

Morphology

The morphology of cataracts offers important clues to their age of onset and visual prognosis. In addition, it provides insights into the etiology of a cataract. When possible, a slit-lamp examination is invaluable in identifying the morphology. Refinements in the morphology can be obtained intraoperatively.[3] The morphology is largely determined by the anatomy of the lens, its embryology, and the timing and nature of the insult that caused it (Box 36.1).

Some morphological types of cataracts have a better prognosis than others. Anterior polar (Fig. 36.1), lamellar (Fig. 36.2), sutural (Fig. 36.3), and posterior lentiglobus (Fig. 36.4) cataracts are associated with the best visual prognoses, whereas dense, central, and posterior cataracts have poorer visual prognoses.[4] Acquired cataracts generally have a more favorable visual prognosis than congenital cataracts.

Certain types of cataracts are frequently associated with other ocular abnormalities. For instance, nuclear cataracts are often associated with microphthalmos (Fig. 36.5) while autosomal dominant anterior polar cataracts (Fig. 36.6) are more commonly associated with corneal guttata or astigmatism. Anterior subcapsular and anterior capsular cataracts are often associated with severe skin diseases (syndermatotic cataract).

Box 36.1

Morphological classification of infantile cataract

Fetal nuclear Opaque lens material between anterior and posterior "Y" suture that may spread into the surrounding (especially posterior) cortex and often associated with posterior capsule plaque

Cortical Anterior and/or posterior cortical opacity not involving the fetal nucleus and often associated with posterior capsule plaque

Persistent fetal vasculature A combination of one or more of the following: retrolental membrane with or without visible vessels, patent or non-patent persistent hyaloid vessel, or stretched ciliary processes

Isolated posterior capsule plaque (posterior polar) Opacity of the posterior capsule without overlying opacity in the cortex or nucleus

Posterior lentiglobus Posterior bowing of the posterior capsule with or without a pre-existing posterior capsule defect

Total Entire lens is white

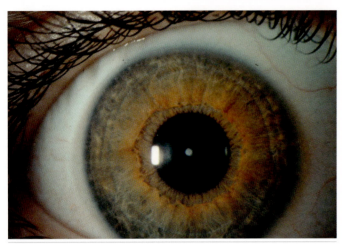

Fig. 36.1 Anterior polar cataract. A small anterior polar cataract generally results in minimal visual deprivation, but is commonly associated with anisometropic amblyopia.

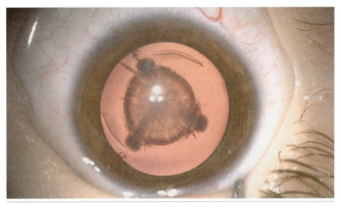

Fig. 36.2 Lamellar cataract.

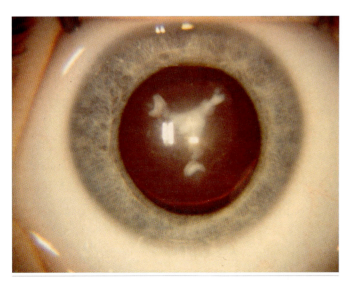

Fig. 36.3 Sutural cataract.

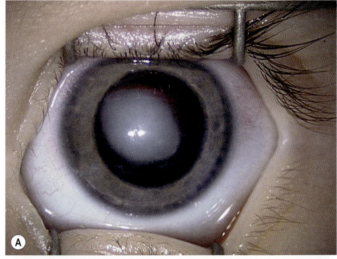

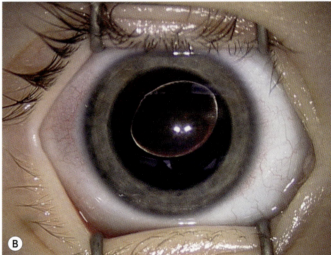

Fig. 36.4 Bilateral posterior lentiglobus. This 8-month-old child presented with lentiglobus in both eyes. (A) There is a dense cataract overlying the lentiglobus in the left eye. (B) The lens cortex is still clear over the lentiglobus in the right eye.

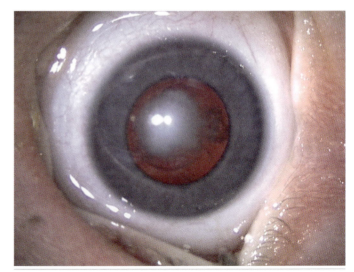

Fig. 36.5 Nuclear cataract. This child underwent a lensectomy and anterior vitrectomy in the right eye when 4 weeks of age. The lens was normal in the left eye. Both eyes had corneal diameters of 10 mm, but the axial length was only 15.74 mm in the right eye compared to 17.32 mm in the left eye.

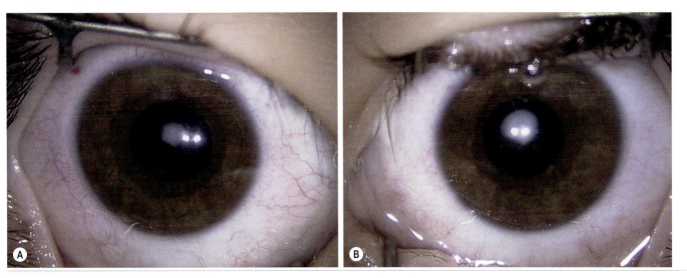

Fig. 36.6 **Autosomal dominant anterior polar cataracts.** The child's mother, sister, and brother also had bilateral anterior polar cataracts.

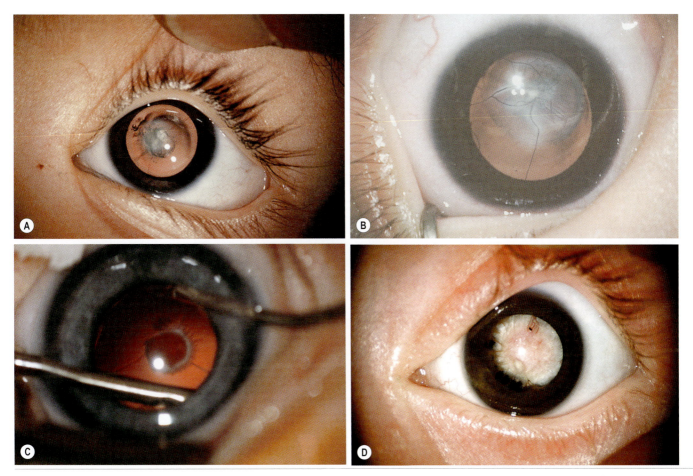

Fig. 36.7 **Persistent fetal vasculature (PFV).** (A) Mild PFV with a hyaloid vessel attaching to a retrolenticular plaque. (B) Moderate PFV with prominent iridohyaloid vessels and a large retrolenticular plaque. (C) Small vascular PFV with a "blood lake" representing a low-flow shunt centrally in an eye with PFV. (D) Severe PFV with stretching of the ciliary processes.

Partially reabsorbed cataracts in an infant boy are suggestive of Lowe's syndrome or Hallermann-Streiff syndrome. Wedge-shaped or sectional cataracts may occur with Stickler's syndrome and Conradi's syndrome and may be due to lyonization.

Persistent fetal vasculature

The term persistent fetal vasculature (PFV) describes a wide spectrum of congenital anomalies which commonly consist of a retrolental plaque (Fig. 36.7) in a microphthalmic eye

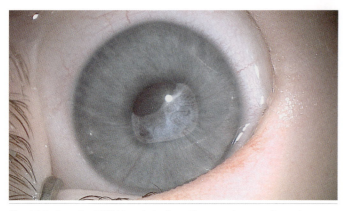

Fig. 36.8 Anterior PFV. Vascularized pupillary membrane and prominent iridohyaloid vessels in an infant with microcoria.

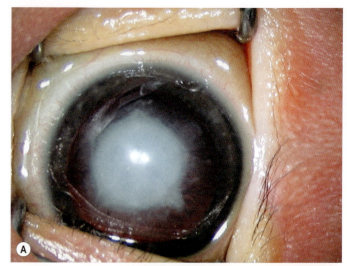

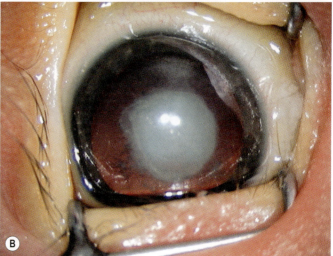

Fig. 36.9 Trisomy 21. Dense cataracts in an infant with trisomy 21.

with prominent blood vessels on the iris, a shallow anterior chamber, elongated ciliary processes, and occasionally intra-lenticular hemorrhages.[5] Less commonly, these patients may present with a vascularized pupillary membrane, microcoria, and an anterior capsular cataract (Fig. 36.8).[6] PFV is unilateral in 90% of patients. Although the lens may be clear initially, over time they usually become cataractous. The lens may undergo spontaneous absorption. In others, it becomes swollen, with loss of the anterior chamber and glaucoma. The fibrovascular plaque may bleed if cut. The retrolental plaque may contract with traction on the vitreous base and periph-eral retina. Usually the posterior pole is normal, but fibrous tissue from the hyaloid remnants may cause peripapillary tractional retinal detachment. Conditions that can mimic PFV include retinoblastoma, retinopathy of prematurity, retinal dysplasia, and posterior uveitis. The presence of microphthal-mos, a shallow anterior chamber, elongated ciliary processes, a cataract, and a retrolental opacity with a persistent hyaloid artery are all helpful in distinguishing PFV from these conditions.

Etiology

Bilateral

An etiology can be established in about 50% of children with bilateral congenital cataracts. The most common etiology in Europe and the US are autosomal dominantly inherited cata-racts. Less frequently, cataracts can be associated with trisomy 21 (Fig. 36.9), Lowe's syndrome (Fig 36.10) and Hallerman-Streiff-Francois syndrome (Fig. 36.11) (Box 36.2). Congenital rubella syndrome is a cause of cataracts where rubella immu-nization rates are low.[7]

Acquired cataracts may arise secondary to poorly controlled diabetes mellitus, the use of corticosteroids, or external beam radiation therapy (Fig. 36.12).

Unilateral

Many eyes with unilateral congenital cataracts have PFV.[8] They are infrequently associated with systemic disorders. Trauma is the most common cause of an acquired unilateral cataract in a child. Findings such as iris sphincter tears or a corneal scar can suggest the traumatic etiology (Fig. 36.13). They also may develop after laser photoablative therapy for retinopathy of prematurity (Fig. 36.14) or after intraocular surgery.[9]

History

The history should include a family history of childhood cata-racts (and an examination of both parents and any siblings), exposure to corticosteroids or radiation therapy, and ocular trauma. Comorbidities may suggest systemic disease. The age the child was first noted to squint or to have leukocoria should be noted. In children with bilateral cataracts, the parents should be asked when they first noted abnormal visual behav-ior or nystagmus. Reviewing photographs of the child is par-ticularly helpful in children with unilateral cataracts because the abnormal red reflex can be compared to the normal red reflex in the fellow eye (Fig. 36.15). The most helpful photo-graphs are taken indoors with a flash and the child looking slightly eccentrically.[10]

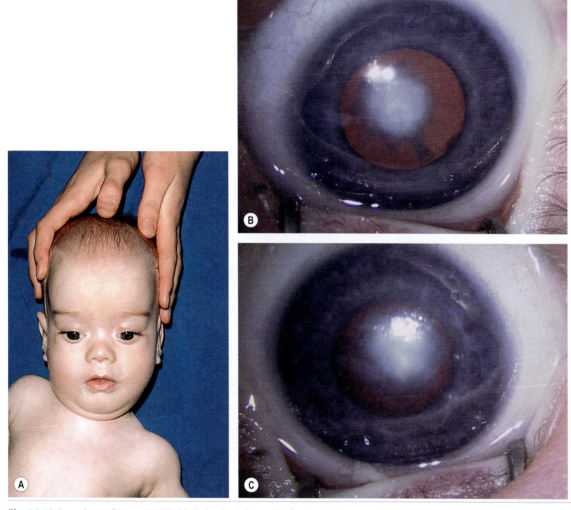

Fig. 36.10 Lowe's syndrome. (A) "Chubby" cheeks and rounded forehead. Dense nuclear cataracts in right (B) and left (C) eyes.

Ocular examination

The visual acuity of older children should be assessed using optotypes. In younger children, the ability to fix and follow with each eye should be assessed. The pupillary reflexes should be evaluated for an afferent pupillary defect suggesting a poor visual prognosis. A slit-lamp examination should be performed to evaluate the cornea, iris, and morphology of the cataract. Slit-lamp examination of the parents sometimes will identify asymptomatic cataracts that may establish the heredity (Fig. 36.16). The retina and optic disc should be assessed using indirect ophthalmoscopy. If the density of the cataract precludes an adequate view of the fundus, an ultrasound examination should be performed prior to surgery.

Laboratory work-up

A systemic investigation is not usually indicated for children with unilateral cataracts since most are isolated ocular problems, but it can be helpful with bilateral cataracts. Where rubella vaccination is not routinely performed, infants with bilateral congenital cataracts should be screened for rubella IgM titers. Male infants with cataracts, hypotonia, problems with weight gain, delayed milestones, and feeding difficulties should be screened for Lowe's syndrome by assaying urine amino acids and serum electrolytes and can be confirmed by an enzyme assay (inositol polyphosphate 5-phosphatase OCRL-1) in cultured skin fibroblasts and *OCRL* gene testing. Most cases of galactosemia are detected neonatally by routine metabolic screening; however false negatives may occur. Infants with cataracts and signs of galactosemia, such as failure-to-thrive, should undergo detailed metabolic testing. Children with cataracts and systemic findings of an intrauterine infection should be evaluated by a pediatrician (Fig. 36.17). Children with cataracts and dysmorphic features or suspected metabolic disease should be referred to a geneticist. It may be appropriate to screen children with a family history of congenital or early onset cataracts for one of the 20+ mutations known to cause autosomal dominant cataracts (http://cat-map.wustl.edu/),[11] but this is not widely available and may not influence management. Most mutations are on genes for crystallins and connexins.[12] There can be marked heterogeneity in autosomal dominant cataracts (Fig. 36.18).

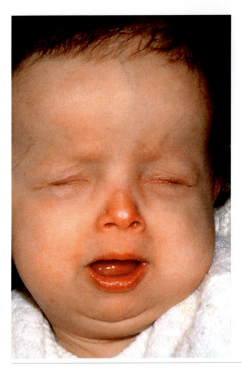

Fig. 36.11 Hallerman-Streiff-Francois syndrome. Note the receding hairline and the vascular, small, upturned nose.

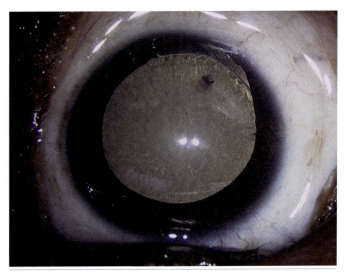

Fig. 36.12 Posterior subcapsular cataract. This 4-year-old child was diagnosed with bilateral retinoblastoma when age 10 months. After treatment with chemotherapy, external beam radiation, and cryotherapy he developed a dense posterior subcapsular cataract in his right eye. After cataract extraction with implantation of an intraocular lens his visual acuity improved from counting fingers to 20/60 in his right eye.

Box 36.2

Etiology of cataracts in childhood

Idiopathic

Intrauterine infection

Rubella

Varicella

Toxoplasmosis

Herpes simplex

Uveitis or acquired infection

Pars planitis

Juvenile idiopathic arthritis

Toxocara canis

Drug-induced

Corticosteroids

Chlorpromazine

Metabolic disorders

Galactosemia

Galactokinase deficiency

Hypocalcemia

Hypoglycemia

Diabetes mellitus

Mannosidosis

Hyperferritinemia

Trauma

Accidental

Laser photocoagulation

Non-accidental

Radiation-induced

Other diseases

Microphthalmia

Aniridia

Retinitis pigmentosa

Persistent hyperplastic primary vitreous

Retinopathy of prematurity

Endophthalmitis

Inherited

Autosomal dominant

Autosomal recessive

X-linked

Mental retardation

See text

Inherited with systemic abnormalities

Chromosomal

Trisomy 21

Turner's syndrome

Trisomy 13

Trisomy 18

Cri du chat syndrome

Craniofacial syndromes

Cerebro-oculofacial skeletal syndrome

Renal disease

Lowe's syndrome

Alport's syndrome

Hallermann-Streiff-François

Skeletal disease

Smith-Lemli-Opitz

Conradi's syndrome

Weill-Marchesani syndrome

Stickler's syndrome

Syndactyly, polydactyly, or digital anomalies

Bardet-Biedl syndrome

Rubinstein-Taybi syndrome

Neurometabolic disease

Zellweger's syndrome

Meckel-Gruber syndrome

Marinesco-Sjögren syndrome

Infantile neuronal ceroid-lipofuscinosis

Muscular disease

Myotonic dystrophy

Dermatological

Crystalline cataract and uncombable hair

Cockayne's syndrome

Rothmund-Thomson

Atopic dermatitis

Incontinentia pigmenti

Progeria

Congenitals ichthyosis

Ectodermal dysplasia

Werner's syndrome

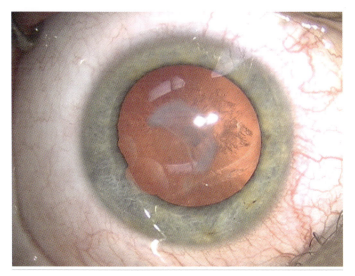

Fig. 36.13 Traumatic cataract. This teenager developed a hyphema, iris sphincter tears, and an anterior subcapsular cataract in his right eye after a paintball injury.

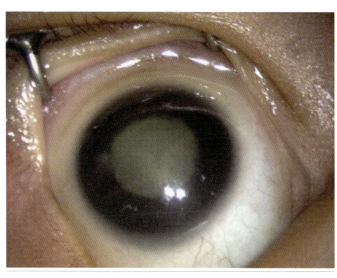

Fig. 36.14 Cataract following diode laser retinal photoablation. This 4-month-old baby developed a dense cataract immediately following diode laser photoablation of the peripheral retina to treat retinopathy of prematurity.

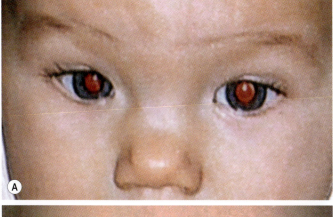

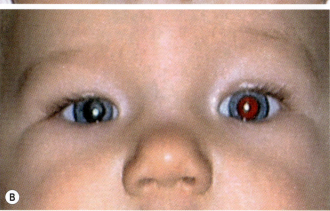

Fig. 36.15 (A) Personal photograph of an infant taken when 4 months of age showing normal red reflexes in both eyes. (B) Personal photograph of the same infant 2 months later showing loss of the red reflex in the right eye. At the time of cataract surgery, the right eye was found to have a dense central cataract and persistent fetal vasculature.

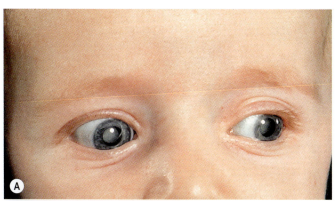

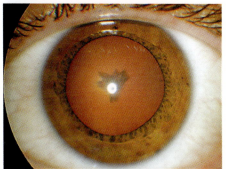

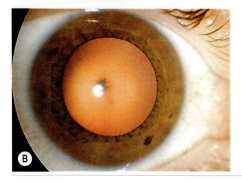

Fig. 36.16 Autosomal dominant cataracts. (A) Three-month-old infant with bilateral dense cataracts. (B) His mother has mild cataracts that have never been operated on.

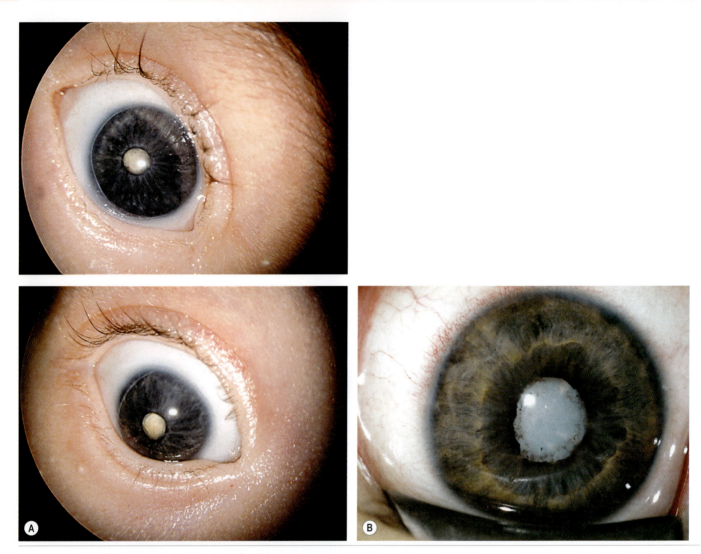

Fig. 36.17 Congenital cataract in intrauterine infections. (A) Bilateral cataracts and microphthalmos in a child with congenital toxoplasmosis syndrome. (B) Congenital cataract in a child with congenital varicella syndrome. If there is a cataract in a child with an intrauterine infection, it is very likely that there is severe intraocular disease.

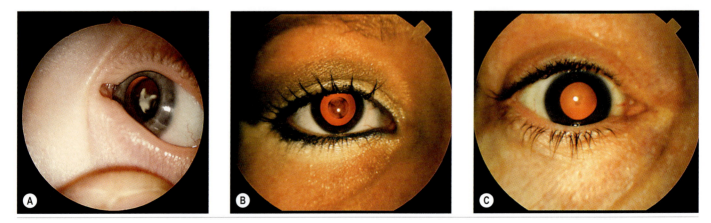

Fig. 36.18 Heterogeneity in autosomal dominant cataracts. (A) A dense central cataract in an infant who presented with leukocoria in both eyes. (B) His asymptomatic mother had mild lamellar cataracts in both eyes. Her vision is good enough to drive a car. (C) His grandmother had visually insignificant lamellar cataracts in both eyes.

Management

Non-surgical: patching, dilation

Although dense bilateral congenital cataracts should be removed during infancy, partial cataracts should only be removed after assessment of their morphology and the visual behavior. Conservative management is indicated until the child's visual acuity can be accurately assessed (Fig. 36.19). The visual prognosis of bilateral incomplete cataracts correlates better with the density than with the size of the opacity. Nuclear cataracts, although smaller in size than lamellar cataracts, have a worse visual prognosis. If major blood vessels in the fundus cannot be distinguished through the central portion of the cataract, significant visual deprivation can be expected.

Surgical

Surgery for visually significant congenital cataracts should be performed during infancy. Most surgeons prefer to wait until 4 weeks of age since there is evidence that cataract surgery during the first month of life is associated with an increased risk of glaucoma.[13] Simultaneous bilateral cataract surgery may

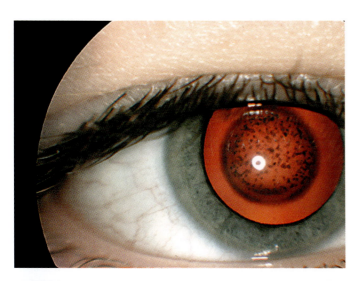

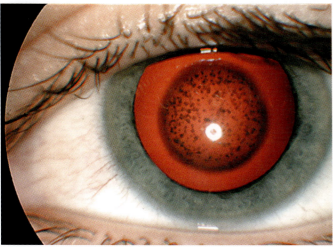

Fig. 36.19 Bilateral symmetrical lamellar cataracts in retroillumination.
The acuity is 20/30 in both eyes.

be considered in neonates and infants particularly if they have comorbidities that increase the risk of general anesthesia.[14] However, the risk of bilateral endophthalmitis should be discussed. Precautions should be taken to reduce this risk by using different trays of instruments for each eye, disposable cannulas, redraping between eyes, and using different lots of irrigating solution and medications for each eye. If sequential bilateral cataract surgery is performed, only a short interval should elapse between the removal of the two lenses to reduce amblyopia in the second operated eye.

Surgical techniques

A lensectomy and anterior vitrectomy should be performed in infants with a closed eye system. By creating a primary posterior capsulotomy and anterior vitrectomy, the number of secondary operations can be greatly reduced and the clear visual axis facilitates retinoscopy. In children 6 months of age or older, I recommend lens aspiration, a primary posterior capsulotomy, anterior vitrectomy, and implantation of an intraocular lens (Fig. 36.20). In older children, who are less susceptible to amblyopia and in whom posterior capsular opacification may be delayed for several years, a primary posterior capsulotomy and anterior vitrectomy may be omitted if it is possible to follow the child at regular intervals and the child will cooperate with a YAG laser capsulotomy. Phacoemulsification is not necessary to remove a pediatric cataract.

Optical correction

One of the major obstacles in children following cataract surgery is optical correction of the induced aphakia.

Contact lenses

Contact lenses remain the standard method of optically correcting infant aphakia (Fig. 36.21). Rigid gas-permeable contact lenses are well suited during infancy because of the wide range of available powers, low cost, ability to correct large astigmatic errors, and ease of insertion and removal.[15] The biggest obstacle is the greater expertise required to fit them. Silicone lenses have the advantage of being worn on an extended wear basis, but are more expensive and are only available in a limited range of powers and sizes. The frequent loss of lenses and the need to change the lens power as the eye elongates necessitates frequent lens replacements. Parents are advised to remove the lenses if the eye becomes inflamed or irritated, or if excessive discharge develops. Inadequate care can result in keratitis and corneal scarring. Poor compliance with contact lens wear is commonly due to reduced vision in the aphakic eye or poor patient cooperation, rather than complications from their use.

Spectacles

Aphakic spectacles (Fig. 36.22) are better tolerated than contact lenses by some children with bilateral aphakia especially between 18 months and 4 years of age. Aphakic spectacles have the cosmetic advantage of improving the appearance of microphthalmic eyes because of the magnification they induce which also helps those with low vision. Secondary strabismus may be reduced by the prismatic effect of spectacles.

Intraocular lenses

Intraocular lens (IOL) use in young children is complicated by the increased number of additional intraocular operations

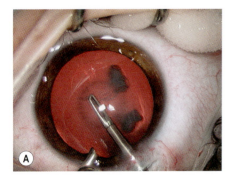
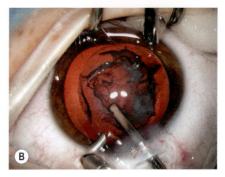
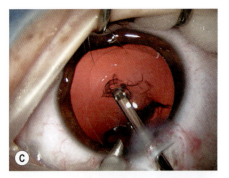
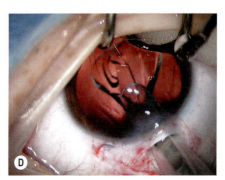
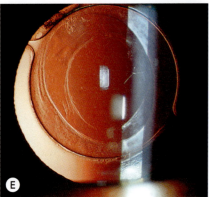
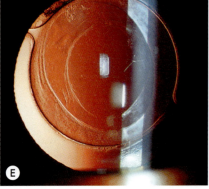

Fig. 36.20 Extracapsular cataract extraction and intraocular lens implantation in a 3-year-old child with a lamellar cataract. After (A) performing a manual anterior capsulorrhexis, (B) the lens cortex is aspirated, (C) a primary posterior capsutomy and anterior vitrectomy is performed, and (D) a foldable acrylic lens is then implanted in the capsular bag. (E) PMMA intraocular lens (IOL) in an infant's eye. The central posterior capsulotomy is smaller than the anterior capsulotomy which facilitated in-the-bag fixation of the IOL.

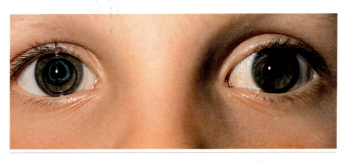

Fig. 36.21 Aphakic contact lenses. The child has successfully worn contact lenses since undergoing lensectomies at 3 weeks of age.

required to remove visual axis opacities and the difficulty of predicting the lens power.[16,17] In most young children, an IOL power is chosen that undercorrects the eye in anticipation of a myopic shift developing.[18] While it is better to implant an IOL "in the bag" when the cataract is removed (Video 36.1), IOLs can be implanted as a secondary procedure in the sulcus or the capsular bag. If there is a large Soemmerring's ring, the IOL can be implanted into the capsular bag by opening the

Soemmerring's ring, aspirating its contents, and positioning the IOL between the capsular leaflets (Video 36.2).[19] It is important to leave a 360 degree rim of capsule at the time of the lensectomy to facilitate secondary IOL implantation into the capsular bag later in childhood. If there are insufficient capsular remnants available for in-the-bag fixation, the IOL can be implanted into the sulcus if there is a continuous rim of lens capsule. IOLs offer the advantage of a constant optical correction. An overcorrection with spectacles or contact lenses is usually needed to fully focus the eye.

Management of amblyopia

Whatever the aphakic correction, frequent re-examinations are necessary. Each examination includes assessment of fixation behavior or grating acuity in preverbal children and optotype acuity in verbal children to detect or manage amblyopia. With amblyopia, occlusion therapy of the preferred eye should be initiated. Frequent retinoscopy and adjustments in the refractive correction are imperative. The importance of encouragement and support for the parents is vital to a successful rehabilitation program.

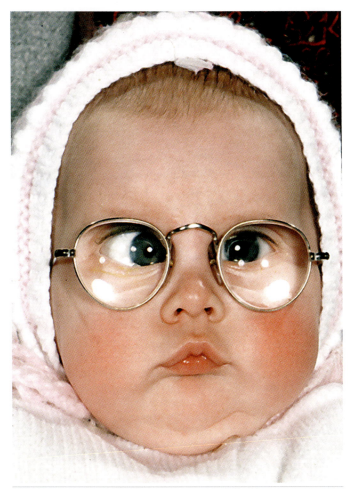

Fig. 36.22 Aphakic spectacles. Aphakic spectacles are safe and the power can be easily changed, but they have optical and cosmetic disadvantages.

Unilateral cataract

The management of a unilateral congenital cataract is challenging. Although such eyes may be successfully rehabilitated, many do not achieve a visual acuity compatible with reading[20] and the importance of occlusion to the visual goal should be emphasized to the parents.

If a decision is made to perform surgery on a unilateral congenital cataract, prompt surgical intervention is important. Surgery after the first 6 weeks of life is less likely to result in good visual outcome.[21] Immediate and continued optical correction of the aphakic eye and monitored occlusion therapy of the fellow eye is crucial.

Occluding the fellow eye 50–70% of all waking hours throughout early childhood is associated with the best visual outcomes in aphakic eyes.[22] Excessive patching may result in the development of subtle visual deficits in the fellow eye and impaired binocularity. Although "binocular vision" is rare in children treated for unilateral congenital cataracts, it can be achieved.[23]

Bilateral and traumatic cataracts

Occlusion therapy is not usually necessary in older children with bilateral congenital cataracts or children with unilateral traumatic cataracts who are treated promptly.

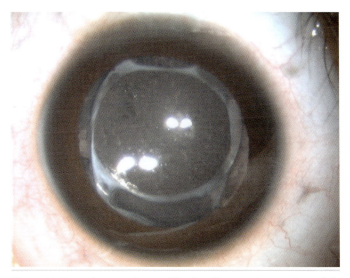

Fig. 36.23 Posterior capsular opacification. The posterior capsule was left intact at the time of cataract surgery and IOL implantation. The posterior capsule was too thickened to open with a YAG laser so a membranectomy was performed.

Postoperative complications

Complications after cataract surgery in children are more common than in adults. Some are preventable by careful attention to surgical technique and postoperative care; others arise due to the intrinsic abnormalities in these eyes or the more exuberant inflammatory response with surgery on an immature eye.

Visual axis opacities

Visual axis opacities may arise from fibrin forming a pupillary membrane, opacification of the residual posterior lens capsule or lens re-proliferation extending into the visual axis. It is particularly common after IOL implantation (Fig. 36.23). Because of the high incidence in children, a primary posterior capsulotomy and anterior vitrectomy is recommended. In older children, the posterior capsule can be left intact and a YAG laser capsulotomy can be used to open the posterior capsule when it opacifies,[24] typically about 2 years after cataract surgery. The procedure should not be delayed because of amblyopia and the increased difficulty of opening a thickened posterior capsule. If the posterior capsule is too dense for a YAG laser, a membranectomy may be performed with a vitrector. A variable Soemmerring's ring develops in all children's eyes after cataract surgery. In most cases, the reproliferating lens material is confined to the retro-iridial space, but it may extend into the pupil. The IOL prevents the pupillary margins of the anterior and posterior capsular leaflets from fusing together allowing reproliferating lens material to extend into the pupillary space. In these instances, intraocular surgery may be necessary to clear the visual axis. Anterior capsulorrhexes that are too small may also undergo phimosis (Fig. 36.24), which can be treated with intraocular surgery or a YAG laser capsulotomy.

Amblyopia (see Chapter 70)

Amblyopia is nearly universal in children with congenital cataracts and common in children with developmental cataracts

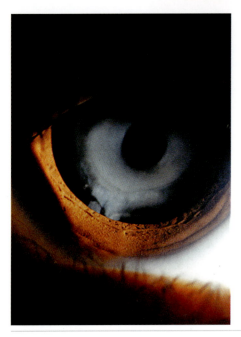

Fig. 36.24 Anterior capsular phimosis. The capsulorrhexis has undergone progressive phimosis which makes it difficult to perform retinoscopy.

during the first 7 years of life, particularly in children with unilateral congenital cataracts. It arises as a result of the retina receiving a defocused image during the critical period of visual development. Uncorrected aphakia or induced anisometropia can exacerbate amblyopia even after the removal of a cataract. It can be treated by part-time patching or optical defocus of the preferred eye. Optical defocus in a child with bilateral aphakia wearing contact lenses can be achieved by delaying insertion of the contact lens in the preferred eye for a specified time each day.

Glaucoma (see Chapter 37)

Glaucoma may arise during the early postoperative period or years later. It is a serious problem and is difficult to manage.

Pupillary block glaucoma has a higher incidence in neonates following lensectomy due to vitreous prolapse into the anterior chamber or pupillary membrane formation. It can be prevented by performing an anterior vitrectomy (ideally one-third of the vitreous) and atropinizing the pupil postoperatively. Affected patients usually have ocular pain, corneal edema, and iris bombé but some infants do not have the pain. Glaucoma is one of the most common late complications of pediatric cataract surgery, particularly in children undergoing cataract surgery during early infancy and in eyes with PFV. The risk of glaucoma increases twofold by performing cataract surgery at 1 month compared to 2 months of age.[25] Unlike infantile-onset glaucoma, which is usually associated with readily detectable signs and symptoms, juvenile-onset glaucoma is usually more subtle in its onset and the intraocular pressure should be assessed at each outpatient examination. Rebound tonometry is better tolerated by young children than applanation tonometry.[26] Attention should be paid to cupping of the optic disc, an increase in axial length or the corneal diameter, or a rapid myopic shift.

Strabismus

Strabismus is often the presenting sign of a child with a unilateral cataract and is also common in bilateral cataracts. Esotropia is more commonly observed in children with congenital cataracts, while exotropia is more frequently observed in children with acquired cataracts. Even more children develop strabismus after surgical and optical treatment of cataracts. Strabismus is particularly troubling to older children with acquired cataracts if there is a delay in the removal of the cataract or optical correction; they can develop diplopia even after the eyes are surgically aligned due to a disturbance of central fusion.

Irregular pupil

An irregular pupil is sometimes a complication of infantile cataract surgery. The iris sphincter may be damaged by the vitreous cutter. In other instances, the iris may prolapse through the scleral incision during surgery and become atrophic often due to faulty wound construction, most noticeable in children with lightly colored irides.

Strands of vitreous extending to the surgical incision may cause peaking of the pupil. This may be averted by turning off the infusion line before removing the vitreous-cutting instrument from the eye, maintaining a low flow of irrigating solution, and minimizing the number of times the vitreous-cutting instrument is inserted and removed from the eye. Even when the pupil is round after cataract surgery, it frequently is less reactive to light and pharmacological dilation. Rigid pupils are common in children who undergo a lensectomy during infancy.

Heterochromia iridis

Cataract surgery during infancy is commonly associated with increased iris pigmentation in the operated eye (Fig. 36.25). This is likely due to the release of prostaglandins following cataract surgery.[27]

Endophthalmitis

Bacterial endophthalmitis is an uncommon, but devastating complication after cataract surgery.[28] A concurrent nasolacrimal duct obstruction, upper respiratory infection, or periorbital skin disease increases the risk. The most common organisms causing it in children are *Staphylococcus aureus* and *Streptococcus pneumoniae*.

Even though most cases are diagnosed during the early postoperative days, the visual prognosis is poor. In one series, 65% of affected eyes ended up with no light perception despite aggressive treatment with intravitreal and systemic antibiotics.[28] This complication can be minimized by using strict sterile techniques and delaying surgery for children with ocular infections. Intracameral or subconjunctival antibiotics at the end of cataract surgery may reduce the incidence of this complication.

Retinal hemorrhages and detachments

A hemorrhagic retinopathy develops in some infants after a lensectomy and anterior vitrectomy. In most cases, this consists of flame-shaped hemorrhages in the posterior pole that resolve without sequelae in weeks.[29] Occasionally, a hemorrhage may

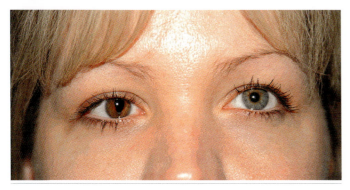

Fig. 36.25 Heterochromia iridis. This 32-year-old woman underwent a lensectomy in her right eye when 1 year of age. The iris tends to become darker in the operated eye.

occur in the fovea and result in a severe reduction of vision. In these cases, even after the hemorrhage has resolved, the visual acuity may remain reduced by amblyopia.

Retinal detachments are infrequent and usually occur decades after the removal of a congenital cataract. They are particularly common in developmentally delayed children following cataract surgery due to self-inflicted trauma. Retinal detachments are frequently bilateral, and the visualization of the retinal breaks may be hampered by miotic pupils and Soemmerring's rings.

Cystoid macular edema

Cystoid macular edema is rare in children.

Corneal edema

Corneal edema after cataract surgery usually resolves in a few days. In most cases it is probably caused by prolongation of the surgical procedure. It may occur secondary to detergent or chemicals left on the surgical instruments or cannulas.[30] Disposable cannulas should be used whenever possible and toxic chemicals such as formaldehyde should not be used to clean instruments used for intraocular surgery.

Visual outcomes

The visual results after the surgical removal of pediatric cataracts have improved dramatically. Improvements in visual results may be attributed to improved screening, better surgical techniques, and the increased use of IOLs.

The visual results depend on a number of factors, including:

1. The age of onset of the cataracts
2. The age when surgery is performed
3. Associated ocular and systemic conditions
4. Compliance with optical and patching therapy.

Children who develop cataracts after full visual development usually have an excellent visual prognosis.

Many children with early onset bilateral cataracts have an excellent visual outcome with immediate treatment. However, if treatment is delayed, many remain visually impaired due to amblyopia.

Early onset unilateral cataracts have the worst visual prognosis, although they can be associated with a good visual outcome if treatment is initiated early and patching and optical correction is maintained throughout early childhood.

Concomitant ocular abnormalities such as corneal opacities, glaucoma, retinal abnormalities, and nystagmus worsen the visual prognosis. Gross stereopsis may develop on rare occasions in a child after unilateral congenital, especially unilateral, cataract surgery.

References

1. Rahi JS, Dezateux C. Measuring and interpreting the incidence of congenital ocular anomalies: lessons from a national study of congenital cataract in the UK. Invest Ophthalmol Vis Sci 2001; 42: 1444–8.
2. Lambert SR, Lynn MJ, Reeves R, et al. Is there a latent period for the surgical treatment of children with dense bilateral congenital cataracts? J AAPOS 2006; 10: 30–6.
3. Wilson ME, Trivedi RH, Morrison DG, et al. Infant Aphakia Treatment Study: Video evaluation of cataract morphology in eyes with monocular cataracts. J AAPOS 2011; 15: 421–6.
4. Amaya L, Taylor D, Russell-Eggitt I, et al. The morphology and natural history of childhood cataracts. Surv Ophthalmol 2003; 48: 125–44.
5. Goldberg MF. Persistent fetal vasculature (PFV): an integrated interpretation of signs and symptoms associated with persistent hyperplastic primary vitreous (PHPV). LIV Edward Jackson Memorial Lecture. Am J Ophthalmol 1997; 124: 587–626.
6. Lambert SR, Lenhart PD, Buckley EM, Zhang Q. Recurrence of congenital fibrovascular pupillary membranes following surgical excision. Ophthalmology 2010; 199: 634–41.
7. Lambert SR. Congenital rubella syndrome: the end is in sight. Br J Ophthalmol 2007; 91: 1418–19.
8. Mullner-Eidenbock A, Amon M, Moser E, Klebermass N. Persistent fetal vasculature and minimal fetal vascular remnants: a frequent cause of unilateral congenital cataracts. Ophthalmology 2004; 111: 906–13.
9. Lambert SR, Capone A, Jr., Cingle KA, Drack AV. Cataract and phthisis bulbi after laser photoablation for threshold retinopathy of prematurity. Am J Ophthalmol 2000; 129: 585–91.
10. Sawhney GK, Hutchinson AK, Lambert SR. The value of serial personal photographs in timing the onset of unilateral cataracts in children. J AAPOS 2009; 13: 459–62.
11. Shiels A, Bennett TM, Hejtmancik JF. Cat-Map: putting cataract on the map. Mol Vis 2010; 16: 2007–15.
12. Hejtmancik JF. Congenital cataracts and their molecular genetics. Semin Cell Dev Biol 2008; 19: 134–49.
13. Vishwanath M, Cheong-Leen R, Taylor D et al. Is early surgery for congenital cataract a risk factor for glaucoma? Br J Ophthalmol 2004; 88: 905–10.
14. Dave H, Phoenix V, Becker ER, Lambert SR. Simultaneous vs sequential bilateral cataract surgery for infants with congenital cataracts: visual outcomes, adverse events, and economic costs. Arch Ophthalmol 2010; 128: 1050–4.
15. Amos CF, Lambert SR, Ward MA. Rigid gas permeable contact lens correction of aphakia following congenital cataract removal during infancy. J Pediatr Ophthalmol Strabismus 1992; 29: 243–5.
16. Lambert SR, Buckley E, Drews-Botsch C, et al. A randomized clinical trial comparing contact lens with intraocular lens correction of monocular aphakia during infancy: grating acuity and adverse events at age 1 year. Arch Ophthalmol 2010; 128: 810–18.
17. VanderVeen DK, Nizam A, Lynn M, et al. Predictability of IOL calculation and early refractive status in the Infant Aphakia Treatment Study. Arch Ophthalmol Arch Ophthalmol 2012; 130: 293–9.
18. Plager DA, Kipfer H, Sprunger DT et al. Refractive change in pediatric pseudophakia: 6-year follow-up. J Cataract Refract Surg 2002; 28: 810–15.

19. Wilson ME, Jr., Englert JA, Greenwald MJ. In-the-bag secondary intraocular lens implantation in children. J AAPOS 1999; 3: 350–5.

20. Birch EE, Cheng C, Vu C, Stager DR, Jr. Oral reading after treatment of dense congenital unilateral cataract. J AAPOS 2010; 14: 227–31.

21. Birch EE, Stager DR. The critical period for surgical treatment of dense congenital unilateral cataract. Invest Ophthalmol Vis Sci 1996; 37: 1532–8.

22. Lambert SR, Plager DA, Lynn MJ, Wilson ME. Visual outcome following the reduction or cessation of patching therapy after early unilateral cataract surgery. Arch Ophthalmol 2008; 126: 1071–4.

23. Gregg FM, Parks MM. Stereopsis after congenital monocular cataract extraction. Am J Ophthalmol 1992; 114: 314–17.

24. Hutcheson KA, Drack AV, Ellish NJ, Lambert SR. Anterior hyaloid face opacification after pediatric Nd:YAG laser capsulotomy. J AAPOS 1999; 3: 303–7.

25. Beck AD, Freedman SF, Lynn MJ, Bothun E, Neely NE, Lambert SR for the Infant Aphakia Treatment Study Group. Glaucoma-related adverse events in the Infant Aphakia Treatment Study. Arch Ophthalmol 2012; 130: 300–5.

26. Lundvall AH, Svedberg H, et al. Application of the ICare rebound tonometer in healthy infants. J Glaucoma 2011; 20: 7–9.

27. Lenart TD, Drack AV, Tarnuzzer RW, et al. Heterochromia after pediatric cataract surgery. J AAPOS 2000; 4: 40–5.

28. Wheeler DT, Stager DR, Weakley DR, Jr. Endophthalmitis following pediatric intraocular surgery for congenital cataracts and congenital glaucoma. J Pediatr Ophthalmol Strabismus 1992; 29: 139–41.

29. Christiansen SP, Munoz M, Capo H. Retinal hemorrhage following lensectomy and anterior vitrectomy in children. J Pediatr Ophthalmol Strabismus 1993; 30: 24–7.

30. Lambert SR. Toxic anterior segment syndrome after pediatric cataract surgery. J AAPOS 2010; 14: 381–2.

CHAPTER **37**

Childhood glaucoma

Maria Papadopoulos · John L Brookes · Peng T Khaw

Introduction

Glaucoma in children is a rare, potentially blinding condition characterized by elevated intraocular pressure (IOP) and optic disc cupping. Successful control of IOP is crucial but challenging and most often achieved surgically, with medical therapy playing a supportive role. To maximize vision, the correction of ametropia and amblyopia therapy are integral in management.

Classification

There are many classifications of childhood glaucomas. However, they can simply be classified as *primary*, where a developmental abnormality of the anterior chamber angle only exists, and *secondary*, where aqueous outflow is reduced due to congenital or acquired ocular diseases or systemic disorders (Box 37.1). Classification will change as we learn more about the genetic and biologic basis of each condition.

Clinical findings

A child suspected of having glaucoma will usually present in one of three ways:

1. Signs of elevated IOP (e.g. buphthalmos)
2. With a predisposing condition (e.g. aphakia), or
3. As part of screening where there is a family history of pediatric glaucoma.

The clinical manifestations are highly variable and largely determined by the magnitude of the elevated IOP and the age of onset. Very high IOP can present dramatically in a newborn with cloudy, enlarged corneas. A slower rise in IOP results in a less acute presentation with buphthalmos but no corneal clouding or photophobia. The timing of the pressure rise influences the clinical features owing to the limited potential of the young eye to deform.

Glaucoma from any cause in a neonate and infant is associated with the *classic triad of lacrimation, blepharospasm, and photophobia* due to corneal edema from elevated IOP. These signs are not specific but are suggestive of glaucoma and may appear before the hazy cornea (most frequent physical sign) and buphthalmos become obvious. Beyond the age of 3 years, children are more likely to present with progressive myopia, strabismus, or after having failed school vision testing.

Unique features of glaucoma in infancy

Generalized ocular enlargement

Buphthalmos refers to a prominent, enlarged eye due to elevated IOP from any cause in infancy (Fig. 37.1). The young eye is vulnerable to the effects of increased IOP due to corneal and scleral collagen immaturity. The potential for corneal enlargement usually ceases by the age of 3 although the sclera remains deformable until the age of 10. As the IOP rises, Descemet's membrane eventually ruptures with one edge usually retracting as a scroll to form a ridge known as *Haab's striae* (Fig. 37.2). As the underlying endothelium is torn, localized or diffuse corneal edema results from aqueous influx into the stroma causing a sudden cloudiness (Fig. 37.3). With successful lowering of IOP, corneal clouding clears first in the periphery (Figs 37.4 and 37.5). Photophobia may persist for several years with normalization of IOP due to the Haab's striae.

Reversible optic nerve cupping

Glaucomatous optic disk cupping in infants differs from that in adults in two ways:

1. It occurs *earlier and more rapidly*, with severe excavation possible at birth.
2. It is often *reversible* if IOP reduction occurs before irreversible nerve atrophy. The younger the child is the greater the potential for disk cupping reversal.

Box 37.1

Classification of childhood glaucomas

1. Primary

(a) Primary congenital glaucoma (isolated trabeculodysgenesis)

(b) Juvenile open angle glaucoma

(c) Angle closure glaucoma

2. Secondary

Anterior segment dysgenesis

Axenfeld-Rieger anomaly

Peters' anomaly

Iris hypoplasia

Congenital ectropion uveae

Microcornea

Lens related

Congenital cataract surgery

   (i) Aphakia

   (ii) Pseudophakia

Ectopia lentis et pupillae

Microspherophakia

Lenticonus

Other ocular disease/treatment

Aniridia

Persistent hyperplastic primary vitreous

Retinopathy of prematurity

Microphthalmos

Trauma related – hyphema, angle recession

Postretinal detachment surgery

Oculodermal melanocytosis (nevus of Ota)

Sclerocornea

Posterior polymorphous dystrophy

Phacomatoses

Sturge-Weber syndrome (complete = facial *and* leptomeningeal hemangioma) (incomplete = facial *or* leptomeningeal hemangioma)

Klippel-Trenaunay-Weber syndrome

Neurofibromatosis (von Recklinghausen's disease)

von-Hippel-Lindau syndrome

Inflammatory/infective disease

Juvenile idiopathic arthritis

Idiopathic uveitis

Sarcoidosis

Congenital rubella

Congenital syphilis

Cytomegalovirus

Herpes simplex disease

Ocular tumors

Benign – iris cysts, juvenile xanthogranuloma

Malignant – retinoblastoma, leukemia, medulloepithelioma

Metabolic disease

Oculocerebrorenal syndrome (Lowe's syndrome)

Homocystinuria

Mucopolysaccharidoses, e.g. Hurler's syndrome

Cystinosis

Chromosomal disorders

Down's syndrome (trisomy 21)

Patau's syndrome (trisomy 13–15)

Turner's syndrome (XO)

Prader-Willi syndrome

Connective tissue abnormalities

Marfan's syndrome

Weill-Marchesani syndrome

Homocystinuria

Ehler-Danlos syndrome

Sulphite oxidase deficiency

Osteogenesis imperfecta

Stickler's syndrome

Other systemic congenital disorders

Rubinstein-Taybi syndrome

Pierre Robin syndrome

Cutis marmorata telangiectasia congenita

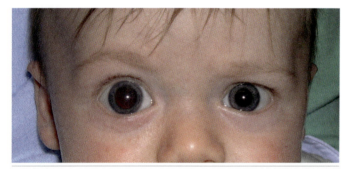

Fig. 37.1 Infant with right buphthalmos.

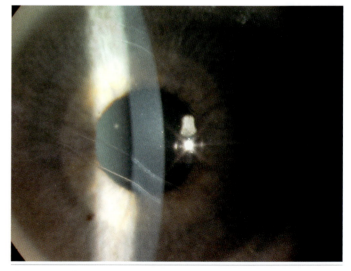

Fig. 37.2 Haab's striae – pathognomonic of glaucoma in infancy in the presence of enlarged corneas.

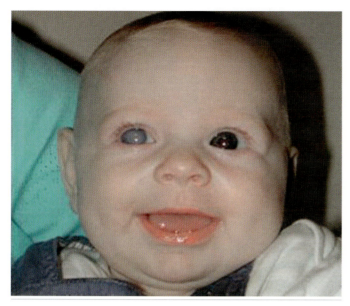

Fig. 37.3 Right stromal edema from ruptured Descemet's membrane due to elevated IOP.

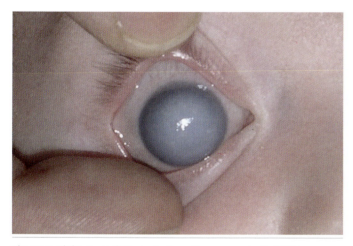

Fig. 37.4 Right corneal stromal edema from uncontrolled IOP before surgery.

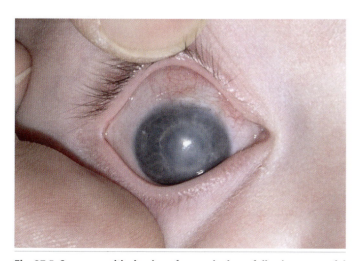

Fig. 37.5 Same eye with clearing of corneal edema following successful lowering of IOP with trabeculectomy.

Box 37.2

Differential diagnosis of childhood glaucoma

Corneal enlargement

(no Descemet's membrane splits, corneal edema, non-progressive, symmetrical)

Megalocornea (optic disk and axial length are normal, follow-up necessary to exclude glaucoma and refractive amblyopia)

Megalophthalmos

Axial myopia (physiologic cupping associated with tilted disk, peripapillary scleral crescent)

Osteogenesis imperfecta

Connective tissue disorders

Corneal splits

(no corneal enlargement, normal optic nerve)

Birth trauma (history)

Hydrops (history)

Corneal edema or opacity

(usually no corneal enlargement unless associated with glaucoma, which is rare)

Birth trauma

Congenital corneal dystrophies e.g. CHED

Sclerocornea

Metabolic, e.g. mucopolysaccharidoses, cystinosis

Infective, e.g. congenital rubella, herpes simplex keratitis

Watering and 'red eye'

(no Descemet's membrane splits, corneal edema or enlargement, normal optic nerve)

Conjunctivitis

Nasolacrimal duct obstruction

Corneal epithelial defect, very occasionally dystrophy

Ocular inflammation

Optic nerve abnormalities

Congenital optic nerve pits

Optic disk colobomata

Physiologic cupping in large optic disks

Differential diagnosis

The differential diagnosis of glaucoma in children is broad. Remember that the IOP is normal and the signs will not be progressive in non-glaucoma cases. A list of differential diagnoses is outlined in Box 37.2.

Classification

Primary childhood glaucoma

Primary congenital glaucoma

Primary congenital glaucoma (PCG) is bilateral in 70–80% and usually manifests in the first year of life. Diagnosis is based on the finding of *isolated trabeculodysgenesis*.

Demographics

PCG is the commonest glaucoma in infancy but has an incidence of only about 1 in 10 000–20 000 live births in Western countries.[1] The highest reported incidence is 1 : 1 250 in Slovakian gypsies. Parental consanguinity is responsible for the higher prevalence in certain ethnic and religious groups. PCG occurs more frequently in males than females at a ratio of between 2 : 1 and 2.5 : 1.

Genetics

Most cases of PCG are sporadic. A family history of glaucoma is reported in 10–40% of cases associated with autosomal recessive inheritance and variable penetrance ranging from 40% to 100%.

GCL3A is the major locus for PCG, accounting for 85–90% of all familial cases. It has been mapped to the short arm of chromosome 2p21, the GLC3B locus to chromosome 1p36 and GLC3C to chromosome 14q24.3 with more loci speculated to exist.[2] The primary molecular defect underlying the majority of cases of PCG is related to mutations of the *CYP1B1 gene* associated with the GLC3A locus[3] but its frequency varies according to populations, ranging from 100% in Slovakian Roma to 20% in the Japanese. It encodes for enzyme cytochrome P4501B1 which is postulated to participate in the development and function of the eye. Genotype–phenotype correlations have been reported with specific mutations possibly associated with certain angle abnormalities.

The risk of PCG in siblings and offspring in patients with no history of parental consanguinity is low (<5%), but it is prudent to examine the siblings and offspring of patients, especially in the first 6 months of life.

Pathogenesis

The pathogenesis of PCG remains uncertain. The *immature angle* appearance results from the developmental arrest of tissues derived from cranial neural crest cells in the third trimester of gestation. Obstruction to outflow was thought to be due to the presence of an impermeable membrane (*Barkan's membrane*); this has never been verified histopathologically. It is now thought to be due to thick, compacted trabecular sheets.[4]

Gonioscopic findings

The characteristic gonioscopic appearance includes a flat iris insertion and the absence of an angle recess. Changes seen due to the physical stretching of structures from elevated IOP include:

1. A thin and hypopigmented iris stroma
2. Peripheral scalloping of the posterior pigmented iris layer
3. Easily visible, hyperemic iris vessels with circumferential vessels running tortuously in the peripheral iris or on the ciliary body (Fig. 37.6).

In unilateral disease, the fellow eye usually shows gonioscopic findings of PCG with a large corneal diameter and axial length, but the disk is normal and the unilaterality may represent drainage angles that have opened late leading to *spontaneous arrest* of the disease. The fellow eye of "unilateral" cases must be followed as closely as the affected eye as it may relapse at any stage. Parents need to be warned that surgery may eventually be needed for both eyes even in what appears to be a "unilateral" case.

Treatment

The principal of treatment is to restore the aqueous drainage pathway. Conventional angle surgery, goniotomy and trabeculotomy, are the procedures of choice in PCG but require an experienced surgeon. Often more than one operation is

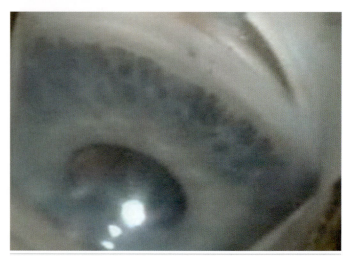

Fig. 37.6 Classic immature angle appearance with scalloped posterior iris pigment epithelium.

required to achieve IOP control. They enjoy a similar high rate of success in favorable cases such as unoperated eyes between 3 and 12 months of age. Our preference is for goniotomy as it spares the conjunctiva, an important point since further surgery is often required in the child's lifetime. If trabeculotomy is performed, we recommend it be performed inferotemporally, where it does not reduce the success rate of future surgery. The options in children that fail angle surgery are antimetabolite trabeculectomy or tube drainage surgery.

Juvenile open angle glaucoma

Juvenile open angle glaucoma (JOAG) refers to patients who have no anterior segment abnormalities and usually present with glaucoma late in childhood but up to the age of 35. Often there is a strong family history of glaucoma. Up to 20% of patients have mutations of the *myocilin/TIGR (trabecular meshwork inducible glucocorticoid response) gene* at the GLC1A locus on chromosome 1q23.[5] These patients typically have high pressures (40–50 mmHg) and respond well to prostaglandin analogs but often require an antimetabolite trabeculectomy.

Secondary childhood glaucoma

With conditions that predispose to secondary glaucomas it is important to be mindful of the potential risk of glaucoma. Those at risk need lifelong annual IOP review to prevent devastatingly late presentations of glaucoma that are usually associated with a poor long-term visual prognosis.

Anterior segment developmental anomalies
(see Chapter 32)

Anterior segment developmental anomalies (ASDAs) represent a spectrum of developmental disease involving neural crest mesenchyme. *Axenfeld-Rieger anomaly* is now recognized to be a spectrum of disease with overlapping clinical features. It is no longer divided as it was traditionally into the distinct entities of:

Axenfeld's anomaly [posterior embryotoxon (anteriorly displaced, prominent Schwalbe's line) with attached iris strands] and

Rieger's anomaly [these peripheral changes plus iris changes such as corectopia or iris thinning (Fig. 37.7)] and

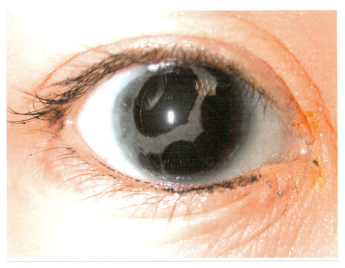

Fig. 37.7 Axenfeld-Rieger anomaly with corectopia and posterior embryotoxon.

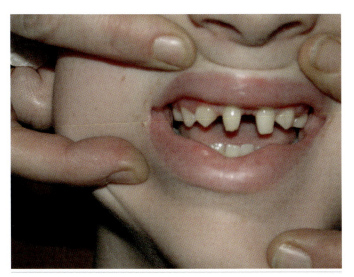

Fig. 37.8 Axenfeld-Rieger syndrome with small conical widely spaced teeth.

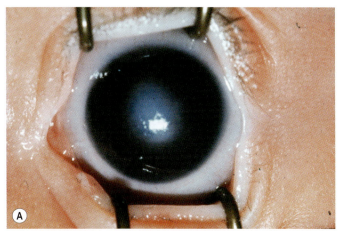

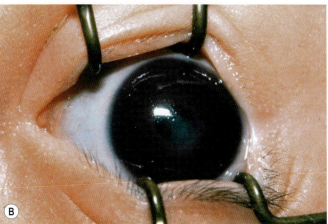

Fig. 37.9 (A) Uncontrolled IOP and dense central corneal opacification before antimetabolite trabeculectomy. (B) Same eye with controlled IOP in low teens and improved corneal clarity after surgery.

Axenfeld-Rieger syndrome refers to these ocular features in association with systemic anomalies such as hypertelorism, periumbilical skin folds, and dental abnormalities (Fig. 37.8). It is usually bilateral, asymmetric and inherited as an autosomal dominant trait. It shows genetic heterogeneity: several genes cause similar clinical phenotypes and, conversely, a single mutation may cause different phenotypes (variable expressivity). Several genes have been identified, the most common being *RIEG1* at chromosome 4q25. It is also associated with FOXC1, RIEG2, and PAX6 gene mutations.

Peters' anomaly is characterized by a congenital central corneal opacity with underlying defects in stroma, Descemet's membrane, and endothelium with iris strands and sometimes lens attachment to the periphery of this opacity. It is usually bilateral (80%) and sporadic. Peters' anomaly may result from abnormalities of the PAX6 gene, RIEG1/PITX2 and FOXC1 genes. *Iris hypoplasia* refers to a condition with distinctive hypoplastic iris stroma and is probably part of the ASDA

spectrum. It is associated with a characteristic maldevelopment of the anterior stromal layer of the iris, early onset glaucoma, a strong family history, and can have the same systemic features as Axenfeld-Rieger syndrome. Autosomal dominant iris hypoplasia is associated with RIEG1/PITX2 gene mutations.

The risk of glaucoma with ASDA is 50%, so lifelong surveillance is indicated. Glaucoma usually occurs in childhood or young adulthood, very rarely in infancy and is due to an underlying trabeculodysgenesis. The IOP is often labile. The cause of outflow obstruction is due to the arrested maturation of angle structures. Medical therapy is indicated on diagnosis but surgery is required in the majority of cases, usually antimetabolite trabeculectomy. It is our impression that the more disorganized the anterior segment, the greater the risk of failure and the more potent the anti-scarring agent required. A potent antimetabolite is more likely to achieve IOP in the low teens and so significantly reduce corneal opacification (Fig. 37.9). Primary tube drainage surgery may be indicated in the most severe cases.

Chronic pupil dilation or an optical iridectomy (via a scleral approach to prevent further corneal scarring) should be considered rather than penetrating keratoplasty, which is associated with disappointing results.[6] In Axenfeld-Rieger anomaly and iris hypoplasia where inheritance is often dominant, it is important to examine the patient's parents and siblings.

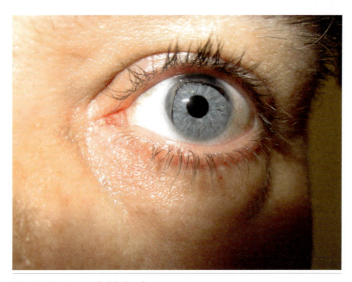

Fig. 37.10 Cosmetic iris implant.

Aniridia

Aniridia is characterized by bilateral variable absence of iris (see Chapter 32). Visual deficit in infancy is usually due to optic nerve and foveal hypoplasia. Later, loss of vision is due to glaucoma, cataract, ectopia lentis, and corneal surface abnormalities due to corneal epithelial stem cell dysfunction. Aniridia results from abnormal neuroectodermal development secondary to PAX6 gene mutations at chromosome 11p13. Inheritance is usually autosomal dominant although recessive transmission is possible; 30% of sporadic aniridia cases are associated with nephroblastoma (Wilm's tumor), genitourinary abnormalities and mental retardation (WAGR) related to large deletions of 11p13, which encompasses PAX6 and the adjacent Wilm's tumor locus. All sporadic cases must be screened regularly for renal abnormalities.

Glaucoma occurs in 50% of cases usually presenting in pre-adolescence or early adulthood. It may be due to progressive angle closure from the iris stump or be associated with an open angle. Medical therapy should always be first line treatment as this is safest but surgery is often inevitable. Goniotomy, both as therapy and prophylaxis, has been described but the latter is not widely practiced due to the potential risk of intraocular trauma. In the presence of a clear lens, we perform antimetabolite trabeculectomy with mitomycin C (MMC). If significant cataract is present or trabeculectomy fails, tube drainage surgery is indicated and can be associated with favorable results.[7] Hypotony should be avoided due to the danger of lens-corneal touch, which will cause both cataract and corneal decompensation. Symptomatic relief of photophobia can be achieved with tinted spectacles, iris contact lenses, or a cosmetic iris implant inserted at the time of cataract surgery (Fig. 37.10).

Phakomatoses

The commonest phakomatosis associated with glaucoma is *Sturge-Weber syndrome (encephalotrigeminal angiomatosis)*, a sporadic condition with a facial cutaneous angioma (port wine stain) present at birth, which affects the regions innervated by the first and second divisions of the trigeminal nerve (see Chapter 65). Choroidal hemangiomas occur in 40% of patients of whom 90% develop glaucoma. They are usually diffuse and can be easily missed on examination but identified by comparing the red reflex of both eyes or by ultrasound.

Glaucoma can occur at any time from birth to adulthood and arises from elevated episcleral venous pressure. There may be an element of goniodysgenesis with infantile presentations. Contralateral and bilateral glaucoma with unilateral cutaneous hemangioma have been reported so it is important to monitor both eyes.

Other phakomatoses can be associated with glaucoma although with a lower incidence than Sturge-Weber syndrome (see Chapter 65):

1. *Klippel-Trenaunay-Weber syndrome*: triad of cutaneous hemangioma and varicosities involving one limb along with hypertrophy of bone and soft tissue. Most cases with glaucoma also have a facial nevus.
2. *Neurofibromatosis*: may present with iris abnormalities, e.g. ectropion uveae and glaucoma, before the systemic disease is apparent, especially if there is an ipsilateral lid plexiform neuroma.

Surgery is indicated when medical treatment fails particularly with congenital or infantile presentations. Angle surgery may be successful if there is goniodysgenesis, but they respond less well than PCG with a higher failure rate. With a choroidal hemangioma, the potential for serious complications is high; it may give rise to expulsive choroidal hemorrhage if rapid decompression of the globe occurs or to choroidal effusions if there is prolonged hypotony. As the risk of hypotony is high with filtering surgery in children, an antimetabolite trabeculectomy is our treatment of choice when there is no choroidal hemangioma. If the hemangioma is very thick (>5 mm), preoperative radiotherapy should be considered. Our preference, when a choroidal hemangioma coexists, is for tube drainage surgery with measures against hypotony, i.e. an extraluminal occlusive suture and an intraluminal stent. We have noticed that choroidal effusions occur at a relatively higher IOP than expected in these patients. All surgery in these patients must be coupled with measures to minimize hypotony.

Aphakic glaucoma

Aphakic glaucoma is the commonest secondary childhood glaucoma and one of the most serious causes of late visual loss following successful congenital cataract surgery. Glaucoma can occur at any time. The diagnosis can be easily missed as patients are often asymptomatic; the signs may be subtle and examining these patients is difficult. One must remain vigilant for the onset of raised IOP.

Its pathogenesis is uncertain. Both chemical (inflammatory cells, lens remnants, and vitreous derived factors) and mechanical theories (lack of ciliary body tension and trabecular meshwork collapse) have been proposed, combined with developmental reasons, i.e. arrest of postnatal angle maturation due to surgical insult. The incidence of glaucoma following childhood cataract surgery varies with duration of follow-up, ranging from 5% with simple aspiration[8] to as high as 41% with lensectomy and vitrectomy with at least a 5-year follow-up.[9] Risk factors for aphakic glaucoma such as microcornea, poor pupil dilation, early surgery, the need for secondary surgery and nuclear cataract are well documented. The role of posterior capsule integrity and intraocular lens implantation is still debated. Lifelong surveillance for glaucoma is crucial. If IOP measurement is difficult, monitor the optic disk appearance for progressive cupping frequently. Excessive loss of hyperopia or contact lens intolerance may be useful signs.

Aphakic glaucoma is refractory to treatment. Medical treatment is first line but only controls IOP in 50% of cases. Angle surgery does not provide good long-term control. Filtration surgery with MMC not only has a poor success rate[10] but often excludes postoperative contact lens use in the presence of a thin, avascular cystic bleb due to the risk of endophthalmitis. Cyclodiode laser provides temporizing treatment with occasional long-term control after multiple treatments.[11] However, it is difficult to titrate with marked inflammation and phthisis possible especially in microphthalmic eyes, in which case less energy should be considered. Furthermore, it may prejudice future surgery to failure or be associated with chronic hypotony. Drainage tube implants have the highest chance of long-term success and allow contact lens use.[12] However, aphakic eyes have higher rates of complications, especially suprachoroidal hemorrhage, if hypotony occurs particularly if buphthalmic. Techniques to avoid catastrophic hypotony are mandatory.

Inflammatory glaucoma

Glaucoma may arise following inflammation from any cause but is most common in juvenile idiopathic arthritis (30%) usually 2–3 years after presentation. Uveitic glaucoma is multifactorial due to chronic cellular trabecular obstruction, trabeculitis, peripheral anterior synechiae, pupil block secondary to cataract removal, and following chronic topical steroid usage. Children with uveitis develop more severe glaucoma than adults and they progress rapidly to severe visual loss. The principles of management are to aggressively treat the uveitis with topical or systemic steroids and other immunosuppressives, while avoiding the temptation to adjust the steroids to control the IOP. After this, attention may be directed to controlling IOP control.

This glaucoma is refractory to treatment, especially medical treatment. Angle surgery often requires medical treatment to control IOP.[13] Antimetabolite trabeculectomy with MMC can be considered but recurrent ocular inflammation may compromise long-term success. Our preference is for primary tube drainage surgery especially if lensectomy is anticipated, or if aphakia is present. With any surgery, the risk of postoperative hypotony is high even in the absence of overdrainage due to potentially brittle aqueous production. Therefore, we prefer a smaller surface area drainage implant, e.g. Baerveldt implant (250 mm²) or Ahmed implant (184 mm²). It is essential that you operate on a "quiet" eye so these patients must be adequately immunosuppressed systemically before surgery. Cyclodiode treatment is associated with poor success rates as primary treatment.[14] We avoid cyclodiode treatment because it is aimed at an already compromised ciliary body so there is significant risk of hypotony.

Miscellaneous conditions

A wide variety of other, rare conditions are associated with childhood glaucoma and there is little precedent in the literature as to the appropriate treatment (see Box 37.1). Determining the mechanism of the glaucoma by a thorough history and examination, along with an assessment of risk factors for surgical failure, results in the best treatment plan. For instance, diseases such as *Marfan's syndrome*, *Weill-Marchesani syndrome*, *homocystinuria*, and *high myopia* may give rise to childhood glaucoma which is usually associated with lens displacement

and secondary pupil block. A prophylactic iridectomy and chronic miosis may be required to prevent pupil block glaucoma or dislocation of the lens into the anterior chamber.

Childhood tumors such as *leukemia* or *retinoblastoma* may give rise to glaucoma from outflow obstruction by tumor cells or secondary hemorrhage. The diagnosis of these rare conditions is important as inadvertent surgery may worsen the prognosis for life. The treatment is generally conservative: treat the primary disorder and use topical medical treatment or cyclodestruction.

Management

Assessment

The suspicion of glaucoma in a child should always be treated seriously and with urgency to minimize visual impairment. This requires examination in the clinic or under anesthesia depending on the child's ability to cooperate. A neonate who is feeding can be thoroughly examined in the clinic. Most infants and young children (<5 years) require an examination under anesthesia (EUA).

The initial consultation is an absolutely vital part of management as it is the beginning of what may be a lifetime relationship between the ophthalmologist, patient, and their parents. The aim of the initial assessment is to rule out glaucoma or establish that enough evidence for glaucoma exists to justify an EUA for a more complete examination and surgery if indicated. If there is any doubt as to the diagnosis, it is advisable to proceed with an EUA.

History

In a neonate or infant enquire about a history of epiphora, photophobia, blepharospasm, and change in ocular appearance. It is important to determine:

1. The age at clinical onset for prognosis
2. Associated systemic problems for anesthetic risk
3. Problems during pregnancy (rubella) or labor (forcep use)
4. A family history of pediatric glaucoma
5. Parental consanguinity.

In older children a history of trauma, ocular surgery or corticosteroid use may be relevant.

Examination

Following the determination of visual acuity, the ambient illumination can be reduced to allow the infant to open their eyes, permitting a more complete examination. It may be possible to assess the presence of corneal edema, lacrimation, photophobia, blepharospasm, and the relative and actual size of both eyes. It is important to examine the patient's parents as the subtle signs of anterior segment dysgenesis may change the genetic advice given and the management of subsequent siblings.

Intraocular pressure measurement
Measuring IOP in children can be challenging. The gold standard for measuring IOP is with Goldmann applanation tonometry. In Peters' anomaly a Tono-pen® measures the IOP more accurately in the peripheral cornea than over the central corneal opacity which may give a falsely high IOP. However, a Tono-pen® overestimates the IOP compared to a Perkins applanation

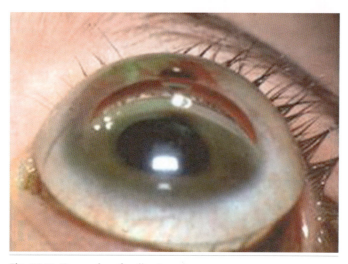

Fig. 37.11 Koeppe lens for direct gonioscopy.

tonometer in both normal children and those with glaucoma.[15,16]

The iCare portable rebound tonometer can measure IOP without the installation of topical anesthetic in both supine and upright positions, and may be better tolerated than non-contact methods. It has a similar reliability to a Tono-pen® with a tendency to overestimate IOP in known or suspected glaucoma cases compared to applanation tonometry.[17,18] Regardless of the instrument used, lid squeezing and crying may falsely elevate the IOP.

The gold standard for tonometry in children undergoing an EUA is the Perkins hand held tonometer with a blue filter after installation of fluorescein. Avoid the use of a lid speculum and pressure on the eye. The eyes should be in the primary position and motionless as pressure readings may be altered by eye movements. The IOP should be measured several times in both eyes. Accurate IOP measurement under EUA can be difficult as the type of anesthetic, instrumentation, corneal thickness, and opacities affect it. Tonometry under anesthesia provides us only with an approximation of the true tension. *It should never be the sole method by which the presence or control of glaucoma is assessed.*

Anterior segment examination

The cornea must be examined for the presence of posterior embryotoxon, edema, opacities, and Haab's striae. Oblique illumination and magnification are necessary as the signs can sometimes be subtle. Under an EUA, a portable slit-lamp should be used. The presence of *corneal enlargement with splits, with or without edema, indicates raised IOP at some stage in infancy.* Persistent corneal edema may be a sign of poorly controlled glaucoma.

When a deep anterior chamber in a neonate or young infant is associated with an enlarged cornea, glaucoma should be strongly suspected. Detecting iris, pupil abnormalities, or co-existing lens opacities is important. The latter may require treatment and influence the choice of glaucoma surgery. Furthermore, lens subluxation should be identified as it increases the likelihood of vitreous prolapse during surgery.

Corneal diameter measurement

The normal horizontal neonatal diameter is up to 10.5 mm increasing by about 1 mm in the first year of life. *A corneal diameter greater than 11 mm in a newborn and 12 mm in an infant less than 1 year is suggestive of raised IOP; with Haab striae it is diagnostic.* A measurement of greater than 13 mm in a child of any age and asymmetric corneal diameters is abnormal. During EUA, the horizontal corneal diameter is measured with calipers from limbus to limbus and checked with a graduated ruler with estimation to the nearest 0.25 mm. An increasing corneal diameter in a vulnerable eye suggests inadequate control of IOP requiring further treatment.

Corneal thickness

Patients with PCG have thinner corneas and, in theory, a tendency for under reading the IOP. Conversely an increase in corneal thickness, as is found in patients with aphakia and aniridia, may lead to an over reading of IOP. Pachymetry may be indicated to avoid unnecessary treatment. However, children with aphakia and markedly thickened corneas, regardless of the theoretical overestimation of the IOP, do develop glaucomatous cupping and visual field defects.[21] This may be due to altered biomechanical properties in children with glaucoma.[22] The role of pachymetry in childhood glaucoma is uncertain; standard correction factors cannot be used and regardless of corneal thickness the emphasis remains on the optic disk appearance.

Gonioscopy

Gonioscopy is crucial in making the correct diagnosis, which determines the most appropriate operation and prognosis. In an EUA, direct gonioscopy can be performed with a variety of lenses including a *Koeppe* lens (direct gonioscopy) (Fig. 37.11).

Posterior segment examination

The appearance of the optic disk is the most important and sensitive parameter for both diagnosis and progression of glaucoma. It is influenced neither by anesthesia nor the effect of growth. The optic disk and the nerve fiber layer should be examined through a dilated pupil and carefully recorded with a drawing or photograph. Examining the optic disk in infants may only be possible after the corneal haze or edema has cleared.

Prior to an EUA, the pupil is not dilated as this may alter the angle appearance, spuriously increase IOP, and increase the risk of lens damage if surgery is required. An indirect ophthalmoscope with a small pupil facility can be useful in obtaining a view of the disc. Richardson noted a cup-to-disk ratio (CDR) of greater than 0.3 in only 3% of 468 *normal* newborn eyes,[19] in contrast to Shaffer who found a CDR of greater than 0.3 in 61% of 85 eyes in infants less than 1 year with *congenital glaucoma.*[20] *A CDR >0.3 in an infant less than 1 year or >0.5 in a Caucasian child and disk asymmetry should increase suspicion of glaucoma.* An increase in disk cupping is definite evidence of poorly controlled glaucoma and the need for further treatment, regardless of IOP measurement obtained. Optic disk photographs can be taken while under EUA.

The remainder of the fundus should be examined for any associated abnormalities such as foveal hypoplasia associated with aniridia, choroidal hemangiomas in Sturge-Weber syndrome, and pigmentary retinopathy associated with rubella.

Refraction

Loss of hypermetropia or the presence of myopia is often evidence of glaucoma. Progressive myopia may suggest inadequate IOP control. If satisfactory cycloplegic refraction is not possible in the outpatient setting, retinoscopy will need to be performed during the EUA if corneal clarity allows.

Examination under anesthesia

Anesthesia

Anesthetics usually lower the IOP with the exceptions of ketamine and chloral hydrate. Inhalation anesthetics, such as sevofluorane, may substantially lower the IOP by 10–30 mmHg; the amount is idiosyncratic and unpredictable. This makes an appropriate anesthetic vital in the assessment of these patients; in subtle cases it can have a profound impact on the timing of the diagnosis and the visual prognosis. The finding of a normal IOP with the use of agents known to reduce IOP does not exclude glaucoma. *Whichever agent is used, it is important to have a consistent approach and to measure the IOP first.*

Although it is not universally practiced, it is our preference to use ketamine hydrochloride which results in IOP measurements that are commensurate with those taken in awake infants.[23] It is given intravenously following the use of local anesthetic patches. Children are premedicated with atropine, which reduces bronchial secretions, and oral midazolam which acts as a sedative and an amnesic. Its duration usually lasts 10 to 15 minutes.

While the patient is under anesthesia, a general examination and venesection for laboratory investigation (e.g. screening for infective agents and chromosome studies) can be performed.

Examination findings

It is important to record IOP, corneal diameters, axial lengths, and cup-to-disk ratio along with other clinical findings such as corneal clarity at every EUA.

Investigations

Ultrasound

A-scan Serial axial lengths can be useful in children when the eye is still distensible. In glaucoma, axial length measurements are usually asymmetric in contrast to megalocornea and normal eyes. There usually is a decrease in axial length following successful lowering of IOP. Anterior chamber depth is usually increased in infants with glaucoma.

B-scan A high-resolution B-scan may be useful in an eye with opaque media to detect severe cupping or exclude posterior segment pathology such as choroidal hemangioma.

Visual fields

Visual fields are usually possible in mid-childhood but (see Chapter 4) need to be repeated to confirm any defects. Due to significant functional reserve, children may have normal visual fields in the presence of severe disc damage.

Optic disk and nerve fiber layer analysis

Differences have been reported between normal and glaucomatous eyes in children using optical coherence tomography.[24] A prospective, observational study in children with glaucoma revealed retinal nerve fiber layer and macular thickness measurements declined with increasing severity of glaucomatous disk damage as seen in stereophotographs.[25] However, along with other quantitative measurements of the optic nerve and nerve fiber layer such as confocal scanning laser ophthalmoscopy and scanning laser polarimetry, respectively, further testing in children is warranted. Results should be interpreted with caution.

Interpretation of findings

The diagnosis of glaucoma and the assessment of glaucoma control are based on clinical findings and investigation results which vary depending on the age of the child. The most important clinical sign is the state of the optic disk.

In a young child whose eye is still vulnerable to the effects of elevated pressure but the IOP measurement may be inaccurate, the appearance and diameter of the cornea along with the axial length provide useful information. When the IOP reading is discordant with other findings, one should remember that it may be unreliable. If the IOP is normal, but buphthalmos, corneal enlargement with Haab's striae, and pathologic optic cupping are present, it may be a case of falsely low IOP related to anesthesia or "arrested" glaucoma. If the diagnosis is unclear and there is a high risk of glaucoma, further examinations under anesthesia are necessary to confirm pathology before committing the patient to surgery. If the cornea is normal sized but hazy and the IOP is normal, suspect Congenital hereditary endothelial dystrophy (see Chapter 34).

As the child gets older, the IOP can be measured more accurately on the slit-lamp and the optic disk and the nerve fiber layer can be better assessed with greater magnification. The corneal diameter and axial length become less useful measurements as the sclera and cornea mature. Visual fields become possible to assess functional vision especially in advanced cases.

If glaucoma is confirmed explain to the parents the chronic nature of the condition, the possible need for surgery, and definite lifelong follow-up as glaucoma can relapse at any stage and may develop in the fellow eye of "unilateral glaucoma".

Treatment

The treatment of primary and secondary pediatric glaucoma differs in two major ways. In secondary glaucoma, medical treatment is usually first line followed promptly by surgery when ineffective. Furthermore, angle surgery is usually associated with limited success.

Medical therapy

Long-term medical therapy is sometimes necessary if surgery is significantly high risk or not possible due to risk of anesthesia. Do not persist with prolonged, suboptimal medical treatment; it results in ongoing optic nerve damage and has a deleterious effect on conjunctival wound healing after glaucoma filtration surgery.

Great care must be exercised when prescribing glaucoma drugs. Children are at a higher risk of systemic, potentially fatal side-effects from topical administration. Blood levels from drops can approach or even exceed oral therapeutic levels. Warn parents of potential systemic side-effects and instruct them on punctal occlusion.

Beta-blockers

Use in premature or newborn infants and children with asthma or any cardiac problems including arrhythmias should be avoided. It is important to inquire about asthma symptoms, which may manifest with nocturnal cough in children rather than wheezing. *Timolol 0.1%* and *timolol gellan 0.25%* are the beta-blockers of choice as first line treatment due to their superior risk profile.

Prostaglandin analogs

Latanoprost is the first drug to be licensed for use in children. In a prospective randomised trial comparing its efficacy with Timolol 0.5% in patients with pediatric glaucoma, it was similarly effective to Timolol.[26] It may be less effective in Sturge-Weber patients. Heterochromia in children has been reported. Patients with JOAG may respond particularly well and it should be considered first line in these patients.

Carbonic anhydrase inhibitors

Although *oral acetazolamide* is more potent in reducing IOP than dorzolamide, its use in children is limited by serious systemic side-effects such as failure to thrive, disturbed hyperactive behavior, and bed-wetting. It should be considered for short-term use prior to surgery. *Brinzolamide* is less irritating than *dorzolamide*: both are useful as second line drugs or when beta-blockers are contraindicated.

Sympathomimetics

Brimonidine crosses the blood–brain barrier and can cause drowsiness to the point of coma and apnea in infants. We avoid it in children less than the age of 6 years. The use of *apraclonidine* in children is theoretically safer as it is less lipophilic. It should be considered when beta-blockers are contraindicated.

Parasympathomimetics

Parasympathomimetic agents are useful in the post-operative management of PCG after angle surgery as they may enhance aqueous outflow and prevent anterior synechiae formation. They have a role in aphakic glaucoma.

Surgical therapy

The principal treatment modality of childhood glaucoma is surgical. The surgical procedures have varying indications with both advantages and disadvantages and potentially good success rates, especially when performed at referral centers where there is sufficient volume to ensure skillful surgery and safe anesthesia. Lack of familiarity with buphthalmic eyes can lead to severe complications related to difficult access in small orbits, distorted limbal anatomy, thin sclera with low rigidity, lens subluxation from stretched zonules, and syneretic vitreous. The procedure of choice is largely determined by type of glaucoma and may be further influenced by age of onset, corneal clarity, degree of optic nerve damage, associated ocular disease, history to previous surgery, and the surgeon's experience.

As repeat surgery is often inevitable, making the right choice initially is paramount as the first operation has the greatest chance of success. In eyes that have undergone multiple procedures it is important to make the next operation the definitive one. Once the procedure has been chosen, surgery must be meticulous to minimize complications.

Angle surgery

Goniotomy

Goniotomy is the treatment of choice in PCG where the cornea allows satisfactory visualization of the angle. The exact

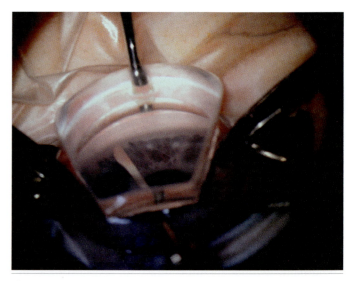

Fig. 37.12 Goniotomy performed in primary congenital glaucoma.

mechanism of action remains unknown. The advantages and disadvantages of goniotomy are summarized in Box 37.3.

Although goniotomy is simple in concept and brief in execution, it is a difficult procedure to perform requiring considerable experience and rare surgical skills. *Adequate visualization of the angle is the key to successfully performing this procedure.* Epithelial debridement with absolute alcohol provides an adequate view of the angle to allow goniotomy in more than 90% of Caucasian patients.[27] To be performed safely, general anesthesia, an operating microscope, a contact lens (e.g. Barkan lens), and a tapered goniotomy blade are required[28] (Fig. 37.12). If there has been a reasonable but suboptimal lowering of IOP after the first goniotomy, it can be repeated in the non-operated part of the angle. Direct visualization of the angle allows precise location of the incision making it less traumatic than trabeculotomy. Potential complications include lens and corneal damage, inadvertent iridodialysis, or cyclodialysis and scleral perforation.

Goniotomy is a very effective operation, with success following multiple goniotomies usually ranging from 70% to 90% with medium term follow-up.[27,29] However, these eyes are at risk of relapsing at any stage. Russell-Eggitt et al. reported a

Box 37.4

Advantages and disadvantages of trabeculotomy

Advantages
- Can be performed even when cornea is opaque
- Many components of technique similar to trabeculectomy

Disadvantages
- Damages conjunctiva and prejudices success of future filtering surgery
- Angle not directly visualized leading potentially to significant complications
- Requires special trabeculotomy probes
- When combined with trabeculectomy may be technically more difficult
- Converting a trabeculotomy entry site to trabeculectomy places the sclerostomy very close to the iris root predisposing to iris incarceration
- Undesirable external filtration is possible

Box 37.5

Advantages and disadvantages of trabeculectomy (with antimetabolites)

Advantages
- Postoperative pressures "titratable" compared with angle surgery by using techniques such as adjustable, releasable sutures and postoperative antimetabolites
- Lower pressures achievable with antimetabolites
- Trabeculectomy with antimetabolites may significantly clear cloudy corneas

Disadvantages
- Greater risk of hypotony with choroidal effusion and hemorrhage than angle surgery particularly with MMC
- Greater risk of endophthalmitis than angle surgery particularly with small treatment areas of MMC and limbus based flaps
- Poor results in aphakic glaucoma even with MMC

20% relapse rate over a 30-year period with no peak age of relapse,[27] emphasizing the importance of lifelong follow-up. The surgical prognosis of goniotomy is influenced by the age of manifestation; infants presenting between the ages of 3 to 6 months have the best prognosis.

Trabeculotomy

Since corneal opacification does not prevent the performance of trabeculotomy it has greater application than goniotomy. The advantages and disadvantages of trabeculotomy are summarized in Box 37.4.

An operating microscope and special trabeculotome are essential for conventional trabeculotomy.[28] *Accurate localization of Schlemm's canal is the key to the successful performance of this operation.* However, abnormally stretched limbal anatomy in buphthalmic eyes makes it difficult to identify and it may not be found at all in 4–20% of patients, especially if the anterior chamber is inadvertently entered before the canal is found. Beck and Lynch have described a 360° suture trabeculotomy using a blunted 6/0 polypropylene, with results suggesting greater success than goniotomy.[30] However, success is not always possible with a single incision and severe hypotony along with misdirected (subretinal) sutures have been reported. In cases with severe corneal edema it may not be possible to view the suture gonioscopically, although a recently described fine fiber-optic probe with light emission from the tip may be useful in these cases.[31]

Complications are uncommon but can include stripping of Descemet's membrane, iris prolapse, iridodialysis, cyclodialysis with persistent hypotony, lens subluxation, false passages, significant hyphema, bleb formation, and prolonged flat anterior chambers.

Success rates and prognostic factors in PCG are similar to those of goniotomy.[32,33]

Trabeculotomy combined with trabeculectomy

Trabeculotomy has the added advantage of being combined with trabeculectomy to provide two major outflow pathways and so improve results. In practice, the clinical benefit is unclear; some authors report greater success than with either procedure performed alone, especially in populations at high risk of failure such as in East Asia and the Middle East.[34,35] Others have found no difference in success between the three procedures.[36] Technically, it is a more complex procedure with significant complications especially with antimetabolite use.

Filtering surgery

Trabeculectomy

One of the main indications for trabeculectomy is failed angle surgery. It may be the primary procedure of choice when:

1. The surgeon has limited experience with angle surgery
2. The patient is unlikely to respond to angle surgery (very early or late presentation)
3. Very low target pressures are required (improved corneal clarity, advanced disk cupping)
4. In most secondary glaucomas.

The advantages and disadvantages of trabeculectomy are summarized in Box 37.5.

Technically it is a more demanding procedure and more likely to fail in children than adults. A superior fornix based conjunctival flap with a wide area of antimetabolite treatment (the Moorfields Safer Surgery System) allows adequate exposure, reduces surgical trauma to the conjunctiva and episclera, and improves bleb morphology thus reducing blebitis and endophthalmitis.[37] It is vital, in buphthalmic eyes, that the scleral flap is large and as thick as possible to control flow and avoid sutures from "cheesewiring." Scleral flap closure should be very tight; these eyes are prone to develop hypotony. Intraoperative hypotony can be minimized with the use of pre-placed scleral flap sutures before the sclerostomy is performed and with an anterior chamber maintainer. For a summary of technique see Table 37.1. Complications with antimetabolites include moderate hyphema, shallow or flat anterior chamber, iris incarceration, lens dislocation, choroidal effusions, vitreous loss, vitreous and suprachoroidal hemorrhage, staphyloma, retinal detachment, phthisis, chronic bleb leak, and endophthalmitis. If significant conjunctival inflammation is present at the drainage site, subconjunctival 5-fluorouracil (5FU) (0.2–0.3 ml of 5FU 50 mg/ml) and steroids such as betamethasone can be injected adjacent to the bleb during an EUA.

Table 37.1 – Important surgical points in pediatric trabeculectomy

Point	Action	Rationale
Exposure	Corneal traction suture (7/0 mersilk) Fornix based conjunctival flap	Allows adequate exposure Allows better visualization of limbal anatomy Easier placement of sutures in scleral flap Less likely to limit posterior flow
Hemostasis	Corneal traction suture Wet field cautery	Avoids hemorrhage from superior rectus suture Avoids scleral shrinkage (very important in thin sclera)
Prevention of scarring	Antimetabolites	See text
Scleral flap	Anterior placement Large and thick (5 × 3–4 mm) Small radial cuts (1–2 mm) not all the way to limbus	Avoids iris, ciliary body, and vitreous incarceration Easier to suture without cheese-wiring thin sclera Greater resistance to aqueous outflow (vital in buphthalmic eyes, especially with antimetabolites) Directs aqueous posteriorly to prevent cystic blebs Valve effect to prevent hypotony
Paracentesis for anterior chamber (AC) maintainer	Oblique, long tunnel (21G needle)	Reduces risk of inadvertent lens damage during maneuver and less likely to leak Allows reformation of the AC postoperatively
Maintenance of intraoperative IOP	Anterior chamber maintainer	Prevents eye from becoming hypotonous and choroidal effusions forming during surgery Can be used to gauge flow through the scleral flap and ensure adequate flap closure
Sclerostomy	Small (500 μm bite) with special punch Anterior as possible	Increased control of aqueous outflow intra- and postoperatively Quick therefore less intraoperative hypotony Prevents iris, ciliary body, vitreous incarceration
Scleral flap closure	Preplaced sutures before sclerostomy Tight releasable, and fixed sutures (apices) Releasable loop buried in cornea	Easier to place with formed globe Faster to tie therefore reduced period of intraoperative hypotony Allow control of opening pressures (vital with antimetabolite use) Sutures can be left indefinitely Allow tight closure but can be loosened or removed under anesthetic without need for laser
Conjunctival closure (fornix based)	10/0 nylon purse string at edges	Retains tension longer than dissolvable sutures Minimal associated inflammation Ends of nylon buried under conjunctiva
Postoperative prevention of hypotony	Viscoelastic in anterior chamber	May be necessary if flow rate too high despite maximal suturing

Trabeculectomy without antimetabolites is associated with poor long-term success[38,39] due to the aggressive healing response seen in children. As a primary procedure the results are better.[40,41] Most recent reports of pediatric trabeculectomies include the use of adjunctive MMC, a potent cytotoxic agent which kills fibroblasts, resulting in moderate cumulative success rates of 59–90% at 2 years reducing to 51% at 5 years.[42-44] Poor prognostic factors are age less than 1 year and aphakia.[43,45]

Non-penetrating surgery for congenital glaucoma has been performed in an attempt to avoid potential trabeculectomy-related complications but there is a high learning curve with a high complication rate.[46] There is a significant rate of conversion to trabeculectomy.

Antimetabolite treatment
The long-term success rate of glaucoma filtering surgery in children is reduced compared to adults because of a more vigorous wound healing response due to a thicker Tenon's capsule which impedes filtration and contains a large reservoir of fibroblasts responsible for scarring. This is further compounded by difficult postoperative management in the very young, which may delay the implementation of adjunctive measures that prolong bleb survival. Hence, the use of intraoperative antimetabolites to enhance success in refractory or difficult cases is unavoidable. In children a single application of the more potent MMC is preferable to 5FU.

The potential for intraoperative and postoperative complications after trabeculectomy, especially with MMC, cannot be overstated in children.[42,45,47] Early postoperative complications usually relate to hypotony whereas late complications largely relate to progressive bleb thinning putting the child at a significant lifetime risk of endophthalmitis,[42,43,48] chronic leak, and hypotony. However, modifications to the intraoperative application of MMC and surgical technique have resulted in more favorable bleb morphology[37] (Fig. 37.13). If patients develop thin cystic blebs they should be given antibiotics to keep at home and start half hourly if they develop a sticky eye and then immediately seek ophthalmologic help.

Box 37.6

Advantages and disadvantages of tube surgery

Advantages

- Very effective in reducing IOP long term even if previously failed antimetabolite trabeculectomy
- Most likely to survive future intraocular surgery, e.g. penetrating keratoplasty, lensectomy, vitrectomy, therefore best drainage option in these circumstances
- Contact lens wear possible in aphakic glaucoma

Disadvantages

- Longest surgical time
- Highest short term complication rate, particularly hypotony related complications including sight threatening complications
- Longest rehabilitation period

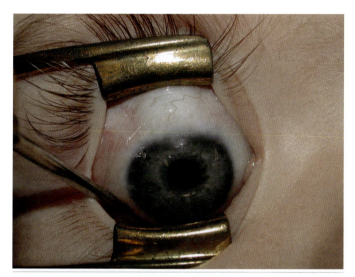

Fig. 37.13 Mitomycin C trabeculectomy in a child following fornix based conjunctival flap and large antimetabolite treatment area.

Tube drainage surgery

Tube drainage surgery remains an important part of the therapeutic repertoire in pediatric glaucoma as it offers the best chance of long-term IOP control in a small proportion of patients whose disease relentlessly progresses despite conventional surgical treatment. It is indicated if future intraocular surgery such as cataract extraction is contemplated, as it is more likely to control IOP postoperatively than filtering surgery. The prevailing current opinion is that tubes are best implanted sooner rather than later in the hope of achieving early, definitive IOP control and in doing so optimizing long-term visual prognosis. The advantages and disadvantages of tube drainage surgery are summarized in Box 37.6.

Common to all studies, regardless of the implant, is the ongoing decline in success with duration of follow-up and the requirement for adjunctive topical medication to control IOP. Plate encapsulation is a major cause of late failure. Success rates of 80% are reported with a mean follow-up of 2 years or less,[49-51] falling to 50% with longer term follow-up.[52-55] The use of adjunctive MMC has been reported but there are no prospective studies in children.

Box 37.7

Advantages and disadvantages of diode laser cyclodestruction

Advantages

- Short surgical time
- Rapid rehabilitation
- Good short-term response rate
- Very useful where surgery has high risks particularly in only eyes
- Technically less demanding than other procedures in difficult eyes

Disadvantages

- Often needs to be repeated in more than 50% of cases due to recovery of ciliary body
- Most patients remain on medical therapy
- Pressure control is worse than drainage surgery (pressures in the low teens usually not achieved)
- Danger of long-term phthisis with recurrent treatment due to recurrent damage to ciliary body
- ? May affect future drainage surgery: hypotony due to hyposecretion and fibrotic failure due to destruction of blood–aqueous barrier releasing stimulatory cytokines into aqueous and drainage site

Drainage devices offer the most effective long-term treatment for IOP control but they have a high complication rate. The problems relate to hypotony or to the tube itself (e.g. occlusion, retraction, corneal or iris touch) with an associated high surgical revision rate. Buphthalmic eyes are especially prone to hypotony-related complications because reduced scleral rigidity allows leakage around the tube at its entry site making subsequent problems such as choroidal effusions and suprachoroidal hemorrhage more likely, even with the use of valved implants. Modifications to protect from intra- and postoperative hypotony (mandatory when using MMC in a buphthalmic eye) include the following:

1. An anterior chamber maintainer (Lewicky cannula)
2. A relatively long and "snug" limbal tunnel incision (25 gauge needle for Molteno and Baerveldt implants)
3. The use of an intraluminal suture (3/0 Supramid)
4. An external ligating suture (6/0 vicryl) with a venting "Sherwood" slit[56]
5. Viscoelastic or intraocular gases such as 20% C_3F_8 in the anterior chamber.

Cyclodestruction

The indications for cyclodestruction are blind painful eyes, those with poor visual potential, or in whom surgery has a poor prognosis or is technically impossible (e.g. severely scarred conjunctiva). The advantages and disadvantages of diode laser cyclodestruction are summarized in Box 37.7.

Contact trans-scleral semi-conductor diode laser (810 nm) is more popular than Nd:YAG laser and cyclocryotherapy as a method of ciliary body ablation because it is better tolerated and associated with fewer complications. As buphthalmic eyes often have distorted anatomic landmarks, transillumination of the eye is essential to ensure accurate placement of the laser burns (Fig. 37.14). Care must be taken to avoid areas of

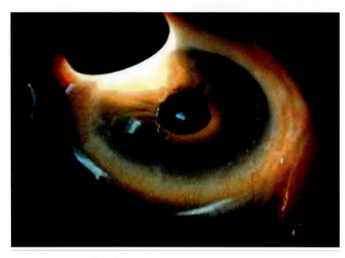

Fig. 37.14 Cyclodiode laser. Transillumination is crucial for correct placement of burns on the ciliary body.

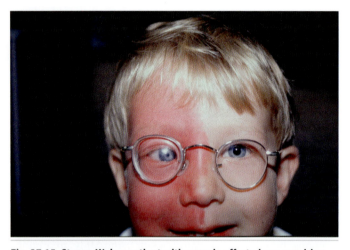

Fig. 37.15 Sturge-Weber patient with myopic-affected eye requiring optical corrections.

pigmentation, hemorrhage, and scleral thinning as scleral perforation in a buphthalmic eye has been reported.[57]

Diode laser is moderately effective in the short term with a success rate over 50% on medical therapy. These results have been achieved with total energy doses of between 74 and 113 J and a variable retreatment rate of 33–70%.[11,58] These results are similar to those achieved with endoscopic diode with a lower re-treatment rate. Overall visual loss rates of up to 18% have been reported, usually in eyes with pre-existing poor vision.[59]

Refractive correction and amblyopia therapy

The ultimate aim of preserving lifelong vision in children with glaucoma is dependent not only on IOP control but also the treatment of ametropia and amblyopia (Fig. 37.15). All children with glaucoma should be examined regularly for the presence of amblyopia. Refraction should be part of the periodic examination, with glasses prescribed as appropriate when the cornea clears. Occlusion therapy for amblyopia should be attempted in all patients in whom there is potential for visual improvement.

The role of penetrating keratoplasty

The results of penetrating keratoplasty in children with glaucoma are poor.[60,61] Erlich et al. advised against attempting penetrating keratoplasty in congenital glaucoma,[62] and Ariyasu et al.[63] only recommended penetrating keratoplasty when there was bilateral, visually disabling congenital glaucoma and a dedicated, reliable caregiver to deal with the postoperative management. Descemet stripping endothelial keratoplasty may be a safer procedure.[64] The use of antimetabolites can achieve lower IOP to levels that can clear corneal opacities (see Fig. 37.9).

Prognosis

Visual prognosis depends on many factors but the most important are:

1. The age and severity at presentation: early, severe cases do less well
2. The time elapsed between the first clinical manifestations and surgery
3. Successful control of IOP
4. Correction of ametropia and amblyopia therapy.

There will be some patients in whom, despite all efforts, the prognosis for long-term vision is poor. However, it is worth persisting because the longer the child is kept seeing, the better they will function as an adult. Biglan in a review of children with glaucoma found that 28% achieved 6/12 or better and that 50% were legally blind. The best prognosis was in children with PCG (40% 6/12 or better) and the worst in aphakic glaucoma (10% 6/12 or better).[65]

Periodic examination must continue throughout life, not only because an increase in IOP can occur at any stage, but also because complications can occur many years after a seemingly successful operation.[66] Parents and patients should be warned that minor blunt trauma in buphthalmic eyes may result in severe visual loss. Protective eyewear should be prescribed, especially in monocular patients.

Acknowledgments

Our work and research with children has been supported by: NIHR Biomedical Research Centre at Moorfields Eye Hospital and UCL Institute of Ophthalmology, UCL Partners, Academic Health Science Centre, Michael & Isle Katz Foundation, Helen Hamlyn Trust in memory of Paul Hamlyn, Fight for Sight, Moorfields Trustees, Hobson Foundation, Freemasons Grand Charity, Michael and Ilsa Katz foundation, Ron and Liora Moskovitz.

References

1. Papadopoulos M, Cable N, Rahi J, Khaw PT, BIG Eye Investigators. The British Infantile and Childhood Glaucoma (BIG) Eye Study. Invest Ophthalmol Vis Sci 2007; 48: 4100–6.
4. Anderson DR. The development of the trabecular meshwork and its abnormality in primary infantile glaucoma. Trans Am Ophthalmol Soc 1981; 79: 458–85.

5. Wiggs JL. Genetic etiologies of glaucoma. Arch Ophthalmol 2007; 125: 30–7.

9. Simon JW, Mehta N, Simmons ST, et al. Glaucoma after pediatric lensectomy/vitrectomy. Ophthalmology 1991; 98: 670–4.

10. Mandal AK, Bagga H, Nutheti R, et al. Trabeculectomy with or without mitomycin-C for paediatric glaucoma in aphakia and pseudophakia following congenital cataract surgery. Eye 2003; 17: 53–62.

11. Kirwan JF, Shah P, Khaw PT. Diode laser cyclophotocoagulation: role in the management of refractory pediatric glaucomas. Ophthalmology 2002; 109: 316–23.

16. Garcia-Resua C, Gonzalez-Meijome JM, et al. Accuracy of the new ICare rebound tonometer vs. other portable tonometers in healthy eyes. Optom Vis Sci 2006; 83: 102–7.

19. Richardson KT. Optic cup symmetry in normal newborn infants. Invest Ophthalmol 1968; 7: 137–40.

20. Shaffer RN. New concepts in infantile glaucoma. Can J Ophthalmol 1967; 2: 243–8.

22. Kirwan C, O'Keefe M, Lanigan B. Corneal hysteresis and intraocular pressure measurement in children using the Reichert ocular response analyzer. Am J Ophthalmol 2006; 142: 990–2.

23. Blumberg D, Congdon N, Jampel H, et al. The effects of sevoflurane and ketamine on intraocular pressure in children during examination under anesthesia. Am J Ophthalmol 2007; 143: 494–9.

24. Hess DB, Asrani SG, Bhide MG, et al. Macular and retinal nerve fiber layer analysis of normal and glaucomatous eyes in children using optical coherence tomography. Am J Ophthalmol 2005; 139: 509–17.

25. El-Dairi MA, Holgado S, Asrani SG, et al. Correlation between optical coherence tomography and glaucomatous optic nerve head damage in children. Br J Ophthalmol 2009; 93: 1325–30.

27. Russell-Eggitt IM, Rice NSC, Jay B, Wyse RKH. Relapse following goniotomy for congenital glaucoma due to trabecular dysgenesis. Eye 1992; 6: 197–200.

35. Al-Hazmi A, Awad A, Zwaan J, et al. A. Correlation between surgical success rate and severity of congenital glaucoma. Br J Ophthalmol 2005; 89: 449–53.

37. Wells AP, Cordeiro MF, Bunce CV, Khaw PT. Cystic bleb formation and related complications in limbus versus fornix-based conjunctival flaps in pediatric and young adult trabeculectomy with mitomycin C. Ophthalmology 2003; 110: 2192–7.

40. Burke JP, Bowell R. Primary trabeculectomy in congenital glaucoma. Br J Ophthalmol 1989; 73: 186–90.

44. Giampani J Jr, Borges-Giampani AS, Carani JC, et al. Efficacy and safety of trabeculectomy with mitomycin C for childhood glaucoma: a study of results with long-term follow-up. Clinics (Sao Paulo) 2008; 63: 421–6.

45. Freedman SF, McCormick K, Cox TA. Mitomycin C-augmented trabeculectomy with postoperative wound modulation in pediatric glaucoma. J AAPOS 1999; 3: 117–24.

46. Lüke C, Dietlein TS, Jacobi PC, et al. Risk profile of deep sclerectomy for the treatment of refractory congenital glaucomas. Ophthalmology 2002; 109: 1066–71.

48. Waheed S, Ritterband DC, Greenfield DS, et al. Bleb-related ocular infection in children after trabeculectomy with mitomycin C. Ophthalmology 1997; 104: 2117–20.

49. Fellenbaum PS, Sidoti PA, Heuer DK, et al. Experience with the Baerveldt implant in young patients with complicated glaucomas. J Glaucoma 1995; 4: 91–7.

55. Rolim de Moura C, Fraser-Bell S, Stout A, et al. Experience with the baerveldt glaucoma implant in the management of pediatric glaucoma. Am J Ophthalmol 2005; 139: 847–54.

58. Hamard P, May F, Quesnot S, Hamard H. Trans-scleral diode laser cyclophotocoagulation for the treatment of refractory pediatric glaucoma. J Fr Ophthalmol 2000; 23: 773–80.

59. Bock CJ, Freedman SF, Buckley EG, Shields MB. Transscleral diode laser cyclophotocoagulation for refractory pediatric glaucomas. J Pediatr Ophthalmol Strabismus 1997; 34: 235–9.

60. Yang LL, Lambert SR. Peters' anomaly: a synopsis of surgical management and visual outcome. Ophthalmol Clin North Am 2001; 14: 467–77.

61. Frueh BE, Brown SI. Transplantation of congenitally opaque corneas. Br J Ophthalmol 1997; 81: 1064–9.

62. Erlich CM, Rootman DS, Morin JD. Corneal transplantation in infants, children and young adults: experience of the Toronto Hospital for Sick Children, 1979–88. Can J Ophthalmol 1991; 26: 206–10.

65. Biglan AW. Glaucoma in children: are we making progress? J AAPOS 2006; 1: 7–21.

66. de Silva DJ, Khaw PT, Brookes JL. Long-term outcome of primary congenital glaucoma. J AAPOS 2011; 15: 148–52.

Access the complete reference list online at

http://www.expertconsult.com

Part 5
The uvea

The uveal tract

Michael O'Keefe

Anatomy

The uveal tract consists of the iris, the ciliary body, and the choroid. The iris stroma is composed of pigmented and non-pigmented cells, collagen fibers, and a hyaluronic acid matrix. The crypts vary in size, shape, and depth and the surface is covered by an interrupted layer of connective tissue cells that merges with the ciliary body. Differences in color are related to the pigmentation in the anterior border layer and the deep stroma: the stroma of blue irises is more lightly pigmented than brown irises.

The ciliary body has the functions of aqueous humor production, lens accommodation, and trabecular and uveoscleral outflow of aqueous humor. It extends 6 mm from the iris root to the anterior area of the choroid, the anterior 2 mm with the ciliary processes, and the smoother and flatter posterior 4 mm, the pars plana. It has an external pigmented and an internal non-pigmented epithelial layer. The ciliary muscle has longitudinal radial and circular portions. The ciliary processes are composed mainly of large fenestrated capillaries that leak fluorescein and veins that drain to the vortex veins.

The choroid lies between the retina and the sclera. It is composed of blood vessels which are bounded by Bruch's membrane internally and the avascular suprachoroid externally. It is 0.25 mm thick with three layers of vessels supplied by the long and short posterior ciliary arteries and from the anterior ciliary arteries. The choriocapillaris is the innermost layer with a middle layer of small vessels and an outer layer of large vessels. The middle and outer choroidal vessels are non-fenestrated. The choriocapillaris is a continuous layer of large capillaries lying beneath the retinal pigment epithelium nourishing the outer portion of the retina; their endothelium is fenestrated and leaks fluorescein. Bruch's membrane has three layers: an outer elastic, a middle collagenous, and an inner circular layer, the basement membrane of the retinal pigment epithelium. The choroid firmly attaches to the margin of the optic nerve and extends to the ora serrata anteriorly joining the ciliary body.

Embryology

The uveal tract develops from the neural ectoderm, neural crest, and mesoderm. The iris sphincter and dilator muscles and posterior iris epithelium is formed from the neural ectoderm. Pigment differentiation and migration continues into the second and third trimesters. The smooth muscle of the iris, choroidal stroma, and ciliary body develop from the neural crest. Iris formation starts with the closure of the fetal cleft at 35 days' gestation. The sphincter muscle first appears at the optic margin at 10 weeks' gestation becoming myofibrils at 10–12 weeks. The dilator muscle forms at 24 weeks' gestation. The neuroectoderm differentiates into both pigmented and non-pigmented ciliary epithelium at 10–12 weeks' gestation. The smooth muscle in the ciliary body is present at 4 months' gestation, before the iris stroma develops; it connects to the ciliary spur in the fifth month. Neural crest cells form the pigmented cells of the uvea, which are complete at birth. The blood vessels are from the mesoderm and neural crest. The choroidal vasculature first differentiates from mesenchymal elements at 2 weeks' gestation and develops over the next 3–4 months. The pupillary membrane disappears shortly before term birth. The pupil is small at birth but, as the iris dilator muscle develops, it enlarges. The ciliary muscle's role in accommodation increases between 3 and 6 months. Three-quarters of the final adult ciliary body length is achieved by 2 years of age. Pigmentation in all races is complete by 1 year; irises normally get darker, never lighter, in the first year of life.

Symptoms of uveal disease

Symptoms of uveal disease depend on the site of the disease process. Pain and photophobia are features of iritis, but not of choroidal disease. The choroid's close contact to the retina means it usually affects the latter, and, if the macula is affected, there is decreased acuity with floaters and haze from vitreous cells.

Congenital structural and developmental abnormalities of the pupil include iridodonesis, aniridia, micro pupil, polycoria, corectopia, ectopia, coloboma, iris sphincter atrophy, and dilated oval pupils (Box 38.1, Figs 38.1 and 38.2). Acquired abnormalities include trauma (Fig. 38.3), ischemia, hemorrhage, or involvement with tumors such as lymphoma, leukemia, juvenile xanthogranuloma, leiomyoma, and neurofibromas.

Anisocoria is a difference in the size of the pupils. It occurs in up to 20% of the normal population. It may be transmitted as an autosomal dominant trait with variable expression.[1]

Congenital idiopathic microcoria, an abnormality of development of the pupillary membrane, is usually unilateral with an almost absent eccentric pupil. It may be an autosomal dominant trait. It is associated with myopia and corectopia.[2] Deformed pupils may be caused by unequal growth of neural crest cells in parts of the iris stroma. Bilateral microcoria has been reported in association with microphthalmos and posterior anomalies.[3] Early surgical treatment and occlusion therapy can result in useful vision.[4]

Box 38.1
Congenital pupil abnormalities
Aniridia
Ectopia
Micro pupil
Coloboma
Polycoria
Microcoria
Corectopia
Anisocoria

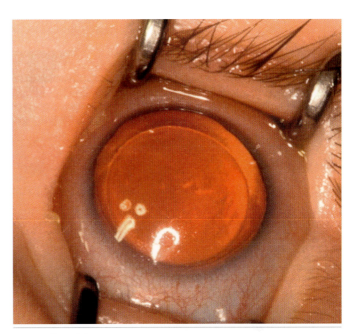

Fig. 38.2 **Aniridia.**

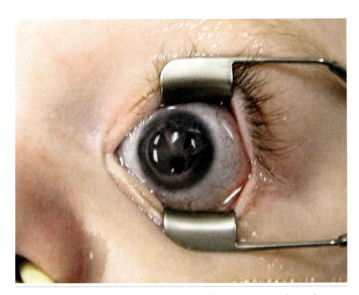

Fig. 38.1 **Child with Peters' anomaly showing corectopia through a corneal transplant.**

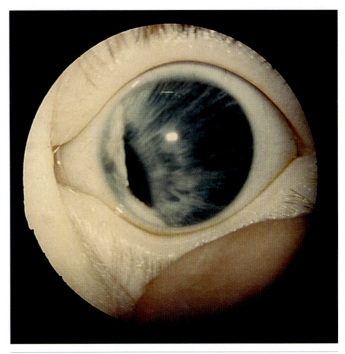

Fig. 38.3 **Iris incarceration in a penetrating injury.**

Box 38.2

Congenital iris abnormalities

Brushfield's spots

Iris melanosis

Iris ectropion

Lisch nodules

Iris stromal cyst

Juvenile xanthogranuloma

Heterochromic iridis

Persistent pupillary membranes

Colobomas

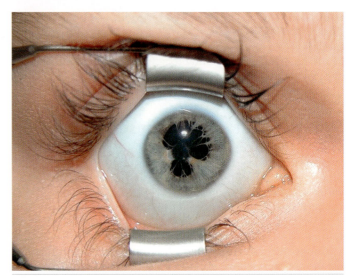

Fig. 38.5 Right eye in child bilateral pupillary membranes.

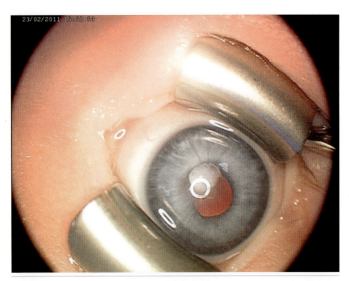

Fig. 38.4 Persistent pupillary membrane.

Persistent pupillary membranes

Congenital persistent pupillary membranes result from incomplete involution of the tunica vasculosa lentis which does not involute until the third trimester and is seen in premature babies. They are mostly sporadic. They are formed by buds from the annular iris vessels growing centrally to form the anterior vascular tunic of the lens.[5] They may span the entire pupil and be attached to the anterior capsule of the lens with or without a cataract. They may occur with microcornea, megalocornea, microphthalmos, and coloboma. Persistence of extensive membranes is uncommon. Most are asymptomatic and require only a mydriatic or no treatment.[6] However, it is sometimes difficult to assess whether a membrane is amblyogenic. Removal involves surgery with viscoelastics and excision with microscissors[7] or a vitrector. A cataract may be induced if the lens is damaged, and the surgeon must avoid cutting the iris or creating an iridodialysis.[8,9] Laser lysis uses a Nd:YAG laser to disrupt the adhesions between the strands of the membrane and the normal iris.[10] Pigment dispersion and hyphema are potential complications. The visual prognosis can be good,[11] but poor initial visual acuity is an indication of a poor outcome. Myopic and hyperopic anisometropia is more prevalent in eyes with more severe hyperplastic persistent pupillary

membranes. A 5-week-old baby presented with persistent pupillary membranes in her left eye (Fig. 38.4). They seemed amenable to medical treatment so we used pupil dilation and patching. At 4 months, she was intolerant of patching. We removed the membranes through a small incision using viscoelastics and capsulotomy scissors. She had a clear visual axis postoperatively and tolerated patching. She now has equal vision in both eyes. A 10-year-old child presented with pupillary membranes in both eyes (Fig. 38.5). He was photophobic and had reduced vision. His pupils dilated poorly and it was impossible to see his fundi or assess his refraction. Surgical removal was performed using viscoelastics and a capsulotomy scissors. Four years later he has a corrected vision of logMAR 0.3 (6/12, 20/40, 0.50) and is moderately myopic.

Congenital iris and stromal cysts

Iris cysts may be congenital resulting from an accumulation of fluid in an epithelium lined cyst.[12] They can be in the pigment epithelium or stroma and have a squamous epithelial or neuroepithelial lining.[13] Iris pigment cysts are usually stationary and have a transparent wall with a vascular lining and occur at the pupillary margin. Stromal cysts are progressive, in the anterior surface of the iris. Whilst some advocate a conservative approach, many require surgery.[13] The main treatment options are aspiration with or without cryotherapy applied to the base of the cysts near the limbus, injection of sclerosant (risky), surgical excision with sector iridectomy, Nd:YAG or argon laser, or irradiation.[14,15] The differential diagnosis of congenital iris cysts includes cysts from epithelial implantation due to surgery, trauma, and iris or ciliary body tumors.[16] Complications include glaucoma,[17] cataract,[18] and spontaneous detachment to become free-floating.[19] Ciliary body cysts are less common; they may be solid or filled with fluid and may cause astigmatism and amblyopia. A neonate presented with a large iris stromal cyst encroaching on the visual axis (Fig. 38.6). At 6 weeks it was drained and partially excised. Three years later it remained small and he has excellent vision in the eye.

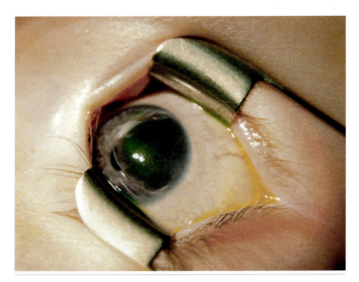

Fig. 38.6 **Large stromal cyst involving the visual axis.**

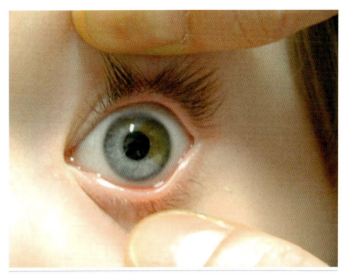

Fig. 38.8 **Heterochromia.**

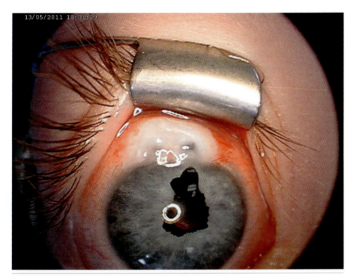

Fig. 38.7 **Ectropion uveae and a cystic drainage bleb.**

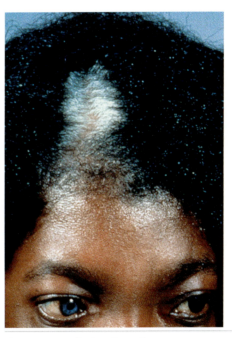

Fig. 38.9 **Waardenburg's syndrome.**

Iris ectropion or ectropion uveae

This is when the posterior pigment epithelium of the iris extends to the front of the iris. It may be congenital or acquired.[20] It is sometimes associated with glaucoma, neurofibromatosis type 1 (NF1), or anterior segment dysgenesis. Iris flocculi are excrescences of the pigment epithelium at the pupil margin. They may be a marker of familial aortic dissection.[21] A 2-year-old girl was referred with raised intraocular pressure (IOP) and a grossly cupped disk. She had ectropion uveae. She had a mitomycin-enhanced trabeculectomy which controlled her IOP to 8 mm, bleb revision 1 year later, and her vision improved to logMAR 0.48 (6/18, 20/60, 0.33) equivalent with Sheridan Gardner (Fig. 38.7).

Heterochromia iridis

A difference in iris color can be congenital or acquired (Fig. 38.8). In congenital heterochromia the involved iris is

darker, an indicator of ocular melanocytosis, oculodermal melanocytosis, or a sector hamartoma syndrome. Congenital Horner's syndrome (see Chapter 63) results in ipsilateral hypopigmentation, miosis, and ptosis. Waardenberg's syndrome (WS) (Fig. 38.9) is an autosomal dominant condition with sensorineural deafness, white forelock, and heterochromia iridis. Type 1 WS includes lateral displacement of the inner canthi, prominent root of the nose, and unusual brows. It is caused by a mutation in the PAXax 3 gene.[22] Type 2 WS does not include facial dysmorphism: the gene has been located to 3p12-p141.[23] Other types are rarer.

Iris sector heterochromia and Hirschsprung's disease is an autosomal recessive condition representing a neural crest cell lineage abnormality.[24,25]

In acquired heterochromia the iris is darker. It results from such infiltrative processes as nevi, melanomatous tumors, and deposition of material within the iris such as iron (siderosis).[26] Hemosiderosis results from iron deposition derived from a long-standing hyphema.[27] In an acquired lighter colored iris, Fuchs' heterochromic iridocyclitis should be considered. Infiltrations such as juvenile xanthogranuloma, metastatic malignancy, and leukemia must also be considered. Acquired Horner's syndrome infrequently leads to heterochromia.

Williams' syndrome is a rare autosomal dominant disorder. Associated systemic features include aortic valve disease, hypercalcemia, elfin facial features, prominent lips, hyperacusis, and developmental delay.[28,29] It has a unique iris stellate pattern appearance.[30] Other ocular features include strabismus, hyperopia, and retinal vein tortuosity.[31,32]

Juvenile xanthogranuloma

Juvenile xanthogranuloma is a benign condition of unknown etiology occurring in infancy and early childhood.[33] There is a proliferation of non-Langerhans' histiocytes, plasma cells, occasional eosinophils with Touton's giant cells. The skin lesions are accompanied by ocular involvement or ocular lesions occur alone, usually on the iris,[34] but they can occur in the choroid, orbit, cornea, conjunctiva, and sclera.[35] They are localized or diffuse yellow iris lesions, mostly unilateral. They may be vascular and can cause hyphema giving rise to glaucoma and corneal edema. Risk factors for the development of eye disease include the number of skin lesions and age under 2 years. Diagnosis is usually made on clinical examination. They are more common in children with neurofibromatosis.[36] If there is skin involvement, it can be biopsied to show typical giant cells, or the child may present with unexplained hyphema. The differential diagnosis includes xanthogranuloma, retinoblastoma, rubeosis secondary to persistent hyperplastic primary vitreous, and iris-corneal malformation. Biopsy of the iris carries the risk of hyphema. Treatment should be individualized for different presentations. Options include topical, subconjunctival and systemic steroids, low dose radiotherapy, and surgical excision.[37,38,39] Surgical excision should be the last option because of the risk of bleeding.

Lisch nodules are dome-shaped lesions on the anterior surface of the iris (Fig. 38.10). They are brown/orange in color, round, uniformly distributed on the iris, and bilateral. Their size varies from being microscopic to involving a segment of the iris.[40] Histologically, they are melanocytic hamartomas. In NF1 they are present in one-third of 2.5-year-olds, half of 5-year-olds, three-quarters of 15-year-olds, and 100% of patients over 21 years.[41] They may also occur in patients with NF2.[42] In dark irises they appear lighter than the background.

Brushfield's spots

Originally described in a normal individual,[43] Brushfield's spots represent areas of normal or hypercellular iris tissue with surrounding stromal hypoplasia. Thomas Brushfield considered them to be characteristic of Down's syndrome.[44] They are found in 86% of patients with trisomy 21. However, a quarter of normal individuals have similar spots. They differ from normal spots or freckles because they are more central and more numerous.

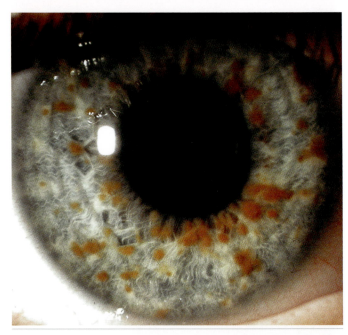

Fig. 38.10 Multiple Lisch nodules in a 10-year-old with NF1 and an optic nerve glioma.

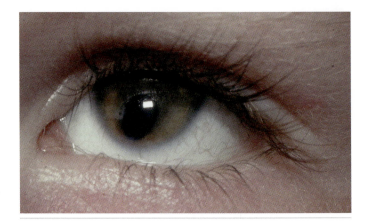

Fig. 38.11 Coloboma ("keyhole pupil").

Colobomas

Iris colobomas may be typical or atypical depending on their location. They may be complete or partial. Typical colobomas, caused by failure of fetal fissure closure, are found in the inferior nasal quadrant and are referred to as a "keyhole" pupil (Fig. 38.11). They may involve the iris, ciliary body, choroid, retina, and optic nerve (Fig. 38.12). Atypical colobomas are those found anywhere except at the inferior nasal quadrant and are usually restricted to the iris. Colobomas are part of a continuum that includes microphthalmos and anophthalmos. Autosomal dominant colobomas can be isolated lesions or manifestations of microphthalmia and anophthalmos.[45,46]

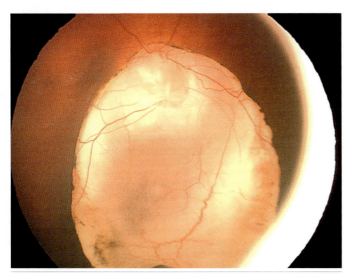

Fig. 38.12 Choroidal coloboma.

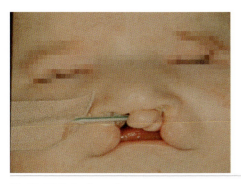

Fig. 38.13 Patau's syndrome.

Box 38.3

Chromosomal disorders associated with coloboma

Trisomy 13 ("cat eye" syndrome)
4P   11q   13q   18q   18f   18r
Trisomy 18

Several chromosomal disorders are associated with ocular colobomas (Box 38.3). Trisomy 13 or Patau's syndrome (Fig. 38.13) are most frequent and best known. Several syndromes are associated with ocular colobomas (Box 38.4). In CHARGE syndrome, coloboma is associated with heart disease, choanal atresia, mental retardation, genital hypoplasia, and deafness.[47] There is also an association between uveal colobomas and teratogens such as thalidomide.[48] Children with colobomas should have a complete eye examination, medical examination, and a family history and examination of relatives. The affected child should be followed for amblyopia, anisometropia, and retinal detachments.

Iris melanosis and iris mammillations

Iris melanosis is rare: the iris is hyperpigmented. It is associated with scleral pigmentation and choroid hyperpigmentation. It may be familial, usually an autosomal dominant trait.[49]

Box 38.4

Some syndromes associated with colobomas

Aicardi's syndrome
CHARGE syndrome
Goldenhar's syndrome
Goltz's syndrome (focal dermal hypoplasia)
Median facial cleft syndrome
Warburg's syndrome
Rubienstein-Taybi syndrome
Linear nevus sebaceous syndrome
Meckel's syndrome
Klinefelter's syndrome
Turner's syndrome

Box 38.5

Tumors of the uveal tract

Iris nevi
Medulloepithelioma
Leiomyomas
Hemangiomas
Choroidal osteoma
Iris melanomas
Choroidal melanomas

Iris mammillations are villiform protuberances that can cover much of the anterior surface of the iris and are sometimes associated with an iris nevus.[50] There is a risk of glaucoma with both conditions.

Cogan-Reese syndrome is a unilateral iris nevus which occurs with peripheral anterior synechiae in young people with ocular hypertension.

Tumors of the uveal tract (Box 38.5)

Leiomyomas of the iris and ciliary body are rare, benign, slow growing tumors of smooth muscle, more common in females. They appear pale pink. Presentation is with pupillary distortion and hyphema that can lead to secondary glaucoma and cataract. They can be indistinguishable from melanomas.[51] If they enlarge, excision is necessary.

Iris hemangioma

Iris hemangiomas (Fig. 38.14) are rare, usually grow inferiorly and may cause spontaneous hyphema. The differential diagnosis includes juvenile xanthogranulomas, iris hemangiomas, or an iris foreign body. They are isolated lesions, or part of generalized diffuse neonatal hemangiomas or associated with lid hemangiomas.[52]

Choroidal hemangiomas present in an adult as a circumscribed hemangioma without systemic manifestations, or with a diffusely red appearance ("tomato ketchup") within two disk diameters, usually temporally, of the optic disk.[53] The latter occur in 40% of infants with Sturge-Weber syndrome (see Chapter 65).[54] If the hemangioma grows and threatens

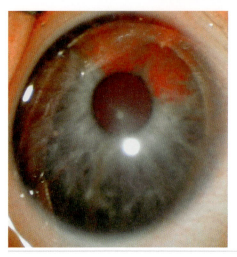

Fig. 38.14 Iris hemangioma.

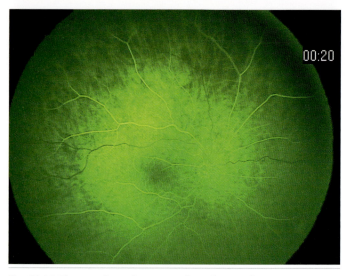

Fig. 38.16 Fluorescein angiogram confirms hemangioma.

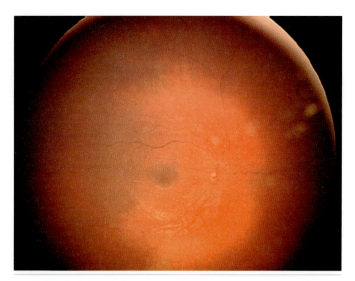

Fig. 38.15 Fundus with no obvious hemangioma.

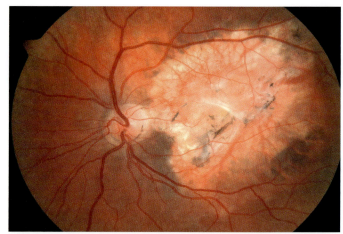

Fig. 38.17 A typical choroidal osteoma with loss of central vision.

vision, photocoagulation and cryotherapy are used to treat it.[55] A neonate was diagnosed with Sturge-Weber syndrome. He was referred at age 5 years for management of the glaucoma. The fundal appearance does not show a choriohemangioma (Fig. 38.15), but a fluorescein angiogram confirms its presence (Fig. 38.16).

Medulloepitheliomas (diktyomas) are usually unilateral, solid, or cystic tumors occurring in the non-pigmented ciliary body epithelium or iris. They appear in infancy or early childhood. They present as glaucoma, leukocoria, abnormal shaped pupil, glaucoma, or hyphema. They are composed of membranes, tubes, and rosettes and may undergo malignant transformation. However, the potential for spread is low. If the tumor is well localized anteriorly, local resection or cryotherapy is the treatment.[56] However, if diagnosis is late, there is a risk of extraocular extension and enucleation is the recommended treatment.

Choroidal osteomas are unilateral benign ossifying tumors whose pathogensis is unknown. They are yellow white and mostly peripapillary (Fig. 38.17). Complications include visual loss secondary to foveal extension with subfoveal neovascular membrane formation or serous detachment.[57,58]

Iris melanomas are rare in children and are clinically benign. They usually occur in the iris inferiorly[59] and may present as a hyphema. They differ from choroidal and ciliary body melanomas with 60% being spindle cell, 33% mixed or epitheloid cells.[60] The differential diagnosis includes juvenile xanthogranuloma, iris rhabdomyosarcoma, and iris foreign body.

Figure 38.18 shows the eye of a baby who presented at 6 months with an iris nevus. Normal vision remains after 14 years follow-up.

Choroidal melanomas

Choroidal melanomas are rare in childhood and represent between 0.6% and 1% of all patients with choroidal melanomas,[61] but we need to consider this potentially fatal tumor,[62] which may occasionally be congenital. The clinical and histopathologic features in children are similar to adults. Visual symptoms include metamorphopsia, blurred vision, photophobia, field loss, and leukocoria.[63] Many are asymptomatic, found on routine examination, usually unilateral, with equal predilection for either eye, and without gender bias. Fifty-four percent affect the choroid, 25% the iris. The differential

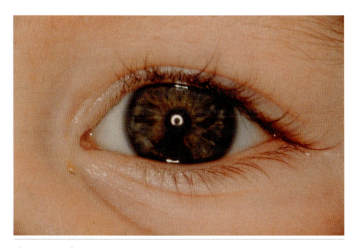

Fig. 38.18 Iris nevus.

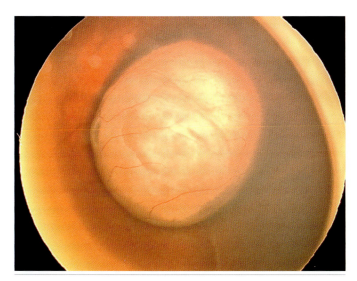

Fig. 38.19 Childhood choroidal melanoma.

diagnosis includes medulloepithelioma, hematoma, and melanocytoma. Associations include ocular melanocytomas, NF1, familial melanomas, and cutaneous dysplastic nevus syndrome.[64] The risk for metastatic disease is related to tumor size and cell type, ciliary body involvement, epithelioid cell type, extraocular extension, and high mitoses count. Cytogenetics may show chromosomal denaturation, a major prognostic indicator.[65] Patients with monosomy 3 have a 5-year survival of less than 50%.[66] Treatment is based on the tumor size and location. Treatment options include brachytherapy, proton beam therapy, stereotactic radiotherapy, local scleral resection, and enucleation. A 7-year-old girl presented with a left upper temporal fundus mass (Fig. 38.19). She had a trans-scleral local resection. Histology identified an amelanotic spindle cell melanoma with a high number of mitoses. Multiplex ligation-dependent probe amplification analysis showed two copies of chromosome 3, three copies of the short arm of chromosome 6, and two copies of chromosome 8, indicating a good prognosis. Three years later, she had no visible tumor, a flat retina, and vision of "counting fingers".[67]

Spontaneous hyphemas

Spontaneous hyphemas may be caused by anomalous iris capillary loops, tumors such as juvenile xanthogranuloma, medulloepithelioma or retinoblastoma, retinopathy of prematurity, persistent hyperplastic vitreous and blood dyscrasias, and, in older children, scurvy and iris rubeosis. Direct leukemic infiltration of the iris may cause hyphema, glaucoma, and hypopyon. Studies to determine the underlying cause include eye ultrasound, CT scanning, and general physical examination. Hematological screening for blood disorders is also necessary.

References

5. Merin S, Crawford JS, Cardarelli J. Hyperplastic persistent pupillary membranes. Am J Ophthalmol. 1971; 72: 717–9.
7. Cibis GW, Tripathi RC, Tripathi BJ. Surgical removal of congenital pupillary iris lens membrane. Am J Ophthalmol 1997; 123: 839–41.
8. Reynolds JD, Hiles DA, Johnson BL, Biglan AW. Hyperplastic persistent pupillary membranes surgical management. J. Pediatr Ophthalmol Strabismus 1983; 20: 149–52.
11. Lee SM, Yu YS. Outcome of hyperplastic persistent pupillary membrane. J Pediatr Ophthalmol Strabismus 2004;41:163–71.
12. Shields JA, Kline MUS, Augsburger JJ. Primary iris cysts a review of the literature and report of 62 cases. Br J Ophthalmol 1984; 68: 152–66.
20. Wilson ME. Congenital iris ectropion and new classification for anterior segment dysgenesis. J. Pediatr Ophthalmol Strabismus 1990; 27: 48–55.
21. Lewis RA, Merin LM. Iris flocculi and familial aortic dissection. Arch Ophthalmol 1995; 113: 1330–1.
22. Tassabehi M, Read AP, Newton VE, et al. Mutations in the PAX3 gene causing Waardenburg syndrome type 1 and type 2. Nat Genet 1993; 3: 26–30.
24. Brazel SM, Sullivan TJ, Thorner PS, et al. Iris sector heterochromia as a marker for neural crest disease. Arch Ophthalmol 1992; 110: 233–5.
25. Liang JC, Juanrez CP, Goldberg MR. Bilateral bicoloured irides with Hirschsprung's disease: a neural crest syndrome. Arch Ophthalmol 1983; 101: 69–73.
31. Greenberg F, Lewis RA. The Williams syndrome: spectrum and significance of ocular features. Ophthalmology 1988; 95: 1608–12.
33. Zimmerman LE. Ocular lesions of juvenile xanthogranuloma (nevoxanthogranuloma). Trans Am Acad Ophthalmol Otolaryngol 1965; 69: 412–42.
34. Gass JD. Management of juvenile xanthogranuloma of the iris. Arch Ophthalmol 1964; 71: 344–7.
35. Sanders TE. Infantile xanthogranuloma (nevoxanthogranuloma) survey of 20 cases. Trans Am Ophthalmol Soc 1960; 58: 59–74.
37. Casteels I, Olver J, Malone M, Taylor D. Early treatment of juvenile xanthogranuloma of the iris with subconjunctival steroids. Br J Ophthalmol 1993; 77: 57–60.
39. Harley RD, Romayanoida N, Chan GH. Juvenile xanthogranuloma. J Pediatr Ophthalmol Strabismus 1982; 19: 33–9.
41. Lubs ML, Bauer MS, Formas ME, Dyokic B. Lisch nodules in neurofibromatosis type 1. N Engl J Med 1991; 324: 1264–6.
42. Charles SJ, Moore AT, Yates JRW, Ferguson-Smith MA. Lisch nodules in neurofibromatosis type 2: case report. Arch Ophthalmol 1989; 107: 1571–2.
45. Duke-Elder S. System of Ophthalmology Normal and Abnormal Development Congenital Deformities Vol III. Part 2. London: H Kimpton; 1964.
46. Savell J, Cook JR. Optic nerve colobomas of autosomal dominant heredity. Arch Ophthalmol 1976; 94: 395–400.

47. Davenport SLH, Hefner MA, Mitchell JA. The spectrum of clinical features in CHARGE syndrome. Clin Genet 1986; 14: 290–8.

53. Anand R, Augsburger JJ, Shields JA. Circumscribed choriodal hemangiomas. Ophthalmology 1989; 107: 1338–42.

54. Phelps CD. Glaucoma in Sturge Weber syndrome. Ophthalmology 1978; 85: 276.

56. Broughton WL, Zimmerman LE. A clinicopathologic study of 56 cases of intraocular medulloepitheliomas. Am J Ophthalmol 1978; 85: 407–18.

58. Eting E, Savir H. An atypical fulminant course of choriodal osteoma in two siblings. Am J Ophthalmol 1992; 113: 52–5.

59. Arentsen JJ, Green WR. Melanoma of the iris: report of 72 cases treated surgically. Ophthal Surg 1975; 6: 23–37.

62. Singh AD, Shields CL, Shields JA, Sato T. Uveal melanoma in young patients. Arch Ophthalmol 2000; 118: 918–23.

66. Meir T, Zeschnigk M, Masshöfer L, et al. The spatial distribution of monosomy 3 and network vasculogenic mimicry patterns in uveal melanoma. Invest Ophthalmol Vis Sci 2007; 48: 1918–22.

67. Russo A, Coupland SE, O'Keefe M, Damato BE. Choroidal melanoma in a 7-year-old child treated by trans-sceral local resection. Graefes Arch Clin Exp Ophthalmol 2010; 248: 747–9.

Access the complete reference list online at
http://www.expertconsult.com

SECTION 4
**Systematic pediatric
ophthalmology**

CHAPTER **39**

Part 5
The uvea

Uveitis

Clive Edelsten

Box 39.1

**Differential diagnosis of childhood
intraocular inflammation**

Unreported trauma or intraocular foreign body

Neoplasia

> Diffuse retinoblastoma
>
> Juvenile xanthogranuloma
>
> Relapse of leukemia
>
> Rosai-Dorfman disease

Photoreceptor dystrophy, especially where retinal pigmented
epithelium (RPE) changes have not yet developed or where RPE
changes resemble choroiditis

Retinochoroidal dysgenesis

Hereditary vitreoretinal degeneration

Retinal vascular abnormalities that leak or bleed: Coats' disease,
vasoproliferative tumors

Congenital disk abnormalities especially with secondary vascular
complications

Infection, especially in the congenitally or iatrogenically
immunodeficient

Introduction

This chapter will include endogenous childhood ocular inflammation including uveitis and the vasculitides. The differential
diagnosis of childhood uveitis includes infection, hereditary
anatomic abnormalities, and degenerations that may be
accompanied by inflammation and tumors of childhood (Box
39.1). Ocular inflammation also accompanies systemic vasculitides; following infection ("reactive uveitis"); and accompanying congenital immunodeficiency syndromes and systemic
autoinflammatory diseases.

Uveitis is a relatively common feature of several localized
autoinflammatory diseases that have both unique and shared
genetic associations (Table 39.1). There is often a family
history of a wide range of autoimmune and autoinflammatory
conditions in children with idiopathic uveitis unaccompanied
by systemic disease. However, despite the wide variety of identified genetic associations, uveitis patients only rarely cluster
in families, other than those with a high prevalence of HLA-
B27, and there must be many environmental triggers and other
genetic causes that remain unidentified.

Experimental models of uveitis have concentrated upon
antigen-specific autoimmune mechanisms of inflammation.
Sympathetic ophthalmia and phacoanaphylaxis may be examples of ocular organ-specific autoimmunity but the majority of
childhood uveitis syndromes are secondary to localized or
generalized disorders of the control of inflammation. The phenotypes of human uveitis are more varied than the range of
available animal models of autoimmunity; there is increasing
interest in the variety of mechanisms, other than antigen-
specific autoimmunity, that may underlie ocular inflammation. Advances in genetics and study of the differential response
to treatment with non-specific and lymphocyte-specific or
cytokine-specific immunosuppressants has led to a continuing
reappraisal of disease classifications and the therapeutic implications of newly discovered genetic associations.

General considerations

When considering ocular inflammation in childhood one
needs to ask:

Table 39.1 – Inflammatory disease associated with childhood uveitis

Systemic autoinflammatory diseases

Disease	Systemic disease	Ocular disease	Gene	Inheritance
Familial Mediterranean fever	Peritonitis, rash, arthritis	Uveitis	MEFV	Recessive
Hyperimmunoglobulin D syndrome	Peritonitis, rash, arthralgia		MVK	Recessive
Tumor necrosis factor receptor-associated periodic syndrome	Rash, myalgia	Conjunctivitis	TNFRSFIA	Dominant
Chronic infantile neurologic cutaneous articular syndrome	Rash, arthritis, hepatosplenomegaly, deafness, chronic meningitis	Disk edema, uveitis	CIAS1	Dominant
Muckle-Wells syndrome	Rash, arthralgia, deafness	Conjunctivitis, disk edema	CIAS1	Dominant
Blau's syndrome	Rash, arthritis	Panuveitis	CARD15	Dominant

Localized autoinflammatory diseases

Disease	Systemic disease	Common type of uveitis	Gene associations	Ethnicity
Juvenile idiopathic arthritis	Joint	Chronic anterior	DRB*0801, 1101, 1301, DPB1*02	
Behçet's disease	Mucosa, skin, vasculitis	Pan	B51	Eastern Mediterranean to Orientals
Enthesis-related arthritides	Joint	Acute anterior	B27	N. Europeans
Sarcoidosis	Skin, joints, lung	Pan	DR3	N. Europeans, Afro-Caribbeans
Ulcerative colitis	Colon, joints	Acute anterior	DRB1*150 2, 0103	
Crohn's disease	Bowel, joints	Acute anterior	CARD15	
Vogt-Koyanagi-Harada syndrome	Skin, CNS	Pan	DRB1*04	Native Americans, Orientals, Asians
Tubulointerstitial nephritis and uveitis syndrome	Kidney	Chronic anterior	DRB1*0102	
Multiple sclerosis	CNS	Intermediate	DR1501	N. Europeans
Psoriasis	Skin, joints	All	Cw6, CARD15	

1. Why has the inflammation started in childhood rather than adulthood?
2. Will the age of onset influence the disease phenotype?
3. Is there a genetic disorder of the control of inflammation?
4. Is there a disorder of immunity predisposing to autoimmunity?
5. Is the inflammation secondary to a genetic degenerative process?

Familial clustering of unusual disease patterns suggests rare or novel mutations. The immune system develops through childhood and adolescence when most infections are first encountered. An unusual ocular inflammatory response to infection may be the first expression of a congenital systemic immune disorder (Box 39.2).

Organization of service

Childhood uveitis requires an organizational approach:

1. Early therapeutic decisions have to be made.
2. Effective management depends on primary care, pediatricians, and long-term social and educational planning.

Box 39.2

Immunodeficiency diseases associated with uveitis

Cyclic neutropenia
Chronic granulomatous disease of childhood
X-linked lymphoproliferative disease with Epstein-Barr virus and hypogammaglobulinemia
Common variable immunodeficiency
IgG_2 deficiency
Hyper IgM disease with hypogammaglobulinemia
Hypocomplementemic vasculitis

3. Multiple surgical and medical specialties may be required.
4. Outcomes depend on public health measures as well as drugs and surgery.
5. General ophthalmologists need information about the threshold for tertiary referral. Late presentation and chronicity are common leading to high complication rates compared to similar conditions in adulthood.
6. In children, amblyopia, postsurgical glaucoma and fibrosis, the growth effects of parenteral steroids, and immunosuppressants pose special problems.

7. Compliance with treatment may be problematic for children and families.

Evaluation for systemic disease

Ocular inflammation may herald systemic disease (see Table 39.1). Physicians and ophthalmologists best work as teams. Symptoms of systemic disease may occur later than the ocular disease in oligoarticular juvenile idiopathic arthritis (JIA), sarcoidosis, Behcet's disease, and Vogt-Koyanagi-Harada (VKH) syndrome.

Associated central nervous system (CNS) inflammation is difficult to diagnose if it presents with behavioral changes, deafness, retrobulbar optic neuritis, headaches, or movement disorders in preverbal toddlers. Optic disk edema is frequent in childhood uveitis and scleritis and should not invariably require the exclusion of raised intracranial pressure (ICP) by lumbar puncture and neuroimaging. However, the diagnosis of optic disk changes (Figs 39. 1 and 39. 2) may be challenging and raised ICP can occur in pediatric sarcoidosis, systemic lupus erythematosus (SLE),[1] chronic infantile neurologic

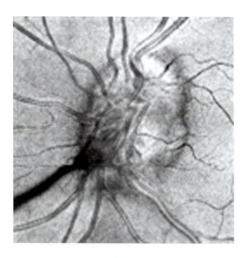

Fig. 39.1 Persistent optic disk edema with anterior inferonasal vitreous band to disk, 1 year after remission of intermediate uveitis.

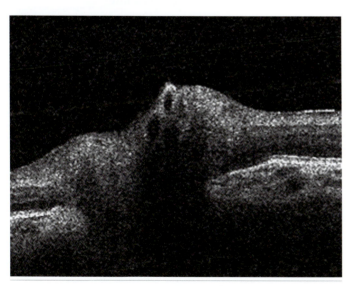

Fig. 39.2 Optical coherence tomography of persistent optic disk edema 15 years after onset of JIA-uveitis.

cutaneous and arthritis (CINCA) syndrome, venous sinus thrombosis, and steroid use. Other causes of optic disk swelling include hypotony and optic neuritis.

Epidemiology of pediatric uveitis

Childhood uveitis is uncommon; rising with age. In 0- to 4-year-olds, the incidence is 3/100 000, in 10- to 14-year-olds 6/100 000, and in adults aged 17–25/100 000. It comprises 5% of most series of uveitis patients.[2]

The most common type of pediatric uveitis at a population level is idiopathic. The most common pattern in young children is chronic anterior uveitis; in those aged 8–16 it is intermediate uveitis. After age 16, the pattern of uveitis types is similar to that in adulthood (Box 39.3). Idiopathic chronic painful bilateral anterior uveitis, idiopathic anterior and intermediate uveitis, and idiopathic panuveitis are also not uncommon in children. Specific uveitis syndromes, such as birdshot retinochoroidopathy, are exceptionally rare in children.[3]

Juvenile idiopathic arthritis (JIA) is the most common extraocular disease reported in tertiary referral series followed by those with no systemic disease (idiopathic uveitis), enthesitis related arthritis (ERA), sarcoidosis,[4] inflammatory bowel disease (IBD), and Behçet's disease. Even in countries with high rates of Behçet's disease, Behçet's uveitis is uncommon in childhood.[5] VKH[6] and tubulointerstitial nephritis and uveitis syndrome (TINU)[7] can begin in childhood. Behçet's disease and VKH syndrome are 10–100 times more common in some Oriental, Asian, and Mediterranean groups than in Caucasians.

HLA-B27 related diseases, multiple sclerosis (MS), and sarcoidosis are more common in North Europeans; there are also high rates of sarcoidosis in Afro-Caribbeans and high rates of ERA in Middle America. MS-associated uveitis is very rare in this age group although children with intermediate uveitis may well have the same genotype predisposing to the development of MS.

Epidemiology of vasculitis

The commonest type of childhood systemic vasculitis is Henoch-Schonlein purpura which does not have ocular involvement;[8] giant cell arteritis does not occur in childhood. The incidence of SLE is 0.8/10 000 and juvenile dermatomyositis 0.4/100 000. Childhood polyarteritis nodosa (PAN) is the fourth most common and ocular involvement is not uncommon. Wegener's granulomatosis, Behçet's disease, and microscopic polyangiitis are very rare – each less than 0.1/100 000.

Takayasu's disease and Kawasaki's disease are more common in Asians and Orientals. In Japan, the incidence of Kawasaki's

Box 39.3	
Commonest types of uveitis by age	
0–6 years	JIA-CAU
7–12 years	Idiopathic CAU, IU
13–16 years	IU, B27-associated AAU
Adult	B27-associated AAU

For abbreviations, see text.

disease in under 5s is 110/100 000: in the UK it is about a hundred times less frequent.

Clinical types of uveitis

Idiopathic uveitis

Classification is best made on the basis of the site of visible inflammation: unilateral or bilateral, acute or chronic, painful or painless and redness present or not (Fig. 39.3). The anatomic classification and terms for clinical activity of uveitis have been revised.[9] Patients with significant cell counts in both the anterior chamber and vitreous should be classified as "anterior and intermediate uveitis." This describes some cases of JIA-uveitis and some previously classified as intermediate uveitis. Chronic unilateral uveitis suggests an infective cause but should not preclude a search for systemic disease. Twenty percent of JIA-uveitis remains unilateral.

Although acute and chronic are classifying terms, they rely on a history and are less helpful in children. It is more practical to introduce a distinction between red and painful eyes, at presentation, as distinct from inflammation associated with white and painless eyes at presentation.

Painful anterior uveitis

Unilateral, painful, acute anterior uveitis (AU) is most frequently associated with HLA-B27-related diseases. They present in later childhood, rarely under 6 years; an infective or posterior segment cause is likely in this age group. Bilateral painful AU is the most frequent uveitis type following infection or severe systemic inflammation and is a common pattern of uveitis in otherwise healthy 7- to 14-year-olds where it can persist for a couple of years. Complications, other than ocular hypertension, are uncommon in chronic painful AU despite the length of disease when compared to the chronic painless AU of JIA.

Painless anterior uveitis

Chronic painless AU, without systemic disease, is common in young children. The arthritis of JIA may develop up to 7 years after the onset of chronic painless AU (Fig. 39.4). Investigation of renal function, for TINU syndrome, sarcoidosis, and possible immunodeficiency is also indicated. Skin rashes are a common manifestation of sarcoid, Blau's early onset sarcoidosis syndrome and CINCA: they are easier to biopsy. Fuchs' heterochromic cyclitis is very rare in early childhood

Intermediate uveitis

This refers to vitritis with a variable retinal inflammation and a minimal anterior segment inflammation (Table 39.2). The average age of onset is 9–13 years. Young children present late, and there may be extensive retinal complications rarely seen in adults. Children are less likely to develop macular edema but it is more difficult to resolve. Optic disk edema with chronic vitritis is more common than in adults. Peripheral vascular abnormalities are difficult to detect and may only be suspected when they cause hemorrhage. Neovascularization of the optic disk and retina may be caused solely by inflammation and subside with immunosuppression.[10]

Changing signs in the inferior fundus are useful to monitor disease progression as the level of vitritis is difficult to monitor in children and visual acuity may be maintained despite progressive extramacular damage. Sarcoidosis produces aggregates of white cells in the inferior vitreous ("snowballs") rather than pars planitis ("snow bank") and multifocal choroiditis is characteristic. IU associated with MS rarely produces vitreous opacities. Focal retinal pigment epithelial scars can develop inferiorly at sites of previous retinal inflammation and do not necessarily indicate the development of choroiditis. Retinal vascular leakage and periphlebitis may be marked in acute IU but are not diagnostic of any specific cause.

Panuveitis and multifocal choroiditis

Unifocal, unilateral choroiditis suggests infection such as toxoplasmosis. Multifocal, bilateral disease suggests systemic disease or a white spot syndrome, both rare in childhood. Many children with multifocal choroiditis and vitritis resemble

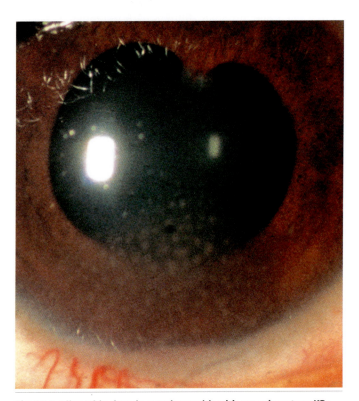

Fig. 39.3 Idiopathic chronic anterior uveitis with granulomatous KPs and limbal inflammation.

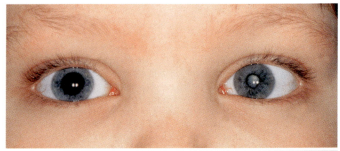

Fig. 39.4 Idiopathic chronic anterior uveitis in white eyes presenting with left cataract in a 4-year-old. JIA developed 7 years later.

Table 39.2 – Structural complications of JIA-uveitis and IU

JIA-uveitis	Intermediate uveitis
Anterior segment changes	
AC cells and flare	AC signs only in "anterior and intemediate uveitis," and usually confined to cells only
Band keratopathy	
Extensive posterior synechiae	
Progressive anterior synechiae	
Iris hyperemia and rarely vascularization	
Unexplained hyphema	
Iris vascularized membrane	
Pupillary membrane	
Early irreversible ciliary body damage with chronic hypotony and phthisis	Hypotony rare
high risk glaucoma	Low risk glaucoma
Early cataract formation	Late developing despite persistent inflammation
Persistent diffuse vitreous flare and opacities with minimal vitritis	Vitritis necessary for diagnosis Opacities tend to be dependent and aggregate – snowballs, snowbanks
Diffuse macular and disk edema and subretinal fluid with minimal vitritis	Disk edema can be marked in absence of macular edema
Disk neovascularization	Disk and peripheral retinal neovascularization
Vitreous hemorrhage	Vitreous hemorrhage
Retinal detachment rare without	
Coexisting hypotony	Retinal detachment, pars plana cysts, localized peripheral detachments Retinoschisis
Postoperative complications	
IOL membrane formation	Usually tolerates IOL
Universal posterior capsular opacification	
Membrane formation following capsulotomy	

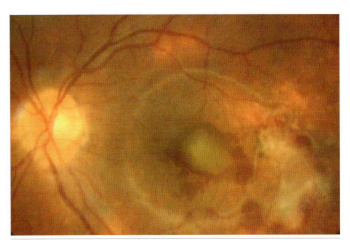

Fig. 39.5 Idiopathic panuveitis and multifocal choroiditis complicated by cataract, glaucoma, and choroidal neovascular membranes.

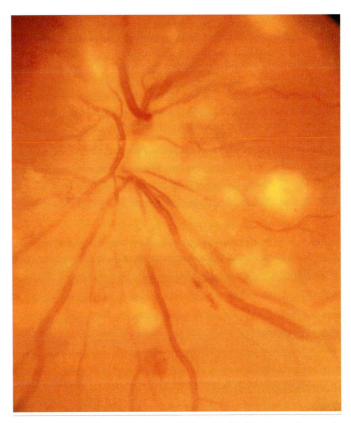

Fig. 39.6 Postviral retinitis with multiple retinal infiltrates and normal acuity.

sarcoidosis, with no evidence of extraocular disease. Some infections such as brucellosis, borreliosis, and varicella may also mimic sarcoid choroiditis. Multifocal choroiditis and panuveitis rarely occurs in childhood. It can be complicated by severe visual loss from secondary choroidal neovascularization and warrants aggressive control of inflammation (Fig. 39.5). If the fundus cannot be seen in children with AU it must be assumed they have panuveitis. Ultrasound may disclose scleritis or focal infection or tumor.

Retinitis

Focal infiltrates of the inner retina with little overlying vitritis are typical of acute viral infections (Fig. 39.6). They are more discrete and persistent and yellower than cotton-wool spots.

Retinal infiltrates in Behçet's disease always have signs of retinal vasculitis.

Neuroretinitis

In neuroretinitis, swelling of the neuroretina, maximal at the optic disk, is out of proportion to signs of posterior segment inflammation (see Chapter 53). Exudates around the fovea form a macular star. Children are more likely to develop edema in response to infections that trigger optic neuritis and neuroretinitis. Cat-scratch disease typically involves the posterior segment in this manner.

Post-traumatic uveitis

Trauma may provoke an autoimmune response to ocular antigens. Children are as prone as adults to these rare conditions.

Sympathetic ophthalmia

There is a bilateral chronic panuveitis with peripheral multifocal choroiditis with many clinical and histologic similarities to VKH and sarcoidosis. Vitritis may be severe. It follows unilateral penetrating trauma, cycloablation, or intraocular surgery. It may coexist with lens-induced uveitis.

Lens-induced uveitis

This is a granulomatous panuveitis that may occur hours to months after the release of lens material and can complicate severe uveitis from other causes.

Paraysinfectious uveitis

Childhood is a time when airborne pathogens are first encountered and transient ocular inflammation may result. Varicella and streptococcal infections are frequent causes of reactive uveitis. Reported associations may be coincidental and identification of intraocular viruses in specific uveitis types remains rare. Clusters of severe acute panuveitis in children have been reported from Tanzania and Nepal; in the former the incidence was 540/100 000 in the under 9s.[5–8]

Acute anterior uveitis (AAU) is the most common ocular inflammation following varicella but mild retinal vasculitis, a self-limiting retinitis, and multifocal choroiditis can occur, usually within 4 weeks (Fig. 39.6). Chronic inflammation and progressive retinitis is an absolute indication for antiviral treatment, not usually necessary for AAU.

Enteric infections triggering reactive arthritis may cause a reactive uveitis: HLA-B27 positivity is a risk factor. Reactive arthritis with urethritis and uveitis is very rare in children.

Localized autoinflammatory diseases

Juvenile idiopathic arthritis

JIA describes chronic joint inflammation starting before 16 years and lasting more than 6 weeks. Early onset rheumatoid arthritis, vasculitides, and ERA are extremely rare causes of arthritis under the age of 7.

Epidemiology

The incidence of juvenile arthritis is 10/100 000. Only half are patients with oligoarticular or polyarticular JIA, and the incidence of JIA-uveitis is 1/100 000 (Table 39.2).

JIA types associated with CAU

The ILAR classification of arthritis starting before the age of 16 years uses a personal or family history of psoriasis, a family history of HLA-B27-related disease and rheumatoid factor to aid classification. The classification was designed primarily to aid the epidemiologic study of arthritis. Antinuclear antibody (ANA) and age at onset are not used in the classification but are major independent risk factors for uveitis.

Genetic studies suggest similarities between oligoarticular and polyarticular JIA in the youngest groups.[11] Older children with ANA-negative polyarticular JIA may have a distinct pattern of disease and appear to be at a much lower risk of CAU. JIA is found in all races; JIA-uveitis may be more common in Caucasians.

Several genes, including HLA, are associated with different clinical types of JIA.[13,14] Oligoarticular onset JIA is associated with HLA genes common to polyarticular JIA (DRB1*08), psoriatic arthropathy (DRB1*1301), and systemic onset JIA (DRB1*11), as well as unique associations such as DPB1*02. Uveitis appears to be associated primarily with the DRB1*13 haplotype, which is most frequent in oligoarticular JIA, and DPB1*02. ERA and early onset rheumatoid arthritis are clinically and genetically distinct from the types of JIA associated with CAU.

Oligoarticular JIA is defined by the involvement of less than five joints at the onset of disease. If more joints are later involved it is classified as extended oligoarticular JIA. If more than five joints are involved at onset it is classified as polyarticular. The cut-off is artificial and age at onset of arthritis and ANA status are as important as the number of joints in defining JIA phenotypes.

All children with chronic painless AU are screened for joint abnormalities and to exclude other systemic diseases. Uveitis is associated with oligoarticular, ANA-positive JIA of early onset: the highest risk groups may have a frequency of uveitis of over 50%. The risk of uveitis diminishes to zero in those whose arthritis starts after age 13, and the cut-off may be much younger in those with polyarticular ANA-negative JIA. ANA status does not change the risk sufficiently to alter screening policy.

In those developing uveitis, arthritis typically starts at 28 months and uveitis 13 months later: 86% have oligoarticular onset JIA, 75% are female, and 80% are ANA-positive.[10,12]

Investigation of CAU

Routine laboratory testing in CAU can be limited to white count, serum angiotensin converting enzyme (sACE), ANA, immunoglobulins, antistreptolysin titers, electrolytes, and C-reactive protein. Other autoantibodies, such as double-stranded DNA, anticardiolipin and perinuclear antineutrophil cytoplasmic, as well as raised ASO titers, may occur in JIA. Raised sACE, immunoglobulins, and a lymphopenia suggest sarcoid which may present with arthritis indistinguishable from JIA.

Other JIA types

Systemic onset JIA involves the eye in only 1–2% of cases and occurs within months of presentation.

Psoriasis is associated with ERA, IBD, and Behçet's disease. It may also be an independent risk factor for uveitis.[9] Psoriasis present in a family member changes the rheumatologic classification, but the accompanying arthritis may initially be indistinguishable from oligoarticular JIA; some have a distinctive pattern of arthritis-psoriatic arthritis with dactylitis and nail changes. Eight percent of children with psoriatic arthritis develop uveitis.

Psoriasis may develop years after the onset of arthritis and uveitis. Psoriasis in the patient or relative of a patient with oligoarticular JIA does not alter the risk or nature of uveitis and patients should undergo the normal screening.

ERA presents with peripheral arthritis and enthesitis (inflammation where tendons or ligaments attach to bone) in children, rather than sacroiliitis. In younger children it may be indistinguishable from JIA and patients need to be screened until a definite clinical diagnosis of ERA is made – which is usually after the age of 7 years. A family history of ERA is highly suggestive of the diagnosis. The usual form of uveitis is AAU as in adults and screening has no role. AAU with ERA very rarely occurs before the age of 10 years.

Early onset rheumatoid arthritis starts around the age of 11 years and is not associated with uveitis. The presence of a positive rheumatoid factor in children with JIA does not equate to a diagnosis of juvenile rheumatoid arthritis; it should not alter screening in oligo/polyarticular JIA.

IBD related arthropathy may also be associated with uveitis. Patients may develop arthritis first and be diagnosed as JIA. Uveitis may be a CAU-like JIA but may also suffer AAU and retinal vasculitis.

Screening

The period of risk of developing uveitis depends on the age at onset of the arthritis. Those developing arthritis below the age of 3 years remain at risk for 7 years. Those developing arthritis after the age of 6 years are at risk for 3 years. In those regularly screened the development of uveitis after the age of 13 years is rare. The optimal screening interval is not known. There seems little value in screening at intervals of more than 3 months. These considerations are incorporated into the UK screening programme (2006) and can be found at http://www.bspar.org.uk/pages/clinical_guidelines.asp.

Screening is the most easily achievable method for reducing visual loss. The majority of those with JIA-uveitis will unfortunately develop CAU prior to the onset of screening, or before they develop arthritis. The efficacy of various screening regimens has not been tested. Screening involves the exclusion of anterior chamber cells and keratic precipitates by a slit-lamp. Younger children require experienced ophthalmologists; frequent checks may be needed at the onset until the child is happy to cooperate. When patients are old enough to cooperate with slit-lamp examination and can reliably report blurring and floaters, monitoring can be devolved to less specialist practitioners. The age at which this is possible depends on each individual child and local facilities.

Rheumatologists should be encouraged to dilate new cases and check for posterior synechiae and media opacities in order for severe uveitis to be detected early.

Monitoring

Subclinical and clinical uveitis may develop whilst on systemic arthritis treatment; the former may only be apparent when the effective dose is reduced through growth or when the arthritis is in remission. Uveitis may recur vigorously when systemic immunosuppression is reduced, especially abruptly, and patients should be checked within a few weeks of dose reductions. In remission and off all treatment, monitoring needs to be maintained. This should continue for 3 years.

Patients also require screening for glaucoma. To reduce the need for examination under anesthetic, children need to be trained to accept contact tonometry soon after the diagnosis of uveitis. Air-puff tonometry is less well tolerated. Disk appearances must be documented at the initial visit and changes photographed. There should be a low threshold for examination under anesthesia as inflammatory glaucoma can progress rapidly.

Clinical signs

The course of uveitis has a wide range of aggressiveness, severity, and chronicity (see Table 39.2). Late presentation has a profound effect on the severity and risk of long-term complications. Mild disease is a painless CAU; severe disease may cause a chronic AU and IU or a red, painful eye. A red eye occurring at each relapse warrants reconsideration of the diagnosis.

Minimal disease may produce "dusting" of the corneal endothelium only. A severe cellular reaction with 4+ cells, hypopyon, or fibrin is unusual. Band keratopathy accompanying mild uveitis is characteristic, not universal. Progression of keratopathy on treatment indicates aggressive disease (Figs 39.7 to 39.9). Persistent flare, iris hyperemia (may be mistaken for rubeosis), and an intraocular pressure (IOP) less than 10 are signs of severe disease, reversible if treated aggressively

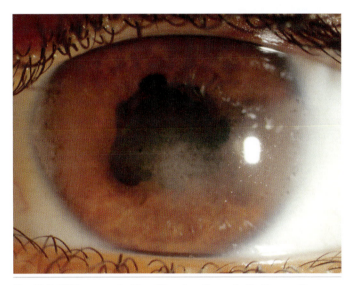

Fig. 39.7 Mild paracentral band keratopathy not affecting acuity.

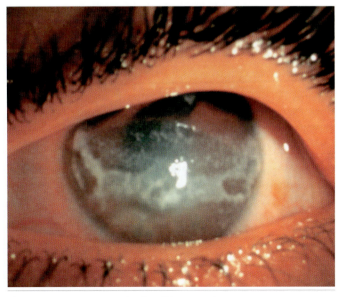

Fig. 39.8 Severe progressive band keratopathy.

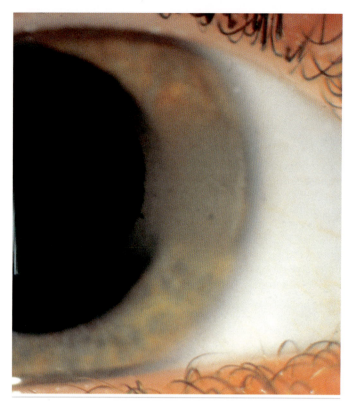

Fig. 39.9 **Clear central cornea following excimer laser removal of band keratopathy.**

early. Fibrovascular sheets may cover the pupil and impede a view of the posterior segment despite a clear lens. Iris bombé is not uncommon. Sometimes posterior synechiae are not obvious without mydriasis as they are present at the pupil margin.

AC cells rarely "spill over" into the vitreous in significant numbers as with adult AAU, but a dense vitreous haze with fibrin clumps that takes several weeks of systemic steroids to clear may occur in untreated disease. Posterior segment edema occurs with severe CAU: hypotony may contribute. Macular edema can be more extensive than in adults. Disk edema can be profound and persistent and mimic papilledema.

There is a close association between anterior segment complications and macular edema; optic disk edema and hypotony also cluster together.[13]

Course

Patients take several weeks to develop irreversible complications even with aggressive disease: the inflammation changes slowly compared to other forms of uveitis. Relapses are usually unaccompanied by redness or pain. Complications are present near onset from untreated disease. Complications may arise as secondary phenomena such as aphakic glaucoma or because of the length of active disease. The majority of those entering remission will have done so after 12 years.

The risk and nature of complications may therefore change through the course of the disease and the benefits of treatment regimens may alter over time. This is especially true when steroid treatment is used and where complete remission has not been achieved. Twenty-five percent of complications occur more than 10 years after disease onset in those who have not achieved a significant period of complete remission. The risks of new severe visual loss continue for more than 15 years after disease onset.[12,14]

Indications for treatment

With such a wide range of outcomes it is important that treatment risks and costs are matched to the risk of patient-centered quality outcomes such as functional visual loss, surgical interventions, and frequent hospital attendance (see Box 39.4).

As complete remission is not associated with the development of new inflammatory complications it is thus the aim of treatment. Prolonged periods of low activity may precede complete remission. It is not known what level of AC activity leads to complications. Cell counts may have limited value as a prognostic indicator. Cataracts form at similar rates in those with a trace of AC cells and those with 2+ of cells. AC cell counts are of less importance than AC flare in increasing risk of complications.[15,16] The persistence of activity is more significant than the level of activity. Complications are more likely in males, non-Caucasians, and those with prior episodes of macular edema and hypotony or frequent relapses. Cataract surgery increases the risk of complications.[17-21]

The level of disease activity one aims to achieve with immunosuppression depends on the relative risk of that eye developing further inflammatory complications. As the affected eye develops more risk factors for losing vision, the need for tighter disease control grows. The range of risk is great: females with no complications at diagnosis may have an 80% chance of complete, complication free remission within 15 years. Males with cataract at presentation may have 50% risk of blindness over 15 years. It would seem sensible to aim to prevent persistent flare, ocular hypertension, and visually significant lens opacities in those with no complications at presentation. Whether this requires systemic immunosuppression in all patients is unknown.

Alternative treatments to topical steroids

At some point the risks of cataract and glaucoma with continuous topical steroid treatment are sufficiently high to justify changing to immunosuppression.

Topical steroids cannot treat adequately the posterior segment complications even when AC activity is controlled. A frequent cause of avoidable complications is the failure to treat vitreous haze, disk and macular edema, and hypotony with systemic treatment in patients presenting with these signs.

The aim of treatment is to achieve a sufficiently long remission that withdrawal of treatment is not followed by a recurrence. This differs in different types of uveitis but is likely to be of the order of 12–18 months in JIA-uveitis and it may be best to achieve 3 years of remission before tailing off treatment in those who are at most risk. About half of patients given methotrexate (MTX) for JIA arthritis will relapse on withdrawal of treatment. Only half of patients with JIA-uveitis started on MTX will be off the drug after 7 years.[22-24]

Alternatives to methotrexate

MTX is in widespread use because of trial data in arthritis and the long-term safety data. It has not been compared to other immunosuppressive monotherapy in any form of uveitis. Other single immunosuppressive agents have been tried.[25-27] JIA-uveitis may respond less well to MTX than other forms of uveitis.

Inadequate control of arthritis with MTX usually leads to the addition of another drug such as an anti-TNF (tumor necrosis factor) agent and subsequent failure may lead to further combinations of biologic agents with no strong evidence and as yet unknown long-term risks.[28-30]

The management of severe uveitis requires a clear understanding of the treatment goals, the need for occasional revision of those goals, and the knowledge that many complications are not amenable to immunosuppression. Where there is no trial data, there is only opinion and parents must understand that expert opinion may vary.

Glaucoma

Glaucoma occurs in 13% of recent studies, less than earlier reports. Steroid-induced ocular hypertension (OHT) and aphakia are major risk factors; inflammatory glaucoma may contribute and usually develops after 2 or 3 years of CAU, not at presentation. Steroid-induced OHT is expected in 5% and is usually evident within a few months. Angle-closure glaucoma can occur if the early presentation was complicated by iris bombé but is rarely the sole cause in late-developing glaucoma. The cause of IOP changes is usually complex in severely damaged eyes as outflow obstruction may be combined with severe ciliary body damage with aqueous hyposecretion.

Other localized autoinflammatory diseases

Behçet's disease

Systemic features

Recurrent, painful, oropharyngeal, and genital ulceration with uveitis are major criteria for the diagnosis. Ulceration may precede the full expression of disease by 2 years. Mild symptoms such as arthralgia, erythema nodosum, gastrointestinal inflammation, and ulceration are non-specific. Acne, folliculitis, epididymitis, and intestinal ulcers are more specific. Spondylitis may occur in one-third of cases.

Vascular thrombosis and CNS disease are the major causes of morbidity. Thrombosis is more common in veins than in arteries. CNS inflammation can be primary, with demyelination, or secondary to thrombosis. The pyramidal brain stem is commonly involved but there may be diffuse, acute meningoencephalitis with behavioral changes.

Children may have milder disease and more delay to the complete syndrome: arthritis may be more common and ulceration less common.[31] Neonatal onset has been reported.

Ocular features

There is a panuveitis with explosive relapses, hypopyon, and sudden small and large retinal vein occlusion with white patches of retinitis. Retinal arteries may be involved; macular edema occurs in a minority. Retinal ischemia frequently leads to neovascularization complications.

A non-granulomatous CAU may occur but chronic intermediate uveitis is unusual. Conjunctivitis and episcleritis or scleritis may occur. Choroidal involvement is rare. The optic nerve may be involved by inflammatory optic neuropathy, and papilledema from CNS involvement, particularly sinus venous thrombosis. Secondary optic atrophy is common. The natural course of retinal vasculitis and ischemia leads to a high risk of bilateral blindness and a quarter of eyes may eventually lose vision.

Sarcoidosis

Systemic features

There is a chronic granulomatous inflammation that can affect any part of the body. Histology shows a non-caseating epithelioid cell granuloma with an accumulation of CD4+ T-lymphocytes. In adults, sarcoid involves the lung in 90% of cases. In two-thirds of patients, the disease remits, usually within 2 years, the majority requiring no treatment.

Sarcoidosis presents differently in those under 8 as it rarely involves the lung. Skin, joint, and eye involvement are the common sites of presentation and therefore it can sometimes mimic JIA, and an aggressive biopsy policy is warranted. Diagnostic biopsies are most frequently obtained from skin, synovium, and liver. Joints develop synovial hypertrophy with little pain or restriction in early stages. Skin involvement consists of a persistent follicular or nodular rash. Renal involvement is not uncommon. In one series of childhood sarcoid arthritis, 44/53 developed uveitis. sACE may be elevated in a third of cases and gallium-67 scanning can aid the diagnosis. CNS involvement is common in those with posterior segment inflammation and may require cerebrospinal fluid (CSF) analysis and neuroimaging to detect meningeal involvement.

Childhood sarcoidosis is more common in Caucasians. Familial disease occurs in 4%, and this must be distinguished from Blau's syndrome, which is also familial and lung involvement also does not occur.

Ocular features

Anterior uveitis may start with pain and redness and become chronic and painless. Iris and angle granulomas may distinguish the CAU from JIA-uveitis; band keratopathy is less common and inflammatory ocular hypertension more common than other types of CAU.

Sarcoid rarely causes chronic intermediate uveitis without other features. Panuveitis can develop with multifocal choroiditis that may be very widespread (Fig. 39.10). Visual loss may result from choroidal neovascular membranes arising from macular scars. Optic disk swelling is frequent and may have multiple causes including a granulomatous optic neuropathy, raised intracranial pressure, or secondary to uveitis. There may be a necrotizing vasculitis. Unilateral posterior segment or optic nerve disease may occur.

As young children with sarcoid may present with uveitis, disease may be very advanced at presentation and blindness frequently results. Uveitis frequently requires more prolonged and intensive immunosuppression than extraocular sarcoid. Sarcoid may involve the lid margins and cornea more frequently in childhood (Fig. 39.11).

Inflammatory bowel disease

Crohn's disease and ulcerative colitis are associated with ocular inflammation in a minority of patients. Both may present with a mild arthritis in childhood: IBD arthropathy. A family history of IBD is not uncommon in children with idiopathic uveitis (see Fig. 39.11).

AAU and episcleritis are the most frequent presentations: 6% of children with Crohn's disease were found to have AAU, but none of those with ulcerative colitis. Rarely, there may be a severe retinal vasculitis, and anterior uveitis may produce an acute hypopyon.

Vogt-Koyanagi-Harada syndrome

Systemic features

There is an acute onset meningoencephalitis with headache, vitiligo, poliosis, tinnitus, and dysacusia. The skin may be painful to touch in the acute phase. Some cases begin in childhood and most of those present with painful panuveitis with vitiligo developing later.

Ocular features[32]

There is a painful bilateral panuveitis with granulomatous anterior uveitis. Ciliary body edema may shallow the anterior chamber and increase or lower the IOP. Scleral perforation may occur. Serous retinal detachments are characteristic, especially inferiorly. Disk edema and peripheral choroiditis are frequent and angiography may demonstrate widespread pinpoint sites of leakage at the retinal pigmented epithelium (RPE). After repeated inflammation, depigmentation of the RPE and choroid leads to a "sunset glow fundus."

Children are more likely to have severe ocular disease because of late presentation with 61% of eyes losing sight compared to 26% in adults.

Tubulointerstitial nephritis and uveitis syndrome

Systemic features

Acute tubulointerstitial nephritis and uveitis (TINU) occur within a few weeks. The commonest symptoms are fever, malaise, and weight loss: a third have signs of ocular inflammation. Twenty percent present with uveitis occurring up to 2 months before renal involvement. The median age of onset is 15 years: the youngest is 9 years. Renal disease consists of an eosinophilic and mononuclear infiltrate but granulomas can also be found in the lymph nodes and marrow. Interstitial nephritis occurs in other conditions associated with uveitis such as sarcoidosis, Behçet's disease, Sjögren's syndrome, and postviral syndromes. Uveitis has also been reported with IgA nephropathy.

Ocular features[33,34]

There is a CAU with pain at onset; there may be granulomatous features. Posterior involvement occurs in one-fifth with retinal periphlebitis, hemorrhages, disk edema, and multifocal

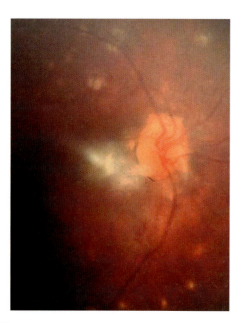

Fig. 39.10 Sarcoid multifocal choroiditis.

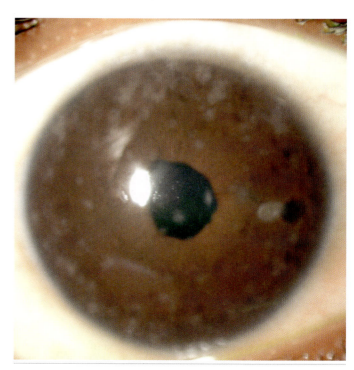

Fig. 39.11 Sarcoid multifocal keratitis.

choroiditis. The mean length is 2 years and visual outcome is usually good.

Multiple sclerosis

MS is rare in childhood. It can occasionally present with uveitis, usually a mild intermediate uveitis.

Rasmussen's syndrome

This is chronic unilateral epilepsy associated with an ipsilateral chronic uveitis that may present in childhood. It has been associated with cytomegalovirus infection.[35]

Systemic autoinflammatory disorders and familial granulomatous diseases

There are several familial disorders presenting with periodic fevers, urticarial rashes, and that may be accompanied by intermittent or persistent joint and ocular inflammation. There are two groups: those associated with cryopyrin mutations and those associated with other gene variants.[36]

Familial granulomatous syndromes such as Blau's syndrome and familial sarcoidosis may also present in childhood with fevers, rashes, joint, and eye involvement. Sporadic granulomatous diseases share some genetic abnormalities with the familial diseases.

Although single gene disorders of inflammation, some of these conditions may manifest in localized sites.

Cryopyrin associated periodic fever syndromes

These are disorders of innate immunity with a prevalence of 3/million. Mutations of the NLRP3 gene lead to uncontrolled activation of inflammasomes, multimolecular intracellular complexes composed of cryopyrin, leading to increased production of active IL-1-beta, IL-18, and inteferon-gamma.

Severity ranges from those suffering transient, non-destructive rashes and fevers (familial cold autoinflammatory syndrome) to those with more persistent inflammation and significant rates of renal failure from amyloid, deafness, chronic uveitis, and arthropathy (CINCA). Muckle Wells' syndrome describes patients with intermediate levels of severity. Forty percent of CINCA patients do not have a recognized genetic abnormality; some may be mosaics. There are overlap syndromes within the three groups.

Treatments targeting IL-1-beta can be very effective.

Chronic infantile neurologic, cutaneous, arthritis syndrome

Systemic

A persistent neonatal onset migratory urticarial rash occurs on the trunk and limbs and a destructive arthritis of the large joints with endochondral ossification. There may also be chronic meningoencephalitis with developmental delay and papilledema. There is frequent sensorineural deafness from cochlear inflammation. Renal failure may result from amyloidosis. CINCA commonly arises from de novo mutations – hence the severity whereas the milder syndromes are

usually familial. Cases have previously been misdiagnosed as systemic JIA.

Ocular

The chronic meningitis is associated with a cellular CSF and raised intracranial pressure, with chronic disk swelling and optic atrophy.[37] A mild CAU develops around 7 years of age without synechiae formation or redness: band keratopathy may occur.[38]

Familial granulomatous disease

The gene CARD15 encodes the NOD2 receptor and 40% of patients with Crohn's disease have one of three gene variants. CARD15 variants may act as disease modifying genes with IBD5 risk alleles in ulcerative colitis. Mutations may lead to inappropriate inflammation in response to bacterial peptidoglycan and result in IL-1 overproduction. The CARD15 mutations associated with Blau's syndrome are in a separate area of the gene from those associated with Crohn's disease. The type of mutation may influence the severity of ocular involvement in Blau's syndrome.[39] Other CARD15 mutations may be associated with early onset sarcoidosis and psoriatic arthritis. Blau's syndrome (familial) and early onset sarcoidosis (sporadic) are sometimes grouped as "pediatric granulomatous arthritis."

Blau's syndrome

Systemic features

Blau's syndrome is a familial, early onset granulomatous disorder with many features resembling childhood sarcoidosis. There is a transient punctate erythematous rash and a non-erosive arthropathy with giant synovial cysts starting in the first 3 years. Granulomas are found on synovial or tendon biopsy. The hands may show curving of the little fingers: camptodactyly. Hepatic and renal involvement may occur but not the lung. A vasculopathy may develop involving small and large vessels. There is earlier onset in successive generations and incomplete forms may occur.

Ocular features

Uveitis develops at 8 years, 4 years after arthritis; the youngest recorded is 18 months.[40] A JIA-like CAU with band keratopathy is the most frequent presentation. Evanescent subepithelial corneal opacities are said to be diagnostic. Multifocal choroiditis is common later. The vasculopathy may affect the optic nerve, retina, and cranial nerves. The outcome can be severe: in one series 11/16 had cataracts, 6/16 developed glaucoma, and half required immunosuppression.

Vasculitides

Vasculitis is uncommon in childhood and ocular involvement in most types is rare. However, they are life-threatening diseases which may present with ophthalmic signs and sight-threatening disease may require rapid and intensive treatment. Their treatment may require prolonged immunosuppression, which may result in drug-associated ocular complications (e.g. hydroxychloroquine and steroids) and an increased risk of infection. Some infections may predispose to vasculitis such as streptoccocal and hepatitis B infections.

Some congenital immunodeficiencies such as CGD may predispose to vasculitis.

Classification

Primary vasculitides involve inflammation of the arteries and are classified by the size of the vessel.[41] They occur in connective tissue disorders, autoinflammatory diseases, and malignancy.

Ocular involvement in vasculitis

There are few diagnostic signs as the pathologic processes may be common to different vasculitis syndromes. Vasculitis occurs in 2% of adults with uveitis and is usually a monoepisodic or recurrent AAU. In adults, prolonged uveitis accompanying vasculitis is most uncommon: ocular involvement secondary to vasculitis is usually an inflammatory or ischemic optic neuropathy, sclerokeratitis, or orbital inflammation.

An acute red eye in children with vasculitis needs full evaluation although it may appear to be of low priority when life-threatening disease is present. Episcleritis appears more likely to be accompanied by systemic disease in childhood than in adults; in contrast most childhood posterior scleritis is idiopathic.

Types of ocular involvement

1. Bilateral signs of severe systemic disturbance: conjunctivitis, episcleritis, scleritis, anterior uveitis, retinopathy, and optic disk edema.
2. Localized ocular vasculitis: peripheral ulcerative keratitis, scleritis, episcleritis, retinal vasculitis, choroidopathy, optic neuropathy, orbital inflammation.
3. CNS inflammation, which may be diffuse (e.g. lupus encephalopathy) or focal and secondary to cerebral vasculitis.
4. Hypertensive retinopathy secondary to renal vasculitis.
5. Acute and chronic ischemic complications within the eye and CNS.

Large vessel

Takayasu's disease

Systemic

This is an inflammation of the aorta and its major branches. It is 100 times more common in East Asia, nine times more common in females and, in one-third, starts before the age of 20. Phases of systemic inflammation may precede chronic occlusive vasculopathy by several years. Cardiac failure may result.[42]

Ocular

Ocular symptoms are secondary to chronic carotid and vertebral artery occlusion and collateral formation.

Medium vessel

Polyarteritis nodosa

Systemic

PAN is a necrotizing segmental vasculitis of small and medium arteries with frequent aneurysm formation. Diagnosis requires tissue biopsy or abdominal angiography when the clinical picture is unclear. Thrombosis of involved arteries is frequent.

It can be secondary to infections such as hepatitis and streptococci as well as neoplasia. Disease may be limited to the skin but half of children with PAN present with fever, rashes, and musculoskeletal pain, neuropathy and renal impairment. The main age of onset is 7–11 years. Seizures from CNS involvement are more frequent than peripheral nerve involvement.

Ocular

Conjunctivitis, episcleritis and necrotizing scleritis, and peripheral ulcerative keratitis are found in up to 20%. AAU and bilateral panuveitis are rare. Choroidal vasculitis is a common histologic change but is usually asymptomatic; retinal involvement is usually an arteriolitis but veins may also be involved.

Kawasaki's disease

Systemic

There is an acute conjunctivitis, a red tongue and lips, and erythema of the trunk, palms, and soles. There may be marked edema of hands and feet. The skin of the soles and hands desquamate on recovery. Later 20% develop coronary artery aneurysms some of which may resolve with treatment, but there may be long-term cardiac sequelae. CNS involvement is uncommon.

Ocular

AAU and conjunctivitis occur in the majority in the acute phase and appear to be benign: disk edema and congested retinal vessels may occur.[24]

Small vessel, ANCA associated vasculitides

Wegener's granulomatosis

Systemic

Diagnosis requires three of six criteria: involvement of kidneys; upper airways; laryngotracheobronchial system; lung parenchyma; biopsy or classic antineutrophil cytoplasmic antibody (cANCA) positive.

Tissue damage from respiratory tract granulomas can be extensive. Subglottic stenosis and nasal deformity are more common in children. Limited forms without cANCA positivity can occur, including cases limited to the CNS.

Ocular

Ocular involvement may occur eventually in most patients and is the presenting site in 10%. Focal, necrotizing scleritis with adjacent keratitis is the most common presentation. Orbital inflammation may be diffuse or from adjacent sinus involvement. A panuveitis or AAU can occur rarely.

Urticarial vasculitis

There is a leukocytoclastic vasculitis that mostly occurs in middle-aged women; half have reduced complement. It has been associated with uveitis, scleritis, and idiopathic intracranial hypertension.

Vasculitis accompanying connective tissue disease

Systemic lupus erythematosus

Systemic

The vasculopathy involves small arteries, arterioles, and capillaries, resulting in fibrinoid necrosis. A hypersensitivity vasculitis occurs in 28%. Thrombosis is more likely in the presence of anticardiolipin antibodies, and these may also occur as an independent phenomenon in the antiphospholipid syndrome, or precede the development of SLE for several years. CNS disease may be caused by diffuse vasculopathy and localized thrombosis exacerbated by the presence of anticardiolipin antibodies. It may originate from abnormal DNA methylation in T cells leading to autoreactivity.

Ocular

Five percent of children with SLE have ocular involvement. The most frequent ocular involvement is dry eye: chronic inflammation is unusual. Lupus retinopathy is a sign of severe systemic vasculopathy and may be complicated by hypertensive changes. AAU, scleritis, episcleritis, and keratitis are uncommon and may indicate uncontrolled systemic disease.

Scleroderma

Systemic

Limited forms start with skin involvement of the extremities but may progress to the diffuse form with proximal limb and organ involvement (systemic sclerosis). The mean age of onset in childhood is 9 years; most are female. Localized scleroderma is more common in young females and may involve isolated patches of skin (morphea) or a linear patch on the face (en coup de sabre).

Ocular

Thirteen percent of those with localized scleroderma have eye involvement, and it is not always related to the site of skin disease.[43] Uveitis may occur, especially in scleroderma en coup de sabre. Choroidopathy is relatively common, arising from choroidal capillary closure and perivascular mucopolysaccharide deposition. The retinal circulation is usually spared but hypertensive changes may occur.

Sjögren's syndrome

Very rare in childhood, this usually presents with dry eyes and mouth and is associated with several connective tissue disorders.

Dermatomyositis and polymyositis

Dermatomyositis is the commonest inflammatory myopathy of childhood presenting with gradual muscle weakness. A heliotrope rash on the eyelids commonly precedes the myopathy. Extramuscular features are more common in children, including subcutaneous calcification and vasculitis. A retinal microangiopathy may occur.

Relapsing polychondritis

Systemic

There is recurrent inflammation of cartilage in the ear, nose, trachea and larynx, and joints with an adjacent dermal vasculitis. One-quarter of patients have other connective tissue disease, particularly rheumatoid arthritis. It is rare in childhood.

Ocular

Up to 60% have ocular involvement and 25% present with ocular symptoms. Episcleritis and scleritis are the most frequent patterns with keratitis, uveitis, and retinal vasculitis occurring rarely. A CNS vasculitis may occur.

Other vasculitides

Cogan's syndrome

Systemic features[44]

Typically, acute interstitial keratitis, deafness, and systemic vasculitis occur in the third decade. Acute hearing loss and keratitis can occur in many inflammatory syndromes and infections. Atypical Cogan's syndrome needs to be distinguished from systemic autoinflammatory syndromes. There is aortitis in classic disease, other vessels are more frequently involved in atypical disease including CNS vasculitis. There may be an autoantigen shared between the cornea, large vessels, and the inner ear. Childhood onset occurs with delays in diagnosis from difficulties in distinguishing progressive inflammatory sensorineural from congenital hearing loss.

Ocular

Interstitial keratitis is found in two-thirds of cases. Episcleritis and scleritis are found in 36% and retinal vasculitis in 24%. Uveitis and conjunctivitis may be the sole manifestation in a minority. Keratitis can be severe, leading to corneal perforation and extensive neovascularization (Figs 39.12 and 39.13).

Medical treatment of ocular inflammation

Treatment of uveitis

Visually significant uveitis needs as aggressive management as severe arthritis but families need to participate with full knowledge of the efficacy of treatment on reducing visual loss and the side-effects of treatment.

Symptoms or acuity can rarely guide disease control and, because of the long periods of asymptomatic disease in childhood chronic uveitis, treatment is more often required to

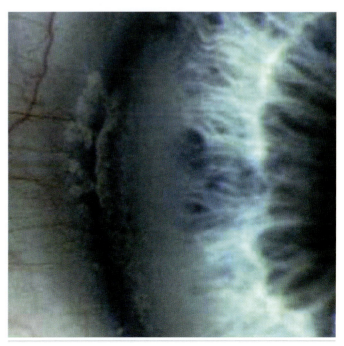

Fig. 39.12 Cogan's keratitis. Early limbal deposits.

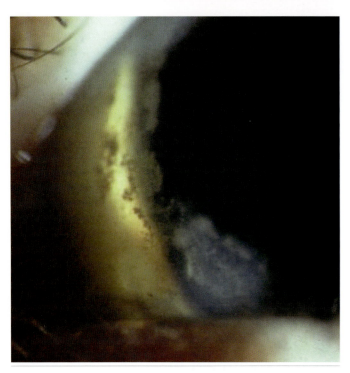

Fig. 39.13 Cogan's keratitis. Later paralimbal deposits.

prevent future complications rather than react to symptomatic relapse.

The initial treatment of most patients with endogenous uveitis is with topical and systemic steroids and cycloplegic agents. Steroids are especially effective at rapidly controlling inflammation causing tissue edema from vascular leakage and some cases of neovascularization. Their short-term disadvantages must be balanced against their ease of administration and dosage. Complications include steroid-induced ocular hypertension, behavioral changes, infection (especially varicella), diabetes, and weight gain.

Steroid-sparing immunosuppressants may be indicated when long-term, high-dose steroids are needed to control disease. They have potential side-effects whose frequency may vary between patients, they rarely have proven superiority to steroids in achieving initial disease control, and head to head comparisons of efficacy are not available for most ocular disease.

MTX has been most frequently used because of its use in JIA. It may not control disease in 25% and half of patients in whom control is achieved relapse on its withdrawal.

Azathioprine has a low rate of side-effects in children compared to ciclosporin and mycophenolate mofetil and has been used in JIA-uveitis.[25] Mycophenolate has also been used in pediatric uveitis and vasculitis.[45]

Cyclophosphamide may be useful in uveitis unresponsive to less toxic immunosuppressants. A variety of monoclonal antibodies used in pediatric arthritis and vasculitis have also been used in resistant cases of pediatric uveitis, but evidence of their effectiveness remains anecdotal.

In the absence of formal treatment trials in childhood ocular inflammation, one must use information from comparable adult disease as well as the experience in those systemic diseases associated with uveitis; however, analogies are not always reliable. There is no adult equivalent of JIA-uveitis and the safety profile, dosage, and tolerability of some drugs such as MTX are very different in adults. Diseases such as multiple sclerosis and ankylosing spondylitis often have uveitis that responds well to short courses of steroids, whereas the chronic course of extraocular disease is unaffected. Ciclosporin may be far more effective in neuro-ophthalmic sarcoidosis than in pulmonary disease. Some anti-TNF agents appear to have a profound effect on the course of chronic arthritis, yet minimal effect on the uveitis associated with these conditions.

Treatment of vasculitis

The treatment of the various vasculitides has tended to be similar. When steroid-unresponsive cyclophosphamide is used to induce remission. Maintenance therapies have moved from continuing cyclophosphamide to less toxic therapies using antimetabolites such as azathioprine and mycophenolate. Anti B cell monoclonal antibody treatment may be as effective as cyclophosphamide as an induction agent.

Ocular inflammation is usually controlled by the treatments required for control of the systemic vasculitis. On occasions, ocular involvement may drive the treatment and, rarely, limited ocular disease such as idiopathic orbital inflammation and severe sclerokeratitis may be the sole indication for a vasculitic drug regimen.

Surgical treatment

Cataracts

The indications for cataract surgery are:

1. The prevention of amblyopia
2. To allow the management of posterior segment disease
3. To improve visual function with an acceptable risk.

It should not be embarked upon lightly. Children with mild bilateral cataracts and persistent inflammation may easily complete their education with 6/18 vision and surgery deferred until disease activity subsides. A single aphakic amblyopic eye rarely adds to the visual function, but failing to quickly remove a rapidly forming unilateral cataract during the first years of life will not only produce amblyopia, but also prevent adequate monitoring of posterior segment disease. In these circumstances the family must be informed that in some circumstances all that cataract surgery might achieve is an eye of normal appearance but little visual function.

Disease activity must be rigorously controlled as postoperative inflammation can be unpredictable and severe. When cataract surgery appears likely, patients should be started on systemic immunosuppression in order to see whether disease can be completely controlled without topical medication. Treatment should be increased before and at the time of surgery and for at least 2 months thereafter. Some patients with preoperative macular edema require 4 or 5 months of systemic steroids as well as second-line immunosuppression before maximum postoperative acuity is achieved. Operating soon after presentation may occasionally be necessary to avoid amblyopia; it can take some years of management to determine what level of long-term immunosuppression is required in each case. When planning surgery in cases with a short history, one should assume that inflammation may become more difficult to control for some years afterwards. Periocular or intraocular steroids given intraoperatively reduce the load of systemic steroid in the perioperative period.

Visibility may be compromised by band keratopathy and preoperative excimer laser, or EDTA scrub may be performed prior to intraocular surgery. Posterior synechiae can be more extensive than is apparent on slit-lamp examination. Pupillary membranes may be vascularized and bleed intraoperatively but may be simply peeled off the anterior capsule without jeopardizing the capsulorrhexis.

Techniques of lens removal depend on the possibility of capsulorrhexis, visibility, and hardness of the lens. Often the lens is aspiratible, even if white. Occasionally there are calcified lumps at sites of synechiae.

Posterior capsule opacification is universal and a posterior capsulorrhexis is advisable especially if the child needs laser treatment under general anesthetic. An anterior vitrectomy may reduce the risk of posterior IOL membrane formation but a more extensive vitrectomy may add other risks.

Intraocular lenses are easy to put in but are very difficult to take out. JIA-uveitis is an inflammation unlike most other uveitis syndromes with a high rate of IOL "cocooning," synechiae, and membrane formation. Some patients develop unexpected postoperative complications despite adequate preoperative systemic immunosuppression and uncomplicated surgery. It may be prudent to delay IOL implantation until months after lens extraction. The drawbacks of aphakia are trivial compared to the profound visual loss that may result from complications of IOL implantation so families should be fully informed of the added risk to the visual outcome that IOL implantation provides.

In contrast, late developing cataract in JIA-uveitis may be uncomplicated. The outcomes of unilateral cataract surgery in children prone to amblyopia are poor and this is also the case in JIA-uveitis.[19,46]

Treatment of glaucoma

Glaucoma occurs in up to 70% following cataract surgery, and has multiple causes including steroid use, persistent inflammation, aphakia, and perhaps age at cataract surgery. When glaucoma develops some months after the use of steroids it is usually not simply steroid-related but every effort should be made to minimize steroid use. Many standard surgical treatments have been tried as well as goniotomy and cycloablation. As patients may have compromised aqueous production, despite raised IOP, all procedures need caution when the eye has been severely inflamed due to the great risk of postoperative hypotony.

The use of tube drainage devices has greatly improved the prognosis of aphakic glaucoma. Steroid-induced glaucoma in a quiet eye may respond well to conventional assisted trabeculectomy.

References

1. Dave S, Longmuir R, Shah VA, et al. Intracranial hypertension in systemic lupus erythematosus. Semin Ophthalmol 2008; 23: 127–33.
2. Edelsten C, Reddy MA, Stanford MR, Graham EM. Visual loss associated with pediatric uveitis in English primary and referral centers. Am J Ophthalmol 2003; 135: 676–80.
3. Smith JA, Mackensen F, Sen HN, et al. Epidemiology and course of disease in childhood uveitis. Ophthalmology 2009; 116: 1544–51.
4. Choi DE, Birnbaum AD, Oh F, et al. Pediatric uveitis secondary to probable, presumed, and biopsy-proven sarcoidosis. J Pediatr Ophthalmol Strabismus 2010: 1–6. Epub 2010/05/29.
5. Soylu M, Ozdemir G, Anli A. Pediatric uveitis in southern Turkey. Ocular immunology and inflammation 1997; 5: 197–202.
6. Garcia LA, Carroll MO, Garza Leon MA. Vogt-Koyanagi-Harada syndrome in childhood. Int Ophthalmol Clin 2008; 48: 107–17.
7. Mackensen F, Billing H. Tubulointerstitial nephritis and uveitis syndrome. Curr Opin Ophthalmol 2009; 20: 525–31.
8. Gardner-Medwin JM, Dolezalova P, Cummins C, Southwood TR. Incidence of Henoch-Schonlein purpura, Kawasaki disease, and rare vasculitides in children of different ethnic origins. Lancet 2002; 360(9341): 1197–202.
9. Jabs DA, Nussenblatt RB, Rosenbaum JT. Standardization of uveitis nomenclature for reporting clinical data: results of the First International Workshop. Am J Ophthalmol 2005; 140: 509–16.
10. de Boer J, Berendschot TT, van der Does P, Rothova A. Long-term follow-up of intermediate uveitis in children. Am J Ophthalmol 2006; 141: 616–21.
11. Hollenbach JA, Thompson SD, Bugawan TL, et al. Juvenile idiopathic arthritis and HLA class I and class II interactions and age-at-onset effects. Arthritis Rheum 2010; 62: 1781–91.
12. Edelsten C, Lee V, Bentley CR, et al. An evaluation of baseline risk factors predicting severity in juvenile idiopathic arthritis associated uveitis and other chronic anterior uveitis in early childhood. Br J Ophthalmol 2002; 86: 51–6.
13. Holland GN, Denove CS, Yu F. Chronic anterior uveitis in children: clinical characteristics and complications. Am J Ophthalmol 2009; 147: 667–78, e5.
14. Ayuso VK, Ten Cate HA, van der Does P, et al. Male gender and poor visual outcome in uveitis associated with juvenile idiopathic arthritis. Am J Ophthalmol 2010; 149: 987–93.
15. Holland GN. A reconsideration of anterior chamber flare and its clinical relevance for children with chronic anterior uveitis. Trans Am Ophthalmol Soc 2007; 105: 344–64.
16. Thorne JE, Woreta FA, Dunn JP, Jabs DA. Risk of cataract development among children with juvenile idiopathic arthritis-related uveitis treated with topical corticosteroids. Ophthalmology 2010; 117: 1436–41.
17. Woreta F, Thorne JE, Jabs DA, et al. Risk factors for ocular complications and poor visual acuity at presentation among patients with uveitis associated with juvenile idiopathic arthritis. Am J Ophthalmol 2007; 143: 647–55.
18. Thorne JE, Woreta F, Kedhar SR, et al. Juvenile idiopathic arthritis-associated uveitis: incidence of ocular complications and visual acuity loss. Am J Ophthalmol 2007; 143: 840–6.
19. Sijssens KM, Los LI, Rothova A, et al. Long-term ocular complications in aphakic versus pseudophakic eyes of children with juvenile idiopathic arthritis-associated uveitis. Br J Ophthalmol 2010; 94: 1145–9.
20. Kalinina Ayuso V, Ten Cate HA, van der Does P, et al. Male gender as a risk factor for complications in uveitis associated with juvenile idiopathic arthritis. Am J Ophthalmol 2010; 149: 994–9, e5.
21. Sijssens KM, Rothova A, Van De Vijver DA, et al. Risk factors for the development of cataract requiring surgery in uveitis associated with juvenile idiopathic arthritis. Am J Ophthalmol 2007; 144: 574–9.
22. Kalinina Ayuso V, van de Winkel EL, Rothova A, de Boer JH. Relapse rate of uveitis post-methotrexate treatment in juvenile idiopathic arthritis. Am J Ophthalmol 2011; 151: 217–22.
23. Foell D, Wulffraat N, Wedderburn LR, et al. Methotrexate withdrawal at 6 vs 12 months in juvenile idiopathic arthritis in remission: a randomized clinical trial. JAMA 2010; 303: 1266–73.
24. Southwood TR, Foster HE, Davidson JE, et al. Duration of etanercept treatment and reasons for discontinuation in a cohort of juvenile idiopathic arthritis patients. Rheumatology (Oxford) 2011; 50: 189–95.
25. Goebel JC, Roesel M, Heinz C, et al. Azathioprine as a treatment option for uveitis in patients with juvenile idiopathic arthritis. Br J Ophthalmol 2011; 95: 209–13.

26. Tappeiner C, Roesel M, Heinz C, et al. Limited value of cyclosporine A for the treatment of patients with uveitis associated with juvenile idiopathic arthritis. Eye (Lond) 2009; 23: 1192–8.

27. Daniel E, Thorne JE, Newcomb CW, et al. Mycophenolate mofetil for ocular inflammation. Am J Ophthalmol 2010; 149: 423–32.

28. Tynjala P, Lindahl P, Honkanen V, et al. Infliximab and etanercept in the treatment of chronic uveitis associated with refractory juvenile idiopathic arthritis. Ann Rheum Dis 2007; 66: 548–50.

29. Heiligenhaus A, Miserocchi E, Heinz C, et al. Treatment of severe uveitis associated with juvenile idiopathic arthritis with anti-CD20 monoclonal antibody (rituximab). Rheumatology (Oxford) 2011. Epub 2011/03/08.

30. Kenawy N, Cleary G, Mewar D, et al. Abatacept: a potential therapy in refractory cases of juvenile idiopathic arthritis-associated uveitis. Graefe's Arch Clin Exp Ophthalmol 2011; 249: 297–300.

31. Atmaca L, Boyvat A, Yalcindag FN, et al. Behcet disease in children. Ocular Immunol Inflamm 2011; 19: 103–7.

32. Abu El-Asrar AM, Al-Kharashi AS, Aldibhi H, et al. Vogt-Koyanagi-Harada disease in children. Eye (Lond) 2008; 22: 1124–31.

33. Mandeville JT, Levinson RD, Holland GN. The tubulointerstitial nephritis and uveitis syndrome. Surv Ophthalmol 2001; 46: 195–208.

34. Jahnukainen T, Ala-Houhala M, Karikoski R, et al. Clinical outcome and occurrence of uveitis in children with idiopathic tubulointerstitial nephritis. Pediatr Nephrol 2011; 26: 291–9.

35. Fukuda T, Oguni H, Yanagaki S, et al. Chronic localized encephalitis (Rasmussen's syndrome) preceded by ipsilateral uveitis: a case report. Epilepsia 1994; 35: 1328–31.

36. Rigante D, Stabile A, Minnella A, et al. Post-inflammatory retinal dystrophy in CINCA syndrome. Rheumatol Int 2010; 30: 389–93.

37. Prieur AM, Griscelli C, Lampert F, et al. A chronic, infantile, neurological, cutaneous and articular (CINCA) syndrome: a specific entity analysed in 30 patients. Scand J Rheumatol Suppl 1987; 66: 57–68.

38. Goldbach-Mansky R. Current status of understanding the pathogenesis and management of patients with NOMID/CINCA. Curr Rheumatol Rep 2011; 13: 123–31.

39. Okafuji I, Nishikomori R, Kanazawa N, et al. Role of the NOD2 genotype in the clinical phenotype of Blau syndrome and early-onset sarcoidosis. Arthritis Rheum 2009; 60: 242–50.

40. Punzi L, Furlan A, Podswiadek M, et al. Clinical and genetic aspects of Blau syndrome: a 25-year follow-up of one family and a literature review. Autoimmunity Rev 2009; 8: 228–32.

41. Ozen S, Ruperto N, Dillon MJ, et al. EULAR/PReS endorsed consensus criteria for the classification of childhood vasculitides. Ann Rheum Dis 2006; 65: 936–41.

42. Hong CY, Yun YS, Choi JY, et al. Takayasu's arteritis in Korean children: clinical report of seventy cases. Heart Vessels Suppl 1992; 7: 91–6.

43. Zannin ME, Martini G, Athreya BH, et al. Ocular involvement in children with localised scleroderma: a multi-centre study. Br J Ophthalmol 2007; 91: 1311–4.

44. Pagnini I, Zannin ME, Vittadello F, et al. Clinical features and outcome of Cogan syndrome. J Pediatr 2011. Epub 2011/09/17.

45. Chang PY, Giuliari GP, Shaikh M, et al. Mycophenolate mofetil monotherapy in the management of paediatric uveitis. Eye (Lond) 2011; 25: 427–35.

46. Grajewski RS, Zurek-Imhoff B, Roesel M, et al. Favourable outcome after cataract surgery with IOL implantation in uveitis associated with juvenile idiopathic arthritis. Acta Ophthalmol 2011. Epub 2011/02/12.

Part 5
The uvea

Albinism

Isabelle M Russell-Eggitt

More than 100 genes influence pigmentation of the hair, skin, and eyes of mice. It is likely that as many genes are involved in man. Mutation of these genes produces generalized or localized hypopigmentation. A disorder is only classified as albinism if there is associated underdevelopment of the retina and visual pathways. This is usually associated with nystagmus.

The main pigmentation genes

- Genes controlling development and differentiation of pigment cells (melanocytes). Mutation of these genes, such as MITF, may be associated with deafness, but not usually with ocular defects.
- Genes encoding components of melanosomes (pigment producing organelles within melanocytes). Mutation of these genes affects skin pigmentation and vision pathways producing albinism.
- Genes controlling biogenesis of lysosome related organelles (LROs) including melanosomes. Mutations cause Hermansky-Pudlak (HPS) and Chediak-Higashi (CHS) syndromes which have ocular features of albinism.

- Genes involved in organelle transport, including LROs. Mutations cause Griscelli's immunodeficiency syndromes and Elejalde's syndrome, both with normal eyes.
- Genes involved in switching between eumelanin (brown and black pigment) and pheomelanin (red and yellow pigment) such as melanocortin 1 receptor protein alter the phenotype of albinism but mutation does not cause albinism.

What is albinism?

In albinism, production or transport of melanin pigments is defective in association with anomalous development of the retina and higher visual pathways.

Albinism is not a single condition, but a group of disorders caused by mutation of one or more genes involved in the function of the melanosome – a specialized organelle involved in melanin pigmentation.[1] In man, there are specialized melanosomes in cerebral astrocytes and melanolysosomes in retinal pigment epithelium and iris. Individuals with albinism are distinguished from blondes by their ocular features.

Albinos usually are hypopigmented due to deficiency of melanin pigments, not due to a deficiency in melanocytes. Not all individuals with albinism are hypopigmented. However, they are lighter in coloring than unaffected family members and have ocular and vision pathway features and may have dysfunction of related organelles such as platelet dense granules and lysosomes.

Why a diagnosis is important

It is important to make the diagnosis of albinism as early as possible to:

- Avoid concern that a child will be blind. Delayed vision maturation is common in albinism (see Chapter 4). Nystagmus is often misinterpreted as roving eye movements. The prognosis for many children with albinism is of severe vision impairment, with corrected distance acuity of logMAR 1.0. However, they will see to read, even small print, albeit at a reduced distance and be able to navigate well. Except in one very rare form albinism is not degenerative.

- Avoid concern that nystagmus is a sign of neurologic or progressive retinal disease. The majority will be healthy and have no intellectual impairment.
- Give advice on promotion of best vision outcome, ocular comfort in bright lighting, and skin protection.
- Be aware of the subtypes that may be associated with impaired platelet and immune function. Rarely, an infant will present with features of albinism and retinal hemorrhages after minimal head trauma, even birth, with Hermansky-Pudlak albinism. Standard coagulation screening may miss this diagnosis.[2]

Classification of albinism

Tyrosinase is a key enzyme in the melanin pathway and deficiency is the cause of albinism in many animals. Whilst this is a common cause of albinism in man (oculocutaneous albinism type 1; OCA1) other parts of the pathway can be disrupted. The OCA2P' protein stabilizes melanosome pH allowing melanin to form. Tyrosinase and tyrosinase related protein TYRP1 (defective in OCA3) interact; mutation in one influences the maturation and stability of the other. Mutation of TYRP1 alone probably does not result in full ocular phenotype of nystagmus and chiasmal misrouting. The MATP protein (OCA4) is important for normal function of tyrosinase and maturation of melanosomes. Many other proteins, some not unique to the melanosome, that also occur in related organelles (LROs) are involved in mammalian melanin production and transport from the organelle.

The most useful classification of albinism is where the defect is of a gene product expressed only in the melanosome or where other related organelles also malfunction (Table 40.1). The former individuals have a non-progressive ocular disorder and lack photoprotection, yet the latter may have serious systemic problems.

Albinism affects all ethnic groups, but prevalence is variable due to the founder effect. Prevalence of HPS1 in Puerto Rico is 1:1800, and may be as low as 1 in 1 000 000 in other communities. About 1 in 70 northern Europeans have one abnormal allele for OCA1. OCA2 is prevalent in southern and central African populations where there is a frequent 2.7 Kb deletion that removes one exon of the gene. OCA4 is rare outside Japan where it accounts for 25% of albinism. The genotypes OCA1, OCA2, OCA3, OCA4, OA1, and HPS1 account for more than 90% of cases of albinism in most populations and together give a prevalence of albinism in the USA of about 1 in 17 000.

Inheritance of albinism and gene product interaction

All forms of albinism are inherited as autosomal recessive except for OA1 which is X-linked. The expression of the Mendelian gene defect is modified by interaction with other genes in the pathway.

In the future, there may be gene-specific treatments. At present, the primary reason to differentiate between genotypes that do not affect other organelles is for genetic counseling. Genes interact to produce a wide variety of pigmentation, in normal individuals and those with albinism. Albinism phenotype varies with ethnic group. If an individual with albinism

due to two mutant OCA1 alleles has children with an albino partner with two OCA2 mutant alleles, all their children will carry both types of disorder, but none will have albinism as they are distinct non-allelic conditions. If an individual has a null mutation of one allele for OCA1 and the second allele is a polymorphism with reduced enzyme activity, they will have normal eyes unless they also have a mutation in MITF which is in the same pathway. This additive effect of two genes in a pathway is an example of digenic inheritance. In Puerto Rico, there is an increased incidence due to a founder effect of not one but two distinct types of HPS; individuals homozygous for one type may be carriers of the other and they may have a more severe phenotype. Individuals with OCA2 who form some melanin may have brown hair or ginger hair. Their pigmentation is modified by their genotype for the melanocortin receptor (MC1R) gene.

Contiguous gene syndromes

Deletion of a portion of the X chromosome in the Xp22.3 region results in OA1 and loss of function of other genes in this region. The phenotype in affected males varies with the site and extent of the deletion.

Genes and loci in this region and features include:

- NLGN4X Neuroligin 4: autism, learning difficulties
- STS Steroid sulfatase: ichthyosis
- ARSE arylsulfatase E: chondrodysplasia punctata
- OA1 albinism
- KAL1 Kallmann's syndrome
- (hypogonadotropic hypogonadism and anosmia)
- LECD Lisch's epithelial corneal dystrophy
- OASD albinism and deafness of late onset
- SHOX short stature homeobox

Rare types of albinism

- *Oculocerebral syndrome with hypopigmentation (Cross' syndrome, OMIM 257800):* features are silver grey hair, skin hypopigmentation, nystagmus, corneal opacities, microphthalmia, peripapillary pigmented "scars," psychomotor retardation, spasticity, and extrapyramidal movements. There is a case report of absent electroretinogram.
- *Oculocerebral hypopigmentation syndrome of Preus (OMIM 257790):* features are growth retardation, dolichocephaly, cataracts, nystagmus, iris translucency, highly arched palate, small widely spaced teeth, generalized hypopigmentation, psychomotor retardation, and hypochromic anemia.
- *Elejalde's neuroectodermal melanolysosomal syndrome (OMIM 256710):* silvery hair and frequent occurrence of fatal neurologic episodes. May be allelic with Griscelli's syndrome.

Confusing terminology

"Partial albinism" should be avoided as it is used both for disorders such as piebaldism, where there is localized absence

Table 40.1 – The classification of albinism

(a) Albinism types where the defect is thought to be confined to melanosomal organelles

Abbreviation	Phenotypic names	Gene product	Locus	Inheritance pattern
OCA1	Oculocutaneous Tyrosinase negative Tyrosinase dependent Minimal pigment Yellow variant Thermolabile pigment type	Tyrosinase	11q14–q21	Autosomal recessive
OCA2	Oculocutaneous "Tyrosinase positive" Minimal pigment Brown albinism	P gene	15q11.2–q12	Autosomal recessive
OCA3		TRP tyrosinase related protein	9p23	Autosomal recessive
OCA4		MATP membrane associated transport protein (also called SLC45A2/AIM1)	5p13.3	Autosomal recessive
OA1	X-linked ocular albinism	GPR143	Xp22.3	X-linked recessive

(b) Albinism where the defect is not only of melanosomes but also of other related organelles (autosomal recessive inheritance and platelet storage pool deficit and bleeding tendency)

Abbreviation	Long name	Gene product	locus	Phenotype distinctions
HPS1	Hermansky-Pudlak syndrome	HPS1	10q23	Commonest type of HPS, ceroid deposition lungs & gut, severe restrictive lung disease, founder effect in NW Puerto Rico
HPS2		ADTB3A	5q13	Neutropenia, frequent respiratory infections, impaired lymphocyte function, congenital dislocation of hips (dysplastic acetabulae), poor balance, conductive hearing loss, hemophagocytic lymphohistiocytosis
HPS3		HPS3	3q24	
HPS4		HPS4	22q11–q12	Ceroid deposition lungs & gut, mild to severe restrictive lung disease
HPS5		HPS5	11p15–p13	Hypercholesterolemia & hypertriglyceridemia
HPS6		HPS6	10q24	Respiratory and urinary tract infections, urinary and rectal incontinence, hearing loss, global developmental delay
HPS7		DTNBP1 dysbindin	6p22	Mild lung disease
HPS8		BLOS3	19q13.32	
CHS1	Chediak-Higashi syndrome	LYST	1q42.1–q42.2	Immunodeficiency, hemophagocytic lymphohistiocytosis, neurologic defects, hepatosplenomegaly

of melanocytes and no visual pathway features of albinism, and also for cases of true albinism where some pigment is present.

"*Ocular albinism*" is used both for albinism with X-linked inheritance, OA1, where the abnormality of melanosomes is not confined to the eye, and for autosomal recessive forms of albinism where hypopigmentation is not marked.

The division between *eponymous syndromes* on the basis of early phenotypic descriptions can be misleading now that there is a better understanding of the underlying mechanisms: for example, HPS2 is associated with neutropenia, and impaired lymphocyte function similar to CHS1 and CHS1 is associated with platelet deficit, not just immune dysfunction.

Ocular features of albinism

The ocular features of albinism are common to all genetic types with variable expression dependent mostly upon whether the mutant gene product has some function rather than which gene is affected:

- Reduced visual acuity with delayed vision maturation
- Nystagmus
- Foveal hypoplasia
- Iris, globe, and retinal hypopigmentation (Fig. 40.1)
- Photophobia, glare, and dazzle due to ocular stray light

- Strabismus
- Reduced stereoacuity
- Refractive error (astigmatism, myopia, hypermetropia)
- Anomalous chiasmal and higher visual pathways
- *Anomalous auditory pathways?*
- Behavioral problems, *autism association?*

Some individuals with OCA2 and OCA4 may be as deficient in pigment as OCA1 as individuals homozygous for a null mutation in tyrosinase and phenotypically indistinguishable. Some individuals with OCA2 and OCA4 have an indistinguishable ocular phenotype from OA1 and HPS with mild bleeding disorder.

Visual acuity is reduced due to the anatomy of the fovea, reduced foveation time due to nystagmus, refractive error, disability glare due to ocular stray light, and amblyopia.

Marked improvement in behavioral acuity occurs at 3 to 5 months of age coincident with development of the fast phase of nystagmus. Final acuity varies from near normal to more commonly about logMAR 1.0 corrected distance acuity (20/30–20/400). Acuity of albinos who develop pigment may improve into teenage years. Even in severe phenotypes near acuity is good, albeit at reduced working distance for short periods. Demands on eyes increases with age, particularly at school, and they have difficulty using convergence and very near fixation as their accommodation declines. Children with an eccentric null point of nystagmus, or who prefer a shortened near vision distance aided by their uncorrected myopia, may reject glasses. Early detection and correction of refractive error with glasses or contact lenses may reduce amblyopia. The waveform of the nystagmus changes with development and may be modified by eye muscle surgery,[3] drugs, and biofeedback from rigid contact lenses (see Chapter 90). Albinism is not associated with retinal dystrophy and progressive vision loss, except for a rare variant of CHS.

Albinos often suffer from ocular stray light (loss of retinal image contrast as a result of intraocular light scatter), as more light enters the eye through a translucent iris and globe wall and less light is absorbed by the retinal pigment epithelium.

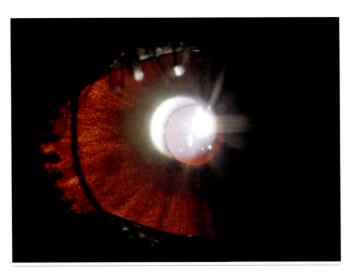

Fig. 40.1 **Iris translucency.**

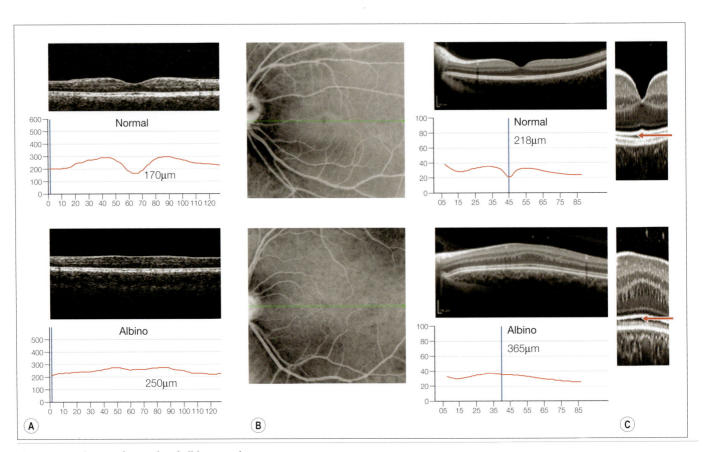

Fig. 40.2 **OCT image of normal and albino macula.**

Transmitted light can be reduced by the use of hats with a long brim with a matt dark fabric interior. The Legionnaire style protects the neck and bonnets side shield. Photochromatic lenses are often not dark enough. Neutral grey fixed tinted glasses with light transmission factor (LTF) 20% are a good starting point. Darker tint of LTF 5% requires side shielding to see through the lens. Contact lenses can be evenly tinted but change the appearance of the eyes. A blue lens with grey pupil may be more acceptable.

The macula region is underdeveloped to a variable degree. The vascular pattern may be anomalous with a vessel coursing across the fovea. Optical coherence tomography (OCT) imaging is helpful in addition to visual evoked potential testing in distinguishing albinism from idiopathic nystagmus[4] (Fig. 40.2):

- Reduced foveal pit with a thicker fovea and presence of multiple inner retinal layers normally absent at the center of the fovea.
- Thin photoreceptor nuclear layer at the fovea compared to normal subjects and lower macular volume.

Visual evoked potential (VEP) crossed asymmetry is a feature of all forms of albinism (Fig. 40.3).[5] Visual pathway misrouting of retinal ganglion cell axons can be detected by recording the VEP with uniocular stimulation and comparing the response from electrodes either side of the midline and comparison of projections with hemifield stimulation. There is reduction in the size and disruption of laminar structures of the lateral geniculate body nucleus in cats with OCA1 and HPS. There is a severe disruption of binocular driven neurons in cortical areas 17, 18, and 19. Functional MRI scanning of normal individuals during binocular stimulation results in activation of the two hemispheres from the occipital pole to deep in the calcarine fissure. In albinos, there is some asymmetry between the occipital lobes.[6]

Generally individuals with albinism have normal or even above normal levels of intelligence. Relationships with other children may be challenging due to their different appearance, not allowing "personal space" as they approach others closely to see, and not recognizing friends at a distance (see Chapter 60). Early education may be difficult as some young children with albinism have a shorter attention span. Later in childhood, individuals with albinism are often high achievers at school. Case reports suggest a rare association with autism.

Interaction of P gene with other genes

In both Angelman's syndrome (AS) and Prader-Willi syndrome (PWS) hypopigmentation of the hair skin and eyes occurs where the P gene is deleted. Albinism occurs if the other P gene is mutant.

Prader-Willi syndrome (PWS) is characterized by infantile hypotonia, hyperphagia with obesity, hypogonadism, mental retardation, short stature with small hands and feet, and is due to a gene defect on the long arm of chromosome 15 in the region of the P gene. There is a deletion of a portion of the paternally derived chromosome, mutation of the imprinting control center, chromosomal translocation, or uniparental disomy of the maternal chromosome 15. Many individuals have translucent irides and hypopigmented skin.

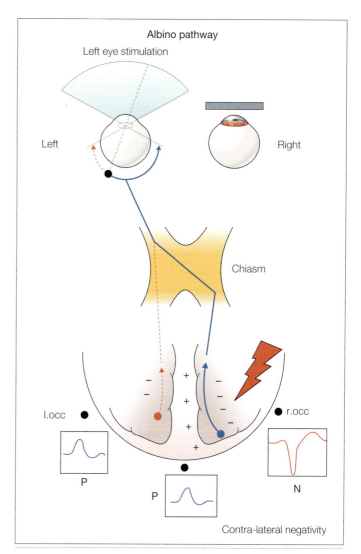

Fig. 40.3 Albino pathway. "Crossed asymmetry" of the visually evoked potential recording in albinism results from a larger than normal proportion of crossing fibers in the chiasm. When the left eye is stimulated, the majority of the resulting electrical activity takes place in the right visual cortex with the largest positivity detected over the left occiput. When the right eye is stimulated, the opposite occurs. (Marmor MF, Choi SS, Zawadzi RJ, Werner JS. Visual insignificance of the foveal pit: reassessment of foveal hypoplasia as fovea plana. Arch Ophthalmol 2008; 126(7): 907–913. Mohammad S, Gottlob I, Kumar A, et al. The functional significance of foveal abnormalities in albinism measured using spectral-domain optical coherence tomography. Ophthalmology 2011; 118: 1645–1652.)

Angelman's syndrome (AS) is characterized by severe developmental delay, speech impairment, ataxia, microcephaly, seizures, and frequent inappropriate laughing. VEP evidence of chiasm misrouting has been reported without other ocular features of albinism.[5] AS is caused by deletion of a portion of the maternally derived chromosome in the same region that is affected in PWS, uniparental disomy, an imprinting defect, or mutation of the UBE3A gene.

Diagnosing OA1

Carriers of OA1 may have diaphanous irides and normal acuity. Affected males do not always have iris translucency and may be misdiagnosed as X-linked idiopathic infantile

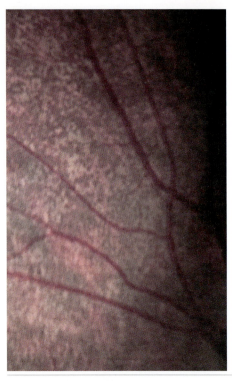

Fig. 40.4 X-linked ocular albinism. Peripheral retina of female carrier of X-linked ocular albinism (OA1) with "mud splattered" pigmentation.

nystagmus (see Chapter 90). Examination of the fundus of the mother and other female relatives may aid diagnosis. Typical mosaical fundus pigmentation, "mud splattered" appearance, is present in more than 90% of obligate heterozygotes (Fig. 40.4). The pattern can be highlighted using autofluorescence. OA1 males and some carriers have giant spherical macro-melanosomes within their skin. They occur in some cases of HPS and CHS but not in OCA1, OCA2, OCA3, and OCA4. Macromelanosomes are also found in a wide variety of non-albino disorders including neurofibromatosis.

How to diagnose the rare types of albinism with malfunction of other lysosomal related organelles

Lysosome related organelles (LROs) are organelles that are specialized for the type of cell they are in, but have common factors in their generation and how they traffic substances (see Fig. 40.4). They include melanosomes, platelet dense granules (gamma storage pool diseases δ SPD), lytic granules, major histocompatibility complex MHC class II compartments, and basophil granules.

Melanosome function is abnormal leading to ocular features of albinism. In CHS1 there are macromelanosomes and hair color is often silver gray rather than blond.

Platelet dense bodies (granules) are important for the formation of a hemostatic plug.

- Ask about ancestry, especially Puerto Rican or Turkish in view of founder effect.
- Ask each visit about easy bruising.

- Look for bruising especially in unusual sites.
- When suspected, ask the advice of a hematologist and perform electron microscopy of platelets to look for reduction in dense granules.
- Test platelet ADP and ATP content and release (not platelet numbers which usually are normal).[7]
- Many will have a normal "coagulation screen."

Lysosomes are important for the breakdown of proteins and lipids in cells. Abnormal giant lysosomes occur in CHS1. Defective killer cell function and neutropenia are features of CHS1 and HPS2. Partially degraded proteolipids accumulate in lysosomes (ceroid lipofuscinosis), damaging cells and leading to restrictive pulmonary fibrosis and granulomatous colitis in HPS1 and HPS4. Kidneys may be damaged by ceroid accumulation.

- Recurrent bacterial infections.
- "Accelerated phases" that mimic leukemia and can be fatal (hemophagocytic lymphohistiocytosis).

Additional features of LRO disorders include:

- Progressive neurologic dysfunction in CHS1.
- Congenital dislocation of hips in HPS2.

It is probable that further disorders in this group are yet to be identified. Data from the study of mouse mutants with similar LRO dysfunction suggest that it is likely that some will have neurologic dysfunction.

Griscelli's syndrome has three phenotypes that may be allelic genetic disorders of immune dysfunction. They belong to the LRO group but whilst Griscelli patients may have silver hair and impaired melanosome transfer to keratinocytes, this is not associated with the ocular features of albinism or with lack of platelet dense bodies.

Mutation and polymorphism data on the genes are available on the International Center Albinism Database website (http://www.cbc.umn.edu/tad).

Support groups

National Organization for Albinism and Hypopigmentation: NOAH (http://www.albinism.org)
UK Albinism Fellowship (http://www.albinism.org.uk)
Hermansky-Pudlak syndrome (http://www.hermansky-pudlak.org and http://www.hpsnetwork.org)

References

1. Schiaffino MV. Signalling pathways in melanosome biogenesis and pathology. Int J Biochem Cell Biol 2010; 42: 1094–104.
2. Russell-Eggitt I, Thompson DA, Khair K, et al. Hermansky-Pudlak syndrome presenting with subdural haematoma. J R Soc Med 2000; 93: 591–2.
3. Hertle RW, Anninger W, Yang D, et al. Effects of extraocular muscle surgery on 15 patients with oculo-cutaneous albinism (OCA) and infantile nystagmus syndrome (INS). Am J Ophthalmol 2004; 138: 978–87.
4. Mohammad S, Gottlob I, Kumar A, et al. The functional significance of foveal abnormalities in albinism measured using spectral-domain optical coherence tomography. Ophthalmology 2011; 118: 1645–52.

5. Thompson DA, Kriss A, Cottrell S, et al. Visual evoked potential evidence of albino-like chiasmal misrouting in a patient with Angelman syndrome with no ocular features of albinism. Dev Med Child Neurol 1999; 41: 633–8.

6. Wolynski B, Kanowski M, Meltendorf S, et al. Self-organisation in the human visual system: visuo-motor processing with congenitally abnormal V1 input. Neuropsychologia 2010; 48: 3834–45.

7. Sandrock K, Zieger, B. Current strategies in diagnosis of inherited storage pool defects. Transfus Med Hemother 2010; 37: 248–58.

Vitreous

Michel Michaelides • Anthony T Moore

Introduction

The vitreous, a transparent gelatinous structure that fills the posterior four-fifths of the globe, is firmly attached to the pars plana and loosely to the retina and optic nerve posteriorly. In childhood there is a firm attachment to the lens.

The development of the vitreous body and zonule can be divided into three stages:

1. The *primary* vitreous is formed during the first month of gestation and is a vascularized mesodermal tissue separating the developing lens vesicle and the neuroectoderm of the optic cup. It contains branches of the hyaloid artery that later regress.
2. The *secondary* vitreous starts at 9 weeks and develops throughout embryonic life. It forms the vitreous body, is avascular and transparent, and displaces the primary vitreous, which becomes Cloquet's canal, running from the optic disc to the lens. By the third month, the secondary vitreous fills most of the developing vitreous cavity.
3. The *tertiary* vitreous lies between the ciliary body and lens, separated from the secondary vitreous as well-formed fibrils, which later develop into the zonule.

Developmental anomalies of the vitreous

Persistence of the primary vitreous or part of its structure may give rise to a number of congenital abnormalities.

Persistent hyaloid artery (see Chapter 35)

Persistence of all of or, more frequently part of, the hyaloid artery is a common congenital abnormality. Hyaloid artery remnants occur in 3% of full-term infants but are commonly seen in premature infants, with most regressing. Rarely, the whole artery may run from the disc to the lens. Posterior remnants may give rise to a single vessel running from the center of the disc or to an elevated bud of glial tissue – Bergmeister's papilla. Anterior remnants of the hyaloid system may be seen as a small white dot on the posterior lens capsule – Mittendorf's dot. They are non-progressive and do not interfere with vision.

Vitreous cysts

Acquired cysts occur with inflammatory disease and, rarely, with juvenile X-linked retinoschisis.

Congenital cysts are usually found in otherwise normal eyes. Their origin is unknown but, as blood vessels are sometimes seen within them, they may develop from hyaloid artery remnants.

Cysts may lie in the vitreous immediately behind the lens (Fig. 41.1) or in the posterior vitreous. They may be mobile or attached to the lens or optic disc. Mostly, intervention is not required; occasionally laser treatment (Nd : YAG or argon laser) may be used to collapse the cyst if it is symptomatic. However, repeat Nd : YAG therapy of an anterior pigmented cyst has resulted in a cataract.[1]

Persistent fetal vasculature (persistent hyperplastic primary vitreous) (see Chapter 35)

Persistent fetal vasculature (PFV) persistent hyperplastic primary vitreous (PHPV) is caused by failure of the primary vitreous to regress. Most cases are sporadic and unilateral; there may be minor abnormalities in the fellow eye. Bilateral and familial cases have been reported but these are likely to represent cases of vitreoretinal dysplasia (see Vitreoretinal dysplasia).

For anterior PFV, see Chapter 35.

In posterior PHPV, the ocular abnormality is confined to the posterior segment, and may present with leukocoria,

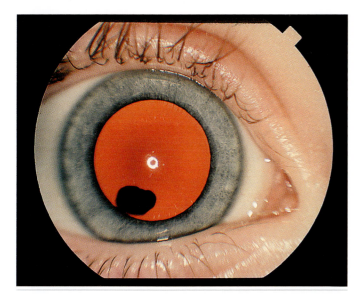

Fig. 41.1 Anterior vitreous cyst seen with retroillumination.

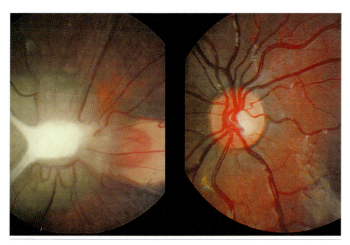

Fig. 41.2 Posterior PHPV. A fold of condensed vitreous running from the optic disc can be seen. The left optic disc is normal.

strabismus, microphthalmia, or nystagmus. The lens is usually clear. There is often a fold of condensed vitreous and retina running from the optic disc to the ora serrata or lens (Fig. 41.2), often associated with a retinal detachment. Ultrasound and CT imaging help in differentiating PHPV from retinoblastoma (see Chapter 42).

Enucleation should be avoided because a prosthesis may be less acceptable cosmetically, and there may be decreased growth of the orbit giving facial asymmetry. A limbal or pars plicata approach may be used to remove the lens and retrolental tissue to clear the visual axis, improve cosmesis, deepen the anterior chamber, and prevent angle closure glaucoma caused by anterior chamber shallowing. However, in many cases, surgical intervention is not required.

Vitreoretinal dysplasia

Maldevelopment of the vitreous and retina, vitreoretinal dysplasia, is seen either as an isolated abnormality or associated with systemic abnormalities.[2] Syndromes such as Norrie's disease and Warburg's syndrome may have bilateral

vitreoretinal dysplasia. It also occurs in trisomy 13, trisomy 18, triploidy, and in association with cerebral malformations.

There appears to be no relationship between the histologic findings and the various syndromes in which retinal dysplasia is reported. The dysplastic retina contains rosettes that resemble retinoblastoma rosettes but contain Müller cells with an abnormal relationship between the retina and retinal pigment epithelium (RPE).

Norrie's disease

Clinical and histologic findings

Norrie's disease is an X-linked recessive disorder; affected males are blind at birth or in early infancy. Twenty-five percent of affected males are developmentally delayed; one-third later develop cochlear deafness. A more severe systemic phenotype is seen in patients with large chromosomal deletions which encompass the Norrie's gene locus. Ocular findings include bilateral cataracts, bilateral retinal folds, retinal detachment, vitreous hemorrhage, and bilateral vitreoretinal dysplasia (Fig. 41.3). The retinal detachments are usually of early onset and have been observed *in utero* by ultrasonography. Most cases progress to an extensive vitreoretinal mass and bilateral blindness.

Angle closure glaucoma may develop; this is best managed by lensectomy. Late signs include corneal opacification, band keratopathy, and phthisis bulbi (see Fig. 41.3).

Carrier females do not usually show any ocular abnormality and electroretinography (ERG) is normal. An affected female has been reported, born to a carrier mother, who had a retrolental mass in the right eye and a retinal fold with a tractional retinal detachment in the left. Molecular genetic testing confirmed that she was a manifesting heterozygote. She showed skewed X-inactivation in her peripheral blood lymphocytes suggesting non-random inactivation, with inactivation occurring more frequently in the normal rather than the mutant X chromosome. A female with Norrie's disease, with an X autosome translocation has also been described.[3]

Histopathology of a vitreoretinal biopsy suggested an arrest of normal retinal development during the third or fourth month of gestation, but the eyes of an aborted 11-week fetus with Norrie's disease showed no evidence of primary neuroectodermal maldevelopment of the retina, suggesting a later disorder of development, probably related to abnormal retinal vascular development (see below).

Molecular genetics and pathogenesis

More than 100 mutations have been identified in the Norrie's disease gene, *NDP*. The gene is expressed in the neural layers of the retina, throughout the brain, and in the spiral ganglion and stria vascularis of the cochlea. The encoded protein, Norrin, is a component of the Wnt signaling pathway, a key regulator of various stages of ocular development, including retinal field establishment, maintenance of retinal stem cells, vasculogenesis in the retina, formation of the ciliary body, and cornea and lens development.[4] Wnt-signaling is important in retinal development: uncontrolled, it may cause other retinal diseases including familial exudative vitreoretinopathy, the osteoporosis-pseudoglioma syndrome, and Norrie's disease. The association of Norrie's disease with peripheral vascular disease is evidence for a role of the Norrin gene in extraocular angiogenesis.

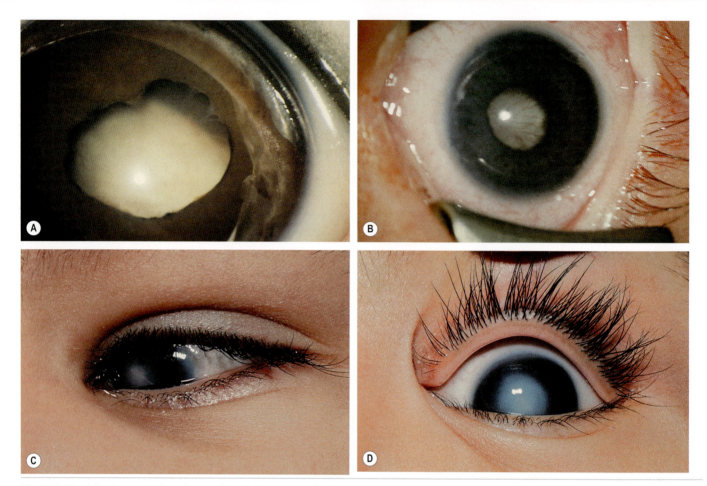

Fig. 41.3 Norrie's disease. (A) Posterior synechiae, shallow anterior chamber, and retrolental white mass. (B) Brother of patient in (A) showing vascularized white retrolental mass. (C,D) Flat anterior chambers and lens–cornea adhesions.

The identification of the Norrie's disease gene allows molecular genetic diagnosis of the carrier state and prenatal diagnosis. Norrie's disease may be associated with chromosomal deletions involving the *NDP* locus, the adjacent monoamine oxidase genes *MAOA* and *MAOB*, and additional genetic material. Children with such deletions have a more severe ("atypical") phenotype.[5] In addition to the characteristic retinal dysplasia, the "atypical" phenotypes may include: severe learning difficulties, involuntary movements, atonic seizures, hypertensive crises, and hypogonadism.[5]

Mutations of the Norrie's disease gene may be responsible for another rare vitreoretinal disorder, X-linked familial exudative vitreoretinopathy (see below).

Coats' disease may be caused by somatic mutations in *NDP* only in the retina of affected eyes; the somatic mutations result in deficiency of Norrin with consequent abnormal retinal vascular development, the hallmark of Coats' disease.[6]

The role of the *NDP* gene in ROP is controversial. Some case–control studies have suggested that sequence variants in the *NDP* gene may predispose to stage 5 ROP; other studies have been negative. The controversy will not be resolved until larger studies have been performed.

NDP knock-out mouse models have a similar ocular phenotype to humans, with fibrous masses in the vitreous cavities, disorganization of retinal ganglion cells, and sporadic degeneration of other retinal cell types. The retinal vasculature is abnormal by postnatal day 9, with abnormal vessels in the inner retina and few vessels in the outer retina. This is further evidence for disordered retinal vascular development being the primary cause of the retinal detachment in Norrie's disease. As in humans, these mice have progressive hearing loss leading to profound deafness, with abnormal vasculature and eventual loss of most of the vessels in the stria vascularis (the main vasculature of the cochlea), suggesting a principal function of Norrin in regulating the interaction of the cochlea with its vasculature.

Trisomy 13

Clinical and histologic findings

Trisomy 13 (Patau's syndrome) is the chromosomal abnormality most consistently associated with severe ocular defects. Systemic abnormalities include microcephaly, cleft palate, congenital cardiac defects, polydactyly, skin hemangiomas, umbilical hernia, and malformation of the central nervous system. Most children die within the first few months of life.

Bilateral ocular abnormalities are seen in almost all cases of trisomy 13; the common ocular findings are detailed in Box 41.1. Affected infants often show total disorganization of the vitreous and retina. Histology shows extensive retinal dysplasia. Intraocular cartilage is frequent and may be characteristic.

Box 41.1

Ocular abnormalities in trisomy 13

- Microphthalmos
- Coloboma of the uveal tract
- Cataract
- Corneal opacities
- Retinal dysplasia
- PHPV
- Dysplastic optic nerves
- Cyclopia

Incontinentia pigmenti (Bloch-Sulzberger syndrome)

Clinical and histologic findings

Incontinentia pigmenti (IP) is an uncommon X-linked dominant disorder affecting the skin, bones, teeth, central nervous system, and eyes, which is usually lethal *in utero* in males, leading to a marked female preponderance. The characteristic skin lesions appear soon after birth with a linear eruption of bullae predominantly affecting the extremities (Fig. 41.4A). The bullae gradually resolve to leave a linear pattern of pigmentation (Fig. 41.4B).

Ocular abnormalities are common including amblyopia, strabismus, nystagmus, optic atrophy, and retinal changes.[7] The retinal changes are the cause of severe visual impairment that may be seen in IP. Corneal abnormalities include whorl-like epithelial keratitis with epithelial microcysts, mild mid-stromal "haziness," and corneal subepithelial anterior stromal opacities.

The most serious complication is retinal detachment, which may lead to severe visual impairment. Retinovascular abnormalities are common and include retinal vascular tortuosity, capillary closure, and peripheral arteriovenous shunts (Fig. 41.4C–E). These are most marked in the temporal periphery and may be associated with retinal neovascularization. Fluorescein angiography demonstrates areas of non-perfusion in the temporal periphery (Fig. 41.4E). Retinal neovascularization, if left untreated, may lead to tractional retinal detachment.

An ophthalmologist should regularly assess affected females soon after diagnosis and during infancy, in order to detect those cases of retinal vascular non-perfusion requiring treatment, usually occurring in the first 2 to 3 years of life. We undertake a retinal examination in affected infants every 2 months for the first year of life then, if normal, 4 monthly for the next 12 months then 6 monthly. If any peripheral retinal abnormality is seen or if a view of the retinal periphery is not obtained after repeated examination, examination under anesthetic is indicated. We combine this with RETCAM fluorescein angiography to document peripheral retinal non-perfusion and neovascularization. Laser treatment is indicated when there is significant capillary non-perfusion (Fig. 41.4F). Established retinal detachment is difficult to manage and has a poor visual outcome (Fig. 41.4G). It is rarely bilateral.

Strabismus, refractive errors, and amblyopia are common in patients with IP and clinic visits for retinal examination are an opportunity for examination of visual behavior, refraction, ocular alignment, and treatment of amblyopia where necessary.

Molecular genetics and pathogenesis

IP is caused by mutations in the ubiquitously expressed gene, *NEMO* (NF-κB essential modulator). The NEMO protein is the regulatory component of the IκB kinase (IKK) complex, a central activator of the NF-κB transcriptional signaling pathway.[8] In IP, loss-of-function mutations in *NEMO* lead to a susceptibility to cellular apoptosis in response to TNF-α.[8]

A recurrent genomic deletion within *NEMO* accounts for 90% of mutations. This deletion eliminates exons 4 to 10 (*NEMOΔ4-10*) and abrogates protein function. The remaining mutations are small duplications, substitutions, and deletions. Most *NEMO* mutations caused premature protein truncation, which is predicted to eliminate NEMO function and thereby cause cell death. Expression analysis of human and mouse *NEMO/nemo* has shown that the gene becomes active early during embryogenesis and is expressed ubiquitously, suggesting a vital role in embryonic and postnatal development.

Irrespective of the mutation causing IP, X-inactivation is likely to modulate the severity in females and account for some of the phenotypic variation. Some females carry the common deletion but are clinically normal, suggesting that selection against mutant cells commenced very early in prenatal development, as in mouse models, in which surviving *nemo*[+/-] female mice show marked skewing of X-inactivation. Although X-inactivation may account for the female phenotypic variation, a role for modifier genes cannot be excluded. In males, X-inactivation is not an issue, and most *NEMO* mutations are lethal because they abolish NF-κB activity, making cells susceptible to TNF-α-induced apoptosis, a finding also demonstrated in *nemo*-null male mice.

Less deleterious mutations can give rise to surviving males and an ectodermal dysplasia-like phenotype with immunodeficiency. Males with skin, dental, and ocular abnormalities typical of those seen in female patients with IP are rare. To date, all carried the common deletion *NEMOΔ4-10*, normally associated with male death *in utero*. Survival in one patient was explained by a 47,XXY karyotype and skewed X-inactivation. The three other patients had a normal 46,XY karyotype, with both wild-type and deleted copies of the *NEMO* gene, and thereby represent somatic mosaics for the common mutation: they acquired the deletion at a post-zygotic stage. There are, therefore, three mechanisms for survival of males carrying a *NEMO* mutation: mild mutations, a 47,XXY karyotype, and somatic mosaicism.

Walker-Warburg syndrome (HARD ± E) and related syndromes

Clinical findings

The acronym HARD ± E stands for hydrocephalus, agyria, retinal dysplasia with or without encephalocele (Fig. 41.5). This autosomal recessive syndrome is characterized by type II lissencephaly (absence of cortical gyri) (see Chapters 56 and 62), retinal dysplasia, cerebellar malformation, and congenital muscular dystrophy. Hydrocephalus is common, which is helpful in prenatal diagnosis by ultrasonography. Other variable features of the Walker-Warburg syndrome (WWS) include Dandy-Walker malformation and encephalocele. Neonatal death is common and survivors are severely developmentally delayed. The ocular features in this disorder are variable and

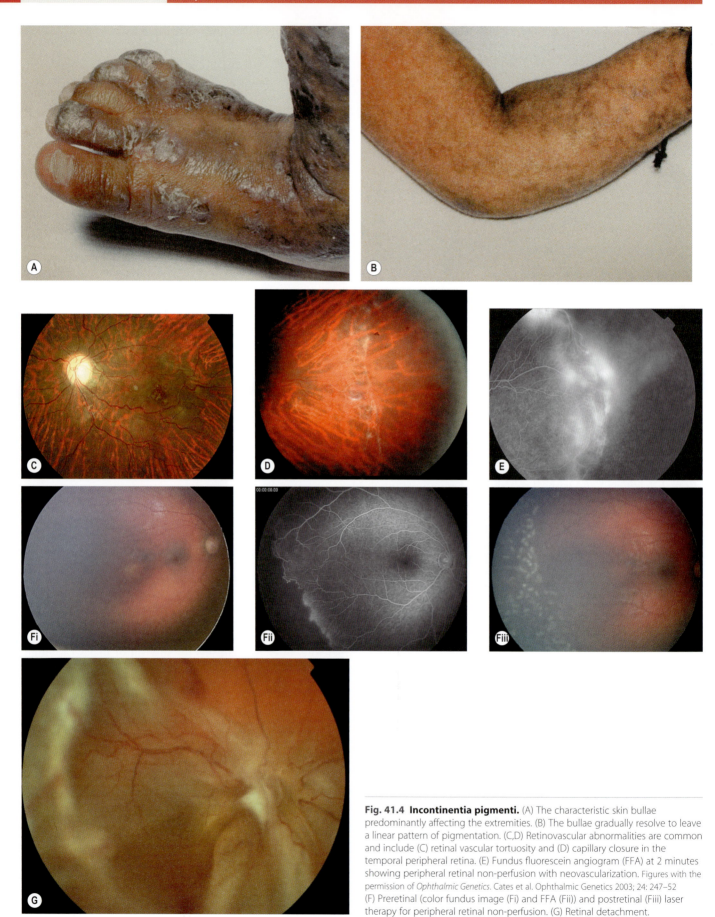

Fig. 41.4 Incontinentia pigmenti. (A) The characteristic skin bullae predominantly affecting the extremities. (B) The bullae gradually resolve to leave a linear pattern of pigmentation. (C,D) Retinovascular abnormalities are common and include (C) retinal vascular tortuosity and (D) capillary closure in the temporal peripheral retina. (E) Fundus fluorescein angiogram (FFA) at 2 minutes showing peripheral retinal non-perfusion with neovascularization. Figures with the permission of *Ophthalmic Genetics*. Cates et al. Ophthalmic Genetics 2003; 24: 247–52 (F) Preretinal (color fundus image (Fi) and FFA (Fii)) and postretinal (Fiii) laser therapy for peripheral retinal non-perfusion. (G) Retinal detachment.

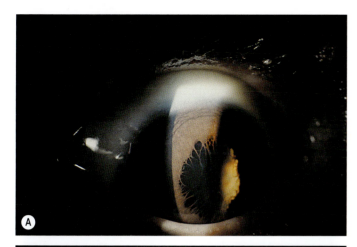

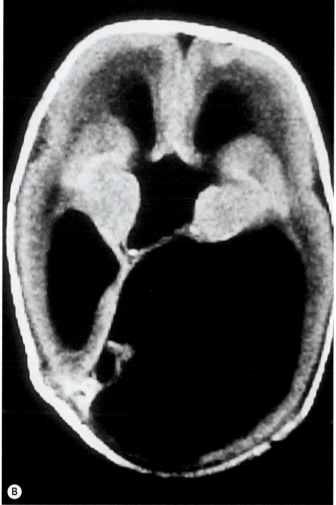

Fig. 41.5 Walker-Warburg syndrome. (A) Shallow anterior chamber and a retrolental mass. (B) CT scan showing hydrocephalus, lissencephaly, and colpocephaly.

include microphthalmia, Peters' anomaly, cataract, retinal coloboma, and retinal dysplasia.

There are two other rare autosomal recessive disorders characterized by the combination of congenital muscular dystrophy and brain malformations, including a neuronal migration defect: muscle–eye–brain (MEB) disease and Fukuyama congenital muscular dystrophy (FCMD) (see Chapter 56). Ocular abnormalities are a constant feature in MEB and WWS, but not in FCMD.[9] The distinction between MEB and WWS is difficult due to the overlap in their clinical characteristics.[6] Survival past 3 years of age is far more likely in MEB; death in infancy is more usual in WWS. MRI findings can also be helpful in differentiating between MEB and WWS: an absent corpus callosum suggests WWS.[9]

Genetic linkage studies have shown that WWS is not allelic to MEB.[9] The molecular genetics of these three disorders is likely to be helpful in distinguishing between them when the clinical diagnosis is unclear.

Molecular genetics and pathogenesis

The causative genes have been identified in MEB and FCMD, with the encoded proteins involved in protein glycosylation. Mutations in the gene *POMT1*, encoding *O*-mannosyltransferase 1, have been identified in WWS. Immunohistochemical analysis of muscle from patients with *POMT1* mutations corroborated the *O*-mannosylation defect, as judged by the absence of glycosylation of α-dystroglycan, with lack of such glycosylation believed to be sufficient to explain the muscular dystrophy in WWS. The brain and eye phenotypes in WWS may involve defective glycosylation of other proteins. Further genetic heterogeneity in WWS is likely since only 20% of patients with WWS harbor *POMT1* mutations.

Autosomal recessive vitreoretinal dysplasia

Vitreoretinal dysplasia may occur as an isolated abnormality in a healthy child. The inheritance is presumed to be autosomal recessive. In male infants, mutations in the Norrie's disease gene (*NDP*) must be excluded. Presentation is with bilateral poor vision in early infancy, a shallow anterior chamber, and white retrolental mass. Progressive shallowing of the anterior chamber may lead to pupil-block glaucoma which, following failure to respond to medical therapy, may require lensectomy.

Osteoporosis–pseudoglioma syndrome

Clinical findings

This autosomal recessive syndrome is characterized by osteoporosis, severe learning difficulties, and vitreoretinal dysplasia (Fig. 41.6). Multiple fractures, often after minor trauma, are commonplace. Affected children present in infancy with bilateral nystagmus and severe visual impairment; the systemic features occur in later infancy and childhood. Ocular features include vitreoretinal dysplasia with retrolental masses, microphthalmia, anterior chamber anomalies, cataract, and phthisis bulbi. Most patients are blind from birth but a few patients have useful vision into their teenage years.

Molecular genetics and pathogenesis

Mutations have been identified in the gene encoding the low-density lipoprotein receptor-related protein 5 (LRP5). Mutations in *LRP5* have also been shown to be associated with both autosomal recessive and autosomal dominant familial exudative vitreoretinopathy (FEVR). These patients have also been shown to have reduced bone mineral density, suggesting that osteoporosis-pseudoglioma syndrome and LRP5-associated FEVR are part of a single phenotypic spectrum with both ocular and bone manifestations.[10]

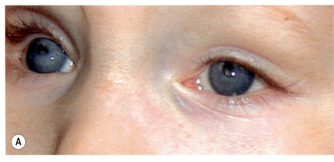

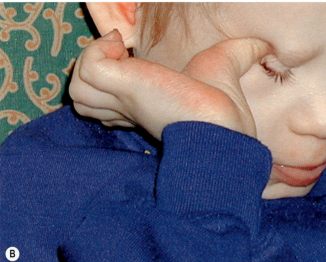

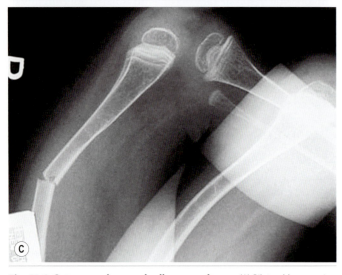

Fig. 41.6 Osteoporosis–pseudoglioma syndrome. (A) Bilateral leucocoria secondary to retrolental masses. (B) Eye poking in children with blindness due to retinal disease is common. (C) X-ray of femur showing fracture and bone demineralization. (Figures reproduced with the permission of the *British Journal of Ophthalmology*. From Wilson G, Moore A, Allgrove J. Bilateral retinal detachments at birth: the osteoporosis psedoglioma syndrome. Br J Ophthalmol 2001; 85: 1139.)

Studies of LRP5 indicate that it affects bone accrual during growth by regulating osteoblastic proliferation. Furthermore, LRP5 is a component of the Wnt-signaling pathway, regulating retinal development and angiogenesis, thereby accounting for the resulting retinopathy when LRP5 function is perturbed.[4,11]

Oculopalatal–cerebral dwarfism

Three siblings of consanguineous parents were described with vitreoretinal dysplasia and systemic abnormalities including microcephaly, mental retardation, cleft palate, and short stature.[12] The ocular abnormalities, similar to those seen in PHPV, were bilateral in one child and unilateral in the others. It is probably autosomal recessive.

Unilateral retinal dysplasia

Lloyd et al. reported a family in which three affected members had unilateral retinal dysplasia without any systemic abnormalities.[13]

Genetic counsellng in the vitreoretinal dysplasias

The vitreoretinal dysplasias are genetically heterogeneous disorders which result in a similar ocular abnormality; it is often not possible to subdivide them on the clinical or pathologic ocular findings alone, so the diagnosis depends on the systemic findings or molecular genetics, although the family history may suggest the mode of inheritance.

For the purposes of genetic counseling, families fall into two groups.

Group 1

The diagnosis and hence the mode of inheritance of the affected child is clear. When one child has been born with a trisomy, the risk of a similar affected child in a future pregnancy is 1%, but may be higher if one of the parents has a structural chromosome abnormality or mosaicism.[14] Such parents may be offered prenatal diagnosis.

In children with the systemic features of Walker-Warburg syndrome or the osteoporosis–pseudoglioma syndrome the inheritance is autosomal recessive.

In Norrie's disease there are no detectable clinical abnormalities in the carrier female to aid counseling. When there is another affected male relative the mother can be assumed to be a carrier. In isolated boys, the status of the mother is uncertain, but can usually be resolved by molecular genetics. If the mutation has been identified in the affected child, the mother and other at-risk female members can be screened for the mutation. Most mothers will be identified as carriers. However, some mothers will not carry the identified Norrie's gene mutation: their affected child may have a new mutation. Germ line mosaicism is possible but rare. In this situation, the mother will need to be counseled that there is an increased, but low, risk of having a further child with Norrie's disease.

Group 2

Counseling a family with an otherwise normal child with bilateral retinal dysplasia is more difficult. Isolated retinal dysplasia is rare so there are insufficient empirical data to aid counseling. If the affected child is female, retinal dysplasia may be autosomal recessive or non-genetic. Autosomal recessive dysplasia is rare; if there is no parental consanguinity, the recurrence risk is likely to be low. In an affected male child, retinal dysplasia may be autosomal recessive, X-linked, or non-genetic. Most affected males will have Norrie's disease which can be confirmed by molecular genetics. In the small minority without identifiable mutations in the *NDP* gene, if there is no parental consanguinity and other multisystem disorders have been excluded, the recurrence risk is probably low.

Inherited vitreoretinal dystrophies

Wagner's syndrome

Clinical findings

Wagner's syndrome is an autosomal dominant vitreoretinal dystrophy with low myopia and vitreous and retinal abnormalities, without systemic abnormalities. The vitreous appears optically empty apart from scattered translucent membranes: there is usually a posterior vitreous detachment with a thickened posterior hyaloid. Peripheral vascular sheathing is common and normally associated with perivascular RPE atrophy and pigment deposition. The ERG is subnormal and parallels the chorioretinal pathology and poor night vision. Cataract develops after the second decade and is the usual cause of visual loss. Rhegmatogenous retinal detachment is infrequent, whereas peripheral tractional retinal detachment occurs in most of the elderly affected.

Wagner's disease and erosive vitreoretinopathy share some clinical features; they both have subnormal ERGs, poor night vision, and field defects which are not found in *COL2A1*-associated Stickler's syndrome. The vitreoretinal phenotype is different, as neither of the recognized vitreous abnormalities in Stickler's syndrome are present in Wagner's syndrome (see below). In addition, retinal detachment is less common in Wagner's syndrome, but occurs in the majority of patients with Stickler's syndrome and erosive vitreoretinopathy.

Molecular genetics and pathogenesis

Wagner's syndrome and erosive vitreoretinopathy are linked to 5q13–14 and are likely to be allelic disorders, distinct from Stickler's syndrome. Heterozygous mutations in the gene encoding chondroitin sulfate proteoglycan-2 (CSPG2), a proteoglycan present in the vitreous body, have been identified in Wagner's syndrome.

A phenotypically distinct vitreoretinopathy with early onset retinal detachments and anterior segment developmental abnormalities, without systemic features, has been described which also maps to 5q13–q14, to a 5-cM region already implicated in both Wagner's syndrome and erosive vitreoretinopathy.

Erosive vitreoretinopathy

Clinical findings

Erosive vitreoretinopathy is characterized by autosomal dominant inheritance, night-blindness, progressive field loss, vitreous abnormalities, progressive RPE atrophy, and combined tractional and rhegmatogenous retinal detachment.[15] ERG shows widespread rod and cone dysfunction. Peripheral RPE atrophy, field loss, and ERG abnormalities are evident in childhood. The vitreous is syneretic with areas of condensation but without the inflammatory signs seen in autosomal dominant neovascular inflammatory vitreoretinopathy. There are no systemic abnormalities.

Dragged retinal vessels and macular ectopia may occur, with tractional or rhegmatogenous retinal detachment in most

affected adults. Twenty percent of affected eyes become blind from retinal detachment.[15]

Molecular genetics and pathogenesis

The syndromes referred to above have been mapped to 5q13–q14 suggesting they may be allelic.

Stickler's syndrome (see also Chapter 50)

Clinical findings

In Stickler's syndrome, abnormalities of vitreous gel architecture are a pathognomonic feature, usually associated with congenital and non-progressive high myopia. Other eye features include paravascular pigmented lattice degeneration, cataracts, and retinal detachment. Non-ocular features are very variable: deafness, a flat mid-face with depressed nasal bridge, short nose, anteverted nares, and micrognathia that can become less pronounced with age. Midline clefting, if present, ranges from a submucous cleft to Pierre-Robin sequence, whilst joint hypermobility declines with age. Osteoarthritis may develop after the third decade. Stature and intellect are normal.

Molecular genetics and pathogenesis

The *COL2A1* gene encodes type II procollagen, a precursor of components of secondary vitreous and articular cartilage; several mutations occur in families with Stickler's and Kniest's syndrome. There is phenotypic variability with presence or absence of systemic features and locus heterogeneity with about two-thirds of families showing linkage to *COL2A1*.

Stickler's syndrome can be divided into two types by slit-lamp biomicroscopy of the vitreous, facilitating prioritization of molecular screening:

1. Type 1: with retrolental vitreous anomaly and is associated with mutations of the *COL2A1* gene.
2. Type 2: no retrolental vitreous anomaly and does not harbor *COL2A1* variants. Mutations in *COL11A1* (encoding α1 chain of type XI collagen) and *COL11A2* (encoding α2 chain of type XI collagen) have been identified in type 2 families.

Mutations in exon 2 of the *COL2A1* gene may produce a Stickler's phenotype with predominantly ocular manifestations.

Myelinated nerve fibres, vitreoretinopathy, and skeletal malformations

Severe vitreoretinal degeneration, high myopia, myelinated nerve fibers, and skeletal abnormalities were described in a mother and daughter that were distinct from those seen in Stickler's syndrome. Both had severe visual impairment and roving eye movements, and electrophysiologic testing in the mother showed an abnormal scotopic and photopic ERG.

Juvenile X-linked retinoschisis

See Chapter 49

Clinical and histologic findings

This X-linked disorder is almost exclusive to males. The characteristic fundus abnormality is a cystic spokewheel-like maculopathy (foveal schisis), present in about two-thirds of males (Fig. 41.7A–C). Fifty percent of affected males show additional peripheral retinal changes (Fig. 41.7D). Foveal retinoschisis may occur in early infancy, but most children present between 5 and 10 years either with reading difficulties or when they fail the school eye test. The visual acuity is 6/12–6/36 at presentation and strabismus, hypermetropia, and astigmatism are common. If the macular changes are subtle, it may be misdiagnosed as strabismic or ametropic amblyopia or functional visual loss (see Chapter 60).

Familial exudative vitreoretinopathy

FEVR describes a group of inherited disorders with abnormal retinal vascularization often associated with exudation, neovascularization, and tractional retinal detachment. In advanced disease there are some clinical similarities to cicatricial ROP. The clinical appearance varies considerably, even within families, with severely affected patients often registered as blind during infancy and mildly affected patients having few or no visual problems.

FEVR can be inherited as an autosomal recessive, autosomal dominant, and X-linked disorder, with all the genes identified to date being components of the Wnt-signaling pathway.[4,11] There appears to be no correlation between mode of inheritance, particular mutations, or mutation types and phenotype. LRP5 mutation carriers (autosomal dominant and autosomal recessive FEVR) remain the only subset of FEVR patients that can be clinically distinguished by the presence of low bone-mass density.[4,10,11]

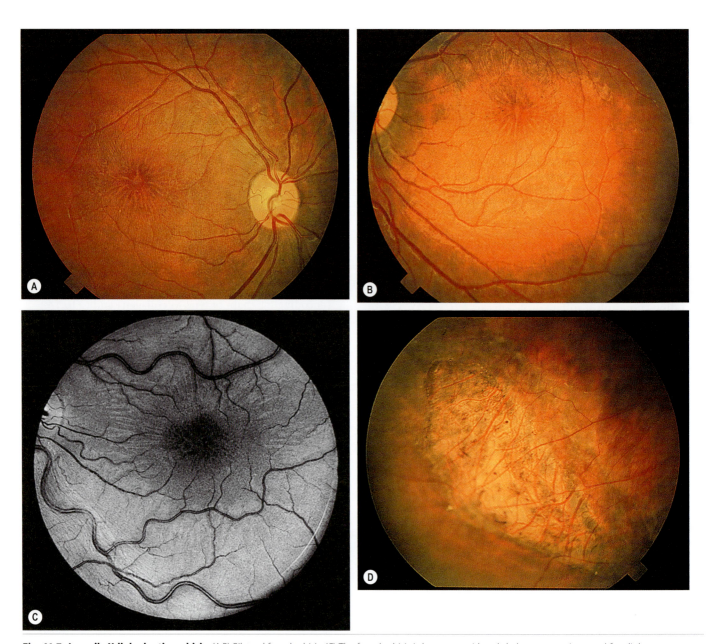

Fig. 41.7 Juvenile X-linked retinoschisis. (A,B) Bilateral foveal schisis. (C) The foveal schisis is best seen with ophthalmoscopy using a red free light. (D) Peripheral pigmentary changes in an area of schisis.

Autosomal dominant familial exudative vitreoretinopathy

Clinical findings

Early reports were of a progressive vitreoretinopathy like cicatricial ROP, autosomal dominant inheritance, and a variable clinical expression (Box 41.2).

There is a widespread abnormality of the retinal vasculature, due to arrest of normal vasculogenesis.[3,8] In the asymptomatic form, fundoscopy and fluorescein angiography reveals peripheral retinovascular abnormalities, particularly temporally, although fundus findings may be subtle (Fig. 41.8). These include vascular dilatation and tortuosity, arteriovenous shunting, capillary closure, and peripheral retinal neovascularization (Fig. 41.9). Optic disc neovascularization is less common. Vitreoretinal adhesions are frequently seen at the border between vascularized and non-vascularized retina, and other peripheral retinal changes include retinal pigmentation and intraretinal white deposits.

More advanced cases show vascular leakage, cicatrization with macular ectopia, tractional retinal detachment, and macular edema (Fig. 41.10). Vitreous hemorrhage and secondary rhegmatogenous retinal detachment are complications. The retinal changes may progress throughout childhood, rarely after the age of 20. In children who show progression from stage I disease (Box 41.2), laser ablation of peripheral ischemic retina may be indicated. In advanced cases, vitreoretinal surgery may be beneficial.

The majority of FEVR gene carriers are asymptomatic and have only minor retinovascular abnormalities. The gene is highly penetrant. It is important to perform a careful fundoscopic examination, preferably with fluorescein angiography, before excluding carrier status.

Molecular genetics and pathogenesis

Mutations in *FZD4* and *LRP5* have been detected in affected individuals.[4,11] *FZD4* and *LRP5* encode the receptors Frizzled-4 and low-density lipoprotein receptor-related protein-5, respectively, with these two proteins acting as co-receptors for Wnts and Norrin.[4,11] Mutations in *TSPAN12* have also been identified, which encodes a protein that facilitates the binding of Norrin to the aforementioned receptor.

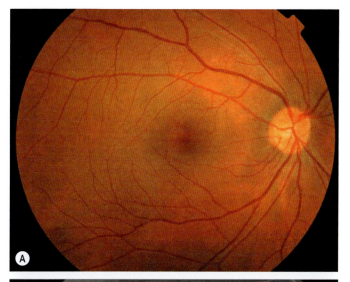
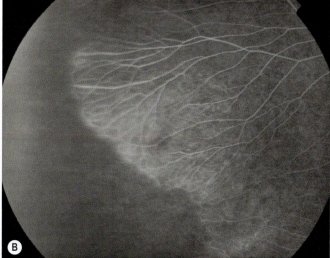

Fig. 41.8 Autosomal dominant familial exudative vitreoretinopathy. (A,B) An asymptomatic carrier with a normal examination of the posterior pole (A). The importance of fundus fluorescein angiography (FFA) can be seen in helping to determine status, with marked temporal retinal capillary closure observed on FFA.

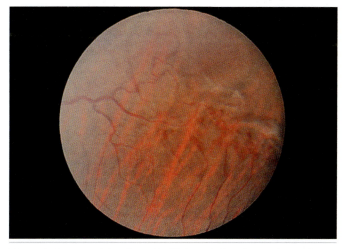

Fig. 41.9 Autosomal dominant familial exudative vitreoretinopathy. Peripheral vascular dilatation, tortuosity, and shunting with some preretinal changes.

Box 41.2

Classification of autosomal dominant familial exudative vitreoretinopathy

Stage I

  Mild peripheral retinal changes with abnormal vitreous traction but no evidence of retinal vascular or exudative change

Stage II

  Dilated tortuous vessels between the equator and ora serrata with subretinal exudates and localized retinal detachment. Dragging of disc vessels and macular ectopia is often present

Stage III

  Advanced disease with total retinal detachment and extensive vitreoretinal traction. There may be secondary cataract and rubeosis iridis

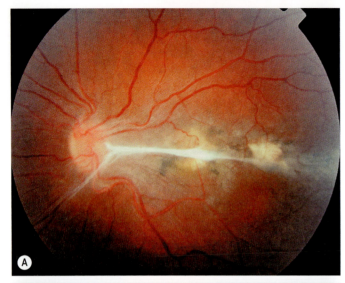

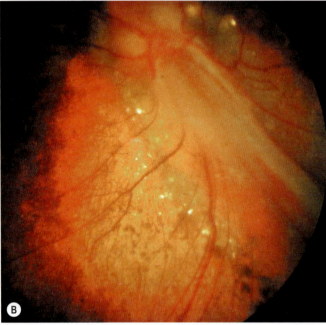

Fig. 41.10 Autosomal dominant familial exudative vitreoretinopathy.
(A) Cicatrization with macular ectopia. (B) Severe retinal fold secondary to FEVR.

X-linked familial exudative vitreoretinopathy

Clinical findings

The phenotype may be similar to the severe form of dominant exudative vitreoretinopathy and may also resemble congenital falciform retinal folds. Affected males often have severe early onset visual impairment, and prominent retinal folds from the disc to the ora serrata are characteristic.

Molecular genetics and pathogenesis

Point mutations in *NDP* have been identified. X-linked FEVR (XL-FEVR) and Norrie's disease are thereby allelic disorders (different mutations of the same gene giving rise to a different but well-defined phenotype).

Autosomal recessive familial exudative vitreoretinopathy

Autosomal recessive FEVR (AR-FEVR) has been identified less commonly compared to AD- and XL-FEVR. AR-FEVR is usually more severe than the dominant form of the disorder (Fig. 41.11).

Molecular genetics and pathogenesis

Biallelic mutations in *LRP5* have been detected in affected individuals.[4,11]

Autosomal dominant vitreoretinochoroidopathy

Clinical and histologic findings

This rare dystrophy has abnormal chorioretinal pigmentation in a 360° circumference between the vortex veins and the ora serrata which is present in childhood and usually progresses. There are areas of hypo- and hyperpigmentation and scattered yellow dots may be seen in the peripheral retina and at the posterior pole. There are usually retinovascular changes with arteriolar narrowing, venous occlusion, and widespread leakage. A demarcation line is seen between the normal and abnormal retina. The vitreous is liquefied with peripheral condensation. Presenile cataract occurs frequently. Fluorescein angiography shows areas of capillary dilatation and diffuse vascular leakage; peripheral neovascularization may develop in a few cases.

Visual symptoms are rare in childhood but may occur in adults from cataract, macular edema, vitreous hemorrhage, and retinal detachment. Nyctalopia is not prominent and the ERG is normal, sometimes becoming abnormal with age. The EOG usually suggests a widespread RPE defect but can be normal. There are no consistent systemic abnormalities.

Light and electron microscopy showed similar findings in a young and an old patient suggesting that ADVIRC is an early onset peripheral retinal dystrophy with minimal subsequent progression, characterized by a RPE response that includes marked intraretinal migration and extracellular matrix deposition.

Molecular genetics and pathogenesis

Mutations have been found in the bestrophin-1 gene (*BEST1*). Sequence variants have also been identified in *BEST1* in several other retinal phenotypes,[16] including Best's disease (see Chapter 46), autosomal recessive bestrophinopathy, adult vitelliform macular dystrophy, MRCS (microcornea, rod–cone dystrophy, cataract, and posterior staphyloma), and retinitis pigmentosa (see Chapter 44).

Autosomal dominant neovascular inflammatory vitreoretinopathy

Clinical findings

This rare autosomal dominant disorder is characterized by panocular inflammation, peripheral retinal pigment deposition, retinal vascular occlusion and neovascularization, vitreous hemorrhage, and tractional retinal detachment. Presenile cataract is common. The single bright white flash ERG shows early selective loss of the b-wave ("negative-ERG"),

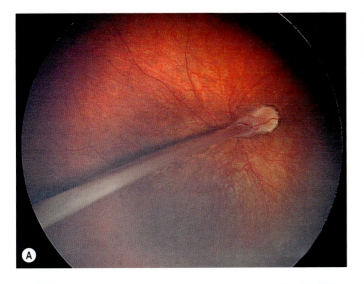

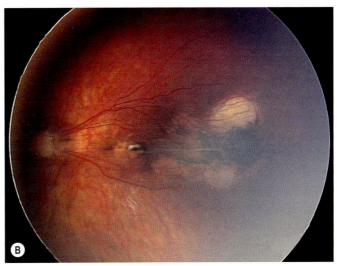

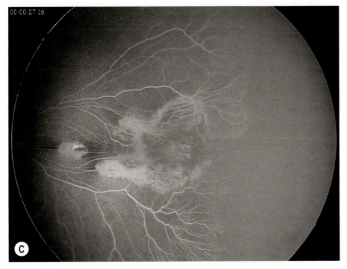

Fig. 41.11 Autosomal recessive familial exudative vitreoretinopathy. A marked retinal fold involving the macula is seen in the right eye (A) and temporal dragging of retinal vessels with retinal fibrosis and scarring in the left eye (B), with corresponding temporal capillary non-perfusion (C).

which differentiates it from the other vitreoretinopathies with vascular closure. Night-blindness is a late feature; the ERG may become totally extinguished in advanced disease. There are no reported systemic abnormalities.

The earliest signs are vitreous cells, mild peripheral retinal ischemia, and reduced b-wave amplitudes on ERG. It cannot be reliably detected in childhood.

Molecular genetics

It has been mapped to 11q close to the 11q locus for autosomal dominant familial exudative vitreoretinopathy (*FZD4* and *LRP5*); the causative gene has not been identified.

Autosomal dominant snowflake degeneration

This disorder is characterized by extensive "white-with-pressure" change in the peripheral retina, multiple minute "snowflake" retinal deposits, and sheathing of the peripheral retinal vessels. Later, there may be peripheral vascular occlusion and retinal pigmentation. The vitreous is degenerate and liquefied. Psychophysical studies show abnormal rod and cone function and although ERG may be normal initially, the b-wave amplitude is later reduced. There is an increased risk of retinal tears

and detachment. The retinal changes may be seen in childhood, more often in the teens or later. There are no systemic abnormalities.

Molecular genetics and pathogenesis

A missense mutation has been identified in *KCNJ13*, which encodes an inwardly rectifying potassium channel. Null mutations in this gene have been implicated in a rare form of Leber's congenital amaurosis (see Chapter 44).

Acquired disorders of the vitreous

Acquired disorders of the vitreous are uncommon in childhood and generally occur when there is vitreous opacification caused by hemorrhage or, less commonly, inflammation. Tumor or infection may involve the vitreous cavity.

Vitreous hemorrhage (Box 41.3)

The management of vitreous hemorrhage is relatively straightforward in children who have reached the age of visual maturity. A conservative approach is preferred with surgery only

Box 41.3

Some causes of vitreous hemorrhage in children

- Trauma
  - Blunt
  - Penetrating
- X-linked juvenile retinoschisis
- Vitreoretinal dystrophies
  - FEVR
  - ADVIRC
  - ADNIV
- Stickler's syndrome
- ROP
- PHPV
- Retinal dysplasias
- Retinal hemangioblastoma
- Cavernous hemangioma
- Eales' disease
- Coats' disease
- Non-accidental injury/Child abuse
- Birth-related hemorrhages
- Hematological disorders
  - Leukemia
  - Thrombocytopenia
  - Hemophilia
  - Von Willebrand's disease
  - Protein C deficiency

indicated if the hemorrhage is persistent or if there is an associated retinal detachment. In infants and young children, vitreous hemorrhage may lead to amblyopia and affect emmetropization. If, after a short period of observation, there is no resolution and if there is no underlying retinal abnormality that may herald a poor prognosis, early lens-sparing vitrectomy may be considered. Occlusion needs to be started as soon as possible.

Inflammatory disease of the vitreous

See Chapter 39

Vitreous opacity due to tumor

Vitreous seeding may complicate retinoblastoma; clumps of tumor cells float in the vitreous but rarely give rise to diagnostic problems as there is usually a typical retinoblastoma. When there are clumps of cells in the anterior vitreous in an inflamed eye with an opaque vitreous there may be doubt as to whether

the underlying etiology is inflammatory or neoplastic. Ultrasound or CT scan usually demonstrates a retinoblastoma, but not in the rare diffuse infiltrating forms.

Tumor cells may be found in the vitreous in leukemia but there is almost always associated retinal infiltration (see Chapter 64). Other intraocular tumors are rare.

References

1. Gupta R, Pannu BK, Bhargav S, et al. Nd:YAG laser photocystotomy of a free-floating pigmented anterior vitreous cyst. Ophthal Surg Lasers Imaging 2003; 34: 203–5.
2. Edwards AO. Clinical features of the congenital vitreoretinopathies. Eye 2008; 22: 1233–42.
3. Ohba N, Yamashita T. Primary vitreoretinal dysplasia resembling Norrie's disease in a female: associated with X autosome chromosomal translocation. Br J Ophthalmol 1986; 70: 64–71.
4. Lad EM, Cheshier SH, Kalani MY. Wnt-signaling in retinal development and disease. Stem Cells Dev 2009; 18: 7–16.
5. Suarez-Merino B, Bye J, McDowall J, et al. Sequence analysis and transcript identification within 1.5 MB of DNA deleted together with the NDP and MAO genes in atypical Norrie disease patients presenting with a profound phenotype. Hum Mutat 2001; 17: 523.
6. Black GC, Perveen R, Bonshek R, et al. Coats' disease of the retina (unilateral retinal telangiectasis) caused by somatic mutation in the NDP gene: a role for norrin in retinal angiogenesis. Hum Mol Genet 1999; 8: 2031–5.
7. Holmström G, Thorén K. Ocular manifestations of incontinentia pigmenti. Acta Ophthalmol Scand 2000; 78: 348–53.
8. Aradhya S, Nelson DL. NF-kappaB signaling and human disease. Curr Opin Genet Dev 2001; 11: 300–6.
9. Cormand B, Pihko H, Bayes M, et al. Clinical and genetic distinction between Walker-Warburg syndrome and muscle-eye-brain disease. Neurology 2001; 56: 1059–69.
10. Qin M, Hayashi H, Oshima K, et al. Complexity of the genotype-phenotype correlation in familial exudative vitreoretinopathy with mutations in the LRP5 and/or FZD4 genes. Hum Mutat 2005; 26: 104–12.
11. Warden SM, Andreoli CM, Mukai S. The Wnt signaling pathway in familial exudative vitreoretinopathy and Norrie disease. Semin Ophthalmol 2007; 22: 211–7.
12. Frydman M, Kauschansky A, Leshem I, Savir H. Oculo–palato–cerebral dwarfism. Clin Genet 1985; 27: 414–19.
13. Lloyd I, Colley A, Tullo A, Bonshek R. Dominantly inherited unilateral retinal dysplasia. Br J Ophthalmol 1993; 77: 378–80.
14. Steve J, Steve E, Mikkelson M. Risk for chromosome abnormality at amniocentesis following a child with a non-inherited chromosome aberration. Prenat Diagn 1984; 4: 81–5.
15. Brown DM, Kimura AE, Weingest TA, et al. Erosive vitreoretinopathy: a new clinical entity. Ophthalmology 1994; 101: 694–704.
16. Boon CJ, Klevering BJ, Leroy BP, et al. The spectrum of ocular phenotypes caused by mutations in the BEST1 gene. Prog Retin Eye Res 2009; 28: 187–205.

CHAPTER **42**

Retinoblastoma

Brenda L Gallie • Mandeep S Sagoo • M Ashwin Reddy

Retinoblastoma is an uncommon malignant ocular tumor of childhood, occurring in 1 : 18 000 live births.[1] Late diagnosis globally results in up to 70% mortality; where optimal therapy is accessible, more than 95% of children are cured. An integrated team approach of clinical specialists (ophthalmologists, pediatric oncologists and radiotherapists, nurses, geneticists) with imaging specialists, child life (play) specialists, parents, and others is an effective way to manage retinoblastoma. National guidelines can bring the whole health team up to developed standards and set the stage for audits, studies, and clinical trials to continuously evolve better care and outcomes.[2] The tumor(s) arises from embryonic retinal cells so the majority of cases occur under the age of 4 years. Primary treatments include enucleation and chemotherapy with laser and cryotherapy. Patients with a constitutional mutation of the *RB1* tumor suppressor gene are at increased life-long risk of developing other cancers, which is increased with exposure to radiation (Figs 42.1 and 42.2).[3,4] Therefore, radiation is no longer a primary therapy to save an eye, and screening for extraocular and trilateral retinoblastoma is performed with MRI and ultrasound, not CT scan.

The study of retinoblastoma has been seminal in the understanding of cancer in general. Studies of retinoblastoma have revealed that hereditary and non-hereditary tumors are initiated by the loss of both alleles of the tumor suppressor gene, *RB1*.[5,6] The existence of specific genes that act to suppress cancer was predicted from clinical studies of retinoblastoma.[7,8] The *RB1* gene was the first tumor suppressor gene to be cloned,[5] and has been found to have a critical role in many types of cancer.

Pathogenesis of retinoblastoma

Heritable and non-heritable retinoblastoma

All children with retinoblastoma tumors in both eyes (bilateral) have an *RB1* gene mutation on one of their chromosomes (13) that predisposes them to develop retinal tumors in infancy and other cancers throughout life (see Figs 42.1 and 42.2). While 90% have no family history of retinoblastoma and are the first affected in their family with a *new* germ line mutation,[9] 50% of their offspring will inherit the mutant *RB1* gene and develop tumors. Most children without a family history with retinoblastoma in only one eye have normal constitutional *RB1* alleles, but the eye tumor(s) loses both functional alleles, similar to hereditary tumors. Fifteen percent of persons who had unilateral retinoblastoma have constitutional *RB1* mutations that can be transmitted to their offspring. Molecular and clinical genetics is an integral part of the management of all families affected by retinoblastoma.

Loss of both *RB1* alleles induces retinoblastoma

The observation that the children with bilateral retinoblastoma tend to be diagnosed at a younger age than those with non-hereditary retinoblastoma led to Knudson's prediction that two mutational events were required to initiate retinoblastoma tumors.[7] His analysis suggested that in the presence of a predisposing constitutional mutation a single second mutation in one developing retinal cell initiated tumor development (heritable retinoblastoma), but both alleles were mutated in the single developing retinal cell in non-heritable unilateral retinoblastoma. The two events could be mutations of both alleles of a gene that would "suppress" tumor formation in the retina.[8] The chance of losing the second *RB1* allele from developing retinal cells with only one normal *RB1* allele is sufficiently high that multiple tumors are common in hereditary retinoblastoma (see Fig. 42.1). However, it is virtually impossible for children without constitutional *RB1* mutations to lose

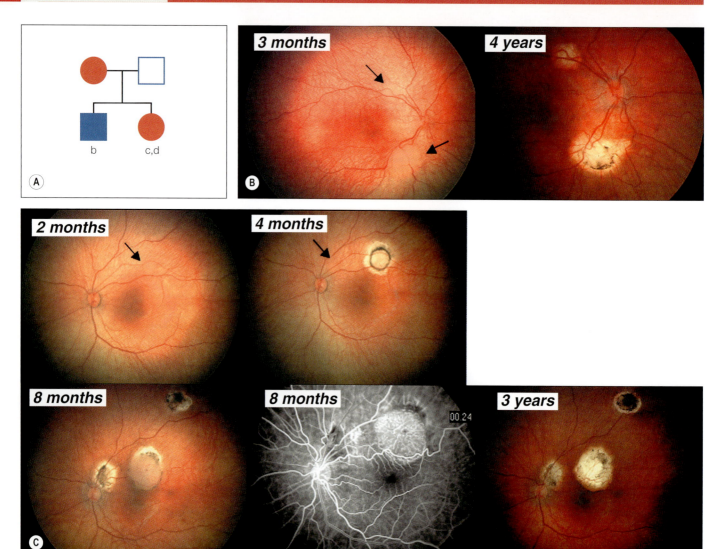

Fig. 42.1 (A) Family tree: mother was cured of bilateral retinoblastoma by enucleation of one eye and external beam radiation of the other eye. Forty-two years later, she developed metastatic hemangiosarcoma in the path of the exit beam of radiation (red*). Both children were delivered at 36 weeks' gestation to facilitate early treatment of tumors and developed bilateral tumors. Mother and both children carry a germline *RB1* mutation (M1, deletion of ATTTC starting at bp 778, reading to a STOP, 9 codons away) that results in no pRB when the normal *RB1* allele is lost (M2) from a developing retinal cell, initiating a tumor. (B) RetCam® images: prior to treatment, right eye (IIRC group A, more than 1.5 mm from optic disk) of the boy at 3 months, showing two tumors; stable right eye of boy age 4 years after laser, two cycles of CEV (carboplatin, etoposide, and vincristine) with cyclosporin A chemotherapy, and more laser treatments. (C) RetCam® images: prior to treatment, left eye (IIRC group B, tumor less than 3 mm from fovea) of the girl at 2 months; laser scar and new tumor above nerve at 4 months of age; recurrence in original scar extending toward fovea, with tumor vascularization showing on fluorescein angiography; flat scars at age 2.5 years after laser, two cycles of CEV with cyclosporin A chemotherapy to control recurrence threatening vision chemotherapy and more laser. (Images by Leslie MacKeen, Cynthia VandenHoven and Carmelina Trimboli.)

both alleles from several retinal cells so they develop only one, unilateral tumor (Fig. 42.3), and tend to be diagnosed at an older age than children with hereditary retinoblastoma.

Function of the retinoblastoma protein

The product of the *RB1* gene (pRB) is a 110 kDa phosphoprotein that interacts with many proteins in the regulation of the cell cycle, differentiation, and control of genomic stability.[10] DNA tumor viruses that induce cancer, such as human papilloma virus, do so in part by binding to pRB through the "pocket" region of pRB.

Germ line mutation of *RB1* leads to a 40 000-fold relative risk (RR) for retinoblastoma, a 500-fold RR for sarcoma that is increased up to 2000-fold by therapeutic radiation, but no

increase in the RR for leukemia.[11] Although pRB is key to all cycling cells, its function in development is highly tissue-specific. A subset of developing retinal cells may be uniquely dependent on pRB in order to differentiate terminally into adult, functioning retina. Loss of pRB promotes genomic changes and instability, leading to further mutations in oncogenes and other tumor suppressor genes that result in a retinal tumor.[12,13]

Spectrum of *RB1* mutations

The majority of *RB1* mutations are unique to each family, and are distributed throughout the *RB1* gene with no real hot spots.[9] Sensitive mutation identification requires determination of the copy number of each exon and the gene promoter

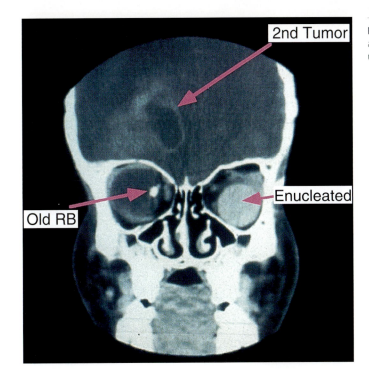

Fig. 42.2 Glioblastoma multiforme arising within the radiation field, 10 years after enucleation of the left eye and irradiation of the right eye for bilateral retinoblastoma (RB).

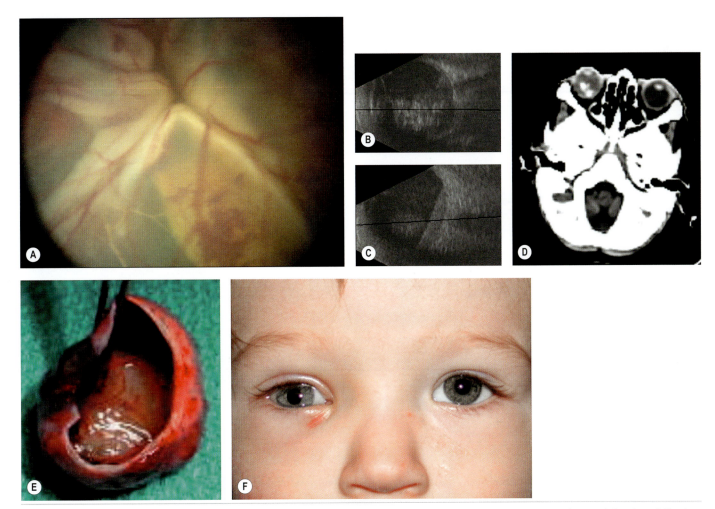

Fig. 42.3 (A) Exophytic retinoblastoma (IIRC group D) with retinal detachment in a unilaterally affected 3-year-old boy. (B) B-scan ultrasound showing calcification in a single tumor beside the optic nerve. (C) B-scan ultrasound showing subretinal hemorrhage and no tumor involvement of optic nerve. (D) CT scan showing intraocular calcification, normal sized optic nerve. (E) The eye was opened immediately after enucleation, in order to obtain live tumor cells and the two RB1 mutations (homozygous exon 16 deletion C-1450, insertion AT) defined. The mutant RB1 allele was not detected in the child's blood, eliminating risk for his siblings. His future offspring will be checked for the mutant allele of the tumor, since he could still be mosaic. (F) The child 2 days after enucleation, wearing the temporary prosthetic conformer inserted at the time of surgery. The exon 16 RB1 mutation of the tumor was not detected in blood, indicating high likelihood that the retinoblastoma is not heritable, eliminating risk for siblings. Due to the remaining possibility that the affected child is mosaic for the RB1 mutation, his future offspring will be tested for this mutation. (Images by Cynthia VandenHoven and Carmelina Trimboli.)

to reveal large deletions and duplications, sequencing for point mutations, examination of the mRNA to confirm or detect intronic mutations altering exon splicing, and assay for the methylation status of the promoter in tumor samples (Fig. 42.4). Application of these techniques, combined with a retinoblastoma-specific focused expertise in interpreting the data, identifies over 95% of the *RB1* mutations[9,14] (see Figs 42.1–42.4).

Other manifestations of *RB1* mutant alleles

Mutation of *RB1* also predisposes to benign retinal tumors, retinoma,[15] ectopic intracranial retinoblastoma (trilateral retinoblastoma),[16,17] and second non-ocular malignancies.[18,19]

Retinoma

A retinoma is a non-malignant manifestation of the *RB1* mutation.[15] Three features characterize these non-progressive lesions: an elevated grey retinal mass, calcification, and surrounding retinal pigment epithelium (RPE) proliferation and pigmentation (Fig. 42.5). These features are also seen after radiation treatment for retinoblastoma. If documented in childhood, which is very rare, retinoma is a quiescent tumor that has not progressed to malignancy. Occasional cases occur where a retinoma progresses to active retinoblastoma. However, retinoma commonly underlies active retinoblastoma and can be discovered on pathologic examination of an enucleated eye.[12] A distinctive feature is fleurette formation and absence

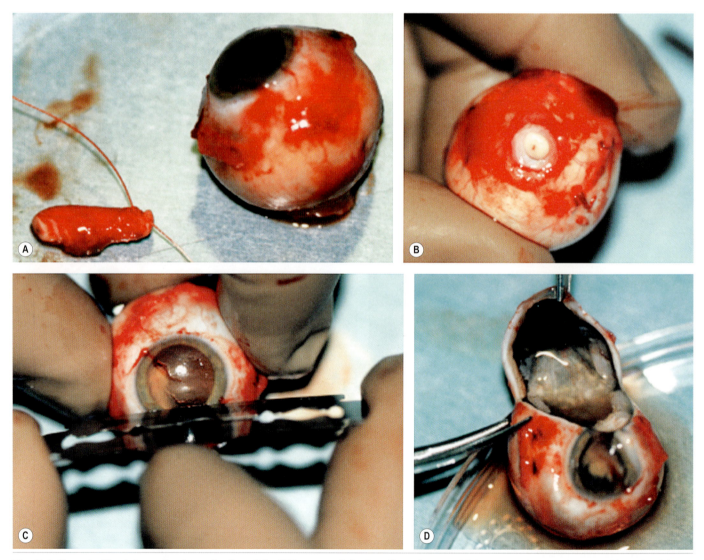

Fig. 42.4 Harvest of fresh tumor for determination of the *RB1* mutant alleles in unilateral tumor. (A) Optic nerve (8–12 mm) is excised from the globe and the distal end marked with a suture. The nerve is submitted as a separate specimen in a separate formalin container so that it is not contaminated by tumor from the opened eye. (B) Optic nerve just beyond the cribriform plate appears normal on gross inspection, to be confirmed microscopically. (C) Globe is opened with a razor incision in a pupillary-optic nerve plan, superior or inferior, at the limbus, in order to access intraocular live tumor. (D) Superior or inferior callotte allows harvest of large amount of intraocular tumor for adequate molecular studies. Optic nerve and choroid are not interfered with, since these are important for pathologic assessment for risk of extraocular spread. Tumor for molecular studies is sent to the lab in sterile tissue culture medium. The *RB1* mutations (M1 and M2) in this unilateral tumor were a heterozygous exon 14 CGA to TGA (R445X) and a heterozygous intron 16 G to A (cDNA 1498+5) causing a splice mutation. Neither M1 nor M2 were detected in blood of the child. (Images by Cynthia VandenHoven.)

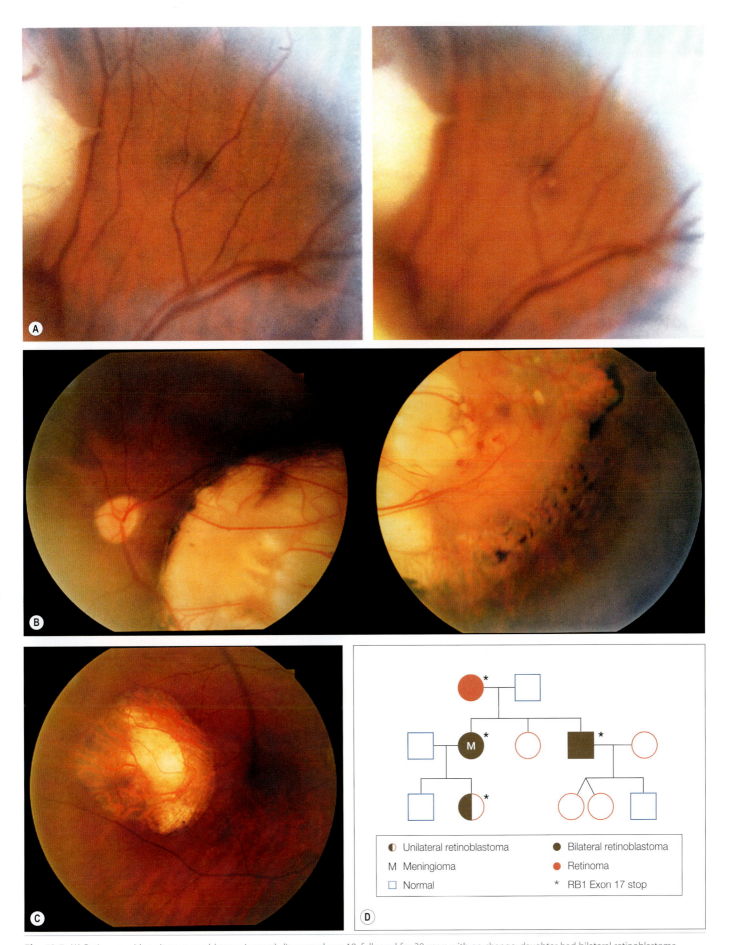

Fig. 42.5 (A) Retinoma with a vitreous seed (stereo images) discovered age 18, followed for 30 years with no change; daughter had bilateral retinoblastoma. (B, C) Multifocal bilateral retinoma discovered in the grandfather when his grand-daughter developed unilateral retinoblastoma. His daughter had bilateral retinoblastoma and meningioma at age 40. (D) All affected members carry a "null" germline RB1 mutation (heterozygous point mutation in exon 17 resulting in a STOP codon).

of proliferative markers. Both *RB1* alleles are mutant in the retinoma and genomic instability is detectable, which progresses in degree and number of genes involved in the adjacent highly proliferative retinoblastoma.[12] Discovery of retinoma on retinal examination of a relative of a patient with retinoblastoma indicates that they carry the *RB1* mutant allele (see Fig. 42.5).

Ectopic intracranial (trilateral) retinoblastoma

Trilateral retinoblastoma is a midline intracranial tumor or a primary pineal tumor associated with heritable retinoblastoma that is not related to a metastasis.[16] The tumors are neuroblastic and resemble a poorly differentiated retinoblastoma. Pineal tumors arise in 5% of children with an *RB1* mutation but should not be confused with pineal cysts which occur in 2% of all children and require no treatment.[20] Affected children may present with raised intracranial pressure and are found to have a pineal or parasellar mass on MRI.[17] Routine screening by MRI for intracranial tumors may detect pineal tumors at a stage when they can be cured.[16,17]

Multiple different malignancies

Persons with *RB1* gene mutant alleles are at increased risk of developing second non-ocular malignancies[4,18,19] which may occur within or outside the radiation field (see Fig. 42.2). Radiation, particularly of infants under 1 year of age, increases the risk of sarcomas and other cancers within the radiation field. Osteosarcoma is the commonest second primary tumor in persons with *RB1* mutations, but a wide variety of other neoplasms have been reported. Since these radiation-induced tumors are very difficult to treat, in the past more children with *RB1* mutations have died of their second tumor than have died of uncontrolled retinoblastoma. Radiation is now restricted to salvage of the remaining eye in children with retinoblastoma.[21]

Genetic counseling for retinoblastoma

The most accurate way to predict who in a family will develop retinoblastoma is to test them for the precise *RB1* mutant allele found in the proband. In the absence of precise knowledge of the *RB1* mutant alleles in tumor or blood, the empiric risk for the relatives of retinoblastoma patients to be affected can be estimated.[22] Offspring of patients with a family history of retinoblastoma or bilateral tumors have a 50% risk of inheriting the mutant allele and a 45% risk of developing retinoblastoma, due to incomplete penetrance. When two affected children are born to apparently normal parents, one parent must be carrying but not expressing the mutant allele. Hence, there is also a 45% risk that any subsequent child born will develop retinoblastoma. The risk that other relatives have inherited the mutant allele depends on the number of intervening "apparently normal" individuals, each of which have a 10% chance of carrying but not expressing the mutant allele. The risk falls by a factor of 0.1 for each intervening unaffected generation. Since 15% of patients with unilateral retinoblastoma have a germinal mutation, the offspring of individuals with unilateral retinoblastoma have a 7.5% risk of carrying the abnormal gene. The probability of other relatives developing retinoblastoma falls by a factor of 0.1 for each intervening unaffected generation.[22]

Infants born with a risk of developing retinoblastoma need to be examined immediately after birth and then at regular intervals to detect early tumors that can be treated to obtain the best visual result (see Fig. 42.1). Infants proven to carry the family's *RB1* mutant allele can be delivered a few weeks early, to optimize the chance to keep good vision with minimally invasive therapy. Examination of the retina starts at birth, and continues at frequent intervals depending on the child's risk. Up to 3 months of age, examination may be done without general anesthetic, greatly facilitated by the RetCam® camera on video mode. After 3 months, anesthetic is necessary to get an accurate view of the retina to detect tiny tumors up to the ora serrata.

Timely and sensitive molecular diagnosis of *RB1* mutations has a strong positive effect on quality of outcomes: early treatment of retinoblastoma achieves lower risks and better health outcomes, allows families to make informed family-planning decisions, and costs less than conventional surveillance.[9,23] The savings when at risk children avoid repeated examinations substantially exceeds the one-time cost of molecular testing. Moreover, health care savings continue to accrue as succeeding generations avoid the unnecessary examinations and often do not need molecular analysis because their parents do not carry the family's mutant allele.

The *RB1* mutations usually result in unstable or absent protein. Such mutations show high penetrance (>95% of offspring affected) and expressivity (average of seven tumors per child). More uncommon *RB1* mutations cause lower penetrance and expressivity:[23] "In frame" deletions or insertions that result in a stable but defective pRB;[24] promoter mutations that result in a reduced amount of otherwise normal protein;[23] and splice mutations that may be additionally altered by unlinked "modifier genes".[25]

Presentation

The majority of children with retinoblastoma without a family history are first noticed because of leukocoria (Table 42.1).[26] Parents observe an odd appearance in their child's eye. Too often primary health care personnel are unaware of the importance of what the parents are saying and diagnosis is delayed.

Table 42.1 – Presenting symptoms and signs of retinoblastoma (Ellsworth 1969)

White reflex	56%
Strabismus	20%
Glaucoma	7%
Poor vision	5%
Routine examination	3%
Orbital cellulitis	3%
Unilateral mydriasis	2%
Heterochromia iris	1%
Hyphema	1%
Other	2%

Ellsworth RM. The practical management of retinoblastoma. Trans Am Ophthalmol Soc 1969; 67: 462–534.

Health care professionals should respond to a parent's description of a "cat's eye reflex" by referring the child for full investigation of the eyes (Fig. 42.7).

Retinoblastoma family support groups have embarked upon awareness campaigns to educate the lay public in the importance of a "white pupil" (Figs 42.6 and 42.7). Digital images of the baby with retinoblastoma frequently show a white pupil, "photoleukocoria," in contrast to the red eye reflex of the flash picture of a normal eye.[27] While retinoblastoma is the most important and dangerous condition to cause leukocoria, various conditions also show unusual appearance on flash images, such as congenital cataract, myelinated nerve fibers, optic nerve coloboma, high myopia, astigmatism, and normal optic nerves when the camera angle is directed at the optic nerve.[28]

The second most common presenting sign of retinoblastoma is strabismus (esotropia or exotropia).[26] The red reflex test should be applied to any child with strabismus or suspected strabismus, with prompt, urgent referral from the primary health level to an ophthalmologist if the red reflex test is abnormal.[2] Other presenting symptoms and signs (see Table 42.1) include a painful red eye (due to glaucoma), orbital cellulitis secondary to extensive necrosis of the intraocular tumor (Figs 42.8–42.10),[29] unilateral mydriasis, heterochromia, hyphema, hypopyon, uveitis, and "searching" nystagmus (due to blindness from bilateral macular involvement).[26] In countries with limited medical services, many children present with extensive unilateral or bilateral proptosis with orbital extension and/or metastatic disease due to delayed access to care (see Figs 42.8 and 42.9).

Retinoblastoma in babies and children that are relatives of patients with heritable retinoblastoma should be looked for specifically by screening examinations, before any symptoms occur unless genetic testing rules out the mutant allele in that individual (see Fig. 42.1). For most families, it is possible to detect the precise *RB1* mutation of the proband, check the relatives for that mutation, identify those carrying the mutant allele, and diagnose and initiate treatment early when the tumors are small and can often be cured by laser therapy alone, or with short cycles of chemotherapy in order to obtain the best visual outcome.

Diagnosis

The initial examination of the child presenting as possible retinoblastoma will provide a short-list of differential diagnoses, including Coats' disease (Fig. 42.11), persistent hyperplastic primary vitreous, toxocara (Fig. 42.12), medulloepithelioma (Fig. 42.13), and others (Box 42.1).[26] Referral of a child with possible retinoblastoma is urgent, generally requiring examination within 1 week.[2]

Ultrasound is a readily available tool to confirm the diagnosis, with the demonstration of a calcified mass in the eye with leukocoria, and also to check a "normal" other eye for possible tumor. To rule out trilateral retinoblastoma and evaluate the optic nerve, MRI is standard in many units, since CT scans incur significant radiation which is to be avoided in children with *RB1* mutant alleles. If chemotherapy is indicated,

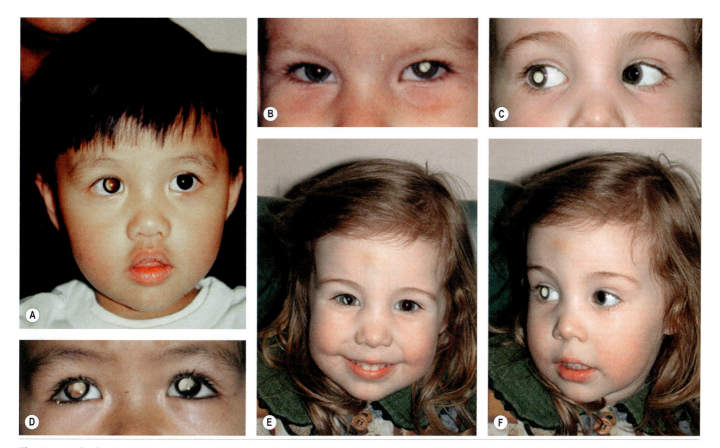

Fig. 42.6 Leukoria. (A–C) Unilateral leukoria. (D) Bilateral leukoria. (E,F) Right unilateral leukoria, more obvious in right gaze due to the anterior temporal location of tumor. (Images by Leslie MacKeen.)

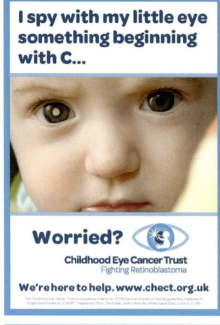

Fig. 42.7 Childhood Eye Cancer Trust awareness campaign poster (UK). (This image is part of a campaign run by the Childhood Eye Cancer Trust UK.)

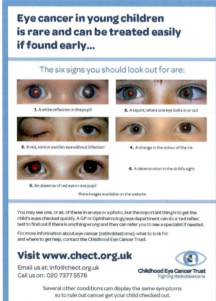

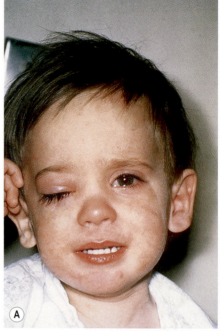

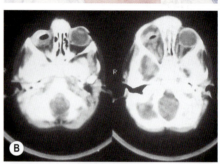

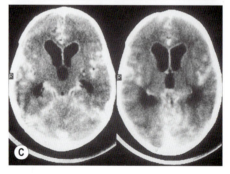

Fig. 42.8 (A) Unilateral retinoblastoma that presented as orbital cellulitis (IIRC group E, suggestive of extraocular tumor). (B) Extensive intraocular necrosis and replacement of the optic nerve with tumor. (C) Despite therapy, the brain was covered with meningeal retinoblastoma 4 months later and the child died.

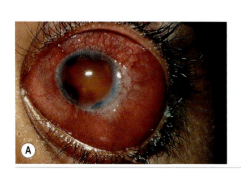

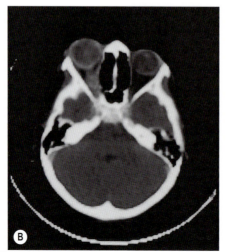

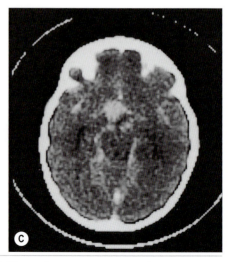

Fig. 42.9 (A) Extraocular retinoblastoma with iris invasion, glaucoma, subconjunctival and orbital extension. (B) CT scan showing optic nerve involvement. (C) CT scan showing suprasellar and cerebral extension from optic nerve invasion.

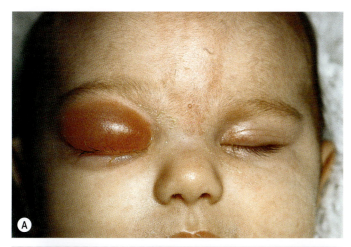

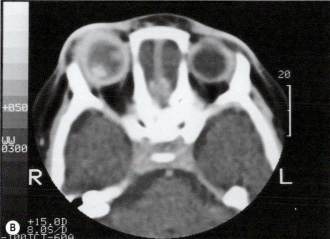

Fig. 42.10 Retinoblastoma presenting as orbital cellulitis (IIRC group E). (A) At referral the patient was ill but not apyrexial. The globe could not be seen due to lid swelling, which reduced after 2 days of systemic steroid treatment. A small non-calcified tumor was present in the left eye and a calcified retinoblastoma was present in the right eye, (B) shown on CT scan.

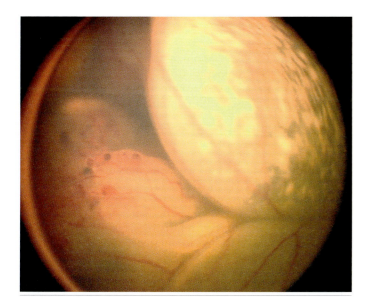

Fig. 42.11 Coats' disease. Presenting with leukocoria, with a yellow appearance (xanthocoria), not white like retinoblastoma, total retinal detachment and the characteristic aneurysmal vascular malformations in the peripheral retina.

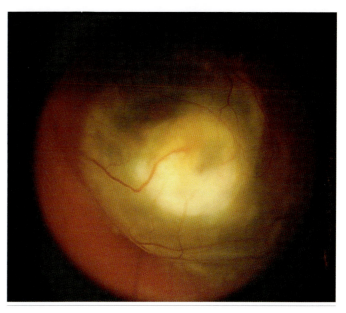

Fig. 42.12 Solitary toxocara granuloma in the macular, with a cilioretinal arteriole, masquerading as a retinoblastoma.

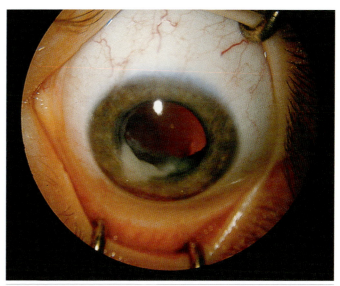

Fig. 42.13 Medulloepithelioma (diktyoma) presenting as a felt-like structure arising in the ciliary body and involving the iris.

a central venous line needs to be placed. The whole multidisciplinary team should be aware of the patient since each will play a role throughout the course of care.

Examination under anesthesia

For full assessment of the eye with retinoblastoma, including anterior segment examination and complete fundus examination, examination under anesthesia (EUA) is required. The pupils must be widely dilated and scleral depression used to visualize the retina to the ora serrata. Retinoblastoma appears as a creamy white mass (Figs 42.14 and 42.15) projecting into the vitreous with large irregular blood vessels running on the surface and penetrating the tumor. Hemorrhage may be present on the surface of the tumor. Clumped tumor cells in the vitreous ("seeding") are pathognomonic of retinoblastoma (see

Box 42.1

Differential diagnosis of retinoblastoma

Hereditary conditions
Norrie's disease
Warburg's syndrome
Autosomal recessive retinal
  dysplasia
Dominant exudative
  vitreoretinopathy
Juvenile X-linked retinoschisis
Orbital cellulitis

Developmental anomalies
Persistent hyperplastic primary
  vitreous
Cataract
Coloboma
Congenital retinal fold
Myelinated nerve fibers
High myopia
Morning glory syndrome

Others
Coats' disease
Retinopathy of prematurity
Rhegmatogenous retinal
detachment
Vitreous hemorrhage
Leukemic infiltration of the iris

Inflammatory conditions
Toxocariasis
Toxoplasmosis
Metastatic endophthalmitis
Viral retinitis
Vitritis

Tumors
Astrocytic hamartoma
Medulloepithelioma
Choroidal hemangioma
Combined hamartoma

Modified from Shields JA, Augsburger JJ. Current approaches to diagnosis and management of retinoblastoma. Surv Ophthalmol 1981; 25: 347–72.

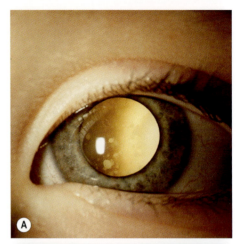

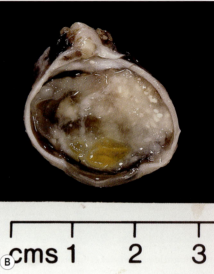

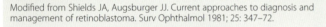

Fig. 42.14
Endophytic retinoblastoma. (A) The tumor has invaded the vitreous and seeds can be seen on the back of the lens (IIRC group E). (B) Calotte of enucleated eye with tumor filling the eye (same patient).

Fig. 42.15). Some tumors are surrounded by a halo of proliferating retinal pigment epithelium, suggesting that they may be slow-growing and have a retinoma component. Calcification within retinoblastoma is common and resembles "cottage cheese" (Figs 42.16, and 42.17). Such tumors leave no doubt as to the diagnosis of retinoblastoma.

Less commonly, retinoblastoma presents as an avascular white mass in the periphery of the retina. The tumor may be obscured by vitreous opacity or extensive retinal detachment (see Fig. 42.3). Calcification of a mass shown on ultrasound, formerly by CT (see Figs 42.3 and 42.10) and MRI, may be critical in establishing the diagnosis of retinoblastoma.

The presence of tumors in the second eye confirms the diagnosis of heritable, bilateral retinoblastoma. If no tumors are seen on clinical exam, the second eye cannot be assured to be normal until examined under anesthetic.

Unusual presentations such as heterochromia, hypopyon (see Fig. 42.9), uveitis, or orbital cellulitis (see Fig. 42.10) may delay and mask the diagnosis of retinoblastoma. It is important that retinoblastoma is considered as a differential diagnosis early as it can be lethal with delay. Diffusely infiltrating retinoblastoma is uncommon, and can masquerade as uveitis. Since there is no solid, calcified tumor mass or retinal detachment, diagnosis is difficult.

When the inner limiting membrane of the retina breaks, "seeds" float in the vitreous cavity, where they are hypoxic and relatively resistant to therapy and cannot be treated by laser or cryotherapy. When the seeds fall onto the retinal surface, they can attach and grow (see Fig. 42.15) and, if caught early, successfully treated with laser and cryotherapy.

Bone marrow aspiration and lumbar puncture to screen for metastatic disease are performed only when there is a suggestion of extraocular extension and can be performed later if adverse pathologic features are discovered on the enucleated eye.

Conditions which may simulate retinoblastoma are detailed in Box 42.1. In North America, Coats' disease, toxocariasis, and persistent hyperplastic primary vitreous are the three commonest conditions confused with retinoblastoma.[30]

Images for retinoblastoma management

The RetCam® wide-angle camera provides wide-field imaging of the retina and anterior segment, including the anterior chamber angle (Figs 42.1, 42.15, 42.16, 42.19–42.21). Some small retinoblastomas, obscuring the clarity of the choroidal vessels, and vitreous seeds, may be better seen on RetCam® images than with indirect ophthalmoscopy (Figs 42.1 and 42.21). Sequential images are useful to determine if the tumors are growing or regressing. The anterior segment and anterior chamber angle can also be well visualized with the RetCam®.

Fluorescein angiography using the RetCam® can assess vascularity, residual tumor activity, and recurrences within laser scars (Figs 42.1 and 42.18). Occasionally, focal laser and cryotherapy to control tumor results in islands of ischemic retina that can be clearly demarcated by fluorescein angiogram and

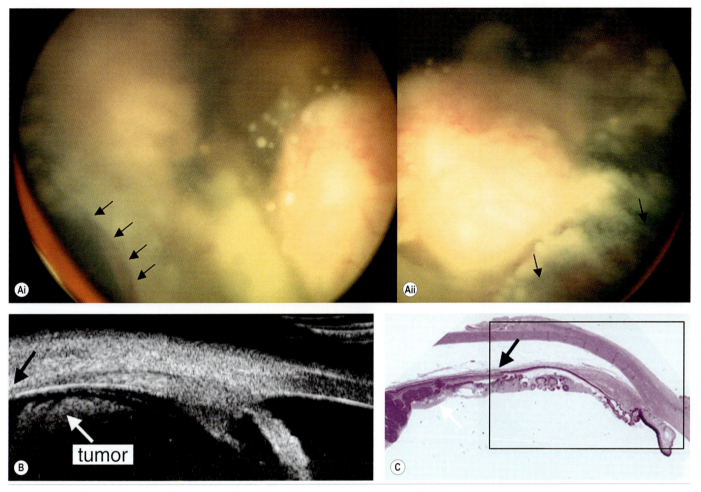

Fig. 42.15 Unilateral endophytic IIRC group E retinoblastoma. RetCam® images showing (Ai) massive vitreous seeding (left); and (Aii) (right) extension of tumor for 180° inferiorly, anterior to the ora serrata (arrows) to lie on the pars plana. (RetCam® images by Carmelina Trimboli.) (B) Ultrasound biomicroscopy of tumor on pars plana and pars plicata of ciliary body. (C) H&E section of ciliary region showing tumor anterior to ora serrata (arrow); box corresponds to area imaged in (B).

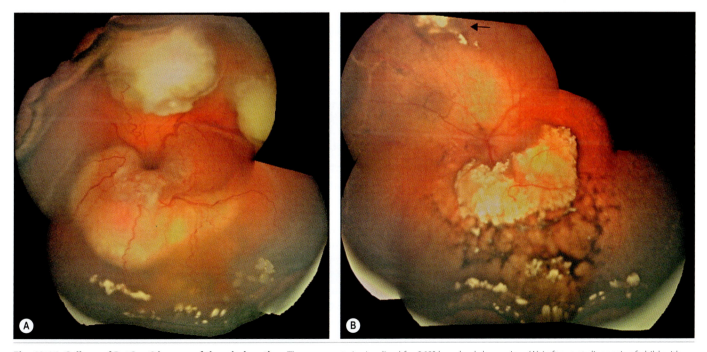

Fig. 42.16 Collage of RetCam® images of the whole retina. The ora serrata is visualized for 360° by scleral depression. (A) Left eye at diagnosis of child with bilateral multifocal exophytic IIRC group D retinoblastoma, no family history, and a "null" *RB1* mutation (heterozygous deletion of exons 18 to 23) in blood. (B) Excellent regression after 3 of 7 cycles of CEV with cyclosporin A chemotherapy, with arrow indicating residual tumor treated by laser and cryotherapy. Similar appearance of residual tumor and tented retina near the macula was not treated to optimize vision and has not changed over 1 year off treatment. This child had excellent response in both IC group D eyes. (Images and collage by Cynthia VandenHoven.)

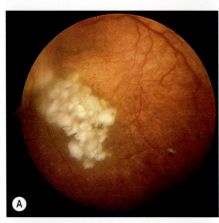

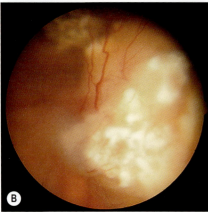

Fig. 42.17
Retinoblastoma regression following external beam radiation. (A) Calcified "cottage cheese" appearance. (B) Mixed, suspicious regression, but after 4 years follow-up, no recurrence occurred.

treated prophylactically with panretinal photocoagulation to prevent ischemic angiogenesis.

Ultrasound biomicroscopy is the only way to detect disease anterior to the ora serrata in the ciliary body, behind iris, and touching lens (see Fig. 42.12). These parts of the eye cannot be viewed by indirect ophthalmoscopy, RetCam®, or conventional ultrasonography. It is critical to detect anterior disease (IIRC group E), which requires immediate enucleation, since we have no accurate focal therapy in the anterior part of the eye.

Optical coherence tomography (OCT) is also very useful when performed at the time of EUA. Small tumors are very clear in the inner nuclear layer, so that suspicious retinal spots can be confirmed or eliminated as tumors by OCT in infants at risk (i.e. they carry a mutant *RB1* allele). OCT is also useful to monitor response to laser therapy, identify edge recurrences, localize precisely sensitive structures for treatment planning, and identify secondary pathologies such as cystoid macular edema that may affect visual prognosis.

Since the survival of patients is normal if retinoblastoma remains intraocular (96% of cases), but cure is very difficult once retinoblastoma becomes extraocular, the biopsy of retinoblastoma is strictly contraindicated due to the risk for tumor spread outside the eye. In rare cases, when the diagnosis remains unclear despite all investigations, an aqueous tap through clear cornea may be cautiously performed for a cytologic diagnosis followed by cryotherapy to the injection site, after very carefully considering the risk–benefit in full discussion with the interprofession team of experts and with the parents.

Treatment

The optimal treatment of retinoblastoma depends on collaboration between all those involved in the care of the child. Specialized centers with interprofessional teams have developed expertise, resources and equipment, and specific treatment protocols that are increasingly evidence-based. This cancer is too uncommon for ophthalmologists and oncologists in non-specialized units to remain up-to-date, or to have acquired the expertise necessary to optimize outcomes for the children and their families. Overall outcomes will only improve over time if each affected child is treated systematically on carefully defined protocols, such that the knowledge gained can be used in the design of more effective future protocols.

Classification

Optimized care and outcome for intraocular retinoblastoma balances the morbidity of treatment with the likelihood to cure the cancer. Classification of cancer severity/extent is the standard way to categorize eyes/patients best suited to particular therapies most likely to succeed, based on current evidence.[31,32]

The Reese-Ellsworth (R-E) classification was devised to predict prognosis when intraocular retinoblastoma was treated with external beam radiotherapy. Since radiotherapy is no longer a primary treatment for retinoblastoma, the International Intraocular Retinoblastoma Classification (IIRC) was developed to predict outcomes from current therapies (predominantly chemotherapy and focal therapy, with radiation as a salvage modality for refractory recurrence) (see Figs 42.1, 42.3, 42. 4, 42.8, 42.10, 42.14, 42.16, 42.18, 42.19, 42.21).[31] The TNM cancer staging system has been developed for all types of cancer, and the 7th edition includes extensive revision for retinoblastoma.[32] The two eyes are staged for clinical intraocular disease (IIRC and cTNM) (Box 42.2) and pathology (pTNM). The stage of the worst eye, or extraocular disease, determines the whole patient TNM stage. At diagnosis, it is valuable to record all three classifications: the R-E and IIRC groups and the TNM stage. Major journals now request the TNM stage for publications (http://www.daisyseyecancerfund.org/Files/StagingSystems/Staging_TNM.pdf).

IIRC

Group A eyes: small tumors not threatening vision – are treated primarily with focal therapy (see Fig. 42.1); often this is the only treatment modality, but repeated treatments are necessary.

Group B eyes: medium-sized tumors or tumors near the macula and the optic nerve – may be first consolidated with a small number of chemotherapy cycles to optimize the visual potential, and then treated definitively with focal therapy (see Fig. 42.1).

Group C eyes: large tumors with limited vitreous and/or subretinal seeding – are primarily treated with chemotherapy followed by focal therapy.

Group D eyes: large tumors with extensive vitreous and/or subretinal seeding – are also primarily treated with chemotherapy and focal therapy (see Figs 42.1, 42.3, 42.4, 42.16,

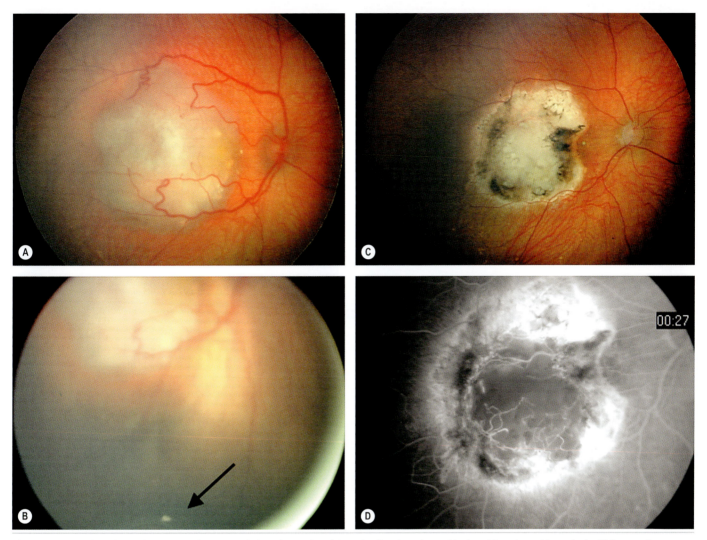

Fig. 42.18 (A) Unilateral retinoblastoma at diagnosis. (B) The subretinal seed (arrow) inferiorly at the 6 o'clock position places this eye in the IIRC group D (subretinal seeding more than 3 mm from the tumor). (C) Response to chemotherapy (4 cycles of CEV with high-dose cyclosporin) and laser and cryotherapy. (D) Fluorescein angiography shows active tumor vessels in the scar, which were successfully ablated by 532 nm and 810 nm laser treatments. (Images by Leslie MacKeen and Cynthia VandenHoven.)

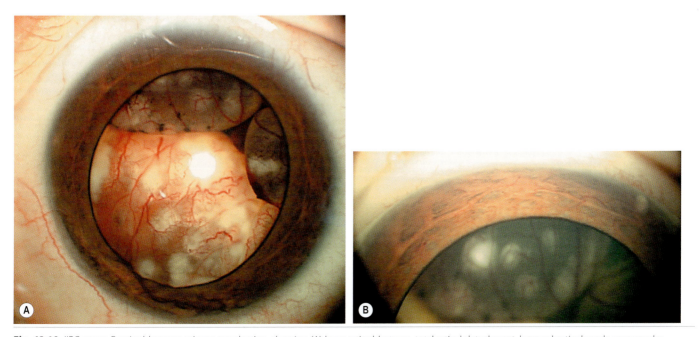

Fig. 42.19 IIRC group E retinoblastoma prior to enucleation, showing (A) large retinoblastoma, total retinal detachment, large subretinal seeds, neovascular glaucoma and (B) anterior chamber seeding visualized by RetCam® anterior segment and anterior chamber angle photography through gel. (Images by Leslie MacKeen.)

International intraocular retinoblastoma classification

Group A: Small intraretinal tumors away from foveola and disk

- All tumors 3 mm or smaller in greatest dimension, confined to the retina *and*
- All tumors located further than 3 mm from the foveola **and** 1.5 mm from the optic disk

Group B: All remaining discrete tumors confined to the retina

- All tumors confined to the retina not in group A
- Any tumor-associated subretinal fluid less than 3 mm from the tumor with no subretinal seeding

Group C: Discrete local disease with minimal subretinal or vitreous seeding

- Tumor(s) discrete
- Subretinal fluid, present or past, without seeding, involving up to 1/4 retina
- Local subretinal seeding, present or past, less than 3 mm (2 DD) from the tumor
- Local fine vitreous seeding close to discrete tumor

Group D: Diffuse disease with significant vitreous or subretinal seeding

- Tumor(s) may be massive or diffuse
- Subretinal fluid, present or past, without seeding, involving up to total retinal detachment
- Diffuse subretinal seeding, present or past, may include subretinal plaques or tumor nodules
- Diffuse or massive vitreous disease may include "greasy" seeds or avascular tumor masses

Group E: Presence of any one or more of these poor prognosis features

- Tumor touching the lens
- Neovascular glaucoma
- Tumor anterior to anterior vitreous face involving ciliary body or anterior segment
- Diffuse infiltrating retinoblastoma
- Opaque media from hemorrhage
- Tumor necrosis with aseptic orbital cellulitis
- Phthisis bulbi

42.21). External beam irradiation is only considered as a salvage modality for groups B, C, and D eyes that have failed chemotherapy and focal therapy.

Group E eyes (Figs 42.8, 42.10, 42.14): high-risk features such as tumor touching the lens, neovascular glaucoma, orbital cellulitis (see Figs 42.6, 42.8), anterior segment, anterior chamber (see Fig. 42.17), iris or ciliary involvement (see Fig. 42.15), total hyphema, suspected choroid, or optic nerve or orbital involvement (see Fig. 42.9) on ultrasonography and MRI – are enucleated immediately.

Enucleation

Immediate enucleation is indicated for all group E eyes since a trial of chemotherapy (whether systemic or intra-arterial) prior to enucleation may create a sense of false security by obscuring pathologic adverse factors that put the child's life at risk.[33] Such adverse risk factors may be indications for further intensive therapy such as bone marrow or peripheral stem cell transplantation. Enucleation is an excellent way to cure retinoblastoma confined to the eye. When only one eye is involved,

or when the other eye is group A for which chemotherapy is not necessary, the group D eye is enucleated to avoid giving the child chemotherapy. Enucleation of group C eyes is more controversial as the risks of chemotherapy must be weighed against the potential for vision. A frank discussion with the family is essential. Enucleation is also indicated for recurrent tumor that has failed all other treatment modalities.

Bilateral retinoblastoma commonly presents with one eye full of tumor, with smaller tumors in the fellow eye. Both eyes may be primarily treated with chemotherapy for groups B, C, or D disease (see Figs 42.16 and 42.21).

If both eyes are group E, bilateral enucleation may be indicated, since attempts to save severely involved group E eyes puts the child's life in jeopardy from difficult-to-treat, poor-prognosis systemic metastasis.[33] Even if group E eyes can be cured, vision is very poor in such severely damaged eyes. The short- and long-term morbidities of chemotherapy and radiation may not be in the best interest of a child with bilateral group E eyes.

Enucleation should be performed with great care so as not to penetrate the eye and spill tumor. A long optic nerve (8 to 12 mm) is important to ensure that the surgical margin is tumor-free. For unilaterally affected children, the tumor is very important for *RB1* mutation studies, since this is the best way to determine whether the child has heritable or non-heritable retinoblastoma (see Fig. 42.4).

While expensive porous implants have been widely used to give good movement of the prosthesis, they frequently acquire a deep chronic infection that is challenging to treat. A randomized study evaluated polymethyl methacrylate implants and prosthesis movement after enucleation using the myoconjunctival technique versus a porous implant with muscle imbrication in the standard manner.[34] In the myoconjunctival technique, the four rectus muscles are sutured to the conjunctival fornices rather than in front of the implant, and provide excellent movement by directly acting on the edges of the prosthesis (see http://www.youtube.com/watch?v=YXi1oMvFPOo). A conformer is placed under the eyelids to retain the fornices for the prosthetic eye. We use a "stock" prosthetic eye as a conformer, so that when the patch is removed 24–48 hours later, the child looks quite normal, a psychologic benefit to child and family[35] (see Fig. 42.4). This temporary artificial eye allows healing to be completed over several months before fittings for the final artificial eye are made. Where there is no access to custom prosthetic eyes, these prostheses and the myoconjunctival approach may be a solution.

Histopathology

Retinoblastomas are poorly differentiated malignant neuroblastic tumors, composed of cells with large hyperchromatic nuclei and scanty cytoplasm. Mitotic figures are common. In some tumors, differentiated cells form typical Flexner-Wintersteiner rosettes[36] in which columnar cells are uniformly arranged in spheres around a lumen containing hyaluronic acid. Homer-Wright rosettes also occur, characteristic of many neuronal tumors, with centrally located neurofibrils.

Retinoblastoma cells often outgrow their blood supply leading to cell necrosis. True spontaneous regression of retinoblastoma is rare, but is probably due to extensive tumor necrosis and central retinal artery occlusion, resulting in phthisis bulbi.[15,29] Programmed cell death or apoptosis is also evident in the retinoblastoma. Calcification is almost pathognomonic of retinoblastoma, but its etiology is not known.

The most important component of histopathology of eyes enucleated for retinoblastoma is accurate assessment of risk that the tumor has become extraocular and life-threatening. The pTNM for retinoblastoma provides this evaluation (see Box 42.2).[32] The most common routes of dissemination are through the optic nerve to brain and through the choroid to bone marrow. Tumor extending into the optic nerve beyond the cribriform plate carries a significant risk of direct extension to brain and seeding into cerebrospinal fluid. Good sections through the optic nerve showing the relationship of the lamina cribrosa to the tumor are essential. Extensive tumor invasion of choroid and/or sclera carries high risk of hematogenous spread, usually to bone marrow. Post-enucleation adjuvant chemotherapy may still cure, if given when detected by surveillance bone marrow/lumbar puncture, prior to clinical presentation of extraocular retinoblastoma.

If retinoblastoma metastasizes, it generally becomes evident within 18 months of the last active tumor in the eye, and is rare beyond 3 years without evidence of tumor activity in the eye.[37] The most common and dangerous route of metastasis of retinoblastoma is direct extension into the optic nerve. The tumor can grow towards the optic chiasm and beyond, or into the subarachnoid space with leptomeningeal involvement (see Figs 42.8 and 42.9). Direct extension via the choroidal vessels, or spread along the ciliary vessels and nerves into the orbit, may occur in advanced cases (see Figs 42.8 and 42.9).[38,39] Systemic metastases may occur via the choroidal circulation or aqueous drainage, particularly if glaucoma is present. Bone marrow is the preferred site for retinoblastoma metastasis, and only terminally are bone, lymph node, and liver involved. Lung metastases are rare and late.

Chemotherapy

Systemic chemotherapy has become the standard primary treatment for IIRC groups B, C, and D. Following an initial response to the first few cycles of chemotherapy, focal therapy with cryotherapy or laser therapy is initiated to destroy residual or recurrent tumor[40] (Figs 42.1, 42.20–42.22). Chemotherapy is best given on a rigorous protocol. The most commonly used chemotherapy drugs include carboplatin, etoposide, and vincristine (CEV) given every 3 weeks through a central venous access line.[41]

The Toronto Multicenter Clinical Trial is studying the efficacy and toxicity of short 3-hour infusions of high-dose cyclosporin A (achieving high cyclosporin peak levels of >20 000 ng/ml for a very short time) to block P-glycoprotein that mediates multidrug resistance by acting as a plasma membrane drug-efflux pump, which is commonly overexpressed in retinoblastoma tumors.[42] Cyclosporin may also act through the circumvention of other non-P-glycoprotein drug resistance mechanisms, such as by the reduction of carboplatin induction of expression of c-fos or c-myc oncogene,[43,44] or genes required for repair of drug-induced DNA damage.[45]

Increased intraocular concentrations of the chemotherapy drugs (e.g. carboplatin) may be induced in eyes with vitreous seeding by the application of a single-freeze cryotherapy ("pre-chemo-cryotherapy") at the peripheral retina in the vicinity of the seeds.[46] The concurrent usage of high-dose cyclosporin can further increase the intraocular concentrations of chemotherapy,[46] possibly by inhibiting the P-glycoprotein expressed in the blood–eye barrier.

On the Toronto protocol, group C and D eyes are treated with four cycles of CEV chemotherapy modulated with high-dose cyclosporin, and group B eyes with two cycles. With a good response, consolidation is followed by frequent (q 3–4 weeks) focal cryotherapy and laser therapy (see Fig. 42.19). We observe more than 55% salvage of group D eyes without using radiation (see Figs 42.3, 42.16, 42.18, 42.22),[47,48] and better results with less severely affected eyes. We have not seen a significant increase in the toxicity of chemotherapy with high-dose cyclosporin. Final conclusions await completion of the international multicenter clinical trial.

The Toronto protocol has successfully salvaged eyes that have already failed previous chemotherapy and/or radiotherapy, and uses higher than usual carboplatin and etoposide dosages with standard dose vincristine, with high-dose cyclosporin, and cytokine granulocyte-stimulating factor support of the myeloid bone marrow. Local recurrence is expected approximately 2 to 6 months after finishing the chemotherapy, best controlled by focal therapy given when recurrence first appears. EUAs with appropriate focal therapy every 4 to 6 weeks are important for at least 1 year after tumor activity.

The addition of high-dose cyclosporin does not significantly increase the toxicity due to chemotherapy. Unlike radiation, chemotherapy is not associated with long-term cosmetic deformity of the orbit and upper face, radiation-induced cataracts, or ocular complications. Although chemotherapy is used in order to avoid the large risk of induction of the second primary tumor by radiation (estimated to be as high a 51% risk at 50-year follow-up),[49] we recommend caution in use of

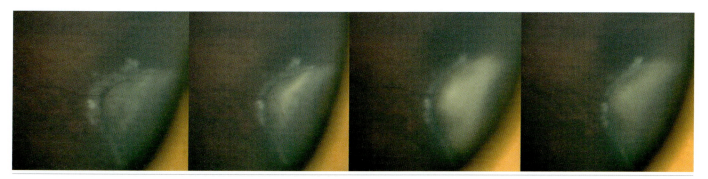

Fig. 42.20 Sequential RetCam® images of the first freeze of triple freeze-thaw cryotherapy applied to a small peripheral retinoblastoma after placement of a 532 nm laser barrier line to limit serous effusion.

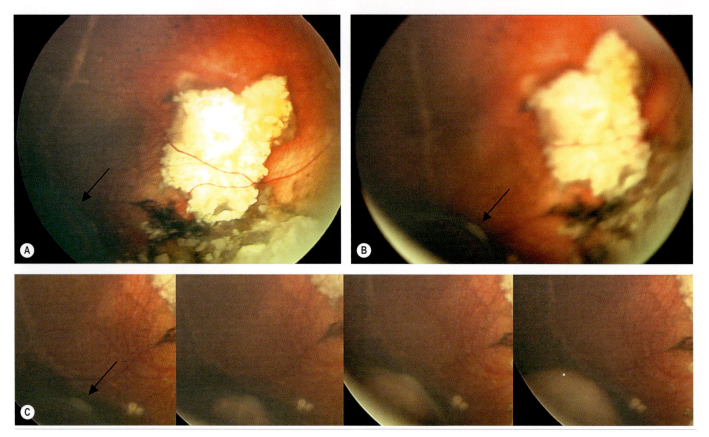

Fig. 42.21 New tumor in a previously treated eye. (A) Arrow indicates no tumor 8 months after initiation of CEV chemotherapy with cyclosporin for IIRC group D retinoblastoma in the right eye of the child whose left eye is shown in Figure 42.7. (B) New peripheral small tumor 2 months later, 10 months after diagnosis. (C) Triple freeze-thaw cryotherapy for the small new tumor, encasing the tumor in ice, thawing for one minute, and refreezing. (RetCam® images by Cynthia VandenHoven.)

chemotherapy, particularly etoposide, which carries a small risk of induction of a specific type of acute myelogenous leukemia. The cumulative dosage of etoposide used for treating retinoblastoma is less than the higher dosages that have been estimated to carry a 2–3% risk of inducing leukemia, generally in the first 2 years after completion of etoposide chemotherapy.[50]

Paraocular chemotherapy

To avoid systemic chemotherapy, carboplatin and topotecan have been given subconjunctivally to treat retinoblastoma. Local chemotherapy with instillation of carboplatin into Tenon's space achieves increased vitreous concentrations,[51] but has significant local orbital toxicity, including orbital fat necrosis that may limit ocular motility and cause enophthalmos, and fibrosis that may complicate any subsequent enucleation.[52]

Topotecan given paraocularly at the usual systemic dose has no local orbital toxicity and no bone marrow toxicity.[53] For small volume tumors often diagnosed around birth because children carry a mutant *RB1* allele, topotecan given in a fibrin clot gains significant tumor control to allow vision-sparing focal therapy.

Cryotherapy

Cryotherapy is used for small anteriorly placed tumors (IIRC groups A and B eyes), or more posterior tumors when visual damage will not result.[54] Since the tumor cells are killed when they thaw, a triple freeze-thaw technique is used, with a full minute for thawing between the successive freezes (see Figs 42.20 and 42.21). Cryotherapy is repeated at several EUAs 4 weeks apart, until no residual active tumor remains. Cryotherapy may be used as a primary procedure for small tumors, or to treat residual or recurrent tumors. When moderately sized tumors are treated with cryotherapy, a laser barrier placed posterior to the tumor may protect the retina from detachment by the serous exudate of the acute freeze (see Fig. 42.20).

Laser

Laser coagulation is used for small tumors (groups A and B eyes) (see Fig. 42.1), for tumors that have been initially shrunk by chemotherapy, or for recurrences following chemotherapy. Small tumors (group A eyes) behind the equator are treated by encircling the tumor with a double row of contiguous laser burns. The small avascular tumor can be directly coagulated, starting with power/duration settings that barely blanch or opacify the tumor, and gradually increasing the power to make the tumor turn opaque white. Larger or visually threatening tumors (groups B and C eyes) treated first with chemotherapy and recurrent tumors after cessation of chemotherapy are treated with laser coagulation. For group D eyes, laser is used only after a good response has occurred with chemotherapy, to eliminate recurrence before the tumor has a chance to regrow (see Fig. 42.16).

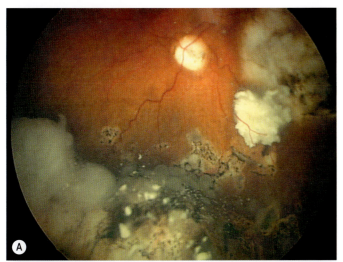

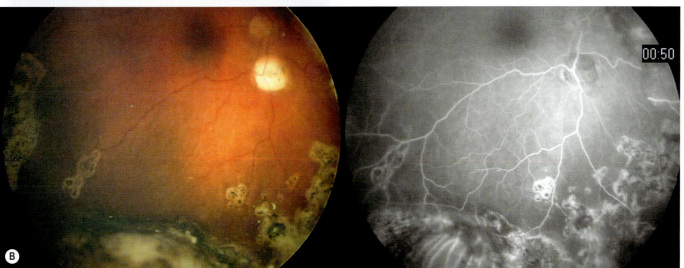

Fig. 42.22 Bilateral retinoblastoma was treated with enucleation of the left eye and CEV chemotherapy without cyclosporin for the right eye with IIRC group D disease. (A) Extensive recurrence with vitreous seeding. (B) No detectable active tumor 3 months after 4 cycles of CEV chemotherapy with cyclosporin A with pre-chemo-cryotherapy and sub-Tenon's carboplatin; fluorescein angiogram showing bare sclera in the location of recurrent tumor. (RetCam® images by Cynthia VandenHoven.)

The diode 810 nm laser is most widely available but causes more scarring and traction that may progress than the green frequency-doubled YAG at 532 nm. Thermotherapy has been promoted widely, using a 810 nm laser to gently heat tumors over a long period of time, but clear efficacy awaits clinical trials.[55,56] For group A small tumors, 532 nm is effective without drifting of the scars. Infrared lasers (diode 810 nm or 1064 nm long duration YAG) can be applied after chemotherapy to larger, thicker tumors with good effect. With all lasers, it is important NOT to use too much power at any one treatment, and retreat at frequent intervals until only flat scars remain. Fluorescein angiography is useful for identifying early potential spots of recurrences in a laser scar (see Figs 42.1 and 42.18).

Focal irradiation

Solitary tumors less than 15 mm in diameter which are not adjacent to the disk or macula may be treated with an episcleral radioactive plaque,[125]iodine, or [106]ruthenium.[57] Plaques are useful to treat single recurrences after chemotherapy or whole eye radiation has failed. A second course of radiation to the whole eye (external beam radiation) is prohibited because it will lead to severe radiation retinopathy and/or optic neuropathy, and potential increase in the already high risk of late induced cancers. Under general anesthesia, the tumor is localized, and the plaque is sutured to the sclera apposed to the tumor and left *in situ* until the prescribed dose of radiation has been delivered to the apex of the tumor.

External beam irradiation

Radiation was the first approach that cured intraocular retinoblastoma, saving many eyes with useful vision, but with severe consequences of inducing second cancers and severe cosmetic deformities. Most commonly, there is significant calcification ("cottage cheese-like") or a combination of calcification and translucent residual tumor after radiation (see Fig. 42.17). The risk of second primary cancers within the radiation field in children with a germline *RB1* mutation is significant; most children die of these induced cancers[3,4] (see Fig. 42.2). The risk may be greatest when infants are irradiated under 1 year of age.[58] Additional complications of external beam irradiation include cosmetic deformity due to growth retardation of the orbit (worse the younger the child is at the time of irradiation), cataract (reduced by lens sparing radiation portals, unless tumor is "missed"), reduced lacrimation, and dry-eye syndromes. Recurrences following irradiation are commonly seen with large tumors and vitreous seeding.

External beam radiotherapy is mostly used for treatment of postchemotherapy recurrences that are too large or extensive for focal therapy, or unresponsive to focal therapy. Focused radiation such as stereotactic radiation may avoid radiation of adjacent tissues for treatment of localized disease. However, whole eye radiation may be the only choice in chemoresistant retinoblastoma with extensive vitreous or subretinal seeding.

A total dose of 3500–4000 cGy has been traditionally given for primary or secondary irradiation of eyes with retinoblastoma, in divided fractions over a 3–4 week period.[59] A temporal portal excluding the lens (lens sparing) is used whenever possible to avoid a radiation-induced cataract,[60] but when it is important to irradiate the ora serrata, or when vitreous seeds are present, an anterior approach must be used despite the certainty of cataract induction. Corneal damage can be reduced by irradiating with the eyelid opened with a speculum, to move the increased entry dose 5 mm below the surface, deeper into the eye.

Intra-arterial chemotherapy

Local treatment of retinoblastoma with chemotherapy is an attractive idea as the child would not be subjected to the complications of systemic drugs. Injection of a chemotherapeutic agent (melphalan) into the carotid artery/ophthalmic artery has been performed for over 20 years in Japan, but the single outcome study is inconclusive about efficacy and safety.[61] Despite lack of outcome data, intra-arterial (IA) chemotherapy has been widely adopted in the last few years because of the predictions that all eyes with retinoblastoma might be saved by this approach. Without formal rigorous follow-up of clinical trials, initial studies were very encouraging. A retrospective study suggests that IA chemotherapy is most successful as primary therapy, but not as effective for tumors refractory to previous therapies.[62] Local side effects, such as third cranial nerve palsy, retinal pigment epithelial changes and retinal detachment can occur, though external beam radiotherapy or enucleation can be avoided for some eyes.[63] Most risky, however, is the use of IA chemotherapy for group E retinoblastoma. The IA chemotherapy results in a sometimes dramatic local shrinking of intraocular tumor, but tumor leaving the eye into the nerve, choroid, and blood remains unacknowledged. As a result a child may be responding well until an extraocular relapse is identified and the child dies. Such a child might have been cured by enucleation of the group E eye and adjuvant therapy for the high-risk pathologic features. Such stories abound on parent blogs, but are not yet acknowledged in the medical literature.

Extraocular retinoblastoma

Extraocular retinoblastoma results in a precipitous drop in the prognosis for life (see Figs 42.8 and 42.9). Until recently, metastatic retinoblastoma was considered fatal. Local orbital recurrence is generally treated with 40–50 Gy orbital radiation and systemic chemotherapy. Metastatic retinoblastoma to bone marrow or other sites may be treated with intensive chemotherapy, with cyclosporin to counter multidrug resistance, and, if remission is attained, supralethal chemotherapy and peripheral stem cell transplantation are performed. Meningeal spread of retinoblastoma is treated additionally with intrathecal and intraventricular chemotherapy via an Ommaya reservoir. Long-term follow-up suggests that such approaches can achieve cure.[64]

Prophylactic radiation is considered when histopathologic examination of the enucleated globe shows involvement of the cut end of the optic nerve with high risk of orbital recurrence. When marked choroidal invasion and involvement of the optic nerve past the cribriform plate are noted on histopathology (pT3), adjuvant therapy may be advised to treat potential tumor spread beyond the eye. However, tumor into or minimally past the lamina cribrosa may be managed by surveillance with regular MRI, bone marrow, and cerebrospinal fluid examinations, treating only when disease is documented. Otherwise, many children may be treated unnecessarily. Evidence to support these treatment recommendations is pending a multicenter trial of prophylactic treatment for adverse histology.

Prognosis

With modern methods of diagnosis and treatment, the prognosis for retinoblastoma is excellent. The 3-year survival for both unilateral and bilateral retinoblastoma approaches 96%.[37] More patients with germline *RB1* mutations die of their second primary cancer than from uncontrolled retinoblastoma.[4]

The prognosis for vision is excellent in unilateral retinoblastoma (for the normal eye), but depends on the size and location of the tumors in bilateral cases. Awareness and prompt diagnosis, with good results with chemotherapy and focal therapy means that bilateral enucleation is now rare. Extrafoveal tumors have a good visual prognosis but, when the macular region is directly involved, the visual results may be poor, despite tumor control. The most important impact on further improving visual outcome for retinoblastoma children lies in the earlier recognition of the presenting signs by the primary caregivers.

Long-term follow-up

Following the initial management and resolution of active tumor, assessment of the response to treatment will require frequent general anesthesia, especially in the first year following diagnosis with completion of chemotherapy when recurrence or new tumors are most likely to occur. Regular EUAs will be necessary until the child is old enough to co-operate for a full-dilated eye examination in the clinic, variably at about 3 years of age. Follow-up can then be continued on an outpatient basis. However, children with groups C and D eyes may need a much longer follow-up with EUA in order to assess peripheral tumors for recurrence.

Life-long implications of retinoblastoma

Retinoblastoma patients who carry a mutant *RB1* allele are at risk of other cancers throughout their lives, many years after their initial treatment for retinoblastoma. Anecdotal reports demonstrate that some adults who were treated as children (often by enucleation or radiation) are not aware that they had cancer and have been lost to follow-up. They may, however, present to their local ophthalmologists with ocular and/or orbital problems. It is important that ophthalmologists are aware of the long-term systemic problems associated with retinoblastoma as they may be the only secondary care physician seen by the patient.

Everybody in the Western world has a lifetime risk of approximately 1 in 3 of developing cancer. Patients with an abnormal *RB1* gene reach this risk by the age of about 50 years of age. The non-ocular cancers that have increased incidence include bone and soft tissue sarcomas during adolescence and early adulthood, malignant melanoma, epithelial cancers, bladder, esophagus, and probably breast cancer. These risks are increased significantly by radiation exposure.

All patients with a past history of retinoblastoma should be offered molecular *RB1* gene analysis for counseling with regard to the risk of retinoblastoma in their offspring, and their own increased risk of developing a non-ocular cancer. This is particularly important for the patients with unilateral disease who may carry a mutation of the *RB1* gene and are unaware of this fact. Emphasizing the dangers of known carcinogenic factors such as smoking, radiation, obesity and excess UV light is particularly important. As radiation is associated with an increased risk of cancers, routine X-rays and CT scans are not advised.

Likewise, patients who have been treated with chemotherapy and/or radiation will require oncologic follow-up for early detection and appropriate management of possible long-term complications. It is important for retinoblastoma patients to retain contact with their oncologist because of the risk of secondary malignancies, whether sporadic or induced by radiation or chemotherapy. It is also important to ensure that accurate genetic counseling is available to the parents, and to the child when he or she reaches maturity.

References

1. Kivela T. The epidemiological challenge of the most frequent eye cancer: retinoblastoma, an issue of birth and death. Br J Ophthalmol 2009; 93: 1129–31.
2. National Retinoblastoma Strategy Canadian Guidelines for Care. Stratégie thérapeutique du rétinoblastome guide clinique canadien. Can J Ophthalmol 2009; 44: S1–88.
5. Friend SH, Bernards R, Rogelj S, et al. A human DNA segment with properties of the gene that predisposes to retinoblastoma and osteosarcoma. Nature 1986; 323: 643–6.
7. Knudson AG. Mutation and cancer: statistical study of retinoblastoma. Proc Natl Acad Sci USA 1971; 68: 820–3.
9. Richter S, Vandezande K, Chen N, et al. Sensitive and efficient detection of RB1 gene mutations enhances care for families with retinoblastoma. Am J Hum Genet 2003; 72: 253–69.
12. Dimaras H, Khetan V, Halliday W, et al. Loss of RB1 induces non-proliferative retinoma: increasing genomic instability correlates with progression to retinoblastoma. Hum Mol Genet 2008; 17: 1363–72.
13. Corson TW, Gallie BL. One hit, two hits, three hits, more? Genomic changes in the development of retinoblastoma. Genes Chromosomes Cancer 2007; 46: 617–34.
14. Rushlow D, Piovesan B, Zhang K, et al. Detection of mosaic RB1 mutations in families with retinoblastoma. Hum Mutat 2009; 30: 842–51.

18. MacCarthy A, Bayne AM, Draper GJ, et al. Non-ocular tumours following retinoblastoma in Great Britain 1951 to 2004. Br J Ophthalmol 2009; 93: 1159–62.
20. Rodjan F, de Graaf P, Moll AC, et al. Brain abnormalities on MR imaging in patients with retinoblastoma. AJNR 2010 Apr 22.
21. Chan HS, Gallie BL, Munier FL, et al. Chemotherapy for retinoblastoma. Ophthalmol Clin North Am 2005; 18: 55–63.
24. Bremner R, Du DC, Connolly-Wilson MJ, et al. Deletion of RB exons 24 and 25 causes low-penetrance retinoblastoma. Am J Hum Genet 1997; 61: 556–70.
28. Muen W, Hindocha M, Reddy M. The role of education in the promotion of red reflex assessments. JRSM Short Rep 2010; 1: 46.
30. Shields JA, Parsons HM, Shields CL, Shah P. Lesions simulating retinoblastoma. J Pediatr Ophthalmol Strabismus 1991; 28: 338–40.
32. Finger PT, Harbour JW, Murphree AL, et al. Retinoblastoma. In: Edge SB, Byrd DR, Carducci MA, Compton CC, editors. AJCC Cancer Staging Manual. New York, NY: Springer; 2010: 561–8.
34. Shome D, Honavar SG, Raizada K, Raizada D. Implant and prosthesis movement after enucleation: a randomized controlled trial. Ophthalmology 2010; 117: 1638–44.
38. Palma J, Sasso DF, Dufort G, et al. Successful treatment of metastatic retinoblastoma with high-dose chemotherapy and autologous stem cell rescue in South America. Bone Marrow Transplant 2011 May 23.
39. Dimaras H, Heon E, Budning A, et al. Retinoblastoma CSF metastasis cured by multimodality chemotherapy without radiation. Ophthalmic Genet 2009; 30: 121–6.
40. Gallie BL, Budning A, DeBoer G, et al. Chemotherapy with focal therapy can cure intraocular retinoblastoma without radiation. Arch Ophthalmol 1996; 114: 1321–9.
42. Chan HSL, Lu Y, Grogan TM, et al. Multidrug resistance protein (MRP) expression in retinoblastoma correlates with rare failure of chemotherapy despite cyclosporine for reversal of P-glycoprotein. Cancer Res 1997; 57: 2325–30.
46. Wilson TW, Chan HSL, Moselhy GM, et al. Penetration of chemotherapy into vitreous is increased by cryotherapy and cyclosporin in rabbits. Arch Ophthalmol 1996; 114: 1390–5.
47. Chan H, Heon E, Budning A, Gallie B, editors. Long term outcome from retinoblastoma treated with cyclosporine-modulated chemotherapy. Paris: 14th International Symposium for Genetic Eye Diseases (ISGED) and 11th International Symposium on Retinoblastoma (ISR); 2003.
49. Wong FL, Boice JD, Jr., Abramson DH, et al. Cancer incidence after retinoblastoma: radiation dose and sarcoma risk [see comments]. JAMA 1997; 278: 1262–7.
51. Abramson DH, Frank CM, Dunkel IJ. A phase I/II study of subconjunctival carboplatin for intraocular retinoblastoma. Ophthalmology 1999; 106: 1947–50.
52. Mulvihill A, Budning A, Jay V, et al. Ocular motility changes after subtenon carboplatin chemotherapy for retinoblastoma. Arch Ophthalmol 2003; 121: 1120–4.
53. Mallipatna AC, Dimaras H, Chan HS, et al. Periocular topotecan for intraocular retinoblastoma. Arch Ophthalmol 2011; 129: 738–45.
55. Deegan WF. Emerging strategies for the treatment of retinoblastoma. Curr Opin Ophthalmol 2003; 14: 291–5.
57. Shields CL, Shields JA, Cater J, et al. Plaque radiotherapy for retinoblastoma: long-term tumor control and treatment complications in 208 tumors. Ophthalmology 2001; 108: 2116–21.
61. Suzuki S, Yamane T, Mohri M, et al. Selective ophthalmic arterial injection therapy for intraocular retinoblastoma: the long-term prognosis. Ophthalmology 2011; 10: 2081–7.
64. Chan H, Pandya J, Valverde K, et al. Metastatic retinoblastoma in the CSF that responded to intensive systemic and intraventricular multidrug resistance-reversal chemotherapy. Proc Am Assoc Cancer Res 2002; 43: 3720.

Access the complete reference list online at

http://www.expertconsult.com

Part 6
Retinal & vitreous disorders

Retinopathy of prematurity

Graham E Quinn • Alistair R Fielder

Retinopathy of prematurity (ROP) was first reported by Terry.[1] This condition, then known as retrolental fibroplasia, is a disorder of the immature retinal vasculature. It was extremely rare before the 1940s.[2] The retinopathy developed after a normal fundus examination at birth.[3] Clinical and experimental evidence supported a toxic effect of oxygen on the immature retinal vasculature[4,5-7] which led to the restriction of oxygen use in preterm neonates.[8] This resulted in a dramatic fall in the incidence of ROP, but even though oxygen plays a central role, many other factors contribute to the pathogenesis,[8-11] which has been comprehensively reviewed.[9,11-16]

Retinal vascular development

Retinal vasculature develops to meet retinal metabolic demand except at the fovea which has a different vascular pattern.[17] Early in development the retina receives all its nutrients from the choroid which is vascularized from about 6 weeks' gestational age;[18] vascularization of the retina begins at 14–15 weeks of gestation. Vascular endothelial cells, microglia, pericytes, and astrocytes migrate centrifugally from the optic disk, proliferate, and become aligned into vascular cords that develop lumina and differentiate into capillaries. The capillaries remodel and form a mature retinal vascular network with capillary-free areas.[19] The retinal tissue responds to excessive or insufficient oxygen by trimming or inducing growth in microvasculature to match the retina's metabolic requirements.[20]

Oxygen-dependent vascular endothelial growth factor (VEGF) plays a part in all stages of vascular development; other factors are also involved.[10,16,21-24] One is oxygen-independent insulin-like growth factor (IGF-1) that controls VEGF activation of the Akt endothelial cell survival pathway; low levels result in reduced survival and growth of vascular endothelial cells.[21-23]

The nasal retina is vascularized by 32 weeks gestational age, the temporal retina just after term.[25] The retinal vessels in the preterm infant are slender, relatively straight, and taper as they terminate toward the gray, avascular periphery (Fig. 43.1). The foveal region is differentiated ophthalmoscopically at around 40 weeks.[26]

Pathogenesis

Oxygen restriction does not abolish ROP; believing it would "seems naive in light of our current understanding."[24,27-29] At present, ROP is treatable, but not preventable.

According to the first – "classic" – theory,[7,8] ROP consists of two phases of equal importance:

1. A hyperoxic phase leading to retinal arteriolar constriction.
2. Vaso-obliteration with death of retinal capillary endothelial cells on removal from a hyperoxic environment.

The second – "gap junction" – theory is based on the activity of mesenchymal spindle cell retinal capillaries precursors.[30a] Mesenchymal spindle cells migrate centrifugally from the optic disk and form capillaries just behind the advancing vanguard. In the relative hyperoxic extrauterine condition, tight bonds or gap junctions appear between adjacent spindle cells, interfering with normal cell migration and vessel formation. The angiogenic factors secreted by gap-junctioned spindle cells trigger the neovascular response.

Current concepts of ROP pathogenesis encompass both classic and gap junction theories.[10,31b] VEGF is secreted in response to physiologic hypoxia of the maturing avascular retina. Hyperoxia causes cessation of vessel growth and

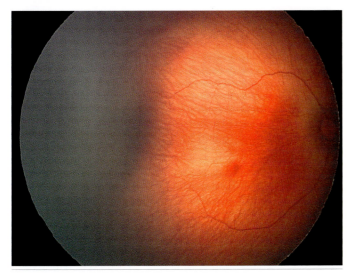

Fig. 43.1 Normal retinal vasculature and optic disk of a preterm baby without retinopathy. Note the straightness and fine caliber of retinal vessels; – the arterioles are hardly visible. The vessels taper into the gray non-vascularized periphery. Macular area is poorly defined. This and many other figures were obtained using wide-field digital imaging (RetCam 130).

apoptosis of parts of the retinal vasculature and capillary regression with consequent retinal ischemia stimulating VEGF. This results in neovascularization known as ROP.[10,31b-33]

There are two VEGF-A phases:

1. A vessel sustaining role, reduced by hyperoxia, leading to downregulation of VEGF-A with cessation of vessel growth and capillary regression.
2. Subsequent upregulation of VEGF-A induced by hypoxia, with vasoproliferation known as ROP.

There are two VEGF-A receptors in the mouse retina: VEGFR-1 supports retinal vessel survival (phase 1), and VEGFR-2 supports endothelial permeability and vasoproliferation.[34]

IGF-1, a somatic growth factor, controls VEGF activation: when IGF-1 is low, vessels do not grow.[35] The levels of placenta-derived IGF-1 rise in the second and third trimesters and fall after preterm birth. Oxygen-independent IGF-1 and oxygen-dependent VEGF are synergistic, and IGF-1 permits VEGF to function maximally at low levels. A slow recovery to "normal" levels of serum IGF-1 may predict phase 2 proliferative ROP;[10,15,21,23] causality has not been established[35] but evolves[36] with a number of exciting therapeutic options.[37]

The classic and gap junction theories have similarities with VEGF theory. In all three, normal vasculogenesis is impeded, and all require an oxidative insult. Thus, hyperoxia is important initially and vascular shutdown results from VEGF downregulation not direct cytotoxic action on retinal vessels. Not all of the early theories of ROP pathogenesis can be incorporated into current concepts: the separation of the "oxygen" and "room air" phases cannot be applied to the current model.

Risk or associated factors

The major ROP risk factor is the degree of immaturity as measured by either birth weight or gestational age,[38,39] the first being the more powerful predictor.[27,30b,40,41]

Clinical studies confirmed the relationship between oxygen and ROP,[42-44] and the duration of transcutaneous PO_2 over 80 mmHg and its incidence and severity.[45-47] Oxygen levels are particularly critical for ROP development, within the first few weeks after birth.[44,48] Safe levels of oxygen usage for clinical practice have yet to be detailed.[48,49]

ROP may develop in preterm infants who never received oxygen and in premature those with cyanotic heart disease.[9] A relationship between neonatal hypoxia and ROP is suggested.[9,49,50,51] That hyperoxia and hypoxia may be associated with ROP is not entirely contradictory.[52a] Relative hyperoxia may, via VEGF, lead to initial retinal capillary damage; subsequent ischemia stimulates VEGF overproduction and vasoproliferation explaining the association of recurrent apnea and cerebral ischemic events with ROP.[53]

The STOP-ROP trial tested the efficacy and risks of supplemental oxygen therapy for prethreshold disease but failed to show a beneficial effect.[54] A meta-analysis noted that "late" (≥32 weeks PMA) high oxygen was associated with reduced incidence of severe ROP.[44] Oxygen still plays a central role in ROP.[55] Babies with target saturation levels of 94–98% (but not measured) had a much higher incidence of ROP requiring treatment compared to those with target oxygen levels of 70–90%, with no increase in neurologic morbidity in the latter.[49,56] Looking at higher levels, a randomized controlled trial, comparing oxygen saturation ranges of 91–94% against 95–98%, reported no difference in infant growth, neurodevelopment, or rates of ROP.[52b] The risk of ROP should not be considered in isolation, but in the context of the wellbeing of the baby. Lower oxygen levels reduced the incidence of ROP blindness but at the expense of reduced survival, and higher morbidity.[8,50]

Acidosis is a risk factor for ROP,[53] whereas hypercarbia is not.[57,58] High PCO_2, PaO_2, and low pH in the first 3 days after birth were associated with severe ROP[48] and hyperglycemia is a risk factor,[59,60] perhaps related to insulin resistence. Antenatal steroids may be protective for ROP,[61,62] but not when given after birth.[63,64]

There is no difference in ROP incidence in Hispanic compared to White non-Hispanic infants,[65] while Indo-Pakistani infants are more likely to develop severe ROP than Caucasians.[66,67] Afro-Caribbean infants may be less,[40,68] or more,[67] likely to develop ROP.

There is high concordance for ROP in monozygotic twins.[69] ROP-associated mutations are all in the Wnt signaling pathway,[70] which also encompasses the Norrie's gene[71-73] and familial exudative vitreoretinopathy; the importance of this is not yet understood.[74]

Multiple birth, per se, does not increase the risk but concordant twins behave similarly.[75] In discordant twins, the smaller baby has the greater risk.[76,77] Male gender is a risk factor[78] as is assistive reproductive technology, the latter probably independent of multiple births.[79]

The antioxidant vitamin E[31a] is found at low levels in preterm neonates;[81] initially, supplementation did not appear to reduce the frequency of ROP but reduced its severity.[82,83] Due to side-effects of vitamin E its use prophylactically is not now recommended,[80,84] although Raju et al.,[85] in a meta-analysis of vitamin E prophylaxis, reported a reduction in the incidence of stage 3+ ROP, and suggested re-evaluation. Anemia is frequent in preterm infants; they may be transfused adult hemoglobin which binds oxygen less avidly than fetal hemoglobin so that more oxygen is delivered to the tissues giving hyperoxia, theoretically increasing the risk of ROP. There is a suggested association between ROP and blood transfusion,[86-89] but it has not been confirmed.[90,91] Recombinant erythropoietin, a cytokine which regulates fetal erythropoiesis and is important in angiogenesis, may now be used to treat neonatal anemia. Its role in ROP has yet to be clarified,[92,93] including its timing.[94,95]

Surfactant has reduced mortality, the severity of respiratory distress syndrome, and chronic lung disease in very immature neonates[96] but its effect is less clear with regard to ROP.[97-99]

Early exposure to light was suggested to be a risk factor.[1,100,101] Studies by Hepner et al.[10] and Locke and Reese[102] did not provide supportive evidence; later studies did not support this[10,102] at a time when supplemental oxygen could have swamped any effect of light. Light could, by damaging retinal tissues, generate free radicals and cause ROP. A reduction in neonatal unit illumination reduced the incidence and severity of ROP[103] but this was not confirmed by the LIGHT-ROP study[104] and another study.[105]

Antenatal exposure to infection and inflammation *individually* are not associated with ROP but, *together*, they carry an increased risk for severe ROP;[106] postnatal systemic fungal infection is a risk factor for both ROP development and severity.[107]

Many factors are active simultaneously and differently according to the standard of neonatal care. Thus, the characteristics of babies developing ROP in some countries are different from those in others: larger and more mature infants are at risk in less developed countries,[108] where the unrestricted use of oxygen and sepsis also need consideration.[109]

Classification

The international classification of acute ROP[110] was expanded to include retinal detachment and ROP sequelae[111] replacing the Reese et al. classification.[112] All stages of ROP are now covered by a single classification (Table 43.1) allowing direct comparison between centers and countries. A revision was published,[113] expanding two concepts, pre-plus disease and aggressive posterior ROP (AP-ROP).

The classification involves describing ROP by four parameters:

1. *Severity* by stage describing the retinopathy at the junction between the vascularized and avascular retina.
2. *Location* by zone describing the anterior–posterior position of the retinopathy.
3. *Extent* by clock hour of circumferential retinal involvement at the junction between the vascularized and avascular retina.
4. *Plus disease*, describing abnormally dilated or tortuous vessels of the posterior pole.

The normal fundus of the extremely premature baby can be difficult to visualize in detail (Figs 43.1 to 43.3). The retinal blood vessels are thin and straight. Later, they increase in caliber and tortuosity, but abnormally so with active ROP.

Severity of disease

The peripheral changes at the leading edge of the developing retinal vessels have been divided into five stages.

Stage 1

A flat gray-white demarcation line separates the vascularized from non-vascularized retina. Often faint, it can be difficult to identify. Retinal vessels run up to the line but do not cross it (Figs 43.4 and 43.5).

Stage 2

The demarcation line has increased in volume and extends out of the plane of the retina (Figs 43.5–43.7). The color of the ridge may be white or pink and small neovascular tufts may

Table 43.1 – International classification of retinopathy of prematurity – revisited (2005)

Severity	Stage of ROP	• Stage 1: demarcation line
		• Stage 2: ridge
		• Stage 3: ridge with extraretinal vascular proliferation
		• Stage 4: subtotal retinal detachment
		  • 4A: extrafoveal detachment
		  • 4B: foveal detachment
		• Stage 5: total retinal detachment

	Aggressive posterior ROP (ROP)	• Severe dilation and tortuosity of posterior pole vasculature • Innocuous appearance of ROP at junction between vascularized and avascular retina • Zone I or zone II
Anterior-posterior location		• Zone I: retina within a circle centered on the disk with a radius of twice the disk–foveal distance • Zone II: a doughnut-shaped area that extends from the edge of zone I to a circle which has a radius of the distance from the disk to the nasal ora serrata • Zone III: crescent-shaped retinal area peripheral to zone II
Extent of disease		• 30-degree sectors (clock hours) of ROP along the circumference of the vascularized retina
Posterior pole vessel abnormality	Pre-plus disease	Abnormal vascular dilation and tortuosity insufficient for diagnosis of plus disease (at least 2 quadrant involvement required)
	Plus disease	Dilated and tortuous vessels of the posterior pole (at least 2 quadrant involvement required)

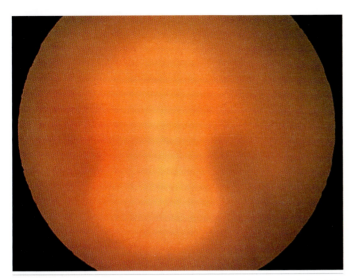

Fig. 43.2 Immature retinal vessels in an extremely immature baby. The view is hazy. Note how thin and straight are the retinal vessels.

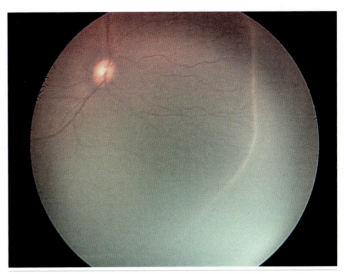

Fig. 43.5 ROP stages 1 and 2. Stage 1 in its lower part, but the line becomes thicker (ridge) toward the top of the image. Differentiating stages 1 and 2 is not always easy – or necessarily important.

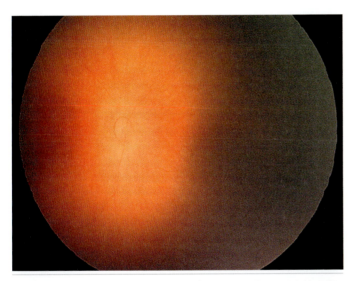

Fig. 43.3 Immature retinal vessels 1 week after image in Figure 43.2. No ROP.

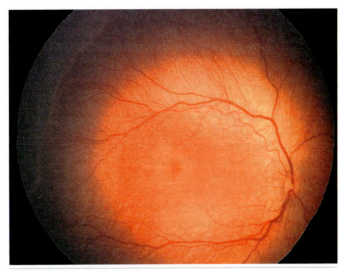

Fig. 43.6 Stage 2 ROP.

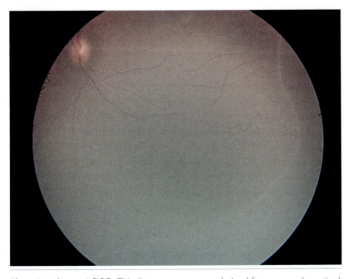

Fig. 43.4 Stage 1 ROP. Thin line separates vascularized from avascular retinal regions. The bluish tint is due to dark fundus.

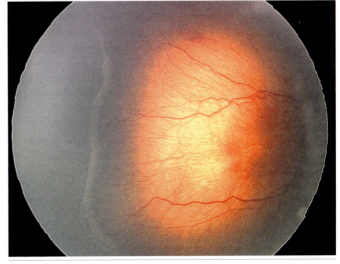

Fig. 43.7 Stage 2 and stage 3 ROP. Stage 2 at top and bottom of the image with about 1 clock hour of mild stage 3 disease that curls away from the ridge at its lower edge.

be seen posterior to the ridge. Differentiating stage 1 and early stage 2 is difficult but usually not prognostically important.

Stage 3

Stage 3 has the features of stage 2, but is characterized by extraretinal neovascularization (Figs 43.7 and 43.8). The new vessels may be continuous with, or disconnected from, the posterior border of the ridge, or extend into the vitreous. The extraretinal neovascularization may extend from the region of the ridge into the vitreous or, typically in more posterior disease, lies back across the surface of the vascularized retina.

Stage 4

This is characterized by subtotal exudative or tractional retinal detachment that is extrafoveal (stage 4B), or involves the foveal region (stage 4A).

Stage 5

There is a funnel-shaped total retinal detachment (Fig. 43.9). This stage is further defined according to the anterior and posterior characteristics of the funnel.

Aggressive posterior ROP (AP-ROP)

This severe form of ROP[113] is characterized by a posterior location (zone I or posterior zone II) and a prominence of plus disease out of proportion with the rather innocuous appearance of the vascular abnormality at the vascular/avascular junction. The severity often makes it difficult to distinguish arterioles and venules (Fig. 43.10). Over time, the progression from stage 1 to stage 2 and stage 3 is not apparent; the flat network of new vessels can easily be missed.

Plus disease

The first signs of plus disease (Figs. 43.11) are tortuosity of the retinal arterioles and congestion of the retinal veins close to the optic disk. Later, the vessels of the iris become engorged and the pupil fails to dilate to mydriatics. The vitreous becomes hazy. Signs of plus disease may appear at any ROP stage and

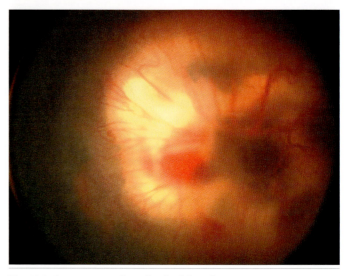

Fig. 43.9 Acute stage 5 funnel retinal detachment.

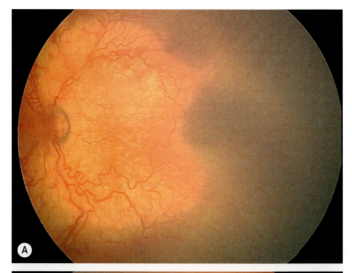

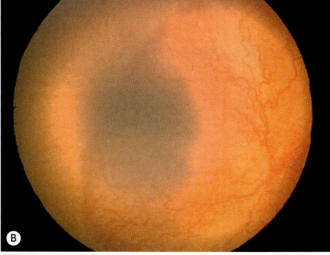

Fig. 43.10 Examples of aggressive posterior retinopathy of prematurity (AP-ROP). (A) View of AP-ROP – note the posterior locations, prominence of plus disease, and the modest appearance of the peripheral retinopathy. (B) AP-ROP image showing plus disease with a brushlike neovascular proliferation at junction between vascular and avascular retina. (Reproduced with permission from Arch Ophthalmol 2005; 123: 991–9.)

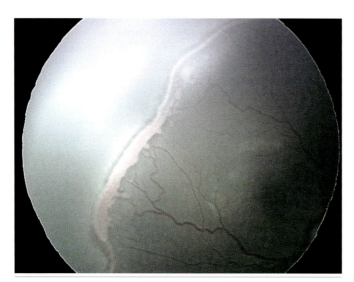

Fig. 43.8 Stage 3 ROP that has developed in the eye with stage 2 disease shown in Figure 43.6. Note the peripheral tortuosity and dilation as the vessels become close to the ROP lesion (compare with Figure 43.6). The shadow, just behind the lesion, indicates that the lesion is off the retinal surface.

occasionally as a precursor. The diagnosis is clinical comparing with a reference photograph; at least two quadrants must be involved and the peripheral changes of ROP must be present. Plus disease does not refer to vascular changes in the retinal periphery. The diagnosis of plus disease is critical; it is an

indicator of severe ROP[114] that may require treatment,[115] and increased likelihood of an unfavorable outcome.[66]

Pre-plus disease

The posterior vascular abnormalities that occur in ROP with plus disease are the most severe. The term "pre-plus"[113] indicates posterior vascular abnormalities with insufficient arteriolar tortuosity and venular dilation to be termed plus disease although still abnormal (Fig. 43.12). It alerts to the possibility of peripheral retinopathy.

Location

The retina is divided into three zones centered on the optic disk, in contrast to retinal neural organization, which centers on the fovea:

Zone I is a circle that has a radius twice the disk–foveal distance – about 30°.

Zone II extends from the edge of zone I to the ora serrata on the nasal side and encircles the anatomic equator.

Zone III includes all retina temporally, superiorly, and inferiorly anterior to zone II. With no anatomic landmarks identifying zone III, only when the directly nasal retina is fully vascularized can it be stated that zone III has been entered.

Extent

The extent of disease is described in clock hours or by 30° sectors. As the examiner looks at the eyes, the 3 o'clock position is on the right for both eyes, i.e. on the nasal side of the right eye and temporal side of the left eye.

Regression and resolution

Resolution of acute retinopathy has been less well studied, because, once the need for surgical intervention has passed, there is less need for surveillance and recording.[111] The rate of regression reflects PMA;[116] the first signs are failure to progress and the lessening of any signs of plus disease. The ridge thins and breaks up. Later, vessels grow through the ridge into the peripheral avascular retina.[117] Involution is characterized by vascular remodeling with gradual movement of vessels toward the periphery: in some eyes, vascularization to the ora serrata does not occur. The acute ROP lesion becomes white and vessels may be seen extending beyond the lesion into the periphery. Vasoproliferative lesions become fibrotic.[109,111] All

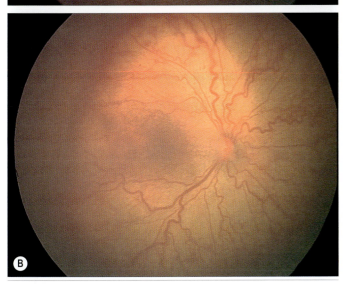

Fig. 43.11 Two examples of plus disease. Note the different appearance with different magnification and field of view between (A) and (B). (Reproduced with permission from Arch Ophthalmol 2005; 123: 991–9.)

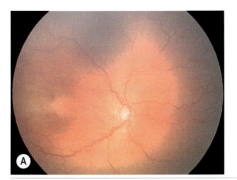 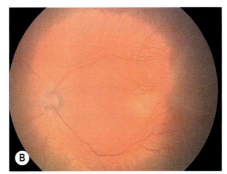 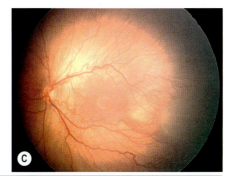

Fig. 43.12 Examples of pre-plus disease showing increased tortuosity and dilation compared to normal, but insufficient to be designated plus disease. (Reproduced with permission from Arch Ophthalmol 2005; 123: 991–9.)

exclusively stage 1 and 2 ROP undergo complete resolution. Stage 3 may or may not resolve, depending on severity. A sign of incomplete resolution is retinal dragging (Figs 43.13 and 43.14). The mean time of onset of signs of involution in children with birth weights of less than 1251 g was 38.6 weeks; 74% of all ROP had begun to involute by 40 weeks of PMA 90% by 44 weeks.[116]

Advanced cicatricial changes involving the anterior vitreous and retina (Table 43.2) may push the lens/iris diaphragm forward and cause shallowing of the anterior chamber, glaucoma, and corneal decompensation. In such cases, lensectomy is indicated to relieve narrow angle glaucoma.

Incidence and prevalence

Acute phase ROP

Early publications[15,66,118,119,120] were mostly from single centers, but prospective geographic studies[40,121] were undertaken, one of which was carried out after treatment was introduced.[122]

The multicenter study of cryotherapy for retinopathy of prematurity (CRYO-ROP study) was conducted in 23 nurseries in the USA.[70] Over 4000 children with birth weights of less than 1251 g had serial eye examinations. ROP was observed in one or both eyes of 65.8% of these infants, with ROP observed in 90% of children with birth weights of less than 750 g, in 78% of those with birth weights of 751–1000 g, and in 47% of those with birth weights of 1001–1250 g. The CRYO-ROP study reported on the residua of ROP (the cicatricial phase in the eyes of 2759 children at age 1 year). None of these eyes had undergone cryotherapy. There was advanced scarring involving the posterior pole in approximately 4%, with 2% likely to have severe visual loss due to posterior pole scarring or retinal detachment.[123]

ROP may have declined in incidence,[49,123-125] but not universally.[126,127] The overall incidence of ROP in an intensive care nursery[128] in infants with birth weights of less than 1251 g was 34% compared to 65.8% for CRYO-ROP study patients. For infants with birth weights of less than 1000 g, there was an incidence rate for ROP of 46%, compared to 81.6% for CRYO-ROP patients in the same birth weight group. However, there are several biases in single-center studies,[129] including survival rates,[130] ethnicity, and standard of care.

The ETROP study enrolled babies with birth weights of less than 1251 g in 26 neonatal intensive care unit (NICU) systems

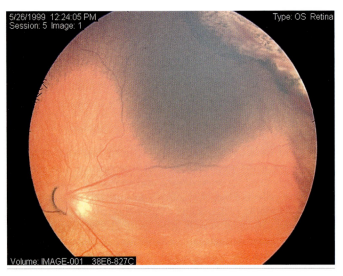

Fig. 43.13 Mild dragging of the retinal vessels. Note response to cryotherapy on upper border of picture.

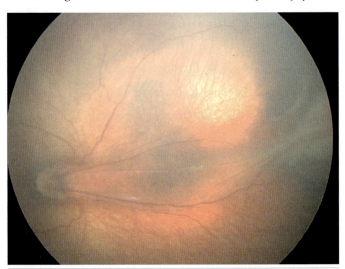

Fig. 43.14 Fundus photograph showing late cicatricial changes including stage 4B retinal detachment with extensive temporal dragging of vessels and macula. (Reproduced with permission from Arch Ophthalmol 2005; 123: 991–9.)

Table 43.2 – Cicatricial changes in retinopathy of prematurity

Peripheral changes		Posterior changes	
Vascular	• Failure to vascularize peripheral retina abnormal, non-dichotomous branching of retinal vessels • Vascular arcades with circumferential interconnection • Telangiectatic vessels	Vascular	• Vascular tortuosity • Straightening of vessels in temporal arcade • Decrease in angle of insertion of major temporal arcade
Retinal	• Pigmentary changes • Vitreoretinal interface changes • Thinning of the retina • Peripheral folds • Vitreous membranes with or with traction on the retina • Lattice-like degeneration • Retinal breaks • Traction/rhegmatogenous retinal detachment	Retinal	• Pigmentary changes • Distortion or ectopia of macula • Stretching and folding of retina in macular region leading to periphery • Vitreoretinal interface changes • Vitreous membrane • Dragging of retina over disk • Traction/rhegmatogenous retinal detachment

Adapted from Committee of Classification of Retinopathy of Prematurity (Arch Ophthalmol 1987).

in the USA and imposed a rigorously controlled examination technique and frequency. The incidence of ROP in the ETROP study was 68% among infants of 1251 g birth weight, which is a very similar incidence to that for the CRYO-ROP study (65.8% among infants of similar birth weights). However, in the ETROP study, the incidence of more severe prethreshold ROP was 36.9% among infants with ROP while the incidence was 27.1% for patients in the CRYO-ROP study. The mean birth weight and gestational age for babies developing prethreshold ROP in the ETROP study were less than those in the CRYO-ROP study (740 vs. 831 g and 25.6 vs. 26.5 weeks),[14] indicating that prethreshold ROP occurred among smaller and younger infants in the ETROP study cohort than in the CRYO-ROP study cohort.

Despite these caveats, in countries with well developed NICU systems, both the incidence and severity of ROP rise with the degree of prematurity, and more than 50% of babies under 1000 g at birth develop some stage of ROP; babies under

1251 g birth weight have an incidence of stage 3 ROP of around 18%. Approximately 6–8% of babies under 1251 g birth weight will develop ROP sufficiently severe to require treatment with peripheral retinal ablation.[131]

In industrialized countries, severe ROP is largely confined to infants with birth weights of less than 1000 g and gestational age of 31 weeks or less, and blinding disease is rare in larger babies.[132] However, the prevalence in developing and industrializing countries appears to be increasing and blinding ROP is not confined to very low birth weight infants. When the infant mortality rates fall between 10 and 50 per 1000 births in an industrializing country, the risk for blindness due to ROP increases dramatically. The risk is very low in those countries with infant mortality rates of more than 50 per 1000 births[133] (Fig. 43.15 and Table 43.3). In settings where only the premature babies with higher birth weights survive (e.g. the ROP epidemic of the 1940–1950s), extent of prematurity and low birth weight have minimal contributions because oxygen

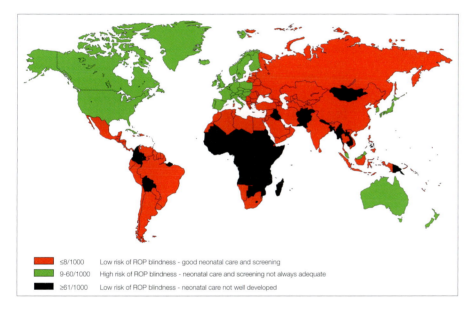

Fig. 43.15 Likely distribution of blindness in children due to retinopathy of prematurity as a public health problem, using infant mortality rates as an indicator. (Reproduced with permission from Eye 2007; 21: 1338–43.)

≤8/1000	Low risk of ROP blindness - good neonatal care and screening	
9-60/1000	High risk of ROP blindness - neonatal care and screening not always adequate	
≥61/1000	Low risk of ROP blindness - neonatal care not well developed	

Table 43.3 – Risk factors for retinopathy of prematurity: an historical perspective

		First epidemic (1940–1950s)	Second epidemic (1970–1980s)	Current: regions with well developed neonatal care systems	Current: regions with developing neonatal care systems (third epidemic)
Risk factors	Prematurity	+	++	++++	+ to ++++
	Low birth weight (BW)	+	++	++++	+ to ++++
	Excessive oxygen supplementation	++++	+++	+	++++
	Illness	+	+	+/−	+/−
BW < 1000 g	Survival rate	+	++	++++	+ to +++
	Risk of ROP	+	++	+++	+ to ++++
BW 1000–1500 g	Survival rate	+++	++++	++++	+ to +++
	Risk of ROP	+++	+	+/−	+ to +++
BW >1500 g	Survival rate	++	+++	++++	++ to ++++
	Risk of ROP	+++	+	0	0 to +++
Ocular outcome		Poor	Moderate	Good	Poor to good

Adapted from Gilbert C. Retinopathy of prematurity: A global perspective of the epidemics, population of babies at risk and implications for control. Early Human Development 2008; 84: 77–82.

supplementation as a surrogate for the level of neonatal care is the prominent risk factor. Now that more babies with the lowest birth weights survive due to improvements in neonatal and perinatal care (as in the nurseries of the 1990s and 2000s), the extent of the infant's prematurity becomes more important.

ROP disability: the three epidemics

There have been three ROP epidemics:[108,133-137]

1. The first in the 1940s was due to unrestricted, unmonitored oxygen and was brought to an end by oxygen restriction. The survival of neonates of < 1000 g birth weight was 5–8%, and most of the babies blinded during this period were of heavier birth weight. ROP was largely eliminated by advances in neonatal care.[138]

2. In the late 1960s, in countries with well developed neonatal intensive care services, the increased survival of the very immature neonate who did not previously survive (now around 50–60% < 1000 g birth weight) resulted in a second epidemic.

   In retrospect, the first epidemic could be considered preventable, whereas the second is not preventable at our current level of neonatal care.

3. The term "third epidemic" describes the prevalence of ROP-induced visual disability worldwide and provides insights and opportunities for preventive interventions.[108]

Countries can be subdivided according to health–socioeconomic criteria into high-, middle-, or low-income according to the health provision (Fig. 43.16). There may be diverse health–socioeconomic communities within a single country. In high-income countries, where wealth and technology permit generally high-quality health care and neonatal intensive care, ROP-induced disability accounts for 3–8% of childhood vision impairment.[139-142] In middle-income communities, technology permits increased survival of preterm babies, but limited health resources may limit the standard of care.[133] Consequently, babies with higher birth weights and gestational ages are at risk of severe ROP; ROP-induced blindness contributes up to 39% of childhood vision impairment due to increased survival and associated limited resources with poor quality neonatal care[108,143] (see Table 43.3). In low-income countries, very few preterm babies survive to develop ROP.[108,109]

The evidence that ROP-induced disability has been reduced by treatment comes from two sources. First, from studies such as the CRYO-ROP study, which demonstrated that the beneficial effects of treatment are maintained at least 15 years after treatment.[144] Second, epidemiologic studies such as the report from the UK which showed that, between 1976 and 1985, ROP contributed 5% of childhood vision impairment; this proportion rose to 8% between 1986 and 1990[140] and subsequently fell to 3% by 2000.[145] Given the increase in survival of the most immature babies,[143] in the absence of treatment, a considerable increase would have been anticipated.

Natural history

The natural history of ROP provides clues to underlying mechanisms and is vital for screening and management. There are

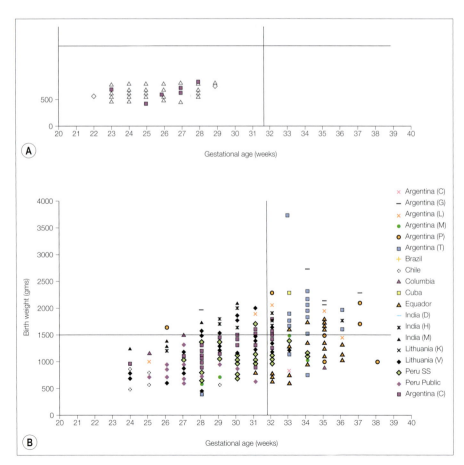

Fig. 43.16 (A) Birth weights and gestational ages of babies treated for threshold ROP in Canada, the USA, and UK (2000 to 2004). (B) Birth weights and gestational ages of babies with severe retinopathy of prematurity in low- and middle-income countries between 2000 and 2004. (Reproduced with permission from Pediatrics 2005; 115: 518–25 by the American Academy of Pediatrics.)

five important elements to the natural history of ROP, which are outlined below.

1. Age at onset and rate of progression

ROP affects only immature retinal vessels and cannot develop after retinal vascularization is complete. One would expect the most premature, often ill, neonate with a very immature retinal vascular system to develop ROP sooner postnatally than a larger and more mature baby. However, this is not so (Fig. 43.17); ROP develops over a relatively narrow PMA range.[40,119,146,147] The time of ROP onset is linked more to the stage of development of the infant, by PMA, than neonatal events such as oxygen therapy or illnesses,[40,119] acknowledging that the latter contribute to ROP occurrence and severity. The time during which ROP can develop is governed by PMA, but is terminated by complete retinal vascularization (also related to PMA). The narrowness of this "window" is exhibited by the occasional example of a baby of >33 weeks gestational age and >2000 g body weight (by which time the time remaining to develop ROP is very limited) who has received prolonged and excessive 100% oxygen and has reached stage 5 by 37 weeks PMA.

As with onset, the rate of progression is also governed predominantly by the stage of development (PMA) rather than by postnatal age, or neonatal events. Data[119,130,132,148] show remarkable consistency in the behavior of ROP. The median PMA at which the various ROP stages and features develop is as follows:

1. Stage 1, 34.1 weeks
2. Stage 2, 35.1 weeks
3. Stage 3, 36.6 weeks

4. Plus, 36.0 weeks
5. Prethreshold, 36.1 weeks
6. Threshold ROP, 37.3 weeks

In the CRYO-ROP study, babies were randomized for treatment (i.e. within 72 hours of diagnosis of threshold ROP) at a mean age of 37.7 weeks PMA (range 32–50 weeks).[149] The mean age at treatment for prethreshold and threshold eyes in ETROP was 35.2 weeks and 37.0 weeks, respectively. The extremes of the age range at which eyes require treatment are notable, the earliest being 31 weeks PMA,[119,130,149] Yet, almost all babies (99%) that develop severe ROP will have done so by 46.3 weeks PMA.[148] The literature cited so far has all come from countries with high standards of neonatal care.

In countries with more variability in the standard of care, sight-threatening disease affects more mature and larger babies.[108,109,150] In regions developing neonatal care systems, ROP progression also behaves according to PMA.

2. Zone of involvement

The propensity for severity of ROP is governed by the state of retinal vascularization, so that zone is the most important predictor of outcome.[42,131] Incomplete vascularization in zone I carries a 54% risk of reaching threshold, but this risk falls to 8% when vessels have reached zone II. For ROP developing in zone III the risk of an adverse outcome is almost nil.[151]

3. Site of onset

ROP commences in the temporal retina in the more mature neonates when the nasal retina is already vascularized. However, in the immature neonate ROP commences preferentially in the nasal retina and later extends to other regions.[39,152] The zones of vascular development were depicted by the international classification as being circular, but when this was revised in 2005[113] their elliptical shape was recognized; retinopathy in the nasal retina is frequently closer to the optic disk than ROP in the temporal retina.[153] The vertical retinal regions are less likely to be involved at onset and are only involved when ROP involves most of the circumference. The finding of ROP in these regions early in the course of the disease is a useful indicator of the possibility of future severity. The more premature the neonate, the more posterior by zone the location of the retinopathy and the greater the potential for progression. Thus, zone I disease is very likely to progress to stage 3, but ROP confined entirely to zone III rarely does.[119]

4. Plus disease

Plus disease is a critical sign of ROP activity and is now the main driver for treatment.[132] Plus disease may be superimposed on any ROP stage and is a sign that ROP is, or is about to become, severe.[40,114] Advanced plus disease is obvious, but if mild, is the least robust diagnostic aspect of ROP. To overcome this, attempts are being made to quantify some components of plus disease by digital imaging.

5. Regression

How ROP regresses is less well documented than its onset and progression, but proceeds according to PMA rather than postnatal age. This is not surprising because the process of regression, unless it fails to occur, does not require clinical decisions.

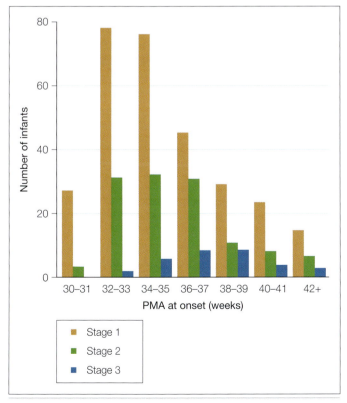

Fig. 43.17 ROP developing over narrow postmenstrual age.

ROP detection programs

Severe ROP can be successfully treated.[131] The ophthalmologist has a duty to examine babies to detect development of ROP requiring treatment. Understanding its natural history provides the basis for a logical and simple ROP examination protocol that is cost-effective in countries with well developed NICU systems.[154-159]

Although it takes time for advances to be incorporated into national guidelines, we believe that ROP detection programs must be implemented in communities of the world that have significant differences in their neonatal populations. The purpose of ROP examinations is to identify severe, potentially treatable ROP. Apart from the need to diagnose ROP requiring treatment, babies with stage 3 ROP have a high risk of developing strabismus, myopia, and various vision deficits and thus merit ophthalmic surveillance.

Which infants should undergo ROP examinations?

In high-income countries, severe ROP (stage 3 or more) is largely confined to infants of birth weight <1501 g and <32 weeks gestational age.[159] Thus, in the UK, these are the current guidelines for those babies who require ROP examinations. In the USA, ROP examinations are recommended for all babies <1501 g or with a gestational age of <30 weeks and for babies between 1500 and 2000 g birth weight who had an unstable clinical course and are considered at risk of ROP.[158]

For high-income countries, the UK criteria include most, if not all, babies who develop severe ROP (stage 3 or more).[160-165] Can we safely reduce the number of babies screened for ROP? Many of the larger and more mature babies who currently undergo examination are at very low risk of developing severe ROP. Of 16 000 babies, there was only one baby over 1200 g with severe ROP.[166] Two studies from the UK have shown that the criteria of <1251 g birth weight and/or <30 weeks gestational age included all babies with stage 3;[160,161] however, three US studies have reported stage 3 in larger babies.[162,163,167]

For low- and middle-income countries, larger babies also develop severe ROP, and the UK and US criteria may not include all babies at risk.[133] It is essential in these communities for ROP examination guidelines to be based on local data.

Timing of examinations

Examinations can be timed on the principle that the onset and progression of ROP are predominantly determined by PMA rather than by neonatal events. While most guidelines recommend commencing ROP examinations between 4 and 7 weeks, Reynolds et al.[148] developed an algorithm for examining the most immature baby later postnatally than the more mature baby. Timing of examinations is critical; there is only a narrow, imperfectly determined window for treatment. Onset of any stage of ROP is rare before 30 weeks PMA, and ROP commencing once vascularization has entered zone III and/or after 36–38 weeks PMA is most unlikely to reach severe disease.

After the initial ROP examination, weekly or every other week examinations are indicated, but as ROP progresses, more frequent examinations will be required. A weekly visit to the NICU allows examination of those babies likely to be discharged home soon and decreases the need for babies to be recalled, decreasing the likelihood of missed examinations and their potentially disastrous consequences.[168] For the baby transferred to another hospital while still at risk, arrangements must be made for the continuation of ROP examinations.

ROP examinations can cease when the retinal vessels have grown well into zone III. This can only be ascertained with certainty when the nasal retina is vascularized so that there is no doubt of the extent of vascularization. It is safer to require vascularization into zone III on two occasions.

ROP detection protocol

The next paragraph is written with developed countries in mind; it is not generalizable to all preterm populations.

All infants determined to be at risk for ROP should be examined at 30–32 weeks PMA and then every 1–2 weeks at least until 36–38 weeks PMA or until vascularization has progressed into zone III and the risk of severe ROP requiring treatment has passed. Some larger babies may be discharged before an initial ROP examination. In such situations, an examination before discharge is recommended. This can indicate the potential for ROP and frequently obviate the need for later examination.

Methods of examination

Eye examinations are stressful for the preterm baby,[169-173] but this can be reduced by supportive neonatal care. Infants should be handled gently. It is helpful if a trained nurse is in attendance to help and to monitor the infant's wellbeing. The ophthalmic examination should be performed using the indirect ophthalmoscope, with a 28- or 20-diopter lens, through dilated pupils, achieved by instilling dilating drops well prior to examination. A child's lid speculum and scleral indenter (for ocular rotation rather than indentation), after anesthetic eye drops, may be used to permit complete evaluation of the peripheral retina. Although it can be argued that very peripheral disease so observed is of no clinical importance, identifying peripheral nasal retinopathy can be a clue to later progression. Only by observing the state of vascularization of the nasal retina can the ophthalmologist determine whether zone III has been entered.

Clinical findings

The ophthalmoscopic appearance of the neonate is different from that of the older infant.[172] Before examining the retina it is important to use the indirect lens as a simple magnifier to examine the anterior segment, for instance, to see the amount of regression of the tunica vasculosa lentis as an indicator of maturity (regressing between 28 and 34 weeks gestational age).[173]

The retinal periphery is white-gray in its non-vascularized regions; the extent of this depends on the degree of immaturity (see Fig. 43.1). The optic disk frequently has a grayish and a double-ring appearance but the disk is a normal size. The macular area is relatively ill defined, there being no macular or foveolar reflexes until 36 and 42 weeks PMA, respectively.[26] The retinal arterioles in the early neonatal period are not tortuous, tending to become so later, in part related to ROP severity.[39]

Acute phase retinopathy of prematurity

The purpose of ROP examinations is to identify severe ROP which might require treatment. The four parameters by which

ROP is classified, according to the international classification, should be noted at each location at every examination:

1. Zone
2. Severity by stage
3. Extent by clock hour or sector
4. The presence of plus disease.

The extent of retinal vascularization and ROP location indicate the likelihood of future progression. The more posterior the retinopathy, the greater the likelihood of progression to severe retinopathy. In the CRYO-ROP study, eyes that were initially observed to have vascularization only in zone I were very likely to progress to severe disease.[119] Only if the advancing edge of the peripheral retinal vessels can be visualized, can one determine whether ROP is present. Another diagnostic aid indicating the presence of ROP is vessels that dilate slightly rather than taper as they traverse the retina toward the periphery. Abnormal arborization and circumferential arcading are often seen in the vessels running up to the ridge.

Start by observing the posterior pole vessels to look for signs of plus disease. This alerts the clinician that ROP is likely present and active in the retinal periphery and may require treatment.

ROP screening in the future

Predicting severe ROP through postnatal weight gain

Both VEGF and IGF-1 are critical for normal retinal vascular development. IGF-1 is a somatic growth factor which is correlated with birth weight and postnatal growth. IGF-1 levels rise during the last trimester of pregnancy so promoting, through VEGF activation, normal retinovascular development.[174-176] Following preterm birth, IGF-1 levels fall, inhibit retinovascular development, and set the scene for subsequent ROP. When IGF-1 increases some time after birth, VEGF is maximally stimulated and ROP results. Being a somatic growth factor birth weight and postnatal growth can to be used as surrogate for retinal vascular development and assessing the potential for ROP. The decrease in IGF-1 levels after preterm birth is manifested by a corresponding decrease in postnatal weight gain; its magnitude indicates the severity of retinovascular hypoxia. As this postnatal weight gain dip precedes clinical ROP by weeks, this concept has been developed into a computer-based algorithm for ROP screening (WINROP)[175-178] in which an alarm is triggered when postnatal weight gain decreases, compared to controls. In one study, WINROP correctly identified all 28 babies who developed severe ROP, the alarm being activated at a median 9 weeks for ROP diagnosis, although the alarm was also activated for 53 who did not.[179] The study by Wu et al. is important as it had a racially mixed cohort, in contrast to previous studies.[175-177] In Brazil, WINROP was not quite so sensitive; it failed to identify 9.5% of stage 3 ROP and the alarm was set off by 44% of babies with less than stage 3 ROP.[180]

A clinical,[181] not computer-based, prediction model can be based on postnatal weight gain. This model triggered an alarm when the predicted probability of severe ROP was >0.085 and identified 66 of 67 babies with severe ROP. It is not known[181] how well WINROP, or any algorithm based on postnatal weight gain, will work in centers where neonatal care is sub-optimal. Excessive oxygen is used and ROP may develop in larger and more mature babies.

The use of postnatal weight gain as a predictor of severe ROP and eyes which need to be screened could reduce the number of babies screened by 30% or more. How it will work across the range of neonatal care has yet to be determined.

Digital imaging

Another exciting development has been wide and narrow field digital imaging of the neonatal retina. This provides a range of opportunities for the study of ROP and the developing retina and contributed to the revised ROP classification.[113] Images can be obtained by anyone suitably trained: ophthalmologists, pediatricians, nurses, or ophthalmic photographers.[182-186] The image presented on a monitor at the cotside can be viewed by several observers reducing the need for multiple examinations. The retinal picture can be seen by the neonatal team and the parents. Digital ocular imaging provides high-quality retinal images and has several important features:

1. Examinations can be performed by non-ophthalmologists.
2. It is probably less, certainly not more, painful than indirect ophthalmoscopy.[187,188]
3. Images can be transmitted via the internet to local or distant centers for expert opinion (telemedicine).
4. Images can be stored for analysis, permitting quantification of changes.
5. Image details can be objectively analyzed and quantified.

Quantifying retinal vessels

Retinal parameters of digital imaging has permitted measurement.[189] For instance, ROP zones were considered to be circular until digital imaging showed that they were not and that ROP in the nasal retina is closer to the optic disk compared to ROP in the temporal retina.[153]

All methods of retinal vessel measurement use image segmentation to detect various parameters of the image. Various techniques of retinal image segmentation are used to localize retinal blood vessels for quantification: vessel tracking, neural networking, and morphologic processing.

Vessel analysis software includes: Retinal Image multiScale Analysis (RISA),[190-194] ROPtool,[195,196] Computer-Aided Image Analysis of the Retina (CAIAR),[197,198] IVAN,[199] and others.[200,201] Applied to ROP, all methods reliably measure vessel tortuosity, some less robustly than others.

Currently, the analysis times are long, and, being semi-automated, require some manual input. Completely automated methods, which can speedily analyze images, may soon be introduced.

As an adjunct or replacment for binocular indirect ophthalmoscopy

While binocular indirect ophthalmoscopy is the current gold standard, it is a qualitative assessment of the retinal appearance and each parameter cannot be objectively analyzed or measured. Experts do not always agree when advanced ROP is present. In the CRYO-ROP study,[148] research-trained ophthalmologists disagreed at the point when the decision to treat was being made in 12% of eyes. Moreover, the indirect ophthalmoscopic examination is a malpractice issue.[202]

Several studies[182,183,185,203-207] compared the sensitivities of RetCam® digital imaging to indirect ophthalmoscopy in the detection of any ROP. Several of these studies[204-207] and others[182,208-212] compared the RetCam imaging and indirect ophthalmoscopy in the identification of moderate and severe ROP. RetCam has high sensitivities for detecting moderate and severe ROP. The sensitivities and specificities for RetCam identifying mild ROP are lower, but it is possible to fail to see peripheral ROP by either method. Because of this a confirmatory examination by indirect ophthalmoscopy prior to discharging a baby from the screening program performed by RetCam should be considered.

The topic of wide and narrow field digital imaging for ROP screening[213] is still the subject of current research but used by many for routine ROP screening. It presents new opportunities for clinical research including image analysis.[214]

Quantifying plus disease

The main feature differentiating type I ROP, which requires treatment, from type II ROP, which does not, is the presence of plus disease.[115] Plus disease close to the optic disk, rather than assessment of the entire retina, is a current driver for treatment. The diagnosis of plus disease is a dichotomous decision based on subjective comparison to two reference images, the first from the international classification of 1984[111] and the second from clinical trials, e.g. CRYO-ROP[131] and ETROP.[115] The vascular abnormalities of ROP represent a spectrum rather than a simple dichotomy, so the additional category of pre-plus was added in 2005.[113] The majority of eyes with pre-plus subsequently require laser treatment.[215] However, clinicians have difficulty in diagnosing plus disease with an alarmingly low rate of inter-clinician agreement.[193,205,216,217] This is a major dilemma and we are in a more difficult situation than when threshold (as defined in the CRYO-ROP study[131]) was the treatment criterion.

The vascular changes of plus disease can be quantified by semi-automated analysis[192,193,203,217-221] which can probe the dynamics of the vascular changes which culminate in plus disease.

Telemedicine

Telemedicine for ROP screening has attracted considerable interest,[205,211,222] with good interphysician agreement.[205,208,223] Digital imaging raised this to another level by the reporting of good agreement between physician and image-based interpretation[224] and moderate agreement between physician and semi-automated analysis.[212] ROP should be an ideal topic for telemedicine as the location of the babies at risk is known, and because ROP's natural history and the appropriate time for screening are also well defined. Where ophthalmic expertise is sparse, nurses can obtain and upload the images for remote analysis by experts.[186] The images can be analyzed automatically in the NICU or remotely to identify the baby requiring an examination by an ophthalmologist. Non-contact narrow field imaging is attractive. It does not permit imaging of the peripheral retina, but plus disease can be assessed clinically[186] or quantified by semi-automated analysis.[212] Telemedicine may be utilized in a number of ways. The wide-field digital images from a detailed retinal examination (using a 5-image protocol [Photo-ROP 2008]) could enable a remote reader to make a detailed diagnosis. From these images, a decision could be made about the need for an in-person ophthalmic assessment (referral-warranted ROP[208]). By non-contact narrow, or contact wide-field, imaging plus disease may be remotely evaluated either clinically or by semi-automated methods. The last two uses would not permit a precise diagnosis, but they would identify the vast majority of babies without sight-threatening ROP who need not undergo a full examination.

An automatic objective measure of plus disease may soon be obtained from one digital image of the vessels close to the optic disk. Screening could be undertaken by non-medical personnel[225] and the expert ophthalmologist consulted only, via telemedicine, when plus disease is present.

Remoteness is relative. The baby with sight-threatening ROP who is only a mile or so from a too-busy ophthalmologist is as equally remote from care as one many miles away. To have a real and sustainable effect, telemedicine needs not only to work afar, but must also contribute to routine medical care enabling local teams to work better than they do currently.[226]

Treatment[157,227,228]

Prophylaxis

There is no obvious prophylactic treatment. There are a number of factors that might minimize the incidence and severity of ROP or reduce the rate of progression, improving outcome. These include improving standards of obstetric and neonatal care, oxygen administration, and nutrition of the premature baby.

Acute phase retinopathy of prematurity

Cryotherapy and xenon arc photocoagulation were first used for acute ROP[228,229] with argon laser later. However, it was not until 1988 that retinal ablative therapy was proven to have a beneficial effect on severe retinopathy.[154]

The CRYO-ROP study

The Multicenter Trial of Cryotherapy for Retinopathy of Prematurity (CRYO-ROP) set out to determine prospectively whether cryotherapy is effective in the treatment of severe acute ROP and to study its natural history.[149,154] 9751 infants of less than 1251 g birth weight were enrolled at 23 centers in the USA over a 23-month period. This was approximately 15% of infants of less than 1251 g birth weight born in the USA during this period. Ophthalmic examinations using indirect ophthalmoscopy started at 4–6 weeks postnatally and were continued at least every 2 weeks until vascularization was complete. A total of 291 infants participated in a trial in which eyes were randomly allocated to treatment with cryotherapy or observation. Infants who had bilateral threshold ROP (defined as 5 continuous or 8 cumulative clock hours of stage 3 in zone I or II with plus disease) at the same time had one eye randomized to treatment and the fellow eye to observation (control). If an infant had threshold ROP in one eye and less severe or no ROP in the fellow eye, the threshold ROP eye was assigned to either treatment or observation. "Threshold" severity of ROP had been selected since the risk of blindness if untreated is 50%. Cryotherapy was to be performed within 72 hours.

Cryotherapy produced a significant reduction in the unfavorable structural outcome of threshold ROP of 49.3% at 3 months[131,149] and 45.8% at 12 months,[230] as judged by fundus photographs and clinical examination. The beneficial effect of cryotherapy has persisted[231-237] with a 42.2% reduction in unfavorable structural outcomes at the 15-year follow-up study examinations.[144]

Visual acuity was added as an outcome in this trial beginning at the 1-year study examinations. At 1 year, treated infants had significantly better visual acuity (using acuity cards) than controls.[238] At the final 15-year study examination, the rates of unfavorable visual acuity outcomes (a Snellen score of 20/200 or worse using the ETDRS chart) were 44.7% in the treated group and 64.1% in controls. At 15 years, 23% of the eyes in the control group and 23% of eyes in the treated group had a visual acuity of 20/40 or better. There was a similar number of both treated and control eyes that developed retinal detachments from the 1 year exam to the 15 year exam.[144]

The CRYO-ROP study showed that cryotherapy for threshold ROP produced a significant benefit for structural status of the eye and for vision.[131,144,230-237,239,240] However, retinal ablation in eyes with severe ROP did not necessarily result in normal retinal structure or the development of visual acuity in the normal range.

Further clinical trials

Since the CRYO-ROP trial, two large clinical trials have addressed the timing and mode of treatment for sight-threatening ROP. The first STOP-ROP involved the use of supplemental oxygen to determine whether progression from moderate (prethreshold) stages to severe (threshold) stages of ROP could be affected.[54] At the diagnosis of prethreshold disease in one or both eyes, the infants were randomly assigned to receive conventional oxygen treatment with pulse oximetry targets of 89% to 94% saturation or to receive supplemental oxygen treatment with pulse oximetry targets of 96% to 99%. With 649 infants enrolled during the 5-year study, the rate of progression to threshold disease was not different between children assigned to conventional oxygen treatment or the supplemented oxygen group (48% treated, 41% supplemented, p = NS). Supplemental oxygen treatment increased the risk of adverse pulmonary events including pneumonia and chronic lung disease.[54]

A second study examined the possibility that some eyes with ROP of less than threshold severity might benefit from treatment. The multicenter Early Treatment for Retinopathy of Prematurity Randomized Trial (ETROP)[115] was conducted at 26 clinical sites in the USA. This study used a risk model (RM-ROP2, based on data from the CRYO-ROP study) including patient demographic characteristics, pace of disease, and severity of retinopathy to predict the likelihood of eyes with prethreshold ROP going on to retinal detachment.[241] Prethreshold ROP was defined as:

1. Zone 1, any ROP less than threshold.
2. Zone 2, stage 2 with plus disease and stage 3 without plus disease.
3. Stage 3 with plus disease but less than threshold.

Eyes found to have a risk of 0.15 or greater of progressing to unfavorable structural outcome were randomized to receive peripheral retinal ablation (with laser photocoagulation since it was now in general use) at the diagnosis of "high-risk prethreshold" or to conventional management. Conventional management consisted of observation with treatment only if threshold ROP developed. Four hundred and one infants with high-risk ROP in one or both eyes participated.

The initial report showed that early treatment of high-risk prethreshold eyes significantly reduced unfavorable outcomes.[115] At 9 months, grating acuity was assessed and showed a reduction in unfavorable visual acuity outcomes from 19.5% to 14.5% (p = 0.01). Structural outcomes also benefited from early treatment with a reduction in unfavorable structural outcomes from 15.6% of conventionally treated eyes to 9.1% for earlier-treated eyes (p<0.001). The ETROP investigators developed a clinical algorithm based on the ROP status of an eye that provides the clinician with indications of whether an eye should be considered for treatment. Two types of prethreshold disease are defined:

Type 1 should be considered for earlier treatment.
Type 2 can be followed conservatively and treated if progression to type 1 or threshold is observed.

Using this algorithm, approximately 38% fewer high-risk eyes would be treated with no increase in unfavorable outcomes. At the final ETROP 6-year examinations,[242] there continued to be a benefit to ocular structure in early-treated eyes compared to conventionally managed eyes (8.9% vs 15.2%, p<0.001), but there was no statistically significant visual benefit from earlier treatment of high-risk prethreshold eyes. Among early treatment eyes, 24.6% had unfavorable visual acuity compared to 29% of conventionally managed eyes. However, when the results at 6 years were classified using the type 1 or type 2 algorithm, visual acuity was significantly better in the group of eyes with type 1 compared to the eyes with type 2 ROP (25.1% vs. 32.8%, p = 0.02). Furthermore, there is a significant benefit to the extent of visual field, measured using white-sphere double arc perimetry, for the group of eyes with type 1 ROP that received early treatment compared to the group of type 2 eyes.[243]

Current treatment of ROP

Treatment details change rapidly.[157,244-247]

Rationale and criteria for treatment

The aim of treatment is to remove the stimulus for vessel growth by ablating the peripheral avascular retina. Either cryotherapy or laser can be used, and, although both are effective,[244,248-251] laser is the modality of choice by most ophthalmologists (93% in STOP-ROP study).[54] Although treatment is usually applied to the entire 360° of the retina, partial ablation is sometimes considered for highly localized disease.[252]

Indications for treatment

After the ET-ROP study,[115] the recommendation for treatment of severe acute phase ROP is now laser photocoagulation within 48–72 hours for eyes that have type 1 ROP and close observation for progression of eyes that develop type 2 ROP (Table 43.4).

Type 1 ROP is defined as:

1. Zone 1, any stage of ROP with plus disease.
2. Zone 1, stage 3 with or without plus disease.
3. Zone 2, stage 2 or 3 with plus disease.

These eyes have highly active ROP and should be considered for early treatment.

Table 43.4 – Treatment algorithm based on results of the ETROP study

	Zone	Stage of ROP	Plus disease
Type 1 ROP: treatment indicated	Zone I	Any stage ROP	+
	Zone I	Stage 3 ROP	−
	Zone II	Stage 2 or 3	+
Type 2 ROP: observe closely for progression	Zone I	Stage 1 or 2	−
	Zone II	Stage 1	+
	Zone II	Stage 1, 2, or 3	−
Other ROP: observe for progression	Zone III	Any ROP	+/−

Type 2 is defined as:

1. Zone 1, stage 1 or 2 with no plus disease.
2. Zone 2, stage 3 with no plus disease.

These eyes should be followed conservatively and treated should they progress to type 1 ROP.

The window for treatment probably is a *maximum* of 1 week; treatment should be undertaken as soon as possible. Determining the urgency of treatment requires clinical judgment; some eyes with posterior ROP with severe plus disease require very urgent treatment, some eyes progress more slowly and the urgency is less. Treatment should ideally be performed in the NICU where there are neonatal support facilities.

Cryotherapy is painful and systemic complications can occur.[253] Laser treatment can take an hour to perform. Both can be performed under sedation or full anesthesia, but the important components are good analgesia and facilities for artificial ventilation. A neonatologist, or a neonatal anesthetist, will help in this decision. Resuscitation equipment must be available, and an intravenous line must be in place before starting the administration of sedation or anesthetic agents.

Laser

Interest in using laser for treatment of acute phase ROP was facilitated by the introduction of portable diode and argon lasers delivered through an indirect ophthalmoscope. Had the clinical trial of treatment for ROP been delayed until after this development, laser rather than cryotherapy may have been employed.[254] Portable indirect laser is now the treatment of choice.[248-251,255-257] No large randomized trial comparing the outcomes after cryotherapy or laser treatment is likely to be undertaken due to the large sample needed. Laser can be accurately placed, is simpler than cryotherapy to administer in experienced hands, and may be easier to deliver and more effective in zone 1 disease. Whether laser lesions should be confluent or one burn-width apart is debated.[246] Complications of laser include corneal, iris, and lens burn; the tunica vasculosa lentis may absorb energy. Cataract formation has been reported.[258] Retinal or vitreous hemorrhage may occur, but is probably not laser-specific. Diode red (810 nm) may be preferable to argon green (514 nm) laser for ROP.[244] The former is more portable and requires less power. It causes less tissue destruction and, as energy is less likely to be taken up by other ocular tissues, complications are fewer.

Laser can be applied by a trans-scleral probe, not dissimilar to the cryoprobe, to the external scleral surface, which induces retinal blanching as with transpupillary laser.[259]

Cryotherapy

Cryotherapy is applied trans-sclerally to the avascular zone anterior to the acute ROP lesion, avoiding it. Using a retinal probe or one specially designed, the cryotherapy lesions are applied confluently. The endpoint of cryotherapy is the appearance of whitening of the retina due to freezing. It is not necessary to open the conjunctiva unless the lesion is so posterior that the posterior section of the avascular zone cannot be reached.

In the absence of active ROP it is not necessary to re-treat all skip areas. Ocular complications of cryotherapy include eyelid edema, lacerations, and hemorrhage of the conjunctiva, and preretinal and vitreous hemorrhage.

Postoperative management

Postoperative eyedrops (steroid and antibiotic) are often instilled for a few days postoperatively. The response to treatment becomes visible by 6–7 days with the subsidence of plus disease, regression of the ROP lesion, and the appearance of pigmented lesions. Should treatment fail to induce regression, re-treatment should be considered within 7–14 days. If left much later, the fibrotic process will have begun and outcome will be compromised. Assessing whether ROP will resolve or require re-treatment is one of the most difficult management problems.

Retinal detachment surgery

The benefit of surgical intervention for stage 5 ROP is unclear. 67–70% of stage 4 and 40% of stage 5 eyes can be surgically reattached.[260] Lens-sparing vitrectomy for partial retinal detachment has been advocated,[261] but others used a variety of surgical procedures including scleral buckle and vitrectomy.[262] For older infants both "open sky"[263] and closed vitrectomy[264-265] approaches have been used, anatomic reattachment being achieved in 40–50% of cases. Infants who developed retinal detachment in the CRYO-ROP study were managed conservatively (71 eyes) or by vitrectomy (58 eyes).[266] Reattachment was achieved in 28% of the former and none of the latter. Only two eyes (both in the vitrectomy group) had any pattern vision, and that at the lowest measurable spatial frequency. A follow-up report provided structural and functional results on the same cohort at age 5½ years.[267] All except one of the 128 eyes in 98 children had vision limited to light perception or no light perception, regardless of whether a vitrectomy had been performed. Significantly better acuities were reported in a small number of infants following surgery for stage 5 ROP.[268] A series of eyes that had initially responded successfully to vitrectomy were reviewed:[269] retinas that were attached after surgery re-detached and the visual results were disappointing, although they concluded that "there is some evidence that vitrectomized eyes function better than non-vitrectomized eyes." With such dismal results, surgical management cannot be recommended.[270] It is critical that parents are made aware of the difference between structural and functional success.

The situation for patients with regressed ROP who develop vitreoretinal complications in adult life is different; most eyes can be successfully treated.[271-272] With such a variable clinical picture, the functional improvement in many cases is quite modest; however, the stability of the eye is improved.

Other potential therapies for severe ROP

The BEAT-ROP (bevacizumab eliminates the angiogenic threat of retinopathy of prematurity) study[273] provides evidence that anti-VEGF treatment may result in outcomes at least as good as, or better than, those currently achieved with laser photocoagulation. This trial follows a series of case reports and case series reporting the use of anti-VEGF as a primary treatment, rescue therapy, and as an adjunctive therapy.[274-281]

The BEAT-ROP trial[273] was a prospective, controlled, randomized, multicenter trial that compared the outcome of babies who had stage 3+ ROP in zone I or zone II and who were randomized to receive intravitreal bevacizumab (0.625 mg in 0.025 ml of solution) or undergo conventional laser photocoagulation. From the sample of 150 babies (300 eyes), 143 survived to PMA 54 weeks when the primary outcome measure of recurrence of ROP requiring re-treatment could be determined. When both zone I and zone II eyes were considered, 6 of the 140 eyes (4%) of the bevacizumab group required re-treatment compared to 32 of the 146 eyes (22%) in the laser treated group (p = 0.002). This effect was largely driven by eyes with zone I disease. Seven of the enrolled babies died before the PMA 54 week endpoint, five in the bevacizumab group and two in the laser group. These results should be viewed with caution; long-term follow-up is planned. The study sample was inadequate to determine longer term ocular and systemic safety. The editorial accompanying the article was more emphatic in recommending bevacizumab for zone I ROP.[282]

There have been a series of Letters to the Editor[283-287] and articles[288-291] raising concerns about components of this study including the dosage used, the choice of primary outcome, how long the baby would have to be followed, and whether the findings can be generalized, as well as concerns about systemic and ocular safety. More work is needed in this promising area. Randomized clinical trials need to be undertaken to determine ocular and systemic adverse effects. These studies must have sufficient follow-up to determine visual function and neurodevelopmental outcomes.

Involving parents

The parents of a very preterm infant have much to cope with and they have a right to know what ocular problems may befall their baby. Providing sensitive, balanced written information is important, but face-to-face discussion is essential to enable parents to be part of the decision-making process.[291a] Information is required at several stages. It is important to discuss the possibility of ROP early during the baby's hospital stay even though serious disease may not develop until near discharge. Such a discussion will eliminate the need to discuss surgical intervention at the first contact from the examining ophthalmologist.

Written information should be available at three levels for:

1. All babies who are to undergo ROP examination: A general description of ROP is required, which emphasizes that, although ROP is a frequent occurrence, over 90% of cases of acute retinopathy spontaneously resolve without adverse sequelae. Generally, the ophthalmologist does not personally counsel the parents of all babies who have ROP examinations, but the ophthalmologist should be available to speak to any parent requiring more information.

2. The parents of babies with ROP that might become severe: Written information that emphasizes that treatment is available and may need to be considered should be supplied. The ophthalmologist should discuss the situation with parents, mindful of the fact that severe ROP often occurs just when the baby is nearing discharge. When severe ROP develops, always keep parents fully and frequently informed.

3. The parents of the baby with end-stage disease: Not all eyes with ROP respond satisfactorily to treatment and blindness still occurs. Ophthalmologists should not lose contact with the family. Most accept that treatment carefully performed sometimes fails, but they cannot accept what is perceived as lack of interest or care.[14] The ophthalmologist must ensure that the child gains early access to the services for the visually impaired with registration as blind or partially sighted. Encouraging the family to contact social and educational services is essential.

Outcome

Premature birth can affect the developing visual system by refractive changes (see Chapter 5), strabismus, neurologic damage (see Chapters 57 and 58), and retinopathy of prematurity. Most infants with ROP undergo complete resolution without adverse effects, and mild ROP (stages 1 and 2) has no additional adverse effect on vision.[291b] Severe ROP may impact acuity[220,292] and contrast sensitivity.[293] It was the less than ideal response following cryotherapy that generated the Early Treatment Study. Color vision does not seem to be affected by preterm birth alone, although the CRYO-ROP study noted an increased prevalence of blue–yellow deficits not related to ROP severity.[294,295] Visual field area measured at 10 or 11 years in children who had significant acute phase ROP was reduced regardless of whether the eyes underwent cryotherapy.[296,297] Both visual acuity and visual field benefitted from treatment of Type I but not Type II.[242,243]

The prevalence of strabismus is increased by preterm birth and by ROP stage (even mild ROP). The incidence of strabismus is raised from around 6% to over 30%,[298-307] and this increases as acute phase ROP increases.[307-309]

The direct consequences of ROP are more frequent in severe and posterior disease, but occasionally occur in mild acute ROP.[131] Retinal detachment can occur at any time of life, including after peripheral retinal ablation for severe ROP, although this is infrequent.[271,310,311] Large punched-out macular lesions are infrequent sequelae of severe ROP. When they develop is unknown, but they have been observed during infancy. Originally thought to be the consequence of cryotherapy,[312] they may occur in eyes that have not been treated.[313]

Anterior segment sequelae of severe ROP have been described.[313-314] Microcornea/microphthalmos may be the consequence of reduced growth during the acute phase or later shrinkage due to advanced cicatrization. Other changes are due to changes in the anterior vitreous causing anterior displacement of the iris-lens diaphragm, causing shallowing of the anterior chamber[131] and, if severe, corneal opacity and cataract.

Children who were preterm have an increased prevalence of all refractive errors, especially myopia.[294,310,315-321] Myopia is a consequence of low birth weight even in the absence of ROP. The myopia is low and has the following characteristics: steep corneal curvature, shallow anterior chamber, thick lens, and an axial length shorter than expected for the degree of myopia.[294,318,322,323] Myopia is a well-known complication of severe ROP. In contrast to myopia of prematurity, which has its onset in school years, myopia associated with severe ROP has its onset in infancy with progression during the first year after birth but with relative stability thereafter, unlike most forms of myopia not associated with ROP.[317,322] There is no significant difference in myopia between eyes with severe ROP that were treated compared to those that were not.[324]

References

8. Cross CW. Cost of preventing retrolental fibroplasia. Lancet 1973; 2: 954–6.

10. Smith LE. Through the eyes of a child: understanding retinopathy through ROP. The Friedenwald Lecture. Invest Ophthalmol Vis Sci 2008; 49(12): 5177–82.

23. Hellström A, Peruzzi C, Ju M, et al. Low IGF-1 suppresses VEGF-survival signalling in retinal endothelial cells: direct correlation with clinical retinopathy of prematurity. Proc Natl Acad Sci USA 2001; 98: 5804–8.

27. Darlow BA, Horwood LJ, Clemett RS. Retinopathy of prematurity: risk factors in a prospective population-based study. Paediatr Perinatal Epidemiol 1992; 6: 62–80.

41. Schaffer DB, Palmer EA, Plotsky DF, et al. on behalf of the Cryotherapy for Retinopathy of Prematurity Cooperative Group. Prognostic factors in the natural course of retinopathy of prematurity. Ophthalmology 1993; 100: 230–7.

50. Stenson B, Brocklehurst P, Tarnow-Mordi W; UK BOOST II trial; Australian BOOST II trial; New Zealand BOOST II trial. Increased 36-week survival with high oxygen saturation target in extremely preterm infants. N Engl J Med 2011; 364: 1680–2.

78. Darlow BA, Hutchinson JL, Henderson-Smart DJ, et al. Australian and New Zealand Neonatal Network: Prenatal risk factors for severe retinopathy of prematurity among very preterm infants of the Australian and New Zealand Neonatal Network. Pediatrics 2005; 115: 990–6.

101. Hepner WR, Krause AC, Davis ME. Retrolental fibroplasia and light. Pediatrics 1949; 3: 824–8.

108. Gilbert C, Fielder A, Gordillo L, et al. on behalf of the International NO-ROP Group. Characteristics of infants with severe retinopathy of prematurity in countries with low, moderate and high levels of development: Implications for screening programs. Pediatrics 2005; 115: e518–25.

110. Committee for the Classification of Retinopathy of Prematurity. The international classification of retinopathy of prematurity. Br J Ophthalmol 1984; 68: 690–7.

111. Committee for the Classification of Retinopathy of Prematurity II. The classification of retinal detachment. Arch Ophthalmol 1987; 105: 106–12.

113. An International Committee for the Classification of Retinopathy of Prematurity. The International Classification of Retinopathy of Prematurity – Revisited. Arch Ophthalmol 2005; 123: 991–9.

115. Early Treatment for Retinopathy of Prematurity Cooperative Group. Revised indications for the treatment of retinopathy of prematurity. Arch Ophthalmol 2003; 121: 1684–96.

119. Palmer EA, Flynn JT, Hardy RJ, The Cryotherapy for Retinopathy of Prematurity Cooperative Group. Incidence and early course of retinopathy of prematurity. Ophthalmology 1991;98: 1628–40.

131. Cryotherapy for Retinopathy of Prematurity Cooperative Group. Multicenter trial of cryotherapy for retinopathy of prematurity: preliminary results. Arch Ophthalmol 1988; 106: 471–9.

144. Cryotherapy for Retinopathy of Prematurity Cooperative Group. Multicenter Trial of Cryotherapy for Retinopathy of Prematurity: Fifteen-year outcomes following threshold retinopathy of prematurity: final results from the Multicenter Trial of Cryotherapy. Arch Ophthalmol 2005; 123: 311–18.

148. Reynolds JD, Dobson V, Quinn GE, et al. on behalf of the CRYO-ROP and LIGHT-ROP Cooperative Groups. Evidence-based screening for retinopathy of prematurity: natural history data from CRYO-ROP and LIGHT-ROP Studies. Arch Ophthalmol 2002; 120: 1470–6.

158. Section on Ophthalmology. American Academy of Pediatrics, American Academy of Ophthalmology, American Association for Pediatric Ophthalmology and Strabismus. Screening examination of premature infants for retinopathy of prematurity. Pediatrics 2006; 117(2): 572–6. Erratum in: Pediatrics 2006; 118(3): 1324.

159. Wilkinson AR, Haines L, Head K, Fielder AR. UK retinopathy of prematurity guideline. Early Hum Dev 2008; 84: 71–4. In full http://www.rcpch.ac.uk/ROP.

177. Lofqvist C, Andersson E, Sigurdsson J, et al. Longitudinal postnatal weight and insulin-like growth factor I measurements in the prediction of retinopathy of prematurity. Arch Ophthalmol 2006; 124(12): 1711–18.

181. Binenbaum G, Ying GS, Quinn GE, et al. Premature Infants in Need of Transfusion Study Group. A clinical prediction model to stratify retinopathy of prematurity risk using postnatal weight gain. Pediatrics 2011; 127: e607–14.

198. Wilson CM, Cocker KD, Moseley MJ, et al. Computerized analysis of retinal vessel width and tortuosity in premature infants. Invest Ophthalmol Vis Sci 2008; 49: 3577–85.

226. Fielder AR, Gilbert C, Ells A, Quinn GE. Internet-based eye care. Lancet 2006; 367: 300–1.

233. Quinn GE, Dobson V, Hardy RJ, et al., for the CRYO-ROP Cooperative Group. Visual fields measured with double-arc perimetry in eyes with threshold retinopathy of prematurity (ROP) from the CRYO-ROP trial. Ophthalmology 1996; 103: 1432–7.

240. Quinn GE, Dobson V, Barr CC, et al. Visual acuity of eyes after vitrectomy for ROP: follow-up at 5½ years. Ophthalmology 1996; 103: 595–600.

273. Mintz-Hittner HA, Kennedy KA, Chuang AZ, for the BEAT-ROP Cooperative Group. Efficacy of intravitreal bevacizumab for stage 3+ retinopathy of prematurity. N Engl J Med 2011; 364: 603–15.

287. Moshfeghi DM, Berrocal AM. Retinopathy of prematurity in the time of bevacizumab: Incorporating the BEAT-ROP results into clinical practice. Ophthalmology 2011; 118: 1227–8.

322. Quinn GE, Dobson V, Kivlin J, et al. Prevalence of myopia between three months and 5½ years in preterm infants with and without retinopathy of prematurity. Ophthalmology 1998; 105: 1292–300.

Access the complete reference list online at
http://www.expertconsult.com

Inherited retinal disorders

Michel Michaelides • Graham E Holder • Anthony T Moore

Chapter contents

Introduction

The inherited retinal disorders are a clinically and genetically heterogeneous group of conditions: many become symptomatic in childhood, occurring as an isolated abnormality in an otherwise healthy child. Some are associated with systemic abnormalities (see Chapter 45). Most of the genes causing the major childhood retinal dystrophies have been identified: the genotype–phenotype relationship is complex. There is considerable genetic heterogeneity for individual clinical disorders, and mutations in a single gene may give rise to several different phenotypes. Despite this, these disorders can be usefully divided clinically according to whether they:

1. Are stationary or progressive

2. Exhibit predominantly rod or cone involvement.

Stationary disorders present at birth or in the early months of life and are best referred to as dysfunction syndromes. Progressive conditions, which typically present later, are termed dystrophies.

Stationary retinal dysfunction syndromes

These include the forms of stationary night-blindness (rod dysfunction syndromes) and the cone dysfunction syndromes (stationary cone disorders).

Stationary night-blindness (rod dysfunction syndromes)

There are three main forms of stationary night-blindness; in congenital stationary night-blindness (CSNB) the fundus is normal or shows myopic changes. Fundus albipunctatus and Oguchi's disease have a distinctive fundus appearance.

Congenital stationary night-blindness

Clinical findings

CSNB is characterized by night-blindness, variable visual loss, and a normal fundus. It may be inherited as an autosomal dominant (AD), autosomal recessive (AR), or X-linked (XL) disorder.

The visual acuity is usually normal or mildly reduced in the AD form, whereas mild to moderate central visual loss is common in the AR and XL subtypes. Other features of XL and AR CSNB include moderate to high myopia, nystagmus, strabismus, and paradoxical pupil responses. Fundus examination is usually normal but some patients have myopic fundi and pale or tilted optic disks (Fig. 44.1). Patients with AD CSNB usually present with symptomatic night-blindness, but in XL and AR CSNB, patients usually present in infancy with nystagmus, strabismus, and reduced vision. Nystagmus is not invariable and some patients are not diagnosed until late childhood or adulthood. The diagnosis is easily missed without

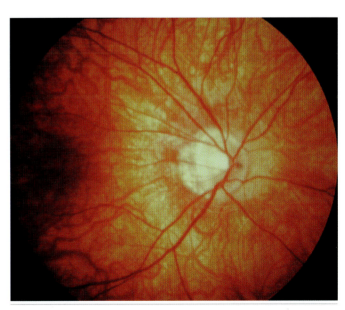

Fig. 44.1 X-linked congenital stationary night-blindness. Tilted optic disk with myopic fundus.

electroretinography (ERG). XL and AR CSNB may be further subdivided into *complete* and *incomplete* forms. This differentiation was originally proposed in XL disease using electrophysiologic and psychophysical criteria and was subsequently shown to reflect genetically distinct disorders.

Electrophysiology

International Society for Clinical Electrophysiology of Vision (ISCEV) standard ERGs should be performed. This may not be possible in infants in whom a modified protocol is used (see Chapter 8). Four main responses are defined: a rod-specific ERG and a bright flash response performed under scotopic conditions, and two measures of cone function, a 30 Hz flicker ERG and a single flash photopic ERG. Both complete and incomplete CSNB show a "negative ERG": the photoreceptor-derived a-wave in the bright flash response is normal, but there is selective reduction in the inner nuclear derived b-wave, such that it is smaller than the a-wave, indicating predominantly inner retinal dysfunction. In complete CSNB there is no detectable rod-specific ERG and a profoundly negative bright flash response. Cone ERGs show subtle abnormalities reflecting ON bipolar cell dysfunction (Fig. 44.2). There is a detectable rod-specific ERG in incomplete CSNB, and a profoundly negative bright flash response. Cone ERGs are much more abnormal than in complete CSNB, reflecting involvement of both ON- and OFF bipolar pathways. They show the characteristic triphasic appearance in the flicker response (see Fig. 44.2).

ERG evidence of inner retinal rod system dysfunction may also occur in AD CSNB but in association with normal ISCEV cone ERGs. In other cases of AD CSNB, ERG rod responses are attenuated with normal cone responses, but the standard bright flash response does not have a negative waveform.

Molecular genetics and pathogenesis

Autosomal dominant CSNB Mutations in the genes encoding three components of rod-specific phototransduction have been reported in AD CSNB: rhodopsin, the α-subunit of rod transducin and the rod cyclic guanosine monophosphate (cGMP) phosphodiesterase β-subunit (PDEβ).

X-linked CSNB Two causative genes (*CACNA1F* and *NYX*) have been identified accounting for most families with XL CSNB. Incomplete CSNB is associated with mutation in *CACNA1F*, which encodes the retina-specific α_{1F}-subunit of the voltage-gated L-type calcium channel. The expression of *CACNA1F* appears limited to photoreceptors and is prominent in the synaptic terminals. Most mutations are inactivating truncation sequence variants. The loss of functional channels impairs the calcium flux into rod and cone photoreceptors required to sustain tonic neurotransmitter release from presynaptic terminals. This results in the inability to maintain the normal transmembrane potential of bipolar cells, so the retina remains in a partially light-stimulated state, unable to respond to changes in light-levels.

Complete CSNB is associated with mutation in *NYX*, the gene encoding the leucine-rich proteoglycan nyctalopin. Leucine-rich repeats are believed to be important for protein interactions, with many of the mutations identified within these repeats. Nyctalopin is expressed in photoreceptor inner segments, outer and inner nuclear layers, and ganglion cells. Nyctalopin may guide and promote the formation and function of the retinal ON- pathway.

Several genotype–phenotype studies have been performed in individuals with either *CACNA1F* or *NYX* mutations. There is considerable inter- and intra-familial phenotypic variability associated with *CACNA1F* mutations, even with an identical sequence variant,[1] suggesting that other genetic or environmental factors modify the phenotype. Although most patients with XL CSNB have non-progressive disease, Nakamura et al. reported two brothers with a *CACNA1F* mutation and progressive decline in vision with eventually undetectable rod and cone ERGs.[2] We have also infrequently observed slow progression in patients with XL CSNB. Patients with complete CSNB (*NYX* mutations) are invariably myopic and have more pronounced night-blindness.[3]

Autosomal recessive CSNB Mutations in *GRM6* and *TRPM1* lead to complete CSNB. *GRM6* encodes a metabotropic glutamate receptor (mGluR6) located on the dendrites of rod and cone ON bipolar cells, mediating the sign inversion that occurs at the first synapse, such that glutamate release in the dark by photoreceptors causes hyperpolarization of the ON bipolar cell membrane. TRPM1, a transient receptor potential cation channel, subfamily M, member 1, is probably involved in effecting the membrane voltage change in ON bipolar cells in response to glutamate.

Mutations in *CABP4* have been associated with incomplete CSNB. CABP4, a member of the calcium-binding protein (CABP) family, is specifically located in photoreceptor synaptic terminals, where it is directly associated with the C-terminal domain of CACNA1F.

Sequence variants have been identified in *SLC24A1*, in patients with AR CSNB without a negative ERG; in the standard scotopic bright flash response, both the a- and b-waves are equally reduced.[4] SLC24A1 is a member of the solute carrier protein superfamily located in inner segments, outer and inner nuclear layers, and ganglion cells.

Åland Island eye disease

Åland Island eye disease (AIED) is an X-linked recessive disorder similar to incomplete CSNB, characterized by reduced visual acuity, nystagmus, nyctalopia, mild red–green dyschromatopsia, and myopia. Affected males may show iris translucency, foveal hypoplasia, and decreased fundus pigmentation. The clinical appearance may resemble X-linked ocular albinism (XLOA) but in XLOA color vision is usually normal and patients with AIED do not show the typical optic nerve fiber misrouting seen in albinism.[5]

The symptoms of night-blindness and the psychophysical and the ERG changes seen in AIED are similar to those in the incomplete form of the XL CSNB. Both disorders map to the same region of Xp: they are probably allelic but mutations in *CACNA1F* have not been identified in AIED.

Other related phenotypes

Patients with a contiguous gene syndrome (which includes glycerol kinase deficiency, congenital adrenal hypoplasia, Duchenne's muscular dystrophy (DMD), and ocular abnormalities known as Oregon eye disease), with a deletion of Xp21, have ocular features in common with affected males with AIED and have similar predominantly inner retinal ERG abnormalities. Furthermore, some males with isolated DMD (mutations of the dystrophin gene at Xp21) have ERG abnormalities similar to those of CSNB. All these multisystem

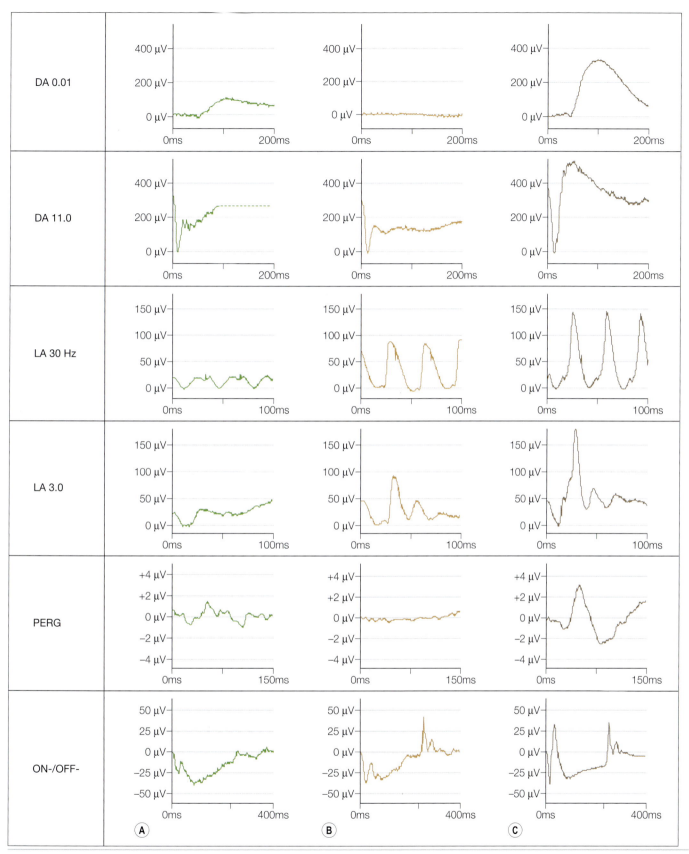

Fig. 44.2 Congenital stationary night-blindness. The left hand column traces (A) show data from a patient with "incomplete" CSNB (iCSNB); the center traces (B) are from a patient with "complete" CSNB (cCSNB); the right hand column traces (C) are from a representative normal subject. In iCSNB the rod ERG (DA 0.01) is mildly subnormal. The bright flash response (DA 11.0) is electronegative, with a normal a-wave confirming normal photoreceptor function, but a profoundly reduced b-wave. The 30 Hz flicker ERG (LA 30 Hz) is markedly subnormal and clearly shows the delayed double peak characteristically seen in iCSNB. The photopic single flash ERG (LA 3.0) shows marked reduction in the b : a ratio with simplification of the waveform and loss of the photopic oscillatory potentials, shown on ON-/OFF- response recording (200 ms orange stimulus on a green background) to reflect involvement of both ON- (depolarizing) and OFF- (hyperpolarizing) cone bipolar cell pathways. The PERG (pattern electroretinogram) is mildly subnormal in keeping with mild macular dysfunction. In cCSNB there is no detectable DA 0.01 response and the profoundly electronegative DA 11.0 ERG confirms the site of the dysfunction to be post-phototransduction. The LA 3.0 response shows a distinctive broadened a-wave and a sharply rising b-wave with a reduced b : a ratio and lack of photopic oscillatory potentials. This appearance indicates marked dysfunction of cone ON- bipolar cell pathways but preservation of the OFF- pathways. The profoundly negative ON- response, with preservation of the ON- a-wave and loss of the ON- b-wave, accompanied by a normal OFF- response supports this proposal. The broadened trough of the 30 Hz flicker ERG with a sharply rising peak is a manifestation of the same phenomenon. The PERG is almost undetectable. Overall, the findings in cCSNB are those of loss of ON- pathway function in both rod and cone systems.

disorders have a non-progressive form of predominantly rod retinal dysfunction.

Oguchi's disease

Clinical findings

Oguchi's disease is a rare autosomal recessive stationary night-blindness with a greyish or green-yellow discoloration of the fundus at the posterior pole or extending beyond the arcades, which reverts to normal on prolonged dark adaptation (Mizuo phenomenon) (Fig. 44.3). Exposure to light then usually leads to the gradual reappearance of the abnormal discoloration in 10–20 minutes.

Most patients present with poor night vision. Visual acuity is normal or mildly reduced and photopic visual fields and color vision are normal. Although most cases are from Japan it occurs in other races.

Electrophysiology and psychophysics

There are two types of Oguchi's disease depending on the dark adaptation findings:

Type 1: rod adaptation is markedly slowed; full recovery of sensitivity takes several hours and the absolute threshold is normal or only minimally elevated.

Type 2: there is no recognizable rod adaptation; the abnormal retinal appearance is less marked and the Mizuo phenomenon may be absent.

Most patients with Oguchi's disease have a "negative" bright flash ERG, confirming the site of dysfunction to be post-phototransduction, as in XL CSNB. As opposed to fundus albipunctatus (below), the ERG remains abnormal even after prolonged dark adaptation.

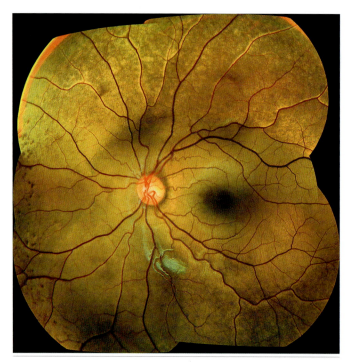

Fig. 44.3 Oguchi's disease. Greyish or green-yellow discoloration of the fundus, which reverts to normal on prolonged dark adaptation (Mizuo phenomenon).

Molecular genetics and pathogenesis

There is a truncating deletion in *SAG*, encoding arrestin, in patients with Oguchi's disease. Reduced activity of arrestin is likely to result in prolonged activation of transducin and rod phosphodiesterase following light exposure. cGMP levels would thereby be maintained at a low level in even dim light exposure and the outer segment cation channels would remain closed resulting in prolonged rod hyperpolarization. The rods would behave as if they were light adapted and would be unresponsive to light at low levels of illumination, explaining the psychophysical abnormalities.

Null mutations in *GRK1*, encoding a second component of the rod phototransduction pathway, rhodopsin kinase (RK), have also been identified in Oguchi's disease. The key function, of both RK and arrestin, in the normal deactivation and recovery of the photoreceptor after exposure to light, explains the delayed recovery in Oguchi's disease. The consequences of these reported RK mutations have been assessed by expression studies in COS7 cells of wild-type and human mutant RK. The markedly reduced mutant RK activity supported their pathogenicity.[6]

Evidence from knockout mice models suggests that patients with *SAG* or *GRK1* mutations may be more susceptible to light-induced retinal damage; it may therefore be advisable for patients to wear tinted spectacles.[7,8]

Fundus albipunctatus

Clinical findings

This autosomal recessive form of stationary night-blindness has a characteristic fundus appearance with multiple white dots throughout the retina. Patients either present with night-blindness or an abnormal retinal appearance on routine fundoscopy. The visual acuity is usually normal and the condition non-progressive.

The deposits are discrete dull white lesions at the level of the retinal pigment epithelium (RPE). They are most numerous in the mid-periphery and are usually absent at the macula; the optic discs and retinal vessels are normal. Fluorescein angiography shows multiple areas of hyperfluorescence, which may not directly correlate to the deposits seen clinically. In some patients there is good correlation between the white dots and increased autofluorescence on fundus autofluorescence imaging, but not in others. The differential diagnosis is from other causes of flecked retina (see Chapter 48).

Electrophysiology and psychophysics

Dark adaptation is severely delayed in fundus albipunctatus (FA), reflecting abnormal regeneration of rhodopsin. The rod-cone break is delayed and full rod adaptation may take many hours. Rod ERGs are markedly abnormal, with the rod-specific ERG (DA 0.01) being undetectable under standard conditions, but becoming normal following prolonged dark adaptation (Fig. 44.4). The dark-adapted bright flash ERG (DA 11.0), which after standard dark adaptation arises in dark-adapted cones, can have a low b : a ratio; a red flash stimulus under dark adaptation shows a normal cone component but an undetectable rod component and prevents confusion with a form of CSNB associated with a negative ERG. To confirm the diagnosis of FA it is necessary to exceed the ISCEV ERG standard recommendations for dark adaptation considerably. Most but not all patients with *RDH5* mutations show full recovery of rod function with extended dark adaptation. This contrasts with the findings in retinitis punctata albescens (see below),

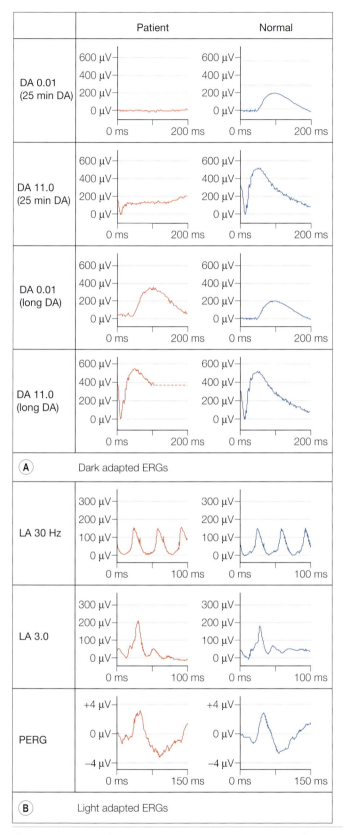

Fig. 44.4 Fundus albipunctatus. The DA 0.01 ERG is undetectable following a standard period of dark adaptation and the DA 11.0 response is reduced with additional reduction in the b:a ratio. However, following an extended period of dark adaptation both DA 0.01 and DA 11.0 responses are completely normal in keeping with delayed regeneration of rhodopsin.

related to mutation in *RLBP1*, and usually allows the distinction between the two disorders.

There are two forms of FA, one in which cone ERGs are normal, and a rarer form described as fundus albipunctatus with cone dystrophy and negative ERG.[9]

Molecular genetics and pathogenesis

Mutations in three genes (*RDH5*, *RLBP1*, and *RPE65*), encoding components of the visual cycle, have been identified to date. The gene *RDH5* encodes 11-cis-retinol dehydrogenase, a component of the visual cycle. Recombinant mutant 11-cis retinol dehydrogenases have reduced activity compared with recombinant enzyme with wild-type sequence.[10] The phenotype of patients with *RDH5* mutations is variable, including normal or reduced cone responses.[11] The function of the protein product of *RDH5* is consistent with the delay in the regeneration of photopigments characteristic of the disorder.

Mutations have also been reported in *RLBP1*, encoding the cytosolic cellular retinaldehyde binding protein (CRALBP). Retinitis punctata albescens is usually associated with *RLBP1* mutations (see below). CRALBP has been localized to the RPE Müller cells, and ciliary epithelium. It can select 11-cis-retinaldehyde from a mixture of retinoids and protect it from photoisomerisation, suggesting a possible role in the generation of 11-cis-retinoids in the visual cycle; in keeping with the phenotypic features of FA.

Sequence variants in *RPE65* have also been identified in patients with a retinal appearance similar to FA.[12] Reduced fundus autofluorescence has been observed in patients with *RPE65* and *RDH5* mutations,[11,12] supporting the belief that disruption of retinoid recycling in the RPE is essential for the development of FA.

Stationary cone disorders (cone dysfunction syndromes)

The cone dysfunction syndromes include congenital color vision disorders where there is normal visual acuity but defective color vision, and the various forms of cone dysfunction associated with reduced central vision and often nystagmus and photophobia (Table 44.1).[13]

Disorders of color vision with normal visual acuity

Color vision in humans is trichromatic; there are three classes of cone photoreceptor that contain visual pigments maximally sensitive at 560 nm (L-cones (red)), 535 nm (M-cones (green)) and 440 nm (S-cones (blue)). The genes for the protein component (opsin) of the red and green cone pigments are on the long arm of the X chromosome, and the blue cone opsin gene on chromosome 7. About 8% of men and 0.5% of women have a red–green color vision defect, which is associated with abnormalities of the red and green cone opsin genes. Tritanopia is an uncommon autosomal dominant disorder in which there is a specific deficiency of blue cone sensitivity associated with mutations of the blue cone opsin gene.

This group of disorders, their clinical characteristics, and the molecular pathology are reviewed elsewhere.[14]

Achromatopsia

Achromatopsia is genetically heterogeneous and characterized by an absence of functioning cones in the retina.[13] It may occur in complete (typical) and incomplete (atypical) forms.

Table 44.1 – Summary of the cone dysfunction syndromes

Cone dysfunction syndrome	Alternative names	Mode of inheritance	Visual acuity	Refractive error	Nystagmus	Color vision	Fundi	Mutated gene(s) or chromosome locus
Complete achromatopsia	Rod monochromatism Typical achromatopsia	Autosomal recessive	6/36– 6/60	Often hypermetropia	Present	Absent	Usually normal	CNGA3 CNGB3 GNAT2 PDE6C
Incomplete achromatopsia	Atypical achromatopsia	Autosomal recessive	6/24– 6/60	Often hypermetropia	Present	Residual	Usually normal	CNGA3 PDE6C
Oligocone trichromacy	Oligocone syndrome	Autosomal recessive	6/12– 6/24	Equal incidence of myopia and hypermetropia	Often absent	Normal	Normal	–
RGS9/R9AP retinopathy	Bradyopsia	Autosomal recessive	6/12– 6/24	Equal incidence of myopia and hypermetropia	Often absent	Normal	Normal	RGS9 R9AP
Cone monochromatism	-	Uncertain	6/6	–	Absent	Absent or markedly reduced	Normal	–
Blue cone monochromatism	X-linked atypical achromatopsia X-linked incomplete achromatopsia	X-linked	6/24– 6/60	Often myopia	Present	Residual tritan discrimination	Usually normal or myopic	(i) Deletion of the LCR (ii) Single inactivated L/M hybrid gene
Bornholm eye disease	–	X-linked	6/9– 6/18	Moderate to high myopia with astigmatism	Absent	Deuteranopia Protanopia	Myopic	Xq28

Complete achromatopsia (rod monochromatism)

Clinical and histopathologic findings

The usual presentation is with reduced vision, nystagmus, and marked photophobia in infancy. The incidence is approximately 1 in 30 000. Parents often comment that vision is much better in dim illumination. Pupil reactions are sluggish or may show paradoxical constriction in the dark. High hyperopic refractive errors may be present and the fundi are normal. The nystagmus and photophobia, marked in infancy, may improve with age.

The visual acuity is usually 6/60 and there is complete color blindness. Peripheral visual fields are normal but a small central scotoma can often be detected. Achromatopsia is generally a stationary disorder but slow deterioration and macular atrophy may occur.[15,16]

Histopathologic studies have demonstrated cone-like structures in the retina,[17,18] which have also been observed *in vivo* using adaptive optics imaging, albeit to a variable degree.[16] This is promising with regard to gene replacement therapy.

Electrophysiology and psychophysics

The dark adaptation curve is monophasic with no evidence of a cone contribution and spectral sensitivity studies show that rods mediate threshold under both photopic and scotopic conditions; there is no evidence of a Purkinje shift. Electroretinography (Fig. 44.5) shows normal rod-derived ERGs but no detectable cone-derived responses.

Molecular genetics and pathogenesis

Achromatopsia is recessively inherited and genetically heterogeneous. Four genes have been identified, CNGA3, CNGB3, GNAT2 and PDE6C; all encoding components of cone phototransduction.

CNGA3 and CNGB3 code for the α- and β-subunits of the cGMP-gated (CNG) cation channel in cone cells, respectively. In the dark, cGMP levels are high in cone photoreceptors, therefore enabling cGMP to bind to the α- and β-subunits of CNG channels, resulting in them adopting an open conformation and permitting influx of cations, with consequent cone depolarization. When light is applied, activated photopigment interacts with transducin, a three-subunit guanine nucleotide binding protein, stimulating the exchange of bound GDP for GTP. The cone α-transducin subunit (encoded by GNAT2), which is bound to GTP, is then released from its β- and γ-subunits and activates cGMP-phosphodiesterase by removing the inhibitory γ-subunits from the active site of this enzyme, which is formed by two α-subunits (encoded by PDE6C). cGMP-phosphodiesterase lowers the concentration of cGMP in the photoreceptor, which results in closure of cGMP-gated cation channels.

More than 60 disease-causing mutations in CNGA3 have been identified in patients with achromatopsia; with four mutations (Arg277Cys, Arg283Trp, Arg436Trp, and Phe-547Leu) accounting for approximately 40% of all mutant CNGA3 alleles.[19] By comparison, far fewer mutations have

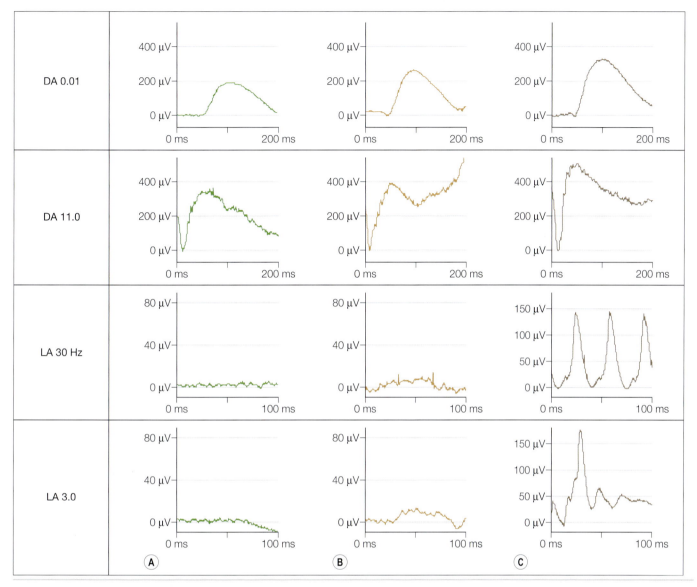

Fig. 44.5 ERGs from a patient with rod monochromacy (A), a patient with S-cone monochromacy (B), and a representative normal (C). The rod-specific (DA 0.01) and bright flash ERGs (DA 11.0) show no definite abnormality in either of these cone dysfunction syndromes. The 30 Hz flicker ERG (*LA 30 Hz) is undetectable in both, but the single flash photopic ERG (LA 3.0) is small and late, typical of S-cone origins. Note that the scale for the photopic ERGs in the two patients differs from that in the normal subject better to illustrate the low amplitude LA 3.0 response in the S-cone monochromat.

been identified in *CNGB3*; with the 1 base-pair frameshift deletion, 1148delC (Thr383fs), accounting for up to 80% of *CNGB3* mutant disease chromosomes.[20,21] The majority of *CNGA3* mutations identified to date are missense mutations, indicating that there is little tolerance for substitutions with respect to functional and structural integrity of the channel polypeptide. In contrast, the majority of *CNGB3* alterations are nonsense mutations.

About 70% of achromatopsia results from mutations of *CNGA3* and *CNGB3*, with *GNAT2* and *PDE6C* each accounting for less than 1%;[19,20,21] further causative genes remain to be discovered.

Incomplete achromatopsia

Clinical findings

The presentation and clinical findings in infancy are similar to the complete form of achromatopsia, but the visual prognosis may be better. Visual acuity is often in the range 6/24–6/36 and there may be some residual color perception. This form is also inherited as an autosomal recessive trait.

Molecular genetics and pathogenesis

As in the complete form, mutations in *CNGA3* have been identified in individuals with incomplete achromatopsia.[19] The mutations identified are all missense mutations, located throughout the channel polypeptide including the transmembrane domains, ion pore, and cGMP-binding region. Only three of these, Arg427Cys, Arg563His, and Thr565Met, are exclusively found in patients with incomplete achromatopsia.[19] Therefore, in the majority of cases of incomplete achromatopsia, other factors may influence the phenotype such as modifier genes or environmental factors. The missense variants identified in incomplete achromatopsia must be compatible with residual channel function since the phenotype is milder than in complete achromatopsia. Mutations in *PDE6C* have also been identified in incomplete achromatopsia.[22]

Mutations in *CNGB3* or *GNAT2* have not been reported in association with incomplete achromatopsia. However all *GNAT2* mutations to date, and the vast majority of *CNGB3* mutants, result in premature termination of translation, and thereby truncated and probably non-functional phototransduction proteins. Therefore an incomplete achromatopsia phenotype is unlikely to be compatible with these genotypes, which are predicted to encode mutant products lacking any residual function.

S-cone monochromatism (blue cone monochromatism)

Clinical findings

Blue cone monochromatism (BCM) is an X-linked recessive disorder, affecting approximately 1 in 100 000 individuals, in which affected males have normal rod and blue (S) cone function but lack red (L) and green (M) cone function. The clinical features are similar to complete achromatopsia but less severe. Affected infants have photophobia and develop small amplitude rapid nystagmus in early infancy. They are usually myopic, in contrast to achromatopsia (Fig. 44.6). The nystagmus reduces with time.

BCM is generally accepted to be a stationary disorder but deterioration and the development of macular atrophy may occur.[23,24,25,26]

Electrophysiology and psychophysics

Achromatopsia and BCM may be differentiated by the mode of inheritance, findings on psychophysical testing and electrophysiology. There is some preservation of the single flash photopic ERG (LA 3.0) in BCM (Fig. 44.5), and specialised spectral ERG techniques to measure S-cone ERGs can also be used (see Fig. 44.5). Female carriers of X-linked BCM may have abnormal cone ERGs and mild anomalies of color vision.

Color vision tests that probe the tritan color axis, such as the Hardy, Rand and Rittler® (HRR) plates, are necessary in order to distinguish between achromatopsia and BCM; with relative preservation of tritan discrimination in BCM. Blue cone monochromats display fewer errors along the vertical axis in the Farnsworth 100-hue test (fewer tritan errors), and may display protan-like patterns on the Farnsworth D-15.

Molecular genetics and pathogenesis

Mutation analyses have established the molecular basis for BCM.[24] The mutations in the L- and M-opsin gene array cause BCM to fall into two main classes:

1. A normal L- and M- pigment gene array is inactivated by a deletion in the locus control region (LCR), located upstream of the L-pigment gene. A deletion here abolishes transcription of all genes in the pigment gene array and therefore inactivates both L- and M-cones.

2. The LCR is preserved but changes within the L- and M-pigment gene array lead to loss of functional pigment production. The most common genotype in this class consists of a single inactivated L/M hybrid gene. The first step in this second mechanism is unequal crossing over reducing the number of genes in the array to one, followed in the second step by a mutation that inactivates the remaining gene. The most frequent inactivating mutation that has been described is a thymine-to-cytosine transition at nucleotide 648, which results in a cysteine-to-arginine substitution at codon 203 (Cys203Arg), a mutation known to disrupt the folding of cone opsin molecules.

The data suggest that 40% of BCM genotypes are a result of a one-step mutational pathway that leads to deletion of the LCR. The remaining 60% of BCM genotypes comprise a heterogeneous group of multi-step pathways. Studies have not detected the genetic alteration that would explain the BCM phenotype in all assessed individuals.[24] In one study the structure of the opsin array did not reveal the genetic mechanism for the disorder in 9 of 35 affected patients[24] which may suggest genetic heterogeneity yet to be identified in BCM.

Oligocone trichromacy

Oligocone trichromacy is characterized by reduced visual acuity (6/12 to 6/24), mild photophobia, normal fundi, reduced cone ERGs with normal rod responses, and normal color vision.[13] Patients have been described both with and without nystagmus. These patients may have a reduced number of normal functioning cones (oligocone) with preservation of the three cone types in the normal proportions, thereby permitting trichromacy. High-resolution quantitative retinal imaging supports this.[27]

Color vision testing either reveals normal or slightly elevated color discrimination thresholds. Slightly elevated discrimination thresholds are compatible with a reduction in cone numbers.

Oligocone trichromacy is inherited as an autosomal recessive trait; the molecular genetic basis is unknown. Patients with either *RGS9/R9AP* mutations ("bradyopsia"; see below) or oligocone trichromacy have very similar clinical phenotypes, characterized by stationary cone dysfunction with normal color vision.[28] The distinctive electrophysiologic features associated with *RGS9* and *R9AP* mutations enable directed genetic screening.

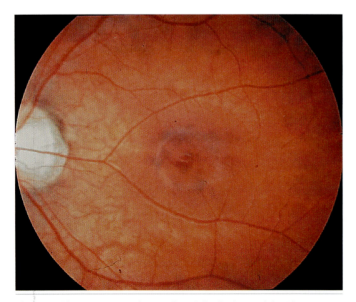

Fig. 44.6 Blue cone monochromatism. Pale tilted optic disk with myopic fundus.

RGS9/R9AP retinopathy (bradyopsia)

Clinical findings

Bradyopsia is a stationary cone dysfunction syndrome with onset in early childhood; it is characterized by mild photophobia, markedly delayed dark and light adaptation, moderately reduced visual acuity, normal color vision, and normal fundi. Some patients report difficulty seeing moving objects. It is not possible clinically to distinguish bradyopsia from oligocone trichromacy; however there are pathognomonic findings on extended electrophysiologic assessment.[28]

Electrophysiology

The rod-specific ERG (DA 0.01), the red flash ERG under dark adaptation (which has both a cone and rod component), and the single bright white flash (DA 11.0) with inter-stimulus interval (ISI) of 2 minutes are normal. The DA 11.0 ERGs with an ISCEV standard ISI of 20 seconds show amplitude reduction, which becomes progressively less severe with increasing ISI, consistent with delayed recovery following the flash. The pattern electroretinogram (PERG) and standard 30 Hz flicker ERG (LA 30 Hz) are usually undetectable. A residual low amplitude standard photopic single flash ERG (LA 3.0) is usually recorded.

The electrophysiologic findings are distinctive for the disorder, needing more extended testing than in the ISCEV ERG standard protocol which shows normal dark-adapted responses, an undetectable 30 Hz flicker ERG, and a severely reduced LA 3.0 ERG suggesting incomplete achromatopsia. However, ERGs to a red flash under dark adaptation, which in a normal subject gives an early cone system derived response and a later rod system derived response, show that dark-adapted cones retain good function and rule out achromatopsia.

Molecular genetics and pathogenesis

Mutations in both *RGS9* and *R9AP* have been associated with bradyopsia, with no sequence variants in either of these genes identified in subjects with oligocone trichromacy.[28]

To turn off the visual response, each of the activated phototransduction molecules has to be deactivated; α-transducin and cGMP-phosphodiesterase are simultaneously deactivated by the hydrolysis of the α-transducin bound GTP to GDP. This GTPase activity is substantially accelerated by RGS9, a GTPase activating protein that binds to the Gβ5 subunit and to R9AP, a membrane anchor protein. RGS9 and R9AP have a critical role in the recovery phase of visual transduction. RGS9 is anchored to photoreceptor outer segment disk membranes by R9AP; required for the correct targeting and localization of RGS9 in photoreceptors and enhances RGS9 activity up to 70-fold.

Bornholm eye disease

Clinical findings

Bornholm eye disease is an X-linked disorder with moderate to high myopia and astigmatism, impaired visual acuity, moderate optic nerve hypoplasia, thinning of the RPE in the posterior pole with visible choroidal vasculature, and abnormal cone ERGs.[29] Affected members in this single family were all deuteranopes, with a stationary natural history; however a similar phenotype has also been published in association with protanopia.[30,31] This disorder is therefore best characterized as an X-linked cone dysfunction syndrome with myopia and dichromacy.

Molecular genetics and pathogenesis

Linkage analysis has mapped the locus to Xq28, in the same chromosomal region as the L/M opsin gene array. Perhaps molecular genetic analysis of the opsin array will reveal mutations accounting for both the cone dysfunction and the color vision phenotype or rearrangements within the opsin gene array may be found to account for the color vision findings, whilst the cone dysfunction component of the disorder may be ascribed to mutation within an adjacent but separate locus.

Progressive retinal dystrophies

Rod–cone dystrophies

The rod–cone dystrophies (retinitis pigmentosa (RP)) are a clinically and genetically heterogeneous group of disorders with progressive loss of rod and later cone photoreceptor function leading to severe visual impairment. RP usually occurs as an isolated retinal abnormality, but it may also be seen with systemic abnormalities (see Chapter 45).

Leber's congenital amaurosis

Clinical findings

Leber's congenital amaurosis (LCA) is a severe congenital or early infant-onset non-syndromic retinal blindness described by Theodore Leber in 1869. He characterized the disorder by a searching nystagmus, abnormal pupil responses, minimal if any vision beyond infancy, and a normal fundus appearance initially, followed by the development of pigmentary changes. He later described a milder form of the same disease which has had several names, including early onset severe retinal dystrophy (EOSRD), severe early childhood onset retinal dystrophy (SECORD), and early onset retinitis pigmentosa. LCA/EOSRD is the most common inherited cause of severe visual impairment in children, accounting for 10–18% of children in institutions for the blind.

Severe visual impairment is from birth or the first few months of life with roving eye movements or nystagmus and poor pupillary light responses. Eye-poking, the "oculodigital" sign, is common (Fig. 44.7). Fundus examination may be normal but a variety of abnormal fundus appearances may be present such as disk pallor, vessel attenuation, or mild peripheral pigmentary retinopathy. There may also be disk drusen,

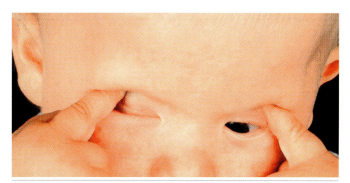

Fig. 44.7 Leber's congenital amaurosis. Eye-poking, the "oculodigital sign" is very common but of unknown cause; it results in atrophy of orbital fat and enophthalmos.

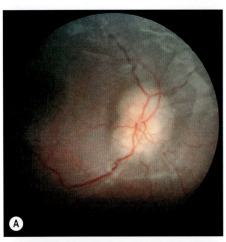

Fig. 44.8 Leber's congenital amaurosis. High hypermetropia and pseudopapilloedema.

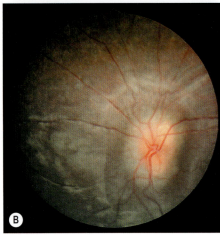

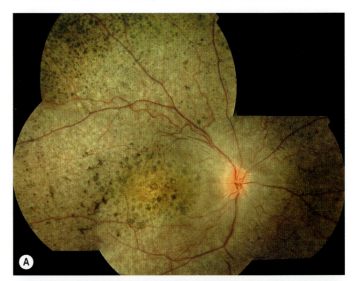

Fig. 44.9 Leber's congenital amaurosis. *RDH12*-associated disease characterized by bone spicule pigmentation and maculopathy.

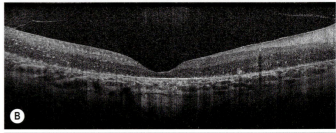

Fig. 44.10 Leber's congenital amaurosis. *CRB1*-associated disease which is characterized by (A) nummular pigmentation, maculopathy, relative preservation of para-arteriolar RPE, with (B) retinal thickening and loss of lamination observed on optical coherence tomography.

optic disk edema or pseudopapilledema (Fig. 44.8), a flecked retina, maculopathy, or nummular pigmentation. Affected infants often have high hyperopia, or less commonly high myopia, suggesting some interference with emmetropization.

Although most patients have normal fundi in infancy, signs of a pigmentary retinopathy appear in later childhood with optic disk pallor and retinal arteriolar narrowing. Other late signs, which may be related to eye-poking, include enophthalmos, keratoconus, and cataract. Eventual vision is in the region of 3/60 to perception of light, with progression not observed in all cases.

Following the discovery of many disease-causing genes (below) it has sometimes been possible to identify characteristic associated phenotypes (Figs 44.9 to 44.12): *RDH12*-associated disease is characterized by bone spicule pigmentation and maculopathy (Fig. 44.9) and *CRB1*-associated disease has nummular pigmentation, maculopathy, relative preservation of para-arteriolar RPE, with retinal thickening and loss of lamination on optical coherence tomography (Figs 44.10 and 44.11).

Electrophysiology

The ERG is undetectable or severely abnormal in infants with LCA. It is important to distinguish LCA from CSNB and achromatopsia, which may also present in infancy with nystagmus and poor vision. The visual evoked potential is often undetectable, but can be preserved, despite an undetectable ERG: it may indicate a better visual prognosis.

Non-ocular features

Most cases of LCA occur in otherwise normal infants and any non-ocular symptoms or signs should be investigated for syndromic retinal dystrophies or neurometabolic disease, usually in conjunction with a pediatrician (see Chapters 45 and 62).

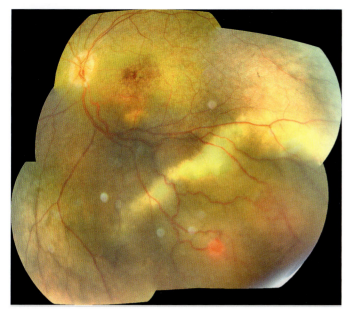

Fig. 44.11 Leber's congenital amaurosis. *CRB1*-associated disease can be complicated by a Coats-like exudative retinopathy.

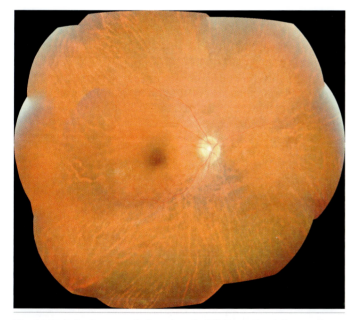

Fig. 44.12 Leber's congenital amaurosis. *RPE65*-associated disease often characterized by mild peripheral RPE mottling and white dots at the level of the RPE, usually with relatively normal vessel caliber and optic disk.

Molecular genetics and pathogenesis

LCA and EOSRD are extremely genetically heterogeneous, being caused by more than 16 genes (including *AIPL1*, *CEP290*, *CRX*, *CRB1*, *GUCY2D*, *IMPDH1*, *LCA5*, *LRAT*, *MERTK*, *RD3*, *RDH12*, *RPGRIP1*, *RPE65*, *SPATA7*, *KCNJ13*, and *TULP1*).[32] All exhibit autosomal recessive inheritance except *CRX*, where certain *de novo* mutations result in an autosomal dominant trait.[32] These genes are expressed preferentially in the retina or the RPE. Their putative functions are quite diverse and include retinal photoreceptor development (*CRX*), photoreceptor cell structure (*CRB1*), phototransduction (*GUCY2D*), protein trafficking (*AIPL1*, *RPGRIP1*), and vitamin A metabolism (*RPE65*).

Molecular genetic testing can now define the diagnosis in approximately 50–60% of patients, facilitating advice about prognosis. For example, patients with *RPE65* mutations have a better prognosis than those with *GUCY2D* mutations.[32] Identification of disease-causing mutations in LCA patients allows improved genetic counseling, the potential for prenatal diagnosis, and, in the future, may be used to select patients for gene-specific therapies.

Therapeutic intervention

Animal models of retinal blindness from deficiency of *RPE65* have either been engineered via targeted disruption of the gene in the mouse, or are available due to a natural mutation in the Briard dog. Pharmacologic bypass of the metabolic block, using synthetic retinoids has resulted in rapid restoration of visual pigment and function in the mouse. Gene replacement, using a normal copy of the gene in an adeno-associated virus (AAV) vector administered subretinally, has successfully restored ERGs and retinal function in both the murine and the canine model resulting in substantial, durable, recovery of vision as determined by ERGs, pupillary responses, and behavioral measures. This success has led to human clinical trials, in the USA and UK, involving a subretinal injection of AAV-vector delivering a wild-type copy of *RPE65*. These have all reported good safety with early results of varying degrees of efficacy.[33,34,35]

Further forms of LCA/EOSRD will likely become amenable to gene replacement therapy.

Retinitis pigmentosa

Retinitis pigmentosa (RP) is a term used for a genetically heterogeneous group of disorders characterized initially by night-blindness and visual field loss. ERGs are either undetectable or show the rod system to be more severely affected than the cone system, with dysfunction of photoreceptors. Dysfunction confined to the rod system is unusual but can occur early in the course of the disorder. Onset is often in childhood and inheritance can be autosomal recessive (AR), autosomal dominant (AD), and X-linked (XL). The disease may be confined to the eye or it may be part of a more widespread systemic disorder (see Chapter 45).

Clinical findings

Children with RP may present with night-blindness or with symptoms associated with extensive field loss or central retinal involvement. The age of onset is extremely variable. In some, there may be no symptomatic night-blindness and the child is referred after routine fundoscopy. When a close relative has RP, children may be referred early for investigation to exclude the disease.

In most cases, the visual acuity is initially normal; later, visual loss may occur from posterior subcapsular cataract, macular edema, or macular involvement. Early visual field changes are small scotomata in the mid-periphery, commonly in the upper visual field. These gradually coalesce to give the classical peripheral ring scotoma. Visual fields become very constricted in time, often leaving an island of preserved field in the far temporal periphery. In sector RP, which commonly involves the lower nasal quadrant, bilateral upper temporal field loss may lead to unnecessary investigation to exclude a chiasmal lesion – but the temporal field defect in RP does not follow the midline.

The appearance of the fundus in the early stages of RP is variable and, in young children, subtle. The earliest change may be mild pigment epithelial disturbance in the mid-periphery often with small white dots at the level of the RPE (Fig. 44.13). Later, pigment deposition is seen in the equatorial retina and there may be arteriolar narrowing and optic disk pallor. Abnormal pigment may be lacking in some children (RP sine pigmento) and, less commonly, there may be multiple white deposits throughout the retina (retinitis punctata albescens). The classical fundus appearance of optic disk pallor, retinal arteriolar attenuation, and peripheral pigment epithelial atrophy and intra-retinal "bone corpuscle" pigmentation is present in advanced disease (Fig. 44.14). Other possible changes include vitreous cells, posterior subcapsular cataract, optic disk drusen and macular edema. Occasionally, retinovascular changes similar to Coats' disease are seen.

The retinal phenotype is similar in most forms of RP although there may be marked variation in severity between affected individuals. There are, however, some gene-specific phenotypes. AD sector RP is usually associated with mutations in the rhodopsin gene, and the uncommon AR form of RP (RP12) with preserved para-arteriolar RPE, is associated with *CRB1* mutations. Two early onset forms of AR RP caused by mutations in the *RLBP1* gene are associated with multiple white deposits at the level of the RPE (Newfoundland rod-cone dystrophy and Bothnia dystrophy).[36,37]

Electrophysiology and psychophysics

The ERG in RP shows a rod–cone pattern of dysfunction such that the rod-derived responses are more affected than the cone-derived responses. There is marked variation in severity, partly related to the nature of the mutation, the inheritance pattern, and the subject's age. The ERG may be undetectable in the late stages of RP, or small residual cone responses may be found. There is reduction in the amplitude of the rod a- and b-waves in mild disease or early RP and the rod-mediated b-wave peak-time may be prolonged. The 30 Hz cone flicker ERG is usually both delayed and reduced, in keeping with generalized cone system dysfunction.

The electro-ocuologram (EOG) provides little further information than the ERG and is difficult to perform in young children. The macula may be spared and central retinal function tests, such as the PERG or multifocal ERG, may show minimal involvement despite almost complete loss of the full-field ERG. PERG may also be helpful in demonstrating central retinal involvement prior to the development of visible abnormalities.

Sector retinitis pigmentosa

The term sector RP should be reserved for those forms of RP (usually autosomal dominant) where functional testing suggests restricted loss of function; pigmentary abnormalities are usually confined to the inferior retina (Fig. 44.15). A similar sectorial involvement may occasionally be seen in the female

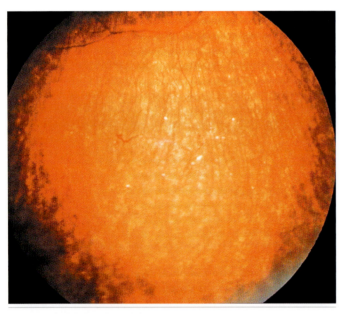

Fig. 44.13 Retinitis pigmentosa. Pigment epithelial atrophy in the mid-periphery with small white dots at the level of the RPE.

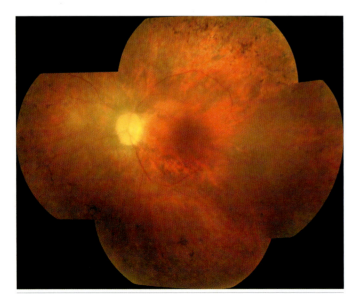

Fig. 44.14 Retinitis pigmentosa. "Bone spicule" formation, arteriolar narrowing, and optic nerve pallor.

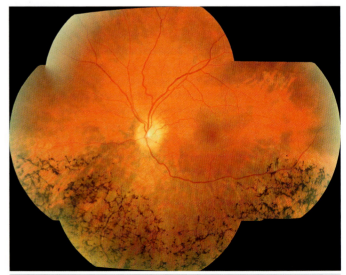

Fig. 44.15 Sector retinitis pigmentosa. Retinal pigmentary changes confined to the lower quadrants.

carriers of X-linked RP or as an early stage in generalized RP. The ERG in true sector RP usually shows amplitude reduction but no peak-time changes; the presence of marked peak-time shift suggests generalized dysfunction even though the pigmentary changes may be restricted. It is important in isolated cases to examine other family members, as the disorder is often asymptomatic. Dominant sector RP is often associated with mutations of the rhodopsin gene. Children with sector RP are usually asymptomatic and are referred when an abnormal fundus appearance is noted on routine fundoscopy or they are ascertained during family surveys.

Field loss on Goldmann perimetry is confined to the sector corresponding to the clinically involved retina. However, dark-adapted perimetry may show mild rod and cone threshold elevation in the apparently uninvolved retina indicating dysfunction outside the clinically evident region. Rod dark adaptation may be extremely delayed. The ERG is usually relatively well preserved with mild or moderate reductions in both rod and cone amplitudes. Disease progression is slow and usually confined to the clinically involved sector. The visual prognosis is good.

Autosomal dominant retinitis pigmentosa with incomplete penetrance

Variability of expression is common in autosomal dominant RP but true incomplete penetrance is unusual. However, incomplete penetrance is notable and common in some families, where the disease is of early onset and severe. There is genetic heterogeneity in autosomal dominant RP with incomplete penetrance, with mutations identified in several genes including RP9 and PRPF31.

Genetic counseling in families showing incomplete penetrance may be problematic because of the high incidence of asymptomatic gene carriers, but molecular genetic diagnosis is now possible in some families.

X-linked retinitis pigmentosa

X-linked RP is severe with onset of night-blindness usually by 10 years and progression to blindness by the third to fourth decade. They are often myopic and show fundus abnormalities and ERG changes early (Fig. 44.16). If there is a family history of other affected males the diagnosis is usually straightforward. Examination of close female relatives is helpful in the absence of a family history, as the recognition of the XL carrier state confirms the diagnosis.

The carrier state for XL RP can be diagnosed with certainty in females who have affected sons or fathers and are therefore obligate gene carriers, or where they can be shown by molecular genetic testing to carry the causative mutation. In other female family members, carrier detection depends upon recognition of the heterozygote's abnormal fundus appearance or on the results of electrophysiologic or psychophysical testing.

Fundus abnormalities are common in XL heterozygotes: a prominent "tapetal" reflex may be seen at the posterior pole (Fig. 44.17) or a mild equatorial pigment epithelial thinning and pigmentation. The ERG is usually abnormal and asymmetric in heterozygotes (see Fig. 44.16). Delay in the 30 Hz flicker response is probably the most frequent abnormality, but reduced rod amplitude may also occur. XL carriers can be identified in most cases using a combination of fundoscopy and electrophysiology. Molecular genetic diagnosis is possible in many families and is increasingly the method of choice for identification of heterozygotes.

The retinal dysfunction in some XL carriers can be progressive as older carriers may report symptoms of night-blindness and have detectable field loss and more extensive retinal pigmentation. Some carrier females may be severely affected at a relatively young age; however, there is considerable intra- and interfamilial variability. Skewed X inactivation, with the X chromosome having the mutant allele active in most cells, may account for severely affected females.

Unilateral "retinitis pigmentosa"

Fundus changes of unilateral RP have been described but only one case from an extended family with RP. The patient with unilateral RP in this family[38] harbored a common nonsense mutation in RP1, a common cause of AD RP. Thus, a somatic mutation might have occurred in a progenitor cell during the development of the unaffected retinal tissue that ameliorates the effect of the RP1 mutation.[38]

Most other cases are probably not genetically determined and may be postinflammatory, post-traumatic, or follow retinal ischemia. Some individuals with RP have an asymmetric fundus appearance at presentation so that one eye appears clinically unaffected, but psychophysical testing and ERG demonstrate abnormal function bilaterally.

Differential diagnosis of retinitis pigmentosa

Other disorders may be confused with RP either because there is symptomatic night-blindness or because of a similar fundus appearance (Table 44.2) (Fig. 44.18). The other inherited dystrophies can usually be differentiated from RP by the clinical

Table 44.2 – Differential diagnoses of retinitis pigmentosa

Pigmentary retinopathy	Night-blindness
Blunt trauma	**Genetic disorders**
Retained intraocular FB	Congenital stationary night-blindness
Congenital infection	Oguchi's disease
Rubella	Fundus albipunctatus
Varicella	Choroideraemia
Herpes simplex	Gyrate atrophy
Syphilis	Progressive cone–rod dystrophy
	Enhanced S-cone syndrome
Acquired infection	
Measles	
Onchocerciasis	
Metabolic	**Acquired**
Cystinosis	Vitamin A deficiency
Oxalosis	Desferrioxamine toxicity
Drugs	
Phenothiazines	
Chloroquine	
Desferrioxamine	
Resolved retinal detachment	
Ophthalmic artery occlusion	
Other retinal dystrophies	
Cone–rod dystrophy	
Inherited vitreoretinal dystrophies	
Enhanced S-cone syndrome	
Unknown etiology	
Pigmented paravenous chorioretinal atrophy	

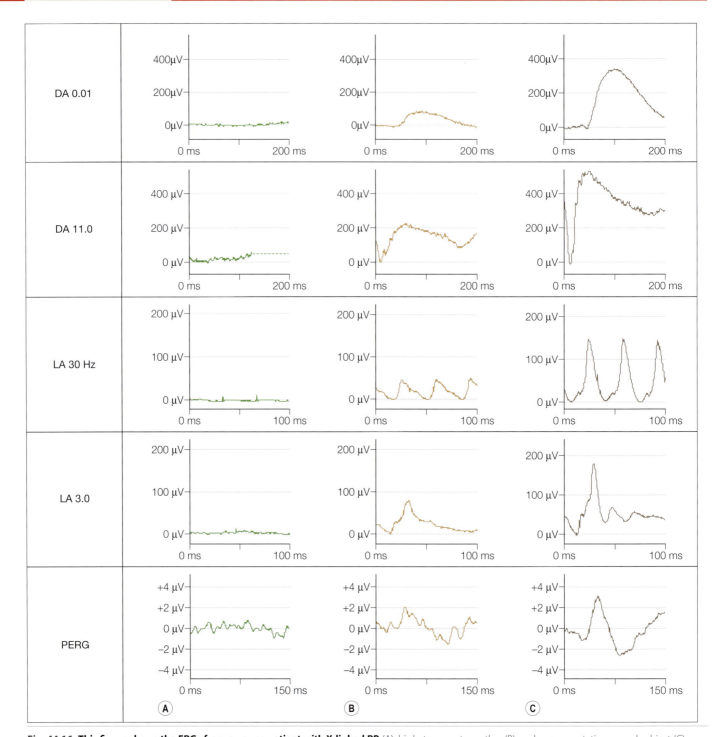

Fig. 44.16 This figure shows the ERGs from a young patient with X-linked RP (A), his heterozygote mother (B), and a representative normal subject (C). There is only residual ERG activity detectable in the patient. The ERGs in his mother are mildly subnormal under all stimulus conditions, the subnormal a-wave of the bright flash response (DA 11.0) confirming the abnormality to be at the level of the photoreceptor. ERG abnormalities are usually present in heterozygotes, and can vary from mild to severe.

findings and electrophysiology. Although history and examination may exclude many of the acquired causes of pigmentary retinopathy it is likely that some cases of apparently sporadic RP are due to acquired retinal or pigment epithelial disease.

Genetics of retinitis pigmentosa
RP may be inherited as an autosomal dominant (AD), autosomal recessive (AR), or X-linked (XL) recessive disorder. There is genetic heterogeneity within these subtypes. The relative frequency of the different modes of inheritance differs widely in the different series, but 50% of patients have no family history of RP or parental consanguinity. It is unlikely that all such cases have AR disease. Some males may have XL disease transmitted via asymptomatic female carriers; other cases may represent new AD mutations or AD disease in a family with reduced penetrance. Some sporadic patients may not have genetic disease. Similar retinal dystrophies may be seen in association with mutations of mitochondrial DNA but

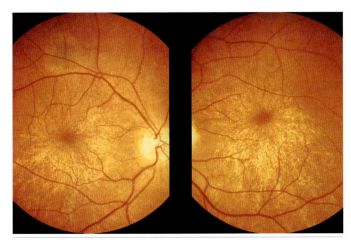

Fig. 44.17 X-linked RP carrier female showing the "tapetal reflex."

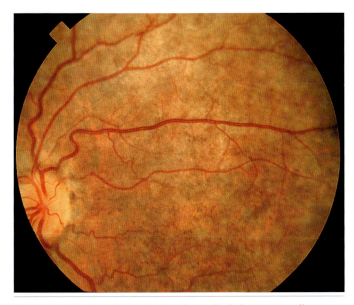

Fig. 44.18 Rubella retinopathy showing retinal pigment mottling.
Retinal function is usually good and the ERG normal, whereas most retinal dystrophies with deafness have severely abnormal ERGs.

there are usually other systemic abnormalities (see Chapters 45 and 62).

XL and AR RP tend to have an earlier onset and are more severe than dominant disease. The clinical findings should be taken into account, particularly when counseling those patients with apparently sporadic disease. A severely affected female is more likely to have AR disease, whereas a severely affected male may have XL or AR disease. A significant number of patients with sporadic RP, however, have mild disease and some of these probably have new AD mutations. Prior to counseling it is important to examine other family members, especially the mothers of severely affected males who may show the fundus or electrophysiologic abnormalities of an X-linked heterozygote.

Accurate genetic counseling depends upon identification of the causative mutation. Much progress has been made, and molecular genetic diagnosis is now possible in many forms of RP. More than 50 genes have been identified in non-syndromic RP; encoding proteins of the phototransduction cascade, proteins involved in vitamin A metabolism and cell–cell interaction, photoreceptor structural proteins and transcription factors, intracellular transport proteins, and splicing factors.[39,40,41]

Molecular genetics

Autosomal dominant retinitis pigmentosa There is considerable genetic heterogeneity within AD RP. Mutations in more than 20 genes have been identified, accounting for approximately 60–70% of patients with AD RP, with mutations in the rhodopsin gene (*RHO*) being commonest. Sequence variants in *RP1* and *PRPF31* are the next commonest causes of AD RP.

Mutations of the rhodopsin gene account for about 25% of patients with AD RP and more than 80 different mutations have been identified. There is considerable variation in the ocular phenotype seen with the different mutations which have also been reported in dominant forms of CSNB and AR RP. The phenotypic variability is more marked with mutations of the gene *PRPH2* (formerly *RDS/peripherin*), where the clinical picture may resemble RP, cone–rod dystrophy, cone dystrophy, a fleck retina syndrome, or macular dystrophy (see Chapters 46 and 48). *PRPH2* mutations account for about 5% of cases of AD RP.[39,40,41]

In an unusual form of RP, showing digenic inheritance, mutations of both the *PRPH2* and *ROM1* (rod outer segment protein 1) genes are present within the same family. Individuals with a mutation of one gene but not the other are clinically unaffected. Affected individuals are double heterozygotes with mutations of both *ROM1* and *PRPH2*. Peripherin is located in rod and cone outer segment disks, whilst ROM1 is only found in rods. In the rod outer segment, interaction of the two proteins is important for outer segment structure: and some mutations in the *PRPH2* gene may be insufficient to cause significant photoreceptor disease unless accompanied by a defective ROM1 protein.

Splice factors have increasingly been identified as being associated with AD RP, including mutations in *PRPF31*, *PRPF3*, *PRPF6*, and *PRPF8*.[39,40] An insufficiency in splicing function may be disease-causing only under conditions of elevated splicing demand. With the need to replenish disk proteins daily, such conditions exist in rod photoreceptors, which may explain the paradox of isolated retinal disease caused by ubiquitously expressed splice-factor genes.

See references 39, 40, and 41 for AD RP phenotype–genotype correlations.

Autosomal recessive retinitis pigmentosa Mutations in more than 30 genes have been identified to date in AR RP, accounting for approximately 40–50% of patients with AR RP: the commonest being *USH2A* (10–15% of AR RP), with more severe mutations causing Usher's syndrome type 2 (see Chapters 45 and 105).[39,40,41]

Mutations in genes encoding many components of the rod phototransduction cascade have been identified[39,40,41] including:

1. The rhodopsin gene
2. The genes coding for the α-subunit and the β-subunit of the rod cGMP-phosphodiesterase
3. The genes for the α- and β-subunits of rod cGMP-gated cation channels
4. In *SAG*, encoding arrestin
5. Genes coding for components of the visual cycle involved in recycling vitamin A have been implicated in AR RP; including *RPE65*, *ABCA4*, *LRAT*, and *RLBP1*.

X-linked retinitis pigmentosa Mutations in two genes have been identified in X-linked RP, *RPGR* (RP3) and *RP2* (RP2). Sequence variants in *RPGR* cause approximately 75% of all XL RP.[39,40,41] Three other loci have been reported: Xp22 (RP23), Xp21.3–p21.2 (RP6), and Xq26–27 (RP24).

RPGR mutations are usually associated with typical rod–cone degeneration, but in a few patients, retinal dystrophy, deafness, and abnormalities in respiratory cilia have been noted.[42] The majority of mutations may result in premature termination of translation. Exon ORF15 is a "hot spot" for mutation responsible for 80% of cases of XL RP.[43] RPGR may act as a regulator of a specific type of membrane transport or trafficking which is particularly active in the retina or RPE.

Mutations in *RP2* account for up to 15% of XL RP.[39,40,41] RP2 is a novel protein of unknown function, which is targeted to the plasma membrane by dual *N*-terminal acyl-modification. Dual-acylated proteins are targeted to lipid rafts, suggesting a potential role for the protein in signal transduction.

Management of retinitis pigmentosa

Most forms of RP are not amenable to specific treatment. In some rare disorders where the biochemical basis of the disorder is better elucidated, the deterioration may be slowed by diet (chapter 45 and 62).

In one randomized controlled trial of vitamin A supplementation in RP there was a small effect on the rate of decline of the cone flicker ERG; the effect was however marginal and no beneficial effect was found on visual acuity or visual field loss.[44] This form of treatment has not gained widespread acceptance.

Despite the lack of effective treatment for RP, the ophthalmologist has an important role to play in the management of both the child and the family. Once the diagnosis is established, it is important that the parents and the child (if old enough) are given a full and sympathetic explanation; they can be reassured that most children complete their education at a normal school as central vision is preserved until later.

Parents are often concerned that other children may be at risk of developing the disease; they should be offered genetic counseling and it may be appropriate to examine other family members. It is also helpful to have available the addresses of patient self-help groups such as their national RP association.

Practical help can also be given when there are visual difficulties. Many patients with RP have poor vision in bright sunlight and have problems in adapting from bright to dim illumination; tinted lenses may be helpful. Significant refractive errors should be corrected. A trial of oral acetazolamide, topical dorzolamide, orbital floor or intravitreal steroids, or intravitreal bevacizumab or ranibizumab should be considered if there is macular edema. Low vision aids may be helpful in established edema or macular atrophy. Visual loss may also develop secondary to posterior subcapsular cataract and, although cataract surgery is often successfully performed in adults with RP, it is rarely necessary in childhood.

Prognosis

The prognosis in RP varies according to the type of disease and the causative mutation. Ideally, prognosis should be inferred by the identification of the specific genetic mutation. Advice on prognosis can also be given by phenotyping to establish the diagnosis and a full family history to establish the mode of inheritance. It is helpful to carry out an examination of all affected members to establish changes of disease severity with increasing age. However intrafamilial variability of disease expression occurs: the visual outcome of older affected family members is not necessarily a good guide to the likely prognosis in younger children.

In XL RP affected males are night-blind in early childhood, usually show extensive field loss by their teens and central visual loss in their twenties. By the fourth decade most have visual acuity reduced to less than count fingers. AR RP is such a heterogeneous condition that accurate prognosis is difficult. The disease is usually of early onset and severe. Most patients have a severely constricted visual field by their teens and may have marked central visual loss by their late twenties. Some with recessive disease follow a more benign course.

The prognosis is better in AD RP. Although night-blindness and field loss may develop in childhood, central vision may remain normal throughout life. Many patients maintain reasonable visual acuity until the fifth or sixth decade, although they may have extremely constricted visual fields. There is, however, wide variation even in RP caused by mutations at the same locus.[39,40,41] Severe, early onset forms are unusual.

True sector RP has the best prognosis of any form of the disease. Although there may be severe upper visual field loss, severe involvement of the macula is uncommon.

Pigmented paravenous chorioretinal atrophy

This is a rare chorioretinal atrophy in which there is paravenous RPE atrophy and pigment clumping (Fig. 44.19). It is more common in males, most cases are sporadic, and it is usually diagnosed on routine examination in asymptomatic patients. The ERG shows a spectrum of abnormalities and in contrast to most retinal dystrophies may show marked interocular asymmetry. Retinal function may be relatively stable, or may show slow deterioration.

It is uncertain whether this disorder may have a genetic basis, with only one report of a heterozygous *CRB1* mutation of uncertain significance identified in a family with

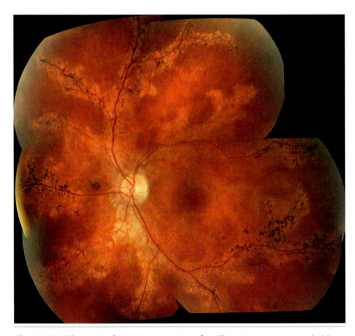

Fig. 44.19 Pigmented paravenous atrophy. The veins are surrounded by a band of retinal pigment atrophy and clumping.

dominantly inherited PPCRA with variable expressivity.[45] In one report the monozygotic twin of an affected adult was unaffected, suggesting that at least some cases are non-genetic.[46]

Acquired rod–cone dysfunction

Vitamin A deficiency

Worldwide, vitamin A deficiency is the most common cause of blindness in childhood. In developing countries it is usually caused by a combination of malnutrition and malabsorption associated with frequent gastrointestinal infection. In developed countries, vitamin A deficiency is rare and usually seen in association with liver disease or malabsorption; rarely an unusual diet may be the cause.

Vitamin A is an essential component of rhodopsin and cone opsins; night-blindness is an early symptom of deficiency. In early deficiency there is slowing of rod dark adaptation and, later, rod and cone thresholds are elevated. Peripheral fields may be constricted and in some patients white dots at the level of the pigment epithelium are seen throughout the periphery. Rod ERGs are undetectable with cone responses usually being well preserved.

The ocular abnormalities are reversible with vitamin A supplementation if this is started before the disease is too advanced.[47] The recovery of retinal function is extremely rapid and accurate early diagnosis is important since vitamin A deficiency is a treatable cause of night-blindness.

Vitamin A and vitamin E supplementation may be curative in abetalipoprotein deficiency, Bassen-Kornzweig disease, a malabsorption diarrhea syndrome of infancy (see Chapter 62).

Desferrioxamine toxicity

Desferrioxamine is a chelating agent used in the treatment of iron storage disorders such as transfusion siderosis. Ocular side-effects include cataract, optic neuropathy, and retinal degeneration.[48] Patients with retinal toxicity develop night-blindness, peripheral field loss, and a peripheral pigmentary retinopathy; dark adaptation is abnormal and the rod ERG shows reduced amplitude.[48] Some improvement occurs on stopping the drug.

Histologically, the RPE is predominantly affected.

Isotretinoin toxicity

Isotretinoin (13-*cis*-retinoic acid) is a treatment for acne vulgaris which has several potential severe adverse effects including liver toxicity and dysregulation of lipid metabolism, necessitating regular blood testing whilst on therapy. Ocular side-effects include photophobia, meibomian gland dysfunction, blepharoconjunctivitis, corneal opacities, keratitis, and reversible decreased night vision.[49]

Inherited chorioretinal dystrophies

Choroideremia

Clinical and histopathologic findings

Choroideremia is an X-linked recessive disorder characterized by progressive atrophy of the RPE and choriocapillaris. Affected males usually present in early childhood with night-blindness and progressive field loss, but central vision is usually preserved until late in the disease. A longitudinal study reported a slow rate of visual acuity loss and good retention of central vision until the seventh decade.[50] There is a wide variation in clinical expression.[51] Female carriers, usually asymptomatic,

have a widespread fine peripheral RPE atrophy and granular pigment deposition (Figs 44.20 and 44.21). Cases with deafness, hypopituitarism, and mental retardation probably represent a contiguous gene defect.

Affected males usually present between the ages of 5 and 10 years with night-blindness and mild myopia. The earliest fundus signs are fine pigment epithelial atrophy and pigmentation in the equatorial retina; the clinical appearance may then be confused with RP. Focal areas of atrophy of the RPE and choriocapillaris, well demonstrated on fluorescein angiography or autofluorescence imaging (Figs 44.22 and 44.23), develop as the disease progresses. These coalesce to give a widespread atrophic appearance throughout the equatorial retina spreading to involve the peripheral and more posterior retina; the macula is spared until late in the disease.

Visual fields initially show small mid-peripheral scotomata corresponding to areas of atrophy. Marked constriction of the visual field develops with disease progression, often with a preserved island of field in the far periphery.

Histologic examination of eyes with early disease[52] showed marked degeneration of the outer retina with loss of RPE, Bruch's membrane, and choriocapillaris. Biochemical studies showed reduced levels of interphotoreceptor retinal binding protein (IRBP) and increased levels of cAMP in the RPE and choroid. These observations, if typical, may limit current gene replacement therapy trials.

Electrophysiology

The ERG is markedly abnormal at an early stage and may be undetectable. Rod and cone amplitudes are reduced in those with ERG preservation. Peak-time changes are less prominent, but may be present later in the disease process.

Female heterozygotes

Most female carriers are asymptomatic but the fundus appearance is characteristic. The EOG and ERG are usually normal. Some elderly heterozygotes may develop nyctalopia and show more extensive RPE atrophy with an abnormal ERG and

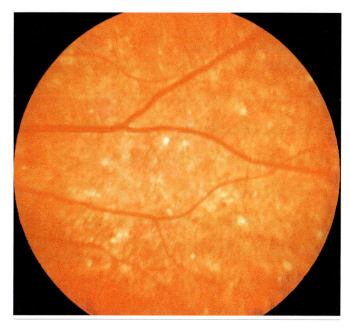

Fig. 44.20 Choroideremia carrier. Granular pigmented and depigmented areas in the peripheral retina.

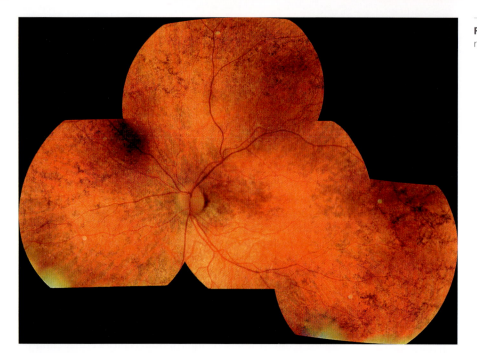

Fig. 44.21 **Choroideremia carrier.** Peripheral retinal pigmentation.

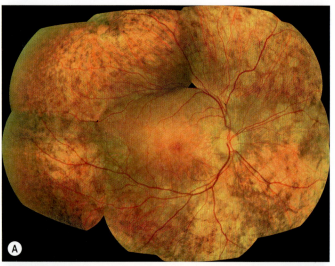

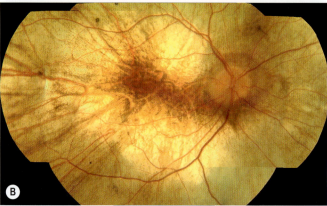

Fig. 44.22 **Choroideremia.** Chorioretinal changes with scalloped edges: (A, early disease; B, advanced).

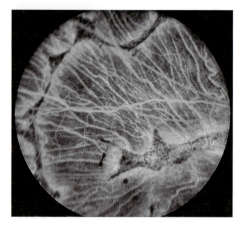

Fig. 44.23 **Choroideremia.** Fluorescein angiogram showing characteristic scalloped appearance given by the surviving retinal pigment epithelium and loss of the choriocapillaries.

elevated rod thresholds on psychophysical testing. Molecular genetic diagnosis is now possible.

Molecular genetics and pathogenesis

The choroideremia gene (*CHM*) has been mapped to Xq21, with many mutations in *CHM* identified. An intronic mutation remote from the exon–intron junctions has been reported in *CHM*, creating a strong acceptor splice site and leading to the inclusion of a cryptic exon into the *CHM* mRNA. Intronic sequence is often not screened in inherited retinal dystrophy mutation investigations, which suggests that a significant proportion of disease-causing variants are being missed.

CHM is widely expressed and the product of this gene, Rab escort protein (REP)-1, is involved in the post-translational lipid modification and subsequent membrane targeting of Rab proteins, small GTPases that play a key role in intracellular trafficking.

Gyrate atrophy of the choroid and retina

Clinical and histopathologic findings

Gyrate atrophy of the choroid and retina is a rare, autosomal recessive, disorder with progressive chorioretinal dystrophy, hyperornithinemia, and a deficiency of the mitochondrial enzyme ornithine aminotransferase (OAT). The level of OAT activity in obligate carriers of the gene is about 50% of normal.

Children may present with night-blindness, progressive myopia, or field loss but the diagnosis of gyrate atrophy may be made in early infancy when a raised level of plasma ornithine is found in a child with a family history. The earliest fundus changes are small discrete areas of choroidal and RPE atrophy in the mid- and far-peripheral fundus. The adjacent fundus may show diffuse depigmentation of the RPE and atrophic areas. The atrophic areas coalesce and enlarge toward the posterior pole with a characteristic scalloped leading edge.

Most patients have moderate to high myopia and posterior subcapsular cataracts develop in early adult life. Some develop visual loss secondary to macular edema or atrophy. Most patients maintain a reasonable level of visual acuity until their forties or fifties, although with a constricted field. There are early small mid-peripheral scotomata but progression leads to marked peripheral constriction.

Light and electron microscopy (EM) from a patient with a pyridoxine-sensitive form of gyrate atrophy showed focal areas of photoreceptor and RPE atrophy at the posterior pole; in the mid-periphery there were areas of abrupt transition from near-normal to atrophic areas of retina.[53] EM showed abnormal mitochondria in the cornea, ciliary epithelium, ciliary muscle, and in the photoreceptors. Similar mitochondrial abnormalities in other tissues of patients with gyrate atrophy are likely to be a secondary effect of the biochemical disturbance.

Electrophysiology and psychophysics

The ERG relates to the severity of disease; early in the course of the disorder rod and cone amplitudes are reduced; later, the ERG is undetectable. EOG reduction parallels the reduction in the rod ERG. Dark adaptation shows markedly elevated rod thresholds in areas of field corresponding to involved retina.

Non-ocular features

Although patients with gyrate atrophy show no muscle weakness, muscle biopsy shows atrophy of type 2 fibers with accumulation of tubular aggregates. Other reported abnormalities include structural abnormalities of the hair, electroencephalographic abnormalities and mild developmental delay, peripheral neuropathy, and mitochondrial abnormalities in a variety of tissues.

Molecular genetics and pathogenesis

The human ornithine-Δ-aminotransferase gene was cloned in 1988. A large number of mutations of the OAT gene have been identified in patients with gyrate atrophy including some in which the OAT is pyridoxine-responsive. Expression studies have demonstrated reduced mutant OAT activity.

Can chronic reduction of ornithine prevent the retinal degeneration of gyrate atrophy? Using an arginine-restricted diet in a mouse model of OAT deficiency (oat$^{-/-}$),[54] it was found that plasma ornithine levels were substantially reduced and completely prevented retinal degeneration in oat$^{-/-}$, suggesting that ornithine accumulation is important in the pathophysiology of the retinal degeneration and that restoration of OAT activity in the retina may not be required for effective treatment.

Biochemical findings and treatment

Patients with gyrate atrophy have a deficiency of the pyridoxal phosphate-dependent mitochondrial enzyme OAT which is responsible for the conversion of ornithine to glutamic acid. The major dietary source of ornithine is arginine, which may be converted to ornithine by the arginase reaction of the urea cycle or by the glycine transamidase reaction. Ornithine, an intermediary in the urea cycle is necessary for the production of polyamines and in the synthesis of proline and glutamate.

It is not clear whether high levels of ornithine or the reduced levels of proline and glutamate that accompany OAT deficiency cause the retinal abnormalities. Not all patients with raised ornithine levels develop gyrate atrophy and one patient with gyrate atrophy has been reported who had normal ornithine levels and low plasma proline levels suggesting that reduced availability of proline may be a contributory factor.[55]

Three different approaches to treatment have been used:

1. A few patients are responsive to pyridoxine (B$_6$) supplements and show reduced plasma ornithine levels and improvement in the ERG. Vitamin B$_6$ should be used initially in all patients and continued in those who show a positive response.
2. In non-responders, adhering to an arginine-restricted diet may reduce plasma ornithine levels.
3. Proline supplementation may slow the progress of retinal degeneration in some patients.[55,56]

Children with gyrate atrophy need to be managed in collaboration with a clinical biochemist. Although present treatment regimens are promising, more long-term studies are needed to assess whether such treatment will prevent retinal deterioration.

Cone and cone–rod dystrophies

The inherited cone dystrophies are a heterogeneous group of progressive disorders characterized by photophobia, reduced central vision, abnormal color vision, and abnormal cone ERGs.[57] Autosomal recessive (AR), autosomal dominant (AD), and X-linked recessive (XL) inheritance has been reported and there is heterogeneity even amongst these subtypes.[57]

The functional deficit is confined to the photopic system in some forms of cone dystrophy but in most there is later evidence of rod dysfunction (cone–rod dystrophy). The distinction between cone and cone–rod dystrophies may be difficult, particularly during childhood and is dependent upon good electrophysiology. Most forms of cone and cone–rod dystrophy are seen in otherwise normal individuals; those associated with systemic abnormalities are discussed in Chapter 45.

Progressive cone dystrophy

Clinical findings

In contrast to the stationary cone disorders, which present in early infancy, the progressive cone dystrophies are not usually symptomatic until later childhood or early adult life.[57] The age of onset of visual loss and the rate of progression shows wide variability but visual acuity usually deteriorates eventually to the level of 6/60 or to an ability to count fingers only. Photophobia is a prominent early symptom with progressive loss of visual acuity and color vision. Since all three classes of cone photoreceptor can be affected, the color vision defects are along all three color axes, often progressing to complete loss

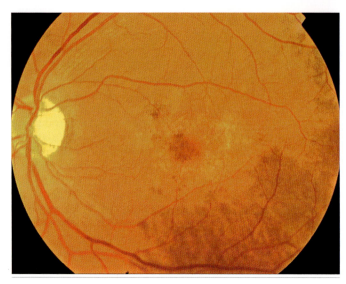

Fig. 44.24 Progressive cone dystrophy with bull's eye maculopathy.

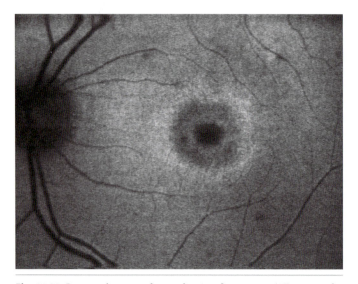

Fig. 44.25 Progressive cone dystrophy. Autofluorescence (AF) images of bull's eye maculopathy.

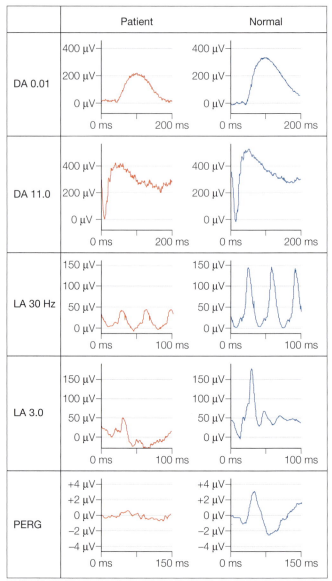

Fig. 44.26 The rod-specific (DA 0.01) and bright flash dark-adapted ERGs (DA 11.0) fall within the normal range. The 30 Hz flicker ERG (LA 30Hz) is both delayed and reduced, typically present in most cone dystrophies. The photopic single flash ERG (LA 3.0) is markedly subnormal with particular reduction in the b-wave. The PERG is profoundly subnormal in keeping with marked macular involvement.

of color vision. Some cases have a predominant early involvement of L-cones leading to a protan color vision phenotype.[58,59] AD cone dystrophy pedigrees with early tritan color vision defects have also been reported.[60,61] High frequency, low amplitude nystagmus may be seen. A small central scotoma is frequently detected on visual field testing; peripheral fields may be normal in the early stages and constricted later.

Fundus examination may show a typical "bull's eye" maculopathy (Figs 44.24 and 44.25) (Box 44.1). In some cases there may only be minor macular pigment epithelial atrophy. The optic disks show variable temporal pallor. The retinal periphery is usually normal although, rarely, white flecks may be seen. Fluorescein angiography shows typical "window" defects at the macula in the majority of cases and the so-called dark choroid sign (see Chapter 46) may be seen.

Electrophysiology and psychophysics

Electroretinography shows normal rod responses but substantially abnormal cone responses (Fig. 44.26). The 30 Hz flicker

Box 44.1

Bull's eye maculopathy in childhood

Stargardt's disease
Progressive cone dystrophy
Cone–rod dystrophy
Batten's disease
Hallervorden-Spatz disease
Bardet-Biedl syndrome
Mucolipidosis IV
Fucosidosis
Drug toxicity (e.g. chloroquine)
Benign concentric macular dystrophy
Fenestrated sheen dystrophy

ERG is usually of increased peak-time but rarely, such as in the cone dystrophy related to GCAP1 mutation,[57] the peak-time is normal and amplitude reduction is the only abnormality. A small subgroup of patients with cone dystrophy may show supernormal rod responses or rod responses within the normal range but with distinctive and specific abnormal characteristics[57] (see below).

Dark adaptation studies show either a monophasic curve with no recognizable cone component, or a biphasic curve with elevated cone thresholds; rod-mediated thresholds are normal. Spectral sensitivity studies show variable abnormalities of the photopic responses. In some families there is generalized depression of sensitivity across all wavelengths tested, whilst others show more specific functional deficits in the early stages of the disease. In advanced disease a typical rod sensitivity curve may be seen under both scotopic and photopic conditions.

Obligate carriers of X-linked cone dystrophy may show evidence of cone dysfunction on electrophysiologic or psychophysical testing.

Cone dystrophy with supernormal rod ERG

Clinical findings

An unusual AR disorder has been described with abnormal photopic responses associated with supernormal and delayed rod ERG b-waves.[57] Patients have generalized loss of cone vision, clinical evidence of progression, and nyctalopia.[62] Cone ERGs are reduced and delayed; with a bright flash the dark-adapted b-wave is of high amplitude (and may be supernormal), but at low stimulus strengths the rod b-wave is smaller than normal and is profoundly delayed.[62] Some cases have supernormal rod ERGs without nyctalopia, suggestive of reasonable rod function despite an abnormal scotopic ERG.[63]

Several clinical features may suggest the diagnosis.[57] Onset of symptoms of reduced central vision and marked photophobia is in the first and second decades of life. Patients are usually myopic and often have severely reduced red–green color discrimination with relative preservation of tritan color vision. Onset of nyctalopia and presence of nystagmus is variable.

There is often RPE disturbance at the macula with a normal retinal periphery. Autofluorescence (AF) imaging reveals a perifoveal ring of increased AF; in older subjects an area of increased AF may be seen centrally. By the fifth decade there is usually marked central atrophy and hypofluorescence.

Electrophysiology

The PERG is often absent, indicative of marked macular dysfunction. Rod ERG amplitudes are found to be subnormal at the lowest flash energies, but a characteristic abnormality seen in all published cases is a profound and rapid increase in the amplitude of a delayed b-wave despite only a relatively small increase in stimulus intensity. At higher flash strengths the b-wave may exceed the upper limit of normal (supernormal). The initial phase of the bright flash dark-adapted ERG a-wave is well formed, suggesting that the kinetics of phototransduction are within normal limits. The shape of the dark-adapted bright flash ERG (that to a flash strength greater than the routine ISCEV standard flash) is characteristic with a normally commencing a-wave which then plateaus, shows a small dip, and is then followed by a very sharply rising b-wave.

Molecular genetics and pathogenesis

Recessive mutations have been identified in KCNV2, encoding a voltage-gated potassium channel subunit.[64] In situ hybridization has demonstrated KCNV2 expression in human rod and cone photoreceptors.[64] KCNV2 mutations might perturb or abrogate the potassium current within vertebrate photoreceptor inner segments shown previously to set their resting potential and voltage response.[64]

Progressive cone–rod dystrophy

Clinical findings

In this disorder, affected patients develop the typical findings of a cone dystrophy in early life but later develop rod involvement with night-blindness. Most present in the first two decades of life, with the retinal dystrophy either being isolated or associated with systemic abnormalities. AD, AR, or XL inheritance has been reported.

Fundus examination shows macular atrophy in the early stages of the disease, with peripheral RPE atrophy, retinal pigmentation, arteriolar attenuation, and optic disk pallor in the late stages (Figs 44.27 and 44.28). A bull's eye maculopathy may also be seen.

Electrophysiology and psychophysics

Both rod and cone thresholds are elevated on psychophysical testing and the ERG shows reduced rod and cone amplitudes. Generalized abnormalities of rod and cone responses are seen, with the cone ERGs being more abnormal than the rod ERGs. The 30 Hz cone flicker ERG peak-time is usually delayed. The bright flash dark-adapted ERG (*DA 11.0) a-wave is subnormal in keeping with rod photoreceptor involvement.

Molecular genetics of cone and cone–rod dystrophies

Most cases of progressive cone and cone–rod dystrophy are sporadic, with the majority of these probably representing AR inheritance, but some may represent new AD mutations, and in severely affected males, X-linked disease.

Several loci and causative genes have been identified in the progressive cone dystrophies.[57] Mutations in ABCA4, CNGA3, CNGB3, and PDE6C have been identified in autosomal recessive cone dystrophies, GUCA1A mutations have been reported in autosomal dominant pedigrees, and RPGR and OPN1LW/OPN1MW sequence variants in XL disease.[22,57]

More than eight genes have been associated with AD cone–rod dystrophy,[57] including CRX, GUCY2D, RIMS1, PRPH2, GUCA1A, PROM1, and AIPL1. Ten genes have been associated with AR disease,[57] including ABCA4, CNGA3, CNGB3, ADAM9, and RPGRIP1. Mutations in ABCA4 have been shown to be the commonest cause of AR cone–rod dystrophy.[57] Mutations in RPGR, the gene encoding the protein that interacts with RPGRIP1, have been associated with XL CORD families.[57]

Goldmann-Favre syndrome and enhanced S-cone syndrome

Clinical findings and electrophysiology

Goldmann-Favre is a rare AR disorder characterized by gradual visual loss or night-blindness with liquefaction of the vitreous, macular retinoschisis and peripheral RPE atrophy and pigmentation. Peripheral retinoschisis and cataract may also occur. The retinal dystrophy is progressive, resulting in extensive visual field loss and variable central visual loss. Fluorescein

Fig. 44.27 **Cone–rod dystrophy.** (A,B) Bilateral macular atrophy. (C,D) Autofluorescence (AF) images showing decreased AF at the maculae corresponding to the atrophy seen ophthalmoscopically with an abnormal mottled appearance of the surrounding retina, with areas of relative increased and decreased AF.

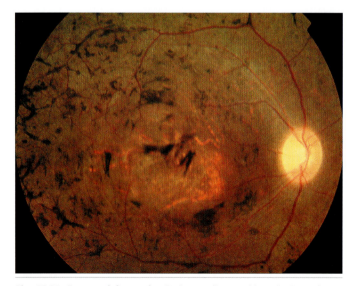

Fig. 44.28 **Cone–rod dystrophy.** End-stage disease with marked macular atrophy, retinal pigmentation, and arteriolar narrowing.

angiography may show evidence of peripheral capillary closure and vascular leakage. ERG is markedly abnormal or undetectable. Studies of patients with the Goldmann-Favre syndrome using spectral ERG have demonstrated that S-cones are less affected than the mid-spectral cones.

There is overlap between Goldmann-Favre syndrome and enhanced S-cone syndrome (ESCS) where there are no rods but increased numbers of cones, mostly short wavelength sensitive. Patients usually present with nyctalopia and are found to have foveal schisis/cysts (Figs 44.29 and 44.30). Since mutations have been identified in *NR2E3* in both disorders, Goldmann-Favre syndrome probably represents severe ESCS. Although the macular appearance may be similar, the vitreous changes, peripheral retinopathy, ERG abnormalities, and mode of inheritance help differentiate this condition from X-linked juvenile retinoschisis and inherited forms of isolated foveal schisis (see Chapter 49).

The characteristic pigmentary deposition in ESCS is at the level of the RPE rather than intra-retinal, has a nummular appearance and tends to be around the arcades (see Fig. 44.30). Despite this typical appearance, patients are often mistaken for RP. The ERG in ESCS is diagnostic (Fig. 44.31). The rod-specific ERG, to a dim flash under dark adaptation (DA 0.01), is

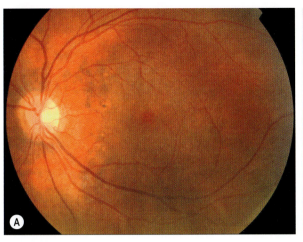

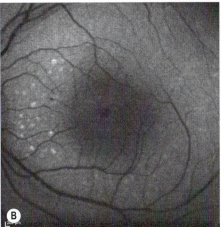

Fig. 44.29 Enhanced S-cone syndrome. (A) White dots are seen at the level of the RPE in early disease, which are more readily seen on autofluorescence imaging (B).

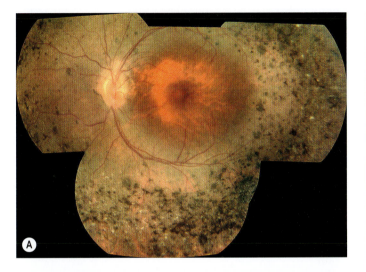

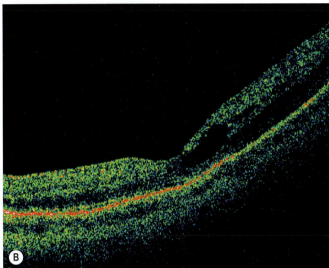

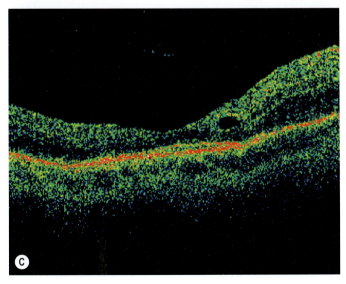

Fig. 44.30 Enhanced S-cone syndrome. (A) Typical pigment clumps (including nummular pigmentation) seen at the posterior pole and macular atrophy (advanced disease). (B,C) Optical coherence tomography images showing bilateral foveal cysts.

undetectable. The responses to the same flash strength under photopic (LA 3.0) and scotopic conditions (DA 3.0) are of similar waveform, being simplified and very delayed. In addition, the amplitude of the 30 Hz flicker ERG, which in a normal subject falls between that of the LA 3.0 response a- and b-waves, is usually of lower amplitude than the photopic a-wave..

Molecular genetics and pathogenesis

Mutations in *NR2E3* (encoding a transcription factor) have been identified in ESCS and Goldmann-Favre syndrome; a gene believed to play a role in determining cone cell fate.[65] In ESCS there is evidence of a greater than normal number of S-cones, with mutation in *NR2E3* thought to cause disordered

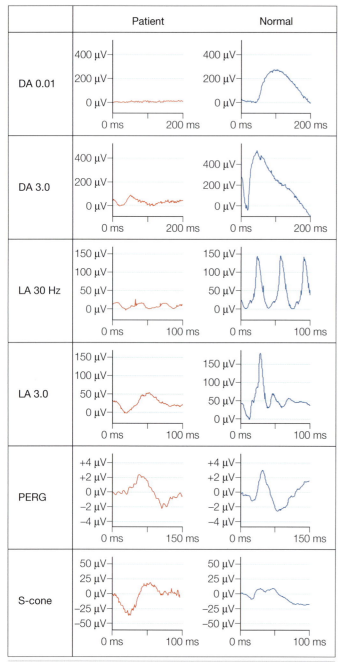

Fig. 44.31 Enhanced S-cone syndrome (ESCS). The rod-specific ERG (DA 0.01) is undetectable in keeping with the known absence of rods in this disorder. However, the two main diagnostic features are, firstly, the similarity in waveform between the photopic (LA 3.0) and scotopic (DA 3.0) ERG to the same stimulus, both of which show a simplified grossly delayed waveform, and, secondly, the amplitude of the grossly delayed 30 Hz flicker ERG being lower than that of the photopic a-wave. In a normal subject, the 30 Hz flicker ERG amplitude always falls between that of the photopic a-wave and the photopic b-wave. Note the profoundly delayed PERG, often present when the PERG is detectable in this disorder, and the increased sensitivity to short wavelength stimulation revealed by specific S-cone ERG recording (5 ms blue stimulus on a bright orange background). In a normal subject, the S-cone ERG consists of two components: a late S-cone specific component at ~50 ms and an L-/M- cone component at ~30 ms. The earlier component is not present in the patient, and the later component is enhanced.

cone cell differentiation, possibly by encouraging default to the S-cone pathway and thereby altering the relative ratio of cone subtypes. A small number of cones coexpress L-/M- and S-opsins.[65]

Management

There is currently no specific treatment for the vast majority of these inherited retinal disorders. Nevertheless, it is important that the correct diagnosis is made at an early stage, in order to be able to provide accurate information on prognosis and for informed genetic counseling. Obtaining a molecular genetic diagnosis often facilitates genetic counseling and advice on prognosis.

The provision of appropriate spectacle correction, low vision aids, and educational support is also very important. Photophobia may be a prominent symptom, especially in the cone dysfunction syndromes, and therefore tinted spectacles or contact lenses may be beneficial in both improved comfort and vision. Macular edema or foveal schisis may be amenable to treatment with topical or oral carbonic anhydrase inhibitors.

Conclusions

Inherited retinal disorders are a common cause of childhood blindness and most are not currently amenable to specific forms of treatment. Advances in molecular biology have led to the identification of many causative genetic mutations and it is likely that over the next few years the molecular pathology of most disorders will be known. This is the first stage in understanding the mechanisms that lead to photoreceptor cell death.

Treatment strategies aimed at prolonging photoreceptor survival or improving function are currently being investigated in animal models and in limited human clinical trials, and include the use of exogenous growth factors, pharmacologic intervention, gene therapy, and stem cell based therapies.[33,34,35,66,67,68,69] Another approach for more advanced disease is the development of retinal implants, which are also being investigated in clinical trials.[70]

There is cautious optimism that these multiple avenues of research will yield meaningful treatments for various forms of genetic retinal disease in the near future.

References

1. Boycott KM, Pearce WG, Bech-Hansen NT. Clinical variability among patients with incomplete X-linked congenital stationary night-blindness and a founder mutation in *CACNA1F*. Can J Ophthalmol 2000; 35: 204–13.
3. Jacobi FK, Andreasson S, Langrova H, et al. Phenotypic expression of the complete type of X-linked congenital stationary night blindness in patients with different mutations in the *NYX* gene. Graefes Arch Clin Exp Ophthalmol 2002; 240: 822–8.
5. van Dorp DB, Eriksson AW, Delleman JW, et al. Åland eye disease – no albino misrouting. Clin Genet 1985; 28: 526–31.
7. Chen J, Simon MI, Matthes MT, et al. Increased susceptibility to light damage in an arrestin knockout mouse model of Oguchi disease (stationary night blindness). Invest Ophthalmol Vis Sci 1999; 40: 2978–82.

8. Chen CK, Burns ME, Spencer M, et al. Abnormal photoresponses and light-induced apoptosis in rods lacking rhodopsin kinase. Proc Natl Acad Sci U S A. 1999; 96: 3718–22.

11. Sergouniotis PI, Sohn EH, Li Z, et al. Phenotypic variability in rdh5 retinopathy (fundus albipunctatus). Ophthalmology 2011; 118: 116–70.

12. Schatz P, Preising M, Lorenz B, et al. Fundus albipunctatus associated with compound heterozygous mutations in RPE65. Ophthalmology 2011; 118: 888–94.

13. Michaelides M, Hunt DM, Moore AT. The cone dysfunction syndromes. Br J Ophthalmol 2004; 88: 291–7.

14. Neitz M, Neitz J. Molecular genetics of color vision and color vision defects. Arch Ophthalmol 2000; 118: 691–700.

16. Genead MA, Fishman GA, Rha J, et al. photoreceptor structure and function in patients with congenital achromatopsia. Invest Ophthalmol Vis Sci 2011; 52: 7298–308.

18. Glickstein M, Heath GG. Receptors in the monochromat eye. Vision Res 1975; 15: 633–6.

20. Johnson S, Michaelides M, Aligianis IA, et al. Achromatopsia caused by novel mutations in both CNGA3 and CNGB3. J Med Genet 2004; 41: e20.

26. Michaelides M, Johnson S, Simunovic MP, et al. Blue cone monochromatism: a phenotype and genotype assessment with evidence of progressive loss of cone function in older individuals. Eye (Lond) 2005; 19: 2–10.

30. Michaelides M, Johnson S, Bradshaw K, et al. X-linked cone dysfunction syndrome with myopia and protanopia. Ophthalmology 2005; 112: 1448–54.

32. den Hollander AI, Roepman R, Koenekoop RK, Cremers FP. Leber congenital amaurosis: genes, proteins and disease mechanisms. Prog Retin Eye Res 2008; 27: 391–419.

33. Bainbridge JW, Smith AJ, Barker SS, et al. Effect of gene therapy on visual function in Leber's congenital amaurosis. N Engl J Med 2008; 358: 2231–9.

34. Cideciyan AV, Aleman TS, Boye SL, et al. Human gene therapy for RPE65 isomerase deficiency activates the retinoid cycle of vision but with slow rod kinetics. Proc Natl Acad Sci USA 2008; 105: 15112–7.

35. Hauswirth WW, Aleman TS, Kaushal S, et al. Treatment of Leber congenital amaurosis due to RPE65 mutations by ocular subretinal injection of adeno-associated virus gene vector: short-term results of a phase I trial. Hum Gene Ther 2008; 19: 979–90.

38. Mukhopadhyay R, Holder GE, Moore AT, Webster AR. Unilateral retinitis pigmentosa occurring in an individual with a germline mutation in the RP1 gene. Arch Ophthalmol 2011; 129: 954–6.

39. Ayuso C, Millan JM. Retinitis pigmentosa and allied conditions today: a paradigm of translational research. Genome Med 2010; 2: 34.

40. Berger W, Kloeckener-Gruissem B, Neidhardt J. The molecular basis of human retinal and vitreoretinal diseases. Prog Retin Eye Res 2010; 29: 335–75.

42. Zito I, Downes SM, Patel RJ, et al. RPGR mutation associated with retinitis pigmentosa, impaired hearing, and sinorespiratory infections. J Med Genet 2003; 40: 609–15.

44. Berson EL, Rosner B, Sandberg MA, et al. A randomized trial of vitamin A and vitamin E supplementation for retinitis pigmentosa. Arch Ophthalmol 1993; 111: 761–72.

48. Lakhampal V, Schockett SS, Jiji R. Desferrioxamine (Desferol) induced toxic retinal pigmentary degeneration and presumed optic neuropathy. Ophthalmology 1984; 91: 443–51.

50. Roberts MF, Fishman GA, Roberts DK, et al. Retrospective, longitudinal, and cross sectional study of visual acuity impairment in choroideraemia. Br J Ophthalmol 2002; 86: 658–62.

51. Karna J. Choroideremia: a clinical and genetic study of 84 Finnish patients and 126 female carriers. Acta Ophthalmol 1986; 176 (Suppl.): 1–68.

55. Tada K, Saito T, Hayasaha S, Mizuno K. Hyperornithinemia with gyrate atrophy: pathophysiology and treatment. J Inherit Metab Dis 1983; 6: 105–6.

57. Michaelides M, Hardcastle AJ, Hunt DM, Moore AT. Progressive cone and cone-rod dystrophies: phenotypes and underlying molecular genetic basis. Surv Ophthalmol 2006; 51: 232–58.

62. Gouras P, Eggers HM, MacKay CJ. Cone dystrophy, nyctalopia, and supernormal rod responses: a new retinal degeneration. Arch Ophthalmol 1983; 101: 718–24.

67. Smith AJ, Bainbridge JW, Ali RR. Prospects for retinal gene replacement therapy. Trends Genet 2009; 25: 156–65.

 Access the complete reference list online at http://www.expertconsult.com

473

Part 6
Retinal & vitreous disorders

Pediatric retinal degeneration in systemic inherited diseases

Hélène Dollfus

Children affected by retinal degeneration associated with extraocular manifestations define the inherited systemic retinitis pigmentosa (RP) syndromes (retinal dystrophies related to inborn errors of metabolism are covered in Chapter 62) (Tables 45.1 and 45.2). The gene or the group of genes involved in the syndrome belong to a specific biologic network whose mutations lead to retinal degeneration associated with manifestations in other organs defined by the specific biologic role of the protein. Retinal degeneration in these syndromes illustrates the biologic complexity of the retina. The photoreceptor cell is remarkably sensitive to alterations in many biologic pathways but the clinical presentation is often indistinguishable between syndromes with the classical features of retinal degeneration: night-blindness, visual field constriction,

Table 45.1 – Main extraocular features found and the corresponding systemic retinitis pigmentosa syndrome

Extraocular clinical feature associated with RP in a child		Key feature found in systemic syndrome
Stature	Nanism	Cockayne's syndrome (cachectic), spondylometaphyseal dysplasia or spondyloepiphyseal dysplasia associated with cone dystrophy
	Obesity	Bardet-Biedl syndrome (BBS) Alström's syndrome, Cohen's syndrome (truncal), MORM (**m**ental retardation, truncal **o**besity, **r**etinal dystrophy, and **m**icropenis)
Skeletal abnormality	Polydactyly	BBS, Joubert's syndrome, Jeune's syndrome
	Short ribs with abnormal thorax	Jeune's syndrome
	Various abnormal skeletal development	Spondylometaphyseal dysplasia or spondyloepiphyseal dysplasia
Deafness	Deafness	Usher's syndrome (variable severity according to types), Alström's syndrome (progressive starting in childhood)
CNS malformations	Cerebellar agenesis (molar tooth)	Joubert's syndrome
Kidney dysfunction	Polyuria-polydipsia	BBS, Alström's syndrome, Jeune's syndrome, Senior-Loken syndrome, Joubert's syndrome
	Kidney failure	
Endocrine dysfunction	Type 2 juvenile	Alström's syndrome
	Pituitary deficiency	Oliver-McFarlane
Cardiomyopathy		Alström's syndrome
Cognitive impairment		Classical: Cohen's syndrome, Joubert's syndrome Occasional: BBS, Alström's
Teeth	Amelogenesis imperfecta	Jalili's syndrome
	Prominent incisors	Cohen's syndrome
Skin/hair	UV sensitivity	Cockayne's syndrome
	Alopecia – early hair loss	Hypotrichosis with juvenile macular dystrophy; EEM (ectodermal dysplasia, ectrodactyly, macular dystrophy) syndrome
	Long eye lashes	Oliver-McFarlane

Table 45.2 – Main systemic retinitis pigmentosa syndromes

Name of the syndrome with retinal degeneration	Main diagnostic extraocular signs	Identified gene(s)	Pathogenesis
Usher's syndrome type 1	Deafness congenital and profound Vestibular dysfunction	MYO7A, cadherin-23 *(CDH23)* Harmonin protocadherin-15 *(PCDH15), SANS*	Stereocilia and photoreceptor development and function. Network of Usher proteins
Usher's syndrome type 2	Deafness congenital moderate to severe No vestibular deficit	*GPR98, Ush2A, PDZD7*	Stereocilia and photoreceptor development and function. Network of Usher proteins
Usher's sydnrome type 3	Late onset rod–cone dystrophy Late onset progressive deafness	*USH3A*	Stereocilia and photoreceptor development and function. Network of Usher proteins
Bardet-Biedl syndrome	Polydactyly Obesity Cognitive impairment Kidney dysfunction Urogenital malformation	*BBS1 to BBS16*	Ciliopathy
Alström's syndrome	Obesity Type 2 diabetes mellitus Deafness Dilated cardiomyopathy Kidney dysfunction Liver dysfunction Growth and endocrine deficiency Occasional developmental delay	*ALSM1*	Ciliopathy
MORM	Mental retardation Truncal obesity Micropenis	*INPP5E*	Ciliopathy
Senior-Loken syndrome	Nephronophtysis	*NPHP1 to 6, SDCCAG8*	Ciliopathy
Joubert's syndrome	Cerebellar vermis hypoplasia Ataxia Cognitive impairment Tachypnea Abnormal eye movements Kidney dysfunction Polydactyly	*INPP5E, CRPGRIP1L, CC2D2A, ARL13B, TMEM67, AHI1, NPHP1, NPHP6, CXORF5* (X-linked)	Ciliopathy
Jeune's syndrome	Severe constricted thorax Chondrodysplasia with short bones Kidney dysfunction Liver fibrosis	*ATD1, DYNC2H1, TTC21B, IFT80*	Ciliopathy
Cohen's syndrome	Myopia Facial gestalt Truncal obesity Prominent upper incisors Intermittent granulocytopenia Long tapered fingers Joint laxity Mental retardation	*VPS13B*	Presumed vesicular transport
Cockayne's syndrome	Cachectic darwfism Deafness Optic atrophy Cataract UV sensitivity Neurodegeneration	*CSA, CSB*	Transcription factor related
Jalili's syndrome	Amelogeneisis imperfecta	*CNNM4*	Metal transport protein
Hypotrichosis with juvenile macular dystrophy	Early hair loss	*CDH3*	Cadherin family
Ectodermal dysplasia, ectrodactyly, macular dystrophy (EEM) syndrome	Early hair loss Lobster-claw hands	*CDH3*	Cadherin family
Oliver-McFarlane syndrome	Long eye lashes Early hair loss Short stature – pituitary deficiency Developmental and neurologic impairment	Not known	
Spondylometaphyseal dysplasia or spondyloepiphyseal dysplasia associated to cone dystrophy	Short stature Limb abnormalities	Not known	

and reduced visual acuity. In the early phases of the retinal degeneration, the fundus may appear normal although the electroretinogram (ERG) is altered. Later, the fundus will denote the usual aspects observed in retinal degeneration: pigment mottling, pigment migration with spicules, optic disk pallor, narrowed vessels, and macular changes which are prominent and inaugural in the cone–rod dystrophies.

All the conditions are rare inherited diseases; the most frequent syndromes are Usher's syndrome (USH) and Bardet-Biedl syndrome (BBS).

During the last two decades, a considerable number of genes responsible for these conditions have been identified. This field will continue to greatly benefit from new genome exploration especially high-throughput sequencing.[1-5] Molecular diagnosis and genetic counseling are constantly improving especially for those syndromes that are highly heterogeneous. The classical syndromes illustrating this group of diseases are described, but a growing number of overlapping phenotypes are revealed as molecular investigations improve. Moreover, different mutations in the same gene may lead to different syndromes of the same clinical spectrum (see section on the ciliopathies). Major clinical variability in each syndrome has been described. For some genes, specific mutations may lead to isolated features such as isolated RP (e.g. Usher's syndrome gene *USH2A* or Bardet-Biedl gene *BBS8* and *BBS3*).[6-8]

A child with RP should be evaluated for extraocular associated feature. These conditions require multidisciplinary follow-up and management.

Usher's syndrome: a deaf child who loses vision

Usher's syndrome (USH) is the association of sensorineural deafness with progressive retinal degeneration. Usher's syndrome occurs in 1 of every 10 deaf children (5% of all cases of congenital deafness). It is the most frequently inherited syndrome with deafness and is the most common syndrome among the deaf–blind.[9-11] The syndrome is subdividied into three groups: Usher's type 1 (USH1), type 2 (USH2), and type 3 (USH3). USH1 and 2 are usually diagnosed in early or late childhood, respectively, but may be diagnosed later in life as the visual impairment may be overlooked in a deaf child. Vestibular dysfunction is classically associated with USH1. Each type of Usher's syndrome is autosomal recessive but genetically heterogeneous. For each type, a number of genes have been identified[12-16] (Table 45.1). Molecular studies have shown clinical overlap between the classical types USH1 and USH2.[17] Some Usher's genes can be involved in either isolated deafness or isolated RP (USH2A).[6,16]

Cochlear implantation is highly recommended for these children (especially in USH1). No therapy is yet available for the retinal degeneration[18,19] (Fig. 45.1A–C).

Usher's syndrome type 1: the most severe form

The child with USH1 is affected with congenital severe to profound sensorineural hearing loss associated with delayed sitting and walking due to abnormal vestibular function. Retinal degeneration occurs early in childhood. As early as 2 or 3 years old, the ERG can confirm the diagnosis of retinal degeneration although the fundus appears to be normal.[20,21] Five causative genes are known and mutated in various proportions according to the studied population: MYO7A (recognized to be the main USH1 gene mutated in half of the cases and also responsible for non-syndromic deafness), USH1C, CDH23, PCDH15, and USH1G.[14,16] Although always severe, the course of disease may vary according to the type of mutation.[22]

Usher's syndrome type 2: later onset retinal degeneration in a deaf child

Congenital mild to severe sensorineural stable hearing loss with major impairment in high frequencies and normal vestibular function are the main characteristics of USH2. The retinal degeneration occurs later than in USH1, usually during puberty or after. USH2 and USH3 are not usually symptomatic in the first decade and initially have a normal fundus appearance. Many patients retain good visual acuity in spite of constricted visual fields. The ERG may initially be normal; however, ERG changes may be detected in presymptomatic young children. During the second decade, night-blindness and loss of peripheral vision become evident and inexorably progress (Fig. 45.1D). Three genes have been identified: USH2A (Usherin found also mutated in isolated RP), GPR98, and DFNB31.[14,16]

Usher's syndrome type 3: the later onset, variable form

The onset of RP in USH3 is variable and is often recognized after the second decade of life, but can be confused with the two other types. Sensory hearing loss is postlingual (as opposed to the prelingual loss in USH1 and USH2) with patients acquiring normal speech, but it evolves progressively to profound deafness. Vestibular dysfunction of variable intensity occurs in half of the patients.

The USH3A gene has been identified in particular in Askenazi Jews and Finns. USH3 has also been found mutated in patients with USH1 and USH2.[14,16]

Pathogenesis of Usher's syndromes

Progress has been made in understanding the pathogenesis of this disease affecting the inner ear stereocilia and photoreceptor cells of the retina.[23-26] The USH1 gene products form a network, the Usher's interactome, which plays a key role in the early hair bundle development. They are also key components of the mechanoelectrical transduction machinery necessary for hearing. In the retina, the Usher interactome acts at the level of the ciliary/periciliary region of the connecting cilia of the photoreceptor cells. It is important in the transport of proteins between the outer and the inner segments.[27] Alteration of the USH proteins lead to early dysfunction of the inner ear and of the retina simultaneously (Fig. 45.1E).

The ciliopathies: a novel systemic retinal dystrophies group

A single non-motile cilium ("primary cilium") is present in almost every vertebrate cell; motile cilia are present only

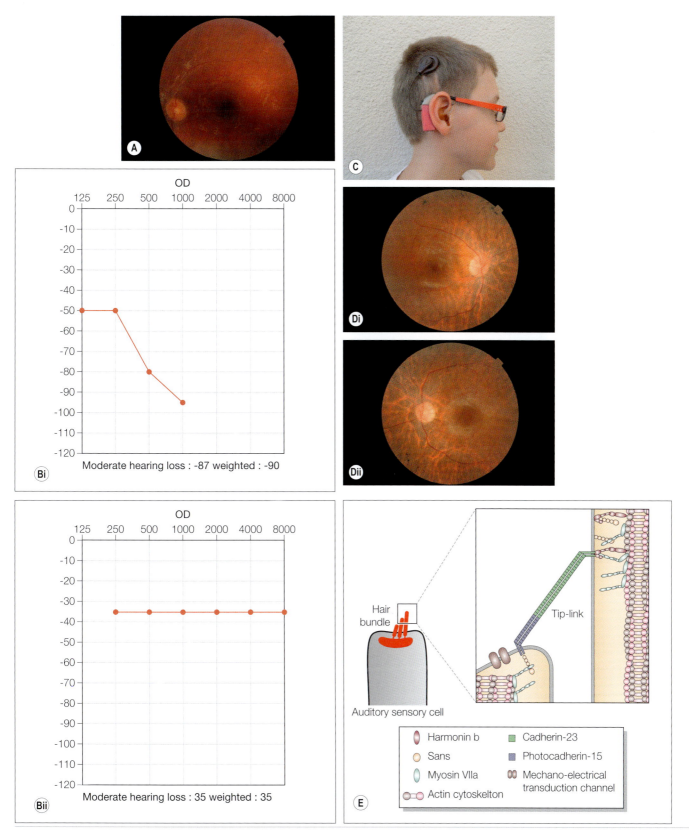

Fig. 45.1 Usher's syndrome. (A) Fundus photograph of a 5-year-old patient with Usher's syndrome type 1 mutated in MYO7A. The patient walked at age 24 months. The fundus shows very mild pigment epithelium heterogeneity and the ERG is extinguished. (Bi) Audiogram of the same patient before implantation showing profound deafness. (Bii) Audiogram after cochlear implantation showing dramatic hearing improvement. (C) Profile photograph of the patient showing the cochlear implantation device. (Di) Fundus photograph of the right eye of a patient affected by Usher's syndrome type 2 C (carrying mutations in VLGR1). (Dii) Fundus photograph of the left eye of the same patient showing retinitis pigmentosa. (Ei) Schematic representation of an auditory sensory cell and of the tip link molecular complex. (Eii) Disorganized hair bundles of auditory sensory cells in Ush1 mutant mice (scanning electron microscopy). In the control mouse (left), the three rows of stereocilia (small, middle, and tall) form the V-shaped hair bundle. In a mutant mouse that lacks one of the Ush1 proteins (right), the hair bundle is fragmented. (Fig. 45.1E courtesy of Professor Christine Petit, Institut Pasteur, Inserm, UPMC, Collège de France, Paris, France.)

in specific organs such as the respiratory or the reproductive system (Fig. 45.2A). The primary cilium is the central "antenna" of the cell allowing transduction of sensorial information from the extracellular environment to the cell. The photoreceptor cell has a connecting cilium and is, therefore, a ciliated cell.

Ciliopathies are rare genetic disorders characterized by primary cilium dysfunction, frequently affecting photoreceptors and causing retinal degeneration either as an isolated condition (e.g. Leber's congenital amaurosis with CEP290 mutations) or as a ciliopathy syndrome affecting more than one organ system.[28-30] Ciliopathies involve many target organs that have in common an important role of the primary cilia.

Overlapping phenotypes have been reported, as well as high clinical variability on the number of affected organs among patients with the same syndrome. The most common ciliopathies are schematically represented in Fig. 45.2B.

Molecular investigations have revealed major genetic heterogeneity for each syndrome and also allelic variability (different mutations in the same gene may lead to different syndromes). For instance, CEP290-*NPHP6* truncating mutations have been identified in Joubert's syndrome and hypomorphic mutations in Leber's congenital amaurosis (LCA). Moreover, CEP290-*NPHP6* is mutated in several distinct disorders (nephronophthisis, Senior-Loken syndrome, Joubert's syndrome, BBS and the lethal Meckel syndrome).[31]

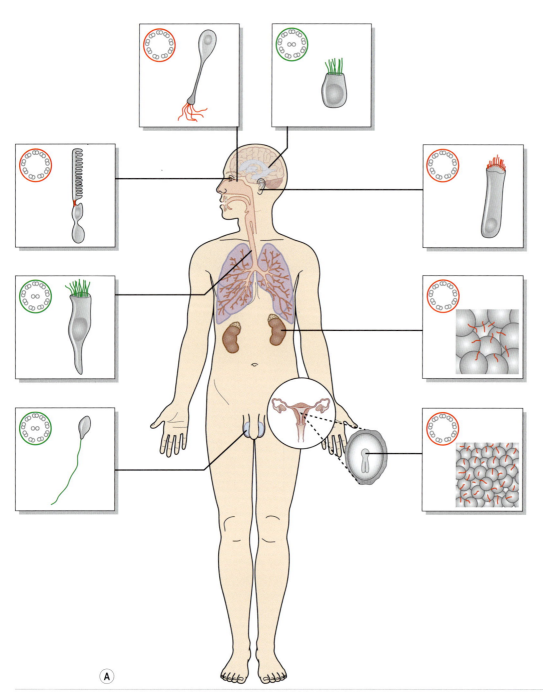

Fig. 45.2 Ciliopathies. (A) Schematic representation of cilia in various cells in the human being. In green: motile cilia; in red: primary cilia.

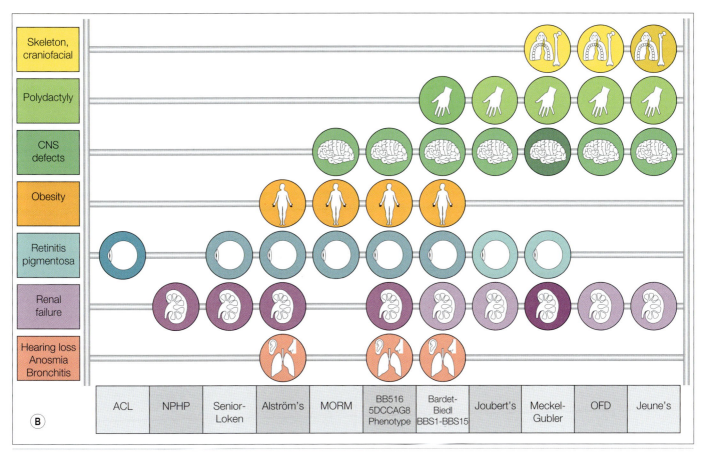

	ACL	NPHP	Senior-Loken	Alström's	MORM	BB516 5DCCAG8 Phenotype	Bardet-Biedl BBS1-BBS15	Joubert's	Meckel-Gubler	OFD	Jeune's

Fig. 45.2 *Continued* (B) Schematic representation as an abacus (adding various target organs) of syndromes recognized as ciliopathies.

Supplementary genetic factors such as a third mutated allele in a BBS gene (known as oligogenism – a third mutation occurring in addition to the two main mutations found in recessive inheritance) or other genetic modifiers can influence the phenotype.[32,33]

A yearly multidisciplinary follow-up is recommended for these children with special attention given to kidney function and prevention of obesity.

Bardet-Biedl syndrome

The cardinal features of the BBS syndrome are early onset retinal degeneration, obesity, polydactyly, renal failure, hypogonadism, and cognitive impairment (Fig. 45.3A–D). Secondary features may include anosmia, diabetes, cardiac anomalies, hepatic fibrosis, brachydactyly, and Hirschprung's disease.[34,35] The retinal dystrophy is early in onset leading to severe visual handicap before adulthood. Profound ERG abnormalities can be detected as early as 3 years old. Legal blindness usually results before the second decade of life.[36-42] Retinal dystrophies in BBS are mainly a rod–cone dystrophy or a cone–rod dystrophy,[34] usually classified as a global retinal degeneration because both rods and cones are affected[29] (Fig. 45.3E).

Obesity is the second major feature, present in 72–96% of BBS patients, usually beginning in early childhood and worsening with age. The origin of obesity is both central (the hypothalamic eating control) and peripheral (the adipose tissue).[43-45] Limb anomalies are found in almost 95% of BBS patients, usually a postaxial polydactyly (69%). Other

limb malformations such as brachydactyly or syndactyly are frequently reported for both hands and feet and have a diagnostic value. Abnormalities of the genitalia are common: hypogonadism in males or vaginal atresia in females. Rarely, there is hydrometrocolpos, a neonatal vaginal malformation leading to a massive abdominal tumor.[46,47] Renal dysfunction can occur in late childhood and may lead to kidney failure.[48]

Neuropsychiatric symptoms can include developmental delay, mental retardation, learning difficulties, speech deficit, and behavioral problems.[34] Intellectual function ranges from severe mental retardation (29%) through weak intelligence and average intelligence (29%). Slow ideation and hyperemotive status are common.

BBS is an autosomal recessive heterogeneous condition with 16 genes identified accounting for about 85% of cases.[49] All the genes have been related to cilium biogenesis and/or function. BBS1 and BBS10 are the two most common, each accounting for about 20% of the cases. Implication of the other BBS genes ranges from a unique family to a few percentage of mutated families. The classical autosomal recessive inheritance model has been challenged by molecular and functional investigations with the oligogenic model and the effect of additional genetic modulators on the phenotype.[33]

Alström's syndrome

Alström's syndrome (ALMS) manifestations include RP in early childhood, hearing impairment, and metabolic defects

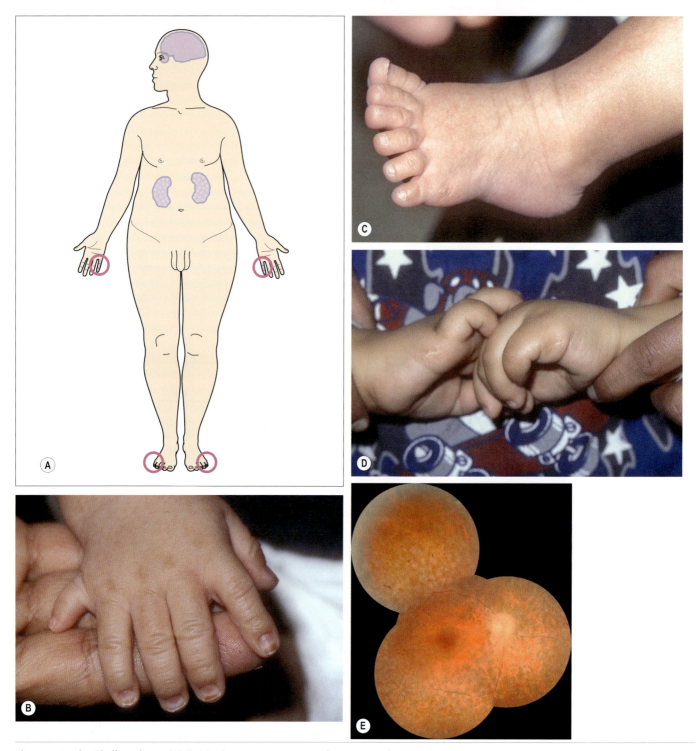

Fig. 45.3 Bardet-Biedl syndrome (BBS). (A) Schematic representation of the BBS with five major manifestations: obesity, polydactyly, renal dysfunction, retinitis pigmentosa, and cognitive impairment. (B) Polydactyly of the hand of a patient aged 6 months old carrying mutations in the BBS1 gene. (C) Polydactyly of the foot of a patient aged 6 months old carrying mutations in the BBS1 gene. (D) Bilateral scarring resulting of the surgical removal of the extra digits in the eldest brother of the previous case. (E) Fundus photograph of a teenager patient carrying mutations in the *BBS16* gene showing widespread retinal degeneration.

leading to hyperinsulinemia and type 2 diabetes mellitus and obesity in childhood. Polydactyly does not occur. Dilated cardiomyopathy, often fatal, in infancy or later in life and renal dysfunction are reported in half of ALMS cases.[50] Developmental or motor delays occur, but most children have normal intelligence.

The first manifestation of ALMS is severe early onset cone–rod retinal dystrophy, sometimes mimicking Leber's congenital amaurosis with very early visual impairment, photophobia, and nystagmus (Fig. 45.4). Children usually become truncally obese during their first year. Sensorineural hearing loss presents in the first decade in up to 70%; it may progress to the

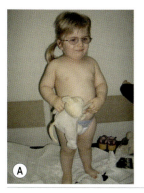
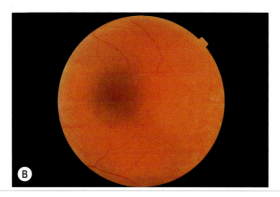
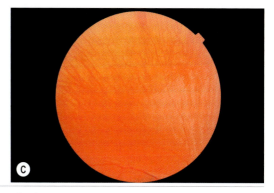

Fig. 45.4 Alström's syndrome. (A) The patient is 26 months old, referred for photophobia and overweight. She carries mutations in the ALS gene. (B) Fundus photograph of the patient's macular region showing marked heterogeneity of the macula confirmed by major photopic impairment on ERG (complemented by scotopic impairment at a lesser degree). (C) Peripheral photograph of the fundus showing retinal thinning and heterogeneous pigmentation.

moderately severe range (40–70 db) by the end of the first to second decade. Insulin resistant type 2 diabetes mellitus often presents in the second decade and is accompanied by acanthosis nigricans (pigmentation mostly in body folds). Other endocrine and metabolic abnormalities include hypothyroidism, diabetes insipidus, growth hormone deficiency, hyperuricemia, hyperlipidemia, hypothyroidism, and hypogonadotrophic hypogonadism. Hepatic and renal dysfunction can be present in the second decade. This syndrome requires a multidisciplinary follow-up to detect complications once the diagnosis is confirmed.[50,51]

A single gene is involved in all the cases, *ALMS1*.[52,53] ALMS1 protein is found at the base of cilia.[54]

MORM syndrome

MORM syndrome (**m**ental retardation, truncal **o**besity, **r**etinal dystrophy, and **m**icropenis) is very rare.[55] A congenital nonprogressive retinal dystrophy with poor night vision occurs within the first year of life with reduced visual acuity by 3 years that remains stable thereafter. The identified gene, *INPP5E* (inositol polyphosphate-5-phosphatase), classifies this syndrome as a ciliopathy. It is related to Joubert's syndrome.[56]

Senior-Loken syndrome

Senior-Loken syndrome (SLS) combines nephronophthisis (NPH) and retinal degeneration. NPH, the most common cause of inherited renal failure in childhood, is characterized by initial normal kidney size that will eventually shrink, tubulo-interstitial nephritis, and a loss of corticomedullary differentiation leading to cyst formation.[30,57,58] The first symptoms are polyuria and polydipsia caused by a urinary concentration defect. The end-stage of the renal failure is variable – infantile, juvenile, or adolescent. The occurrence of the retinal dystrophy is higher in the juvenile form of NPH. The early retinal dystrophy usually occurs years before the kidney involvement is detected. The retinal dystrophy may be very early, mimicking isolated LCA or may have a later onset. Thus, clinical diagnosis of LCA should lead to clinical and molecular testing for LCA-SLS associated genes and, according to the results, annual kidney follow-up may be indicated.

SLS is a ciliopathy and the kidney involvement is explained by the role of the *NPHP* proteins at the level of the tubular epithelial renal cells that each carry a primary cilium in contact with the urinary flow.

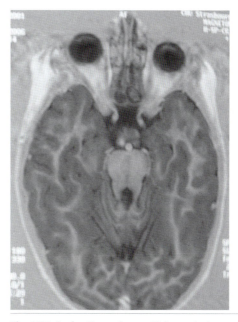

Fig. 45.5 Joubert's syndrome. Molar tooth sign on the MRI of a child with Joubert's syndrome carrying mutations in the *NPHP6/CEP290* gene.

Eleven genes (*NPHP1* to *NPHP11*) are known to be involved in NPH, and for all of them, except *NPHP7*, cases of SLS associated with RP have been reported.[30,58-61] Mutations in *NPHP5*[62] and *NPHP6*[63] are more often linked to severe and early RP. A milder retinal phenotype is observed with mutations in other *NPHP* genes.

Joubert's syndrome

Joubert's syndrome may be autosomal recessive or inherited as an X-linked pattern.[64] This syndrome is a combination of cognitive impairment, ataxia, tachypnea, eye movement abnormalities with frequent retinal degeneration, and kidney manifestations. Cerebellar vermis hypoplasia is a pathognomonic finding on MRI named "the molar tooth" sign (Fig. 45.5).[65,66] Multiple other features can be associated with this midbrain–hindbrain malformation leading to the denomination of Joubert's syndrome and associated disorders (JSAD). Kidney manifestations are cystic dysplasia, caused by multiple cysts of different sizes, or NPH. More than 30% of Joubert's patients develop kidney failure. Hepatic fibrosis occurs in 10%

of patients. Skeletal findings are rarer and include polydactyly and cone-shaped epiphyses. The ocular phenotype is broad and may include abnormal motility, nystagmus, and ocular motor apraxia (saccade initiation failure; see Chapter 90).[67] Coloboma has been reported rarely. RP occurs in a third of patients with either very early onset (mimicking LCA) or later onset night-blindness.[65] Ten genes have been identified to be mutated in JSAD: *INPP5E, AHI1, NPHP1, CEP290/NPHP6, MKS3, RPGRIP1L, ARL13B, CC2D2A, TMEM216,* and *OFD1* (oral-facial-digital syndrome 1).[66]

The RP phenotype varies with the mutated gene. Eighty percent of *AHI1* mutated patients present with a retinal dystrophy and NPH-related renal disorder but no hepatic defects. RP has been observed in one family out of two mutated in *ARL13B*.[68] *CC2D2A* is found mutated in JSAD patients with or without RP.[69] The same mutation in *TMEM216* was identified in eight JSAD-related families presenting psychomotor retardation and frequent retinopathy.[70]

Jeune's syndrome

Jeune's asphyxiating dystrophy or Jeune's syndrome is an autosomal recessive chondrodysplasia. The phenotype is highly variable and can lead to death in early infancy because of a severely constricted thoracic cage and respiratory insufficiency.[71,72] Patients present with a long narrow thorax due to short ribs (Fig. 45.6), shortened long bones, and sometimes polydactyly. Kidney cysts, hepatic fibrosis, and RP may occur as early as 5 years old. Two genes reported in patients with no retinal dystrophy have been identified: *IFT80* (intraflagellar transport 80 homolog Chlamydomonas) and *DYNC2H1* (dynein, cytoplasmic 2, heavy chain 1).[73-75]

Pathogenesis of the ciliopathies

The retinal degeneration in ciliopathies is related to dysfunction of the connecting cilium, a major site of transport and transit for proteins synthesized in the inner segment and necessary for phototransduction taking place in the outer segment[29] (Fig. 45.7). The ciliary-specific transport machinery is known as the intraflagellar transport (IFT) machinery and is composed of molecular motors linked to IFT protein complexes that organize anterograde and retrograde transport. Jeune's

syndrome is the only ciliopathy known to be related to IFT gene mutations, namely *IFT80*, a potential regulator of IFT particles[74,76] and *DYNC2H1*, a retrograde motor. To regulate cargo delivery to the cilium, two main regulatory pathways occur: vesicular sorting from the Golgi to the ciliary base and selective transport along the cilium. BBS proteins (the BBSome complex) are involved in these regulatory processes.[77]

The extraocular manifestations are linked to specific roles of ciliary proteins involved in the development or function of many organs. As an example, the kidney epithelial cells' primary cilia are mechanosensors.[78] Primary cilia are implicated in major developmental processes and especially in planar cell polarity, body asymmetry, or limb development.[79]

Other rare syndromes with retinal dystrophy

The following syndromes with retinal degeneration may correspond to a well defined biologic system (e.g. Cockayne's syndrome and DNA repair); others are still under investigation (e.g. Cohen's syndrome).

Cohen's syndrome

Cohen's syndrome is a rare worldwide autosomal recessive disorder, common in Finland where the phenotype is well defined, with clinical variability.[80-83] It is characterized by mental retardation, postnatal microcephaly, intermittent granulocytopenia, and facial dysmorphism with downslanting and wave-shaped palpebral fissures, short philtrum, heavy eyebrows, and a prominent nasal base (Fig. 45.8A,B). Long tapered fingers and joint laxity are common as well as prominent upper central incisors (Fig. 45.8C,D).[81,84] There may be a history of neonatal hypotonia with poor feeding and delay in motor milestones with speech delay, and stridor secondary to laryngomalacia. Truncal obesity is common, but not invariable, by 5 years of age. Early onset retinal dystrophy with myopia is classical.[85] The onset of myopia is usually under 5 years of age and exceeds 7 diopters by the second decade. The macula may develop a "bull's eye" appearance (Fig. 45.8E) in the first decade evolving toward a cone–rod dystrophy. The first

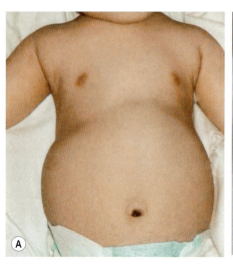
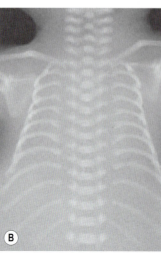

Fig. 45.6 Jeune's syndrome. (A) Photograph of the narrow thorax of a young patient with Jeune's syndrome. (B) X-ray of a patient with Jeune's syndrome showing short ribs. (Courtesy of Professor Valerie Cormier-Daire, Medical Genetics Department, IMAGINE Foundation, Hôpital Necker-Enfants Malades, Paris, France.)

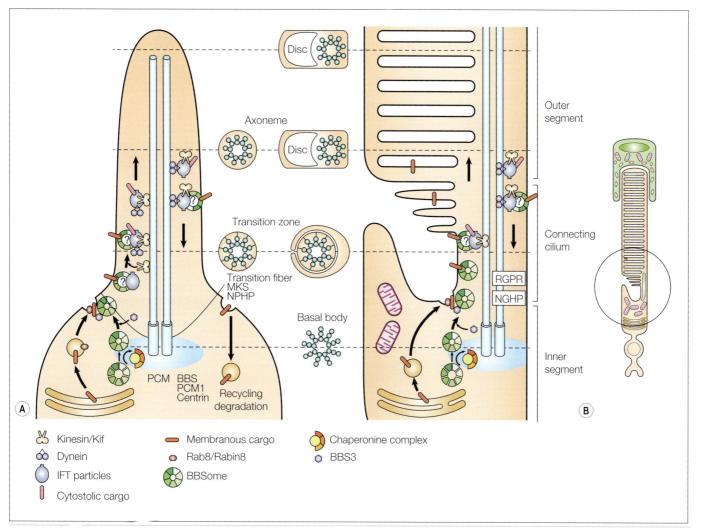

Fig. 45.7 Ciliary structure. The photoreceptor connecting cilium is structurally very similar to the classical primary cilium which are compared in the picture. Schematic representation of the ciliary protein complexes especially the BBS proteins and noticeably the BBSome. (From Mockel A, Perdomo Y, Stutzmann F, et al. Retinal dystrophy in Bardet-Biedl syndrome and related syndromic ciliopathies. Prog Retin Eye Res 2011; 30: 258–74.)

symptoms are of myopia and night-blindness followed by reduced acuity, visual field, generalized pigmentary retinopathy with bone spicules, or lacunar RPE atrophy in the mid-periphery by the second decade.

One gene has been identified which encodes for Vps13B that could have a role in vesicle-mediated sorting and transport of proteins within the cell.[86] Many mutations and intragenic deletions have been reported.[87,88]

Cockayne's syndrome and DNA repair

Cockayne's syndrome is a DNA repair disorder due to a dysfunction of the transcription-coupled DNA repair genes.[89,90] All the cells are hypersensitive to effects of UV light, which is used as the basis for the diagnostic cellular tests of cultured fibroblasts from a skin biopsy.

The main characteristics of the disease are UV skin sensitivity and severe physical and mental retardation (cachetic dwarfism) with progressive neurologic deterioration, sensorineural deafness, and retinal degeneration[91,92] (Fig. 45.9Ai–Aiii).

The retinal dystrophy is characterized by a "salt and pepper" pigmentation with optic disk pallor and progressive deterioration in the rod and cone ERG.[93,94] The progression is usually rapid. Cataracts may be present from birth and are often associated with poorly developed iris dilator muscle (the children are difficult to dilate and examine). Corneal changes may occur associated with lagophthalmos as well as chronic blepharitis that can make aphakic contact lens wear difficult[95] (Fig. 45.9(Aii)). Cachexia may lead to massive orbital fat atrophy.

Early death can occur especially if early onset cataracts are observed.[96] However, a spectrum of severity has been reported ranging from an early onset severe form, the cerebro-ocular-facial syndrome,[97,98] to severe, moderate, and mild forms diagnosed in adulthood as UV sensitivity only[99] (Fig. 45.9Bi–Biv). Mutations in two genes have been identified: CSA (group 8 excision-repair cross-complementing protein; ERCC8) and CSB (group 6 excision-repair cross-complementing protein; ERCC6).[100,101,102] The latter is more frequently mutated (60–80%).[103]

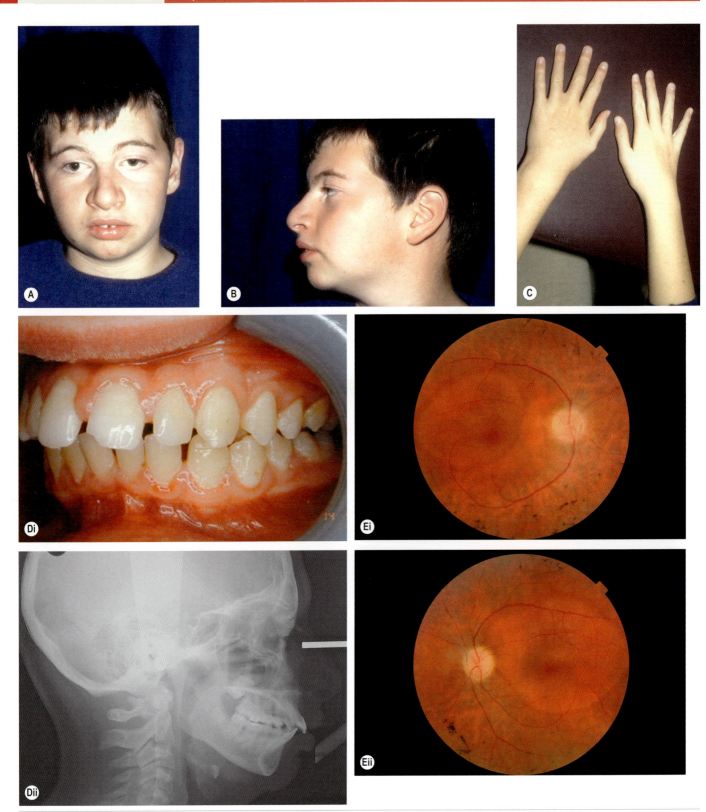

Fig. 45.8 Cohen's syndrome. (A) Photograph of the face of a patient with Cohen's syndrome carrying mutations in the *COCH* gene. (B) Profile photograph of the same patient. (C) Hands of the patient showing long tapered fingers. (Di) Prominent upper incisors seen on clinical dental photograph and (Dii) on X-ray. (Courtesy Dr Y. Bollender, Strasbourg, France.) (Ei,Eii) Fundus photographs of the patient showing retinal degeneration and a bull's eye appearance in constitution.

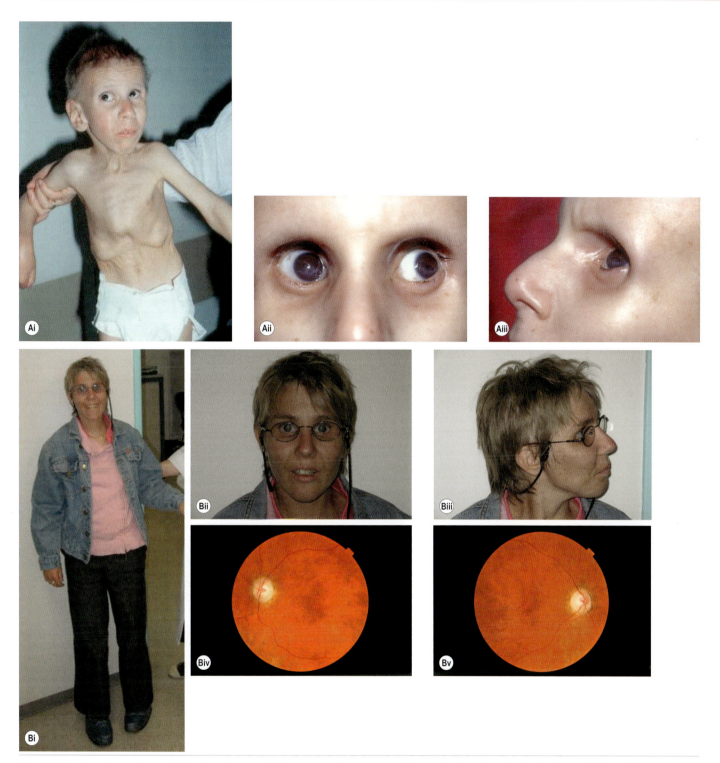

Fig. 45.9 Cockayne's syndrome. (Ai) Patient with severe Cockayne's syndrome carrying *CSB* mutation showing cachetic dwarfism and UV sensitivity after a very short sun exposure coming into the clinic. (Aii) Close-up photograph of the same patient a couple of years later with melting of the periocular fat and sunken eye appearance. Both pupils are miotic; he has chronic blepharitis and corneal involvement. (Aiii) Profile picture of the sunken eye appearance. (Bi) Patient with moderate Cockayne's syndrome with growth delay, carrying mutations in the *CSB* gene. (Bii) Facial close-up. Notice miotic pupils. (Biii) Profile close-up showing sunken eye appearance. (Biv,Bv) Fundus photographs showing retinal dystrophy and optic atrophy.

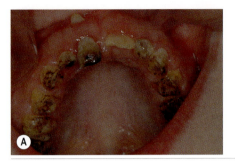
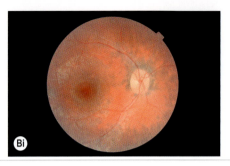
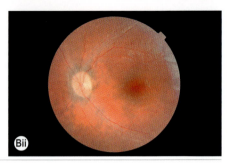

Fig. 45.10 Jalili's syndrome. (A) Amelogenesis imperfecta (abnormal enamel development) observed in the upper jaw of a patient carrying mutations in Jalili's syndrome gene. (Courtesy of Professor A. Bloch Zupan, Center for Rare Dental Diseases, Strasbourg, France.) (Bi,Bii) Fundus photographs of both eyes of the patient showing macular changes related to the cone dystrophy manifestations.

Pediatric syndromes with retinal degeneration and features of the ectodermal spectrum (hair, skin, teeth)

Retinal degeneration observed in children with abnormalities related to the ectodermal dysplasia spectrum (affecting hair, skin, nails, or sweat glands or teeth) is rare.

Hypotrichosis with juvenile macular dystrophy

Congenital hypotrichosis associated with juvenile macular dystrophy (HJMD, OMIM 601553) is an autosomal recessive condition with early hair loss and juvenile macular degeneration in the first decade that can show phenotypic variability.[104-106] The retinal involvement becomes widespread and is a cone–rod dystrophy.[107] Mutations have been identifed in a P-cadherin gene, *CDH3*, that encodes an integral membrane glycoprotein responsible for calcium-dependent cell–cell desmosomal adhesion.[108]

Ectodermal dysplasia, ectrodactyly, macular dystrophy syndrome

The ectodermal dysplasia, ectrodactyly, macular dystrophy (EEM) syndrome inherited as an autosomal recessive entity is a specific ectodermal entity because of the unusual associated retinal features.[109,110] The retinal involvement has a typical severe macular onset with geographic atrophy that has a peripheral progression. The patients are characterized by hypotrichosis with sparse and short hair, eyebrows and eyelashes, partial anodontia, and limb defects with syndactyly or "lobster-claw" hands.[110] The syndrome shares features with the HJMD syndrome and the *CHD3* gene is mutated, showing allelic variability.[111]

Interestingly, cadherins constitute a superfamily of genes found mutated in various genetic disorders including Usher's syndrome type 1 (USH1). For the latter, there is a crucial role of transient fibrous links formed by cadherin 23 and protocadherin 15 in the cohesion of the developing hair bundle as well as the involvement of these cadherins in the formation of the tip link, a key component of the mechanoelectrical transduction machinery.[112] This illustrates that proteins of the same superfamily may have different roles in inherited systemic retintal degenerative syndromes.

Uncombable hair with retinal pigmentary dystrophy, brachydactyly, and dental anomalies

This is a very rare ectodermal dysplasia with RP and is reported to be autosomal dominant.[113,114]

Oliver-McFarlane syndrome, trichomegaly, and chorioretinopathy with pituitary dysfunction

The Oliver-McFarlane syndrome is extremely rare, possibly autosomal recessive, and most often reported as sporadic cases with long eye lashes, hair abnormalities such as early alopecia, and short stature due to pituitary deficiency. Developmental and neurologic impairment with cerebellar ataxia may occur.[115-117] The retinal degeneration occurs as early as 5 years of age with night-blindness and rapid panretinal dysfunction. Vision is very reduced and there is extensive atrophy of the retinal pigment epithelium and choriocapillaris with an undetectable ERG.[118]

Retinal dystrophy and dental abnormalities: Jalili's syndrome

Jalili's syndrome is a very rare autosomal recessive condition with early onset cone–rod dystrophy and *amelogenesis imperfecta* (abnormal tooth biomineralization). The *CNNM4* gene has been identified as responsible. It encodes for a metal transport protein important for the retina and teeth[119,120] (Fig. 45.10).

RP syndrome with prominent skeletal involvement

Retinal degeneration may rarely be associated with inherited skeletal dysplasias. A child with spondylometaphyseal/epiphyseal dysplasia should undergo systematic ocular checkup. Genes and pathogenesis remain unknown although theories linking them to ciliopathies have been suggested.[121]

Spondylometaphyseal dysplasia short stature with cone dystrophy

This autosomal recessive condition has postnatal growth deficiency, profound short stature, platyspondyly (flattened vertebral bodies) and rhizomelic foreshortening of the limbs and early bowing of the long bones of the legs with shortening of all the tubular bones.[122] The retinal degeneration occurs in early childhood; it initially involves the macula with a cone–rod evolution. A phenotypically less severe skeletal axial spondylometaphyseal dysplasia with features of retinal dystrophy has been reported.[123-126]

Spondyloepiphyseal dysplasia with cone–rod dystrophy

Another skeletal dysplasia with short stature characterized by spondyloepiphyseal dysplasia has been described with cone–rod dystrophy[127,128] and associated with growth hormone deficiency.[121]

Conclusion

Retinitis pigmentosa can be part of a syndrome particularly when it presents in childhood. Extraocular manifestations may appear later or be already present at the time of diagnosis. Follow-up of a child affected with syndromic RP is multidisciplinary. The molecular diagnosis of these conditions is continuously improving, facilitating diagnosis and genetic counseling. The understanding of the pathogenesis is important and opens avenues for specific treatment for the retinal degeneration, such as gene therapy or pharmacologic approaches.

References

1. Biesecker LG. Exome sequencing makes medical genomics a reality. Nat Genet 2010; 42: 13–4.

15. Yan D, Liu XZ. Genetics and pathological mechanisms of Usher syndrome. J Hum Genet 2010; 55: 327–35.

23. Reiners J, Nagel-Wolfrum K, Jürgens K, et al. Molecular basis of human Usher syndrome: deciphering the meshes of the Usher protein network provides insights into the pathomechanisms of the Usher disease. Exp Eye Res 2006; 83: 97–119.

26. Richardson GP, Boutet de Monvel J, Petit C. How the genetics of deafness illuminates auditory physiology. Annu Rev Physiol 2011; 73: 311–4.

28. Baker K, Beales PL. Making sense of cilia in disease: the human ciliopathies. Am J Med Genet C Semin Med Genet 2009; 151C: 281–95.

29. Mockel A, Perdomo Y, Stutzmann F, et al. Retinal dystrophy in Bardet-Biedl syndrome and related syndromic ciliopathies. Prog Retin Eye Res 2011; 30: 258–74.

30. Hildebrandt F, Benzing T, Katsanis N. Ciliopathies. N Engl J Med 2011; 364: 1533–43.

33. Zaghloul NA, Katsanis N. Mechanistic insights into Bardet-Biedl syndrome, a model ciliopathy. J Clin Invest 2009; 119: 428–37.

34. Beales PL, Elcioglu N, Woolf AS, et al. New criteria for improved diagnosis of Bardet-Biedl syndrome: results of a population survey. J Med Genet 1999; 36: 437–46.

50. Marshall JD, Bronson RT, Collin GB, et al. New Alstrom syndrome phenotypes based on the evaluation of 182 cases. Arch Intern Med 2005; 165: 675–83.

52. Collin GB, Marshall JD, Ikeda A, et al. Mutations in ALMS1 cause obesity, type 2 diabetes and neurosensory degeneration in Alstrom syndrome. Nat Genet 2002; 31: 74–8.

54. Girard D, Petrovsky N. Alström syndrome: insights into the pathogenesis of metabolic disorders. Nat Rev Endocrinol 2011; 7: 77–88.

57. Salomon R, Saunier S, Niaudet P. Nephronophthisis. Pediatr Nephrol 2009; 24: 2333–44.

66. Sattar S, Gleeson JG. The ciliopathies in neuronal development: a clinical approach to investigation of Joubert syndrome and Joubert syndrome-related disorders. Dev Med Child Neurol 2011; 53: 793–8.

67. Khan AO, Oystreck DT, Seidahmed MZ, et al. Ophthalmic features of Joubert syndrome. Ophthalmology 2008; 115: 2286–9.

71. Tuysuz B, Baris S, Aksoy F, et al. Clinical variability of asphyxiating thoracic dystrophy (Jeune) syndrome: evaluation and classification of 13 patients. Am J Med Genet 2009; 149A: 1727–33.

74. Beales PL, Bland E, Tobin JL, et al. IFT80, which encodes a conserved intraflagellar transport protein, is mutated in Jeune asphyxiating thoracic dystrophy. Nat Genet 2007; 39: 727–9.

75. Dagoneau N, Goulet M, Genevieve D, et al. DYNC2H1 mutations cause asphyxiating thoracic dystrophy and short rib-polydactyly syndrome, type III. Am J Hum Genet 2009; 84: 706–11.

81. Kivitie-Kallio S, Norio R. Cohen syndrome: essential features, natural history, and heterogeneity. Am J Med Genet 2001; 102: 125–35.

82. Kolehmainen J, Wilkinson R, Lehesjoki AE, et al. Delineation of Cohen syndrome following a large-scale genotype-phenotype screen. Am J Hum Genet 2004; 75: 122–7.

83. Chandler KE, Kidd A, Al Gazali L, et al. Diagnostic criteria, clinical characteristics, and natural history of Cohen syndrome. J Med Genet 2003; 40: 233–41.

85. Kivitie-Kallio S, Summanen P, Raitta C, Norio R. Ophthalmologic findings in Cohen syndrome: a long-term follow-up. Ophthalmology 2000; 107: 1737–45.

90. Egly JM, Coin F. A history of TFIIH: Two decades of molecular biology on a pivotal transcription/repair factor. DNA Repair (Amst) 2011; 10: 714–21.

91. Rapin I, Lindenbau Y, Dickson DW, et al. Cockayne syndrome and xeroderma pigmentosum. Neurology 2000; 55: 1442–9.

94. Dollfus H, Porto F, Caussade P, et al. Ocular manifestations in the inherited DNA repair disorders. Surv Ophthalmol 2003; 48: 107–22.

96. Nance MA, Berry SA. Cockayne syndrome: review of 140 cases. Am J Med Genet 1992; 42: 68–84.

103. Laugel V, Dalloz C, Durand M, et al. Mutation update for the CSB/ERCC6 and CSA/ERCC8 genes involved in Cockayne syndrome. Hum Mutat 2010; 31: 113–26.

108. Sprecher E, Bergman R, Richard G, et al. Hypotrichosis with juvenile macular dystrophy is caused by a mutation in CDH3, encoding P-cadherin. Nat Genet 2001; 29: 134–6.

117. Haimi M, Gershoni-Baruch R. Autosomal recessive Oliver-McFarlane syndrome: retinitis pigmentosa, short stature (GH deficiency), trichomegaly, and hair anomalies or CPD syndrome (chorioretinopathy-pituitary dysfunction). Am J Med Genet 2005; 138A: 268–71.

119. Parry DA, Mighell AJ, El-Sayed W, et al. Mutations in CNNM4 cause Jalili syndrome, consisting of autosomal-recessive cone-rod dystrophy and amelogenesis imperfecta. Am J Hum Genet 2009; 84: 266–73.

 Access the complete reference list online at
http://www.expertconsult.com

Inherited macular dystrophies

Michel Michaelides • Anthony T Moore

Chapter contents

Introduction

The inherited macular dystrophies are characterized by bilateral central visual loss and symmetrical macular abnormalities. Most present in the first two decades of life with a wide range of clinical, electrophysiological, psychophysical, and histological findings. The molecular basis of inherited macular disease is now well understood, providing insights into the pathogenesis (Table 46.1).

We review pediatric macular dystrophies and not those that present later, such as Sorsby's fundus dystrophy, dominant drusen, and adult vitelliform macular dystrophy. Systemic disorders with macular dystrophy will be discussed in Chapters 45 and 62.

Autosomal recessive inheritance

Stargardt's disease and fundus flavimaculatus

Clinical and histological findings

Stargardt's macular dystrophy (STGD) is the most common inherited macular dystrophy with a prevalence of 1 in 10 000; it is inherited as an autosomal recessive trait. Most cases present with central visual loss in early teens. There is typically macular atrophy with yellow-white flecks at the level of the retinal pigment epithelium (RPE) at the posterior pole

Table 46.1 – Chromosomal loci and causative genes in inherited macular dystrophies

Macular dystrophy; OMIM number	Mode of inheritance	Chromosome locus	Mutated gene
Stargardt's disease/fundus flavimaculatus; 248200	Autosomal recessive	1p21–p22 (STGD1)	ABCA4
Stargardt's-like macular dystrophy; 600110	Autosomal dominant	6q14 (STGD3)	ELOVL4
Stargard's-like macular dystrophy; 603786	Autosomal dominant	4p (STGD4)	PROM1
Autosomal dominant 'bull's-eye' macular dystrophy; 608051	Autosomal dominant	4p (MCDR2)	PROM1
Best's macular dystrophy; 153700	Autosomal dominant	11q13	BEST1
Pattern dystrophy; 169150	Autosomal dominant	6p21.2-cen	PRPH2
Doyne's honeycomb retinal dystrophy; 126600	Autosomal dominant	2p16	EFEMP1
North Carolina macular dystrophy; 136550	Autosomal dominant	6q14–q16.2 (MCDR1)	Not identified
Autosomal dominant macular dystrophy resembling MCDR1; 608850	Autosomal dominant	5p15.33–p13.1 (MCDR3)	Not identified
North Carolina-like macular dystrophy associated with deafness	Autosomal dominant	14q (MCDR4)	Not identified
Progressive bifocal chorioretinal atrophy; 600790	Autosomal dominant	6q14–q16.2	Not identified
Sorsby's fundus dystrophy; 136900	Autosomal dominant	22q12.1–q13.2	TIMP3
Central areolar choroidal dystrophy; 215500	Autosomal dominant	6p21.2-cen; 17p13	PRPH2; GUCY2D
Juvenile retinoschisis; 312700	X-linked	Xp22.2	XLRS1

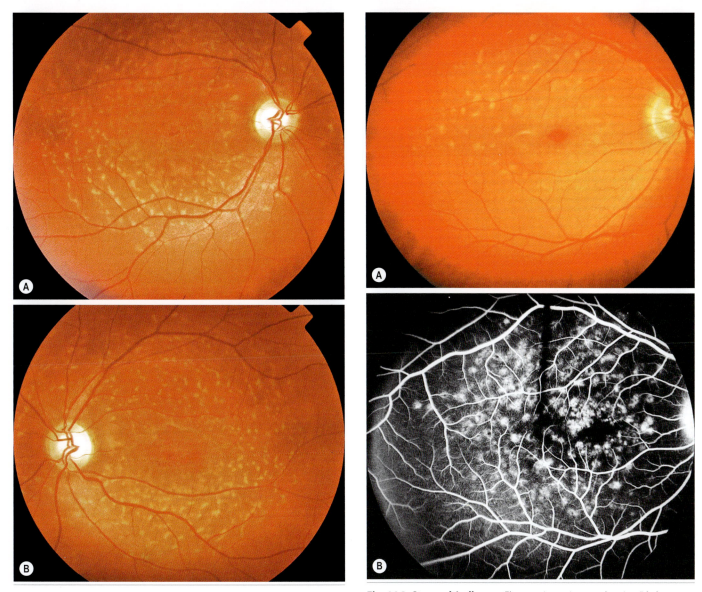

Fig. 46.1 Stargardt's disease. Yellow-white flecks at the level of the retinal pigment epithelium at the posterior pole. There is early macular atrophy.

Fig. 46.2 Stargardt's disease. Fluorescein angiogram showing "dark choroid" and transmission defects with a color fundus photograph above for comparison.

(Fig. 46.1). The flecks may be "fish-shaped" (pisciform), round, oval, or semilunar. The oval area of macular atrophy may, in the early stages, have a "beaten bronze" appearance (see Fig. 46.1). However, there may be no evidence of flecks at presentation, with the only abnormality being macular atrophy; but usually flecks develop over time. Fundus flavimaculatus (FFM) is when the retinal flecks occur without macular atrophy. STGD and FFM are caused by mutations in the same gene; both patterns may be seen in the same family. Most patients who present with FFM develop macular atrophy.

In both STGD and FFM, fluorescein angiography classically reveals a dark or masked choroid (Fig. 46.2) in the early phase. This is due to excess lipofuscin accumulation in the RPE, which obscures fluorescence from choroidal capillaries. The retinal flecks appear hypofluorescent on FFA early in their evolution, but later they appear hyperfluorescent due to RPE atrophy. Autofluorescence (AF) imaging, using the intrinsic fluorescence from lipofuscin in the RPE, has superseded FFA in confirming the diagnosis. The abnormal accumulation of

lipofuscin, the presence of active and resorbed flecks, and RPE atrophy are characteristic on fundus AF imaging.[1] (Fig. 46.3). In children with normal fundoscopy and visual loss from macular dysfunction, FFA is still helpful; a subtle window defect in the central macula or a dark choroid helps confirm the diagnosis.

Optical coherence tomography (OCT) often reveals loss, or marked disruption, of central outer retinal macular architecture with relative preservation of peripheral macular structure (Fig. 46.4).

Electrophysiology

Electrophysiological abnormalities in STGD are variable. An abnormal electro-oculogram (EOG), suggestive of generalized RPE dysfunction, is common. The pattern electroretinogram (PERG) and focal ERG are usually abolished or markedly reduced, suggesting macular dysfunction. The full-field ERG may be normal at diagnosis (group 1) or suggest widespread retinal dysfunction (group 2 or 3):[1]

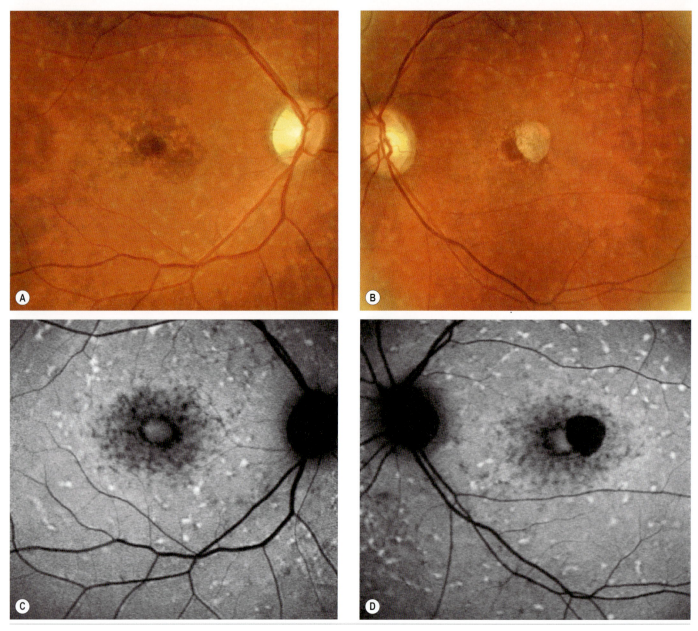

Fig. 46.3 Stargardt's disease. Characteristic appearance on fundus autofluorescence imaging showing abnormal accumulation of lipofuscin, the presence of active and resorbed flecks, and RPE atrophy. Color fundus photographs (above) are shown for comparison.

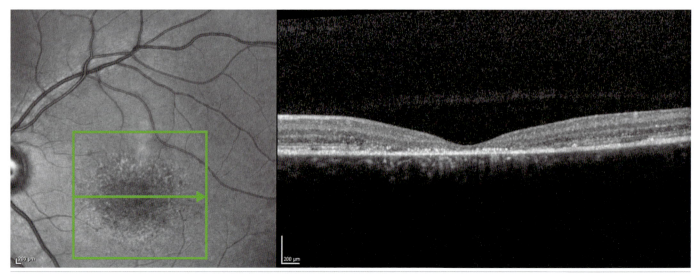

Fig. 46.4 Stargardt's disease. Spectral domain optical coherence tomography (SD-OCT) showing loss of central outer retinal macular architecture with relative preservation of peripheral macular structure. Outer retinal debris can be seen at the fovea.

Group 1: severe pattern ERG abnormality with normal full-field ERG.

Group 2: additional generalized cone dysfunction.

Group 3: generalized cone and rod dysfunction.

These groups are not explained by differences in age of onset or duration of disease; these electrophysiological groups may represent different phenotypic subtypes and thereby be helpful in informing prognosis. Patients in group 1 have better visual acuity, more restricted distribution of flecks, and macular atrophy; those in group 3 have the worst visual acuity, more widespread flecks, and macular atrophy is universal.

Molecular genetics and pathogenesis

Mutations in the gene *ABCA4* underlie STGD/FFM, and have also been implicated in retinitis pigmentosa (RP) and cone–rod dystrophy. *ABCA4* encodes a transmembrane rim protein in the outer segment discs of rod and cone photoreceptors involved in transport of retinoids from photoreceptor to RPE. Failure of this transport results in deposition of a lipofuscin fluorophore, A2E (*N*-retinylidene-*N*-retinylethanolamine), in the RPE,[2] which is deleterious to the RPE and leads to secondary photoreceptor degeneration.

More than 500 sequence variations in *ABCA4* have been reported, demonstrating the high allelic heterogeneity and highlighting the difficulties in assigning disease-causing status to sequence variants detected when screening such a large (50 exons) and polymorphic gene. Nonsense mutations with a major effect on the encoded protein can be confidently predicted to be disease-causing. A major problem occurs with missense mutations since sequence variants are common in controls; therefore, establishing pathogenicity may be problematic. Direct evidence of pathogenicity can only be established by functional analysis of the encoded mutant protein. The most common *ABCA4* mutation seen in STGD is Gly-1961Glu; Ala1038Val is also seen frequently.

Correlation between the type and combination of *ABCA4* mutations with the severity of the phenotype is often possible.[3] For example, biallelic null mutations usually lead to a cone–rod dystrophy phenotype rather than STGD. Variable retinal phenotypes within families may be explained by different combinations of *ABCA4* mutations segregating within a single family; it is likely that other modifier genes or environmental factors may also influence intra-familial variability.

Accumulation of lipofuscin-related products in the RPE, such as A2E, occurs in STGD and in *ABCA4* knockout mice (*abca4–/–*), resulting in free radical generation, release of pro-apoptotic mitochondrial proteins, and lysosomal dysfunction.[2] This leads to RPE dysfunction and cell death and subsequent photoreceptor cell loss.

A2E synthesis can be reduced by raising *abca4–/–* mice in total darkness, and is increased by feeding the mice supplemental vitamin A. It seems reasonable to advise STGD patients to avoid vitamin A supplementation and to wear ultraviolet light-blocking sunglasses. We also recommend an antioxidant rich diet which slows photoreceptor cell death in animal models of retinal dystrophies. Affected children may be helped by low vision aids and educational support.

There is a 1% risk of an affected individual having an affected child (higher if the partner is a close relative). The carrier frequency of STGD is 1 in 50; there is a 1 in 50 chance that an asymptomatic partner carries a disease-associated sequence change in *ABCA4*.

Future therapies

New therapeutic interventions for STGD include drugs that target the ATP dependent transport mechanism thereby augmenting ABCA4-related retinoid transport, or slow the visual cycle, reducing the production of A2E. Directly inhibiting the toxic effects of A2E may prove more effective. Pharmacological agents aimed at these three targets have been developed and are likely to progress to a human clinical trial in the near future.[2,4] Such agents may also be helpful in other macular degenerations associated with lipofuscin accumulation, such as Best's disease.

Other interventions include gene supplementation (http://www.clinicaltrials.gov), and cell-based or stem cell-based strategies aimed at providing supportive growth factors or RPE/photoreceptors for transplantation, respectively. It is likely that cell/stem cell-based clinical trials will be undertaken soon.

Autosomal dominant inheritance

Autosomal dominant Stargardt's-like macular dystrophy

Clinical and histological findings

Compared to the recessive disorder, individuals with autosomal dominant (AD) STGD-like dystrophy have a milder phenotype with good vision and minimal color vision defects. Individuals usually present in the first or second decades with visual loss which may precede retinal changes. Temporal optic disc pallor may precede retinal findings. The "dark choroid" sign on fluorescein angiography is uncommon in the dominant form. Histopathological findings are similar to autosomal recessive STGD, with widespread accumulation of lipofuscin throughout the RPE.

Electrophysiology

Individuals with AD-STGD-like dystrophy often have no significant EOG or ERG abnormalities.

Molecular genetics and pathogenesis

Inheritance patterns may distinguish the two forms of STGD but pseudodominance is a confounding factor – the carrier frequency of autosomal recessive STGD is sufficiently common (1 in 50) for an affected individual to have an asymptomatic partner carrying a disease-associated sequence change in *ABCA4*. Pseudodominance is also common in consanguineous families.

Two chromosomal loci have been identified: 6q14 (STGD3) and 4p (STGD4). Two mutations, a 5-bp deletion and two 1-bp deletions separated by four nucleotides, in the gene *ELOVL4* have been associated with STGD3 and other macular dystrophies, including pattern dystrophy. *ELOVL4* is expressed in rod and cone photoreceptor inner segments and may be involved in retinal fatty acid metabolism.

A missense mutation, p.Arg373Cys, in *PROM1* co-segregates with disease in STGD4. *PROML1* encodes human prominin 1 which has a role in outer segment disc formation and maintenance. The same *PROM1* missense mutation, p.Arg373Cys, occurs in patients with an early-onset autosomal dominant "bull's-eye" macular dystrophy (MCDR2).

Autosomal dominant "bull's-eye" macular dystrophy (MCDR2)

Clinical and histological findings

Onset is from the end of the first to the sixth decade, most presenting with reading difficulties.[5] RPE mottling in younger subjects progresses to a bull's-eye maculopathy (BEM) and, later, macular atrophy. Some patients have typical features of RP (see Chapter 44). Patients have a mild to moderate reduction in visual acuity, except when associated with RP where markedly reduced central vision is common.

Electrophysiology

Electrophysiological findings range from isolated macular dysfunction without generalized photoreceptor dysfunction, to a very severe rod–cone dysfunction.

Molecular genetics and pathogenesis

A distinct missense mutation, p.Arg373Cys, in *PROM1* has been identified.[5] Recessive nonsense mutations have also been reported in *PROM1* that cause a severe form of autosomal recessive RP, not associated with BEM.

Best's disease (vitelliform macular dystrophy)

Clinical and histological findings

Best's disease (BD) is an autosomal dominantly inherited macular dystrophy with a round or oval yellow subretinal macular deposit that is highly autofluorescent on AF imaging (Fig. 46.5). Although most gene carriers show a reduced light rise on EOG, the retinal phenotype is variable. Some gene carriers have a completely normal fundus. The phenotype is classified into five stages (Table 46.2):

Stage 0: pre-vitelliform – a normal fundus in an asymptomatic gene carrier with an abnormal EOG.

Stage I: minor RPE changes.

Stage II: classical "egg yolk" macular lesion (Fig. 46.6A). FFA shows a corresponding area of blocked choroidal fluorescence (Fig. 46.6B). This appearance is usually seen during the first or second decades, often with near normal visual acuity.

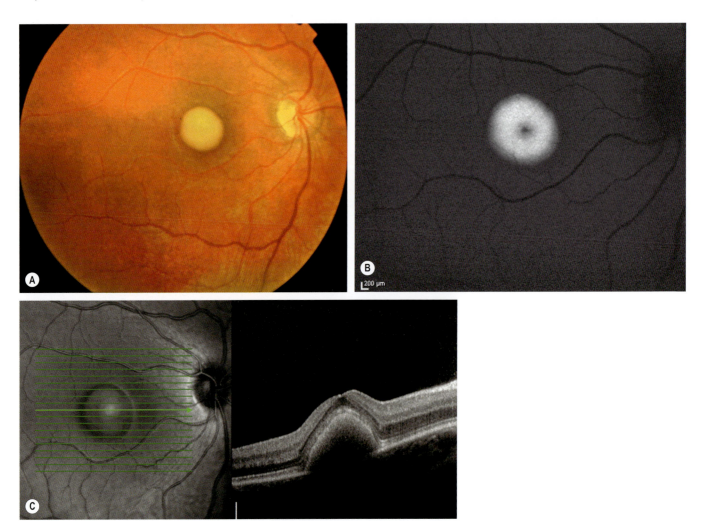

Fig. 46.5 Best's disease. Classical vitelliform lesion (stage II) (A), which is highly autofluorescent on AF imaging (B), and appears as a homogeneous subretinal deposit on SD-OCT (C).

Stage IIa: the "egg yolk" begins to break up secondary to resorption of the yellow material lying between the RPE and sensory retina, usually associated with noticeable visual impairment (Fig. 46.7).

Stage III: pseudohypoyon – part of the lesion is resorbed leaving the appearance of a "fluid level" at the macula.

Stage IVa: the yellow material is completely resorbed, leaving RPE atrophy.

Stage IVb: subretinal fibrosis.

Stage IVc: choroidal neovascularization (Fig. 46.6C,D).

Histopathology shows accumulation of lipofuscin throughout the RPE. Although the ophthalmoscopic abnormality is usually in the macular region, more widespread retinal involvement is present. The visual prognosis is good; most patients retain reading vision beyond the fifth decade. Carriers who have minimal macular abnormality or a normal fundus appearance (but abnormal EOG) in early adult life, usually retain good visual acuity.

Electrophysiology

Full-field ERG is normal; the EOG shows a reduced or absent light rise indicating widespread RPE dysfunction. Most individuals carrying mutations in the gene associated with BD, *BEST1*, have an abnormal EOG, but the macular appearance may be normal. True non-penetrance is rare.

Molecular genetics and pathogenesis

Best's disease is caused by mutations in *BEST1*, encoding the protein bestrophin, localized to the basolateral plasma membrane of the RPE. It forms a calcium-activated chloride channel that maintains chloride conductance and regulates fluid transport across the RPE. OCT studies suggest that impaired fluid transport in the RPE secondary to abnormal chloride conductance leads to accumulation of fluid and/or debris between RPE and photoreceptors and between RPE and Bruch's membrane, leading to detachment and secondary photoreceptor degeneration.[6] The variable expression of BD remains unexplained: additional genes and/or environmental influences may play a role in the wide range of clinical expression.

Recessive mutations have been identified in *BEST1* in a condition associated with multiple vitelliform retinal deposits and maculopathy: autosomal recessive bestrophinopathy (ARB).[7] Hyperopia is common and there is an increased incidence of angle-closure glaucoma. In childhood, the retinopathy is characterized by bilateral multifocal subretinal yellow deposits seen most clearly on AF imaging. Retinal edema and subretinal fluid may be observed clinically and on OCT (Fig. 46.8). The EOG light rise is absent or severely reduced. In contrast to the dominant form, the parents of patients with ARB have a normal EOG. Adults with ARB have an abnormal EOG and reduced rod and cone responses on full-field ERG.

Table 46.2 – Classification of vitelliform dystrophy

Stage	Macular appearance
0	Normal fundus (abnormal EOG)
I	Minor retinal pigment epithelial changes
II	Typical vitelliform lesion
IIa	"Scrambled egg" appearance
III	Pseudohypopyon phase
IVa	Atrophic retinal pigment epithelium
IVb	Fibrous scar tissue
IVc	Choroidal neovascularization

Modified from Mohler CW, Fine SL. Long-term evaluation of patients with Best's vitelliform dystrophy. Ophthalmology 1981; 88: 688–92.

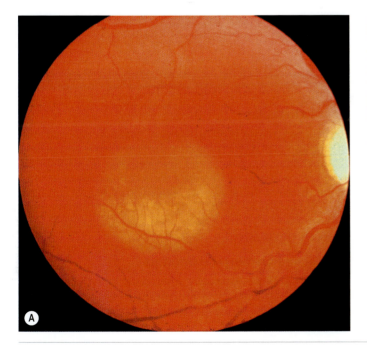

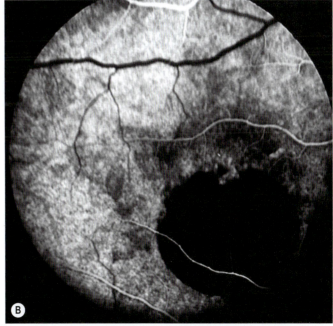

Fig. 46.6 Best's disease. (A) Classical vitelliform lesion (stage II) resembling an egg yolk "sunny-side up". (B) Fluorescein angiogram shows a corresponding area of blocked choroidal fluorescence.

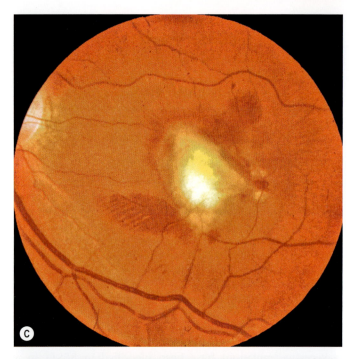

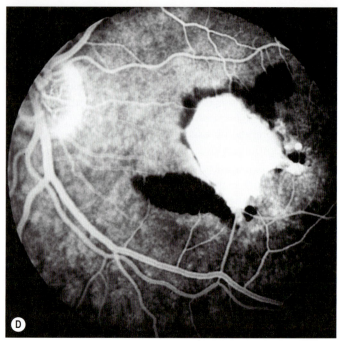

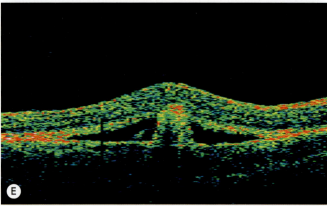

Fig. 46.6 *Continued* (C) Vitelliform lesion with choroidal neovascularization and subretinal hemorrhage (stage IVc). (D) Fluorescein angiogram. (E) OCT showing a choroidal neovascular membrane elevating the overlying retina.

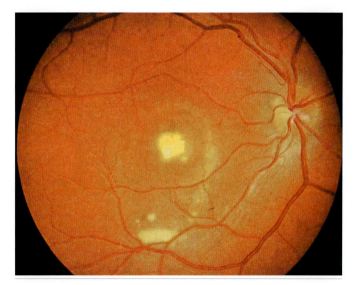

Fig. 46.7 Best's disease. A partially resorbed yellow subretinal macular deposit (stage IIa).

In children with ARB the ERG is usually normal. The prognosis for central vision is worse than in BD.

Future therapies

Future interventions may include gene-based therapies or therapeutic agents that either improve the function of the calcium-activated chloride channel and fluid exchange across the RPE, or slow the visual cycle to reduce the accumulation of lipofuscin, or directly inhibit the toxic end-product A2E, as has been described for STGD.[4]

Pattern dystrophies

Clinical and histological findings

Pattern dystrophies are usually dominantly inherited disorders of the RPE, with bilateral symmetrical yellow-orange deposits at the macula in various distributions, including butterfly or reticular patterns. There is increased AF (Fig. 46.9). On FFA, the macular deposits appear hypofluorescent secondary to blockade of underlying choroidal fluorescence. The macular deposits represent the accumulation of lipofuscin in RPE cells

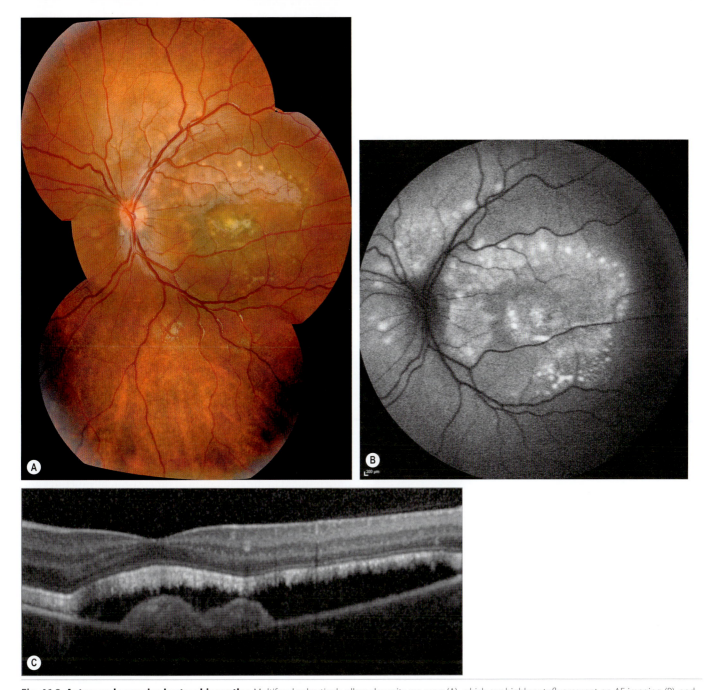

Fig. 46.8 Autosomal recessive bestrophinopathy. Multifocal subretinal yellow deposits are seen (A), which are highly autofluorescent on AF imaging (B), and often associated with retinal edema and subretinal fluid that may be observed clinically and on OCT (C).

and within the sub-RPE space, seen histopathologically. However, the RPE accumulation is not restricted to the macular region.

The macular changes are often associated with good vision although a slowly progressive loss of central vision may occur with atrophic macular changes. The age at presentation is between the second to fifth decades: it is rarely symptomatic in childhood. Examination of at-risk young family members may show mild macular changes.

Three main pattern dystrophy phenotypes have been described–butterfly-shaped dystrophy, reticular dystrophy, and fundus pulverulentus:

Butterfly-shaped dystrophy is inherited as an autosomal dominant trait, first evident in late childhood, characterized by normal or mildly reduced visual acuity and normal color vision, peripheral visual fields, and dark adaptation.

Reticular dystrophy is inherited as an autosomal dominant or recessive trait first appearing in early childhood. First, there is an accumulation of pigment granules at the fovea, later a typical reticular pattern extends to the periphery. Visual acuity is usually normal.

Fundus pulverulentus is a rare non-progressive disorder characterized by normal visual acuity and a symmetrical granular mottled pigmentation at the posterior pole (Fig. 46.10).

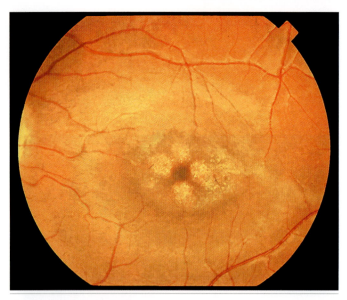

Fig. 46.9 **Pattern dystrophy.**

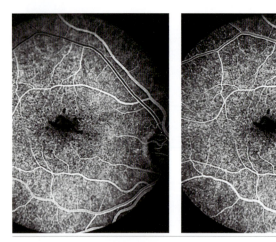

Fig. 46.10 **Fundus pulverulentus.** Fluorescein angiogram showing mottled and clumped pigment epithelium at the posterior pole. (Courtesy of Professor A.C. Bird.)

Electrophysiology

Usually, the pattern ERG and the EOG are abnormal, with variable full-field ERG ranging from normal to generalized cone and rod system dysfunction, suggesting widespread RPE-photoreceptor dysfunction.

Molecular genetics and pathogenesis

Mutations in the gene *PRPH2* (previously *peripherin/RDS*) have been described. Further genes remain to be identified.

The *PRPH2* gene was identified in mice with a photoreceptor degeneration known as "retinal degeneration, slow" (rds). Subsequently, the orthologous human *PRPH2* gene was shown to cause autosomal dominant RP. Mutation in codon 172 of *PRPH2* has been implicated in autosomal dominant macular dystrophy.[8] Weleber et al described a 3-bp deletion in *PRPH2* that resulted in retinitis pigmentosa, pattern dystrophy, and FFM in different individuals.[9]

The PRPH2 protein is a membrane-associated glycoprotein restricted to photoreceptor outer segment discs in a complex

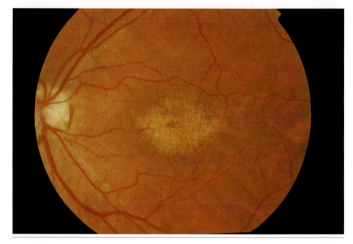

Fig. 46.11 **North Carolina macular dystrophy (MCDR1).** Small yellow drusen-like lesions at the central macula (grade 1).

with ROM1. It may function as an adhesion molecule involved in the stabilization and maintenance of a compact arrangement of outer segment discs. It interacts with the GARP domain (glutamic acid- and proline-rich region) of the beta-subunit of rod cGMP-gated channels, in a complex including the Na/Ca–K exchanger. This interaction may anchor the channel-exchanger complex in the rod outer segment plasma membrane. The rds mouse (homozygous for a null mutation in *PRPH2*), fails to develop photoreceptor discs and outer segments with down regulation of rod opsin expression; resulting in apoptotic loss of photoreceptor cells. Subretinal injection of recombinant adeno-associated virus encoding a *PRPH2* transgene in these mice resulted in the generation of outer segment structures and formation of new stacks of discs containing both PRPH2 and rhodopsin with electrophysiological function preserved.[10] Ultrastructural improvement depended on the age at treatment, but a single injection may be long-lasting. Thus, gene therapy in patients with photoreceptor defects may need early intervention and accurate control of transgene expression.

North Carolina macular dystrophy

Clinical and histological findings

North Carolina macular dystrophy (MCDR1) is a non-progressive autosomal dominant disorder with complete penetrance and a variable macular phenotype. Presentation is usually during the first or second decade. The disorder is a failure of development of the macular region. Bilaterally symmetrical fundus appearances in MCDR1 range from a few small (less than 50 μm) yellow drusen-like lesions in the central macula (grade 1) (Fig. 46.11) to larger confluent lesions (grade 2) and well-demarcated macular chorioretinal atrophy (grade 3) (Fig. 46.12). Peripheral retinal drusen-like deposits have been described. The severity of visual loss is grade-dependent; vision is poorest with grade 3 lesions. Color vision is usually normal. Occasionally MCDR1 is complicated by subretinal neovascular membrane formation (SRNVM).

Histopathology shows accumulation of lipofuscin in the RPE within the atrophic macular lesion.

Electrophysiology

EOG and ERG are normal.

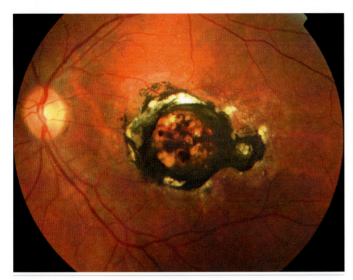

Fig. 46.12 North Carolina macular dystrophy (MCDR1). Macular atrophy and hyperpigmentation with surrounding drusen-like deposits (grade 3).

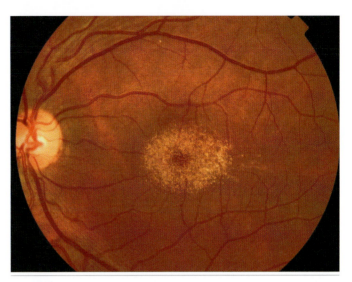

Fig. 46.13 Autosomal dominant macular dystrophy (MCDR3) resembling North Carolina macular dystrophy. Characteristic drusen-like deposits at the macula.

Molecular genetics and pathogenesis

MCDR1 is linked to a locus on chromosome 6q16. There is no genetic heterogeneity.[11] The identification of the gene may improve our understanding of the pathogenesis of drusen and SRNVM.

A dominantly inherited macular dystrophy has been mapped to chromosome 6q14, adjacent to, but probably distinct from the MCDR1 locus.[12] It has a highly variable phenotype; an autosomal dominant drusen disorder with macular degeneration (DD). Most young adults had fine macular drusen and good vision. Patients who were symptomatic from infancy or early childhood had poorer vision with an atrophic maculopathy and drusen. There was also evidence of progression in late adulthood. The DD disease interval overlaps with that of STGD3 and an autosomal dominant atrophic macular degeneration (adMD),[13] suggesting an allelic disorder. However, the phenotype of DD differs from that of STGD3 and adMD. Macular drusen are a hallmark of DD, whilst RPE atrophy and subretinal flecks are prominent features of STGD3 and adMD.

North Carolina macular dystrophy-like phenotypes

Three North Carolina macular dystrophy-like phenotypes map to different genetic loci than MCDR1 suggesting further genetic heterogeneity in the MCDR1 phenotype.

Autosomal dominant macular dystrophy (MCDR3) resembling North Carolina macular dystrophy

Clinical and electrophysiological findings

A pedigree has been described with an early-onset autosomal dominant macular dystrophy (MCDR3).[14] Visual acuity ranged from 6/5 to 6/60. The retinal changes, confined to the macular region, varied from mild RPE pigmentary change to atrophy. Drusen-like deposits were present to varying degrees and were characteristic of the phenotype (Fig. 46.13). Choroidal neovascular membrane formation was a complication. The only significant differences between this phenotype and MCDR1 is that in MCDR3 color vision is abnormal in the majority of

affected individuals and there was evidence of disease progression in a single case.

A phenotype similar to MCDR3 mapping to the same locus has been recently reported.[15]

Molecular genetics

Linkage to chromosome 5p13.1–p15.33, but excluding the MCDR1 locus,[14,15] has been reported. The gene is unidentified.

North Carolina-like macular dystrophy and progressive sensorineural hearing loss

Clinical and electrophysiological findings

A non-progressive MCDR1-like macular dystrophy in association with progressive sensorineural hearing loss has been reported (MCDR4).[16] Visual acuity ranged from 6/9 to hand movements. The EOG and full-field ERG were normal. Progressive sensorineural deafness was present in all adult affected individuals.

Molecular genetics

Genotyping excluded linkage to the MCDR1 locus and established linkage to chromosome 14q.

North Carolina-like macular dystrophy and digital anomalies (Sorsby's syndrome)

Clinical findings

A dominantly inherited condition with bilateral macular dysplasia and apical dystrophy or brachydactyly has been reported (Fig. 46.14).[17,18] Visual acuity ranged from 6/12 to 4/60. The maculopathy was non-progressive and variable in severity, ranging from mild RPE pigmentary changes to excavated chorioretinal atrophic lesions. There was no generalized retinal dysfunction.

Molecular genetics

The MCDR1, MCDR3, and MCDR4 loci have all been excluded providing evidence of further genetic heterogeneity associated with the North Carolina macular dystrophy-like phenotype.[19] This is in keeping with the established heterogeneity in the genetic mechanisms underlying split-hand and split-foot malformations (microdeletions being common) and the developmental macular dystrophies.

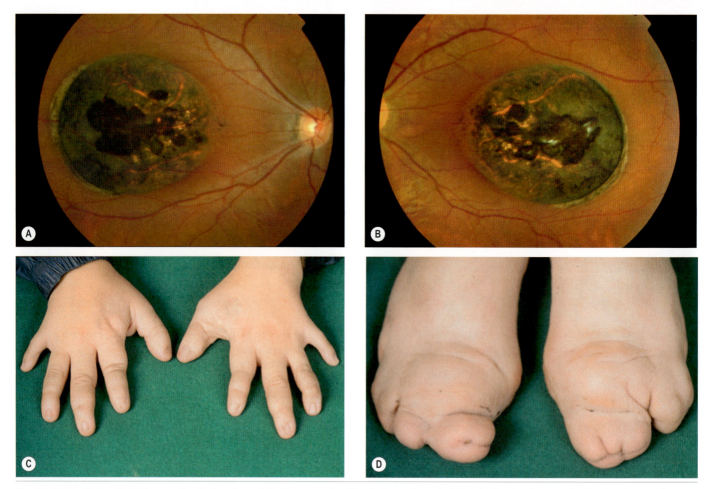

Fig. 46.14 North Carolina-like macular dystrophy and digital anomalies (Sorsby's syndrome). (A,B) Color fundus photographs showing the typical bilateral macular dysplasia. (C,D) In this individual there is shortening and deformity of the fingers and toes due to aplasia and hypoplasia of middle and terminal phalanges. There is skin syndactyly in association with bifurcation of the terminal phalanx of the hallux causing severe deformity of the foot.

Progressive bifocal chorioretinal atrophy

Clinical findings

Progressive bifocal chorioretinal atrophy (PBCRA) is an early-onset autosomal dominant disorder characterized by infantile onset nystagmus, myopia, poor vision, and slow progression.[20] A large atrophic macular lesion and nasal subretinal deposits present soon after birth. An atrophic area nasal to the optic disc appears in the second decade and enlarges progressively (Fig. 46.15). Marked photopsia in early/middle age and retinal detachment extending from the posterior pole are complications. FFA and indocyanine green angiography (IGA) demonstrate a large circumscribed area of macular choroidal atrophy with staining of deposits in the peripheral retina.

Electrophysiology

Unlike MCDR1, both ERG and EOG are abnormal, reflecting widespread abnormality of photoreceptors and RPE.

Molecular genetics and pathogenesis

PBCRA has been linked to 6q14–q16.2; the disease locus overlaps with the established MCDR1 interval. These two autosomal dominant macular dystrophies have some phenotypic similarities; both result from a failure of normal macular development. PBCRA differs significantly from MCDR1 in several important respects, including slow progression, abnormal color vision, extensive nasal as well as macular atrophy, and abnormal ERG and EOG. If allelic, it is likely that different mutations are involved in their etiology. An alternative explanation is that PBCRA and MCDR1 are caused by mutations in two different adjacent developmental genes.

Central areolar choroidal dystrophy

Clinical and histological findings

Central areolar choroidal dystrophy (CACD) is characterized by bilateral, symmetrical, subtle mottling of the RPE at the macula in the second decade, which progresses to atrophy of the RPE and choriocapillaris. The round or oval macular lesion is well demarcated. CACD has been divided into four stages:[21]

Stage I: slight parafoveal changes of the RPE.
Stage II: RPE mottling encircling the fovea;
Stage III: additional atrophy of the choriocapillaris without central involvement.
Stage IV: stage III plus central involvement.

Color vision is abnormal and central scotomata are present with normal peripheral visual fields. FFA and IGA reveal RPE atrophy and various degrees of choriocapillaris loss.

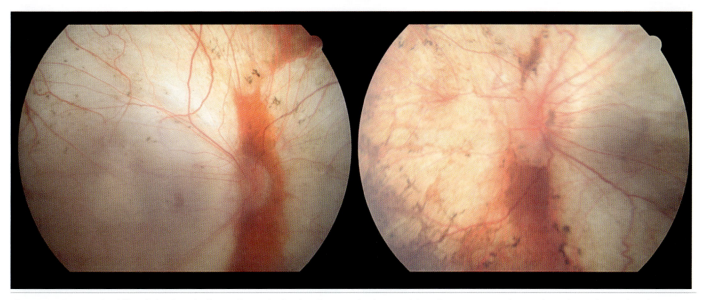

Fig. 46.15 Progressive bifocal chorioretinal atrophy. Color fundus photographs showing bilateral extensive macular atrophy and atrophy nasal to the optic nerve head.

Electrophysiology

Full-field ERGs are normal in the early stages, but may become abnormal in advanced stages.

Molecular genetics and pathogenesis

A p.Arg142Trp mutation in *PRPH2* has been implicated as one cause of this rare autosomal dominant macular dystrophy. Sporadic cases of CACD have been described but no mutations have been found in *PRPH2* suggestive of further genetic heterogeneity. A locus at 17p13 has also been identified, with a novel mutation in *GUCY2D* recently reported.

X-linked inheritance

X-linked juvenile retinoschisis (XLRS)

See Chapter 41.

Foveal hypoplasia

Clinical findings

This presents in infancy with reduced vision, nystagmus and a poorly developed fovea; there is no recognized foveal pit or luteal pigment and blood vessels may cross the presumed foveal region. These changes can be demonstrated using OCT and fundus autofluorescence imaging (Fig. 46.16). Foveal hypoplasia may be an isolated abnormality or associated with aniridia or albinism (see Chapter 40).

Molecular genetics

Isolated foveal hypoplasia is most commonly sporadic, but two dominant pedigrees have been reported, with a *PAX6* missense mutation identified in one of these families.[21,22] The mutation occurred in the C-terminal part of the paired domain.[21] However, *PAX6* has been screened in some reported isolated cases, with no mutations identified.[23] It is likely that further cases will be identified with OCT and will allow a more detailed study of the incidence of *PAX6* mutations in isolated foveal hypoplasia.

Bull's-eye maculopathy

The term "Bull's-eye" maculopathy (BEM) first described the characteristic appearance of chloroquine retinopathy. Bull's-eye lesions have since been reported in cone dystrophy, cone–rod dystrophy, rod–cone dystrophy, *ABCA4*-retinopathy, and in some dominantly inherited macular dystrophies, including Benign concentric annular dystrophy, Fenestrated Sheen macular dystrophy, and in association with the p.Arg373Cys *PROM1* variant.[5,24] BEM is a frequent finding in neurodegenerative disorders, especially Batten's disease, Hallervorden-Spatz disease, and olivopontocerebellar atrophy (see Chapters 45 and 62).

The pathogenesis of BEM is poorly understood. The annular RPE atrophy and central sparing may correspond to the pattern of lipofuscin accumulation in the RPE, which in healthy individuals is highest at the posterior pole and shows a depression at the fovea (Fig. 46.17). The initially spared center usually becomes involved as the disease advances. BEM is not a discrete macular disorder but describes a retinal phenotype that may be seen in a wide variety of macular dystrophies at an early stage of their evolution.

Conclusions

The inherited macular dystrophies are clinically and genetically heterogeneous with well-characterized phenotypes; and many causative genes identified. Although in some inherited macular dystrophies the disease is confined to the macula, in the majority there is electrophysiological, psychophysical or histological evidence of widespread retinal dysfunction.

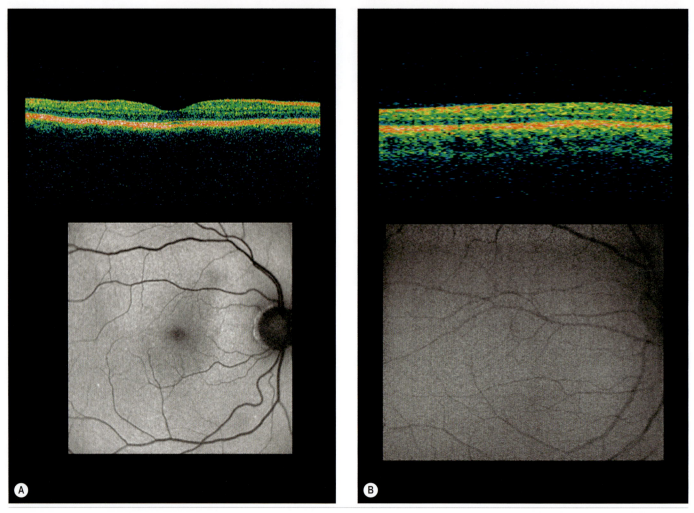

Fig. 46.16 Foveal hypoplasia. Autofluorescence imaging demonstrating a lack of macular pigment and optical coherence tomography revealing an absence of a foveal pit. A normal patient is shown for comparison.

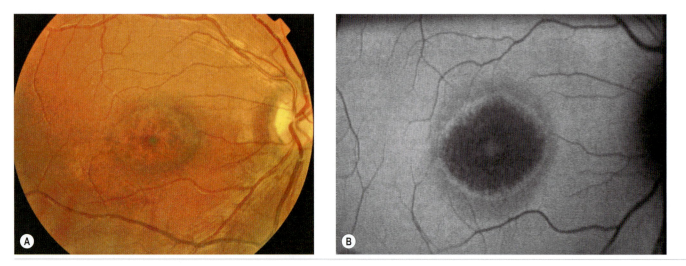

Fig. 46.17 Bull's-eye maculopathy (BEM). (A) Characteristic ophthalmoscopic appearance in which there is annular RPE atrophy and central sparing. (B) Typical autofluorescence image of BEM.

There is no established treatment but treatment trials have begun for STGD: others are anticipated over the next decade. It is important that the correct diagnosis is made to provide accurate information on prognosis and to offer informed genetic counseling. Prenatal diagnosis is possible when the mutation(s) causing disease in the family is known.

Although there is no specific treatment available for these disorders research is resulting in clinical trials. There is cautious optimism that effective interventions will be available soon. The provision of best refractive correction, appropriate low vision aids, and educational support is very important. Photophobia may be prominent and tinted spectacles or contact lenses and a sunhat may improve comfort and vision.

References

1. Lois N, Holder GE, Bunce C, et al. Phenotypic subtypes of Stargardt macular dystrophy-fundus flavimaculatus. Arch Ophthalmol 2001; 119: 359–69.
2. Tsybovsky Y, Molday RS, Palczewski K. The ATP-binding cassette transporter ABCA4: structural and functional properties and role in retinal disease. Adv Exp Med Biol 2010; 703: 105–25.
3. Gerth C, Andrassi-Darida M, Bock M, et al. Phenotypes of 16 Stargardt macular dystrophy/fundus flavimaculatus patients with known ABCA4 mutations and evaluation of genotype-phenotype correlation. Graefes Arch Clin Exp Ophthalmol 2002; 240: 628–38.
4. Travis GH, Golczak M, Moise AR, Palczewski K. Diseases caused by defects in the visual cycle: retinoids as potential therapeutic agents. Annu Rev Pharmacol Toxicol 2007; 47: 469–512.
5. Michaelides M, Gaillard MC, Escher P, et al. The PROM1 mutation p.R373C causes an autosomal dominant bull's eye maculopathy associated with rod, rod-cone, and macular dystrophy. Invest Ophthalmol Vis Sci 2010; 51: 4771–80.
6. Schatz P, Bitner H, Sander B, et al. Evaluation of macular structure and function by OCT and electrophysiology in patients with vitelliform macular dystrophy due to mutations in BEST1. Invest Ophthalmol Vis Sci 2010; 51: 4754–65.
7. Boon CJ, Klevering BJ, Leroy BP, et al. The spectrum of ocular phenotypes caused by mutations in the BEST1 gene. Prog Retin Eye Res 2009; 28: 187–205.
8. Downes SM, Fitzke FW, Holder GE, et al. Clinical features of codon 172 RDS macular dystrophy: similar phenotype in 12 families. Arch Ophthalmol 1999; 117: 1373–83.
9. Weleber RG, Carr RE, Murphy WH, et al. Phenotypic variation including retinitis pigmentosa, pattern dystrophy, and fundus flavimaculatus in a single family with a deletion of codon 153 or 154 of the *peripherin/RDS* gene. Arch Ophthalmol 1993; 111: 1531–42.
10. Ali RR, Sarra GM, Stephens C, et al. Restoration of photoreceptor ultrastructure and function in retinal degeneration slow mice by gene therapy. Nat Genet 2000; 25: 306–10.
11. Yang Z, Tong Z, Chorich LJ, et al. Clinical characterization and genetic mapping of North Carolina macular dystrophy. Vision Res 2008; 48: 470–7.
12. Stefko ST, Zhang K, Gorin MB, Traboulsi EI. Clinical spectrum of chromosome 6-linked autosomal dominant drusen and macular degeneration. Am J Ophthalmol 2000; 130: 203–8.
13. Griesinger IB, Sieving PA, Ayyagari R. Autosomal dominant macular atrophy at 6q14 excludes CORD7 and MCDR1/PBCRA loci. Invest Ophthalmol Vis Sci 2000; 41: 248–55.
14. Michaelides M, Johnson S, Tekriwal AK, et al. An early-onset autosomal dominant macular dystrophy (MCDR3) resembling North Carolina macular dystrophy maps to chromosome 5. Invest Ophthalmol Vis Sci 2003; 44: 2178–83.
15. Rosenberg T, Roos B, Johnsen T, et al. Clinical and genetic characterization of a Danish family with North Carolina macular dystrophy. Mol Vis 2010; 16: 2659–68.
16. Francis PJ, Johnson S, Edmunds B, et al. Genetic linkage analysis of a novel syndrome comprising North Carolina-like macular dystrophy and progressive sensorineural hearing loss. Br J Ophthalmol 2003; 87: 893–8.
17. Sorsby A. Congenital coloboma of the macula, together with an account of the familial occurrence of bilateral macular coloboma in association with apical dystrophy of the hands and feet. Br J Ophthalmol 1935; 19: 65–90.
18. Thompson EM, Baraitser M. Sorsby syndrome: a report on further generations of the original family. J Med Genet 1988; 25: 313–21.
19. Kalhoro A, Puech V, Puech B, et al. A molecular genetic investigation of two families with macular dysplasia in association with digit abnormalities. ARVO Meeting Abstracts 2008; 49: E456. http://abstracts.iovs.org//cgi/content/abstract/49/5/456?sid=8c4d2 027-ef12-4200-9b18-6d0793b28480.
20. Godley BF, Tiffin PA, Evans K, et al. Clinical features of progressive bifocal chorioretinal atrophy: a retinal dystrophy linked to chromosome 6q. Ophthalmology 1996; 103: 893–8.
21. Azuma N, Nishina S, Yanagisawa H, et al. PAX6 missense mutation in isolated foveal hypoplasia. Nat Genet 1996; 13: 141–2.
22. O'Donnell FE Jr, Pappas HR. Autosomal dominant foveal hypoplasia and presenile cataracts: a new syndrome. Arch Ophthalmol 1982; 100: 279–81.
23. Querques G, Bux AV, Iaculli C, Delle Noci N. Isolated foveal hypoplasia. Retina 2008; 28: 1552–3.
24. Michaelides M, Chen LL, Brantley MA Jr., et al. ABCA4 mutations and discordant ABCA4 alleles in patients and siblings with bull's eye maculopathy. Br J Ophthalmol 2007; 91: 1650–5.

Congenital and vascular retinal abnormalities

Susmito Biswas • Graeme C M Black

Congenital hypertrophy of the retinal pigment epithelium

Congenital hypertrophy of the retinal pigment epithelium (CHRPE) lesions are pigmented lesions of the retinal pigment epithelium (RPE) that are flat or very slightly raised, round or oval, and predominantly located at the mid-periphery as well as in the peripapillary or macular regions (Fig. 47.1). A pigmented and non-pigmented halo may surround lesions with multiple depigmented lacunae within the lesion. Depigmented CHRPEs are less common.[1] Optical coherence tomography (OCT) demonstrates lack of photoreceptors overlying the lesion[2] while absent autofluorescence shows a lack of lipofuscin. Fluorescein angiography demonstrates choroidal masking.[3]

Prevalence

CHRPEs have a prevalence of 1.2% in the population.[4]

Associations

Vascular sheathing, vessel attenuation and microangiopathy, drusen, adjacent white-without-pressure, and adjacent

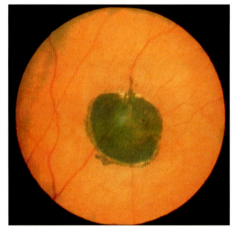

Fig. 47.1
Congenital hypertrophy of the retinal pigment epithelium (CHRPE). Slightly raised jet black lesion in the mid-periphery with an associated small visual field defect. (Professor A. C. Bird's patient.)

depigmented linear RPE streaks are found on or around lesions. Lesions gradually enlarge in diameter; 83% of lesions enlarged at a rate of 2 μm/mm lesion-base per month.[1] Flat CHRPE are rarely associated with visual loss. A small proportion (1.5%) contain nodules. Visual loss may occur due to macular edema. Exceptionally, malignant transformation occurs within nodular lesions.[5]

CHRPE associated with adenomatosis polyposis of the colon

The majority of CHRPEs have neither visual nor health implications. However, multiple (more than three), bilateral, mixed pigmented, and depigmented CHRPEs are specific and sensitive markers of adenomatous polyposis of the colon (APC), or familial adenomatous polyposis (FAP). In APC, CHRPEs may be ovoid, pisciform or irregular in shape and may be surrounded by a pale gray halo or an adjacent depigmented linear streak (Fig. 47.2). They vary in size, from dot-like lesions to multiple disk diameters and position.

Genetics

APC is an autosomal dominant disorder, with an incidence of 1 in 8300[7] that predisposes to malignancy and accounts for ~1% of all colorectal cancers. CHRPEs are associated with Gardner's syndrome (APC with extracolonic manifestations such as osteoma and desmoid tumors) and Turcot's syndrome (co-occurrence of FAP and medulloblastoma), and are found in APC families without extracolonic manifestations.[7] All are

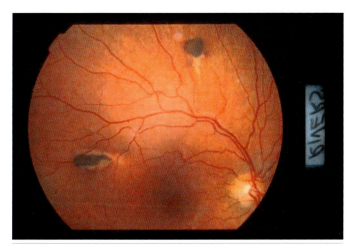

Fig. 47.2 CHRPE lesions in a patient with familial adenomatous polyposis.

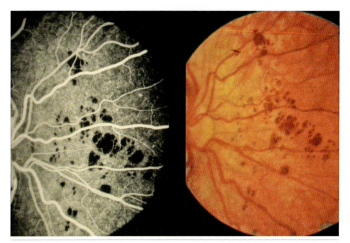

Fig. 47.3 Congenital grouped pigmentation ("bear track"). Unilateral, multiple brown patches in the retinal pigment epithelium of no functional significance. Fluorescein angiography shows masking of the underlying choroidal fluorescence. (Professor A. C. Bird's patient.)

caused by mutations within the APC gene on chromosome 5q21–22.[8] CHRPEs are not seen in all individuals with the APC phenotype and when present suggest a mutation between codons 463 and 1387. In families where CHRPEs are present they are highly penetrant.

Most affected individuals with APC develop multiple adenomatous colorectal polyps between the second and fourth decades.[9] Malignant transformation occurs in over 90% of patients by age 50 years. Tumor surveillance for gene carriers by colonoscopy begins from around 12 years and usually leads to elective colectomy. Polyps may also develop in the stomach, small bowel, and duodenum, the last being associated with a risk of malignant transformation. Ten percent of patients develop desmoid tumors: benign, locally invasive fibrous tissue tumors. Osteomas of the mandible and dental anomalies, such as missing or supernumerary teeth, are common.

Congenital grouped pigmentation of the RPE

Congenital grouped pigmentation of the RPE is characterized by small, darkly pigmented, flat, circumscribed lesions at the level of the RPE that generally increase in size as they approach the retinal periphery. The lesions resemble animal tracks ("bear tracks") (Fig. 47.3). They do not affect vision; electrodiagnostic and color vision testing are normal. Mostly, lesions are unilateral and sectoral. Occasionally, the entire fundus may be involved.[10] A depigmented variant ("polar bear tracks") has been described in a sibling of a girl with normal bear tracks.[11]

Prevalence

Prevalence is around 0.12% in the ophthalmic clinic population.[12]

Associations

Grouped pigmentation is usually isolated. Presumed chance associations include: retinoblastoma, café-au-lait spots and hairy nevus, persistent fetal vasculature, microcephaly, Rieger's anomaly, and macular coloboma.

Congenital simple hamartoma of the retina

These solitary, rare lesions differ from congenital hypertrophy of the RPE and RPE hyperplasia. They are typically located close to the fovea. They are circumscribed, nodular, and heavily pigmented, arising from the RPE and projecting into the vitreous through the full thickness of the retina. A feeder arteriole and venule are usually present. Subtle surrounding retinal traction may reduce visual acuity. Ultrasound shows a nodular echogenic mass with moderate to high internal reflectivity. Fluorescein angiography demonstrates non-fluorescence with a late, variable, surrounding ring of hyperfluorescence.[13] The lesion blocks indocyanine green choroidal fluorescence. OCT shows elevation of the retina at the lesion with enhanced reflectivity of the vitreous face of the lesion and optical shadowing of the retina and choroid.[14] The lesions are congenital, stable, and asymptomatic throughout life; intraretinal hemorrhage adjacent to the lesion and intraretinal exudation can occur.[13]

Torpedo maculopathy

Torpedo maculopathy, or paramacular coloboma, is characterized by an ovoid, sharply defined, non-pigmented lesion in the temporal region of the macula, centered on the horizontal raphe (Fig. 47.3). Lesions are longer horizontally (2–3 mm) than vertically (1 mm) with a characteristic point aimed toward the fovea and either a frayed, pigmented tail or rounded temporal margin (Fig. 47.4). Usually unilateral and solitary, satellite lesions may occur. The margins are sharply defined by a hyperpigmented border.

OCT reveals absent RPE, overlying retinal disorganization and thinning, irregularity and degenerate photoreceptor outer segments.[15] Autofluorescence imaging shows hypoautofluorescence within the lesion.[16] The foveal architecture and visual acuity are normal.

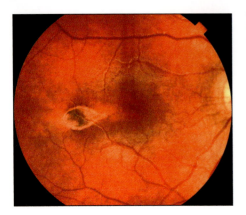

Fig. 47.4 "Torpedo" maculopathy. Sharply defined, non-pigmented lesion in the temporal region of the macula with a characteristic point aimed toward the fovea.

Prevalence

Torpedo maculopathy is rare, but of unknown prevalence.

Associations

Usually isolated, torpedo maculopathy may coexist with kidney disease, blepharophimosis, situs inversus, and choroidal nevus.

Retinal astrocytic hamartoma

Retinal astrocytic hamartomas are benign glial tumors of the retinal nerve fiber layer frequently associated with tuberous sclerosis (see Chapter 65). Calcification can cause diagnostic confusion with retinoblastoma, although the mean age at diagnosis of retinoblastoma is around 2 years, whilst that of astrocytoma is 14.5 years.[17] Progression from flat to nodular lesions can occur. Most lesions range from 0.5 to 5 mm in diameter. They are slow growing, but very occasionally exhibit more aggressive growth resulting in retinal exudation, vitreous hemorrhage, retinal detachment, retinochoroiditis, neovascular glaucoma, vitreous seeding,[18] and globe perforation.[19]

TSC is associated with mutations in one of two tumor suppressor genes, Hamartin (TSC1) and Tuberin (TSC2). The encoded proteins form a cytoplasmic molecular complex that controls cell growth and survival signals conveyed through the P13K signal transduction pathway.[20]

Retinal capillary hemangioma

Retinal capillary hemangiomas (RCH), more correctly hemangioblastomas, are circumscribed, orange–red, round, vascular tumors with a prominent feeding and draining vessel (see Chapter 65). When sporadic, they are usually unilateral and unifocal. RCHs are a frequent association with von Hippel-Lindau syndrome (VHL, see Chapter 65), a multisystem, autosomal dominant, familial, cancer-predisposition syndrome. In VHL, the RCHs are often bilateral and multifocal.[21] Fluorescein angiography shows early hyperfluorescence, late leakage, and distinguishes feeder vessels from draining venules; it highlights small peripheral RCHs, otherwise undetectable.[22] B-scan ultrasound detects a mass lesion, measures basal dimensions, and detects subretinal fluid. A-scans show medium to high internal reflectivity.[23] OCT can measure retinal thickness at the macula and monitor treatment response.[24]

RCHs are mostly located anterior to the equator usually superotemporally or, less frequently (10–15%), in the juxtapapillary region.[25] Peripheral RCHs increase in size gradually with surface glial proliferation resulting in striae and traction. Visual loss occurs from leakage and exudation leading to cystoid macular edema, exudative and tractional retinal detachment.[26] Neovascular glaucoma or cataract may occur.

Juxtapapillary hemangiomas are typically located temporal to the optic nerve. They may be sessile, usually endophytic or sometimes exophytic;[27] they may remain stable for prolonged periods. This, together with close proximity to the optic nerve and the high likelihood of visual loss from nerve damage as a result of treatment, has led to many advocating observation until the macula is threatened by exudation and visual loss.[27]

Genetics

VHL is an autosomal dominant disorder with an estimated prevalence of 1 in 39 000–53 000. Tumors associated with VHL can occur sporadically; 20% of VHL patients represent de novo mutations. Thus, the diagnosis of VHL depends on a positive family history or the presence of two typical tumors. Organs affected include CNS (hemangioblastomas), pancreas (cysts), kidney (renal cell carcinoma), liver, and adrenal glands (pheochromocytoma). The VHL gene encodes two VHL proteins which regulate proteolytic degradation of hypoxia inducible factors HIF-1 and HIF-2.[28]

In VHL, onset of hemangioblastomas occurs around 4 years of age and the probability of developing RCHs increases with age often causing visual symptoms by the second decade. Annual screening, beginning at 10 years, is recommended. Manifestation of RCHs mostly occurs by 30 years; adults with normal retinal examination after this age are unlikely to develop tumors.[26,29]

Management

Treatment for RCHs includes laser photocoagulation, photodynamic therapy (PDT), cryotherapy, plaque radiotherapy, trans-scleral penetrating diathermy, vitreoretinal surgery, and systemic and intravitreal bevacizumab. For small (<1.5 mm in diameter), posteriorly located lesions, laser photocoagulation applied directly to the RCH and the feeder vessels is highly effective.[30] More anteriorly located lesions and those with subretinal fluid may best be treated with cryotherapy.[30] PDT with verteporfin has been used in both peripheral and juxtapapillary RCHs. PDT has a moderate effect using standard parameters as used in the TAP study.[31] Complications include vitreous hemorrhage, subretinal hemorrhage, ischemic optic neuropathy, vascular occlusion, increase in subretinal fluid, and retinal detachment. PDT shows a relatively better outcome in juxtapapillary RCHs; more than one treatment may be required.[31]

Anti-VEGF (vascular endothelial growth factor) treatments, systemic or intravitreal, provide mixed results with a transient reduction in retinal edema but no significant reduction in tumor size or new tumor development.[32,33]

Cavernous hemangioma

This rare congenital vascular malformation (hamartoma) of the retina is usually sporadic, occasionally autosomal dominant with incomplete penetrance. Retinal lesions are unilateral

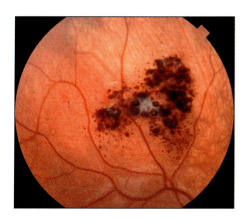

Fig. 47.5 Cavernous hemangioma of the retina showing the "grape-like" clusters of saccular aneurysms.

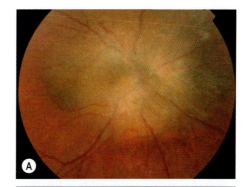

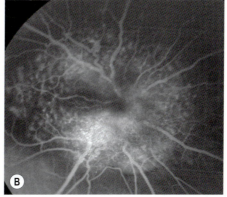

Fig. 47.6 Combined hamartoma of the retina and retinal pigment epithelium (CHRRPE). (A) Elevated, very slowly progressive right optic disk lesion presenting in a 6-year-old child with visual loss to 0.7 LogMAR at 11 years old. Note the pigmentation, aneurysmal vessels and pale "glial" tissue. (B) Fluorescein angiogram showing widespread telangiectatic vessels.

and unifocal and, while often isolated, can be associated with intracranial or cutaneous cavernous hemangiomas: a neuro-oculocutaneous phakomatosis.[34] Cavernous hemangiomas consist of saccular aneurysms resembling a cluster of grapes anywhere in the inner retina following the course of a retinal vein (Fig. 47.5). Visual loss may occur due to recurrent vitreous hemorrhage or macula involvement. Those located at the optic disk may compress nerve fibers.[35] Fluorescein angiography demonstrates delayed filling with hyperfluorescent capping of the saccules. No leakage or exudation occurs.[36]

Genetics

Autosomal dominant inheritance has been described; it is recommended to examine first-degree relatives. The coexistence of retinal cavernous hemangioma with cerebral cavernous malformations (CCM) may be associated with three genetic loci (CCM1-3). The three encoded proteins interact in a protein complex involved in the regulation of endothelial cell morphogenesis.[37]

Management

Neuroimaging is recommended to rule out intracranial involvement. Lesions do not progress with age, frequently have an overlying preretinal glial membrane, and are managed conservatively. Traction may cause spontaneous vitreous hemorrhage.[38] Photocoagulation and cryotherapy have been used; regression with intravenous inflixamab has been reported.[39]

Combined hamartoma of the retina and retinal pigment epithelium

Combined hamartomas of the retina and retinal pigment epithelium (CHRRPEs) are rare benign, usually solitary, unilateral lesions, occasionally bilateral.[40] They are congenital, described in infants as young as 2 weeks old.[41] Many are non-progressive, but most present with reduced vision, metamorphopsia or strabismus, particularly with macular involvement.

Lesions are slightly elevated with a variable amount of pigment (Fig. 47.6). Retinal vascular tortuosity is typical, as is an overlying epiretinal membrane (ERM). Lesions are classified according to the most prominent element within them: melanocytic, vascular, or glial. Glial subtypes, associated with ERM, are most amenable to surgery.[42]

Fluorescein angiography demonstrates hypofluorescence of the background choroid during the arterial phase, retinal vascular tortuosity, and capillary dilatation within the lesion, and intralesional vascular leakage. OCT demonstrates a hyper reflective ERM with underlying retinal folds. Spectral domain OCT can demonstrate disorganization and thickening of the underlying retina with obscuration of the outer retina and photoreceptor layers due to high internal reflectivity.[43]

Histopathology

Histopathology reveals thickened, disorganized retina and optic nerve, abundant hyperplastic and dysplastic glial cells, reduplicated sheets, and cords of proliferating retinal pigment epithelium infiltrating the overlying tissue.[44]

Associations

The most notable associations are:

1. Neurofibromatosis type 1
2. Gorlin's syndrome (nevoid basal cell carcinoma syndrome)
3. Tuberous sclerosis.

Management

Aside from treatment of amblyopia, management is conservative. Progressive traction from ERM may require intervention but careful selection of patients is key.[42,45] Complications include retinal hemorrhages, vitreous hemorrhages, retinal and choroidal neovascularization, retinal holes, retinoschisis, retinal detachment (usually exudative), and macular edema.[41]

Coats' disease

Described by Coats as "characterized by the presence in some part of the fundus of an extensive mass of exudation" and by "some very peculiar forms of vascular disease."[46] The clinical hallmarks are vascular telangiectasia (Fig. 47.7), aneurysmal retinal vessel dilation ("light-bulbs", Fig. 47.8), and capillary microaneurysms with associated subretinal and intraretinal exudation. The exudate is yellow-white, located at the posterior pole in patches and beneath the retinal vessels which may be sheathed with cholesterol deposits. The equatorial and peripheral retina is usually affected with the temporal side involved first, although any quadrant may be affected. It generally progresses to retinal detachment (Fig. 47.9), glaucoma, cataract, and phthisis bulbi. Preschool-age children usually present with strabismus or leukocoria; reduced vision on vision screening was responsible for ascertaining 16%.[47] Rarer presentations such as cholesterolosis bulbi have been described. Older children or adults can present with visual loss; poor vision in over half of cases is a result of exudative retinal detachment or macular involvement.[47,48] Macular pathologies include telangiectasia, exudation and edema, macular fibrosis, or full thickness hole.[49] The staging of Coats' disease is given in Table 47.1.[50] Most eyes present at stage 2 or 3, rarely at stage 1 or 5. Younger patients tend to present at stage 3.

Incidence

Coats' disease has a male : female ratio of 17:3. Eighty percent of cases are unilateral, with no racial or ethnic predilection and an estimated population incidence of 0.09/100 000.

Median age at presentation was 8 years, the majority in the first 15 years of life. Earlier onset disease signals a more rapid progression.[47]

Histopathology

Vascular changes include vessel thickening and hyalinization, thinning and loss of endothelium, and plasma leakage into vessel walls due to breakdown of the blood–retinal barrier. This leads to necrosis, disorganization, dilation, and telangiectasias. Leakage into the intraretinal and subretinal spaces leads to exudates, hemorrhage, cysts, edema, lymphocytic infiltration, and deposition of fibrin. The neural retina undergoes secondary degeneration and RPE cells phagocytose lipid, transforming them into lipid laden "ghost cells".[51,52]

Genetics

Many cases appear sporadic although Coats' disease may represent a somatic mutation in the *NDP* gene (mutated in Norrie's disease) within the retina at a stage of development that results in a segment of the retina carrying the mutant allele.[53] Coats' disease-like changes occur in retinitis pigmentosa (RP), and in RP with preserved para-arteriolar retinal pigment epithelium phenotype associated with CRB1 gene mutations.[54] Children have been described with Coats' disease

Table 47.1 – The staging of Coats' disease

Stage	Description
0	Regressed; no telangiectasia/exudation
1	Retinal telangiectasia only
2	Telangiectasia and exudation
2A	Extrafoveal exudation
2B	Foveal exudation
3	Exudative retinal detachment
3A1	Extrafoveal detachment only
3A2	Foveal detachment
3B	Total retinal detachment
4	Total retinal detachment with glaucoma
5	Endstage disease (phthisis bulbi)

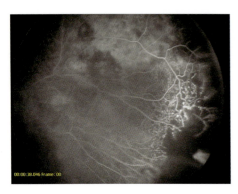

Fig. 47.7 Coats' disease. The "hallmark" is vascular telangiectasia, shown in this peripheral fluorescein angiogram, and aneurysmal dilation of the retinal vessels.

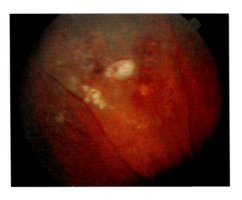

Fig. 47.8 Coats' disease. Aneurysmal dilatation of retinal vessels, exudates – few in this case – and microaneurysms.

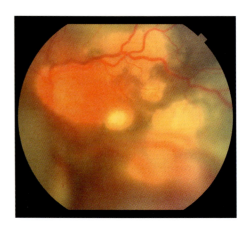

Fig. 47.9 Coats' disease. Serous retinal detachment with massive subretinal cholesterol accumulation.

in association with a presumed autosomal recessive condition characterized by intracerebral calcification, cerebral microangiopathy, sparse hair, dystrophic nails, intrauterine growth retardation, bone marrow involvement, and postnatal growth failure.[55] Other associations include facioscapulohumeral muscular dystrophy (where it is often bilateral), plasminogen deficiency type 1, Cornelia de Lange syndrome, Hallerman-Streiff syndrome, Senior-Loken syndrome, and multiple glomus tumors.[56-61]

Management

The diagnosis of Coats' disease is often straightforward. An important differential diagnosis is retinoblastoma, in particular the diffuse infiltrating tumors that are flat and ill-defined, uncalcified and present at an older age. The inability to exclude retinoblastoma still leads to enucleation.[62] Other differential diagnoses include persistent fetal vasculature, vitreoretinal dysplasia, retinopathy of prematurity, pars planitis, X-linked retinoschisis, toxocariasis, and VHL disease.

Coats' disease progresses slowly with ~64% of patients progressing to retinal detachment over a 5-year period, especially in patients 4 years or younger. Poor prognostic features include: post-equatorial involvement, diffuse and superior retinal location of telangiectasias and exudates, retinal macrocysts, failed resolution of fluid after treatment, and retinal detachment at presentation.[48,63]

Most cases stabilize or improve with treatment (98% in one study).[64] In milder cases, the goal of treatment is to preserve vision. In more advanced cases the goal is ocular comfort and cosmesis.

Early ablation of peripheral telangiectasia and aneurysms is more effective because there is little or no exudate and fewer quadrants are involved. Treatments include cryotherapy, argon laser, or a combination. Green diode laser (532 nm) has been used in the presence of subretinal fluid.[65] Complications include cataract, retinal detachment, and proliferative vitreoretinopathy.

In cases of retinal detachment, apposition of the retina by drainage of subretinal fluid, with or without scleral buckling, helps with laser application. Vitrectomy with drainage of subretinal fluid and encirclement may maintain visual function.[66] Adjunctive intravitreal therapy with steroid, anti-VEGF antibody, or a combination has varying success. However, tractional retinal detachment due to development of contractile vitreoretinal fibrosis has been documented.[67] Intraocular steroid also risks development of cataract and glaucoma.

Familial retinal arteriolar tortuosity

Familial retinal arteriolar tortuosity is an autosomal dominant disorder with progressive tortuosity of second and third order retinal arterioles associated with retinal hemorrhages.[68] The venules and major arterioles are normal. The arterioles around the macula region are most obviously affected. The youngest patient reported was 6 years old.[68] The vessels are of a normal caliber, without aneurysmal dilation or arteriolar–arteriolar anastamoses. Fluorescein angiography shows no vessel leakage. Retinal hemorrhages cause transient visual disturbance or loss when involving the macula, or if extensive, and can arise following exertion or valsalva maneuver.[68]

Associations

None.[68]

Inherited retinal venous beading

Inherited venous beading is a rare, dominant disorder of unknown etiology, with an unusual pattern of ocular vascular abnormalities comprising saccular, aneurysmal changes of the conjunctival vessels, and prominent sausage-like retinal venous beading. Retinal arterioles may show narrow caliber. Acute vascular decompensation with areas of capillary non-perfusion, neovascularization, and vitreous hemorrhage may occur. Intraretinal lipid, leakage of fluorescein, and intraretinal microvascular changes including microaneurysms and telangiectasias may be observed. Families have been described with nephritis, neutropenia, and deafness.[69]

Congenital retinal macrovessel

Congenital retinal macrovessel is a large vessel, typically a vein which crosses the macula and has large tributaries extending on both sides of the horizontal raphe and, sometimes, almost encircling the fovea. Visual acuity is not normally affected.[70,71] Occasionally, the retinal macrovessel is an artery or combined artery and vein.[72] Vessels may branch off the inferotemporal vessels, superotemporal vessels, or infero/superotemporal aspect of the optic nerve.

Retinal macrovessel is rare; in a series of 3506 eyes, seven eyes of six patients had branches coming off the inferotemporal artery; none had a branch off the superotemporal artery or vein.[73]

Fluorescein angiography may demonstrate arteriovenous communications with filling of the venous vessel during the arterial phase. Communication between a cilioretinal artery and macrovessel has been described.[74] Areas of capillary non-perfusion in the perifoveal or perivenular region have also been described. During the late phase of the angiogram the retinal macrovessel remains preferentially hyperfluorescent. Fluorescein angiography may show a disturbance of the foveal capillaries with poorly defined or enlarged avascular zones or microaneurysms. OCT demonstrates high reflectivity of the vessel and blood attenuating the OCT beam beneath the vessel. Macular thickening may occur.[75]

Complications include serous retinal detachment[76] and exudation, valsalva retinopathy[74] (possible coincidental), and intraretinal cyst.[71]

Racemose retinal hemangioma

These rare, unilateral congenital vascular malformations do not usually cause visual loss in themselves, but they can be associated with brain vascular malformations which can hemorrhage and cause strokes (Fig. 49.10). They are usually discovered at routine examination or when the patient has presented with a neurological episode. They usually require no treatment.

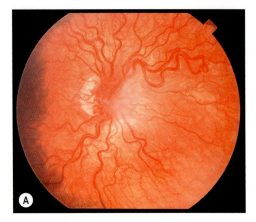
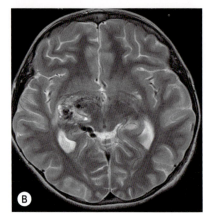
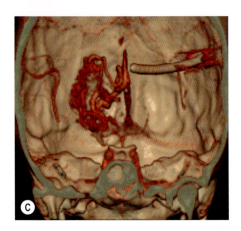

Fig. 47.10 (A) Racemose hemangioma. Large loop vein in upper nasal quadrant of the right eye. Normal visual acuity. (B) MRI showing right sided vascular malformation from which a sudden hemorrhage occurred at 10 years old causing obtundation (from which the child recovered) and a left homonymous hemianopia (which did not recover). (C) MR angiogram reconstruction showing anteroposterior view with a right sided vascular malformation and a shunt on the left.

Inherited familial retinal macroaneurysms

Three sets of siblings from three unrelated often consanguineous families had multiple, bilateral retinal arterial macroaneurysms and beading affecting first order arterioles and progressing to affect second and third order peripheral vessels.[77] They had signs and symptoms of disease in childhood, as early as 3 months. The macroaneurysms arose from areas of retinal arterial beading. This was accompanied by intraretinal and subretinal exudate and reactive changes including pigmentary changes at the level of the RPE and subretinal scarring, atrophy, and vascular sheathing.[77] Complications included recurrent sub-ILM hemorrhages and leakage from the macroaneurysms demonstrated on fluorescein angiography, with areas of exudative retinal detachment. Leakage resolved spontaneously and green argon laser photocoagulation favorably influenced the clinical course.[77]

References

2. Shields CL, Materin MA, Walker C, et al. Photoreceptor loss overlying congenital hypertrophy of the retinal pigment epithelium by optical coherence tomography. Ophthalmology 2006; 113: 661–5.

3. Shields CL, Pirondini C, Bianciotto C, et al. Autofluorescence of congenital hypertrophy of the retinal pigment epithelium. Retina 2007; 27: 1097–100.

5. Shields JA, Eagle RC Jr, Shields CL, et al. Malignant transformation of congenital hypertrophy of the retinal pigment epithelium. Ophthalmology 2009; 116: 2213–16.

9. Petersen GM, Slack J, Nakamura Y. Screening guidelines and premorbid diagnosis of familial adenomatosis polyposis using linkage. Gastroenterology 1991; 100: 1658–64.

14. Lopez JM, Guerrero P. Congenital simple hamartoma of the retinal pigment epithelium: optical coherence tomography and angiography features. Retina 2006; 26: 704–6.

15. Tsang T, Messner LV, Pilon A. Torpedo maculopathy: in-vivo histology using optical coherence tomography. Optom Vis Sci 2009; 86: 1380–5.

20. McCall T, Chin SS, Salzman KL, Fults DW. Tuberous sclerosis: a syndrome of incomplete tumour suppression. Neurosurg Focus 2006;20:1–9.

23. Shields CL, Shields JA, Barrett J, et al. Vasoproliferative tumours of the ocular fundus: classification and clinical manifestation in 103 patients. Arch Ophthalmol 1995; 113: 615–23.

25. Kreusel K-M, Bechrakis NE, Krause L, et al. Retinal angiomatosis in von Hippel-Lindau disease: a longitudinal study. Ophthalmology 2006; 113: 1418–24.

26. Webster AR, Maher ER, Moore AT. Clinical characteristics of ocular angiomatosis in von Hippel-Lindau disease and correlation with germline mutation. Arch Ophthalmol 1999; 117: 371–8.

28. Maxwell PH, Wiesner MS, Chang GT-W, et al. The tumor suppressor protein VHL targets hypoxia-inducible factors for oxygen dependant proteolysis. Nature 1999; 399: 271–5.

29. Webster AR, Richards FM, MacRonald FE, et al. An analysis of phenotypic variation in the familial cancer syndrome von Hippel-Lindau disease: evidence for modifier effects. Am J Hum Genet 1998; 63: 1025–35.

30. Singh AD, Shields CL, Shields JA. von Hippel-Lindau Disease. Surv Ophthalmol 2001; 46: 117–42.

32. Wackernagel W, Lackner E-M, Pilz S, et al. von Hippel-Lindau disease: treatment of retinal haemangioblastomas by targeted therapy with systemic bevacizumab. Acta Ophthalmol 2010; 88: 271–2.

33. Wong WT, Liang KJ, Hammel K, et al. Intravitreal ranibizumab therapy for retinal capillary hemangioblastoma related to von Hippel-Lindau disease. Ophthalmology 2008; 115: 1957–64.

37. Faurobert E, Albiges-Rizo C. Recent insights into cerebral cavernous malformations: a complex jigsaw puzzle under construction. FEBS J 2010; 277: 1084–96.

38. Pringle E, Chen S, Rubenstein A, et al. Optical coherence tomography in retinal cavernous haemangioma may explain the mechanism of vitreous haemorrhage. Eye 2009; 23: 1242–3.

39. Japiassú RM, Moura Brasil OF, de Souza EC. Regression of macular cavernous hemangioma with systemic infliximab. Ophthal Surg Lasers Imaging 2010; 9: 1–3.

41. Shields CL, Thangappan A, Hartzell K, et al. Combined hamartoma of the retina and retinal pigment epithelium in 77 consecutive patients: visual outcome based on macular versus extramacular tumor location. Ophthalmology 2008; 115: 2246–52.

45. Cohn AD, Quiran PA, Drenser KA, et al. Surgical outcomes of epiretinal membranes associated with combined hamartoma of the retina and retinal pigment epithelium. Retina 2009; 29: 825–30.

47. Morris B, Foot B, Mulvahill A. A population-based study of Coats disease in the United Kingdom I: Epidemiology and clinical features at diagnosis. Eye 2010; 24: 1797–801.

50. Shields JA, Shields CL, Hanovar SG, et al. Classification and management of Coats disease. The 2000 Proctor Lecture. Am J Ophthalmol 2001: 131: 572–83.

53. Black GC, Parveen R, Bonshek R, et al. Coats' disease of the retina (unilateral retinal telangiectasis) caused by somatic mutation in the NDP gene: a role for Norrin in retinal angiogenesis. Hum Mol Genet 1999; 8: 2031–5.

54. den Hollander AI, Heckenlively JR, van den Born LI, et al. Leber congenital amaurosis and retinitis pigmentosa with coats-like exudative vasculopathy are associated with mutations in the Crumbs Homologue 1 (CRB1) gene. Am J Hum Genet 2001; 69: 198–203.

55. Crow YJ, McMenamin J, Haenggeli CA, et al. Coats' plus: a progressive familial syndrome of bilateral coats' disease, characteristic cerebral calcification, leukoencephalopathy, slow pre- and post-natal linear growth and defects of bone marrow and integument. Neuropediatrics 2004; 35: 10–19.

57. Patrassi GM, Sartori MT, Piermarocchi S, et al. Unusual thrombotic-like retinopathy (Coats' disease) associated with congenital plasminogen deficiency Type I. J Intern Med 2009: doi: 10.111/j.1365–2796.

63. Morales AG. Coats' disease: natural history and results of treatment. Am J Ophthalmol 1965; 60: 855–65.

65. Shapiro MJ, Chow CC, Karth PA, et al. Effects of green diode laser in the treatment of pediatric Coats disease. Am J Ophthalmol 2011; 151: 725–31.

67. Ramasubramanian A, Shields CL. Bevacizumab for Coats' disease with exudative retinal detachment and risk of vitreoretinal traction. Br J Ophthalmol 2011 Jun 7. [Epub ahead of print].

68. Sutter FKP, Helbig H. Familial retinal arteriolar tortuosity: a review. Surv Ophthalmol 2003; 48: 245–55.

Access the complete referece list online at
http://www.expertconsult.com

Flecked retina disorders

Panagiotis Sergouniotis • Peter J Francis • Anthony T Moore

Introduction

"Flecked retina" describes disorders characterized by multiple yellow-white retinal lesions of various size and configuration.[1,2] A number of inherited or acquired conditions, associated with a variable degree of retinal dysfunction, correspond to this definition. This chapter reviews the differential diagnosis of flecked retina in childhood; some disorders predominantly seen in adults are also included.

Clinical evaluation

It is important to enquire about visual symptoms such as blurred vision, nyctalopia, or hemeralopia and obtain a full family history. Examination of relatives can be helpful, as other affected family members may remain asymptomatic. Current or previous systemic drug administration and dietary habits should be enquired after. Careful note should be taken of any other medical disorders particularly those associated with malabsorption (e.g. cystic fibrosis).[3]

When examining the child, the distribution of retinal deposits, their depth in the retina and whether they are crystalline in nature should be noted. Investigations that may be helpful include spectral-domain optical coherence tomography (SD-OCT), fundus autofluorescence imaging (FAF), and, in some cases, psychophysical and electrophysiologic (electroretinogram [ERG] and electro-oculogram [EOG]) testing. Molecular diagnostic testing can be useful to confirm the diagnosis.

Yellow-white retinal lesions in primary ocular disease

Stargardt's disease and fundus flavimaculatus
(See Chapter 46)

Stargardt's disease is a typically autosomal recessive retinal dystrophy, associated with mutations in the *ABCA4* gene.[4] Pseudo-dominant inheritance where an affected parent (whose partner is unknowingly a carrier of the disorder) may have an affected child can be observed particularly in consanguineous families.[5] In such cases, it is important for counseling to distinguish *ABCA4*-related disease from phenotypically similar autosomal dominant disorders due to mutations in *ELOVL4*[6] or *RDS*.[7] Stargardt's disease is characterized by the presence of yellow-white flecks that are scattered throughout the posterior pole (Fig. 48.1). Macular atrophy is common and affected individuals typically present with reduced visual acuity in the second decade of life. Some patients have good central vision with minimal or no macular involvement at presentation, and may be diagnosed as fundus flavimaculatus.[8] Stargardt's disease and fundus flavimaculatus are parts of the phenotypic spectrum of the same disorder and the same genetic etiology is frequently observed. Patients rarely complain at presentation of poor night vision or field constriction although rod function can be abnormal.[9-10]

FAF is very useful in diagnosing individuals with Stargardt's disease; it allows detection of the abnormal phenotype even in cases when it is not otherwise evident. Abnormalities in the form of a speckled hyper- and hypo-autofluorescence pattern and/or focal areas of increased signal, spatially correlating with flecks on fundoscopy, can be identified even in the early stages.[11] SD-OCT, in particular the degree of preservation of the line corresponding to the inner/outer segment junction, allows more accurate assessment of disease severity. A "dark choroid" has been classically described on fluorescein angiography, although this is now not a commonly used diagnostic tool for Stargardt's disease, particularly in children.[12]

Electrophysiologic testing reveals an abnormal pattern ERG and attenuated central macular responses on the multifocal

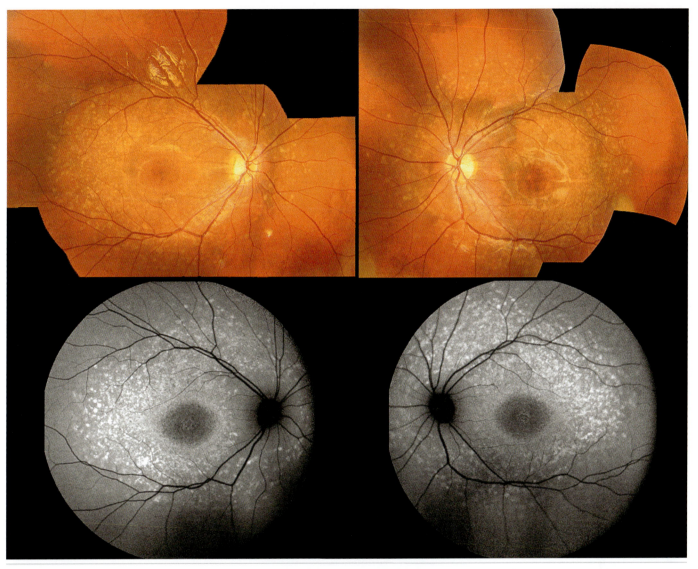

Fig. 48.1 Stargardt's disease. Fundus photograph of the left and right eyes of a 9-year-old individual with Stargardt's disease (top row). Fundus autofluoresence imaging (bottom row) revealed hyperautofluorescent lesions corresponding to the flecks and abnormal autofluorescence at the foveal region.

ERG. The results of full-field electroretinography are variable and often normal in the early stages of disease. Full-field ERGs may be prognostically useful since individuals with early evidence of rod and/or cone photoreceptor dysfunction are at more risk of severe and progressive disease.[9]

Benign fleck retina

Benign fleck retina is an autosomal recessive condition associated with a distinctive retinal appearance and no apparent visual or electrophysiologic deficits.[13] Affected individuals are asymptomatic, but fundus examination reveals a striking pattern of diffuse, yellow-white flecks extending to the far periphery, sparing the foveal region (Fig. 48.2).[14-16] The flecks are located at the level of the retinal pigment epithelium (RPE) and can be present in early infancy.

FAF reveals multiple hyperautofluorescent lesions corresponding in location with the flecks. On SD-OCT, discrete deposit accumulation located posterior to the photoreceptor inner/outer segment junction but without disrupting it is observed. Normal full-field and pattern ERGs confirm the diagnosis;[15] multifocal ERG may be slightly subnormal in some isopters.[16]

Recessive mutations in the gene encoding group V phospholipase A_2 (*PLA2G5*) and mildly elevated low-density lipoprotein and total cholesterol levels have been identified in some individuals with benign fleck retina.[17]

Benign fleck retina should not be confused with "fleck retina of Kandori." The latter is associated with large white lesions, possibly atrophic changes, and night-blindness.[18] It is not clear if "fleck retina of Kandori" is a genetic condition or even an independent clinical entity.

Fundus albipunctatus (See Chapter 44)

Fundus albipunctatus is an autosomal recessive condition associated with night-blindness and numerous widespread yellow-white punctate lesions at the level of the RPE (Fig. 48.3).[19-20] Patients are either noted to have an abnormal retinal appearance on a routine eye test or present with nyctalopia.

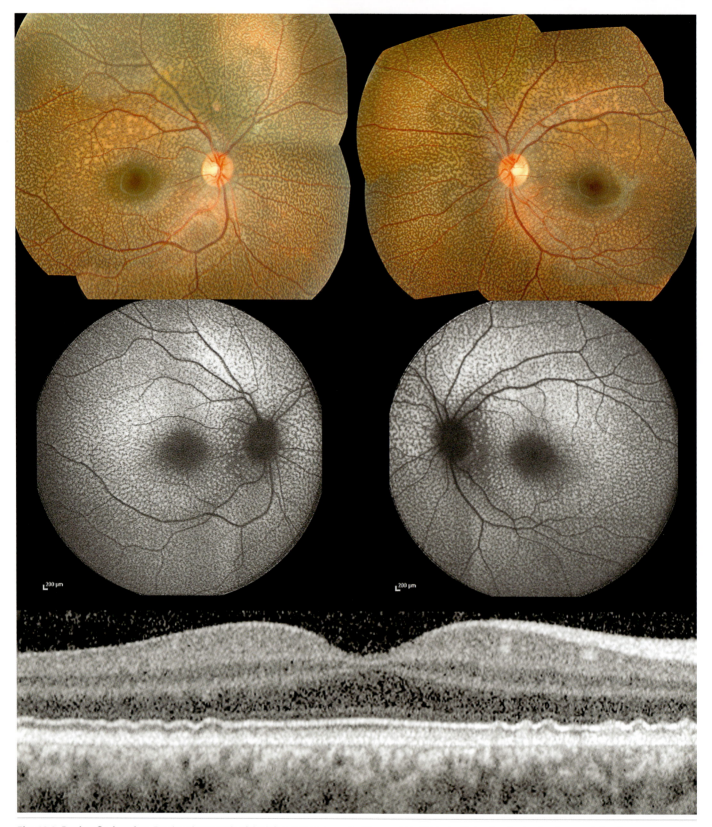

Fig. 48.2 Benign fleck retina. Fundus photograph of the left and right eyes of a 10-year-old individual with benign fleck retina (top row). Fundus autofluorescence (middle row) and optical coherence tomography (horizontal, centerd on the fovea, linear scan of the right eye; bottom row) revealed endogenously fluorescent lesions at the level of the retinal pigment epithelium.

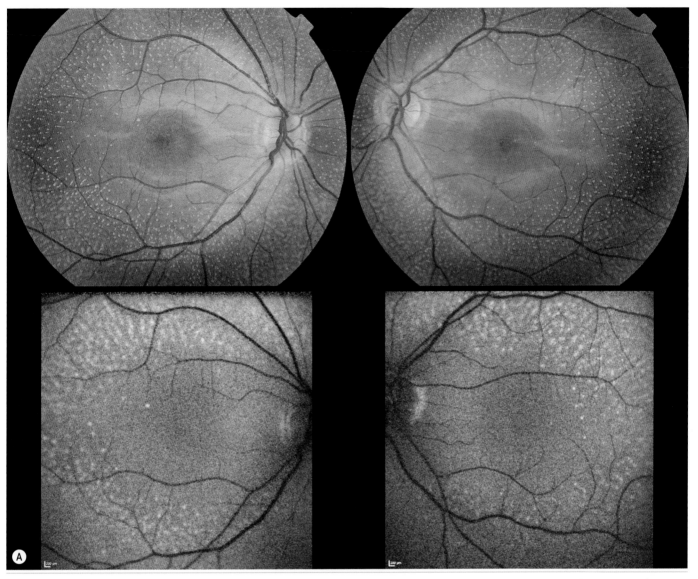

Fig. 48.3 Fundus albipunctatus. (A) Fundus photograph of the left and right eyes of an 18-year-old, *RDH5*-mutation positive, individual (top row). Fundus autofluorescence imaging (bottom row) revealed hyperautofluorescent lesions.

Affected individuals describe night-blindness from birth and delay in dark adaptation after exposure to bright light.[19] Visual acuities and visual fields are usually normal.

FAF in individuals with fundus albipunctatus often reveals a low autofluorescent signal; digital enhancement artefacts such as autofluorescence from the optic disk and large vessels may be observed.[21] In young subjects, high-density foci partially associating with the white dots on fundoscopy can be observed (Fig. 48.3A).[19] Hyper reflective lesions at the level of the RPE are detected on SD-OCT (Fig. 48.3B).[19]

Characteristic abnormalities on electrophysiology and dark adaptometry facilitate the diagnosis (see Chapter 44). Notably, dark-adapted ERG responses are subnormal following conventional dark adaptation but partially recover or normalize following extended dark adaptation.[19,22] Light-adapted ERGs and pattern ERGs can be normal or abnormal.[19,23,24]

Molecular testing can be useful: fundus albipunctatus is commonly associated with recessive mutations in *RDH5*, a gene encoding an enzyme with 11-*cis*-retinol dehydrogenase activity.[25] This enzyme catalyzes the oxidation of 11-*cis*-retinol

to 11-*cis*-retinaldehyde, the universal vertebrate chromophore of visual pigments, in human RPE.[26-27] Mutations in the *RPE65*[28] and *RLBP1*[29] genes have also been described in patients with some features of fundus albipunctatus.

Retinitis punctata albescens, Bothnia and Newfoundland retinal dystrophies

Retinitis punctata albescens is a variant of retinitis pigmentosa characterized by multiple retinal white dots rather than pigment deposition.[30] Patients have family history consistent with autosomal recessive inheritance and present with nyctalopia and/or peripheral vision problems; decreased visual acuity may also occur.[31] On fundoscopy, white spots similar to the ones observed in fundus albipunctatus are observed (Fig. 48.4). These spots spare the foveal region and may evolve to give rise to a more classical pigmentary retinopathy. It is important to differentiate early retinitis punctata albescens from fundus albipunctatus: the prognosis for daytime vision is considerably better in the latter and the

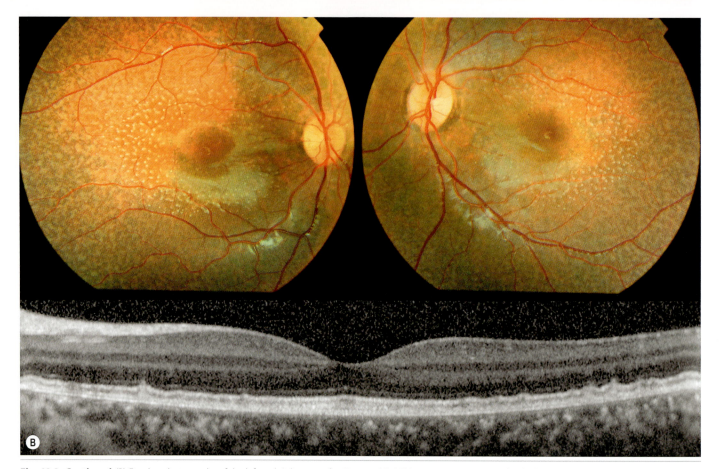

Fig. 48.3 *Continued* (B) Fundus photographs of the left and right eyes of a 10-year-old, *RDH5*-mutation positive, individual (top row). Optical coherence tomography (horizontal, centered on the fovea, linear scan of the left eye; bottom row) revealed hyper-reflective lesions at the level of the retinal pigment epithelium.

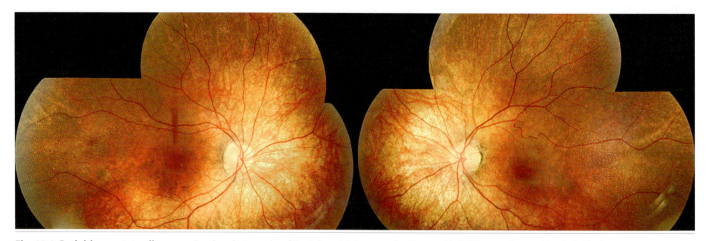

Fig. 48.4 Retinitis punctata albescens. Fundus photographs of the left and right eyes of a 15-year-old, *RLBP1*-mutation positive, individual.

former features more severe and progressive retinal degeneration. Vascular attenuation, visual field loss, and a more severe electrophysiologic phenotype are key distinguishing features (see Chapter 44).[31]

Retinitis punctata albescens is primarily associated with recessive mutations in the cellular retinal binding protein-1 gene (*RLBP1*; see Chapter 44).[32] Mutations in the RDS[33] and

the rhodopsin[34] genes have also been described in rare cases of dominantly inherited retinitis punctata albescens.

Newfoundland rod–cone dystrophy[35] and Bothnia dystrophy[36] are two early-onset forms of retinal disease that have high prevalence in the genetic isolate populations of northeastern Canada and northern Sweden, respectively. Both share genetic etiology (*RLBP1* mutations) and key phenotypic features (multiple white dots, night-blindness) with recessive retinitis punctata albescens[35,37,38] and are parts of the phenotypic spectrum of the same disorder.

Enhanced S-cone syndrome and Goldmann-Favre syndrome

Small subretinal white dots can be an early feature of a progressive retinopathy named "enhanced S-cone syndrome" (ESCS).[39-42] Patients typically present with night-blindness and/or visual acuity loss in the first or second decade of life; a hyperopic refractive error is often noted.[40] ESCS has been associated with various fundoscopic features: the most typical are retinoschisis and deep nummular pigmentary deposition with or without yellow-white spots, primarily along the vascular arcades.[43,44] White dots have been described in pediatric patients (Fig. 48.5); those tend to progress to a pigmentary retinopathy in later adulthood.[41,42,45]

FAF reveals abnormal signal, in particular beyond the vascular arcades; mid-peripheral hyperautofluorescent spots only partially corresponding to fleck-like abnormalities on fundoscopy are often observed in young subjects.[42,44] A hyperautofluorescent ring has also been described.[40] Cystic spaces, rosette-like lesions, and/or schisis may be observed on OCT.[40,42-44]

ESCS is unique among retinal dystrophies: there is both retinal degeneration resulting in visual loss and an increased function in a subset of photoreceptors, the S-cones.[46-49] A distinctive electophysiologic phenotype is observed.[40]

ESCS is associated with recessive mutations in the NR2E3 gene, encoding a retinal nuclear receptor with a role in activating rod development and repressing cone development.[49,50]

Goldmann-Favre syndrome was initially described as an autosomal recessive vitreoretinopathy characterized by night-blindness, pigmentary degeneration, macular and peripheral retinoschisis, cataract, and degenerative vitreous changes.[51,52]

Many of these features are shared with ESCS and appropriate electrophysiologic and genetic testing revealed that they are not distinct entities but two identifiable phenotypes in a wide spectrum of clinical expression of the same retinal degeneration.[41,52,53]

Miscellaneous reports of retinal flecks associated with inherited retinal disease

Small yellow-white fleck-like lesions have been reported in association with a number of other retinal disorders including early-onset retinal dystrophy due to RPE65 mutations[54,55] and juvenile retinoschisis.[56-58] In the former, the dots tend to be more fine and peripheral; in the latter, they are usually within the posterior pole. Additionally, autosomal recessive bestrophinopathy, a condition associated with biallelic BEST1 mutations, may present in childhood with small yellow-white subretinal deposits in the fovea and around the vascular arcades.[59,60]

Drusen-like deposits in inherited retinal disease

Drusen deposition at the macula is the hallmark of age-related maculopathy. Similar lesions may be seen in young adults affected with Sorsby's fundus dystrophy (mutation in the TIMP3 gene[61,62]) or autosomal dominant drusen, also known as Doyne's honeycomb retinal dystrophy[63] or malattia leventinese[64] (mutation in the EFEMP1 gene[65]) – two dominantly inherited maculopathies. Rarely, drusen-like lesions are observed in asymptomatic children as an incidental finding.[1]

Drusen-like deposits can be observed in children with North Carolina macular dystrophy. North Carolina macular dystrophy (see Chapter 46) is an autosomal dominant condition characterized by macular drusen that are present

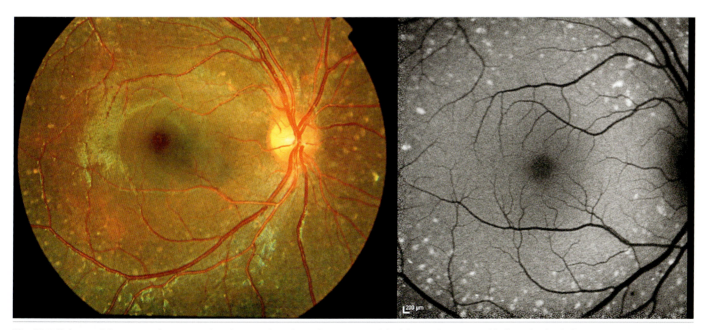

Fig. 48.5 Enhanced S-cone syndrome. Fundus photograph and autofluorescence of the left eye of a 13-year-old affected individual.

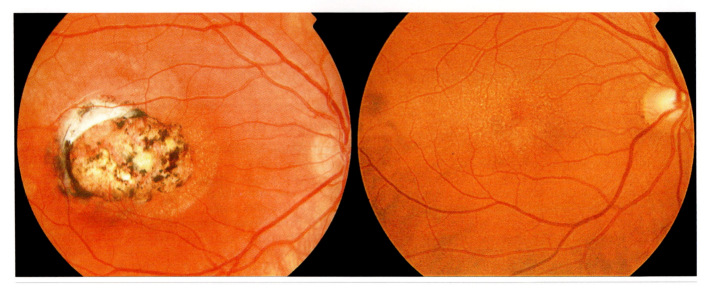

Fig. 48.6 North Carolina macular dystrophy. Fundus photograph of the right eyes of a 12-year-old boy (left panel) and his 40-year-old father (right panel). Both are affected with North Carolina macular dystrophy.

from birth.[66,67] Fundoscopic findings are highly variable (Fig. 48.6) and tend to be more dramatic than one would predict from visual acuity measurements. Affected individuals may have:

1. Only a few drusen in the fovea (grade I)
2. Confluent drusen with or without RPE changes (grade II), or
3. Central macular chorioretinal atrophy with hypertrophic fibrous tissue (grade III).[66,68]

The condition rarely progresses; the grading does not reflect successive stages of progression.[68-70] Visual acuity is stable and generally well-preserved except in those with central atrophic lesions. Development of choroidal neovascularization is uncommon but can result in fibrosis and late visual loss.[66,70]

Although the genetic defect is not known, the disease-causing gene has been mapped to the long arm of chromosome 6.[70-72] A number of macular dystrophies that do not map to chromosome 6 but share features with North Carolina macular dystrophy (including macular drusen) have been described.[73-75]

Bietti's crystalline corneoretinal dystrophy

Bietti's crystalline dystrophy is an autosomal recessive disorder characterized by progressive chorioretinal degeneration, nyctalopia, reduced visual acuity, visual field constriction, and multiple yellow-white crystalline deposits at the retina, in circulating lymphocytes and, occasionally, at the corneoscleral limbus.[76,77] Retinal crystals are observed predominantly at the posterior pole, in the superficial and deep retinal layers (Fig. 48.7). They are associated with multiple, sharply demarcated areas of RPE atrophy and tend to disappear as the disease advances.[76,78,79] Affected individuals typically become symptomatic after the second decade of life.[79,80] However, some pediatric cases have been described.[81] Lesions partially corresponding to the crystals may or may not be evident on FAF imaging.[82] SD-OCT reveals hyperreflective lesions throughout the retina;

many of these lesions do not spatially associate with retinal crystals on fundus photography.[82-84] When full-field ERG testing is performed, both cone and rod systems are found affected even in the early stages of disease.[81,85,86]

Bietti's corneoretinal dystrophy is associated with defects in *CYP4V2* (cytochrome P450, family 4, subfamily V, polypeptide 2),[77] a gene encoding an enzyme with a role in fatty acid metabolism.[87] A high heterozygous carrier frequency for *CYP4V2* mutation, and therefore, relatively high prevalence of the condition, has been reported in East Asia, especially in Chinese and Japanese populations.[80]

A dominantly inherited retinopathy (with incomplete penetrance and variable expressivity) with clinical features similar to the ones observed in Bietti's crystalline dystrophy has been described.[88]

Yellow-white retinal lesions in acquired disease

Vitamin A deficiency

Deficiency of the fat-soluble vitamin A (hypovitaminosis A) limits growth, weakens innate and acquired host defenses, and increases the risk of infectious morbidity.[89-92] Ocular manifestations of hypovitaminosis A account for approximately 500 000 cases of childhood blindness worldwide usually as a result of corneal scarring (xerophthalmia).[3,93] Vitamin A deficiency can be due to malnutrition (commonest cause of vitamin A deficiency in developing countries), malabsorption, or impaired metabolism of vitamin A associated with liver disease or cystic fibrosis.[94]

Chronic vitamin A deficiency may lead to visual symptoms as a result of reduced photoreceptor visual pigment formation.[95] Night-blindness is a common complication and an early symptom of the disorder; visual field loss, abnormal color vision, and visual acuity loss may occur in later stages. Fundus examination often reveals multiple gray-white punctate spots at the level of the RPE and scattered in the

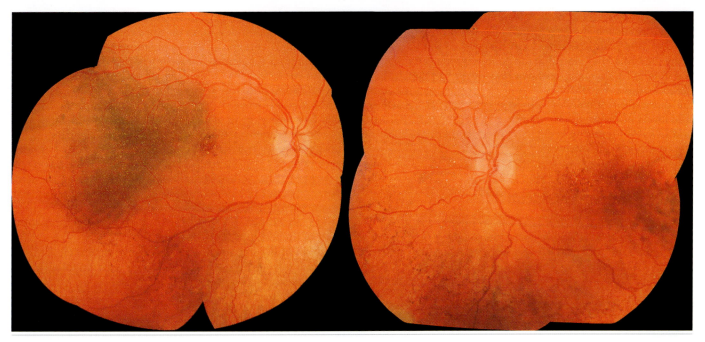

Fig. 48.7 Bietti's crystalline corneoretinal dystrophy. Fundus photographs of the left and right eyes of a 16-year-old, *CYP4V2*-mutation positive, individual showing crystalline deposits.

peripheral retina.[96-98] Atrophic and pigmentary changes may occur with disease progression. Dark adaptometry demonstrates elevated rod and cone thresholds, with rods more severely affected.[99] Electrophysiology reveals reduced or undetectable rod-specific ERGs and reduced amplitude cone-flicker ERGs of normal implicit time.[98,99] The flecked retinopathy, visual field, psychophysical, and electrophysiologic abnormalities usually resolve completely upon prompt vitamin A supplementation.[100]

Inflammatory chorioretinopathies

A heterogeneous group of rare inflammatory chorioretinopathies is associated with multiple yellow-white macular lesions of various size. These conditions are more commonly seen in adults, are broadly termed "white dot syndromes" and include:

1. Acute posterior multifocal placoid pigment epitheliopathy
2. Multiple evanescent white dot syndrome
3. Serpiginous choroiditis
4. Birdshot chorioretinopathy
5. Multifocal choroiditis with panuveitis
6. Punctate inner choroidopathy.[101,102]

Drug induced crystalline retinopathies

A number of disorders, acquired (mainly due to medication side effects) or inherited (for example, Bietti's crystalline dystrophy described above or primary hyperoxaluria type I and Sjogren-Larsson syndrome discussed later in this chapter), can give rise to yellow-white retinal lesions that are crystalline in nature.[103] Acquired, drug induced disorders include methoxyflurane anesthesia, tamoxifen therapy, canthaxantine therapy, and talc retinopathy.[104] These are generally seen in adults rather than in children.

Yellow-white retinal lesions in systemic disease

Abetalipoproteinemia (Bassen-Kornzweig syndrome)

Abetalipoproteinemia is a rare autosomal recessive metabolic disorder that affects absorption of cholesterol, dietary fats, and fat-soluble vitamins from the small intestine.[105-108] The condition is associated with a number of multisystem manifestations including fat malabsorption, absence of serum betalipoprotein, abnormally shaped red blood cells (acanthocytosis), and ataxic neuropathy.[109,110] Ophthalmic involvement in abetalipoproteinemia is variable and a wide range of symptoms has been reported. These include ophthalmoplegia, ptosis, nystagmus, anisocoria, cataract, angioid streaks, and a progressive retinal dystrophy characterized by white dots at the level of the RPE and pigmentary changes.[111-113]

The disorder is associated with recessive mutations in *MTTP*, the gene encoding the microsomal triglyceride transfer protein.[107,108] Treatment with vitamins A and E slows the course or prevents the development of the retinal degeneration.[114,115]

Alport's syndrome

Alport's syndrome is a genetically heterogeneous inherited disorder that can be associated with X-linked semidominant (~85% of cases; *COL4A5* gene), autosomal recessive (~15% of cases; *COL4A3* and *COL4A4* genes), or autosomal dominant (rare; *COL4A3* gene) inheritance.[116,117] It is a disorder of the basement membrane that results in progressive renal failure due to glomerulonephropathy, high-tone sensorineural hearing loss and variable ocular abnormalities including cataract, anterior lenticonus, corneal dystrophy, and a dot-and-fleck retinopathy.[116,118] Retinal changes in the latter, typically occurring in affected adult males, comprise numerous yellow-white perimacular flecks at the level of the RPE; these spare the fovea, may extend to the periphery, and can resemble the dots in fundus albipunctatus (Fig. 48.8).[119] Though there are exceptions, visual function and electrophysiologic testing are generally normal.[119,120] Alport's syndrome is caused by mutations in collagen biosynthesis genes (COL4A3, COL4A4, and COL4A5) resulting in defective production or assembly of the type IV collagen network.[121-123]

Pseudoxanthoma elasticum

Pseudoxanthoma elasticum (PXE) is an inherited disorder of the connective tissue associated with characteristic skin findings (lax, redundant, and relatively inelastic skin in flexural areas) as well as retinal and cardiovascular complications.[124] Recessive mutations in the ABCC6 gene are identified in the majority of affected individuals.[125,126] Nevertheless, pseudodominance is relatively common due to an unexpectedly high prevalence of heterozygous carriers in the population; this has important consequences for genetic counseling of PXE patients.[127]

The most frequent retinal abnormalities in PXE are RPE irregularities, primarily temporal to the fovea (peau d'orange) and angioid streaks originating from the optic disk.[124] The latter develop in almost all PXE patients and often lead to choroidal neovascularization, fibrovascular scarring of the posterior pole, and visual loss.[128] The peau d'orange appearance precedes angioid streaks and can be observed in younger patients as fine, yellow-white, drusen-like lesions in the temporal posterior or midperipheral fundus (Fig. 48.9).[124,129] FAF is very useful in assessing PXE patients and it reveals the extent of RPE alterations.[130,131] OCT reveals pathologic features at the level of the RPE/Bruch's membrane complex.[129,132,133] Early recognition of the PXE phenotype is important, alerting the ophthalmologist and prompting referral to a dermatologist and cardiologist.

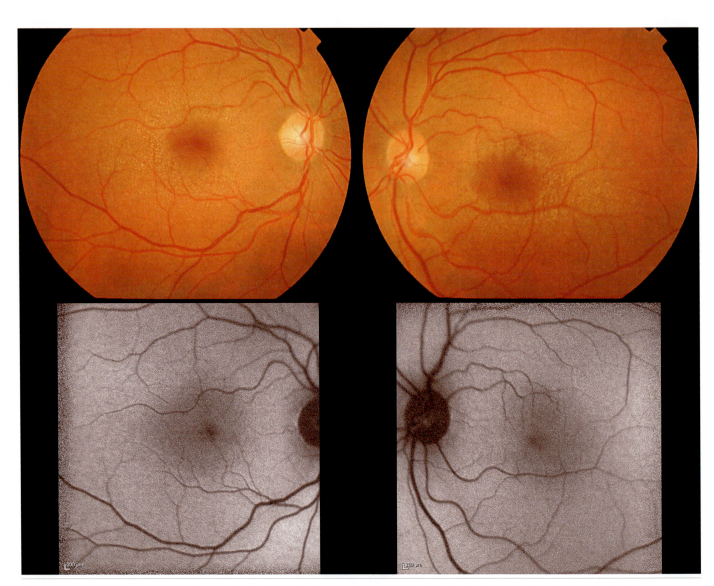

Fig. 48.8 Alport's syndrome. Fundus photograph of the left and right eyes of a 28-year-old individual with Alport's syndrome (top panel); fundus autofluorescence imaging (bottom panel) was normal. (Courtesy of Dr Andrew R. Webster.)

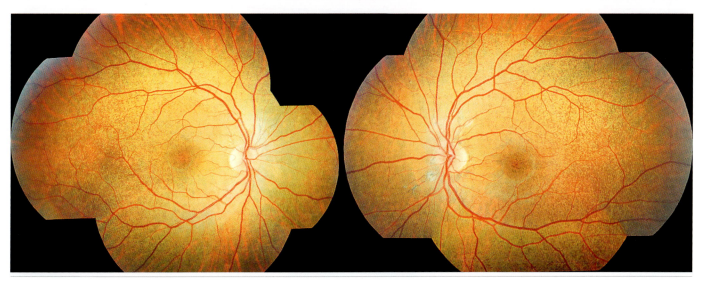

Fig. 48.9 Pseudoxanthoma elasticum. Fundus photograph of the left and right eyes of a 16-year-old affected individual.

Type II membranoproliferative glomerulonephritis

Membranoproliferative glomerulonephritis type II is a rare form of glomerulonephritis characterized by the presence of dense deposits within the glomerular basement membrane.[134] Deposits of similar composition and structure may occur along the choriocapillaris–Bruch's membrane–RPE interface of affected individuals.[134,135] Drusen-like lesions, often detectable at the posterior pole in the second decade of life, can develop.[134] These tend to vary in distribution among patients and SD-OCT findings suggests that they have a different composition and a more detrimental effect compared to age-related macular degeneration-associated drusen.[136] There are usually no symptoms and visual acuity remains good.[137] Over time, however, specialized tests of retinal function such as EOG and ERGs may become abnormal.[134]

Primary hyperoxaluria

Primary hyperoxaluria is a rare inborn error of glyoxylate and oxalate metabolism resulting in increased serum and urinary levels of oxalate.[138] As serum levels rise, calcium precipitates with oxalate to form insoluble crystals that are then deposited in a number of tissues, primarily in the kidney.[139] Renal involvement leading to chronic renal failure is a major cause of premature death.

Three different types of the disorder have been described.[140,141] Type I hyperoxaluria, the most common form, is caused by a deficiency of the liver-specific peroxisomal enzyme alanine : glyoxylate aminotransferase (AGT)[142] and has been associated with ocular abnormalities.[143] Primary hyperoxaluria usually presents in early childhood. Affected individuals may show multiple yellow crystals deposited at the level of the RPE, more numerously at the posterior pole and along the vascular arcades (Fig. 48.10).[144] Atrophic macular lesions may develop and patches of pigment may be observed.[145,146] FAF reveals hyperautofluorescent dots; SD-OCT shows hyperreflective lesions below the level of the RPE ("dome-shaped elevated RPE").[145] Retinal oxalate crystal deposition has been reported

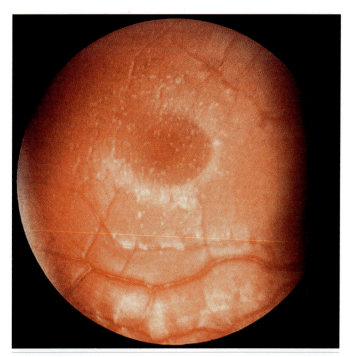

Fig. 48.10 Primary hyperoxaluria type I. Fundus photograph of the right eye of an affected individual. (Courtesy of Professor Alistair Fielder.)

in adults with secondary hyperoxaluria resulting from methoxyflurane anesthesia.

Sjögren-Larsson syndrome

Sjögren-Larsson syndrome is an autosomal recessively inherited neurocutaneous disorder of childhood caused by deficiency of the microsomal enzyme fatty aldehyde dehydrogenase (*FALDH*).[147] Pathologic features include congenital ichthyosis, mental retardation, and spasticity.[148] Most patients are born preterm and exhibit a characteristic crystalline childhood-onset maculopathy characterized by

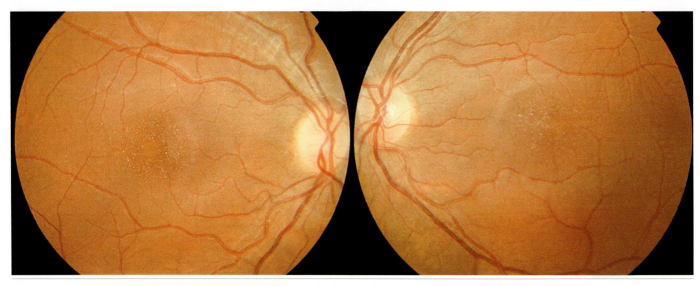

Fig. 48.11 Sjögren-Larsson syndrome. Fundus photograph of the left and right eyes of a 22-year-old affected individual. (Courtesy of Dr Andrew R. Webster.)

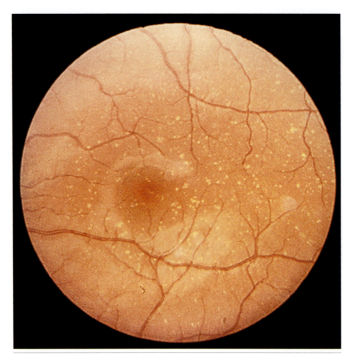

Fig. 48.12 Flecked retina syndrome and ring chromosome 17. Fundus photograph of the left eye of an affected individual.

photophobia and visual acuity loss. Yellow-white glistening macular deposits (Fig. 48.11) and possible atrophic RPE changes have been described.[149-151] Generalized retinal function is preserved.[152-154]

Miscellaneous reports of retinal flecks associated with syndromic eye disease

A number of other systemic disorders can give rise to yellow-white retinal lesions. They include:

1. Kjellin's syndrome (recessive mutations in SPG11 or SPG15)[155-158]

2. Breadcrumb-flecked retina syndrome[159]
3. Sensorineural hearing loss, dental abnormalities, and flecked retina[160]
4. Flecked retina syndrome and ring chromosome 17 (Fig. 48.12)[161-163]
5. Peroxisomal bifunctional enzyme complex deficiency.[164-166]

References

1. Krill AE, Klien BA. Flecked retina syndrome. Arch Ophthalmol 1965; 74: 496–508.
2. Walia S, Fishman GA, Kapur R. Flecked-retina syndromes. Ophthalmic Genet 2009; 30: 69–75.
9. Lois N, Holder GE, Bunce C, et al. Phenotypic subtypes of Stargardt macular dystrophy-fundus flavimaculatus. Arch Ophthalmol 2001; 119: 359–69.
14. Sabel Aish S, Dajani B. Benign familial fleck retina. Br J Ophthalmol 1980; 64: 652–59.
19. Sergouniotis PI, Sohn EH, Li Z, et al. Phenotypic variability in RDH5 retinopathy (fundus albipunctatus). Ophthalmology 2011; 118: 1661–70.
32. Morimura H, Berson EL, Dryja TP. Recessive mutations in the RLBP1 gene encoding cellular retinaldehyde-binding protein in a form of retinitis punctata albescens. Invest Ophthalmol Vis Sci 1999; 40: 1000–4.
39. Khan AO, Aldahmesh M, Meyer B. The enhanced S-cone syndrome in children. BMJ Case Rep 2009.
41. Sharon D, Sandberg MA, Caruso RC, et al. Shared mutations in NR2E3 in enhanced S-cone syndrome, Goldmann-Favre syndrome, and many cases of clumped pigmentary retinal degeneration. Arch Ophthalmol 2003; 121: 1316–23.
54. Weleber RG, Michaelides M, Trzupek KM, et al. The phenotype of Severe Early Childhood Onset Retinal Dystrophy (SECORD) from mutation of RPE65 and differentiation from Leber congenital amaurosis. Invest Ophthalmol Vis Sci 2010; 52: 292–302.
57. van Schooneveld MJ, Miyake Y. Fundus albipunctatus-like lesions in juvenile retinoschisis. Br J Ophthalmol 1994; 78:659–61.
60. Borman AD, Davidson AE, O'Sullivan J, et al. Childhood-onset autosomal recessive bestrophinopathy. Arch Ophthalmol 2011; 129: 1088–93.
66. Small KW, Killian J, McLean WC. North Carolina's dominant progressive foveal dystrophy: how progressive is it? Br J Ophthalmol 1991; 75: 401–6.

76. Wilson DJ, Weleber RG, Klein ML, et al. Bietti's crystalline dystrophy: a clinicopathologic correlative study. Arch Ophthalmol 1989; 107: 213–21.

81. Chaker N, Mghaleth F, Baccouri R, et al. [Clinical and angiographic characteristics of Bietti's corneoretinal dystrophy: a case study of an 8-year-old girl.] J Fr Ophtalmol 2007; 30: 39–43.

88. Miyauchi O, Murayama K, Adachi-Usami E. A family with crystalline retinopathy demonstrating an autosomal dominant inheritance pattern. Retina 1999; 19: 573–4.

98. Genead MA, Fishman GA, Lindeman M. Fundus white spots and acquired night blindness due to vitamin A deficiency. Doc Ophthalmol 2009; 119: 229–33.

101. Matsumoto Y, Haen SP, Spaide RF. The white dot syndromes. Compr Ophthalmol Update 2007; 8: 179–200; discussion 203–4.

103. Drenser K, Sarraf D, Jain A, Small KW. Crystalline retinopathies. Surv Ophthalmol 2006; 51: 535–49.

113. Cogan DG, Rodrigues M, Chu FC, Schaefer EJ. Ocular abnormalities in abetalipoproteinemia: a clinicopathologic correlation. Ophthalmology 1984; 91: 991–8.

119. Colville DJ, Savige J. Alport syndrome. A review of the ocular manifestations. Ophthalmic Genet 1997; 18: 161–73.

124. Finger RP, Charbel Issa P, Ladewig MS, et al. Pseudoxanthoma elasticum: genetics, clinical manifestations and therapeutic approaches. Surv Ophthalmol 2009; 54: 272–85.

129. Charbel Issa P, Finger RP, Gotting C, et al. Centrifugal fundus abnormalities in pseudoxanthoma elasticum. Ophthalmology 2010; 117: 1406–14.

134. Appel GB, Cook HT, Hageman G, et al. Membranoproliferative glomerulonephritis type II (dense deposit disease): an update. J Am Soc Nephrol 2005; 16: 1392–403.

144. Meredith TA, Wright JD, Gammon JA, et al. Ocular involvement in primary hyperoxaluria. Arch Ophthalmol 1984; 102: 584–7.

149. Willemsen MA, Cruysberg JR, Rotteveel JJ, et al. Juvenile macular dystrophy associated with deficient activity of fatty aldehyde dehydrogenase in Sjogren-Larsson syndrome. Am J Ophthalmol 2000; 130: 782–9.

158. Frisch IB, Haag P, Steffen H, et al. Kjellin's syndrome: fundus autofluorescence, angiographic, and electrophysiologic findings. Ophthalmology 2002; 109: 1484–91.

159. Protzko EE, Schatz H, Raymond WR, et al. Bread crumb-flecked retinopathy. Retina 1992; 12: 21–3.

160. Innis JW, Sieving PA, McMillan P, Weatherly RA. Apparently new syndrome of sensorineural hearing loss, retinal pigment epithelium lesions, and discolored teeth. Am J Med Genet 1998; 75: 13–17.

162. Kumari R, Black G, Dore J, Lloyd IC. Flecked retina associated with ring 17 chromosome. Eye (Lond) 2009; 23: 2134–5.

166. Al-Hazzaa SA, Ozand PT. Peroxisomal bifunctional enzyme deficiency with associated retinal findings. Ophthalmic Genet 1997; 18: 93–9.

Access the complete referece list online at

http://www.expertconsult.com

Acquired and other retinal diseases (including juvenile X-linked retinoschisis)

David A Hollander • Jay M Stewart

Diabetic retinopathy

Diabetic retinopathy, while uncommon in children, is strongly correlated with duration of diabetes and overall glycemic control (percentage of glycosylated hemoglobin). The prevalence of diabetic retinopathy rises steadily following puberty, with a 4.8 times greater risk of postpubescent adolescents developing retinopathy relative to pubescent or prepubescent children with the same duration of diabetes.[1] The progression of diabetic retinopathy associated with puberty is a combination of metabolic changes as well as decreased patient compliance.

Until recently, pediatric diabetes was almost exclusively the type 1 insulin-dependent form. With increasing obesity in the pediatric population, however, type 2 diabetes and insulin resistance is an emerging epidemic in children and adolescents, comprising 8–45% of all juvenile diabetes.[2] Initial screening of diabetic children by an ophthalmologist 3–5 years following diagnosis remains critical; in a cohort aged 13–17

years intensive insulin therapy delayed the onset and reduced the progression of diabetic retinopathy.[3]

Retinopathy is slowly progressive, affecting between 5% and 44% of insulin-dependent diabetic children after 5 years of systemic disease and nearly 100% within 20 years.[4-6] Longitudinal studies demonstrate clinically significant macular edema after 7 years of systemic disease, with a linear yearly cumulative risk as high as 6.7% between 10 and 20 years of duration.[7] Proliferative diabetic retinopathy (Fig. 49.1), though extremely rare in the pediatric population, has been observed in children as young as 13 years old with an 8-year history of diabetes.[8]

Sickle cell retinopathy

Ocular manifestations of sickle cell (SC) disease are most commonly seen in hemoglobin SC disease, homozygous SC disease, SC thalassemia, and heterozygous SC trait. Under conditions of hypoxia, dehydration, acidosis, and hyperviscosity, the abnormal hemoglobins polymerize, resulting in sickled erythrocytes.[9] Sickled erythrocytes are less pliable and cannot easily migrate through small capillaries or pores of the

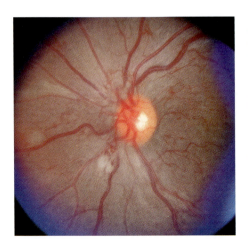

Fig. 49.1 Diabetic retinopathy. Proliferative diabetic retinopathy in a young adult. Neovascularization of the disc is present, in addition to multiple cotton-wool spots and intraretinal hemorrhages.

trabecular meshwork. Retinal non-perfusion initiates a cascade of vascular remodeling at the junction of perfused and non-perfused retina. Arteriovenous anastomoses may develop, eventually giving rise to "sea fan" proliferative retinopathy (Fig. 49.2), most commonly seen in SC and SC thalassemia disease.[10-12] Intraretinal salmon patch hemorrhages are often observed, which upon resorption may result in refractile spots of hemosiderin deposition beneath the internal limiting membrane. Black "sunburst" lesions, the sequela of subretinal hemorrhage, are focal areas of retinal pigment epithelial hypertrophy and hyperplasia.[13]

Proliferative SC retinopathy may lead to vitreous hemorrhage, tractional and rhegmatogenous retinal detachments, but more frequently undergoes spontaneous regression.[14,15] Suggested mechanisms for autoinfarction include feeder arteriolar occlusion, capillary occlusion, or hemodynamic alterations induced by vitreous traction.[16,17] Peripheral scatter photocoagulation may induce regression and reduce the risk of vitreous hemorrhage.[18] In the event of retinal detachment, caution should be taken to minimize the risk of anterior segment ischemia as reported with encircling scleral buckles.[19]

Traumatic hyphema in children with SC hemoglobinopathies poses an increased risk of complications, including raised intraocular pressure as a result of aqueous outflow obstruction by sickled erythrocytes.[20,21] Even mild elevations in intraocular pressure may produce sludging in the vascular supply to the optic nerve and retina, leading to central retinal artery occlusion or optic atrophy.[22] Therefore, surgical intervention or antifibrinolytic therapy with aminocaproic acid may be necessary. Additionally, there is an increased risk of rebleeding after the initial hyphema in pediatric SC patients.[23]

Radiation retinopathy

Radiation retinopathy[24,25] is seen in children secondary to focal plaque (brachytherapy) and external beam treatments for retinoblastoma and orbital tumors.[26,27] The total dose and the fraction size of radiation are the key elements predisposing to radiation retinopathy, with retinal vascular damage occurring at lower doses with external beam than with plaque therapy.[26] The threshold for retinopathy is a total dose of 3000–3500 cGy with external beam radiotherapy, but retinopathy has been reported with as little as 1500 total cGy.[26,28] Radiation

retinopathy most commonly develops between 6 months and 3 years following treatment; retinal changes have been observed as early as 1 month following both plaque and external beam.[29-31]

Radiation induces a cascade of changes in the retinal vascular architecture, predominantly in the macula, which lead to vascular non-perfusion, incompetence, and proliferation. Histologic studies demonstrate a preferential loss of vascular endothelial cells with a relative sparing of the pericytes, a distinct contrast to the early loss of pericytes in diabetic retinopathy.[29] Progressive endothelial cell loss results in capillary occlusion and irregular dilatations, telangiectasias, and microaneurysms of the neighboring capillary bed.[32] More severe and extensive radiation retinopathy is associated with diabetes mellitus and the administration of chemotherapeutic agents.[26,33,34]

Bone marrow transplant retinopathy

An ischemic retinopathy, similar to that observed with radiotherapy, is seen following bone marrow transplantation (BMT) for hematologic malignancies and aplastic anemia. The retinopathy is decreasing in prevalence as better chemotherapy makes BMT less necessary and stem cell transplants reduce the immunologic complications. The retinal manifestations include capillary non-perfusion, cotton-wool spots, and intraretinal hemorrhages (Fig. 49.3).[35] The vasculopathy generally develops within 6 months of BMT, with histologic changes resembling those of early radiation retinopathy.[35,36] While the majority of ocular complications associated with BMT are cataract and dry eye, the incidence of ischemic retinopathy and disc swelling ranges from 6.9% to 13.5%.[35,37-40] In a study of children undergoing bone marrow transplantation, 95.7% of eyes retained visual acuity of 20/40 or better, with poor visual outcomes associated with cytomegalovirus retinitis, a presumed submacular *Nocardia* abscess, corneal ulcers secondary to dry eye syndrome, and cataracts.[40]

The pathogenesis of the retinopathy in BMT patients remains unclear, confounded by the conditioning regimens prior to transplantation which typically involve total body radiation and chemotherapy, as well as the administration of agents following transplantation designed to suppress graft-versus-host disease. The chemotherapeutic agents may be directly toxic to the retinal vasculature, potentially increasing the susceptibility to retinopathy, as retinopathy develops with relatively low doses of total radiation[40,41] as well as in its absence.[42]

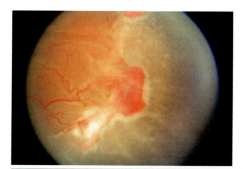

Fig. 49.2 Sickle cell retinopathy. Proliferative SC retinopathy in a young male with hemoglobin SC disease. Proliferative retinopathy is seen at the border of perfused and non-perfused retina. The patient subsequently developed a tractional retinal detachment.

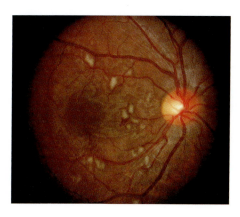

Fig. 49.3 Bone marrow transplant retinopathy. Multiple cotton-wool spots and a small perifoveal hemorrhage occurring 3 months after bone marrow transplant.

Retinal vasculitis

Retinal vasculitis may occur secondary to a systemic disease or an infectious agent, or as an isolated retinal etiology. Posterior segment manifestations include vascular sheathing, intraretinal hemorrhages, retinal exudates, vitritis, as well as macular edema. Both vascular incompetence and ischemia may be seen on fluorescein angiography; vessel staining or leakage are common findings. Non-perfusion may produce cotton-wool spots (Fig. 49.4), intraretinal whitening, and proliferative retinopathy. Fundus features are often non-specific, and other ocular or systemic features may aid in the diagnosis of the underlying etiology.

Causes of retinal vasculitis in the pediatric population include collagen vascular disorders,[43] Behçet's disease,[44] Eales' disease,[45] acquired toxoplasmosis,[46] multiple sclerosis,[47] human immunodeficiency virus, human T-cell lymphotropic virus type-1,[48] common variable immunodeficiency syndrome,[49] Henoch-Schönlein purpura,[50] and the syndrome of idiopathic vasculitis, aneurysms and neuroretinitis.[51] Treatment is tailored to the underlying etiology and retinal pathology.

Frosted branch angiitis

Frosted branch angiitis is a syndrome of acute, often bilateral, vision loss in otherwise healthy patients, commonly children and young adults.[52] Fundus examination reveals thick inflammatory sheathing surrounding the veins (and arteries to a lesser extent), extending from the optic nerve to the periphery (Fig. 49.5). The visual acuity is often reduced to counting fingers, but may be relatively unaffected in mild cases.[53] Intraretinal hemorrhages, serous macular detachment, optic disc swelling, conjunctival injection, anterior uveitis, and vitreous inflammation may be present.[54,55] Fluorescein angiography demonstrates late staining and leakage from the veins without any evidence of stasis or occlusion.

Systemic corticosteroids remain the mainstay of treatment, with prompt resolution of perivascular infiltrates and recovery of vision in the majority of cases.[54-57] A similar recovery with topical or subconjunctival steroids alone has been reported.[53,57,58] Visual recovery, however, may be limited by macular scarring, branch retinal vein occlusions, and diffuse retinal fibrosis.[54,59]

The origin of frosted branch angiitis is uncertain, though the efficacy of corticosteroids suggests an underlying immune response. Frosted branch-like appearances have been associated with cytomegalovirus retinitis in immunosuppressed patients,[60-63] and with autoimmune diseases such as systemic lupus erythematosus[64] and Crohn's disease.[65]

Angioid streaks

Angioid streaks are irregular linear streaks of variable pigmentation which may radiate in all directions from the peripapillary retina (Fig. 49.6). The streaks taper as they approach the optic disc, producing a circumferential peripapillary ring. The lesions are typically bilateral and vary in coloration depending on the pigmentation of the fundus. Angioid streaks are not seen at birth and only rarely have been observed in children, with earliest observations at 8 years of age.[66,67] Angioid streaks have been noted to increase in length and width over time. The incidence of angioid streaks increases with age, especially in the sickle hemoglobinopathies in which angioid streaks are typically observed only after the age of 25 years.[68,69]

The term angioid streak was originally coined by Knapp, reflecting the prevailing notion that this fundus abnormality had a vascular etiology.[70] Subsequent clinical and histopathologic studies have demonstrated that the streaks represent localized breaks at the level of Bruch's membrane.[80] Indocyanine green has proven to be a useful diagnostic tool in identifying angioid streaks and their associated ocular pathology.[71]

Angioid streaks, in up to 50% of cases, are associated with a systemic condition, most commonly pseudoxanthoma elasticum (PXE) (Fig. 49.7), Paget's disease of bone, and sickle hemoglobinopathies.[72] Extensive calcification of Bruch's membrane has been demonstrated in cases of Paget's disease and PXE, potentially rendering Bruch's membrane more brittle and subject to breaks. In hereditary spherocytosis, iron deposition may predispose Bruch's membrane to breaks.[73] The distribution of angioid streaks may represent the effects of biomechanical forces and the traction exerted by the extraocular muscles.[74]

Choroidal neovascularization, though a rare phenomenon in children, may develop secondary to the breaks in Bruch's membrane, resulting in serous detachments, subretinal

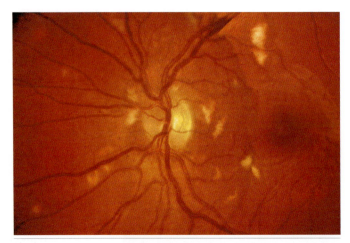

Fig. 49.4 Retinal vasculitis in a child with systemic lupus erythematosus. Shows multiple cotton-wool spots.

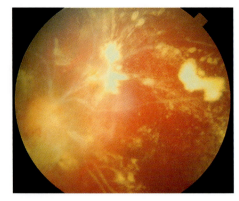

Fig. 49.5 Frosted branch angiitis. Unilateral frosted branch angiitis in a 10-year-old girl, of no known cause. Sheathed retinal vessels and subretinal exudates.

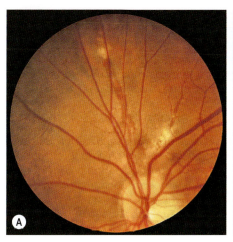

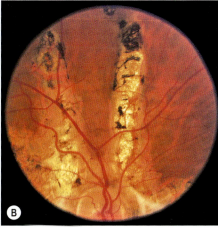

Fig. 49.6 Angioid streaks. (A) Angioid streak above the left optic disc in a 10-year-old girl with abetalipoproteinemia. (B) Marked angioid streaks in an adult with PXE. They taper away from the optic disc where they have formed a confluent ring around the disc. Neovascularization and hemorrhage occur at the margins of the streaks.

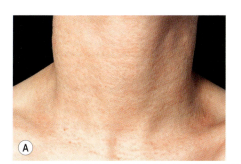

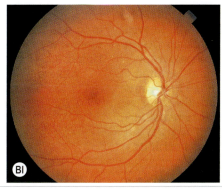

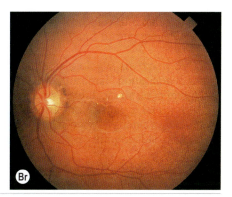

Fig. 49.7 Pseudoxanthoma elasticum. (A) The skin lesions of PXE consist of small, yellowish bumps in rows or a lacy pattern, which may join to make large patches. The skin is soft, lax, and slightly wrinkled or pebbly in appearance, which has been described as cobblestoned. The neck is often affected. (B) A 14-year-old child with PXE. "Peau d'orange" pigment speckling in the RPE at the posterior pole, yellow deposits in the RPE in both eyes, and angioid streaks at 12 and 6 o'clock in the right eye (Br) and 3 o'clock in the left (Bl).

hemorrhage, and disciform scarring. Fundus precursors to angioid streaks may be seen in children with PXE, and include a peau d'orange pigment speckling in the posterior pole (Fig. 49.7), as well as peripheral salmon spots, yellow deposits in the retinal pigment epithelium (RPE).[66,67] Subretinal hemorrhages following blunt ocular trauma have been observed in eyes with angioid streaks.[75] Identifying angioid streaks necessitates a work-up for an underlying systemic disorder as well as close follow-up for potential ocular complications.

Idiopathic epiretinal membrane

Epiretinal membrane formation (macular pucker, premacular gliosis, premacular fibrosis, cellophane maculopathy) in young adults is often associated with an underlying etiology such as ocular trauma,[76] posterior segment inflammation,[77] combined hamartoma of the RPE and retina,[78] Coats' disease,[79] and neurofibromatosis type II.[80] Unlike in adults, idiopathic epiretinal membrane (Fig. 49.8) is rare in children and adolescents.[81] Histopathologic studies demonstrate that epiretinal membranes consist of glial and retinal pigment epithelial cells, with a greater proportion of myofibroblasts and collagen formation observed in the epiretinal membranes of adolescents than in those of the elderly.[82]

The etiology of idiopathic epiretinal formation in young adults remains unknown, with cases of epiretinal membranes in both the presence and absence of an attached posterior vitreous.[82,83] The congenital persistence of primary vitreous has been proposed, supported by reports of epiretinal membranes in young patients with both a Mittendorf dot and a Bergmeister papilla.[84] In contrast, epiretinal membrane formation in young adults may be an acquired abnormality, with reported cases of epiretinal membrane in eyes with previous normal funduscopic examinations.[85]

Many young adults with epiretinal membranes can be followed conservatively without surgical intervention.[85-87] Epiretinal membranes in young adults tend to be thicker, more adherent, and associated with a higher recurrence rate than in adults, particularly those overlying retinal blood vessels.[82,83,88] Spontaneous separation of idiopathic epiretinal membrane in young patients, even in the absence of a posterior vitreous detachment, has been reported.[89,90] Banach et al. demonstrated that patients with a visual acuity of 20/50 or better have favorable outcomes with observation alone, while those with 20/60 vision or worse had significant improvement following vitrectomy and membrane peeling.[91] In cases in which spontaneous peeling occurs, long-term follow-up is warranted until posterior vitreous detachment is complete as delayed cases of macular hole have been reported.[92]

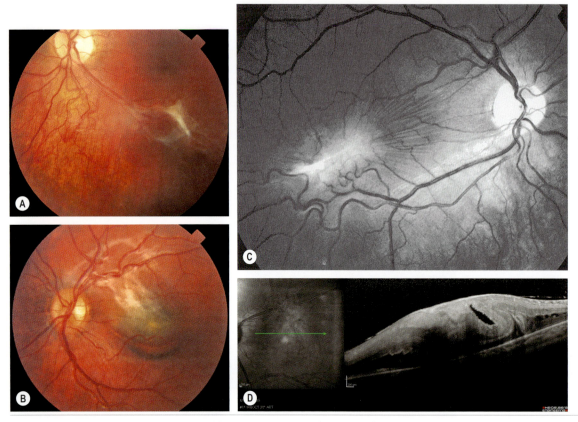

Fig. 49.8 Epiretinal membranes. (A) Preretinal fibrosis in a child with neurofibromatosis type 2. It is distorting the inferior vascular arcade and puckering the macula. (B) Macular epiretinal membrane causing traction on the superior and inferior arcades and a subretinal disturbance. (C) Idiopathic epiretinal membrane in a 15-year-old leading to retinal folds and macular distortion. (Photo courtesy of Professpr Alain Gaudric, from Benhamou N, Massin P, Spolaore R, et al. Surgical management of epiretinal membrane in young patients. Am J Ophthalmol 2002; 133: 358–64.) (D) Epiretinal membrane in a 10-year-old boy with pars planitis. Optical coherence tomography demonstrates severe retinal distortion and swelling with preretinal gliosis.

Lipemia retinalis

Lipemia retinalis is a rare ocular manifestation of hypertrigly-ceridemia.[93] With serum triglyceride levels greater than 1000–2500 mg/dl (normal <200 mg/dl), the retinal arteries and veins appear uniform creamy white in color, distinguishable only by vessel caliber.[94] Earliest fundus changes are seen in the periphery, with posterior involvement correlating with pro-gressively higher triglyceride levels.[95] The background fundus may also appear lightened or salmon colored as a result of elevated triglycerides in the choroidal circulation.

Lipemia retinalis may occur in neonates[96] and children[97] as a result of a primary familial lipid disorder (hyperlipoproteine-mia types I, III, IV, and V), in hyperchylomicronemia (Fig. 49.9) and very low-density lipoproteins, the lipoproteins which transport triglycerides, or as an acquired abnormality. Secondary hyperlipidemia has been associated with diabetes mellitus,[97] biliary obstruction, nephrotic syndrome, pancreati-tis, hypothyroidism, alcoholism, medications (estrogens, beta-blockers, protease inhibitors), and acquired immunodeficiency syndrome.[98]

Visual acuity typically remains unaffected, though retinal vein sludging secondary to hyperchylomicronemia has been demonstrated,[99] and a significant lipid exudative response has been observed following vein occlusion.[100] Reversible electro-physiologic changes have been demonstrated even in cases in

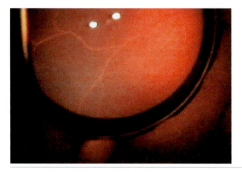

Fig. 49.9 Lipemia retinalis. Indirect ophthalmoscopic view of the retinal vessels, which stand out pale against the background, in a child with hyperchylomicronemia.

which there were no changes in visual acuity.[101] Recognition of lipemia retinalis may facilitate the earlier detection and treat-ment of hyperlipidemia in order to prevent complications such as pancreatitis and accelerated atherosclerosis. Treating the underlying systemic condition may simply require instituting insulin therapy or thyroid supplementation,[97] or discontinu-ing particular medications. Dietary modifications alone, including fat restriction[102] and the use of medium-chain trig-lyceride milk for neonates,[103] are often sufficient to reverse the ocular findings.

Cystoid macular edema

Cystoid macular edema (CME) may occur in children secondary to chronic ocular inflammation,[104] retinitis pigmentosa,[105] diabetes,[7] radiation,[29] Coat's disease,[79] Letterer-Siwe disease,[106] retinoschisis,[107] an autosomal dominant hereditary dystrophy,[108] and following cataract extraction.[109] Hoyt and Nickel observed cystoid macular edema in 10 of 27 eyes (37%) which underwent lensectomy and anterior vitrectomy;[109] a much lower incidence (0–4%) has been reported by others.[110-113] Explanations for the lower incidence of postoperative CME in children than adults include a healthier vitreous body and vasculature, a lack of systemic disease, and possible differences in prostaglandin physiology.[113] Different surgical techniques do not pose any additional risk for developing postoperative CME in children.[111,114]

Choroidal neovascularization

Choroidal neovascularization (CNV) is rare in children and adolescents. It is most commonly associated with intraocular inflammation and infection.[115] Patients may be asymptomatic or complain of metamorphopsia and blurring of vision. Fundus findings may include a deep grayish membrane, subretinal or intraretinal hemorrhage, and pigmentary changes, most commonly in the macula or peripapillary region.[116] Reported associations in the pediatric population, listed in Box 49.1, include congenital toxoplasmosis,[117] presumed ocular histoplasmosis syndrome,[118] congenital rubella (Fig. 49.10),[119] Best's disease,[120] optic nerve head drusen,[121] traumatic choroidal rupture,[122] and choroidal coloboma.[123]

Box 49.1

Associations with CNV in children and adolescents

Inflammatory/infectious
Presumed ocular histoplasmosis syndrome
Toxocara canis
Toxoplasmosis
Rubella retinopathy
Chronic uveitis
Trauma
Choroidal rupture
Inherited retinal disorders
Best's vitelliform macular dystrophy
Choroideremia
Fundus flavimaculatus
Miscellaneous
Congenital optic pits
Optic nerve head drusen
Angioid streaks
Myopia
Choroidal osteoma
Choroidal hemangioma
Combined retinal pigment epithelium: retinal hamartomas
Photocoagulation
Idiopathic

CNV in children has a more favorable prognosis than in adults with age related macular degeneration. Goshorn et al. reported spontaneous involution of CNV in 11 of 19 (58%) untreated eyes in children; nine patients achieved visual acuity better than or equal to 20/50.[115] Laser photocoagulation, photodynamic therapy with verteporfin,[124] and submacular surgery[125] have been employed successfully. Repeated injections with anti-vascular endothelial growth factor (anti-VEGF) agents[126,127] or a combination of intravitreal injections of corticosteroids and anti-VEGF have been employed, though the long-term effects of suppressing VEGF in children remains unclear.[128]

Chronic granulomatous disease

Chronic granulomatous disease (CGD) is a group of rare, inherited disorders of the immune system that are caused by defects in phagocytes giving rise to often severe recurrent bacterial and fungal infections and chronic inflammatory conditions such as gingivitis, lymphadenopathy, or granulomas. Two-thirds of people with CGD inherit the disease as an X-linked trait, one-third are autosomal recessive. The eye is affected with chorioretinal lesions in 23.7–35.3% of patients with CGD.[129,130] The chorioretinal lesions include RPE atrophy or pigment clumping (Fig. 49.11); vision loss may occur secondary to retinal ischemia, neovascular membranes, subretinal fibrosis, and macular edema.[130,131]

Juvenile X-linked retinoschisis

Juvenile X-linked retinoschisis (JXLRS) is an hereditary disease characterized by vision loss in males due to splitting of the retina within its inner layers. The condition is caused by a mutation in the RS1 gene at Xp22.1 and occurs at a frequency of up to 1 in 15 000 to 1 in 30 000.[132] RS1 encodes an extracellular photoreceptor secreted cell adhesion protein, retinoschisin. Visual impairment initially presents in infancy or at school age and can remain stable for a number of years.[133] Typical features include a characteristic cyst-like maculopathy as well as schisis in the inferotemporal periphery of the retina (Figs 49.12 and 49.13). Vitreous hemorrhage may be the presenting feature. Pathologically, the retina is disorganized at its

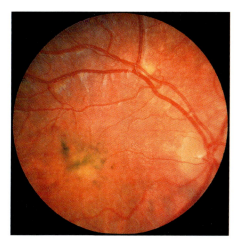

Fig. 49.10
Choroidal neovascularization. This 7-year-old with congenital rubella had a congenital cataract in the left eye and noted a reduction in the vision in the right eye. Background pigment mottling is present as well as serous detachment and a disciform lesion. The acuity fell to 6/60 but recovered to 6/12 over 4 months.

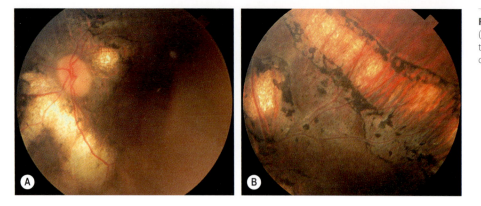

Fig. 49.11 Chronic granulomatous disease.
(A) Chorioretinal atrophy and pigment clumping in the retinal arcades. (B) Linear peripheral chorioretinal atrophy and pigment clumping.

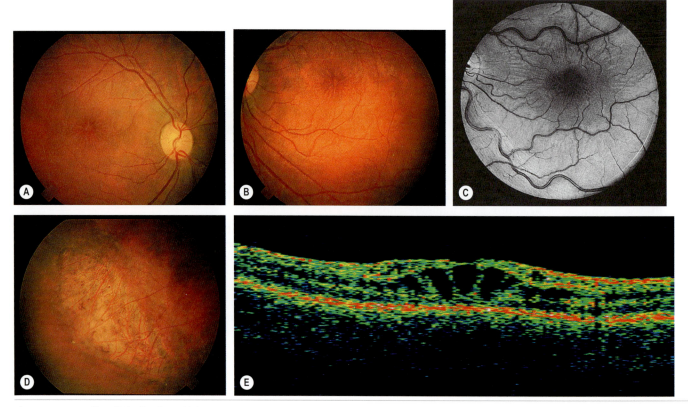

Fig. 49.12 Juvenile X-linked retinoschisis. (A,B) Bilateral foveal schisis. (C) The foveal schisis is best seen with ophthalmoscopy using a red free light. (D) Peripheral pigmentary changes in an area of schisis. (E) OCT study of retinoschisis demonstrating the optically empty spaces in the macula. (Image courtesy of Dr Dorothy Thompson.)

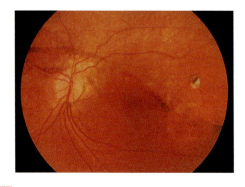

Fig. 49.13 Juvenile X-linked retinoschisis.
Fundus appearance after a bullous retinoschisis cyst involving the macula has resolved, leaving a flat retina with a pigment demarcation line.

inner aspect with splitting at the level of the ganglion cell and nerve fiber layers[134] with intraretinal filaments from defective Müller cells.

The diagnosis of JXLRS is made through a combination of clinical examination an electronegative ERG, and fundus imaging. OCT is helpful in distinguishing classic cystic changes in younger patients from collapsed, thinned tissue in older patients.[135] Carbonic anhydrase inhibitors reduce fluid in the macula, but have not consistently improved vision.[136] Surgery is not indicated except for retinal detachment or vitreous hemorrhage associated with the schisis.[137]

References

7. Vitale S, Maguire MG, Murphy RP, et al. Clinically significant macular edema in type I diabetes: incidence and risk factors. Ophthalmology 1995; 102: 1170–6.

8. Kimmel AS, Magargal LE, Annesley WH, Donoso LA. Diabetic retinopathy under age 20: a review of 71 cases. Ophthalmology 1985; 92: 1047–50.

11. Fox PD, Dunn DT, Morris JS, Serjeant GR. Risk factors for proliferative sickle retinopathy. Br J Ophthalmol 1990; 74: 172–6.

18. Farber MD, Jampol LM, Fox P, et al. A randomized clinical trial of scatter photocoagulation of proliferative sickle cell retinopathy. Arch Ophthalmol 1991; 109: 363–7.

21. Lai JC, Fekrat S, Barron Y, Goldberg MF. Traumatic hyphema in children: risk factors for complications. Arch Ophthalmol 2001; 119: 64–70.

32. Hayreh SS. Post-radiation retinopathy: a fluorescence fundus angiographic study. Br J Ophthalmol 1970; 54: 705–14.

34. Gragoudas ES, Li W, Lane AM, Munzenrider J, Egan KM. Risk factors for radiation maculopathy and papillopathy after intraocular irradiation. Ophthalmology 1999; 106: 1571–7.

40. Suh DW, Ruttum MS, Stuckenschneider BJ, et al. Ocular findings after bone marrow transplantation in a pediatric population. Ophthalmology 1999; 106: 1564–70.

56. Sakanishi Y, Kanagami S, Ohara K. Frosted retinal angiitis in children. Jpn J Clin Ophthalmol 1984; 38: 803–7.

72. Clarkson JG, Altman RD. Angioid streaks. Surv Ophthalmol 1982; 26: 235–46.

74. Pruett RC, Weiter JJ, Goldstein RB. Myopic cracks, angioid streaks, and traumatic tears in Bruch's membrane. Am J Ophthalmol 1987; 103: 537–43.

76. Khaja HA, McCannel CA, Diehl NN, Mohney BG. Incidence and clinical characteristics of epiretinal membranes in children. Arch Ophthalmol 2008; 126: 632–6.

82. Smiddy WE, Michels RG, Gilbert HD, Green WR. Clinicopathologic study of idiopathic macular pucker in children and young adults. Retina 1992; 12: 232–6.

97. Martinez KR, Cibis GW, Tauber JT. Lipemia retinalis. Arch Ophthalmol 1992; 110: 1171–1171.

111. Kirwan C, O'Keeffe M. Cystoid macular oedema in paediatric aphakia and pseudophakia. Br J Ophthalmol 2006; 90: 37–9.

116. Wilson ME, Mazur DO. Choroidal neovascularization in children: report of five cases and literature review. J Pediatr Ophthalmol Strabismus 1988; 25: 23–9.

127. Sisk RA, Berrocal AM, Albini TA, Murray TG. Bevacizumab for the treatment of pediatric retinal and choroidal diseases. Ophthalmic Surg Lasers Imaging 2010; 41: 582–92.

132. Sikkink SK, Biswas S, Parry NR, Stanga PE, Trump D. X-linked retinoschisis: an update. J Med Genet 2007; 44: 225–32.

135. Menke MN, Feke GT, Hirose T. Effect of aging on macular features of x-linked retinoschisis assessed with optical coherence tomography. Retina 2011; 31: 1186–92.

 Access the complete reference list online at

http://www.expertconsult.com

Retinal detachment in childhood

Martin P Snead

Rhegmatogenous retinal detachment (RRD) is uncommon in childhood but the prognosis is often poor due to aggressive proliferative vitreoretinopathy (PVR) and late presentation with or without second eye involvement at the time of diagnosis. The majority of cases of RRD in childhood are associated with trauma, developmental abnormalities, or the inherited vitreoretinopathies.

Rhegmatogenous retinal detachment associated with trauma

Traumatic retinal detachment is seen mostly in older children, usually caused by blunt trauma where retinal tears may be found in 2–5%.[1] Penetrating injuries and retained intraocular foreign bodies are less frequent causes[2,3] but are frequently associated with severe PVR.

Blunt ocular trauma

Retinal dialysis

Retinal detachment due to blunt trauma is mostly caused by a disinsertion at the ora serrata in older children. Sudden antero-posterior compression of the globe with a violent coronal expansion leads to retinal avulsion (Fig. 50.1A) characterized by a festoon of non-pigmented pars plana epithelium in the vitreous cavity. This is the hallmark of traumatic retinal dialysis. There may be signs of related orbital injury (Fig. 50.2) or, more frequently, subtle signs of collateral trauma to the iris, lens, or drainage angle. Superior quadrant involvement is more frequent than the lower temporal quadrant involvement seen in non-traumatic dialysis (Fig. 50.1B and see below). Although the disinsertion may exceed 90° and resemble a giant retinal

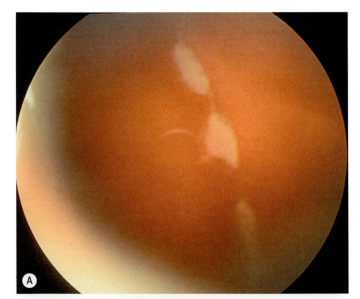

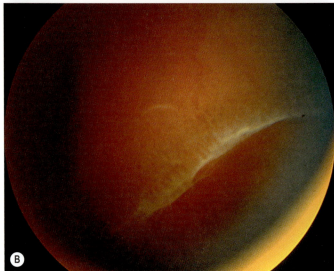

Fig. 50.1 Retinal dialysis. (A) Traumatic 180° "bucket handle" avulsion non-pigmented pars planar epithelium from patient in Figure 50.2. (B) Non-traumatic retinal dialysis. Note characteristic associated cystic oral frill and transdialysis tissue bridges.

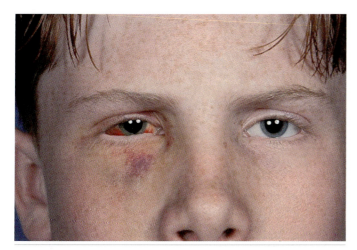

Fig. 50.2 Blunt injury with associated traumatic retinal dialysis. Vision logMAR 0.0 (6/6, 20/20, 1.0) unaided. Note enophthalmos. Fundus findings illustrated in Figure 50.1A.

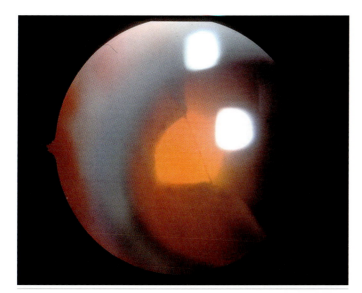

Fig. 50.3 Gravity induced radial extension at apex of giant retinal tear.

tear, the vitreous characteristically remains attached to the posterior flap so that independent mobility is not a feature. Dialyses, therefore, respond very well to conventional scleral buckling techniques – an accurately positioned 3 mm sponge being all that is required. Further distinguishing features are the absence of radial extensions, which frequently occur at the apices of true giant retinal tears (GRTs) (Fig. 50.3) and the normal compact healthy vitreous architecture. GRTs in childhood are typically associated with abnormal vitreous and inherited vitreoretinopathies (see below). Subretinal fluid recruitment in dialyses is typically slow, so that unless the ora serrata is routinely inspected after blunt trauma, the diagnosis may be delayed by weeks or months until macular involvement causes poor acuity.[3]

Ragged impact necrosis breaks account for about one-fifth of the retinal breaks in blunt trauma.[3] Retinal vessel and retinal pigment epithelial disruption may be confirmed on fundus fluorescein angiography and retinal detachment usually presents within 6 weeks.[3] These breaks are often large, post-equatorial, and irregular, making closure by external buckling

problematic so that an internal approach is more usually required.

Giant retinal tears

True GRTs account for a minority of retinal breaks due to blunt trauma.[4] They are best managed with vitrectomy and internal tamponade although the visual prognosis is often limited by associated collateral ocular damage.[5]

Penetrating ocular trauma

Penetrating injury is an uncommon cause of retinal detachment in childhood and may rarely follow inadvertent perforation of the globe at strabismus surgery. More common causes include accidental sharp penetrating injuries. Intraocular foreign bodies are rarely seen in very young children, although penetrating injuries from air-gun pellets may be seen in older children and adolescents, usually with a poor prognosis because of the associated damage and aggressive PVR. Retinal perforation or incarceration from penetrating trauma rarely causes acute rhegmatogenous retinal detachment. The corneo-scleral wound provides access for extrinsic fibroblasts so that the more common sequel is late tractional and rhegmatogenous retinal detachment.[5] Vitrectomy and internal tamponade with or without retinal relieving incisions may be required.

Non-traumatic retinal dialysis

Non-traumatic retinal dialysis accounts for approximately 10% of all juvenile retinal detachment[2,4] and in 97% affects the inferotemporal quadrant (Fig. 50.1B). Examination of the entire retinal periphery may reveal two or more separate dialyses in the same eye. There is a 2:3 male propensity and the majority are hypermetropic or emmetropic.[6,7] Detachments associated with dialyses progress slowly and present either as an incidental finding or when the macula becomes detached. They can be managed routinely with conventional buckling. The use of a small (typically 3 mm) circumferential sponge reduces postoperative motility problems. Although the anatomic success rate of surgery is high, visual recovery may remain poor if there has been chronic macular involvement. Familial dialyses are rare, but consideration should be given to sibling examination because (1) the patients are asymptomatic and (2) visual recovery once macular involvement has occurred may be poor. Examination of the fellow eye under anesthesia is important as retinal dialysis may be bilateral and abnormalities of the ora serrata, in the form of a "frill" or flat dialysis, are found in the fellow eye in up to 30%. Prophylactic retinopexy can be applied to avert detachment with potential macular involvement requiring formal repair.

Rhegmatogenous retinal detachment associated with developmental abnormality

Ocular coloboma

Eyes with colobomas are at increased risk of detachment and account for approximately 0.5% of pediatric retinal detachments[8,9] forming part of the spectrum of wider systemic developmental abnormality (Fig. 50.4). GRTs are seen with lens

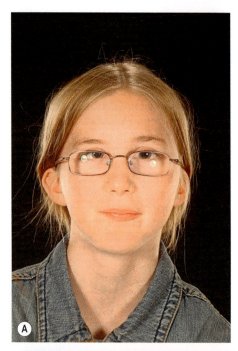

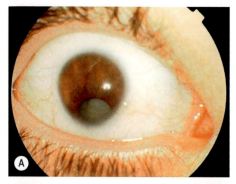

Fig. 50.5 Bilateral coloboma associated with microphthalmos, nystagmus, and cataract. Intercalary membrane simulating detachment on b-scan ultrasonography.

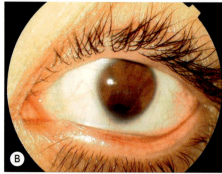

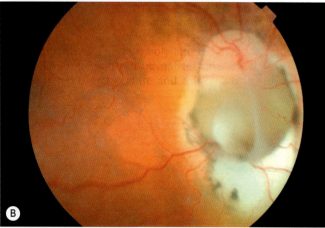

Fig. 50.4 Optic disk coloboma associated with macular-off retinal detachment in CHARGE syndrome. (© Addenbrookes Hospital.)

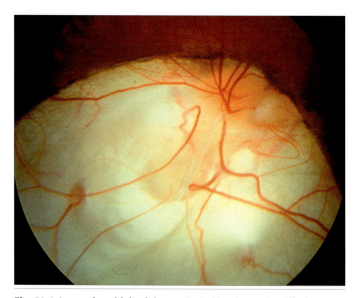

Fig. 50.6 Large choroidal coloboma. Retinal breaks may be difficult to identify preoperatively, but visualization of schlieren during vitrectomy can assist localization.

colobomas[10] and rhegmatogenous detachment may also develop in eyes with choroidal coloboma, when small retinal breaks may be found in the hypoplastic retina overlying the coloboma. Assessment of vision can be difficult and the diagnosis of detachment can be further impaired by restricted pupil dilation, nystagmus, microphthalmos, and cataract (Fig. 50.5). The intercalary membrane stretched across the coloboma cavity can simulate a retinal detachment on ultrasound examination. The clinician should be alert to this and assess the retinal mobility on dynamic examination before surgery. The intercalary membrane consists of hypoplastic inner retina with reversal and duplication of outer neuroblastic layers at the coloboma margin.[11] This marginal duplication has been proposed as a "locus minoris resistentiae" providing adhesion. Both retinal pigment epithelium and Müller cells are vestigial or absent within the coloboma; thus, effective retinopexy may be impossible unless applied outside the margin.

Where retinal breaks occur away from the coloboma, they may be managed by conventional buckling provided the sclera

is of sufficient quality and the break can be adequately closed. More usually, the retinal break lies within the coloboma so that identification and closure with retinopexy may be impossible without an internal approach. Retinal breaks over a coloboma are often small and multiple. Their localization can be very difficult preoperatively against the pale scleral background (Fig. 50.6), but may be confirmed peroperatively by the visualization of proteinaceous schlieren (optical variations and inhomogeneities in the transparency of the subretinal fluid) during internal drainage. Laser may be applied around the border of the colobomatous area and where this includes the papillomacular bundle it may be applied prior to retinal reattachment to minimize thermal damage to the nerve fiber layer. Maintenance of tamponade throughout the retinopexy can be compromised by the abnormal configuration of the colobomatous globe and recurrent detachment may occur in up to 30%,[12] necessitating permanent internal tamponade.

Optic disk pits and macular detachment

The association of serous macular detachment and optic disk pits and coloboma is well recognized and similar findings with the morning glory disk abnormality suggest that these conditions are variations of the same abnormality (Fig. 50.7). The vitreous is characteristically attached. It has been suggested that up to 45% of optic disk pits may be complicated by serous retinal detachment.[13,14] Although cases of spontaneous resolution have been reported, the visual prognosis is poor if the detachment persists beyond 6 months.[14]

Although natural history studies have shown eventual spontaneous reattachment in 25% of cases[14] and photocoagulation alone has mixed success, the combination of argon laser photocoagulation with internal tamponade, either with or without vitrectomy, may offer a greater chance of successful retinal reattachment, albeit at greater risk of operative morbidity.

Rhegmatogenous retinal detachment associated with inherited vitreoretinopathies

Inherited vitreoretinopathies are the basis for the majority of rhegmatogenous retinal detachments in childhood and are classified according to Meredith and Snead[15] as follows:

1. Vitreoretinopathies with skeletal abnormalities
2. Vitreoretinopathies with progressive retinal dysfunction
3. Vitreoretinopathies with abnormal retinal vasculature
4. Vitreoretinopathy with corneal changes

The detachments are often complex and frequently associated with GRTs.

Vitreoretinopathies with skeletal abnormalities

Vitreoretinopathies associated with skeletal abnormalities form the largest subgroup (Table 50.1). Of these, Stickler's syndromes in various guises account for the majority.

The Stickler's syndromes

The Stickler's syndromes form part of the spectrum of type II/XI collagenopathies, which include Kniest's dysplasia (MIM 156550) and spondyloepiphyseal dysplasia congenita (SEDC, MIM183900). So far, at least six clinically different subgroups have been identified (Table 50.1) and further genetic heterogeneity remains to be resolved.

Most cases seen by an ophthalmologist are type 1 Stickler's syndrome, inherited in an autosomal dominant fashion. However, a significant minority result from de novo mutations so there will be no diagnostic help from a family history. Furthermore, there are "ocular-only" variants which have too few systemic features to suggest the possible diagnosis[16] – clinician beware!

Diagnosis
Before routine molecular genetic analysis, diagnosis was wholly reliant on the combination of major and minor clinical criteria.[17] Notwithstanding, the assignment of clinical pheno-

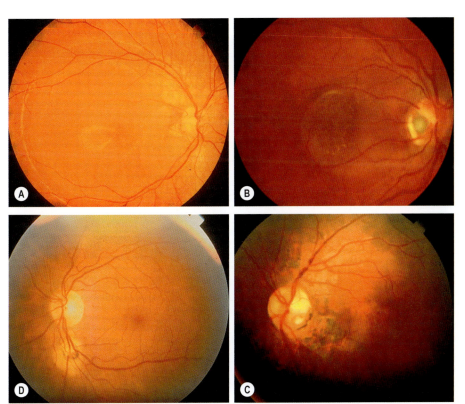

Fig. 50.7 Optic disk coloboma associated with macular detachment. Child (C) and parent (D) illustrating inherited etiology in some cases.

Table 50.1– Vitreoretinopathies associated with skeletal abnormalities

Syndrome		Gene	Distiguishing features	MIM No.
Stickler's syndrome				
	Type 1	COL2A1	Membranous congenital vitreous anomaly, congenital megalophthalmos, deafness, arthropathy, cleft palate	108300
	Type 2	COL11A1	Beaded congenital vitreous anomaly, congenital megalophthalmos, deafness, arthropathy, cleft palate	604841
	Type 3	COL11A2	Normal vitreous and ocular phenotype, deafness, arthropathy, cleft palate	215150
	Type 4	COL9A1 COL9A2	Recessive inheritance, sensorineural deafness, myopia, vitreoretinopathy, epiphyseal dysplasia	120210
	Ocular only	COL2A1	Membranous congenital vitreous anomaly (usually), congenital megalophthalmos. No systemic features.	108300
	Other	unknown	Hypoplastic vitreous, deafness, arthropathy, cleft palate	Not assigned
Kniest's Dysplasia		COL2A1	Severe arthropathy, short stature, phalangeal dysplasia	156550
Spondyloepiphyseal dysplasia congenital (SEDC)		COL2A1	Severe short stature, Rhizomelic limb shortening, barrel chest	183900
Marshall's syndrome		COL11A1	Sparse hair, reduced sweating, congenital / juvenile cataract	154780
Knobloch's syndrome		COL18A1	Occipital encephalocele, renal abnormalities, abnormal palmar creases	267750
Marfan's syndrome		FBN1	Cornea plana, ectopia lentis, arachnodactyly, aortic root dilatation	154700

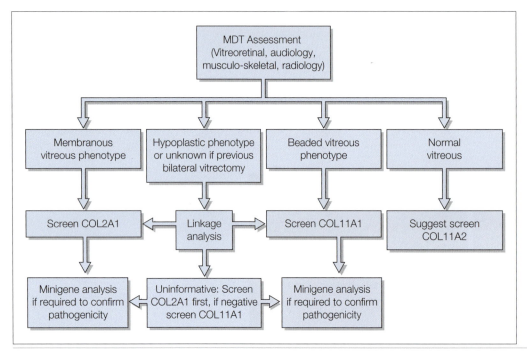

Fig. 50.8 Screening algorithm for assessment and molecular genetic analysis of Stickler's syndrome.

type assists substantially in directing molecular genetic analysis according to the algorithm shown in Fig. 50.8.

Clinical features

Ocular features The fundamental feature of Stickler's syndrome is a congenital abnormality in vitreous development, which manifests as an abnormal architecture visible on slit-lamp examination (Fig. 50.9). This pathognomonic feature is important for the clinical diagnosis of the ocular-only subgroups which have no systemic features to suggest the diagnosis. The

majority of patients presenting to an ophthalmologist will have either type 1 or type 2 Stickler's syndrome and are frequently myopic.[16] Autosomal recessive Stickler's syndrome due to mutations in type IX collagen is rare.[16]

The refractive error is congenital, of high degree, and often associated with a significant astigmatism (Fig. 50.10). In some series almost a quarter of patients have no refractive error. The association with congenital cataract is well recognized and some patients exhibit a characteristic quadrantic lamellar cortical lens opacity, which can be a useful diagnostic sign (Fig. 50.11). It does not, however, differentiate between subgroups, being present in both type 1 and type 2 Stickler's syndrome.

The risk of retinal detachment in Stickler's syndrome in the UK and USA is over 50% of patients with a clinical diagnosis of one of the Stickler's syndromes.[18] In the genetically confirmed type 1 subgroup, this figure rose to over 70% of which almost half had bilateral involvement.[19] The risk in type 2 Stickler's syndrome is slightly less, but unquantified, perhaps between 40% and 50%.[16]

Patients with type 1 Stickler's syndrome are prone to developing retinal detachment as a result of a GRT, defined as a circumferential break at the pars plana junction caused by a separation of the posterior hyaloid membrane (PHM) much more anteriorly than would normally be the case (Fig. 50.12). In such instances (with or without GRT), the PHM will sit behind the pre-existing type 1 anomaly resulting in a double membrane (Fig. 50.13A,B).). The clinician should be alert to posterior vitreous detachment in type 2 Stickler's syndrome resulting in the (single) detached posterior hyaloid membrane in a child masquerading as the type 1 anomaly. Prophylactic retinopexy designed and positioned specifically to prevent GRT progression substantially reduces the risk of retinal detachment and blindness from this type of break in type 1 Stickler's syndrome.[19] Detachment due to more posterior breaks can occur unpredictably in position making effective prophylaxis impractical.

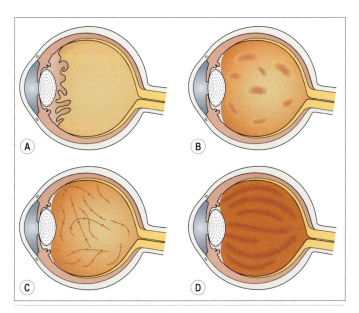

Fig. 50.9 **Schematic illustration of vitreous phenotypes in Stickler's syndrome.** (A) Membranous congenital vitreous anomaly. (B) Beaded congenital vitreous anomaly. (C) Hypoplastic congenital vitreous anomaly. (D) Normal vitreous architecture: compact lamellar array.

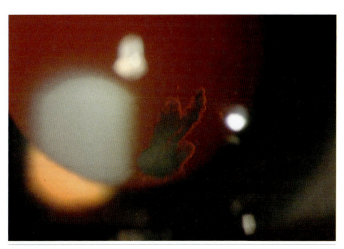

Fig. 50.11 **Classic quadrantic lamellar cataract found in both type 1 and type 2 subgroups of Stickler's syndrome.**

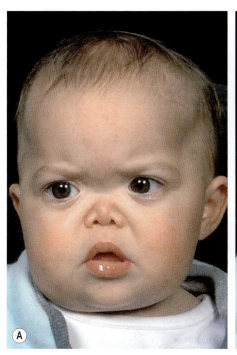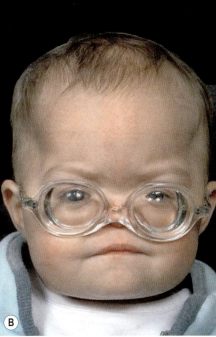

Fig. 50.10 **Stickler's syndrome.** Marked nasal hypoplasia and congenital high myopia revealed with refraction under cycloplegia.

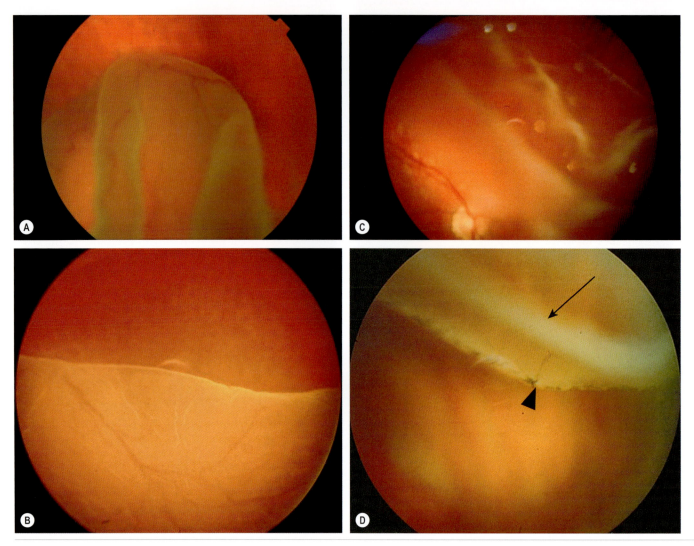

Fig. 50.12 Giant retinal tear detachments in type 1 Stickler's syndrome. Note previous laser prophylaxis too posterior to prevent detachment in (D). Arrow shows giant retinal tear; arrowhead indicates equatorial laser prophylaxis.

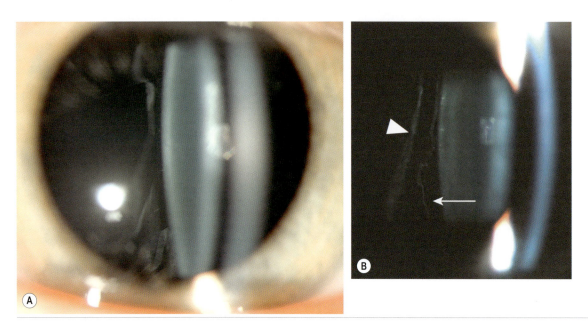

Fig. 50.13 (A) Type 1 Stickler's syndrome – typical membranous congenital vitreous anomaly. (B) PVD in type 1 Stickler's syndrome. The posterior hyaloid membrane (solid triangle) now visible behind the pre-existing type 1 anomaly (arrow) resulting in a double membrane.

Systemic features All subgroups of Stickler's syndrome exhibit clefting of the hard or soft palate distinct from other causes of midline clefting which are often associated with cleft lip. Stickler's syndrome patients do not usually have cleft lip. Abnormalities of the hard and soft palate are frequently associated with Eustachian tube dysfunction and middle ear impairment. In those patients without a history of palate repair, direct examination and palpation will help identify those with subclinical clefts (Fig. 50.14) – another easily overlooked diagnostic sign.

Mid-line clefts are frequently associated with middle ear hearing impairment, but many patients also exhibit a subtle, subclinical high-tone sensorineural hearing defect due to cochlear abnormalities.

Over 80% of children with the Stickler's syndromes report musculoskeletal symptoms, which may have a considerable impact on their quality of life. Some children have bony joint enlargement due to epiphyseal dysplasia. Joint hypermobility is common (Fig. 50.15) and although it may be asymptomatic, it can lead to knock knees, flat feet, joint subluxation or dislocation, and widespread joint pain. Patients are occasionally given an erroneous diagnosis of Perthe's disease as the appearances can be similar radiologically. It is also common for adolescent Stickler's syndrome patients to receive a diagnosis of Osgood-Schlatter's disease, but since this is a clinical rather than a radiologic diagnosis (and it is common in adolescence generally to have anterior tibial pain) the true nature of this association remains to be clarified.

Kniest's dysplasia (MIM 156550)

Kniest's dysplasia is an autosomal dominant disorder that shares many similarities with Stickler's syndrome and the same genetic locus. Mutations are found in the same gene as for type 1 Stickler's syndrome (COL2A1), but result in dominant-negative effects rather than haploinsufficiency with consequently more severe arthropathy. It typically presents at birth with shortened trunk and limbs, congenital megalophthalmos, and flattened nasal bridge (Fig. 50.16). The joints are often large at birth and the fingers long and knobbly. Motor

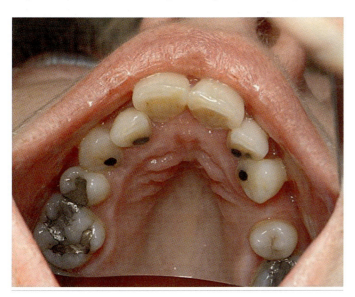

Fig. 50.14 Stickler's syndrome. Even in the absence of a history of cleft palate repair, remember to examine the palate. This patient thought their palate was normal.

milestones can be delayed by joint deformities, and disuse muscle atrophy may result. Both conductive and sensorineural hearing loss may be present as with the Stickler's syndromes. The intellect is normal, and myopia, retinal detachment, and GRT are the major ophthalmic complications.

Spondyloepiphyseal dysplasia congenita (MIM 183900)

Spondyloepiphyseal dysplasia congenita (SEDC) presents at birth with shortening of the trunk and, to a lesser extent, the extremities (rhizomelic limb shortening) (Fig. 50.17). It is an autosomal dominant disorder and characteristically results from dominant-negative mutations in the gene for type II collagen (COL2A1). In common with other type II collagenopathies, they exhibit congenital abnormalities of vitreous development, both conductive and sensorineural hearing loss and cleft palate. Patients develop a barrel-shaped chest and an exaggerated lumbar lordosis, which may compromise respiratory function. Odontoid hypoplasia may be present, predisposing to cervicomedullary instability and imaging of the cervical spine should be considered prior to general anesthesia. In parallel with the other type II/XI collagenopathies, patients with SEDC are at significant risk of rhegmatogenous retinal detachment.

Marshall's syndrome (MIM 154780)

There remains considerable uncertainty as to whether or not Marshall's syndrome and type 2 Stickler's syndrome are separate entities. Many features are shared, such as midfacial hypoplasia, spondyloepiphyseal abnormalities, cleft palate, and sensorineural hearing loss, but patients with Marshall's syndrome also have ectodermal dysplasia with hypertrichosis and hypohydrosis, calvarial thickening, and ocular hypertelorism. The term Marshall-Stickler syndrome is best avoided until Marshall's syndrome is better characterized.[15]

Knobloch's syndrome (MIM 267750)

Knobloch's syndrome is an automosomal recessive disorder which features high myopia, nystagmus, congenital vitreoretinopathy, retinal detachment, congenital occipital encephalocoele, unusual palmar creases, nail hypoplasia, and dental caries (Fig. 50.18). Molecular genetic analysis most commonly implicates homozygous splice site changes in the gene encoding the α1 chain of type XVIII collagen (COL18A1; 21q22.3; 46kb;41 exons), although compound heterozygotes have also been identified. COL18A1 is expressed in two distinct isoforms, the longer isoform in the retina with a putative role in retinal structure as well as in the closure of the neural tube. It is highly expressed in kidney and liver, but no patients reported have had any major kidney or liver defects. Mice which are col18a1 knockouts show abnormalities in the uveal tract.

Marfan's syndrome (MIM 154700)

Marfan's syndrome is an autosomal dominant connective tissue disorder associated with an abnormal vitreous architecture, myopic astigmatism, and characteristic skeletal features of increased height with disproportionately long limbs and digits, scoliosis, lumbar lordosis, joint laxity, a crowded, high-arched (but not cleft) palate, and anterior chest deformity. It is a disorder of fibrillin, a high-molecular-weight extracellular glycoprotein. Mutations in the fibrillin gene on chromosome

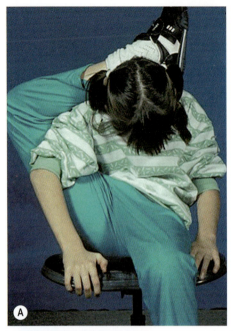

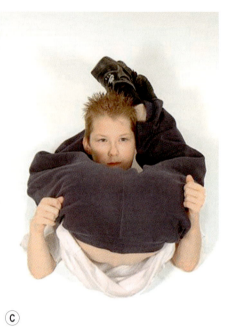

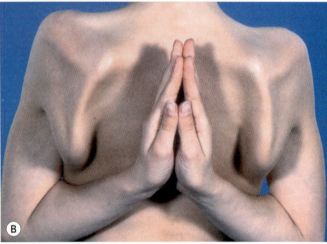

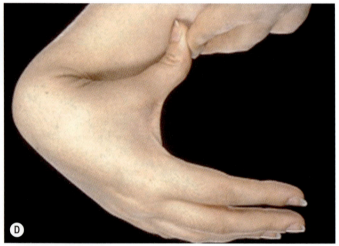

Fig. 50.15 Stickler's syndrome. Joint hypermobility can be assessed in a variety of ways. (Part (C) © Addenbrookes Hospital.)

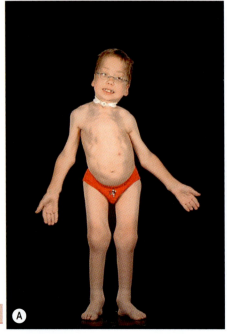

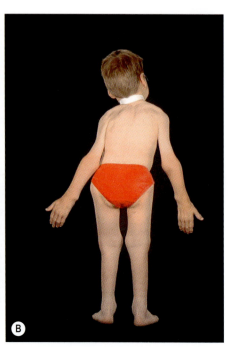

Fig. 50.16 Kniest's dysplasia. Note high myopia and severe arthropathy, particularly spine, knees, elbows, and phalangeal dysplasia. (© Addenbrookes Hospital.)

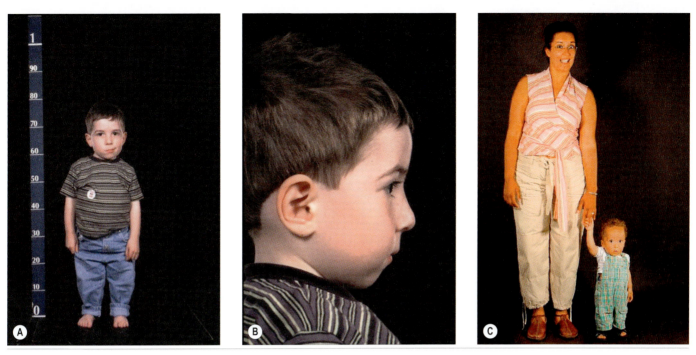

Fig. 50.17 Spondyloepiphyseal dysplasia congenita. Note short stature, barrel chest, and rhizomelic (proximal) limb shortening. Patients typically exhibit the membranous congenital vitreous anomaly. (Part (C) © Addenbrookes Hospital.)

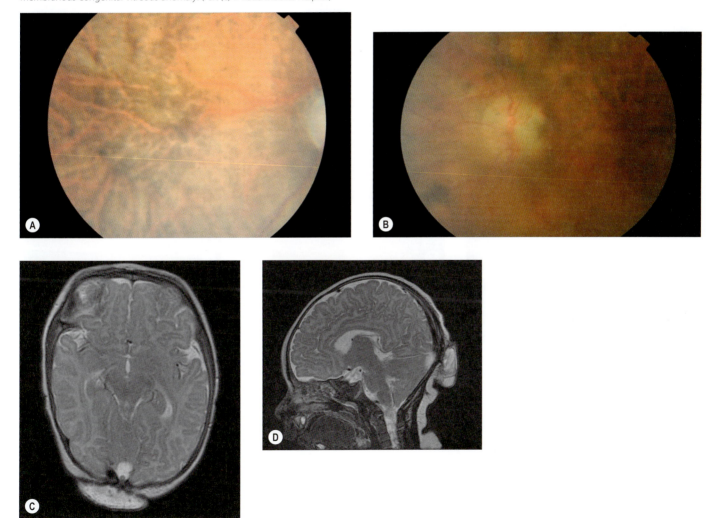

Fig. 50.18 Knobloch's syndrome. Macular-off detachment left eye associated with high myopia and occipital encephalocele.

15 (FBN1) cause both Marfan's syndrome and dominant ectopia lentis. Other ocular features include retinal detachment, myopia, megalophthalmos, cornea plana, hypoplastic iris, glaucoma, and early nuclear sclerotic cataract.

The association with rhegmatogenous retinal detachment has been reported in 8–50% of cases; approximately 75% of these occur before 20 years of age. The myopia is characteristically developmental as no case of myopia was found under 3 years of age in one large series, in contrast to the congenital non-progressive myopia found in type 1 Stickler's syndrome. In Marfan's syndrome the pupils dilate poorly because of a structural iris abnormality, and when combined with lens subluxation and weak scleral architecture the repair of retinal detachment becomes a formidable surgical challenge. Pars plana lensectomy and internal tamponade are often required.

Cardiovascular associations include mitral valve prolapse, mitral regurgitation, dilation of the aortic root, and aortic regurgitation, with aneurysm of the aorta and aortic dissection being the major life-threatening complications.

Vitreoretinopathies associated with progressive retinal dysfunction

Wagner's vitreoretinopathy (MIM 143200)

Wagner's syndrome features autosomal dominant inheritance, low myopia (−3.00 diopters or less), fluid vitreous, cortical cataract, inconstant and variably affected dark adaptation, and retinal detachment. The cardinal features are absence of the normal vitreous architecture and thickening and incomplete separation of the posterior hyaloid membrane, which tends to occur in a circular band. A large range of chorioretinal abnormalities have been described with the typically chorioretinal atrophy with pigment migration into the retina (Fig. 50.19) and gradual progressive visual loss without retinal detachment. Electroretinographic responses are progressively subnormal and visual-field testing demonstrates ring scotomas with eventual loss of central visual acuity. The phenotype at the end-stage is referred to as erosive vitreoretinopathy. The lenses typically develop anterior and posterior cortical opacities in puberty with rapid progression to "complicated cataract" during the fourth decade. The anterior lens capsule is tough and elastic which can make capsulorrhexis difficult. Rhegmatogenous retinal detachment and glaucoma were not reported by Wagner, but are now recognized. Wagner's syndrome is also associated with large angle kappas indicative of an ectopic fovea (Fig. 50.19). The prognosis is poor with progressive visual loss. The risk of rhegmatogenous retinal detachment, although higher than normal, is not as high as in the Stickler's syndromes. The term Jansen's syndrome has been used to describe a hereditary vitreoretinopathy with clinical features consistent with Wagner's syndrome and it shows linkage to the same locus.

Goldmann-Favre syndrome/enhanced S-cone dystrophy (MIM 268100)

Patients with Goldmann-Favre syndrome have liquefaction and fibrillar changes of the vitreous, night-blindness, equatorial chorioretinal atrophy and pigment clumping, peripheral

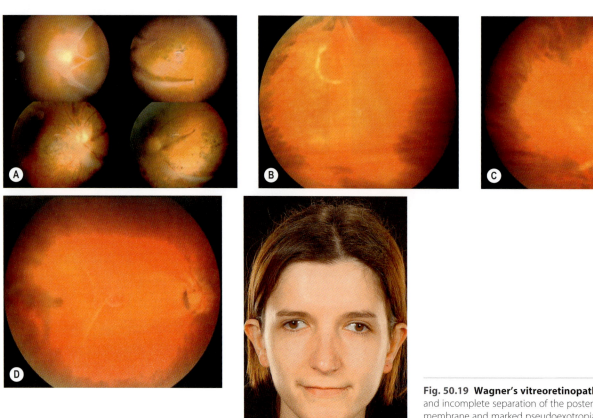

Fig. 50.19 Wagner's vitreoretinopathy. Note thickening and incomplete separation of the posterior hyaloid membrane and marked pseudoexotropia. (Reproduced from Meredith S, Snead MP. Inherited vitreoretinopathies. In: Besharse JC, Bok DP, editors. The Retina and its Disorders. Elsevier (Academic Press); 2011: 252–62. Part (E) © Addenbrookes Hospital.)

and macular schisis, cortical lens opacities, rod–cone dysfunction, and diffuse vascular leakage on fluorescein angiography. Goldmann-Favre syndrome is inherited as an autosomal recessive disorder and is caused by a mutation in the same gene (the NR2E3 gene) that causes enhanced S-cone syndrome (ESCS). ESCS is the only inherited retinal disease that exhibits a gain in photoreceptor function. Patients show enhanced sensitivity to blue (short wavelength) light, night-blindness, and loss of sensitivity to long and medium wavelengths. The ERG findings in this group demonstrate undetectable rod-isolated responses and reduced combined rod–cone responses.

Vitreoretinopathies associated with abnormal retinal vasculature

Familial exudative vitreoretinopathy (MIM 133780, 601813, 305390)

Familial exudative vitreoretinopathy is believed to be a premature arrest of retinal angiogenesis and vascular differentiation resulting in incomplete vascularization of the peripheral retina. The failure to fully vascularize the retina may be asymptomatic, but secondary changes can include neovascularization, retinal exudate, peripheral snowflake vitreous changes, and tractional or combined tractional and rhegmatogenous retinal detachment. Epiretinal membranes can cause severe retinal distortion and macular ectopia, which may be the presenting feature of poor vision in children (Fig. 50.20). The prognosis is highly variable with some individuals blind by age 10 and others asymptomatic throughout adult life. Vascular abnormalities in individuals with milder phenotypes may only be visible on fluorescein angiography. It is an autosomal dominant condition.

Autosomal dominant vitreochoroidopathy (MIM 193220)

Autosomal dominant vitreochoroidopathy is characterized by vitreous syneresis with or without peripheral vitreous changes. Peripheral pigmentary changes typically occur at the equatorial region with a discrete posterior boundary (Fig. 50.21) associated with diffuse retinal vascular leakage, cystoid macular edema, and early-onset cataract. The peripheral pigmented band extends from the ora serrata to the equator for 360° of the retina. Other features are rhegmatogenous retinal detachment, punctate retinal opacities, choroidal atrophy, and early nuclear sclerosis. The ERG responses are normal although the electrooculogram is abnormal.

Vitreoretinopathy associated with corneal changes

Snowflake vitreoretinal degeneration (MIM 193230)

The pathognomonic feature of snowflake vitreoretinal degeneration is the association with corneal guttata, and disk pallor which is not a feature of any of the other hereditary vitreoretinopathies. The vitreous has a fibrillar appearance and small snowflake-like opacities in the retina may not be immediately obvious. Minor vascular abnormalities of small retinal vessels have been reported.

X-linked retinoschisis (MIM 312700)

X-linked retinoschisis is an uncommon cause of retinal detachment in childhood accounting for 2.5–5% of all pediatric retinal detachments. The incidence of retinal detachment varies in the different series, but it may occur in up to 16% of affected males. Vitreous hemorrhage is another cause of visual

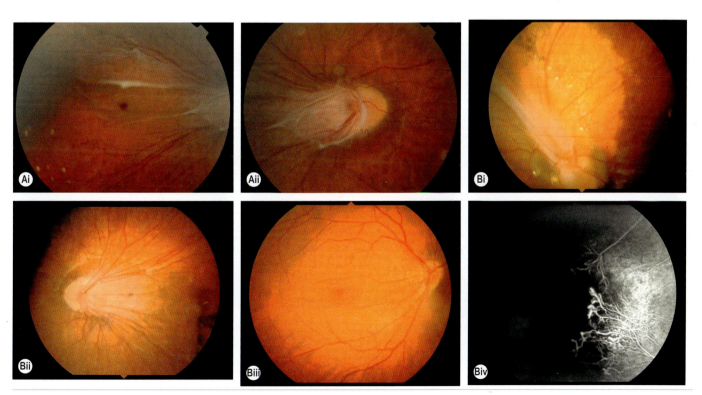

Fig. 50.20 Familial exudative vitreoretinopathy. Epiretinal surface membrane can cause severe retinal distortion and macular ectopia.

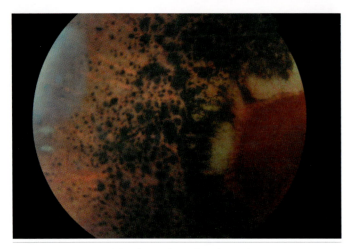

Fig. 50.21 Autosomal dominant vitreochoroidopathy. Peripheral pigmentary changes typically occur at the pre-equatorial region with a characteristically sharp posterior boundary.

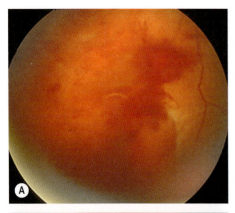

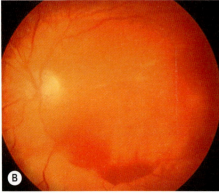

Fig. 50.22 Non-accidental injury? This was the initial diagnosis in X-linked retinoschisis with bilateral vitreous hemorrhage presenting in a 10-year-old boy.

loss (Fig. 50.22). Peripheral retinoschisis is found in approximately 50% of cases and can be complicated by retinal detachment by various mechanisms. A full-thickness retinal break occurring de novo, or a communication between outer and inner leaf defects in the schisis wall, may lead to rhegmatogenous retinal detachment. Full-thickness breaks may be managed by scleral buckling procedures provided complete break closure can be achieved. Where communication exists between inner and outer leaf breaks an internal approach may be required to effect and maintain closure.

Occasionally, X-linked retinoschisis can be complicated by cyst formation, hemorrhaging into the cavity, or even be so bullous as to obscure the visual axis. Spontaneous resolution can occur but prolonged delay may compromise the visual prognosis so that some advocate surgical drainage and internal deroofing of the cyst.

References

1. Eagling EM. Ocular damage after blunt trauma to the eye: its relationship to the nature of the injury. Br J Ophthalmol 1974; 58: 126–40.
2. Verdaguer J. Juvenile retinal detachment. Arch Ophthalmol 1982; 93: 145–56.
3. Johnson PB. Traumatic retinal detachment. Br J Ophthalmol 1991; 75: 18–21.
4. Hagler WS. Retinal dialysis: a statistical and genetic study to determine pathogenic factors. Trans Am Ophthalmol Soc 1980; 78: 686–733.
5. Aylward GW, Cooling RJ, Leaver PK. Trauma-induced retinal detachment associated with giant retinal tears. Retina 1993; 13: 136–41.
6. Scott JD. Retinal dialysis. Trans Ophthalmol Soc UK 1977; 97: 33–5.
7. Chignell AH. Retinal dialysis. Br J Ophthalmol 1973; 57: 572–7.
8. Daniel R, Kanski JJ, Glasspool MG. Retinal detachment in children. Trans Ophthalmol Soc UK 1974; 94: 5–34.
9. McDonald HR, Lewis H, Brown G, et al. Vitreous surgery for retinal detachment associated with choroidal coloboma. Arch Ophthalmol 1991; 109: 1399–402.
10. Hovland KR, Schepens CL, Freeman HM. Developmental giant retinal tears associated with lens coloboma. Arch Ophthalmol 1968; 80: 325–31.
11. Schubert HD. Schisis-like rhegmatogenous retinal detachment associated with choroidal colobomas. Graefe's Arch Clin Exp Ophthalmol 1995; 233: 74–9.
12. Gopal L, Kini MM, Badrinath SS, et al. Management of retinal detachment with choroidal coloboma. Ophthalmology 1991; 98: 1622–7.
13. Cox MS, Witherspoon CD, Morris RE, et al. Evolving techniques in the treatment of macular detachment caused by optic nerve pits. Ophthalmology 1988; 95: 889–96.
14. Sobol WM, Blodi CF, Folk JC, et al. Long-term visual outcome in patients with optic nerve pit and serous retinal detachment of the macula. Ophthalmology 1990; 97: 1539–42.
15. Meredith S, Snead MP. Inherited vitreoretinopathies. In: Besharse JC, Bok DP, editors. The Retina and its Disorders. Elsevier (Academic Press), Oxford; 2011: 252–62.
16. Snead MP, McNinch AM, Poulson AV, et al. Stickler syndrome. Ocular only variants and a key diagnostic role for the ophthalmologist. Eye 2011; 25: 1389–400.
17. Snead MP, Payne SJ, Barton DE, et al. Stickler syndrome: correlation between vitreo-retinal phenotypes and linkage to COL 2A1. Eye 1994; 8: 609–14.
18. Stickler GB, Hughes W, Houchin P. Clinical features of hereditary progressive arthro-ophthalmopathy (Stickler syndrome): a survey. Genet Med 2001; 3: 192–6.
19. Ang A, Poulson AV, Goodburn SF, et al. Retinal detachment and prophylaxis in type 1 Stickler syndrome. Ophthalmology 2008; 115: 164–8.

Part 7
Neural visual systems

Congenital optic disk anomalies

Michael C Brodsky

Introduction

A comprehensive evaluation of congenital anomalies of the optic disk needs an understanding of the ophthalmoscopic features, associated findings, pathogenesis, and ancillary studies for each anomaly.[1] New ocular and systemic associations and theories of pathogenesis for many optic disk anomalies have emerged. Subclassification of excavated optic disk anomalies previously lumped together as colobomatous defects has further refined our ability to predict associated central nervous system (CNS) anomalies based on the appearance of the optic disk. High-resolution neuroimaging has refined prediction of subtle neurodevelopmental and endocrinologic associations of CNS anomalies.[1]

Four concepts are helpful in the management of congenital optic disk anomalies:

1. Children with bilateral optic disk anomalies present in infancy with poor vision and nystagmus: unilateral cases present during preschool years with sensory esotropia.
2. CNS malformations are common in patients with malformed optic disks.

a. Small disks are associated with malformations involving the cerebral hemispheres, pituitary infundibulum, and midline intracranial structures (e.g. septum pellucidum, corpus callosum).
b. Large optic disks (i.e. morning glory) are associated with trans-sphenoidal basal encephaloceles.
c. Colobomatous optic disks are associated with systemic anomalies in a variety of syndromes.[1]
3. Any structural ocular abnormality that reduces visual acuity in infancy may lead to amblyopia.[2] A trial of occlusion is warranted in a child with asymmetric optic disk anomalies and decreased vision.
4. The finding of a discrete V- or tongue-shaped zone of infrapapillary retinochoroidal depigmentation with an anomalous optic disk should prompt a search for a trans-sphenoidal encephalocele.[3]

Optic nerve hypoplasia

Optic nerve hypoplasia is unquestionably the most common optic disk anomaly encountered in ophthalmologic practice in many countries.[1] Many cases previously went unrecognized or were misconstrued as congenital optic atrophy. Parental drug and alcohol abuse, more widespread in recent years, contributes to an increasing prevalence of optic nerve hypoplasia.[1,4] Teratogenic agents and systemic disorders associated with optic nerve hypoplasia are summarized in Box 51.1.

Ophthalmoscopically, optic nerve hypoplasia appears as an abnormally small optic nerve head, pink, gray or pale in color, and is often surrounded by a yellowish mottled peripapillary halo, bordered by a ring of increased or decreased pigmentation (the "double-ring" sign) (Fig. 51.1).[4] The major retinal

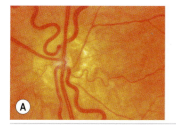 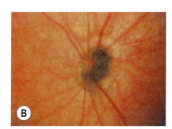 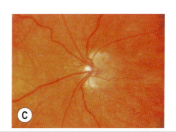 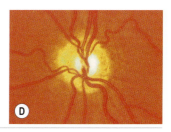

Fig. 51.1 Variants of optic nerve hypoplasia. (A) Double-ring-sign. (B) With congenital optic disk pigmentation. (C) With choroid and retinal pigment epithelium eclipsing temporal disk. (D) Double-ring sign simulating normal disk despite vision of NLP. (From Brodsky MC, Glasier CM, Pollock SC. Optic nerve hypoplasia: identification by magnetic resonance imaging. Arch Ophthalmol 1990; 108:1562–7.)

Systemic and teratogenic associations with optic nerve hypoplasia

Systemic associations	Risk factors
Albinism	Young maternal age
Aniridia	Maternal insulin-
Duane's syndrome	dependent diabetes
Median facial cleft syndrome	Fetal alcohol syndrome
Klippel-Trénauney-Weber syndrome	Maternal use of illicit
Goldenhar's syndrome	drugs
Linear sebaceous nevus syndrome	
Meckel's syndrome	
Hemifacial atrophy	
Blepharophimosis	
Osteogenesis imperfecta	
Chondrodysplasia punctata	
Aicardi's syndrome	
Apert's syndrome	
Trisomy 18	
Potter's syndrome	
Chromosome 13q-	
Neonatal isoimmune thrombocytopenia	
Fetal alcohol syndrome	
Dandy-Walker syndrome	
Delleman's syndrome	
Frontonasal dysplasia	
Kallmann's syndrome	
Congenital retinal arterial malformations	

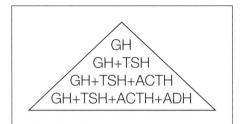

Fig. 51.2 Pyramid of pituitary hormone deficiencies in optic nerve hypoplasia.

veins are often tortuous which may be helpful in establishing the diagnosis.[5]

Histopathologically, optic nerve hypoplasia is a subnormal number of optic nerve axons with normal mesodermal elements and glial supporting tissue.[6,7] The double-ring sign consists of the normal junction between the sclera and lamina cribrosa, corresponding to the outer ring, and an abnormal extension of retina and pigment epithelium over the outer portion of the lamina cribrosa, corresponding to the inner ring.[6,7]

Visual acuity in optic nerve hypoplasia ranges from logMAR 0.0 (6/6, 20/20, 1.0) to no light perception with localized visual field defects, often with a generalized constriction.[8] Since visual acuity is determined primarily by the integrity of the papillomacular nerve fiber bundle, it does not necessarily correlate with the overall size of the disk. There is a strong association of astigmatism with optic nerve hypoplasia.[9]

Amblyopic eyes have smaller optic disks and smaller axial lengths compared to fellow eyes, suggesting that vision impairment in amblyopia may be caused by optic nerve hypoplasia with relative microphthalmos.[10] This might be due to amblyopia being correlated with hyperopia and anisometropia[11] but when axial length was measured, the optic disk areas of eyes with hyperopic strabismus with and without amblyopia were significantly reduced compared with hyperopic eyes without amblyopia or esotropia.[12]

Except when amblyopia develops in one eye, visual acuity usually remains stable throughout life. However, mild optic nerve hypoplasia occurs in children with congenital suprasellar tumors. A confusing diagnostic picture of acquired visual loss in the child with optic nerve hypoplasia may result.[13]

Optic nerve hypoplasia is often associated with CNS abnormalities. Septo-optic dysplasia (de Morsier's syndrome) is the constellation of small anterior visual pathways, absence of the septum pellucidum, and thinning or agenesis of the corpus callosum;[14] it may be associated with pituitary dwarfism.[15] Isolated growth hormone, thyrotropin, corticotropin, or antidiuretic hormone deficiency may occur (Fig. 51.2).[1,16] Hypothyroidism, panhypopituitarism, diabetes insipidus, and hyperprolactinemia may result.[17-19] Growth hormone deficiency may be clinically inapparent in early life because high prolactin levels stimulate normal growth.[20] Puberty may be precocious, or delayed, in children with hypopituitarism.[21] Subclinical hypopituitarism can manifest as acute adrenal insufficiency following general anesthesia. It may be prudent to treat children who have optic nerve hypoplasia with perioperative corticosteroids.[22]

In an infant with optic nerve hypoplasia, a history of neonatal jaundice suggests congenital hypothyroidism, while neonatal hypoglycemia or seizures suggests congenital panhypopituitarism.[4] Because of difficulties in measuring normal growth hormone levels that vary diurnally, most patients with optic nerve hypoplasia are followed clinically and investigated biochemically if growth is subnormal. However, when MRI shows posterior pituitary ectopia, or when a clinical history of neonatal jaundice or neonatal hypoglycemia is obtained, anterior pituitary hormone deficiency is probable, and more extensive endocrinologic testing becomes mandatory.[23]

Children with septo-optic dysplasia and corticotropin deficiency are at risk for sudden death during febrile illness,[24] which may be caused by an impaired ability to increase corticotropin secretion in response to the stress of infection. They may have diabetes insipidus that contributes to dehydration during illness and hastens the development of shock. Some also have hypothalamic thermoregulatory disturbances signaled by hypothermia during well periods and high fevers during illnesses; they usually have had multiple hospital admissions for viral illnesses which can precipitate hypoglycemia, dehydration, hypotension, or fever of unknown origin.[24] Because corticotropin deficiency represents the pre-eminent threat to life in children with septo-optic dysplasia, a complete anterior pituitary hormone evaluation, including provocative serum cortisol testing and assessment for diabetes insipidus, should be performed in children who have clinical symptoms (history of hypoglycemia, dehydration, or hypothermia) or neuroimaging signs (absent pituitary infundibulum with or without posterior pituitary ectopia) of pituitary hormone deficiency.

MRI delineates associated CNS malformations in patients with optic nerve hypoplasia.[25] MRI provides high-contrast resolution and multiplanar imaging capability, allowing the anterior visual pathways to be visualized as distinct, well-defined structures.[25] Coronal and sagittal T1-weighted MR images shows thinning and attenuation of the corresponding prechiasmatic intracranial optic nerve (Fig. 51.3). Coronal

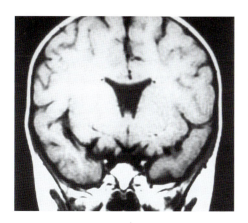

Fig. 51.3 Optic nerve hypoplasia. Coronal MR image showing absence of the septum pellucidum, normal right optic nerve, and hypoplasia of the left optic nerve.

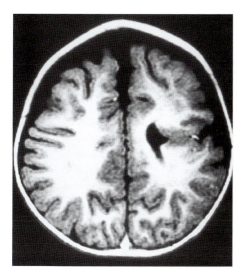

Fig. 51.4 Schizencephaly involving the left cerebral hemisphere. (From Brodsky MC, Glasier CM. Optic nerve hypoplasia: clinical significance of associated central nervous system abnormalities on magnetic resonance imaging. Arch Ophthalmol 1993; 111: 66–74.)

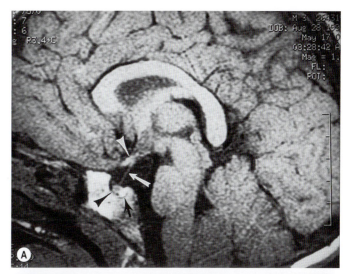

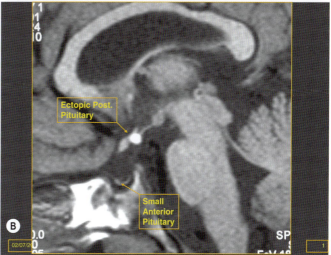

Fig. 51.5 Posterior pituitary ectopia. (A) Normal pituitary infundibulum, and posterior pituitary gland. (B) Absence of the pituitary infundibulum, absence of posterior pituitary gland, with ectopic posterior pituitary gland adjacent to optic chiasm. (From Brodsky MC, Glasier CM. Optic nerve hypoplasia: clinical significance of associated central nervous system abnormalities on magnetic resonance imaging. Arch Ophthalmol 1993; 111: 66–74.)

T1-weighted MRI shows diffuse thinning of the optic chiasm in bilateral optic nerve hypoplasia and focal thinning or absence of the side of the chiasm corresponding to the hypoplastic nerve in unilateral optic nerve hypoplasia.[25] MRI may show a decrease in intracranial optic nerve size accompanied by other features of septo-optic dysplasia assisting in the diagnosis.[25]

Cerebral hemispheric abnormalities are evident in approximately 45% of patients with optic nerve hypoplasia (Fig. 51.4). They may consist of hemispheric migration anomalies (e.g. schizencephaly, cortical heterotopia), intrauterine or perinatal hemispheric injury (e.g. periventricular leukomalacia, encephalomalacia).[26] Evidence of perinatal injury to the pituitary infundibulum (seen on MRI as posterior pituitary ectopia) is found in approximately 15% of patients with optic nerve hypoplasia.[26] Normally, the posterior pituitary gland appears bright on T1-weighted images, because of the composition of the vesicles within it.[23,26] In posterior pituitary ectopia, MRI demonstrates absence of the normal posterior pituitary bright spot and the pituitary infundibulum, and an ectopic posterior pituitary bright spot where the upper infundibulum is normally located (Fig. 51.5).[23,26]

In optic nerve hypoplasia, posterior pituitary ectopia usually suggests anterior pituitary hormone deficiency; cerebral hemispheric abnormalities are predictive of neurodevelopmental deficits.[26] Absence of the septum pellucidum does not portend neurodevelopmental deficits or pituitary hormone deficiency.[27]

Thinning or agenesis of the corpus callosum predicts neurodevelopmental problems by association with cerebral hemispheric abnormalities. The finding of unilateral optic nerve hypoplasia does not preclude coexistent intracranial malformations.[26] Therefore, MRI is used to provide prognostic information in the child with optic nerve hypoplasia.[26]

Segmental optic nerve hypoplasia

Some forms of optic nerve hypoplasia are segmental.[28] "Superior segmental optic hypoplasia" (SSOH) with an inferior visual field defect occurs in some children of insulin-dependent diabetic mothers (Fig. 51.6).[29,30] SSOH is usually an isolated anomaly[31] and has an incidence of approximately 8%. The inferior visual field defects in superior segmental optic hypoplasia differ from typical nerve fiber bundle defects perhaps due to a regional impairment in retinal development.[30] SSOH also occurs in patients whose mothers were not diabetic; it, therefore, is not pathognomonic for maternal diabetes.[32] The mechanism by which insulin-dependent diabetes mellitus interferes

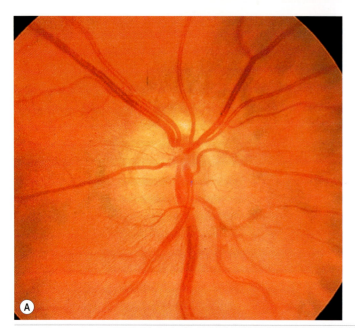

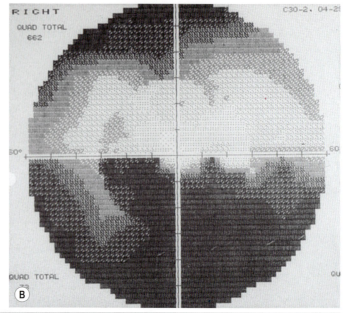

Fig. 51.6 Superior segmental optic hypoplasia. (A) Right optic disk shows superior entrance of central retinal vessels, relative pallor, superior peripapillary crescent, and selective loss of superior nerve fiber layer. (B) Corresponding visual field showing characteristic inferior loss. (Reproduced with permission from Brodsky MC, Schroeder GT, Ford R. Segmental optic nerve hypoplasia in identical twins. J Clin Neuro-Ophthalmol 1993; 13: 152–4.)

with the early gestational development of superior retinal ganglion cells or their axons remains elusive.[33] Mice lacking EphB receptor guidance proteins exhibit guidance defects in axons originating from the dorsal or superior part of the retina,[34] which may explain this segmental hypoplasia.[34]

Congenital lesions of the retina, optic nerve, chiasm, tract, or retrogeniculate pathways are associated with segmental hypoplasia of the corresponding portions of the optic nerve (Fig. 51.7).[28] Chiasmal hypoplasia produces focal loss of the nasal and temporal nerve fiber layer with hypoplasia of corresponding portions of the optic nerve (see Fig. 51.7). "Homonymous hemioptic hypoplasia" is an asymmetric form of segmental optic nerve hypoplasia seen in patients with unilateral congenital lesions of the postchiasmal afferent visual pathways.[35] The nasal and temporal aspects of the optic disk contralateral to the hemispheric lesion show segmental hypoplasia and loss of the corresponding nerve fiber layer. There may be a central band of horizontal pallor across the disk. The ipsilateral optic disk may be normal in size or hypoplastic.[28] Homonymous hemioptic hypoplasia results from transsynaptic degeneration of the optic tract that is usually seen in congenital hemispheric lesions.[28,35a] Congenital suprasellar tumors can rarely produce a horizontal "bow-tie" cupping with selective loss of the nasal and temporal nerve fiber layer.[35b]

Periventricular leukomalacia and optic nerve hypoplasia

Periventricular leukomalacia (PVL) produces another form of optic nerve hypoplasia. PVL can be associated with abnormally large optic cups and a thin neuroretinal rim contained within normal-sized optic disks (Fig. 51.8).[36] This may be due to intrauterine injury to the optic radiations with retrograde trans-synaptic degeneration of retinogeniculate axons after the

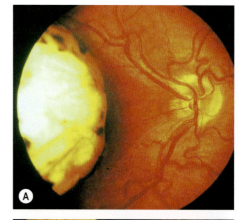

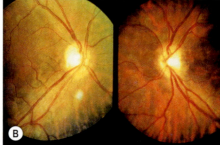

Fig. 51.7 Segmental optic nerve hypoplasia. (A) Macular "coloboma" produces selective temporal nerve fiber loss and corresponding temporal hypoplasia of the optic disk. (From Novakovic et al. Localizing patterns of optic nerve hypoplasia-retina to occipital lobe. Br J Ophthalmol 1988; 72: 176–82.) (B) Achiasmia. Left eye showing horizontal band hypoplasia with preservation of the superior and inferior poles of the optic disc.

scleral canals had established normal diameters. The large optic cups can simulate glaucoma, but the history of prematurity, normal intraocular pressure, and characteristic symmetric inferior visual field defects distinguish PVL from glaucoma.[37] This may be a form of segmental optic nerve hypoplasia, although some believe it is a prenatal form of optic atrophy because of its normal optic disk diameter.[37]

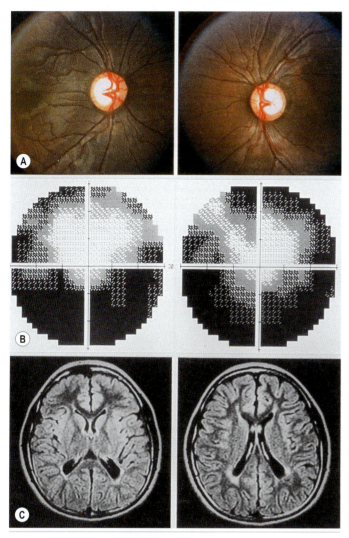

Fig. 51.8 Periventricular leukomalacia. (A) Enlarged optic cups with greater thinning of superior than inferior neuroretinal rim. (B) Characteristic inferior visual field defects. (C) MRI showing causative lesions involving optic radiations. (From Brodsky MC. Periventricular leukomalacia: an intracranial cause of pseudoglaucomatous cupping. Arch Ophthalmol 2001; 119: 626–7.)

The embryogenesis of optic nerve hypoplasia

At least two mechanisms may be operative in the embryogenesis of optic nerve hypoplasia:

1. A primary failure of retinal ganglion cell differentiation at the 13–15 mm stage of embryonic life (4–6 weeks of gestation).[38]
2. A deficiency of axon guidance molecules at the optic disk.

Netrin-1 is an axon guidance molecule expressed by neuroepithelial cells at the developing optic nerve head. Retinal ganglion cells in vitro respond to netrin-1 as a guidance molecule. Mice with a targeted deletion of the netrin-1 gene exhibit pathfinding errors at the optic disk. Retinal ganglion cells fail to exit into the optic nerve and optic nerve hypoplasia results.[39-41] The lack of netrin-1 also results in abnormalities in other parts of the CNS (agenesis of the corpus callosum and axonal guidance defects in the hypothalamus).[40] The timing of the CNS injuries suggests optic nerve hypoplasia results from intrauterine encephaloclastic destruction of a normally developed structure, whereas others represent a primary failure of

axons to develop.[16] In human fetuses, Provis et al. found a peak of 3.7 million optic axons at 16–17 weeks of gestation, with a subsequent decline to 1.1 million axons by the 31 weeks of gestation.[42] This massive apoptotic loss of supernumerary axons may establish the correct functional topography of the visual pathways.[4] Toxins or CNS injury could augment the processes by which superfluous axons are eliminated from the developing visual pathways.[4,16,26] The association of optic nerve hypoplasia with periventricular leukomalacia[26] cannot be reconciled with a deficiency of axon guidance molecules at the optic disk. It suggests retrograde trans-synaptic degeneration in the development of some forms of optic nerve hypoplasia.[36,37]

Cases of optic nerve hypoplasia in siblings[43,44] are rare, and subsequent siblings of a child with optic nerve hypoplasia are at little additional risk. While genetic mutations in the human netrin-1 and *DCC* genes have not been described, homozygous mutations in the *HESX1* gene have been identified in two siblings with optic nerve hypoplasia, absence of the corpus callosum, and hypoplasia of the pituitary gland.[45] Five additional mutations in *HESX1* have been observed in children with sporadic pituitary disease and septo-optic dysplasia[46] which have clustered in the DNA-binding region of the protein consistent with a presumed loss in protein function. Examination of homeobox genes with expression patterns similar to *HESX1*, such as Six3 and Six6, may yield additional genes responsible for both sporadic and familial septo-optic dysplasia.[47] Optic nerve hypoplasia may accompany other ocular malformations in patients with mutations in the PAX6 gene.[48]

Excavated optic disk anomalies

Excavated optic disk anomalies include optic disk coloboma, morning glory disk anomaly, peripapillary staphyloma, megalopapilla, optic pit, and the optic disk anomalies associated with periventricular leukomalacia and papillorenal syndrome.

Morning glory disk anomaly

In the morning glory disk anomaly and peripapillary staphyloma, an excavation of the posterior globe surrounds and incorporates the optic disk. In the other conditions, the excavation is contained within the optic disk. It is clear that optic disk colobomas, morning glory optic disks, and peripapillary staphylomas are distinct anomalies, each with a specific embryologic origin and not phenotypic spectrum variants.[49]

The morning glory disk anomaly is a congenital, funnel-shaped excavation of the posterior fundus that incorporates the optic disk[49] which resembles a morning glory flower.[50] The disk is markedly enlarged, orange or pink and may appear to be recessed or elevated centrally within a funnel-shaped peripapillary excavation (Fig. 51.9).[49] A wide annulus of chorioretinal pigmentary disturbance surrounds the disk[49] and a white glial tuft overlies its central portion. The blood vessels appear increased in number and arise from the periphery of the disk,[49] curving abruptly as they leave the disk to run an abnormally straight course over the peripapillary retina. It is often difficult to distinguish arterioles from venules. Small peripapillary arteriovenous communications may occur.[51] The macula may be incorporated into the excavation ("macular capture").[52] Neuroimaging shows a funnel-shaped enlargement of the distal optic nerve at its junction with the globe.[1]

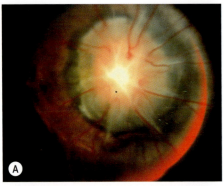

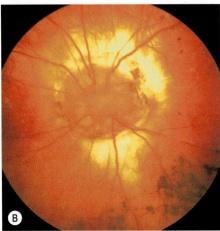

Fig. 51.9 Morning glory disk anomaly.
(A) Without transsphenoidal encephalocele. (From Pollock S. The morning glory disk anomaly: Contractile movement, classification, and embryogenesis. Doc Ophthalmol 1987; 65: 439–60, with permission.)
(B) With V-shaped infrapapillary depigmentation signifying transsphenoidal encephalocele. (From Brodsky MC, Hoyt WF, Hoyt CS, et al. Atypical retinochoroidal coloboma in patients with dysplastic optic disks and transsphenoidal encephalocele. Arch Ophthalmol 1995; 113: 624–8.)

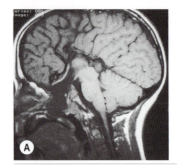

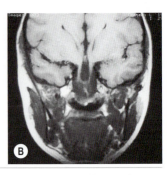

Fig. 51.10 MRI of trans-sphenoidal encephalocele. (A) Sagittal image showing encephalocele extending down through the sphenoid bone into the nasopharynx. (B) Coronal image showing third ventricle and chiasm extending inferiorly into the encephalocele. (From Brodsky MC, Hoyt WF, Hoyt CS, et al. Atypical retinochoroidal coloboma in patients with dysplastic optic disks and transsphenoidal encephalocele. Arch Ophthalmol 1995; 113: 624–8.)

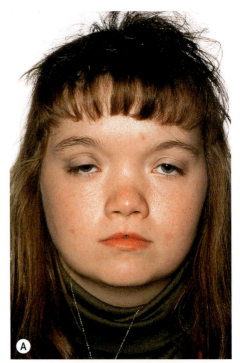

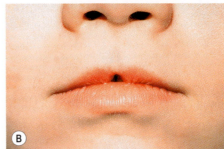

Fig. 51.11 Midfacial anomalies associated with trans-sphenoidal encephalocele.
(A) Facial photograph showing hypertelorism, flat nasal bridge, widened bitemporal diameter.
(B) Closer photograph showing midline cleft in the upper lip. (From Brodsky MC, Glasier CM. Optic nerve hypoplasia: clinical significance of associated central nervous system abnormalities on magnetic resonance imaging. Arch Ophthalmol 1993; 111: 66–74.)

The morning glory disk anomaly is usually unilateral, but several bilateral cases have been reported.[49,52] Visual acuity usually ranges from logMAR 1.0 (6/60, 20/200, 0.1) to "finger counting," although cases with 20/20 vision as well as no light perception have been reported. Amblyopia may contribute to visual loss[2] and a trial of occlusion therapy is warranted in children. Optic disk colobomas have no racial or gender predilection: morning glory disks are more common in females and rare in black people.

The morning glory disk anomaly is associated with a transsphenoidal basal encephalocele.[52-54] It may be accompanied by a V- or tongue-shaped zone of infrapapillary depigmentation, a sign suggesting a trans-sphenoidal encephalocele (see Fig. 51.9).[3] Trans-sphenoidal encephalocele is a rare midline congenital malformation in which a meningeal pouch, often containing the chiasm and adjacent hypothalamus, protrudes through a defect in the sphenoid bone (Fig. 51.10). Children with this basal meningocele have a wide head, a flat nose, mild hypertelorism, a midline notch in the upper lip, and sometimes a midline cleft in the soft palate (Fig. 51.11). The meningocele protrudes into the nasopharynx and may obstruct the airway. Symptoms including rhinorrhea, nasal obstruction, mouth breathing, or snoring[55,56] may be overlooked unless the morning glory disk anomaly or the facial configuration is recognized. A trans-sphenoidal encephalocele may appear as a pulsatile posterior nasal mass or as a "nasal polyp" high in the nose. Surgical biopsy or excision can be lethal.[55] Associated brain malformations include agenesis of the corpus callosum and posterior dilatation of the lateral ventricles. Absence of the chiasm (achiasmia) is seen in approximately one-third of patients. Most of the affected children have no overt intellectual or neurologic deficits, but panhypopituitarism is

common.[55] Surgery for trans-sphenoidal encephalocele may be contraindicated, since herniated brain tissue can include vital structures.[1,3]

The morning glory disk anomaly can be associated with hypoplasia of the ipsilateral intracranial vasculature.[57-59] With MR angiography, ipsilateral intracranial vascular dysgenesis (with or without Moyamoya syndrome) is seen in some patients with morning glory disk anomaly (Fig. 51.12).[57-59]

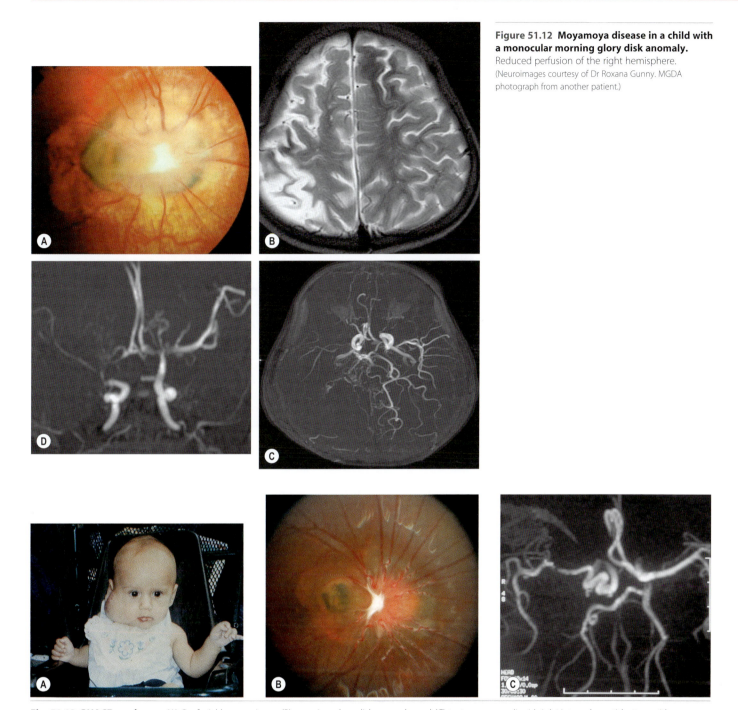

Figure 51.12 **Moyamoya disease in a child with a monocular morning glory disk anomaly.**
Reduced perfusion of the right hemisphere.
(Neuroimages courtesy of Dr Roxana Gunny. MGDA photograph from another patient.)

Fig. 51.13 PHACE syndrome. (A) Orofacial hemangioma, (B) morning glory disk anomaly, and (C) tortuous supraclinoid right internal carotid artery with hypoplasia of the ipsilateral middle cerebral artery on MR angiography. (From Kniestedt C, Landau K, Brodsky MC, et al. Infantile orofacial hemangioma with ipsilateral peripapillary excavation in girls: a variant of PHACE syndrome. Arch Ophthalmol 2004 ; 122: 413–15, with permission from the American Medical Association.)

This suggests that the morning glory disk anomaly results from a primary vascular dysgenesis as part of a regional mesodermal dysgenesis.[60]

Usually, the morning glory disk anomaly is not part of a genetic disorder[1,50] but it has been associated with ipsilateral orofacial hemangioma.[61] This association may fall within the spectrum of the PHACE syndrome (posterior fossa malformations, large facial hemangiomas, arterial anomalies, cardiac anomalies and aortic coarctation, and eye anomalies) which occurs only in girls.[62] Associated ipsilateral intracranial vascular dysgenesis (Fig. 51.13) supports this.[63] Atypical morning glory disk anomalies have also rarely been reported in patients with neurofibromatosis 2.[64]

Serous retinal detachments develop in 26–38% of eyes with morning glory optic disk anomalies;[49] they originate in the peripapillary area and extend through the posterior pole, occasionally progressing to total detachments. Small retinal tears adjacent to the optic nerve in patients with morning glory disk-associated retinal detachments have been identified,[65] and subretinal neovascularization may develop adjacent to a morning glory disk.[66] Contractile movements occur in morning glory optic disks,[49] perhaps due to fluctuations in subretinal fluid volume altering the degree of retinal separation within the excavation.[49] One patient had episodes of amaurosis with transient dilation of the retinal veins in an eye with a morning glory disk.[67]

The embryologic defect leading to the morning glory disk anomaly is widely disputed.[68] Unlike optic disk coloboma (discussed below), it does not result from defective closure of the embryonic fissure.[68-70] The central glial tuft, vascular anomalies, and a scleral defect, together with the histologic findings of adipose tissue and smooth muscle within the peripapillary sclera perhaps signify a primary mesenchymal abnormality. The midfacial anomalies in some patients support a primary mesenchymal defect: most of the cranial structures are derived from mesenchyme.[68] The basic defect may be mesodermal, but some features may result from a dynamic disturbance between the relative growth of mesoderm and ectoderm.[61]

The symmetry of the fundus excavation with respect to the disk implicates an anomalous funnel-shaped enlargement of the distal optic stalk at its junction with the primitive optic vesicle, as the primary embryologic defect.[49] This hypothesis suggests that the glial and vascular abnormalities that characterize the morning glory disk anomaly are secondary effects of a primary neuroectodermal dysgenesis on the formation of mesodermal elements that arise later in embryogenesis.[49]

Optic disk coloboma

The term coloboma (kolobma in Greek) means curtailed or mutilated.[71] In optic disk coloboma, a sharply delimited, glistening white, bowl-shaped excavation occupies an enlarged optic disk (Fig. 51.14). The excavation is decentered inferiorly, reflecting the position of the fetal fissure relative to the primitive epithelial papilla.[49] The inferior neuroretinal rim is thin or absent while the superior neuroretinal rim is relatively spared. Rarely, the entire disk may appear excavated; however, the colobomatous nature of the defect can still be appreciated since the excavation is deeper inferiorly.[49] The defect may extend further inferiorly to involve the adjacent choroid and retina, in which case microphthalmia is frequently present.[72] Iris and ciliary colobomas often coexist. Axial scanning shows a crater-like excavation of the posterior globe at its junction with the optic nerve.[69]

Visual acuity may be decreased and is difficult to predict from the appearance of the disk.[1] Unlike the morning glory disk anomaly, which is usually unilateral, optic disk colobomas occur equally unilaterally or bilaterally.[49] Optic disk colobomas may arise sporadically or be inherited in an autosomal dominant fashion. They may be accompanied by multiple

systemic abnormalities in a myriad of conditions including the CHARGE association,[73] Walker-Warburg syndrome, Goltz' focal dermal hypoplasia, Aicardi's syndrome, Goldenhar's syndrome, and linear sebaceous nevus syndrome.[1] Rarely, large orbital cysts occur in conjunction with atypical excavations of the disk. These are probably colobomatous.[72,74] The cyst may communicate with the excavation.[74,75] Intrascleral smooth muscle strands oriented concentrically around the distal optic nerve[76] may account for the contractility of the optic disk seen rarely in optic disk colobomas.[77]

Eyes with isolated optic disk colobomas can develop serous macular detachments in contrast to the rhegmatogenous retinal detachments that complicate retinochoroidal colobomas,[78,79] perhaps from diffusion of retrobulbar fluid into the subretinal space.[79] Treatment includes patches, bedrest, corticosteroids, vitrectomy, scleral buckling procedures, gas-fluid exchange, and photocoagulation.[80,81] Spontaneous reattachment may occur.[81]

Coronal T1-weighted MRI confirms that the intracranial portion of the optic nerve is reduced in size.[81] Many uncategorizable dysplastic optic disks are indiscriminately labeled as optic disk colobomas.[82] This complicates the nosology of coloboma-associated genetic disorders. It is crucial that the diagnosis of optic disk coloboma be reserved for disks that show an inferiorly decentered, white-colored excavation with minimal peripapillary pigmentary changes.[1,49] In striking contrast to the numerous well-documented reports of morning glory optic disks occurring in conjunction with basal encephaloceles, cases of optic disk coloboma with basal encephalocele are conspicuous by their absence.[83,84]

Although the phenotypic profiles of optic disk coloboma and the morning glory disk anomaly may overlap, the ophthalmoscopic features of optic disk coloboma (Table 51.1) are most consistent with a primary structural dysgenesis involving the proximal fetal fissure, as opposed to an anomalous dilatation confined to the distal optic stalk in the morning glory disk anomaly.[49] The differences in associated ocular and systemic findings between the two anomalies (Table 51.2) support this hypothesis.[1] Anomalous optic disks with features of both are occasionally seen: they may represent early embryonic injury involving both the proximal fetal fissure and the distal optic stalk. However, the great majority of colobomatous and morning glory optic disks are distinct.

Colobomas are most often sporadic but may be autosomal dominant, autosomal recessive, or X-linked recessive. One study found a 10% recurrence rate, but the true percentage of

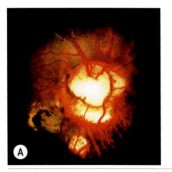
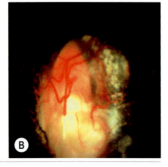

Fig. 51.14 Variants of optic disk coloboma. (Courtesy of William F. Hoyt, MD.)

Table 51.1 – Ophthalmoscopic findings that distinguish the morning glory disk anomaly from optic disk coloboma

Morning glory disk	Optic disk coloboma
Optic disk lies within the excavation	Excavation lies within the optic disk
Symmetrical defect (disk lies centrally within the excavation)	Asymmetrical defect (excavation lies inferiorly within the disk)
Central glial tuft	No central glial tuft
Severe peripapillary	Minimal peripapillary
Pigmentary disturbance	Pigmentary disturbance
Anomalous retinal vasculature	Normal retinal vasculature

Table 51.2 – Associated ocular and systemic findings that distinguish the morning glory disk from isolated optic disk coloboma

Morning glory disk	Optic disk coloboma
More common in females; rare in Blacks	No sex or racial preference
Rarely familial	Often familial
Rarely bilateral	Often bilateral
No iris, ciliary, or retinal colobomas	Iris, ciliary, and retinal colobomas common
Rarely associated with multisystem genetic disorders	Often associated with multisystem genetic disorders
Basal encephalocele common	Basal encephalocele rare

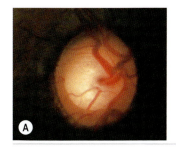
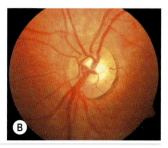

Fig. 51.16 Two cases of megalopapilla. (A) illustrates pseudoglaucomatous cupping.

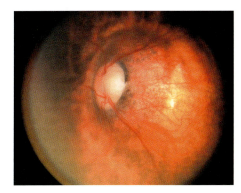

Fig. 51.15 Peripapillary staphyloma. (From Brodsky MC. Congenital optic disk anomalies. Surv Ophthalmol 1994: 89–112.)

colobomas that are inherited is probably higher.[85] A wide variety of mutations have been documented in patients with colobomas. Except for the *CHD7* mutation, which accounts for 60% of cases of CHARGE syndrome,[86] no mutations predominate and no "genetic panel" exists. For this reason, genetic testing is probably unwarranted unless there are other dysmorphic features.

Peripapillary staphyloma

Peripapillary staphyloma is an extremely rare, usually unilateral, anomaly in which a deep fundus excavation surrounds the optic disk.[87,88] The disk is at the bottom of the excavated defect and may appear normal or show temporal pallor (Fig. 51.15).[88] The walls and margin of the defect may show atrophic pigmentary changes involving the RPE and choroid.[88] There is no central glial tuft overlying the disk and the retinal vascular pattern is normal. The staphylomatous excavation is deeper than that in the morning glory disk anomaly. Several cases of contractile peripapillary staphyloma have been documented,[89-91] sometimes with transient visual obscurations.[92]

Visual acuity is usually reduced, but normal acuity has been reported.[93] Affected eyes are usually emmetropic or slightly myopic.[87] Eyes with decreased vision frequently have centrocecal scotomas.[87] Although peripapillary staphyloma is usually unassociated with systemic or intracranial disease, it has been reported in association with trans-sphenoidal encephalocele,[94] PHACE syndrome,[62,95] linear nevus sebaceous syndrome, and 18q- syndrome.[96]

The relatively normal appearance of the optic disk and retinal vessels in peripapillary staphyloma suggests that the

development of these structures is complete prior to the onset of the staphylomatous process.[49] The clinical features of peripapillary staphyloma are consistent with diminished peripapillary structural support, perhaps resulting from incomplete differentiation of sclera from posterior neural crest cells. Staphyloma formation presumably occurs when establishment of normal intraocular pressure leads to herniation of unsupported ocular tissues through the defect.[49] Peripapillary staphyloma and the morning glory disk anomaly appear to be pathogenetically distinct both in the timing of the insult (5 months' gestation vs. 4 weeks' gestation) as well as the embryologic site of structural dysgenesis (posterior sclera versus distal optic stalk).

Megalopapilla

Megalopapilla[97] is a generic term for an abnormally large optic disk that lacks the inferior excavation of optic disk coloboma or the features of the morning glory disk anomaly.

Megalopapilla comprises two phenotypic variants:

1. The optic disk is greater than 2.1 mm in diameter but has an otherwise normal configuration.[87,97] This relatively common form is usually bilateral and often associated with a large cup-to-disk ratio suggesting glaucoma (Fig. 51.16).[1] The optic cup is usually round or horizontally oval with no vertical notching or encroachment, in contradistinction to glaucoma. Because the axons are spread over a larger surface area, the neuroretinal rim may be pale, mimicking optic atrophy.[98]

2. A unilateral form of megalopapilla is seen in which the normal optic cup is replaced by a grossly anomalous non-inferior excavation that obliterates the adjacent neuroretinal rim. It is distinct from coloboma. Cilioretinal arteries are more common in megalopapilla.[99] A high prevalence of megalopapilla has been observed in the Marshall Islands.[100]

Two reports have documented large optic disks in patients with optic nerve hypoplasia associated with a congenital homonymous hemianopia.[101,102] This rare combination of findings suggests that a prenatal loss of optic nerve axons leading to optic nerve hypoplasia may not always alter the genetically predetermined size of the scleral canals.[102]

Visual acuity is usually normal but may be mildly decreased. Visual fields are usually normal except for an enlarged blind spot. Colobomatous disks are distinguished from megalopapilla by their predominant excavation of the inferior optic disk. The differential diagnosis of megalopapilla includes orbital optic glioma, which in children can cause progressive enlargement of a previously normal-sized optic disk.[103]

Most cases of megalopapilla may represent a variant of normal, but it is likely that it results from altered optic axonal migration early in embryogenesis, as evidenced by megalopapilla occurring in a child with basal encephalocele.[53] The rarity of this association suggests that neuroimaging is unwarranted unless midfacial anomalies coexist.

Optic pit

An optic pit is a round or oval, gray, white, or yellowish depression in the optic disk (Fig. 51.17). Optic pits commonly involve the temporal optic disk but may be in any sector.[104] Temporally located, pits are often accompanied by adjacent peripapillary pigment epithelial changes. One or two cilioretinal arteries are seen to emerge from the bottom or the margin of the pit in greater than 50% of cases.[87,105] Although optic pits are typically unilateral, they are bilateral in 15% of cases.[87] Optic pits are herniations of dysplastic retina into a collagen-lined pocket extending posteriorly, often into the subarachnoid space, through a defect in the lamina cribrosa.[87] Reports of familial optic pits suggest autosomal dominant transmission.[106-108]

In unilateral cases, the disk is slightly larger than the normal disk.[87] Visual acuity is normal in the absence of subretinal fluid. Visual field defects are variable and often correlate poorly with the pit location. The most common defect is a para-central arcuate scotoma from an enlarged blind spot.[104] Optic pits rarely portend additional CNS malformations.[109] Acquired depressions in the optic disk, indistinguishable from optic pits, have been documented in normal tension glaucoma.[110]

Serous macular elevations develop in 25–75% of eyes with optic pits[104] and become symptomatic in the third and fourth decade of life. Vitreous traction on the margins of the pit and tractional changes in the roof of the pit may lead to late-onset macular detachment.[105]

All optic pit-associated macular elevations were thought to be serous detachments, but stereoscopic examination of the macula in conjunction with kinetic perimetry[111] demonstrates the following events (see Fig. 51.17):

1. A schisis-like inner-layer retinal separation forms in communication with the optic pit, producing a relative centrocecal scotoma.

2. An outer-layer macular hole develops beneath the boundaries of the inner-layer separation and produces a dense central scotoma.

3. An outer-layer retinal detachment develops around the macular hole (presumably from influx of fluid from the inner-layer separation); this detachment resembles an RPE detachment but fails to hyperfluoresce on fluorescein angiography.

4. The outer-layer detachment may enlarge and obliterate the inner-layer separation when it is no longer ophthalmoscopically or histopathologically distinguishable from a primary serous macular detachment.

The histopathologic finding of a sensory macular detachment in eyes with optic pits presumably represents the end-stage, but whether this sequence of events leads to all optic pit-associated macular detachments is unclear.

The risk of optic pit-associated macular detachment is greater in eyes with large, temporally located pits.[104] Perhaps because of age differences in vitreopapillary traction, optic pit-associated serous maculopathy in children may spontaneously resolve.[112,113] Spontaneous reattachment is seen in approximately 25% of cases.[104,114,115] Most optic pit-associated macular detachments result in permanent visual loss in untreated patients, even when spontaneous reattachment occurs.[114,116] Bedrest and bilateral patching leads to retinal reattachment in some patients, presumably by decreasing vitreous traction.[79,11] Laser photocoagulation to block the flow of fluid from the pit to the macula has been largely unsuccessful, perhaps due to the inability of laser photocoagulation to seal a retinoschisis cavity.[111,117] Vitrectomy with internal gas tamponade laser photocoagulation has produced long-term improvement in acuity.[79,111,118] The source of intraretinal fluid in eyes with optic pits is controversial.[119] Possible sources include:

1. Vitreous cavity via the pit.
2. The subarachnoid space.
3. Blood vessels at the base of the pit.
4. The orbital space surrounding the dura.

Although fluorescein angiography shows early hypofluorescence of the pit followed by late hyperfluorescent staining, optic pits do not generally leak fluorescein, and there is no extension of fluorescein into the subretinal space toward the macula.[104] Late hyperfluorescence correlates strongly with cilioretinal arteries emerging from the pit.[105] Slit-lamp biomicroscopy often reveals a thin membrane overlying the pit[104] or a persistent Cloquet's canal terminating at the margin of the pit.[120] Active flow of fluid from the vitreous cavity through the pit to the subretinal space has been demonstrated in dogs. This mechanism has not been demonstrated in humans.[121]

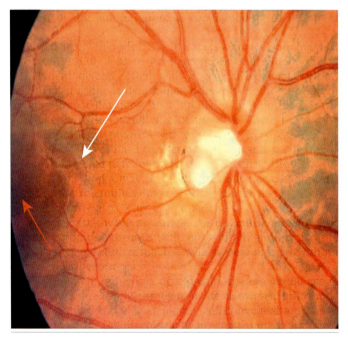

Fig. 51.17 This patient has an optic disk pit at 8 o'clock in the right optic disk. The white arrow points to an area of previous damage by subretinal fluid, the red arrow points to the fovea.

The pathogenesis of optic pits is unclear. The majority of authors view them as a variant of optic disk colobomas.[1] However:

1. Optic pits are usually unilateral, sporadic, and unassociated with systemic anomalies. Colobomas are often bilateral, commonly autosomal dominant, and may be associated with multisystem disorders.

2. It is rare for optic pits to coexist with iris or retinochoroidal colobomas.

3. Optic pits usually occur in locations unrelated to the fetal fissure.

Papillorenal (renal–coloboma) syndrome ("the vacant optic disk")

The papillorenal syndrome (renal–coloboma syndrome) was first described by Rieger.[122] It is a rare autosomal dominant disorder consisting of bilateral optic disk anomalies associated with hypoplastic kidneys.[123] Retinal detachments are associated, as is renal failure. There are sometimes mutations in the PAX2 gene in affected families.[124,125]

Renal abnormalities include hypoplasia, variable proteinuria, vesiculoureteral reflux, recurrent pyelonephritis, microhematuria, echogenicity on ultrasound, or high resistance to blood flow on Doppler ultrasound. It is characterized by a distinct optic disk malformation:[123] the excavated optic disk is normal in size, and may be surrounded by pigmentary disturbance.[123] Unlike colobomatous defects, the excavation is central (Fig. 51.18). A defining feature is the multiple cilioretinal vessels emanating from the periphery of the disk, and variable attenuation or atrophy of the central retinal vessels (see Fig. 51.18).[123] Color Doppler imaging has confirmed the absence of central retinal circulation.[123] Visual acuity is usually good but may be severely diminished by choroidal and retinal hypoplasia and later-onset serous retinal detachments.[123,126] Peripheral visual field defects corresponding to areas of retinal hypoplasia are often present. The central optic disk excavation and peripheral field defects can simulate coloboma as well as normal tension glaucoma. Follow-up examination has shown renal disease in some patients who were originally reported as having isolated familial autosomal dominant "coloboma."[127,128]

This malformation is attributed to a primary deficiency in angiogenesis.[123] There is a failure of the hyaloid system to convert to normal central retinal vessels analogous to a feline pattern of circulation.[123] Some patients with papillorenal syndrome have detectable mutations in the PAX2 gene.[123,126]

Congenital tilted disk syndrome

The tilted disk syndrome is a non-hereditary bilateral condition in which the superotemporal optic disk is elevated and the inferonasal disk is posteriorly displaced, resulting in an oval optic disk, with its long axis obliquely oriented (Fig. 51.19)[1] accompanied by situs inversus of the retinal vessels, congenital inferonasal conus, thinning of the inferonasal RPE and choroid, and bitemporal hemianopia.[129] The anomalous optic disk appearance is secondary to a posterior ectasia of the inferonasal fundus and optic disk. Because of the regional fundus ectasia, affected patients have myopic astigmatism, with the plus axis oriented parallel to the ectasia. Corneal topography indicates that an irregular corneal curvature contributes to the astigmatism.[130] The cause is unknown, but the inferonasal or inferior location of the excavation suggests a relationship to coloboma.[131]

Affected patients may present with bitemporal hemianopia or optic disk elevation that simulates papilledema.[1,131] The bitemporal hemianopia is typically incomplete and confined primarily to the superior quadrants. It is a refractive scotoma, secondary to regional myopia localized to the inferonasal retina. Unlike in chiasmal lesions, these field defects fail to respect the vertical meridian on kinetic perimetry. Furthermore, the superotemporal depression is selectively confined to the midsize isopter, while the large and small isopters remain fairly normal, due to the marked ectasia of the mid-peripheral fundus. Repeat perimetry after addition of a –4.00 lens often eliminates the visual field abnormality. In some cases retinal sensitivity may be decreased in the area of the ectasia, and the defect persists to some degree despite appropriate refractive correction.[129]

The tilted disk syndrome has been associated with true bitemporal hemianopia in several patients who were found to harbor a congenital suprasellar tumor. This may reflect the disruptive effect of the suprasellar tumor on optic axonal migration during embryogenesis.[13] This makes neuroimaging mandatory in any patient with a tilted disk syndrome whose bitemporal hemianopia either respects the vertical meridian or fails to preferentially involve the mid-peripheral isopter on kinetic perimetry.[132,133] Tilted disks without retinal ectasia occur in patients with trans-sphenoidal encephalocele.[3] The tilted disk syndrome has also been reported in X-linked congenital stationary night-blindness.[83,119,134] Anomalies at the junction of the staphyloma or at the junction between peripapillary retina and the altered disk margin may cause serous macular detachments.[135-137]

Optic disk dysplasia

The term "optic disk dysplasia" is a descriptive term that connotes a markedly deformed optic disk that fails to conform to any recognizable diagnostic category (Fig. 51.20). The distinction between an uncategorizable "anomalous" disk and a "dysplastic" disk is arbitrary and based upon the severity of the lesion. The term optic disk dysplasia was applied to cases of the morning glory disk anomaly[53,138] or which were indiscriminately labeled as optic disk colobomas.[1] Additional variants of optic disk dysplasia will likely be recognized as distinct anomalies.

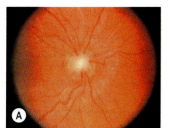
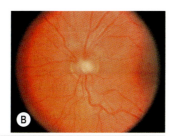

Fig. 51.18 Papillorenal syndrome. This 9-year-old girl with chronic renal failure secondary to interstitial fibrosis had vacant optic disks with an exclusive cilioretinal circulation. (Photographs courtesy of Erika M. Levin, MD.)

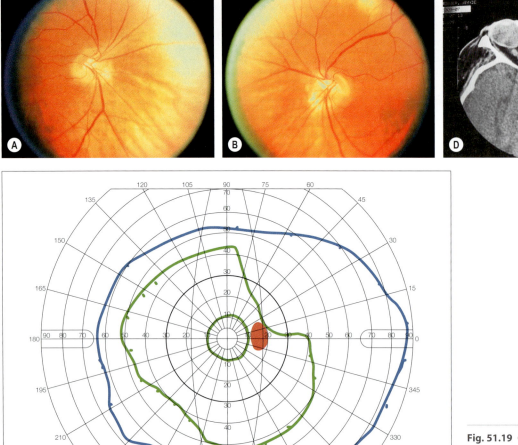

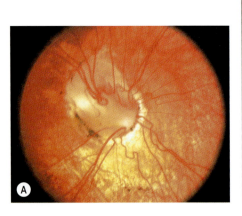
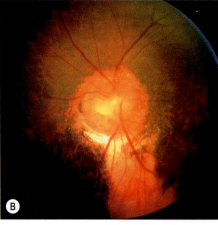

Fig. 51.19 Congenital tilted disk syndrome.
(A) Right optic disk. (B) Left optic disk. (C) Right visual field showing superotemporal defect confined to the mid-peripheral isopter that does not respect the vertical meridian. (D) CT scan showing increased curvature of the posterior sclera nasally and flattening of the posterior sclera temporally nasally. (Brodsky MC. Congenital optic disk anomalies. Surv Ophthalmol 1994: 89–112.)

Fig. 51.20 Optic disk dysplasia with and without trans-sphenoidal encephalocele.
(A) Without trans-sphenoidal encephalocele. (B) With tongue-shaped infrapapillary depigmentation signifying trans-sphenoidal encephalocele. (From Brodsky MC, Baker RS, Hamed LF. Pediatric Neuro-Ophthalmology. Springer Verlag 1996, with permission. © 1996 Springer Verlag.)

Dysplastic optic disks can occur with trans-sphenoidal encephalocele.[3] An infrapapillary zone of V- or tongue-shaped retinochoroidal depigmentation has been described in five patients with anomalous optic disks and trans-sphenoidal encephalocele (Fig. 51.20). These juxtapapillary defects differ from retinochoroidal colobomas, which widen inferiorly and are not associated with basal encephalocele. Moreover, there is minimal scleral excavation and no disruption in the integrity of the overlying retina. In patients with anomalous optic disks, the finding of this V- or tongue-shaped infrapapillary retinochoroidal anomaly should prompt neuroimaging.[3]

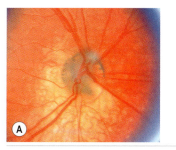
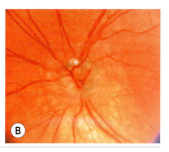

Fig. 51.21 Congenital optic disk pigmentation. (Brodsky MC, Buckley EG, Rosell-McConkie A. The case of the gray optic disk! Surv Ophthalmol 1989; 33: 367–72.)

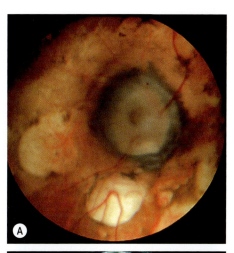

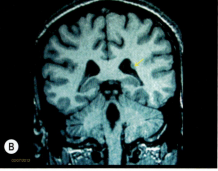

Fig. 51.22 Aicardi's syndrome.
(A) Peripapillary chorioretinal lacunae are clustered around the optic disk. (With permission from Williams and Wilkins.) (B) MRI shows agenesis of the corpus callosum. (From Brodsky MC, Baker RS, Hamed LF. Pediatric Neuro-Ophthalmology, Springer Verlag 1996, with permission. © 1996 Springer Verlag.)

Congenital optic disk pigmentation

Congenital optic disk pigmentation is a condition in which melanin deposition anterior to or within the lamina cribrosa imparts a gray appearance to the optic disk (Fig. 51.21).[139] True congenital optic disk pigmentation is extremely rare, but it has been described in a child with an interstitial deletion of chromosome 17 and in Aicardi's syndrome.[139] Congenital optic disk pigmentation is compatible with good visual acuity but may be associated with coexistent optic disk anomalies that decrease vision.[139] In developing mice and rats, a transient zone of melanin in the distal developing optic stalk influences migration of the earliest optic nerve axons.[140] The effects of abnormal pigment deposition on optic nerve embryogenesis could explain the frequent coexistence of congenital optic disk pigmentation with other anomalies.

Most patients with gray optic disks do not have congenital optic disk pigmentation. Some optic disks of infants with delayed visual maturation and albinism may have a diffuse gray tint which disappears in the first year of life without visible pigment migration. Beauvieux observed gray optic disks in premature and albino infants who were apparently blind, but who later developed good vision.[141,142] Gray optic disks may be seen in normal neonates and are, therefore, a nonspecific finding of little diagnostic value.

Despite their fundamental differences, "optically gray optic disks" and congenital optic disk pigmentation have been lumped together in many reference books. These two conditions can usually be distinguished ophthalmoscopically since melanin deposition in true congenital optic disk pigmentation is discrete, irregular, and granular in appearance.[20]

Aicardi's syndrome

Aicardi's syndrome is a cerebroretinal disorder of unknown etiology. Its clinical features are infantile spasms, agenesis of the corpus callosum, an electroencephalographic pattern termed hypsarrhythmia, and multiple depigmented "chorioretinal lacunae" clustered around the disk (Fig. 51.22).[143,144] Histologically, chorioretinal lacunae consist of well-circumscribed, full-thickness defects limited to the RPE and choroid. The overlying retina remains intact but is often histologically abnormal.[144]

Optic disk coloboma, optic nerve hypoplasia, and congenital optic disk pigmentation, may accompany chorioretinal lacunae.[144,145] Other ocular abnormalities include microphthalmos, retrobulbar cyst, pseudoglioma, retinal detachment, macular scars, cataract, pupillary membranes, iris synechiae, and iris colobomas.[143,145] The most common systemic findings are vertebral malformations (e.g. fused vertebrae, scoliosis, spina bifida) and costal malformations (e.g. absent ribs, fused or bifurcated ribs),[143–145] muscular hypotonia, microcephaly, dysmorphic facies, and auricular anomalies. Severe mental retardation is almost invariable.[143,144] Choroid plexus papilloma has been documented in five patients.[146]

CNS anomalies in Aicardi's syndrome include agenesis of the corpus callosum, cortical migration anomalies (e.g. pachygyria, polymicrogyria, cortical heterotopias), and multiple structural CNS malformations (e.g. cerebral hemispheric asymmetry, Dandy-Walker variant, colpocephaly, midline arachnoid cysts) (see Fig. 51.22).[144] An overlap between Aicardi's syndrome and septo-optic dysplasia has been recognized.[144]

Aicardi's syndrome may result from an X-linked mutational event that is lethal in males.[145,147] Parents should be asked about a previous history of miscarriages. All cases of Aicardi's syndrome probably represent fresh mutations since cases of affected siblings are rare.[145] Aicardi's syndrome in two sisters suggests parental gonadal mosaicism for the mutation.[148] Although early CNS infections can lead to severe anomalies, tests for infectious agents have been consistently negative. No teratogenic drug or other toxin has yet been associated with Aicardi's syndrome.[144] The pattern of cerebroretinal malformations suggests a CNS insult between the fourth and eighth week of gestation.[14] Most children have intractable seizures and 91% attain milestones no higher than 12 months.[149] Intraocular malformations include microphthalmos, persistent pupillary membrane, persistent hyperplastic primary vitreous, vascular loops on the optic disk, and epiretinal glial tissue.[150]

Doubling of the optic disk

Doubling of the optic disk is a rare anomaly in which two disks appear to be in close proximity to one another.[151] This is presumed to result from a duplication or separation of the distal optic nerve into two fasciculi.[151] Most reports describe a "main" disk and a "satellite" disk, each with its own vascular system (Fig. 51.23). It is usually unilateral and associated with decreased vision in the involved eye.[151]

The majority of clinical reports antedate the era of high resolution neuroimaging and have relied upon the roentgenographic demonstration of two optic nerves in the same orbit, results of fluorescein angiography, synchronous pulsations of each major disk artery, dual blind spots, and angioscotomas to provide indirect evidence of optic nerve diastasis.[151] In some cases, an apparent doubling of the optic disk results from a focal, juxtapapillary retinochoroidal coloboma that displays an abnormal vascular anastomosis with the optic disk.[151]

Separation of the optic nerve into two or more is rare in humans but common in lower vertebrates.[151] Separation of portions of an intracranial or orbital optic nerve occurred in a handful of autopsy cases.[152-155] MRI should confirm optic nerve diastasis in doubling of the optic disk.

Optic nerve aplasia

Optic nerve aplasia is a rare non-hereditary malformation usually seen in a unilaterally malformed eye of an otherwise healthy person.[156] Optic nerve aplasia is the complete absence of the optic nerve and disk, retinal ganglion and nerve fiber layers, and retinal vessels.[157] Histopathologic examination usually demonstrates a vestigial dural sheath entering the sclera in its normal position, as well as retinal dysplasia with rosette formation (Fig. 51.24).[156] Some reports of optic nerve aplasia are cases of severe hypoplasia, incorrectly diagnosed.[157,158]

Ophthalmoscopically, optic nerve aplasia may have the following appearances:[159]

- Absence of an optic nerve head without central blood vessels or macular differentiation.
- A whitish area corresponding to the optic disk, without central vessels or macular differentiation.
- A deep avascular cavity in the site corresponding to the optic disk, surrounded by a whitish annulus.

Optic nerve aplasia is distinct from optic nerve hypoplasia; it is unilateral and frequently associated with malformations confined to the involved eye (microphthalmia, malformations in the anterior chamber angle, hypoplasia or segmental aplasia of the iris, cataracts, persistent hyperplastic primary vitreous, colobomas, and retinal dysplasia), as opposed to the brain.[159-162] The pathogenesis is unknown. When it occurs bilaterally, it is usually associated with other CNS malformations.[163-167]

Myelinated (medullated) nerve fibers

Myelination of the afferent visual pathways begins at the lateral geniculate body at 5 months of gestation and terminates at the lamina cribrosa at about term.[168] Oligodendrocytes, responsible for myelination of the CNS, are not normally present in the human retina.[168] Histologic studies have confirmed the presence of presumed oligodendrocytes and myelin in areas of myelinated nerve fibers and their absence in other areas.[169] Myelinated retinal nerve fibers are found in approximately 1% of autopsy eyes and in 0.3–0.6% of routine ophthalmic patients.[168]

Myelinated nerve fibers usually appear as white striated patches at the upper and lower poles of the disk (Fig. 51.25). They may simulate papilledema, both by elevating the involved portions of the disk and by obscuring the disk margin and the

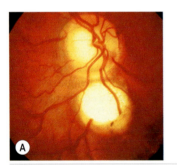
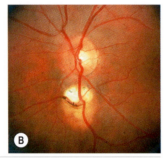

Fig. 51.23 "Doubling of the optic disk" produced by infrapapillary chorioretinal coloboma. (A, courtesy of Klara Landau, MD; B, courtesy of Anthony C. Arnold MD.)

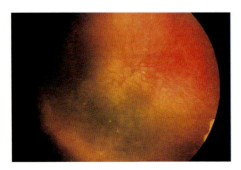

Fig. 51.24 Optic nerve aplasia. (Brodsky MC, Atreides SP, Fowlkes JL, Sundin OH. Optic nerve aplasia in an infant with hypopituitarism and posterior pituitary ectopia. Arch Ophthalmol 2004; 122: 125–6.)

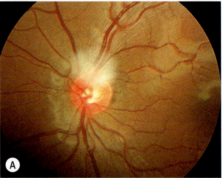
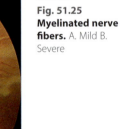

Fig. 51.25 Myelinated nerve fibers. A. Mild B. Severe

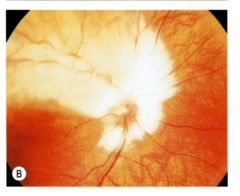

underlying retinal vessels.[168,170] Distally, they have an irregular fan-shaped appearance. Small slits or patches of normal-appearing fundus color are occasionally visible within an area of myelination.[168] Myelinated nerve fibers are bilateral in 17–20% of cases. They are discontinuous with the optic nerve head in 19%. Isolated patches of myelinated nerve fibers in the peripheral retina are rarely found nasal to the optic disk.[170]

The pathogenesis of myelinated nerve fibers remains speculative,[170] but animals with little or no lamina cribrosa tend to have deep physiologic cups and extensive myelination of retinal nerve fibers, while animals with a well-developed lamina cribrosa show fairly flat nerve heads and no retinal myelination suggesting several possible mechanisms:[170]

1. A defect in the lamina cribrosa may allow oligodendrocytes to access the retina and produce myelin there.
2. There may be fewer axons relative to the size of the scleral canal, producing enough room for myelination to proceed into the eye. In eyes with remote, isolated peripheral patches of myelinated nerve fibers, an anomaly in the timing or formation of the lamina cribrosa permits access of oligodendrocytes to the retina which migrate through the nerve fiber layer until they find a region of relatively low nerve fiber layer density where myelination proceeds.
3. Late development of the lamina cribrosa may allow oligodendrocytes to migrate into the eye.

Extensive unilateral (or rarely bilateral) myelination of nerve fibers can be associated with high myopia and refractory amblyopia[171] (Fig. 51.26). In such patients, myelin envelops most if not all of the circumference of the disk. The macula (although unmyelinated) usually appears abnormal, showing a dulled reflex or pigment dispersion.[172] The appearance of the macula may be the best direct correlate of response to occlusion therapy.[172]

Myelinated nerve fibers occur in association with the Gorlin's (multiple basal cell nevi) syndrome,[173] and an autosomal dominant vitreoretinopathy characterized by congenitally poor vision, bilateral extensive myelination of the retinal nerve fiber layer, severe vitreal degeneration, high myopia, a retinal dystrophy with night-blindness, and limb deformities.[174]

Myelinated nerve fibers may be inherited in an autosomal dominant fashion.[175] Isolated cases of myelinated nerve fibers have been described in association with abnormal length of the optic nerve (oxycephaly),[176] effects in the lamina cribrosa (tilted disk),[177] anterior segment dysgenesis,[170] and NF-2 (neurofibromatosis 2).[178] Although myelinated nerve fibers may be associated with neurofibromatosis,[178] many feel that this is questionable.[168]

Rarely, areas of myelinated nerve fibers may be acquired after infancy and even in adulthood.[179,180] Trauma to the eye (a blow to the eye in one patient and an optic nerve sheath fenestration in the other) seems to be a common denominator in these cases. Perhaps there is sufficient damage to the lamina cribrosa to permit oligodendrocytes to enter the retina.[170] Myelinated nerve fibers may disappear as a result of axonal insult.[168]

The optic disk in albinism

The optic disks of albinos have a number of ophthalmoscopic appearances. They often have a diffuse gray tint in the first few years of life. This discoloration may be related to optical effects resulting from surrounding chorioretinal depigmentation since it is no longer evident in older children and adults.

Five persistent ophthalmoscopic findings characterize albino optic disks:[181]

1. Small disk diameter.
2. Absence of the physiologic cup.
3. Oval shape with long axis oriented obliquely.
4. Origin of the retinal vessels from the temporal aspect of the disk.
5. Abnormal course of retinal vessels consisting of initial nasal deflection followed by abrupt divergence and reversal of direction to form the temporal vascular arcades (Fig. 51.27).

Pseudopapilledema

Anomalous elevation of the optic disk is a primary diagnostic consideration in the child referred for papilledema.[183] Buried drusen within the optic disk is the most common form of pseudopapilledema and must be distinguished from other causes of pseudopapilledema, such as hyperopia, myelinated nerve fibers, epipapillary glial tissue, and hyaloid traction on the disk.[184]

Optic disk drusen

The word drusen, of Germanic derivation, originally meant tumor, swelling, or tumescence.[185] It was used in mining 500

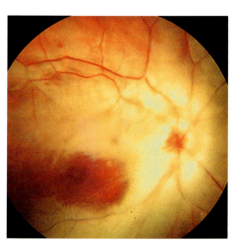

Fig. 51.26 Unilateral high myopia with myelinated nerve fibers. (From Brodsky MC, Baker RS, Hamed LF. Pediatric Neuro-Ophthalmology. Springer Verlag 1996, with permission. © 1996 Springer Verlag.)

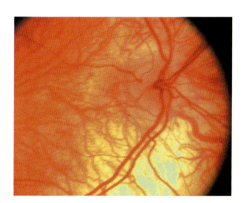

Fig. 51.27 Albinotic optic disk (Pollock's sign). (From Brodsky MC, Baker RS, Hamed LF. Pediatric Neuro-Ophthalmology. Springer Verlag 1996, with permission. © 1996 Springer Verlag.)

years ago to indicate a crystal-filled space in a rock.[185] Other terms used occasionally are hyaline bodies and colloid bodies.[186]

Drusen may closely simulate papilledema and be associated with visual field defects and solitary hemorrhages. This complicates the diagnostic problem.[187] If buried drusen go unrecognized, the elevated optic disks may precipitate inappropriate diagnostic studies.[188]

The viewing of drusen as the cause rather than the effect of an underlying configurational anomaly of the disk carries over into our analysis of associated complications (e.g. the lack of correspondence between visual field abnormalities with the position of visible drusen on the disk has puzzled many). The time course of evolution of optic disk drusen and the histopathologic findings suggest that disk drusen result from axonal degeneration, a chronic, low-grade optic neuropathy measured over decades.

Lorentzen examined 3200 children from an ophthalmologic practice and found that 11 had drusen of the optic disk (a prevalence of 0.34%).[185] This prevalence increased by a factor of 10 in family members of patients with disk drusen. Friedman et al. examined 737 cadavers and found disk drusen in 15.[186] Drusen are often minute and situated deep within the optic nerve.[189] Familial drusen are transmitted as an autosomal dominant trait.[190-192] Disk drusen are rare in African-Americans.[188] That disk drusen are associated with hyperopia has not been substantiated.[188,192,194] Visible disk drusen are bilateral in two-thirds of cases: buried drusen in 86% of cases.[188,193] Clumsiness, learning disabilities, and neurologic problems were reported in children with drusen,[195] but subsequently unsubstantiated.

Ophthalmoscopic appearance in children

Most childhood cases present with pseudopapilledema secondary to buried drusen (Fig. 51.28). The disk is elevated and its margins are blurred or obscured.[186] The elevated disk may have a gray or a yellow-white discoloration. Disk drusen tend to become more conspicuous with age.[196] Discrete hyaline bodies are first noted at a mean age of 12.1 years;[197] in older children, there is often a scalloped contour to the disk margins, due to partially buried drusen protruding from the edge of the disk into the peripapillary retina.[186]

Buried drusen are most visible at the margin of the disk, where they impart an irregular "lumpy-bumpy" contour (see Fig. 51.28). Exposed drusen are more frequent on the nasal side of the optic disk. Surface drusen appear as yellowish, globular, translucent bodies often in larger or smaller conglomerations[185] (Fig. 51.29). They may occur singly, in grape-like clusters, or as fused conglomerations, varying in size from small dots to several vein widths in diameter.[186] By direct illumination, the central portion of each shines uniformly, while the border may be a glistening ring. With indirect illumination from light focused on the peripapillary retina, the drusen shine uniformly, except for a brighter, semicircular marginal zone on the side opposite from the spot of light ("inverse shading"). In addition to the small size of the optic disk and the absence of a physiologic cup, the disk vasculature is anomalous. The major retinal vessels are increased in number and often tortuous (see Fig. 51.28). They tend to branch early and may trifurcate or quadrificate. The prevalence of cilioretinal arteries is increased, with estimates ranging from 24.1%[194] to 43%.[195] Peripapillary atrophy or pigment epithelial derangement occurs in a third of eyes.[194] Retinal venous loops or anomalous retinociliary shunt vessels are occasionally seen. Unlike in papilledema, the retinal vessels overlying the optic disk are not obscured. However, the retinal veins may appear slightly dilated, and spontaneous venous pulsations are absent in 75% of children with pseudopapilledema.[198]

Distinguishing buried disk drusen from papilledema

The distinction between pseudopapilledema associated with buried drusen from papilledema (or other forms of optic disk edema) can be difficult, but there are several clinical signs that serve to distinguish these two conditions (Table 51.3).[183] In papilledema, the swelling extends into the peripapillary retina and obscures the peripapillary retinal vasculature. In pseudopapilledema, there is a discrete, sometimes grayish or straw-colored elevation of the disk without obscuration of vessels or opacification of peripapillary retina. There is a graying or

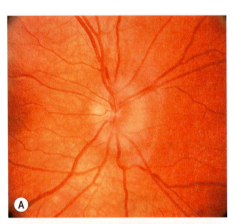
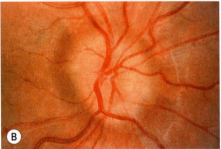

Fig. 51.28 (A) Pseudopapilledema with buried disk drusen. (B) Note cupless disks with elevation confined to the disk, increased retinal vessels that overlie the disk without obscuration, and clear circumpapillary light reflex from the internal limiting membrane.

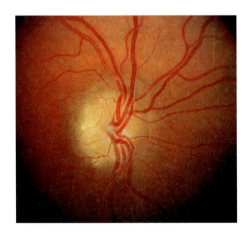

Fig. 51.29 **Visible disk drusen.** (From Brodsky MC, Baker RS, Hamed LF. Pediatric Neuro-Ophthalmology. Springer Verlag 1996, with permission. © 1996 Springer Verlag.)

Table 51.3 – Ophthalmoscopic features useful in differentiating optic disk edema from pseudopapilledema associated with buried drusen

Optic disk edema	Pseudopapilledema with buried drusen
Disk vasculature obscured at disk margins	Disk vasculature remains visible at disk margins
Elevation extends into peripapillary retina	Elevation confined to optic disk
Graying and muddying of peripapillary nerve fiber layer	Sharp peripapillary nerve fiber
Venous congestion	No venous congestion
+/– Exudates	No exudates
Loss of optic cup only in moderate to severe disk edema	Small cupless disk
Normal configuration of disk vasculature despite venous congestion	Increased major retinal vessels with early branching
No circumpapillary light reflex	Crescentic circumpapillary light reflex
Absence of spontaneous venous pulsations	Spontaneous venous pulsations may be present or absent

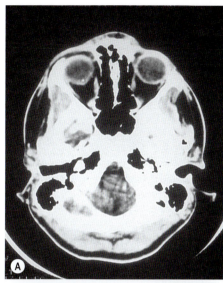

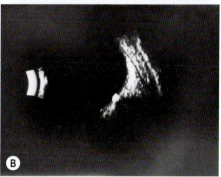

Fig. 51.30 Ancillary studies showing calcifications in patients with pseudopapilledema and buried disk drusen. (A) CT scan. (Courtesy of Stephen C. Pollock, MD.) (B) B-scan ultrasonography. (Courtesy of Laurie Barber, MD.) (From Brodsky MC, Baker RS, Hamed LF. Pediatric Neuro-Ophthalmology. Springer Verlag 1996, with permission. © 1996 Springer Verlag.)

muddying of the peripapillary nerve fiber layer that occurs with swelling of the optic disk from papilledema or other causes.[199] With buried drusen, light reflexes of the peripapillary nerve fiber layer appear sharp, and the elevated disk is often haloed by a crescentic peripapillary ring of light that reflects from the concave internal limiting membrane surrounding the elevation (see Fig. 51.28). This crescentic light reflex is absent in papilledema, due to diffraction of light from distended peripapillary axons.[195,199] Single splinter or subretinal optic disk hemorrhages are occasionally seen with disk drusen, but exudates, cotton-wool spots, hyperemia, and venous congestion are conspicuously absent.[200]

Fluorescein angiography

Prominent drusen (see Fig. 51.29) may exhibit autofluorescence in the preinjection phase.[186] This is followed by a true nodular hyperfluorescence corresponding to the location of the drusen. Hyperfluorescence, typically mild, begins in the arteriovenous phase and continues into the late phases. The superficial disk capillary network may show prominence in areas overlying buried drusen.[186] The late phases are characterized by minimal blurring of the drusen that may either fade or maintain fluorescence (staining). Unlike papilledema, there is no visible leakage along the major vessels.[187,193] Venous anomalies (venous stasis, venous convolutions, and retinociliary venous communications) and staining of the peripapillary vein walls are occasionally seen.[201]

Neuroimaging of pseudopapilledema

The distinction between papilledema and pseudopapilledema with buried drusen has been aided by CT scanning and ultrasonography which show calcifications within the elevated optic disk (Fig. 51.30).[202-205] B-scan ultrasonography is superior to CT scanning (or to photography to look for autofluorescence) in the detection of disk drusen.[205]

Histopathology

Optic disk drusen are anterior to the lamina cribrosa; they occur nowhere else in the brain. They consist of homogeneous, globular concretions, often collected in larger, multilobulated agglomerations. Individual drusen usually exhibit a concentrically laminated structure, which is not encapsulated and contains no cells or cellular debris.[185] Drusen are often most concentrated within the nasal portion of the disk. The optic disk axons are atrophic adjacent to large accumulations of drusen.[185,206,207]

Pathogenesis

The primary developmental expression of the genetic trait for drusen may be a smaller-than-normal scleral canal.[208,209] The peripapillary sclera forms after the optic stalks are complete.[209] Mesenchymal elements from the sclera then invade the glial framework of the primitive lamina, reinforcing it with collagen.[209] An abnormal encroachment of sclera, Bruch's membrane, or both upon the developing optic stalk would narrow the exit space of optic axons from the eye. The absence of a central cup in affected eyes is consistent with the existence of axonal crowding. Drusen are often first detected at the margins of the optic disk, which raises the possibility that the rigid edge of the scleral canal may be an aggravating factor in producing a relative mechanical interruption of axonal transport.[210-214] The lower prevalence of optic disk drusen in African-Americans, who have a larger disk area with less potential for axonal crowding, is noteworthy.[208]

Ocular complications

Despite the gradual attrition of optic axons that occurs throughout life, most patients with pseudopapilledema remain asymptomatic. Most develop visual field defects (measurable in 71–87% of eyes).[182] Other rare, but recognized, defects include superficial and deep hemorrhages in or adjacent to the disk peripapillary subretinal neovascularization, ischemic optic neuropathy, peripapillary central serous choroidopathy, and acute loss of central acuity.[182]

Associated systemic conditions

Systemic disorders associated with pseudopapilledema include Down's syndrome, Alagille's syndrome, Denny's syndrome, Leber's hereditary optic neuropathy, mucopolysaccharidosis, linear sebaceous nevus syndrome, orbital hypotelorism and trisomy 13q-.[182] Systemic disorders associated with visible optic disk drusen include retinitis pigmentosa, pseudoxanthoma elasticum, megalencephaly, migraine headaches, and pigmented paravenous retinochoroidal atrophy.[182]

References

1. Brodsky MC. Congenital optic disk anomalies. Surv Ophthalmol 1994; 39: 89–112.

3. Brodsky MC, Hoyt WF, Hoyt CS, et al. Atypical retinochoroidal coloboma in patients with dysplastic optic discs and transsphenoidal encephalocele. Arch Ophthalmol 1995; 113: 624–8.

16. Skarf B, Hoyt CS. Optic nerve hypoplasia in children: association with anomalies of the endocrine and CNS. Arch Ophthalmol 1984; 102: 255–8.

24. Brodsky MC, Conte FA, Taylor D, et al. Sudden death in septo-optic dysplasia: report of five cases. Arch Ophthalmol 1997; 15: 66–70.

26. Brodsky MC, Glasier CM. Optic nerve hypoplasia: clinical significance of associated central nervous system abnormalities on magnetic resonance imaging. Arch Ophthalmol 1993; 111: 66–74.

28. Novakovic P, Taylor DS, Hoyt WF. Localizing patterns of optic nerve hypoplasia-retina to occipital lobe. Br J Ophthalmol 1988; 72: 176–82.

30. Kim RY, Hoyt WF, Lessell S, et al. Superior segmental optic hypoplasia: a sign of maternal diabetes. Arch Ophthalmol 1989; 107: 1312–5.

36. Jacobson L, Hellström A, Flodmark O. Large cups in normal-sized optic discs. Arch Ophthalmol 1997; 115: 1263–9.

39. Deiner MS, Kennedy TE, Fazeli A, et al. Netrin-1 and DCC mediate axon guidance locally at the optic disc: loss of function leads to optic nerve hypoplasia. Neuron 1997; 19: 575–89.

40. Oster SF, Sretavan DW. Connecting the eye to the brain: the molecular basis of ganglion cell axon guidance. Br J Ophthalmol 2003; 87: 639–45.

42. Provis JM, Van Driel D, Billson FA, et al. Human fetal optic nerve: overproduction and elimination of retinal axons during development. J Comp Neurol 1985; 238: 92–100.

52. Beyer WB, Quencer RM, Osher RH. Morning glory syndrome: a functional analysis including fluorescein angiography, ultrasonography, and computerized tomography. Ophthalmology 1982; 89. 1362–4.

55. Pollack JA, Newton TH, Hoyt WF. Transsphenoidal and transethmoidal encephalocele: a review of clinical and roentgen features in 8 cases. Radiology 1968; 90: 442–53.

63. Kniestedt C, Brodsky MC, North P, et al. Infantile orofacial hemangioma with ipsilateral peripapillary excavation in girls: a variant of the PHACE syndrome. Arch Ophthalmol 2004; 122: 413–415.

73. Pagon RA. Ocular coloboma. Surv Ophthalmol 1981; 25: 223–36.

87. Brown G, Tasman W. Congenital Anomalies of the Optic Disc. New York, NY: Grune & Stratton; 1983: 31–215.

104. Brown GC, Shields JA, Goldberg RE. Congenital pits of the optic nerve head. II. Clinical studies in humans. Ophthalmology 1980; 87: 51–65.

110. Javitt JC, Spaeth GL, Katz LJ, et al. Acquired pits of the optic nerve. Ophthalmology 1990; 97: 1038–44.

121. Brown GC, Shields JA, Patty BE, et al. Congenital pits of the optic nerve head. I. Experimental studies in collie dogs. Arch Ophthalmol 1979; 97: 1341–4.

123. Parsa CF, Silva ED, Sundin OH, et al. Redefining papillorenal syndrome: an underdiagnosed cause of ocular and renal morbidity. Ophthalmology 2001; 108: 738–49.

128. Parsa CF, Attie-Bitach T, Salomon R, et al. Papillorenal ("renal-coloboma") syndrome. Am J Ophthalmol 2002; 134: 301–2.

129. Young SE, Walsh FB, Knox DL. The tilted disc syndrome. Am J Ophthalmol 1976; 82: 16–23.

131. Apple DJ, Rabb MF, Walsh PM. Congenital anomalies of the optic disc. Surv Ophthalmol 1982; 27: 3–41.

132. Keane JR. Suprasellar tumors and incidental optic disc anomalies: diagnostic problems in two patients with hemianopic temporal scotomas. Arch Ophthalmol 1977; 95: 2189–93.

133. Osher RH, Schatz NJ. A sinister association of the congenital tilted disc syndrome with chiasmal compression. In: Smith JL, editor. Neuro-Ophthalmology Focus 1980. New York, NY: Masson; 1979: 117–23.

139. Brodsky MC, Buckley EG, Rosell-McConkie A. The case of the gray optic disc! Surv Ophthalmol 1989; 33: 367–72.

143. Hoyt CS, Billson F, Ouvrier R, et al. Ocular features of Aicardi's syndrome. Arch Ophthalmol 1978; 96: 291–5.

151. Donoso LA, Magargal LE, Eiferman RA, et al. Ocular anomalies simulating double optic disc. Can J Ophthalmol 1981; 16: 84–7.

169. Straatsma BR, Foos FY, Heckenlively JR, et al. Myelinated retinal nerve fibers. Am J Ophthalmol 1981; 91: 25–38.

195. Erkkila H. Optic disc drusen in children. Acta Ophthalmol 1977; 129 (Suppl): 7–44.

Access the complete referece list online at

http://www.expertconsult.com

Hereditary optic neuropathies

Nancy J Newman • Valérie Biousse

Chapter contents

The hereditary optic neuropathies comprise a group of disorders in which the cause of optic nerve dysfunction appears to be hereditary, based on familial expression or genetic analysis. Clinical variability, both within and among families with the same disease, often makes recognition and classification difficult.[1-3] Inherited optic neuropathies are often classified by pattern of transmission, most commonly autosomal dominant, autosomal recessive, and maternal (via mitochondrial DNA (mtDNA)). The same genetic defect may not be responsible for all pedigrees with optic neuropathy inherited in a similar fashion. Similarly, different genetic defects may cause identical or similar phenotypes – some inherited in the same manner, others not. Alternatively, the same genetic defect may result in different clinical expression, although the pattern of inheritance should be consistent. Also, single cases are often presumed or proven to be caused by inherited genetic defects, making the pattern of familial transmission unavailable as an aid to classification.

The inherited optic neuropathies typically manifest as symmetric, bilateral, painless, central visual loss. In many of these disorders, the papillomacular nerve fiber bundle is affected, with resultant central or cecocentral scotomas. The exact location of initial pathology along the ganglion cell and its axon, and the pathophysiologic mechanisms of optic nerve injury remain unknown, but mitochondrial dysfunction plays a central role in the pathogenesis of most, if not all, of the inherited optic neuropathies.[2,3] Optic nerve damage is usually permanent and may be progressive. Once optic atrophy is observed, substantial nerve injury has already occurred.

In some of the hereditary optic neuropathies, optic nerve dysfunction is isolated. In others, various neurologic and systemic abnormalities are regularly observed and inherited diseases with primarily neurologic or systemic manifestations, such as the multisystem degenerations, can include optic atrophy. In this chapter the hereditary optic neuropathies are a classified into three major groups:[1]

1. Those that occur primarily without associated neurologic or systemic signs.
2. Those that frequently have associated neurologic or systemic signs.
3. Those in which the optic neuropathy is usually recognized as secondary in the overall disease process.

As more specific genetic defects are discovered, our concept of the phenotypes of these disorders will likely change, as will our classification.

Monosymptomatic hereditary optic neuropathies

Leber's hereditary optic neuropathy

Leber's hereditary optic neuropathy (LHON) is one of the first diseases to be etiologically linked to specific mtDNA defects.[1-3] It has a minimum point prevalence of 1 in 31 000 in the northeast of England, 1 in 39 000 in The Netherlands and 1 in 50 000 in Finland.[3] Age of onset typically occurs between 15 and 35, but may range from 1 to 87 years. LHON is expressed predominantly in males of the lineage, a feature not expected from mtDNA inheritance. Between 25% and 50% of male and 5% and 10% of female LHON carriers will have vision loss during their lifetimes. Visual loss is bilateral, painless, central, and usually abrupt in onset. In about 50% of cases, the vision loss is recognized as occurring sequentially, with one eye affected weeks to months before second eye involvement. Within 1 year, both eyes are invariably affected. Vision worsens in each eye over weeks or months, and usually deteriorates to acuities of 20/200 or worse. Color vision is affected early and severely, and visual fields typically show central or cecocentral defects. Funduscopic abnormalities may be seen in patients with LHON and in their asymptomatic maternal relatives. Especially during the acute phase of visual loss, there may be hyperemia of the optic nerve head, dilation and tortuosity of vessels, hemorrhages, circumpapillary telangiectatic microangiopathy, or circumpapillary nerve fiber layer swelling (pseudoedema) (Fig. 52.1). Eventually, the only fundus findings will be optic atrophy with nerve fiber layer dropout, especially in

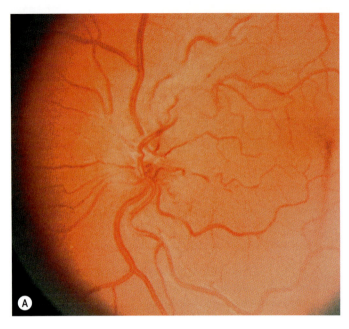

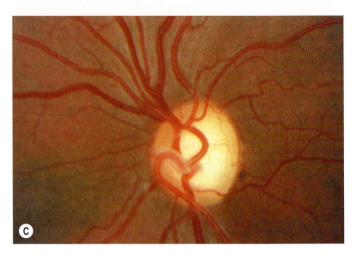

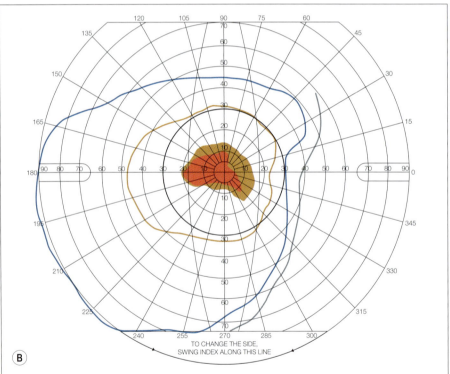

Fig. 52.1 Leber's hereditary optic neuropathy. (A) Left fundus at the time of visual loss showing mild hyperemia of the optic disc with peripapillary telangiectasias. (B) Goldmann visual field demonstrating a central scotoma in the left eye. (C) Left optic disc pallor with cupping 5 months after visual loss in a patient with Leber's hereditary optic neuropathy.

the papillomacular bundle. There may be non-glaucomatous cupping of the disc and arterial attenuation. In most LHON patients, visual loss is the only manifestation of the disease. Some pedigrees have family members with associated cardiac conduction abnormalities, especially pre-excitation syndromes. Minor neurologic and skeletal abnormalities have been reported in some patients, as has multiple sclerosis-like disease.

Ancillary tests in LHON are of limited clinical value. Fluorescein angiography may help distinguish the LHON optic disc from true disc edema. Electrocardiograms may show cardiac

conduction abnormalities. Optical coherence tomography has demonstrated initial thickening of the peripapillary nerve fiber layer, followed by thinning as optic atrophy ensues. Visual evoked responses are predictably abnormal when there is visual loss. Standard flash electroretinograms, electroencephalograms, cerebrospinal fluid, and brain CT and MRI are generally normal. Rarely, MRIs have shown anterior visual pathway enhancement acutely in affected LHON patients and bright T2 lesions in the late phases. Phosphorus-31 magnetic resonance spectroscopy has suggested impaired mitochondrial

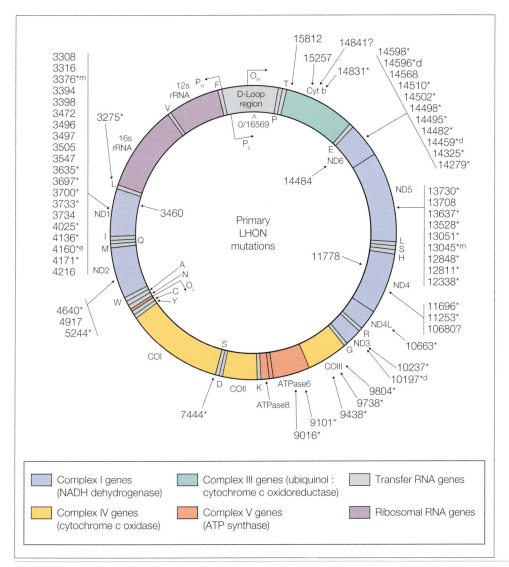

Fig. 52.2 Mitochondrial genome showing the point mutations associated with Leber's hereditary optic neuropathy. Over 90% of all cases of LHON are associated with the three primary mutations located inside the genome (circle), and the other mutations are shown outside the genome. These other mutations vary markedly in their prevalence, degree of evolutionary conservation of the encoded amino acids altered, and frequency among controls. Mutations marked * may be primary, but they each account for only one or a few pedigrees worldwide. Mutations marked ** are primary mutations associated with LHON and dystonia. (Adapted from Newman NJ. Hereditary optic neuropathies. In: Miller NR, Newman NJ, Biousse V, et al. editors. Walsh and Hoyt's Clinical Neuro-Ophthalmology, Vol I, 6th ed. Baltimore, MD: Williams & Wilkins; 2005: 465–501.)

metabolism within several LHON patients' limb muscles and occipital lobes. Deficiency in respiratory chain complex I function has been demonstrated in muscle and blood samples of some LHON patients.

LHON pedigrees follow a maternal inheritance pattern, and the disease has been linked to point mutations in the mtDNA[1-4] (Fig. 52.2). Three point mutations in the mtDNA, known as the "primary LHON mutations," cause about 90% of cases of LHON worldwide. They are located at mtDNA nucleotide positions 11778 (69% of cases), 3460 (13% of cases), and 14484 (14% of cases) (see Fig. 52.2). Other point mutations have been found with a greater frequency in LHON patients than controls, but caution must be taken in assuming a causal significance for these secondary mutations. Some may truly be primary mutations, but each accounts for only a few pedigrees worldwide. Others' pathogenic significance remains unclear. Screening for LHON in a patient with visual loss should begin with the three primary mutations. In those

primary mutation-negative patients in whom suspicion remains high, testing for the other mtDNA mutations associated with LHON is probably warranted, especially for those mutations deemed likely to be causal in a few pedigrees. Alternatively, since the majority of these other mtDNA mutations reside in genes encoding subunits of complex I, complete sequencing of complex I, perhaps beginning with the so-called "hot spot" ND6 gene, might also be considered. Finally, sequencing the entire mitochondrial genome is possible, although labor intensive. This should be performed only in those cases of high suspicion, and interpreted by someone versed in the complexities of mitochondrial genetics.

Among the primary mutations, the LHON clinical phenotype is remarkably similar. The only consistent differentiating feature is the better prognosis for visual outcome in those patients with the 14484 mutation.[1] Up to 70% of patients with the 14484 mutation will have some degree of visual improvement compared to only 5% of patients with the 11778 mutation. Patients with the 3460 mutation may have a better chance of visual recovery than those with the 11778 mutation, but the numbers of patients are too small for meaningful analysis. Patients with an age of onset of visual loss of less than 20 years, especially less than 10 years, have a much better visual prognosis.[2,3]

The genetic defects, however, cannot fully explain the determinants of expression in this disease. The presence of a mtDNA mutation is necessary for phenotypic expression, but it is not sufficient.[1-3] The presence of heteroplasmy (the co-existence of both mutant and normal mtDNA) may be a factor in expression. In heteroplasmic pedigrees, individuals with a greater amount of mutant mtDNA may be at higher risk for visual loss. However, many individuals with 100% mutant mtDNA never suffer visual loss. The interaction of genetic (mitochondrial or nuclear) and environmental factors may complicate the issue of assigning a pathogenic role to individual mtDNA mutations. Other mitochondrial or nuclear DNA factors may modify expression of the disease, including X-linkage as an explanation for the prominence of male expression. Various environmental triggers for the development of visual loss in LHON have been suggested. Systemic illnesses, nutritional deficiencies, and medications or toxins that stress the organism's mitochondrial energy production might be detrimental to those individuals already genetically at risk for mitochondrial energy deficiency. Smoking, probably by its deleterious effect on mitochondrial function, has been associated with a higher expression of visual loss among carriers of the LHON primary mutation; only heavy alcohol intake has been similarly associated.[5]

The pathophysiology of LHON remains unknown.[2-4] It may involve abnormal oxidative phosphorylation and deficient generation of ATP, either directly or indirectly related to free radical production, resulting in irreversible damage to the ganglion cells and their axons. The reason these mechanisms result in selective damage to the optic nerve remains uncertain. Histochemical studies of the optic nerve in animals have shown a high degree of mitochondrial respiratory activity within the unmyelinated, prelaminar portion of the optic nerve, suggesting a particularly high requirement for mitochondrial function in this region. Of great interest is the recent identification of genetically induced rodent models of complex I deficiency that show histopathological features of optic nerve degeneration similar to those seen in LHON patients.[4] Further development of animal models for mitochondrial diseases should better facilitate the understanding of the pathogenesis of human mitochondrial disorders.

Therapies tried in the treatment of LHON include coenzyme Q10, idebenone, L-carnitine, succinate, dichloroacetate, vitamin K1, vitamin K3, vitamin C, thiamine, vitamin B2, and vitamin E.[1-4] A randomized, controlled study of idebenone in the treatment of LHON patients within 5 years of visual loss suggested that patients with a disparity in their visual function between the two eyes (i.e. those likely earlier in the course of their disease) may have a better visual outcome with treatment.[6] However, irreversible damage makes optic atrophy an unlikely candidate for a good response to any therapy. Avoiding agents that might stress mitochondrial energy production is a non-specific recommendation with no proven benefit. However, we suggest that LHON patients and maternal relatives at risk avoid tobacco, cyanide-containing products, excessive alcohol, and environmental toxins. Symptomatic therapies include pacemakers in those patients with heart block or serious cardiac conduction defects and low-vision aids for the patient with severe visual loss. As the specific genetic and biochemical abnormalities are better defined, more directed therapies may be created to replace or bypass the genetic or metabolic deficiencies in patients with the disease and in their relatives at risk. A promising form of gene therapy known as allotypic expression may play a future role in the therapy of LHON and other mitochondrial diseases.[4] Meanwhile, one should not underestimate the importance of informed genetic counseling regarding maternal inheritance among family members.

Dominant optic atrophy

Autosomal dominant ("Kjer type") optic atrophy (DOA) is the most common of the autosomal hereditary optic neuropathies, with an estimated disease prevalence in the northeast of England of 1 in 35 000 individuals, and as high as 1 in 12 000 in Denmark.[1-3]

Although it is difficult for patients to identify a precise onset of reduced vision, the majority of affected patients date the onset of visual symptoms between 4 and 10 years of age, with 58–84% of patients reporting visual impairment by age 11. Rarely, severely affected individuals have visual difficulties and sensory nystagmus prior to schooling. Many patients are unaware of a visual problem and are discovered to have optic atrophy as a direct consequence of examination of other affected family members. These phenomena attest to the usually imperceptible onset in childhood, mild degree of visual dysfunction, absence of night-blindness, and absence of dramatic progression.[1,2] Visual acuity is usually reduced to the same mild extent in both eyes. Acuities range from 20/20 to 20/800, with only about 15% of patients with vision of 20/200 or worse. Hand motion or light perception vision is extremely rare. There is considerable interfamilial and intrafamilial variation in acuities. Although not as rapid and devastating as LHON, DOA results in visual impairment severe enough to preclude safe motor vehicle operation in about 50% of affected adults. Blue-yellow color defects are classic in patients with dominant optic atrophy, but a mixed color deficit is most common. Visual fields in patients with dominant optic atrophy characteristically show central, paracentral, or cecocentral scotomas. A bitemporal depression may mimic chiasmal compression. The optic atrophy in patients with dominantly inherited optic neuropathy may be subtle, temporal only, or involve the entire disc (Fig. 52.3). The most characteristic change is a striking triangular excavation of the temporal portion of the disc, sometimes leading to the erroneous diagnosis of glaucoma. Insidious progressive decline in visual function occurs in about 50–75% of patients.

Dominant optic atrophy is believed to be a primary degeneration of the retinal ganglion cells. The majority of cases of DOA (50–60%) are the result of mutations in the OPA1 gene, located on the long arm of chromosome 3 (3q28–q29).[1-3] This nuclear gene is widely expressed in mitochondria and encodes a dynamin-related protein anchored to the inner membrane of mitochondrial cristae, abundantly represented in the retina. More than 200 pathogenic mutations in the OPA1 gene have been identified, including missense, nonsense, deletion/insertion, and splicing mutations. However, the monosymptomatic DOA phenotype is genetically heterogeneous, and other genetic loci have been implicated. In a single family of German

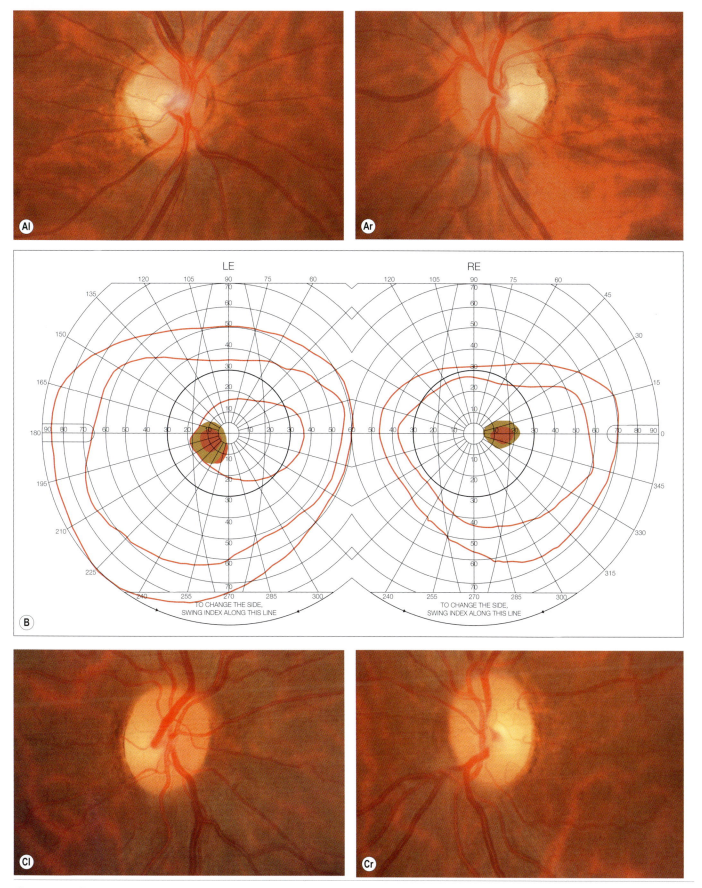

Fig. 52.3 Dominant optic atrophy. (A) Funduscopy showing bilateral temporal pallor with excavated appearance. (B) Goldmann visual field showing bilateral cecocentral scotomas (depression). (C) Funduscopy of the above patient's mother who is asymptomatic. Note the temporal pallor of both optic discs.

descent with DOA, the causative OPA4 locus was mapped to chromosome 18 (18q12.2–12.3), and in two unrelated French families the OPA5 locus was mapped to chromosome 22 (22q12.1–13.1).[2,3] Neither of the gene products nor their function have been characterized further. Interestingly, linkage analysis of patients with normal tension glaucoma has shown an association with polymorphisms of the OPA1 gene.[2]

Classically, DOA presents with monosymptomatic optic atrophy and no other neurologic or systemic manifestations. However, it has long been known that some pedigrees with individuals manifesting classic DOA, have also included affected family members with other clinical features such as sensorineural hearing loss and even chronic progressive external ophthalmoplegia, ataxia, myopathy, peripheral neuropathy, and, rarely, phenotypes suggestive of hereditary spastic paraplegia. Most of these families are not genetically distinct from pedigrees with monosymptomatic DOA, and, indeed, OPA1 gene mutations have been confirmed as the causative genetic defects in many of these syndromic forms of DOA, so-called "DOA Plus".[7] In these patients, a severely dysfunctional OPA1 protein may result in aberrant replication of mtDNA and multiple large-scale deletions of the mtDNA, and hence a more dramatic phenotype suggestive of mitochondrial disease. While these new observations emphasize the common final pathway of mitochondrial dysfunction in the hereditary optic neuropathies, they also blur the classic classification distinctions of the non-syndromic from the syndromic forms of hereditary optic neuropathy.

Autosomal recessive optic atrophy

This form of optic atrophy is present at birth or develops at an early age and is usually discovered before the patient is 3 or 4 years of age.[1] It is presumed to have autosomal recessive transmission and there is often consanguinity between parents. The visual acuity is so severely affected that the patient may be blind with sensory nystagmus. The visual fields show variable constriction, and there are often paracentral scotomas. The optic discs are completely atrophic and often deeply cupped. By funduscopy alone, it is difficult to differentiate this entity from infantile retinal degeneration, making electroretinography essential. In one consanguineous family of French origin, isolated autosomal recessive optic atrophy was linked to chromosome 8 (8q21–q22)[8] and the gene was designated OPA6, although the gene product and its function have yet to be determined. In a number of consanguineous North African families with autosomal recessive optic atrophy both with and without mild (often asymptomatic) sensorineural hearing loss, defects were found in a gene designated OPA7 on chromosome 11 (11q14.1–q21) which codes for a transmembrane mitochondrial protein.[9]

X-linked optic atrophy

Pedigrees with optic atrophy inherited in a documented sex-linked fashion are extremely rare, especially with the primary manifestation of only monosymptomatic optic atrophy. In two families, linkage to the X chromosome at the same locus (Xp11.4–Xp11.2) has been established and the gene designated OPA2, although the gene product and its function have yet to be determined.[10] Other families with presumed X-linked optic atrophy more consistently have other neurologic and systemic signs.

Hereditary optic atrophy with other neurologic or systemic signs

Autosomal dominant optic atrophy and sensorineural hearing loss

Several pedigrees with autosomal dominant optic atrophy (DOA) and hearing loss have been described. In many of these pedigrees, there are no other systemic or neurologic abnormalities. Some, but not all, of these pedigrees have now been shown to harbor OPA1 mutations that in other pedigrees cause only optic neuropathy.[1-3] In one Italian family, a new locus on chromosome 16 (16q21–q22) was designated OPA8, and preliminary studies suggest its pathogenesis may also be via mitochondrial dysfunction.[11]

In a Dutch pedigree with DOA and deafness, OPA1 mutations were excluded, but a novel missense mutation was found in the WFS1 gene on chromosome 4 (4p16.1), a common locus for mutations typically causing the autosomal recessive DIDMOAD or Wolfram's syndrome, a syndromic optic neuropathy with diabetes mellitus, diabetes insipidus, and hearing loss (see below).[12] Similarly, in another DOA pedigree with hearing impairment and impaired glucose regulation, mutation analysis excluded mutations within the OPA1, OPA3, OPA4, and OPA5 genes, but identified a novel missense mutation in the WFS1 (Wolfram) gene.[13]

In other pedigrees with DOA and deafness, there may be associated ataxia, limb weakness, or polyneuropathy. The hearing loss in these pedigrees may be severe at birth with poor speech development, or may be only moderate and slowly progressive. The acronym CAPOS (cerebellar ataxia, areflexia, pes cavus, optic atrophy, and sensorineural deafness) has been suggested, but is as yet genetically undefined.[1] "DOA Plus" with OPA1 mutations may ultimately account for many of these more complicated syndromic pedigrees, but clearly the syndromic combination of DOA and hearing loss is genetically heterogeneous.

Autosomal dominant optic atrophy, deafness, ophthalmoplegia, and myopathy

The combination of autosomal dominant optic atrophy, deafness, ptosis, ophthalmoplegia, dystaxia, and myopathy should raise suspicion for "DOA Plus" and prompt testing for mutations in the OPA1 gene on chromosome 3.[7] Visual loss usually occurs in the first decade and progresses to the 20/30 to 20/400 range, mostly on the basis of optic neuropathy, but electroretinograms may be abnormal. Hearing loss is sensorineural and progressive, with onset in the first or second decade. Ophthalmoplegia and myopathy occur in midlife. This disorder represents mitochondrial disease secondary to nuclear genetic abnormalities (see above under DOA).

Autosomal dominant optic atrophy with premature cataracts

Two French families manifest optic atrophy and premature cataract in an autosomal dominant mode of inheritance. Mutations in the OPA1 gene were excluded and pathogenic mutations were found in the OPA3 gene on chromosome 19 (19q13.2–q13.3), a locus for mutations which typically cause

Costeff's syndrome, an autosomal recessively inherited syndromic optic neuropathy (see below). Screening for OPA3 mutations as a cause of monosymptomatic DOA cases in multiple other pedigrees has failed to identify any pathogenic OPA3 variants, suggesting that OPA3 mutations as a cause of DOA are likely very rare.[14]

Autosomal recessive optic atrophy with progressive neurodegeneration and type III 3-methylglutaconic aciduria (Costeff's syndrome)

In this autosomal recessive syndrome most commonly seen in Iraqi Jewish pedigrees, severe optic atrophy is associated with extrapyramidal signs, cognitive impairment, increased urinary levels of 3-methylglutaconic acid, and elevated plasma levels of 3-methylglutaric acid. The causative gene is located on chromosome 19 (19q13.2–q13.3), and has been designated OPA3.[2,3]

Autosomal recessive optic atrophy with juvenile diabetes mellitus, diabetes insipidus, and hearing loss (Wolfram's syndrome)

This syndrome consists of of juvenile diabetes mellitus and progressive visual loss with optic atrophy, almost always associated with diabetes insipidus, neurosensory hearing loss, or both (hence, the eponym DIDMOAD for diabetes insipidus, diabetes mellitus, optic atrophy, and deafness).[3,15] Diabetes mellitus develops within the first or second decade of life and usually precedes the development of optic atrophy. In several cases, however, visual loss with optic atrophy is the first sign of the syndrome. In the early stages, visual acuity may be normal despite mild dyschromatopsia and optic atrophy. In later stages, visual loss becomes severe. Visual fields have shown both generalized constriction and central scotomas. Optic atrophy is uniformly severe (Fig. 52.4), and there may be mild to moderate cupping of the disc. Both hearing loss and diabetes insipidus begin in the first or second decade of life and may be quite severe. Atonia of the efferent urinary tract is present in half of patients and is associated with recurrent

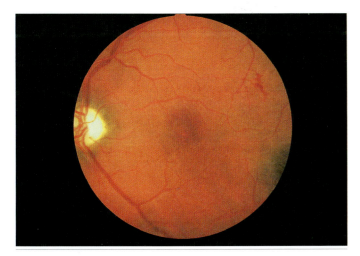

Fig. 52.4 DIDMOAD. The optic disc is atrophic and there is retinal hemorrhage associated with the diabetes mellitus.

urinary tract infections, neurogenic incontinence, and even fatal complications. Other systemic and neurologic abnormalities include ataxia, axial rigidity, seizures, startle myoclonus, tremor, gastrointestinal dysmotility, vestibular malfunction, central apnea, neurogenic upper airway collapse, ptosis, cataracts, pigmentary retinopathy, iritis, lacrimal hyposecretion, Adie's pupil, ophthalmoplegia, convergence insufficiency, vertical gaze palsy, nystagmus, mental retardation, psychiatric abnormalities, short stature, primary gonadal atrophy, other endocrine abnormalities, anosmia, megaloblastic and sideroblastic anemia, abnormal electroretinography, and elevated CSF protein. Neuroimaging and pathology in some patients reveal widespread atrophic changes and malformations of cortical development, and suggest a diffuse neurodegenerative disorder, with particular involvement of the midbrain and pons. When the syndrome is accompanied by anemia, treatment with thiamine may ameliorate the anemia and decrease the insulin requirement.

Linkage analysis in several families has shown localization of a Wolfram gene to chromosome 4 (4p16.1). The gene responsible at this locus has been designated WFS1, in which multiple point mutations and deletions have been identified. The gene product, wolframin, is an endoplasmic reticulum protein, which plays a role in the regulation of intracellular calcium. A second causative Wolfram gene on the other arm of chromosome 4 (4q22–24) has been identified and designated CISD2. The affected patients showed a bleeding tendency and peptic ulcers. Knockout of the CISD2 gene in mice results in a Wolfram-type syndrome associated with mitochondrially mediated premature aging. Indeed, many of the associated abnormalities reported in Wolfram's syndrome are commonly encountered in patients with presumed mitochondrial diseases, especially those patients with the chronic progressive external ophthalmoplegia syndromes. This has led to speculation that the Wolfram phenotype may be non-specific, reflecting a variety of underlying nuclear or mitochondrial genetic defects with a final common pathway of mitochondrial dysfunction.[2,3] Indeed, most cases of Wolfram have been classified as sporadic or recessively inherited, the latter usually concluded from sibling expression (which is now known to also be consistent with maternal transmission).

Spastic paraplegia, optic atrophy, and neuropathy (SPOAN syndrome)

An autosomal recessive neurodegenerative disorder was clinically defined by: non-progressive congenital optic atrophy; infantile-onset spastic paraplegia; childhood-onset of progressive motor and sensory axonal neuropathy; dysarthria starting in the third decade of life; exaggerated acoustic startle response; and progressive joint contractures and spine deformities.[16] Linkage is to chromosome 11q13, but the responsible gene has not yet been detected.[17]

Congenital cerebellar ataxia, mental retardation, optic atrophy, and skin abnormalities (CAMOS)

Non-progressive autosomal recessive congenital ataxia was associated with optic atrophy, severe mental retardation, and structural skin abnormalities; it was linked to a locus on chromosome 15 (15q24–q26), but the gene is not yet detected.

Table 52.1 – Optic neuropathy as a manifestation of hereditary degenerative or developmental diseases

Condition name	Onset	Locus gene product inheritance	Clinical course	References
Hereditary ataxias				
Friedreich's	2nd decade	9q13–q21 FRDA/x25 Frataxin AR	Ataxia, dysarthria, scoliosis, diabetes mellitus, cardiac disease, pes cavus, cerebellar abnormality. Progressive to death in 5th decade. Optic neuropathy very common but usually asymptomatic	1, 19, 20
Spinocerebellar ataxias	Varies	30+ varieties SCA1→ SCA31 AD	Signs & symptoms of cerebellar degeneration & neurologic dysfunction. Optic neuropathy variable. Some have retinal degeneration	1, 18, 19
Hereditary polyneuropathies				
Charcot-Marie-Tooth disease	1st & 2nd decades	30+ mutations AD or AR	Commonest hereditary neuropathy. Pes cavus, progressive peripheral motor weakness & wasting. 75% have optic neuropathy, often sub-clinical, some severe but a few recover	1, 2, 3
Familial dysautonomia (Riley-Day syndrome)	Birth	Ch 9 *IKBKAP* AR	Optic atrophy very common, usually mild, after 1st decade. 50% die by 30 years	1
Hereditary spastic paraplegias				
Hereditary spastic paraplegias (Strümpell-Lorrain)	3rd decade	40+ mapped loci AD, AR, X-LR	Progressive spasticity of lower limbs. AR form with prominent OA	2, 3
Hereditary muscular dystrophies				
Myotonic dystrophy	20+ years	DM1 DMPK Ch 9 DM2 ZNF9 Ch3 AD	Progressive myopathy, ptosis, cataracts, cardiomyopathy with conduction defects, frontal balding, bifacial weakness, and diabetes mellitus. External ophthalmoplegia, pigmentary retinopathy, and optic atrophy	1, 19
Storage diseases and cerebral degenerations: see Chapter 62 & Box 52.1				
Mitochondrial disorders				
Leigh's disease (subacute necrotizing encephalomyopathy)	2 months to 6 years	Complex disorders of mitochondrial metabolism AR, X-LR, maternal	Progressive deterioration of brainstem functions, ataxia, seizures, peripheral neuropathy, intellectual deterioration, impaired hearing, and poor vision. Optic atrophy + retinal degeneration	Chapter 45 1–3
MELAS	Variable 20+ years	Mitochondrial tRNA gene MT-TL1 Maternal	Mitochondrial myopathy, encephalopathy, lactic acidosis, and stroke-like episodes. Retinal degeneration. Optic atrophy	Chapter 45 1–3
MERFF	Childhood	tRNA gene MT-TK Maternal	Myoclonic epilepsy and ragged red fibers. Cardiac disease retinal degeneration. Optic atrophy	Chapter 45 1–3
Kearns-Sayre	<20 years	tRNA & rRNA mutations Maternal	Retinal degeneration & cardiac conduction abnormalities	Chapter 45 1–3

MELAS: mitochondrial myopathy, encephalopathy, lactic acidosis, and stroke-like episodes.
MERRF: myoclonic epilepsy and ragged red fibers.

Deafness, dystonia, and optic neuropathy (DDON, Mohr-Tranebjaerg syndrome)

In this X-linked disorder, sensorineural deafness, dystonia and ataxia present in late childhood, followed by optic atrophy by age 20, and cognitive decline and psychiatric manifestations before age 50.[2] The visual prognosis is poor with most patients blind by age 40. The disorder is caused by mutations in the TIMM8A gene on the X chromosome (Xq22) whose gene product localizes to the mitochondrial intermembrane space. Mitochondrial biochemical dysfunction has been demonstrated.

Complicated hereditary infantile optic atrophy (Behr's syndrome)

The designation of Behr's syndrome reflects optic atrophy beginning in early childhood, associated with variable pyramidal tract signs, ataxia, mental retardation, urinary incontinence, and pes cavus. Both sexes are affected and the syndrome is usually inherited as an autosomal recessive trait. Visual loss usually manifests before age 10 years, is moderate to severe, and is frequently accompanied by nystagmus. In most cases, the abnormalities do not progress after childhood. Neuroimaging may demonstrate diffuse symmetric white matter abnormalities. Clinical findings in some patients with Behr's syndrome may be similar to those in cases of hereditary ataxia. Behr's syndrome is likely heterogeneous, reflecting different etiologic and genetic factors.[1]

Progressive encephalopathy with edema, hypsarrhythmia, and optic atrophy (PEHO syndrome)

A progressive encephalopathy with onset in the first 6 months of life, followed by severe hypotonia, convulsions with hypsarrhythmia, profound mental deterioration, hyper-reflexia, transient or persistent facial and body edema, and optic atrophy has been described. Optic atrophy is usually noted by the first or second year of life and nystagmus is common. A metabolic defect has yet to be determined and an autosomal recessive mode of inheritance is likely.[1] This could be considered a form of Behr's syndrome, which likely represents a heterogeneous group of disorders (see above).

Optic neuropathy as a manifestation of hereditary degenerative or developmental diseases

Optic neuropathy may be associated with a variety of hereditary degenerative or developmental systemic disorders. Table 52.1 and Box 52.1 summarize the important findings in the more common such disorders.

Acknowledgments

This study was supported in part by a departmental grant (Department of Ophthalmology) from Research to Prevent Blindness, Inc., New York, NY, and by Core Grant P30-EY06360 (Department of Ophthalmology) from the National Institutes of Health, Bethesda, MD. Dr Newman is a recipient of a Research to Prevent Blindness Lew R. Wasserman Merit Award.

Box 52.1

Familial storage diseases and cerebral degenerations of childhood associated with optic neuropathies

Mucopolysaccharidoses (MPS IH, IS, IHS, IIA, IIB, IIIA, IIIB, IV, VI)

Lipidoses (infantile and juvenile GM1-1 and GM1-2, GM2, infantile Niemann-Pick disease)

Metachromatic leukodystrophy

Krabbe's disease

Adrenoleukodystrophy

Zellweger's syndrome

Pelizaeus-Merzbacher disease

Infantile neuroaxonal dystrophy

Hallervorden-Spatz disease

Menkes' syndrome

Canavan's disease

Cockayne's syndrome

COFS

Allgrove's syndrome ("4A")

Smith-Lemli-Opitz syndrome

GAPO syndrome

Blepharophimosis-mental retardation syndromes

Cerebral palsy

MPS IH: Hurler's; MPS IS: Sheie's; MPS HIS: Hurler-Sheie; MPS IIA and IIB: Hunter's; MPS IIIA and IIIB: Sanfilippo's; MPS IV: Morquio's; MPS VI: Maroteaux-Lamy.

GM1-gangliosidoses: GM1-1 and GM1-2.

GM2-gangliosidoses: Tay-Sachs disease, Sandhoff's disease, late infantile, juvenile and adult GM2-gangliosidose.

COFS: Cerebro-oculo-facio-skeletal syndrome.

"4A": alacrima, achalasia, autonomic disturbance, and ACTH insensitivity.

GAPO: growth retardation, alopecia, pseudoanodontia, and optic atrophy.

References

1. Newman NJ. Hereditary optic neuropathies. In: Miller NR, Newman NJ, Biousse V, et al., editors. Walsh and Hoyt's Clinical Neuro-Ophthalmology, vol I, 6th ed. Baltimore, MD: Williams & Wilkins; 2005: 465–501.

2. Yu-Wai-Man P, Griffiths PG, Chinnery PF. Mitochondrial optic neuropathies: disease mechanisms and therapeutic strategies. Progr Retin Eye Res 2011; 30: 81–114.

3. Fraser JA, Biousse V, Newman NJ. The neuro-ophthalmology of mitochondrial disease. Surv Ophthalmol 2010; 55: 299–334.

4. Koilkonda RD, Guy J. Leber's hereditary optic neuropathy – gene therapy: from benchtop to bedside. J Ophthalmol 2011; 2011: 179412. Epub 2010 Dec 26.

5. Kirkman MA, Yu-Wai-Man P, Korsten A, et al. Gene-environment interactions in Leber hereditary optic neuropathy. Brain 2009; 132: 2317–26.

6. http://lhon.ncl.ac.uk/

7. Yu-Wai-Man P, Griffiths PG, Gorman GS, et al. Multi-system neurological disease is common in patients with OPA1 mutations. Brain 2010; 133: 771–86.

8. Barbet F, Gerber S, Hakiki S, et al. A first locus for isolated autosomal recessive optic atrophy (ROA1) maps to chromosome 8q. Eur J Hum Genet 2003; 11: 966–71.

9. Hanein S, Perrault I, Roche O, et al. TMEM126A, encoding a mitochondrial protein is mutated in autosomal-recessive

nonsyndromic optic atrophy. Am J Hum Genet 2009; 84: 493–8.

10. Katz BJ, Zhao Y, Warner JEA, et al. A family with X-linked optic atrophy linked to the OPA2 locus Xp11.4-Xp11.2. Am J Med Genet 2006; 140A: 2207–11.

11. Carelli V, Schimpf S, Fuhrmann N, et al. A clinically complex form of dominant optic atrophy (OPA8) maps on chromosome 16. Hum Mol Genet 2011; 20: 1893–905.

12. Hogewind BF, Pennings RJ, Hol FA, et al. Autosomal dominant optic neuropathy and sensorineural hearing loss associated with a novel mutation of WFS1. Mol Vis 2010; 16: 26–35.

13. Eiberg H, Hansen L, Kjer B, et al. Autosomal dominant optic atrophy associated with hearing impairment and impaired glucose regulation caused by a missense mutation in the WFS1 gene. J Med Genet 2006; 43: 435–40.

14. Yu-Wai-Man P, Shankar SP, Biousse V, et al. Genetic screening for OPA1 and OPA3 mutations in patients with suspected inherited optic neuropathies. Ophthalmology 2011; 118: 558–63.

15. Chaussenot A, Bannwarth S, Rouzier C, et al. Neurologic features and genotype-phenotype correlation in Wolfram syndrome. Ann Neurol 2011; 69: 501–8.

16. Macedo-Souza LI, Kok F, Santos S, et al. Spastic paraplegia, optic atrophy, and neuropathy: new observations, locus refinement, and exclusion of candidate genes. Ann Hum Genet 2009; 73: 382–7.

17. Delague V, Bareil C, Bouvagnet P, et al A new autosomal recessive non-progressive congenital cerebellar ataxia associated with mental retardation, optic atrophy, and skin abnormalities (CAMOS) maps to chromosome 15q24-q26 in a large consanguineous Lebanese Druze family. Neurogenetics 2002; 4: 23–7.

18. Pula JH, Gomez CM, Kattah JC. Ophthalmologic features of the common spinocerebellar ataxias. Curr Opin Ophthalmol 2010; 21: 447–53.

19. Lynch DR, Farmer JF. Practical approaches to neurogenetic disease. J Neuro-Ophthalmol 2002; 22: 297–304.

20. Fortuna F, Barboni P, Liguori R, et al. Visual system involvement in patients with Friedreich's ataxia. Brain 2009; 132: 116–23.

Access the complete reference list online at

http://www.expertconsult.com

Other optic neuropathies in childhood

Philip G Griffiths • Patrick Yu-Wai-Man

Childhood optic neuritis

Childhood optic neuritis presents the ophthalmologist with many difficulties. First, diagnosis may be difficult. Second, the evidence base for our therapeutic decisions is based on adult studies.

Optic neuritis must be distinguished from neuromyelitis optica (NMO) and neuroretinitis. These are separate entities rather than part of the same spectrum and each requires different investigation and treatment.

Pediatric neurologists must be involved in the management of childhood optic neuritis.

Optic neuritis

Although optic neuritis is diagnosed in children using the same clinical criteria as in adults (subacute visual loss, pain with eye movements, visual field defects, and a relative afferent pupil defect), diagnosis may be more difficult. Children find it difficult to articulate the typical history of optic neuritis and may not present until they are profoundly affected. They may complain that it is dark all the time or insist on keeping the house lights on even in daylight because of impaired brightness sense (Fig. 53.1). Perimetry or fields to confrontation often reveal a central scotoma (Fig. 53.2). The abnormal vision and difficulty navigating may be interpreted as poor gait. Input from a pediatric neurologist is important, because transverse myelitis may be the presenting feature of neuromyelitis optica (NMO) – see below. The conversion rate to multiple sclerosis in children is unclear due to a lack of adequately powered long-term studies. However, as with adults, T2 lesions on MRI scan are associated with an increased risk of developing MS.[1-3]

Factors that are associated with a reduced risk of developing MS include young age, bilateral optic neuritis, disk swelling (Fig. 53.3), and antecedent infection.

Neuromyelitis optica

Neuromyelitis optica (NMO) or Devic's disease is a central nervous system inflammatory disorder that predominantly

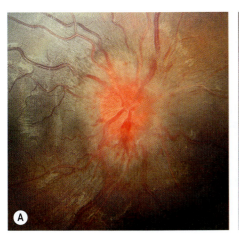
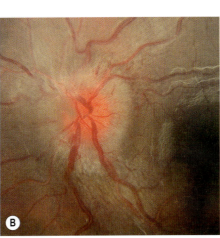

Fig. 53.1 Bilateral optic neuritis. The severely swollen right (a) and left (b) eye of a 7-year-old girl with bilateral optic neuritis. When she presented she was blind: after 6 weeks her acuities were 0.3 right, 0.4 left.

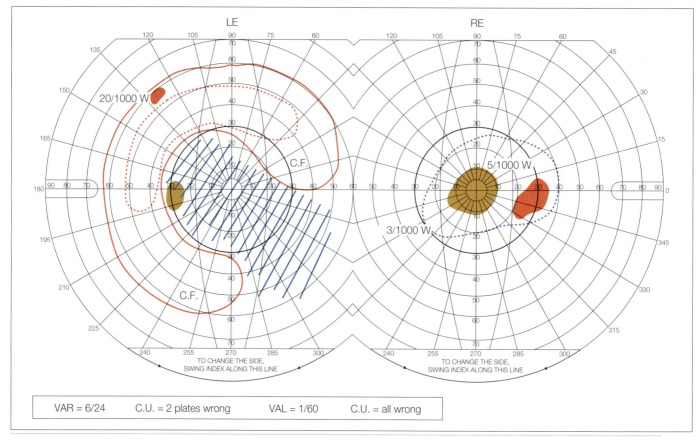

Fig. 53.2 Optic neuritis in a 7-year-old boy. Sudden onset of visual loss to 6/24 acuity right eye, 1/60 left eye. Central scotomas and color vision loss.

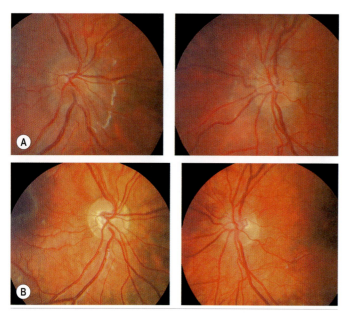

Fig. 53.3 Bilateral optic neuritis. (A) Bilaterally swollen optic disks. (B) Normal optic disks 2 months later. Complete visual recovery. Same patient as in Figure 53.2.

affects the optic nerves and spinal cord. It is a distinct entity, and in about 70% of cases it is associated with an NMO-IgG autoantibody which targets aquaporin-4 channels. AQP4 is expressed in the collecting duct cells in the kidneys and in astrocytes. It is upregulated by direct insult to the central

nervous system. Aquaporins are involved in the conduction of water through cell membranes.[4] The NMO-IgG antibody is not present in MS. Standard MS immunomodulatory treatment may not be effective. Plasmapheresis may be required if immunosuppression is ineffective. The primary goal of therapy is to prevent future attacks.

NMO should be considered in any case with severe bilateral optic neuropathy particularly with evidence of transverse myelitis. Not all of the features of NMO may be present at the first presentation. The term NMO spectrum disorder is used for those cases with some, but not all, of the disease defining features. The remaining diagnostic features may develop over time.

MRI does not usually show the periventricular white matter lesions seen in typical MS. It is important to specifically request imaging of the spinal cord to detect longitudinal myelitis involving ≥three segments (Fig. 53.4).

The diagnostic criteria for NMO are summarized in Box 53.1.

The disease is more prevalent in females than males (greater than 4:1 ratio). It is more prevalent among the Black, Asian, and Indian populations. In Europe NMO is very rare and the majority of cases are not associated with NMO-IgG autoantibodies.[5]

In the absence of AQP4 antibodies, the disease is more likely to be monophasic and long-term treatment with azothioprine, mycophenolate, or rituximab is usually not required.[5]

Because a diagnosis of NMO is not always established until well after the presenting illness, rescue treatment with

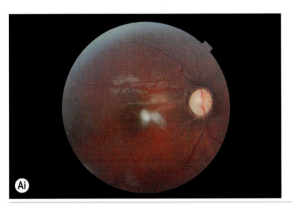
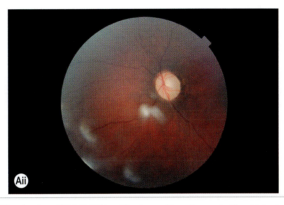
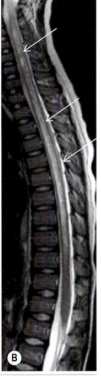

Fig. 53.4 (A) Optic atrophy and (B) spinal cord changes in a child with relapsing NMO (AQP4) antibody positive, demonstrating high signal lesions within the cervical and lower thoracic regions. The patient has been relapse free for 2 years after commencing treatment with aziothioprine and oral prednisolone. (Courtesy of Dr Michael Absoud, Clinical Research Fellow and Dr Evangeline Wassmer, Consultant Paediatric Neurologist, Birmingham Childrens Hospital.)

Box 53.1

Diagnostic criteria for definite neuromyelitis optica

Optic neuritis

Acute myelitis

Two of three supporting criteria:

　Contiguous spinal cord MRI lesions ≥3 vertebral segments

　Brian MRI does not meet diagnostic criteria for MR

　NMO seropositivity (aquaporin 4 antibodies)

plasmapheresis should be considered in all cases of severe optic neuritis refractory to steroids.

Neuroretinitis

Neuroretinitis is usually unilateral, occasionally bilateral. It is an inflammatory disorder characterized by optic disk edema and formation of a macular star (Fig. 53.5). The primary abnormality is inflammation and increased permeability of the optic disk vasculature, causing leakage of fluid into the peripapillary retina.[6] The cause of this vasculitis is not clear: some cases have an infectious etiology, most commonly *Bartonella henselae* (cat scratch disease), also syphilis, tuberculosis, Lyme disease, leptospirosis, and toxoplasmosis.[7]

Because a macular star can occur in papilledema, symptoms and signs of raised intracranial pressure should be sought and further investigations, including a lumbar puncture and an MRI scan, may be required. Malignant hypertension should also be excluded.

Fluorescein angiography discloses an arteriolar vasculitis on the optic disk. The diagnosis is established by serologic testing, enzyme immunoassays, or indirect immunofluorescence.

The evidence base for treatment is poor and spontaneous recovery is common. Nevertheless most ophthalmologists treat neuroretinitis associated with cat scratch disease with antibiotics.

Postimmunization optic neuritis

A link between optic neuritis and inoculation with a number of different vaccines including measles, rubella,[8,9] rabies,[10] meningococcus,[11] and influenza has been reported, based on vaccine administration a few days prior to the onset of optic neuritis. There is no conclusive evidence of an epidemiologic association between routine childhood immunization and optic neuritis.[12] Caution is needed when advising parents, given the clear evidence linking the natural diseases to neurologic impairment.

Infectious optic neuropathy

Many infectious agents can cause an optic neuropathy. If there is anterior involvement affecting the optic disk vasculature, it may be termed neuroretinitis (see above) while posterior involvement causes retrobulbar neuritis. Perineuritis is sometimes seen in syphilis and is characterized by disk swelling without gross optic nerve dysfunction.

Other spirochaetes associated with optic neuropathy include *Borrelia burgdorferi* causing Lyme disease and *Treponema pallidum*. A fungal optic neuropathy may occur in

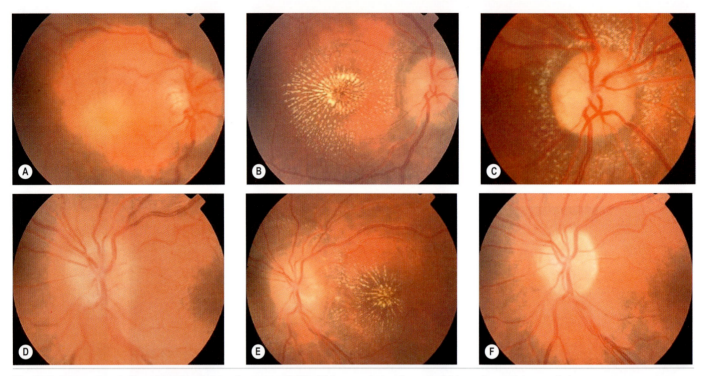

Fig. 53.5 Stages of evolution of fundus changes in neuroretinitis. (A) At presentation the optic disk is swollen and the macula has an opaque appearance. (B) 3 weeks later there is a well-formed macular star. (C) Further resolution leading later to optic atrophy. (D–F) Neuroretinitis in the left with resultant optic atrophy in the fellow eye. (Picture reproduced with permission of Valerie Purvin Midwest Eye Institute USA. From Journal of Neuro-Ophthalmology 2011; 31: 58–68. Neuroretinitis: Review of the Literature and New Observations.)

immunosuppressed patients – most commonly due to *Cryptococcus neoformans*.

Although cytomegalovirus optic neuropathy is usually associated with juxtapapillary retinitis, cases with optic neuropathy in the absence of retinitis have been described,[13] presumably due to direct invasion of the retrolaminar optic nerve. Other causes of pos viral optic neuropathy include varicella-zoster[14] characterized by a delayed onset optic disk edema and spontaneous recovery.

Optic neuropathy may occur primarily due to HIV-1 infection rather than secondary to opportunistic infections.[15]

Distant malignancy and the optic nerve

Leukemic infiltration (see Chapter 64)

Leukemic retinopathy is a manifestation of the acute forms of leukemia. It is characterized by tortuous vessels, dilated veins, retinal hemorrhages, and cotton-wool spots. Optic disk infiltration tends to be associated with central nervous system relapses and it may be the presenting feature of relapses among patients in prolonged remission. About 90% of the cases of optic nerve involvement are in the acute forms of leukemia.

The optic nerve is a pharmacologic sanctuary where leukemic cells are resistant to systemic chemotherapy. Even intrathecal chemotherapy may not penetrate well into the optic nerve. Consequently, radiotherapy is often required for optic nerve involvement in leukemia.[16]

The affected nerves appear swollen and may have surface hemorrhages. However, there is no disk appearance that is diagnostic. MR scanning may show perioptic nerve infiltration.[17]

Optic nerve involvement in leukemia is an emergency. Without prompt diagnosis and treatment, permanent and catastrophic loss of vision may occur.

Optic neuropathy and other systemic neoplasms

Solid neoplasms such as neuroblastoma or pinealoblastoma can metastasize to the orbit or sphenoethmoidal region causing visual loss. Neuroblastoma is the commonest extracranial solid tumor of childhood. Although it typically causes orbital metastases that can compress the optic nerves, neuroblastoma causing visual loss due to intracranial deposits has been described.[18,19] Visual loss in the setting of neuroblastoma requires urgent investigation and treatment.

Fibrous dysplasia and osteopetrosis

Fibrous dysplasia is a benign, but slowly progressive disorder, in which normal cancellous bone is replaced by immature woven bone and fibrous tissue. It is not inherited and the pathogenesis is poorly understood. In most cases, a single location is affected – "monostotic fibrous dysplasia." When the craniofacial bones are involved, significant deformity and visual impairment can result (Fig. 53.6).

The visual impairment may be due to stenosis of the optic canal with compression of the optic nerve. However, other mechanisms may be more important, including cystic degeneration of dysplastic bone in the anterior clinoid process,

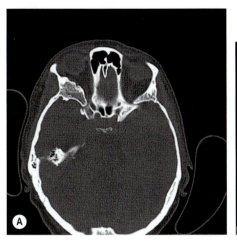
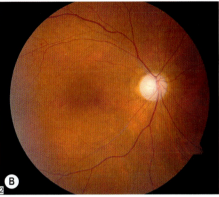

Fig. 53.6 Patient with fibrous dysplasia affecting the right orbit. The right disc is pale with attenuated arterioles. The vision had remained stable in the right eye 6/60 for 5 years. The CT scan reveals dysplastic bone involving the optic canal as well as the anterior clinoid process.

retinal ischemia, exophthalmos induced optic nerve traction, and sinus mucocele formation.[20]

Surgical decompression of the optic canal has been attempted and bisphosphonates may help to stabilize the condition.[21] Radiotherapy is associated with an increased risk of malignant transformation and should be avoided.

Osteopetrosis is a rare autosomal recessive disorder in which bones harden due to excessive mineralization. It has been associated with loss of the CIC-t chloride channel in experimental animals and man. Cranial nerve dysfunction occurs when the bones of the skull base are involved. Two mechanisms of optic nerve dysfunction have been described in osteopetrosis. Firstly, there may be raised intracranial pressure due to cerebral venous outflow obstruction, which may respond to optic nerve sheath fenestration.[22] Secondly, bony stenosis of the optic canal may compress the optic nerve. This may respond to surgical decompression.[23]

A primary retinal degeneration is associated with some cases of osteopetrosis and electrodiagnostic testing is necessary to differentiate it.

It is noteworthy that enlargement of the optic canal has been noted following bone marrow transplantation.[24]

Optic neuropathy of malnutrition

Optic neuropathy associated with malnutrition is frequently multifactorial. Poor diet with deficiency of B vitamins, particularly thiamine, purging, alcohol abuse, and smoking may be contributory factors. Although rare, nutritional optic neuropathy is sometimes seen in children or adolescents with anorexia nervosa.[25] An epidemic of bilateral optic neuropathy, linked with poor nutrition, affecting Tanzanian children of secondary school age has been described.[26] A central or cecocentral scotoma is found and in the acute stages there may be mild nerve fiber layer swelling (Fig. 53.7) and temporal optic atrophy.

Hypotensive anterior ischemic optic neuropathy

The typical adult presentation of anterior ischemic optic neuropathy on waking, presumably linked to nocturnal drops in blood pressure, is not seen in children. Anterior ischemic optic neuropathy in children is usually associated with more

severe dips in blood pressure, for example with hemodialysis, peritoneal dialysis, or overly aggressive treatment of severe hypertension.[27] In these settings uremia and diabetes may also be contributory (Fig. 53.8).

Toxic optic neuropathy

Antituberculous agents

Streptomycin, isoniazid and, more frequently, ethambutol are implicated in optic nerve toxicity (Fig. 53.9). Age, duration of treatment, and dose are correlated with toxicity.[25] Ethambutol can trigger or accelerate visual loss in patients harboring mutations associated with Leber's hereditary optic neuropathy and autosomal dominant optic atrophy[28] (see Chapter 52).

Antibiotics

Systemic administration of chloramphenicol is associated with an optic neuropathy.[29] In our experience, this is characterized by mild disk swelling and central/cecocentral scotomas with partial resolution on discontinuing treatment. Chloramphenicol results in depletion of mitochondrial DNA implicating a mitochondrial toxic effect as a cause of the optic neuropathy.

Linezolid is a synthetic antibiotic used in the treatment of serious Gram-positive infections. Prolonged treatment is associated with a reversible optic neuropathy and usually with a peripheral neuropathy that has been linked to mitochondrial toxicity.[29,30]

Immunomodulatory agents

Infliximab is an anti-tumor necrosis factor alpha antagonist. Optic nerve toxicity has been reported following its use in the treatment of Crohn's disease, ulcerative colitis, and psoriatic arthropathy[31] (Fig. 53.10).

Antineoplastic agents

Vincristine disrupts neurofilament organization resulting in a reversible optic neuropathy.[32]

Traumatic optic neuropathy

Traumatic optic neuropathy (TON) is classified according to the site of injury (optic nerve head, intraorbital,

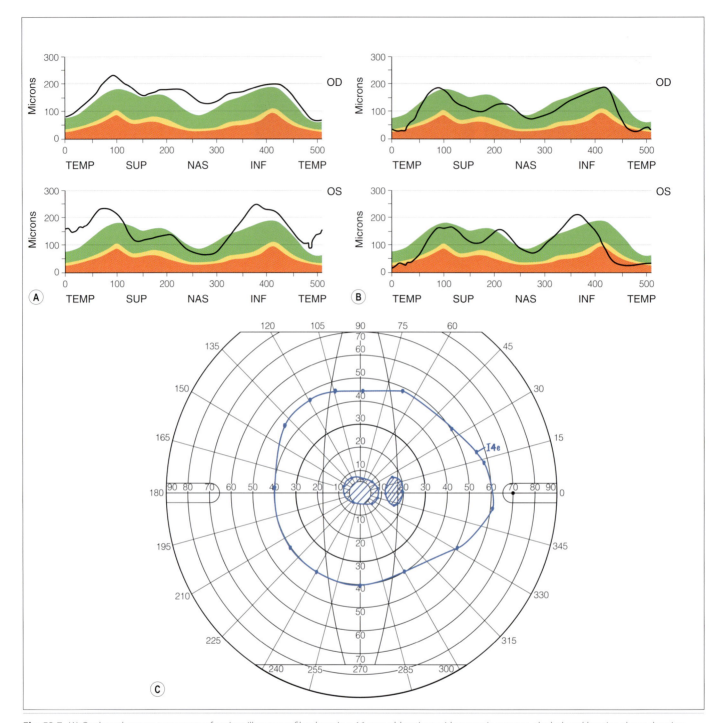

Fig. 53.7 (A) Ocular coherence tomogram of peripapillary nerve fiber layer in a 16-year-old patient with anorexia nervosa, alcohol, and laxative abuse showing thickening in the acute phase. (B) Normalization of nerve fiber layer thickness occurred with re-feeding and vitamin supplementation coincident with improvement in the visual acuity from 6/60 each eye to 6/12 each eye. (C) Goldmann visual field, at presentation, of the right eye showing central scotoma to I4e target.

intracanalicular, and intracranial), or according to the mode of injury (direct and indirect). It is an uncommon cause of visual loss with a reported incidence of 0.7–2.5% following blunt or penetrating head trauma, and a prevalence of about 1 in 1 000 000 in the general population.[33] Bilateral optic nerve involvement is rare (5%). Although most patients are young adult males in their thirties, 20% occur during childhood. In children, the most common causes of TON are falls, road traffic accidents, and sporting injuries.[34]

A diagnosis of TON is based on the clinical history and examination findings indicative of an optic neuropathy. The assessment can be difficult when the patient's mental status is impaired due to severe trauma. It is essential to exclude other reversible causes of visual loss such as a retrobulbar hemorrhage.[35,36] TON frequently results in profound loss of central vision with 50-60% of patients presenting with visual acuities of light perception or worse. The optic disk usually looks normal in the acute phase (Fig. 53.10), but with injuries

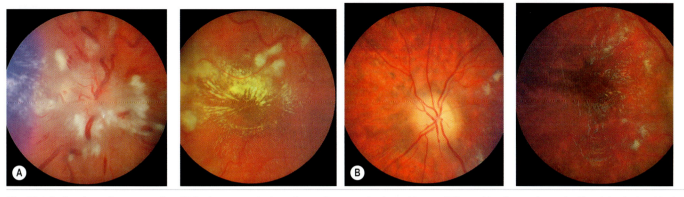

Fig. 53.8 Ischemic optic neuropathy. (A) Optic neuropathy in malignant hypertension in an 11-year-old boy with reflux nephropathy. The vision had suddenly dropped associated with a gut hemorrhage: this was the presenting symptom. (B) Same patient showing the profound optic atrophy that subsequently occurred.

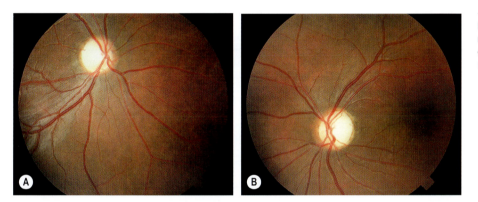

Fig. 53.9 A patient with tuberculosis meningitis. Bilateral optic neuropathy. The organism was only sensitive to ethambutol, which may cause a toxic optic neuropathy.

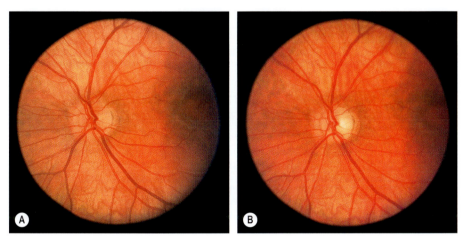

Fig. 53.10 Traumatic optic neuropathy. (A) Right optic disk 4 hours after the eye was blinded by a billiards cue being accidentally thrust into the orbit of a 10-year-old boy. (B) Same patient 6 weeks later at the first appearance of optic atrophy.

anterior to the entry point of the central retinal vessels, edema of the optic nerve head and retinal hemorrhages can be observed. In cases of optic nerve avulsion, the optic disk is absent and there is a surrounding ring of hemorrhage. The visual outcome in TON is largely dictated by the patient's initial visual acuities. For those individuals with light perception or worse at baseline, limited or no visual recovery can be expected. Other poor prognostic factors include loss of consciousness, no improvement in vision after 48 hours, and the absence of visual evoked responses. Optic canal fractures have been associated with a worse visual prognosis in some case series.

The management of TON remains controversial. Some clinicians favor observation alone, whilst others treat with systemic steroids (in various doses, duration, and mode of administration), surgical decompression of the optic canal, or both. An optic canal fracture with a bone fragment impinging on the optic nerve is an indication to some clinicians for prompt surgical intervention. The evidence base for these treatments is weak. Recent reviews have not supported the routine use of high-dose steroids or surgery in TON.[36] There is a high rate of spontaneous visual recovery (40–60%) among patients managed conservatively, and the adverse effects of intervention need to be carefully considered. It is essential to be vigilant about the possibility of delayed visual loss in TON. If this is secondary to the development of an optic nerve sheath hematoma, urgent decompression with sheath fenestration is indicated.

References

1. Bonhomme GR, Waldman AT, Balcer J, et al. Pediatric optic neuritis: brain abnormalities and the risk of multiple sclerosis. Neurology 2009; 72: 881–5.

2. Absoud M, Cummins C, Desai N, et al. Childhood optic neuritis clinical features and outcome. Arch Dis Child 2011; 96: 860–2.

3. Cakmakli G, Kurne A, Guven A, et al. Childhood optic neuritis: the pediatric neurologist's perspective. Eur J Paediatr Neurol 2009; 13: 452–7.

4. Lennon VA, Wingerchuk DM, Kryzer TJ, et al. A serum autoantibody marker of neuromyelitis optica: distinction from multiple sclerosis. Lancet 2004; 364: 2106–12.

5. Huppke P, Bluthner M, Stark BW, et al. Neuromyelitis optica and NMO-IgG in European pediatric patients. Neurology 2010; 75: 1740–4.

6. Kitamei H, Suzuki Y, Takahashi M, et al. Retinal angiography and optical coherence tomography disclose focal optic disc vascular leakage and lipid-rich fluid accumulation within the retina in a patient with Leber idiopathic stellate neuroretinitis. J Neuroophthalmol 2009; 29: 203–7.

7. Purvin V, Sundaram S, Kawasak AI. Neuroretinitis: review of the literature and new observations. J Neuroophthalmol 2011; 31: 58–68.

8. Arshi S, Sadeghi-bazargani H, Ojaghi H, et al. The first rapid onset optic neuritis after measles-rubella vaccination: case report. Vaccine 2004; 22: 3240–2.

9. Stevenson VL, Acheson T, Ball J, et al. Optic neuritis following measles/rubella vaccination in two 13-year-old children. Br J Ophthalmol 1996; 80: 1110–1.

10. Gupta V, Bandyopadhyay S, Baspuraj JR, et al. Bilateral optic neuritis complicating rabies vaccination. Retina 2004; 24: 179–81.

11. Laria C, Gonzalez C. [Optic neuritis after meningococcal vaccination.] Arch Soc Esp Oftalmol 2006; 81: 479–82.

12. Nass M. Data vs conclusions in the optic neuritis vaccination investigation. Arch Neurol 2006; 63: 1809–10; author reply 1810.

13. Cackett P. Optic neuropathy without retinopathy in AIDS and cytomegalovirus infection. J Neuroophthalmol 2004; 24: 94–5.

14. Selbst RG, Selhorst JB, Harbison JW, et al. Parainfectious optic neuritis. Report and review following varicella. Arch Neurol 1983; 40: 347–50.

15. Golnik, KC. Infectious optic neuropathy. Semin Ophthalmol 2002; 17: 11–7.

16. Lin YC, Wang AG, Yen MY, Hsu WM. Leukaemic infiltration of the optic nerve as the initial manifestation of leukaemic relapse. Eye (Lond) 2004; 18: 546–50.

17. Madani A, Christophe C, Ferster A, Dan B. Peri-optic nerve infiltration during leukaemic relapse: MRI diagnosis. Pediatr Radiol 2000; 30: 30–2.

18. Lau JJ. Metastatic neuroblastoma presenting with binocular blindness from intracranial compression of the optic nerves. J Neuroophthalmol 2004; 24: 119–24.

19. McGirt MJ, Cowan JA, Gala V, et al. Surgical reversal of prolonged blindness from a metastatic neuroblastoma. Childs Nerv Syst 2005; 21: 583–6.

20. Michael CB, Lee AG, Patrinely JR, et al. Visual loss associated with fibrous dysplasia of the anterior skull base. Case report and review of the literature. J Neurosurg 2000; 92: 350–4.

21. Chao K, Katznelson L. Use of high-dose oral bisphosphonate therapy for symptomatic fibrous dysplasia of the skull. J Neurosurg 2008; 109: 889–92.

22. Allen RC, Nerad JA, Kattah JC, Lee AG. Resolution of optic nerve edema and improved visual function after optic nerve sheath fenestration in a patient with osteopetrosis. Am J Ophthalmol 2006; 141: 945–7.

23. Vanier V, Miller NR, Carson BS. Bilateral visual improvement after unilateral optic canal decompression and cranial vault expansion in a patient with osteopetrosis, narrowed optic canals, and increased intracranial pressure. J Neurol Neurosurg Psychiatry 2000; 69: 405–6.

24. Kerr NC, Wang WC, Mohadier Y, et al. Reversal of optic canal stenosis in osteopetrosis after bone marrow transplant. Am J Ophthalmol 2000; 130: 370–2.

25. Moschos MM, Gonidakis F, Varsou E, et al. Anatomical and functional impairment of the retina and optic nerve in patients with anorexia nervosa without vision loss. Br J Ophthalmol 2010; Published online.

26. Bourne RR, Dolin PJ, Mtanda AT, et al. Epidemic optic neuropathy in primary school children in Dar es Salaam, Tanzania. Br J Ophthalmol 1998; 82: 232–4.

27. Jackson TL, Farmer CK, Kingswood C, Vickers S. Hypotensive ischemic optic neuropathy and peritoneal dialysis. Am J Ophthalmol 1999; 128: 109–11.

28. Guillet V, Chevrollier A, Cassereau J, et al. Ethambutol-induced optic neuropathy linked to OPA1 mutation and mitochondrial toxicity. Mitochondrion 2010; 10: 115–24.

29. Godel V, Nemet P, Lazar M. Chloramphenicol optic neuropathy. Arch Ophthalmol 1980; 98: 1417–21.

30. Rucker JC, Hamilton SR, Bardenstein D, et al. Linezolid-associated toxic optic neuropathy. Neurology 2006; 66: 595–8.

31. Chan JW, Castellanos A. Infliximab and anterior optic neuropathy: case report and review of the literature. Graefes Arch Clin Exp Ophthalmol 2010; 248: 283–7.

32. Weisfeld-Adams JD, Dutton GN, Murphy DM. Vincristine sulfate as a possible cause of optic neuropathy. Pediatr Blood Cancer 2007; 48: 238–40.

33. Lee V. Surveillance of traumatic optic neuropathy in the UK. Eye (Lond) 2010; 24: 240–50.

34. Mahapatra AK, Tandon AK. Traumatic optic neuropathy in children: a prospective study. Pediatr Neurosurg 1993; 19: 34–9.

35. Yu-Wai-Man P, Griffiths PG. Steroids for traumatic optic neuropathy. Cochrane Database Syst Rev 2011: CD006032.

36. Yu Wai Man P, Griffiths PG. Surgery for traumatic optic neuropathy. Cochrane Database Syst Rev 2005: CD005024.

Part 7
Neural visual systems

The optic chiasm

Michael C Brodsky

Introduction

The chiasm is so named because it is shaped like the Greek letter chi.[1] Over 2 million nerve fibers pass through it: most are visual but some non-visual fibers project from the optic chiasm to hypothalamic nuclei, forming the retinohypothalamic tract subserving circadian rhythms.[2] The ratio of crossed to uncrossed fibers in the human chiasm is about 53:47.[3]

Evolutionary considerations

The chiasm provides the major route for the juxtaposition of corresponding parts of the visual field in each eye. It is important for binocular vision. To establish fusion, it is necessary to have overlapping visual fields, congruence of corresponding retinal elements, and extraocular muscles to maintain alignment of the visual axes.[4] In lateral-eyed animals, optic fibers from each eye decussate entirely to the contralateral hemisphere. The percentage of uncrossed fibers increases as the orbits rotate anteriorly and the frontal field of single binocular

vision increases.[5] The reason that our visual system is crossed is controversial[5,6] (Fig. 54.1).

In humans, there is more retina nasal to the fovea than temporally so the right eye covers more right visual field than left visual field. The primordial nasal retinas are concerned with a phylogenetically older "panoramic" function. The temporal retinas have entered into a phylogenetically younger "binocular" function.

Our foveas are placed where nasal (panoramic) and temporal (binocularity providing) retinas meet.[6] This allows vision to subserve its elemental functions:

- Exploration (mobility).
- Detail (foveas).
- Stereopsis (binocularity).[6]

Exploration of the surround is a primordial panoramic function of the nasal retinas, while binocular vision, stereopsis, and convergence concern the temporal retinas.

Anatomy

The optic nerves, chiasm and optic tracts extend posteriorly and upwards 45 degrees from the optic canals in adults and children.[7] The chiasm lies in the suprasellar cistern several millimeters above the diaphragma sellae. The anterior cerebral arteries and the anterior communicating arteries lie anteriorly and above the chiasm and optic nerves. The carotid arteries lie laterally with the posterior communicating artery passing underneath the optic tracts. The chiasm lies in the floor of the anterior end of the third ventricle. Expansion of the third ventricle may cause chiasmal compression. Posteriorly lies the hypothalamus and the pituitary stalk, the tuber cinereum, and the mamillary bodies. The optic nerves emerge from the optic canals. The length of the intracranial optic nerve varies so the position of the chiasm in relation to other structures also varies. When the optic nerves are short, the chiasm is "prefixed", when long it is "postfixed". Von Willebrand's knee is an artefact.[8]

Embryology

The chiasm appears in the first month of life,[9] arising from a thickening of the floor of the forebrain. Retinal ganglion cells grow down the optic stalks and enter the floor of the third

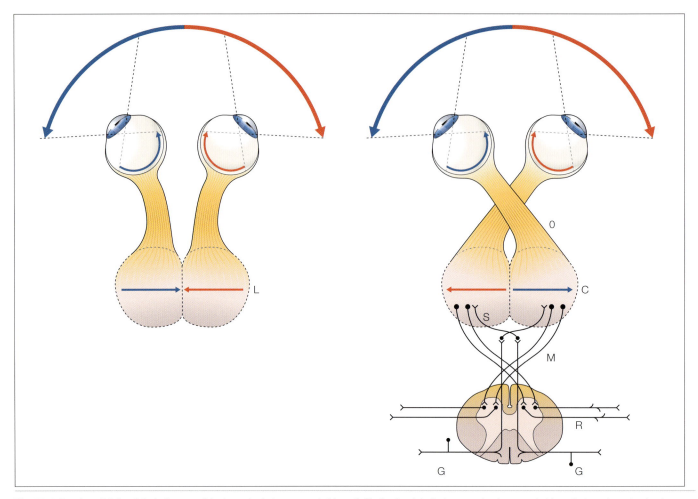

Fig. 54.1 Ramón y Cajal's original diagram of the hypothetical uncrossed chiasm (left). On the right is the completely crossed chiasm in lateral-eyed animals. (With permission from Polyak S. The Vertebrate Visual System. Edited by Heinrich Kluver. © 1957 University of Chicago Press.)

ventricle where they decussate to form the optic chiasm. The pattern of axon crossing occurs in two phases.[10] The first retinal axons meet in the midline at the ventral diencephalon forming an X-shaped chiasm; subsequent axons grow into either the ipsilateral or contralateral optic tract.[11]

A morphological specialization of the axon called a growth cone allows the axon to sense and respond to signals in the embryonic brain environment.[12] Neuronal and glial cells provide guidance information to ingrowing RGC axon. Histologic evidence suggests that uncrossed axons are confined within the lateral portion of the optic nerve and do not approach the chiasmal midline.[13] Neurons and radial glial cells in the ventral diencephalon serve a role in retinal ganglion cell axon guidance during chiasm formation. Growth associated proteins in retinal growth cones enable RGC axons to progress and perform path finding tasks. In the mouse, neurons at the site of the future chiasm are required for its formation by retinal ganglion cell axons. A growth associated protein essential for chiasm formation has been identified.[14] There is substantial overproduction of neurons which later die back by apoptosis.[15] The chiasm reaches its definitive form by the fourth month of gestation.

Transcription factors that pattern the developing chiasm have been identified.[16-19] Foxd1 expressed in the developing temporal retina and its downstream effectors (tyrosine kinase membrane proteins) are involved in patterning of the optic chiasm in chicks and mammals.[17,18] Foxd1 imprints axons ipsilaterally. Foxd1 is expressed in progenitors of Zic2 positive retina ganglion cells and is the determinant of temporal retinal identity.[17,18] Neuropilin molecules, transmembrane proteins, serve as receptors for axonal guidance to regulate axon divergence at the chiasm in mammals.[19] Neuropilin 1 (NRP1) is expressed at the chiasm midline and acts on contralateral retinal ganglion cells to provide growth-promoting and chemoattractive signals for commissural axon crossing at the chiasm.[19]

Signs and symptoms

Developmental defects and suprasellar tumors are common in children (Box 54.1). Most chiasmal syndromes result from neoplastic disorders, developmental derangements, radiation injury, inflammation, infection, demyelination, infarction, transection, or hypoplasia.[20] Dominant optic atrophy may present with a bitemporal hemianopia simulating a chiasmal disorder.[20]

In young children, chiasmal disease often presents late because the child compensates and is not suspected of having poor vision until there is substantial bilateral visual loss.

The hallmark of chiasmal disease is a bitemporal hemianopia. Some form of visual field testing is essential. Inferior lesions have to grow large before signs of chiasmal compression appear. They compress the lower nasal fibers first and tend to give an upper bitemporal field defect. Lesions from above tend to cause an inferior defect. By the time a compressive lesion has caused defects, there is usually thinning of the chiasm and the pattern of the field defect is not always clear-cut.

There is often an acuity defect. Chiasm splitting lesions, such as trauma, do not affect acuity greatly because the nasal field and the nasal half of the fovea is not affected, but involvement of the optic nerve or widespread involvement of both crossed and uncrossed fibers in the chiasm give rise to an acuity

Box 54.1

Signs and symptoms of chiasmal disease

Loss of stereopsis
Postfixational blindness
Loss of motor fusion
Hemifield slide
Bitemporal hemianopia
Band atrophy
See-saw nystagmus
"Spasmus nutans"

defect. Frequently, one eye has a very severe acuity defect and the other is relatively spared, except for a field defect. In chronic lesions, there is often preservation of a high level of acuity despite funduscopic evidence of a profound loss of neurons.

With optic nerve involvement there is significant color vision defect. Stereoacuity tests and Bagolini striated lens are useful tests in patients with suspected chiasmal compression.[4] Decreased stereoacuity is common with chiasmal lesions, even when no visual field abnormalities are detectable.[4] Stereopsis can be elicited with complete chiasmal transection by haploscopic stimulation of the intact temporal retinas.[21] This shows the sensory capacity for stereopsis is retained in chiasmal transection but the absence of motor fusion precludes stereopsis.[22] Bagolini striated lens testing reveals a binocular "mountain" pattern in chiasmal lesions.[23] Children with early-onset chiasmal disease may present with nystagmus. The classic form is see-saw nystagmus, but most patients have a compound nystagmus with vertical, horizontal, and rotary components (see Chapter 90).

Optic atrophy frequently occurs in chiasmal disease. There may be a generalized loss of neurons, or a pattern of band atrophy due to the loss of the fibers subserving the temporal fields and the preservation of fibers subserving the intact nasal field (Fig. 54.2). In developmental chiasmal defects and tumors

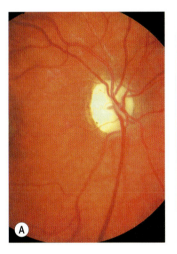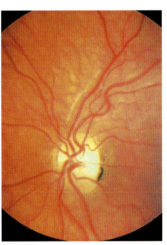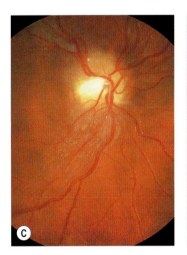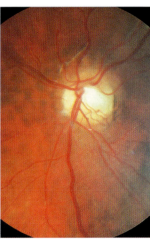

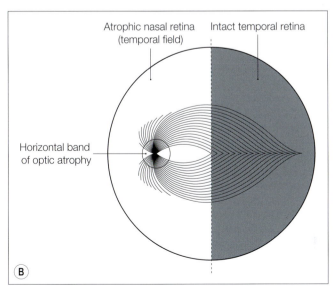

Fig. 54.2 Craniopharyngioma. (A) The right eye has bare perception of hand movements. The left eye has an absolute temporal hemianopia, normal color vision, and a visual acuity of −0.1logMAR (6/4.8, 20/16, 1.25). The left optic disc shows band atrophy: there is loss of the nerve fibers that subserve the temporal visual field but preservation of those that subserve the nasal field which are inserted into the upper and lower segments of the disc. (B) The origin of the band of atrophy is due to the fact that the horizontal band or bow-tie area is the visible area of atrophy where temporal field fibers alone are inserted into the disc. (C) Craniopharyngioma showing "bi-lobed" papilledema during a period of raised intracranial pressure. Since papilledema occurs only when the retinal ganglion cell axons are swollen and only the superior and inferior (nasal field) axons survive in chiasmal compression, the papilledema occurs only in the upper and lower poles giving bi-lobed or "twin peaks" papilledema.

there are often optic disc anomalies (Figs 54.3 and 54.4), e.g. hypoplasia.[24,25] Congenital suprasellar tumors can produce horizontal "bow-tie" cupping with selective loss of the nasal and temporal nerve fiber layer.[26] Papilledema in these optic discs occurs predominantly in the superior and inferior poles (Fig. 54.2C).

Because of the proximity of the hypothalamus and pituitary gland, endocrine and growth defects may occur. Infants with hypothalamus-involving tumors may develop Russell's diencephalic syndrome: emaciation with loss of subcutaneous fat (Fig. 54.5), accelerated growth in length relative to weight (Fig. 54.6), and personality changes with euphoria and hyperactivity. One must examine and measure the infant's general body habitus and inquire about weight gain.

In bitemporal hemianopia the hemifield slide phenomenon may occur (Fig. 54.7). Since only the nasal portion of each visual field is functioning fully, corresponding retinal points between the two eyes no longer exist. Sensory fusion becomes impossible, and motor fusion cannot maintain alignment. A previous heterophoria becomes a manifest deviation. Esodeviations lead to letters or words appearing deleted. Exodeviations produce letters or words appearing duplicated. A vertical hemifield slide causes the child to lose track of which line of text they are reading. These children do not complain of diplopia but rather a duplication of the middle of words or objects. The hemifield slide phenomenon does not require a complete

bitemporal hemianopia and can occur as the initial symptom.[27a] Signs and symptoms of chiasmal disease are summarized in Table 54.1. Rarely, chiasmal tumors can produce photophobia as their presenting symptom.[27b]

Further investigations

Further investigations consist of endocrine studies, neurophysiological evaluation (see Chapter 8) and neuroimaging. Neurophysiological studies may detect a crossover defect (particularly in a preverbal child) and quantitatively and qualitatively assess the visual defect. Magnetic resonance imaging (MRI)[28,29] provides neuro-anatomical detail of the chiasm and surrounding structures. Computed tomography (CT) scanning may provide important information about tumor and bony changes involving the parasellar area.

Developmental defects

Developmental derangements of the optic chiasm include:

- Albinism.
- Achiasmia.
- Aplasia.
- Anophthalmia.

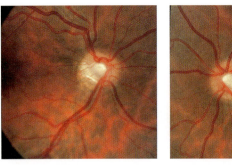
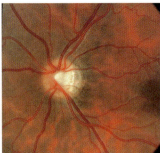

Fig. 54.3 Craniopharyngioma. Bilateral segmental hypoplasia or "tilted" optic disc. Bitemporal hemianopia with a visual acuity of −0.1logMAR (6/4.8, 20/16, 1.25) right eye (refraction: −4.0 D) and −0.22 (6/3.6. 20/12, 1.67) left eye (−4.50 D).

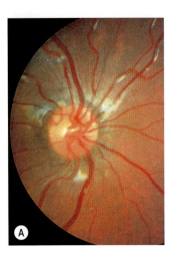
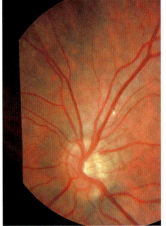
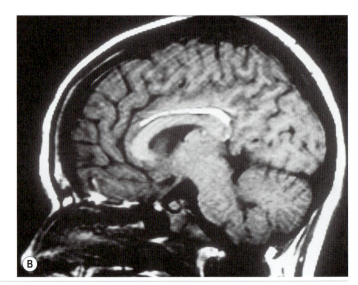

Fig. 54.4 Midline facial defect. (A) Dysplastic tilted left optic disc in a patient with a midline facial defect. (B) MRI of corpus callosum lipoma in a patient with a midline facial defect.

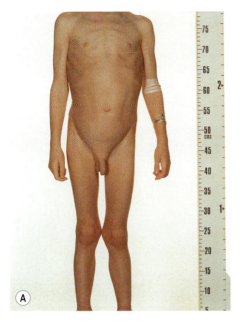

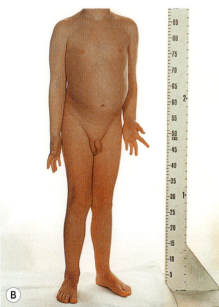

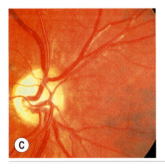 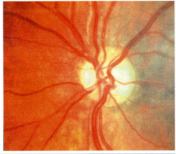

Fig. 54.5 Chiasmal glioma. (A) This boy presented with poor vision and recent weight loss. Photograph on 12 February 1973. (B) Photograph on 31 January 1974 showing rapid growth in weight and height. Weight and growth rate fluctuation are common in chiasmal glioma. (C) Bilateral band atrophy (same patient).

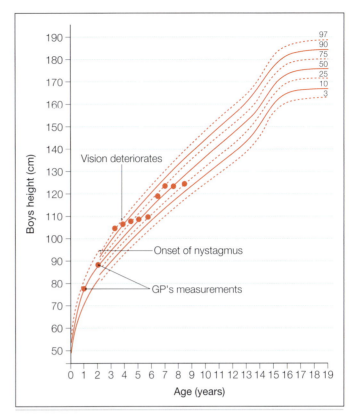

Fig. 54.6 Height growth record of a child with chiasmal glioma showing height growth rate fluctuation. Pediatric ophthalmology clinics need to have these charts available.

Albinism (see Chapter 40)

Anomalous decussation of chiasmal projections occurs in albinos.[23] Retinogeniculate axons arising from ganglion cells in the portion of the temporal retina within 20 degrees of the vertical meridian decussate abnormally in the optic chiasm to synapse in the contralateral lateral geniculate nucleus.[30-32] The human optic chiasm retains a predominance of crossed fibers. MRI shows smaller optic nerves, chiasm, and tracts, with a wider angle between the two optic nerves and the two optic tracts.[33] The crossed predominance can be diagnosed electro-physiologically by asymmetrical hemispheric visual evoked potentials[34,35] (Fig. 54.8; see Chapters 8 and 40). Pigment around the optic disc plays an important role in axonal guidance, suggesting that loss of retinal epithelial pigment could be the source of chiasmal misrouting in albinism.[36] Recently, the role of the transcription factor Zic2 has been implicated in the chiasmal misrouting in albinism.[37]

Achiasmia

Belgian sheep dogs with achiasmia have congenital nystagmus and see-saw nystagmus.[38,39] Two unrelated girls with achiasmia had normal visual fields and no stereoacuity.[40] Eye movement recordings showed congenital nystagmus in the horizontal plane and see-saw nystagmus in the vertical and torsional planes. MRI showed absence of the chiasm with each optic nerve projecting entirely to the ipsilateral hemisphere. The polarity of the visual evoked potential (VEP) distribution across the occiput was the reverse of the crossed asymmetry

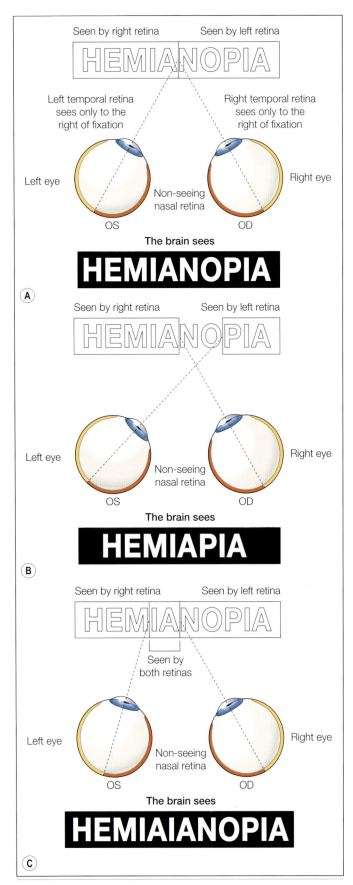

Fig. 54.7 Hemifield slide phenomenon. (Fritz KJ, Brodsky MC. Elusive neuro-ophthalmic reading impairment. American Orthoptic Journal 1992; 42: 159–164. Reprinted by permission of The University of Wisconsin Press.)

Table 54.1 – Chiasmal diseases in children

Developmental defects	Albinism
	Achiasmia
	Aplasia
	Anophthalmia
Tumors	Chiasmal glioma
	Craniopharyngioma
	Pituitary adenoma
	Dysgerminoma
	Retinoblastoma ("trilateral")
Trauma	Transection
	Hematoma
	Contusion
	Traction
Infiltration	Langerhans' cell histiocytosis
	Sarcoidosis
	Juvenile xanthogranuloma
Chiasmal neuritis	Postviral
	Postimmunization
	Multiple sclerosis
Optochiasmatic arachnoiditis	Tuberculosis
	Neurosyphilis
	Fungal
	Cysticercosis
Vascular anomalies	Arteriovenous malformation
	Cavernous angioma
Radiation	Acute visual loss months to years after radiation
Empty sella	Third ventricular distension secondary to aqueductal stenosis
	Downward traction on chiasm secondary to surgical scarring on pituitary apoplexy

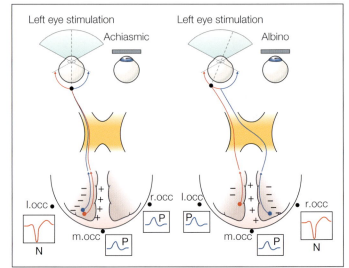

Fig. 54.8 Schematic comparing the visual pathway and VEP distribution in albino and achiasmic patients for flash stimulation of the left eye. Stimulation of the right eye produces the mirror image distribution for either condition. In the achiasmic subject, all the visual fibers from the left eye project to the left occipital cortex, and at 80–100 milliseconds a positivity is recorded over the right scalp and a negativity over the left. In contrast, most of the fibers from one eye cross at the chiasm in albinism, and the VEP distribution is the opposite, with a positivity recorded over the left scalp, and negativity over the right. (Courtesy of Dr. Dorothy Thompson.)

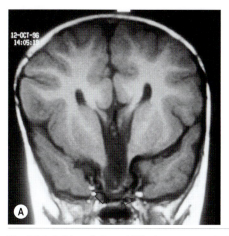
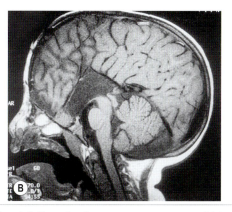
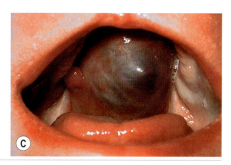

Fig. 54.9 Achiasmia in a child who presented with a cleft lip and palate: see-saw nystagmus. (A) Coronal MRI and (B) sagittal MRI showing a large encephalocele completely dividing the chiasm. (Photographs courtesy of Dr. Dorothy Thompson.) (C) The encephalocele protruding through the hard palate.

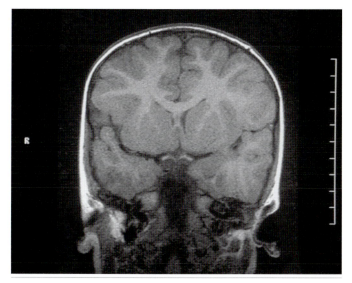

Fig. 54.10 Chiasmal hypoplasia. The chiasm is divided into two halves which are joined by a fragment of tissue. Electrophysiologically the patient was achiasmic. (Photograph courtesy of Dr. Dorothy Thompson.)

that has been described in albinism (see Fig. 54.8).[41] Altered expression of transcription factors such as NRP1, which promotes contralateral axon projection in mammals, may be found to produce achiasmia.[18]

Achiasmia may be complete (Fig. 54.9) or partial (Fig. 54.10). Patients with bilateral optic nerve hypoplasia invariably have chiasmal hypoplasia; those with unilateral optic nerve hypoplasia have selective hypoplasia of the ipsilateral side of the chiasm.[42] Patients with isolated chiasmal hypoplasia may have segmental optic nerve hypoplasia confined to the nasal and temporal sectors of the optic discs.[43,44] Chiasmal anomalies have been described in patients with midline defects, e.g. septo-optic dysplasia, or midfacial defects, or basal encephaloceles. The chiasm may be abnormal in midline facial and skull clefting syndromes associated with hypertelorism and encephalocele.[45-47]

Aplasia and anophthalmia

Unilateral anophthalmos or optic nerve aplasia produces an asymmetrical chiasm.[48] Bilateral anophthalmia or optic nerve aplasia is usually associated with absence of optic nerves, chiasm, and lateral geniculate bodies:[49-51] some show remnants of the optic nerve and chiasm.[52] Bilateral optic nerve aplasia is also associated with an absent chiasm. In mice, prenatal removal of one eye produces a preponderance in crossed fibers from the other eye, whereas postnatal removal of one eye produces an increase in the surviving uncrossed component.[32] Patients with unilateral optic nerve aplasia may show crossed hemispheric VEP asymmetry.[48]

Trauma

Following closed head trauma a child may develop an absolute bitemporal hemianopia and poor acuity and color vision if there is also damage to the non-crossing fibers or optic nerve.[53] Damage to surrounding structures may lead to diabetes insipidus, anosmia, cerebrospinal fluid rhinorrhea, growth defects, and mood changes. Traumatic enucleations can produce tractional injury to the optic chiasm and a temporal hemianopic defect in the other eye.[54]

Tumors

The peculiar geometry of the optic chiasm may render its midportion more vulnerable to deformation stress exerted from below. Despite its anatomical vulnerability to compression by suprasellar tumors, the optic chiasm is surprisingly resistant to compression.[55] Frisén and Jensen found an elevation of 6 mm is necessary to produce visual field defect in 50% of patients, and an additional elevation of 5 mm to produce visual field defects in 90% of patients.[56]

Chiasmal glioma

Chiasmal, optic nerve, and hypothalamic gliomas are closely related; they may show common histopathological features and clinical behavior. All occur with increased frequency in neurofibromatosis (NF). Up to 50% of patients with chiasmal or optic glioma have this disease.[57] It may occur in Beckwith-Wiedemann syndrome – macrosomia, macroglossia, encephalocele, hemihypertrophy, hepatomegaly, and advanced bone age.[58]

Infants with large chiasmal-hypothalamic glioma can present with Russell diencephalic syndrome. The main features are emaciation despite a normal or only slightly diminished caloric intake, alert appearance, hyperkinesis or increased vigor, euphoria, skin pallor, irritability, and normal or accelerated linear growth (see Fig. 54.5). These infants usually have large chiasmal gliomas. Radiation therapy can induce dramatic tumor shrinkage and long-term regression of clinical abnormalities.[59,60]

Small children often present with a compound nystagmus, typically see-saw in nature (see Chapter 90). Any child with a compound nystagmus with rotary, vertical and horizontal elements should be suspected of having a chiasmal lesion.[61] Visual loss is often profound before it is noticed, but in older children the visual defect may be noticed by the child or detected by school visual testing. Some large optic gliomas may have no gross visual defect.[62] Chiasmal gliomas may affect growth and development. An unusual presentation is the "bobble-headed doll syndrome." This is usually an indication of hydrocephalus.

The diagnosis can be suggested by visual field testing or multi-focal visual evoked cortical potential testing. Plain X-rays are seldom used, but the classical finding is an expanded and pear-shaped sella turcica (Fig. 54.11) with chronic bone changes without calcification. One or both optic foramina may be enlarged, especially if there is an optic nerve component to the tumor. CT scanning shows three diagnostic patterns (Fig. 54.12):[63]

1. A tube-like thickening of optic nerve and chiasm.
2. A suprasellar tumor with contiguous optic nerve expansion.
3. A suprasellar tumor with optic tract involvement.

Cystic or "globular" suprasellar tumors are not characteristic and may require histological confirmation.[51] MRI scanning better delineates the extent and nature of the tumor.[64] CT and MRI scanning will both diagnose hydrocephalus. Tumors may evolve in areas thought to be normal on initial CT and even MRI scans.[65]

The histopathology of optic gliomas has long been the subject of a discussion because it is relevant to treatment decisions. Optic gliomas are benign tumors that often behave similarly to hamartomas.[66] They undergo enlargement by an accumulation of mucosubstance, local invasion, induction of hyperplasia in adjacent glial cells, or growth of cell "rests" present in adjacent optic nerve or chiasm.[67] Malignant gliomas rarely occur and mainly in adults. Meningeal spread in children, however, is not unknown[68,69] and spread through a ventriculoperitoneal shunt has been recorded.[70]

The clinical course of 36 optic gliomas (29 chiasmal) were reviewed:[66] some were reviewed in 1971,[71] others in 1986.[57] The 1971 follow-up showed a very stable course but the later follow-up showed that 57% of the 29 patients with chiasmal gliomas were dead, although only 18% from the direct effects of the glioma. The patients were more at risk from other tumors associated with neurofibromatosis type 1 (NF1). Twelve survivors had not had radiation therapy, whereas 11 of 16 patients who died had.[57]

Early studies reported that NF had no influence on the prognosis of optic pathway gliomas. It now appears that NF acts as a protective factor, both visually and neurologically.[72-74] In one study, the most common site of visual pathway involvement in NF was the orbital optic nerve (66%) followed by the chiasm (62%). This contrasted to patients without NF in which the chiasm was the most common site of involvement (91%) and the orbital optic nerves were involved in only 32%. Extension beyond the optic pathway at diagnosis was uncommon in the NF group (2%) but frequent in the non-NF group (68%). In the NF group, the tumor was smaller and the original shape of the optic pathways was preserved (91% vs. 27% in the non-NF group). The presence of a cystic tumor was significantly more common in non-NF patients 66% vs. 9% in the NF group). The tumors in half the NF patients remained stable, in contrast to 5% of the non-NF group. Hydrocephalus as a presenting symptom was found only in the non-NF group.

In children with NF and optic pathway gliomas, the likelihood of visual loss is dependent on the extent and location of the tumor and is particularly associated with involvement of postchiasmal structures.[75] Complete spontaneous regression can occur in both NF and non-NF associated gliomas.[76] Spontaneous visual improvement can also take place in the absence of MRI changes.[77] Many authors have reported a reasonable long-term prognosis that does not seem to be improved by treatment.[57,78,79] Radiotherapy may decrease the size of tumors[51] and may improve vision, but[80-84] its use should be avoided, except in the Russell diencephalic syndrome, because of its serious side-effects, especially in young children.[85-87] Chemotherapy[68,88,89] is as yet of uncertain benefit. Newer agents are promising and may allow deferment of damaging radiotherapy in the young child.[89]

Surgery is not indicated except to treat obstructive hydrocephalus in large chiasmal/hypothalamic gliomas,[90] or if there is a cystic tumor with doubts about its pathology. A biopsy and cyst aspiration may be indicated.

Follow-up usually involves periodic review of the visual fields, acuity, color vision and optic discs, neurophysiological studies, where available, and CT or MRI scanning.

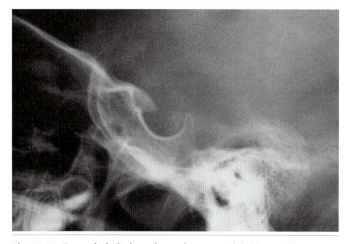

Fig. 54.11 Expanded pituitary fossa shown on plain X-ray with some calcification due to a craniopharyngioma.

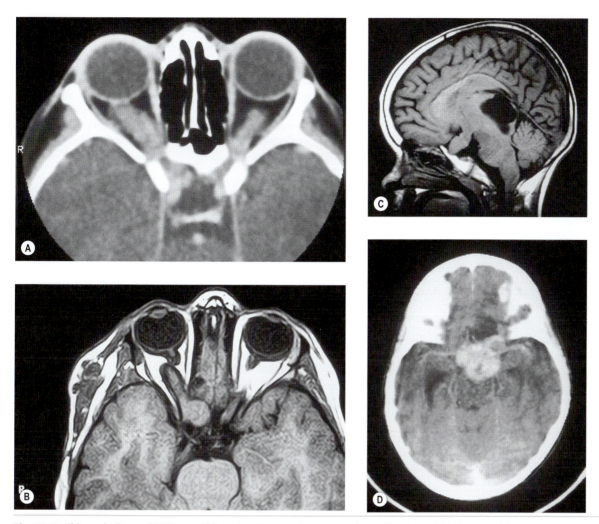

Fig. 54.12 Chiasmal glioma. (A) CT scan of bilateral optic nerve gliomas extending to the chiasm. (B) MRI scan of left optic nerve glioma extending to the chiasm and kinking the intra-orbital optic nerve. (Courtesy of Dr. Kling Chong, Great Ormond Street Hospital, London and Dr. Bob Zimmerman of the Children's Hospital, Philadelphia.) (C) Sagittal MRI of an optic nerve and chiasmal glioma. (D) CT scan with contrast of a cystic chiasmal glioma.

Craniopharyngioma

These cystic tumors grow slowly and do not usually present until after 3 or 4 years of age. They may present even in old age. Their origin is from the pituitary stalk and they compress the chiasm, classically from behind and above. Hypothalamic disturbances are frequent and loss of vision may be profound. Young children tend to develop hypothalamic disturbances or hydrocephalus, whilst older children (first decade) are more likely to present with visual disturbance, strabismus or nystagmus (Figs 54.11 and 54.13). The diagnosis is made by CT or MRI scanning (Fig. 54.13). Calcification occurs in virtually every case in childhood and the tumors are often cystic. Endocrine assessment and management is essential. The tumors are usually treated by surgery with or without radiotherapy; total removal is sometimes possible.

Pituitary adenomas

Pituitary tumors are relatively uncommon in childhood, but can occur in adolescence.[7] In the pubertal period, they are more likely to show extrasellar extension and hemorrhage.[91,92] Children with macroadenomas may develop pituitary apoplexy, characterized by sudden headache, visual deterioration, ophthalmoplegia, and depressed consciousness consequent to hemorrhage into the tumor.[93,94]

Dysgerminoma

Diabetes insipidus is a common symptom of dysgerminomas together with chiasmal defects, including acuity and visual field loss and hypothalamic or pituitary disturbances.[95,96] They are often not large[97] and occur in older children or young adults.[98]

Other chiasmal tumors

Trilateral retinoblastoma is the association of bilateral retinoblastomas and ectopic intracranial primitive neuroectodermal tumor. These midline intracranial tumors most commonly occur in the pineal region, but can occur in the suprasellar area involving the chiasm.[99] The suprasellar tumors can present before the diagnosis of ocular retinoblastoma.[100] Other rare tumors, such as metastatic neuroblastoma, arachnoid cysts, choristomas,[101] ependymomas, epidermoid tumors, leukemic deposits, ectopic pinealomas, and teratomas can occur.[102]

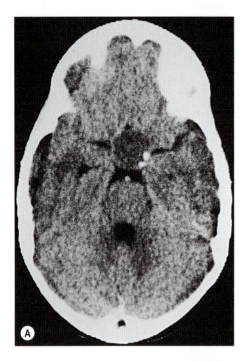

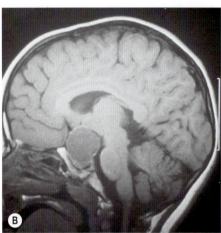

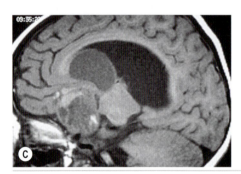

Fig. 54.13 Craniopharyngioma. (A) CT scan of a small cystic craniopharyngioma with calcification in its wall. (B) Sagittal MRI of small craniopharyngioma. (C) MRI scan of a large cystic craniopharyngioma with calcification in its wall. There is hydrocephalus.

Granulomas and chronic inflammatory disorders

The chiasm and surrounding structures may be involved in abnormalities of the skull base as Langerhans' cell histiocytosis (see Chapter 27). A variant of this condition tends to present with diabetes insipidus and visual defects. Sarcoidosis, juvenile xanthogranulomas, and pseudotumors may also affect the chiasmal area.

Sphenoid sinus disease

A chiasmal syndrome, or even rapid blindness, may result from the formation and expansion of a mucocele,[103] even in the absence of symptomatic sinus disease.[104]

Chiasmal neuritis

Chiasmal neuritis is characterized by visual loss and bitemporal hemianopia.[93] Most cases are associated with demyelinating disease,[105] although Purvin et al. described a boy with infectious mononucleosis and chiasmal neuritis.[106] MRI shows swelling and enhancement of the chiasm.[105]

Optochiasmatic arachnoiditis

Optochiasmatic arachnoiditis with localized thickening of the arachnoid at the base of the brain may surround and compress the optic nerves and chiasm. Tuberculous meningitis, hydatid disease, cysticercosis, and fungal disorders (especially in debilitated, immune deficient children) may affect the suprasellar cistern with damage to the chiasm and surrounding structures.[107-109] Although the diagnosis has come to imply that surgical lysis of intracranial adhesions may be necessary to restore vision, the efficacy of surgical treatment remains unproven. Corticosteroids and cytotoxic agents are reportedly effective in some instances.[110] Modern neuroimaging seems to have rendered the diagnosis of optochiasmatic arachnoiditis an anachronism.

Third ventricle distension

In hydrocephalus, distension of the third ventricle may cause chiasmal damage with visual field defects[111] and profound vision loss due to stretching or compression of the optic nerves and chiasm. Unilateral visual loss from compression of one optic nerve against the internal carotid artery has been reported.[112]

Vascular malformations

Aneurysm is an extremely rare cause of chiasmal defects in children.[113,114] In children intracranial aneurysms may be large and associated with polycystic kidneys, coarctation of the aorta, and Marfan's and Ehlers-Danlos syndromes. Multiple aneurysms (usually small) may also occur in "mycotic" aneurysms with subacute bacterial endocarditis and moya moya disease:[115-117] these mostly affect cerebral hemispheres.

Arteriovenous or cavernous malformations localized to the chiasm may hemorrhage to produce the sudden-onset chiasmal visual deficit accompanied by headache (termed *chiasmal apoplexy*).[118]

Radionecrosis

Radiation injury to the optic chiasm is uncommon, but a serious complication of radiation treatment. When vision becomes impaired, enhancement of the chiasm after gadolinium injection is a consistent finding. Chiasmal enlargement may also be present. These neuroimaging abnormalities may antedate visual loss by several months.[119] The pathogenesis involves damage to the capillary beds. The risk of radionecrosis appears to be increased by the concomitant use of chemotherapy.

Empty sella syndrome

Empty sella syndrome is where the subarachnoid space extends into the sella turcica, and the pituitary gland is flattened against the sellar floor or walls.[120,121] Chiasmal visual field defects occasionally occur.[121,122] Chiasmal prolapse can be caused by a distended third ventricle pushing the chiasm down into the sella, or by scarring and contracture pulling the chiasm into the sella. Aqueductal stenosis is particularly prone to produce ballooning of the third ventricle with downward herniation of the chiasm.[123] Pituitary apoplexy or sellar surgery can produce adhesions and cause downward traction of the chiasm into the sella.[122] Although pseudotumor cerebri is the most common cause of empty sella,[121] it does not seem to be associated with chiasmal prolapse into the empty sella.[122]

References

2. Lubkin V, Beizai P, Sadun AA. The eye as metronome of the body. Surv Ophthalmol 2002; 47: 17–26.

4. Hirai T, Ito Y, Arai M, et al. Loss of stereopsis with optic chiasmal lesions and stereoscopic tests as a differential test. Ophthalmology 2002; 109: 1692–702.

5. Polyak S. The Vertebrate Visual System. Chicago: University of Chicago Press; 1957: 779–89.

6. Linksz A. On Writing, Reading and Dyslexia. New York: Grune and Stratton; 1973.

7. Hoyt WF. Correlative functional anatomy of the optic chiasm. Clin Neurosurg 1970; 17: 189–208.

8. Horton JC. Willebrand's knee of the primate optic chiasm is an artefact of monocular enucleation. Trans Am Ophthalmol Soc 1997; 95: 579–609.

11. Guillery RW, Mason CA, Taylor JS. Developmental determinants of the mammalian optic chiasm. J Neurosci 1995; 15: 4727–37.

12. Sretavan DW, Pure E, Siegel MW, et al. Disruption of retinal axon ingrowth by ablation of embryonic mouse optic chiasm neurons. Science 1995; 269: 98–101.

15. Provis JM, van Driel P, Billson FA, et al. Human fetal optic nerve: overproduction and elimination of retinal axons during development. J Comp Neurol 1985; 238: 92–100.

16. Neveu MM, Jeffery G. Chiasm formation in man is fundamentally different from that in the mouse. Eye 2007; 21: 1264–70.

17. Herrera E, Marchus R, Li S, et al. Foxd1 is required for proper formation of the optic chiasm. Development 2004; 131: 5727–39.

18. Carreres MI, Escalante A, Murillo B, et al. Transcription factor Foxd1 is required for the specification of the temporal retina. J Neurosci 2011; 31: 5673–81.

19. Erskine L, Reijntjes S, Pratt T, et al. VEGF signaling through neuropilin 1 guides commissural axon crossing through the optic chiasm. Neuron 2011;70:951–65.

21. Blakemore C. Binocular depth perception and the optic chiasm. Vision Res 1970; 10: 43–7.

23. Hirai T, Kondo M, Takai Y, et al. Bagolini striated glasses test and lesions of the optic chiasm. Binoc Vis Strabis Q 2005; 20: 82–7.

24. Taylor D. Congenital tumors of the anterior visual system dysplasia of the optic discs. Br J Ophthalmol 1982; 66: 455–63.

30. Guillery RW, Kaas JH. A study of normal and congenitally abnormal retinogeniculate projections in cats. J Comp Neurol 1971; 143: 73–100.

32. Guillery RW. Why do albinos and other hypopigmented mutants lack normal binocular vision, and what else is abnormal in their central visual pathways? Eye 1996; 10: 217–21.

34. Creel D, Witkop CJ Jr, King RA. Asymmetric visually evoked potentials in human albinos: evidence for visual system anomalies. Invest Ophthalmol 1974; 13: 430–40.

37. Herrera E, Brown LY, Aruga I, et al. Zic2 patterns binocular vision by specifying the uncrossed retinal projection. Cell 2003; 114: 545–557.

40. Apkarian P, Bour LJ, Barth PG, et al. Non-decussating retinal-fugal fiber syndrome: an inborn achiasmatic malformation associated with visuotopic misrouting, visual evoked potential ipsilateral asymmetry and nystagmus. Brain 1995; 118: 1195–216.

44. Novakovic P, Taylor DS, Hoyt WF. Localizing patterns of optic nerve hypoplasia: retina to occipital lobe. Br J Ophthalmol 1998; 72: 176–82.

46. Thompson DA, Kriss A, Chong K, et al. Visual-evoked potential evidence of chiasmal hypoplasia. Ophthalmology 1999; 106: 2354–61.

56. Frisén L, Jensen C. How robust is the optic chiasm? Perimetric and neuro-imaging correlates. Acta Neurol Scand 2008; 117: 198–204.

59. Russell A. A diencephalic syndrome of emaciation in infancy and childhood. Arch Dis Child 1951; 26: 274–9.

63. Fletcher WA, Imes RK, Hoyt WF. Chiasmal gliomas: appearance and long-term changes demonstrated by computerized tomography. J Neurosurg 1986; 65: 154–9.

76. Parsa CF, Hoyt CS, Lesser RL, et al. Spontaneous regression of optic gliomas. Arch Ophthalmol 2001; 119: 516–29.

77. Liu GT, Lessell S. Spontaneous visual improvement in chiasmal gliomas. Am J Ophthalmol 1992; 114: 193–201.

89. Petronio J, Edwards MS, Prados M, et al. Management of chiasmal and hypothalamic gliomas of infancy and childhood with chemotherapy. J Neurosurg 1991; 74: 701–8.

118. Maitland CG, Abiko S, Hoyt WF, et al. Chiasmal apoplexy: report of four cases. J Neurosurg 1982; 56: 118–22.

123. Osher RH, Corbett JJ, Schatz NJ, et al. Neuro-ophthalmological complications of enlargement of the third ventricle. Br J Ophthalmol 1978; 62: 536–42.

Access the complete reference list online at

http://www.expertconsult.com

Raised intracranial pressure

Nor Fadhilah Mohamad • James F Acheson

Introduction

Raised intracranial pressure (RICP) may be caused by space-occupying lesions including intracranial tumors, obstructed circulation and readsorption of cerebrospinal fluid (CSF) resulting in hydrocephalus, or pseudotumor cerebri syndromes. These conditions generate frequent clinical questions in the eye clinic. For example, patients in primary eye care may have physical signs which point toward RICP and which require urgent neurologic evaluation; other specialists frequently request ophthalmic assessment when there is known or suspected RICP and patients with treated RICP need to be followed carefully to be sure that vision remains stable.

General features of raised intracranial pressure

Headache (see Chapter 108)

Headache is the most common symptom of a brain tumor causing RICP by the time of hospital admission, but is a rare presenting symptom. Because headache is such a common symptom it accounts for many referrals because of concerns about the possibility of RICP. Brain tumor headaches may be intermittent, non-specific, and indistinguishable from tension headaches. A number of features are suggestive of RICP:

1. Headaches that wake the patient at night or are worse on awakening.
2. Headache associated with visual obscuration associated with changes in posture.
3. Supratentorial tumors typically produce frontal headaches.
4. Posterior fossa tumors usually produce occipital headache or neck pain.
5. Nausea and vomiting may be features of RICP (or fourth ventricle tumors).

Brain tumors cause RICP by a variety of mechanisms. They may grow so large, so quickly that they cause stretching of pain-sensitive intracranial structures by a direct mass effect or by an effect on the microvasculature leading to cerebral edema. Tumors may also cause RICP by producing large cysts. Smaller tumors, particularly those in the posterior fossa, may cause headaches by obstructing cerebrospinal fluid circulation and producing hydrocephalus. Headaches with migrainous features are rarely due to an underlying tumor. Occipital tumors may produce occipital seizures, similar in some respects to migraine.

RICP may lead to gradual deterioration in cognition, intermittent drowsiness, and eventually coma. Progressive herniation of the medial temporal lobe across the tentorium causes an ipsilateral third nerve palsy; herniation of the cerebellar tonsils through the foramen magnum leads to coma and death.

Non-visual features of raised intracranial pressure

Infants and younger children may present with vague symptoms including poor feeding, mood changes, lethargy, irritability, and somnolence. Other symptoms include failure to thrive, behavioral disturbances, drowsiness, posturing, and seizures. Physical findings may include bulging fontanelles, rapid growth of head circumference, and distended scalp veins. In older children and teenagers, abnormal signs may be confined to the eyes.

Ophthalmic features of raised intracranial pressure

Pupils

Examination of the pupils using a bright light will help to exclude partial third nerve palsy and the pupillary light-near dissociation of a pretectal syndrome.

Eye movements

Abnormalities may include supranuclear vertical gaze palsies in pretectal syndromes, horizontal gaze palsies and nystagmus in posterior fossa masses, and skew deviation in a pretectal syndrome. Single infranuclear cranial nerve palsies may be a false localizing sign of raised pressure, especially sixth or fourth nerve palsy; third nerve palsy may be due to uncal herniation. Childhood comitant esotropia with a deviation larger for distance than near may originate from central nervous system (CNS) lesions. Tumors involving the anterior visual pathways (e.g. optic pathway glioma and craniopharyngioma) may present with a sensory deviation in one eye with advanced visual loss and optic atrophy combined with RICP.

Fundoscopy

Great care is needed when a good view for fundoscopy is difficult to obtain, in patients with high refractive error and with buried optic disk drusen.

Visual function

Acute papilledema does not usually reduce vision (apart from blindspot enlargement), but as secondary atrophy develops, peripheral field loss may develop with preserved central acuity. Acuity is only lost after major field loss, and is not usually recoverable. Monitoring visual field (VF) is mandatory. Monitoring disk swelling alone is not sufficient.

Hydrocephalus and shunts

Hydrocephalus is RICP associated with dilated lateral ventricles. This is due to an imbalance between secretion of CSF in the choroid plexus within the lateral ventricles, and reabsorbtion from the arachnoid villi in the subarachnoid space. Causes are classified as:

1. Obstructive: there is a block preventing CSF circulation within the ventricular system.
2. Communicating: when reabsorption in the subarachnoid space is impaired.

Hydrocephalus may be congenital or acquired. Congenital hydrocephalus is one of the most frequent congenital abnormalities of the CNS and a common complication of spina bifida and neural tube defects. Other causes include cerebral aqueduct stenosis, Chiari malformation, and Dandy-Walker syndrome. Common causes of acquired hydrocephalus include meningitis and intraventricular hemorrhage in preterm infants.

The features of hydrocephalus depend on the age of the child and whether the RICP is acute in onset. When the cranial sutures have not closed, there is a progressive increase in skull growth with separation of the sutures. The fontanel is tense and scalp veins are dilated due to compression of the cortical veins and sinuses. If the ventricles are greatly enlarged, the skull may transilluminate. There may be failure to thrive and developmental delay. Papilledema is uncommon but the "setting-sun" sign – upper-lid retraction and downwardly deviated eyes due to upgaze paresis – may be seen in infants. In later childhood, papilledema is typically present often accompanied by unilateral or bilateral sixth nerve paresis and upgaze impairment.

Ventriculo-peritoneal shunt insertion is the most commonly performed pediatric neurosurgical procedure. In a series from the United States, 69 000 discharges and 36 000 procedures related to shunts were performed in 1995. The population with hydrocephalus has grown considerably since that study due to improved survival of very premature infants. The morbidity due to complications remains significant. In one UK series, there was a 11% mortality rate during a 10-year follow-up study of 155 children.[1]

In addition to shunts, some children are managed with endoscopic third ventriculostomy. There continues to be a significant failure rate of up to 40% in the first year. One cause of failure is obstruction, with recurrent RICP. Ophthalmologists may be involved in assessing these children. However, visual assessment, is complicated by pre-existing optic disk atrophy from previous papilledema. Recurrent RICP may not cause the optic disks to swell. Moreover, afferent visual deficits (acuity and field) do not always reflect isolated optic atrophy secondary to papilledema. Chiasmal compression by a dilated third ventricle or cortical visual impairment causes visual dysfunction: this is particularly important in preterm infants with periventricular leukomalacia and intraventricular hemorrhage.

Ocular ultrasound is useful in assessing dilatation of the retrobulbar optic nerve sheath. This correlates with acute ICP rises and is a non-invasive, well-tolerated, technique allowing an indirect measure of shunt function. Some cases still require lumbar puncture or ICP monitoring by an indwelling intracranial device

Idiopathic intracranial hypertension (pseudotumor cerebri)

Introduction

Idiopathic intracranial hypertension (IIH) is characterized by elevated ICP in the absence of any identifiable etiology. The modified Dandy criteria include:

"High-pressure" headache and papilledema

CSF opening pressure of >25 cmH$_2$O

An awake and alert patient

No localizing signs other than lateral rectus paresis

Normal CSF constituents

Normal brain imaging with no evidence of venous or CSF obstruction

No other cause of RICP

Drugs	Metabolic and endocrine	Systemic disorders and infections
Tetracyclines	Obesity and recent weight gain	Iron deficiency
Vitamin A analogs	Hypo/ hyperthyroidism	Aplastic anemia
Nalidixic acid	Cushing's disease	Sickle cell anemia
Sulphonamides	Adrenal insufficiency	Systemic lupus
Corticosteroid therapy or withdrawal	Menarche	Lyme disease
Growth hormone		Sarcoidosis
Oral contraceptives		Guillain-Barre

IIH is uncommon in children.[2-5] It classically occurs in obese adult women of childbearing age. The annual incidence of IIH in children is 0.9 in 100 000 and increases to 1.5 in 100 000 in adolescents aged 12–15 years.[2] In reproductive age women over 10% above ideal body weight it is 13/100 000. There is no sex predilection and obesity is less significant in prepubertal children.[2,4] After puberty, there is a higher incidence of obesity and female preponderance.[4,5]

Etiology

In contrast to adults, many children will demonstrate associated conditions. This "secondary" IIH accounts for the majority of pediatric cases. Some of the associations with IIH are listed in Box 55.1. Cerebral venous outflow obstruction due to thrombosis or dural arteriovenous shunting are important causes, which may only be diagnosed by specific investigations including CT venography and angiography.

Clinical presentation

Children with RICP often present with non-specific features. There are a subset of children who do not have headache, and other children who have headache, but who do not have papilledema.[6] Headache is often accompanied by nausea and vomiting, is progressive, occurs daily, may be diffuse, pulsatile or non-pulsatile, and is aggravated by Valsalva maneuver or change in posture. Transient visual obscurations occur several times a day in the majority of patients who develop papilledema.

Visual acuity loss is present in up to 20% of cases and VF loss in up to 91% of pediatric patients. Field deficits include enlarged blind spot, nasal field defects especially inferonasal, disk-related arcuate scotomata, and global constriction. Other ophthalmic presentations are double vision and squint secondary to abducens palsy, retro-orbital pain, and photophobia especially in prepubertal children.

Course and prognosis

Rapid resolution of disk swelling and improvement of visual function is expected in patients with mild to moderate papilledema following prompt diagnosis and treatment. Residual visual acuity deficits and VF defects are present in 0–10% and 17–33% of patients, respectively, after treatment. Chronic papilledema, optic disk infarction, chorioretinal folds, macular edema, subretinal and peripapillary hemorrhages, or neovascular membrane may cause progressive impairment of vision despite treatment. Some patients run a malignant course with rapid and fulminant visual failure.[7]

Neuroimaging

Magnetic resonance imaging (MRI) is the preferred imaging technique and can detect most mass lesions and hydrocephalus. Non-localizing changes seen on MRI scans include flattening of the posterior sclera, distension of perioptic subarachnoid space, intraocular protrusion of pre-laminar optic nerve, tortuosity of optic nerve, and empty sella.

In selected cases with progressive visual failure, recent otitis media or sinus infection, magnetic resonance venography (MRV) and/or CT venography is advisable to rule out cerebral venous sinus thrombosis.

Lumbar puncture

Lumbar puncture should only be performed after a space-occupying lesion has been ruled out on neuroimaging. Several factors artificially raise the pressure readings including Valsalva maneuver, (crying), flexion, hypercarbia, and general anesthesia. The opening pressure should be measured and CSF sent for biochemistry and cytology.

Ophthalmic assessment

All suspected cases of IIH must undergo ophthalmologic assessment. Visual acuity, color vision, pupillary light reflexes, and ocular motility should be recorded. Dilated fundoscopy allows careful assessment of the optic nerve head. Fundus photography can be used to monitor changes over time. Ultrasonography can differentiate true papilledema from pseudopapilledema due to disk drusen by characterizing pathologic optic nerve sheath dilatation.[8] Buried optic disk drusen can coexist with pathologic disk swelling due to RICP, and assessment of thickening of the peripapillary retinal nerve fiber layer by optical coherence tomography is useful.

Early visual loss is best detected by VF assessment. VF is used not only to diagnose but also to monitor progress and treatment. Children aged 8 or more can reliably perform field tests. Manual kinetic perimetry remains useful in younger and less cooperative patients.

Management

The goal of treatment is to relieve symptoms and preserve vision. A multidisciplinary team involving ophthalmology, pediatric neurology, neuroradiology, and neurosurgery is essential. In obese children, usually older, managed weight reduction may help. Some patients are cured after a single diagnostic lumbar puncture. However, serial lumbar punctures are poorly tolerated and only indicated in the very short-term when visual failure is progressive and a shunt is required.

Medical therapy begins with diuretics. Acetazolamide is the drug of choice as it reduces CSF production. Common dose-related side effects include paresthesia of the lips, fingers and toes, gastrointestinal upset, electrolyte imbalance, fatigue, depression, anorexia, and nausea, which may limit compliance. Thiazide and loop diuretics including bendrofluazide and furosemide may be used. Topiramate, an anticonvulsant drug with secondary carbonic anhydrase inhibitory properties, may be useful. In addition to its effects on reduced CSF production and reducing papilledema, some obese patients may experience beneficial weight loss.

When headache cannot be controlled or when visual failure progresses in spite of optimal medical management, CSF diversion surgery is indicated. Options include ventriculoperitoneal and lumboperitoneal shunting, as well as optic nerve sheath decompression (ONSD).[9] There are no true comparative studies to evaluate these methods. Shunting alone will normalize raised pressure and is usually preferred when headache is the dominant feature. However, if visual failure is prominent without significant headache, especially in one eye, ONSD may be preferred, especially if the optic nerve sheath is large on MRI scanning.

Illustrative cases

Case 1 (Figs 55.1–55.3)

A 15-year-old schoolgirl presented with a 2-week history of headache, visual disturbance, and neck pain. Fundoscopy revealed chronic papilledema with atrophy of the right optic disk. She had extensive VF loss in both eyes with preservation of her acuities and reasonable color vision. MRI showed no space-occupying lesion with normal sized ventricles, and MRV confirmed the patency of the major dural sinuses and evidence of fluid distension of both perioptic subarachnoid space and intraocular protrusion of the optic nerve head. BMI (body mass index) 27 kg/m^2. There was no relevant medical history or medications.

The opening CSF pressure was more than 40 cmH$_2$O. Her symptoms improved soon after the procedure, but vision continued to deteriorate. She was started on acetazolamide 250 mg

qds. There was persistent high CSF pressure despite the acetazolamide being increased to 500 mg qds.

She underwent bilateral optic nerve fenestration. A lumbar puncture showed opening pressure of 40 cmH$_2$O; therefore, a lumboperitoneal shunt was inserted. The vision stabilized at RVA 6/9, LVA CF with bilateral field loss.

Key point: RICP due to IIH may present with advanced visual loss. Aggressive management including CSF diversion surgery may be required to stabilize vision and prevent further loss.

Case 2 (Fig. 55.4)

A 14-year-old boy had blurred vision and variable diplopia on reading. Examination showed normal visual acuities and fundi. He had an exodeviation, greater at near thought to represent convergence insufficiency. Four weeks later he had increasing symptoms including headache. He had sluggish direct pupillary light reactions, absent upwardly directed saccades in response to the rotating optokinetic drum, convergent-retraction nystagmus on attempted upwardly directed saccades, and optic disk swelling. Imaging revealed an enhancing pineal region tumor with dilated lateral and third ventricles consistent with obstructive hydrocephalus. After third ventriculostomy a biopsy revealed a germinoma without ventricular seeding. He was referred for radiotherapy.

Key point: Pretectal mass lesions with obstructive hydrocephalus may present with dysfunction of the near-triad.

Case 3

A 4-year-old boy developed a left comitant convergent squint and had bilateral papilledema on examination. An MRI brain scan showed dilated optic nerve sheaths and normal intracranial appearances; CSF opening pressure was over 40 cmH$_2$O. Medical evaluation was initially unremarkable and IIH was

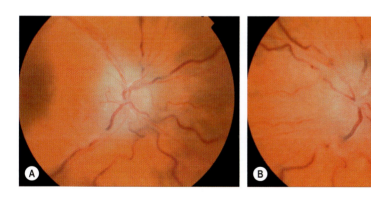

Fig. 55.1 Right and left fundi showing acute papilledema.

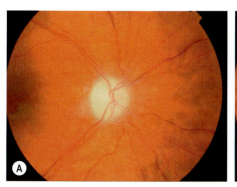
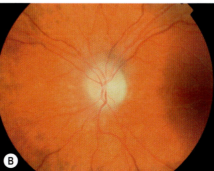

Fig. 55.2 Right and left fundi showing subsequent secondary optic atrophy.

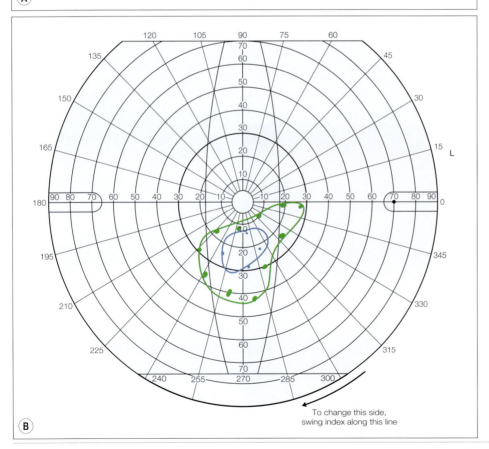

Fig. 55.3 Right and left visual fields showing bilateral visual field loss by time vision had stabilized. Green = V/4e isopter. Blue = I/4e isopter.

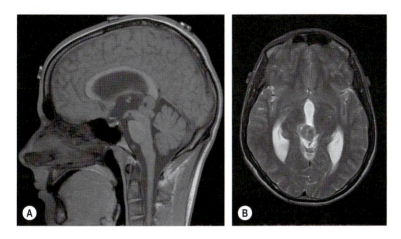

Fig. 55.4 Sagittal non-contrast T1-weighted and axial contrast enhanced T2-weighted MR images of pretectal tumor with secondary obstructive hydrocephalus.

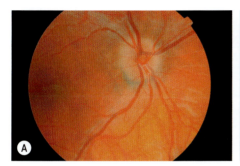
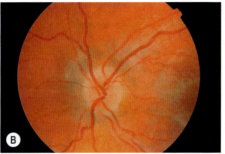

Fig. 55.5 Left and right fundi showing subtle optic disk swelling.

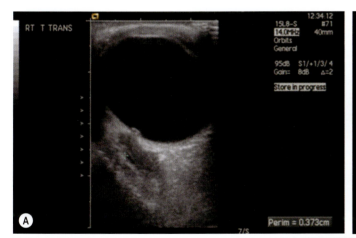
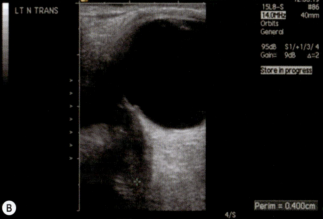

Fig. 55.6 B-mode ultrasound showing dilated optic nerve sheath on right and left and no drusen.

diagnosed. He was treated with oral acetazolamide 500 mg bd, but this did not control the papilledema. His headaches became more prominent. Further evaluation yielded a diagnosis of multisutural synostosis and after vault expansion surgery the headaches and papilledema resolved.

Key point: IIH is always a diagnosis of exclusion and underlying causes must be sought.

Case 4 (Figs 55.5 and 55.6)

A 10-year-old boy had mild bilateral optic disk elevation with subtle optic disk margin blurring. The referral diagnosis was optic disk drusen. Ultrasound showed dilated optic nerve sheaths and no evidence of drusen. Further investigations showed chronic RICP due to IHH.

Key point: Optic disk drusen require confirmation by ultrasound or neuroimaging and their presence does not exclude the possibility of true papilledema due to RICP.

References

1. Casey A, Kimmings EJ, Kleinlugtebeld AD, et al. The long-term outlook for hydrocephalus in childhood: a ten year cohort study of 155 patients. Pediatr Neurosurg 1997; 27: 63–70.

2. Gordon K. Paediatric pseudotumor cerebri: descriptive epidemiology. Can J Neurol Sci 1997; 24: 219–21.

3. Cinciripini GS, Donahue S, Borchert MS. Idiopathic intracranial hypertension in prepubertal pediatric patients: characteristics, treatment, and outcome. Am J Ophthalmol 1999; 127: 178–82.

4. Kesler A, Fattal-Valevski A. Idiopathic intracranial hypertension in the pediatric population. J Child Neurol 2002; 17: 745–8.

5. Youroukos S, Psychou F, Fryssiras S, et al. Idiopathic intracranial hypertension in children. J Child Neurol 2000; 15: 453–7.

6. Lim M, Kurian M, Penn A, et al. Visual failure without headache in idiopathic intracranial hypertension. Arch Dis Child 2005; 90: 206–10.

7. Thambisetty M, Lavin PJ, Newman N, Biousse V. Fulminant idiopathic intracranial hypertension. Neurology 2007; 68: 229–32.

8. Newman WD, Hollman AS, Dutton GN, Carachi R. Measurement of optic nerve sheath diameter by ultrasound: a means of detecting acute raised intracranial pressure. Br J Ophthalmol 2002; 86: 1109–13.

9. Thuente D, Buckley E. Pediatric optic nerve sheath decompression. Ophthalmology 2005; 112: 724–7.

Part 7
Neural visual systems

The brain and cerebral visual impairment

Creig S Hoyt

Numerous congenital and acquired disorders of the central nervous system affect children's vision and many directly affect vital visual structures with varying disability. Others do not, but are associated with structural eye defects. In many parts of the world, especially in more developed countries, the prevalence of visual impairment in children due to brain disorders equals or exceeds that related to purely ocular disease. Many children with visual impairment due to brain disorders are multi-handicapped and their long-term potential for successful rehabilitation, education, employment, and independent-living is limited. Nevertheless, it is essential that their visual deficits and potential be carefully assessed in order that appropriate medical, rehabilitation, and educational services can be provided for them.

Developmental defects

Embryological errors

Cephalocele (encephalocele)

During the first month of embryogenesis, a neural plate is formed which invaginates into the neural groove and then fuses into a neural tube. Cephaloceles (defects in the skull and dura mater with extracranial extension of intracranial structures) are probably the result of a disturbance in the closure of the neural groove. Alternatively, they may occur as a post-neuralation event with brain tissue herniating through the mesenchyme that will give rise to the cranium and dura. Three of the four major types of cephaloceles are of interest to ophthalmologists.

1. *Occipital cephaloceles.* In these portions of the occipital cortex and the occipital horn of the lateral ventricle herniate into the defect. Severe visual defects are associated both with the anomaly and the results of any surgical correction.

2. *Frontal ethmoidalcephaloceles.* These do not usually impinge on any visual structures, but ipsilateral optic nerve dysplasia may be associated with them.

3. *Nasal pharyngeal cephaloceles.* These are uncommon, but visual function is almost always affected. The optic nerves and chiasm may be compromised as they are stretched when they extend into the sac of the defect. Optic nerve hypoplasia and retinal dysplasia and coloboma are frequent associations.

Holoprosencephaly

During the second month of gestation the forebrain (prosencephalon) is cleaved transversely into the telencephalon and diencephalon and sagittally into the cerebral hemispheres and lateral ventricles. Failure of differentiation and cleaving of the prosencephalon results in a group of disorders referred to as "the holoprosencephalies." These are caused by both teratogens and genetic factors. Maternal diabetes is the most common recognized teratogen. Holoprosencephaly can be seen in a number of syndromes including Patau's syndrome (trisomy 13), Edwards' syndrome (trisomy 18), and de Morsier's syndrome. Facial dysmorphism (hypotelorism and midline clefts) and numerous central nervous system anomalies are frequently associated (Fig. 56.1). Corpus callosum dysgenesis is common; unsurprisingly, therefore, so is optic nerve hypoplasia (see Chapter 51). Indeed, a significant subset of patients with septo-optic dysplasia may have a mild form of lobar holoprosencephaly.

Malformations of cortical development

Between the second and fourth gestational months, the neurons in the ventricular and subventricular zones of the lateral ventricles proliferate and migrate to the cortical plates. This area of cell proliferation is known as the germinal matrix; here, stem cells give rise to the neurons and glial cells that will form the mature brain. Neurons in early embryogenesis migrate relatively short distances; neurons later in development migrate long distances across the intermediate zones. Neurons arriving first in the cortical mantle assume the deepest locations while later arriving neurons assume a more superficial location. Migration is facilitated by radial glial cells

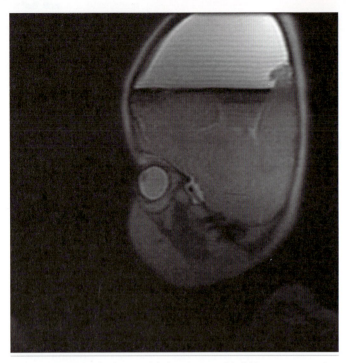

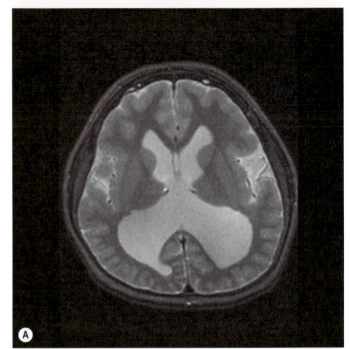

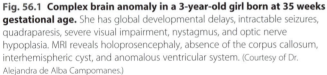

Fig. 56.1 Complex brain anomaly in a 3-year-old girl born at 35 weeks gestational age. She has global developmental delays, intractable seizures, quadraparesis, severe visual impairment, nystagmus, and optic nerve hypoplasia. MRI reveals holoprosencephaly, absence of the corpus callosum, interhemispheric cyst, and anomalous ventricular system. (Courtesy of Dr. Alejandra de Alba Campomanes.)

acting as guidelines. After arriving in the cortex neurons form discrete lamina and begin to establish synaptic connection with local and distant neurons. Aberrations in this normal migration and development process result in important neural abnormalities.[1] In general, the resulting malformations can be divided into three categories – those due to:

1. Abnormal neuronal and glial proliferation, or apoptosis.
2. Abnormal neuronal migration.
3. Abnormal cortical organization.

Lissencephaly (smooth brain) occurs when neurons fail to migrate normally to the cortical mantle but remain in deeper layers. Over 90% of children with lissencephaly have seizures. Cobblestone lissencephaly occurs in at least three muscular dystrophy syndromes with important ocular features:

a. Fukuyama-type congenital muscular dystrophy: affected children develop high myopia and a retinal degeneration (Fig. 56.2).
b. The muscle–brain–eye syndrome: this is associated with myopia and early-onset glaucoma and cataracts.
b. The Walker-Warburg syndrome: this comprises microphthalmos, glaucoma, optic nerve anomalies, and retinal dysplasia and non-attachment.

Pachygyria is related to lissencephaly, but occurs at a later stage resulting in reduced numbers of gyri that are thick and underpopulated with neurons. Pachygyria of the occipital cortex may be associated with congenital hemianopia (see below). Pachygyria of the perirolandic and occipital areas is a prominent feature of Zellweger's syndrome.

Polymicrogyria is the most common malformation of cortical development. It occurs as the result of the interruption of the

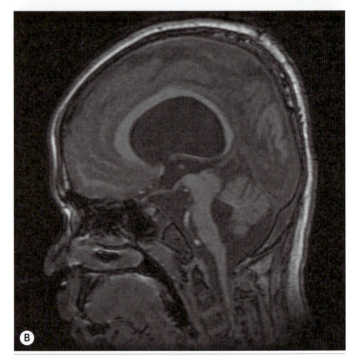

Fig. 56.2 A 10-year-old Vietnamese girl with severe developmental delays and hypotonia presents with bilateral cataracts, glaucoma, retinal detachments, and vitreous hemorrhages. (A). Axial MRI reveals dilated ventricles and pachygyria of the frontal cortex. (B) Sagittal MRI reveals pachygyria and polymicrogyria of frontal cortex, partial agenesis of the septum pellucidum, and hypoplasia of the brainstem. A diagnosis of Fukuyama's disease was made. (Courtesy of Dr. Alejandra de Alba Campomanes.)

late stages of neuron migration during the stages of cortical organization. The neurons reach the cortical mantle, but the deep layers are distributed which results in disorganized, multiple, and small gyri. Its effect on neurological function is less severe than the proliferation and migration anomalies. It may occur as an isolated focal anomaly of little consequence. The most common area is around the Sylvian fissure. However, it may also occur as a diffuse disorder affecting the entire brain. As an isolated and focal disorder it has been associated with congenital hemianopia (occipital cortex) and dyslexia (left frontal and temporal cortex). It is an important feature of several genetic syndromes including Aicardi's syndrome, Joubert's syndrome, Zellweger's spectrum, Sturge-Weber syndrome, X-linked hydrocephalus, and 22q11.2 deletion syndrome. It is also associated with numerous metabolic disorders.[2]

Schizencephaly (agenetic porencephaly) is characterized by full thickness clefts spanning the wall of the cerebral hemispheres that are lined by gray matter and often surrounded by polymicrogyric cortex. The pathogenesis is incompletely understood although it is thought to represent an in utero injury to the germinal matrix during the second trimester before the hemispheres form. Previous reports that schizencephaly may be associated with mutations of the EMX2 homeobox gene, located on chromosome 10q26, and expressed in the germinal matrix has been challenged.[3] The clefts may be unilateral or bilateral; the lips of the clefts may be open or closed. Seizures, hemiplegia, and mental retardation are the most common symptoms. Involvement of the occipital cortex is unusual but, when it occurs, especially when the cleft's lips are fused, a homonymous hemianopia may occur. In contrast, patients with bilateral clefts are more likely to be severely retarded, severely limited by motor problems and blindness. The blindness is not usually cortical in origin, but due to optic nerve hypoplasia, a frequent accompanying anomaly in all forms of schizencephaly.

Congenital hemianopia

Children with congenital hemianopia show little evidence of visual dysfunction; the visual field defect is often discovered later in life on a routine eye examination. There may be a history of frequent bicycle or auto accidents, but many patients experience little effect on their daily lives. Therefore, the history may not be helpful in suspecting the presence of a congenital hemianopia. However, there are certain associated ophthalmologic and systemic findings that should alert the ophthalmologist to the possibility of a congenital hemifield defect.[4]

Most children with a congenital, but not acquired, hemianopia, turn their face toward the defective field when fixing on a target straight ahead of them (see Chapter 81). It is not clear how this compensates for the field defect, although the intact field is "centered" on the body by this maneuver. In any case, a persistent face turn in a child without incomitant strabismus or nystagmus with a null zone (the more common ocular causes of such a turn) should prompt an evaluation of the visual fields. In some cases, the face turn is accompanied by a constant, non-alternating exotropia;[5] the exotropic eye is ipsilateral to the field defect (see Chapter 78). Theoretically, a large angle exotropia might significantly expand the binocular visual field with the appropriate sensory adaptation (harmonious anomalous retinal correspondence) although the evidence that it does so is incomplete. The frequent occurrence of exodeviations in neurologic disorders raises the question of the specificity of this finding. However, the unique combination of a face turn and exotropia ipsilateral to the face turn is highly suggestive of congenital hemianopia.

In addition to the visual field defect, face turn, and possible exodeviation, the most prominent ophthalmological finding in these children is localized changes in the optic disc and

nerve fiber layer – "homonymous hemioptic atrophy" (hypoplasia). There is loss of retinal nerve fibers in the retinal sectors nasal and temporal to the disc in the eye contralateral to the field defect; in the ipsilateral eye the loss is superior and inferior. This subtle pattern of nerve fiber loss can be seen ophthalmoscopically or with OCT (optical coherence tomography).[6] Examination of the optic discs will reveal a band-shaped atrophy of the contralateral disc and temporal atrophy of the ipsilateral disc. Since the lesions causing congenital hemianopia are almost always posterior to the lateral geniculate body, this points to transsynaptic degeneration of the retinogeniculate striate pathways. This has been thought to only occur with prenatal or perinatal insults, but recent experiments in non-human primates and OCT studies in patients with acquired hemianopias suggest that this is not the case.[7]

Children with congenital homonymous hemianopia may show an afferent pupil defect in the eye contralateral to the field defect. However, it is usually very subtle and rarely useful diagnostically.

Isolated congenital hemianopias are typically caused by developmental anomalies of the occipital cortex.[8] These include:

- Occipital lobe dysplasia: abnormality of neuronal/glial proliferation
- Occipital lobe pachygyria: abnormality of neuronal migration
- Occipital lobe polymicrogyria: abnormality of cortical organization
- Porencephaly with or without polymicrogyria
- Gangliogliomas: neoplastic abnormality of neuronal/glial proliferation
- Cerebral hemiatrophy
- Vascular malformations.

The more extensive the cortical anomaly, the more likely there will be other neurological disorders including hemiplegia, seizures, and developmental delays. The majority of patients with congenital hemiplegias will have an accompanying hemianopia. Syndromes in which congenital occipital cortex lesions with hemianopia occur include the Sturge-Weber syndrome, retinocephalic vascular malformation syndrome (Wyburn-Mason), and familial porencephaly.

Asymmetric injury to the periventricular ventricular white matter (periventricular leukomalacia, PVL) can present as an isolated congenital hemianopia, or, more commonly, with hemiparesis. The vast majority of cases of PVL present with bilateral involvement (see below). Rarely, congenital hemianopia associated with absence of the optic tract has been reported. It is unclear how this defect might occur.

Patients with congenital hemianopia are less visually disabled than those with acquired hemianopia. Our understanding of their adaptations and compensations accounting for their minimal disability is incomplete. The possibility that a face turn and/or exotropia could be compensatory has been cited above. A unique saccadic strategy limited to patients with congenital hemianopia allows them to search the blind field. This is distinctly more efficient than the multiple hypometric saccades made by the patient with an acquired hemianopia, but it can occur in congenital lesions (Video 56.1). Moreover, in children with acquired hemianopias the reaction time to initiate a saccade to explore the blind field is prolonged; this is not the case in congenital hemianopia.[9] Some have suggested that the extra-geniculostriate pathways may be playing a compensatory role; others have theorized that re-wiring of the uninjured brain allows it to assume the functions of the injured portion. Convincing evidence for the latter two theories is wanting.

Patients with isolated congenital hemianopias require very little in the way of special ophthalmologic care except to communicate with schools, employers, and government agencies (especially the driving authorities) to reassure them that many of these children are little affected by their visual field defect. If the child has a constant, non-alternating exotropia, strabismus surgery may be contraindicated.

Acquired hemianopia

Children with acquired hemianopia present in a similar fashion to adults with comparable acquired lesions. Visual acuity is usually normal, but the field defect is easily detected and the disability associated with it declared in the history. Trauma and tumor are the most important causes of acquired hemianopia in children. In contrast to congenital hemianopia where the lesion is usually cortical, in children with acquired hemianopia the most common site of injury is the optic radiations. A significant number of children with acquired hemianopias show some spontaneous improvement in the visual field.[10]

Perinatal insults

There are many causes of perinatal brain injury but the vast majority of them are metabolic. They may occur as the result of inherited defects in metabolic pathways or from transient ischemia-reperfusion events. It is the latter group that accounts for most of the visual disability related to brain disorders in infancy. Although these disorders are referred to as hypoxic-ischemic in nature, there are multiple factors that contribute to the pathophysiology. Nevertheless, cerebral hypoperfusion is the primary problem with hypoxia playing an ancillary role in the genesis of the brain damage. The pattern of brain injury and the nature of the resulting visual deficits are determined largely by the age of the infant at the time of the insult as well as the duration and severity of the hypoperfusion event.

The premature infant

Several types of brain injury may occur in premature infants due to a mild to moderate episode of hypoxia and hypoperfusion. These include PVL, periventricular hemorrhagic infarct, germinal matrix hemorrhage, intraventricular hemorrhage, and cerebellar infarction. PVL is the predominant form of brain injury and the leading cause of cerebral palsy and cognitive defects in premature infants.

Periventricular leukomalacia

Advances in neonatology have improved the long-term survival of premature infants and simultaneously reduced the overall incidence and severity of white matter injury in surviving preterm infants, especially those with a birth weight of more than 1500 g. Nevertheless, PVL remains the major brain pathology in preterm infants. It accounts for cognitive/behavioral deficits in 25–50% and cerebral palsy in 5–10% of infants with a birth weight less than 1500 g.[11] It has significant

visual consequences and is a major cause of visual disability in many parts of the world.

The pathogenesis of PVL is complex, but most likely involves ischemia/reperfusion in a critically ill premature infant with impaired regulation of cerebral blood flow. The lack of autoregulation of cerebral blood flow in premature neonates and the high incidence of lung immaturity contributes to the hypoxic perfusion difficulties. In light of these pathogenetic events, the frequent coexistence of PVL and retinopathy of prematurity (see Chapter 43) should not be surprising. The association of maternal infection with PVL suggests that inflammatory mechanisms play an important secondary role in this type of brain injury. The primary cells vulnerable to hypoxic-ischemic injury in the immature brain are the premyelinating oligodendrocytes, oligodendrocyte progenitor cells and subplate neurons. Subplate neurons only appear transiently during brain development, but they are essential to the formation of the connections between the thalamus and visual cortex. As a result, the pathology of PVL consists of periventricular necrosis and diffuse gliosis in the cerebral white matter and neuronal loss in the thalamus, corpus callosum, and globus pallidus.[12] In long-term survivors with PVL, neuroimaging studies may show reduced cerebral white matter volume, impaired myelination, ventriculomegaly, and reduced volume in the corpus callosum (especially posterior portion) and thalamus (Fig. 56.3). Although PVL is primarily a disorder of ill, preterm babies it does occur in near-term infants.[13]

The motor and visual pathways course through the periventricular white matter that is affected. As a result motor (commonly "spastic diplegia") and visual impairment are the most

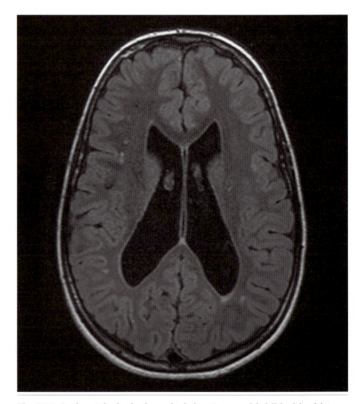

Fig. 56.3 Periventricular leukomalacia in a 9-year-old child with a history of premature birth at 25 weeks gestational age. Axial MRI reveals multiple small foci of high FLAIR signal seen in the periventricular and subcortical white matter representing ischemic changes or gliosis. The ventricles are markedly enlarged with adjacent white matter loss. (Courtesy of Dr. Stacy Pineles.)

common neurologic findings in PVL. The motor fibers serving the lower extremities course more medial than those of the upper extremity and thus are more likely to be injured by the periventricular injury. However, the consequences for the motor system may range from a mild spastic diplegia to a severe quadraparesis. Other neurologic symptoms may include athetosis, seizures, and cognitive and attention disorders.

Visual impairment is equally variable in its severity, ranging from nearly blind to minor field defects. The inferior visual fields appear to be more affected than superior in most patients.[14] A normal-sized optic nerve with an enlarged optic cup ("pseudo-glaucomatous") is seen in many patients. It is probable that this anomalous optic nerve is not an independent contributing factor to the visual disability, but simply a "marker" for the upstream damage to the optic radiations. This implies that retrograde transsynaptic degeneration has occurred, similar to the case of congenital hemianopia described above. However, the importance of recognizing that a large optic cup in a premature infant is far more likely to indicate PVL and not glaucoma cannot be overemphasized. Tonic downward gaze is a common finding in young infants with PVL. That it is not an upgaze palsy (as in hydrocephalus) can be easily demonstrated on doll's head maneuver. It is usually accompanied by a moderate to large angle esotropia, much less frequently an exotropia. The tonic downward gaze usually resolves, but the esotropia persists. It is tempting to attribute the downward deviation and esotropia to the thalamic damage, but there are, as yet, no correlative neuroimaging or pathologic studies addressing this issue. Unlike in adult thalamic injury, the pupils are usually not miotic in infants with PVL. Infantile nystagmus and manifest-latent and latent nystagmus have all been observed in children with PVL; most of the children with nystagmus will also have strabismus. As in all cases of cerebral palsy, reduced accommodative facility may occur in PVL and it should be specifically sought and corrected with glasses, if found.

The long-term visual disability of children with PVL is frequently underestimated by analyzing only the visual field deficits. A visuo-perceptual impairment related to PVL has been defined.[15] It consists of a deficit in eye–hand coordination and a constructional dyspraxia thought to reflect damage to the "dorsal stream" of the occipital-parietal pathways (see Chapter 57). Less well studied, but perhaps more important, is the question concerning the visual consequences of the thalamic damage resulting from the injury to the subplate neurons. Cognitive deficits occur in 30–50% of very preterm (<32 gestational weeks) survivors.[12] Injury to two specific subnuclei of the thalamus is found in many of them. The mediodorsal nucleus through its reciprocal connections with the prefrontal lobe plays an essential role in working memory. The mediodorsal nucleus in consort with several cortical centers is vital for attention mechanisms, especially visual attention. Further studies are needed to understand the full range of visual disabilities in PVL.

There is no known treatment for PVL. The role of the ophthalmologist is to assess the visual deficits as fully as possible and counsel the child's parents, other physicians, rehabilitation specialists, and teachers about them. Refractive errors and poor accommodation, if present, should be corrected even in severely handicapped children. Strabismus surgery may be indicated if the child's general health would not be compromised by an anesthetic. Many trials are underway to see whether PVL can be prevented or lessened in its severity. Pre-myelinating oligodendroglia are highly vulnerable to death caused by glutamate, free radicals, and pro-inflammatory cytokines. Pharmacological interventions that target these toxic molecules may be useful in diminishing the severity of PVL.[16]

Periventricular and intraventricular hemorrhage

Despite advances in neonatal care, intraventricular hemorrhage remains a major complication of prematurity. It characteristically originates from the periventricular germinal matrix, a highly vascular site where glial and neuronal precursor cells are located at the head of the caudate nucleus beneath the ventricular ependyma. The vessels within the germinal matrix have very thin walls and are especially sensitive to changes in blood flow and pressure. Most intraventricular hemorrhages are an extension of a germinal matrix hemorrhage which usually occurs within the first 48 hours after birth.[17] Periventricular and intraventricular hemorrhages in premature babies have been divided into four grades:

Grade I: germinal matrix hemorrhage with little or no intraventricular hemorrhage.

Grade II: germinal matrix hemorrhage with extension into the ventricle, but normal ventricle size.

Grade III: intraventricular hemorrhage with ventricular enlargement.

Grade IV: periventricular hemorrhagic infarction.

Grade I and II hemorrhages have a good prognosis for survival and good neurological outcome. Grade III and IV hemorrhages have a significant risk of early death or significant neurological sequelae in the survivors. The neurological complications with important visual consequences include post-hemorrhagic hydrocephalus (see Chapter 55) and infarction, and porencephalic cyst formation in the areas of the occipital-parietal cortex. Significant visual loss may occur even in vigorously treated hydrocephalic neonates as a result of direct damage to the visual cortex and secondary optic atrophy (see Chapter 55).[18] Periventricular hemorrhagic infarctions are associated with significant brain damage and more than 50% of the neonates affected have serious neurological sequelae. In many of these neonates porencephalic cysts will develop in the area of infarction.

Porencephalic cysts are focal cavities within the cortex which have smooth walls and minimal surrounding glial reaction (Fig. 56.4). They are the result of focal brain destruction from any cause prior to the 26th week of gestation when the potential for glial reactivity is minimal. Porencephalic cysts associated with periventricular hemorrhagic infarction commonly involve the optic radiations and occipital cortex and result in homonymous hemianopia and homonymous hemioptic atrophy (hypoplasia) (see above).

The term infant

Neonatal encephalopathy

Neonatal encephalopathy occurs in 1 to 6 of every 1000 live term births. It is a serious medical problem: 15–20% of affected infants die in the newborn period; 25% develop permanent neurologic deficits, and many of these will have significant visual disability.[19] The terms "neonatal encephalopathy," "hypoxic-ischemic encephalopathy," and "birth asphyxia" are often used interchangeably. This is unfortunate. Although hypoxia and ischemia are a major factor in most cases of

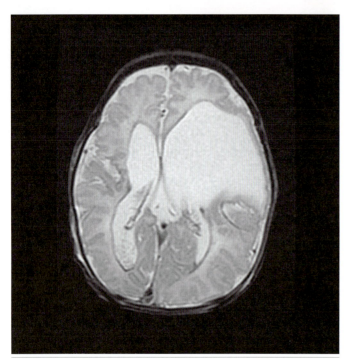

Fig. 56.4 Bilateral hemorrhagic porencephaly seen on MRI in a term infant. The patient has bilateral horizontal gaze palsies and quadraparesis.

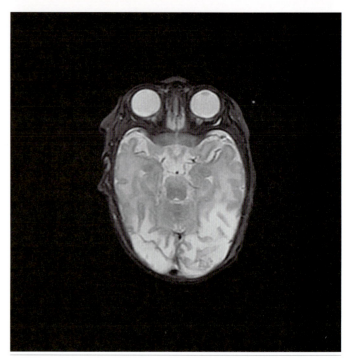

Fig. 56.5 A T2-weighted MRI scan of a term infant with severe hypoxic-ischemic encephalopathy primarily involving the visual cortex.

neonatal encephalopathy, intrauterine inflammation may be an essential co-factor in many cases. Moreover, antepartum risk factors (maternal hypotension, infertility treatment, and thyroid disease) have been identified. However, even if antepartum risk factors are present, prospective MRI studies suggest that at least 80% of term infants who develop neonatal encephalopathy sustain a causative acute brain injury in the perinatal period.[20]

The regions of the brain susceptible to injury due to hypoxia and ischemia change depending on the gestational age of the infant at the time of injury. Unlike the case of immature oligodendrocytes and oligodendrocyte progenitor cells, mature oligodendrocytes are resistant to hypoxic-ischemic damage.[19] Thus, isolated deep white matter injury is not the primary feature of neonatal encephalopathy in the term infant. The main site of damage in the term infant is in the cerebral cortex intervascular boundary zones ("watershed areas"). These are the areas between the anterior and middle cerebral arteries and those between the middle and posterior cerebral arteries. Certain neurons in the deep grey nuclei and perirolandic cortex are most likely to be damaged. As a result, the most common consequence of mild to moderate hypotensive events in the term infant is discrete infarctions in the frontal and parieto-occipital regions of the brain. Watershed cortical damage is the primary site of pathology but, in extensive infarcts, the underlying white matter may be affected. MRI studies may reveal (Fig. 56.5):

1. Wedge-shaped infarctions in the watershed zones.
2. Cortical thinning and diminution of the underlying white matter in the area of infarction.
3. Ex-vacuo dilation of the lateral ventricles.
4. The development of ulegyria (narrow and distorted gyri, a secondary gyrial anomaly) resulting from the cortical shrinkage.

A different pattern of injury is seen in neonates who suffer profound hypotension or cardio-circulatory arrest. They show injury primarily in the lateral thalami, posterior putamen, hippocampi, and corticospinal pathways, regions of the brain most active metabolically and with the highest degree of synaptic construction at birth.[21] Some of the children develop damage in the lateral geniculate nucleus and optic radiations. Many of these infants die in infancy, but if they survive they will manifest a severe seizure disorder, quadriparesis, mental retardation, microcephaly, and blindness.

It is difficult to predict during the neonatal period which infants with signs of encephalopathy will suffer permanent neurological disability. Thirty percent of neonates with moderate encephalopathy have clinically normal outcomes. The most common neurological sequelae of neonatal encephalopathy are motor impairment, developmental delays, mental retardation, seizures, and visual impairment. The motor impairment is often a mixture of spasticity, ataxia, weakness, and athetosis. Neonatal seizures occur in the majority of infants with neonatal encephalopathy. Although they are difficult to treat and a poor prognostic sign, they are a persistent problem in only a minority. Cognitive disability occurs infrequently in moderate encephalopathy, but is a common feature in children with severe encephalopathy. Neuropsychological testing identifies memory and attention/executive disabilities as the most common cognitive consequences of neonatal injury.

Infarction of the occipital cortex may result in a wide range of visual disability depending on the location and size of the infarct. The degree of visual impairment may range from "apparent blindness" to barely detectable isolated visual field defects (see Chapter 57). The majority of these children have detectable residual vision. However, they all have variable and inconsistent visual performance. They function better when well rested and in familiar surroundings. Color perception is frequently superior to perception of form. Detection of motion may be the only consistently documented visual function. When reaching for objects, they frequently turn their face away from the object to apparently use their peripheral vision. They may be able to read isolated letters of varying sizes on an acuity test, but unable to read whole words of a similar size.

Examination of the anterior visual pathways is usually normal. Although there is OCT evidence that transsynaptic degeneration of the geniculostriate pathways does occur with postnatal injuries to the occipital cortex,[5,7] only in a minority of cases of neonatal encephalopathy is mild optic atrophy seen on ophthalmoscopy.[22] Optic atrophy is not a major determinant of visual disability in most cases where it is found. The pupil responses are normal. In contrast to PVL, nystagmus rarely occurs. In a minority of cases exotropia may occur, but large angle esotropias are rarely seen. Supranuclear ocular motor abnormalities that may occur in children with neonatal encephalopathy include horizontal conjugate gaze deviations, horizontal gaze palsies, and difficulties in ocular pursuit movements. These may contribute to the child's visual disability. Accommodation should be specifically evaluated and, if found to be abnormal, treated with spectacles.

The diagnosis of neonatal encephalopathy with visual loss can usually be established on the basis of the history and other neurologic findings. Neuroimaging studies can be helpful in subtle cases with subtle vision loss and minimal neurologic abnormalities (Fig. 56.6). They are also useful to document the anatomic site(s) and extent of brain damage, but correlations with functional disability and outcome have proven to be disappointingly imprecise with these studies. Functional neuroimaging studies such as positron emission tomography and single photon emission tomography may prove to be valuable especially in demonstrating that sites remote from the major anatomic lesions seen on conventional neuroimaging may be contributing to the overall visual disability. Although still a research procedure, diffusion tensor imaging holds promise to be the most definitive way to assess the extent and nature of brain damage in neonates.[23] Pattern visual evoked potential (VEP) studies can be helpful in diagnosing visual cortex damage, but they are imprecise when quantitatively evaluating visual function in these children. Sweep and Step VEPs may be more reliable in quantitative assessments. Vernier acuity VEPs may prove to be the most sensitive electrophysiological technique for quantitative assessment of these injuries.[24]

In caring for the child with neonatal encephalopathy and visual disability, the ophthalmologist's role is twofold:

1. Periodic assessment of the visual disability and residual visual function.
2. Treatment of any co-existing eye disorder.

Clinical assessment of these children is difficult and time-consuming but vital as a part of the habilitation and education programs for them. Behavioral assessment techniques have been developed to assist ophthalmologists in counseling those caring for these children (see Chapter 57). The vast majority of affected children show some improvement over time, so re-evaluation is essential. There are no reliable predictors of long-term visual outcome for any specific child. Parents, educators and other therapists should be encouraged to keep an open mind about the ultimate visual outcome, especially in early infancy when often little or no purposeful visual function

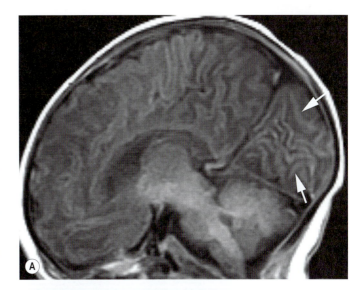

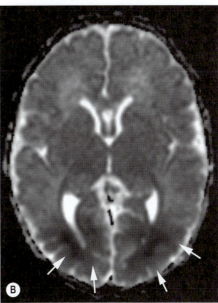

Fig. 56.6 An 8-day-old infant with seizures and profound hypoglycemia. (A) The sagittal T1-weighted image shows abnormal high signal intensity of the occipital cortex. (B) The axial diffusivity map (ADC map) shows markedly reduced diffusion in both occipital lobes (arrows on figures). The child has cortical visual impairment. (Courtesy of Dr. Jim Barkovich.)

can be appreciated. Intensive visual stimulation programs appear to enhance the visual recovery in these children.[25]

Until recently, there has been no available treatment for the brain damage that occurs in neonatal encephalopathy. Recently, techniques for neuroprotection of neonates have been developed. Cerebral hypothermia improves outcome of experimental perinatal hypoxia-ischemia. A multi-centered randomized controlled trial of selective head cooling after neonatal encephalopathy showed a beneficial effect in neonates with moderate brain injury.[26] Subsequent studies have confirmed that hypothermia is effective in reducing death and moderate to severe neurodevelopmental disability in neonatal encephalopathy. Treating neonatal encephalopathy with moderate whole body or selective head hypothermia has become routine clinical practice in many centers.[27] Studies of drugs that might enhance protection or repair in neonatal encephalopathy are ongoing.

Older children

When hypoxia, ischemia, or circulatory arrest occurs in older children, a different pattern of brain injury is seen compared to neonates. The physiological and biochemical differences that account for this are not yet defined. The differences are relatively minor in injuries from mild to moderate hypotension although the older child is less likely to develop deep white matter injury. With profound hypotension, the older child will show basal ganglia involvement (with sparing of the thalamus) and severe diffuse cortical involvement. The relatively modest injuries suffered by many children as the result of near-drowning events probably are due to the protective effect of hypothermia (the water) and the mammalian diving reflex.

Visual recovery in brain disorders

There is considerable evidence to suggest that the capacity of the child's visual system to recover from cerebral injury exceeds that of the adult.[25,28,29] There are several reasons that might explain this improved capacity. First, the child may be able to develop unique strategies to utilize the remaining visual function. Examples of this include the large single saccade and preserved visual search capacity in cases of congenital hemianopia.[9] A second factor may be that the young brain is endowed with endogenous neuroprotection and repair and regeneration capacities superior to the adult brain.[30] A third possibility is that the child can expand the visual functions normally subserved in uninjured cortical areas outside the primary visual cortex. This has been well documented in experimental animals.[22] This might account for why motion detection (Riddoch's phenomenon) is preferentially preserved in so many children with neonatal encephalopathy. Fourth, it is now apparent that the extent of neurological deficit after a focal brain injury cannot be accounted for by the dysfunction attributable just to it. Rather, it is determined by the functional impairment of the connected neural systems that are structurally intact.[31] Diaschisis (inhibition of function in distant portions of the brain anatomically connected to injured brain) is a major factor in determining this, but deactivation, hyperactivity, and hemispheric imbalance also play a role. Children may be more capable of recalibrating these uninjured connected systems. Finally, the possibility that the extrageniculostriate system might be capable of processing vision even in the absence of the visual cortex (blindsight) seems real. There is some evidence that it plays a role in visual recovery in children with visual impairment due to brain injury.[32] Further defining these recovery mechanisms would be extremely useful in designing habilitation and education programs for these children.

References

1. Sun XZ, Takahashi S, Cui C, et al. Normal and abnormal migration in the developing cortex. J Med Invest 2002; 49: 97–110.
2. Hennekam RCM, Barth PG. Syndromic cortical dysplasias: a review. In: Barth PG, editor. Disorders of Neuronal Migration. London: MacKeith Press; 2003: 135–69.
3. Merello E, Swanson E, De Marco P, et al. No major role for the EMX2 gene in schizencephaly. Am J Med Genet 2008; 9: 1142–50.
4. Paysee EA, Coats DK. Anomalous head posture with early-onset homonymous heminanopia. J AAPOS 1997; 1: 209–13.
5. Donahue SP, Haun AK. Exotropia and face turn in children with homonymous hemianopia. J Neuro-Ophthalmol 2007; 27: 304–7.
6. Mehta JS, Plant GT. Optical coherence tomography (OCT) findings in congenital long-standing homonymous hemianopia. Am J Ophthalmol 2005; 140: 727–9.
7. Jindahra P, Petrie A, Plant GT. Retro-grade trans-synaptic retinal ganglion cell loss identified by optical coherence tomography. Brain 2009; 132: 628–34.
8. Barkovich AJ. Pediatric Neuroimaging. Philadelphia: Lippincott William and Wilkins; 2005: 190–3, 292–364.
9. Tinelli F, Guzzetta A, Bertini C, et al. Greater sparing of visual search abilities in children after congenital rather than acquired brain damage. Neurorehabil Neural Repair 2011; doi: 10.1177/1545968311407780.
10. Kedar S, Zhang X, Lynn MJ, et al. Pediatric homonymous hemianopia. J AAPOS 2006; 10: 249–52.
11. Marlow N, Wolfe D, Bracewell M, Samara M. Neurologic and developmental disability at six years after extremely preterm birth. N Engl J Med 2005; 352: 9–19.
12. Ligam P, Haynes RL, Folkerth RD, et al. Thalamic damage in periventricular leukomalacia: novel pathologic observations relevant to cognitive deficits in survivors of prematurity. Pediatr Res 2009; 65: 524–9.
13. Kinney HC. The near-term (late preterm) human brain and risk for periventricular leukomalacia: A review. Seminars in Perinatal 2006; 30: 81–8.
14. Jacobson L, Flodmark O, Martin L. Visual field defects in prematurely born patients with white matter damage of immaturity: a multiple case study. Acta Ophthalmol Scand 2006; 64: 357–62.
15. Fazzi E, Bova SM, Uggetti C, et al. Visual-perception impairment in children with periventricular leukomalacia. Brain Dev 2004; 26: 506–12.
16. Deng W, Pleasure J, Pleasure D. Progress in periventricular leukomalacia. Arch Neurol 2008; 65: 1291–5.
17. Ballabh P. Intraventricular hemorrhage in preterm infants: mechanism of disease. Pediatr Res 2010; 67: 1–8.
18. O'Keefe M, Kafil-Hussain N, Flitcroft I, Lanigan B. Ocular significance of intraventricular haemorrhage in premature infants. Br J Ophthalmol 2001; 85: 357–9.
19. Ferriero DM. Neonatal brain injury. N Engl J Med 2004; 351: 1985–95.
20. Cowan F, Rutherford M, Groenendaal F, et al. Origin and timing of brain lesions in term infants with neonatal encephalopathy. Lancet 2003; 361: 736–42.
21. Miller SP, Ramaswamy V, Michelson D, et al. Patterns of brain injury in term neonatal encephalopathy. J Pediatr 2005; 146: 453–60.
22. Hoyt CS. Brain injury and the eye. Eye 2007; 21: 1285–9.
23. McKinstry R, Miller J, Snyder A, et al. A prospective, longitudinal diffusion tensor imaging study of brain injury in newborns. Neurology 2002; 59: 824–33.
24. Skoezenski AM, Good WV. Vernier acuity is selectively affected in infants and children with cortical visual impairment. Dev Med Child Neurol 2004; 46: 526–32.
25. Malkowicz DE, Myers G, Leisman G. Rehabilitation of cortical visual impairment in children. Int J Neurosci 2006; 116: 1015–33.
26. Gluckman PD, Wyatt JS, Azzopardi D, et al. Selective head cooling with mild systemic hypothermia after neonatal encephalopathy: multicentre randomized trial. Lancet 2005; 365: 663–70.
27. Azzopardi D, Strohm B, Edwards AD, et al. Treatment of asphyxiated newborns with moderate hypothermia in routine clinical practice: how cooling is managed in the UK outside a clinical trial. Arch Dis Child Fetal Neonatal Ed 2009; 94: F260–4.
28. Werth R. Cerebral blindness and plasticity of the visual system in children: a review of visual capacities in patients with occipital lesions, hemispherectomy or hydrancephaly. Restorative Neurol Neurosci 2008; 26: 377–89.

29. Matsuba CA, Jan JE. Long-term outcome of children with cortical visual impairment. Dev Med Child Neurol 2006; 48: 508–12.

30. Kochanek PM, Clark RS, Ruppell RA, et al. Biochemical, cellular, and molecular mechanisms in the evolution of secondary damage and severe traumatic brain injury in infants and children: lessons learned from the bedside. Pediatr Critical Care 2000; 1: 4–19.

31. Corbetta M, Kincade MJ, Lewis C, et al. Neural basis and recovery of spatial attention in spatial neglect. Nat Neurosci 2005; 8: 1603–10.

32. Boyle NJ, Jones DH, Hamilton R, et al. Blindsight in children: does it exist and can it be used to help the child? Observations on a case series. Dev Med Child Neurol 2005; 47: 699–702.

Part 7
Neural visual systems

Perceptual aspects of cerebral visual impairment and their management

Gordon N Dutton • Richard J C Bowman

Introduction

Cerebral visual impairment (CVI) is the commonest cause of visual impairment in children in developed countries.[1,2] Improved perinatal care and survival of young children with profound neurological disease have increased the prevalence of cerebral causes.[3] A large proportion of the brain involves visual processing, and, when affected, visual perception and cognition can be disordered. Affected young children are anosagnostic (unaware) for their perceptual deficits, which cause a range of often disabling visual behaviors.

Retrogeniculate damage to the visual brain can impair visual acuity and contrast sensitivity, and restrict visual fields,[4,5] while damage to the posterior parietal and temporal lobes and their pathways gives rise to perceptual and cognitive visual impairment.

The pathology may primarily affect gray matter, white matter, or as in some cases of cerebral palsy, no anatomical abnormality is found on MRI scanning. Perceptual visual dysfunction in children is common but easily missed. It is not always accompanied by visual field deficits and poor visual acuity. Strabismus is a frequent association, and affected children may not be identified.[6]

Patterns of perceptual and cognitive visual dysfunction vary; many cases manifest unique features. The principal elements of perceptual visual dysfunction include impaired visual search (due to limited visual attention), often associated with inaccuracy of visual guidance of movement of the limbs. Peripheral bilateral lower visual field impairment is a common accompaniment due to posterior parietal pathology. Less commonly, impaired recognition due to disordered image processing of people, shape and objects, frequently associated with disordered orientation and route finding, may occur. The visual system alone may be affected, or associated with cerebral palsy and/or other developmental disorders. Perceptual visual dysfunction also contributes to the features of autistic spectrum disorder,[7] and Williams' syndrome.[8]

The differential diagnosis for perceptual visual dysfunction in children includes cerebellar and labyrinthine disorders (which can cause the horizon to appear tilted), the Pulfrich phenomenon (causing the perception of oncoming targets on the affected side to appear to veer towards them), and the Charles Bonnet syndrome (causing unformed or formed visual hallucinations).

Synesthesia (unformed visual hallucinations while listening to music) is a benign condition, which simply warrants explanation. Normal physiological perceptions can cause concern.[9] These include blurring of print, words "swimming" when reading (relaxing accommodation), seeing double (physiological diplopia), or colors (after-image effect) or spots (vitreous floaters), and things looking smaller or bigger than they should (image size flux with accommodation or cortical adaptation). The history with normal clinical examination allows the child and family to be reassured, without recourse to needless investigation.

A clinical model of the perceptual visual system

Of the many connections to centers for visual processing, the striate cortex has two principal pathways (Fig. 57.1):

1. The dorsal stream linking to the posterior parietal cortex.
2. The ventral stream linking to the inferotemporal cortex.

Both are responsible for discrete, separate but closely interconnected perceptual functions (Fig. 57.2).

The dorsal stream and the result of bilateral damage

The dorsal stream and posterior parietal cortex assimilate incoming visual information to bring about moment-to-moment, immediate ("on line") visual guidance of skilled actions. A constantly refreshed virtual map of the environment is created without conscious awareness. This creates internal, precise, "egocentric coordinates" to continuously stream, coincide with, and emulate the surrounding three-dimensional environment in time and space. This determines the temporal and spatial resolution of body movement and visual search.

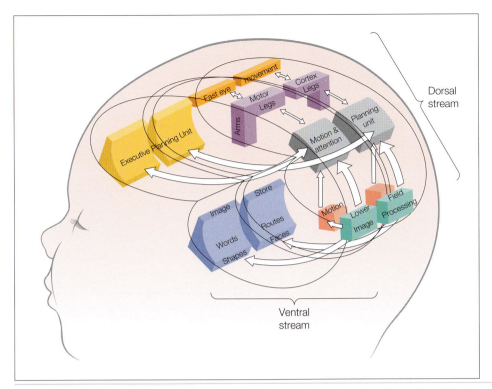

Fig. 57.1 Diagram showing a basic conceptual framework for the areas serving higher visual function, and their connections.

This internal representation of the surrounding image data provides the substrate for frontal areas to appraise and search the visual scene, to make choices, and facilitates accurate visual guidance of movement of the body.

Bilateral damage affecting the dorsal stream and posterior parietal territory causes inaccurate visual guidance of movement (optic ataxia), despite conscious visuospatial awareness afforded by the ventral stream. It commonly impairs perception of movement and limits the number of entities which can be attended to at once, thus impairing visual search. In its severe form (Balint's syndrome), it results in great disability using vision to guide movement (despite intact stereopsis in some cases) accompanied by the disability of being able to identify a limited number of items at once. Although eye movements are intact, there may be an inability to *elect* to move the eyes to visual targets ("egocentric coordinates" – extrageniculostriate vision).

The ventral stream and its damage

The ventral stream and inferotemporal cortices provide a store of previous visual experiences, and serve conscious recognition and understanding of what is seen, by reference to the prior memory base.

Severe focal damage to the inferotemporal cortices and ventral stream pathways impairs visual recognition and route finding, but visual guidance of movement may remain intact. This has been called "travel vision." Such residual perception of the moving image is known as the Riddoch phenomenon,[10] and the intact visual guidance of movement is served by "blindsight."[11]

Less severe bilateral ventral stream dysfunction causes inaccurate recognition of faces, objects, and shapes. Impaired face recognition ranges in severity from inability to recognize close family members, to not being able to recognize people when seen out of context. Incorrect identification of strangers as being known is typical. Children can become adept at recognizing people by voice and other cues. It is only when cues are not available, such as a mother gesturing to her child through a window, that the problem becomes apparent. Difficulties in recognizing shape and form have also been described, and profound alexia may be evident.

Visual memory is commonly impaired in children with ventral stream dysfunction. This is required for copying, drawing, and remembering where things are. Educational strategies are required for these problems.

Unilateral ventral stream damage

Acquired damage to the right temporal lobe impairs recognition of people (prosopagnosia) and their facial expressions. Less commonly, animals may also be difficult to recognize and differentiate. Impairment in the ability to find the way around and be oriented in place (topographic agnosia) is common.

Acquired damage to the left temporal lobe impairs recognition of shape (shape agnosia), objects (object agnosia), letters (literal alexia), and words causing alexia or dyslexia. The deficits can be relative or absolute.

Very early onset damage to ventral stream structures tends to be bilateral, and impairs both form and shape recognition to similar degrees. When there is additional damage to the occipital lobes causing reduced visual acuity, it can be difficult to determine whether lack of recognition relates solely to poor acuity. Memory impairment is a clue to possible additional visual agnosia.

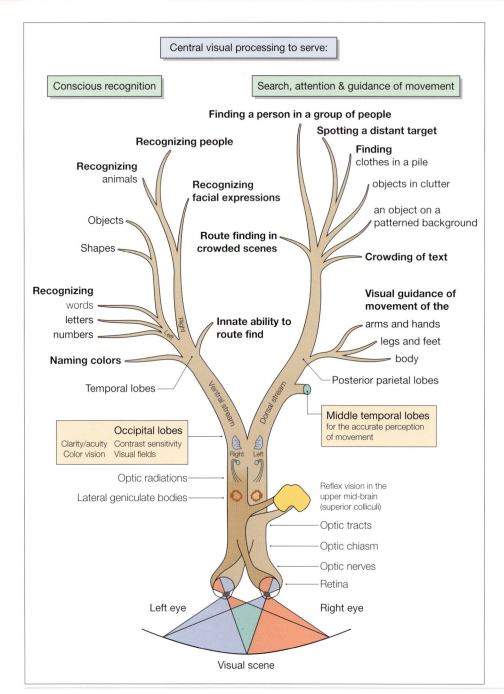

Fig. 57.2 Diagram in the form of a tree, denoting the range of visual functions which can be impaired by focal damage. Damage at a low level of the tree interferes with all the functions above that level. The branching pattern denotes the common groupings of patterns of dysfunction seen in children sustaining damage to the brain impairing vision and perception.

Diagnosis of perceptual visual dysfunction

History taking

Features of cerebral visual impairment in general

CVI covers a wide range of visual impairment and dysfunction, which can be difficult to quantify when co-existing motor or intellectual dysfunction impair communication. Variability in vision related to impaired attention, visual overload, and fatigue is common. Variation in visual field assessment probably relates to attentional and simultanagnostic visual dysfunction. Light gazing and photophobia have both been described with severe visual impairment.

Features of perceptual visual dysfunction

We have found that structured history taking for behaviors typical of perceptual visual dysfunction helps identify the condition and pathology, as well as guiding habilitation. We have developed targeted question inventories.

A 51 item inventory (divided into seven groups of questions) has been devised to seek dysfunction in the following areas: visual field or localized attention; perception of movement; visually guided movement of the body; visual attention; coping with crowded scenes or environments; and recognition and orientation) (Table 57.1). This inventory has good reliability in evaluating mild/moderate CVI.[12] In our experience, the following questions (found to be particularly specific and sensitive) provide a useful, rapid tool for determining the children who warrant more detailed assessment:[13]

1. Does your child have difficulty walking downstairs?
2. Does your child have difficulty seeing things which are moving quickly, such as small animals?
3. Does your child have difficulty seeing something which is pointed out in the distance?
4. Does your child have difficulty locating an item of clothing in a pile of clothes?
5. Does your child find copying words or drawings time-consuming and difficult?

A 12 item inventory has also been tested on a large longitudinal population-based cohort ("normals").[14] Three sets of visual behaviors explained half the overall variance in the visual perceptual question responses obtained:

1. Interpreting cluttered scenes.
2. Visual guidance of movement.
3. Face recognition.

Table 57.1 – Inventory of questions designed to elicit the nature and impact of perceptual and cognitive visual impairment upon daily life

Name:		Hospital number:	
Temporal severity gradings			
All of the time	4	Most of the time	3
Some of the time	2	Occasionally	1
Never	0	Not applicable	N/A (e.g. the child is too young)
Question topics			
Lower visual field		Grade	
Walking over toys and obstacles			
Walking over little children (e.g. brother or sister)			
Tripping over or bumping into low obstacles			
Difficulty going down stairs			
Walking off the end of pavements			
Tripping going up pavements			
Difficulty/fear of going down a slope			
Easier to go up a slope			
Leaving food on the near side of the plate			
School work is easier with a tilted work station			
Unilateral visual field			
Regularly misses traffic on one side		(Which side?)	
Leaving food on one side of the plate		(Which side?)	
Bumping into doorways or obstacles on one side		(Which side?)	
Regularly missing information on one side of a page		(Which side?)	
Difficulty finding the beginning of a line when reading			
Difficulty finding the next word when reading			
Seeing moving things			
Movement of the child – difficulty seeing when moving quickly			
Movement of the environment – difficulty seeing from a moving car			
Movement of targets in the environment – difficulty seeing things which are moving quickly, such as small animals			
Avoid watching fast moving TV			
Choose to watch slow moving TV			
Seeing information when there is a lot to see			
Difficulty seeing something which is pointed out in the distance			
Difficulty identifying a close friend or relative in a group			
Difficulty finding things in a supermarket			

Continued

Table 57.1 *Continued*

Getting lost in places where there is a lot to see	
Difficulty finding clothes in a pile of clothes	
Difficulty finding toys in a toy box	-
Getting close to the television	(How close?)
Reading enhanced by masking off surrounding text	
Copying time consuming and difficult	
Seeing where the feet are	
Late to walk	No / Yes (When?)
Difficulty going down stairs	
Difficulty going up stairs	
Pavements – foot may be lifted too high or too low, too early or too late	
Holding onto clothes of accompanying person, while pulling down	

Inside floor boundaries may be difficult to cross:
    New boundaries
    Well known boundaries	

Exploring a floor boundary with the foot before crossing the boundary	
Exploring outside floor boundaries, e.g. from tarmac onto grass with the foot	
Uneven ground is difficult to walk over	
Likes to push a wheeled vehicle such as a toy pram or pushchair	
Furniture –	Is it bumped into? Is it bumped into if it is moved?
Does moving the furniture cause anger?	
Seeing where the hands are	
Accuracy of reach is inaccurate	
Hand inaccurately positioned to pick an object up	
The gap between fingers to pick up an object is wide and inaccurate	
Attention	
Difficulty engaging visual attention	
Difficulty maintaining visual attention	
Difficulty in breaking visual attenion	
Loss of visual attention when things are moving at the side	
Vision is worse when listening	
Vision is worse when talking	
Vision is worse when day dreaming	
Behavior	
Rooms with a lot of pattern are associated with difficult behavior	
Rooms with a lot of clutter are associated with difficult behavior	
Plain undecorated places are associated with better behavior	
Being in crowds may be associated with difficult behavior	
Quiet places, open countryside may be associated with better behavior	
Behavior in busy supermarkets may be difficult	
Better behavior in quiet corner shops	
Angry reactions when other restless children cause distraction	
Recognition	
Difficulty recognizing a parent through a window	

Table 57.1 *Continued*

Difficulty recognizing close relatives: In real life In photographs
Difficulty recognizing friends and acquaintances: In real life In photographs
Difficulty recognizing people from unusual angles
Incorrect recognition of people who are not known
Difficulty understanding the meaning of facial expressions
Difficulty recognizing and naming different types of animal
Tends to get lost in places which are not well known
Easily gets lost outside because of disorientation
Difficulty locating a chosen room
Difficulty finding things in immediate surroundings
Difficulty naming colors_
Difficulty naming shapes such as squares, triangles, and circles
Difficulty recognizing objects such as the family car
Difficulty with letter and word recognition
Additional question
Do you have other concerns about vision or behavior? If so, what are they?
This list should only be employed once history taking has elicited evidence of such difficulties, and it is important to seek to validate the parental observations.

The cluttered scenes factor had a positive correlation with reading test results, while the guidance of movement factor suggested a positive correlation with mathematics results. This suggests that structured history taking in the clinic may play a role in screening for sub-clinical visual perceptual disorders, potentially affecting school performance. Such screening would obviously only be appropriate should evidence emerge for effective educational strategies for such disorders.

Further refinement of these questions and investigation of how their results correlate with targeted psychometric tests of visual perception are required.

Examination

Neuro-ophthalmological assessment

A neuro-ophthalmological examination is required, including visual acuities for near and distance, color vision (often relatively well preserved in CVI), visual fields, ocular movement assessment (apraxias, gaze palsies, and poor smooth pursuit are all common, more so if there is subcortical involvement), fundoscopy (optic atrophy or retinal abnormalities are often co-existent), and refraction (higher rates of all types of refractive error are seen) including dynamic retinoscopy because impaired accommodation is common in cerebral palsy.[15]

Psychometric evaluation

Reduced psychometric visual perception scores are found in extremely premature children and those with CVI. Children with impaired brain function may score poorly on psychometric tests of visual perception either because of a specific visual perceptual disorder or global impairment due to diffuse brain damage.[16] The results of such tests must be interpreted with caution in children with CVI.

Specific motion processing recognition deficits may occur in preterm children with periventricular leukomalacia.[17,18]

Visual acuities may adversely affect scores of perceptual visual function, although some children with low vision can score well on such tests.[16]

Investigations

Higher visual processing has been investigated electrophysiologically allowing more accurate temporal resolution, but less accurate anatomical localization than MRI and fMRI.

Visual evoked potentials

Investigation of late or event-related visual evoked potentials as an index of higher visual processing has the potential to provide objective validation and monitoring.

MRI

MRI is the neuroimaging method of choice in suspected CVI. Primarily cortical pathology (where specific anatomical lesions may be associated with specific perceptual problems) (Fig. 57.3) can be distinguished from subcortical pathology such as periventricular white matter disorders, typically associated with dorsal stream dysfunction. There is a correlation between radiological lesions and psychometric visual perception performance.[18,19,20] fMRI and diffusion tensor imaging have provided insights into the topography and functional organization of the visual pathways and show promise for better understanding of CVI.

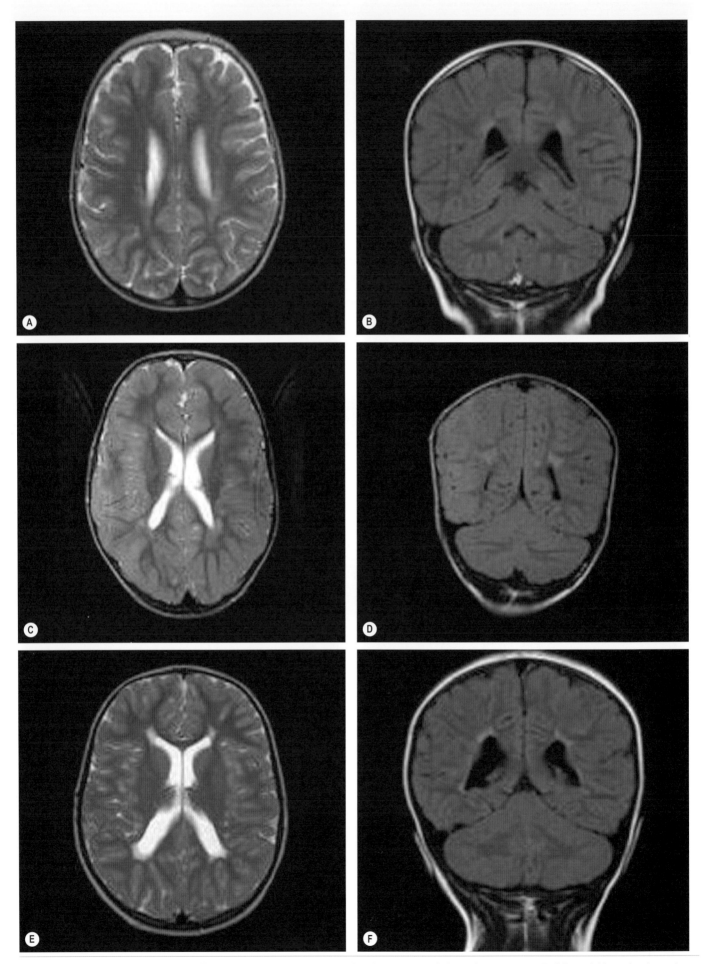

Fig. 57.3 Axial (T2-weighted) and coronal (flair) MRI scans (showing periventricular white matter pathology of varying severity) of three children who showed behavioral features typical of dorsal stream dysfunction associated with lower visual field impairment. (A,B) Patient 1; (C,D) patient 2; (E,F) patient 3.

Management

Visual functions, comprising threshold measurements including visual acuities, visual fields, contrast sensitivity and color vision, are elicited; and functional vision (assessed with both eyes open) describing the impact of the visual perceptual limitations on everyday life are determined in the context of:

- Access to information, both for near and in the distance
- Interacting socially
- Guiding the movement of the upper limbs, lower limbs, and the body

Optimal habilitation and rehabilitation necessitates matching strategies for each of the above requirements in relation to the following approaches:

- Compensation or adaptations to the impairments
- Substitution or the use of environmental modifications and the use of devices
- Restitution or training of the impaired functions

All children with visual and perceptual difficulties need to be understood and optimally catered for both at home and at school, with an understanding of the unique visual profile for each child, and implementation of the appropriate habilitation strategies are needed (Table 57.2).[21]

Table 57.2 – Table highlighting the common behaviors, adaptive strategies described, and approaches that assist children with perceptual visual difficulties

Problem	Solution
Reduced functional visual acuity	Enlarge text Double space text Present text in small sections Reduce distractions Rest when tired
Color vision and contrast sensitivity impairment	Use bright and clear educational material and toys Distinct color boundaries Good contrast
Hemianopia and unilateral inattention/neglect	Trace text with a finger or ruler Turn text vertically or obliquely (for acquired hemianopia) Decenter text to sighted side for unilateral inattention Appropriate seat position in classroom (teacher in sighted area) Turn head and body to check the "hemianopic" side Careful guidance around new environments Train in crossing roads Turn plate to eat food
Lower visual field defect	Regularly look down to check ground ahead Use tactile guide to ground height
Impaired tracking	Move the head Enlarge text Double space text Trace text with a finger or ruler
Impaired movement perception	Television programs with limited movement Educational material with limited movement Careful training or guidance in crossing roads
Finding a toy in a toy box Finding an item of clothing in a pile or wardrobe	Separate storage of favorite items Organized storage systems Always store in same location Avoid clutter Color coding and labeling
Finding an object on a patterned background	Use plain carpets, bedspreads, and decoration
Finding food on a plate	Avoid patterned plates Separate food portions
Seeing a distant object	Share zoom on video/digital camera to view
Reading	Enlarge text Double space text Mask surrounding text Computer programs to present information Use lightly squared paper for arithmetic

Continued

Table 57.2 *Continued*

Problem	Solution
Identifying someone in a group	Wear obvious identifier which can be seen from all directions Always stand in same location Wave Speak
Tendency to get lost	Training in seeking and identifying landmarks Visit new locations at quiet times
Problems with floor boundaries, steps, kerbs, and uneven surfaces	Avoid patterned floor surfaces Bannister Mark edge of stairs Good lighting Tactile guides to gauge the height of the ground Approach obstacles with: "Look–Slow–Check–Go" Activities to improve coordination
Inaccurate visually guided reach	Reach beyond object to gather it Use other hand, or extend little finger of reaching hand to locate object and surface it is on Body contact with work surface Activities to improve coordination Occupational therapy
Difficulty "seeing" when talking at the same time	Limit conversation when walking Look at face before and after speaking Do not say "Look at me when I am talking to you" Identify obstacles by touch or stick
Frustration at being distracted	Limit distraction Reduce background clutter and pattern Reduce background activity Quiet table at school
Difficulty recognizing people and photographs	Use informative introductions Train in identifying voices Wear consistent identifiers visible from all directions Train to recognize identifiers
Difficulty recognizing shapes and objects	Train to identify and recognize identifiers Train in tactile recognition
Difficulty reading facial expression	Train to recognize and reciprocate facial expressions Expression of mood by tone of voice Explanation of mood in words
Getting lost in known locations	Train in orientation Use landmarks on horizon (where clutter is least) Encourage taking the lead Use mnemonics, poems, and songs to sequence landmarks
Difficulty in new environments	Train in orientation Encourage exploration Visit new places to learn about at a quiet time Play hide and seek Devise and play treasure hunts
Visual fatigue after prolonged visual processing	Minimize clutter Reduce distractions Reduce detail and complexity Provide a quiet room to chill out Well earned breaks
Social difficulties	Encourage good school support Identify problems and seek solutions Encourage child to overcome them Well known peer group Find and reward for activities child enjoys and can excel in

References

1. Rahi JS, Cable N. Severe visual impairment and blindness in children in the UK. Lancet 2003; 362: 1359–65.

2. Hatton DD, Schwietz E, Boyer B, Rychwalski P. Babies count: the national registry for children with visual impairments, birth to 3 years. J AAPOS 2007; 11: 351–5.

3. McClelland J, Saunders KJ, Hill N, et al. The changing visual profile of children attending a regional specialist school for the visually impaired in Northern Ireland. Ophthalmic Physiol Opt 2007; 27: 556–60.

4. Good WV, Jan JE, Burden SK, et al. Recent advances in cortical visual impairment. Dev Med Child Neurol 2001; 43: 56–60.

5. Matsuba CA, Jan JE. Long-term outcome of children with cortical visual impairment. Dev Med Child Neurol 2006; 48: 508–12.

6. Muen WJ, Saeed MU, Kaleem MN, et al. Unsuspected periventricular leukomalacia in children with strabismus: a case series. Acta Ophthalmol Scand 2007; 85: 677–80.

7. Braddick O, Atkinson J, Wattam-Bell J. Normal and anomalous development of visual motion processing: motion coherence and "dorsal-stream vulnerability". Neuropsychologia 2003; 41: 1769–84.

8. Atkinson J, King J, Braddick O, et al. A specific deficit of dorsal stream function in Williams' syndrome. Neuroreport 1997; 27:1919–22.

9. Wright JD, Boger WP. Visual complaints from healthy children, Survey of Ophthalmol 1999; 44: 113–21,

10. Zeki S, Ffytche DH. The Riddoch syndrome: insights into the neurobiology of conscious vision. Brain 1998; 121: 25–45.

11. Weiskrantz L, Barbur JL, Sahraie A. Parameters affecting conscious versus unconscious visual discrimination with damage to the visual cortex (V1). Proc Natl Acad Sci USA 1995; 92: 6122–6.

12. Macintyre-Beon C, Young D, Calvert J, et al. Reliability of a question inventory for structured history taking in children with cerebral visual impairment. Presented as an abstract at Royal College of Ophthalmologists Congress, 2009.

13. Dutton GN, Calvert J, Ibrahim H, et al. Impairment of cognitive vision: its detection and measurement. In: Dutton GN, Bax M, editors. Visual Impairment in Children Due to Damage to the Brain. (Clinics in Developmental Medicine No. 186). London: MacKeith Press; 2010: 117–128.

14. Williams C, Northstone K, Sabates R, et al. Visual perceptual difficulties and under-achievement at school in a large community-based sample of children. PLoS One 2011; 21(6): e14772.

15. Leat SJ, Gargon JL. Accommodative response in children and young adults using dynamic retinoscopy. Ophthalmic Physiol Opt 1996; 16: 375–84.

16. Stiers P, Fazzi E. Psychometric evaluation of higher visual disorders: strategies for clinical settings. In: Dutton GN, Bax M, editors. Visual Impairment in Children Due to Damage to the Brain (Clinics in Developmental Medicine No. 186). London: MacKeith Press; 2010: 149–161.

17. MacKay TL, Jakobson LS, Ellemberg D, et al. Deficits in the processing of local and global motion in very low birthweight children. Neuropsychologia 2005; 43: 1738–48.

18. Jakobson LS, Frisk V, Downie AL. Motion-defined form processing in extremely premature children. Neuropsychologia 2006; 44: 1777–86.

19. Guzzetta A, Tinelli F, Del Viva MM, et al. Motion perception in preterm children: role of prematurity and brain damage. Neuroreport 2009; 20: 1339–43

20. Drummond SR, Dutton GN. Simultanagnosia following perinatal hypoxia: a possible pediatric variant of Balint syndrome. J AAPOS 2007; 11: 497–8.

21. McKillop E, Dutton GN. Impairment of vision in children due to damage to the brain: a practical approach. Br Ir Orthop J 2008; 5: 8–14.

Ethics, morality and consent in pediatric ophthalmology

Louise E Allen • Pinar Aydin • Susan H Day

Chapter contents

In this chapter we give an international view of the issues. Since the interpretation of ethical issues has subtle but significant differences between cultures there must be a local interpretation of what we write. The common ethical issues are those concerning consent, confidentiality, and child protection. The guiding principles are that we should:

1. Always act in the child's best interest
2. Treat each child as an individual
3. Respect their views and confidentiality.

What differentiates ethical dilemmas in children is that, though our primary responsibility is to care for the child, it is the surrogates (the parents or carers) who are responsible for the child. Usually, this triangular interdependence works, but when parents' wishes are at odds with our perception of the child's needs or wishes, an ethical dilemma can become a legal one.

Informed consent

Patient empowerment and autonomy lie at the heart of informed consent. As a partner in the consent discussion, we must enable the parent to make a decision about care based on an understanding of the nature of the disease and intervention, including risks and benefits. Consent is a process, not an event or document; the consent form itself is merely a written

record that the discussion has taken place. Assent, on the other hand, is a declaration of acceptance to undergo a medical diagnostic and/or treatment procedure. Even very young children should be asked to assent for medical procedures.

Capacity to give consent (Box 58.1)

The legal position concerning parental responsibility and the capacity of a child to give consent varies from country to country and we need to be familiar with the laws governing consent where we practice. According to the ICD11 of the World Health Organization, the age of adultness is 18. In the USA, the differentiation of "minor" from "adult" is decided according to the each State's law.[1] On the other hand, in countries such as Australia, the age at which a person becomes an adult is 18. The Australian law recognizes that those who are under 18 may have the capacity to consent to their own medical management even without their parents' knowledge, especially in sex-related issues.[2] In some eastern countries, however, it is a preferred practice not to discuss the medical issues in the presence of the subject child.

In most countries, young people over 16 are assumed to have the capacity to consent, as are some mature children

---

Box 58.1

Consent for treatment can be given by different people in different countries and different legal systems

As an example, in England and Wales,[3] it is given by:

- The young person, if over 16
- The child under 16 if they have the capacity to consent, depending on their maturity and understanding
- Mother and father whether married or divorced
- Unmarried father if the child was born after 2003 and he is named on the birth certificate
- Those who have acquired parental responsibility by court order
- Adoptive parents/special guardians
- Local authority representative if the child is in care

under 16. To assess if a young person under 16 has the capacity to consent, the doctor must ensure that the child is able to understand, retain, and weigh up the purpose and consequences of the procedure, as well as the consequences of not having the procedure. Although an adult with parental responsibility should be asked to give consent for a procedure on a younger child's behalf, the child should be involved in the process and be given information in a manner appropriate to his/her age and stage of development.[4]

Points for giving informed consent
(Box 58.2)

Procedures which involve any significant risk, and all research procedures, require written consent. Although it is always preferable for informed consent to be sought by the surgeon performing the procedure, the process may be delegated to a trainee or nurse as long as that person is suitably trained and has sufficient knowledge to enable them to give a full explanation of the risks and benefits of the procedure.[5] Ultimately, however, it is the operating surgeon who must accept such responsibility for a surgical procedure. Information leaflets and procedure-specific consent forms are helpful to *back up* the information given in the clinic. It is also always wise for the surgeon him/herself to check the parents' understanding of the procedure on the day of surgery. In situations where you are uncertain which procedure may be necessary until you perform an examination under anesthesia, discuss the possible outcomes and clarify if there are any procedures to which the parents would not consent.

In an emergency, when no-one may be available to provide informed consent, surgery should proceed without consent if there is a significant risk to the child in delaying treatment.[5]

If the child patient refuses the procedure

The right to refuse treatment made by a competent young person who understands the facts should be respected. However, some may refuse treatment because they lack the maturity and understanding to consider the long-term

---

Box 58.2

Points for giving informed consent

- Tailor your discussion to the individual patient
- Explain the diagnosis, prognosis, and investigation or treatment options, including the option not to treat, without bias
- Discuss the possible side effects or risks of the procedure in a balanced way including serious complications that happen infrequently and more frequent minor complications
- Explain if the procedure involves training or research
- Ensure the parent understands the information given
- Encourage questions from parents and the child; answer them openly and fully
- Give supplementary written information to help with the decision making
- Give time for the parent to make the decision and offer to arrange for a second opinion if necessary
- Accept the decision

---

implications of their choices. Parents can have an important role to play in persuading their child to co-operate with treatment but, in some families, the views of the parents may not influence the young person. A resolution may be enabled by an open and full discussion in a meeting between the ophthalmologist, the young person, an independent advocate, and the parents. The harm caused by failing to treat must be carefully balanced against the potential harm caused by violating a young person's choice and, in cases of doubt, legal advice may be necessary.

Younger children may also refuse treatment. Again, the harm of imposing treatment on a child must be balanced against the importance of the treatment, the urgency of the decision, and whether there are less invasive alternatives available. A child may refuse a procedure because of a particular fear about which they may be unable or unwilling to talk. Parental support is important and the involvement of play therapists and child psychologists can also help to discover and allay the child's fears. Some countries have made into law a physician's responsibility in circumstances where the parents' wishes and the physician's perspective on appropriate care are in conflict. In large part, such laws pertain to circumstances in which life is endangered in the event that treatment is refused. Such laws require the physician to contact and recommend legal override of the parents' decision. Usually, this conflict can be avoided through proper and complete education and explanation to the parents of the risks inherent in non-treatment. As an example, young children with retinoblastoma may require enucleation, sometimes bilateral, in order to spare the child the risk of early death. Physicians in some countries are held accountable to protect such children by requesting court intervention. Conversely, other countries allow complete authority to reject such intervention despite the likelihood of early death.

If the parent refuses the procedure

Refusal of treatment by a person with parental responsibility cannot override the consent of a competent young person to treatment which the ophthalmologist considers is in their best interests. It is, of course, best to have the parents' agreement and, if necessary, discussions should take place involving a patient advocate, the parents, and the young person. Where the child is not competent to give consent, a discussion should take place between a pediatrician with responsibility for child protection, the ophthalmologist, and the parents. Again, it may be necessary to seek legal advice as a last resort.[4]

Consent to research

Research in which children are subjects adds a completely new dimension to the ethics of clinical research not shared by research with adult subjects. Such projects should have potential benefits for children in general, should not infringe the subject's best interests, and should involve only minimal or a low risk of harm. All projects involving children should have approval from the relevant research ethics committee (or Institutional Review Boards).

Children and young people should not be involved in research if they object or appear to object in words or by actions, even if their parents give consent. Although many young people have the capacity to consent to their inclusion in research, it is typically mandatory depending on the country to involve their parents in the decision. No pressure should be placed on a child or his/her parents to consent to research in expectation of therapeutic or financial benefit.[6] Clear distinction must be made between the goals of clinical care and those of research interest when such projects are undertaken, with disclosure of any potential commercial relationship or financial conflict of interest among the team of researchers.

Confidentiality

Respecting confidentiality is an essential part of good medical care and is as important for children and young people as it is for adults. Without the trust that confidentiality brings, young people may not seek medical care and may withhold important information.

Occasionally, children and young children share information with you on the understanding that it is confidential: younger children may fear reprisal or blame if they disclose bullying or abuse, older children may not want their parents to know about their lifestyle. Assure the child or young person that the information given will remain confidential unless you feel that it is essential and in his/her best interests to disclose it: this includes information that the child or a third party was at risk of harm from neglect or abuse, or the young person was involved in high-risk behavior such as drug addiction or self-harm. It can be helpful to have an appropriate advocate for the child involved in the discussion. Try to agree with the child or young person what information needs to be disclosed, how and to whom you will disclose it and document the discussion in the notes.

When communicating patient information in clinical practice, particularly for audit, teaching, and research, identifiable information should be kept to a minimum and personal data anonymized wherever possible. Appropriate arrangements for the security of personal information must be made when it is stored, sent, or received, particularly by fax, computer, or email. Email communication is not regarded as confidential unless encrypted; be aware that your well-meaning communication regarding patients with other medical professionals could be intercepted, and do not email identifiable information. Parents and children should be asked for their consent if identifiable information is to be disclosed to non-medical staff such as optometrists, visual impairment teachers or schools, or if identifiable images are to be used for teaching or research purposes.[7] In the case of images, signed consent should be obtained.

Access to medical records by children, young people, and parents

In many countries, competent young people have a legal right of access to their health records. Parents should also be allowed to access the records with the consent of the child/young person, if is not against the child's best interests. Divorce or separation does not alter parental rights or responsibilities and both parents should be allowed reasonable access to the child's health records. If the records contain information given by the

child or young person in confidence, the records should not be disclosed to the parents without his/her consent.[7]

Child protection

Doctors play a crucial role in protecting children from abuse and neglect. We may notice things or be told things by the child that other people have not, and we may have access to confidential information that raises concern for the safety or well-being of the child. All doctors working with children should have the knowledge and skills to identify abuse and neglect, and know how to proceed if suspicious of it.

Children might not disclose information about neglect or abuse to the social services or police if they think that they will be blamed or made to feel ashamed, or if they fear authority figures. If they disclose such information during the consultation, help them to understand the importance and benefits of sharing information and try to get their consent for you to disclose the information. However, disclosure must not be delayed if you feel the child is at significant risk.

You may have a concern that a child you look after is at risk of neglect or abuse. Sometimes this risk is only identified when a number of clinicians or health professionals with similar concerns share them. If in doubt about taking your concerns further, seek advice from an experienced colleague, the doctor or nurse in charge of child protection, your medical defence organization, or regulatory body. Raising a concern through the appropriate channels is justified, even if later found to be groundless, if the intention is honest and your action is prompt and made on the basis of reasonable belief.[3] Our first concern must always be the safety of children and young people.

References

1. USA Office for Human Research Protections. §46.408 Requirements for permission by parents or guardians and for assent by children. http://www.hhs.gov/ohrp/humansubjects/guidance/45cfr46.html#46.408
2. Bird S. Consent to medical treatment: the mature minor. Defence Update MDA National. Aust Fam Physician 2011; Winter: 18–19.
3. General Medical Council. 0–18 years: Guidance for all Doctors. London: General Medical Council; 2007. http://www.gmc-uk.org/guidance/ethical_guidance/children_guidance_index.asp
4. General Medical Council. Consent Guidance: Patients and Doctors Making Decisions Together. General Medical Council 2008. http://www.gmc-uk.org/guidance/ethical_guidance/consent_guidance_index.asp
5. Dimond B. Legal Aspects of Consent, 2nd ed. London: MA Healthcare Ltd. 2009.
6. British Medical Association. Medical Ethics Today. London: BMJ Books; 2004.
7. General Medical Council. Confidentiality: Protecting and Providing Information. London: General Medical Council; 2009. http://www.gmc-uk.org/guidance/ethical_guidance/confidentiality.asp

Further reading

American Academy of Ophthalmology. Code of Ethics. http://www.aao.org/about/ethics/code_ethics.cfm
International Council of Ophthalmology. Code of Ethics. http://www.icoph.org/downloads/icoethicalcode.pdf

How to help the visually disabled child and family

Creig S Hoyt • James E Jan

For a child with a serious visual problem, the correct diagnosis can usually be established from the history, clinical examination, and electrodiagnostic, neuroimaging, and genetic testing. A more difficult task remains: telling the family, grieving with them, helping them to get appropriate services, and remaining an available sympathetic advocate for them and their child.

Telling the family

Ophthalmologists play a critical role in management of the visually impaired (VI) child; they make the diagnosis and inform the family. The diagnosis of visual impairment in a child is shattering to the family. The manner in which we convey this information can affect the family and child for years. We may expect that families should "accept the situation" but how can parents be expected to "accept" what seems unacceptable about their child? The family may express anger, fear, and resistance; aggressive questioning may follow and needs to be handled calmly and sympathetically. We should not hesitate to show our own feelings.

Parents may be so anxious during the initial office visit that they can remember little afterwards; more than one appointment may be necessary. It is important that both parents be present, if possible, and even better for them to be accompanied by a friend or relative. Most affected children appear to be blind in early infancy; the majority will develop useful vision. The diagnosis of total blindness should be avoided, unless it is absolutely certain. Refer the child **as soon as possible**, if available, to a VI habilitation clinic or to a neurodevelopmental pediatrician. If such services are not available, the ophthalmologist should take the responsibility with available colleagues.

The family

Parents have to cope with heavy physical and emotional demands for years. Instead of being perfect, their new baby has a visual impairment and, perhaps, other disabilities; parents experience persistent feelings of shock, denial, grief, guilt, despair, and anger. It is not unusual for the parents to cry in the office. This is better than when they show little emotion because then they are not moving through the various emotional stages. Most mothers have guilt feelings that they have done something wrong to cause the problem. Even when they do not mention their guilt, we need to strongly state that it is not their fault. Many fathers deal with their grief by seemingly retreating from the problem: the stress on the marriage should not be underestimated.

We can offer practical and easily understood information, to help the parents, on the type of visual disorder and disability but the content and scope of information may be improved.[1] Most parents need repeated explanations. Raising a VI child is very hard work for the entire family and the parents carry out the majority, only aided by the professionals.

Parents often need help to deal with the attitudes of their extended families, the prejudices of the public, and, sometimes, with complex cultural issues.[2] Both mother and father must be involved in the process of habilitation; the needs of the siblings must not be neglected or they may feel ignored. Parent group discussions are helpful for educational, social, and cultural issues. Local and national support groups can be found in most countries and provide invaluable services and support. In the USA, see the National Association for Parents of Children with Visual Impairments (NAPVI) (http://www.FamilyConnect.org).

Early interventions

The habilitation (or rehabilitation) of VI children results from their physical, emotional, and intellectual growth responding to skilled, early intervention.[3] The VI advisors must be trusted by the parents. They must be well trained and are best supported by a multidisciplinary team.

The multidisciplinary team

The interaction of visual loss and other disabilities on development is complex. The multidisciplinary approach is an effective way to deal with VI children. The team may include ophthalmologists, pediatricians, geneticists, nurses, psychologists, speech-language pathologists, audiologists, physiotherapists, and orientation and mobility specialists. Close co-operation between the professionals dealing with the visually impaired is a necessity even if not in a formal team.

When the parents become team members, they are more effective in the management of their children. The parents should receive copies of reports related to their child. In addition, the team are advocates for blind people, educate the community, and participate in research.

Development of the child

Motor development

VI children who are raised in a rewarding, stimulating environment provided by loving, informed parents, who are supported by professionals, develop motor skills faster than when they are understimulated.[4] However, even intelligent infants with severe visual loss, reared under ideal circumstances, may experience motor delays. Crawling and independent walking may begin late, whereas unsupported sitting and standing may be age-appropriate. Understimulated congenitally blind infants frequently develop generalized hypotonia with poor posture, delayed motor skills and poor co-ordination, and walk with a gait disturbance. When intervention is not introduced early, these problems become permanent. Moreover, physical fitness in older VI children is often poor from habitually reduced physical activity.[5]

Blind infants without brain damage are usually quiet, passive, and require encouragement to be mobile. They may not acquire skills through "accidental" learning, as do the sighted. Motor tasks such as sitting, pushing, pulling, jumping, and early aspects of orientation and mobility must be taught. Partially sighted children usually learn to move about normally and cannot be distinguished from the sighted, unless they are required to carry out balance activities.

The development of visual motor skills, arrangement of objects in space, and constructive play are also affected. VI children often avoid activities such as construction toys, puzzles, and drawing. When trying to use their partial sight, they often adopt head tilts or head turns, aimed at improving vision and controlling nystagmus. These and other adaptations should not be discouraged.

Conceptual development

Visual impairment has a noticeable effect on cognition. Severe visual loss forces fragmented processing of information, as only a part of the object can be seen or felt at one time. The relationships to other objects may be lost.

The attention span in VI children is usually shorter than for the sighted. Self-initiated exploration is reduced because they are frequently unaware of their surroundings. They may become passive and understimulated if experiences are not brought to them. Therefore, when they are assessed about their knowledge of their environment, delays are frequent. This does not necessarily indicate poor cognitive ability, but insufficient opportunity to acquire the skills and information which would be normal for a sighted child. Making experiences available, and encouraging them to use their residual vision is essential.

Language development

For VI infants to learn from hearing, structuring of the environment is required: minimizing background noises and encouraging the child to listen to meaningful sounds. They learn to recognize voices and anticipate events through sound, smell, and touch.

Without the full range of sensory information, language concepts and words and phrases retained from overheard conversations are based on auditory memory, not direct experience. Language skills become stilted, more self-oriented, and word meanings are limited.[6] Children with these types of language difficulties sometimes use sophisticated sentences, without fully understanding their meaning. Intervention services minimize this problem.

Social and emotional development

Most young VI infants have poor vision which may improve with maturation. The parents miss the rewarding experiences of mutual gaze and smiling, an important part of bonding. Although these infants smile and respond to voices and touch, the responses are subtle. The early intervention specialist must interpret the infant's signals to the parents and encourage them to keep their babies nearby, talking to them often.

Older VI children have difficulty in sensing their effect on their peers because they may not see "body language." They may not be able to see who is available for play, leading to isolation and persistent egocentric behavior. Because VI children need more structure and predictability in their environments they are often resistant to change; their behavior may appear rigid.

Neurodevelopmental issues and the visually impaired child

Neurodevelopmental disabilities are associated with a number of ocular disorders and seen in most children with cerebral visual impairment.[7] Many VI children have additional disabilities, which make habilitation more complex.[8] For intervention specialists, it is suboptimal to have experience only with visual disorders.

Cognition is frequently affected in VI children.[9] The diagnosis of intellectual deficit is difficult and best made by skilled persons such as child psychologists. Children with severe visual impairment can memorize words and phrases but, with less first-hand experience, they have less understanding of their meaning. The psychologist must separate understimulation from intellectual deficit.

Epilepsy is more common among the visually impaired than in the general population. Uncontrolled seizures may result in visual unresponsiveness, which is temporary if the seizures can be controlled. Sedative anticonvulsant drugs should be avoided since they interfere with attention and learning.

The development and management of the deaf-blind is unique (see Chapter 105).

Blind mannerisms

Many children with severe visual impairment exhibit stereotyped behaviors – body rocking, repetitive handling of objects, hand and finger movements, lying face downwards, and jumping.[10] Blind mannerisms need to be carefully analyzed and appropriately managed. They should not be confused with autism or Tourette's syndrome.[11]

Stereotyped behavior involving the visual system includes eye rubbing, pressing, poking, gazing compulsively at light, staring at hands, flicking fingers in front of the eyes against a light source, pulling on eyelids, tapping or hitting their globes, repeatedly blinking, or rolling the eyes. Rubbing, pressing, and poking the eyes are grouped together as "oculodigital phenomena" but each are different. Eye rubbing is observed in normal or disabled, fatigued children.

Eye pressing occurs with severe bilateral, but usually not total, congenital visual loss. Most commonly, eye pressers have retinopathies. The cause of eye pressing is unknown: it may be stimulatory, requiring functioning retinal ganglion cells. This type of stimulation occurs when the vision cannot provide well-formed, sustained images. It occurs when the child is bored, anxious, or during various activities, such as listening to music. It tends to be prolonged and persistent but is not painful. The orbits may eventually become enlarged and distorted with the eye appearing enophthalmic. Parents must continually keep the child's hands busy and remove them from their eyes during the first years of life, when eye pressing is most intense. Later, the urge to eye press diminishes.

Eye poking is deliberate and harmful. Usually, eye poking causes pain; it is not unusual for them to scream afterwards. Eye poking occurs in severely multidisabled or emotionally disturbed children, who are not necessarily visually impaired. It can cause corneal scarring, infection, retinal detachment, intraocular bleeding, and cataracts; it may lead to blindness. Treatment is difficult.

Compulsive light gazing is one of the signs of cortical visual impairment. VI children who flicker their fingers in front of their eyes against a light source are also light gazers. The urge to light gaze can be mild or so severe that the child may stare at the sun.

Possible behavioral problems?

Professionals not familiar with VI children may draw the wrong conclusions from their mannerisms, speech, posture, facial expressions, and psychological test results. These children may be misdiagnosed as emotionally disturbed or unintelligent. However, behavioral disorders are more common among the visually impaired than among the sighted, especially with additional disabilities.

The assessment of behavioral deviations is complex. It often requires multiple persons and settings. The cause is often simple, but when more complex, the treatment needs to be directed to the family. The psychologist or psychiatrist needs to be familiar with visual impairment and preferably be part of the multidisciplinary team.

Promotion of vision development

Children require constant experience to best develop vision. Normally, this process is spontaneous but infants with VI must be encouraged to use their sight. Visual interaction with the environment can be reduced by severe acuity or field loss, defective eye movements, marked developmental delay, or visual attention disorders. Although visual learning continues throughout life, the rate of acquisition of visual skills is greatest during infancy. The development and structuring of the visual brain is influenced by visual input. The visual environment for young children must be rewarding, meaningful, and increasingly complex; otherwise, there is a loss of opportunity to fully develop their visual potential. Vision stimulation can improve visual potential.[12] It should start immediately after diagnosis. Professionals working with VI infants must first test and understand their visual abilities. It is important to avoid repetitive visual stimuli, such as flashing lights, and to make interactions increasingly meaningful for learning. The facilitation of visual development can be carried out by family members throughout the day when the infant is alert. For parents and siblings to be involved in the visual and neurodevelopmental habilitation is rewarding.

The majority of children with significant congenital visual loss appear to have little or no vision during early infancy but most develop useful sight later. There are two reasons for this:

1. Visual acuity, fields, eye movements, accommodation, perception, and cognitive factors rapidly improve after birth.
2. The vision may be so severely reduced by the combination of physiologic, ocular, or neurologic factors that they cannot use their vision spontaneously and experience delayed visual development.

Because the maturation of the brain and visual system is stimulus-dependent, encouraging these infants to use their sight is critical.

Education

Visual disorders have a major impact on education: normally, learning requires good vision. The education of the blind is a specialized field. Educators are important in the lives of VI children. The teachers who plan the curricula and teach the students require special training and experience. The dedication, time commitment, skills, and attitudes of the teachers impact on the success of VI students in adult life.

In addition to the usual subjects adopted from the sighted curriculum, the education includes concept formation, orientation and mobility, daily living techniques, non-visual communication in reading, writing, speaking, listening, and the use of technical aids. To succeed, educators must understand the ocular or neurologic visual disorders, the cognitive abilities, and the health issues facing their students. This requires good parent–teacher relationships and access to information from treating ophthalmologists. The distance acuity determines where the students should sit in the classroom and how much board work is required. Those with homonymous hemianopia must be seated so that their functioning visual field is directed toward the teacher and the class: someone with a left homonymous hemianopia should sit to the right of the class in order not to have to use an exaggerated head posture to see. Children with severe peripheral field loss but intact acuity function better if they are further away from the blackboard. Students with photosensitivity (as in aniridia, cone dystrophy, or albinism) must not be placed next to a window where the glare is most intense. Appropriate lighting, individually adjusted, is critical. Impaired accommodation, contrast sensitivity, color perception, or eye movements can adversely affect learning. It is helpful for educators to understand the reasons for the head turn or shaking associated with nystagmus. When the visual disorder is progressive, the rate of deterioration determines the timing of introduction of Braille and assistive devices. Visual aids are more effective when the educators are involved in the transition and instructions.

Since many VI children have neurodevelopmental disabilities, educators require detailed information about them. Educators for the visually impaired often accompany students to appointments with ophthalmologists and other physicians; it is helpful when they receive copies of the medical reports. Educators should preferably participate in the multidisciplinary team.

The education of children with cerebral visual impairment (CVI) and ocular visual loss differs.[13] With purely ocular disorders, visual input may be reduced, but neural processing is sound. Thus, visual enrichment and training to scan efficiently are useful. For children with CVI, this approach does not work: visual input must be controlled, to avoid "overloading." Images should be simple and presented in isolation. In their training, teachers for the visually impaired should be exposed to the management of the increasingly common neurologically and visually impaired child.

Previously, severely VI students were educated in segregated schools but now, in many regions of the world, they are "integrated" into classrooms, resulting in benefits and disadvantages.[14,15] Full integration may lead to devaluation of the disability and is often detrimental to the multidisabled visually impaired, who learn best in a carefully controlled classroom.

Orientation and mobility

Orientation is the understanding of one's location; mobility is movement from one area to another. Orientation and mobility (O&M) teaches concepts and skills to children with visual impairment on how to travel safely and efficiently in different environments. O&M specialists need to know about the visual disorders, the cognitive and neurodevelopmental disabilities, and the emotional issues of each VI child. They are members of the multidisciplinary team. Successful O&M starts early when basic sensory awareness of the environment is formed. It is much more than just training to use a white stick or cane!

O&M cannot be taught by words, or by models. It must be experienced in the real world. While it begins in infancy, instruction continues in preschool years. The most common methods of O&M are sighted guides, cane, alternate mobility devices, guide dogs, electronic and ultrasonic travels aids, and computer-generated alternative training.[16]

Assistive technology

Technology has helped the visually impaired.[17] Assistive or adoptive technology has improved the way they are educated or trained and has increased employment opportunities. When assistive technology is offered, the visual and intellectual abilities are evaluated, costs and social issues considered, and devices are selected, adjusted and maintained. The school and home are often modified and the students, parents, and educators are instructed how to use the devices, while the services are co-ordinated with other therapies. Assistive technology is a basic tool, like pencil and paper for sighted students and, as they grow, this is a continuous process.

There are a number of devices listed on the Web, ranging from computer screen magnification, Windows-based tutorials, Braille translation of software, portable note takers, Braille writing equipment, scanners, voice simulation programs, to a variety of video magnifiers or closed-circuit televisions.

It is beneficial to introduce these services before school age, so that young VI children may have a chance to learn how to scribble, draw, or color: early referral is important. Professionals who provide assistive technology should be members of the multidisciplinary team. Low Vision Clinics, operated by ophthalmologists or optometrists, are best integrated with the team and they should be familiar with assistive technology or work with professionals who are.

References

1. Rahi JS, Manaras I, Tuomainen H, Hundt GL. Health services experiences of parents of recently diagnosed visually impaired children. Br J Ophthalmol 2005; 89: 213–18.
2. Nikolaraizi M, De Reybeliel HN. A comparative study of children's attitudes towards deaf children, children in wheelchairs and blind children in Greece and in the UK. Eur J Spec Needs Ed 2001; 16: 167–82.
3. Shonkoff JP, Hauser-Cram P. Early intervention for disabled infants and their families: a quantitative analysis. Pediatrics 1987; 80: 650–8.
4. Fazzi E, Lanners J, Ferrari-Ginerva O, et al. Gross motor development and reach on sound as critical tools for the development of the blind child. Brain Dev 2002; 24: 269–75.
5. Lieberman L, Stuart ME. Health-related fitness of children who are visually impaired. JVIB 2001; 31: 21–9.
6. McConachie HR, Moore V. Early expressive language of severely visually impaired children. Dev Med Child Neurol 1994; 36: 230–40.
7. Mervis CA, Boyle CA, Yeargin-Allsopp M. Prevalence and selected characteristics of childhood visual impairment. Dev Med Child Neurol 2002; 44: 538–42.
8. Sonsken PM, Dale N. Visual impairment in infancy: impact on neurodevelopmental and neurobiological processes. Dev Med Child Neurol 2002; 44: 782–91.

9. Langley MB. ISAVE: Individualized, Systematic Assessment of Visual Efficiency for the Developmentally Young and Individuals With Multihandicapping Conditions, Vols 1 & 2. Louisville, Kentucky: American Printing House for the Blind; 1998.

10. Fazzi E, Lanners J, Danova S, et al. Stereotyped behaviours in blind children. Brain Dev 1999; 21: 522–8.

11. Brown R, Hobson RP, Lee A, Stevenson J. Are there "autistic-like" features in congenitally blind children? J Child Psychol Psychiatry 1997; 38: 693–703.

12. Sonksen PM, Petrie A, Drew KJ. Promotion of visual development of severely visually impaired babies: evaluation of a developmentally based programme. Dev Med Child Neurol 1991; 33: 320–35.

13. Groenveld M, Jan JE, Leader P. Observations on the habilitation of children with cortical visual impairment. JVIB 1990; 84: 11–152.

14. Hatlen PH, Curry SA. In support of specialized programs for blind and visually impaired children: the impact of vision loss on learning. JVIB 1987; 81: 7–13.

15. Hehir T. Eliminating ableism in education. Harvard Ed Rev 2002; 72: 1–33.

16. Inman DP, Loge K. Teaching orientation and mobility skills to blind children using simulated acoustical environments. Proceedings of HCI International, 1999.

17. Saarinen R, Jarvi J, Raisamo R, et al. Supporting visually impaired children with software agents in a multimodal learning environment. Virtual Reality 2006; 9: 108–17.

Visual conversion disorder: fabricated or exaggerated symptoms in children

David Taylor

Features and definitions

Many terms have been used (Table 60.1) and many are useful but none perfectly encapsulates what we refer to as visual conversion disorder (VCD).

Children commonly present to ophthalmologists not only with symptoms that do not fit in with known ophthalmic diseases but that also must be *proved* to have characteristics that *definitely cannot be caused by organic disease*. VCD is not a diagnosis of exclusion but one that is made by positive identification of signs that cannot possibly be due to disease processes. It is safer to assign those without positive diagnosis to an "unknown cause – to be reviewed" category than to assign them an incorrect diagnosis for any reason.

Many of the symptoms that children describe to us are not always understandable. That does not necessarily mean that they are fabricated and we need to be careful not to diagnose a child's description of a normal phenomenon as an abnormal or fabricated one.

The major characteristics of VCD are as follows (modified from The Diagnostic and Statistical Manual (now IV-SR) of the American Psychiatric Association[1]):

Table 60.1 – Alternative terminologies used for children with fabricated or exaggerated symptoms

Terminology	Advantages or disadvantages
Conversion disorder (visual conversion disorder, VCD)	The preferred term of the American Psychiatric Association but it implies certain knowledge of the underlying mechanism
Hysterical blindness/amblyopia	Incorrectly implies instability or "madness" but it is commonly used
Stress-related visual disorder	Many cases are not apparently stressed by any definition
Conversion neurosis	Implies a certain knowledge of the underlying mechanism and instability
Medically unexplained visual loss	Obscures the meaning from parents and patients
Amblyopic schoolgirl syndrome	A sexist and pejorative term
Functional visual loss	Meaningless term designed to obscure the meaning from parents and patients
Malingering	A term correctly used for someone who deliberately feigns a symptom for some form of gain – compensation, avoidance of work, military service, etc.[2] This is usually seen in adults
Factitious disorder	A term correctly used for a person acting as if they have an illness by deliberately producing, feigning, or exaggerating symptoms to gain attention or sympathy. Was known as Munchausen's syndrome
Factitious disorder by proxy	Used to be known as Munchausen's syndrome by proxy. Symptoms or signs produced in a child by a carer to elicit sympathy etc. for the carer
Psychogenic blindness Non-organic visual loss	Terms that are still used and can be helpful

- One or more symptoms or deficits are present that affect voluntary motor or sensory function suggesting a neurologic or other medical condition.
- Psychologic factors are judged by the clinician to be associated with the symptom or deficit because conflicts or other stressing events precede the initiation or exacerbation of the symptom or deficit by a variable time. It is important to understand that it is often difficult or impossible to find any clearly abnormal stressing event.

The symptom or deficit is *not intentionally* produced or feigned (as it is in factitious disorder or malingering):

- The symptom or deficit, after appropriate investigation, cannot be explained fully by a general medical condition, the direct effects of a substance, or as a culturally sanctioned behavior or experience.
- The symptom or deficit causes significant distress or impairment in social, educational, or other important areas of functioning or warrants medical evaluation.
- The symptom or deficit is not limited to pain or, in older children, to sexual dysfunction and is not better accounted for by another mental disorder.

Conversion disorder

Conversion disorder was described[3] as a loss or distortion of neurologic function not fully explained by organic disease. The patient has an internal conflict, of which they are unaware, which becomes converted into a symptom as a means of expression after dissociation, a mental mechanism whereby underlying feelings and the symptoms are separated. Conversion disorder can be distinguished from other psychiatric disorders mimicking organic loss by its absence of conscious or intentional desire to trick the doctor (or parent). The child with the ocular manifestations of a visual conversion disorder (VCD) develops visual loss due to unconscious problems or mental disturbances outside their awareness. Often such children have a history of previous conversion reactions, not necessarily involving the visual system (e.g. non-organic loss of motor function).

Clinical presentation and symptoms

The child with VCD is between 6 and 16 years, most frequently 10 years old; girls are more frequently affected than boys.[4] There may be a family history of illness or of eye disease, such as retinitis pigmentosa.[5] The symptoms come on gradually in most cases, often following a marginal failure at a school eye test. Subsequent examinations reveal varying degrees of acuity and visual field loss, often worsening as time goes on but rarely to the extent that the child becomes bilaterally blind. The remarkable thing is how little most children are inconvenienced by an apparently marked visual loss. Repeated objective examinations and further examinations, including neurophysiology and radiology, are all normal. The condition is usually bilateral,[4] with the most common complaints being "just not seeing," blurred vision, or distorted or small images. Occasionally visual field defects are described, commonly "tunnel vision"; hemianopias are occasionally encountered. Central scotomas are rare and should make one think of associated organic disease. Non-ocular defects occasionally also occur,[6] including spasm of the near reflex, headaches, voluntary nystagmus, and eye movement tics, contraversive eye deviation, and accommodation paralysis.

The symptoms of VCD have some of the following characteristics:[7,8]

1. They conform to the child's concept of a symptom or a disorder.
2. They are definable, if somatic, in terms of positive evidence and, if psychologic, by techniques of clinical examination.
3. They are related to emotional conflict.
4. Despite being profound, the symptoms often cause little concern to the affected child.
5. There is usually only one symptom. It is unusual for this to present like a somatization disorder where the child has multiple symptoms often in more than one organ system.
6. Conversion disorders are rare under 6 years old, and the sex ratio is equal up to 10 years, then females outnumber males by 3 : 1.
7. In children, both visual fields and acuity are affected; adults tend to be monosymptomatic.[8]
8. Family disharmony is common and incestuous relationships should be borne in mind as an underlying cause.[9]
9. Patients tend to have equal difficulty with both large and small letters and to read down the letter chart very slowly (and time-consumingly) from the top to the lowest they can achieve, often getting further down the chart if cajoled or, for some, if the test is done competitively. They read the near vision test excruciatingly slowly, often only to a level far disparate from that achieved at distance.
10. A few children have a history of previous psychiatric or psychologic disease[6] but it is often difficult to elicit the history. Most are perfectly normal children.

Depression

Some children develop somatic complaints in response to depression. Therefore, questions that can elicit signs of depression should be raised when depression is suspected. Depressed children may have sleep and eating disturbances, and may have suicidal thoughts. Their peer relationships may have suffered in the preceding few months, and they may appear irritable. These need to be addressed, usually with help from a pediatrician or psychiatrist.

Association with organic disease

Non-organic symptoms are common amongst children referred to a pediatric ophthalmology service.[10] Their prompt and correct diagnosis, with appropriate management, saves the doctor, the child, and the parents much heartache and time and saves the discomfort and risk of unnecessary investigations.

The fear of missing organic disease means that doctors have become more cautious about diagnosing non-organic disorders. In VCD, misdiagnoses occur particularly with macular disease and hereditary optic atrophy in children, but no disease is exempt!

Organic disease may be associated with non-organic disease; the classic situation is the occurrence of pseudoseizures in epileptics. The same may well be true of children with VCD but, *in childhood*, the symptoms usually occur free of both organic disease and psychiatric disease.[6]

Psychologic background

Enquiry into the background, looking for the underlying stress that produces the symptoms, should center on two main areas:

1. *The home and family.* Conflict between children, sibling rivalry, the child who needs more attention, an unhappy marriage, overcrowding, sexual abuse,[11] harassment by relatives or others, or conflict with neighbors and their children may be predisposing factors.
2. *The school.* In the school it is the slow child who is being overstretched or the bright child who is being understretched who may produce visual symptoms. Unsympathetic or aggressive teachers, teasing or bullying, sexual or non-sexual harassment, or abuse[11] all predispose to non-organic visual loss.

It is of utmost importance to enlist the help of the parents, and to tell them explicitly of the possible underlying problems so that they can best help their own child, because relieving underlying factors best treats the symptoms.

Detection of functional ocular disorders in children

It is of crucial importance that the diagnosis is made positively, with the clear demonstration of signs that are widely outside the bounds of physiologic possibility. Taking a detailed history is essential, if time-consuming, and is often vital to making the correct diagnosis. Certain clinical situations are particularly suggestive of a non-organic disorder as outlined in Box 60.1.

Clinical examination in visual conversion disorders

Total blindness

Bilateral

Although unusual, this severe disturbance is usually easy to detect as being non-organic.

1. Direct threat or throwing a ball on a string at the patient while the eyes are open invariably produces a blink (Fig. 60.1). The string can be concealed before the ball is thrown.
2. When facing a mirror a patient will involuntarily move his eyes when the mirror is rotated about a vertical axis running through the center of the mirror. The velocity of the eye movement is proportional to the velocity of rotation of the mirror. The only way in which the patient

---

Box 60.1

Presentations and progressions suggestive of visual conversion disorders

1. A severe functional defect in the presence of a normal physical examination, especially when there is a severe unilateral defect with normal pupil reactions and no refractive error.
2. The sudden onset of a disorder related to an emotionally significant event or situation.
3. A step-like deterioration, with the patient's acuity becoming one or two lines worse on each examination but with no objective abnormalities.
4. The ability of a patient to achieve a better acuity or better visual fields with coaxing or cajoling.
5. A monotonous and excessively slow reading of all the letters on a letter chart, regardless of whether they are large or small.
6. A single symptom is most frequent in hysterics whereas psychoneurotic patients will tend to have numerous symptoms. Children rarely have substantial ocular complaints.
7. A previous history of hysterical manifestations, ocular or non-ocular, is a recognized predisposing factor to further hysterical disorders.
8. The occurrence of visual problems in other members of the family, especially if serious.

---

can inhibit the eye movement is by "looking through" the mirror, usually easily detected by a change in convergence of the eyes and an associated pupil reaction (Fig. 60.2).
3. An optokinetic drum or tape, subtending a large angle at the eye, can be held in front of the patient and the drum rotated to elicit visual evoked movement (Fig. 60.3). It is possible for the patient to look through the tape or drum giving the impression that he is not seeing it. If a large drum, in which the patient sits, is available (usually in an eye movement laboratory), this provides whole field stimulation and an irresistible source of visual evoked eye movement.
4. A 5 or 25 diopter prism placed base out in front of a seeing eye will normally induce an appropriate, and totally involuntary, fusional movement (Fig. 60.4). This will not occur in severe visual defects.

Unilateral

The same tests as described in the previous section can be used by covering the normal eye. There are several additional, more subtle, tests:

1. A dexterous refractionist can usually manage to confuse the patient into reading with the "blind" eye while he thinks that he is using his good eye. Putting a high plus lens or rotating two cylinders (Fig. 60.5) from a canceling to an additive position to occlude the good eye causes the patient to unsuspectingly read down the chart to a normal level. Polaroid lenses or polaroid projection devices can also be used to trick the patient into reading with the affected eye.
2. Worth's dots (see Chapter 7) in which four illuminated spots, two green, one white and one red, are viewed by the patient wearing a red goggle over the right eye and a green over the left. A normal person will see two spots with the right eye (the red and the white appear red)

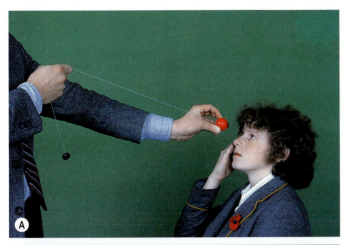

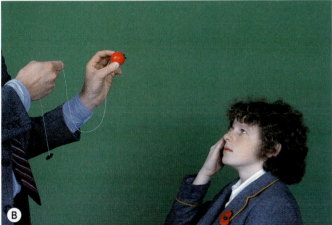

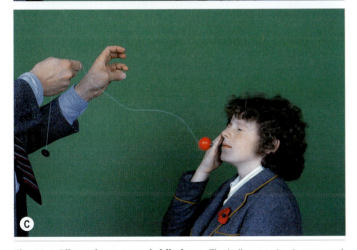

Fig. 60.1 Bilateral non-organic blindness. The ball on a string is measured for distance (A), withdrawn (B), and then thrown at the child, eliciting a blink if they are indeed sighted (C). The first two steps are better performed with the eyes closed.

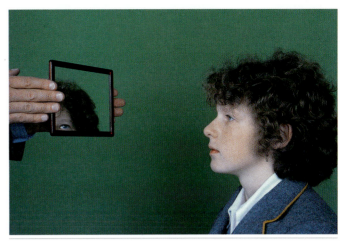

Fig. 60.2 When a blind person looks at a mirror, no movement takes place when the mirror is rotated. The sighted person's eyes will move as the mirror rotates although they believe they are looking straight ahead.

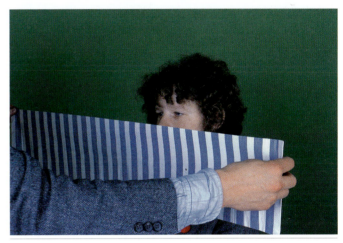

Fig. 60.3 Bilateral non-organic blindness. As long as the patient does not "look through" the tape, the patient's eyes will move with the OKN tape.

through the red filter and three with the left eye (two green and one white all appearing green through the green filter). With both eyes open the patient sees four dots if he is able to fuse the two white dots. If there is a latent or manifest strabismus without suppressions he sees five dots. If the patient sees more than three green or two red he must be using both eyes.

3. The stereoacuity test most useful for this purpose is the Frisby stereotest since this does not require the use of polaroid or red/green glasses to achieve dissociation of the eyes. While the plate shown is held steadily (movement induces parallax and detection of the target) the patient is invited to point out the square containing a circle. It requires quite a high degree of binocular vision to achieve this.

4. Either a horizontal prism, as described in the previous section, or a vertical prism may be placed in front of the apparently defective eye. The vertical prism, if over 5 diopters in power, usually involves diplopia and the patient may report this or terminate the examination.

5. It is in this group that pupil reactions are most useful; if one eye is blind and the other is normal there is always a relative afferent pupil defect.

6. Bar reading is a commonly used technique in orthoptics. To read with a bar placed in an appropriate position between the reading matter and the patient's eyes requires both eyes to work simultaneously in order to read a complete line.

7. A pseudoscope is a device in which a system of mirrors in a box is used to confuse the observer as to which eye he is using. When the patient thinks they are covering one eye he is in fact covering the other.

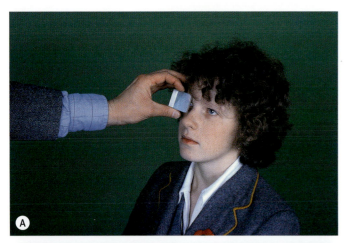

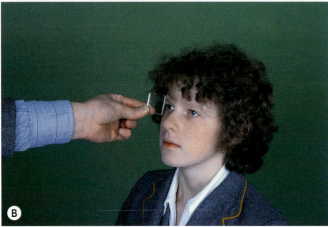

Fig. 60.4 A 25 diopter prism. (A) elicits a movement even with only peripheral vision. A 4 diopter prism (B) requires central vision to elicit a movement.

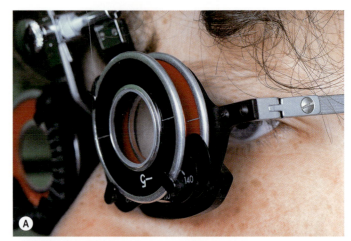

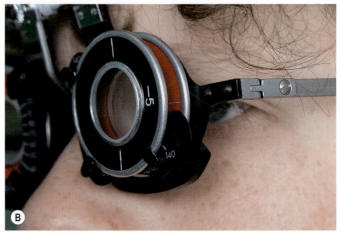

Fig. 60.5 The right eye is suspected of seeing better than the patient indicates. The ophthalmologist puts two canceling cylinders at the same axis in front of the left eye (A), obscures the patient's view of the test type by moving across him, switches the lenses to add to each other (B) and occlude the left eye and as he moves away from the patient urges him to read quickly. The left eye is obscured by the lens combination and the right is forced to be used; the patient does not usually detect the change to being forced to use the right eye.

Partial acuity loss

In partial visual acuity loss it is essential to accept only the most clearly non-organic signs as being true; for instance, a small difference between near and distance acuity is not necessarily non-organic and should not be the basis by itself for such a diagnosis.

Unilateral

In this group the same tests that are used for unilateral complete visual loss are applicable. The results, however, are often much less easy to interpret. Pupil reactions are rarely helpful. Since there are no clear norms for the correlation between acuity and stereoacuity, the stereoacuity tests are difficult to interpret. The pseudoscope and the confusion–refraction test are most useful.

Bilateral

This group is the most difficult to diagnose as non-organic but they nearly always have associated functional field defects that can establish the diagnosis.

1. The finding of an acuity that greatly varies in terms of the angle subtended at different distances is an indicator of VCD. By the use of a second chart with different sized figures or a mirror placed so as to hide the increased distance between the patient and the chart, the patient

may be induced to read letters of a size that they were not previously able to read. Similarly, near vision testers, using Snellen near equivalent letters, may show a disparity.
2. Severe bilateral loss of acuity due to organic disease is not compatible with a high level of stereoacuity: a partial loss may be.
3. It is unusual for a patient to make fusional movement when a 5 diopter prism is placed base out in front of the other eye, if that eye has organically reduced acuity.

Visual field defects

In children, the most common presentation is one in which fine vision (acuity) symptoms are present but peripheral vision (visual fields) symptoms are not. When having their visual fields tested, even normal children may perform in a non-organic manner if the examination is not carefully conducted. Abnormal fields are often associated with an apparently reduced acuity in functional visual loss, or sometimes with other symptoms including reading disability.

Tunnel vision is the most common of the non-organic visual field defects. In tunnel vision the size of the field is the same at all distances; usually the field is also small. Purely constricted fields, as in retinitis pigmentosa, are conical, becoming larger as the patient moves away from the testing screen. The defect is always gross; there is an apparently dense defect involving the whole visual field only a few degrees away from the fixation point and this is the same size whether tested at 1, 2 or more meters away from the screen.

The defect, characterized by the "piling" of isopters (isopters all at or near the same eccentricity), is usually "sharp edged" so that both large and small targets are perceived at the same eccentricity, which is often remarkably constant. This "piling" of the isopters may occur even in the face of gross changes in the contrast between the brightness of the background and the target; a distinctly non-physiologic effect!

The absolute nature of the defect makes it easier to detect as being functional. Only clearly abnormal findings should be accepted as indicating a non-organic disorder.

1. In a confrontation technique, if the patient alternates fixation between the examiner's eye and a fixation point on a stick held by the examiner, and at a time when he is fixing the examiner's eye, the fixation point is moved (Fig. 60.6). If the patient has organic disease with constricted fields, he will have difficulty in relocating the spot, whereas a child with VCD finds it accurately.

2. On parting, the examiner fixes the patient in the eye and, without speaking, raises his hand from the elbow as though to shake hands. Given the variations of social and cultural backgrounds, most patients with organically constricted fields do not see the examiner's hand, while the child with VCD will.

Using large targets, one may obtain a square visual field, the target when moved inwards from one direction being detected in areas previously blind.

On successive testing the field may become smaller. If the target is moved inwards as though around a clock-face the target becomes detectable at an ever decreasing distance from fixation giving rise to "spiraling." This also occurs in patients with organic disease so caution is necessary.

Hemifield defects are rare. A binasal field defect may be a non-organic phenomenon. Functional binasal defects are usually clear-cut, organic ones are not.

In the very rare bitemporal non-organic visual field defect there is a wedge of blindness extending away from the fixation point. Therefore, if the patient fixes the examiner's nose and then fixes a point between the examiner's nose and himself, if the bitemporal hemianopia is complete there will be a loss or blurring of the central features of the examiner's face. This does not occur in a child with VCD.

Blue visual field testing targets are normally detected more peripherally than the red targets of identical size and brightness; the reverse is normal in VCD field testing.

It must be emphasized that an examiner skilled in testing for functional loss should not let his enthusiasm for testing to allow him either to overlook co-existing organic disease, or to encourage the patient to give apparently non-organic results when none are normally present: 9% of 193 normal asymptomatic schoolchildren demonstrated non-organic fields.[12] Visual field testing is best done with a tangent screen.

Confirmatory studies

It is easy to diagnose the condition too late and to overinvestigate.[13] Once the clinician has made a *positive* diagnosis of non-organic visual loss and has not found evidence of any disease, there remains little to do from the point of view of diagnosis. The more one investigates the child the more stress one creates and the more one reinforces his underlying problem. If there is any doubt in the mind of the doctor, parent, or the older child about the possibility of organic disease, detailed neurophysiologic studies, including an electroretinogram (ERG) and pattern visually evoked responses may be very reassuring and may inspire sufficient confidence to base the treatment only on reassurance. Non-organic symptoms may also occur in brain disorders such as Batten's disease or adrenoleukodystrophy, many of which are accompanied by neurophysiologic changes.

Even with the best neurophysiologic studies, it is possible to overlook organic disease, but choosing the optimal test

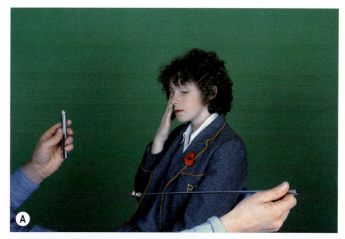

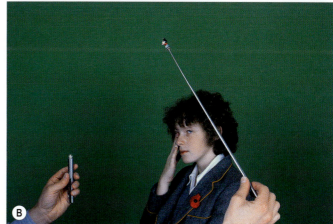

Fig. 60.6 The patient with very constricted visual fields, is asked to look at the light, then at the figure on a stick which is kept still. After doing this a few times, the figure is moved to another part of the apparently blind part of the visual field. If this is done accurately, it is proof that there is a disparity between the tested and the actual visual field and VCD is a likely diagnosis.

helps avoid this pitfall. For instance, in someone with acuity loss and nothing to find clinically, standard ERGs may be normal but a pattern ERG will detect the most common missed diagnosis in many clinics – Stargardt's disease. These are useful confirmatory studies in many cases and are risk-free.

Further investigations such as computed tomography or magnetic resonance imaging are not completely risk-free in children, especially if an anesthetic is needed and they are therefore only indicated if the neurophysiologic tests are abnormal or if there is real doubt in the doctor's mind. Very sophisticated fMRI scanning may demonstrate subtle changes in the responses of VCD patients compared with normal patients.[14]

Management

It is possible to find the underlying psychologic cause in some cases; appropriate and sensitive modification of these underlying predisposing factors will abolish the symptom. It is useful to demonstrate the non-organic nature of the defect to the parents and to reassure them strongly that it is such a common problem that it could be regarded as a "normal stress reaction". There is a very strong need to discuss the condition in full with both child and parents, in language appropriate to both. Most cases can be managed by the ophthalmologist alone. It is important to maintain some contact or follow-up in case the problem does not improve or evolves outside the normal template of non-organic disorders.

The contributions of a psychiatrist or psychologist may be helpful in refractory cases but it is preferable to avoid involvement with too many professionals, because this may reinforce the problem.

The ophthalmologist should maintain a dispassionate approach to the functional patient. Counter-transference problems (doctors' emotional reactions to patients) can be complex, with anger at the patient for "wasting the doctor's time" a common feature.

Prognosis

The prognosis is good[12] and strong reassurance with minimal follow-up is usually indicated. Psychiatric help may be useful in certain cases and it is likely that "integrative" and family therapy may improve the prognosis.[6] Good prognostic factors are younger age, treatment compliance, early intervention, healthy family functioning, lack of psychopathology, insight, and acceptance by the family of the psychologic natures of the illness.[15] If there is any indication of an underlying psychiatric disorder, or of a more widespread psychoneurosis, for instance if the patient has recurrent episodes especially affecting more than one system, the psychiatrist's help is mandatory.

References

1. Yutzy SH, Cloninger CR, Guze SB, et al. DSM-IV field trial: testing a new proposal for somatization disorder. Am J Psychiatry 1995; 152: 97–101.
2. Thompson HS. Functional visual loss. Am J Ophthalmol 1985; 100: 209–13.
3. Marsden CD. Hysteria: a neurologist's view. Psychol Med 1986; 149: 28–37.
4. Yasuna ER. Hysterical amblyopia in children and young adults. Arch Ophthalmol 1951; 45: 70–6.
5. Holden R, Duvall-Young J. Functional visual deficit in children with a family history of retinitis pigmentosa. J Pediatr Ophthalmol Strabismus 1994; 31: 323–4.
6. Catalano RA, Simon JW, Krohel GB, et al. Functional visual loss in children. J Am Acad Ophthalmol 1986; 93: 385–91.
7. Porteous AM, Clark MP. Medically unexplained visual symptoms (MUS) in children and adolescents: an indicator of abuse or adversity? Eye 2009; 23: 1866–67.
8. Lim SA, Siatkowski RM, Farris BK. Functional visual loss in adults and children: patient characteristics, management, and outcomes. Ophthalmology 2005; 112: 1821–8.
9. Editorial. Neurological conversion disorders in childhood. Lancet 1991; 337: 889–90.
10. Schlaegel TF Jr, Quilala FV. Hysterical amblyopia: statistical analysis of 42 cases found in a survey of 800 unselected eye patients at a state medical center. Arch Ophthalmol 1955; 54: 875–84.
11. Roelofs K, Keijsers GP, Hoogduin KA, et al. Childhood abuse in patients with conversion disorder. Am J Psychiatry 2002; 159: 1908–13.
12. Eames TH. A study of tubular and spiral central fields. Am J Ophthalmol 1947; 30: 610–11.
13. Leary PM Conversion disorder in childhood: diagnosed too late, investigated too much? J R Soc Med 2003; 96: 436–8.
14. Werring DJ, Weston L, Bullmore ET, et al. Functional magnetic resonance imaging of the cerebral response to visual stimulation in medically unexplained visual loss. Psychol Med 2004; 34: 577–81.
15. Turgay A. Treatment outcome for children and adolescents with conversion disorder. Can J Psychiatry 1990; 35: 585–9.

Vision, reading and dyslexia

Robert H Taylor

I will outline current thinking about dyslexia, advise about what vision/ocular assessments should be carried out, and discuss the evidence linking dyslexia to the visual system.

Reading

There are diverse causes of poor reading; some are environmental, others have a biological basis. Dyslexia is the most common cause of poor reading. However, abnormalities in the visual and auditory systems can cause a reading problem, and therefore need excluding.

Reading requires the extraction of meaning from print. This is complex, but for most people it is effortless. However, *learning* to read poses a challenge, drawing on a range of language and cognitive skills. In the early stages, children have to learn to convert letter strings to sounds or phonemes. For example, the word "cat" has three phonemes: /k/ /a/ /t/. The ability to draw meaning from these sounds is called semantics; once word meanings are identified, grammatical skills integrate meanings within sentences and beyond.

The orthography conventions of a language consist of the rules and regularities that comprise the writing system. As reading development proceeds, children abstract the mappings between the symbols of the orthography (graphemes) and the sounds of words (phonemes); in turn these sounds make contact with word meanings (semantics).

In an alphabetic language (such as English), poor phonological skills compromise the development of grapheme-phoneme mappings. This is the cornerstone of the current understanding of the term dyslexia.[1,2]

Dyslexia

A definition of the term dyslexia is emerging. This is due to be published in DSM-5 (Diagnostic and Statistical Manual of Mental Disorders, American Psychiatric Association), and is outlined in Box 61.1.[3]

The major change (from the 1994 definition) is the removal of discrepancy between general cognitive ability and reading skills. While a discrepancy between achievement (in reading) and intellectual ability *may* still be present, it is now appreciated that all dyslexic children, irrespective of intellectual ability, have the same poor phonological skills.[?] Furthermore, all groups demonstrate similar improvement as a result of evidence-based phonological interventions.[4,5]

An independent report, authored by Sir Jim Rose, formerly Her Majesty's Inspector and Director of Inspection for the Office for Standards in Education (Ofsted), defined dyslexia as outlined in Box 61.2.[6] Point 2 illustrates the three areas of phonological processing initially described by Wagner and Torgeson:[7]

a. Phonological awareness: the ability to attend to and manipulate sounds in words.

b. Phonological memory: memory for speech-based information – sometimes called verbal memory.

c. Naming (providing the spoken label for visual referent) or verbal processing speed.

Box 61.1

Proposed definition of dyslexia: DSM-5

A. Difficulties in accuracy or fluency of reading that are not consistent with the person's chronological age, educational opportunities, or intellectual abilities

Multiple sources of information are to be used to assess reading, one of which must be an individually administered, culturally appropriate, and psychometrically sound standardized measure of reading and reading-related abilities

B. The disturbance in criterion A, without accommodations, significantly interferes with academic achievement or activities of daily living that require these reading skills

Box 61.2

Definition of dyslexia: Rose Report on Dyslexia 2009

1. Dyslexia is a learning difficulty that primarily affects the skills involved in accurate and fluent word reading and spelling
2. Characteristic features of dyslexia are difficulties in phonological awareness, verbal memory, and verbal processing speed
3. Dyslexia occurs across the range of intellectual abilities
4. It is best thought of as a continuum, not a distinct category, and there are no clear cut-off points
5. Co-occurring difficulties may be seen in aspects of language, motor co-ordination, mental calculation, concentration, and personal organization, but these are not, by themselves, markers of dyslexia
6. A good indication of the severity and persistence of dyslexic difficulties can be gained by examining how the individual responds or has responded to well-founded intervention

Most dyslexic children demonstrate weakness in all three areas. Most educational psychologists agree that one standard deviation from the mean for that age signifies a significant weakness.

Dyslexia is common (5% of the population).[8] It is distributed equally between the sexes,[9,10] is familial, and persistent.

Dyslexia was originally a behavioral description (inaccurate or dysfluent word reading or spelling), but is now based on a defect at a cognitive level (poor phonological processing).[8] Functional MRI findings demonstrate (in adults) activity in the left parietotemporal region during word analysis involving phonemes, and the left occipital temporal region for automatic rapid responding. The latter predominates in skilled reading.[8] There is evidence that children with dyslexia rely on other areas (such as the inferior frontal gyrus and other right hemisphere sites) during reading, possibly as a result of compensatory processes. Anterior cortical areas, involved in articulation, may contribute in developing phoneme awareness (forming the words with the lips and tongue).

Comprehension is not a marker of dyslexia as it is currently defined. Comprehension may be poor as a result of an inability to read, so will often co-exist.

Reading assessment

Phonological processes are examined in a variety of ways (Table 61.1). Most of these tests have been validated in children of different ages.

Dyslexia management

Prospective studies show that 8-year-old dyslexics demonstrated weak letter knowledge in reception classes at school (age 4–5 years) and poor phoneme awareness in year 1.[11,12] It is desirable to identify these children early and to supply early support before these children fail.[4,13]

In primary school, management concentrates on reading development. As dyslexic children develop, they may learn to read, but with a lack of speed. Allowance for this is important – particularly in time-constrained examinations.

Table 61.1 – Tests of phonological processing

Phonological skill	Task	Exemplar test item	Published test
Phonological awareness	Phoneme deletion	What is "bice" without the /b/? ["ice"]	Comprehensive Test of Phonological Processing (CTOPP) Phoneme elision
	Phoneme isolation	Say Bem Now tell me the first sound it makes [/b/]	York Assessment for Reading and Comprehension (YARC) Early Reading
	Spoonerisms	What is cat with /f/ ["fat"]	Phonological Assessment Battery (PhAB)
Verbal memory	Word span	Cat-bun-face-sit (presented 1/sec for immediate recall)	Working Memory Test Battery for Children (WMTB-C)
	Digit span Phonological memory	1-6-8-9 Repeated "dopelate; istrum etc."	CTOPP Children's Non-word Repetition Test (CNRep)
Verbal processing speed	Rapid automated naming (RAN)	Naming sets of colors, letters or digits; matrix of about 50 items timed	CTOPP

Evidence-based reading instruction is administered, based on the three areas of phonemic awareness, phonics, and reading fluency. This is combined with vocabulary and comprehension strategies. Phonemic awareness concentrates on manipulating phonemes with letters, focusing on one or two manipulations rather than multiple types, teaching in small groups, and specific instructions about counting and manipulating the sounds. These strategies work better in younger children, emphasizing the importance of early detection and implementation. Fluency is helped most by guided oral reading, which impacts on fluency, improving comprehension. Large amounts of private reading, with little feedback, are less helpful.

There are many publications (see Snowling[4]) demonstrating reading improvement using phonological based packages. Delay in applying these can lead to harm. Children who fail become disruptive, avoid reading, and cannot access academic material.

The visual system

A working visual system is required to see the script. The areas available to examine and manipulate are up-stream from the pathology of dyslexia, as outlined above. The eye care practitioner's role is to exclude any visual problem. Elucidating whether any visual abnormality coexists and whether it is causative or secondary to poor reading may be difficult (see Handler[14] and the AAO joint statement[15]).

Good communication is essential. Depending on your working environment, the child may be assessed as part of a team, including orthoptists, optometrists, pediatricians, and those connected with education. The child's hearing may need review.

School screening generally examines distance vision. In the context of poor reading, the examiner must concentrate on near tasks (without excluding distance visual acuity).

The clinical work-up

History

The clinician asks about visual symptoms, reading development, and general development. Visual symptoms can be common (depending on how the questions are asked) and can include blurring, movement of the text, and headaches. Developmental delay, cerebral palsy, and prematurity can be associated with poor accommodation and visual perception problems.

It is of great benefit to elucidate any educational work-up, if known. Dyslexic children may have a history of delayed speaking, difficulty in learning rhymes, delay in learning letters, and slow reading. Ask if phonetic testing has been completed. In many areas this may involve an educational psychologist. Older children may have developed coping strategies, but score poorly in time-limited assessments. There may be a family history of dyslexia.

Find out what else has been said to the child and parents, particularly if they have seen any other professionals, for example optometrists, orthoptists, occupational therapists, and teachers. The parents may have read about a number of treatments. One needs to be aware of terms, such as eye teaming, eye tracking, and focusing, and what they mean to the parents (for example, eye tracking often means pursuit movements to parents, which are not used in reading).

Parents may report that their children appear to be daydreaming. Enormous effort is required for some children to read, expending powers of attention and concentration. They may be summoning energy to start again.

Ask about the child's use of hand-held game consoles. It is difficult to think that any near vision abnormality is of much significance if hours are spent playing these devices, unless they are fatiguing their convergence.

Examination

Many aspects of the visual system can be assessed. However, it is inappropriate to keep examining until an abnormality is found. Many of the assessments have not been standardized or validated on sufficiently large populations. Many of them require cooperation and effort from the child. If enough tests are performed, it is relatively easy to find an abnormality in any child. There are limited data to refer to as best practice, or how common many proposed findings should be in any given population. Additionally there is often more than one method

described for many parameters (for example, three ways of examining for accommodative amplitude: the pull away, the push up, and minus lens test). This suggests all have inaccuracies – as is reported.

Care needs to be exercised to avoid spurious findings. A suggested examination profile is outlined in Table 61.2. Some aspects of the examination are discussed below.

Refraction

An accurate refraction is paramount. The decision to perform a "dry" or cycloplegic refraction will depend on a number of factors, including cooperation and age. How much hypermetropic correction one should prescribe, in the absence of esotropia, has not been established. A post-cycloplegic retinoscopy can be a guide.

Near visual acuity

Nearly all near vision tests require reading. Care needs to be exercised in young children who may appear unable to see close, but are, in fact, unable to read. Near chart letter matching may be a more appropriate measure of near acuity. In children who have poor vision, the near threshold is of limited use in the classroom. Of more use is the size needed for comfortable reading. This is usually two grades bigger than threshold. Documenting this in terms of font size translates better to classroom work.

Accommodation

Documentation of normal accommodative function is helpful. It excludes it as an etiological factor and removes any need for low plus glasses. The accommodative amplitude is both active and variable in children. The amount deployed at any given time will depend on interest, effort, target distance, and size. Many children will accommodate to a target for less than a second before moving off, for example re-fixating the examiner. Near point is insufficient to assess the accommodative system, as some children tolerate blur. A combination of near visual acuity, near point distance (amplitude), dynamic refraction (response), and possibly accommodative facility is a reasonable compromise. The prevalence of poor accommodation and insufficiency is low in the children with normal neurological development. However, if there is a true deficiency it is important to detect this as near glasses (or bifocals) may be indicated. Symptoms may include discomfort, blurry near vision, or visual movement. Poor accommodation may be associated with illness, medication, neurotrauma, and functional behavior.

Near point accommodation

Methods described[16] include the push up test (target brought toward the patient as with the RAF rule), the minus lens test, as well as the "pull-away" method. In the pull-away test, the patient wears their distance correction. A fixation stick is held close to the eye to begin the test. The examiner indicates a small letter and the other eye is occluded. The stick is moved away from the eye at about 1–2 cm/second and the patient's task is to say what the letter is as soon as it becomes legible. The test can be done binocularly which is more life-like, although convergence factors will act as confounders. Once the letter is clear, a measurement can be made of accommodative amplitude (inverse of the distance). The statistical power of comparative publications varies.[17,18]

Table 61.2 – Suggested vision and ocular examination in poor readers

Function/structure	Test	Reason	Connection with reading
Visual acuity Distance	• LogMAR or Snellen • Other age appropriate acuity test	To document normal acuity Poor vision associated with refractive error, strabismus, and other ocular pathology	Little evidence of association with difficulty in reading
Visual acuity Near	• Near chart • Font size	To document threshold near vision Could be associated with poor accommodation	Reading comfortable two sizes bigger than threshold Comfortable font size useful for teaching support
Refraction	• Subjective or • Cycloplegic • Post Cyclo Ret	Rule out refractive error Asthenopia	Well accepted cause of asthenopic symptoms Uncorrected hypermetropia common
Sensory fusion	• Worth lights • Bagolini	Documentation	No evidence associated with poor reading
Stereopsis	• Randot • TNO	Documentation Needs normal near vision	No evidence associated with poor reading
Field of vision	• Confrontation • Goldmann • 120 point Humphrey	Rarely present in the absence of neurological disease	Individuals with hemianopia may read better vertically

Accommodation
• Amplitude of accommodation
• Accommodative lag or lead
• Facility of accommodation
	• Pull away
	• RAF rule
	• Dynamic Ret
	  Nott
	  MEM
	  +2.00/−2.00 flippers
		Reduced accommodation leads to poor near VA, variety of symptoms	Associated with certain syndromes (e.g. Down's syndrome), developmental delay, head injury

Ocular alignment	Cover test	Large phoria associated with asthenopic symptoms	May be amenable to treatment, glasses, exercises, Botox, or surgery
Vergence	Near point convergence	Leads to asthenopic symptoms Convergence insufficiency (CI) needs symptoms to make diagnosis and initiate treatment	Responds to home-based convergence exercises
Motor fusion	Fusion range distance and near • Prism bar • Risley prism	Might lead to difficulty with reading. Poor in intermittent strabismus (exotropia usually)	Reduced base out fusion range part of CI spectrum in US
Saccadic function	Refixation in free space	To rule out pathology	Not an established cause of reading disability
Anterior segment	Slit-lamp	To rule out pathology	
Posterior segment	Ophthalmoscopy	To rule out pathology	

Dynamic refraction

Usually the amplitude of accommodation is less than is needed, based on the target distance. This is termed accommodative lag. Accommodative lead describes the situation where too much accommodation is used based on the target distance. The Nott method[19] is recommended. It is quick and requires no lenses other than the child's distance glasses. The child is asked to read down a near acuity stick held at a defined distance (usually 25, 33, or 40 cm). The retinoscope is moved backwards along the line of sight, starting a short distance behind the target. Assuming an accommodative lag, the initial retinoscopic reflex will be "with." As the retinoscope is moved backwards, an end point is reached (before the reflex changes to "against" movement). The measurement from the patient is noted. If for example the stick is held at 33 cm from the patient (should generate 3 D of accommodation) and the retinoscope

is at 40 cm (2.5 D), a lag equal to 0.5 D is measured. Although this test is done binocularly, introducing confounding variables, it is quick. The alternative, the monocular occlusion method (MEM), requires lenses to be introduced to neutralize the reflex, which may stimulate more accommodation.

Accommodative facility

Prevalence reports are conflicting; one publication found the prevalence of reduced accommodative facility to be 1.5% in 1650 children.[14] The usual test uses a +2.00/−2.00 flipper. The subject reads some text one or two lines bigger than their threshold. The lenses are introduced, negative first, and the subject asked to continue reading. The child should continue to read the test type out loud while rotating the flipper. This assumes that they accommodate (for the minus lens) and relax accommodation (positive lens) in order for them to continue reading. It is probably of little value under 8 years of age. If carried out binocularly, convergence acts as a confounder. A complete cycle is one rotation, i.e. clearing the negative lens then the positive lens. Normal values in children from 8 to 12 years old is 5 cycles per minute and in older children up to 10 cycles per minute.[16]

Convergence

Convergence insufficiency (CI) is more common (3–5% prevalence).[14] There is a difference in terminology. In the UK, the term is used to describe a difficulty in obtaining and maintaining convergence (usually defined as to the nose, but less than 6 cm is also accepted), in association with symptoms. In the US the term also includes a near exophoria (usually defined as 4 prism diopters more than any distance exophoria) and reduced base out fusion range (less than 15 prism diopters at near).[20] Symptoms can be varied, and include the symptom questionnaire published in the Convergence Insufficiency Treatment Trial (CITT) trial.[20] CI may be precipitated by illness and increased near work.

Binocular function

There is no causal link between abnormalities in binocular vision and reading and writing and prevalence rates are the same in the two populations.[21] Documentation of sensory binocular function and fusion ranges should be carried out, as they may be a cause of asthenopic symptoms.

Saccadic function

Many studies have demonstrated normal saccadic function in poor readers.[14] Saccadic function changes as reading improves, but there is no evidence to support saccadic training as being beneficial to reading.[16] It is reasonable to clinically assess saccadic function, without progressing to EMG recordings. One method is to hold two objects approximately 40 cm from the patient, about 10 cm either side from the sagittal plane and ask the subject to fixate each alternately. A standard approach has been described by USUCO (Northern State University College of Optometry).[16]

Suggested management

An ocular work-up may open up therapeutic opportunities. Poor visual acuity may be due to refractive error, amblyopia, or a number of other pathologies.

Refractive correction of hypermetropia depends on visual acuity, near and distance, any esophoria, esotropia, and assessment of accommodation, plus background factors (i.e. developmental delay). A post-cycloplegic retinoscopy to assess normal working tonic accommodation will also guide the decision. If there is poor near vision or reduced accommodation, it is logical to give full distance correction before considering giving any near add (addition). Younger children wear the full distance prescription all the time (except when playing violent sports). In older children, glasses use might be more selective, e.g. for close work.

In children with poor accommodation a near add or bifocals work well. A +2.00 add is a reasonable starting point. If bifocal glasses are required, a split pupil large D seg is suggested. This usually results in a rapid improvement in schoolwork.

CI does not interfere with decoding and is not a cause of dyslexia. However, it can affect concentration on near tasks.

Exercises can be performed at home, usually managed by orthoptists. A number of exercises may be used including "pencil push-ups", jump convergence, and stereograms.

Management of phorias and tropias will depend on symptoms and examination findings. Treatments might include glasses, exercises to expand fusion ranges, as well as invasive procedures such as botulinum toxin and surgery. Use of prisms is rare in children.

Field loss is uncommon. Orientating the text vertically can facilitate reading. A left homonymous hemianopia might be helped by reading upwards (rotating the text counter clockwise). For a right hemianopia, often more of a handicap for reading English, the text is read downwards.

Controversial theories and treatments

There are many professional groups who treat or support poor readers. The reader is referred to the reviews published by Handler[14] and Barrett.[22] Visual symptoms are common amongst poor readers and in particular children. Therefore, the temptation to find a unifying "vision theory" has been high. The public needs to develop a degree of skepticism toward vision-related therapies that claim to treat learning disorders and learn to assess carefully the information promoted.

Magnocellular theory

The visual system contains two parallel systems, the magnocellular and parvocellular. The latter is responsible for high spatial frequency vision as used in reading. The magnocellular pathway responds to rapidly changing visual stimuli. The theory[23,24] postulates that the magnocellular pathway is responsible for suppressing vision during saccades, and in dyslexic children this fails in some way, allowing the vision at one end of the saccade to interfere with the vision at the other. This might explain the visual symptoms expressed by some children. The theory and science, in particular the work with contrast sensitivity, has been criticized by many authors.[14,25]

Meares Irlen syndrome

Meares Irlen syndrome (MIS) is a term used to justify the practice of prescribing colored filters (either as overlays or in glasses). The term "visual stress" has now been adopted by some authors and combined with MIS to form the term Meares Irlen syndrome visual stress or MISViS.[26] Visual stress originally linked certain individuals with migraine who have an inability to read for long periods without distortion or discomfort.[27] It is claimed to be prevalent in good and poor readers. Cortical excitability or hypersensitivity has been linked to contrast and pattern glare and it is claimed to be the source of the symptoms.

Neither MIS[28] nor visual stress are acknowledged as identifiable diseases. Many authors have commented that MIS does not exist. A summary or these critical publications is available.[14]

Ocular motor dysfunction

This term encompasses the study of fixation, saccades, and pursuit. The pursuit pathway is redundant in reading. Poor readers exhibit smaller and more numerous saccades. They fixate for longer and they also have more backward saccades (regressions). These improve as their reading progresses. The assumption that these differences are the cause of poor reading is flawed. Many studies have demonstrated that the eye movements of slow readers are normal.[14] In addition, the prevalence of children with reading difficulty is no more common in children with genuine eye movement disorders, such as infantile nystagmus syndrome.[14]

Accommodation exercises and low plus glasses

There is no clear scientific evidence supporting the use of eye exercises for accommodative dysfunction[14,22,29] and little evidence to support low plus glasses if accommodation is normal.[14] If there is a true deficiency in accommodation, a near add may help. Those that improve with exercises may be due to poor accommodation as a result of disinterest in near tasks.

Treatments administered by a number of health professionals are described in the referenced review.[14] Additionally a review concluded that, with the exception of convergence insufficiency, there was little scientific support for the practice of behavioral optometry.[22] In summary, abnormal accommodation, dysmetric saccades, visual-motor dysfunction, binocular instability, perceptual dysfunctions, or difficulties with "crossing the midline" of the visual field remain hypothetical and are, like many other conditions supposedly associated with dyslexia, as common in those who do not have the condition as those that do.

There are numerous tests that children are subjected to in order to find an abnormality. Table 61.3 lists just a few of these.

Table 61.3 – Summary of further tests

Function/ structure	Test	Claimed reason	Comment
Visual stress Susceptibility to Meares Irlen ViS (MISViS)	Colorimeter	To identify a need for colored overlays or tinted glasses	Conflicting published evidence[14]
Rate of reading	Wilkins Rate of Reading	To show improvement in reading with colored filters	No correlation with standard reading assessments
Saccadic function	Developmental eye movement	Test of saccadic function	Disputed relevance to reading
Contrast sensitivity	Pelli Robson	Magnocellular theory	Disputed relevance to reading
Binocular instability	Not clear from the website	Associated with visual stress and magnocellular defects	No published data (in peer reviewed journals)
Pattern glare	IOO (Institute of Optometry) Pattern Glare Test	Designed to diagnose MISViS	Introduced to diagnose MISViS

Summary

Dyslexia is a cognitive defect involving phonetic processing and is not caused by abnormalities in the visual system. Appropriate phonic based teaching should follow early detection. Inappropriate intervention may delay addressing the educational issues and serve to reinforce visual symptoms at a highly suggestible age. Inappropriate intervention may be harmful.

Dyslexic children may improve with all manner of treatments. However, it is important to explain to parents that there is little justification for optometric therapy, or colored overlays/glasses in the face of a normal examination. Much of what may be suggested seems innocuous, and parents must feel free to follow whatever course they perceive to be correct. However, if possible, ophthalmologists should recommend resisting this temptation and avoid hours of inappropriate exercises, when children could be either at school or at home enjoying themselves. It may be helpful to point out that children with known visual problems (poor acuity, poor binocular vision, nystagmus, strabismus) uncommonly have any sort of reading problem.

There is limited healthcare capital in all societies, and inappropriate treatments should not drain the public finance. Communication with the teaching profession, in particular educational psychology, is important.

Parents need to be aware of what is available for reading development and, if problems persist, seek further evaluation. Good results can be achieved with individualized phonemic-based learning programs.

Acknowledgment

I would like to acknowledge Professor Maggie Snowling, Department of Psychology, University of York, for her help and advice.

References

1. Vellutino FR, Fletcher JM, Snowling, MJ, Scanlon DM. Specific reading disability (dyslexia): what have we learned in the past four decades? J Child Psychol Psychiatry 2004; 45: 2–40.
2. Lyon GR, Shaywitz SE, Shaywitz BA. A definition of dyslexia. Ann Dyslexia 2003; 53: 1–14.
3. http://www.dsm5.org/ProposedRevisions/Pages/proposedrevision.aspx?rid=84
4. Snowling M, Duff F, Petrou A, Schiffeldrin J. Identification of children at risk for dyslexia: the validity of teacher judgments using "Phonic Phases" JRIR 2011; 34: 157–70.
5. Report of the National Reading Panel. Teaching Children to Read: An Evidence-Based Assessment of The Scientific Research Literature on Reading and its Implications for Reading Instruction. Bethesda, MD: National Institute of Child Health and Human Development, National Institutes of Health; 2000.
6. https://www.education.gov.uk/publications/eOrderingDownload/00659-2009DOM-EN.pdf
7. Wagner RK, Torgeson JK. The nature of phonological processing and its causal role in the acquisition of reading skills. Psychol Bull 1987; 101: 192–212.
8. Shaywitz SE, Shaywitz BA. The science of reading and dsylexia. J AAPOS 2003;7:158–66.
9. Flynn J, Rahbar M. Prevalence of reading failure in boys compared with girls. Psychol Sci 1994; 31: 66–71.

10. Shaywitz SE, Shaywitz BA, Fletcher JM, Escobar MD. Prevalence of reading disability in boys and girls: results of the Connecticut Longitudinal Study. J Am Med Assoc 1990; 264: 998–1002.

11. Scarborough HS. Very early language deficits in dyslexic children. Child Dev 1990; 61: 1728–43.

12. Snowling MJ, Gallagher A, Frith U. Family risk of dyslexia is continuous: individual differences in the precursors of reading skill. Child Dev 2003; 74: 358–73.

13. Hatcher PJ, Hulme C, Miles JN, et al. Efficacy of small group reading intervention for beginning readers with reading-delay: a randomised controlled trial. J Child Psychol Psychiatry 2006; 47: 820–7.

14. Handler SM, Fierson WM. Learning disabilities, dyslexia, and vision. Pediatrics 2011; 127: e818–56.

15. http://one.aao.org/CE/PracticeGuidelines/ClinicalStatements_Content.aspx?cid=8aa39ca4-039a-4329-beec-42e5a3007329

16. Scheiman M, Wick B. Clinical Management of Binocular Vision: Heterophoric, Accommodative and Eye Movement Disorders, 3rd ed. Philadelphia: Lippincott Williams and Wilkins; 2008: 19–33.

17. Antona B, Barra F, Barrio A, et al. Repeatability intraexaminer and agreement in amplitude of accommodation measurements. Graefes Arch Clin Exp Ophthalmol 2009; 247: 121–7.

18. Rosenfield M, Cohen AS. Repeatability of clinical measurements of the amplitude of accommodation. Ophthalmic Physiol Opt 1996; 16: 247–9.

19. McClelland JF, Saunders KJ. Accommodative lag using dynamic retinoscopy: age norms for school-age children. Optom Vis Sci 2004; 81: 929–33.

20. CITT Group C. Randomized clinical trial of treatments for symptomatic CI in children. Arch Ophthalmol. 2008; 126: 1336.

21. Hertle RW, Kowal LW, Yeates KO. The ophthalmologist and learning disabilities. Focal Points Clinician's Corner 2005.

22. Barrett BT. A critical evaluation of the evidence supporting the practice of behavioural vision therapy. Ophthalmic Physiologic Optics 2009; 29: 4–25.

23. Breitmeyer B. Sensory masking, persistence and enhancement in visual exploration and reading. In: Rayner K, editor. Eye Movements in Reading: Perceptual and Language Processes. New York, NY: Academic Press; 1983: 3–31.

24. Stein J, Walsh V. To see but not to read; the magnocellular theory of dyslexia. Trends Neurosci 1997; 20: 147–52.

25. Skoyles J, Skottun BC. On the prevalence of magnocellular deficits in the visual system of non-dyslexic individuals. Brain Lang 2004; 88: 79–82.

26. Kruk R, Sumbler K, Willows D. Visual processing characteristics of children with Meares-Irlen syndrome. Ophthal Physiol Opt 2008; 28: 35–46.

27. Wilkins AJ. Visual Stress. Oxford: Oxford University Press; 1995.

28. Hoyt CS. Irlen lenses and reading difficulties. J Learn Disability 1990; 23: 624.

29. Rawstron JA, Burley CD, Elder MJ. A systematic review of the applicability and efficacy of eye exercises. J Pediatr Ophthalmol Strabismus 2005; 42: 82–8.

Neurometabolic disease and the eye

Jane L Ashworth • Andrew A M Morris • J Edmond Wraith

Chapter contents

Many neurometabolic diseases present in childhood with ophthalmic manifestations. In some conditions, the characteristic ophthalmic features may lead toward an early diagnosis. In others, the ophthalmic complications present later in the course of the disease but can have significant visual effects for the patient. Findings such as vertical or horizontal gaze palsy, characteristic corneal changes, cherry-red spot, retinopathy, or optic atrophy, particularly in the presence of progressive systemic or neurologic disorders, should alert the ophthalmologist to the possiblity of a neurometabolic disorder.[1]

Although most of the diseases described here are rare, many are now treatable; it is important that the pediatric ophthalmologist is aware of them.

Lysosomal disorders

Lysosomal storage disorders (LSDs) arise as a result of defects in lysosomal enzymes, receptor targets, activator proteins, membrane proteins, or transporters causing accumulation of specific substrates within lysosomes (Table 62.1). This leads to impairment of cellular and tissue function.[2] Most LSDs have central nervous system (CNS) and systemic defects; untreated, many result in death in infancy or childhood. Whilst each type of LSD is rare, their total incidence is 1 per 7000 to 8000 live births. Many have ocular manifestations present early in the course of the disease (Box 62.1). The

Table 62.1 – Classification of LSD by lysosomal function affected

Lysosomal function affected	Disorder
Metabolism of glycosaminoglycans	Mucopolysaccharidoses
Degradation of glycoproteins	Aspartylglucosaminuria, fucosidosis, mannosidosis, Schindler's disease, sialidosis type 1
Degradation of glycogen	Pompe's disease
Degradation of sphingolipids	Fabry's disease, Farber's disease, Gaucher's disease, GM1 gangliosidoses, GM2 gangliosidoses, Krabbe's disease, metachromatic leukodystrophy, Niemann-Pick disease types A and B
Degradation of polypeptides	Pycnodysostosis
Degradation or transport of cholesterol esters or complex lipids	Niemann-Pick type C, Wolman's disease, cholesterol ester storage disease
Multiple deficiencies of lysosomal enzymes	Multiple sulfatase, galactosialidosis, mucolipidosis types I and II
Transport and trafficking defects	Cystinosis, mucolipidosis IV, sialic acid storage disorder, chylomicron retention disease with Marinesco-Sjögren's syndrome, Hermansky-Pudlack syndrome, Chediak-Higashi syndrome, Danon's disease
Unknown defects	Geleophysic dysplasia, Marinesco-Sjögren's syndrome

From Wilcox WR. Lysosomal storage disorders: the need for better pediatric recognition and comprehensive care. J Pediatr 2004; 144: S3–S14.

pediatric ophthalmologist has an important role in facilitating early diagnosis so appropriate treatment can be started early.

All LSDs have autosomal recessive inheritance except for Danon's disease, Fabry's disease and Hunter's disease (mucopolysaccharidosis type II) which are X-linked recessive. Some disorders are more prevalent in a particular geographic area or in certain populations, such as Gaucher's, Tay-Sachs, Niemann-Pick type A, and mucolipidosis IV, which are 50–60 times more prevalent in the Ashkenazi Jewish population.[2]

There is often a wide variation in phenotype, including severity of symptoms, systems affected, and presence of CNS manifestations. In many disorders such as Gaucher's and Tay-Sachs, there are infantile, juvenile, and adult forms. There are characteristic ocular features in some of the LSDs (see Box 62.1) which should alert the ophthalmologist to their possibility, particularly when seen in a child with suggestive systemic features such as organomegaly, skeletal abnormalities or joint stiffness, coarsening of facial features, or a progressive neurologic or muscular deterioration, or unexplained pain.

Diagnosis of LSDs may be made using biochemical assay of blood, urine or skin fibroblasts, and confirmed by molecular genetic testing in many cases.

There have been advances in the availability of treatments for many of the LSDs. Hematopoetic stem cell transplantation provides donor stem cells to produce the deficient enzymes, and is used to treat many LSDs including the mucopolysaccharidoses (MPS) I Hurler's, and MPS VI Maroteaux-Lamy. Enzyme replacement therapy (ERT) provides an exogenous source of enzyme by repeated intravenous infusions, and is available for several LSDs including MPS I (Laronidase), MPS II (idursulfase), MPS VI (galsulfase), Gaucher's disease (Imiglucerase and Velaglucerase) Fabry's disease (Agalsidase alfa and Agalsidase beta) and Pompe's disease (alglucosidase

alpha). However, ERT does not cross the blood–brain barrier, limiting its effect on CNS manifestations. Drug therapy may be helpful in LSDs by reducing substrate production or increasing the activity of residual enzyme. N-Butyldeoxynojirimycin (Miglustat) reduces the production of glycosphingolipids and is effective in treating Gaucher's disease and Nieman-Pick C. Gene therapy for LSDs has been successful in animal models but has not yet been successfully applied in human LSD. Medical and surgical management of the multiple systemic and neurologic manifestations requires a multidisciplinary approach.

Mucopolysaccharidoses

The mucopolysaccharidoses (MPSs) are a heterogeneous group of disorders resulting from accumulation of glycosaminoglycans within ocular and systemic tissues. There is a wide spectrum of phenotypes with a range of skeletal, cardiac, respiratory, gastrointestinal, and neurologic manifestations. The MPSs have been classified according to phenotype, and result from mutations in different lysosomal enzymes (Table 62.2). They are all inherited in an autosomal recessive manner apart from MPS II (Hunter's) which is X-linked.

Early hematopoietic stem cell transplantation and ERT have improved the prognosis for many MPS patients. Visual impairment is common, and can be due to corneal opacification, optic neuropathy, retinopathy, or cortical visual impairment.[3]

Corneal clouding in MPS

Corneal clouding is a characteristic feature of several of the MPS disorders (MPS I Hurler's, Hurler/Scheie and Scheie's, MPS IV Morquio's, MPS VI Maroteaux-Lamy, and MPS VII Sly's), and may help facilitate the diagnosis when present at an early stage. Deposition of glycosaminoglycans (GAGs) within the corneal stroma leads to progressive diffuse corneal opacification, described as having a "ground-glass" appearance (Fig. 62.1). Corneal opacification is milder in the less severely effected MPS I phenotype Scheie's, and is not a feature of MPS III Sanfillipo.

Box 62.1

Ocular manifestations of lysosomal storage disorders

Cornea – diffuse corneal clouding
Corneal verticillata
Lens – characteristic cataract
Macula – cherry red spot
Bull's-eye maculopathy
Vasculature – retinal and conjunctival vascular tortuosity
Optic neuropathy
Ocular motor apraxia (saccadic initiation failure)

Table 62.2 – Mucopolysaccharidoses and underlying enzyme deficiencies

Type	Eponym	Stored material	Enzyme deficiency
MPS IH	Hurler's	DS, HS	Iduronidase
MPS IS	Scheie's	DS, HS	Iduronidase
MPS IH/S	Hurler-Scheie	DS, HS	Iduronidase
MPS II	Hunter's (X-LR) sulfatase	DS, HS	Iduronidase sulfatase
MPS IIIA	Sanfillipo's	HS	Heparan N-sulfatase
MPS IIIB		HS	N-Acetylglucosaminidase
MPS IIIC		HS	Acetyl-CoA-glucosaminidase-acetyltransferase
MPS IIID		HS	N-Acetylglucosamine-6-sulfatase
MPS IVA	Morquio's		Galactosamine-6-sulfatase
MPS IVB			α-Galactosidase
MPS VI	Maroteaux–Lamy	DS	N-Acetylgalactosamine-4-sulfatase
MPS VII	Sly's	HS, CS, DS	α-Glucuronidase
MPS IX	Natowicz	Hyaluronic acid	Hyaluronidase

DS = dermatan sulfate; HS = heparan sulfate; CS = chondroitin 6-sulfate or chondroitin 4,6-sulfate.

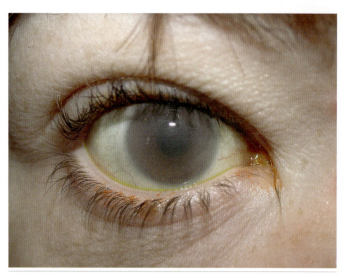

Fig. 62.1 **Corneal clouding in a patient with MPS I (Hurler's).**

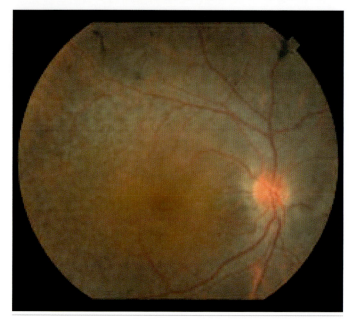

Fig. 62.4 **Retinal pigment epithelial changes in a patient with MPS I.** Vision was 6/60 despite minimal corneal clouding.

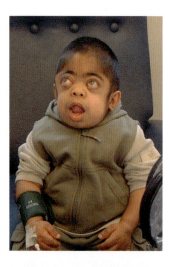

Fig. 62.2 **Pseudoexophthalmos due to shallow orbits in a 17-year-old patient with MPS VI.**

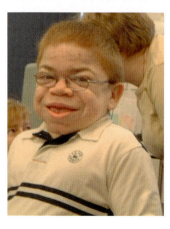

Fig. 62.3 **Coarsening of facial features in a 16-year-old patient with MPS II.**

Patients with MPS may have coarsening of facial features with pseudoexophthalmos (Figs 62.2 and 62.3), which can result in corneal exposure and subsequent vascularization.

A patient with mild corneal clouding may be asymptomatic, but photophobia and reduced vision occur as the opacification worsens. GAG deposition can increase corneal thickness[4,5] and affect corneal hysteresis,[6] thus affecting the accuracy of intraocular pressure measurements. Corneal transplantation

(penetrating keratoplasty or deep lamellar keratoplasty) may result in improvement in vision when severe corneal opacification causes visual loss[7,8] with no reopacification of the graft in up to 11 years follow-up.[7] However, an assessment of potential benefits of corneal transplantation must consider the presence of coexistent retinopathy, optic nerve dysfunction, and cortical visual impairment, as well as the significant anesthetic risks for a patient with MPS.

Hypermetropia and strabismus in MPS

The majority of patients with MPS are hypermetropic due to changes in corneal refraction and reduced axial length.[3,9] Strabismus and amblyopia are common.[3]

Retinopathy in MPS

Progressive retinopathy occurs in MPS I, II, III but is not usually a feature of MPS VI.[10] The patient may experience night-blindness and problems with peripheral vision, but this may go unnoticed due to the visual loss associated with corneal opacities. Signs of retinopathy include retinal pigment epithelial (RPE) atrophy and pigment clumping (Fig. 62.4), arteriolar narrowing, optic disk pallor, and macula changes. Serial electroretinography (ERG) may show initial deterioration of rod mediated responses, followed by involvement of cones. Choroidal folds have occurred in MPS II associated with a ring scotoma; optical coherence tomography demonstrated extrafoveal photoreceptor loss and cystoid spaces within retinal layers.[11]

Optic disk swelling and atrophy

The optic nerve often has a "full" appearance in patients with MPS (Fig. 62.5A,B). GAG deposition occurs in the ganglion cells and within surrounding sclera causing an enlargement of the nerve and thickening of the sclera[12] (Fig. 62.5C,D). The consequent nerve compression can lead to optic atrophy. In addition, patients with MPS may develop raised intracranial pressure and the resultant optic nerve compromise may lead to profound visual loss. Visual evoked potential may be useful

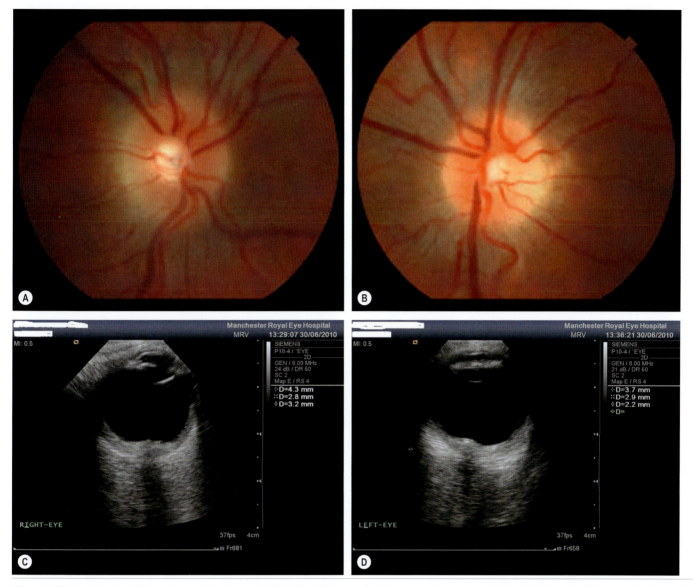

Fig. 62.5 (A,B) "Full" optic disks in a 14-year-old patient with MPS II. (C,D) Ultrasound of the same optic nerves as in (A) and (B), showing thickening of sclera and increase in diameter of the optic nerve (courtesy of Mr Vishwanath, MREH).

in monitoring optic nerve function and in assessment prior to consideration of corneal transplant.

Glaucoma

Glaucoma may arise in MPS due to accumulations of GAGs within the anterior segment resulting in a narrow angle, and within the trabecular cells leading to open angle glaucoma as a result of outflow obstruction. It has been described in MPS I, II, and VI.[10] Difficulties in diagnosis and assessment of glaucoma arise in patients with MPS due to inaccuracy of intraocular pressure measurements, corneal clouding hampering assessment of the angle and disk, and the presence of coexistent disk pathology.

Punctate lens opacities occur in MPS IV.

Systemic manifestations in MPS

A patient with MPS may present in infancy with recurrent ear infections, inguinal or umbilical hernias, or skeletal changes such as kyphoscoliosis (Fig. 62.6). Other systemic manifestations include obstructive sleep apnea, deposits on the cardiac valves and infiltration of the cardiac muscle, spinal cord compression, and pain and stiffness from skeletal dysplasia. Developmental delay and intellectual impairment occur in MPS I; behavioral problems occur early in MPS III, as a result of CNS deposition of GAG. Management is multidisciplinary, coordinated by a pediatrician with input from cardiology, anesthesia, orthopedics, ENT, neurosurgery, physiotherapy, audiology, speech therapy, and ophthalmology. Children with a diagnosis of MPS should have regular assessments by a pediatric ophthalmologist.

Anesthesia should be undertaken in a department with specialist expertise in the MPS disorders. Children with MPS are difficult to intubate, due to MPS deposition around the airway and vulnerable cervical spinal cords.

Prognosis and treatment of MPS

The prognosis in MPS is variable depending on the phenotype; some children die before their second decade and others survive into their fifth or sixth decade. Early hematopoietic stem cell transplantation using either matched bone marrow or umbilical cord blood cells can improve the systemic prognosis of patients with MPS I and VI. ERT for MPS I (laronidase), MPS II (elaprase), and MPS VI (galsulfase) improves systemic manifestations and can be used prior to early BMT. Ophthalmic manifestations of MPS VI may be stabilized by ERT.[13]

Neuronal ceroid lipofuscinosis

The neuronal ceroid lipofuscinoses (NCLs) are autosomal recessive conditions characterized by progressive neurologic deterioration in children or young adults, epilepsy, and visual deterioration due to retinopathy. All the NCLs are associated with accumulation of an autofluorescent material, ceroid lipofuscin, and degeneration of neuronal cells.[14] There are at least 10 genetically distinct NCLs (Table 62.3). The term Batten's disease refers to the juvenile-onset form of NCL and occurs

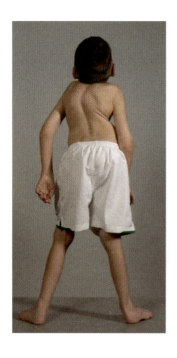

Fig. 62.6 Kyphoscoliosis in MPS I.

most commonly as a result of mutations in CLN3, which maps to chromosome 16p21.

Juvenile NCL must be considered when a child presents with rapidly deteriorating visual function, particularly when associated with behavioral changes, neurologic deterioration, or seizures. The ophthalmologist plays a crucial role in early diagnosis and monitoring of the condition.

Diagnosis of NCLs can be made by demonstration of specific enzyme deficiency in leukocytes, fibroblasts or blood, such as palmitoyl protein thioesterase, which can be used for diagnosis of NCL1.[14] In a school child with retinopathy, CLN3 diagnosis may be confirmed by finding vacuolated lymphocytes in the peripheral blood smears. The more rare NCL variants can be demonstrated by electron microscopic examination of skin biopsy material or isolated blood lymphocytes before proceeding to molecular genetic testing.[14]

There are no specific treatments available for the NCLs, but enzyme replacement, gene and stem cell therapy, and pharmacologic approaches are under investigation.

Specific types of NCL are infantile neuronal ceroid lipofuscinosis, classical late infantile lipofuscinosis, and juvenile neuronal ceroid lipofuscinosis.

Infantile neuronal ceroid lipofuscinosis (CLN1, Haltia-Santavuori disease)

Classical infantile NCL manifests as rapidly progressive neurologic deterioration from approximately 6 months of age with seizures, loss of vision, and brain atrophy, with death in the first decade.

Classical late infantile neuronal ceroid lipofuscinosis (CLN2, Jansky-Bielschowsky disease)

This presents around the third year of life with epilepsy and arrest in development. Visual loss occurs from retinal degeneration.

Juvenile neuronal ceroid lipofuscinosis (CLN3, Batten's disease)

Children with juvenile NCL present with rapid deterioration of vision between 4 and 10 years. Other manifestations such as behavioral problems and cognitive decline and motor deterioration manifest before or after the onset of visual loss.[15-17] There is an increased prevalence in North European

Table 62.3 – Classification of NCLs

Age at onset	Designation	Chromosome location	Deficient protein
Congenital or later	CLN10	11p15	Cathepsin D
Infantile or later	CLN1	1p32	Palmitoyl protein thioesterase 1
Late infantile or later	CLN2	11p15	Tripeptidylpeptidase 1
	CLN5	13q22	Partially soluble protein
	CLN6	15q21	Membrane protein
	CLN7	4q28	Membrane protein
	CLN8	8p23	Membrane protein
Juvenile	CLN3	16p12	Membrane protein
	CLN9		
Adult	CLN4		

Kohlschütter A, Schulz A. Towards understanding the neuronal ceroid lipofuscinosis. Brain Dev 2009; 31: 499-502.

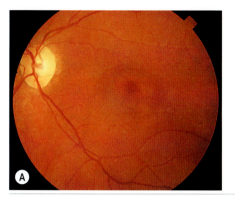 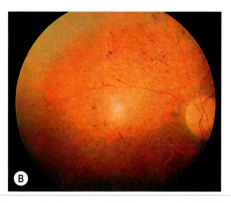 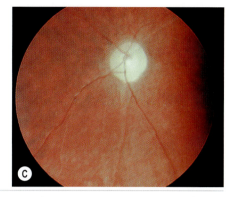

Fig. 62.7 Juvenile Batten's disease. (A) Optic atrophy, arteriolar thinning and bull's-eye maculopathy. (B) Bone-spicule pigmentation, optic atrophy, and arteriolar narrowing. (C) Late retinal changes, including depigmentation, optic atrophy, and extreme arteriolar narrowing.

populations.[15] Night blindness and photophobia may be present in addition to visual loss. Misdiagnosis as macula or retinal dystrophy or even functional visual loss may occcur in the early stages.[16] At presentation, the fundus may be normal or show pigmentary maculopathy, atrophic changes, or bull's-eye maculopathy. Later there is a widespread retinal degeneration with pigment clumping (Fig. 62.7) and sparse bone-spicule pigmentation in the periphery, the disk becomes atrophic and the arterioles thinned (Fig. 62.7C), and the retina becomes avascular. Eccentric viewing or "overlooking" is where children hold their eyes in a raised position whilst attempting to fixate on a target, presumed due to the relative preservation of the superior peripheral retina.[16,17] The children are usually blind within 3 years. Although mental deterioration and behavioral disturbances occur early, often predating the visual deterioration, they are often quite subtle. The disease follows a slow downward path with the onset of fits between 7 and 16 years of age, dementia in the teens, and death sometimes in the second or third decade.

Fluorescein angiography shows diffuse RPE atrophy with stippled hyperfluorescence.[18] ERG may show a photopic and scotopic electronegative waveform, typically in early cases with a markedly reduced b : a ratio in the single flash photopic ERG, consistent with inner retinal dysfunction.[15,19] ERG changes may prompt further investigations to be carrried out at an early stage. Visual field testing may show field constriction.

Glycoprotein disorders

α-Mannosidosis (α-mannosidase deficiency)

α-Mannosidosis is associated with mild facial coarsening (Fig. 62.8), skeletal abnormalities, a variable degree of learning difficulty, and deafness. Ophthalmologic features include cataracts and strabismus.[20] The lens opacities are posterior cortical with multiple discrete clear round vacuoles lying at different depths in the lens, best seen by slit-lamp retroillumination.[21]

Fucosidosis

Fucosidosis is a progressive neurodegenerative disease with seizures, mild coarsening of the facies, skeletal dysplasia, and angiokeratoma. Affected children have conjunctival and retinal vascular tortuosity. A bull's-eye maculopathy and central "lobulated" corneal opacities may occur.[22]

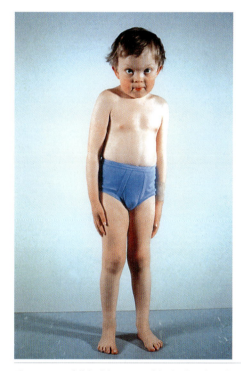

Fig. 62.8 A child with mannosidosis showing the mild coarsening of the features. When older there was an increase in the facial coarsening.

Sialidosis (mucolipidosis type I)

Sialidosis is a result of α-N-acetylneuraminidase deficiency; patients excrete sialyloligosaccharide in the urine.

Type 1 sialidosis "cherry-red spot myoclonus syndrome" presents in late childhood with visual loss associated with a cherry-red spot (Fig. 62.9), myoclonic epilepsy, and ataxia. Type 2 sialidosis has an earlier onset with coarse facies, developmental delay, hepatomegaly, and dysostosis multiplex (Fig. 62.10).

In addition to cherry-red spots, patients with sialidoses may have punctate lens opacities, optic atrophy, corneal clouding, and visual field defects.[23-25]

Sialic acid storage diseases

These result from a block in lysosomal efflux of sialic acid as a result of mutations in SLC17A5, encoding the lysosomal

643

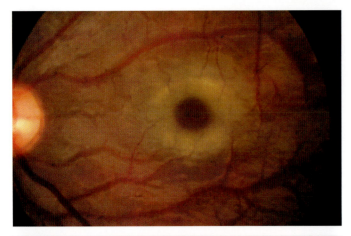

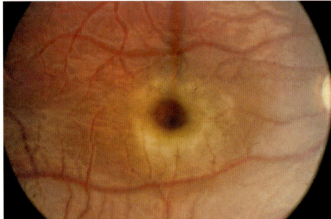

Fig. 62.9 Cherry-red spot in a patient with sialidosis type 1. (Mr M. D. Sander's patient.)

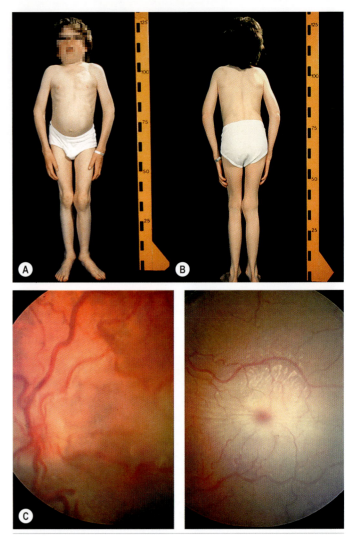

Fig. 62.10 (A,B) Patient with sialidosis type 2. He has kyphoscoliosis and joint changes. (C) Same patient as in (A) and (B), showing a cherry-red spot. The picture is hazy because of corneal clouding.

protein sialin. They range in severity from infantile sialic acid storage disease (ISSD) with coarse facial features and fair complexion, severe developmental delay, hepatosplenomegaly and cardiomegaly, and death in early chidlhood, to Salla's disease with slowly progressive mental retardation, ataxia, spasticity, and epilepsy. In ISSD, children may have albinoid fundi.[26] In Salla's disease strabismus, nystagmus, and optic atrophy may occur.

Mucolipidoses

Mucolipidosis (ML) II and III are autosomal recessive disorders caused by deficiency of *N*-acetylglucosamine-1-phosphotransferase which phosphorylates carbohydrate residues on *N*-linked glycoproteins.

ML II or "I cell" disease presents at an early age with neurologic degeneration, joint stiffening, facial coarsening, and kyphoscoliosis (Fig. 62.11). Death occurs in childhood. There is retinal degeneration and corneal clouding.

ML III is milder, with a slowly progressive course and survival to adulthood. Ophthalmic features include corneal clouding, hypermetropic astigmatism, optic disk swelling, retinal vascular tortuosity, and maculopathy.[27] The ERG is normal.

ML IV is an autosomal recessive disorder resulting from mutations in the MCOLN1 gene, which encodes mucolipin-1. It is seen mainly in Ashkenazi Jews. Clinical features include progressive mental retardation and hypotonia. ML IV patients

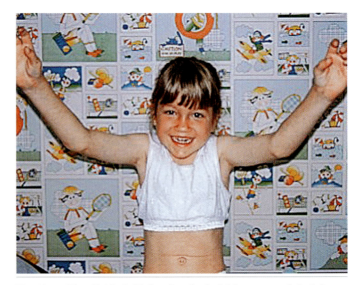

Fig. 62.11 Mucolipidosis III showing the facial features and the joint stiffening which prevents the patient from fully lifting her arms.

have corneal eipthelial haze, retinopathy with optic nerve pallor, vascular attenuation, and RPE change with electronegative ERG.[28,29] Other ophthalmic features include strabismus, corneal erosion and episodic pain, cataract, and ptosis.[28,30] Mild phenotypes have been described with only ocular manifestations of corneal clouding and retinopathy.[31,32]

Sphingolipidoses

Sphingolipidoses are caused by abnormalities of catabolism of sphingolipids, complex membrane lipids which form an integral part of cerebral membranes. There is a wide range of severity and presentations in most of the sphingolipidoses, but progressive neurodegeneration and cherry-red spots are characteristic features.

GM2 gangliosidosis

- *Tay-Sachs disease:* hexosaminidase A deficiency, AR, most common in the Ashkenazi Jewish population.
- *Sandhoff's disease:* hexosaminidase A and B deficiency.

These are severe neurodegenerative disorders, with infantile (most common), juvenile, and adult forms. A cherry-red spot is the typical eye finding.

Tay-Sachs (hexosaminidase A deficiency) usually presents in infancy with progressive neurologic deterioration and spasticity, feeding difficulties, seizures, and deterioration of visual behavior. Macrocephaly is common and death usually occurs by 2–4 years. Sandhoff's disease (hexosaminidase A and B deficiency) follows a similar pattern and most commonly presents in infancy.

A cherry-red spot is apparent at an early stage, due to GM2 ganglioside accumulation in the retinal ganglion cells. As the ganglion cells die the cherry-red spot fades and optic atrophy becomes apparent.[33] The ERG is normal, but the visual evoked potential extinguished.[34] There is no treatment.

Both disorders have a later-onset variety; ataxia and dementia begin in the second year of life and the disease follows a more attenuated form. Late onset Tay-Sachs disease presents in an adult and is associated with abnormalites of saccades: saccadic hypometria, transient decelerations, and premature terminations.[35] A cherry-red spot is less common in the late onset types (Table 62.4).

Table 62.4 – Cherry-red spot in neurometabolic disorders[1]

Disease	Disease frequency of cherry-red spot
Niemann-Pick type A	Occasional
Niemann-Pick type B	Occasional
GM2 gangliosidosis (Tay-Sachs and Sandhoff's)	Frequent
GM1 gangliosidosis, infantile	Occasional
Galactosialidosis	Frequent
Farber's lipogranulomatosis	Occasional
Sialidosis type 1	All
Sialidosis type 2	Frequent
Metachromatic leukodystrophy	Occasional

Metachromatic leukodystrophy (arylsulfatase deficiency)

Metachromatic leukodystrophy may present in infancy, childhood, or adolescence with gait problems, spasticity and loss of reflexes due to neuropathy, behavioral difficulties, and speech and feeding problems. MRI shows central demyelination and cerebellar atrophy. Optic atrophy may occur. No effective treatment exists, but hematopoietic stem cell transplantation (HSCT) may prevent deterioration if done very early in the disease.

Krabbe's disease (galactocerebrosidase deficiency)

This is a severe neurodegenerative disorder with infantile, childhood, and late onset forms. The early onset form develops symptoms in the first few months with irritability and poor feeding, and progresses quickly to spasticity and a vegetative state. Visual impairment is common due to optic atrophy or cortical blindness. There is no treatment. HSCT may have a role very early in the disease.

GM1 gangliosidosis

Infantile GM1 gangliosidosis causes hypotonia from birth. By 6 months, developmental delay and a coarse appearance with puffy skin, maxillary hyperplasia, hypertrophied gums, and macroglossia develop. Affected children have dysostosis multiplex. Ocular motor apraxia (saccadic initiation failure),[36] a cherry-red spot, and corneal clouding may occur. Rapid neurologic deterioration is usual with seizures and swallowing difficulties and death by 2 years. There is no treatment. Juvenile and adult forms occur in which there is neurologic deterioration but no physical changes.

Niemann-Pick disease

Disorders in which there is storage of sphingomyelin were previously termed Niemann-Pick disease types A, B, C, and D. These terms are still used although only types A and B are due to sphingomyelinase deficiency. Types C and D are the same condition where ganglioside and sphingomyelin accumulation is due to a disorder of cholesterol transport within the cell.

Niemann-Pick disease types A and B (sphingomyelinase deficiency)

Niemann-Pick type A presents in infancy with failure to thrive, feeding difficulties, and respiratory infections. Hepatomegaly (Fig. 62.12) is prominent and, in contrast to infantile Gaucher's, is more marked than splenomegaly. Neurologic degeneration starts around 18 months with loss of vision associated with a cherry-red spot (Fig. 62.13) and later optic atrophy. Death usually occurs by 3 years. There may be a brown discoloration of the anterior lens capsule, but minimal corneal opacification.[37]

Niemann-Pick disease type B is less severe and presents later in childhood with hepatosplenomegaly. Usually there are no neurologic symptoms; some patients may have ataxia but are usually of normal intelligence. Massive splenic enlargement, cirrhosis of the liver, and pulmonary infiltration may occur (Fig. 62.14). Eye abnormalities include periorbital fullness, macular granular deposits, and cherry-red spot[38]

Both types are more prevalent in the Ashkenazi Jewish population. There is no treatment for type A; type B may be amenable to bone marrow transplantation.

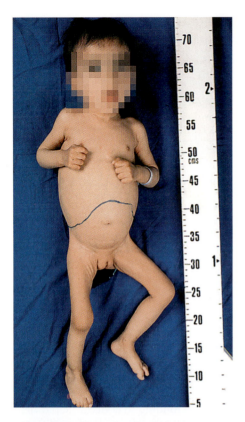

Fig. 62.12 An infant with Niemann-Pick type A showing the hepatomegaly and spastic posture.

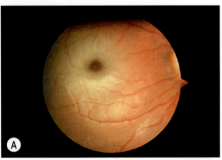

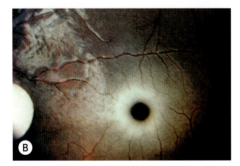

Fig. 62.13 (A) Cherry- red spot in a patient with Niemann-Pick type A: the spot is brownish because of dark pigmentation. (B) Cherry-red spot in a black infant with Niemann-Pick type A. (Professor C. S. Hoyt's patient.)

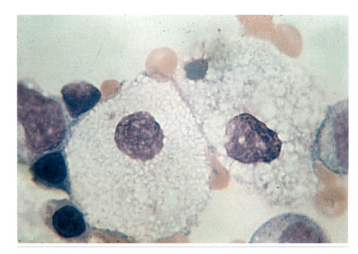

Fig. 62.14 Foam cells. Lipid laden histiocytes seen on bone marrow biopsy in Niemann-Pick disease type B.

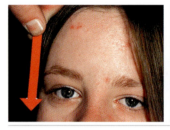
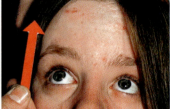

Fig. 62.15 Downgaze palsy in a child with Niemann-Pick type C. The arrow denotes the direction that the child is being told to look. Horizontal and upgaze were normal. (Mr M. D. Sanders patient.)

Niemann-Pick types C and D

Niemann-Pick types C and D are due to impaired intracellular trafficking of cholesterol as a result of mutations in either the NPC1 or NPC2 genes. NPC is pan-ethnic.

Type C has variable presentations including neonatal liver disease, splenomegaly, and neurologic deterioration in late childhood with seizures, dystonia, cerebellar ataxia, and dementia with death by the second decade. A vertical supranuclear gaze palsy (Fig. 62.15) is characteristic of this disorder. There may be horizontal supranuclear eye movement defects or a supranuclear disorder of convergence. A faint cherry-red spot may be seen. Miglustat (an inhibitor of glucosylceramide synthase which catalyzes the first step of glycosphingolipid synthesis) is effective in stabilizing neurologic disease.[39]

Fabry's disease (α-galactosidase deficiency)

Fabry's disease is an X-linked recessive lysosomal storage disease caused by a deficiency of α-galactosidase A, which results in multiorgan failure and premature death. Distinctive ophthalmic manifestations (particularly corneal vertillata, retinal vascular tortuosity) are common although they may not cause any symptoms.[40] Their presence may be helpful in early diagnosis.[41] The symptoms of Fabry's disease occur in males in late childhood or adolesence with pain in the extremities (acroparesthesia) provoked by exertion or change in temperature. Characteristic skin lesions (angiokeratoma corporis diffusum; Fig. 62.16A) are present, with dark red angiectases in the "bathing trunk area" (lower abdomen, buttocks, and scrotum). Patients with Fabry's disease suffer from a chronic progressive neuropathy (Fig. 62.16B), progressive renal dysfunction, heart disease (hypertrophic cardiomyopathy), and stroke. Fabry's disease is treated with ERT with intravenous infusions of recombinant α-galactosidase, agalsidase alfa (Replagal, Shire), or agalsidase beta (Fabrazyme, Genzyme).[42]

Corneal verticillata (whorl-like lines radiating from a single vortex; Fig. 62.16C) occur in both heterozygote and homozygote forms of Fabry's disease and do not affect vision.[43] Corneal involvement includes corneal haze and fine subepithelial brown lines.[44] Conjunctival tortuosity and microaneurysms

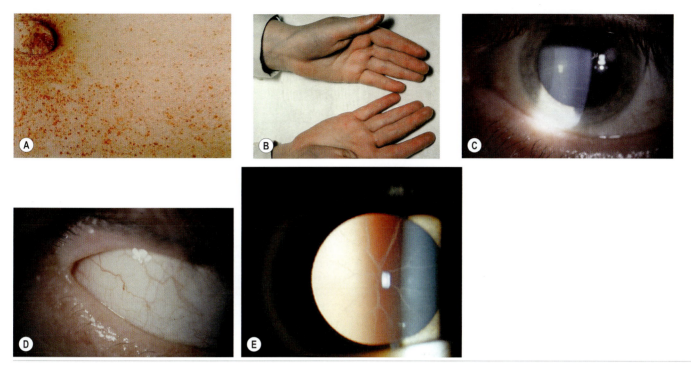

Fig. 62.16 Fabry's disease. (A) Angiokeratoma corporis diffusum. (B) Hypothenar atrophy from peripheral neuropathy. (C) Corneal verticillata. (D) Conjunctival telangectasia. (E) Characteristic spoke-like posterior cortical sutural cataract on retro-illumination.

occur (Fig. 62.16D) and chronic chemosis may occur in an adult with Fabry's disease.[45] Characteristic lens opacities occur less commonly than corneal and vascular changes: a granular, wedge shaped subcapsular cataract, and lines of discrete opacities radiating from the posterior pole of the lens along the sutures[44,46] (Fig. 62.16E). Retinal vascular tortuosity, particularly of veins, occurs in the second decade. The vessels become beaded, with sheathing and may develop arteriovenous anastomoses and thromboses. Vascular tortuosity is more frequently observed in patients with greater impairment of renal and cardiac function.[43] Retinal vascular occlusion may be the initial symptom. Optic disk edema or myelinated nerve fibers may occur. Neuro-ophthalmologic problems include nystagmus, third nerve palsy, and strabismus. Optic atrophy, internuclear ophthalmoplegia, seizures, and strokes occur rarely.

Female heterozygotes may have corneal verticillata, cataract, and conjunctival and retinal vascular tortuosity but are less frequently affected than male homozygotes.[43,46] Females may show clinical features such as acroparesthesia and angiokeratoma. The extent of manifestations in female heterozygotes is determined by X-chromosome inactivation.

Farber's disease

This autosomal recessive disease is characterized by the onset in infancy of multiple subcutaneous nodules, lymphadenopathy, a hoarse cry, and variable involvement of lung, heart, and liver. The course is variable with death between 1 and 18 years. Severely affected children may have a cherry-red spot, nodular corneal opacity, or a pingueculum-like conjunctival lesion. There is no treatment.

Cystinosis

See Chapter 33.

Gaucher's disease (glucocerebrosidase deficiency)

Gaucher's disease (GD) is an autosomal recessive disease which arises from mutations in the glucocerebrosidase (GBA) gene. Gaucher's disease is classified according to severity and neurologic involvement into types 1, 2, and 3. There is a wide phenotypic variation. Ocular motor apraxia (saccadic initiation failure) may be an early manifestation of neurologic involvement.[47,48] Gaucher's disease is no longer treated with HSCT; ERT with recombinant glucocerebrosidase is used in GD types 1 and 3. The dose required is variable but usually not more than 60 units per kg per 2 weeks. Substrate reduction therapy (Miglustat) may be used in patients thought unsuitable for intravenous ERT.

Gaucher's type 1 (non-neurologic)

This is more common in Ashkenazi Jews, and can present in children or adults with hepatosplenomegaly, anemia, thrombocytopenia, and leukopenia. There may be painful splenic and bony infarctions; the distal ends of the femur may develop a typical Erlenmeyer's (a type of conical flask) deformity. Dark brown-yellow pingueculae occur in the nasal bulbar conjunctivae which are characterized by numerous Gaucher's cells on histologic examination. Macular change, choroidal neovascularization, and peripheral retinal vessel leakage occur.[49-51]

Gaucher's type 2 (infantile)

This presents within the first 6 months of life with severe feeding problems, spasticity, neurologic regression, and hepatosplenomegaly. Strabismus is a feature. Affected infants usually die within the first few years.

Gaucher's type 3 (Norrbottnian or chronic neuronopathic)

Type 3 usually presents in childhood with failure to thrive and hepatosplenomegaly (Fig. 62.17). Ocular motor apraxia may

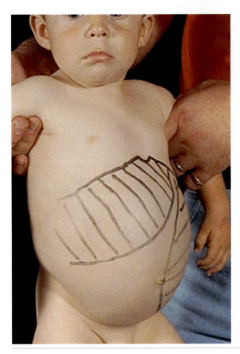

Fig. 62.17 Hepatosplenomegaly in Gaucher's type 3.

be the first sign of neurologic involvement. Intermittent strabismus and vertical gaze palsies may also occur. Progression may be very gradual. Many patients survive into adult life with ERT. Skeletal disease may be problematic with osteopenia and progressive kyphosis being particular problems.

Mitochondrial disorders

Mitochondrial disorders arise as a result of dysfunction of the mitochondrial respiratory chain. They can present at any age and frequently have ocular manifestations such as ptosis, external ophthalmoplegia, optic atrophy, pigmentary retinopathy, cataracts, and cerebral visual impairment.[52-54] Some mitochondrial disorders have only ocular manifestations (e.g. Leber's hereditary optic neuropathy, LHON), but many involve multiple organ systems such as muscle (proximal myopathy), heart (cardiomyopathy), peripheral and central nervous systems (encephalopathy, seizures, dementia, migraine, stroke-like episodes, ataxia, and spasticity), inner ear (sensorineural deafness), and endocrine systems (diabetes mellitus). Several syndromes are described but there is overlap between them. Many patients have an atypical pattern.

Mitochondrial disorders can be caused by mutations of nuclear genes (with Mendelian inheritance) or mitochondrial DNA (mtDNA, which is inherited exclusively from the mother). Many copies of mtDNA are present in each cell. In LHON, mutations affect all copies (homoplasmy). In other conditions, mutant mtDNA usually coexists with wild-type mtDNA (heteroplasmy) and the clinical severity depends on the proportion that is mutated; the proportion varies among members of a pedigree, leading to different symptoms and ages of presentation. If the clinical picture is characteristic of a disorder associated with specific genetic abnormalities (e.g. LHON, NARP, MELAS, or Alpers' syndromes) then the diagnosis can

be confirmed by molecular genetic testing. Many mtDNA point mutations can be detected in blood but mtDNA deletions in Kearns-Sayre syndrome can only be detected in muscle. Other tests include measurement of blood or cerebrospinal fluid (CSF) lactate, and biochemical or histochemical studies of the mitochondrial respiratory chain on a muscle biopsy.

Leber's hereditary optic neuropathy

see Chapter 52.

Kearns-Sayre syndrome

These syndromes are associated with mtDNA "rearrangements" (large deletions or duplications). They are almost always sporadic. The mild end of the spectrum for mtDNA rearrangements is called chronic progressive external ophthalmoplegia (seen in adults).

Kearns-Sayre syndrome has been defined as progressive external ophthalmoplegia and pigmentary retinopathy with onset before 20 years of age and at least one of: heart block, cerebellar syndrome, or CSF protein above 1 g/L. Other features may include hearing loss, dementia, cardiomyopathy and endocrine disorders. The ophthalmoplegia is characterized by ptosis and exotropia but diplopia is rare. The fundus has a "salt and pepper" appearance but visual acuity is seldom severely impaired.[55] Involvement of the orbicularis oculi muscles can lead to exposure keratits and corneal perforation.[56]

MELAS syndrome

MELAS syndrome is characterized by:

M = mitochondrial myopathy
E = encephalopathy
LA = lactic acidosis
S = stroke-like episodes.

The strokes start between 5 and 15 years of age, and may cause visual field defects or cortical blindness and hemiplegia; sometimes the symptoms resolve rapidly. Headaches and vomiting may precede the stroke-like episodes and maternal relatives may have a history of severe migraine. Other ocular manifestations include progressive external ophthalmoplegia, "salt and pepper" pigmentary retinopathy and macular RPE atrophy, optic neuropathy, and non-ischemic central retinal vein occlusion.[57,58] The m.3243A>G mtDNA mutation is present in 80% of patients.

NARP syndrome

This is characterized by:

N = neurogenic weakness
A = ataxia
RP = retinitis pigmentosa.

It is caused by the m.8993T>G or m.8993T>C mutations. The fundus may have a "salt and pepper" or a "bone-spicule" appearance; some patients develop optic atrophy or maculopathy with severe visual loss.

Leigh's disease

See chapter 53.

Alpers' syndrome

This neurodegenerative disorder presents with an explosive onset of seizures in early childhood. Developmental regression is accompanied by cerebral atrophy. Involvement of the occipital cortex is common, leading to cortical visual impairment. Terminally, patients often develop liver failure. The condition is caused by autosomal recessive mutations in POLG1, which is a nuclear gene involved in mtDNA replication.

Sengers' syndrome

Sengers' syndrome is characterized by congenital cataracts, hypertrophic cardiomyopathy, skeletal myopathy, and lactic acidosis.[59] The cardiomyopathy may cause early death or may be milder, in which case patients can survive into their second or third decades.

Autosomal dominant optic atrophy

See Chapter 52.

Peroxisomal diseases

Peroxisomes are organelles involved in the synthesis of plasmalogens (crucial for myelin), bile acids and isoprenoids, and the oxidation of very long chain and branched chain fatty acids (e.g. phytanic acid).

Peroxisomal biogenesis disorders

In these autosomal recessive disorders, peroxisomes cannot be made properly due to mutations in the PEX genes. Peroxisomal biogenesis disorders are classified into the Zellweger's spectrum and rhizomelic chondrodysplasia punctata (RCDP).

Zellweger's spectrum (Zellweger's syndrome, neonatal adrenoleukodystrophy, infantile Refsum's disease)

These disorders vary in severity, with overlap between phenotypes, but with poor vision as a common feature. Zellweger's syndrome is the severe end of the spectrum: patients die within a few months of birth. They are dysmorphic with a large anterior fontanelle, high forehead, shallow supraorbital ridges, and epicanthic folds. Hypotonia, seizures, poor feeding, liver disease, impaired hearing, and ocular abnormalities occur. Neonatal adrenoleukodystrophy is a slightly milder phenotype; some patients survive to mid-childhood, although they become deaf, blind, and profoundly retarded. Infantile Refsum's disease is the "mild" end of the spectrum: patients have little or no dysmorphism but they still have mental retardation, deafness, and pigmentary retinopathy. Diagnosis starts by demonstrating raised plasma concentrations of very long chain fatty acids (VLCFA).

Retinal dystrophy is almost universal[60] (Fig. 62.18). Patients with neonatal adrenoleukodystrophy and infantile Refsum's disease develop macular depigmentation and peripheral pigment clumping, with loss of peripheral vision that often progresses to complete blindness. Patients with Zellweger's syndrome have retinal hypopigmentation and a severely abnormal or absent ERG. They may have corneal clouding,

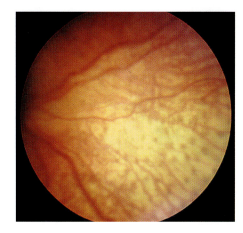

Fig. 62.18 Zellweger's syndrome. Retinal dystrophy with mottled RPE.

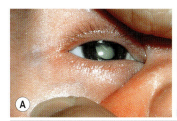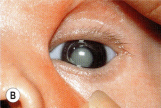

Fig. 62.19 Rhizomelic chondrodysplasia punctata. Bilateral total congenital cataract.

congenital cataracts, and glaucoma. Nystagmus and strabismus are common, secondary to poor vision.

Rhizomelic chondrodysplasia punctata

In Rhizomelic chondrodysplasia punctata (RCDP), there is severe shortening of the humeri and femora and stippled epiphyses. Most patients have facial dysmorphism and severe neurologic abnormalities: few survive beyond 2 years. Cataracts are very common and are usually congenital (Fig. 62.19) though they may appear at a few months of age. Patients with RCDP have normal plasma VLCFA concentrations but erythrocyte plasmalogen levels are abnormally low.

Refsum's disease

Refsum's disease is caused by autosomal recessive deficiency of the peroxisomal enzyme phytanoyl-CoA hydroxylase, leading to accumulation of phytanic acid in blood and tissues. Features of Refsum's disease are cerebellar ataxia, peripheral neuropathy, and retinitis pigmentosa which can be prevented by dietary restriction of phytanic acid.

X-linked adrenoleukodystrophy

In this X-linked recessive disorder, mutations in the ABCD1 gene lead to the accumulation of VLCFAs in blood and tissues. There are two main phenotypes, which may occur in the same pedigree. The childhood cerebral form presents at 4–12 years of age with behavioral, cognitive, and neurologic problems, usually leading to a vegetative state within 3 years. Strabismus, visual field defects, and decreased visual acuity are early symptoms. Later, these patients become blind due to optic atrophy and cortical visual loss[61] (Fig. 62.20). The second phenotype, adrenomyeloneuropathy, presents with paraparesis in adults.

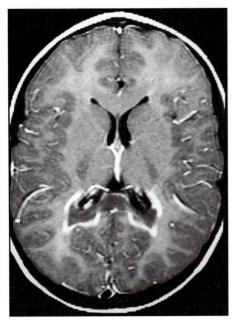

Fig. 62.20 Adreno-leukodystrophy. MRI scan showing characteristically predominant early involvement of the occipital lobes and visual pathway with high signal from the periventricular white matter.

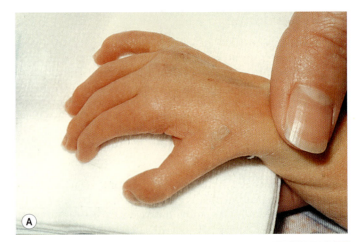

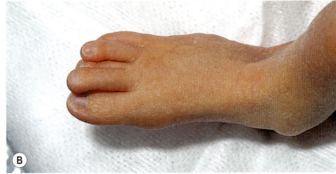

Fig. 62.21 Phosphomannomutase-2 deficiency (carbohydrate-deficient glycoprotein syndrome Ia CDG Ia). (A) Showing long fingers. (B) Showing long toes.

Adrenal failure occurs in both phenotypes, either before or after the onset of neurologic problems.

Lorenzo's oil combined with a low fat diet can normalize plasma VLCFA concentrations, but it does not alter the clinical course once symptoms have started. Bone marrow transplantation can prevent progression of the childhood cerebral disease if undertaken soon after the onset of problems.

Primary hyperoxaluria type I

See Chapter 45.

Congenital defects of glycosylation

Most extracellular and cell surface proteins and some intracellular proteins are glycoproteins. The oligosaccharide may be attached to the amino acid asparagine in the protein (*N*-linked glycosylation) or to a serine or a threonine (*O*-linked glycosylation). Defects of *O*-linked glycosylation cause Walker-Warburg syndrome and muscle-eye-brain disease (see Chapter 56).

Disorders of *N*-linked glycosylation

Phosphomannomutase-2 deficiency is the commonest congenital defect of glycosylation (PMM2-CDG, previously known as CDG Ia). Patients present at birth with hypotonia, esotropia, and dysmorphism – long fingers and toes (Fig. 62.21) – inverted nipples, and fat pads over the buttocks. Death may occur in infancy from sepsis, pericardial effusions, nephrotic syndrome, or liver failure. Those surviving, or presenting later, show delayed development and ataxia, rarely walking without support. At least 50% of patients have esotropia, which is usually present from birth; ocular motor apraxia (saccadic initiation failure) and nystagmus are common. Retinitis pigmentosa appears after 8 years of age but the ERG may be abnormal much earlier. Other problems include delayed visual maturation, visual field loss, and progressive myopia.[62,63]

The other *N*-glycosylation defects are rarer and the ophthalmologic features are less well defined. Nystagmus, poor acuity, optic neuropathy, congenital cataracts, congenital glaucoma, and colobomas of the iris or retina have been reported. Strabismus is common in ALG6-CDG (previously known as CDG Ic).

Walker-Warburg syndrome and muscle–eye–brain disease

See Chapters 41 and 56.

Inborn errors of carbohydrate metabolism

Galactosemia and galactokinase deficiency

Galactosemia is an autosomal recessive disorder caused by a deficiency of the enzyme galactose-1-phosphate uridyltransferase. It presents in neonates with poor feeding, jaundice, and sometimes hepatosplenomegaly or sepsis.[64] Cataract formation occurs due to the accumulation of galactitol within the lens, and can be prevented with early diagnosis and implementation of a galactose-restricted diet.[65,66] "Oil-droplet" cataracts occur at an early stage due to refractive change within the lens nucleus (Fig. 62.22). These may progress to lamellar cataracts in the presence of poor dietary and biochemical control. Galactokinase deficiency causes early-onset juvenile cataracts, which may stabilize or regress with dietary control; mental retardation has been reported in a few patients.[67] Reducing

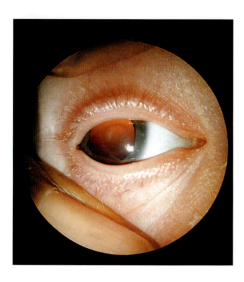

Fig. 62.22 Oil-droplet cataract in galactosemia.

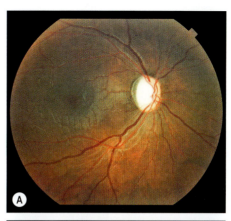

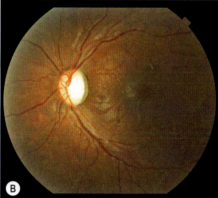

Fig. 62.23 Optic neuropathy in an 11-year-old girl with propionic acidemia. The patient noticed an acute onset of reduced vision in her right eye, and was found to have visions of only counting fingers in the right eye and 1.1 logMAR in the left, with sluggish pupils, a right relative afferent pupil defect, and bilateral optic nerve pallor.

substances are present in the urine in both untreated galactosemia and galactokinase deficiency. The diagnosis is established by enzyme assays of erythrocytes and DNA studies.

Inborn errors of amino acid metabolism

Homocystinuria

See Chapter 35.

Propionic and methylmalonic acidemias

These autosomal recessive conditions result from defects in the catabolism of branched chain amino acids. Neonates or young children present with vomiting, drowsiness, acidosis, and hyperammonemia. Treatment includes carnitine, dietary protein restriction, and prevention of catabolism; some cases of methylmalonic acidemia respond to vitamin B12. Progressive optic neuropathy may occur in propionic acidemia and methylmalonic acidemia due to mutase, CblA, or CblB defects (Fig. 62.23). The onset is generally in older children or adults, independent of metabolic control. The loss of visual acuity is often severe, with central scotomas and optic nerve pallor.[68,69]

CblC (cobalamin C) disease

This autosomal recessive disorder of vitamin B12 metabolism leads to methylmalonic aciduria and homocystinuria. It may present in infancy with failure to thrive, hypotonia, microcephaly, seizures, and nystagmus. A milder form presents later with neurologic deterioration. Visual loss may occur in childhood due to cone–rod retinal degeneration with an early maculopathy[70] and optic atrophy.[71]

Maple syrup urine disease

In this autosomal recessive disorder, branched chain amino-acids accumulate and are neurotoxic. Most cases present with encephalopathy in the first 2 weeks of life. Patients can be treated acutely by hemofiltration and subsequently with dietary management. Ophthalmoplegia may be a prominent feature of the neonatal encephalopathy.[72] In older children,

ataxia is an early feature of encephalopathy and may be accompanied by nystagmus.

Molybdenum cofactor deficiency and isolated sulfite oxidase deficiency

These two autosomal recessive disorders have similar clinical features, with spherophakia and ectopia lentis being common findings. Nystagmus, cortical blindness, enophthalmos, and colobomas may be present.[73] Most patients present in the newborn period with intractable seizures. Subsequently, they develop microcephaly, severe psychomotor retardation, and spastic tetraplegia and early death. Neuroimaging demonstrates multicystic encephalopathy and atrophy. A few patients run a milder course with prolonged survival.

Gyrate atrophy

Gyrate atrophy is an autosomal recessive disorder caused by deficiency of the enzyme ornithine delta-aminotransferase, leading to raised plasma ornithine levels, chorioretinal degeneration, and progressive loss of vision (Fig. 62.24). Myopia and early cataracts may occur.[74] An arginine-restricted diet may slow the rate of deterioration of the chorioretinal degeneration.[75,76]

Tyrosinemia type 2 (Richner-Hanhart syndrome)

This autosomal recessive disorder is caused by deficiency of tyrosine aminotransferase. It may present with ocular signs and symptoms as the initial manifestation in the first years of life with photophobia, pain, and conjunctival injection. There

651

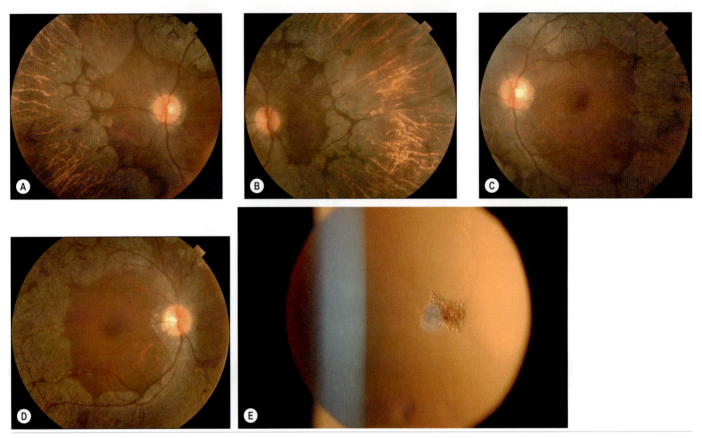

Fig. 62.24 Gyrate atrophy. (A,B) Characteristic sharply demarcated areas of chorioretinal degeneration in the mid-periphery of a myopic patient age 26, with relative sparing of the macula (C,D). The patient had poor dietary control and suffered from significant nyctalopia and had acuities of 6/24 right and 6/36 left. (E) The patient also had bilateral cataract. (Courtesy of Mr IC Lloyd, Manchester Royal Eye Hospital.)

is a bilateral pseudodendritic keratitis which may lead to neovascularization and corneal scarring.[77] Patients may have painful erosions and hyperkeratosis of the palms and soles, and cognitive impairment. Plasma tyrosine concentrations are extremely high and the eye and skin lesions probably result from the intracellular precipitation of tyrosine crystals. Dietary restriction of tyrosine and phenylalanine leads to resolution of these lesions.

Tyrosine concentrations are lower in tyrosinemia types 1 and 3. Type 1 patients treated with nitisinone sometimes complain of sore eyes.

Oculocutaneous albinism

See Chapter 40.

Aromatic L-amino acid decarboxylase deficiency

Eye movement abnormalities are prominent in this rare autosomal recessive disorder, in which the synthesis of catecholamines and serotonin neurotransmitters is impaired. Patients present in infancy with oculogyric crises, hypotonia, and autonomic dysfunction. Convergence spasm, ptosis, and miosis may occur.[78]

Canavan's disease

This is an autosomal recessive disorder prevalent in Ashkenazi Jews. Aspartoacylase deficiency leads to the accumulation of N-acetyl-aspartic acid. Patients with Canavan's disease usually present aged 2–4 months with macrocephaly, hypotonia, and developmental delay. White matter degeneration is seen on neuroimaging. Cortical visual loss, optic atrophy, and nystagmus are common. Most patients die by 3 years of age.[79]

Disorders of fatty acid and fatty alcohol metabolism

Long chain 3-hydroxyacyl-CoA dehydrogenase deficiency

The enzyme long chain 3-hydroxyacyl-CoA dehydrogenase (LCHAD) participates in mitochondrial fatty acid β-oxidation, and the autosomal recessive condition LCHAD deficiency may present in infancy with hypoglycemia, failure to thrive, feeding difficulties, cholestatic liver disease, and hypotonia.[80] Treatment is with dietary restriction of long chain fatty acids, vitamin and mineral supplementation, and avoidance

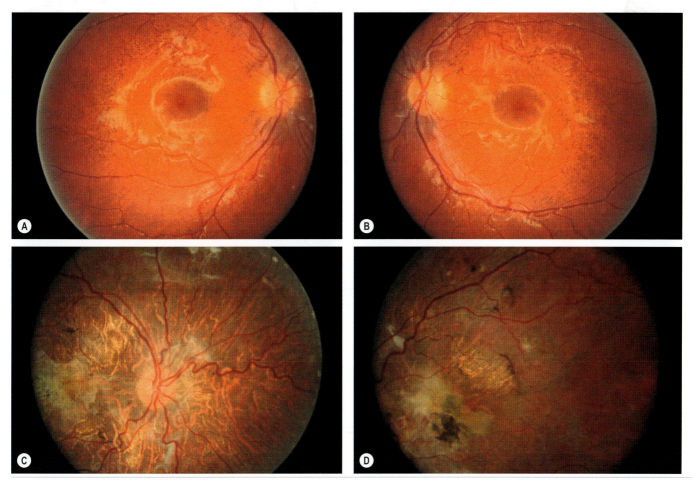

Fig. 62.25 (A,B) Peripapillary and perimacular granular pigmentary changes in an 11-year-old girl with LCHAD deficiency diagnosed neonatally during the first days of life. The acuity was 0.1 logMAR right and left eye with correction for a slight myopia and astigmatism. ERG was of subnormal amplitude. (Courtesy of Kristina Teär Fahnehjelm, St. Erik Eye Hospital, Stockholm.) (C,D) Bilateral areolar chorioretinopathy in a 21-year-old woman with LCHAD deficiency diagnosed at 8 months of age. Bilateral pigmentary retinopathy, exotropia, and bilateral myopia had been present since age 3 years, and by early adulthood the vision deteriorated due to chorioretinal fibrosis. The VA was < 1.0 logMAR with myopic glasses. (Courtesy of Kristina Teär Fahnehjelm, St. Erik Eye Hospital, Stockholm.)

of fasting. LCHAD deficiency causes variable severity of chorioretinal degeneration with visual loss and progressive myopia[81] (Fig. 62.25). Progressive lens opacities may occur.[82] Optimum dietary control may delay the progression of the chorioretinopathy.[83]

Sjögren-Larsson syndrome

See Chapter 45.

Disorders of sterol metabolism

Early onset cataracts are seen in several disorders of sterol metabolism, including defects of cholesterol synthesis and of bile acid synthesis.

Smith-Lemli-Opitz syndrome

Smith-Lemli-Opitz syndrome is caused by deficiency of 7-dehydrocholesterol reductase which catalyzes the final step in cholesterol synthesis, resulting in reduced cholesterol and raised 7-dehydrocholesterol levels. It has a spectrum of phenotypic severity with mental retardation and congenital malformations (microcephaly, ptosis, small upturned nose, micrognathia, polydactyly, syndactyly, genital abnormalities, and malformations of the heart or gut).[84] One-fifth of patients have cataracts (usually congenital). Rarer ophthalmologic abnormalities include strabismus, optic atrophy, and optic nerve hypoplasia. Treatment with cholesterol does not improve intelligence.

Mevalonic aciduria and hyperimmunoglobulinemia D syndrome

Mevalonic aciduria and hyperimmunoglobulinemia D syndrome (HIDS) are caused by deficiency of mevalonate kinase, which catalyzes an early step in cholesterol synthesis. Patients with mevalonic aciduria present in infancy with dysmorphic features (dolichocephaly, down-slanting eyes, and low set ears), mental retardation, failure to thrive, recurrent fevers, cerebellar ataxia, and visual impairment. The febrile episodes are accompanied by hepatosplenomegaly, lymphadenopathy, vomiting and diarrhea, arthralgia, and skin rashes. One-third of patients have cataracts. Uveitis and pigmentary retinopathy occur.[85] Many patients die in the first few years; most survivors have severe psychomotor retardation. Patients with HIDS have similar recurrent fevers with elevated concentrations of IgD, but without the other features of mevalonic aciduria.

X-linked dominant chondrodysplasia punctata 2 (CDPX2, Conradi-Hünermann syndrome)

This is an X-linked dominant condition, lethal in males, in which mutations in the emopamil binding protein (EBP) gene lead to deficiency of 3β-hydroxysteroid Δ^8,Δ^7-isomerase, causing skeletal, cutaneous, and ocular abnormalities. The main features are skeletal dysplasia, stippled epiphyses, neonatal ichthyosis with subsequent atrophic skin changes in a mosaic pattern, and cataracts, which may be congenital or developmental (Fig. 62.26). Microophthalmos, anterior segment dysgenesis, vitreoretinal abnormalities, and optic atrophy occur.[86,87]

Cerebrotendinous xanthomatosis

CTX is caused by mutations in the sterol 27-hydroxylase gene (CYP27A1) leading to the accumulation of cholestanol and cholesterol. Infantile-onset diarrhea may be the earliest clinical manifestation of CTX, followed by juvenile cataracts and neurologic problems (spasticity, ataxia, psychiatric disturbances, dementia, and seizures).[88] Adults develop tendon xanthomas and premature atherosclerosis. Optic neuropathy may occur in addition to cataracts. Treatment with chenodeoxycholic acid prevents deterioration and can reverse some neurologic symptoms.

X-linked ichthyosis (steroid sulfatase deficiency)

X-linked ichthyosis is caused by a deficiency of steroid sulfatase, and results in ichthyosis, usually within the first few months of life, in affected males. Characteristic corneal opacities (fine punctate diffuse opacites in posterior stroma adjacent to Descemet's membrane, or subepithelial granular opacities with epithelial irregularity) are present in 25% of affected males and also in heterozygous females; they have no effect on vision.[89-90]

Lipoprotein disorders

Abetalipoproteinemia (Bassen-Kornzweig syndrome)

This autosomal recessive disorder occurs due to deficiency of microsomal triglyceride transfer protein (MTP), needed for

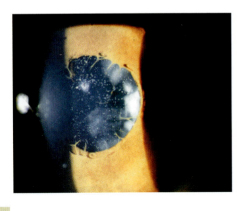

Fig. 62.26 Cataract in a girl with Conradi's syndrome.

the production of lipoproteins, resulting in malabsorption of fat and fat-soluble vitamins. It presents with failure to thrive, developmental delay, and steatorrhea in infancy. If untreated, spinocerebellar degeneration develops. It is associated with a progressive retinal dystrophy which may be stabilized by a low fat diet and combined vitamin A and E supplementation.[91]

Lecithin:cholesterol acyltransferase (LCAT) deficiency and "fish eye" disease (partial LCAT deficiency)

Lecithin-cholesterol acyltransferase (LCAT) catalyzes the formation of cholesterol esters in high density lipoproteins. Complete LCAT deficiency causes adult-onset renal failure, anemia, and corneal opacities. Partial LCAT deficiency ("fish eye" disease) causes no problems except progressive corneal clouding. This is due to extracellular lipid deposition in the corneal stroma. Opacities can be detected in children, though they are often asymptomatic. Some adults require corneal transplantation.

Apo A-I deficiency

Corneal clouding has been reported in a few children with Apo A-I deficiency. Other features of this condition are premature atherosclerosis and xanthomas.

Copper transport disorders

Wilson's disease

Wilson's disease is an autosomal recessive disorder resulting from mutations in ATP7B which transports copper into the Golgi apparatus of hepatocytes. Impaired biliary excretion causes copper accumulation in liver, kidney, cornea, and brain. Wilson's disease usually presents with liver disease at 5–20 years of age or with neurologic problems, typically between 20 and 40 years, but sometimes during childhood. Hepatic manifestations include chronic active hepatitis, cirrhosis, and fulminant hepatic failure. Common neurologic features are dystonia, dysarthria, dysphagia, tremor, and Parkinsonism and psychiatric problems. Rarer problems include hemolysis, arthritis, and Fanconi's syndrome.

Deposition of copper in peripheral Descemet's membrane leads to golden brown pigmentation: the Kayser-Fleischer ring (Fig. 62.27). Slit-lamp examination reveals these rings in 95% of patients with neurologic presentations but they are seldom present in asymptomatic patients and often absent in children presenting with liver disease. Kayser-Fleischer rings may occur with chronic cholestasis from other causes. Retinopathy may occur as a result of dysregulation of photoreceptor copper levels.

Treatment with copper chelators (D-penicillamine, trientine) or zinc results in symptomatic improvement and normal life expectancy. Liver transplantation is occasionally required.

Menkes' disease

Defects in the copper transporter ATP7A cause this X-linked disease. The main features are infantile-onset neurodegeneration, connective tissue disturbances, and characteristic "kinky"

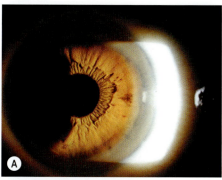

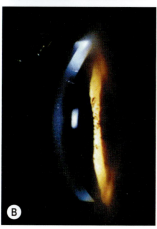

Fig. 62.27 (A) Kayser-Fleischer (K-F) ring in a child with the neurologic presentation of Wilson's disease. A brownish haze can be seen in the peripheral cornea. (B) The K-F ring can be seen in the posterior cornea on slit-lamp examination (arrow).

hair. Affected boys present with hypotonia and seizures at 2–3 months of age. They have "pudgy" cheeks, occipital bossing and sparse, brittle, white hair. Poor visual acuity is common with progressive visual loss due to retinal degeneration and optic atrophy. Early onset myopia, strabismus, blue irides and iris stromal hypoplasia, and aberrant lashes may occur.[92] Patients deteriorate rapidly, with developmental regression, spasticity and lethargy; most die by 3 years of age. Early treatment with parenteral copper-histidine may improve the neurologic prognosis and enhance survival. Occipital horn syndrome (also known as Ehlers-Danlos syndrome type IX or X-linked cutis laxa) is a mild form of Menkes' disease consistent with survival to adulthood.

References

1. Poll-The BT, Maillette de Buy Wenniger-Prick CJ. The eye in metabolic diseases: clues to diagnosis. Eur J Paediatr Neurol 2011; 15: 197–204.

2. Wilcox WR. Lysosomal storage disorders: the need for better pediatric recognition and comprehensive care. J Pediatr 2004; 144: S3–S14.

10. Ashworth JL, Biswas S, Wraith E, et al. Mucopolysaccharidoses and the eye. Surv Ophthalmol 2006; 51: 1–17.

15. Bozorg S, Ramirez-Montealegre D, Chung M, Pearce DA. Juvenile neuronal ceroid lipofuscinosis (JNCL) and the eye. Surv Ophthalmol 2009; 54: 463–71.

16. Collins J, Holder GE, Herbert H, et al. Batten disease: features to facilitate early diagnosis. Br J Ophthalmol 2006; 90: 1119–24.

36. Harris CM, Shawkat F, Russell-Eggitt I, et al. Intermittent horizontal saccade failure ('ocular motor apraxia') in children. Br J Ophthalmol 1996; 80: 151–8.

37. Walton DS, Robb RM, Crocker AC. Ocular manifestations of group A Niemann-Pick disease. Am J Ophthalmol 1978; 85: 174–80.

38. McGovern MM, Wasserstein MP, Aron A, et al. Ocular manifestations of Niemann-Pick disease type B. Ophthalmology 2004; 111: 1424–7.

40. Allen LE, Cosgrave EM, Kersey JP, et al. Fabry disease in children: correlation between ocular manifestations, genotype and systemic clinical severity. Br J Ophthalmol 2010; 94: 1602–5.

41. Samiy N. Ocular features of Fabry disease: diagnosis of a treatable life-threatening disorder. Surv Ophthalmol 2008; 53: 416–23.

43. Sodi A, Ioannidis AS, Mehta A, et al. Ocular manifestations of Fabry's disease: data from the Fabry Outcome Survey. Br J Ophthalmol 2007; 91: 210–4.

48. Harris CM, Taylor DS, Vellodi A. Ocular motor abnormalities in Gaucher disease. Neuropediatrics 1999; 30: 289–93.

52. Morris MA. Mitochondrial mutations in neuro-ophthalmological diseases: a review. J Clin Neuroophthalmol 1990; 10: 159–66.

53. Grönlund MA, Honarvar AK, Andersson S, et al. Ophthalmological findings in children and young adults with genetically verified mitochondrial disease. Br J Ophthalmol 2010; 94: 121–7.

54. Rose LV, Rose NT, Elder JE, et al. Ophthalmologic presentation of oxidative phosphorylation diseases of childhood. Pediatr Neurol 2008; 38: 395–7.

55. Bau V, Zierz S. Update on chronic progressive external ophthalmoplegia. Strabismus 2005; 13: 133–42.

58. Rummelt V, Folberg R, Ionasescu V, et al. Ocular pathology of MELAS syndrome with mitochondrial DNA nucleotide 3243 point mutation. Ophthalmology 1993; 100: 1757–66.

60. Folz SJ, Trobe JD. The peroxisome and the eye. Surv Ophthalmol 1991; 35: 353–68

62. Morava E, Wosik HN, Sykut-Cegielska J, et al. Ophthalmological abnormalities in children with congenital disorders of glycosylation type I. Br J Ophthalmol 2009; 93: 350–4.

64. Bosch AM. Classical galactosaemia revisited. J Inherit Metab Dis 2006; 29: 516–25.

65. Beigi B, O'Keefe M, Bowell R, et al. Ophthalmic findings in classical galactosaemia – prospective study. Br J Ophthalmol 1993; 77: 162–4.

73. Lueder GT, Steiner RD. Ophthalmic abnormalities in molybdenum cofactor deficiency and isolated sulfite oxidase deficiency. J Pediatr Ophthalmol Strabismus 1995; 32: 334–7

75. Kaiser-Kupfer MI, Caruso RC, Valle D, et al. Use of an arginine-restricted diet to slow progression of visual loss in patients with gyrate atrophy. Arch Ophthalmol 2004; 122: 982–4.

77. Macsai MS, Schwartz TL, Hinkle D, et al. Tyrosinemia type II: nine cases of ocular signs and symptoms. Am J Ophthalmol 2001; 132: 522–7.

80. den Boer ME, Wanders RJ, Morris AA, et al. Long-chain 3-hydroxyacyl-CoA dehydrogenase deficiency: clinical presentation and follow-up of 50 patients. Pediatrics 2002; 109: 99–104.

81. Fahnehjelm KT, Holmström G, Ying L, et al. Ocular characteristics in 10 children with long-chain 3-hydroxyacyl-CoA dehydrogenase deficiency: a cross-sectional study with long-term follow-up. Acta Ophthalmol 2008; 86: 329–37.

88. Cruysberg JR, Wevers RA, van Engelen BG, et al. Ocular and systemic manifestations of cerebrotendinous xanthomatosis. Am J Ophthalmol 1995; 120: 597–604

90. Costagliola C, Fabbrocini G, Illiano GM, et al. Ocular findings in X-linked ichthyosis: a survey on 38 cases. Ophthalmologica 1991; 202: 152–5.

 Access the complete reference list online at
http://www.expertconsult.com

Pupil anomalies and reactions

Andrew G Lee • Megan M Geloneck • Derrick C Pau

The anatomy (Fig. 63.1), physiology, and pathophysiology of the pupillary pathways are important to the pediatric ophthalmologist but they are dealt with so excellently elsewhere that only aspects relevant to children will be discussed here.

Development (see Chapter 2)

The pupillary light response is absent in infants of 29 gestational weeks or less, but is usually present by 31 or 32 weeks.[1] At birth the pupil is small. It enlarges in the first months of life and is probably at its largest at the end of the first decade, gradually becoming miotic in old age. The pupil reactions of term or premature infants are often of small amplitude and, because of their small resting size, may be difficult to elicit clinically especially in infants with brown irises. The failure of the pupil grating response in infants under 1 month of age is further evidence of the immaturity of the pupil responses in infancy.[2] Cocaine and hydroxyamphetamine are less potent in infants than in older children, suggesting that miosis of the newborn is due to decreased sympathetic tone.[3] In very premature babies the pupil may not have fully formed; during the seventh month of gestation, the vascular pupillary membrane atrophies and the pupil appears. Before 32 gestational weeks, mydriasis should not be taken as necessarily indicating a central nervous system lesion and an unresponsive pupil does not necessarily indicate an afferent defect.[3]

Dynamic retinoscopy indicates that infants from 6 days to 1 month of age have no accommodation, but that normal function is achieved by 3 to 4 months.[4] The effect of this is defocus of the higher spatial frequencies, the detection of which requires a greater discrimination than the younger infant is capable of. However, photorefraction studies have demonstrated an ability to accommodate of over 1 diopter in the neonate, and this increases rapidly in the first month and to a lesser extent in the first few years of life, with high amplitudes from 4 years onward until presbyopia sets in.

The near synkinesis

When looking from the distance to a near point, the eyes converge, the pupils constrict, and the lens accommodates; these components are separate in origin but linked as a synkinetic response. Disturbances in the relationship between the amount of accommodation and convergence are important aspects of most childhood squints, and the manipulation of that accommodation to convergence ratio is important in management.

In uncooperative children, testing of the near pupil response is more difficult than the response to light. The most important factor in testing is to provide a suitable fixation target, for example a small internally lit toy for an infant, a mobile toy with sufficient detail to stimulate convergence, and letters or numbers for a literate child.

Congenital and structural abnormalities

Congenital, structural, and developmental anomalies in the pupil include the following (many are found in Chapters 32 and 38):

- Aniridia
- Micropupil (congenital idiopathic microcoria)
- Polycoria and corectopia
- Coloboma
- Peninsula pupil (an inherited partial iris sphincter atrophy with dilated oval pupils)
- Persistent pupillary membrane
- Congenital mydriasis and miosis
- Irregular pupils
- Abnormalities of iris color

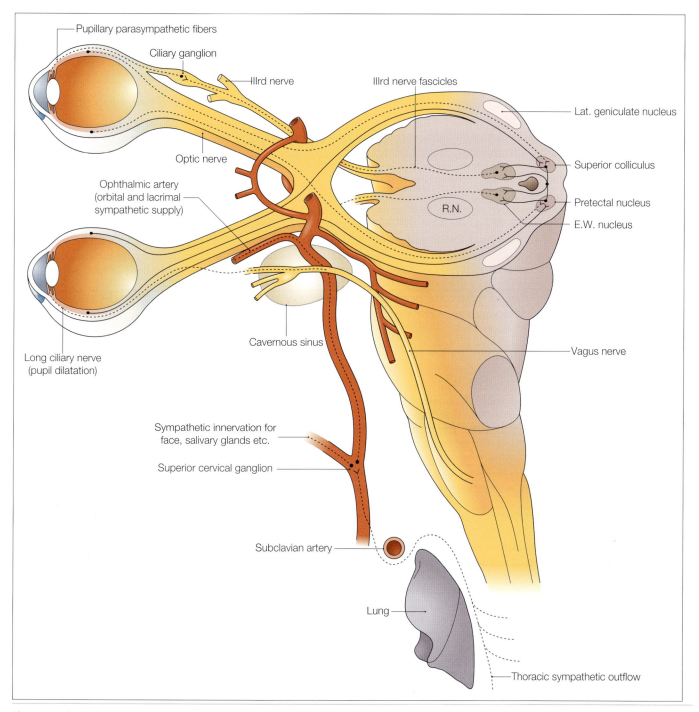

Fig. 63.1 Schematic representation of the efferent and afferent pathways involved in pupillary reactions. Red = blood vessels and parasympathetic. Blue = afferent visual pathways. Green = sympathetic pathway.

Afferent abnormalities of pupil reactivity

Afferent pupil defects

Amaurotic pupils

A totally blind ("amaurotic") eye resulting from ocular disease usually has no pupil reaction to a light shone on it (amaurotic pupil), but a normal near reaction if the efferent side is intact. In monocular blindness, the affected eye has no direct pupil reaction but has an intact consensual response when the light is shifted to the unaffected eye (amaurotic pupil reaction). In cases of binocular blindness due to anterior visual pathway or retinal disease, both pupils are usually dilated, although they may be nearly normal in size in long-standing blindness. If the efferent pupil pathway is intact, then eyes with an amaurotic pupil will still be able to react to near stimuli (light–near dissociation).

Relative afferent pupil defect

When one afferent pathway is affected, or if bilateral afferent pathways are affected asymmetrically, the relative afferent pupil defect (RAPD) in the afferent pupil pathway can be detected clinically with the "swinging flashlight" test (see video 106.1).[5]

Testing for a RAPD

In a dimly lit room, the observer uses a bright light source and shines the light upon each pupil individually. The child should be encouraged to fixate at distance to relax the accommodative pupil response at near. The light is then swung between the two eyes (i.e. "the swinging flashlight test") with one second on each eye and one second between the eyes. If there is a defect in the afferent pupil pathway of one eye, then the direct response will be less than the consensual reaction driven by the fellow eye and the affected pupil will dilate as the light swings from the unaffected to the affected pupil (i.e. a relative afferent pupillary defect). The RAPD can be graded subjectively from I through IV, with IV being an amaurotic pupil. The magnification provided by a slit-lamp may help detect a minimal defect in an older, more cooperative child. In situations in which there is a known unilateral efferent defect or opacity precluding evaluation of the affected pupil, the test for the RAPD can still be performed. In this setting, a second light is held below the unaffected pupil. As the light swings from the affected pupil to the unaffected pupil, the unaffected pupil constricts and when the light swings back to the affected pupil, the pupil in the unaffected eye will dilate and can be seen better with the second light shining indirectly from below. The RAPD is usually attributed to Robert Marcus Gunn who described sequential pupillary assessment with a bright light: the swinging light test is much more sensitive in detecting mild to moderate afferent defects.

The presence of an RAPD is objective evidence for a defect in the afferent pathway from the retina to the optic tract and the intercalated neurons in the midbrain to the efferent pupil pathway. Although uncommon, a small RAPD may occur in deeply amblyopic eyes.[6] In older children, a useful subjective addition to the test for the RAPD is to ask the child which eye sees the light brightest. The child may be asked a question, "if the light in the good eye is worth 1 pound/dollar how much is the other one worth?", which may give a rough subjective quantification.

Light–near dissociation

When the pupil reacts better to a near than to a light stimulus this is referred to as light–near dissociation. Defects in the afferent or efferent pupillary pathway might produce light–near dissociation. In patients with bilateral, but symmetric, afferent disease, an APD might be difficult or impossible to detect. In these situations, it is especially important to look for light–near dissociation of the pupil which might be evidence of afferent disease thereby aiding in localization of the lesion.

Efferent pupillomotor defects

Argyll Robertson pupils

In 1869, Douglas Argyll Robertson described a type of light–near dissociation seen classically with tertiary syphilis. The pupils are small, irregular, and constrict more fully and more briskly to a near stimulus than to light. The iris is often seen to be atrophic on slit-lamp examination. The lesion in the Argyll Robertson pupil is presumed to be located in the dorsal midbrain,[7] and patients with such pupils should undergo serologic testing for syphilis.

Sylvian aqueduct syndrome (Parinaud's dorsal midbrain syndrome)

Expanding lesions dorsal to the Sylvian aqueduct in children include pinealomas, ependymomas, "trilateral" retinoblastoma, granulomas, hydrocephalus, cystic and and other lesions. Compression of the dorsal midbrain produces light–near dissociation that may be associated with a vertical gaze palsy (typically upgaze palsy), lid retraction (Collier's sign), accommodation defects, and convergence–retraction nystagmus. The resting size of the pupils is usually larger than normal. Sometimes, probably in more rapidly enlarging tumors, the pupils may be large and poorly reactive to light or near stimuli.

Adie's syndrome (tonic pupil syndrome)

Adie's syndrome, unusual in young children, is typically idiopathic, but may occur with chicken pox or other viral infections,[8] ophthalmoplegic migraine, and measles vaccination.[9,10] It is more frequent in young female adults.[11] It is usually unilateral but many cases become bilateral.[11] Children rarely have symptoms related to the onset, but they may fail a school near vision test, or complain of blurred near or, if they are hyperopic, distant vision or photophobia. They may develop anisometropic amblyopia. Many patients are asymptomatic and parents may be the first to notice.

The acutely affected pupil is usually larger than the uninvolved eye (Fig. 63.2), but over time the Adie's pupil tends to become miotic ("little old Adie"). There is typically a

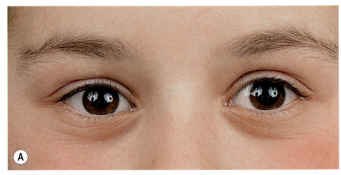

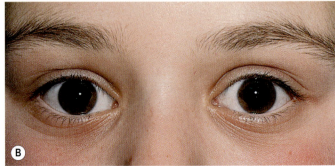

Fig. 63.2 Left Adie's pupil. (A) In light, (B) in dark. The pupil size difference is less in the dark.

segmental paralysis of the iris sphincter which might be more extensive or diffuse. Once constricted, the pupil remains consticted longer (the "tonic" pupil). There may also be a transient defect in accommodation, which is often marked at first but gradually improves over 2 or more years.[11] Corneal sensation may be reduced when tested with an aesthesiometer or even with a wisp of cotton, but is generally asymptomatic. This is probably due to damage to the trigeminal fibers that also pass through the ciliary ganglion. Patients with Adie's pupil may also have hyporeflexia or areflexia in their extremities but no other neurologic findings are usually present. Although the Adie's pupil is a clinical diagnosis, denervation hypersensitivity of the pupil may be demonstrated by finding pupillary constriction compared to the fellow eye 20 minutes after instillation of pilocarpine 0.0625%. Pharmacological hypersensitivity may occur with post- as well as pre-ciliary ganglionic lesions (Fig. 63.3).

Loewenfeld and Thompson proposed that the site of the lesion of the tonic pupil is in the ciliary ganglion and that many of its features can be explained by aberrant regeneration.[12] The cause is unknown but it may be due to a neurotropic virus. Most patients do not require treatment, but they may be helped with their photophobia and occasionally with symptoms due to accommodation paresis by pilocarpine (0.1% three times daily) or another dilute miotic. In distinction to adult patients, young children with Adie's or other tonic pupils should have the unaffected or better eye occluded for a short period each day to avoid amblyopia. Spectacle correction of hyperopia in the affected eye may be necessary to prevent anisometropic amblyopia.

Other causes of tonic pupils

Although Adie's syndrome is the classic idiopathic tonic pupil, other causes of ciliary ganglion damage give rise to a similar syndrome. Congenital or acquired tonic pupils have been described in infants with orbital tumors, traumatic, infectious, or inflammatory diseases or as part of a variety of widespread neuropathies including syphilis, diabetes, Guillain-Barré syndrome, Miller-Fisher syndrome, pandysautonomia, hereditary sensory neuropathy, Charcot-Marie-Tooth disease, and Trilene poisoning. Autonomic neuropathy due to paraneoplastic disease has also caused tonic pupils.

Iris abnormalities

Damage to the iris by trauma, irradiation, uveitis, ischemia or hemorrhage, or involvement with a tumor such as lymphoma, leukemia, juvenile xanthogranuloma, leiomyoma, or neurofibroma, may all give rise to anisocoria, corectopia, and/or impaired pupil reactions (Fig. 63.4). Slit-lamp examination of the iris can demonstrate the disruption of the iris architecture from the underlying cause.

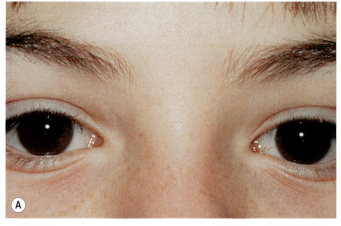

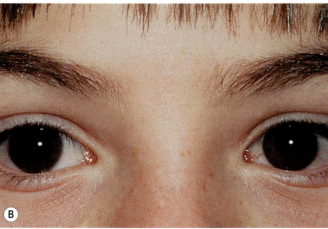

Fig. 63.3 Left Adie's pupil (A) before and (B) after instillation of 0.1% pilocarpine. The right pupil is unchanged while the left constricts due to denervation hypersensitivity.

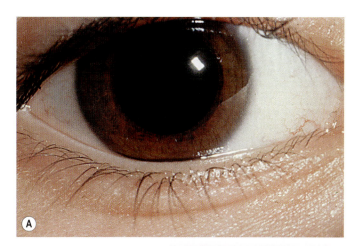

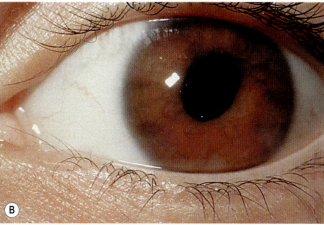

Fig. 63.4 Normal right eye (A) and left iris abnormality with sluggish reactions and small pupil due to leukemic infiltration (B).

Benign episodic unilateral mydriasis ("springing pupil")

The syndrome of idiopathic episodic mydriasis is likely a heterogeneous group of conditions that result in parasympathetic insufficiency of the iris sphincter or sympathetic hyperactivity of the iris dilator.[13] In either case, it results in anisocoria that usually lasts for several hours and then resolves spontaneously. Other signs of oculomotor or sympathetic nerve dysfunction are absent but the syndrome is frequently accompanied by headache or orbital pain.[13] Although it occurs primarily in young women, it has been reported in children.

Midbrain corectopia

Damage to some midbrain pupillary fibers may give rise to unequal upward and inward distortion of the pupil and an unequal, sinuous pupil reaction to light and near stimuli. The patients described were often, but not always, comatose.

Third nerve palsy (see Chapter 82)

In complete third nerve palsy the pupil is unreactive (Fig. 63.5), but in partial or recovering third nerve palsy the ipsilateral pupil reactions may be sluggish or react unevenly. Patients with a poorly reactive pupil or anisocoria should have motility and lid evaluation to exclude third nerve palsy.

Abnormal or aberrant pupillary contractions can occur in aberrant regeneration (Fig. 63.6) following third nerve palsy.[14] The pupil may constrict with activation of extraocular muscles or may be smaller on the ipsilateral side (Fig. 63.7).

Riley-Day syndrome

In the Riley-Day syndrome (familial dysautonomia; see Chapter 98) there is a hypersensitivity to dilute parasympathomimetic agents (i.e. pilocarpine 0.1%).

Iris sphincter or dilator muscle spasms

Spasm of the iris dilator can give rise to "tadpole-shaped" pupils, which usually occurs in otherwise healthy young adults.[15] The pupils are peaked in one direction for a few minutes, which may occur on several, separate occasions. This may represent a subset of patients who carry the diagnosis of springing pupil.

Paradoxical pupils

In some people with retinal disease, a curious phenomenon occurs in which the pupil size in the light is larger than that in the dark despite the other responses being normal.[16] The parents may occasionally remark on this, but it is usually a sign that must be elicited. When present, it is extremely helpful as it usually only occurs in retinal diseases, typically in congenital

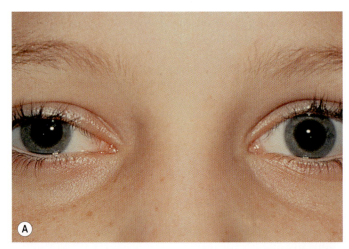

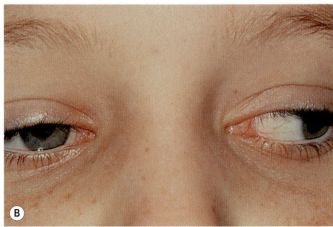

Fig. 63.6 Aberrant regeneration following partial recovery from right traumatic third nerve palsy. The right pupil constricts on attempted adduction.

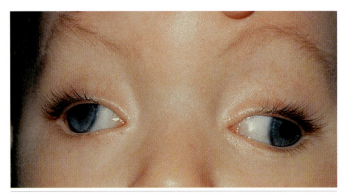

Fig. 63.5 Bilateral congenital third nerve palsy with fixed and unreactive pupils.

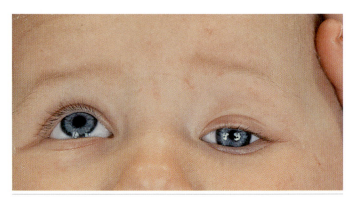

Fig. 63.7 Left congenital third nerve palsy. In long-standing cases the pupil may be small.

stationary night blindness (see Chapter 44), but also with cone dysfunction syndromes, such as achromatopsia;[17] it has also been described in Leber's amaurosis, dominant optic atrophy (see Chapter 52), optic neuritis (see Chapter 53), and amblyopia (see Chapter 70).[18] The pupillary responses are more brisk in patients with lower visual acuity and Ishihara scores.[17]

A good way to record paradoxical pupils is to take a digital photograph of the child in a fully lit room and in a nearly fully darkened room. The photographs may clearly record the difference. It is important to leave the child for at least a minute in the dark; the pupils can be observed there by using a flashlight for a moment, or with an infrared viewing device or video. In the child with nystagmus, the presence of paradoxical pupils suggests that an electroretinogram should be obtained. The mechanism has not been adequately explained, but it is interesting that dark-rearing normal chicks to maturity causes them to have paradoxically constricted pupils in the dark.

Horner's syndrome

Ocular sympathetic denervation in childhood is not uncommon and may be congenital or acquired.

Clinical characteristics

Miosis

The pupils are unequal, with the difference greatest in the dark due to the defect being a failure of the sympathetically innervated dilator pupillae muscle (Fig. 63.8). The difference depends on the completeness of the lesion and the alertness of the child. A drowsy child is more likely to have a small resting pupillary tone and the inequality will be less obvious. There is also a lag in the dilatation of the affected side which results in a greater anisocoria at 5 seconds than at 15 seconds after the lights are turned out. It is best measured by photographs. Pupil reactions to light, near, and accommodation are unaffected.

Ptosis

A 1- to 2-mm ptosis of the upper lid (due to weakness of Müller's muscle) is present but it may be so slight and variable that it escapes notice or may not be present at all (Fig. 63.9). Some children present with miosis without ptosis.[19] Parents should look out for the later development of ptosis as the onset can be asynchronous. Ptosis can also be present without miosis.[19]

The lower lid may also be affected ("reverse ptosis"), giving rise to a more obvious narrowing in the palpebral fissure which gives a false appearance of enophthalmos.

Ipsilateral anhidrosis

Lesions before the superior cervical ganglion, where the sweat and piloerector fibers split off to go with the external carotid artery, will damage these fibers and cause an ipsilateral flushed face and conjunctiva and nasal stuffiness in acute lesions. In longer standing lesions, there is a defect of sweating resulting in a dry, warm side to the face while the unaffected side is cool and sweaty. In chronic lesions, the affected side may be pale due to denervation hypersensitivity to circulating catecholamines. Most children do not complain of anhidrosis, but

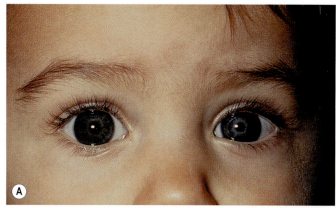
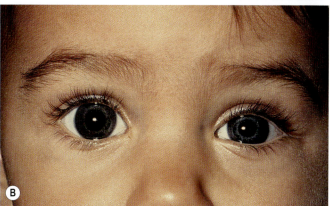

Fig. 63.8 Left Horner's syndrome with mild upper and lower lid ptosis. (A) Photograph taken in the light. (B) Same patient 5 seconds after lights turned out showing dilation lag.

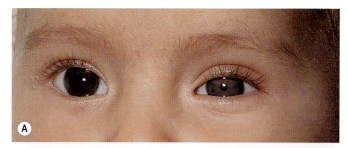
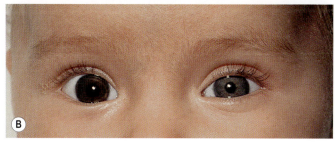

Fig. 63.9 Left congenital Horner's syndrome showing upper and lower lid ptosis and a iris heterochromia with the lighter eye being the affected eye. (A) In bright light and (B) in the dark.

parents may describe that one side of the face does not flush or turn as red with crying.

Heterochromia

In congenital Horner's syndrome, because iris pigmentation is partially dependent upon sympathetic innervation, heterochromia may occur with the lighter iris on the affected side especially in brown irides (Fig. 63.11). Although believed to be a sign of congenital Horner's syndrome, heterochromia has occasionally been described in acquired cases in childhood[20] and adults.[21] In addition, heterochromia is not invariably present in congenital Horner's syndrome especially in already light-colored irides or if insufficient time has elapsed (Fig. 63.10). Histopathologically, in one case, the iris pigment epithelium was normal, there were no iris sympathetic fibers, and the stromal melanocytes were reduced in number, but contained normal melanosomes.[22] The anterior border cells were depleted.

Pharmacological responses

Topical cocaine 10% blocks reuptake of noradrenaline (norepinephrine) by the sympathetic nerve endings. In postganglionic lesions the nerve is damaged and contains no, or reduced, noradrenaline stores. The pupil fails to dilate as well as the fellow eye. It is highly effective as one way of distinguishing

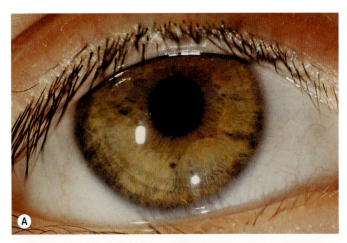

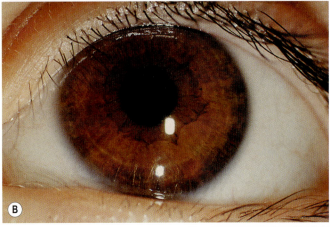

Fig. 63.10 Right congenital Horner's syndrome in a teenager. (A) The right iris was noticed to develop a lighter color at the age of 2 although the ptosis and pupil size were noticed at a few weeks of age. (B) The normal left eye.

between normal or physiological anisocoria and anisocoria due to Horner's syndrome.

Hydroxyamphetamine 1% releases noradrenaline from presynaptic nerve terminal stores; it should be instilled into the conjunctival sac of both eyes at least 24 hours after the use of cocaine. Where the postganglionic neuron is intact, noradrenaline is present and the pupil dilates, but if the postganglionic neuron is "damaged or dead" it contains less norepinephrine (noradrenaline) and does not dilate as well. Hydroxyamphetamine takes about 40 minutes to work. However, trans-synaptic degeneration in children limits the sensitivity and specificity of hydroxyamphetamine for localization purposes and it is not available in many countries.

Low dose adrenaline (epinephrine) 0.1% (1 : 1000) does not normally dilate the pupil, but in postganglionic Horner's syndrome there is denervation hypersensitivity and the pupil dilates. Adrenaline 0.1% has the advantage of being more readily available and is not a proscribed drug.

Apraclonidine 0.5% may be useful in establishing a diagnosis of Horner's syndrome; it causes reversal of anisocoria under both dark and light conditions. Topical apraclonidine is readily available and inexpensive. It is an alpha agonist and the differential effect of alpha 1 and alpha 2 receptors produces dilation in the smaller pupil and constriction in the normal, larger pupil. Apraclonidine's major site of pharmacologic action is postjunctional alpha 2 receptors in the ciliary body that produce lowered intraocular pressure. Up-regulation of alpha receptors that occurs with sympathetic denervation in the Horner's syndrome unmasks the alpha 1 effect and the smaller pupil dilates. In a recent series of Horner's syndrome in children, apraclonidine 0.5% demonstrated excellent sensitivity and specificity with the best observation results obtained under light conditions.[23] It should only be used with caution in infants because of central nervous system depression.

Pharmacological testing is usually not necessary to confirm the Horner's syndrome, but because physiological anisocoria presents sometimes with lid abnormalities and ptosis and miosis can present asynchronously or in isolation it may be helpful. Atypical presentations of Horner's syndrome in children can include miosis only, ptosis only, or even intermittent miosis and ptosis.[19] In these cases, pharmacologic testing may be helpful in the diagnosis.

In children, the main diagnostic difficulty is measuring the inequality and changes in light and dark; this may be aided by photographs. The use of topical testing to differentiate physiologic anisocoria from Horner's syndrome is reasonable for equivocal cases, but most authors believe that children with an unexplained Horner's syndrome should undergo imaging of the ocular sympathetic pathway to exclude treatable and potentially life threatening (e.g. neuroblastoma) causes.

Other characteristics

There have been various reports of ipsilateral accommodative increase or decrease, but the difference does not seem to be reliably present or easy to measure in children. The ipsilateral central cornea may be thicker on the affected side.

Congenital Horner's syndrome (Fig. 63.10)

Weinstein et al. divided congenital Horner syndrome into three causal types:[24]

- Those who suffered obstetric trauma, usually by forceps, to the internal carotid artery and its sympathetic nerve plexus and had a postganglionic Horner's syndrome on drug testing: they did not dilate with 1% hydroxyamphetamine. They had no facial anhidrosis.
- Those who suffered surgical or obstetric trauma to the preganglionic sympathetic pathway including patients with brachial plexus injury (Klumpke's palsy). Cardiothoracic surgery is a common cause in children. The pupil dilates with 1% hydroxyamphetamine.
- Those without a history of birth trauma but with a Horner's syndrome and evidence of a lesion at, or peripheral to, the superior cervical ganglion and anhidrosis. Congenital or early onset Horner's syndrome with a preganglionic lesion and anhidrosis occurs in patients with neuroblastoma.[25,26]

Congenital Horner's syndrome may also be found with hemifacial atrophy, cervical vertebral anomalies, congenital tumors, arachnoidal cysts and holoprosencephaly, and congenital varicella syndrome.

Despite the above list of causes, most children with congenital Horner's syndrome have no other abnormalities.[27]

Postnatally acquired Horner's syndrome

Unexplained acquired Horner's syndrome in children is more significant and usually serious. It may occur in the following:

- "Central" pre-ganglionic lesions due to brain stem trauma, tumors, or vascular malformations, infarcts and hemorrhages, and syringomyelia. Other neurologic dysfunction is usually evident.
- "Preganglionic" lesions, i.e. of the second neuron between the spinal cord and the superior cervical ganglion, due to neck trauma, neuroblastoma, and other tumors (Fig. 63.11).

- "Postganglionic" lesions, i.e. of the final neuron after the superior cervical ganglion, due to cavernous sinus lesions (tumors, aneurysms, or inflammatory disease), neuroblastoma, and trauma.

Management

Congenital Horner's syndrome

Since birth trauma or early cardiothoracic surgery are the most frequent causes of Horner's syndrome, further investigations are not usually necessary.[26] However, the albeit rare occurrence of tumors in children with congenital Horner's syndrome of no obvious cause may still warrant imaging of the oculosympathetic pathway and a 24-hour catecholamine assay. Several children with unexplained Horner's syndrome were found to have neuroblastoma on imaging, but normal urinary catecholamines;[25] this may be due to lower sensitivity of spot urine catecholamine testing as opposed to 24-hour assays and normal urine studies do not necessarily rule out neuroblastoma. The gravity of this diagnosis may demand both imaging and catecholamine assays in initial investigations. However, given the relatively low incidence of neuroblastoma in children with unexplained Horner's syndrome, performing catecholamine assays and a careful physical examination and reserving imaging studies for children with elevated catecholamines or suggestive examination findings or change in clinical findings may be an equally suitable approach.[26]

Acquired Horner's syndrome

Where there is no obvious cause, such as trauma or surgery, a child with acquired Horner's syndrome should be investigated in conjunction with a neurologist, and investigations include imaging of the ocular sympathetic pathway and a 24-hour catecholamine assay (Fig. 63.9).

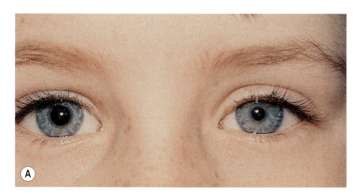
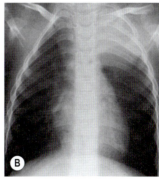
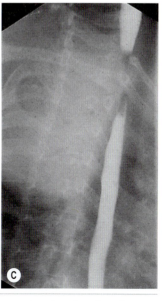

Fig. 63.11 Congenital Horner's syndrome. (A) Left Horner syndrome. This child presented with the complaint of a sudden onset ptosis and small pupil. (B) Chest X-ray showing left apical mass. (C) Barium swallow showing constriction of the esophagus. The cause was a large benign ganglioneuroma.

Pupil changes from high sympathetic "tone"

Cases have been described in which an intermittent dilated pupil, with or without widening of the palpebral fissure, occurs associated with a cervicomedullary syrinx, post spinal cord injury, lung tumors, or seizures or migraine. In seizures and migraine there may well be a lowering of parasympathetic tone at the same time, but sympathetic-induced spasm is suggested by pallor and sweating.

Pupil changes from damage to the parasympathetic system (see Chapter 82)

Internal ophthalmoplegia (paralysis of the sphincter pupillae and accommodation) is occasionally seen without external ophthalmoplegia from nuclear lesions. It is bilateral and often associated with other oculomotor palsies.

Damage to the third nerve in the interpeduncular fossa, where the pupillomotor fibers are confined to the superomedial aspect of the nerve, may occur from aneurysm or tumor and is usually associated with external ophthalmoplegia, but meningitic lesions can cause an isolated internal ophthalmoplegia.

Pharmacological agents

Numerous pharmacological agents affect pupil size and reactivity. Systemic agents usually affect the pupils symmetrically while topical agents are often only instilled into one eye and may be asymmetrical.

Pupil-dilating agents

Parasympatholytic agents

Atropine 0.5–1%, homatropine 2%, cyclopentolate 0.5–1%, and tropicamide 1% are all commonly used agents to dilate the pupil and cause cycloplegia. Homatropine and atropine have a prolonged action and are not often indicated diagnostically or therapeutically unless their long action is desirable as in the case of penalization therapy for amblyopia. Hyoscine 0.5% has an action similar to that of atropine but is less long acting. These agents may cause respiratory failure in children with congenital central hypoventilation. Inadvertent exposure to topical mydriatics can produce pharmacologic dilation in children, and parents should be specifically questioned about these agents. In addition, contact with certain garden or wild plants (e.g. belladonna alkaloids, jimson weed) containing parasympatholytic agents can produce mydriasis.

Sympathomimetics

Adrenaline (epinephrine) 0.1–1% or phenylephrine 2.5–10% may be used to dilate the pupil in association with a parasympatholytic. They have no action on accommodation and are not sufficiently effective to produce good dilation. They must be used with great care, and at lowest dilution, if at all, in premature babies, those with cardiac or vascular disease, or those with hypertension.

Pupil-constricting agents

Cholinergic drugs

Pilocarpine 1–4% is commonly used to constrict the pupil. It is now used occasionally in the treatment of glaucoma and has little effect on infantile glaucoma. Some pet flea and tick treatments or collars contain cholinergic agents that produce miosis.

Anticholinesterases

Phospholine iodide (echothiophate) 0.03–0.125% and eserine 0.5% are infrequently used for the treatment of glaucoma. Phospholine iodide is used to cause peripheral accommodation and "unlink" the association between accommodative convergence and accommodation in some cases of high AC:A ratio strabismus. It may rarely cause cataracts and occasionally reversible iris cysts. It has interactions with some muscle relaxants used in anesthesia.

Sympatholytic agents

Guanethidine 5% (Ismelin) can be used to counter lid retraction in hyperthyroidism. Thymoxamine 1% may also cause pupil constriction. These drugs are rarely if ever used currently in practice.

Systemic agents

Atropine, scopolamine, and benzatropine (benztropine) can cause pupil dilatation and paralysis of accommodation. The seeds of jimson weed, the berries of deadly nightshade, and henbane have all been known to cause a serious or fatal poisoning. The symptoms have been described as "hot as a hare, blind as a bat, dry as a bone, red as a beet, mad as a hatter." When proof of atropine poisoning is needed in the absence of facilities for assay it is said that a few drops of the child's urine put into one eye of a cat suggests the diagnosis. Mydriasis from topical atropine or atropine-like drugs is not counteracted by pilocarpine 1% but in systemic poisoning it may be.

Antihistamines and some antidepressants produce a mydriasis.

Heroin, morphine and other opiates, marijuana, and some other psychotropic drugs cause bilateral pupil constriction.

Abnormalities of the near reflex

Congenital absence

Children may be born with a defect in the near reflex. They have absent accommodation, poor convergence, and the pupil fails to constrict to a near stimulus, but constricts to light.[28]

Familial cases of accommodation defect occur.[29] The cause is unknown but it may be peripheral in origin.

Acquired defects

Sylvian aqueduct (Parinaud's) syndrome

Premature presbyopia is one of the signs of tumors encroaching on the dorsal midbrain. Other more classic signs include retraction nystagmus, vertical gaze defects, eyelid retraction, convergence defect, and pupil light–near dissociation.

Systemic disease

Botulism, diphtheria, diabetes, and head and neck trauma may give rise to accommodation defects either isolated or associated with eye movement and vergence defects. Wilson's disease has been shown to be associated with a defect in the near response in some cases.

Pharmacological agents

See above.

Eye disease

Defective accommodation occurs in children with severe iridocyclitis (see Chapter 39), dislocated lenses (see Chapter 35), large colobomas (see Chapter 32), buphthalmos (see Chapter 37), very high myopia, and direct eye trauma including retinal detachment surgery.

Other neurological causes

Adie's tonic pupil syndrome and third nerve paralysis may cause defective accommodation. Sinus disease, presumably by affecting the short ciliary nerves, may cause cycloplegia and accommodation defect.

Accommodation in school children

One expects a school-aged child to have a high amplitude of accommodation irrespective of refractive error. It has been suggested that there is a causal relationship between a defective near response and some cases of dyslexia.

It is important, however, to distinguish clearly between reading difficulties due to a defective near response, which can be improved by exercises, and dyslexia, which is a specific defect in the perceptual process involved with reading and writing that cannot be remedied by simple exercises.[30]

Spasm of the near reflex

Spasm of the near reflex consists of episodes of:

- Accommodation-induced pseudo-myopia
- Convergence of the eyes
- Miosis.

The symptoms are usually blurred and double vision, and ocular pain or headache. These cases are rarely due to organic disease, although closed head trauma is recognized in a number of cases. Upper brain stem pathology is often suspected, but rarely found. In two cases with closed head trauma, MR studies revealed no abnormalities in the midbrain but both had lesions in the left temporal lobe.[31]

In most cases, it is not possible to demonstrate any organic disease and it is assumed to be psychogenic. The episodes have a sudden onset and can last many hours and may be variable. There is blurred vision and photophobia. The eyes are crossed and may mimic a bilateral sixth nerve paresis. The essential finding is increasing pupillary constriction as the deviation increases. Pupils that become constricted on attempted lateral gaze are also a clue to the functional nature of the complaint. It is unusual in childhood. Occasionally, symptoms may be recurrent over several years.

The treatment is reassurance of the child and parents. Some patients are helped by miotics, but more often by a combination of cycloplegia and bifocal glasses. Unless there are any neurological signs, no investigations are required and the prognosis is good.

References

1. Isenberg S, Molarte A, Vazquez M. The fixed and dilated pupils of premature neonates. Am J Ophthalmol 1990; 110: 168–72.
2. Cocker KD, Moseley MJ, Bissenden JG, et al. Visual acuity and pupillary responses to spatial structure in infants. Invest Ophthalmol Vis Sci 1994; 35: 2620–5.
3. Korczyn AD, Laor N, Nemet P. Autonomic pupillary activity in infants. Metab Ophthalmol 1978; 2: 391–4.
4. Haynes H, White BL, Held R. Visual accommodation in human infants. Science 1965; 148: 528–30.
5. Enyedi LB, Dev S, Cox TA. A comparison of the Marcus Gunn and alternating light tests for afferent pupillary defects. Ophthalmology 1998; 105: 871–3.
6. Donahue SP, Moore P, Kardon RH. Automated pupil perimetry in amblyopia: generalized depression in the involved eye. Ophthalmology 2003; 104: 2161–7.
7. Dasco CC, Bortz DL. Significance of the Argyll Robertson pupils in clinical medicine. Am J Med 1989; 86: 199–202.
8. Goldsmith MO. Tonic pupil following varicella. Am J Ophthalmol 1968; 66: 551–4.
9. Iannetti P, Spalice A, Iannetti L, et al. Residual and persistent Adie's pupil after pediatric ophthalmoplegic migraine. Pediatr Neurol 2009; 41: 204–6.
10. Aydin K, Elmas S, Guzes EA. Reversible posterior leukoencephalopathy and Adie's pupil after measles vaccination. J Child Neurol 2006; 21: 525–7.
11. Thompson HS. Adie's syndrome: some new observations. Trans Am Ophthalmol Soc 1977; 75: 587–626.
12. Loewenfeld IE, Thompson HS. The tonic pupil: a re-evaluation. Am J Ophthalmol 1967; 63: 46–87.
13. Jacobson DM. Benign episodic unilateral mydriasis: clinical characteristics. Ophthalmology 1995; 102: 1625–7.
14. Hamed LM. Associated neurologic and ophthalmologic findings in congenital oculomotor nerve palsy. Ophthalmology 1991; 98: 708–14.
15. Balaggan KS, Hugkulstone CE, Bremmer FD. Episodic segmental iris dilator muscle spasm: the tadpole pupil. Arch Ophthalmol 2003; 121: 744–5.
16. Barricks ME, Flynn JT, Kushner BJ. Paradoxical pupillary responses in congenital stationary night blindness. Arch Ophthalmol 1977; 95: 1800.
17. Ben Simon GJ, Abraham FA, Melamed S. Pingelapese achromatopsia: correlation between paradoxical pupillary response and clinical features. Br J Ophthalmol 2004; 88: 223–5.
18. Frank JW, Kushner BJ, France TD. Paradoxical pupillary phenomena: a review of patients with pupillary constriction to darkness. Arch Ophthalmol 1998; 106: 1564–6.
19. Jeffery AR, Ellis FJ, Repka MX, et al. Pediatric Horner syndrome. J AAPOS 1998; 2: 159–67.
20. Pollard ZF, Greenberg MF, Bordenca M, Lange J. Atypical acquired pediatric Horner syndrome. Arch Ophthalmol 2010; 128: 937–40.
21. Makley LB, Abbott K. Neurogenic heterochromia: a report of an interesting case. Am J Ophthalmol 1965; 59: 297–9.
22. McCartney A, Riordan-Eva P, Howes R, et al. Horner's syndrome: an electron microscopic study of human iris. Br J Ophthalmol 1992; 76: 746–9.
23. Chen PL, Hsiao CH, Chen JT, et al. Efficacy of apraclonidine 0.5% in the diagnosis of Horner syndrome in pediatric patients under low or high illumination. Am J Ophthalmol 2006; 142: 469–74.
24. Weinstein J, Zweifel TJ, Thompson HS. Congenital Horner's syndrome. Arch Ophthalmol 1980; 98: 1074–8.
25. Mahoney NR, Liu GT, Menacker SJ, et al. Pediatric Horner syndrome: etiologies and roles of imaging and urine studies to detect neuroblastoma and other responsible mass lesions. Am J Ophthalmol 2006; 142: 651–9.

26. Smith S, Diehl N, Leavitt J, Mohney B. Incidence of pediatric Horner syndrome and the risk of neuroblastoma: a population-based study. Arch Ophthalmol 2010; 128: 324–9.

27. George ND, Gonzalez G, Hoyt CS. Does Horner's syndrome in infancy require investigation. Br J Ophthalmol 1998; 82: 51–4.

28. Chrousos GA, O'Neill JF, Cogan DG. Absence of the near reflex in a healthy adolescent. J Pediatr Ophthalmol Strabismus 1985; 22: 76–7.

29. Hibbert FG, Goldstein V, Osborne SM. Defective accommodation in members of one family. Trans Ophthalmol Soc UK 1975; 95: 455–61.

30. Shaywitz SE, Shaywitz BA. The science of reading and dyslexia. J AAPOS 2003; 7: 158–66.

31. Montiero ML, Curi AL, Pereira A, et al. Persistent accommodative spasm after head trauma. Br J Ophthalmol 2003; 87: 243–4.

Leukemia

Richard J C Bowman • David Webb

Introduction

Acute lymphoblastic leukemia (ALL) is the most common cancer in childhood, accounting for more than 30% of cases, with 400–500 new children diagnosed annually in the UK. Combination chemotherapy for acute leukemia in children is highly effective; thus, serious ocular involvement is much less common than it was, and routine ophthalmic surveillance is usually unnecessary. Five-year survival rates of over 80% are usual for ALL and up to 60% for acute myeloid leukemia (AML). The majority of treatment failures are due to recurrent leukemia, and treatment-related deaths have become less common with improved supportive care.

Several clinical and biologic criteria adversely affect prognosis and treatment regimens: age (infants under 1 year and children over 10 years suffer higher relapse rates), high presenting white blood cell count, slow response to initial therapy, and chromosomal changes within the leukemic cells. This approach has closed the gap in treatment success rates originally identified between the subgroups of patients.

Almost all children are treated initially with chemotherapy; bone marrow transplantation is reserved for the around 10% of children with initial very poor prognosis, or following relapse. AML accounts for 5% of children's cancers, with only 60–70 new cases in children in the UK each year; treatment is very intensive over 5 or 6 months. Chemotherapy is increasingly effective, and bone marrow transplantation less common. Outcome of therapy correlates with chromosomal changes in the leukemic cells and response to initial treatment which are used to divide children into subgroups in a manner similar to those for acute lymphoblastic disease.

Common sites of disease at presentation are bone marrow, blood, lymph nodes, liver, and spleen. The eye is the only site where the leukemic involvement of nerves and blood vessels can be directly observed and it may act as a "sanctuary" for leukemic cells against chemotherapy. Eye complications may occasionally be the major residual disability[1] but serious eye involvement is unusual.[2] Ophthalmic manifestations may be dramatic, requiring prompt diagnosis and treatment and are more a feature of relapse than of initial presentation. The ocular manifestations of acute leukemia are divided into direct (infiltration of the anterior segment, the orbit, or the CNS) and indirect (secondary to hematologic changes such as hyperviscosity, anemia, thrombocytopenia, and immunosuppression).[3]

Orbital leukemia is a small, but significant cause of proptosis in children[4] and is more likely to be found in uncontrolled disease, in the first decade and with AML. It is associated with higher mortality. Orbital presentation may occur without eye involvement and it may be the only manifestation, especially in AML. Myeloid leukemia may present as an isolated solid tumor mass (granulocytic sarcoma) at a variety of sites, including the orbit (Fig. 64.1). A greenish tinge to the tissue mass led to the term chloroma: this appearance may be due to myeloperoxidase or altered blood products.

Orbital involvement in leukemia may be due to bone or soft tissue infiltration, tumor formation, or hemorrhage; the lacrimal gland, or lacrimal drainage apparatus may be primarily involved, with a more benign diagnosis. Children with orbital involvement present with proptosis, chemosis, and, rarely,

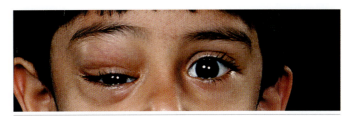

Fig. 64.1 "Chloroma" due to myeloid leukemia.

muscle involvement; these may occur early in the disease. Exposure keratitis may occur. It may be difficult to differentiate between primary leukemic infiltration and complications such as hemorrhage or opportunistic infection; a biopsy may be necessary.[5] A biopsy should be from the center of the abnormal area, not from the periphery where secondary inflammatory changes may occur. Review of the blood count and blood film by a pediatric oncologist, and a thorough clinical assessment prior to biopsy, together with a bone marrow examination at the time of biopsy, are important steps.

Lids

The lids are usually only involved as a part of orbital infiltration, but can be due to direct leukemic infiltration.[4]

Conjunctiva

The conjunctiva may be involved by hemorrhage (Fig. 64.2), infiltration (Fig. 64.3), or hyperviscosity, when the vessels are tortuous or comma-shaped. Conjunctival mass formation, though rare, can be the presenting sign in acute leukemia.[3]

Cornea and sclera

Being avascular, the cornea is not often involved in the leukemias, but it may be involved in herpes simplex or zoster in the immune-compromised child, or by other inflammatory disease. Corneal ulcers may be the presenting sign in acute leukemia[6] and perilimbal infiltrates have been described in acute monocytic leukemia.[7]

Lens

Cataracts occur frequently in patients who have had total body irradiation, related to the total dose and to the rate and fractionation of administration.[8] The use of steroids to treat graft-versus-host disease may cause or exacerbate cataracts.

Anterior chamber, iris and intraocular pressure

Most reported cases have been of relapse in ALL (Fig. 64.4) but, rarely, children present with a leukemic hyphema or hypopyon. In ALL, anterior segment relapse accounts for up to 2% of all relapses; it is very rare in AML.[4,9]

The infiltration is most likely to be blood-borne rather than CNS related[9] and the relatively frequent occurrence of isolated anterior segment relapse supports the concept of the eye as a sanctuary site.[10] Because of the blood–eye barrier, chemotherapeutic agents do not penetrate the eye so well as at many other sites, allowing leukemic cells to survive, causing signs and symptoms after chemotherapy has stopped. Symptoms include redness, watering, photophobia, pain, and visual loss. The parents may notice changes in the shape or reactions of the pupil or in the color and appearance of the iris (Fig. 64.5). Leukemia accounts for 5% of pediatric uveitis[3].

Clinical findings are variable with iritis and hypopyon being the most common. Ciliary injection, keratic precipitates, anterior chamber cells, and flare are frequent. Posterior synechiae

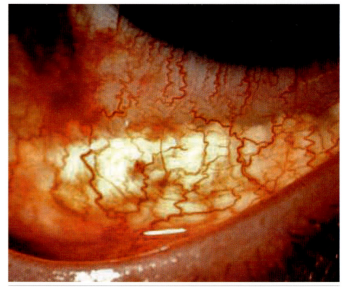

Fig. 64.3 **Conjunctival infiltration with leukemic cells (ALL).**

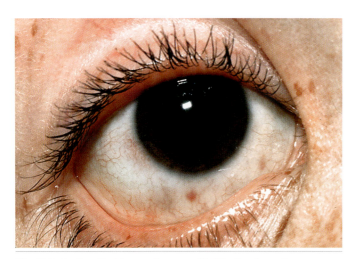

Fig. 64.2 **Conjunctival hemorrhages and infiltration in acute lymphoblastic leukemia.**

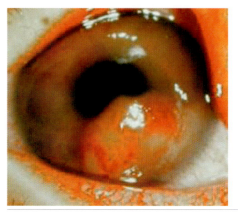

Fig. 64.4 **Anterior chamber relapse (ALL).**

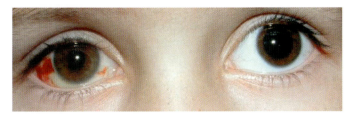

Fig. 64.5 **Anisocoria and mild heterochromia (ALL).**

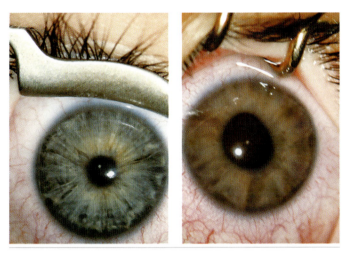

Fig. 64.6 **Iris relapse with heterochromia, infiltrated left iris, and sluggish pupil reactions.**

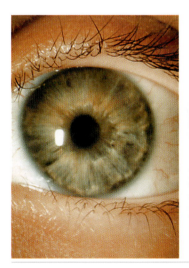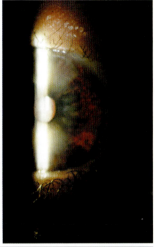

Fig. 64.7 Same patient as in Figure 65.6. After treatment with 2500 cGy there is iris transilluminance. The right eye had become affected.

are unusual, but a grayish hypopyon streaked with blood is common.

Secondary glaucoma is common and is associated with corneal edema, pain, and redness.

The iris may be thickened diffusely (Fig. 64.6) or in the form of one or more nodules or a mass of variable size; the thickening of the iris obliterates the iris crypts and may give a rather featureless iris. The iris may also be thinned with loss of pigment (Fig. 64.7). The iris color may be changed, usually by

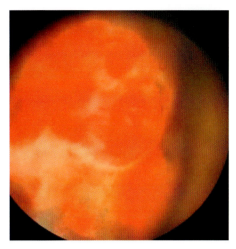

Fig. 64.8 **Choroidal mass in ALL.**

a brownish discoloration. Rubeosis may occur. It is often the failure of standard treatment for uveitis that draws the ophthalmologist's attention to the underlying leukemia. If in diagnostic doubt, perform anterior chamber paracentesis and iridectomy:[9] a paracentesis alone may not be sufficient to give an accurate diagnosis. Pathologic studies show leukemic infiltration of the iris and trabecular meshwork,[4] and the hypopyon consists of leukemic cells, necrotic tissue, and proteinaceous exudate. Leukemic cells may be difficult to find. Patients with glaucoma have leukemic obstruction of the outflow channels and episcleral vessels.

Because children with an apparently localized relapse generally have submicroscopic bone marrow disease, retreatment requires full systemic therapy plus local ocular radiotherapy (at least 2000 cGy) and topical steroid treatment. With this approach, long-term survival and likely cure has been achieved in a substantial proportion of patients.[11]

Choroid

The choroid may be the part of the eye most frequently involved in all types of leukemia,[4,12] but it is only rarely clinically apparent. The clinical manifestations are the result of serous retinal detachment or retinal detachment associated with a subretinal mass (Fig. 64.8). Fluorescein angiography demonstrates myriads of diffuse leakage points at the level of the retinal pigment epithelium.[13] Similar fluorescein patterns are seen in serous detachments with melanoma, metastatic tumor, Vogt-Koyanagi-Harada disease, and posterior scleritis. Leukemic choroidopathy can be detected by ultrasound.

Retina and vitreous

The retina, because of its ready visibility, is the part of the eye most frequently found to be involved clinically. Funduscopy is part of the routine follow-up examination of leukemic patients.

Hyperviscosity changes

Hyperviscosity of the blood occurs in many cases of chronic leukemia with very high blood cell counts, as in monocytic AML. Fluorescein angiography and trypsin digests[3] show capillary saccular and fusiform microaneurysms, and neovascularization, probably related to hyperviscosity,[14] occurs in chronic myeloid leukemia (Fig. 64.9).

Retinal hemorrhages

Hemorrhages occur as a result of hyperviscosity, coagulation defects, infiltration, damage to retinal vessel walls, and vessel occlusion.[15] Sometimes massive, they occur throughout the retina and may involve the vitreous.

Nerve fiber layer hemorrhages are bright red and "flame-shaped." Deeper hemorrhages are less red and usually more rounded. Subhyaloid hemorrhages have sharply defined margins and can form a fluid level with a layer of white cells (Fig. 64.10).

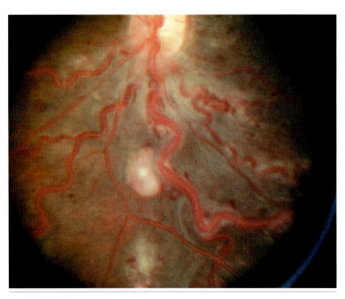

Fig. 64.9 Hyperviscosity changes in chronic myeloid leukemia in a 20-year-old. (Dr. S. Day's patient.)

Some hemorrhages are white centered; this should not be confused with the pinpoint white light reflex from the apex of a hemorrhage, or with hemorrhage around a leukemic deposit. The white area consists of platelet and fibrin deposits that occlude the vessel, or septic emboli. The hemorrhage occurs because of infarction and weakening of the vessel wall, which can also be damaged by leukemic deposits, giving the picture of mixed hemorrhage and infiltration (Fig. 64.11).

Retinal infiltrates and white patches

White areas in the retinas of leukemic children may be caused by the following:

1. Vessel sheathing.
2. Retinal infiltrates: these are leukemic deposits (Fig. 64.12), which, before the era of modern chemotherapy, were commonly seen, often with hemorrhage; they can usually be distinguished from infections by clinical and hematologic examination.[16]
3. Cotton-wool spots: these are retinal nerve fiber layer infarcts (Fig. 64.13) and occur frequently in acute leukemia[4] and transiently after bone marrow transplantation. They occur because of retinal vascular occlusion in patients who have recently received bone marrow transplants, whether or not they have been treated with ciclosporin. They can recover spontaneously and are associated with retinal vascular endotheliopathy.[17]
4. Hard exudates: these small yellowish lesions are seen in relation to vessels that are chronically leaking non-cellular blood elements and are most frequently seen in chronic leukemias with hyperviscosity.
5. Opportunistic infections with cytomegalovirus or fungus in the immunosuppressed.
6. Retinal infarction in the acute stage: this gives rise to large areas of cloudy swelling of the retinal nerve fibers and ganglion cell layer.

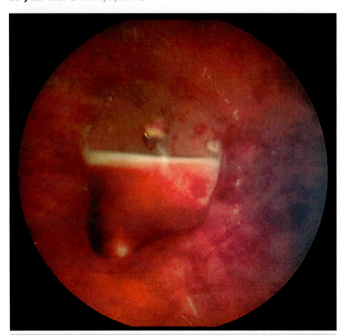

Fig. 64.10 Subhyaloid hemorrhage with a gross leukemic cell content.

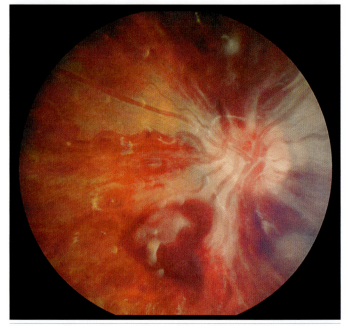

Fig. 64.11 Retinal hemorrhages and infiltrates in acute lymphoblastic leukemia.

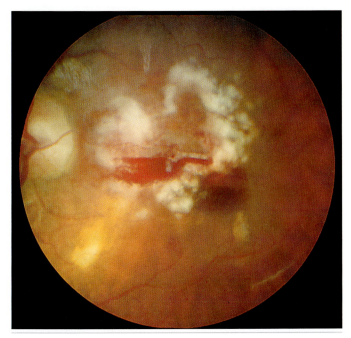

Fig. 64.12 **Retinal infiltrates in acute lymphoblastic leukemia.**

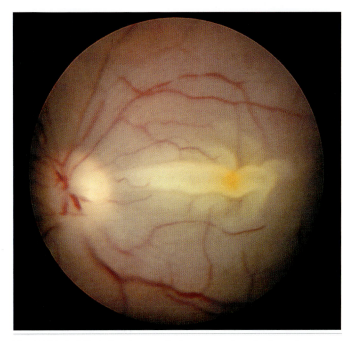

Fig. 64.14 **Ophthalmic artery occlusion as a preterminal event.**

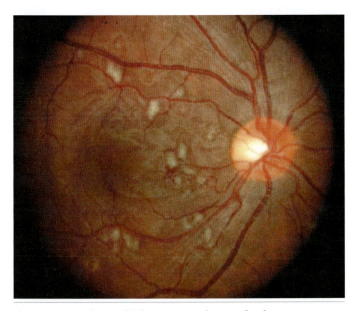

Fig. 64.13 **Transient multiple cotton-wool spots after bone marrow transplant.**

Retinal infarction

Occlusion of larger retinal arterioles or of the ophthalmic artery (Fig. 64.14) occasionally occurs as a preterminal event.[1]

Vitreous cells

Vitreous involvement with leukemic or blood cells is usually secondary to retinal or choroidal infiltration or hemorrhage.[4] Occasionally, vitreous aspiration may be needed for diagnosis, especially if the patient is apparently in remission and there is a possibility of an opportunistic infection. Vitreous organization is an unusual, but serious sequela to widespread retinal or optic nerve infiltration.

Other retinal manifestations

Serous retinopathy[13] and retinal pigment clumping occur as manifestations of choroidal ischemia.

Optic nerve

Optic nerve involvement in postmortem cases occurs in nearly one-fifth of acute or chronic leukemias,[4] although in clinical series it is more frequently seen in ALL.[18] Optic nerve involvement, which used to presage death, is now less frequently seen presumably due to aggressive chemotherapy.[19]

Leukemic optic neuropathy may cause only minimal visual symptoms despite massive involvement, but often marked loss of central vision is observed, especially with infiltration behind the lamina cribrosa.[19] With prelaminar infiltration (Fig. 64.15) there is ophthalmoscopically visible fluffy white infiltration with hemorrhage. On occasion, especially if the infiltration is bilateral, the differentiation from papilledema (which could be caused by idiopathic intracranial hypertension secondary to steroids or steroid withdrawal or CNS infiltration or infection) may be difficult and infectious disease must be remembered. The response to irradiation at 2000 cGy may be dramatic;[20] whatever the treatment, optic atrophy is a frequent sequel. Optic neuropathy may also be caused by vincristine treatment[21] or by radiotherapy.

Other neuro-ophthalmic involvement

CNS involvement with leukemia manifests as meningeal irritation, with headaches and vomiting, or cranial nerve involvement. Vessel occlusion gives rise to various defects from transient deafness to an hypoxic-ischemic encephalopathy. It is usually a feature of leukemia with a very high white blood

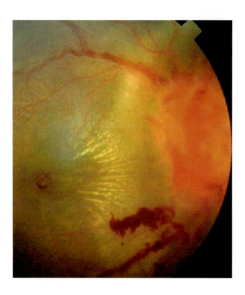

Fig. 64.15 **Prelaminar optic nerve infiltration (AML) with additional retinal nerve involvement.**

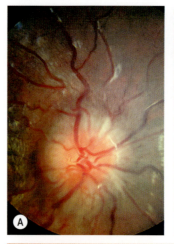
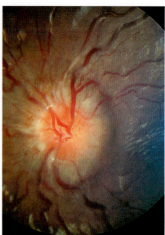

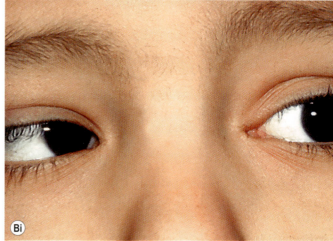

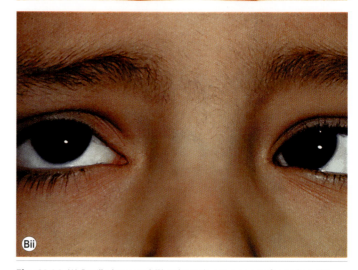

Fig. 64.16 (A) Papilledema and (B) right sixth nerve paresis from idiopathic intracranial hypertension in a patient on withdrawal of steroids in ALL.

cell count and hyperviscosity. Communicating hydrocephalus, chiasmal infiltration, and sixth nerve palsies may occur.

In addition to the disease, many of the drugs and radiotherapy used may have CNS side effects, both short and long term, including fits. Rarely children may develop a leukoencephalopathy due to methotrexate and cranial radiation.

With refinements in therapy, neurologic complications of leukemia and its treatment are now less common. Better supportive care has reduced the incidence of hemorrhage, and refinements in therapy have reduced leukoencephalopathy. Infection by measles, varicella, or mumps has been reduced by vaccination programs and immunoglobulin prophylaxis in children with proven contacts. Bacterial infections of the CNS are rare.

Complications of treatment

Drugs

Vincristine and related drugs may cause corneal hypoesthesia, ptosis, third, sixth and seventh nerve palsies, and optic neuropathy, reversible if the treatment is stopped early. The neuropathy is dose-related and usually starts as a peripheral neuropathy with abnormal deep tendon reflexes. Seizures also occur.

L-Asparaginase may idiosyncratically be associated with a severe, sometimes fatal, encephalopathy.

Cytarabine may cause blurred vision from keratoconjunctivitis (prophylaxis with topical steroids has been tried), corneal epithelial opacities, and microcysts.

Methotrexate is a significant cause of neurologic problems including arachnoiditis from intrathecal administration, seizures, depression, and leukoencephalopathy with ataxia and dementia.

Steroids may cause posterior subcapsular cataracts often not of great visual significance[22] and which have a good prognosis with surgery, if necessary.

Posterior leukoencephalopathy syndrome has been described as a reversible side effect of immunosuppressants such as cyclosporin, usually presenting with seizures, headache, and cortical blindness.[3]

Rapid withdrawal of steroid therapy may cause idiopathic intracranial hypertension (pseudotumor cerebri) (Fig. 64.16).

Chemotherapy, steroids, and radiotherapy contribute to immune suppression, which allows infection by opportunistic bacteria, viruses, fungi, or protozoa, some of which do not usually cause significant infection in humans. These complications are related to the intensity of immune suppression and are most likely following bone marrow transplantation. As broad-spectrum antibiotics have become to be used aggressively for unexplained fever in neutropenic children, uncontrolled bacterial infections have become less frequent, but viruses and fungi have increased. Clinical manifestations may include keratitis, retinitis, endophthalmitis, orbital cellulitis (differentiate from Sweets' febrile neutrophilic dermatosis syndrome[3]), and neuro-ophthalmologic manifestations of CNS infection.

Herpes simplex and zoster affect the cornea (Fig. 64.17), conjunctiva, and lids. Herpes simplex and cytomegalovirus, which have an affinity for neural tissue, may cause a severe necrotizing retinochoroiditis (Fig. 64.18) that may be difficult to differentiate from leukemic infiltrates, a distinction that can be helped by chorioretinal biopsy but can usually be made by culture of urine or saliva.

Yeast and fungal infections are important complications of neutropenia; biopsy is necessary to establish the diagnosis and to plan appropriate treatment. Other infections include mucormycosis, toxoplasmosis, cytomegalovirus, and aspergillosis.

The risk for these infections is related to the severity of immune suppression and, therefore, highest in children who undergo bone marrow transplantation.

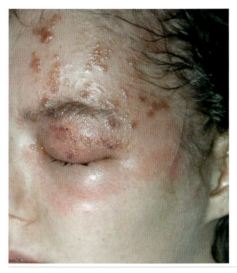

Fig. 64.17 Herpes zoster affecting trigeminal division of the fifth cranial nerve (ALL).

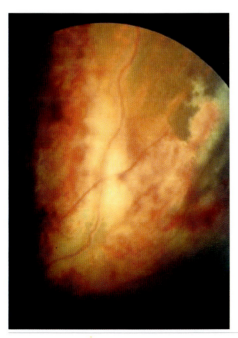

Fig. 64.18 Cytomegalovirus infection in a child with leukemia.

Stem cell transplantation

Bone marrow transplants (BMT) are sometimes necessary in the treatment of childhood leukemia, but as chemotherapy has become increasingly effective, the number of transplants has fallen. Few children now receive BMT as a first-choice therapy, but it is often considered in relapsed disease.

In recent years, the early hemopoietic progenitor cells required for BMT have been obtained from blood or cord blood collections, and term stem cell transplant (SCT) has supplanted BMT. There are two main types of SCT:

1. Allogeneic, when related or unrelated donor stem cells matched by HLA typing are infused.
2. Autologous, when the patient's own stored stem cells are used.

Prior to the SCT, children receive chemotherapy alone or combined with total body irradiation (TBI) as both antileukemia and immune suppressive therapy, to avoid graft rejection. As the marrow regenerates with new stem cells, all blood cell lineages are donor derived. Ocular changes were found in 50% of children treated with BMT for hematologic disorders.[23] The most frequent findings were dry eye (12%), cataracts (23%), and posterior segment complications (13%). These changes did not seriously compromise vision. Another study[24] identified ocular abnormalities in 82% of children, usually in the anterior segment, usually dry eye.

The incidence of eye complications depends on the treatment regimen, especially the use of TBI, the degree of immune suppression with risk of opportunistic infections, and the occurrence of graft-versus-host disease (GvHD). In one series,[25] cataracts were found in 95% of children given TBI, compared with 23% of children on chemotherapy alone. Low dose rates and fractionated rather than single-dose radiotherapy are associated with a lower incidence of cataracts.[26] It is possible these differences reflect alterations in the latent period before diagnosis, rather than a true reduction in eventual prevalence.

Because of failure to recognize the transplant recipient as "self," the transplanted T lymphocytes may attack the recipient and cause GvHD. Acute GvHD is characterized by the occurrence – within 4 months of the transplant – of any combination of fever, rash, diarrhea, and liver dysfunction. If the disorder occurs or persists after this period, it is termed chronic GvHD (cGvHD). Ocular manifestations are common in cGvHD and include dry eye, cicatricial lagophthalmos, sterile conjunctivitis, and uveitis. The eye problems are frequently severe and management testing. At autopsy, the whole eye is affected including the lacrimal gland. About 10% of patients undergoing BMT develop conjunctival involvement with GvHD.[27] Pseudomembranous conjunctivitis was the most frequent manifestation of conjunctival GvHD and carried a poor prognosis for life.

Opportunistic infections are a major risk of BMT, especially in mismatched transplants where depletion of T lymphocytes from the marrow graft in order to minimize GvHD results in delayed immune reconstitution.

An interesting occurrence is the transient appearance of multiple white cotton-wool spots in BMT recipients.[28] Retinal complications including retinal or vitreous hemorrhage, cotton-wool spots, optic disc edema, retinitis, lymphoma, and serous retinal detachments occurred in 12.8% of 397 patients with BMT.[29]

References

1. Taylor DSI, Day SH. Neuro-Ophthalmologic Aspects of Childhood Leukemia. In: Smith JL, editor. Neuro-Ophthalmology Focus. Mosby, St. Louis; 1982: 281–90.

2. Hoover DL, Smith LEH, Turner SJ, et al. Ophthalmic evaluation of survivors of acute lymphoblastic leukemia. Ophthalmology 1988; 95: 151–5.

3. Sharma T, Grewal J, Gupta S, Murray PI. Ophthalmic manifestations of acute leukaemias: the ophthalmologist's role. Eye (Lond) 2004; 18: 663–72.

4. Kincaid MC, Green WR. Ocular and orbital involvement in leukemia. Surv Ophthalmol 1983; 27: 211–32.

5. Rubinfeld RS, Gootenberg JE, Chavis RM, et al. Early onset acute orbital involvement in childhood acute lymphoblastic leukemia. Ophthalmology 1988; 95: 116–20.

6. Wood WJ, Nicholson DH. Corneal ring ulcer as the presenting manifestation of acute monocytic leukemia. Am J Ophthalmol 1973; 76: 69–72.

7. Font RL, Mackay B, Tang R. Acute monocytic leukemia recurring as bilateral perilimbal infiltrates: immunohistochemical and ultrastructural confirmation. Ophthalmology 1985; 92: 1681–5.

8. Bray LC, Carey PJ, Proctor SJ, et al. Ocular complications of bone marrow transplantation. Br J Ophthalmol 1991; 75: 611–4.

9. Novakovic P, Kellie S, Taylor D. Childhood leukaemia: relapse in the anterior segment of the eye. Br J Ophthalmol 1989; 73: 354–9.

10. Ninane J, Taylor D, Day S. The eye as a sanctuary in acute lymphoblastic leukaemia. Lancet 1980; i: 452–3.

11. Somervaille TC, Hann IM, Harrison G, et al. Intraocular relapse of childhood acute lymphoblastic leukaemia. Br J Haematol 2003; 121: 280–8.

12. Leonardy NJ, Rupani M, Dent G, et al. Analysis of 135 autopsy eyes for ocular involvement in leukemia. Am J Ophthalmol 1990; 109: 436–45.

13. Kincaid MC, Green WR, Kelley JS. Acute ocular leukemia. Am J Ophthalmol 1979; 87: 698–702.

14. Rosenthal AR. Ocular manifestations of leukemia: a review. Ophthalmology 1983; 90: 899–905.

15. Kaur B, Taylor D. Fundus hemorrhages in infancy. Surv Ophthalmol 1991; 37: 1–19.

16. Gordon KB, Rugo HS, Duncan JL, et al. Ocular manifestations of leukemia: leukemic infiltration versus infectious process. Ophthalmology 2001; 108: 2293–300.

17. Webster AR, Anderson JR, Richards EM, et al. Ischaemic retinopathy occurring in patients receiving bone-marrow allografts and campath-IG: a clinicopathological study. Br J Ophthalmol 1995; 79: 687–91.

18. Brown GC, Shields JA, Augsburger JJ, et al. Leukemic optic neuropathy. Int Ophthalmol 1981; 3: 111–6.

19. Rosenthal AR. Ocular manifestations of leukemia: a review. Ophthalmology 1983; 90: 899–905.

20. Rosenthal AR, Egbert PR, Wilbur JR, et al. Leukemic involvement of the optic nerve. J Paediatr Ophthalmol 1975; 12: 84–93.

21. Sanderson PA, Kuwabara T, Cogan DG. Optic neuropathy presumably caused by vincristine therapy. Am J Ophthalmol 1976; 81: 146–50.

22. Elliott AJ, Oakhill A, Goodman S. Cataracts in childhood leukaemia. Br J Ophthalmol 1985; 69: 459–61.

23. Suh DW, Ruttum MS, Stuckenschneider BJ, et al. Ocular findings after bone marrow transplantation in a pediatric population. Ophthalmology 1999; 106: 1564–70.

24. Ng JS, Lam DS, Lö CK, et al. Ocular complications of pediatric bone marrow transplantation. Ophthalmology 1999; 106: 160–4.

25. Holmström G, Borgstrom B, Calissendorff B. Cataract in children after bone marrow transplantation. Acta Ophthalmol Scand 2002; 80: 211–5.

26. Leiper AD. Non-endocrine late complications of bone marrow transplant in childhood: Part II. Br J Haematol 2002; 118: 23–43.

27. Jabs DA, Wingard J, Green WR, et al. The eye in bone marrow transplantation III: Conjunctival graft-vs-host disease. Arch Ophthalmol 1989; 107: 1343–9.

28. Gratwahl A, Gloor D, Hann H, et al. Retinal cotton-wool patches in bone-marrow transplant recipients. N Engl J Med 1983; 308: 110–1.

29. Coskuncan NM, Jabs DA, Dunn JP, et al. The eye in bone marrow transplantation VI. Retinal complications. Arch Ophthalmol 1994; 112: 372–9.

Phakomatoses

John R B Grigg • Robyn V Jamieson

Definition

The phakomatoses are systemic disorders with neurologic, ophthalmic, and cutaneous manifestations. A common feature is multiorgan hamartomas. The most common are neurofibromatosis, tuberous sclerosis, Sturge-Weber syndrome, and von Hippel-Lindau syndrome. Others are the Klippel-Trénaunay-Weber, Wyburn-Mason, linear nevus sebaceous, Osler-Weber-Rendu, blue rubber bleb nevus syndromes, ataxia telangiectasia, and diffuse congenital hemangiomatosis. There is increasing understanding of the genetic, molecular, and cellular biology underlying the pathophysiology of the phakomatoses leading to clinical trials with biologic agents.

Neurofibromatoses

The neurofibromatoses (NF) are diverse genetic conditions with a predisposition for tumor development. The two main types are neurofibromatosis type 1 (NF1) and type 2 (NF2).

Neurofibromatosis type 1

NF1 is a progressive disease and the final manifestations are extremely variable. Existing lesions tend to enlarge gradually and new lesions develop. The National Institutes of Health (NIH) diagnostic criteria are listed in Box 65.1.

Genetics

NF1 is the most common single gene disorder affecting the nervous system, occurring in approximately 1 in 3000 people. Inheritance is autosomal dominant with 100% penetrance, but

> **Box 65.1**
>
> **NIH diagnostic criteria for NF1**
> The diagnostic criteria are met if two or more of the following are found:
>
> 1. Six or more café-au-lait macules over 5 mm in greatest diameter in prepubertal individuals and over 15 mm in greatest diameter in postpubertal individuals
> 2. Two or more neurofibromas of any type or one plexiform neurofibroma
> 3. Freckling in the axillary or inguinal regions
> 4. Optic glioma
> 5. Two or more Lisch nodules (iris hamartomas)
> 6. A distinctive osseous lesion such as sphenoid dysplasia or thinning of long bone cortex
> 7. A first degree relative with NF1 by above criteria

highly variable expressivity. The spontaneous mutation rate is up to 42%.[1]

The protein associated with NF1, neurofibromin, down regulates the rat sarcoma viral oncogene homolog (RAS)–mitogen activated protein kinase (MAPK) pathway. Unopposed Ras activity leads to cell growth and activation of downstream signaling intermediates, including the mammalian target of rapamycin (mTOR) protein.[2] NF1 mutations give rise to malignant tumors consistent with the "two hit" hypothesis: a germ-line mutation is the initial "hit"; neurofibromas arise from Schwann cells that undergo loss of heterozygosity at the NF1 gene through somatic mutations (the second "hit").

Clinical presentation

Ocular findings are important in the NF1 diagnostic criteria (see Box 65.1), including Lisch nodules, orbital plexiform neurofibroma, sphenoid wing dysplasia, and optic nerve glioma.

Lisch nodules

Lisch nodules (melanocytic hamartomas) are dome-shaped, discrete lesions on the anterior surface of the iris or in the angle, usually bilateral. They are usually orange-brown (Fig. 65.1), appearing darker than blue irides but paler than brown irides (Fig. 65.2). Most are round and evenly distributed on the iris. Their size varies from a pinpoint to involvement of a segment of iris, sometimes confluent. In NF1, they are present

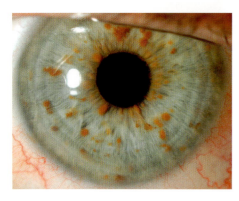

Fig. 65.1 **Multiple Lisch nodules in neurofibromatosis.**

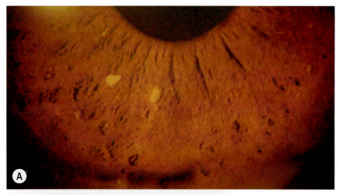

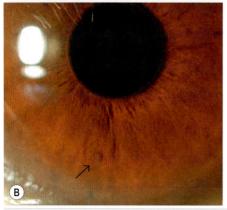

Fig. 65.2 (A) In brown irides, Lisch nodules appear light brown. (Patient of Dr. Shabana Chaudhry.) (B) Lisch nodules may be difficult to see in brown irides.

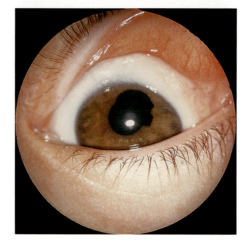

Fig. 65.3 **Ectropion uveae, another iris abnormality occurring in NF1.** (Patient of Dr. Andrew McCormick, University of British Columbia.)

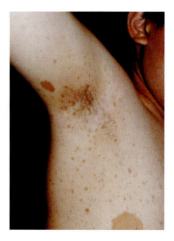

Fig. 65.4 **Café-au-lait patches as well as multiple axillary freckles in a 14 year old boy.**

in one-third of 2.5-year-olds, half of 5-year-olds, three-quarters of 15-year-olds, and almost all adults over 30.[3] They occur earlier than neurofibromas and are, therefore, a useful marker for NF1. They need to be distinguished from iris nevi.

Anterior segment and uvea

Rarely, congenital glaucoma with buphthalmos occurs in NF1, often associated with an ipsilateral upper lid plexiform neurofibroma. Congenital ectropion uveae (Fig. 65.3), iris heterochromia, angle abnormalities, and posterior embryotoxon may predispose to later onset glaucoma. Cataract is not a feature of NF1. Pigmentary hamartomas (choroidal nevi) may involve the posterior uveal tract in up to 35%.

Skin, lids and orbits

Café-au-lait spots are hyperpigmented macular skin lesions, mostly present at birth and all appear by 1 year, enlarging at

puberty. Common on the trunk, they are absent from the scalp, eyebrows, palms, and soles (Fig. 65.4). Histologically, there is melanocytic hyperplasia with increased pigmentation in the basal layer of the epidermis.

Neurofibromas are present in 30–50% of NF1 patients.[4] They are network-like tumor growths involving multiple fascicles of nerve(s); four types are recognized (Table 65.1). The presence and growth pattern of neurofibromas is age related; in infancy and early childhood, diffuse plexiform neurofibromas are most active giving rise to cosmetic and visual problems within the orbit. Cutaneous or subcutaneous neurofibromas develop and grow fastest at puberty, the late teens, and during pregnancy. There is a lifelong risk of malignant transformation with poor prognosis for 5-year survival.[5]

Complete surgical resection of plexiform neurofibromas is difficult due to their large size, location, local invasiveness, or involvement of critical peripheral nerves. Regrowth following subtotal resection is common. Chemotherapy is not effective. Promising clinical trials with biologic agents are underway.[6]

Skeletal anomalies

Hypoplasia of the greater and lesser spenoid wings and widening of the superior orbital fissure may occur. Other osseous abnormalities include abnormal vertebrae, scoliosis, pseudoarthrosis of long bones, and subperiosteal changes (Fig. 65.7). Neurofibromas may interfere with cranial nerve function.

Table 65.1 – Neurofibroma clinical features[4]

Neurofibroma types	Location	Clinical signs
Discrete cutaneous	Epidermis and dermis	Moves with skin, blueish tinge
Subcutaneous	Deep to dermis	Skin moves over, firm and rounded feel, located along peripheral nerves
Nodular plexiform	Localized interdigitation with normal tissues	"Bag of worms" feel (Figs 65.5, 65.6)
Diffuse plexiform	Infiltrate widely and deeply	Smooth, slightly irregular skin thickening

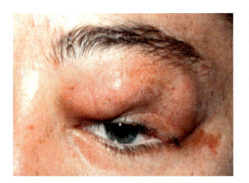

Fig. 65.5 Upper lid plexiform neurofibroma. (Patient of the University of Sydney.)

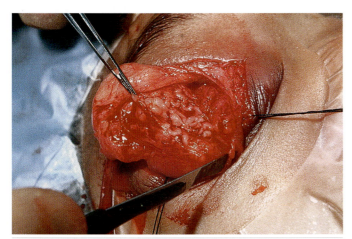

Fig. 65.6 The worm-like consistency of an orbital plexiform neurofibroma can be seen. (Patient of the University of British Columbia.)

Optic disk and central nervous system

Optic pathway gliomas are a significant cause of visual morbidity (see Chapter 23). Optic disk swelling (Fig. 65.8), strabismus (Fig. 65.9), or pallor suggests optic nerve or chiasmal glioma. Retinal manifestations are rare in NF1. The commonest consequence of NF1 in childhood and a major concern of parents is cognitive impairment. Overt mental retardation is rare, but a wide range of learning disabilities, academic underachievement, and behavioral problems may occur.

Other systems

Tumors of the spinal cord, sympathetic nerves, and adrenals may occur. The patient may present with malignant

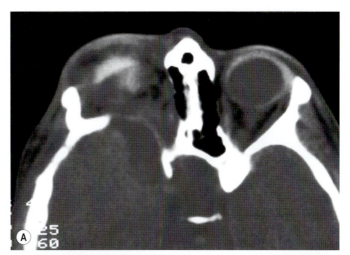

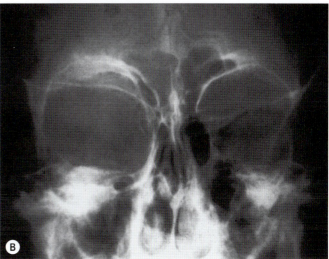

Fig. 65.7 Sphenoid bone dysplasia. (A) Axial CT scan showing absence of greater wing of sphenoid. (B) Plain skull X-ray showing loss of right sphenoid.

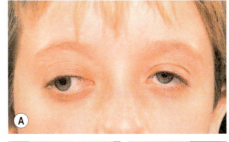

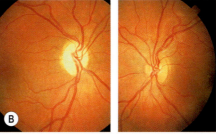

Fig. 65.8 Girl with neurofibromatosis. (A) Right optic nerve glioma, proptosis, and sensory exotropia due to (B) optic atrophy.

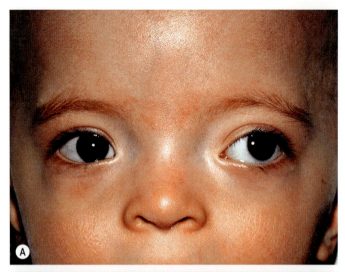

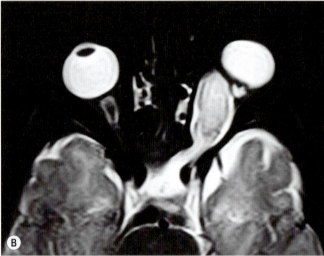

Fig. 65.9 Optic nerve glioma. (A) This 13-month-old girl presented with a history of intermittent exotropia since age 6 months, increasing numbers of café-au-lait spots and increasing proptosis on the left side. She appeared to be blind on the left. (B) T2-weighted MRI showed a fusiform tumor of the optic nerve extending up to and involving the chiasm.

hypertension from pheochromocytoma. There may be multiple neurofibromas of the gastrointestinal tract.

Neurofibromatosis type 2

Neurofibromatosis type 2 (NF2) affects 1 in 35 000 live births and is characterized by bilateral vestibular schwannomas, multiple central nervous system (CNS) tumors, cataracts, and retinal abnormalities. The diagnostic criteria for NF2 are shown in Box 65.2. Two patterns of presentation exist. Mild disease presents late (> 25 years), with few tumors other than bilateral vestibular schwannoma, and slow progression. Those with severe disease have onset before age 25, multiple CNS tumors (at least two of one type), and rapid progression, severe handicap or death before reproductive age. Treatment is multidisciplinary because of the complexities of the multiple and progressive lesions.[7]

Genetics

NF2 is an autosomal dominant condition; half the cases are sporadic mutations. There is an unusually high rate of somatic

mosaics (mutation takes place after conception, resulting in two separate cell lineages). Tumors develop in susceptible organs (i.e. nervous system, eyes, and skin) from cells that lose function of the wild type (normal) *NF2* allele. There is correlation between nonsense and frameshift mutations and the severe early phenotype of NF2.

The NF2 tumor suppressor gene Merlin is localized to the cell membrane–cytoskeletal interface where it indirectly acts through its membrane organization of proteins. Merlin regulates downstream mitogenic signaling pathways. Drugs targeting these pathways (i.e. sorafenib, trastuzumab, lapatinib, LY294002, protein kinase inhibitors, p21-activated kinase inhibitors) and tumor angiogenesis (bevacizumab) are under investigation as potential treatments for NF2.[7]

Systemic findings

The hallmark of NF2 is bilateral vestibular schwannomas ("acoustic neuromas") which may only be evident on gadolinium-enhanced MRI (see Fig. 65.11C). The origin of the trigeminal nerve is another frequent intracranial site for schwannomas; they may occur on multiple cranial nerves. Anti-VEGF (vascular endothelial growth factor) therapy improves hearing and stabilizes tumor growth.[8]

Ocular findings

Most of the ophthalmic findings in NF2 (see Box 65.2) are congenital but may become more symptomatic over time.[9] Visual loss increases morbidity since progressive bilateral hearing loss is so common in this condition.

Anterior segment

The ocular changes of NF2 are early diagnostic markers. 55–87% of affected patients have presenile central posterior subcapsular lens opacities, usually with little effect on vision (Fig. 65.10A,B). Corneal hypoesthesia from trigeminal nerve schwannoma, and decreased tear production, reduced blinking and lagophthalmos from facial nerve palsy may adversely affect the outcome of cataract surgery.

Posterior segment

Epiretinal membranes occur in up to 80% of patients with severe NF2. They are translucent, semitranslucent, or whitish

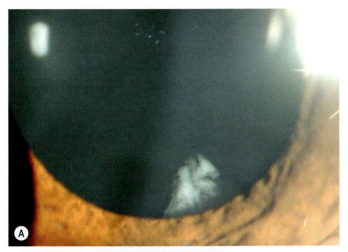

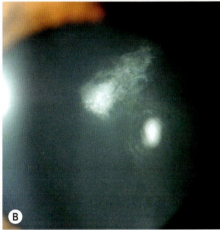

Fig. 65.10 (A) Cortical cataract in a 12-year-old. (B) Posterior subcapsular plaque in a 12-year-old.

gray membranes with prominent whitish edges demarcating their borders. They do not usually cause substantial loss of visual acuity (Fig. 65.11).

Combined retinal and pigment epithelial hamartomas occur in 6–22% of NF2 patients, especially with nonsense mutations.[9] They are slightly raised masses most frequently in the posterior pole (Fig. 65.12), commonly causing reduced vision. Optic nerve sheath meningiomas, sometimes bilateral, can cause visual loss (see Chapter 23). They may be missed on MRI unless fat suppression techniques are used.

Prognosis

Increased understanding of the clinical manifestations and improved precision of genetic tests and imaging studies have improved early diagnosis of patients. Survival is extended because of advances in treatment available at specialized centers and the recognition of mildly affected people with mosaic disease (Box 65.3).

Box 65.3

Recommended intervals for screening children of an affected parent[7]

- Ophthalmologic examination yearly from infancy
- Neurologic examination yearly from infancy
- Audiology with auditory brainstem evoked potentials yearly from infancy
- Presymptomatic genetic testing; one test from 10 years of age[a]
- Cranial MRI at 10–12 years of age[a]
- Spinal MRI at 10–12 years of age[a] (every 2–3 years)

[a]Earlier than age 10 years in severely affected families and families in which early detection of disease would aid family preparation for future events related to NF2.

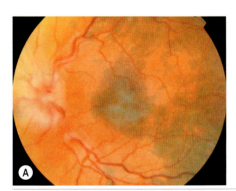

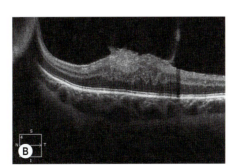

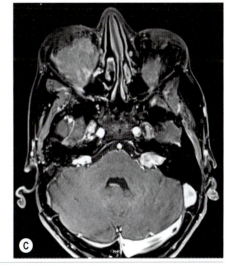

Fig. 65.11 (A) Epiretinal membrane in a 14-year-old NF2 patient. Note also papilledema secondary to optic sheath meningioma. (B) OCT scan of epiretinal membrane. Note loss of internal limiting membrane. (c) Bilateral vestibular schwannomas as well as bilateral optic sheath meningiomas in a 14-year-old boy – same patient as in (A) and (B). (MRI scan courtesy Dr. Mark Dexter, Neurosurgeon.)

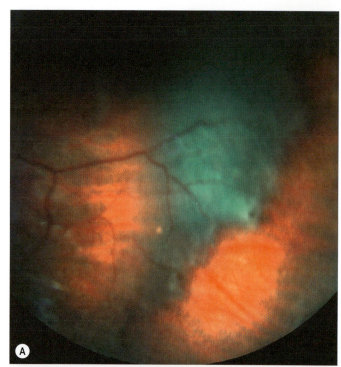

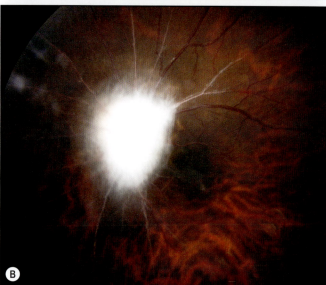

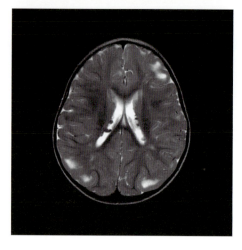

Fig. 65.13 Cortical tubers. These show as hyperintense signals and the calcified subependymal nodules as hypointense signals projecting into lateral ventricles. T2 axial MRI scan.

Fig. 65.12 (A) Combined retinal and pigment epithelial hamartoma of peripheral retina. (B) Combined hamartoma of the retina and retinal pigment epithelium optic disk involvement.

Tuberous sclerosis

Tuberous sclerosis complex (TSC) is a multisystem disorder of cell migration, proliferation, and differentiation characterized by hamartomatous growths commonly affecting the brain, skin, kidneys, eyes, and heart. Malignant tumors are rare, occurring predominantly in the kidney. Incidence is estimated to be 1 in 6000.[10]

Diagnostic criteria

The clinical features are classified into major and minor features (Table 65.2). The presence of two major features or one major plus two minor features constitutes a definitive diagnosis. One major plus one minor feature indicates a probable diagnosis, either one major or two or more minor features suggest possible TSC. Patients with epilepsy, developmental delay, or a learning disability in the absence of other known etiologies should be investigated for TSC.[10]

Specialized TSC clinics enable comprehensive evaluation of the multisystem complications (Table 65.3).

Genetics

TSC is an autosomal dominant condition with a high spontaneous mutation rate; 66% of cases have no family history. TSC results from mutations in two genes, TSC1 or TSC2. TSC2 mutation cases are diagnosed, on average, 9 years before those with TSC1 mutations, and 11 years before those without identifiable mutations (15% of cases).[10] TSC2 mutation patients are more likely to present with infantile spasms, developmental delay, or angiofibromas.[10]

Proteins coded for by TSC1 and TSC2 genes, hamartin and tuberin, respectively, form a heterodimer suppressing the mammalian target of rapamycin (mTOR), a major cell growth and proliferation controller. Increased activation of mTOR kinase results in disorganized cellular overgrowth, abnormal differentiation, and tumor formation. Rapamycin (Sirolimus) normalizes the dysregulated mTOR pathway. Clinical trials have demonstrated it controls various TSC manifestations.[11] Withdrawal of treatment may lead to rebound growth. Everolimus (rapamycin analog) may be an alternative to neurosurgical resection for subependymal giant-cell astrocytoma.[12]

Neurologic features

CNS lesions include tubers in the cerebral cortex, subependymal nodules, and subependymal giant-cell astrocytomas in the ventricular system (Fig. 65.13). Cortical tubers contain atypical glial and neuronal elements with loss of the six-layered structure of the cortex. The large dysplastic neurons show γ-aminobutyric acid (GABA)-transporter defects and low GABAergic inhibition.[13] Tubers are static lesions directly related to the neurologic manifestations of epilepsy, mental retardation, and autism.[14]

The onset of seizures, the most frequent neurologic manifestation, is usually before 2 years of age. Infantile spasms

Table 65.2 – Diagnostic criteria for tuberous sclerosis complex

Major features		Age at onset
1	Facial angiofibromas	Infancy to adulthood
2	Ungal fibroma	Adolescence to adulthood
3	Shagreen patch	Childhood
4	Hypomelanotic macules (more than 3)	Infancy to childhood
5	Cortical tuber	Fetal life
6	Subependymal nodule	Childhood to adolescence
7	Subependymal giant cell astrocytoma	Childhood to adolescence
8	Retinal hamartomas	Infancy
9	Cardiac rhabdomyoscarcoma	Fetal life
10	Lymphangiomyomatosis	Adolescence to adulthood
Minor features		
	Multiple pits in dental enamel	
	Hamartomatous rectal polyps	
	Bone cysts	
	Cerebral white matter radial migration lines	
	Gingival fibromas	
	Retinal achromatic patch	
	"Confetti" skin lesions (very small white macules)	
	Multiple renal cysts	

Table 65.3 – Diagnostic and surveillance screening in tuberous sclerosis complex

	"Asymptomatic" parent, child or first degree relative at time of diagnosis of affected individual	Suspected case or initial diagnostic evaluation	Child — Known case, no symptoms	Known case, symptoms or findings previously documented	Adult — Known case, no symptoms	Known case, symptoms or findings previously documented
Fundus examination	X	X	–	X	X	X[d]
Brain MRI	X[a]	X	X[b]	X	X[c]	X[e]
Brain EEG	–	–[d]	–	X[e]	–	X[e]
Cardiac ECG and ECHO	–[f]	X	–	X[g]	–	X[e]
Renal MRI	X[h]	X	X[i]	X[g]	X[b]	X[g]
Dermatologic screen	X	X	–	X[e]	–	X[e]
Pulmonary CT	–	–	–	X[e]	X[j]	X[e]

Modified from Tuberous Sclerosis Alliance Web site (http://www.tsalliance.org).[a]With negative physical examination MRI and/or CT is recommended.
[b]Every 1 to 3 years.
[c]Probably less frequently in children.
[d]Unless seizures are suspected, generally not useful for diagnosis.
[e]As clinically indicated.
[f]Unless needed for diagnosis.
[g]Every 6 months to 1 year until involution or size stabilizes.
[h]Recent studies recommend MRI as it provides more detail than ultrasound and avoids radiation of CT.
[i]Every 3 years until adolescence.
[j]For women at age 18.

predominate (65%), often preceded by or coexisting with partial seizures. The seizures may increase in frequency and severity with age with grand mal seizures gradually predominating. The treatment of TSC related seizures is difficult. Vigabatrin (GABA agonist) is very effective with complete cessation in up to 95% of cases but risking, in up to 50% of patients treated, bilateral concentric constriction of the visual fields. This commences with nasal loss extending in an annulus over the horizontal midline, with relative sparing of the temporal field.[15]

Moderate to severe learning disabilities occur in 38% to 80% of cases. More severe mental retardation correlates with a larger number of cortical tubers. A TSC child with normal development up to age 5 is likely to continue normally.[16] Multiple behavioral problems include sleep disorders, hyperactivity, attention deficit, aggressiveness, and autism.

Dermatologic manifestations

Hypomelanotic macules (ash leaf spots) are present in 97% of children, from birth in two-thirds of cases and 90% of cases by age 2. They are asymmetrically distributed. A Wood's ultraviolet light aids detection (Fig. 65.14B).

Facial angiofibromas (adenoma sebaceum) are found in up to 75% of patients becoming evident between 5 and 14 years of age and typically distributed in a "butterfly" pattern (Fig. 65.14A).

Shagreen patches occur in approximately 50% of cases. They are flattened yellowish-red or pink with an orange skin texture located on dorsal surfaces particularly the lumbar region (Fig. 65.14C). The forehead fibrous plaque occurs in 25% of cases and may precede facial angiofibromas. They are slightly elevated yellowish-brown or flesh colored plaques that grow slowly rising several millimeters above the skin surface. Periungal fibromas occur in up to 50% of cases. The toe nails are a common site. They arise from the nail bed beneath the nail plate or from the skin of the nail groove. Gingival fibromas are less common.[17]

Visceral features

Cardiac rhabdomyomas (single or multiple) may be present from the neonatal period in up to 45%[17] of TSC patients, identified by echocardiography; they usually do not produce any hemodynamic disturbances and regress.

Renal lesions are found in 92%[17] by age 18. Five different lesions occur: benign angiomyolipomas, malignant angiomyolipomas, cysts, oncocytomas, and renal cell carcinoma. Benign angiomyolipomas occur in 70–80% of older children and adults with TSC. Bleeding is a complication with lesions greater than 4 cm in diameter. Other visceral involvement includes liver angiomyolipomas and lymphangiomyomatosis of the lung[17] predominantly affecting women.

Ocular features

Retinal hamartomas form one of the major diagnostic criteria for TSC. Three types are described:

1. A relatively flat, smooth, non-calcified, gray translucent lesion (Fig. 65.15B,D).
2. An elevated, multinodular, calcified, opaque lesion resembling mulberries (Fig. 65.16A).
3. A transitional lesion having features of both (Fig. 65.16).

They occur in up to 50% of patients; a third are bilateral. Multiple morphologic types are present in a third.

The flat smooth translucent type is the commonest, occurring in 70% of patients with hamartomas.[18] They may be difficult to see, manifesting as an abnormal light reflex, approximately 0.25–2 disk diameters in size, located in the posterior pole frequently superficial to retinal vessels. The classic multinodular "mulberry" occurs in up to 50% of patients with hamartomas. Eighty percent occur on or within 2 disk diameters of the optic disk.[18] The size ranges from 0.25 to 4 disk diameters. Ten percent of patients have a combined lesion with a flat hamartoma and a central area of nodular calcification, located at the posterior pole.

Retinal hamartomas are not calcified in infancy but become so later in life; usually they remain static. Rarely vitreous hemorrhage may occur, presumably from abnormal vessels.

Chorioretinal hypopigmented punched-out lesions occur in up to 40% of patients.[18] They are less than 1 disk diameter in size and are distributed in the mid-peripheral fundus (see Fig. 65.15C).

Ocular management

The management of TSC patients requires a multidisciplinary approach (see Table 65.5). The ophthalmologist's role is in screening, monitoring visual development, progress of lesions, and in the monitoring of ocular complications of systemic therapy, particularly the antiepileptic medication.

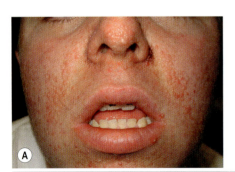
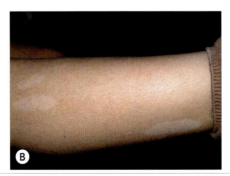
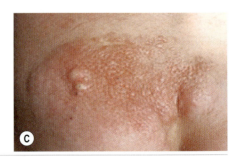

Fig. 65.14 Skin manifestations of tuberous sclerosis. (A) Facial angiofibromas (formerly adenoma sebaceum) are typically distributed in a butterfly pattern. (B) Hypomelanotic macules (ash leaf spots). (C) Shagreen patch on the lower back.

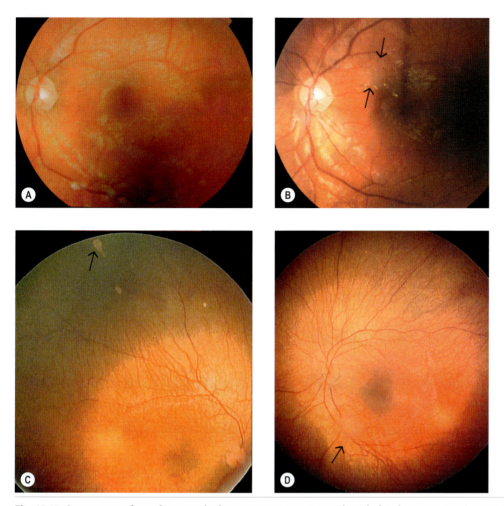

Fig. 65.15 Appearance of translucent retinal astrocytoma over 7-month period. Left superior macular region. (A) No lesion visible. (B) 7 months later astrocytoma present arrows. (C) Hypomelanotic punched-out lesions in midperiphery of right eye. (D) Left translucent retinal astrocytoma along inferior temporal vascular arcade.

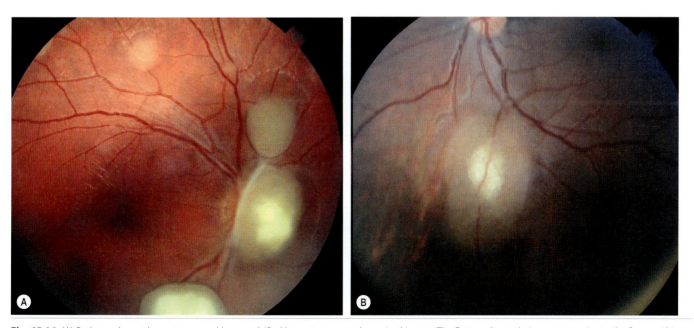

Fig. 65.16 (A) Both translucent hamartomas and larger calcified hamartomas are shown in this case. The flat translucent lesions are superior to the fovea within and above the superior vascular arcade. (B) A combined lesion with a flat hamartoma and a central nodular area.

Vigabatrin monitoring

Monitoring vigabatrin associated visual field defects is challenging. Visual field examination with a Goldmann perimeter (11e or 12e isopter and 14e or V4e isopter) or a Humphrey field analyzer (age related, three zone suprathreshold strategy and the 135 point field) is preferred. For those unable to comply, a full-field ERG (altered cone function) or a multifocal ERG (negative b wave) are useful. Retinal nerve fiber layer assessment with optical coherence tomography can provide an accurate estimate of the extent of vigabatrin toxicity.[19]

von Hippel-Lindau disease

von Hippel-Lindau (VHL) disease is a rare autosomal dominant syndrome causing susceptibility to benign, ocular vascular tumors (retinal capillary hemangioblastomas, RCH) and CNS (angioma or hemangioblastoma), renal cell carcinoma, and pheochromocytoma. Diagnostic criteria have been developed (Table 65.4). VHL affects approximately 1 in 35 000. Symptoms typically develop from the second to fourth decade.

Genetics

VHL disease is caused by germ-line mutation of the VHL tumor-suppressor gene whose product, pVHL, interacts with the hypoxia-inducible factor (HIF). With loss of pVHL activity, HIF is not degraded leading to overproduction of growth factors encoded by HIF target genes, such as VEGF and platelet-derived growth-factor β chain contributing to tumor formation.[20]

Screening (Table 65.5) is important because the lesions are treatable; early detection enables more conservative therapy enhancing the patient's length and quality of life (Table 65.5). There is high penetrance: almost all patients testing positive genetically develop clinically definite disease. Presymptomatic genetic testing is therefore recommended, including at-risk children.

Complete deletions have a lower frequency of RCHs (14.5%) whereas missense mutations (38.0%) and truncating mutations (40.1%) have greater involvement.[21] Almost all missense mutations (98.5%) are located in one of two (the alpha and beta) structural domains of the VHL protein. Alpha-domain mutations are significantly associated with a higher prevalence of RCHs compared with the beta-domain mutations. The prevalence of RCH lesions in the juxtapapillary position is

Table 65.4 – Diagnostic criteria for von Hippel-Lindau

Family history[a]	Required feature
Positive	Any one of the following: • Retinal capillary hemangioma • CNS hemangioma • Visceral lesion[b]
Negative	Any one of the following: • Two or more retinal capillary hemangiomas • Two or more CNS hemangiomas • Single retinal or CNS hemangioma with a visceral lesion[b]

[a]Family history of retinal or CNS hemangioma or visceral lesion.
[b]Visceral lesions include: renal cysts, renal carcinoma, pheochromocytoma, pancreatic cysts, islet cell tumors, epididymal cystadenoma, endolymphatic sac tumor, and adnexal papillary cystadenoma of probable mesonephric origin.

Table 65.5 – Recommended intervals for screening at-risk individuals (adapted from reference [22])

Test	Start age	Frequency
Ophthalmic examination	0 years	Yearly
Neurologic examination	0 years[a]	Yearly
Plasma or 24 hour urinary catecholamines and metanephrines	2 years of age	Yearly and when blood pressure is raised
Imaging of CNS (MRI)	11 years of age	Yearly
CT and MRI of internal auditory canals	Onset of symptoms (hearing loss, tinnitus, vertigo, or unexplained difficulties of balance)	
Ultrasound of abdomen	8 years of age	Yearly MRI as clinically indicated
CT of abdomen	18 years of age or earlier if clinically indicated	Yearly
Audiologic function tests	15 years	Baseline then when clinically indicated

[a]From 0 to 14 years: annual pediatric examinations are recommended.

significantly higher in patients with alpha-domain mutations. Complete absence of the VHL gene has milder disease, suggesting that aberrant VHL function may be more pathogenic in the retina.[21]

Diagnostic criteria and screening

CNS and visceral features

CNS hemangioblastomas occur in up to 70% of patients with VHL. There are three major sites of involvement: cerebellum (Fig. 65.17), spine, and medulla. Pheochromocytomas occur as a principal manifestation in some families and not at all in others. Renal cysts and tumors are present in 60% of patients. Renal cell carcinoma develops in 24–45% of cases.[23] Other systemic involvement includes endolymphatic sac tumors, pancreatic cystic disease, and pancreatic islet cell tumors. CNS hemangioblastomas and renal carcinoma are the main causes of death.

Ophthalmic features

Ocular involvement occurs in approximately 37% of VHL patients with 58% having bilateral involvement.[20] RCHs are hamartomatous malformations; however, they are not usually congenital. RCHs are classified on the basis of retinal location (peripheral and juxtapapillary) (Figs 65.18 and 65.19), morphology (endophytic, exophytic, and sessile), and effect on the retina (exudative or tractional).

RCHs are usually manifested by 30 years of age. Fluorescein angiography visualizes early vascular abnormalities and confirms the diagnosis by revealing the fine vascular pattern. This is particularly helpful for juxtapapillary RCHs and in differentiating the feeder arteriole from the draining vein prior to laser therapy.

Treatments include observation for peripheral small lesions (<500 μm), that are non-vision threatening and have no exudate or subretinal fluid. The juxtapapillary lesions tend to behave differently to peripheral lesions. Treatment is indicated if vision is being lost. Laser photocoagulation is most effective for lesions up to 1.5 mm in diameter. Cryotherapy is most effective for larger lesions up to 4 mm. Photodynamic therapy is also effective for larger lesions.[24] Anti-angiogenesis therapy, in particular VEGF receptor inhibitors, have shown potential. Visual loss is a major complication of VHL; ophthalmic screening is essential to enable early treatments.[25]

Sturge-Weber syndrome

Sturge-Weber syndrome (SWS) is a rare congenital neurocutaneous disorder occurring sporadically in approximately 1 in 40 000–50 000 live births.[26] It is characterized by angiomatous vascular malformations of the face (Fig. 65.20), eye, and CNS, and is classified into three types according to the extent of involvement:

Type I (most common): facial capillary malformation (CM), "port-wine stain," and intracranial leptomeningeal vascular malformation, with or without ocular abnormalities such as glaucoma.
Type II: facial CM and possible glaucoma, but no brain abnormalities.
Type III: leptomeningeal angiomatosis without cutaneous lesion or ocular abnormalities.[27]

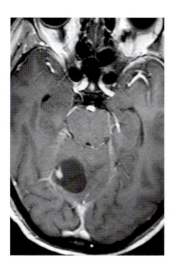

Fig. 65.17 11-year-old von Hippel-Lindau sydrome patient with cerebellar hemangioblastoma. T1 MRI axial scan. (Patient of Dr. Mark Dexter, Neurosurgeon.)

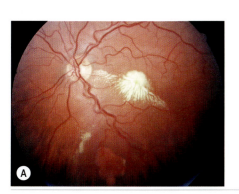
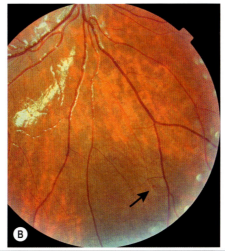
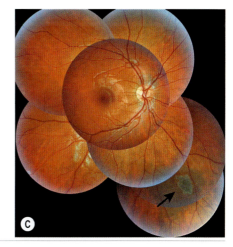

Fig. 65.18 Peripheral retinal capillary hemangioblastomas. (A) Inferior midperipheral hemangioma with dilated arteriole and venule and exudate. (Patient of Professor F. A. Billson.) (B) Pre- and (C) post-laser photocoagulation. (Patient of Professor H. U. Møller.)

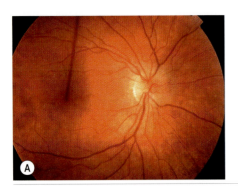
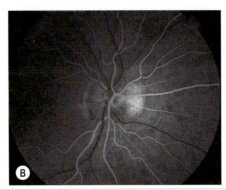
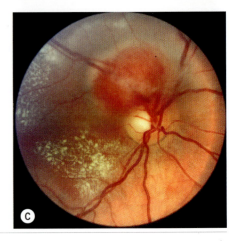

Fig. 65.19 (A) Juxtapapillary retinal capillary hemangioma with (B) fluorescein angiogram. (Patient of Professor A. P. Hunyor.) (C) Large juxtapapillary hemangioma with exudate.

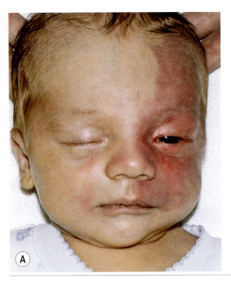
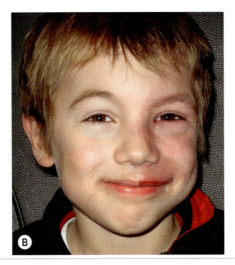
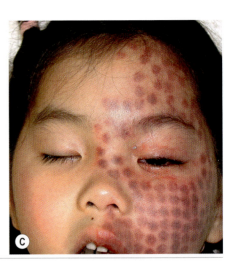

Fig. 65.20 SWS facial capillary malformation "port-wine stain". At age 1 month (A) and after 8 years (B) following multiple laser sessions. (C) Dye laser therapy. Repeat application to fill in untreated areas. Eyelid spared on this occasion due to recent trabeculectomy.

Pathogenesis

The etiology of SWS remains unclear. No inheritance pattern has been identified. The postulated pathogenesis reflects primary venous dysplasia, with failure of regression of primordial embryonic venous plexuses that are normally present at 5–8 weeks of gestation. Other research highlights the ectatic capillaries and venules associated with a reduction in postcapillary venule neural density.[28] Localized primary venous dysplasia, with effects of venous hypertension transmitted to nearby venous passageways and compensatory collateral venous channels is an alternative hypothesis.[29]

These skin lesions are "vascular malformations."[30] In ophthalmology, vascular malformations present in the choroid and conjunctiva are termed "hemangiomas." However, the histology shows diffuse choroidal involvement similar to the skin lesions.[31]

Neurologic features

Neurologic complications include epilepsy, progressive mental retardation, contralateral hemiparesis, hemiplegia, or hemianopsia. Ipsilateral leptomeningeal vascular malformations are the underlying structural lesions. These most commonly affect the occipital and temporal lobes. (Fig. 65.21) The extent and degree of the neurologic symptoms is related to the area and severity of glucose hypometabolism. Mildly affected cortex is associated with epilepsy of a greater severity. A stroke preventative approach is important including good hydration during illness. Low-dose aspirin may reduce the frequency of stroke-like episodes with SWS.

Ophthalmic features and management issues

Glaucoma is the principal ocular complication occurring in 58–71% of cases[26] with a bimodal presentation with an early onset group featuring an angle anomaly with trabeculodysgenesis. The late onset group is related to raised episcleral venous pressure. The early onset group may later worsen as the conjunctival episcleral vascular malformation becomes more apparent.

Choroidal vascular malformations ("hemangiomas") are common. They may be localized to the posterior pole or extend to the whole fundus. Comparison with the other eye

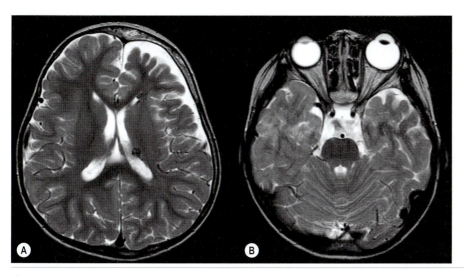

Fig. 65.21 (A) Leptomeningeal enhancement demonstrating the angiomatosis. Associated cerebral atrophy. Post gadolinium T1 axial MRI scan. (B) Left temporal lobe leptomeningeal angiomatosis, cortical atrophy with calvarial skull bone thickening and left buphthalmos. T2 axial MRI image.

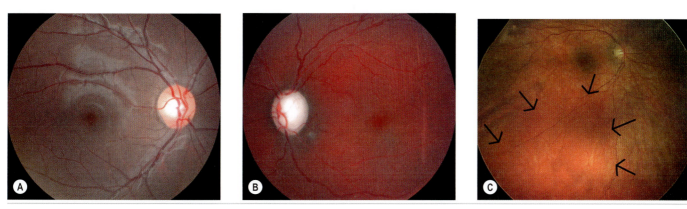

Fig. 65.22 **Choroidal vascular malformation.** (A) Normal right eye. (B) Diffuse posterior pole involvement ("tomato ketchup fundus"), same patient as A. (C) Circumscribed posterior pole choroidal vascular malformation.

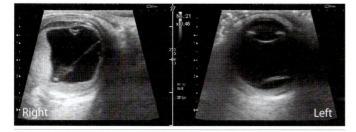

Fig. 65.23 Ultrasound of choroidal vascular malformations ("hemangioma") with associated exudative retinal detachment almost complete in right eye and localized in left eye.

assists in diagnosis. There is loss of the normal choroidal vascular pattern with a diffuse smooth red fundus (Fig. 65.22). Bilateral cases can be difficult to detect. These hemangiomas grow slowly and may lead to degenerative changes of the overlying retina with serous retinal detachment (Fig. 65.23).

Glaucoma management is challenging in SWS. Goniotomy is the procedure of choice in the early onset group. Antiglaucoma medications have an adjunctive role in this group. Medications are the usual initial management option for the late onset group. Filtration surgery, when required, mandates alterations in technique to minimize hypotony and/or hemorrhage. For trabeculectomies this entails preplaced scleral flap sutures (for rapid closure) and either viscoelastic or an anterior chamber maintainer during the procedure. The risk of hemorrhage or effusion is proportional to the size of the choroidal vascular malformation. For tube implants, surgical techniques are required to minimize intraoperative and late hypotony including an anterior chamber maintainer (25 G), and or viscoelastic at time of tube insertion, ligation of tube, and the use of a tube stent. Use of a small gauge needle (25 G) for tube entry into the anterior chamber is advised. If intraoperative choroidal effusions occur, wound closure assisted by elevation of anterior chamber infusion bottle height ± drainage via preplaced sclerostomies is required.

Dermatologic features and management issues

The port-wine stain, present at birth, is a capillary vascular malformation located in the papillary as well as superficial and reticular dermis. In contrast to capillary hemangiomas, they persist without a tendency to resolve and often darken to a violaceous color and become raised by middle age.

Pulsed dye laser is effective in arresting the progressive skin changes, particularly from smooth to lumpy. The laser acts via

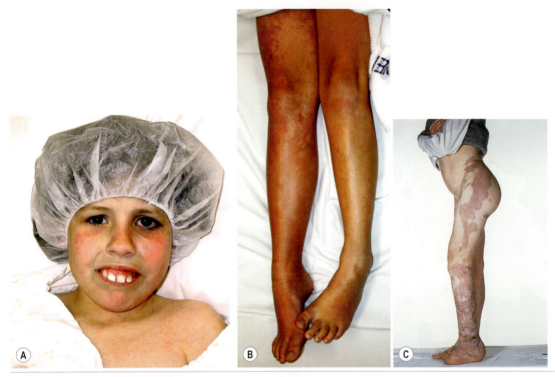

Fig. 65.24 Klippel-Trénaunay-Weber syndrome clinical features. (A) Facial hemihypertrophy, port-wine stain, and buphthalmos. (B) Leg length inequality due to bone hypertrophy (same patient as in (A)). (C) Venous malformations of lower limb.

selective vascular photothermolysis. Multiple treatments may be needed. If a vascular malformation involves the upper lid, intraocular involvement is likely. Dye laser, with the potential to affect alternative episcleral venous drainage, does not lead to increased intraocular pressure or glaucoma.[26,32]

Other conditions sometimes grouped with phakomatoses

Klippel-Trénaunay-Weber syndrome (Fig. 65.24)

Klippel-Trénaunay syndrome (KTS) manifestations can be divided into two groups:

Group A: capillary and venous malformations.
Group B: abnormal growth of girth or length.

Patients require manifestations in both groups for a diagnosis of KTS.[33] The vascular disorder in KTS is a combined capillary, venous, and lymphatic malformation with no evidence of substantial arteriovenous shunting.[34] Ophthalmic features include orbital varix, retinal varicosities, angioma of the choroid, heterochromia iridium, and ipsilateral optic nerve enlargement. Glaucoma, when present, has many features in common with that in the Sturge-Weber syndrome.

Ataxia telangiectasia (Louis-Bar syndrome)

See Chapter 31.

Wyburn-Mason syndrome

See Chapter 47.

References

1. Kissil JL, Blakeley JO, Ferner RE, et al. What's new in neurofibromatosis? Proceedings from the 2009 NF Conference: new frontiers. Am J Med Genet Part A 2010; 152A: 269–83.
2. Brems H, Beert E, de Ravel T, Legius E. Mechanisms in the pathogenesis of malignant tumours in neurofibromatosis type 1. Lancet Oncol 2009; 10: 508–15.
3. Ragge N, Falk R, Cohen W, et al. Images of Lisch nodules across the spectrum. Eye 1993; 7: 95–101.
4. Demestre M, Herzberg J, Holtkamp N, et al. Imatinib mesylate (Glivec) inhibits Schwann cell viability and reduces the size of human plexiform neurofibroma in a xenograft model. J Neuro-Oncol 2010; 98: 11–9.
5. Korf B. Malignancy in neurofibromatosis type 1. Oncologist 2000; 5: 477–85.
6. Jakacki RI, Dombi E, Potter DM, et al. Phase I trial of pegylated interferon-alpha-2b in young patients with plexiform neurofibromas. Neurology 2011; 76: 265–72.
7. Asthagiri A, Parry D, Butman J, et al. Neurofibromatosis type 2. Lancet 2009; 373: 1974–86.
8. Wong H, Lahdenranta J, Kamoun W, et al. Anti-vascular endothelial growth factor therapies as a novel therapeutic approach to treating neurofibromatosis-related tumors. Cancer Res 2010; 70: 3483–93.
9. Sisk RA, Berrocal AM, Schefler AC, et al. Epiretinal membranes indicate a severe phenotype of neurofibromatosis type 2. Retina 2010; 30 (4 Suppl): S51–8.
10. Staley B, Vail E, Thiele E. Tuberous sclerosis complex: diagnostic challenges, presenting symptoms, and commonly missed signs. Pediatrics 2011; 127: e117–25.
11. Napolioni V, Moavero R, Curatolo P. Recent advances in neurobiology of tuberous sclerosis complex. Brain Dev 2009; 31: 104–13.
12. Krueger DA, Care MM, Holland K, et al. Everolimus for subependymal giant-cell astrocytomas in tuberous sclerosis. N Engl J Med 2010; 363: 1801–11.

13. Schwartz RA, Fernandez G, Kotulska K, Jozwiak S. Tuberous sclerosis complex: advances in diagnosis, genetics, and management. J Am Acad Dermatol 2007; 57: 189–202.

14. Borkowska J, Schwartz R, Kotulska K, Jozwiak S. Tuberous sclerosis complex: tumors and tumorigenesis. Int J Dermatol 2011; 50: 13–20.

15. Clayton LM, Devile M, Punte T, et al. Retinal nerve fiber layer thickness in vigabatrin-exposed patients. Ann Neurol 2011; 69: 845–54.

16. Osborne JP, Merrifield J, O'Callaghan FJK. Tuberous sclerosis – what's new? Arch Dis Child 2008; 93: 728–31.

17. Jozwiak S, Schwartz R, Janniger C, Bielicka-Cymerman J. Usefulness of diagnostic criteria of tuberous sclerosis complex in pediatric patients. J Child Neurol 2000; 15: 652–9.

18. Rowley S, O'Callaghan F, Osborne J. Ophthalmic manifestations of tuberous sclerosis: a population based study. Br J Ophthalmol 2001; 85: 420–3.

19. Sergott RC. Recommendations for visual evaluations of patients treated with vigabatrin. Curr Opin Ophthalmol 2010; 21: 442–6.

20. Wong WT, Chew EY. Ocular von Hippel-Lindau disease: clinical update and emerging treatments. Curr Opin Ophthalmol 2008; 19: 213–7.

21. Wong WT, Agron E, Coleman HR, et al. Genotype-phenotype correlation in von Hippel-Lindau disease with retinal angiomatosis. Arch Ophthalmol 2007; 125: 239–45.

22. Alliance VF. VHL screening protocol; 2011. Available from: http://www.vhl.org/handbook/vhlhb4.php.

23. Choyke P, Glenn G, Walter M, et al. von Hippel-Lindau disease: genetic, clinical, and imaging features. Radiology 1995; 194: 629–42.

24. Sachdeva R, Dadgostar H, Kaiser PK, et al. Verteporfin photodynamic therapy of six eyes with retinal capillary haemangioma. Acta Opthalmol 2010; 88: e334–40.

25. Wong WT, Agron E, Coleman HR, et al. Clinical characterization of retinal capillary hemangioblastomas in a large population of patients with von Hippel-Lindau disease. Ophthalmology 2008; 115: 181–8.

26. Sharan S, Swamy B, Taranath D, et al. Port-wine vascular malformations and glaucoma risk in Sturge-Weber syndrome. J AAPOS 2009; 13: 374–8.

27. Roach E, Bodensteiner J. Neurologic manifestations of Sturge-Weber syndrome. In: Bodensteiner J, Roach ES, editors. Sturge-Weber Syndrome. Mt Freedom: Sturge-Weber Foundation; 1999: 27–38.

28. Breugem C, Hennekam R, van Gemert M, van der Horst C. Are capillary malformations neurovenular or purely neural? Plast Reconstruct Surg 2005; 115: 578–87.

29. Parsa C. Sturge-Weber syndrome: a unified pathophysiologic mechanism. Curr Treat Options Neurol 2008; 10: 47–54.

30. Hassanein A, Mulliken J, Fishman S, Greene A. Evaluation of terminology for vascular anomalies in current literature. Plast Reconstruct Surg 2011; 127: 347–51.

31. Witschel H, Font R. Hemangioma of the choroid: a clinicopathologic study of 71 cases and a review of the literature. Surv Ophthalmol 1976; 20: 415–31.

32. Quan SY, Comi AM, Parsa CF, et al. Effect of a single application of pulsed dye laser treatment of port-wine birthmarks on intraocular pressure. Arch Dermatol 2010; 146: 1015–8.

33. Oduber C, van der Horst CM, Hennekam R. Klippel-Trenaunay syndrome: diagnostic criteria and hypothesis on etiology. Ann Plast Surg 2008; 60: 217–23.

34. Jacob A, Driscoll D, Shaughnessy W, et al. Klippel-Trenaunay syndrome: spectrum and management. Mayo Clin Proc 1998; 73: 28–36.

Accidental trauma in children

William V Good

Introduction

Accidental eye trauma in children is a leading public health concern throughout the world. A careful history in cases of eye trauma is important and yet potentially misleading; something unreported could have occurred. Children may try to please adults thereby providing incorrect answers, and may try to deflect blame for an injury with misleading statements. Any history provided by child or parent must fit the physical findings.

Epidemiology

The number of serious eye injuries in children has been estimated at 11.8 per 100 000 per year.[1] At least 35% of serious eye injuries occur in children; the majority occur in children under the age of 12.[2] Eye injuries account for 8–14% of total injuries in children[3] and are the most common cause of unilateral blindness in children. Aside from vision loss, significant disfigurement may accompany a serious eye injury. Several factors place a child at risk for serious accidental eye injury:[4] age between 0 and 5 years, male gender, and a lack of parental supervision. Non-compliance with optical correction and patching is an important factor after childhood perforating anterior eye injury.[5] Amblyopia may limit recovery of vision in children under 7 years of age, even in eye injuries that would carry a good prognosis in older individuals.

Self-inflicted injury

See Chapter 124.

Ophthalmic trauma caused by amniocentesis and birth injury

Eye injuries occur in association with amniocentesis (Fig. 66.1). Of five cases of presumed ophthalmic amniocentesis injury,[6] one had a hemianopia and gaze palsy, two had presumed needle perforation of the eye resulting in a peaked pupil in one case and chorioretinal scar in the other. In the remaining two one showed a small leukoma, and one a limbal scar. After amniocentesis, non-pigmented anterior iris cysts adherent to the posterior cornea and with peripheral anterior synechiae are possibly a result of injury with the amniocentesis needle. Congenital aphakia with retinal scar has also been described following in utero perforation of the globe.

Ocular adnexal injuries occur, albeit rarely, after episiotomy. The possibility of ruptured globe caused by childbirth is discussed below. Forceps should be suspected as the cause of a congenital corneal abnormality in which vertical ruptures in Descemet's membrane (Fig. 66.2) occur with a contralesional occipital depression caused by the other arm of the forceps (Chapter 33).

Eyelid and lacrimal system trauma

In eyelid margin laceration, careful reapproximation of the margins of the eyelid is essential. The etiology is sharp or blunt trauma to the lid margin. Injuries to the canalicular system will occur if the medial eyelid margin is injured, either of the upper or lower lid commonly caused in children by dog bites.[7] They require intubation with silastic tubing passed through both ends of the canaliculus and into the nose or the use of a mono-canalicular stent. With deeper injuries, we close deep edges of

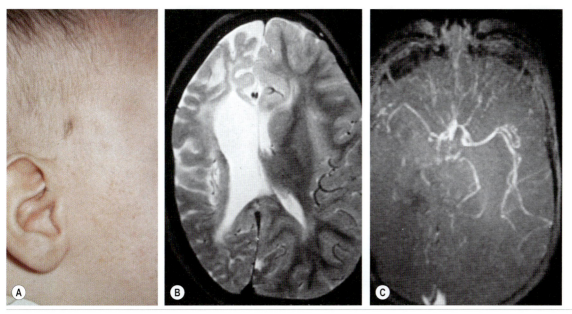

Fig. 66.1 Probable amniocentesis needle injury. (A) A small pigmented dimple on this baby's right temple coincides with radiologic evidence of a needle track. (B) MRI scan showing right cerebral hemiatrophy. (C) MRI angiography showing occlusion of the right middle cerebral artery.

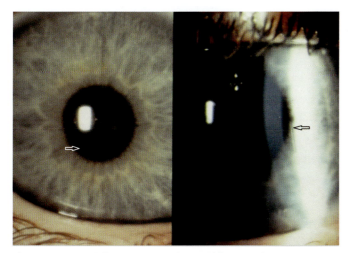

Fig. 66.2 Forceps injury to cornea. The vertically oriented rupture in Descemet's membrane can just be seen to one side of the pupil (arrows).

the wound with fine grade absorbable suture and close the more superficial edges of the wound with fine suture. With dog bite injuries additional problems may be an inferior oblique palsy or restrictive type of ocular motor problem. We close the laceration, as described above, followed later by strabismus management as required.

Anterior segment trauma

Subconjunctival hemorrhage (see Chapter 31)

Despite their dramatic appearance, subconjunctival hemorrhages are of virtually no significance except where enough

swelling occurs near the limbus to interfere with corneal protection by the eyelids and tear film. In this case a delle or some dellen may occur. A delle is a non-inflammatory excavation of the cornea with or without epithelial defect which occurs adjacent to a mass or bump near the corneal scleral limbus. It is probably caused by localized drying.

Subconjunctival hemorrhages associated with trauma indicate the need for a thorough search for a more serious eye injury (Fig. 66.3). The hemorrhage may mask a penetrating injury; look carefully for other signs of penetrating injury (e.g. uvea in a laceration, distorted pupil, lower intraocular pressure).

Corneal abrasion

Corneal abrasions occur when the corneal epithelium is traumatically removed from its underlying basement membrane. Abrasions can occur from blunt or sharp trauma: they are significantly painful. Fluorescein transiently stains the underlying basement membrane and fluoresces in a blue light.

The differential diagnosis for corneal abrasion includes viral (e.g. herpes simplex, adenovirus) keratitis and corneal basement membrane disease and dystrophies. Herpes infection is usually suggested by a dendritic appearance, while basement membrane disease occurs in older children and adults and is recurrent, with no history of trauma (see Chapter 15).

We manage abrasions with a broad spectrum antibiotic ointment, cycloplegia to reduce pain from iridospasm, with or without patching the eye for comfort.

Corneal foreign body

Patients with a corneal foreign body complain of pain and foreign body sensation. We remove the foreign body, usually with irrigation, a rotating "burr," or simply and carefully with a sharp needle brought toward the eye tangentially and used to flick the foreign body away from the surface of the eye. The

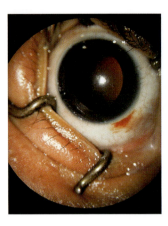

Fig 66.3 Subconjunctival hemorrhage. In this instance associated with shaking, there were severe intraocular injuries.

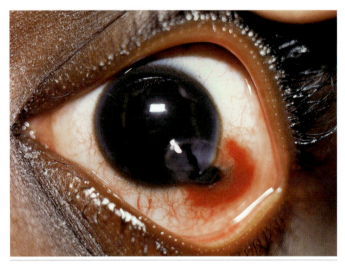

Fig. 66.4 Penetrating injury with iris prolapse and subconjunctival hemorrhage.

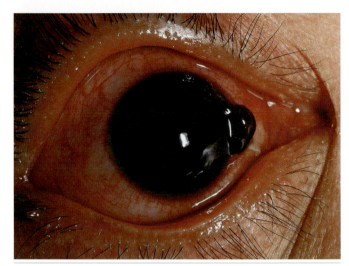

Fig. 66.5 Limbal penetrating injury with iris prolapse.

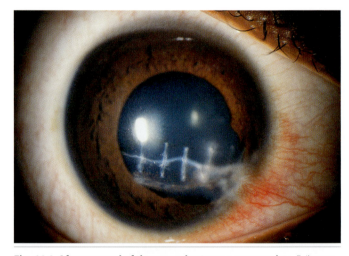

Fig. 66.6 After removal of the corneal sutures a scar persists. Failure to remove suture promptly may cause blood vessel migration and corneal opacification. Note the vessels at the corneoscleral limbus.

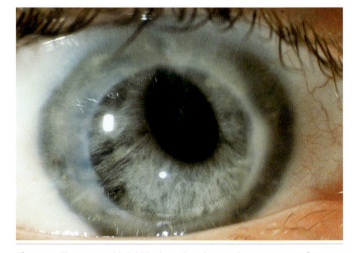

Fig. 66.7 This 5-year-old child had accidental corneal trauma as an infant. Prompt corneal grafting and amblyopia treatment resulted in an acuity of 6/12.

eye is examined carefully for the possibility of a penetrating eye injury and then managed as a corneal abrasion, once the foreign body is gone.

Eye wall injuries

Etiology

Eye wall lacerations can be categorized as either a simple laceration or a rupture, and either anterior laceration or posterior in location.

In simple lacerations, the eye is cut with a sharp object (Figs 66.4–66.7). Very young children usually suffer injury when they fall on a sharp object. Older children may suffer eye wall lacerations from glass (particularly when they wear spectacles), and projectiles.

Predisposition ("brittle corneas")

Certain eyes may be more likely to rupture with relatively minor trauma. In Ehlers-Danlos syndrome, defective collagen cross-linkage leads to scleral and corneal weakness (Fig. 66.8); in Ehlers-Danlos with blue sclera (due to scleral thinning), hyperextensible skin, and hypermobile joints, spontaneous corneal rupture can occur, and in the brittle cornea, blue sclera and joint hyperextensibility syndrome, spontaneous rupture of the globe may occur. Such patients may have red hair and develop keratoglobus, and, unlike Ehlers-Danlos syndrome,

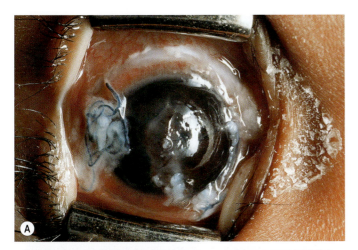

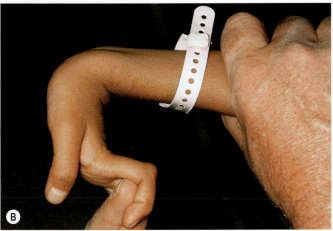

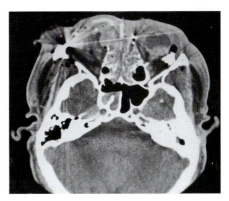

Fig. 66.9 **CT scan showing disrupted right globe following a gunshot wound.** The left eye was also injured from the concussive effect. Note the vitreous hemorrhage.

Fig 66.8 Ehlers-Danlos syndrome. (A) Spontaneous rupture of the cornea. This is an autosomal recessive disease. One of this child's siblings, also affected, had a bilateral corneal rupture at the same time during fisticuffs. (B) Hyperflexible joints.

they have normal levels of lysyl hydroxylase. Osteogenesis imperfecta consists of blue sclera, deafness, and bone fractures. Children with this syndrome may also be more prone to corneal rupture from minor trauma.

Globe rupture

When a globe is ruptured, it is pushed or squeezed so hard that the eye wall breaks under pressure. The results usually are devastating, with partial or complete expulsion of intraocular contents. Expulsion is facilitated due to the increase in intraocular pressure followed by sudden decompression through a hole in the wall of the eye. Events that can cause ruptured globes usually involve encounters with large, blunt objects. In many countries, sporting impacts and automobile crashes (airbag injuries) are major causes of globe rupture in older children.[8] Globe rupture is more common in boys than girls, reflecting the nature of the cause. Eyes are more likely to be ruptured or lacerated in areas where the sclera or cornea are thinnest: under the rectus and superior oblique muscle insertions and the corneoscleral limbus are thin.

Anterior versus posterior laceration

Anterior locations of injuries carry a better prognosis, so long as the injury does not also cut the retina. Injuries anterior to

the pars plana (5 mm posterior to the limbus) will not cut the retina, and therefore carry a better prognosis. If a cataract occurs with an anterior laceration, the prognosis for recovery of vision is not as good.[9] Posterior injuries cut the retina and often result in a complicated retinal detachment, with a far worse prognosis.

Penetrating eye injuries are those in which the causative agent enters the eye but does not pass all the way through. Perforating eye injuries are those that pass through two walls of the eye. The same definition holds true when referring to different parts of the eye. A penetrating corneal injury penetrates the cornea but does not pass all the way through it. A perforating injury passes all the way through the cornea into the anterior chamber or further.

Diagnosis

The diagnosis of penetrating eye injury is obvious when a laceration is apparent. Clues to occult penetration include subconjunctival hemorrhage, distorted pupil, wrinkled lens capsule, and lowered intraocular pressure, particularly compared to pressure in the fellow, uninjured eye, reduced visual acuity, or an afferent pupillary defect.

Management

Prevention

The best form of management for eyeball lacerations is prevention and includes wearing suitable safety glasses or goggles by players who participate in games involving a small ball, and supervision by parents and teachers when sharp objects (fencing, archery, etc.) are used.

The use of safety glasses in monocular children is valuable, especially at times of particular risk.

Treatment

Once the eye laceration or globe rupture is diagnosed, we recommend a protective shield be placed over the eye. Emergency surgery is indicated, but the patient's overall health should not be ignored. The eye laceration may accompany head trauma. We have had the experience of caring for adolescent patients with multiple gunshot wounds, some of which were nearly ignored due to the focus on the eye injury.

Imaging

In many cases, a CT scan of the orbits (Figs 66.9 and 66.10) will help to identify the location of expected or unexpected intraocular foreign bodies, and ultrasound biomicroscopic evaluation also can be helpful to detect zonular deficiency,

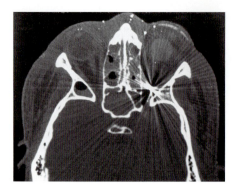

Fig. 66.10 Shotgun injury. CT scanning is particularly helpful in delineating the presence and location of ocular and orbital foreign bodies. This adolescent was shot in the face with a shotgun.

angle recession, iridodialysis, lens dislocation, and irido-corneal adhesions.[10]

Anesthesia

Some advocate avoiding a depolarizing agent for fear that the contraction of extraocular muscles (which initially occurs) could press on the eye and express intraocular contents.

Surgery

With anterior lacerations, prompt closure and re-evaluation of the patient's vision and ocular status in the ensuing several days is advisable. The use of intraocular antibiotics is debatable. The prompt closure of an eye wall laceration would seem to be adequate to greatly reduce the incidence of traumatic endoph-thalmitis. A concurrent traumatic cataract should be removed at the same time as closure of the laceration in young children. Delay in traumatic cataract extraction runs the risk of inducing amblyopia. In older children (>7 years of age), a second opera-tion could be performed and could include intraocular lens implant, so long as the posterior capsule remains largely intact. Although controversial, good results have been reported with combined lensectomy, vitrectomy, and primary intraocular lens implantation as the initial procedure.[11]

Posterior lacerations almost always cut through the retina. Even so, the initial goal of surgery is wound closure. Most authorities do not use cryosurgery or scleral buckling at initial surgery. The trauma alone is enough to cause a retinal scar around a break, and cryosurgery may increase the likelihood of posterior vitreoretinopathy. A posterior vitreous detachment occurs 7–10 days after trauma; after this detachment has taken place, retinal surgery can be undertaken.

Management continues even after successful surgery. Chil-dren under the age of 7 years are at risk for amblyopia. Prompt refractive management with a contact lens over a corneal lac-eration (or spectacles if appropriate), and patching should be started as soon as possible. Corneal sutures in children attract blood vessels and scarring much more quickly than in adults. Sutures may be removed in a few weeks in young children: failure to do this may result in a vascularized cornea, impeding vision.

Prognosis

Anterior lacerations carry a better prognosis than posterior lacerations. But in young children, with the risk of amblyopia, the prognosis may not be good, even with anterior lacerations. When anterior lacerations are combined with cataract, the prognosis worsens. The prognosis is highly dependent upon success in the management of amblyopia.

Traumatic cataracts

Traumatic cataracts can occur as a result of a sharp penetrating injury to the lens capsule and/or lens, or a blunt concussive force. They may take days to years to develop. The diagnosis of traumatic cataracts is based on an abnormality in the red reflex. The cataract problem can be confirmed by examining the lens under magnification, either with loupes or a slit-lamp. In some cases, a Vossius ring may occur, i.e. a ring of pigment forms on the anterior lens capsule as a result of the posterior (pigmented) aspect of the iris striking the capsule. Examina-tion should establish that there are no other ocular injuries.

In partial cataracts, an additional important aspect to the examination is an effort at measuring visual function in the involved eye. In older children this can be done with Snellen acuity. In younger children, an estimate must be made based upon experience with lens clarity and visual functioning. Attempts can be made to measure acuity with forced choice preferential looking techniques, but these may be misleading and probably should not be used as the sole determinant to undertaking surgery.

If there is doubt as to the value of removing a lens with a cataract, then it should be observed. So long as the child is beyond the age when amblyopia can develop, the initial repair of a corneal or scleral laceration can be followed at a later date with removal of the lens. This "wait-and-see" strategy has no deleterious effects on the child other than the necessity for a second general anesthetic.

Children with visually significant traumatic cataracts can have good outcomes if managed appropriately.[12] Surgical man-agement consists of removal of the lens with or without pres-ervation of the posterior capsule. If a lens is removed at the same time that an eye wall laceration is closed, simultaneous lens implant has its advocates. One reason for caution is that the implant could foster survival of bacterial organisms which penetrated the eye as a result of the trauma. Another concerns the choice of power to correct aphakia. In young children, eye growth leads to instability of the refractive power of the eye, making implant power selection problematic.[9] Decisions regarding subsequent implants depend on surgeon preference and the presence or absence of corneal refractive problems. If a child has a significant amount of astigmatism and will require contact lens rehabilitation anyway, then any increased risk of a lens implant can be avoided, since the implant would not avert the need for contact lenses. Contact lenses can be successful in post-traumatic aphakia; rigid gas permeable lenses seem to be most effective if there was a corneal perfora-tion.[13] Combined keratoplasty and lens implantation may have a role in some cases.[14]

A special type of cataract can occur as the result of electrical injury.[15] A characteristic opacity in the posterior aspect of the lens forms as the result of the transmission of electricity to the eye (Fig. 66.11) itself.

Hyphema

An hyphema is a collection of blood in the anterior chamber of the eye and occurs as a result of traumatic avulsion of blood vessels at the base of the iris. Bleeding occurs and then ceases after clot formation or an increase in intraocular pressure. A hyphema may be small enough that it can be identified only with a slit-lamp examination, or it can be so extensive as to fill

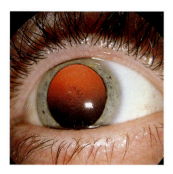

Fig. 66.11 Electric shock. After an electric shock this young man slowly developed a monocular cataract.

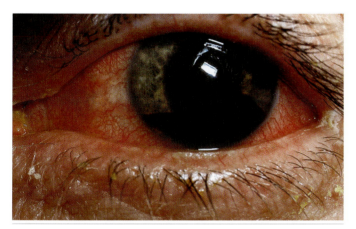

Fig. 66.12 A long-standing hyphema. This is shown by the dark color of the blood in this young man.

the entire anterior chamber with blood ("8-ball hyphema"). In most instances, a superiorly located meniscus develops due to the effects of gravity (Fig. 66.12).

The major cause of hyphema is trauma; it is much more common in boys than in girls[16] but there are other etiologies. Herpes zoster iritis can occasionally cause an hyphema. Spontaneous hyphemas also occur with juvenile xanthogranulomatosis usually in very young children and may or may not be associated with cutaneous lesions. Hyphemas may also occur rarely in association with tumors of the eye, particularly retinoblastoma, but also with iris vascular abnormalities or rubeosis.

In hyphema the clot usually retracts between the third and fifth post-traumatic day, at which point the hyphema may recur. Very small "trickle" hyphemas are less likely to rebleed than larger ones. However, rebleeding cannot be predicted solely on the size of the hyphema if it is visible without magnification. For this reason, most advocate some sort of rest regimen for the child. Whether a child should be hospitalized in order to facilitate resting will certainly depend at least on the child's activity level, the family's ability to supervise the child, and perhaps also on the size of the hyphema.[16] A quick, substantial rise in intraocular pressure (a complication of hyphema) can cause nausea and vomiting, an indication for antiemetics. We use a long-acting cycloplegic agent in order to put the iris and pupil "at rest" and topical steroids if an inflammatory component (iritis) occurs. Systemic steroids or epsilon aminocaproic acid (which blocks fibrinolysis thereby reducing the risk of rebleeding) have been advocated by some. Topical epsilon aminocaproic acid may be effective in reducing rebleeding and is not associated with an increased risk of nausea and vomiting as is the case in its systermic use.[17]

Complications of hyphema are increased intraocular pressure and glaucoma. How much pressure and for how long it can be tolerated safely has not been determined for children. High pressure runs the risk of causing corneal blood staining and optic nerve damage. To prevent these complications, we treat elevated pressure and maintain it below 30 mmHg. Persistent elevation of intraocular pressure is an indication for surgical evacuation of the hyphema. We manage elevated pressure with eye drops such as beta-blockers but avoid acetylcholine agents because they constrict the pupil and may affect fragile blood vessels. We use systemic acetazolamide where necessary.

When a child has sickle cell anemia, the management of glaucoma caused by hyphema is more problematic. The only agent available is a topical beta-blocker, since other agents may either exacerbate the hyphema (e.g. pilocarpine) or lead to sickle cell crisis. Children with sickle cell with an hyphema are candidates for early surgical intervention. We evacuate a clot through a limbal incision. Even in children who do not have sickle cell, but in whom glaucoma remains refractory, surgical evacuation is advisable.

Corneal blood staining occurs when erythrocytes cross the corneal endothelium and Descemet's membrane and stain the cornea when the intraocular pressure is significantly elevated, and when the endothelium is damaged. Corneal blood staining is reversible, but takes several years and may lead to amblyopia.

Months and years later, if the angle of the eye has been traumatized and "recessed," the child may develop "angle recession glaucoma." For that reason, any patient who has had an hyphema probably should have yearly ophthalmology examinations, with intraocular pressure measurements determined.

Posterior segment trauma

Commotio retinae

Commotio retinae, also known as Berlin's edema, frequently occurs after blunt trauma to the front of the eye; in one study it occurred in 35% of cases of contusion or rupture of the globe.[18] The edema, which occurs in the outer retina, has a funduscopic appearance that is white or gray-white. The macula may be involved with or without macular hole formation, in which case central vision will be at least temporarily diminished.[19] Berlin's edema can also involve extramacular areas. In most cases, the edema resolves, but in some cases pigment migration in the macula results in acuity loss. The differential diagnosis consists of retinal infarction, cotton-wool spots, and shallow retinal detachment. No treatment is available for commotio retinae.

Purtscher's retinopathy

Severe trauma to the torso or the head can cause Purtscher's retinopathy. Airbag and seat belt injuries in automobile accidents account for a significant number of cases.[20] Purtscher's disease can be associated with fat or air embolism or pancreatitis.[21] It has the appearance of massive whitening around the optic nerve head associated with hemorrhage. The whitening may represent ischemic areas or exudate. There is no specific treatment for this problem, which may resolve leaving anything from mild to profound vision loss.

Whiplash injury

A macular hole sometimes occurs as a consequence of a severe whiplash injury. Presumably, the head thrusting induces a vitreoretinal interface shearing force which tugs at the fovea and creates a partial or full-thickness hole.

Choroidal rupture

Another complication of blunt injury to the front part of the eye is choroidal rupture, often associated with widespread damage and vitreous hemorrhage (Fig. 66.13). The choroid may be ruptured at the level of the inner choroid and retinal pigment epithelium, and often in the macula. The mechanism is mechanical disruption of tissue. Sometimes the rupture is associated with a serous or hemorrhagic retinal detachment which obscures the nature of the injury. Once the detachment resolves, the patient may be left with diminished vision if there has been scarring or retinal pigment epithelial migration into the area of the macula. Later, choroidal rupture can predispose to choroidal neovascularization, leading to exudate and hemorrhage under the macula, also diminishing vision.

Retinal hemorrhages

Retinal hemorrhages can be caused by direct head or ocular trauma, or by indirect trauma, as in non-accidental trauma (see Chapter 67).

Hemorrhages occur commonly in normal infants in the perinatal period (Fig. 66.14). They usually resolve completely in less than 1 month, occasionally in up to 3 months. Retinal hemorrhages are uncommon in children born by cesarean section.[22] Hemorrhages may occur in any layer of the retina or in the vitreous. Subretinal pigment epithelial hemorrhages appear dark with an amorphous boundary. Intraretinal hemorrhages are red in appearance, usually small and round. Superficial retinal hemorrhages have a splinter appearance because they often occur in the nerve fibre layer. Subhyaloid hemorrhages have a characteristic appearance where blood forms a meniscus in a large cystic filled cavity. Finally, vitreous hemorrhages may also occur in the setting of trauma, and may be localized or diffuse depending on their severity. Preretinal hemorrhages are particularly common in children with subdural or subarachnoid hemorrhages. Since central nervous system (CNS) hemorrhage is frequently caused by trauma in children, a traumatic etiology for preretinal hemorrhages should be suspected.

Prolonged obscuration of vision due to severe vitreous hemorrhage can cause deprivation amblyopia, and is a reason for early vitrectomy, particularly in the first 3–6 months of life.[23]

Traumatic retinal detachment

Blunt trauma to the eye can cause a retinal detachment even if the globe is not cut or ruptured. Typically, the detachment occurs as the result of avulsion of the vitreous base, often in the superonasal quadrant of the eye. Presumably, this location is most vulnerable because a blunt blow to the eye arises from 180° away, in the inferotemporal segment; a blunt object strikes the eye and causes a retinal tear which, days to months later, leads to a retinal detachment.

Self-injury in severely mentally retarded children can also cause retinal detachments by similar mechanisms (see Chapter 124).

In atopy, constant rubbing to relieve itching increases the risk of retinal detachment.

Orbit trauma

Orbital bone fractures

General

Fractures of the orbit frequently involve the eye and demand the involvement of an ophthalmologist.

Blow-out fractures

Blow-out fracture refers to the caving out of one of the orbital bones that surround the eye. In most cases the floor of the orbit is fractured (Fig. 66.15), but the medial wall of the orbit can also be damaged.[24] "Trapdoor" fractures, usually involving the orbital floor, are not uncommon in children. Blow-out fractures are unusual in young children, before the sinuses have formed.

Etiology

Blow-out fractures are caused either by compression of the orbit, increasing the pressure on the orbital contents or by

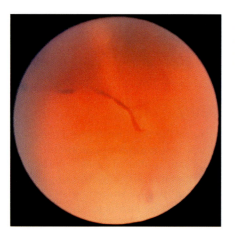

Fig. 66.13 Choroidal rupture. There is a marked vitreous hemorrhage largely obscuring a view of the fundus where a pale organizing clot can barely be made out.

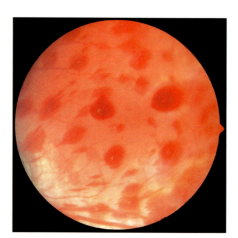

Fig. 66.14 Neonatal retinal hemorrhages in a normal child. (Photograph courtesy of Dr. Andrew Q. McCormick, Vancouver.)

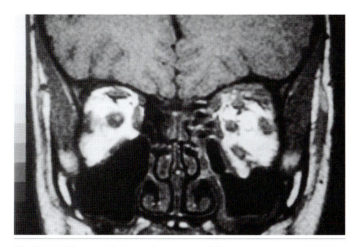

Fig. 66.15 Blow-out fracture. Entrapment of the tissues associated with the inferior rectus in the left orbit.

direct transmission of the force of a blow to the orbital rim, to the bones of the floor, or to the medial wall of the orbit. Experimental injuries to the orbital rim have demonstrated that a posterior orbital floor blow-out fracture can be induced in this fashion.

Complications

Two types of problems can result from a blow-out fracture. Enophthalmos can occur as a result of shifting of intraorbital contents into fractures of the floor or medial wall of the orbit. Enophthalmos may not be apparent immediately after trauma due to edema and swelling but becomes apparent by 5–7 days after injury and should be evaluated then. We manage fractures, if cosmetically significant, by repairing the fracture and replacing orbital contents in order to reconstitute the orbit to its original volume.

A second problem is strabismus, including entrapped or paralysed extraocular muscles, vertical displacement of the globe, Brown's syndrome, and even cranial nerve injury if the force of the blow damage is sufficient. A trapped inferior rectus muscle is the most common cause of strabismus associated with blow-out fracture (Fig. 66.15). The muscle becomes incarcerated in the floor fracture and tethers the eye in a hypotropic position. Most patients experience vertical diplopia, worsening in upgaze.

Traumatic optic neuropathy (see Chapter 53)

Etiology

Traumatic optic neuropathy occurs when head or facial trauma causes direct or indirect injury to the optic nerve. In children it is most commonly associated with motor vehicle accidents or sports injuries.[25] The result is unilateral or bilateral, partial or complete, loss of vision. Frontal bone trauma, occasionally even subtle and apparently insignificant, is most likely to result in optic nerve injury.

One special circumstance bears mentioning. Patients with severe psychiatric disturbances may attempt to enucleate their own eye and in the process sever the optic nerve at some point in its approach to the globe (see Chapter 124). If the severance is posterior near the chiasm, a unilateral blindness may be accompanied by a temporal hemianopia in the fellow eye due to chiasmal damage.[26] Patients who attempt to remove their own eye often experience temporary relief of their psychiatric symptoms if successful; a resurgence of symptoms may lead them to attempt to enucleate their other eye. Such patients should be guarded very closely and their psychotic symptoms should be managed aggressively.

Diagnosis and treatment

The examiner often must rely on signs of unilateral afferent visual dysfunction (afferent pupil defect, diminished color vision, decreased visual acuity). Unfortunately, many patients who experience such trauma may not be able to cooperate with a physical examination. We use high-dose steroids using methylprednisolone at a dose of 30 mg/kg as an intravenous bolus to treat traumatic optic neuropathy. A second option involves surgical intervention. Indications include optic sheath hemorrhage, orbital hemorrhage (focal, diffuse, or subperiosteal), and an optic canal fracture causing compression of the optic nerve. However, there is no convincing evidence that routine medical or surgical treatment alters the long-term visual outcome of patients with traumatic optic neuropathy.[25]

Traumatic retrobulbar hemorrhage

Trauma to the eye or orbit will occasionally cause orbital hemorrhage. Hemorrhage may be the result of blunt trauma, in which case shearing forces on retrobulbar veins or arteries are suspected. Sharp objects can also penetrate behind the eye without actually injuring the globe itself, and may lacerate blood vessels. The affected person will have pain with signs of a rapidly increasing retrobulbar mass: proptosis, an increase in intraocular pressure, chemosis, and diminished eye movements.

Trauma is not the only cause of these retro-orbital signs. Slowly progressive signs may indicate Graves' disease, and conditions such as orbital cellulitis and traumatic carotid-cavernous fistula can also present similarly. Cellulitis may be diagnosed when other signs of infection are present (redness, heat in the area, considerable pain). CT scan usually demonstrates sinusitis extending into the retro-orbital space, and the patient may have fever and leukocytosis. Carotid-cavernous fistula is suspected when there is pulsating exophthalmos and vessels which appear arterialized in the conjunctiva and retina.

Traumatic retrobulbar hemorrhage occasionally is an ophthalmic emergency.[26] When the intraocular pressure is elevated and affecting optic nerve function the pressure must be lowered immediately. We lower intraocular pressure with carbonic anhydrase inhibitors (acetazolamide) and hyperosmotic agents. A lateral canthotomy and inferior cantholysis can relieve retrobulbar pressure almost immediately. We seldom use aqueous paracentesis because it has only a short-term benefit and exposes the patient to the risk of cataract or intraocular infection.

Central nervous system trauma
(see Chapter 56)

Prolonged cortical visual impairment following trauma

Many possible mechanisms can account for prolonged cortical visual impairment after head trauma.[27] A seizure could lead to cortical impaired vision. A cerebral contusion could result in generalized cerebral edema, causing either transient or prolonged cortical visual impairment. Increased cerebral edema can compress the posterior cerebral arteries leading to vascular insufficiency to the visual cortex. CNS hypoxic ischemia could be a sequel to either generalized trauma with blood loss or CNS vasospasm. The occipital region is quite susceptible to hypoxia and may be selectively involved (see Chapter 56).

Post-traumatic transient cortical visual impairment

Cortical visual impairment can be defined as complete, or nearly complete, loss of vision with normal pupillary reflexes, and a normal fundus examination. Cortical visual impairment in children may differ in its manifestations from cortical blindness in adults. Children show fluctuating vision, a preference for observing color (versus black and white), light gazing, and, occasionally, photophobia. A relatively minor blow to the head can cause transient cortical blindness.

Traumatic cranial neuropathy (see Chapter 83)

Thirteen percent of non-fatal head injuries result in cranial neuropathy. The sixth cranial nerve is most commonly traumatized and the most common cause of multiple acquired cranial nerve palsies is trauma.[28] Most cases occur between the ages of 16 and 25 years but even very young children can be affected.

Diagnosis

In sixth nerve palsy, difficulty or inability to abduct the involved eye is noted. The patient demonstrates a large angle esotropia in primary gaze greater for distance than near; they can be bilateral.

Complete third nerve palsies cause dilated pupil, complete ptosis, and inability to abduct, depress or elevate the eye. The resulting eye position is one of exotropia and slight hypotropia. Partial third nerve palsies may occur.

Traumatic fourth nerve palsies may be unilateral or bilateral. Unilateral cases typically show a hypertropia in primary gaze with inferior oblique overaction. Patients may demonstrate excyclotorsion of the eye, and cyclotorsional double vision up to 8°. Bilateral fourth nerve palsies occur in as many as 30% of cases. Bilaterality is suggested by the following physical findings:

- A "V" pattern esotropia greater than 25 prism diopters.
- Alternating hyperdeviation (right hypertropia on right head tilt, and left hypertropia on left head tilt).
- An excyclotorsion in primary gaze which exceeds 15°.

Management

We observe cranial nerve function, since in about 40% of cases it may resolve. Neuroimaging is indicated when a cranial neuropathy is present, particularly when the trauma is slight and would not normally be expected to cause a nerve palsy: tumors present in this way. MRI is probably more sensitive in detecting subtle intraparenchymal lesions or hemorrhages. After 6 months we consider surgical management.

Disorders following concussion

A surprising number of patients will complain of trouble focusing their eyes following head trauma.[29] Other

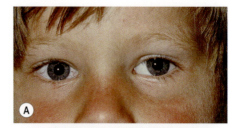
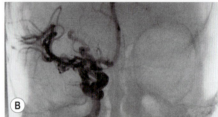
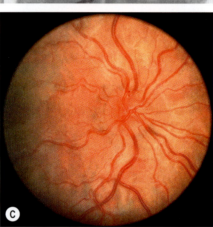
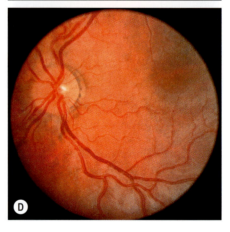

Fig. 66.16 Severe trauma. (A) This 5.5-year-old boy developed right proptosis and a squeaky bruit a week after a severe road traffic accident. (B) Carotid angiogram showing the shunt which was later closed with a balloon catheter. Dilated episcleral veins can be seen on the right. Retinal venous congestion and tortuosity with optic disk edema on the right (C,D).

concussive symptoms include photophobia and convergence insufficiency.

Carotid-cavernous fistulas are rare in children but may occur following severe trauma[30] (Fig. 66.16).

References

1. Morris R, Witherspoon CD, Kuhn F, et al. Epidemiology of Pediatric Injuries from the Injury Registry of Alabama (ERA). Presented at the First International Symposium of Ophthalmology. Bordeaux, France, 9–11 September, 1993.
2. LaRoche GR, McIntyre L, Schertzer RN. Epidemiology of severe eye injuries in childhood. Ophthalmology 1988; 95: 1603–7.

3. Takvam JA, Midelfart A. Survey of eye injuries in Norwegian children. Acta Ophthalmol (Copen) 1993; 71: 500–5.

4. Jethani J, Vijayalaksmi. Eye safety and prevention of visual disability in the paediatric age group. Commun Eye Health J 2005; 18: 58–60.

5. Baxter RJ, Hodgkins PR, Calder I, et al. Visual outcome of childhood anterior perforating eye injuries: prognostic indicators. Eye 1994; 8: 349–52.

6. Naylor G, Roper JP, Willshaw HE. Ophthalmic complications of amniocentesis. Eye 1990; 4: 845–9.

7. Jordan DR, Setareh Z, Gilberg S, Mawn L. Pathogenesis of canalacular lacerations. Ophthalmic Plast Reconstr Surg 2008; 24: 394–8.

8. Kennedy EA, Ng TG, McNally C, et al. Risk factors for human and porcine eye rupture based on projectile characteristics of blunt objects. Stapp Car Crash J 2006; 50: 651–71.

9. Crouch ER, Crouch ER, Jr, Pressman SH. Prospective analysis of pediatric pseudophakia: myopic shift and postoperative outcomes. J AAPOS 2002: 6: 277–82

10. Ozdal MPC, Mansour M, Deschenes J. Ulrasound biomicroscopic evaluation of traumatized eyes. Eye 2003; 17: 467–72.

11. Assi A, Bou C, Cherfan G. Combined lensectomy, vitrectomy, and primary intraocular lens implantation in patients with traumatic eye injury. Int Ophthalmol 2008; 28: 387–94.

12. Reddy A, Ray R, Yen KG. Surgical intervention for traumatic cataracts in children: epidemiology, complications, and outcomes. J AAPOS 2009; 13: 170–4.

13. Titiyal JS, Sinha R, Sharma N, et al. Contact lens rehabilitation following repaired corneal perforations. BMC Ophthalmol 2006; 6: 11–5.

14. Vajpayee RB, Angra SK, Honavour SG. Combined keratoplasty, cataract extraction, and intraocular lens implantation after corneolenticular laceration in children. Am J Ophthalmol 1994; 117: 507–11.

15. Grewal DS, Jain R, Brar GS, Grewal PS. Unilateral electric cataract: Scheimpflug imaging and review of the literature. J Cataract Refract Surg 2007; 33: 1116–19.

16. Rocha KM, Martins EN, Melo LAS, Bueno de Moraes NS. Outpatient management of traumatic hyphema: prospective evaluation. J AAPOS 2004; 8: 357–61.

17. Pieramici DJ, Goldberg MF, Melia M, et al. A phase III, multicenter, randomized, placebo-controlled trial of topical aminocaproic acid (Caprogel) in the management of traumatic hyphema. Ophthalmology 2003; 110: 2106–12.

18. Viestenz A, Kuchie M. [Retrospective analysis of 417 cases of contusion and rupture of the globe with frequent avoidable causes of trauma: Erlangen Ocular Contusion-Registry (EOCR) 1985–1995.] Klin Monatsbl Augenheilkd 2001; 218: 662–9.

19. Youssri A, Young L. Closed-globe contusion injuries of the posterior segment. Int Ophthalmol Clin 2002; 42: 79–86.

20. Shah GK, Penne R, Grand GM. Purtscher's retinopathy secondary to airbag injury. Retina 2001; 21: 68–9.

21. Agrawal A, McKibben M. Purtscher's retinopathy: epidemiology, clinical features and outcome. Br J Ophthalmol 2007; 91: 1445–9.

22. Emerson MV, Pieramici DJ, Stoessel KM, et al. Incidence and rate of disappearance of retinal hemorrhage in the newborn. Ophthalmology 2001; 106: 36–9.

23. Spirin MJ, Lynn MJ, Hubbard GB. Vitreous hemorrhage in children. Ophthalmology 2006; 113: 848–52.

24. Bansagi ZC, Meyer DR. Internal orbital fractures in the pediatric age group: characterization and management. Ophthalmology 2000; 107: 829–36.

25. Goldberg-Cohen N, Miller NR, Repka MX. Traumatic optic neuropathy in children and adolescents. J AAPOS 2004; 8: 20–7.

26. Krauss HR, Yee RD, Foos RY. Autoenucleation. Surv Ophthalmol 1984; 29: 179–87.

27. Poggi G, Calori G, Mancarella G, et al. Visual disorders after traumatic brain injury in developmental age. Brain Injury 2000; 14: 833–45.

28. Holmes JM, Mutyala S, Maus T, et al. Pediatric third, fourth, and sixth nerve palsies: a population-based study. Am J Ophthalmol 1999; 127: 388–92.

29. Ryan LM, Warden DL. Post concussion syndrome. Int Rev Psychiatry 2003; 15: 310–16.

30. Chamoun RB, Jea A. Traumatic intracranial and extracranial vascular injuries in children. Neurosurg Clin North Am 2010; 21: 529–42.

Child maltreatment, abusive head injury and the eye

Patrick Watts

Definitions

- Child maltreatment covers both child abuse and neglect.[1]
- Child maltreatment is defined as any act, or series of acts, of commission or omission by a parent or caregiver that results in harm, potential harm, or threat of harm to a child (Box 67.1).

Epidemiology

Child maltreatment is common with a total of 581 911 cases reported in the year ending March 2008 in England[2] and Wales.[3] In the USA 1 in 58 children suffers from maltreatment.[4] Child maltreatment is often missed or unrecognized and the figures presented may underestimate the problem.

Neglect in various forms is the most common type of child maltreatment (71% in the USA, 41% in Scotland) followed by

---

Box 67.1

Classification of child maltreatment

Child abuse includes acts of commission (words or overt actions) and can be classified as:

- Physical abuse
- Sexual abuse
- Psychological abuse
- Fabricated or induced illness

Child neglect includes acts of omission and can be classified as:

- Failure to provide: physical, emotional, educational, medical/dental neglect
- Failure to supervise: inadequate supervision, exposure to violent environments

---

physical abuse (33% Scotland, 16% USA), sexual abuse (9% USA, 13% Scotland), and emotional abuse (7% USA, 13% Scotland).

The incidence of severe physical abuse is highest (54/100 000) in infants less than a year old and less in older children (9.2/100 000 in children 1–4 years old and 0.47/100 000 in children 5–13 years).[5]

Ophthalmological features are commonly associated with abusive head injury which represent 1.8% of physical abuse.[6] The incidence of abusive head injury varies between 14.2/100 000 and 33.8/100 000 infants in the UK, and is commonest in infants less than 6 months of age.[7,8] Abusive head trauma accounts for the majority of fatal or life-threatening injuries due to abuse in infants.[5]

Risk factors for child maltreatment

The risk factors for child maltreatment include social, family, and community factors. Perpetrators may be those who are responsible for the care and supervision of their victims. Parents either acting alone, or with another person, account for 71% of abuse of children in their care. Though there is no single profile that fits all perpetrators, a number of common characteristics are reported in many studies (Box 67.2).

Presentation of child abuse victims to the ophthalmologist

In the majority of cases the child is referred to the ophthalmologist by pediatricians who suspect an abusive injury. However, it is incumbent on the ophthalmologist to not only recognize cases that occasionally present to them with bruising or unexplained injury who may be maltreated, but to also refer

Box 67.2

Risk factors for child maltreatment

Perpetrator individual risk factors
- Poor parenting skills, lack of understanding of child's needs and development
- Family or parental history of abuse
- Mental health problems, depression, and history of substance abuse
- Young age, low income, single parents
- Mother's boyfriend
- Maltreatment not considered abusive and justified

Children at risk
- Premature babies
- Crying babies
- Siblings of abused children
- Children of previously abused parents
- Handicapped or children with learning difficulties

Family risk factors
- Social isolation
- Broken homes, overcrowding, and domestic violence
- Stress, poor parental bonding

Community risk factors
- Violent neighborhood
- Poverty and unemployment

them on for multiagency assessment of possible abuse or neglect.[9]

The presenting features alerting the professional to child maltreatment include:

a. Physical signs of unusual bruising in non-mobile infants for which there is no explanation (Fig. 67.1). Bruising in non independently mobile infants is very rare (<1%)[10] and bruising that is periocular in infants should be investigated when there is no verifiable explanation. Other signs include bites, burns, and scalds; ligature or strangulation marks and abrasions may accompany a story without a plausible explanation.

b. Anogenital injuries and sexually transmitted diseases in children point to sexual abuse.

c. Clinical presentations include an apparent life-threatening event (where the child presents floppy and apneic), seizures, ingestion of poisonous substances, nasal bleeding, near drowning, and unusual or poor attendance at medical services or school due to ill health.

d. An unkempt child with infestations or tooth decay may signify neglect.

e. Behavioral signs include sexualized behavior, "frozen watchfulness" of a withdrawn child, overt hostility or friendliness of the carers, and a child who acts aggressively.

Protocols for referral to an ophthalmologist vary in different institutes, but are usually governed by the signs and clinical presentations detailed above.

Management

Clinical presentation to an ophthalmologist may be either:

1. The child is referred as part of a multidisciplinary assessment where abusive head injury is suspected.

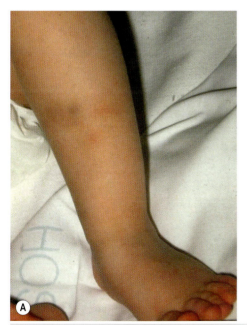 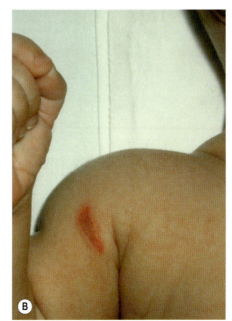 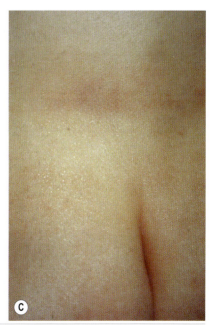

Fig. 67.1 Bruises on the left shin (A), right arm (B), and small of the back (C) in a non-independently mobile infant are suggestive of inflicted injury.

2. An ophthalmologist suspects maltreatment during a consultation for the presenting complaint or presentation of an unkempt dirty child or an unusual injury or pattern of bruising is noticed without an innocent explanation. The ophthalmologist has the duty of care to safeguard the rights of the child by referral to the named child protection lead doctor or a named child protection nurse. This may initiate a multiagency assessment to confirm or rule out maltreatment. Contact details of the child protection team are kept in a prominent and accessible place.

Clinical records

This should contain a detailed history, supplementing information recorded by other medical personnel and a thorough clinical examination. Local protocols for child protection records vary; however, completion of a standardized ophthalmology clinical record supplemented with wide field retinal photography (i.e. Retcam 130) improves documentation, which is helpful when giving evidence in family or criminal courts[11,12] (Fig. 67.2).

There are a number of ways of describing the distribution, location, and types of retinal hemorrhages. Their use in routine clinical practice, however, has not been evaluated.[13,14] Recent systematic reviews of retinal hemorrhages in abusive injury identified the need for consistent and standardized description of retinal findings that would hold under scrutiny in medico-legal cases and help with future research in differentiating patterns of retinal hemorrhages from various causes.

Fluorescein angiography and optical coherence tomography help demonstrate retinal perfusion and vitreo-retinal

RECORDING OF OPHTHAMOLOGICAL FEATURES IN SUSPECTED ABUSE

HISTORY
Continue on reverse

PATIENT DETAILS

Visual Acuity	Right eye	Left eye

SUBCONJUNCTIVAL HEMORRHAGES			
Right eye		Left eye	
Yes	No	Yes	No

ANTERIOR SEGMENT	
Right eye	Left eye

OCULAR MOTILITY
Right eye ☐☐☐ ☐☐☐ Left eye ☐☐☐ ☐☐☐

Pupil size and Pupillary reflexes

Pupils dilated with

PERIOCULAR BRUISING: (mark areas of bruising)

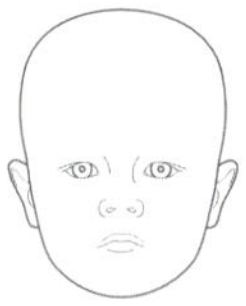

FUNDUS Circle multiple if present	Right eye				Left eye			
Retinal Hemorrhages	Yes		No		Yes		No	
NUMBER. of Retinal hemorrhage	Few (0-10)	Many (10-20)	Too numerous to count		Few (0-10)	Many (10-20)	Too numerous to count	
LOCATION of retinal hemorrhages	Pre retinal	Intraretinal	Subretinal	Multilayered	Pre retinal	Intraretinal	Subretinal	Multilayered
DISTRIBUTION of retinal hemorrhages	Posterior Pole Few/many/ too numerous to count (Zone 1 - ROP classification)		Periphery Few/many/ too numerous to count (outside Zone1)		Posterior Pole Few/many/ too numerous to count (Zone 1 - ROP classification)		Periphery Few/many/ too numerous to count (outside Zone1)	
SIZE of retinal hemorrhages	Small (<1dd)	Medium 1-2dd	Large >2dd		Small (<1dd)	Medium 1-2dd	Large >2dd	
MORPHOLOGY of hemorrhages White centered or other								
Macula Retinoschisis								
Perimacular folds								
Optic disc								
OTHER findings								

Name and signature

Date and time of examination

Fundus examined with
Indirect ophthalmoscope (and 20d / 28d / 30d / 2.2d)
Retcam images ☐
Photography ☐
OCT ☐

Fig. 67.2 Ophthalmology clinical record in suspected abusive head injury.

interface pathology, but their use is yet to be established in practice.[15,16]

Each page of the clinical record should be identified with the child's name and date of birth. The entry should include the clinician's name, designation, signature, date, and time of examination. It should include a differential diagnosis, suggesting appropriate further investigations. A standard list of investigations in suspected abusive head injury has been suggested along with a multidisciplinary assessment involving medical teams, social services, and the police.[17]

A date for a follow-up examination should be clearly indicated on the clinical record.

History

It is often the case that the ophthalmologist is reliant on the history taken by other health care professionals as the carers of the child may not be present at the time. When present, the history of the presenting condition should be confirmed and whether any prior eye disease (e.g. retinopathy of prematurity) or visual concern had been expressed about the child prior to presentation. A family history of an eye disease or a bleeding disorder should be ruled out.

In abusive head injury the history may not be consistent when taken by a number of health care professionals. The injury sustained may be incompatible with the explanation given.

Examination

- External eye examination should include descriptions, drawings, and photography of any periocular injury or subconjunctival hemorrhages.
- If the condition of the child permits, assessment of visual acuity and ocular motility should be noted.
- An assessment of the pupillary reactions, anterior chamber, and lens position should be undertaken before the pupils are dilated for assessment of the fundus. Poor pupillary responses are strongly associated with increased mortality and poor visual outcomes.[18]
- Examination of the retina with an indirect ophthalmoscope and a wide field lens following dilation of the pupils with short-acting mydriatics (phenylephrine 2.5% and tropicamide 1%) is standard practice. Pupillary dilation affects neurological observations and should only be undertaken following discussion with the physicians under whose care the child is admitted. Descriptions of retinal findings should include their distribution, location in terms of the retinal layers, morphology, and severity in terms of number and size.

Medico-legal issues[19]

These issues may vary with different legal systems; however, the underlying principle concerning the welfare of the child remains the same.

The case considered may be subject to:

1. Care proceedings in a civil or family court: a verdict reached by the court based on the "balance of probability."

2. Criminal court proceedings: a verdict is reached when it satisfies the statement of "beyond reasonable doubt."

Expert witness

When writing a report or giving expert evidence as a witness it must be remembered that the expert's duty is to the court and not to any side or to the lawyers who commissioned the report. Common threads of enquiry include the causes of positive findings, the differential diagnosis, the forces required to produce the injuries sustained, the mechanisms of injury, the timing of injury, and the role of confounding issues such as seizures, cardiopulmonary resuscitation (CPR), apparent life-threatening events, and coughing, which frequently coexist in a child with traumatic brain injury. The report should take into account all material sent to the witness and should be well researched. A summary of publications addressing pertinent issues is often useful in providing a balanced view of the literature.[20,21]

The court will look for clarity in presentation and conclusions. The following issues are required by the court in any expert report:[19]

1. Issues it has asked the expert to address.
2. The material the expert has considered.
3. The conclusions reached.
4. Reasons for reaching these conclusions.

Evaluation of child maltreatment literature

Ophthalmology literature frequently lacks strict definitions of abuse. This introduces circular reasoning where the certainty of the findings being truly due to abusive injury cannot be confirmed. Evaluation of the literature should be supported by the use of a ranking system of various levels of certainty of abuse based on criminal or family court proceedings, perpetrator confessions, multidisciplinary team assessments, and defined clinical criteria. The various levels of certainty of child abuse may be defined as definite, probable, or possible, or ranked 1 to 5 where rank 1 represents the highest level of certainty and 5 the least[22,23] (Table 67.1). This does not eliminate circularity, but makes it less likely if cases of "definite" or a high ranking (1 or 2) abuse represent the cases of the studies we need to rely on.

Table 67.1 – Ranking of abusive injury

Ranking	Criteria used to define abuse[23]
1	Abuse confirmed at case conference *or* civil *or* criminal court proceedings *or* admitted by perpetrator *or* independently witnessed
2	Abuse confirmed by stated criteria including multidisciplinary assessment (social services/law enforcement/medical)
3	Abuse defined by stated criteria
4	Abuse stated but no supporting detail given
5	Suspected abuse

Ophthalmic features of physical abuse

Direct injury

Early literature suggested that direct injury to the eye and orbit may manifest with periocular swelling and bruising (Fig. 67.3), burns, lid lacerations, hyphema, cataracts, retinal dialysis, and retinal detachments.[24,25]

Indirect injury

A number of synonyms have been used to describe the presence of intraocular injury associated with brain and skeletal injury. These include whiplash syndrome, battered baby syndrome, shaken baby syndrome, and shaken impact syndrome. Abusive head trauma (AHT) or injury is the currently accepted terminology as the previous names suggest a mechanism, which may or may not be established.

1. Subconjunctival hemorrhages. These may be present in AHT with or without intraocular injury.[26] The presence of subconjunctival hemorrhages in cases of suspected child abuse should prompt a full child protection and ophthalmology assessment (Fig. 67.4).

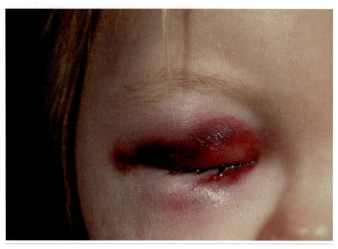

Fig. 67.3 Periocular bruising in a child with direct abusive orbital injury.

2. Retinal hemorrhages. The presence of retinal hemorrhages is not necessary to establish the diagnosis of AHT though they are highly suggestive. There is no pathognomic type (flame shaped, dome shaped, dot, blot, white-centered), size, distribution, or location of retinal hemorrhages seen exclusively in abusive head injury[27] (Fig. 67.5). Bilateral hemorrhages are reported in 74% of cases (sensitivity of 75% and specificity of 94%) of abusive head injury.[28]

   Retinal hemorrhages in the presence of head injury have a 71% positive predictive rate of abusive injury[29] (Fig. 67.6). The prevalence of retinal hemorrhages in AHT varies between 77% and 83%.[18] Preretinal hemorrhages, dome-shaped hemorrhages, situated in the posterior pole are seen commonly in AHT[27] (Fig. 67.7). Retinal hemorrhages may range from a few scattered hemorrhages to widespread hemorrhages extending from the posterior pole to the periphery and situated in multiple layers of the retina[30] (Fig. 67.8). Extensive retinal hemorrhages correlate with severe intracranial injury and poor visual outcome.[31] A recent systematic review reported that in the presence of head injury retinal hemorrhages have a 91% probability of abusive etiology (odds ratio 14.7).[32]

3. Retinal folds. Perimacular folds, an important sign, are seen in 6% to 8% of live AHT cases (Fig. 67.9) and 23% of postmortem cases[18,28,33] (Fig. 67.10). There are also isolated case reports in Terson's syndrome in adult patients[34] and accidental head injury.[35-38]

4. Retinoschisis. Cystic intraretinal cavities (Fig. 67.11) in the macular area are recognized by vessels coursing over the surface or an electronegative electroretinogram. Schisis cavities are seen in 14% to 23% of case studies involving live and postmortem findings. It has been stated that traumatic hemorrhagic macular schisis in not seen in any other condition except AHT;[39] however, recent case reports suggest similar cavities are seen with severe trauma or crush injury.[37,38]

5. Vitreous hemorrhage. Hemorrhage in the vitreous occurs in 14% of cases and is more frequent in autopsy specimens.[18] It is believed to occur with break-through of the dome shaped preretinal hemorrhages into the

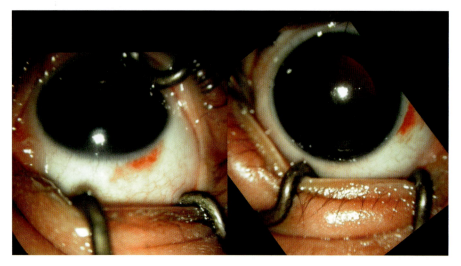

Fig. 67.4 Bilateral subconjunctival hemorrhage in an infant with abusive head injury.

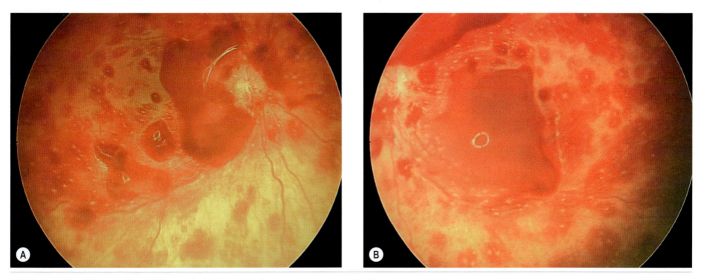

Fig. 67.5 Retinal hemorrhage. Bilateral (A, right eye; B, left eye) multilayered retinal hemorrhages in the posterior pole and periphery in a 3-month-old child with abusive head injury who presented with an apneic episode during feeding.

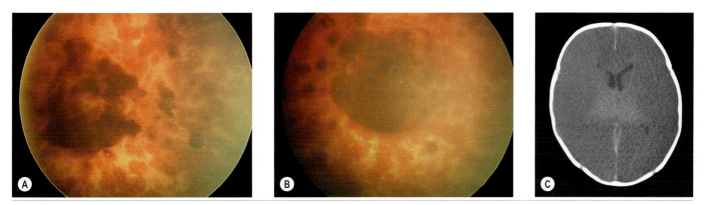

Fig. 67.6 Retinal hemorrhage. Extensive retinal hemorrhages in abusive head trauma in the right (A) and left (B) eye in a 2-month-old infant who was previously well presented with opisthotonus and seizures. The CT scan (C) showed widespread edema, loss of gray–white matter differentiation, and interhemispheric blood. (Courtesy of Dr. A. Liu.)

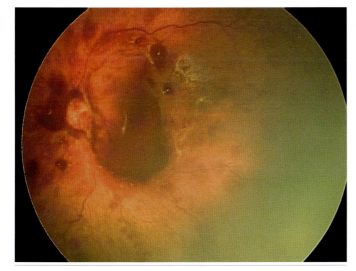

Fig. 67.7 Retinal hemorrhage. Unilateral dome-shaped retinal hemorrhages in the left eye of a 6-month-old infant who presented with an apparent life-threatening event.

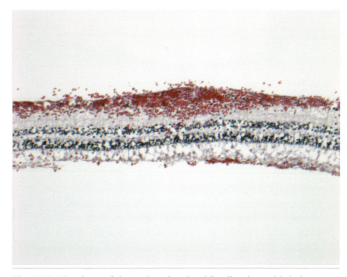

Fig. 67.8 Histology of the retina showing bleeding in multiple layers. (Courtesy of Dr. R. Bonsek.)

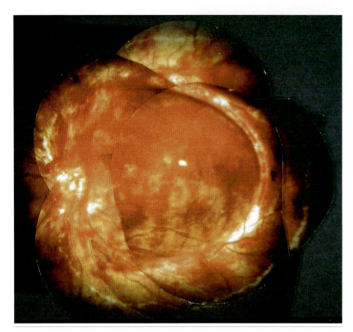

Fig. 67.9 Photomontage of a child with abusive head trauma showing a perimacular retinal fold with extensive retinal hemorrhages.

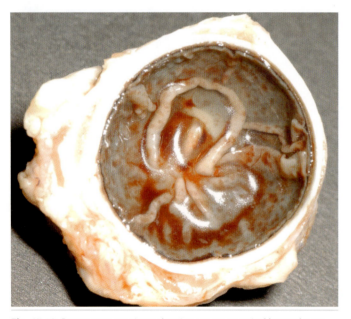

Fig. 67.10 Postmortem specimen showing numerous retinal hemorrhages and postmortem retinal folds.

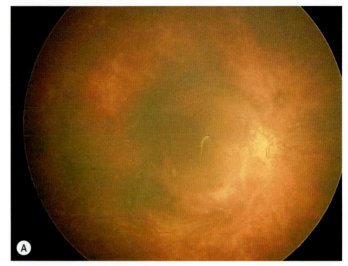

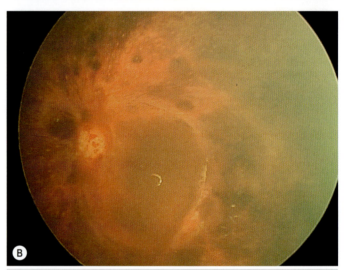

Fig. 67.11 Schisis cavities in the posterior pole in the right (A) and left (B) eye with extensive retinal hemorrhages.

vitreous cavity (Fig. 67.12). Vitreous hemorrhages carry a poor prognosis for visual recovery as they are frequently associated with cerebral visual impairment. Surgery to remove a non-clearing vitreous hemorrhage brings minimal visual improvement.[40]

6. Optic disc edema. This is rare in clinical reports of abused children as the severity of retinal hemorrhages frequently prevents a clear evaluation of the disc. Histopathologically, optic disc swelling is common in postmortem studies.[41] Delayed papilledema in abusive head injury has been reported in a case that developed systemic hypertension and another that developed hydrocephalus weeks after the initial presentation.[42]

7. Orbital and optic nerve sheath hemorrhage. Hemorrhages have been demonstrated in the optic nerve sheath (Fig. 67.13), the orbital fat, the extraocular muscles, and ocular motor nerve sheaths (Fig. 67.14). These findings have not been seen in non-AHT.[41,43]

8. Cranial nerve palsies. The development of acute third, fourth, and sixth cranial nerve palsies as a result of intracranial injury has been reported in abusive head injury.[18]

Ophthalmology outcome on follow-up of abusive head injury

1. Visual acuity. The prognosis for visual acuity is poor for those with severe hemorrhagic retinopathy, vitreous hemorrhage, and poor pupillary responses. Fifty percent of those followed up have severe visual impairment due to retinal scarring, optic atrophy, or cerebral visual impairment.[18]

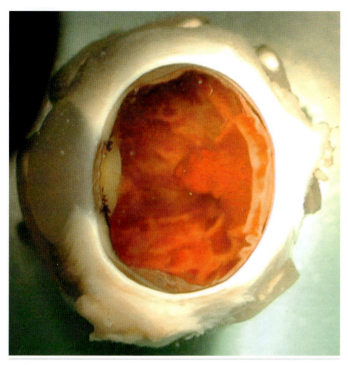

Fig. 67.12 Postmortem specimen of a child with abusive head injury demonstrating retinal blood extending into the vitreous and Cloquet's canal. (Courtesy of Dr. R. Bonsek.)

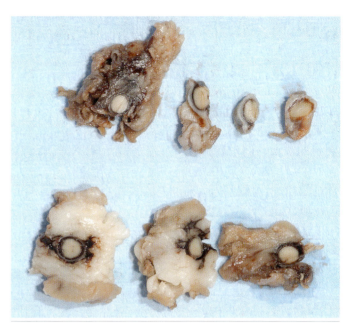

Fig. 67.14 Cross-section of the orbit from behind the globe showing optic nerve, orbital fat, and extraocular muscle hemorrhage.

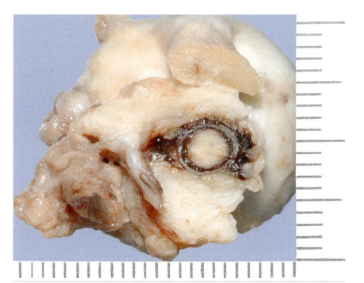

Fig. 67.13 Cross-section of optic nerve behind the globe showing intra-sheath hemorrhage.

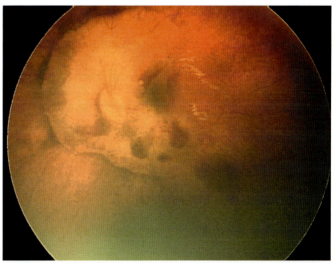

Fig. 67.15 Retinal folds and scarring with residual vitreous and retinal hemorrhage seen 3 months after absorption of extensive retinal and vitreous hemorrhage.

Differential diagnosis of retinal hemorrhages

With unexplained retinal hemorrhages in an infant or young child, an ophthalmologist involved in suspected child abuse cases should be aware of the causes of retinal hemorrhages that may have overlapping features of AHT. To safeguard the child suspected of abusive injury and prevent wrongful conviction it is vital that all relevant etiologies are considered and eliminated clinically or through investigation by the child protection team. This includes conditions that are used by defense teams to explain the retinal findings.

2. Ocular motility. This may be impaired due to nystagmus, nerve palsies, or secondary strabismus due to visual loss.

3. Retina and optic nerve. Macular holes, epiretinal membranes, giant retinal tears, retinal detachment, optic atrophy, neovascularization of the disc, retinal scarring, and choroidal atrophy have been observed after the retinal hemorrhages have cleared[44-46] (Fig. 67.15).

Clinical entities or disease states

1. Birth-related hemorrhages. Retinal hemorrhages are seen in 30% of normal vaginal deliveries, 50% of vacuum-assisted deliveries, and 6% of cesarean sections. Prolonged second stage of labor correlates with an increasing frequency of retinal hemorrhages. They are usually intraretinal, situated in the posterior pole, and may be unilateral or bilateral. They may be flame shaped or dot or blot in shape. The majority resolve completely within 2 weeks of birth[47,48] (Fig. 67.16). Macular retinal hemorrhages may persist for 4 to 5 weeks. An exceptional case of intraretinal hemorrhage persisting for 58 days has been reported.[48]

2. Accidental trauma. There is no pattern of retinal hemorrhages that consistently suggests accidental injury. The hemorrhages tend to be unilateral, few in number, and limited to the posterior pole.[49-54] Retinal hemorrhages have been reported in 5% of accidental injuries where the predominant mode of injury were falls involving a height of less than 4 feet.[32] Retinal folds and retinoschisis are rare in accidental injury: there are single case reports of a crush injury and a fall.[35-38]

3. Metabolic disorders[55,56]
   - (a) Galactosemia
   - (b) Glutaric aciduria
   - (c) Methylmalonic aciduria

4. Bony disorders[57]
   - (a) Osteogenesis imperfecta

5. Bleeding disorders
   - (a) Leukemia
   - (b) Anemia
   - (c) Thrombocytopenia
   - (d) Protein C deficiency
   - (e) Hemorrhagic disease of newborn
   - (f) Platelet dysfunction in Hermansky-Pudlak syndrome
   - (g) Low fibrinogen levels

6. Vascular disorders[42,58]
   - (a) Intracranial aneurysms with Terson's syndrome
   - (b) Fibromuscular dysplasia
   - (c) Hypertension
   - (d) Spinal cord arteriovenous malformations

7. Infections/infestations[59-61]
   - (a) Meningitis
   - (b) Malaria

8. Carbon monoxide poisoning

A recent systematic review reported a group of nine conditions that have overlapping features with abusive injury[62] (Table 67.2).

Pre-existing eye disease

Retinal hemorrhages have been described in the vascularized retina of retinopathy of prematurity, following CPR, and in a premature infant following a screening examination with a contact retina camera. Hence, due consideration to pre-existing retinal disease should be given when evaluating infants with retinal hemorrhages.

Confounding conditions

Children who have sustained AHT frequently present either collapsed with apnea (apparent life-threatening event) and require CPR, or with an encephalopathy or seizures. In addition they may have acute coagulation abnormalities that resolve over a period of a few days. These events are often proposed in court as explanations for retinal hemorrhages introducing uncertainty in the diagnosis of abusive head injury.

1. Apparent life-threatening event.[63]
2. Prolonged coughing.
   Studies of apparent life-threatening events or prolonged coughing have not reported retinal hemorrhages.
3. Seizures. Retinal hemorrhages are rarely reported with seizures. One study revealed 2 of 218 cases with retinal hemorrhages, one case with tonic–clonic seizures for 5 minutes had unilateral hemorrhages around the disc, and the second case with hyponatremia had multiple bilateral hemorrhages in the posterior pole.[64-66]
4. Cardiopulmonary resuscitation (CPR). A well-conducted prospective study of 43 cases reported a 1-month-old infant who had received 60 minutes of open heart massage with co-existing coagulation defects. The retinal hemorrhages were bilateral, small, multiple dot hemorrhages.[67] Three other cases reported: a 6-week-old infant after 75 minutes of CPR had bilateral retinal hemorrhages; a 2-year-old after 40 minutes of CPR with a large unilateral hemorrhage next to the optic disc; and an 18-month-old infant with coagulation abnormalities and arterial hypertension had a retinal hemorrhage. Hence, isolated prolonged CPR is rarely associated with retinal hemorrhages.
5. Use of extracorporeal membrane oxygenation (ECMO). Retinal hemorrhages are rare in infants subjected to ECMO, with one study reporting a prevalence of 5%; however, may of these children are premature and birth-related hemorrhages cannot be ruled out.[68]
6. Coagulopathy of AHT. Head injury is associated with acute coagulation abnormalities with prolonged

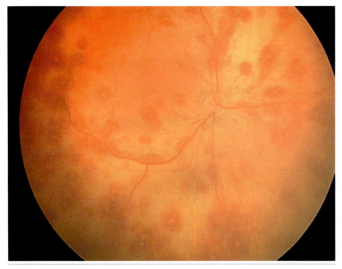

Fig. 67.16 Retinal hemorrhages. Seen with white centered hemorrhages in a full-term child born vaginally with the aid of vacuum extraction.

Table 67.2 – Retinal hemorrhages in conditions with clinical overlap for child abuse[62]

Condition	Features of abuse	Retinal hemorrhage description			
		Severity	Location	Layer	Laterality
Glutaric aciduria	ICH	Multiple	Posterior pole	Intraretinal and vitreous hemorrhage	Bilateral and unilateral
Methylmalonic aciduria with homocysteinuria (cobalamin C deficiency)	ICH	Scattered	Posterior pole and postequatorial	Intraretinal and vitreous hemorrhage	Bilateral
Osteogenesis imperfecta	ICH, bruise, fracture	Multiple	Posterior pole	Preretinal, intraretinal vitreous hemorrhage	Bilateral and unilateral
Platelet function defect (Hermansky-Pudlak syndrome)	ICH	Few	Posterior pole	Subretinal, intraretinal, and subhyaloid	Bilateral
Protein C deficiency	ICH, bruise	Florid and minor	N/A	Subretinal with vitreous hemorrhage	Bilateral and unilateral
Low fibrinogen levels	ICH, bruise	N/A	N/A	Intraretinal, subretinal	Bilateral
Hemorrhagic disease of the newborn	ICH, bruise	Multiple	N/A	Intraretinal, vitreous hemorrhage	Bilateral
Fibromuscular dysplasia	ICH	Extensive	Widespread	Intraretinal and subhyaloid	Bilateral
Spinal cord arteriovenous malformation	ICH	N/A	N/A	Intraretinal and preretinal	Bilateral

ICH = intracranial hemorrhage; N/A = not available.

prothrombin time, and decreased platelets and fibrinogen levels. These abnormalities are accentuated in children with parenchymal brain injury where 54% have a prolonged prothrombin time. In children who die with AHT with parenchymal brain injury, 94% display prolonged prothrombin time.[69] These abnormalities in coagulation seen in abusive head injury are not due to a pre-existing hemorrhagic diathesis. The abnormalities are temporary and do not explain retinal hemorrhages, which are also seen in children without coagulation abnormalities.[8]

Systemic features of abusive head injury

Neurological

Injury to the brain may manifest acutely as simply a general malaise with drowsiness and lethargy to a critically ill infant with impaired consciousness and death.[8] Brain injury includes the presence of extra-axial blood (subdural, subarachnoid), intraparenchymal hemorrhage, diffuse axonal injury, hypoxic ischemic injury, or any combination of the above. Both apnea and retinal hemorrhages have a high positive predictive rate of inflicted brain injury (Fig. 67.17). Although seizures and skull fractures are seen in abusive head injury, they are not discriminatory for abuse.[29] Neurological sequelae of parenchymal brain injury manifest later as cognitive and behavioral disturbances, cerebral palsy, seizures, and blindness with a severe disability reported in 61% of children. Neuroradiological features suggestive of an abusive injury are multiple complex wide fractures (diastatic), multiple site subdural hematomas,

interhemispheric blood, and loss of gray–white matter differentiation. The finding of blood around the spinal cord on MRI and postmortem (Fig. 67.18) in AHT suggests scanning of the spine should be included in the investigations.

Fractures

Fractures from abuse are recorded throughout the skeleton. A child less than 3 years of age with multiple fractures suggests an abusive injury. Abusive fractures involving the femur and fractures of the humerus involving the mid shaft rather than the supracondylar region are more likely to be seen in non-ambulant children. Fractures that have the highest probability of abuse are posterior rib fractures.[70] Rib fractures are rare with CPR in children and are usually located anteriorly at the costochondral junction.[71]

Bites

A human bite is a sign where identifying the perpetrator by the dental imprint and salivary DNA is possible.[72] The hallmark of a human bite is the compression of tissue in two opposing concave arcs. The size of the arcs is measured by the intercanine distance – usually 3 to 4.5 cm in an adult and 2.5 to 3.0 cm in a child. An intercanine distance of less than 2.5 cm identifies a child's deciduous teeth. Animal bites usually tear the flesh, unlike human bites which compress the flesh leaving an imprint.

Burns and scalds

Burns and scalds are less common than other forms of physical abuse. Intentional scalds (immersion into hot water) are seen more frequently in abusive injuries. When intentional they are

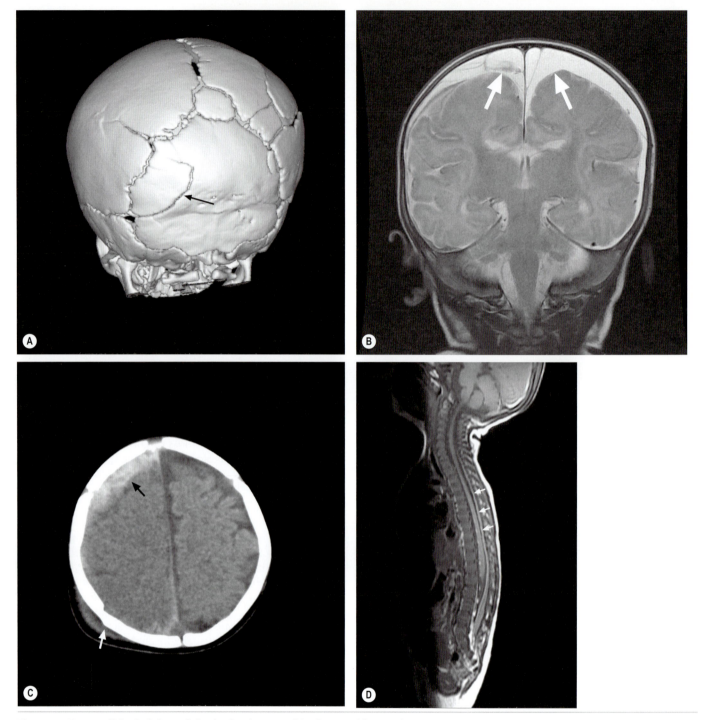

Fig. 67.17 Neuroradiological signs of abusive head trauma. (A) Left occipital fracture shown on 3D CT scan reconstruction. (B) Bilateral subdural hemorrhage on MRI T2 scan (white arrows). (C) Subdural (black arrow) interhemispheric bleeding with scalp hematoma (white arrow). (D) MRI scan showing blood around the spinal cord (white arrows). (Courtesy of Dr. A. Liu.)

usually symmetrical. If they involve the extremities, they have a clear upper margin and may have a glove or stocking-like pattern. If they involve the buttock, sparing of the perineal fold is seen.[23]

Unintentional cigarette burns are usually superficial as contact with the lighted end, for example a child walking into a cigarette, initiates a prompt withdrawal response. Superficial burns should be observed over a period of 3 weeks as they heal without a scar. Deep burns require a contact time of more than

2 seconds; they heal with a scar and are more likely to be intentional (Fig. 67.19).

Bruises

Bruising is the commonest presenting sign in abusive injury. Certain patterns of bruising help to distinguish abusive from accidental bruises. Bruising in non-independently mobile infants, bruising away from bony prominences (e.g. face), and

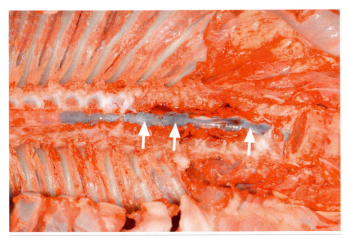

Fig. 67.18 Postmortem dissection of the spine. White arrows indicate subdural blood.

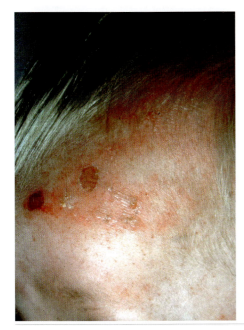

Fig. 67.19 Abusive cigarette burns on the left side of forehead.

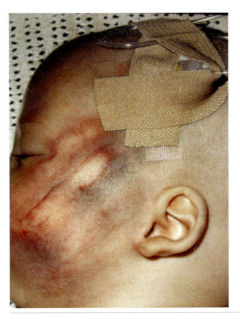

Fig. 67.20 An abusive bruise left cheek demonstrating the imprint of fingers.

large, multiple bruises occurring in clusters and bearing the imprint of an implement are highly suggestive of abusive injury[10] (Fig. 67.20).

Biomechanics of retinal hemorrhages

Theoretic considerations:

- Vitreoretinal traction.
- Impaired retinal venous return.
- Hypoxic ischemia of retina.

Though controversies still exist as to whether a shaking injury alone or one with impact exceeds the threshold of force required to produce head injury, retinal hemorrhages are seen in both impact and non-impact head injuries.[73,74] Experiments with primates demonstrate that angular and rotational accelerations of the head rather than linear acceleration cause brain injury.[75,76] Until recently the evidence for retinal injury was

extrapolated from mechanisms underlying brain injury which have been reviewed.[20,22] Current research lacks conclusive evidence for an underlying mechanism of retinal hemorrhages in abusive injury. Experimental and naturally occurring animal models have failed to replicate the findings seen in AHT in infants.[77-79] Computer modeling using finite element analysis to demonstrate that most forces during simulated shaking cycles are exerted on the posterior retina or the vitreoretinal interfaces suggests that vitreous traction on the retina causes retinal hemorrhages.[80,81] In addition, clinical and postmortem studies and the use of optical coherence tomography demonstrated that vitreous attached to schisis cavities and folds in the retina, suggesting that vitreoretinal traction may cause retinal hemorrhages.[82,83] Postmortem studies have suggested that retinal ischemia may explain the retinal findings in abusive head injury.[84] It is likely that all the theoretic mechanisms contribute to the retinal findings and are not mutually exclusive.

Prevention

Programs have been developed to address a broad segment of society which should include: parents and other child carers (primary prevention); targeted programs which involve populations at higher risk of abusive injury that include parents or carers from lower socioeconomic groups; young parents; those with previous social services contact (secondary prevention); and programs directed at perpetrators to prevent recidivism (tertiary prevention). These programs are predominantly educational and have demonstrated a lower prevalence of abuse in defined populations after interventions.[85]

Munchausen's syndrome by proxy

This is a form of child maltreatment where an illness is fabricated by the caregiver of the child for personal gain or

711

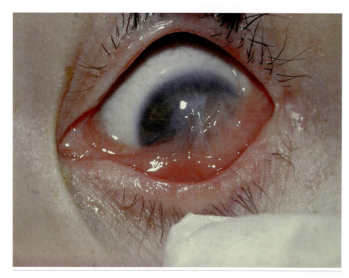

Fig. 67.21 Munchausen's syndrome by proxy. Keratoconjunctivtis with vascularization and pseudo pterygium of the inferior cornea seen in a child from repeated toxin instillation by her caregiver.

attention. The perpetrator, often the mother, simulates or induces an illness in a child not capable of or unwilling to identify the offender. The offender may fabricate the history, cause physical signs by exposing the child repeatedly to infectious agents, toxins or physical trauma, or alter laboratory tests by tampering with the child's specimens. The following should alert the clinician to establish a diagnosis.

1. Over attentive caregiver, or caregiver not as worried about the child as medical staff.
2. Investigations do not tally with clinical signs.
3. Clinical signs do not respond to treatment.
4. Child's condition improves when isolated from the caregiver and recurs in their presence.

Ophthalmic manifestations are rare. There are case reports of recurrent conjunctivitis,[86] unilateral orbital cellulitis, and keratoconjunctivitis[87,88] induced by toxins (Fig. 67.21).

The ophthalmologist and child maltreatment

When confronted with suspected cases of child abuse or neglect, the ophthalmologist's overriding duty is to safeguard the rights of the child. Ophthalmic evaluation should never be considered in isolation but in conjunction with the findings of other specialties, fostering a close working relationship with multidisciplinary teams and child maltreatment experts. The evaluation should be meticulously documented and supplemented where possible with photography. It is to be remembered that there are no pathognomonic ocular signs of child abuse.

As an expert witness, it is important to be well versed with all the documentation provided and with current literature. Do not be drawn by the counsel into giving opinions outside your area of expertise. Evidence is presented for the court and not for a particular side.

References

6. Minns RA, Jones PA, Mok JY. Incidence and demography of non-accidental head injury in southeast Scotland from a national database. Am J Prev Med 2008; 34(4 Suppl): S126–33.
8. Jayawant S, Rawlinson A, Gibbon F, et al. Subdural haemorrhages in infants: population based study. BMJ 1998; 317: 1558–61.
10. Maguire S, Mann MK, Sibert J, Kemp A. Are there patterns of bruising in childhood which are diagnostic or suggestive of abuse? A systematic review. Arch Dis Child 2005; 90: 182–6.
17. Kemp AM. Investigating subdural haemorrhage in infants. Arch Dis Child 2002; 86: 98–102.
18. Kivlin JD, Simons KB, Lazoritz S, Ruttum MS. Shaken baby syndrome. Ophthalmology 2000; 107: 1246–54.
20. The Ophthalmology Child Abuse Working Party. Child abuse and the eye. Eye (Lond) 1999; 13 (Pt 1): 3–10.
21. Adams G, Ainsworth J, Butler L, et al. Update from the Ophthalmology Child Abuse Working Party: Royal College of Ophthalmologists. Eye (Lond) 2004; 18: 795–8.
28. Bhardwaj G, Chowdhury V, Jacobs MB, et al. A systematic review of the diagnostic accuracy of ocular signs in pediatric abusive head trauma. Ophthalmology 2010; 117: 983–92, e17.
29. Maguire S, Pickerd N, Farewell D, et al. Which clinical features distinguish inflicted from non-inflicted brain injury? A systematic review. Arch Dis Child 2009; 94: 860–7.
30. Mungan NK. Update on shaken baby syndrome: ophthalmology. Curr Opin Ophthalmol 2007; 18: 392–7.
31. Morad YK, Armstrong YM, Huyer DC, et al. Correlation between retinal abnormalities and intracranial abnormalities in the shaken baby syndrome. Am J Ophthalmol 2002; 134: 354–9.
35. Lantz PE, Sinal SH, Stanton CA, Weaver RG, Jr. Perimacular retinal folds from childhood head trauma. BMJ 2004; 27(328): 754–6.
36. Lueder GT, Turner JW, Paschall R. Perimacular retinal folds simulating nonaccidental injury in an infant. Arch Ophthalmol 2006; 124: 1782–3.
37. Watts P, Obi E. Retinal folds and retinoschisis in accidental and non-accidental head injury. Eye (Lond) 2008; 22(12): 1514–6.
38. Reddie IC, Bhardwaj G, Dauber SL, et al. Bilateral retinoschisis in a 2-year-old following a three-storey fall. Eye (Lond) 2010; 24: 1426–7.
39. Levin AV. Ophthalmology of shaken baby syndrome. Neurosurg Clin North Am 2002; 13: 201–11, vi.
43. Wygnanski-Jaffe T, Levin AV, Shafiq A, et al. Postmortem orbital findings in shaken baby syndrome. Am J Ophthalmol 2006; 142: 233–40.
47. Emerson MV, Pieramici DJ, Stoessel KM, et al. Incidence and rate of disappearance of retinal hemorrhage in newborns. Ophthalmology 2001; 108: 36–9.
48. Hughes LA, May K, Talbot JF, Parsons MA. Incidence, distribution, and duration of birth-related retinal hemorrhages: a prospective study. J AAPOS 2006; 10: 102–6.
49. Buys YM, Levin AV, Enzenauer RW, et al. Retinal findings after head trauma in infants and young children. Ophthalmology 1992; 99: 1718–23.
50. Pierre-Kahn V, Roche O, Dureau P, et al. Ophthalmologic findings in suspected child abuse victims with subdural hematomas. Ophthalmology 2003; 110: 1718–23.
51. Bechtel K, Stoessel K, Leventhal JM, et al. Characteristics that distinguish accidental from abusive injury in hospitalized young children with head trauma. Pediatrics 2004; 114: 165–8.
52. Vinchon M, Defoort-Dhellemmes S, Desurmont M, Dhellemmes P. Accidental and nonaccidental head injuries in infants: a prospective study. J Neurosurg 2005; 102(4 Suppl): 380–4.
53. Trenchs V, Curcoy AI, Morales M, et al. Retinal haemorrhages in head trauma resulting from falls: differential diagnosis with non-accidental trauma in patients younger than 2 years of age. Childs Nerv Syst 2008; 24: 815–20.
54. Gnanaraj L, Gilliland MG, Yahya RR, et al. Ocular manifestations of crush head injury in children. Eye (Lond) 2007; 21: 5–10.

56. Kafil-Hussain NA, Monavari A, Bowell R, et al. Ocular findings in glutaric aciduria type 1. J Pediatr Ophthalmol Strabismus 2000; 37: 289–93.

57. Ganesh A, Jenny C, Geyer J, et al. Retinal hemorrhages in type I osteogenesis imperfecta after minor trauma. Ophthalmology 2004; 111: 1428–31.

58. Bhardwaj G, Jacobs MB, Moran KT, Tan K. Terson syndrome with ipsilateral severe hemorrhagic retinopathy in a 7-month-old child. J AAPOS 2010; 14: 441–3.

73. Duhaime AC, Gennarelli TA, Thibault LE, et al. The shaken baby syndrome: a clinical, pathological, and biomechanical study. J Neurosurg 1987; 66: 409–15.

74. Cory CZJ, Jones MD. Can shaking alone cause fatal brain injury? A biomechanical assessment of the Duhaime shaken baby syndrome model. Med Sci Law 2003; 43: 317–33.

75. Ommaya AK, Faas F, Yarnell P. Whiplash injury and brain damage: an experimental study. JAMA 1968; 204: 285–9.

88. Taylor D. Unnatural injuries. Eye (Lond) 2000; 14(Pt 2): 123–50.

Access the complete reference list online at
http://www.expertconsult.com

Refractive surgery in children

Evelyn A Paysse

Introduction

Excimer laser surgery for high refractive error associated with amblyopia has been performed for over 15 years with good visual acuity and refractive results and minimal complications.[1-26] Intraocular refractive procedures have been performed in smaller numbers for higher refractive errors for up to 7 years, also with good visual and refractive outcomes and few complications.

Conventional amblyopia therapy consists of the following:

1. Clearing the ocular media of visual obstructions such as leukoma, cataract, or vitreous hemorrhage.
2. Correcting significant refractive errors either with spectacles or contact lenses.
3. Encouraging use of the amblyopic eye through occlusion or pharmacologic and/or optical penalization of the fellow eye (see Chapter 70).[27-29] This conventional therapy is successful in the majority of young amblyopes.

There are, however, subsets of children with amblyopia that often fail this standard therapy. These groups are:

1. Children with bilateral high ametropia (isoametropia) who are spectacle non-compliant or intolerant.

2. Children with severe anisometropia who are non-compliant or intolerant of spectacle and contact lens wear.
3. Children with high ametropia, either anisometropia or isoametropia, who have other special circumstances such as craniofacial anomalies, ear deformities, or neck hypotonia that preclude the proper use of refractive correction.

There are many reasons for poor compliance with spectacles or contact lenses. Spectacles for the treatment of extreme myopia or hyperopia can cause prismatically induced optical aberrations, a narrow visual field, and social ostracism due to unattractive thick lenses. Group 1, above, consists primarily of former premature infants with severe retinopathy of prematurity and high myopia, children with genetic mutations, or with autism spectrum disorder. They are often non-compliant or ill-suited for spectacle wear or contact lenses due to tactile aversion. Their visual impairment may impede their attention and social interaction, exacerbating significant behavioral and social problems and impeding the development of normal skills. In group 2, spectacle-induced aniseikonia and anisovergence impede stereopsis and binocular vision, and may cause asthenopia.[30]

Contact lenses more than spectacles improve the quality of vision, reduce the minification effect of high myopic spectacles, give better contrast sensitivity, and reduced social discomfort. Contact lenses, however, in children are often impractical due to difficulty of insertion, cost, intolerance to extended wear, and non-compliance.

In the past, no other treatment options existed. The result was variable visual impairment in the affected eye(s). If the condition was bilateral, severe visual impairment was the result. Refractive surgery reduces refractive error in these children and opens up a whole new world to them.

A new mindset is needed when we think about the management of severe refractive error in children. Untreated high refractive error in young children can result in severe levels of amblyopia akin to that found with a dense congenital cataract or leukoma. We should approach this form of amblyopia aggressively. Surgery is an effective and safe surgical procedure to treat the high refractive error when standard therapy fails.

Types of refractive surgery used in children

Corneal and intraocular procedures can change refractive error. The corneal procedures are performed with the excimer laser and include photorefractive keratectomy (PRK), laser-assisted sub-epithelial keratectomy (LASEK) (these two procedures together will be referred to as advanced surface ablation (ASA)) and laser-assisted in situ keratomileusis (LASIK). ASA has been used to treat up to 10–12 diopters of myopia, 6 diopters of hyperopia, and 4 diopters of astigmatism. These numbers are typically reduced by about one-third for treatment using LASIK. PRK and LASEK are surface ablations, with minor differences between them, that permanently change the shape of the cornea using the excimer laser to ablate (by vaporization) tissue from the anterior corneal stroma, just under the corneal epithelium.

1. In PRK, epithelium is removed and Bowman's membrane and anterior stroma are treated with laser.
2. In LASEK, the epithelium is not removed, but an alcoholic solution is used to loosen the epithelial cells; the surgeon folds the epithelial layer out of the treatment field, performs the laser ablation, and then replaces the epithelial layer.
3. In LASIK, a partial-thickness corneal flap is created using either a mechanical microkeratome or a femtosecond laser microkeratome. A hinge is left at one end of this flap. The flap is folded back and the laser ablation performed on the deeper stroma. The LASIK flap is then repositioned. The flap remains in position by natural adhesion until healing is completed.

Current intraocular refractive procedures change the existing lens power and include phakic intraocular lenses (phIOLs), refractive lens exchange (RLE), and clear lens extraction (CLE). These procedures are used to treat higher refractive errors that fall outside the treatment parameters for the excimer laser, or in cases where the cornea is too thin for the excimer laser. phIOL procedures add or reduce lens power.[31] An intraocular lens (IOL) is placed into the anterior or posterior chamber preserving the natural crystalline lens. Anterior or posterior chamber phIOLs can be used to treat severely high myopic refractive errors if the anterior chamber is deep enough to tolerate the lens (minimum 3.2 mm).

The other procedures that change lens power are RLE and CLE. They are technically identical to pediatric cataract surgery except the crystalline lens being removed is clear. In RLE, an appropriately powered IOL is placed in the eye after removing the crystalline lens; in CLE, the eye is left aphakic. Currently, both corneal and intraocular refractive procedures are utilized "off-label" in children.

Safety of ASA versus LASIK

Box 68.1 outlines the risks of ASA and LASIK. While LASIK has been shown to be effective in children to correct refractive error, ASA holds several advantages. First, no corneal flap is created so there is no risk of flap loss, epithelial in-growth, or

Box 68.1

Risks of ASA versus LASIK

ASA	LASIK
Dry eyes	Dry eyes
Mild to moderate discomfort for 3–4 days	Flap dislocation
Corneal haze	Flap loss
Long healing time	Epithelial ingrowth
	Keratectasia
	Posterior vitreous detachment
	Retinal detachment

ASA = advanced surface ablation; LASIK = laser-assisted in situ keratomileusis.

flap striae as with LASIK. Second, since ASA is performed on the surface of the cornea, the posterior stroma remains thicker, with less risk of keratectasia. Because most children treated with excimer laser procedures require a large excimer treatment dose, there is significant corneal ablation. There have been no reported cases of keratectasia following ASA in children. The main long-term risk of ASA is corneal haze, but, in our experience, it is uncommon and, typically when the topical steroid (fluorometholone) was discontinued too early. Fluorometholone must be used for 6–12 months following PRK. Corneal haze can be further reduced by limiting ablation treatments to within the Federal Drugs Administration (in the USA) approved parameters and by the child taking vitamin C 250–500 mg daily for a year. The other issue with excimer laser procedures is which causes a reduction in the effect of the procedure or refractive regression. Most of the regression occurs in the first year but it can continue longer; it is more severe with higher excimer treatment doses.

Phakic intraocular lens safety

Phakic IOL implantation is not subject to refractive regression and may be the preferred surgical correction of pediatric myopia and hyperopia beyond the range of ASA.[32] Another major advantage is reversibility. The anterior chamber depth required for an "iris-enclaved" IOL precludes the use of this lens in some children. Children who have high lenticular myopia after retinopathy of prematurity may be unsuitable because of shallow chambers.[33] The major concern with a phIOL in a child is the long-term effect on corneal endothelium. Experience indicates however, that endothelial cell loss is low,[32,34,42] no greater than in adult implantation. Accurate endothelial cell counts are difficult to obtain in the children who may benefit most from implantation.[32] Any refractive surgical procedure, including ASA, LASIK, and RLE/CLE, can cause some reduction of endothelial cell density. We still need to know the comparative loss. Posterior chamber phIOLs have also been implanted in children:[38,39,41] Because they lie adjacent to the iris pigment and lens, they risk pigment dispersion and cataract formation. These potential risks are important, but they must be weighed against the certainty of permanent blur-induced visual impairment if the children continue uncorrected. These potential complications may occur many years later.

Refractive lens exchange and clear lens extraction safety

Refractive lens exchange (RLE) and clear lens extraction (CLE) can be used in children who have refractive error beyond the range of effective ASA who have anterior chambers that are too shallow for phIOLs.[43,44] Removing the natural lens abolishes accommodation. This can be rectified by implantation of a multifocal IOL, but these have their own risks and complications. The major long-term risk of RLE/CLE is retinal detachment, with an estimated prevalence of approximately 3%. If the axial length exceeds approximately 29 mm, prophylactic diode laser therapy may be considered to reduce the risk,[45,46] which itself must be weighed against the certainty of severe blur-induced amblyopia in the affected eye(s) if continued uncorrected.

Strategy for pediatric refractive surgery

Children with hyperopic isoametropia or anisometropia of 3 to 6 diopters or myopic isoametropia or anisometropia of 3 to 10 diopters can be treated with ASA if they fail standard therapy. Children with refractive errors beyond this range can be treated with a phIOL if the anterior chamber depth is 3.2 mm or greater. The remainder of the children can undergo RLE or CLE. These procedures usually require general anesthesia.

Improvements in visual acuity and visual function

Is refractive surgery effective in children? Yes, with qualification. One must remember that the measure of effectiveness in children non-compliant with spectacles is uncorrected visual acuity (UCVA). Substantial gains in UCVA and best corrected visual acuity (BCVA) have been demonstrated using ASA, LASIK, phIOLs, or RLE/CLE in children.

Impressive visual gains have been achieved in isoametropic children for both high hyperopia and high myopia[3-6,21,22,32,44,47] (Tables 68.1 and 68.2). More modest but consistent gains have been achieved in the amblyopic eyes of anisometropic children using ASA, LASIK, phIOLs, and RLE/CLE.[2,6,8,9,15,18,22,23,37,48-51] (Tables 68.1 and 68.3). Most reports on pediatric refractive surgery have used ASA to treat anisometropic amblyopia.[1-3,5-7,9,14,15,17,18,22,23,26,52-54] These series show an initial correction of refractive error to ±1.5 diopters of emmetropia in approximately 90% of treated eyes. The qualification for all pediatric refractive visual acuity results is that tolerances are wider than in adult refractive surgery; seldom does one achieve the precision commonplace in adult refractive surgery. The goal in children is the prevention of high levels of refractive amblyopia. The gains in UCVA or BCVA range from mild to excellent (2–7 lines improvement), with no reported losses of acuity. Half, or more, of the children treated have improved binocular fusion and stereopsis.[2,9,15,18,23]

Beyond the gains in acuity or binocularity, refractive surgery has positive effects on children's day-to-day visual function.[32,47] Enhanced visual awareness, attentiveness, and social interactions have been reported in approximately 80% of children treated for high isoametropia. When measured using Likert scale visual function questionnaires, before and after refractive surgery, scores for eye contact, tracking, observing and reacting, judging depth and distance, and reading improved by an average 73% in isoametropic children and 58% in anisometropic children.[32,55,56] The developmental quotient, calculated as the mental age divided by the biological age ×100, has also been shown to improve in children with neurobehavioral disorders and severe isoametropia following PRK.[47]

Controversies in pediatric refractive surgery

Controversies exist about pediatric refractive surgery even among its advocates. The main concern is the age at which to perform refractive surgery and what procedure is optimal. Most experts recommend the procedure early in the visual neuroplastic years when reversal or even prevention of amblyopia is greatest, after failing all attempts at traditional therapy. The disadvantages of doing the procedure at an early age are similar to those with placing an IOL in a child. The eye is still growing and determination of the proper treatment dose can be difficult as the refractive error may change with eye growth. Another disadvantage is difficulty with centration as young children require general anesthesia. However, in the majority of studies, the refractive error treated was greater than 9 diopters of myopia or 4 diopters of hyperopia, so the risk of overtreatment is low and centration was not found to be problematic.[4-6,8,10,11,13,14,16,18-20,22-25,31]

Summary

Refractive surgery for children with high refractive error and amblyopia unresponsive to standard therapy appears to be effective. Interventional case series and case-control studies of excimer laser refractive surgery, phIOLs, and RLE or CLE in children have improved visual acuity and developmental, social functioning and reduced refractive error with few complications. While the majority of children with refractive error, either unilateral or bilateral, do well with contact lenses or spectacles, for the small subset who do not, refractive surgery is a useful addition to our treatment armamentarium and a reasonable last option to prevent a lifetime of visual impairment. Randomized clinical trials must further validate efficacy.

Table 68.1 – Refractive surgery for high bilateral hyperopia and hyperopic anisometropic amblyopia

Author(s)	Year	Procedure	No. of patients	Age range (years)	Disorder treated	Preoperative SE (D)[a]	Postoperative SE (D)[a]	Mean preoperative BCVA[a]	Mean postoperative UCVA[b]	Follow-up (months)	Complications
Astle et al.[4]	2010	LASEK	47	0.8 to 17	Bilateral hyperopia and hyperopic anisometropia	3.42	0.59	NR	NR. States 41% improvement in BCVA	12	2 patients with mild ring-shaped haze and 1 with severe ring-shaped haze outside visual axis
Yin et al.[25]	2007	LASIK	42	6 to 14	Hyperopic anisometropia	6.41	0.60	20/100	NR. (BCVA 20/40)	17	None
Utine et al.[49]	2008	LASIK	32	4 to 15	Hyperopic anisometropia	5.17	1.39	20/100	20/60	20	NR
Tychsen et al.[29]	2008	PhIOL	2	NR	Bilateral hyperopia	10.5	1.0	NR for this patient, was part of larger group	NR for this patient, was part of larger group	9	None

[a]Mean unless range is given.

[b]These studies include patients treated for anisometropia in the same study.

BCVA = best corrected visual acuity; D = diopters; LASEK = laser subepithelial keratomileusis; NR = not reported; PRK = photorefractive keratectomy; SE = spherical equivalent; UCVA = uncorrected visual acuity.

Table 68.2 – Refractive surgery for high bilateral myopia

Author(s)	Year	Procedure	No. of patients	Age range (years)	Preoperative SE (D)[a]	Postoperative SE (D)[a]	Mean preoperative BCVA[a]	Mean postoperative UCVA[6]	Follow-up (months)	Behavior	Complications
Astle et al.[3,b]	2002	PRK	10	1 to 6	−10.7	−1.4	20/70	NR	12	Improved in 2/3 of patients	40% mild to moderate haze
Astle et al.[5,b]	2004	LASEK	11	1 to 17	−8	−1.2	20/80	NR	12	Improved in 50% to 83% of patients	22% mild haze
Astle et al.[6]	2006	LASEK	1	7	−7.5	−3.3	3/200	NR	12	Improved	None
Tychsen et al.[29]	2006	RLE/CLE	13	1 to 18	−19.1	0.8	20/76	20/38	54	Improved by questionnaire	1 dislocated IOL and 1 posterior capsule opacity
Tychsen and Hoekel[22]	2006	LASEK	9	3 to 16	Range: −3.8 to −11.5	89% within 1 D of goal	20/133	20/60	17	Improved in 88% of patients	35% mild haze

[a]Mean unless range is given.
[b]These data include patients treated for anisometropia in the same study.
BCVA = best corrected visual acuity; D = diopters; IOL = intraocular lens; LASEK = laser subepithelial keratomileusis; NR = not reported; PRK = photorefractive keratectomy; SE = spherical equivalent; UCVA = uncorrected visual acuity.

Table 68.3 – Refractive surgery for high myopic anisometropia

Author(s)	Year	Procedure	Age range (years)	No. of patients	Preoperative SE (D)[a]	Postoperative SE (D)[a]	Preoperative BCVA[a]	Postoperative UCVA[b]	Mean follow-up (months)	Complications
Singh[53]	1995	PRK	10 to 15	6	−12.1	−2.9	20/82	20/44	1	Haze
Nano et al.[52]	1997	PRK	11 to 14	5	−8	−1.6	20/400	20/72	12	Mild haze
Alio et al.[1]	1998	PRK	5 to 7	6	−9.6	−2	20/114	20/35	24	Severe haze (1)
Rashad[20]	1999	LASIK	7 to 12	14	−7.9	−0.6	20/50	20/25	12	None
Agarwal et al.[54]	2000	LASIK	5 to 11	16	−14.9	−1.4	20/37	20/37	12	Free Flap
Nucci and Drack[26]	2001	PRK/LASIK	9 to 14	14	−8	−0.07	20/125	20/121	20	None
Nassaralla and Nassaralla[14]	2001	LASIK	8 to 15	9	−7.2	−0.2	NR	NR	12	None
Astle et al.[3,b]	2002	PRK	1 to 6	27	−10.7	−1.4	20/70	20/40	12	Mild haze
Aurata and Rehurek[9]	2004	PRK/LASEK	4 to 7	27	−8.3	−1.6	20/95	20/26	24	Mild haze (3)
Astle et al.[5,b]	2004	LASEK	1 to 17	13	−8	−1.2	20/80	20/50	12	Minimal haze
Phillips et al.[51]	2004	LASIK	8 to 19	17	−9.06	−3.74	20/25	20/20	18	None
Tychsen et al.[23]	2005	PRK/LASIK	4 to 16	35	−11.5	−3	20/87	20/47	29	Minimal haze (3)
Paysse et al.[17]	2006	PRK	2 to 11	11	−13.8	−3.6	20/316	20/126	31	Minimal haze
Yir et al.[25]	2007	LASIK	6 to 14	32	−10.1	−2.2	20/50	20/33	17	Minimal haze
Ali et al.[45]	2007	RLE/CLE	4 to 20	7	−16.7	NR	NR (UCVA 20/2550)	NR (UCVA 20/130)	4	Posterior capsule fibrosis (1)
Pirouzian and Ip[28]	2010	PhIOL	5 to 11	7	−14.28	−1.1	20/4000	NR (BCVA 20/40)	35	None
Lesueur et al.[27]	2002	PhIOL	3 to 16	11	−12.7	NR (range −0.75 to +2.00)	NR (range CF to 20/63)	NR (BCVA 20/63)	21	None

[a]Mean unless range is given.
[b]These data include patients treated for bilateral high myopia and high myopia after penetrating keratoplasty in the same study.
BCVA = best corrected visual acuity; D = diopters; LASEK = laser subepithelial keratomileusis; LASIK = laser in situ keratomileusis; NR = not reported; PRK = photorefractive keratectomy; RLE/CLE = refractive lens exchange/clear lens extraction; SE = spherical equivalent; UCVA = uncorrected visual acuity.

References

1. Alio JL, Artola A, Claramonte P, et al. Photorefractive keratectomy for pediatric myopic anisometropia. J Cataract Refract Surg 1998; 24: 327–30.
2. Astle WF, Fawcett SL, Huang PT, et al. Long-term outcomes of photorefractive keratectomy and laser-assisted subepithelial keratectomy in children. J Cataract Refract Surg 2008; 34: 411–6.
4. Astle WF, Huang PT, Ereifej I, Paszuk A. Laser-assisted subepithelial keratectomy for bilateral hyperopia and hyperopic anisometropic amblyopia in children: one-year outcomes. J Cataract Refract Surg 2010; 36: 260–7.
6. Astle WF, Papp A, Huang PT, Ingram A. Refractive laser surgery in children with coexisting medical and ocular pathology. J Cataract Refract Surg 2006; 32: 103–8.
8. Autrata R, Rehurek J. Clinical results of excimer laser photorefractive keratectomy for high myopic anisometropia in children: four-year follow-up. J Cataract Refract Surg 2003; 29: 694–702.
9. Autrata R, Rehurek J. Laser-assisted subepithelial keratectomy and photorefractive keratectomy versus conventional treatment of myopic anisometropic amblyopia in children. J Cataract Refract Surg 2004; 30: 74–84.
12. Lin XM, Yan XH, Wang Z, et al. Long-term efficacy of excimer laser in situ keratomileusis in the management of children with high anisometropic amblyopia. Chin Med J (Engl) 2009; 122: 813–7.
14. Nassaralla BR, Nassaralla JJ, Jr. Laser in situ keratomileusis in children 8 to 15 years old. J Refract Surg 2001; 17: 519–24.
15. Paysse EA. Photorefractive keratectomy for anisometropic amblyopia in children. Trans Am Ophthalmol Soc 2004; 102: 341–71.
16. Paysse EA. Pediatric excimer refractive surgery. Int Ophthalmol Clin 2010; 50: 95–105.
17. Paysse EA, Coats DK, Hussein MA, et al. Long-term outcomes of photorefractive keratectomy for anisometropic amblyopia in children. Ophthalmology 2006; 113: 169–76.
18. Paysse EA, Hamill MB, Hussein MA, Koch DD. Photorefractive keratectomy for pediatric anisometropia: safety and impact on refractive error, visual acuity, and stereopsis. Am J Ophthalmol 2004; 138: 70–8.
19. Paysse EA, Hamill MB, Koch DD, et al. Epithelial healing and ocular discomfort after photorefractive keratectomy in children. J Cataract Refract Surg 2003; 29: 478–81.
21. Tychsen L. Refractive surgery for special needs children. Arch Ophthalmol 2009; 127: 810–13.
22. Tychsen L, Hoekel J. Refractive surgery for high bilateral myopia in children with neurobehavioral disorders: 2. Laser-assisted subepithelial keratectomy (LASEK). J AAPOS 2006; 10: 364–70.
23. Tychsen L, Packwood E, Berdy G. Correction of large amblyopiogenic refractive errors in children using the excimer laser. J AAPOS 2005; 9: 224–33.

25. Yin ZQ, Wang H, Yu T, et al. Facilitation of amblyopia management by laser in situ keratomileusis in high anisometropic hyperopic and myopic children. J AAPOS 2007; 11: 571–6.
26. Nucci P, Drack AV. Refractive surgery for unilateral high myopia in children. J AAPOS 2001; 5: 348–51.
31. Huang D, Schallhorn SC, Sugar A, et al. Phakic intraocular lens implantation for the correction of myopia: a report by the American Academy of Ophthalmology. Ophthalmology 2009; 116: 2244–58.
32. Tychsen L, Hoekel J, Ghasia F, Yoon-Huang G. Phakic intraocular lens correction of high ametropia in children with neurobehavioral disorders. J AAPOS 2008; 12: 282–9.
36. Saxena R, van Minderhout HM, Luyten GP. Anterior chamber iris-fixated phakic intraocular lens for anisometropic amblyopia. J Cataract Refract Surg 2003; 29: 835–8.
38. BenEzra D, Cohen E, Karshai I. Phakic posterior chamber intraocular lens for the correction of anisometropia and treatment of amblyopia. Am J Ophthalmol 2000; 130: 292–6.
39. Lesueur LC, Arne JL. Phakic intraocular lens to correct high myopic amblyopia in children. J Refract Surg 2002; 18: 519–23.
42. Pirouzian A, Ip KC. Anterior chamber phakic intraocular lens implantation in children to treat severe anisometropic myopia and amblyopia: 3-year clinical results. J Cataract Refract Surg 2010; 36: 1486–93.
43. Ali A, Packwood E, Lueder G, Tychsen L. Unilateral lens extraction for high anisometropic myopia in children and adolescents. J AAPOS 2007; 11: 153–8.
44. Tychsen L, Packwood E, Hoekel J, Lueder G. Refractive surgery for high bilateral myopia in children with neurobehavioral disorders: 1. Clear lens extraction and refractive lens exchange. J AAPOS 2006; 10: 357–63.
47. Paysse E, Gonzalez-Diaz M, Wang D, et al. Developmental improvement in children with neurobehavioral disorders following photorefractive keratectomy for bilateral high refractive error. J AAPOS 2011; 15: 111.
50. Utine CA, Cakir H, Egemenoglu A, Perente I. LASIK in children with hyperopic anisometropic amblyopia. J Refract Surg 2008; 24: 464–72.
51. Phillips CB, Prager TC, McClellan G, Mintz-Hittner HA. Laser in situ keratomileusis for treated anisometropic amblyopia in awake, autofixating pediatric and adolescent patients. J Cataract Refract Surg 2004; 30: 2522–8.
54. Agarwal A, Agarwal T, Siraj AA, et al. Results of pediatric laser in situ keratomileusis. J Cataract Refract Surg 2000; 26: 684–9.

 Access the complete reference list online at
http://www.expertconsult.com

A vision of the present and future of strabismus

Carlos R Souza-Dias

Pharmacologic treatment of strabismus

Pharmacologic treatment of the deviation

Botulinum toxin A

Scott introduced pharmacologic treatment in the management of eye deviations.[1] Initially, he presented his results of botulinum injection for the treatment of strabismus,[2-4] later those for the treatment of blepharospasm.[5] The safety and effectiveness of this treatment was subsequently documented.[6] In 1989, Botox was approved by the US Food and Drug Administration (FDA) for the treatment of strabismus, blepharospasm, and hemifacial spasm in patients over 12 years old.

The drug is effective not only in strabismus, but also in several other specialties: neurology, urology, cosmetics, and orthopedics. Botulinum toxin now has specific indications in the treatment of strabismus. In our experience, the best indication is in recent sixth nerve paralysis, in order to avoid medial rectus contracture. This treatment is definitively part of the present management of strabismus.

Crotoxin

In the last few years, colleagues in Brazil have tested crotoxin, the major toxin of the venom of the South American rattlesnake. It causes a blockade of the neurotransmitters at the neuromuscular junction, just like botulinum toxin. It has been tested in ocular motor muscles of animals,[7] and human beings. In the treatment of strabismus and blepharospasm, it provides similar results to botulinum toxin.[8] No patient has shown any systemic effect due to crotoxin injection. The data suggest that crotoxin may be a useful and less expensive new option for the

treatment of strabismus and blepharospasm, as well as in other medical areas.

It will be good if, in the future, someone discovers a drug with this effect which can be administered by mouth or intramuscular injection, in order to avoid the unpleasant "injections in the eye."

Bupivacaine

Bupivacaine injection of muscle in animals produces immediate and massive degeneration of muscle fibers with dissolution of myofibrils at the Z-band.[9,10] Other structures around them are unchanged, including the satellite cells, which form the muscle fibers.[11] Inflammatory cells and macrophages remove the degenerated muscle fibers in a few days.[10,11] Two days after injection, satellite cells are activated and regeneration begins with the muscle reaching preinjection size and strength; continued growth is seen for about 180 days,[12,13] with the final muscle size exceeding the initial size. Goldchmit et al. suggested that strabismus after cataract surgery with retrobulbar anesthesia results from muscle hypertrophy induced by bupivacaine.[14] Fibrosis and scarring, the current suggested causes for such strabismus, has not been documented by biopsy, or found in animal studies.

Based on this observation, Scott et al. employed bupivacaine for correcting strabismus, thus enhancing the force of a weak muscle[15] or of the muscle opposite to the deviation in comitant strabismus,[16] the inverse effect of the botulinum toxin. They injected 1.0 to 4.5 mL of bupivacaine into the lateral rectus muscles of six patients with esotropia.[16] The drug improved alignment in four of the six patients. They observed a positive correlation between the improved eye alignment and the increase in muscle size. Clinical and laboratory studies are underway to determine optimal dosages and its effects in other strabismus conditions.

Scott et al. have injected botulinum toxin into the antagonist muscle of that which was injected with bupivacaine.[17] They treated seven patients with comitant horizontal strabismus; the treatment corrected an average of 19.7Δ, about twice the correction reported from bupivacaine alone. The muscle injected with bupivacaine increased its size by 5.8%. This approach may be a useful option in the treatment of strabismus.

Pharmacologic treatment of amblyopia

For more than a century, the treatment of amblyopia has been limited to occlusion of the dominant eye, except for a short usage of pleoptics and the restricted, but growing, use of penalization. Because occlusion treatment is not always effective and depends on several factors, including age of onset of the treatment, etiology of the amblyopia (anisometropia, strabismus, or deprivation), its "deepness", and the presence of eccentric fixation, a pharmacologic treatment has been sought.

Levodopa is a precursor of the catecholamines, dopamine and noradrenalin, both neurotransmitters. Levodopa is used in the treatment of Parkinson's disease to compensate for reduced dopamine in the brain. Dopamine cannot cross the blood–brain barrier: levodopa is used because it can. It is then transformed to dopamine in the brain. Carbidopa, a peripheral inhibitor of decarboxylase, reduces the systemic side effects of levodopa and increases its availability in the brain.

Some studies suggest the possibility that dopamine is effective in the treatment of amblyopia.[18-22] The reduction of the size of the scotoma as documented by Gottlob and Stangler-Zuschott[18] is thought-provoking. The theory is that levodopa enhances the plasticity of the visual cortex and hence supplements occlusion therapy in children who are older than the sensitive period.

In Brazil, Procianoy et al. studied four groups of patients with strabismic amblyopia, aged 7 to 17 years, who had already been treated without improvement with occlusion or penalization. Treatment failure was attributed to patient age or poor compliance.[22] In children less than 40 kg they gave levodopa/carbidopa (4 : 1) in doses of 5 mg (group I), 10 mg (group II), and 20 mg (group III) or a placebo, three times a day after meals. For patients who weighed 40 kg or more, they gave 10, 20, or 40 mg or placebo. Patients were randomly allocated to these treatment groups or the placebo group after stratification by body weight. All patients had the dominant eye occluded for 3 hours per day. At the end of 7 days, visual acuity improved at least 1 line of Snellen chart in 31.3% of the patients from the placebo group, in 60% of group I, in 40% of group II, and 68% of group III (Pearson's χ^2 statistic: P = 0.082).

Bhartiya et al.[23] studied 40 amblyopic children (19 with strabismus with or without anisometropia of less than 3 D and 21 with only anisometropia), 6 to 18 years old (mean age 10.9). Each subject received either levodopa/carbidopa (4 : 1 ratio) or placebo, three times a day after meals over a 4-week period, combined with "full-time" occlusion. Occlusion was continued for the study duration of 3 months (last 2 months without medication). Two strengths of levodopa/carbidopa were used: single strength, 10 mg/2.5 mg of levodopa/carbidopa and double strength, 20 mg/5 mg of levodopa/carbidopa. Children less than 20 kg were given 30 mg of levodopa per day; those whose weight was 21 to 30 kg were given 50 mg of levodopa per day and those whose weight was more than 30 kg were given 60 mg of levodopa per day. The average dose was 1.86 mg/kg/day. The results suggested that levodopa/carbidopa supplementation (in an average dose of 1.8 mg/kg/day) as an adjunct to conventional occlusion in treating amblyopia has no additional benefit over occlusion therapy alone. They did not find any differences in response between strabismic and anisometropic amblyopes. They did demonstrate, however, changes in contrast sensitivity in the occluded eye suggesting that levodopa/carbidopa has some role in modifying the plasticity of the visual system.

These studies show that there is no unanimity as to the utility of levodopa combined with occlusion in the therapy of amblyopia. We hope that in the future a more clearly efficacious pharmacologic treatment for amblyopia will be found. This goal seems extremely difficult when we look at the extent of cortical pathology in amblyopia, but further studies are warranted.

It is possible that any efficacious treatment of strabismic amblyopia will be developed in parallel with a cure of anomalous retinal correspondence (ARC) and achievement of normal fusion. This is another problem related to strabismus that is waiting for cure or prevention. Is ARC always congenital? Can it be acquired?

Some reports have suggested that acupuncture is effective in the treatment of anisometropic amblyopia in children 7 to 12 years old.[24,25] Acupuncture provides an afferent signal to the brain, which may influence certain aspects of neurotransmitter chemistry (including dopamine and acetylcholine) within the central nervous system.[26] Its cost-effectiveness has not been proven[27] but it is one more piece of evidence suggesting the possibility of extending the sensitive period of the developing visual system.

Surgical treatment of strabismus

Strabismus surgery

Strabismus surgery has not evolved much recently. One development is noteworthy. This improvement occurred when strabismologists started to pay more attention to passive forces that oppose active forces (elasticity, tonus or stiffness of antagonist muscle, fascias, orbital fat, conjunctiva, optic nerve, and adherences). For a thorough examination of the passive forces it is necessary to eliminate the active forces. This has led to the concept that the surgical plan must be confirmed or modified in the surgical room. Passive ductions and the "spring-back balance test" must be done at each stage of the operation. These tests allow the surgeon to recognize and compensate for restrictions of globe movement.

A good example is Hummelsheim's muscle transposition for sixth nerve paralysis. At the end of surgery, the passive forces must be balanced to place the eye in slight abduction because when the patient wakes, the restored tonus of the medial rectus brings the eye toward adduction. In contrast, when correcting a large angle exotropia with amblyopia, the eye position at the end of surgery must be in primary position for it will tend to remain there.[28]

Adjustable sutures have improved the prognosis of some types of surgery, but some unpredictability in the strabismus surgery persists. The immediate surgical prognosis depends on the surgeon's skill in planning and executing the surgery. We hope that in the future we will develop more exact surgical planning based on more informative semiology or new surgical techniques.

The long-term surgical result is a very complicated issue, depending on the long-term reaction of a muscle to surgery, the influence of vision on eye position, the evolution of the AC/A relation, and refraction.

Chemical or biologic adhesives

An option for strabismus surgery may be the substitution of adhesives for sutures, reducing the time of surgery and inflammatory reaction and avoiding the possibility of perforating the sclera. Adhesives, once in contact with tissue, polymerize and fix the tissues together. Improvements in their quality have reduced tissue reactions to them. Available and widely utilized in ophthalmology and in other medical specialties, there are various available adhesives and others are being developed. They are grouped according to their chemical characteristics:

1. Fibrin sealants.
2. Compounds of albumin.
3. Compounds of gelatin–resorcinol–formaldehyde–glutaraldehyde.
4. Cyanoacrylate.
5. Hydrogels.
6. Compounds of collagen.

In ophthalmology, the most common are cyanoacrylate (chemical) and fibrin (biologic) adhesives. Cyanoacrylates have been used in experiments with extraocular muscles in rabbits[29] and in strabismic human beings.[30,31]

Fibrin, composed of fibrinogen and thrombin, was first used to close corneal wounds in rabbits.[32] It has been used in various experimental and ophthalmologic procedures[33,34] and in strabismus surgery.[35]

Corrêa and Bicas[34] compared the efficacy of sutures of poliglatin-910, cyanoacrylate, fibrin, albumin and glutaraldehyde, and gelatin–resorcinol–formaldehyde–glutaraldehyde. In rabbits, they disinserted the superior rectus and reinserted it with Vicryl® or one of the biologic adhesives. They analyzed:

a. Time of operation.
b. The force required to rupture the muscle–scleral junctions 10 minutes after reinsertion.
c. Postoperative edema, hyperemia, and secretion.
d. Histologic alterations: inflammation, necrosis, granuloma, and fibrosis.

Surgery time was shorter with the biologic adhesives. In resisting rupture of the muscle–scleral junctions, the sutures were best, followed by the adhesive of fibrin and then cyanoacrylate (65%). All the others were deemed not acceptable. On histopathologic examination the fibrin adhesive was best, followed by sutures and then cyanoacrylate. It should be noted that the polymerized product of cyanoacrylate is solid and not absorbable. It may act as an extraneous body that can be extruded. It appears that the fibrin adhesive is the best biologic adhesive for extraocular muscle surgery. However, Moreira et al.[32] reported technical difficulties with its preparation and application. In eyes where the superior rectus was reinserted with the adhesive, limitation of elevation was seen. Perhaps this was due to adherence of the muscles belly to sclera, thus shortening the arc of contact. Another disadvantage is that it is very expensive.

We hope that the technical problems and high price will be solved because of the advantages of biologic adhesives.

Implantable functional electrical stimulation devices to correct strabismus and nystagmus

Replacement of lost ocular rotational forces

The main goal of strabismus treatment is to achieve fusion in primary gaze and in as large as possible field of versions. Cosmetic appearance and stereopsis are secondary goals. In ocular motor palsies, incomitance makes this goal difficult.

An incurable paralysis of the lateral rectus can be improved surgically, eliminating the torticollis, but without satisfactory comitance. Bicas has sought to restore the lost force of such muscles. He tested implantable materials such as silicone elastic bands.[36-40] This was unsuccessful because the elastic resistance to traction increases exponentially as force increases. In the normal physiologic condition, restriction decreases as the opposite muscle contracts. To obviate this problem, he tested the forces generated by magnetic fields. In this situation restriction decreases as the antagonist muscle contracts. This is similar to the normal physiologic mechanics.[40-42]

The magnetic forces act without contact with the eye or the source of generating force. The magnets are made of neodymium, iron, and boron and they generate relatively intense magnetic forces despite their small size. The magnets are fixed to the internal region of the orbital periosteum edge and a metallic plaque is fixed to the sclera (under conjunctiva and Tenon's capsule). This technique appears promising but is still under development.[43]

Velez et al. described an electrical device that can provide direct functional electric stimulation (FES) to a paralyzed muscle.[44] This method has been tested in other situations: paraplegia[45-47] and in axial muscles, such as those in larynx.[48] The principle is to use a normally innervated muscle as a "master" to control a paralyzed "slave" muscle.[43,48] The authors delivered FES to a denervated lateral rectus muscle in cats. They paralyzed a lateral rectus with botulinum toxin and then used the electrical activity of its contralateral synergistic muscle, the contralateral medial rectus, to supply stimulation to the denervated muscle. The authors concluded that artificial stimulation of the lateral rectus muscle is feasible. They demonstrated that eye position can be modified and controlled by modulating stimulation parameters. We hope that in the future patients with lateral rectus palsy can achieve fusion and a broad diplopia free versional field (comitance) with such devices.

A new method for treating nystagmus

Bicas developed a new method to treat nystagmus without impeding eye rotations and without operating on the ocular motor muscles. He concluded that the best method is to employs forces generated by magnetic fields.[49-52] The principle of his method is the implantation of magnets in the periosteum of the orbit underneath its edges, as well as metallic plaques on the sclera in a corresponding position to the magnets. In this way two opposing horizontal forces are created and the eye movement is dampened. In human beings he has eliminated the nystagmus movements without crippling the versions. The method is better than large recession of the four horizontal rectus muscles, which never eliminates totally the movements and often creates an exotropia. Complications involving inflammation and extrusion need to be addressed.

The genetics of strabismus

Strabismus may have a genetic origin, be part of a syndrome, or have an environmental etiology. The identification of its etiology is essential for genetic counseling. In evaluating strabismus it is important to know if it is congenital or acquired in infancy, or later. Is it associated with physical malformations or mental deficiency? Strabismus can be isolated, or a part of a syndrome. There are more than 200 syndromes in which strabismus is an associated finding. One can investigate all the anomalies of genetic origin according to their clinical picture (http://www.ncbi.nlm.nih.gov/omim) or investigate if there is a molecular test for a specific condition (http://www.genetests.org).

Hereditary diseases can be classified according to their etiology as chromosomal, genetic (autosomal dominant, autosomal recessive, X-linked dominant, and X-linked recessive), mitochondrial, or multifactorial. Numeric alterations of chromosomes can occur in any fetus increasing the risk of recurrence in other children. They are associated frequently with maternal advanced age. Several numeric chromosomopathies have strabismus as a component, e.g. Down's syndrome (trisomy 21) or trisomy 8 mosaicism. The structural chromosomopathies (deletions, insertions, duplications, and translocations) may have strabismus as an associated component. It is important to identify a chromosomopathy at the karyotype of the parents, since it may come from a translocation in equilibrium in one of the parents, bringing a risk of chromosomal alteration in future offspring. Structural alterations involving chromosome 8 are frequently associated with strabismus, including Duane's retraction syndrome.

Some examples of genetic anomalies associated with strabismus are spinocerebellar ataxia, CCDD (congenital cranial dysinnervation disorders), Duane's retraction syndrome, and craniosynostosis. Most forms of isolated strabismus are multifactorial: they combine genetic and environmental factors.

Comitant strabismus

The heredity of comitant strabismus can be observed in the varying incidence of each type of strabismus among different races. The prevalence of strabismus is 2–4% in the White population[53-56] and 0.6% among Africans[53,57] and Asiatics.[58,59] Esotropia is more common among North-American and European White people[54,60] and exotropia is more common among North-American and African Blacks and Asiatics.[58-60]

Family and twin studies support the hereditability of comitant strabismus, which shows concordance in 73–82% among monozygotic twins and 35–47 % among dizygotic twins.[60,61] The greater concordance among dizygotic twins compared to siblings likely reflects the importance of environmental factors.[62] In our experience, the incidence of monozygotic twins with esotropia and with exotropia is similar.

In 7100 squint patients from 12 published familial studies 30.6% of them had a close relative with strabismus.[60] Families are generally concordant as to esotropia or exotropia. These data suggest the presence of two common genes, with variable expressivity.[63,64] The relative risk of a first degree relative to be strabismic was estimated to be between 3% and 5%.[65-68] This is the estimated risk of recurrence of multifactorial anomalies for affected first degree relatives.

Some maternal factors can increase the risk of strabismus in her children: advanced maternal age, smoking during pregnancy, and low birth weight (less than 1500 g).[66]

Incomitant strabismus

The congenital cranial dysinnervation disorders

These refer to congenital forms of strabismus, restrictive and not progressive. The most typical is the so-called congenital fibrosis of the extraocular muscles (CFEOM).

The CFEOMs

CFEOM is congenital restrictive ophthalmoplegia affecting mainly the extraocular muscles innervated by the third nerve. There are different forms of CFEOM (CFEOM 1, CFEOM 2, and CFEOM 3), according to their phenotypes and their heredity, which can be autosomal dominant or recessive.

The most typical example is generalized fibrosis (CFEOM 1), with dominant heredity and complete penetrance. There are many examples of families with one of the parents and all offspring affected. The patient presents with congenital non-progressive bilateral ophthalmoplegia and bilateral blepharoptosis. The eyes are infraducted with inability to elevate above the midline. The horizontal position of the eyes can be orthotropia, esotropia or exotropia; the horizontal movements can be normal or restricted.

An autopsy study of CFEOM 1 (with the most common KIF21A mutation) revealed absence of the superior division of the third nerve[69] and hypoplasia of the superior rectus and the levator palpebrae superioris. There were decreased numbers of motor neurons in all the third nerve's subnuclei and the sixth nerve, a decreased diameter of the inferior division of the third nerve, and an increase in central nuclei within myofibers of all oculomotor muscles.[70] These anomalies result from mutations of genes controlling development of oculomotor neurons and their axonal connections which led them to be included in the group of congenital cranial dysinnervation disorders (CCDDs).[71]

The phenotype is variable. In some patients attempted supraversion initiates convergence, probably the result of tentative contraction of the superior recti against the inelastic inferior recti.[72] Perhaps, there is an element of primary muscle fibrosis in addition to the dysinnervation.

Duane's syndrome

Duane's syndrome is the most common of the CCDDs; it represents 1–5% of cases of strabismus.[73] Among 1450 of our consecutive strabismic patients, we found 29 cases of Duane's syndrome (2%).[74] Most cases of Duane's syndrome are sporadic. Two responsible loci have been identified (DURS1 and DURS2). The DURS1, in chromosome 8q13, is associated with sporadic occurrence and other anomalies. Cytogenetic alterations in chromosome 8, including trisomy and translocations, have been reported. DURS2, in 2q31, is associated with cases with autosomal dominant inheritance.[71]

The embryologic molecular basis allows us to understand the interaction between genes and their protein products in the formation of the extraocular nerves and muscles. Prenatal genetic counseling is possible for some genotypes.[71] Engle has stated our hope for the future:[62] "Future studies are also likely to define the genetic defects that place individuals at risk for the common forms of comitant strabismus, since these disorders appear to be inherited as complex genetic traits. Insight into the genetic basis of common strabismus should lead to an improved ability to detect and prevent loss of binocular vision and amblyopia."

Stem cells and strabismus

One of the greatest advances of science in the last few years is the increased understanding of the biology of stem cells. The potential for stem cells to be used for treatment of various disorders is exciting. In ophthalmology, stem cells have been used to treat ocular surface disorders. New clinical and surgical therapies have been developed, resulting in functional recovery of eyes previously untreatable.[75] Advances have also been made in the use of stem cells in the treatment of retinal degenerations in experimental models. Current investigations suggest that stem cells may be useful in treating some human retinal degenerations.[76,77]

A subpopulation of precursor myogenic cells in the extraocular muscles may account for why these muscles are spared from pathology in aging and Duchenne's muscular dystrophy.[78,79] This suggests that this subpopulation of cells is a potential candidate for stem therapy to treat some cases of ocular motor disorders.[79]

In the case of amblyopia, the current lack of knowledge about the precise pathogenic mechanisms and the neural substrates involved is a major obstacle to stem cell therapy being used in its treatment.[76]

References

7. Ribeiro GB, Almeida HC, Velarde DT, et al. Efeito da crotoxina na indução de paralisia muscular em cães. Arq Bras Oftalmol 2009; 72(4 Suppl): 16.

8. Almeida HC, Ribeiro GB, Velarde DT. Estudo da ação da crotoxina aplicada em seres humanos nos músculos extraoculares e faciais. Arq Bras Oftalmol 2009; 72(4 Suppl): 17.

14. Goldchmit M, Scott AB. Avaliação da motilidade extrínseca ocular de pacientes facectomizados sob anesthesia retrobulbar. Arq Bras Oftalmol 1994; 57: 114–6.

15. Scott AB, Alexander DE, Miller JM. Bupivacaine injection of eye muscle to treat strabismus. Br J Ophthalmol 2007; 91: 146–8.

17. Scott AB, Miller JM, Shieh KR. Treating strabismus by injecting the agonist muscle with bupivacaine and the antagonist with botulinum toxin. Trans Am Ophthalmol Soc 2009; 107: 104–9.

18. Gottlob I, Stangler-Zuschrott E. Effect of levodopa on contrast sensitivity and scotomas in human amblyopia. Invest Ophthalmol Vis Sci 1990; 31: 776–80.

20. Leguire LE, Rogers GL, Bremer DL, et al. Levodopa/carbidopa for childhood amblyopia. Invest Ophthalmol Vis Sci 1993; 34: 3090–5.

22. Procianoy E, Fuchs FD, Procianoy L, Procianoy F. The effect of increasing doses of levodopa on children with strabismic amblyopia. J AAPOS 1999; 39: 337–40.

23. Bhartiya P, Sharma P, Biswas NR, et al. Levodopa-carbidopa with occlusion in older children with amblyopia. J AAPOS 2002; 6: 368–72.

28. Rayner JW, Jampolsky A. Management of adult patients with large angle exotropia and amblyopia. Ann Ophthalmol 1973; 5: 95–9.

31. Dunlap EA, Dunn M, Rossomondo R. Adhesives for sutureless muscle surgery. Arch Ophthalmol 1969; 82: 751–5.

33. Moreira ATR, Torres LFB, Scarpi RJ, et al. Uso do adesivo biologico de fibrina para reinserção de músculos retos superiores em coelhos. I – Estudo clinico. Rev Bras Oftalmol 1998; 57: 501–12.

34. Corrêa B, Bicas HE. A study of the applicability of biologic adhesives to the reinsertion of an external ocular muscle in rabbits – I. Experiment I – Measurements of duration of procedures and clinical and histopathologic studies. Arq Bras Oftalmol 2005; 68: 101–7.

40. Bicas HEA. Replacement of ocular rotational forces. In: Scott AB, editor. Proceedings of the Mechanics of Strabismus Symposium, October 18–19, 1991. San Francisco: The Smith-Kettlewell Eye Research Institute; 1991: 2269–85.

41. Bicas HEA. Studies for obtaining conjugate eye movements in cases of oculomotor paralysis. In: Prieto-Díaz J, editor. XII Congreso del Consejo Latinoamericano de Estrabismo. Buenos Aires; 1996: 551–5.

44. Velez FG, Isobe J, Zealear D, et al. Toward an implantable electrical stimulation device to correct strabismus. J AAPOS 2009; 13: 229–35.

50. Abreu SLD, Bicas HEA. Magnetic forces for stabilization of ocular positions and movements. Experimental studies of a method. In: Scott AB, editor. Festchrift for Arthur Jampolsky. San Francisco: The Smith-Kettlewell Eye Research Institute; 2000: 177.

54. Nordloew W. Squint: the frequency of onset at different ages and the incidence of associated defects in a Swedish population. Acta Ophthalmol (Copenh) 1964; 42: 1015–37.

55. Molnar L. On the heredity of squinting [in German]. Klin Monatsbl Augenheilkd 1967; 150: 557–68.

56. Abrahamsson M, Magnusson G, Sjostrand J. Inheritance of strabismus and the gain of using heredity to determine populations at risk of developing strabismus. Acta Ophthalmol Scand 1999; 77: 653–7.

57. Holm S. Le strabisme concomitant chez les palenegrides au Gabon, Afrique equatoriale francaise. Acta Ophthalmol (Copenh) 1939; 17: 367–87.

58. Ing M, Pang S. The Racial Distribution of Strabismus. New York, NY: Grune & Stratton; 1978.

60. Paul TO, Hardage LK. The heritability of strabismus. Ophthalmic Genet 1994; 15: 1–18.

62. Engle E. Genetic basis of congenital strabismus. Arch Ophthalmol 2007; 125: 189–95.

63. Maumenee I, Alston A, Mets M, et al. Inheritance of congenital esotropia. Trans Am Ophthalmol Soc 1986; 34: 85–93.

65. Scott MH, Noble AG, Raymond WR, Parks MM. Prevalence of primary monofixation syndrome in parents of children with congenital esotropia. J Pediatr Ophthalmol Strabismus 1994; 31: 298–302.

66. Chew E, Remaley NA, Tamboli A, et al. Risk factors for esotropia and exotropia. Arch Ophthalmol 1994; 112: 1349–55.

70. Engle EC, Goumnerov BC, McKeown CA, et al. Oculomotor nerve and muscle abnormalities in congenital fibrosis of the extraocular muscles. Ann Neurol 1997; 41: 314–3.

73. Kirkham TH. Inheritance of Duane's syndrome. Br J Ophthalmol 1970; 54: 323–9.

75. Ricardo JR, Gomes JAP. Use of stem cells cultured ex vivo for ocular surface reconstruction. Arq Bras Oftalmol 2010; 73: 541–7.

79. Kallestad KM, Hebert SL, McDonald AA, et al. Sparing of extraocular muscle in aging and muscular dystrophies: a myogenic precursor cell hypothesis. Exp Eye Res 2011; 317: 873–85.

Access the complete reference list online at
http://www.expertconsult.com

Part 1
The fundamentals of strabismus and amblyopia

Amblyopia management

Michael X Repka

Chapter contents

Amblyopia is the most common cause of visual impairment in children: it often persists into adulthood. The prevalence in childhood is estimated to be 1–4%. It is considered to be the leading cause of monocular vision loss in the 20- to 70-year-old age group.[1] The prevalence of visual loss from amblyopia was 2.9% in one study of adults, indicating the need for improved treatment.[2] Amblyopia is defined as a "decrease of visual acuity caused by pattern vision deprivation or abnormal binocular interaction for which no causes can be detected by the physical examination of the eye and which, in appropriate cases, is reversible by therapeutic measures."[3] Amblyopia may be unilateral or less often bilateral.

Most cases are associated with eye misalignment, usually esotropia in infancy or early childhood, others with anisometropia, or a combination of strabismus and anisometropia (Table 70.1).

Visual loss in amblyopia varies from mild to severe. About 25% of cases have visual acuity worse than 6/30 and about 75% 6/30 or better.[4,6-8] The extent of the deficit may not be equivalent, but vary by cause. Strabismic amblyopia may represent a more severe physiologic deficit than isolated anisometropic amblyopia and combined strabismic and anisometropic amblyopia is a more serious deficit still.[9]

Table 70.1 – Association of amblyopia with strabismus and/or amblyopia

	Woodruff et al.[4]	Shaw et al.[5]
Number of cases	961	1531
Strabismus as the cause	57%	45%
Anisometropia as the cause	17%	17%
Combined strabismus and anisometropia	27%	35%

Precise percentages vary depending on how amblyopia is defined.

Methods of detection

The gold standard for detection is measurement of visual acuity using a crowded or linear letter optotype test. Single optotype presentation and picture optotypes are less sensitive and should be used only when a child is unable to perform a test using surrounded or line optotypes. Tests based on the four letters "H", "O", "T", and "V" in a box or with contour surround bars are the basis of several popular test strategies.[10,11] A defined protocol for testing children with single-surround HOTV has been developed by the Pediatric Eye Disease Investigator Group.[11] The strategy includes a second chance at threshold determination and a portion designed to get the child back on track with some larger above threshold stimuli. It has good testability, test–retest reliability, and has been automated.[12]

For children unable to perform with letter optotypes, clinicians have commonly used picture optotypes. However, standard picture optotypes overestimate the visual acuity of amblyopic eyes and are not recommended for screening or diagnosis of amblyopia. Dr. Lea Hyvärinen designed four picture-like optotypes[13] to have similarities between optotypes and have contours like the Landolt C making them more difficult to successfully recognize. The objects (apple, circle, house, square) chosen are common in Western children's experience and eliminate cultural biases in that population. In one study the single-surrounded Lea tests systematically overestimated acuity by 1.9 lines compared to the crowded Landolt C in normal eyes.[14] A comparison of the Lea symbols to line optotypes in amblyopic eyes has not been thoroughly studied.

Fixation preference testing may be used for children unable to perform any optotype-based testing. For strabismic children the clinician compares the ability to hold fixation with each eye. The child may alternate, be unable to hold fixation after a blink, or be unable to hold fixation. For a patient with no misalignment, the test is performed by placing a 10 diopter prism base down before one eye, having the child fixate a detailed target at distance or near, and assessing fixation preference. If there is a fixation preference for the eye without the prism, switch the prism to the fellow eye and again assess fixation preference. The prism might cause the other eye to be preferred. If the same eye is preferred under each testing condition, then the fellow eye is assumed to have amblyopia. A patient who fixates with the eye without the prism is alternating. Amblyopia therapy may be prescribed for a definite fixation preference as discussed in the sections on treatment. Comparing fixation preference testing to optotype testing has shown fixation preference testing is unreliable as a means of diagnosing amblyopia, generally leading to an over-diagnosis of amblyopia. Optotype testing confirmed only 17 of 52 patients (33%) diagnosed with amblyopia by fixation preference testing.[15] In another study 53 children had two or more lines of difference in visual acuity, yet 45 were graded as normal by fixation preference.

Forced choice preferential looking using Teller acuity cards has been used as an alternative method for infants and non-verbal infants.[16] This test is time consuming and requires an experienced tester to assure reliable results. Unfortunately, this test systematically underestimates amblyopia, reducing its clinical utility as a means of screening or detecting a successful treatment endpoint.[17]

Methods of treatment

There are few data comparing the outcomes of amblyopia treatment to the natural history. Clinicians have noted improvement of acuity when children complied with therapy, but found little improvement when no therapy was actually completed. Simons and Preslan reported that among a case series of amblyopic patients, who were not treated, there was no improvement in visual acuity.[18] However, such a demonstration of improvement in acuity of the amblyopic eye without concurrent untreated or natural history controls is not sufficient to prove a benefit of therapy. This deficiency led to a recommendation in the United Kingdom to stop screening for amblyopia as well as treating it because of a lack of a proven benefit.[19] A recent retrospective, non-randomized study suggested that there is value. A group of strabismic patients with amblyopia were treated with spectacles alone (n=17) or spectacles plus occlusion therapy (n=69).[20] Though both treatments led to improvement, the visual acuity improved more in the patients treated with occlusion.

It is likely that some of the improvement in acuity reported in uncontrolled studies of amblyopia therapy represents a combination of age and learning effects in addition to actual treatment benefit., However, the magnitude of the age and learning effect, which has been reported to be about 0.14 logMAR lines over 6 months in a prospective clinical trial, is far less than the improvement typically reported following treatment of amblyopia.[21]

A randomized clinical trial (Amblyopia Treatment Trial, UK) was undertaken to compare an untreated control group of anisometropic amblyopia with a group of children treated with glasses and a third group treated with glasses and occlusion. This study found slight improvement with about one line between no treatment and treatment with glasses and occlusion.[22] The cause of the visual loss was not known with certainty in each child. In addition, the control group's visual acuity at baseline and at final measurement was without correction, whereas the treatment group was measured with best spectacle correction.

Refractive correction

The initial intervention is always to prescribe any necessary spectacle correction. Logically one should not diagnose amblyopia until refractive correction is prescribed, the glasses obtained, and the visual acuity deficit confirmed with the correction being worn. The precise guidelines for prescribing spectacles for amblyopia vary with clinician's practice and the age of the child, but the clinician should correct any anisometropia of greater than 0.50 D and astigmatism of 1.50 D in any patient in whom amblyopia is suspected. Hypermetropia should be fully corrected in younger strabismic patients and corrected with the plus sphere reduced by up to 1.50 D in orthotropic patients. Myopic errors should be fully corrected during office testing with trial frames to confirm the diagnosis, though the prescribed minus sphere may be cut for infants and toddlers.

When should one start additional therapy such as occlusion? Some clinicians prescribe such therapy immediately, some wait a specified time, others wait until improvement with spectacles alone ceases. Moseley et al. found that 8 of 12 patients prescribed spectacles for the first time improved 3 or more lines in the amblyopic eye.[23] The Pediatric Eye Disease Investigator Group (PEDIG) reported that amblyopia improved in previously untreated anisometropic patients (n=84) with optical correction by at least 2 lines in 77% of the patients and resolved in 27%.[24] Improvement took up to 30 weeks for stabilization. In a pilot project, subjects with strabismic amblyopia experienced similar improvement.

We prefer to prescribe any necessary spectacle correction and then wait for at least 6 weeks to re-evaluate the acuity. A measure of the visual acuity in trial frames when the glasses are prescribed can be helpful in assessing the vision status at the first follow-up visit. As long as the acuity is improving, we continue with just glasses before prescribing additional therapy. This graduated approach is likely to improves patient compliance with each portion of the therapy.

Occlusion therapy

Occlusion therapy has been the mainstay of treatment for a century despite the lack of meaningful data demonstrating its superiority over other modalities. This therapy commonly employs an adhesive patch placed over the fellow eye so that the amblyopic eye must be used. Opinions vary on the number of hours of patching per day that should be prescribed, ranging from a few hours to all waking hours.[1,3,25-28]

Flynn et al. found that the success rates were the same for part-time and full-time occlusion therapy based on reported outcomes in 23 studies.[29] Cleary reported in a very small study that full-time occlusion produced a greater improvement in visual acuity and reduction in interocular difference than part-time occlusion, when the acuity outcome was measured at 6 months.[20]

Several authors have reported significant improvement in visual acuity using brief daily periods of occlusion (20 minutes to 1 hour).[30,31] Campbell et al. noted that 20 minutes per day was effective in improving the vision of 83% of children to 6/12. These authors reported that vision can improve rapidly following brief periods of occlusion, especially when combined with concentration on hard tasks.[32]

The dosages prescribed by clinicians during the last few decades vary greatly and seem to be largely a matter of region or training.[33] For instance, more hours are prescribed in German speaking countries than in the United Kingdom, yet the same outcome is expected.[34] Several clinical trials have evaluated various patching dosages and the outcome of amblyopia treatment.[21,35] These are the Amblyopia Treatment Studies, which are prospective multi-center randomized controlled clinical trials, being conducted by PEDIG in North America. The studies have included only patients with strabismic and anisometropic forms of amblyopia. The first randomized controlled study compared occlusion to atropine treatment. The dosage of occlusion prescribed was a minimum of 6 hours up to full-time, but the investigator chose the actual occlusion dosage. Patients with acuity of 6/24 to 6/30 improved faster when more hours of patching were prescribed, but after 6 months the improvement was not significantly greater than that occurring with fewer hours of patching or with atropine (Fig. 70.1).[35]

Additional prospective randomized trials compared the efficacy of different occlusion dosages. There are two distinct studies, one for moderate amblyopia 6/12 to 6/24, and one for severe amblyopia 6/30 to 6/120, caused by strabismus, anisometropia, or both.[36,37] The studies found that 2 hours of daily patching produces an improvement in visual acuity of similar magnitude to the improvement produced by 6 hours of daily patching in treating moderate amblyopia in children aged 3 to less than 7 years.[36] Each treatment group improved 2.4 lines over 4 months. More interesting was the lack of any benefit in terms of the rate of improvement (Fig. 70.2). The visual acuity gain after 4 months probably does not represent the maximum improvement possible.

The study for severe amblyopia found the improvement in the amblyopic eye acuity from baseline to 4 months averaged 4.8 lines in the 6-hour group and 4.7 lines in the full-time group (P = 0.45).[37] In a recent study, children with severe amblyopia improved a mean of 3.6 lines with just 2 hours of daily patching for 17 weeks.[38]

Children's dislike of occlusion therapy is well known.[39] Reported compliance rates range widely. Parents have used coercion and clinicians have prescribed punitive measures such as elbow splints to enhance compliance. Lack of parental understanding seems to play a large role. In the United Kingdom, failure to comply with the prescribed regimen at least 80% of the time occurred in 54% of patients:[40] the failure to comply related to the parents' lack of understanding that there is a "critical period" for effective therapy.

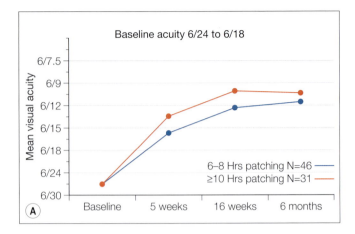

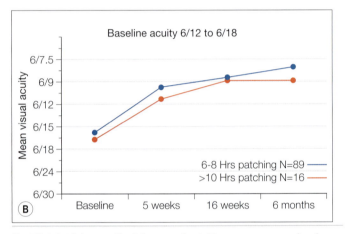

Fig. 70.1 Initial prescribed dosage of patching versus mean visual acuity from a randomized controlled trial.[21] Eighty percent of patients remained on their initial dosage throughout the study. Unsuccessful patients in each subgrouping had patching of 12 or more hours prescribed at the 17-week visit. (A) Patients with amblyopic eye acuity of 6/24 and 6/30. The patients initially treated with 10 or more hours compared to 6 or 8 hours per day had a faster rate of improvement, but by 6 months there was no significant difference in outcome. (B) Patients with amblyopic eye acuity of 6/12 to 6/18. There is no difference in the rate or magnitude of improvement between those initially treated with 10 or more hours compared to those with 6 or 8 hours.

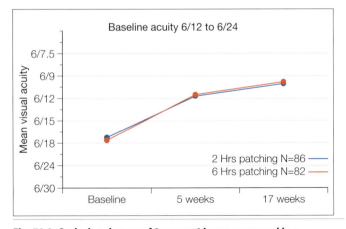

Fig. 70.2 Occlusion dosage of 2 versus 6 hours compared in a randomized controlled trial.[36] No increase in therapy was allowed by the protocol. There was no difference in the rate or magnitude of improvement during the 4 months of prescribed treatment.

Side effects from occlusion are uncommon, usually minor skin irritation or the social stigma of a patch.[21] Adhesive sensitivity to the patches does occur. The clinician should discontinue the patch and treat with an emollient facial cream. Rarely, topical hydrocortisone may be needed.

More serious is occlusion amblyopia, a decrease in vision in the fellow (patched) eye of more than one line. It is more common with more intense therapy and longer treatment intervals, especially if the patient is lost to follow-up. In one prospective study in which the majority of patients were treated with 6 or 8 hours of occlusion per day,[21] only 1 of 204 patients was diagnosed with reverse amblyopia. In most cases occlusion amblyopia is reversible simply by stopping the treatment. Rarely, amblyopia therapy is needed for the originally non-amblyopic eye.

The value of occlusion therapy is well established for anisometropic and strabismic amblyopia. The clinician and the parents should discuss the dosage of occlusion to be prescribed. The number of hours prescribed should be based on many factors including compliance and life-style.

An opaque adhesive patch is the best method currently available. Temperature-sensitive patches to help monitor compliance may be available in the future.[41] Spectacle-mounted patches and non-adhesive patches may be less successful because they are easily removed. Once an occlusion dosage is prescribed, the patient must return for visual acuity monitoring. Traditionally, these intervals have been 1 week per year of age (i.e. a 3-year-old patient would return in 3 weeks). This approach is necessary when full-time occlusion is prescribed, but should be lengthened with part-time occlusion. An initial follow-up interval of 2 months for 2 to 6 hours per day patching is sufficient. If the amblyopic eye has improved and the fellow eye has not been impaired, the treatment interval can be increased. Therapy should be continued until no improvement occurs between two visits. Retesting is warranted to be certain of the lack of improvement.

Most data on the treatment of amblyopia is derived from subjects who have strabismic, anisometropic, or both combined forms of amblyopia. An important group of patients experience form deprivation amblyopia, e.g. from a cataract or media opacity. For these patients, the amblyopia is often severe. Occlusion remains the best choice. The occlusion dosage should be individualized, as there is no treatment trial available to guide the clinician. For patients with unilateral deprivation amblyopia, occlusion dosages of half waking hours are reasonable to avoid damage to the binocular system or to the fellow eye. This dosage can be tapered as the child plateaus to maintain the improvement.

"Penalization" therapy

Penalization is an alternative to occlusion therapy for amblyopia. Both pharmacologic and optical means are used to blur the vision in the better eye for near and/or distance. Penalization was first advocated in 1903 by Worth.[3] However, these approaches have not gained widespread use as a primary treatment modality for amblyopia. Penalization has mainly been employed as a fall-back treatment, for use with occlusion non-compliance, and for post-occlusion maintenance or titration.[3,43-48]

Pharmacologic penalization involves the instillation of a long-acting cycloplegic agent into the fellow eye. Most often atropine has been used, sometimes shorter-acting cycloplegic agents. Cycloplegia prevents accommodation thus blurring the fellow eye at near fixation. The patient uses the amblyopic eye at near. Some clinicians have augmented the therapeutic effect by reducing or removing any plus sphere from the spectacle correction of the fellow eye, effectively blurring the fellow eye at all fixation distances.[49] Pharmacologic penalization has been recommended for moderate amblyopia, but has also been effective for amblyopia 6/30 to 6/60.[44] Compliance with pharmacologic therapy is easier for caregivers: 78% of patients had excellent compliance.[21] The treatment appears to be slower to reach a successful outcome than occlusion, but appears to be equally effective.

Optical penalization involves placement of "plus" fogging lenses over the fellow eye, blurring that eye at near, causing the patient to shift fixation at near to the amblyopic eye. Optical penalization has generally been advocated for only mild amblyopia (20/60 or better).[42,45] The power of the additional plus before the fellow eye may be arbitrarily chosen, usually +2.50 or +3.00 D. It is very convenient for a child wearing bifocals to simply extend the power of the bifocal throughout the entire lens creating an "over-plussed" single vision lens. An alternative is to have the patient fixate a distance vectographic target and increase the plus sphere before the fellow eye until the fixation at distance switches to the amblyopic eye.[42] Compliance is a concern with optical penalization since it is dependent on the child wearing the glasses and not "peeking" around them. For that reason it is a method best reserved for older children and those with milder degrees of amblyopia. The clinician should be prepared to continue this treatment for 2 or more years.

Penalization appears effective because the blur produced selectively removes the high spatial frequency components of the image to the fellow eye, eliminating their suppression of the high spatial frequency components perceived by the cortex responsive to the amblyopic eye.[50] This appears to be critical because amblyopia is a deficit of neuronal responses to high spatial frequencies. With penalization the high spatial frequencies become more dominant in the neurons of the cortex of the amblyopic eye.

Occlusion compared to penalization

Some studies compared penalization and occlusion.[51-53] The first Amblyopia Treatment Study was a randomized controlled trial which enrolled 419 patients comparing occlusion to pharmacologic penalization.[21] Both daily patching (6 or more hours) and daily atropine were effective initial treatments for amblyopia throughout the age range of 3 to less than 7 years old and the acuity range of 20/40 to 20/100. Each method produced nearly the same improvement of about 3 logMAR lines over 6 months. Follow-up through age 10 years found the improvement of the amblyopic eye to be maintained, although residual amblyopia is common.[54] The outcome was similar regardless of initial treatment.

Fogging

An alternative to occlusion or penalization is fogging. This may be done with Bangerter foils, which reduce the visual acuity in the fellow eye. The foils are available in graduated densities. The selected filter may be the one that reduces the fellow eye vision to less than the amblyopic eye. An alternative is to just use the 6/60 (0.1) filter for all patients. A randomized study compared Bangerter filter density of 0.3 (for 6/12–6/18 amblyopic visual acuity) or 0.2 (for 6/24 amblyopic acuity) with patching for 2 hours per day.[55] At 24 weeks, amblyopic eye improvement averaged 1.9 lines in the Bangerter group and 2.3 lines in the patching group. Similar percentages of subjects in each group improved 3 lines (Bangerter group 38% vs. patching group 35%; P = 0.61) or had 6/7.5 amblyopic eye acuity (36% vs. 31%, respectively; P = 0.86).

A readily available and inexpensive alternative is to use an opaque form of adhesive tape placed on the glasses. Each of these is barely visible beyond 0.5 m. This method is ideal for mild visual deficits, long-term maintenance therapy, and in school age children in which compliance with the glasses wear is possible.[56]

Active therapy

Active treatment has been suggested as an important supplement to occlusion therapy. Duke-Elder emphasized the importance of interesting play during occlusion.[57] Physicians have suggested that while patching patients should be involved in some type of activity, which promotes visual interaction. The simplest forms have been home-based activities, performed in conjunction with the occlusion, usually involving activities such as tracing, dot-to-dot tasks, coloring, stringing beads, reading, and playing computer/video games. These therapies may be helpful because they: (1) help overcome compliance problems with occlusion; and (2) may help to improve accommodation and fixation patterns. A study compared 100 patients who were occluded with another 100 who underwent occlusion with active home therapy twice weekly. They achieved the same visual acuities, but the actively stimulated group reached maximum improvement 2 months earlier.[58] Campbell et al. added intensive close work to 20 minutes per day of occlusion and found that 83% of children improved to 6/12.[31] Active therapy has been shown to be helpful when patching alone did not improve the visual acuity. Shippman added 1 hour of video game play to patients previously unsuccessfully treated with occlusion.[59] Fifteen of 19 (78%) had an additional two lines of improvement, and nearly 50% improved by 3 lines of acuity. Similar success in older children has been reported.[60,61] These studies were uncontrolled and do not support or refute the efficacy of this adjuvant therapy.

The Cambridge amblyopic vision stimulator employed more intensive activities.[31] The initial report suggested excellent results. However, subsequent studies included sham visual stimulation arms in which any improvement would be attributed solely to the occlusion. No significant difference in acuity outcomes was found.[62-64]

PEDIG studied adding near activities to a portion of the time patching was prescribed.[65] At 8 weeks, improvement in amblyopic eye visual acuity averaged 2.6 lines in the distance activities group and 2.5 lines in the near activities group.

Systemic therapy

Catecholamine neurotransmitters play a role in maintaining plasticity of the visual cortex during development. The administration of oral levodopa–carbidopa (L-dopa) combination therapy improves the acuity of amblyopic eyes.[66] A standardized dosage regimen is not yet available. When this pharmacologic therapy is combined with occlusion therapy the visual acuity improvement was greater than that with occlusion alone.[67] These studies noted substantial regression after the treatment was stopped, but the outcome acuity was felt to be better when occlusion was combined with L-dopa.[68]

A randomized trial compared L-dopa alone, to L-dopa plus 3 hours per day occlusion, and L-dopa plus occlusion for all waking hours in children with amblyopia.[69] An occlusion only control group was not included. There was no difference in the magnitude of improvement between the three groups. The mean improvement was 1.6 lines. Half of the patients who improved maintained their improvement for 1 year. On the other hand, half of the successful patients experienced a mean 0.8 line regression of acuity after an average of 4 months following treatment. Side effects of nausea, dizziness, decreased respiration, and decreased body temperature have been reported.[70-72]

Citicoline (cytidine-5′-diphosphocholine) may have some success in a study of 50 amblyopic patients.[73] Treatment involved daily intramuscular injections of the medication for 10 days. Both the fellow and amblyopic eyes improved and were stable with 4 months of follow-up. This drug has been less widely used because of the requirement for parenteral administration, but few side-effects have been reported.

The rate of recidivism, the lack of compelling evidence of success greater than that found with conventional treatments, and the use of neuroactive drugs for a condition that does not threaten life or general health make it impossible to recommend systemic therapy at this time.

Combined therapies

Some clinicians simultaneously treat amblyopia with more than one approach. A common approach is to part-time patch and to prescribe topical atropine, thus allowing the child to be continuously treated. The child will use the patch when not in school or at other activities where the patch will not make them self-conscious.

An alternative is to prescribe topical atropine and reduce the plus sphere in the fellow eye to plano (or some other reduction of plus power), thus blurring the fellow eye at all fixation distances.[49] In a randomized trial after 18 weeks of such treatment, amblyopia improvement averaged 2.8 lines in the group that received atropine plus a plano lens and 2.4 lines in the group that received atropine alone.[74] More patients in the group that received atropine plus a plano lens had reduced fellow eye visual acuity at 18 weeks; however, there were no cases of persistent reverse amblyopia. Nonetheless, monitoring these patients for decreased vision in the fellow eye is prudent.

Discontinuation of treatment/ maintenance therapy

Most clinicians stop intensive therapy when the patient no longer shows improvement. However, the duration of treatment before cessation of therapy is unclear but 3 months with no improvement before stopping or reducing therapy is a reasonable approach.

Once therapy is thought to have reached its maximum benefit, I begin to "wean" the patient over months or even a year. I reduce the treatment by 50% every 3 months; this may prevent a recurrence. However, 3 are no data available to prove that weaning is superior to immediate cessation in retaining the treatment benefit. An alternative approach is to carefully follow a child every three months until 7 or 8 years of age without any active treatment besides glasses, but this is inconvenient because of the increased number of visits needed.

The long-term stability of improved acuity in amblyopia therapy is an important public health goal if we are to reduce the high prevalence of amblyopia in adults. The chance of maintaining all, or a portion of, the improvement into adulthood is about 75%.[75-77]

Compliance

Compliance with amblyopia therapy is a key factor in the success of the therapy. However, compliance with occlusion therapy varies widely, from 30% to more than 90%.[20,78-80] The typical reasons for the inability to complete the prescribed occlusion regimen include visual impairment, skin irritation, and psychosocial reasons. Pilot studies of occlusion therapy with occlusion dose monitors have shown the expected correlation of treatment compliance with outcomes.[81,82]

Compliance with topical pharmacologic therapy is simpler, having to put the drop in only once per prescribed day. Compliance was reported to be excellent or good in 96% of patients.[21]

Though children may reject amblyopia therapy, lack of understanding about the disease and the timing of therapy also seem to play a role.[83] Compliance may be improved with better education of the parents and some explanatory materials to take home.[40]

Reverse amblyopia

Reverse amblyopia (occlusion amblyopia) is a form of deprivation amblyopia. It is a reduction of vision in the fellow eye of more than one line due to a treatment prescribed for amblyopia in the fellow eye. Reverse amblyopia has been associated with most forms of therapy of amblyopia. It seems to be most commonly associated with full-time occlusion. It occurs much less often with part-time occlusion and cycloplegic and optical methods of treatment.

Reverse amblyopia generally recovers quickly, though there are reports of permanent visual impairment or change in fixation. Each patient who develops such a reduction in acuity should be reassessed. Confirm that the spectacles are the correct power. Examine the patient for evidence of optic neuropathy including the pupillary light reflex for evidence of an afferent pupil, color vision, and appearance of the optic nerve and nerve fiber layer. Check the refraction with cycloplegia. Retest the vision. If the acuity reduction is confirmed, either stop the active amblyopia therapy and re-examine the patient in several weeks or continue the therapy with careful monitoring of the fellow eye. If the fellow eye is worse than the amblyopic eye, stop therapy and schedule a return visit. If the vision in the fellow eye is still reduced on the subsequent visit, consider treating the formerly fellow eye.

Treatment of adults

Amblyopia therapy is more successful in younger patients, especially when less than 7 years of age. This is consistent with the demonstration of age-specific sensitive periods in neurologic development. Several findings question this tenet. No age effect was found in a retrospective study and in two clinical trials for occlusion and pharmacologic therapy in patients less than 7 years of age.[4,21,25,36] In addition, successful therapy in older patients has been reported,[78] especially in the setting of the loss of vision in the fellow eye from an injury.

PEDIG reported treatment results of older children and adolescents.[84] Improvement with optical correction alone occurred in about a quarter of patients aged 7 to 17 years, although most patients required additional treatment for amblyopia.[84] Most patients were left with a residual visual acuity deficit. For patients aged 7 to 12 years, 2 to 6 hours per day of patching with near visual activities and atropine improved visual acuity even if the amblyopia had been previously treated. For patients aged 13 to 17 years, prescribing patching 2 to 6 hours per day improved visual acuity only when amblyopia had not been previously treated. I conclude that any amblyopic patient who has never been treated should be offered at least one cycle of therapy with this standardized approach of occlusion, pharmacologic, and optical penalization.

References

4. Woodruff G, Hiscox F, Thompson JR, Smith LK. Factors affecting the outcome of children treated for amblyopia. Eye 1994; 8: 627–31.

9. Simons K. Preschool vision screening: rationale, methodology and outcome. Surv Ophthalmol 1996; 41: 3–30.

19. Snowdon SK, Stewart-Brown SL. Preschool vision screening. Health Technol Assess 1997; 1(8)(i-iv): 1–83.

21. Pediatric Eye Disease Investigator Group. A randomized trial of atropine vs patching for treatment of moderate amblyopia in children. Arch Ophthalmol 2002; 120(3): 268–78.

22. Clarke MP, Wright CM, Hrisos S, et al. Randomised controlled trial of treatment of unilateral visual impairment detected at preschool vision screening. BMJ 2003; 327(7426): 1251–55.

24. Pediatric Eye Disease Investigator Group. Treatment of anisometropic amblyopia in children with refractive correction. Ophthalmology 2006; 113(6): 895–903.

28. Scott WE, Stratton VB, Fabre J. Full-time occlusion therapy for amblyopia. Am Orthopt J 1980; 30: 125–30.

35. Pediatric Eye Disease Investigator Group. A comparison of atropine and patching treatments for moderate amblyopia by patient age, cause of amblyopia, depth of amblyopia, and other factors. Ophthalmology 2003; 110(8): 1632–8.

36. Pediatric Eye Disease Investigator Group. A randomized trial of patching regimens for treatment of moderate amblyopia in children. Arch Ophthalmol 2003; 121(5): 603–11.

37. Pediatric Eye Disease Investigator Group. A randomized trial of prescribed patching regimens for treatment of severe amblyopia in children. Ophthalmology 2003; 110(11): 2075–87.

39. Pediatric Eye Disease Investigator Group. Impact of patching and atropine treatment on the child and family in the amblyopia treatment study. Arch Ophthalmol 2003; 121(11): 1625–32.

47. Lithander J, Sjostrand J. Anisometropic and stabismic amblyopia in the age group 2 years and above: a prospective study of the results of treatment. Br J Ophthalmol 1991; 75: 111–6.

49. Kaye SB, Chen SI, Price G, et al. Combined optical and atropine penalization for the treatment of strabismic and anisometropic amblyopia. J AAPOS 2002; 6: 289–93.

54. Pediatric Eye Disease Investigator Group. A randomized trial of atropine vs patching for treatment of moderate amblyopia: follow-up at age 10 years. Arch Ophthalmol 2008; 126(8): 1039–44.

55. Pediatric Eye Disease Investigator Group. A randomized trial comparing Bangerter filters and patching for the treatment of moderate amblyopia in children. Ophthalmology 2010; 117(5): 998–1004.

65. Pediatric Eye Disease Investigator Group. A randomized trial of near versus distance activities while patching for amblyopia in children aged 3 to less than 7 years. Ophthalmology 2008; 115(11): 2071–8.

68. Leguire LE, Komaromy KL, Nairus TM, et al. Long-term follow-up of L-dopa treatment in children with amblyopia. J Pediatr Ophthalmol Strabismus 2002; 39: 326–30.

74. Pediatric Eye Disease Investigator Group. Pharmacological plus optical penalization treatment for amblyopia: results of a randomized trial. Arch Ophthalmol 2009; 127(1): 22–30.

76. Leiba H, Shimshoni M, Oliver M, et al. Long-term follow-up of occlusion therapy in amblyopia. Ophthalmology 2001; 108(9): 1552–5.

80. Parkes LC. An investigation of the impact of occlusion therapy on children with amblyopia, its effect on their families, and compliance with treatment. Br Orthopt J 2001; 58: 30–7.

81. Moseley MJ, Fielder AR, Irwin M, et al. Effectiveness of occlusion therapy in ametropic amblyopia: a pilot study. Br J Ophthalmol 1997; 81: 956–61.

83. Newsham D. Parental non-concordance with occlusion therapy. Br J Ophthalmol 2000; 84: 957–62.

84. Pediatric Eye Disease Investigator Group. A prospective, pilot study of treatment of amblyopia in children 10 to <18 years old. Am J Ophthalmol 2004; 137(3): 581–3.

Access the complete reference list online at

http://www.expertconsult.com

The physiologic anatomy of eye muscles and the surgical anatomy of strabismus

Alejandra de Alba Campomanes

Chapter contents

Introduction

The rational diagnosis of strabismus and its surgical correction requires knowledge of the anatomy of the extraocular muscles and their relationships with other tissues in the orbit. This chapter summarizes the extraocular and orbital anatomy and their surgical applications. Complex theories on the ocular motor physiology and mechanics of the extraocular movements are beyond the scope of this chapter. The traditional, albeit simplistic, description of the extraocular muscle straight-line paths and gaze-determined functions are included because of their didactic value; more modern models of ocular rotations and their clinical applications are briefly reviewed.

The extraocular muscles

The six extraocular muscles (EOMs) form the effector arm of the ocular motor system which is a set of five distinct eye movement control systems (saccades, pursuits, vergences, and vestibulo-ocular and optokinetic reflexes). A common "motor plant" to all these different subsystems comprised the EOMs, motor neurons, the globe, and the orbital connective tissue. The muscles are organized as "yoked pairs" that require precise coordination to maintain binocular fixation on visual targets. These muscles are highly specialized and functionally diverse with distinct biochemical, physiologic, and pathologic properties. The medial rectus (MR) and the lateral rectus (LR) muscles rotate the eye horizontally; adduction is accomplished by the MR and abduction by the LR. The two vertical rectus muscles and the two oblique muscles have more complex actions that depend on the direction of gaze and will be detailed later. The gaze position determines the effect of EOM contraction on the rotation of the globe. When the eye is in the primary position, more than 70% of the ocular motor neurons are active with an average firing rate of approximately 100 Hz;[1] 18% of motor neurons never cease firing for any eye position.[2] This activity level is not common in other motor systems.

During embryogenesis, mesodermal primordia condense around the developing eye and proceed through the same myogenetic steps of other skeletal muscles. However, unlike skeletal muscles, the EOMs retain "developmental" protein isoforms, including embryonic myosin, and fetal acetylcholine receptor. The expression of these alternative proteins may underlie the susceptibility of the EOMs to disorders such as Graves' disease and myasthenia gravis and their resistance to disorders such as muscular dystrophy. The EOMs have an enhanced antioxidant capacity and a substantial calcium sequestration capacity that protects them from toxic agents that act via increases in intracellular calcium concentrations, as well as other distinct functional and metabolic characteristics.[3]

Each EOM comprised two distinct layers subserving different functions (laminar specialization). The global layer is adjacent to the globe in the rectus muscles; in the oblique muscles, it is located in the central core of the muscle. The global layer continues to the terminal tendon of the EOMs that insert on the sclera. The global layer contains three types of muscle fibers. The orbital layer is the outer component, concentric only in the oblique muscles. It does not continue onto the tendon to insert on the sclera. It contains two types of muscle fibers.

The EOMs do not conform to traditional classifications of muscle fiber types which are based on the expression of myosin isoforms. EOMs are unique in that they possess different types of muscle cells. Each muscle cell is composed of groups of myofibrils called sarcomeres. A sarcomere is the major structural and functional unit of striated muscle. Actin and myosin arrangement results in a banding pattern seen by electron microscopy. Muscle contractions take place when myosin and actin filaments are actively moved past each other as a result of release of calcium by the sarcoplasmic reticulum. Fast twitch ("fibrillenstruktur") muscle fibers generate fast eye movements and are composed of well-defined myofibrils with well-developed sarcomeres. "Felderstruktur" muscle fibrils generate slow or tonic eye movements and are composed of poorly developed sarcomeres. Cholinergic motor neurons supply both types of muscle fibers. The innervation of fibrillenstruktur fibrils is thick and heavily myelinated, with a single neuromuscular junction, whereas the innervation of felderstruktur fibrils is thin, with multiple grapelike clusters of neuromuscular junctions. The previous histologic classification of human EOMs has now been replaced by a more complex system based on global and orbital layer distribution, innervation status (single vs. multiple nerve contacts per fiber), and mitochondrial/oxidative enzyme content.[3] Using this classification, five distinct EOM fiber types are identified:

1. Orbital singly innervated fibers (SIFs).
2. Orbital multiply innervated fibers (MIFs).
3. Global red (coarse) SIFs.
4. Global pale (granular) SIFs.
5. Global MIFs.

The predominant fiber in the orbital layer is the fast, twitching-generating, SIF type. These fibers are specialized for intense oxidative metabolism and fatigue resistance and are high in mitochondrial content. Twenty percent of the fibers are multiply innervated non-twitch fibers.[4] It has been proposed that the role of these fibers is proprioception. Many individual muscle fibers do not extend the entire length of the muscle; only a few of the SIFs extend through the entire length of the muscle in the global layer. MIFs run the entire length of the muscle, even extending into the distal tendon. The orbital layer fibers are smaller and shorter than the global layer fibers. All fibers are active at all times and are recruited differentially during different ocular movements.[5] MIFs are responsible for tonic activity; SIFs are responsible for generating most of the force needed to generate a saccade, but they also have roles in fixation and pursuit movements.

The functional heterogeneity of the EOMs is manifest in the myosin heavy chain phenotype of the EOMs. In contrast to skeletal muscles, embryonic myosin isoforms are retained throughout life in orbital layer fibers of the EOMs. In mature EOMs, the fibers of the orbital layer are heterogeneous in their expression of developmental myosin isoforms, with the highest levels in the proximal and distal regions of each fiber.[6] The normal development of the orbital SIFs is dependent on environmental cues during the critical periods of vision development. Early visual stimulus has an important regulatory influence in the myosin expression patterns of the EOMs and shape EOM maturation.[7,8]

Aside from the pulling power that results from the contraction of the EOMs, there are other factors that influence the motility of the eye. The orbital adipose, connective tissue, and the EOMs enable the eye to rotate rapidly, precisely, and in coordination. The nature and arrangement of the non-muscular tissues surrounding the EOMs is essential. It is because of its relationships with the connective tissues that the eye rotates within the orbit instead of shifting. The primary position tone of the horizontal recti is about 8 g; it is 6 g for the vertical recti and 4 g for the obliques.

The EOMs are encased in individual capsules and interconnected by connective tissue (intermuscular septa) and fixed to the orbit at different sites. The annulus of Zinn is the origin of the four rectus muscles. It encircles the optic foramen and a portion of the sphenoid fissure. The medial portion of the annulus of Zinn originates from Lockwood's (superior) tendon that inserts in the body of the sphenoid bone and gives rise to the superior rectus, MR, and portions of the LR. The inferior tendon of Zinn is inserted in the minor sphenoid wing between the optic foramen and the sphenoid fissure, and gives rise to the inferior rectus and parts of the MR and LR muscles. The lateral part of the annulus inserts in the spina rectus lateralis, on the inferior portion of the sphenoid fissure and it is related to the origin of the LR and portions of the superior and inferior rectus. The MR and superior rectus common origin is firmly adhered to the dural sheath of the optic nerve which explains why patients with optic neuritis experience pain with eye movements.

Because strabismus surgery uses millimetric grading, strabismus surgeons pay special attention to the exact location of the insertion sites of the EOMs and their relationship with respect to each other. Starting from the MR the progressive insertion distance with respect to the limbus of the rectus muscle tendons on the sclera has been depicted by a continuous curved line (the spiral of Tillaux). These distances are highly variable[9-13] (Fig. 71.1) and knowledge of normal range rather than a fixed number is essential (Fig. 71.2) (Table 71.1).

Helveston measured the insertion distance of the MR in 114 eyes and found a range between 3 and 6 mm, with an average of 4.4 mm.[18] Kushner and Morton measured the distance from the limbus to the MR insertion in 80 eyes and found the range was between 3.5 and 5.5 mm, with an average of 4.3 mm.[11] Keech measured 40 eyes of patients 10–30 months old with esotropia; the range was 5–6 mm (5.5 average). After

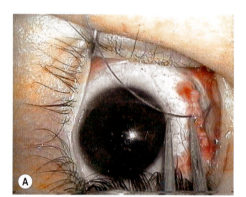
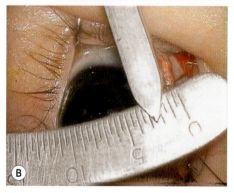

Fig. 71.1 Anterior insertion on the medial rectus.
(Photos courtesy of Dalal Shawky, MD.)

Table 71.1 – Topographic characteristics of the EOMs (all distances are in millimeters)[9,10,14-17]

	Muscle length	Tendon length	Average insertion width (range)	Average insertion distance from limbus	Insertion range	Arc of contact	Relationships
Medial rectus (MR)	39	3.7–4.5	10.5 (9.6–13.3)	5.5	3.0–6.75	6.0–7.0	Distance between inferior edge of MR insertion and nasal edge of IR insertion is 6 mm
Inferior rectus (IR)	40	5.5–7.0	10.2 (8.8–12.8)	6.5*	4.0–7.5	6.5	Distance between the lateral edge of the IR insertion and the inferior edge of the LR insertion is 8 mm
Lateral rectus (LR)	41	7.0–8.8	9.5 (8.3–12.5)	7.0	4.0–8.0	7.0–12.0	Distance between the superior edge of the LR insertion and the temporal edge of the SR insertion is 7 mm
Superior rectus (SR)	41	6.0	11.0 (9.8–14.0)	7.7*	5.0–9.0	6.5	Distance between medial edge of SR insertion and superior edge of MR insertion is 7.5 mm
Superior oblique (SO)	32	26 mm	10.6 (9.0–13)	13.0**	10.5–16	7.0–8.0	Average distance between lateral end of SR and anterior end of SO is 4.0 mm (1.5–7 mm)
Inferior oblique (IO)	38	0–2.0	9.6	15.5***	10–18	15.0	Average distance between inferior insertion of LR and anterior edge of IO insertion is 9.5 mm. The insertion of the IO is 2 mm above the inferior margin of the LR

*From anterior limbus to midpoint of the muscle insertion.
**From limbus to anterior end of superior oblique insertion (limbus to superior rectus insertion + lateral edge of superior rectus to anterior end of superior oblique).
***From limbus to anterior end of inferior oblique (limbus to lateral rectus insertion + inferior end of lateral rectus + to anterior end of inferior oblique).

disinserting the muscle, a movement of 1.2 mm on average toward the limbus was observed (0.5–2 mm).[12]

Axial length and age have been hypothesized as explanatory variables for anatomic variation and response to surgical dosages.[19] Apt studied 100 cadaver eyes and failed to find a relationship between axial length and the EOM insertion distances. However, the age range was 21–90 years (average 60 years) therefore excluding children with immature structures and axial lengths less than 23 mm.[9,15]

The width of the muscle insertions (Table 71.1) is important when considering rectus muscle displacements and transpositions. "Full tendon-width" or "half tendon-width" are terms that are used for the surgical titration of these operations (usually 5 and 10 mm, respectively). However, full width transpositions are practically impossible without impinging on adjacent muscles.[9]

The EOMs are richly vascularized compared to skeletal muscles (Fig. 71.3). Two branches of the ophthalmic artery provide the blood supply to the EOMs: the lateral muscular branch and medial muscular branch. The LR, superior rectus (SR) and the superior oblique (SO) are supplied by the lateral muscular branch; the MR, inferior rectus (IR) and inferior oblique (IO) receive their blood supply from the medial muscular branch. The muscular branches give rise to the anterior ciliary arteries that pass from the muscle to the episclera and are responsible for the blood supply of the anterior segment of the eye. With the exception of the LR, all the EOMs have two ciliary arteries. Supplementary blood supply to the LR comes from the lacrimal artery and the infraorbital artery, which also supplies the IO and IR. When strabismus surgery involves several EOMs, the anterior segment circulation can be compromised. The venous system parallels the arterial system and empties in the superior and inferior orbital veins. The inferior and superior temporal vortex veins are important structures to be aware of during strabismus surgery. The inferior temporal vortex vein is located 8 mm posterior and temporal to the IR insertion. The superior temporal vortex vein is located near the posterior edge of the SO tendon insertion under the SR.

The EOMs are innervated at a ratio of nerve fiber to muscle fiber of up to 10 times that of skeletal muscles. However, sensory innervation of the EOMs is scant. There is no temperature, sharp, or puncture sensation, which allows strabismus surgery under topical anesthesia. However, ischemia and traction are perceived; these maneuvers should be avoided during topical surgery and adjustable strabismus surgery.

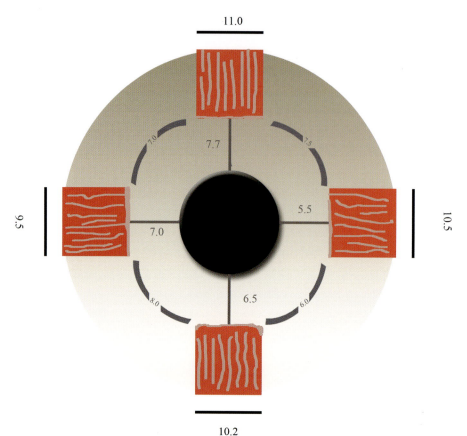

Fig. 71.2 Eye muscle distances.

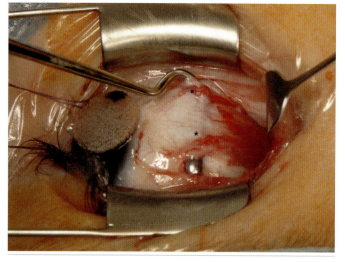

Fig. 71.3 Medial rectus muscle with two robust anterior ciliary arteries.
(Photo courtesy of Tina Rutar, MD.)

Medial rectus muscle

The medial rectus (MR) has its origin at the annulus of Zinn and travels anteriorly along the medial orbital wall to insert in the nasal sclera 3–6 mm posterior to the limbus. Because the MR travels close to the medial orbital wall, it can be injured during ethmoid sinus surgery. The width of the MR insertion is 9–11 mm and its tendon is 4–6 mm long. The total length of the muscle is 40 mm. The MR is innervated by the inferior branch of cranial nerve (CN) III that enters the muscle on its internal surface at the junction of the mid and posterior thirds. In the primary position, the arc of contact of the MR is approximately 5 mm.

Lateral rectus muscle

The lateral rectus (LR) courses 40 mm from the annulus of Zinn along the lateral orbital wall to its insertion on the temporal sclera 6–9 mm from the limbus by means of a very long (8–10 mm) and thin tendon. The width of the insertion ranges between 7 and 9 mm. Its arc of contact with the sclera in the primary position is approximately 7–8 mm. Innervation to the LR is supplied by CN VI.

Superior rectus muscle

The superior rectus (SR) travels from its origin in the annulus of Zinn, 40 mm to its insertion in the superior sclera 7–9 mm from the limbus. The width of the insertion is between 9 and 12 mm, and it is slanted such that the medial edge is closer to the limbus and the lateral insertion is located more posteriorly. The length of its tendon is 6 mm approximately. The SR is innervated by the superior division of the CN III. The muscle trajectory is directed forward, lateral and upward, forming an angle of 23° with respect to the anteroposterior axis of the globe. This angulation explains the variations of the vertical movement of the eye when the SR contracts in different horizontal starting positions, with pure elevation occurring if the movement starts at 23° in abduction. At the theoretical 67° of adduction (the globe usually can only be moved 50° in each horizontal direction) the resulting movement would be of pure intorsion. From the primary position the actions of the

SR are elevation and intorsion, and slight adduction; as the eye moves into adduction the SR becomes more of an adductor and incycloductor and less of an elevator.

The SR is intimately linked to the levator by way of a common fascial sheath. Because of this relationship between the levator and the SR, pseudo-ptosis is frequently associated with hypotropia. Large recessions or resections of the SR can produce retraction of the upper lid or ptosis, respectively.

Inferior rectus muscle

The inferior rectus (IR) courses forward 42 mm from the orbital apex to its insertion on the sclera 6–8 mm from the inferior limbus. Its tendon measures approximately 6 mm and is 8–10 mm wide. Its scleral insertion is also slanted with a difference of 2 mm between the anterior medial insertion and the posterior lateral edge. Since the muscle is directed at a 23° angle with respect to the anteroposterior axis of the globe, pure depression occurs when the muscle contracts at 23° of abduction. Pure extorsion would occur if the eye were rotated to 67° of adduction; between these two points the functions of the IR are depression, adduction, and excyclotorsion. Innervation to the IR is supplied by the inferior division of CN III.

The IR is connected to the lower eyelid tarsus by way of the capsulopalpebral ligament and the eyelid retractors. Recession of the IR can cause widening of the palpebral fissure; resection can elevate the lower lid and narrow the palpebral fissure. The capsulopalpebral fascia of the lower lid arises 5 mm from the insertion of the IR, splits to surround the IO, and condenses anteriorly to it forming Lockwood's ligament. Anterior to Lockwood's ligament the fascia thickens forming the inferior tarsal muscle which inserts into the lower lid tarsus.

Superior oblique muscle

The superior oblique (SO) muscle arises from the periosteum of the lesser wing of the sphenoid bone above the annulus of Zinn. It courses superomedially parallel to the medial wall of the orbit in its own adipose tissue compartment for approximately 40 mm to reach the trochlea. The trochlea is a saddle-shaped cartilage attached to the frontal bone in the superonasal orbit.[20] The SO tendon is reflected and redirected posteriorly at an angle of 55° with respect to the medial wall of the orbit. The SO tendon is the longest of the EOM tendons. It starts 10 mm behind the trochlea and measures approximately 18–20 mm. The reflected tendon becomes sub-Tenon's 2–3 mm nasal to the medial border of the SR muscle and passes beneath the SR 3–5 mm posterior to its medial insertion point when the eye is in primary position. When the globe is rotated downward, the SO tendon moves 8 mm posterior to the SR insertion (Fig. 71.4). The SO tendon spreads like a fan under the SR to insert in the sclera, following a concave line 10–12 mm in length. The anterior end lies 4 mm posterior to the lateral insertion of the SR and its most posterior portion ends 5–6.5 mm from the optic nerve, temporal to the superior temporal vortex vein. This broad insertion would pull the eye down if the starting gaze position is 55° of adduction and incyclotorsion results if the eye movement starts at 39° from abduction. When the movement starts from the primary position there is a combined incyclotorsion and depression plus slight abduction. The extension and angle of the SO insertion are extremely variable. In addition, the SO tendon is often anomalous. It can be redundant or lax, misdirected, absent, or

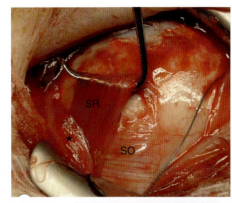

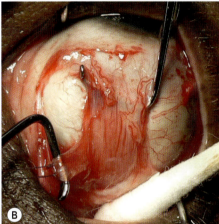

Fig. 71.4 Relationship between superior rectus muscle and superior oblique tendon (surgeon's view). (A) The superior oblique insertion can be seen under the superior rectus muscle (isolated with a muscle hook) of this right eye. (B) The superior rectus and the superior oblique are isolated on muscle hooks and there is a suture on nasal side of the superior oblique tendon.

have anomalous insertion nasal to the SR or into Tenon's capsule.[21,22]

The SO is innervated by CN IV. The insertion of the nerve into the muscle is exceptional in that it is not on the internal surface but on the orbital side of the muscle. The anterior half of the reflected SO tendon has the greatest intorsion function. The posterior half primarily has a depression function. This "division of labor" of the SO fibers is the basis for the surgery described by Harada and Ito that displaces the anterior half of the tendon anteriorly to enhance the intorsion function of the muscle to correct excyclotropia.[23] Conversely, posterior tenotomy of the SO selectively weakens its vertical action. This technique can be used to treat A-pattern deviations without inducing torsional diplopia.

The posterior edge of the SO tendon is intimately linked to the undersurface of the overlying SR muscle by thin, translucent adventitial connections (the SR frenulum).[24] This frenulum is optimally positioned to couple the movement of the SO tendon with that of the SR muscle, causing the SO tendon to move posteriorly when the SR muscle is recessed. It constrains the amount of recession that can be obtained with a suspension technique because the SR does not take up the slack in large recessions (10–14 mm) if the frenulum is left intact.

Inferior oblique muscle

The inferior oblique (IO) arises from the periosteum of the maxillary bone, just posterior to the orbital rim and lateral to the lacrimal fossa in the anterior nasal orbital floor. The tubular muscle travels laterally and posterior underneath the IR to

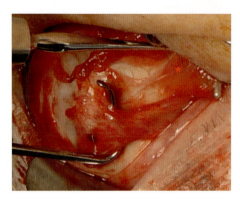

Fig. 71.5 Insertion of the inferior oblique under the lateral rectus muscle (surgeon's view).

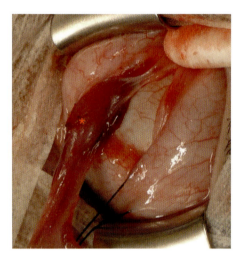

Fig. 71.6 The inferior oblique disinserted from the sclera showing the insertion of the neurofibrovascular bundle in the posterior lateral border (surgeon's view).

insert on the sclera under the LR muscle just anterior to the macula (Fig. 71.5) forming a 51° angle with the anteroposterior axis of the globe in primary position. Contraction of the IO would produce only extorsion if the starting position of the movement is 39° relative to the anteroposterior axis and only elevation if the starting point is 51° of adduction. In primary position, the resulting movement of IO contraction is excyclotorsion, elevation, and slight abduction.

The IO penetrates Tenon's capsule near the ventral surface of the IR. Its length is 37 mm; its short tendon measures 1–2 mm. The IO is innervated by the inferior branch of CN III, which enters the muscle 14–15 mm from its insertion along the posterior lateral border on its global (scleral) side accompanied by an artery and vein (the neurovascular bundle) (Fig. 71.6). The parasympathetic innervation of the pupillary sphincter and the ciliary muscle travels with this branch of the CN III that supplies the IO. These parasympathetic fibers may be injured during IO surgery or orbital floor surgery.

The neurovascular bundle of the IO has a linear course in the orbit, from the apex to the IO muscle, just lateral to the IR. Its anterior portion has a fibrocollagenous capsule with the collagen fibers aligned parallel to the bundle; fibrous bands extend posteriorly to join the IO and IR muscle capsules. This structure has ligamentous characteristics. Stager described the neuro(fibro)-vascular bundle (NFVB) of the IO as its ancillary origin becoming the functional insertion of the IO muscle after anterior transposition and pre-equatorial recessions.[25-28] The NFVB holds the posterior portion of the IO fixed within the orbit; elevation function of the IO is restricted following anterior transposition because of this ligamentous quality. Severing

this bundle causes the muscle to snap forward; denervation is required for total sub-Tenon's dissection of the muscle.

Orbital connective tissue

Although it has been argued that strabismus surgeons regard extraocular connective tissue as a "nuisance" and "mechanically irrelevant,"[29] the importance of the relationship between the eye and other orbital contents for ocular motility has long been recognized.[30,31] Parks and others recognized that "the manner in which muscles are connected between the eye and the orbit and the relationship of their surrounding fascia determine the mechanical features that both produce and limit the motility of the globe."[17] The understanding of the exact role and composition of these structures continues to evolve and it is clear that the study of strabismus and its anatomy should not be limited to the EOMs but should include the biomechanical role of the supporting orbital tissue.[32]

Tenon's capsule (fascia bulbi) is a dense, white, relatively avascular layer composed of collagen, elastic, and smooth muscle fibers. It extends from the limbus to the optic nerve. Tenon's capsule covers the anterior portion of the muscles from their scleral insertion to the posterior edge of the globe where the muscles penetrate Tenon's somewhere between 5 and 15 mm posterior to their insertion. The four rectus muscles penetrate Tenon's capsule posterior to the equator of the globe; the two oblique muscles penetrate it anterior to the equator. The function of Tenon's capsule is essential. The sleeve that it forms around the muscles creates a zone of strong capsular-muscular adherence, which is also suspended to the periosteum of the orbit.[31]

The muscle capsule is a layer of connective tissue firmly adherent to the perimysium. This capsule is essential for the integrity of the muscle's vasculature. The intermuscular septum is an avascular sheet that connects the muscle capsule of adjacent EOMs. Anterior to the muscle insertions, the intermuscular septum lies underneath Tenon's capsule, becoming two distinct layers a few millimeters behind the muscle insertions. It continues posteriorly accompanying the muscle bellies deep into the orbit, and forming the muscle cone. The pulley theory describes the intermuscular septum as a thin anterior extension of the pulley sleeves that forms a sling between the muscles. Anteriorly, within 3 mm from the limbus the intermuscular septum and Tenon's capsule fuse into a single fascial plane which fuses with the conjunctiva 1 mm from the limbus. Consequently, a limbal incision cuts down immediately into bare sclera; incisions away from the limbus will encounter these three tissues in separate layers. A muscle is "slipped" or "lost" after surgery if it recoils through its capsule into the orbit through the penetration in Tenon's capsule. The ligament of Lockwood is the fused muscle capsules of the IR and IO muscles; it has projections to the inferior fornix, the inferior tarsus, the inferior eyelid, and the inferior orbital rim. Posterior to the globe, the intermuscular septum separates the fat cushions inside the muscle cone from the extraconal fat cushions. More posteriorly, the muscular capsule becomes attenuated and the orbital fat cushions attach firmly to the muscles.

The check ligaments ("falsseux tendineux") are small white septal attachments bridging the space between the anterior Tenon's capsule and the muscular capsule of the rectus muscles (at 12 mm from the limbus).[17] True check ligaments (suspensory ligaments) are delicate expansions of the muscle sleeves that extend to the orbital walls inserting in the periosteum.[33] The check ligament of the MR arcs posteriorly to insert in the posterior lacrimal crest behind the medial palpebral ligament. The check ligament of the LR inserts in the lateral orbital tubercle, in the lateral palpebral ligament, and in the conjunctival fornix. Historically, the check ligaments were thought to restrict side-slip of the muscles during normal eye movements and to constrain muscles from "over-contraction"; however recent studies suggest that the sleeves to which the ligaments are attached receive the insertion of nearly 50% of the of the rectus muscle fibers. Thus, they may be displaced by muscle force.[33,34]

Being overlapped by the levator muscle, the SR lacks a direct anchor to the orbital periosteum. Inelastic fibrous extensions of tissue appear as dense adhesions of Tenon's capsule to the IR muscle capsule approximately 7 mm posterior to the IR insertion (Fig. 71.7). These "cords" penetrate Tenon's capsule and insert into the inferior tarsal plate. Dissection of these attachments is important when performing large resections or recessions of the IR muscle to avoid altering the position of the lower lid.

The pulley theory

Not all fibers of the EOMs insert on the globe; half of the fibers insert on Tenon's capsule. A distinct fibroelastic sleeve surrounds the insertion of the orbital layer of each EOM. Located near the equator of the eye, these sleeves have been referred to as "pulleys." Pulleys consist of dense collagen and elastin fibrils and are said to maintain the position of the EOMs relative to the orbit and stabilize the muscle path in different positions of gaze, preventing slide-slipping. This is evident, for example, during vertical ocular rotations, where the pathway of the horizontal relaxed muscles moves radially with respect to the center of the orbit rather than shifting vertically. Posterior to the equator the direction of the muscle changes to a straight path toward the apex.[35] This anterior departure from a straight line is explained by the existence of a structure that couples the muscle to the orbital wall. The pulling direction of the EOMs is not a straight line, but the line segment between the sclera insertion of the global layer of the EOM and its pulley. The pulleys act as functional mechanical origin of the rectus EOMs. Structures coupling the anterior extent of the EOMs have long been recognized (see above description of check ligaments and

intermuscular septum). The pulley theories expand the function of the extraocular connective tissue beyond a passive resistance force. Demer and Miller have emphasized the role that the orbital connective tissue plays during ocular rotations, by using high-resolution MRI images with surface coils to examine patients and experimental animals and cadavers.

In this model, the anterior pulley slings correspond to the intermuscular septum fascia. These tissues play a very minor role in constraining muscle paths. Connective tissue bands (lateral and medial enthesis) that connect the pulleys to bony anchors in the orbital rim are what previously have been known as the true check ligaments. The pulleys are equipped with smooth muscle, distributed in bands, mostly distributed between the MR and IR (inframedial peribulbar muscle), but also located in the Lockwood's ligament region.

During muscle surgery, the orbital layer insertion on the pulley is seen as white fibrous bands (false check ligaments above) after bluntly dissecting the anterior pulley sling (intermuscular septum) lateral to the muscle bellies (Fig. 71.8). The actual pulley sleeves are obscured by the overlying Tenon's capsule. The MR pulley is the densest and longest of the EOM pulleys; it is also anchored to the anterior lacrimal crest via the medial enthesis. The LR pulley is anchored to the orbital wall by the lateral enthesis. The IR pulley is intimately coupled with the pulley of the IO forming part of Lockwood's ligament (see above description). The orbital layer of the IR inserts on this pulley. The orbital layer of the IO inserts on this conjoined pulley and temporally in the sheath of the IO and on the inferior aspect of the LR pulley. The lower lid retractors (Muller's inferior tarsal muscle) are also coupled with this conjoined IR-IO pulley, which synchronizes the lower eyelid position with the vertical eye movements. The SR pulley is the least dense. It is closely related to the pulley of the levator to coordinate upper eyelid position. The SO has an immobile pulley, the trochlea; however, its orbital layer inserts on the medial aspect of the superior rectus pulley. A dense band of collagen and elastin extends between the pulley of the SR and LR and divides the orbital lobe of the lacrimal gland. All four rectus muscle pulleys move anteroposteriorly in coordination with their scleral insertions. The IO pulley shifts anteriorly in supraduction and posteriorly in supraduction because it is coupled with the IR pulley.

The pulley hypothesis was introduced to explain the muscle disposition during eye rotations. The need for alternative theories rises because it is highly unlikely that the central commands for horizontal and vertical eye movements (the nucleus prepositus hypoglossi and the medial vestibular nucleus in the

Fig. 71.7 Inferior rectus muscle and its relation with the lower eyelid retractors that penetrate Tenon's capsule and insert into the inferior tarsal plate.

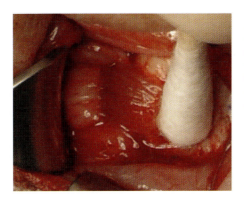

Fig. 71.8 White fibrous bands that mark the insertion of the orbital layer insertion on the medial rectus pulley.

medulla and the interstitial nucleus of Cajal in the midbrain, respectively) can integrate to produce torsion, tertiary eye positions, and non-commutative movements. Mathematical analysis confirms that the rectus muscle pulley positions (observed by MRI) can implement half-angle kinematics required by Listing's law. For primary and secondary gaze positions, the rectus pulleys could be just fixed rigidly to the orbit; however, tertiary gaze positions require the pulleys to actively shift anteroposteriorly within the orbit. The active pulley hypothesis states that these shifts are generated by the contraction of the orbital layer against the elastic resistance of the pulley suspensions.

The finding of smooth muscle in rectus muscle sleeves led Demer et al. to postulate that pulleys modulate small adjustments and refine binocular alignment.[36] Innervation from the superior cervical ganglion, the pterygopalatine ganglion and parasympathetic control of the pulleys confirms these functional properties and their dynamic role in ocular motility.[37] These findings have been contested by other studies.[33,38] Some authors contend that the evidence of independent adjustment of the pulley sleeves is not conclusive.[33] These novel theories suggest much of the extraocular kinematics could be determined by orbital biomechanics rather than by central mechanisms under complex brainstem control.[39]

Pathology of the pulley system has been proposed as the underlying mechanism in several forms of strabismus. Heterotopy (malpositioning) of the rectus pulleys has been described as a cause of incomitant strabismus and oblique dysfunction-like patterns. The "heavy eye syndrome" in patients with and without high myopia may be secondary to an inferior shifting of the LR pulley and degeneration of the LR-SR band, sometimes seen also with older age.[40] Inferior LR pulley shift (pulley instability) in adduction can mimic hypotropia in adduction attributed to SO tendon sheath pathology (Brown's syndrome).[41]

The pulley hypothesis has also been applied to the mechanism underlying several surgical techniques. During transpositions, for example, surface coil MRI has demonstrated that there is no slide-slip of the EOMs and that their paths remain almost fixed in the middle and deep orbit despite large surgical transpositions of their insertions.[35] Larger changes in the pathways of the rectus muscle bellies would have been predicted by conventional modeling. It has been proposed that posterior fixation sutures (fadenoperation) displace the pulley sleeve posteriorly during rotations into the field of action of the involved muscle creating a mechanical restriction rather than a significant change in the muscle tangency with the globe or a decrease in the muscle torque during contraction. It has been proposed that extensive dissection to isolate the muscle belly posteriorly be minimized to avoid surgical destruction of the anterior pulley sling and compromise its ability to mechanically restrict ocular rotations.[42]

Anatomic variations

Anomalous muscular and tendinous structures have been reported in cases of incomitant restrictive strabismus. These structures can insert in different locations on the globe, around the insertion of the EOMs or directly on them. Bands of fibrotic tissue have also been described. Orbital imaging should be considered in patients with unusual patterns of strabismus. Dissinsertion of the anomalous structure should be attempted

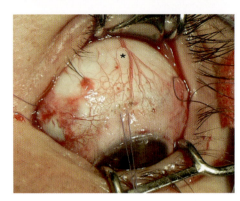

Fig. 71.9 Missing superior rectus muscle in a patient with Apert's syndrome. (Photo courtesy of Nicholas J. Volpe, MD.)

as this usually produces good surgical outcomes. Release of these structures may improve motility.[43]

The absence of the EOMs occurs sporadically in the general population and includes every EOM. The frequency of muscle absence and other abnormalities of the EOMs is high in patients with craniosynostosis syndromes (Fig. 71.9; and see Chapter 28) but can occur in other conditions. This can involve one or both eyes and single or multiple EOMs.

References

1. King WM, Fuchs AF, Magnin M. Vertical eye movement-related responses of neurons in midbrain near intestinal nucleus of Cajal. J Neurophysiol 1981; 46: 549–62.
2. Robinson DL, McClurkin JW, Kertzman C, Petersen SE. Visual responses of pulvinar and collicular neurons during eye movements of awake, trained macaques. J Neurophysiol 1991; 66: 485–96.
3. Andrade FH, Porter JD, Kaminski HJ. Eye muscle sparing by the muscular dystrophies: lessons to be learned? Microsc Res Tech 2000; 48: 192–203.
4. Porter JD, Poukens V, Baker RS, Demer JL. Structure-function correlations in the human medial rectus extraocular muscle pulleys. Invest Ophthalmol Vis Sci 1996; 37: 468–72.
5. Scott AB, Collins CC. Division of labor in human extraocular muscle. Arch Ophthalmol 1973; 90: 319–22.
6. Jacoby J, Ko K, Weiss C, Rushbrook JI. Systematic variation in myosin expression along extraocular muscle fibres of the adult rat. J Muscle Res Cell Motil 1990; 11: 25–40.
7. Brueckner JK, Porter JD. Visual system maldevelopment disrupts extraocular muscle-specific myosin expression. J Appl Physiol 1998; 85: 584–92.
8. Brueckner JK, Ashby LP, Prichard JR, Porter JD. Vestibulo-ocular pathways modulate extraocular muscle myosin expression patterns. Cell Tissue Res 1999; 295(3): 477–84.
9. Apt L. An anatomical reevaluation of rectus muscle insertions. Trans Am Ophthalmol Soc 1980; 78: 365–75.
10. Kushner BJ, Lucchese NJ, Morton GV. Variation in axial length and anatomical landmarks in strabismic patients. Ophthalmology 1991; 98: 400–6.
11. Kushner BJ, Morton GV. A randomized comparison of surgical procedures for infantile esotropia. Am J Ophthalmol 1984; 98: 50–61.
12. Keech RV, Scott WE, Baker JD. The medial rectus muscle insertion site in infantile esotropia. Am J Ophthalmol 1990; 109: 79–84.
13. de Gottrau P, Gajisin S. [Anatomic, histologic, and morphometric studies of the ocular rectus muscles and their relation to the eye globe and Tenon's capsule.] Klin Monatsbl Augenheilkd 1992; 200: 515–6.
14. Fink W. Surgery of the Oblique Muscles of the Eye. St. Louis: Mosby; 1951.
15. Souza-Dias C, Prieto-Diaz J, Uesugui CF. Topographical aspects of the insertions of the extraocular muscles. J Pediatr Ophthalmol Strabismus 1986; 23: 183–9.

16. Parks MM. Ocular Motility and Strabismus. Hagerstown, MD: Harper & Row; 1975.

17. Parks MM. Atlas of Strabismus Surgery. Philadelphia, PA: Harper & Row; 1983.

18. Helveston EM, New Orleans Academy of Ophthalmology. Symposium on Strabismus: Transactions of the New Orleans Academy of Ophthalmology. St Louis: Mosby; 1978.

19. Kushner BJ, Lucchese NJ, Morton GV. The influence of axial length on the response to strabismus surgery. Arch Ophthalmol 1989; 107: 1616–8.

20. Helveston EM, Merriam WW, Ellis FD, et al. The trochlea. A study of the anatomy and physiology. Ophthalmology 1982; 89: 124–33.

21. Helveston EM, Krach D, Plager DA, Ellis FD. A new classification of superior oblique palsy based on congenital variations in the tendon. Ophthalmology 1992; 99: 1609–15.

22. Wallace DK, von Noorden GK. Clinical characteristics and surgical management of congenital absence of the superior oblique tendon. Am J Ophthalmol 1994; 118: 63–9.

23. Harada M, Ito Y. Surgical correction of cyclotropia. Jpn J Ophthalmol 1964; 8: 23–32.

24. Iizuka M, Kushner B. Surgical implications of the superior oblique frenulum. J AAPOS 2008; 12: 27–32.

25. Stager DR. Costenbader lecture. Anatomy and surgery of the inferior oblique muscle: recent findings. J AAPOS 2001; 5: 203–8.

26. Stager DR. The neurofibrovascular bundle of the inferior oblique muscle as its ancillary origin. Trans Am Ophthalmol Soc 1996; 94: 1073–94.

27. Stager DR. The neurofibrovascular bundle of the inferior oblique muscle as the ancillary origin of that muscle. J AAPOS 1997; 1: 216–25.

28. Stager DR, Weakley DR, Jr, Stager D. Anterior transposition of the inferior oblique: anatomic assessment of the neurovascular bundle. Arch Ophthalmol 1992; 110: 360–2.

29. Demer JL. More respect for connective tissues. J AAPOS 2008; 12: 5–6.

30. Koornneef L. Details of the orbital connective tissue system in the adult. Acta Morphol Neerl Scand 1977; 15: 1–34.

31. Roth A, Muhlendyck H, De Gottrau P. [The function of Tenon's capsule revisited.] J Fr Ophtalmol 2002; 25: 968–76.

32. Demer JL, Miller JM, Poukens V, et al. Evidence for fibromuscular pulleys of the recti extraocular muscles. Invest Ophthalmol Vis Sci 1995;36:1125–36.

33. Ruskell GL, Kjellevold Haugen IB, et al. Double insertions of extraocular rectus muscles in humans and the pulley theory. J Anat 2005; 206: 295–306.

34. Demer JL, Oh SY, Poukens V. Evidence for active control of rectus extraocular muscle pulleys. Invest Ophthalmol Vis Sci 2000; 41: 1280–90.

35. Miller JM, Demer JL, Rosenbaum AL. Effect of transposition surgery on rectus muscle paths by magnetic resonance imaging. Ophthalmology 1993; 100: 475–87.

36. Demer JL, Miller JM. Magnetic resonance imaging of the functional anatomy of the superior oblique muscle. Invest Ophthalmol Vis Sci 1995; 36: 906–13.

37. Demer JL, Poukens V, Miller JM, Micevych P. Innervation of extraocular pulley smooth muscle in monkeys and humans. Invest Ophthalmol Vis Sci 1997; 38: 1774–85.

38. McClung JR, Allman BL, Dimitrova DM, Goldberg SJ. Extraocular connective tissues: a role in human eye movements? Invest Ophthalmol Vis Sci 2006; 47: 202–5.

39. Miller JM. Understanding and misunderstanding extraocular muscle pulleys. J Vis 2007; 7: 101–15.

40. Rutar T, Demer JL. "Heavy eye" syndrome in the absence of high myopia: a connective tissue degeneration in elderly strabismic patients. J AAPOS 2009; 13: 36–44.

41. Oh SY, Clark RA, Velez F, et al. Incomitant strabismus associated with instability of rectus pulleys. Invest Ophthalmol Vis Sci 2002; 43: 2169–78.

42. Clark RA, Isenberg SJ, Rosenbaum AL, Demer JL. Posterior fixation sutures: a revised mechanical explanation for the fadenoperation based on rectus extraocular muscle pulleys. Am J Ophthalmol 1999; 128: 702–14.

43. Lueder GT. Anomalous orbital structures resulting in unusual strabismus. Surv Ophthalmol 2002; 47: 27–35.

The clinical approach to strabismus

Anthony J Vivian

Introduction

Strabismus surgery is a sub-specialty in its own right. The provision of high-quality care must be planned and executed strategically. This requires service delivery from primary care through to outcome and satisfaction audits at the end of the management. Although rates of strabismus surgery are declining, the management of strabismus and amblyopia is the majority of the workload of most pediatric ophthalmologists. I will give a few ideas about laying out and managing an efficient and effective strabismus practice. I will stress a friendly, non-threatening environment (both structural and emotional) and the fundamental principles of accurate documentation and audit to ensure clinically effective management.

The clinical setting

Frequently, the structural layout of our clinic space is constrained by immovable walls, doors, and windows, often not ideally placed. Occasionally there is an opportunity to start with a blank piece of paper, giving rise to some fundamental questions. How long should an examination room be? Do all the rooms have to be the same size? How can the most be made of a restricted floor area?

Room layout

The dimensions of an examination room for assessing children with strabismus have been dictated by the need to measure visual acuity at 6 m (20 ft) using Snellen acuity charts. However, tests based on the logarithmic scale of the minimum angle of resolution (logMAR) are more accurate methods for measuring acuity. Many of these tests can be projected or displayed on computer screens and so testing distances are more flexible.

Other factors determining the length of the examination room are the minimum distance required to prevent accommodation affecting the basic deviation measurement and other distance tests such as distance stereopsis and fusion tests. The maximum amount of accommodation when viewing an accommodative target at 6 m is about an eighth of a diopter, which is clinically insignificant. At 4 m accommodation is not completely suspended and could influence the basic deviation measurement (angle of deviation in the primary position for distance with accommodation suspended). At least some rooms should be 6 m in length to best perform accurate motility testing. However, these rooms do not need to be rectangular. To make the best use of limited floor area the rooms can "interlock" so that there is a wide end for the examiner and patient and a thin end for the fixation and acuity targets (Fig. 72.1).

Distance fixation and acuity targets

Obtaining accurate results for the basic deviation measurement in children can be challenging. Failure to achieve an accurate measurement for distance is a common cause of surgical error, as many children with strabismus have a disparity between distance and near deviation. Operating on the near angle (which is easier to measure) may result in an over- or undercorrection for distance. Interesting distance fixation targets are essential in the management of childhood strabismus. The letters of a Snellen acuity chart will not hold the child's attention for long. A variety of fixation targets are necessary, some requiring greater resolution than others. Cartoon characters and soft toys arranged at 6 m provide more interest for the child. DVDs can be displayed on a TV screen and there are many computer based fixation and acuity programs available (including Apps for iPads and mobile phones) (Fig. 72.2).

Tools of the trade

When assessing strabismus, there are a number of useful items (Fig. 72.3). The list is not exhaustive but emphasizes that if the equipment is not at hand, the test will not be done.

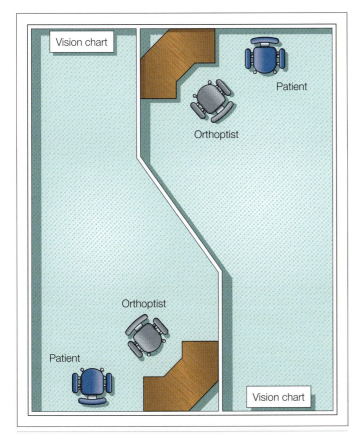

Fig. 72.1 Design for two interlocking 6 m orthoptic rooms making maximum use of available floor space.

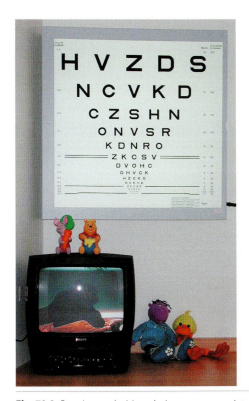

Fig. 72.2 By using a television playing age-appropriate videos, distance fixation is enhanced, allowing better distance measurements.

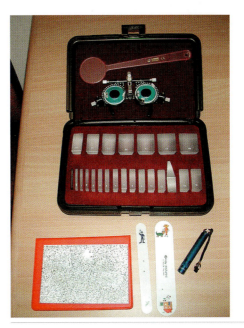

Fig. 72.3 A selection of useful instruments for strabismus assessment.

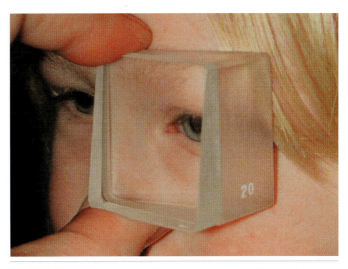

Fig. 72.4 Using single prisms held in one hand, vertical and horizontal deviations can be assessed simultaneously.

1. Occluder for performing cover tests: a transparent (Spielmann) occluder allows visualization of the occluded eye.
2. Single prisms (Berens' square prisms are the most accurate) for performing prism cover tests: single prisms have a number of advantages over prism bars. The larger prism area allows better visualization of the fixation targets by the patient, and allows better visualization of the eye by the examiner. Both horizontal and vertical deviations can be corrected simultaneously in front of the same eye (Fig. 72.4).
3. Near acuity target for determining the near angle as accommodative demand is increased (particularly useful in assessing children with convergence excess esotropia).
4. Near stereoacuity tests (Lang, Frisby, TNO, Wirt).
5. Maddox rods or Bagolini lenses for measuring torsion.
6. Fixation light.

Interaction with the child and parents

First meeting

Children can find their first eye clinic appointment intimidating. They may be too young to understand what is going on and have to wait for a long time to be seen, absorbing the anxiety of their parents. They need to have dilating drops. Make the first visit a positive experience for both the child and the parents; if it has not been too traumatic, subsequent visits will yield more information.

The waiting area should be child-friendly. Play assistants make a significant difference to the overall mood of the waiting area, relieving some of the stress of the parents, which reflects in the behavior of the child.

Several methods for getting the most information out of the first visit can be employed:

1. Observation: this can be performed while talking to the parents or while the child plays. Look at the visual behavior and look for an abnormal head posture or obvious strabismus.
2. Lang stereotest: this can be made into a game, which can be played first by a parent or sibling. It is a good initial test because it is not intimidating (it does not require special glasses to be worn).
3. Distance fixation using DVDs: children's DVDs playing at the far end of the examination room are a useful distance fixation target to enable cover testing and determining fixation preference.
4. Cycloplegic drops: cyclopentolate 1% instilled 30 minutes before refraction is adequate for most children. Best results are obtained if someone other than the examiner, in a separate room, instills them. Topical anesthetic (proxymetacaine 0.5%) reduces the discomfort of the cycloplegic drops considerably and should be considered. Atropine 1% can be used if cycloplegia with cyclopentolate cannot be obtained. If the child finds instillation of drops in the clinic very traumatic, atropine drops or ointment can be instilled at home by the parents prior to the clinic appointment.
5. If a fundus view is not achieved, another attempt should be made at a later date. It is occasionally necessary to physically restrain a child for fundus examination if there is suspicion of fundus pathology.
6. Examination of the optic nerve should include a magnified view. This can be achieved with a direct ophthalmoscope or by slit-lamp biomicroscopy, which gives a much better view. It is important to recheck the fundus and disc appearance in children with amblyopia refractory to treatment to exclude other causes of poor vision such as optic nerve hypoplasia.
7. Hand-held slit-lamp: it is possible to look at children with an adult slit-lamp, but examining small children is easier with a hand-held slit-lamp.

Role of the orthoptist

The orthoptist plays a very important role in the strabismus clinic. However, it is important that the strabismus surgeons are competent at performing a complete examination themselves. Only by examining the patient themselves can they get a feel for the subtleties of strabismus. Strabismus management should involve a multidisciplinary approach. The doctor should be able to perform a sensory and motor examination, and increasingly orthoptists are expanding their role to include parts of the examination traditionally the territory of the ophthalmologist, such as refraction.

Practical history taking: extracting clinically relevant details

A focused assessment of symptoms and past history is mandatory. The history taking does not have to be extensive but should be careful and specific. It is important to find out about:

1. The parents' observations about the strabismus: whether the eyes turn in or out, which eye is most commonly affected, whether the strabismus is intermittent or constant, and changes in the strabismus when the child is tired or unwell.
2. Other ophthalmic symptoms: whether there are any associated abnormalities such as closing one eye in bright light, whether double vision is experienced, and whether the parents have noticed a vertical element to the strabismus or an association with changes in lid height.
3. Past ophthalmic history: whether there is any history of ophthalmic care (including glasses or patching), trauma, or previous strabismus surgery.
4. Past medical history: previous history of systemic or neurologic disease; the pregnancy, delivery and developmental history; and the drug and allergy history.
5. Family history: whether there is a family history of glasses wear in childhood, lazy eyes, or strabismus surgery; and whether there is a family history of either ophthalmic or systemic inherited disease.

Examination

Examination of the strabismus patient should include:

- A sensory examination (acuity, fixation preference, binocular vision, fusion, accommodation, and convergence).
- Ocular motility testing.
- Ocular examination (slit-lamp examination, media and fundus examination).
- Refraction (cycloplegic in children).Further specific examination including a search for dysmorphic or neurologic signs may be necessary.

Sensory examination

Acuity

There are many tests to measure visual acuity in preverbal and verbal children, some more successful than others. They rely on experience in both performing and interpreting the tests. A careful measurement of acuity is essential at each visit. Both near and distance acuity should be measured. In order to maintain reproducible results, acuity measurement techniques and recording should be standardized with specific acuity tests for children at each level of developmental ability. There is a very large range of different acuity tests, each with its own merits. It is important to have a hierarchy of tests that give reproducible results at various ages.

Preferential looking techniques

Preferential looking is a behavioral method of assessing visual acuity, which can be performed from a very young age. The principle is that the child will be more interested in looking at a target with a resolvable pattern on it than looking at a target with no obvious pattern. The resolution of the target can be reduced until the child is unable to make a choice. The point at which the child is unable to make a choice gives an estimate of the visual acuity. For infants and children to the age of about 2 years, grating acuity cards such as Keeler or Teller can be used, and for children between 2 and 3 years of age vanishing optotypes such as Cardiff cards are more appropriate.

Kay pictures

Picture chart acuity tests such as Kay pictures are useful but they tend to overestimate the acuity. They are useful for comparing the acuity of each eye and logMAR versions are available.

logMAR-based matching tests

At about 3½ to 4 years most children will be able to perform a logMAR-based matching test, which can be presented on cards[1] or on a screen.[2] These give accurate and reproducible acuity results.

logMAR

Once the child knows the alphabet, a full logMAR acuity is possible using a logMAR chart (such as a Bailey-Lovie chart). It is important to measure the worst eye first because children have excellent memories.

Fixation preference

Fixation preference is a simple and effective test for detecting amblyopia and can be performed in infants. It is most accurate with strabismus of 10 prism diopters or more. Fixation preference is analyzed by assessing the centrality, steadiness, and maintenance of fixation (CSM method). "Central" fixation requires that the corneal reflex is central in the pupil. "Steady" fixation requires no evidence of nystagmus or oscillatory eye movements. "Maintained" fixation refers to the ability of the non-preferred eye to maintain fixation after occlusion is removed from the preferred eye. This can be graded by determining whether the fixation is maintained through a blink or during a smooth pursuit movement, or by observing the time period through which fixation is maintained by the non-preferred eye when occlusion is removed from the preferred eye.[3]

In orthotropia fixation preference can be assessed by creating a deviation using a 10- or 12-diopter prism either base-up or base-down in front of one eye. The prism is used vertically because vertical fusion is much smaller than horizontal fusion. Fixation should alternate if acuity is equal. If a fixation preference is detected, it can be graded in a similar fashion to strabismic patients.

Binocular single vision, fusion and stereopsis

Amongst the most difficult areas to understand are binocular single vision, fusion, and stereopsis. This is partly the terminology and partly our limited understanding of how the eyes work together. The terminology used by physiologists and ophthalmologists is different, which has contributed to our confusion. Although concepts such as "the horopter" and "Panum's fusional area" are useful for the physiologist, they confound the ophthalmologist who decides the sensory side of strabismus is too much to cope with and leaves it to the orthoptist and the theorist. This is a pity because it is useful and affects management. We must be very clear about our definitions. What follows is a list of definitions, which simplifies the sensory assessment of strabismus patients, and an account of how we use this information in management.

Retinal correspondence

To obtain binocular vision, the images from each eye must be superimposed in the occipital cortex. This superimposition is not done as a complete picture but by piecing together many small parts of a picture, like a jigsaw. Each piece of the jigsaw requires a contribution from both the right and the left retinas. Each retinal area thus has a corresponding point in the other retina that contributes to the same part of the jigsaw in the cortex. Normal retinal correspondence requires that the foveas of each eye contribute to the same piece of cortical jigsaw. Patients with abnormal retinal correspondence have an area of retina adjacent to the fovea of one eye contributing its image to the same piece of jigsaw as the foveal image from the other eye.

Motor and sensory fusion

- Motor fusion: the ability to physically move the eyes so that they are pointing in the same direction, allowing the corresponding areas of the retina in each eye to be pointing at the object of regard.
- Sensory fusion: taking the image from each corresponding retinal area and superimposing them in binocular cells at the level of the occipital cortex.

The two are inextricably linked. It is not possible to have sensory fusion if the eyes are pointing in different directions, and the motor fusion mechanism uses sensory fusion as a feedback. When motor fusion mechanisms have done their job, sensory fusion is possible. If there is no sensory fusion, the motor fusion mechanism has no feedback and may fail, resulting in motor misalignment.

Central (bifoveal) and peripheral fusion

To obtain high-quality single images, the foveal images from each eye must be aligned. Only when this is achieved can stereopsis (depth perception) be obtained. This is called central or bifoveal fusion. A cruder form of single image using both eyes is possible without perfect foveal images (e.g. in patients with an amblyopic eye) and without perfect alignment (e.g. in patients with small angle esotropia). This is called peripheral fusion.

Fusion range (fusion amplitudes)

The fusion range refers to the range over which the motor fusion mechanism is able to pull the eyes together. It is measured by placing progressively more powerful prisms in front of the eyes until the patient experiences diplopia (i.e. the fusional amplitude has been exceeded). The prisms are placed base-in and then base-out to measure both the divergence and convergence fusion range. The vertical fusion range is measured using base-up and base-down prisms.

Binocular vision

Binocular vision means seeing with two eyes but, as ophthalmologists, we take it to mean more. We assume that using two eyes together and gaining a single image is better than using one eye at a time. Even if one eye is amblyopic and no stereopsis (the perception of depth) is measurable, the combined image from two eyes has a quality superior to that of single eye vision. The term binocular single vision is perhaps preferable. It emphasizes that both eyes are being used and a single image is obtained. The fact that binocular single vision is even obtainable if the eyes are not aligned (e.g. in microtropias) shows that the occipital cortex is lenient in terms of what it will accept from corresponding retinal areas and still perceive single vision. Central (foveal) fusion is not a prerequisite for binocular single vision. Fusion of peripheral retinal areas is enough.

Stereopsis

The most advanced form of vision we possess is stereopsis. This is the perception of depth and the impression of three dimensions. This requires perfect alignment of the eyes and good quality of image from each fovea; foveal fusion is a prerequisite for high levels of stereopsis. A low level of stereopsis is possible in microtropias.

Measuring retinal correspondence binocular vision, and fusion

Tests of retinal correspondence

It is not necessary to test retinal correspondence in all patients. The important patients are those who have a manifest strabismus, but have binocular single vision without suppressing one image. In these patients the fovea of the fixing eye has developed a relationship with an extrafoveal area of the non-fixing eye. If the abnormal retinal correspondence is deep-rooted, operating to straighten the eyes results in a return to the original angle postoperatively or diplopia.

Bagolini glasses

Bagolini glasses detect abnormal retinal correspondence without dissociating the eyes. They require a high level of cooperation and understanding and cannot be used in young children. Because the lenses have striations, a point source of light is seen as a straight line. The lenses in front of each eye are arranged at 90° to each other, so with both eyes open a point source of light (at either 33 cm or 6 m) is perceived as a cross. They give information about suppression and are useful in two other situations:

1. The patient with strabismus on corneal reflection, but no movement on cover testing. If the Bagolini glasses result is normal in the presence of an obvious deviation, there must be abnormal retinal correspondence. If this is well established in a patient who is visually mature, surgery could result in intractable diplopia.
2. The patient with microtropia (monofixation syndrome). These patients have ultrasmall deviations (difficult or impossible to detect on cover testing) associated with amblyopia and foveal scotoma. The Bagolini test shows anomalous retinal correspondence with a break in the Bagolini line in the affected eye.

Tests of fusion potential

Strabismus patients with good fusion potential are more likely to maintain alignment after surgery. Testing fusional potential in patients with manifest strabismus is difficult. Fusion potential can be tested using the synoptophore but, because this is a dissociative test, results may be difficult to interpret.

Worth four-dot test

The Worth four-dot test is of limited value in the management of strabismus. It is a very dissociative test (because red and green glasses are used). Patients unable to fuse under the test conditions may have reasonable fusion if the eyes are not dissociated. It measures motor fusion rather than sensory fusion.

The test is composed of four lights – two green, one red, and one white. A red glass is worn over one eye (by convention, the right) and a green glass over the other eye. The test lights are viewed at the appropriate test distance (near or distant, depending on the type of test being used). There are three possible results:

1. Fusion: if four lights are seen, the patient has fusion capability. At the appropriate test distance the lights fall on the fovea so central fusion is being tested. If the test is negative (shows diplopia or suppression) the patient can be moved closer to the test lights so that the lights fall outside of the fovea, and thus peripheral fusion is tested. If the white light appears green, the left eye is dominant, if it appears red or pink the right eye is dominant.
2. Diplopia: if five lights are seen the patient has diplopia and no fusion.
3. Suppression: if only two or three lights are seen, the patient is suppressing one or other of their eyes. If the patient sees two lights and then three, there is alternating suppression.

Testing fusion range (amplitude)

This is best tested using prisms in free space. Prisms are increased in strength until diplopia is reported. If the prisms are placed base-out the eyes must converge to restore binocularity. The prisms are increased in strength until the patient is no longer able to restore binocularity and reports diplopia. The prisms are then placed base-in and the eyes must diverge to restore binocularity. The vertical fusion ranges can be measured in patients with vertical strabismus.

Motor fusion can be estimated in very young children by putting a 20-diopter base-out prism in front of one eye to see whether the patient is able to overcome the prism. If the child has motor fusion potential, a refixation movement will be seen.

Tests of stereopsis

Patients with measurable stereopsis must have sensory fusion. If the stereopsis test is positive, tests of sensory fusion are unnecessary. Stereopsis measurement should be performed before the eyes are dissociated by other tests such as Worth four-dot or cover tests. Patients with obvious manifest deviations are unlikely to have measurable stereopsis (although patients with small angle deviations and good motor fusion may have some stereopsis). The tests are most useful in patients with intermittent deviations or distance/near deviations. Patients who lose stereopsis under either of these conditions need urgent treatment to restore it.

Four commonly used tests of near stereopsis are:

1. Lang stereopsis test: this test is simple, does not involve wearing glasses to dissociate the eyes and can be used for very young children (even 1-year-olds). The disparity of

the images ranges from 1200 to 200 sec of arc and so is only a crude estimation of stereopsis. This test is very useful in the assessment of the sensory status of children with ocular motility disorders and screening children.

2. Titmus stereo test: this test uses polarizing glasses to dissociate the two eyes, and can be used from about the age of 2 to 3 years. There are three separate tests (the fly, circles, and animals) that test stereoacuity down to 40 sec of arc.

3. TNO stereo test: this test uses red and green glasses to dissociate the eyes.

4. Frisby stereo tests: this test does not require any form of glasses, which is advantageous. It is a non-dissociative test. These tests measure near stereopsis. Some patients have distance stereopsis but no near stereopsis. There are distance stereopsis tests available (Frisby distance stereotest) and are useful in children with convergence excess esotropia with a controlled distance deviation but esotropia for near.

Accommodation and convergence

Accommodation and convergence should be measured routinely, when possible, using an accommodative near target. The accommodative convergence/accommodation (AC/A) ratio should be measured in those patients with a distance/near disparity. However, measuring the AC/A ratio is difficult in children younger than about 5 or 6 years of age as it requires participation.

Motor examination

Basic deviation

The basic deviation is the angle of strabismus measured with the eyes in the primary position, having ensured full correction of refractive errors. Fixation should be with the preferred eye on a distance target (6 m) in standard room lighting.

Prism cover tests in nine positions of gaze

A full ocular motility examination involves prism cover tests in nine positions of gaze. However, this is not necessary (and not always possible) in all patients. Nine positions of gaze measurements are most important in patients with vertical deviations and require some patient cooperation. In children with horizontal deviations, it is important to perform prism cover tests in the primary position, but also in up- and downgaze (to exclude "A" and "V" patterns) and in sidegaze to exclude lateral incomitance (especially in patients with exotropia).

The deviation in nine positions of gaze is determined using prism cover tests. Single prisms are used rather than prism bars. Although errors can be introduced during prism cover testing, being aware of the potential pitfalls and avoiding them allows this test to be an accurate measurement method.[4] The patient fixates on a distant target and the head is moved so that the eyes take up the positions of extreme gaze. It is important that the eyes are in extreme gaze positions when performing the prism cover tests to ensure reproducibility. If the nose obscures the vision of one eye, the head can be moved so that vision is just regained. Prisms are held in front of the paretic eye. With single prisms, both the vertical and horizontal elements can be neutralized by holding the appropriate prisms in one hand

in front of the paretic eye. It is inaccurate to stack horizontal prisms and in large deviations it may be necessary to use a prism in front of each eye.

Having performed prism cover tests in nine positions of gaze for distance, the near deviation in the primary position is determined, usually to an accommodative target.

Versions and ductions

Versions are eye movements of each eye tested with both eyes open. The importance of versions is to look at the actions of the six extraocular muscles of each eye for underaction, overaction, or restriction. Versions are tested using a light as a target with both eyes open, and are scored using a nine-point scoring system. Normal versions score 0, overactions are graded from +1 to +4, and underactions are graded from −1 to −4. Sclera should be concealed by the canthus in a normal horizontal version. If sclera is just visible, the version is graded −1 and an inability to abduct or adduct the eye more than halfway into the field of action of the muscle is graded −2. Inability to abduct or adduct an eye more than a quarter-way into the field of action of the muscle is graded −3, and if the eye is unable to move at all from the primary position into the field of action of that muscle the limitation is graded −4. Horizontal rectus overaction is graded according to the amount of cornea covered by the canthus. In extreme overaction half of the cornea is buried, which is graded +4.

Oblique over- and underactions are graded by comparing the height of the inferior limbus of each eye. Overactions are graded from +1, representing a slight overaction, to +4, characterized by abduction of the eye in extreme oblique position. Underactions of the obliques are graded from −1 to −4 (denoting an inability of the eye to move vertically from the midline in the field of action of the oblique being tested). Examples of the four grades of oblique overaction are shown in Fig. 72.5.

Ductions are the excursion of each eye in the direction of each extraocular muscle with the other eye occluded. If an underaction of one eye is noted on versions, the fellow eye is covered and a comparison between the version and duction is made to differentiate a mechanical from a neurogenic strabismus. A mechanical restriction will show equal limitation in both ductions and versions. If there is a nerve paresis, however, the eye will move more in the direction of limitation with the other eye covered (duction movements will exceed versions).

Head tilts

In patients with a vertical deviation, the primary position deviation with the head tilted to the left and right should be measured using single prisms (Bielschowsky head tilt test).

Torsion measurement

Torsion can be measured using the synoptophore and estimated using Hess charts. Both are dissociative and require special instruments. The synoptophore can measure torsion in various positions of gaze. A simple, clinical method of measuring torsion involves using a trial frame with either Maddox rods or Bagolini striated lenses. Torsion should be measured in primary position and downgaze. Both methods can be used in children as young as 5 years of age.

Maddox rods

Two Maddox rods are placed in the trial frame with the cylinders orientated vertically (Fig. 72.6). A patient with torsional

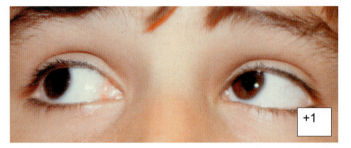

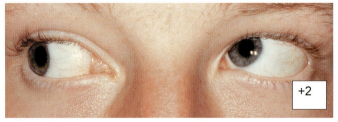

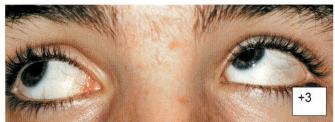

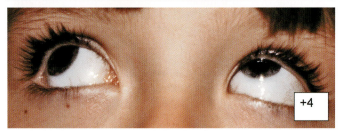

Fig. 72.5 Four grades of inferior oblique overaction.

diplopia perceives two red lines, one horizontal and one tilted. By turning slightly one Maddox rod and then the other it is possible to get an impression of which side the patient feels is the horizontal side and which is the side with torsion. By turning the Maddox rod in the trial frame until the patient sees both lines as being parallel, the amount of torsion can be determined in degrees from the trial frame (Fig. 72.7). If there is a vertical deviation in addition to the torsional deviation (often the case with a fourth nerve paresis), the patient sees two lines, one on top of the other and finds it easy to make the lines parallel. If there is no vertical deviation, patients often find it difficult to be sure that the lines are parallel because they merge with each other. A vertical prism can be put into the trial frame to separate the images, making it easier for the patient to distinguish the lines. Torsional diplopia in downgaze is measured by tilting the patient's head backward and pushing the trial frame down the patient's nose slightly (Fig. 72.8).

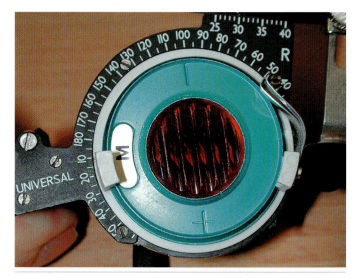

Fig. 72.7 The patient turns one Maddox rod until the lines are parallel and the torsion measurement is read off the trial frame in degrees.

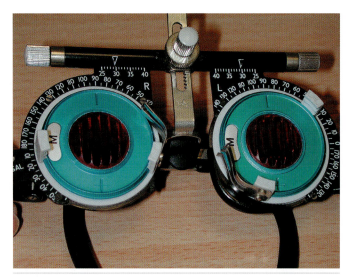

Fig. 72.6 Two Maddox rods aligned vertically in the trial frame are perceived by the diplopic patient as two horizontal lines.

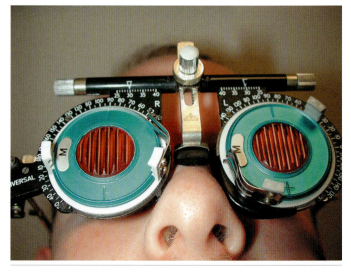

Fig. 72.8 To determine torsion in downgaze, the trial frame is pushed down the nose and the head is tilted back.

Bagolini lenses

Bagolini lenses are used to measure torsion in a trial frame in the same manner as Maddox rods. The patient sees two lines which can be arranged in a parallel orientation. Bagolini lenses have the advantage of being non-dissociative, allowing cyclo-vertical fusion.

Indirect ophthalmoscopy

Information about torsion in various positions of gaze can be obtained by looking at the position of the fovea in relation to the disc using an indirect ophthalmoscope or retinal photography (Fig. 72.9).

Forced duction and forced generation tests

Forced duction tests (FDTs) give important information about restrictive strabismus. In young children, FDTs must be performed under general anesthetic and should be one of the routine procedures at the beginning of each strabismus operation (Fig. 72.10). FDTs can be performed in the clinic using topical anesthetic in older, cooperative children.

Forced generation testing is an essential part of assessment in patients with nerve paresis (including Duane's syndrome). It can only be performed with patient cooperation. This test determines what proportion of the deviation is a result of the nerve paresis, and what proportion is the result of restrictive changes in the antagonist muscle. In a patient with lateral rectus paresis, the eye is held at the temporal limbus with toothed forceps and moved into adduction. The patient is then asked to abduct the eye and the force generated (by the lateral rectus) is estimated (Fig. 72.11).

Abnormal head postures (see Chapter 81)

Abnormal head postures (AHPs) can be in three dimensions: face turns (to the right or left), chin-up or chin-down, and head tilts (to the right or left). They can be measured by using a goniometer (Fig. 72.12).

Ocular examination in strabismus patients

The importance of a detailed ocular examination in patients with strabismus or amblyopia cannot be overemphasized. A number of conditions requiring urgent or prompt treatment present with strabismus or poor vision in one eye that may be misdiagnosed as amblyopia. Conditions such as raised intracranial pressure, retinoblastoma, and congenital cataract can be missed if a careful ocular examination is not performed.

Examination of the lid position and movement may give important information about the underlying strabismus diagnosis. Palpebral aperture changes in Duane's syndrome,

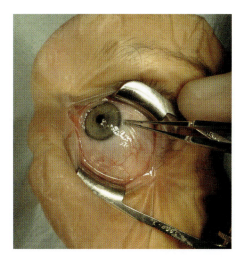

Fig. 72.11 Force generation testing to test lateral rectus power.

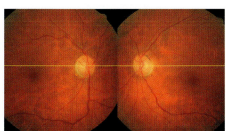

Fig. 72.9 Retinal photography can be used to estimate torsion and gives some idea about whether one eye is contributing more to the torsional diplopia than the other.

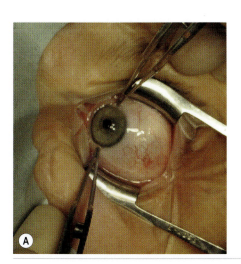
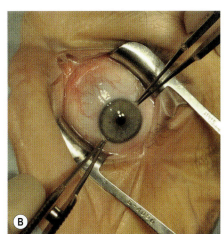
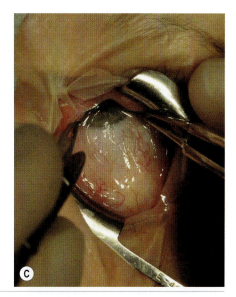

Fig. 72.10 Forced duction testing prior to surgery in an anesthetized child. The eye is moved into adduction (A), abduction (B), and the oblique position (C).

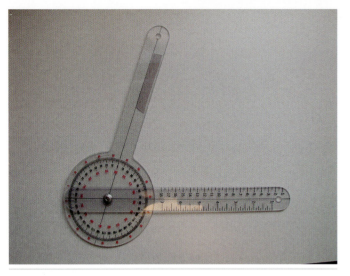

Fig. 72.12 A goniometer. This is used by orthopedic surgeons to measure joint angles, can be used to measure abnormal head postures.

aberrant innervation in congenital third nerve paresis, and seventh nerve paresis in Möbius' syndrome are examples where observation of eyelid changes can help in diagnosis.

The anterior segment is best investigated by slit-lamp, using either a regular slit-lamp or a portable device. Careful examination of the pupils before dilating drops have been given will exclude an afferent pupil defect. Information about media opacities or leukocoria can be gained at the time of refraction. Indirect ophthalmoscopy is an essential part of the examination of all strabismus patients. Further information about media opacities can be obtained, and a detailed examination of the retina and optic nerve will enable diagnosis of other causes of visual impairment such as optic nerve abnormalities, receptor dystrophies, and macular abnormalities. A more magnified view of fundus changes (with the direct ophthalmoscope or slit-lamp biomicroscopy) should be obtained to exclude conditions such as optic nerve hypoplasia, which can easily be missed with indirect ophthalmoscopy.

Special investigations such as visually evoked potentials or electroretinograms (see Chapter 8) may be necessary in unexplained poor vision; neuroimaging and orbital imaging may be necessary in a number of conditions. The use of optical coherence tomograohy (OCT; see Chapter 9) to look at optic nerve and macular architecture is increasingly important (Fig. 72.13).

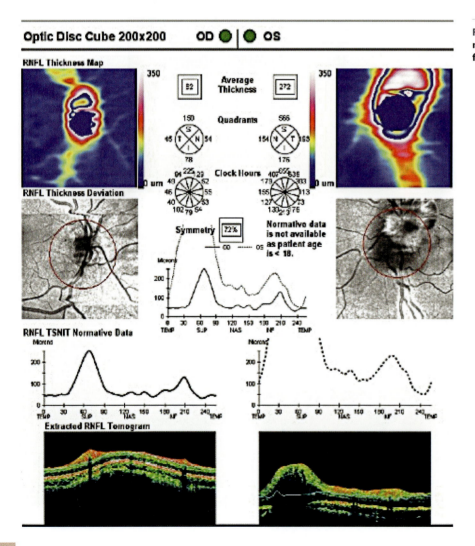

Fig. 72.13 OCT of a patient with right optic nerve hypoplasia and left myelinated nerve fibers at the disk.

Documentation of strabismus findings

Standardization of documentations contributes significantly to the quality of patient care and enables communication within and between departments. Auditing the outcomes of management is much easier with standardized records, and using a numerical rather than a descriptive documentation system has enabled the development of electronic patient records.

Sensory documentation

Figure 72.14 shows an example of a record for documenting sensory findings. This is not all-encompassing and there is still the need for free-text documentation in some cases.

Motor documentation

Documentation of motor findings can be standardized by creating a diagrammatic representation of ocular motor findings.[5] On the same diagrammatic chart, information about prism cover tests, versions and ductions, and abnormal ocular movements can be recorded so that they can be analyzed as if the patient were present. This is a modification of the system by Jampolsky.[6]

Prism cover tests

The basic template is shown in Fig. 72.15. Prism cover test results are recorded using the notation listed in Table 72.1. Horizontal deviations are recorded above the line and vertical deviations below the line. Although it does take a little time to learn the notation language, once fluent it is easy to record quickly a lot of information. For instance, 25(Δ)E is translated as 25(Δ)esophoria, a completely controlled esodeviation, and 25(Δ)ET is translated as 25(Δ)esotropia, a manifest deviation. The use of brackets and underlining conveys further information. For instance, 25(Δ)E(T) is an intermittent esotropia; 25(Δ)$\underline{E}$(T) is an intermittent esotropia that is mainly controlled, whereas 25(Δ)E($\underline{T}$) is an intermittent esotropia, mainly manifest.

Versions

Six version recordings for each eye are recorded corresponding to the direction of principal action of the six extraocular muscles of each eye (Fig. 72.16). Versions are scored using a nine point scoring system where 0 is a normal version, overactions are scored from +1 to +4 and underactions are scored from −1 to −4. The version score for each of the six extraocular muscles of each eye is entered onto the diagram in the appropriate position.

Characteristics of abnormal ocular movements

To further emphasize abnormal ocular movements on the record chart, various symbols can be added (Fig. 72.17). "A" and "V" patterns are emphasized using oblique lines (see example in Fig. 72.18).

Table 72.1 – Notation

Notation for recording the findings of prism cover tests	
E	Esophoria
X	Exophoria
ET	Esotropia
XT	Exotropia
H	Hyperphoria
HT	Hypertropia
Ho	Hypophoria
HoT	Hypotropia
Notation for intermittent deviations	
E(T)	Intermittent esotropia
$\underline{E}$(T)	Intermittent esotropia, mainly latent
E($\underline{T}$)	Intermittent esotropia, mainly manifest

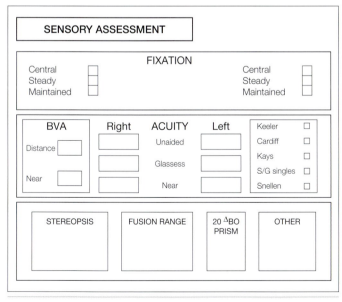

Fig. 72.14 **A simple form for recording the findings of the sensory examination.**

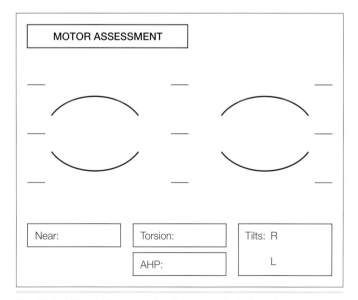

Fig. 72.15 Using this basic template, information including prism cover tests in nine positions of gaze, versions, and abnormalities of ocular movements can be recorded creating a diagrammatic representation of the motility examination findings.

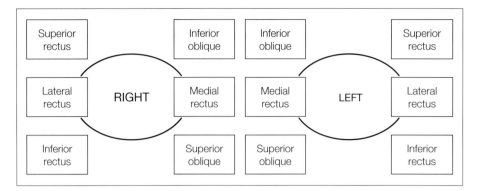

Fig. 72.16 The principal direction of action of the six extraocular muscles of each eye.

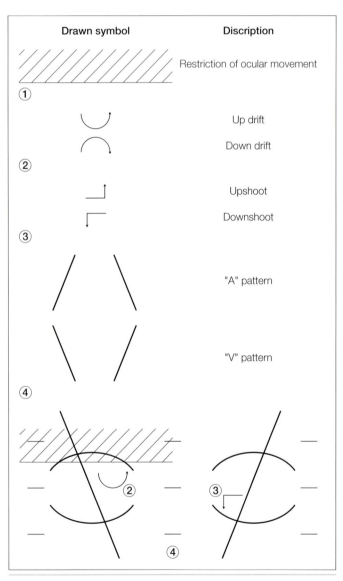

Fig. 72.17 Various characteristics of abnormal ocular movements can be emphasized using a number of symbols. Examples of their use on a basic template are shown.

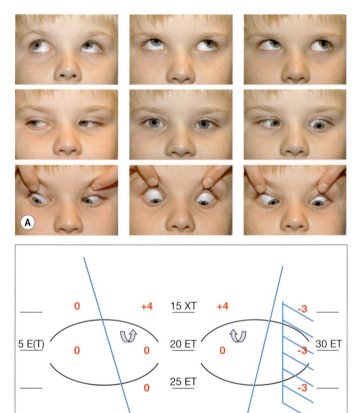

Fig. 72.18 Nine positions of gaze photos (A) and patient eye movement recording chart (B) of a patient with a left sixth nerve palsy and inferior oblique overaction showing restricted left abduction and a "V" pattern.

Electronic patient records and audit in strabismus management

Strabismus surgery is well suited to the application of electronic patient records (EPR). Data are easily recorded in an appropriate format and the EPR can be used to provide a better quality of care.

To allow ease of use and rapid data entry, information must be in a form that is standardized and easily incorporated into drop-down menus. Descriptive terms used in conventional orthoptic reports are not easily adaptable to EPRs, and free-text additions need to be kept to a minimum to prevent data entry from taking too long.

Figures 72.19–72.21 show an example of an EPR developed for strabismus surgery. Figure 72.19 shows the general screen for recording the history, ocular examination, refraction, the final diagnosis, and management plan. Each section has a drop-down menu with a selection of common findings to choose from (although free-text additions can be added).

The screen for entry of sensory and motor findings (see Fig. 72.20) is very similar to the paper version and can be filled in quickly because of the drop-down menus.

The third screen (see Fig. 72.21) is for surgery details. The top portion of the screen is for audit purposes, showing the strabismus type and the preoperative measurements. This enables easy retrieval of operative data to perform an audit of outcomes.

Within each patient's EPR, photographs and videos can be stored. The record automatically creates a diagnostic index.

Computerized clinical records allow more sophisticated data storage and retrieval. With access to better data it is easier to audit surgical outcomes and adjust personal surgical dosage to optimize outcomes.

Satisfaction with the outcome is one aspect that can be measured, but satisfaction with the various elements of the service provision is important. An example of a service satisfaction audit is shown in Fig. 72.22 (available online at http://www.expertconsult.com).

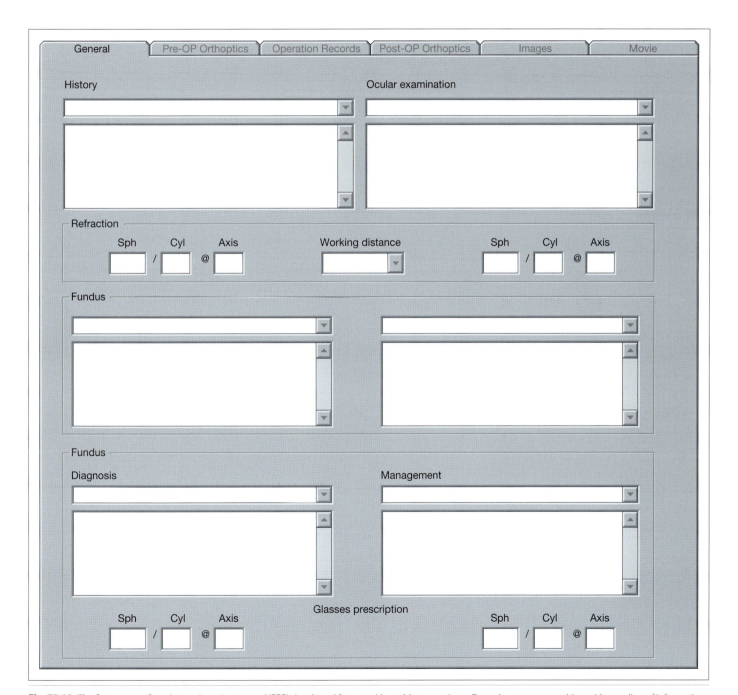

Fig. 72.19 The first screen of an electronic patient record (EPR) developed for use with strabismus patients. Drop-down menus enable rapid recording of information.

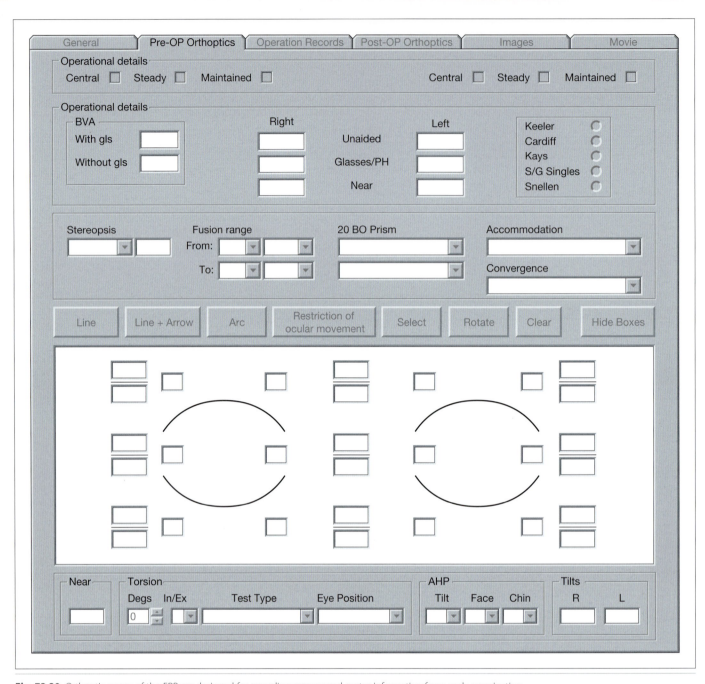

Fig. 72.20 Orthoptic pages of the EPR are designed for recording sensory and motor information from each examination.

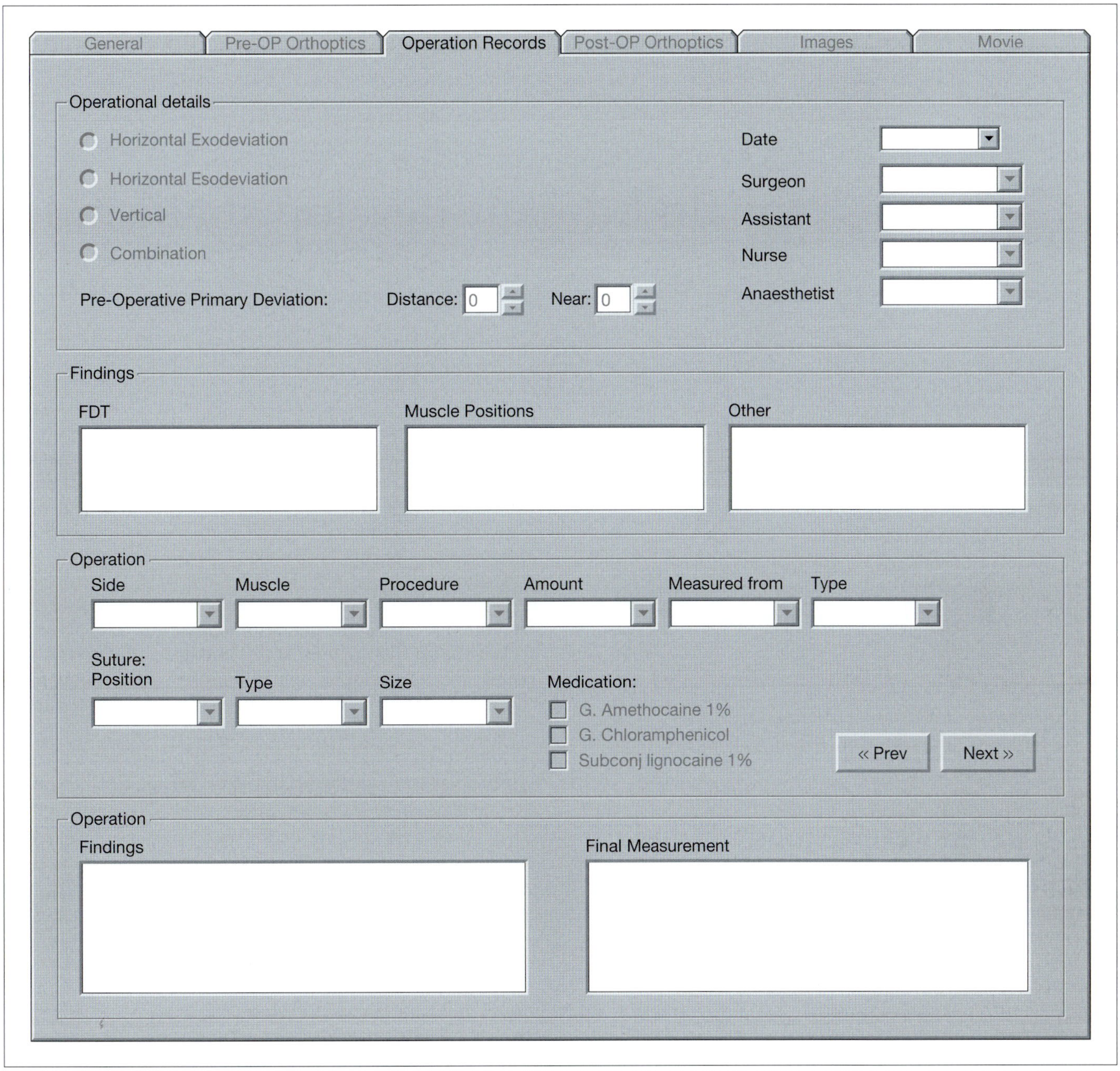

Fig. 72.21 The operation record of the EPR includes data for continuous outcomes audit.

References

1. McGraw PV, Winn B, Gray LS, et al. Improving the reliability of visual acuity measures in the young. Ophthalmic Physiol Opt 2000; 20: 173–84.

2. Holmes JM, Beck RW, Repka MX, et al. Pediatric Eye Disease Investigator Group. The amblyopia treatment study visual acuity testing protocol. Arch Ophthalmol 2001; 119: 1345–53.

3. Sener EC, Mocan MC, Gedik S, et al. The reliability of grading the fixation preference test for the assessment of interocular visual acuity differences in patients with strabismus. J AAPOS 2002; 6: 191–4.

4. Thompson JT, Guyton DL. Ophthalmic prisms: measurement errors and how to minimise them. Ophthalmology 1983; 90: 204–10.

5. Vivian AJ, Morris RJ. Diagramatic representation of strabismus. Eye 1993; 7: 565–71.

6. Jampolsky A. A simplified approach to strabismus diagnosis. Symposium on Strabismus: Transactions of the New Orleans Academy of Ophthalmology. St Louis: Mosby; 1971: 34–51.

Part 1
The fundamentals of strabismus and amblyopia

Why do humans develop strabismus?

Lawrence Tychsen

Developmental non-paralytic strabismus

Developmental strabismus (strabismus with onset in childhood) is a central nervous system (CNS) disorder of the vergence pathways. Epidemiologic and laboratory evidence indicates that the cause is maldevelopment of cerebral visuomotor inputs and outputs: a combination of genetic, intrauterine, and early postnatal factors. Eye rotations are unrestricted (comitant, non-paralytic) in ~98% of cases. Convergent misalignment (esotropia) exceeds divergent misalignment (exotropia) by a ratio of at least 2:1. For constant, as opposed to intermittent, strabismus, the ratio of esotropia to exotropia is 3:1. My discussion is confined to comitant, non-paralytic strabismus. The remaining 2% of childhood-onset cases are paralytic, with limited eye rotation; the cause is cranial neuropathy, myopathy, or orbitopathy.

Early-onset (infantile) esotropia

Esotropia is the leading form of developmental strabismus; it has a bimodal, age-of-onset distribution. The largest peak (~40% of all strabismus) occurs at or before age 12–18 months, with a second, smaller "late-onset" esotropia peak at 3–4 years. Children with early-onset esotropia are predominantly emmetropic:[1] late-onset (accommodative) esotropia is associated with hypermetropia. The most prevalent form of developmental strabismus in humans is comitant, constant, non-accommodative, early-onset esotropia.[2,3] Most cases have onset in the first 12 months of life, i.e. infantile-onset. Infantile esotropia is the paradigm for strabismus in all primates: it is the most frequent type of natural strabismus observed in monkeys.[4]

Early cerebral damage as the major risk factor

What factors contribute to strabismus causation? At highest risk are infants who suffer cerebral maldevelopment from a variety of causes (Table 73.1), especially insults to the parieto-occipital cortex and underlying white matter (geniculostriate projections or optic radiations).[5-8] Periventricular and intraventricular hemorrhage in the neonatal period increases the prevalence of infantile strabismus 50–100 fold.[9] Less specific cerebral insults, e.g. very low birth weight (with or without retinopathy of prematurity) or Down's syndrome, increase the risk by 20- to 30-fold.[8-12]

Table 73.1 – Cerebral damage risk factors for infantile-onset strabismus

Type	Prevalence strabismus	Author(s)
Intraventricular hemorrhage with hydrocephalus	100%	Tamura and Hoyt 1987[5]
Cerebral visual pathway white matter injury	76%	Khanna et al. 2009[9]
Occipitoparietal hemorrhage and/or leukomalacia	54–57%	Pike et al. 1994[6] Hoyt 2003[7]
Very low birth weight infants (<1500 g)	33%*	van Hof-van Duin et al. 1989[8]
Very low birth weight (<1251 g) and prethreshold retinopathy of prematurity	30%	VanderVeen et al. 2006[10]
Very low birth weight (<1251 g) and normal neuroimaging	17%	Khanna et al. 2009[9]
Down's syndrome	21–41%	Hiles et al. 1974[11] Shapiro and France 1985[12]
Healthy full-term infants	0.5–1.0%	PEDIG 2002[23]

*Additional 17% of infants had persistent asymmetric optokinetic nystagmus (OKN).

Cytotoxic insults to cerebral fibers

The occipital lobes in newborns are vulnerable to damage.[7,13-15] Premature infants frequently suffer injury to the optic radiations near the occipital trigone.[9,16] Balanced binocular input requires equal projections from each eye through this periventricular zone. The fibers connect the lateral geniculate laminae to the ocular dominance columns of the striate cortex. The projections are immature at birth and the quality of signal flow is critically dependent upon the function of oligodendrocytes, which insulate the visual fibers. Neonatal oligodendrocytes are especially vulnerable to cytotoxic insult.[17] The striate cortex is also susceptible to hypoxic injury because it has the highest neuron/glia ratio in the cerebrum[18] and the highest regional cerebral glucose consumption.[19]

Genetic influences on formation of cerebral connections

Genetic factors also play a causal role. Large-scale studies show that ~30% of children born to a strabismic parent will develop strabismus.[20] Concordance rates for monozygous twins may be 73%.[21] Less than 100% concordance implies that intrauterine or perinatal ("environmental") factors alter the expression of the strabismic genotype. Pedigree analysis of families containing probands with infantile esotropia[22] suggests a multifactorial or Mendelian co-dominant inheritance pattern. Co-dominant means that both alleles of a single gene contribute to the phenotype but with different thresholds for expression of each allele. These genes could encode cortical neurotrophins, or axon guidance and maturation. Any of these genetically modulated factors could increase susceptibility to

Table 73.2 – Binocular development and visuomotor behaviors in infant primate

Immature behavior	Chief findings before onset of mature behavior	Investigator(s)
Binocular disparity sensitivity absent before ~3–5 months	• Stereo-blindness • Convergent disparity sensitivity emerges earlier than divergent	Fox 1980[26] Birch 1982[27], 1985[28] O'Dell 1997[88]
Binocular sensorial fusion absent before ~3–5 months	• Equal attraction to rivalrous vs. fusible stimuli	Birch 1983[29], 1985[28] Gwiazda 1989[30]
Fusional (binocular) vergence unstable before ~3–5 months	• Binocular alignment errors common despite accommodative capacity	Aslin 1977[36], 1979[37] Birch 1983[29] Hainline 1995[89] Horwood 1993[34], 2004[35]
Nasalward bias of vergence pronounced before ~3–5 months	• Transient convergence errors 4× divergence errors • Convergent disparity sensitivity present earlier than divergent • Convergence fusion range exceeds divergence by 2:1	Riddell 1999[90] Horwood 1993[34], 2004[35]
Nasalward bias of cortically mediated motion sensitivity before ~6 months	• Motion VEP nasotemporal asymmetry • Stronger preferential sensitivity to nasalward motion	Norcia 1991[40], 1996[41] Brown 1997[42] Birch 2000[43] Bosworth 2004[44]
Nasalward bias of pursuit/OKN before ~6 months	• Nasalward motion evokes stronger OKN/pursuit • Nasotemporal asymmetry resolves after onset binocularity	Atkinson 1979[45] Naegele 1982[46] Schor 1983[49] Wattam-Bell 1987[31] Jacobs 1994[47] Tychsen 2001[48]
Nasalward bias of gaze-holding before ~6 months	• Nasalward slow phase drift of eye position • Persists as latent fixation nystagmus with binocular maldevelopment	Schor 1983[49] Tychsen 1985[50] Wong 2003[68]

disruption of visual cortical connections in otherwise healthy infants.

Development of binocular visuomotor behavior in normal infants

Esotropia is rarely present at birth; "infantile esotropia" is a more appropriate descriptor than "congenital esotropia." Constant misalignment of the visual axes appears, typically, after several months, becoming conspicuous between 2 and 5 months.[23-25] To understand visuomotor maldevelopment in strabismic infants it is helpful to understand the development of binocular fusion and vergence in normal infants (Table 73.2) during the 2–5 month postnatal interval.

Development of sensorial fusion and stereopsis

Binocular disparity sensitivity and binocular fusion are absent in infants less than several months of age, as demonstrated by several methods, most notably studies using forced preferential looking (FPL) techniques.[26-30] FPL studies show that stereopsis emerges abruptly in humans during the first 3–5 months of postnatal life, achieving adult-like levels of sensitivity. Sensitivity to crossed (near) disparity appears several weeks before uncrossed (far) disparity.[27] During this interval, infants begin to display an aversion to stimuli causing binocular rivalry, i.e. non-fusable stimuli. Visually evoked potentials (VEPs) in normal infants, recorded using dichoptic viewing and dichoptic stimuli, show comparable results.[31-33] Onset of binocular signal summation occurs after, not before, ~3 months of age.

Development of fusional vergence and an innate convergence bias

Fusional vergence eye movements mature during an equivalent period in early infancy. In the first 2 months of life, alignment is unstable and the responses to step or ramp changes in disparity are often markedly inaccurate[34,35] and cannot be ascribed to errors of accommodation; accommodative precision during this period consistently exceeds that of fusional (disparity) vergence.[35-37]

Studies of fusional vergence development in normal infants reveal an innate bias for convergence.[34,35] Transient large convergence errors exceed divergence errors by 4 : 1. The fusional vergence response to crossed (convergent) disparity is intact earlier and substantially more robust than to divergent disparity. The innate bias favoring fusional convergence in primates persists after full maturation of binocular disparity sensitivity. Fusional convergence capacity exceeds the range of divergence capacity by a mean ratio of 2 : 1.[38,39]

Development of motion sensitivity and conjugate eye tracking (pursuit/optokinetic nystagmus)

The innate nasalward bias of the vergence pathway has analogs in the visual processing of horizontal motion, both for perception and conjugate eye tracking. In the first months of life, monocular VEPs elicited by oscillating grating stimuli (motion VEPs) show a pronounced nasotemporal asymmetry.[40-43] The direction of the asymmetry is inverted when viewing with the right vs. left eye. Monocular FPL testing reveals greater sensitivity to nasalward motion.[44] Monocular pursuit and optokinetic tracking show strong biases favoring nasalward target motion.[31,45-48] Optokinetic after nystagmus (slow phase eye movement in the dark after extinction of stimulus motion) shows a consistent nasalward drift of eye position.[49] These nasalward motion biases are most pronounced before onset of sensorial fusion and stereopsis and diminish thereafter.

Development and maldevelopment of cortical binocular connections

Knowledge of visual cortex development (Table 73.3) is important for understanding the neural mechanisms that cause strabismus:

1. The visual cortex is the initial locus in the CNS at which signals from the two eyes are combined; a combination of visual signals is necessary to generate the vergence error commands that guide eye alignment.
2. The most common form of strabismus (esotropia) appears coincident with maturation of cortically mediated, binocular, sensorimotor behaviors in normal infants.
3. Perinatal insults to the immature visual cortex are linked to subsequent strabismus.
4. The constellation of sensory and motor deficits in infantile strabismus can be explained by known cortical pathway mechanisms.

Persistent nasalward visuomotor biases in strabismic primate

If normal maturation of binocularity is impeded by eye misalignment, the innate nasalward bias of eye tracking does not resolve; it persists and becomes pronounced.[50-53] The bias is evident as a pathologic nasotemporal asymmetry of pursuit/OKN and a nasalward (slow phase) drift of gaze holding (latent nystagmus)[54,55] (see Chapter 88).

Area MST neurons are sensitive to binocular disparity and drive fusional vergence eye movements.[56,57] Eye movement recordings in a primate with infantile esotropia showed inappropriate activation of convergence whenever nasalward monocular OKN was evoked.[58] Analysis of V1 in this monkey showed a paucity of binocular connections and metabolic evidence of heightened interocular suppression. These observations imply that MST neurons promote esotropia, i.e. a bias for nasalward vergence, when binocularity fails to develop in V1. This theory ties together the nasalward biases of vergence, pursuit/OKN, and gaze holding (latent nystagmus) in cortical regions vulnerable to perinatal damage.

Outputs from the cortical areas V1, MT/MST, and related cortical areas descend to brainstem visual relay and premotor neuron pools adjacent to the motor nuclei.[59] Even in the absence of cortical maldevelopments, the vergence system is unbalanced, favoring convergence. Midbrain premotor neurons driving convergence outnumber those driving divergence by 3 : 2.

Repair of strabismic human infants: the historical controversy

Is repair of binocular V1 connections possible, restoring normal fusion and stereopsis, while preventing or reversing the ocular motor maldevelopments? This question was debated by the eminent British strabismologists, Claude Worth and Bernard Chavasse. Worth postulated that esotropic infants suffered "an irreparable defect of the fusion faculty."[60] Their brain

Table 73.3 – Development of neural pathways in normal and strabismic primate

Neurobiological principle	Physiology/anatomy	Investigator(s)
Striate cortex (area V1) is the first CNS locus for binocular processing	• Right eye (RE) and left eye (LE) inputs remain segregated in LGN and input layer (4C) in V1 • Binocular responses recorded from neurons in V1 lamina beyond layer 4C • Neurons in V1 layers 2–6 are sensitive to binocular disparity	Hubel 1977[91], 1982[92] Poggio 1977[93] Wiesel 1982[94]
Binocular structure + function in V1 is immature at birth	• Segregation of RE/LE ODCs immature at birth • Binocular (disparity sensitive) neurons present at birth but tuning poor • Immature binocular neurons have weak excitatory horizontal connections between ODCs and high suppression index	Hubel 1977[95] Levay 1980[96] Chino 1996[97], 1997[98] Horton 1996[99], 1997[100] Endo 2000[101]
Maturation of binocular connectivity in V1 requires correlated RE/LE input	• Absence of correlation causes lack of disparity sensitivity and loss of horizontal connections in V1	Crawford 1979[102], 1984[103], 1996[104] Lowel 2002[105] Trachtenberg 2001[106] Tychsen 1995[107], 2000[108], 2004[73]
V1 feeds forward to extrastriate visual areas MT/MST which control ipsiversive eye tracking and gaze holding	• Extrastriate areas MT/MST mediate pursuit/OKN and receive feed-forward (binocular) projections from V1 lamina 4B • Lesions of MST impair ipsiversive pursuit/OKN and gaze-holding	Pasik 1964[109], 1977[110] Dursteler 1987[111], 1988[112] Ungerleider 1986[113]
V1 feed forward connections to MT/MST at birth are monocular from ODCs driven by the contralateral eye	• Before maturation of binocularity, a nasalward movement bias is apparent when viewing with either eye (RE viewing evokes leftward pursuit/OKN/gaze drift; LE viewing evokes rightward pursuit/OKN/gaze drift) • Nasalward and temporalward neurons are present in equal numbers within V1/MT but nasalward have innate connectivity advantage	Kiorpes 1996[114] Hatta 1998[115] Tychsen 1999[14]
MST inputs from the ipsilateral eye require maturation of binocular V1/MT connections	• If binocularity matures, monocular viewing evokes equal nasalward/temporalward eye movement and stable gaze	Kiorpes 1996[114] Tychsen 1999[14] Wong 2003[68]
MST neurons encode both vergence and pursuit/OKN	• Disparity sensitive neurons in MST also mediate vergence • If binocularity fails to mature, monocular viewing evokes nasalward pursuit/OKN and inappropriate convergence	Maunsell 1983[116] Kawano 1999[56] Yildirim 2000[58] Takemura 2001[57] Wong 2003[68]
Convergence motorneurons are more numerous	• Convergence neurons outnumber divergence neurons 3:2 in the midbrain of normal primates	Mays 1983[117], 1984[82]

was congenitally incapable of achieving substantial binocular vision. Early surgical treatment was therefore futile. Chavasse, nurtured by Sherrington, on the other hand, believed that the neural substrate for fusion was present in esotropic infants, but the development of "conditioned reflexes" for binocular fusion was impeded by factors such as weakness of the motor limb.[61] He postulated that, if the eyes could be realigned during a period of "reflex learning," binocular fusion could be restored.

Repair of high-grade fusion is possible

New knowledge of stereopsis development in the 1980s bolstered the rationale in favor of early surgery.[62,63] This prompted a gradual re-examination of old data and inspired important case studies – on the efficacy of early strabismus surgery.[64-67] These reports showed that, if stable binocular alignment was not achieved until age 24 months, the chances of repairing stereopsis were nil. If stable alignment was achieved by age 6 months, the chances of repairing stereopsis were good. A substantial percentage of infants regained robust stereopsis, i.e. random dot stereopsis with thresholds in the order of 60–400 arc sec.

Early alignment data in infantile esotropia has produced an important conclusion. Figure 73.1A is replotted data on stereopsis outcomes in over 100 consecutive infantile esotropes.[65] The Y axis is prevalence of stereopsis after surgical alignment; the X axis is age of onset or duration of misalignment before surgery. The dashed line at 40% represents the average prevalence of stereopsis when all infants operated upon by 2 years of age are grouped together, without regard to age at correction or duration before correction. The noise in the data is related to the onset of strabismus varying considerably from infant to infant, distributed randomly between 2 to 6 months of age. There is no systematic relationship between age of onset of esotropia and subsequent attainment of stereopsis. However, when the data is re-analyzed with attention to duration of misalignment, a strong correlation is evident between shorter durations of misalignment and restoration of stereopsis (Fig. 73.1B). Excellent outcomes are achievable in infants operated upon within 60 days of onset of strabismus ("early surgery").[65] The conclusion is that age at surgery should be tailored to age of strabismus onset and not chronological age.

Esotropic infants who regain high-grade stereopsis regain robust fusional vergence.[65-67] Clinical observation suggests that they have a lower prevalence of recurrent esotropia (or exotropia), pursuit/OKN asymmetry, motion VEP asymmetry,

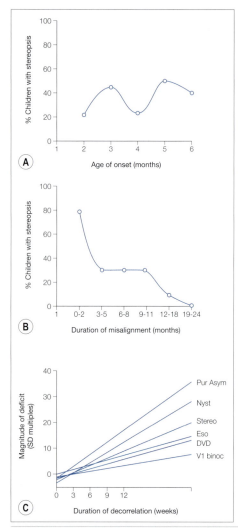

Fig. 73.1 Repair of random dot stereopsis after surgical realignment of the eyes in children with infantile esotropia, and analogous findings in strabismic monkeys. (A) Prevalence of stereopsis as a function of age of onset of strabismus. No systematic relationship is evident. (B) High prevalence (~80%) of stereopsis in infants who were aligned within 2 months of onset of strabismus. Probability of stereopsis was negligible in infants who had durations of strabismus exceeding ~12 months. (Redrawn from data of Birch et al. (2000).) (C) Magnitude of behavioral deficits increases systematically as a function of decorrelation duration in monkeys. One week of monkey visual development is equivalent to 1 month of human. Pur Asym = horizontal pursuit asymmetry; Nyst = velocity of latent nystagmus; Stereo = random dot stereopsis deficit; Eso = angle of esotropia; DVD = magnitude of dissociated vertical deviation; V1 binoc = reduction in binocular connections between RE and LE ODCs in V1 (striate cortex).

latent nystagmus, and dissociated vertical deviation (DVD). However, ocular motor recording is difficult to perform in children and detailed, quantitative information is lacking.

Timely restoration of correlated binocular input: the key to repair

Eye movement studies of strabismic infant monkeys have shown that normal motor and sensory pathway development can be restored when the timing conforms to that of early surgery in humans.[68,69] If binocular image correlation is restored

in strabismic monkeys within 3 weeks of onset of strabismus (the equivalent of 3 months in humans), fusional vergence, pursuit/OKN, and gaze holding return to normal (Fig. 73.1C). The repair of ocular motor behavior occurs with repair of stereopsis and restoration of normal motion responses (motion VEPs). If decorrelation persists in strabismic monkeys until the equivalent of 12 months' duration in humans, esotropia and stereoblindness persist. Prolonged decorrelation animals exhibit latent nystagmus, pursuit/OKN asymmetry, motion VEP asymmetry, and DVD. The quality of behavioral repair correlates with the quality of neuroanatomic repair in V1 (Fig. 73.1C). "Early repair" monkeys, i.e. those who have shorter durations of decorrelation, have a normal compliment of binocular horizontal excitatory connections between ODCs of opposite ocularity and "delayed repair" (longer durations of decorrelation) monkeys a paucity. The restoration of binocular connections in V1 of "early repair" monkeys has equally beneficial effects on downstream areas of extrastriate cortex (MT/MST) driving the ocular motor neurons of the brainstem. The benefit is evident as symmetric nasotemporal eye tracking, stable gaze holding, and more normal fusional vergence.

Visual cortex mechanisms in microesotropia (monofixation syndrome)

Recent data on early correction of infantile strabismus suggests that it is curable, but early surgery is the exception rather than the rule of current practice. The majority of infants with esotropia are corrected 6 or more months after onset of misalignment: the chances of rescuing bifoveal fusion after this interval are slim. Most infants are aligned to within 8 PD (prism diopters) of orthotropia (microesotropia) and regain a degree of subnormal stereopsis and motor fusion: monofixation syndrome.

Monofixation syndrome occurs as a primary disorder (prevalence 1%) or, more commonly, as a secondary phenomenon, after delayed treatment of strabismus.[70,71] The syndrome also occurs in monkeys.[72] The major sensory and motor features of monofixation syndrome are listed in Table 73.4. Neural mechanisms for the first two features listed in Table 73.4 are not difficult to explain. Receptive fields in V1 representing the fovea are tiny and have narrow tolerances. Any defocusing or other decorrelation of one eye's inputs produces a conflict in neighboring V1 columns and promotes suppression of ODCs corresponding to the weaker eye. The fovea subtends ~5 deg of the retinotopic map of V1, thus a suppression scotoma of ≤5 deg makes sense. Subnormal stereopsis could be explained along similar lines. Stereoscopic thresholds increase exponentially from the fovea to more eccentric positions along the retinotopic map of the visual field. If foveal ODCs are suppressed and parafoveal ODCs are left to mediate stereopsis, stereopsis is degraded but not obliterated. Yet, it is the visuomotor features of the monofixation syndrome that are most intriguing. If binocular development is perturbed so that right and left eye foveal ODCs (receptive fields) are not perfectly correlated, why should the "fall back" position of visual cortex be set so predictably ~2–4 deg (~4–8 PD) of microesotropia (Fig. 73.2)? And if the heterotropia exceeds that range, why is fusional vergence typically absent?

Table 73.4 – Monofixation (microstrabismus) syndrome

Clinical feature	Possible neural mechanism
1. Foveal suppression scotoma of 3–5 deg in the non-preferred eye* when viewing binocularly	Inhibitory connection mediated metabolic suppression of decorrelated activity in V1 foveal ODCs of non-preferred eye
2. Subnormal stereopsis (threshold 60–3000 arc sec)	Broader disparity tuning of parafoveal neurons in V1/MT (foveal neurons suppressed)
3. Stable microesotropia** less than ~4–8 PD (~2.5–5 deg)	Small angle ≈ average horizontal neuron length in V1, esotropia by default to convergent disparity coding of major MST population
4. Fusional vergence amplitudes intact for disparities greater than ~2.5–5 deg (~4–8 PD)	V1 excitatory horizontal binocular connections (and V1/MT/MST disparity neurons) intact beyond region of foveal suppression

*Subnormal acuity (amblyopia) in the non-preferred eye in 34% of corrected infantile esotropes and 100% of anisometropes.
**Microexotropia in less than ~10%.

Neuroanatomic findings in area V1 of microesotropic primates

Studies of ODCs and neuronal axons in area V1 have revealed a possible mechanism. The overall pattern and width of ODCs in V1 (~400 microns [0.40 mm]) is the same in normal and strabismic monkeys.[73,74] Horizontal axon length was measured for neurons within the V1 region corresponding to visual field eccentricities of 0 to 10 deg (i.e. the representation of the fovea, parafovea, and macula). The length is similar in both normal and strabismic monkeys, on average ~7 mm.[73,75] In a primate with normal eye alignment, the ODC representing the foveola (or 0 deg eccentricity) of the left eye is immediately adjacent to the column representing the foveola of the right eye. The side-by-side arrangement of the "foveolar" columns in normal V1 is well within the range of horizontal axonal connections needed to allow those ODCs to communicate for high-grade binocular fusion.

In a primate with microesotropia and a right eye fixation preference (Fig. 73.2), a neuron within a foveolar (0 deg) column of the fixating right eye must link up with a non-adjacent column representing the pseudo-foveola of the deviated left eye. Based on retinotopic maps of V1 in a macaque monkey, a horizontal axon ~7 mm in length could join ODCs (and receptive fields) that were up to, but not further than, 2.5 deg (4.4 PD) apart. Figure 73.2B is a two-dimensional map representing V1 from the right cerebral hemisphere (left visual hemi-field) of a microesotropic macaque. The sulci and gyri have been unfolded and the visual field representation super-imposed using standard retinotopic landmarks. One horizontal axon, originating within the foveal representation at 0–1 deg eccentricity, could link to a receptive field shifted 2.5 deg or 4.4 PD distant. Two neurons strung together could join receptive fields 5 deg or 8.7 PD apart. Thus, the 4–8 PD "rule" of the monofixation syndrome is explicable as a combination of innate V1 neuron size and V1 topography. The visuomotor system of the strabismic primate appears to achieve

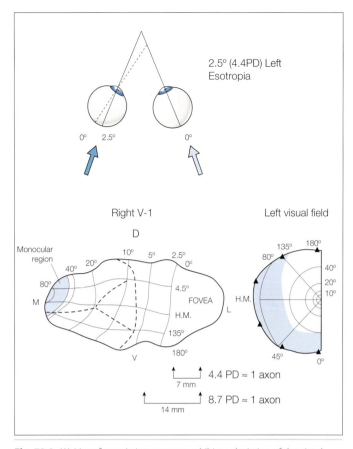

Fig. 73.2 (A) Monofixator/microesotrope exhibits a deviation of the visual axes on cover testing of approximately 4 PD (~2.5 deg), which in this case is a left eye microesotropia (dark arrow = pseudofovea position in deviated eye). When fusional vergence or prism adaptation is tested in such a patient, the angle of deviation tends to persistently return to that 2.3 deg angle. (B) Two-dimensional map representing V1 from the right cerebral hemisphere (left visual hemi-field) of a microesotropic primate. The sulci and gyri have been unfolded and the visual field representation superimposed using standard retinotopic landmarks. One horizontal axon (average length ~7 mm), originating within the foveal representation at 0–1 deg eccentricity, could link to a receptive field shifted 2.5 deg or 4.4 PD distant. Two neurons strung together could join receptive fields 5 deg or 8.7 PD apart. The conclusion is that the 4–8 PD "rule" of monofixation/microesotropia syndrome is explicable as a combination of innate V1 neuron size (one to two axon lengths) and V1 topography.

subnormal but stable binocular fusion if the angle of deviation is confined to a distance corresponding to no more than one to two V1 neurons.[75]

Extrastriate cortex in microesotropia

Neuronal response properties of the vergence-related region of extrastriate visual cortex, MST, may also explain the 2.5 deg microesotropia rule in monofixation syndrome. MST receives downstream projections from disparity-sensitive cells, both in V1 and in MT. The majority of binocular neurons in V1, MT, and MST encode absolute disparity.[57,76] Absolute disparity sensitivity (the location of an image on each retina with respect to the foveola, or 0 deg eccentricity) guides vergence. Relative disparity sensitivity (the location of an image in depth with respect to other images) is necessary for stereopsis but not vergence. The largest population of vergence-related neurons in MST of normal monkeys drives the eyes to ~2.5 deg of convergent (crossed) disparity.[57] Normal primates have the strongest short-latency vergence responses to convergent disparities of ~2.5 deg.[77]

Insults that impair the development of binocular connections in immature V1 would impair the (downstream) development of the population of binocular MST neurons. The probability of surviving an insult would be greatest for the most populous neurons: those encoding ~2.5 deg (~4.4 PD) of convergence. In the presence of a weakened pool of disparity-sensitive neurons, the vergence system may default to the vergence commanded by the surviving population. A stable 2.5 deg convergence angle could be maintained by the next most populous remaining neurons, those encoding 2.5 deg of divergence. These mechanisms account for the direction, approximate magnitude, and stability of microesotropia, with retention of a capacity for fusional (e.g. prism) vergence responses evoked by disparities >2.5 deg.

Acquired (non-infantile) esotropia

Epidemiologic[1-3,78] and animal studies[79,80] indicate that the second most common type of strabismus in humans and monkeys is esotropia linked to accommodation. Onset of accommodative strabismus occurs at ~3 years of age, well beyond the early infantile period of rapid maturation of the visuomotor pathways. The majority of these children regain binocular fusion when the refractive error (and any amblyopia) is corrected. They do not exhibit the eye tracking and gaze holding deficits of infantile esotropia.[50,81] This suggests that cortical binocular connections in this disorder are substantially more abundant than those in children with infantile esotropia. A subtle deficit of binocular connections may be inconsequential until the system, normally biased toward convergence, is taxed by the accommodative demands (most convergence-related neurons in the midbrain of normal primates encode both vergence and accommodation, with a range of different gains).[82-84] Whether accommodative esotropia is intermittent or constant may depend on a multitude of idiosyncratic variables:

1. The ratio of convergence to divergence neurons.
2. The average gain of accommodation-linked convergence neurons.
3. The strength of cortical neuron pools encoding corrective, uncrossed (divergent) disparity.
4. The maturity of excitatory horizontal connections between V1 ODCs mediating fusion.
5. The strength of inhibitory connections between V1 ODCs mediating suppression (and loss of fusion).

Exotropia

Constant exotropia is 3–10 times less prevalent than esotropia. The most common form is intermittent.[20,78] Exotropia does not have a bimodal distribution of age of onset. Onset typically occurs after infancy with slow progression of an exophoria to exotropia, manifest when viewing distant non-accommodative targets. The magnitude of the exotropia tends to increase with age. When the eyes are aligned (exophoria), stereopsis

thresholds tend to be normal. Humans with comitant intermittent exotropia have no evidence of ocular motor nerve dysfunction, midbrain convergence paresis, orbital structural (e.g. pulley) anomaly, or extraocular myopathy.[85] Clinical observations do not point to a single locus in the CNS that would provide a neural mechanism for this disorder. Laboratory studies of CNS function and structure in naturally exotropic monkeys is lacking (as in human, primary exotropia is much less common than esotropia).

The later-onset and progression of the disorder imply that the neural defect promoting exodeviation is present at birth, but controlled by the convergence bias of the infantile visuomotor pathways. As binocularity matures, the nasalward bias of these pathways recedes and the exo-drive gradually manifests. A full normal complement of excitatory horizontal connections between ODCs in V1 would be expected, since stereopsis matured properly during infancy. Normal V1/MT/MST binocularity is also connoted by the robustness of fusional vergence when accommodation is engaged.

Normal primates have transient exodeviations when executing superficially conjugate saccadic eye movements.[86,87] The adducting eye actually lags the abducting eye, necessitating a pulse of short-latency fusional convergence at the end of a saccade. The saccade-related exodeviation in healthy primates appears to represent a "physiologic internuclear ophthalmoplegia," produced by a normal delay in conducting an adduction signal over interneurons, from the abducens nucleus of the pons to the medial rectus subnucleus of the midbrain. It is not known if this behavior is exaggerated in comitant exodeviation. Comitant exodeviation could also be promoted by other brainstem mechanisms, e.g. an abnormally low ratio of convergence to divergence neurons in the midbrain.

Summary of strabismus neuroscience knowledge

- Proper alignment of the eyes requires information sharing (fusion) between monocular visual input channels (ODCs) in the CNS; the first locus for fusion in the CNS of primates is the striate cerebral cortex (area V1).
- Fusion is achieved by excitatory binocular horizontal connections in V1 joining ODCs of opposite ocularity.
- Fusion behaviors and V1 binocular connections are immature at birth, maturing during a brief (critical) period in the first months of life; maturation of fusion (and the V1 binocular connections) requires correlated (synchronized) input from each eye.
- The dominant form of strabismus in primates (esotropia) appears during the period of normal fusion maturation.
- Strabismus can be produced in normal non-human primates by impeding the maturation of fusional connections in V1.
- Strabismus occurs predominantly in humans who have perinatal insults that could directly or indirectly impair maturation of binocular connections in V1.
- Strabismus and related maldevelopments of eye movement conform to innate, directional biases present in the neural pathways of normal primates before maturation of binocularity.

- Therapeutic interventions, applied during the brief period of normal binocular maturation, can achieve functional sensory and motor cures.
- If therapy cannot restore bifoveal fusion, subnormal fusion (monofixation) may be achieved within boundaries set by the properties of neurons in V1 and extrastriate cortex.
- Later-onset forms of strabismus are easier to treat because the fusional connections in V1 matured before the emergence of minor maldevelopments of vergence.

References

2. Christiansen SP, Chandler DL, Holmes JM, et al. Instability of ocular alignment in childhood esotropia. Ophthalmology 2008; 115: 2266–74.

5. Tamura EE, Hoyt CS. Oculomotor consequences of intraventricular hemorrhages in premature infants. Arch Ophthalmol 1987; 105: 533–5.

9. Khanna S, Sharma A, Inder T, Tychsen L. Prevalence of the ocular motor signs of the infantile strabismus complex in children with and without cerebral visual pathway white matter injury. Invest Ophthalmol Vis Sci 2009; 49: 1209.

23. Pediatric Eye Disease Investigator Group. The clinical spectrum of early-onset esotropia: experience of the congenital esotropia observational study. Am J Ophthalmol 2002; 133: 102–8.

25. Birch E, Stager D, Wright K, Beck R, Pediatric Eye Disease Investigator Group. The natural history of infantile esotropia during the first six months of life. J AAPOS 1998; 2: 325–8.

35. Horwood AM, Riddell PM. Can misalignments in typical infants be used as a model for infantile esotropia? Invest Ophthalmol Vis Sci 2004; 45: 714–20.

40. Norcia AM, Garcia H, Humphry R, et al. Anomalous motion VEPs in infants and in infantile esotropia. Invest Ophthalmol Vis Sci 1991; 32: 436–9.

43. Birch EE, Fawcett S, Stager D. Co-development of VEP motion response and binocular vision in normal infants and infantile esotropes. Invest Ophthalmol Vis Sci 2000; 41: 1719–23.

44. Bosworth RG, Birch EE. Direction-of-motion detection and motion VEP asymmetries in normal children and children with infantile esotropia. Invest Ophthalmol Vis Sci 2007; 48: 5523–31.

50. Tychsen L, Hurtig RR, Scott WE. Pursuit is impaired but the vestibulo-ocular reflex is normal in infantile strabismus. Arch Ophthalmol 1985; 103: 536–9.

53. Tychsen L, Rastelli A, Steinman S, Steinman B. Biases of motion perception revealed by reversing gratings in humans who had infantile-onset strabismus. Dev Med Child Neurol 1996; 38: 408–22.

55. Richards M, Wong A, Foeller P, et al. Duration of binocular decorrelation predicts the severity of latent (fusion maldevelopment) nystagmus in strabismic macaque monkeys. Invest Ophthalmol Vis Sci 2008; 49: 1872–8.

58. Yildirim C, Tychsen L. Disjunctive optokinetic nystagmus in a naturally esotropic macaque monkey: interactions between nasotemporal asymmetries of versional eye movement and convergence. Ophthalmic Res 2000; 32: 172–80.

69. Tychsen L, Wong AMF, Foeller P, Bradley D. Early versus delayed repair of infantile strabismus in macaque monkeys: II. Effects on motion visually evoked responses. Invest Ophthalmol Vis Sci 2004; 45: 821–7.

72. Tychsen L, Scott C. Maldevelopment of convergence eye movements in macaque monkeys with small and large-angle infantile esotropia. Invest Ophthalmol Vis Sci 2003; 44: 3358–68.

73. Tychsen L, Wong AMF, Burkhalter A. Paucity of horizontal connections for binocular vision in V1 of naturally-strabismic macaques: cytochrome-oxidase compartment specificity. J Comp Neurol 2004; 474: 261–75.

75. Wong AMF, Lueder GT, Burkhalter A, Tychsen L. Anomalous retinal correspondence: neuroanatomic mechanism in strabismic monkeys and clinical findings in strabismic children. J AAPOS 2000; 4: 168–74.

79. Quick MW, Eggers HM, Boothe RG. Natural strabismus in monkeys: convergence errors assessed by cover test and photographic methods. Invest Ophthalmol Vis Sci 1992; 33: 2986–3004.

80. Quick MW, Newbern JD, Boothe RG. Natural strabismus in monkeys: accommodative errors assessed by photorefraction and their relationship to convergence errors. Invest Ophthalmol Vis Sci 1994; 35: 4069–79.

89. Hainline L, Riddell PM. Binocular alignment and vergence in early infancy. Vision Res 1995; 35: 3229–36.

93. Poggio GF, Fischer B. Binocular interaction and depth sensitivity in striate and prestriate cortex of behaving rhesus monkey. J Neurophysiol 1977; 40: 1392–405.

100. Horton JC, Hocking DR. Timing of the critical period for plasticity of ocular dominance columns in macaque striate cortex. J Neurosci 1997; 17: 3684–709.

106. Trachtenberg JT, Stryker MP. Rapid anatomical plasticity of horizontal connections in the developing visual cortex. J Neurosci 2001; 21: 3476–82.

107. Tychsen L, Burkhalter A. Neuroanatomic abnormalities of primary visual cortex in macaque monkeys with infantile esotropia: preliminary results. J Pediatr Ophthalmol Strabismus 1995; 32: 323–8.

108. Tychsen L, Yildirim C, Anteby I, et al. Macaque monkey as an ocular motor and neuroanatomic model of human infantile strabismus. In: Lennerstrand G, Ygge J, editors. Advances in Strabismus Research: Basic and Clinical Aspects. London, UK: Wenner-Gren International Series, Portland Press Ltd; 2000: 103–19.

111. Dürsteler MR, Wurtz RH, Newsome WT. Directional pursuit deficits following lesions of the foveal representation within the superior temporal sulcus of the macaque monkey. J Neurophysiol 1987; 57: 1262–87.

114. Kiorpes L, Walton PJ, O'Keefe LP, et al. Effects of artificial early-onset strabismus on pursuit eye movements and on neuronal responses in area MT of macaque monkeys. J Neurosci 1996; 16: 6537–53.

115. Hatta S, Kumagami T, Qian J, et al. Nasotemporal directional bias of V1 neurons in young infant monkeys. Invest Ophthalmol Vis Sci 1998; 39: 2259–67.

Access the complete reference list online at

http://www.expertconsult.com

Part 2
Esotropias

Infantile esotropias

Glen A Gole • Jayne E Camuglia

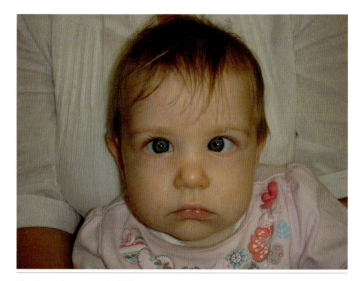

Fig. 74.1 Large angle IET.

"First, we must, I believe, firmly embed strabismus in the matrix where it belongs – an anomaly of neurodevelopment."
John T Flynn[1]

Infantile esotropia (IET) is a constant non-accommodative esotropia (ET) with onset before 6 months of age in a neurologically normal child (Fig. 74.1). The angle is >30 prism diopters with mild or no amblyopia and mild hyperopia. "Congenital esotropia" is often used synonymously but the condition is rarely present at birth. These children may have potential for good binocularity if they are treated early, suggesting the underlying defect is not congenital. It is often accompanied by dissociated vertical deviation (DVD) 50–90%,[2,3] inferior oblique muscle overaction (IOOA) 70%,[4] latent nystagmus 40%, and optokinetic asymmetry. IET and the secondary associations are often grouped under "infantile strabismus complex;" some components may exist in the absence of strabismus.

History

The term infantile esotropia was introduced by Costenbader to include age of onset less than 1 year.[5] He had previously defined "congenital" ET as having an onset less than 6 months.[6] The term congenital ET reflects Claud Worth's theory[7] in which ET is caused by a congenital defect of fusion – *"The essential cause of squint is a defect of the fusion faculty."* Worth's theory implies that the "congenital defect" is irreparable and that surgery can be carried out at leisure, largely for cosmetic reasons. The opposing view, that the infant visual system is normal initially until ET occurs as a result of extrinsic factors, was proposed by Chavasse.[8] Chavasse thought that "most infants with congenital squint are capable of developing fusion if the deviation is fully corrected before the age of two years." This view was accepted by Costenbader,[9] Parks, and his fellows and became widely accepted after the work of Ing.[10] It is not so widely accepted in Europe where surgery is often carried out much later.[11] The evidence supporting Chavasse's view that corrective surgery should be carried out early in infancy appeared in the 1960s and, during the 1980s, there was an explosion of knowledge of vision development in infancy[12-14] and a refinement of surgical techniques. Surgical case series have enabled consolidation of clinical knowledge concerning IET.[15-17] There has been progress in documenting the effects of early surgery on binocular outcomes and motor alignment.

Epidemiology

The prevalence of any ET in a population of 38 000 children aged 1–2½ years was found to be 0.9%.[18] The prevalence of IET in one area of the US was relatively constant at 0.25% of the population.[19] The rate of strabismus surgery in childhood has declined substantially in the UK in recent decades.[20] The decrease may be due to the routine prescribing of the full cycloplegic refraction for strabismus. Despite the decrease in strabismus surgery, Carney et al. stated that the rate of surgery in children under 1 year was unchanged.[21]

IET runs in families so there is a hereditary component and primary monofixation syndrome occurs much more commonly in the parents and families of children with IET than in the general population.[22] Maumenee et al. concluded that the inheritance pattern was most likely Mendelian codominant.[23]

The natural history of the development of ocular alignment

In a study of normal neonates, Sondhi et al.[24] found that 55% had a constant deviation (66% of whom an exodeviation) and 30% were orthotropic. No neonatal esodeviations were seen after 2 months of age and 97.2% of their infants were orthotropic at age 6 months. In another study[25] the same authors concluded that the time of onset of IET was between 2 and 4 months of age. Horwood described "neonatal misalignments" (NMs) as fleeting, large angle, mainly convergent, ocular deviations[26] occurring commonly in the first two months of life (73.2% of infants in the first month of life). The NMs declined to almost zero by 4 months of age except in those children who went on to develop IET where the frequency of misalignment increased.[27] There was no relationship between frequent NMs in the first 2 months of life and the subsequent development of IET. Horwood's report of a high prevalence of convergent misalignments in (older) normal infants is in direct contrast to those of Archer et al.'s[25] high prevalence of divergent deviations (especially in the immediate newborn period). The Sondhi and Archer[24,25] studies used a method which relied on the infant fixating on the examiner's face. This may have had an artifact induced by the large positive angle kappa seen in early infancy and the particular fixation pattern of neonates when looking at a face.[28] Friedrich and de Decker[29] also found a high (50%) incidence of exotropia (XT) in neonates, but only one of 1024 newborn infants developed an ET that was still present at 3 months of age. Children who develop IET begin to be different from normal infants at approximately 4 months of age. Because transient misalignment of the eyes is common parental reports the exact age of onset of strabismus must be viewed with caution.

Birch et al. reported that none of 66 infants with misalignment ≥40 PD of ET and an onset between 2 and 4 months of

age had spontaneous regression suggesting that they were suitable candidates for early surgery.[30] The Congenital Esotropia Observation Study (CEOS)[31] reported that, before 12 weeks of age, the majority of esotropic infants had an intermittent or variable deviation, whereas after 12 weeks of age the deviations were more constant. They concluded that normal infants > 10 weeks old with a constant ET of ≥40 PD and ≤3.00 diopters of hyperopia had very little prospect of spontaneous regression (2%) and could be offered early surgery (Box 74.1).[32,33] However, if the deviation was < 40 PD, intermittent or variable, it usually resolved.

Clinical patterns

Dissociated vertical deviation (alternating sursumduction, occlusion hyperphoria)

In DVD, the eye elevates and extorts and is not associated with a corresponding downwards movement of the other eye when fixation is resumed (Fig. 74.2). DVD does not follow Hering's Law. It can occur spontaneously or only when the fellow eye is occluded. DVD can vary in size and frequency of occurrence. Rarely, the patient adopts a head tilt to the same side. For management purposes, DVD can be quantified with base down prism. The prism is placed in front of the eye with DVD until no more downward movement takes place on alternate cover testing.

Inferior oblique muscle overaction

Inferior oblique muscle overaction (IOOA) is visible in adduction only and associated with fundus excyclotorsion (Fig. 74.3) and a V pattern. DVD and IOOA are usually bilateral, but can be asymmetric. If the eye elevates in adduction and there is a corresponding hypodeviation in the opposite eye, the deviation is due to IOOA. If there is no corresponding hypodeviation, then DVD is present. If the elevation of the adducted

---

Box 74.1

Clinical profile of infants who will benefit most from early surgery, i.e. unlikely to spontaneously resolve

1. Presence or persistence of ET between 10 weeks and 6 months of age
2. Constant ET 40 PD at near (1/3 m) on two examinations 2–4 weeks apart
3. Refractive error ≤+3.00 D
4. Absence of any of the following conditions:
   Gestational age < 34 weeks
   Birth weight ≤1500 g
   Ventilator treatment in the newborn period
   History of meningitis or other major medical event
   Developmental delay
   Incomitant or paralytic strabismus
   Manifest nystagmus or head bobbing
   Prior eye muscle surgery
   Presence of structural ocular anomalies

Adapted from Spontaneous resolution of early-onset esotropia: experience of the Congenital Esotropia Observational Study. Am J Ophthalmol 2002; 133: 109–18 by Wong AMF. Can J Ophthalmol 2008; 43: 643–51.

eye exceeds the hypodeviation in the fellow eye, combined DVD and IOOA are present.

Dissociated horizontal deviation

Dissociated horizontal deviation (DHD) is much less frequent than DVD. Often asymmetric, it can occur simultaneously with DVD. DHD may merely be DVD with a large horizontal component. It can cause confusion with consecutive XT and the two may coexist. The two can be distinguished by a difference in horizontal measurements when measuring with the prism in front of each eye. The treatment is a supramaximal lateral rectus recession of the affected eye.[34]

Latent nystagmus

Latent nystagmus (LN) is common in IET and occurs on monocular occlusion. The fast phase is toward the uncovered eye. The nystagmus is lessened in adduction and worsened in abduction. LN can lower the acuity in the uncovered eye. This can be obviated by fogging the eye not being tested with a +3.00 lens rather than occluding it. Manifest latent nystagmus is "latent" nystagmus which is present in binocular viewing (see Chapter 88).

Optokinetic asymmetry

Infants under 2 months of age show greater sensitivity to objects moving from temporal to nasal than from nasal to temporal. This asymmetry disappears by 4–6 months of age in

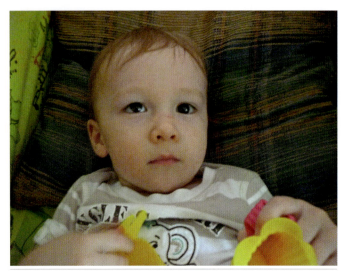

Fig. 74.2 Right dissociated vertical deviation.

normal infants. This nasalward bias persists when infants develop IET and becomes permanent.

Differential diagnosis

The differential diagnosis and clinical forms of IET can be considered as either truly congenital or early in onset (within the first 6 months; Box 74.2). In most cases a thorough history and ophthalmic examination helps to differentiate the subtypes (Fig. 74.4).

Pseudoesotropia is common. It can be confirmed by performing the Brückner, Hirschberg, and cover tests to determine that the eyes are orthotropic (Fig. 74.5). The Brückner test[35] can have false positives in children younger 8 months of age.[36] Examination of photographs with the parents can confirm the diagnosis.

In type 1 Duane's syndrome, the diagnosis is confirmed by limitation of abduction and globe retraction in adduction. Bilateral type 1 Duane's syndrome can be difficult to distinguish from IET, particularly if the child is cross-fixating as the globe retraction in adduction can be quite subtle in infants. Performing a doll's eye maneuver to demonstrate full abduction will exclude Duane's syndrome and congenital sixth nerve palsy (a benign condition which usually resolves by 6 weeks of age).[37] Other techniques to elicit abduction include rotating the child or using monocular occlusion. A sixth and seventh nerve palsy may be due to Möbius syndrome, which may be associated with orofacial and limb abnormalities (Fig. 74.6).

A full ophthalmic examination including cycloplegic refraction will exclude any anterior or posterior segment cause for a sensory ET (see Chapter 72).

Box 74.2

Differential diagnosis of infantile esotropia

True congenital onset ET	Infantile onset ET
(True) Congenital ET	Infantile ET
Pseudoesotropia	Early onset accommodative
Type 1 Duane's syndrome	Sensory ET
Congenital sixth nerve palsy	Ciancia syndrome
Nystagmus blockage syndrome	Associated neurologic – CP, PVL
Congenital fibrosis syndrome	Associated systemic – DS,
Infantile myasthenia gravis	albinism
Möbius syndrome	

CP, cerebral palsy; PVL, periventricular leukomalacia; DS, Down's syndrome.

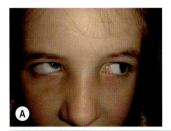 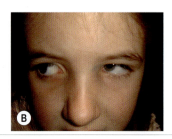 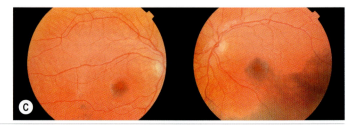

Fig. 74.3 Right IOOA (A), left IOOA (B), and fundus excyclotorsion (C) in the same patient. Note the fovea now lies below a line passing through the inferior edge of the optic discs.

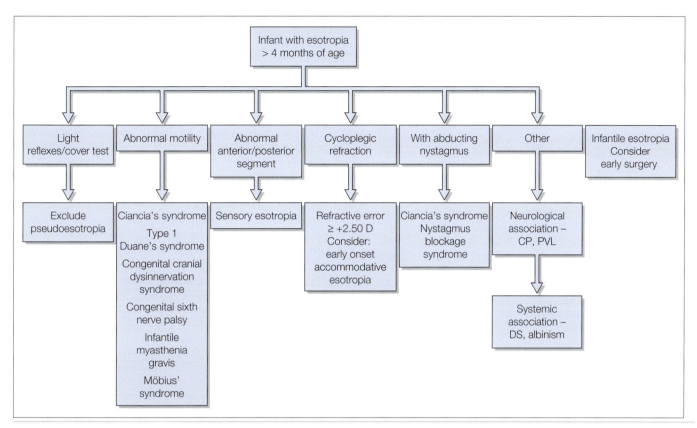

Fig. 74.4 Work-up of infant ≥4 months of age with ET [CP, cerebral palsy; PVL, periventricular leukomalacia; DS, Down syndrome].

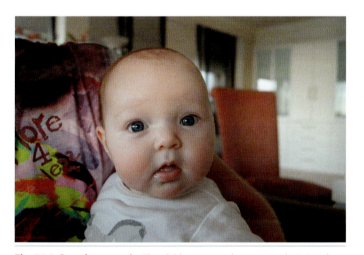

Fig. 74.5 Pseudoesotropia. The child appears to have an esodeviation due to a prominent left epicanthic fold limiting the amount of visible nasal sclera; however, the light reflexes are symmetric and cover test was normal.

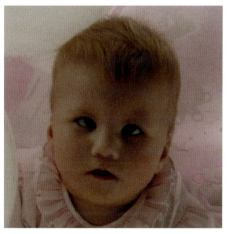

Fig. 74.6 Möbius syndrome.

Ciancia syndrome

Ciancia described a subset of esotropes[38] that others refer to as "cross-fixation congenital esotropia."[17,39]

Ciancia syndrome has the following features:

1. EET of early onset.
2. A large angle of deviation.
3. Bilateral limitation of abduction.
4. Abducting jerk nystagmus with the quick phase toward the fixating eye.

5. Torticollis with face turn toward the fixating eye.
6. Head tilt toward the side of the fixating eye.[40,41]

Nystagmus blockage syndrome

Nystagmus blockage syndrome (NBS) was first described by Adelstein and Cuppers.[42] von Noorden reported a prevalence of between 4.8% and 10.3% of congenital esotropes.[43] The syndrome is characterized by:

1. Nystagmus with early onset large, variable angle ET.
2. Pseudoabducens paralysis.
3. Head turn in direction of fixing eye.

4. Absent nystagmus with the fixing eye in adduction.
5. Increasing magnitude of manifest nystagmus with abduction.

NBS and Ciancia syndrome should be considered in any esotropic child with abducting nystagmus. However, the underlying pathophysiology is different. In Ciancia syndrome, the ET and nystagmus are coincidental,[15] whereas in NBS there is congenital idiopathic nystagmus with the null point in adduction (causing ET). Accommodation/convergence innervation may play a role and pupillary constriction in adduction may assist in making the diagnosis of NBS.[44] With alternating ET and cross-fixation, there is no nystagmus in primary gaze or abduction. The fixating eye is in the primary position and the non-fixating eye adducted (unlike in NBS where both eyes are in adduction). There is often no amblyopia (unlike in NBS).[43] Treatment in all these syndromes is often the same (large bilateral medial rectus recessions (BMRc)) with good motor outcomes[45] in most cases.

The prevalence of strabismus in children with developmental delay is reported to be between 27% and 100%.[46,47] Haugen et al found that strabismus in Down's syndrome occurred in 42% and was predominantly early-onset ET (84%) associated with hyperopia.[48] The rate of strabismus in patients with cerebral palsy is 44% on average (15–62%).[49]

Surgery for ET in developmentally delayed children has variable postoperative outcomes. Some groups report high rates of overcorrections and unpredictable outcomes.[50] Muen et al. reported suboptimal surgical results in seven patients who were unexpectedly diagnosed with periventricular leukomalacia after presenting with strabismus.[51] While some authors decrease the surgical dosage, Yahalom suggested that reduction of standard surgical dosages for ET in Down's syndrome is unnecessary.[50] We follow this practice.

Does stability of preoperative alignment affect outcomes?

Ing showed that the majority of patients observed prior to surgery for IET showed an increase of at least 10 PD with 50% showing an increase of at least 20 PD.[52] When surgery was based on the measurements taken 1 day before surgery, there was no difference in alignment between the group with an increase in angle and those with stable measurements. In a study of infants with IET grouped into stable (<10 PD difference in measurements between visits) or unstable (≥10 PD difference in measurements), Birch et al. demonstrated that there was no difference in postoperative alignment, reoperation rates, rates of prescription of hyperopic or bifocal spectacle or stereoacuity.[53] In a further study, the motor outcomes (alignment) were the same regardless of the stability of measurements before surgery.[54] There is an improvement in measurement stability after 6 months of age.[55]

Measurement uncertainty

Schutte et al. identified sources of human error in strabismus surgery.[56] Half of reoperations were due to inaccuracy in measurement of the angle of strabismus, variability in surgical strategy, or imprecise surgery.

In the Early vs. Late Infantile Strabismus Surgery study (ELISS) pilot study[57] three masked examiners found high intraobserver agreement with the Hirschberg test, but in 10% of cases it exceeded 10° (20 PD). In another study, experienced strabismologists reviewed photographs of strabismic patients and estimated the angle of squint using the Krimsky and Hirschberg tests with an expert examiner prism cover test (PCT) as the "gold standard."[58] The majority of examiners overestimated at least one patient by 10 PD with the Krimsky test. Differences of 5 PD were difficult to distinguish. With the Hirschberg test, each patient was underestimated by 10 PD by at least one examiner, with more inaccuracy for larger angles. The authors concluded that the Krimsky test is more accurate than Hirschberg, but both are less accurate than a cover test. Thompson and Guyton reported that it is impossible to accurately measure extremely large angles of strabismus with prisms.[59] A Pediatric Eye Disease Investigators Group (PEDIG) study[60] looked at interobserver reliability of the prism and alternate cover tests. They concluded that, in childhood ET of more than 20 PD, differences of 12 PD or more are likely to indicate real change, but smaller differences could be due to measurement error. We should be sceptical about the degree of accuracy of our measurements.

The PCT is the "gold standard" for strabismus measurement but can be limited by the child's cooperation. The Krimsky test is easy to perform with the prism split between the two eyes for angles of squint greater ≥40 PD. When the child is uncooperative, we use a combination of the Krimsky and Brückner tests.[61] We use loose plastic prisms for the PCT. Plastic right-angled prisms should be held in the frontal plane position[59] and plastic isosceles prisms should be held close to the position of minimum deviation.[62] This means that for both types of prism, each prism is always held with the base in the sagittal plane. We acknowledge that the prismatic effect of two split prisms is not the arithmetic sum of the two individual prisms,[59] but for most angles of ET the difference is within the measurement error. The measurement of the distance deviation is problematic in small infants, but it is always possible to measure the near angle. We usually base our surgical plan on the near deviation.

Non-surgical management

Refraction is crucial to the management of IET, especially in the postoperative period. Hyperopia occurs in 15% of children with IET.[63,64] At presentation, we treat infants with ≥2.5 D hyperopia with full spectacle prescription[63,65] to determine whether the ET is partially or fully accommodative. This resolves the ET completely in almost 50% of cases, therefore preventing unnecessary surgery.[63,64] However, 20% of infants initially controlled with glasses will decompensate and require surgery.[66] Spectacle correction can reduce a large angle strabismus such that only two muscles might need to be operated on rather than three. Correction of hyperopia is essential to maintain postoperative stability.

Amblyopia can be inferred by the child's fixation pattern. Fixation should be maintained through a blink in both eyes if the vision is equal.[67,68] Cross-fixation occurs when an infant fixes across their nose at the object of interest (Fig. 74.7). As an object of interest is moved from one side to the other, fixation switches at the midline if the vision is equal. If fixation switches

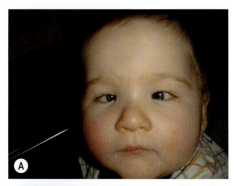

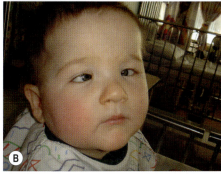

Fig. 74.7 Cross-fixation. Left gaze with right eye fixating (A), right gaze with left eye fixating (B).

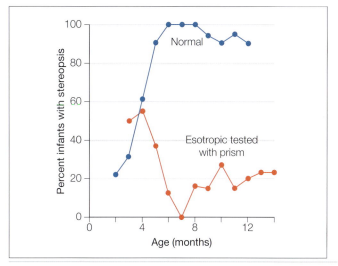

Fig. 74.8 Prevalence of stereopsis as a function of postnatal age in a population of normal versus esotropic infants. Esotropic infants were aligned using prisms and tested before surgery. (Adapted from Stager DR, Birch EE. Preferential-looking acuity and stereopsis in infantile esotropia. J Pediatr Ophthalmol Strabismus 1986; 23: 160–5 by Tychsen L. J AAPOS 2005; 9: 510–21. Reprinted by permission of Slack.)

past the midline, amblyopia is present in the eye towards which the toy is being moved.[69] It would seem logical to treat amblyopia before surgery. However, in one study of older children with untreated amblyopia there was no difference in postoperative alignment compared to those children with amblyopia treated preoperatively. One-sixth of the amblyopic patients had spontaneous resolution of the amblyopia as a result of surgery alone.[70] In a larger series, operating for IET in the presence of mild amblyopia made no difference to outcome, but the results were worse with moderate amblyopia.[71]

Preoperative alternate daily patching of each eye has been recommended to prevent the development of suppression[72] but this has been argued against by Parks.[73] Ing reported no difference in alignment outcome[74] between alternate day preoperative patching with unpatched controls, but the study was underpowered to detect less than a 25% difference in outcome.

Timing of surgery: why early surgery?

Fusion and stereopsis are absent before 2 months of age but develop rapidly between 3 and 5 months of age.[13] Forced-choice preferential looking and visual evoked potential stereoacuity both reach adult levels by 6–7 months of age.[75] Infants with a recent onset of strabismus that had been corrected with prisms had similar stereoacuity to normal infants of the same age[76,77] (Fig. 74.8). The critical period for disruption of stereopsis in IET peaks at 4.3 months of age so the time window for correction of IET with the aim of obtaining high grade stereopsis may be very narrow.[78] Wong reviewed the published data in favor of early surgery.[33] She showed there was a clear trend of declining stereopsis outcomes with increasing age at surgery (Fig. 74.9).

Chavasse argued that infants with IET could develop fusion if the squint was fully corrected before age 2. This was confirmed by Ing[10] who found that there was a significant

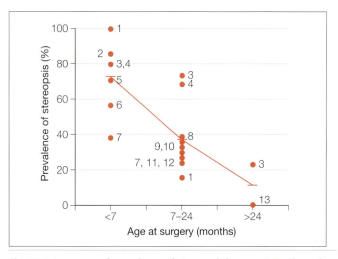

Fig. 74.9 Summary of prevalence of stereopsis by age at the time of surgery. Each circle indicates the prevalence of stereopsis from published studies. Short horizontal dashes represent mean prevalence of stereopsis for different age groups. (From Wong AMF. Timing of surgery for infantile esotropia: sensory and motor outcomes. Can J Ophthalmol 2008; 43: 643–51. Reprinted by permission of Elsevier.)

difference in sensory outcome between infants surgically aligned before and after age 2. Zak and Morin demonstrated that the development of Worth four dot fusion was related to the age at time of surgery.[79] Surgery after age 12 months was related to the development of latent nystagmus, IOOA, amblyopia, and reduced degrees of fusion.

Better sensory outcomes with surgery before age 2 has been confirmed by a controlled prospective multicenter study (ELISS), but the study had a high dropout rate.[11] Birch and Stager compared two groups of infants who had surgery before age 1 year.[80] The first group had surgery at or before 6 months of age and the second between 7 and 12 months of age with a follow-up of 4–17 years. Both cohorts had similar motor outcomes (83–94% had alignment within 6 PD), but the early group had significantly better peripheral and central fusion, Randot stereopsis, and Randot stereoacuity. Even with early surgery, only 38% of infants developed Randot stereopsis and only 20% developed Randot stereoacuity of ≥200 seconds of arc. Birch et al.[81] concluded that the duration of misalignment (not age of onset nor age at alignment) was the significant factor in determining stereopsis outcomes (Fig. 74.10). Patients with Randot stereopsis had fewer reoperations, and a lower prevalence of DVD, but no difference in the prevalence of amblyopia or the need for vertical muscle surgery. Subsequently they reported that patients with absent Randot stereopsis recorded immediately after surgery had 3.6 times more risk of surgery for recurrent ET or consecutive XT than those with measurable stereoacuity.[82] Ing and Okino[83] confirmed that loss of stereopsis was related to the duration of misalignment. In a further paper based on the same patient population, Ing and Rezentes[84] reported there was no significant difference in fusion in subgroups of infantile esotropes who had up to 21 months of misalignment or who were surgically aligned by 6, 12, or 24 months of age. They concluded that the time window for the development of fusion is wider than that for the development of stereopsis.

The importance of Birch et al.'s finding that duration of strabismus is the major determinant of sensory outcomes corresponds to studies of the duration of misalignment required to produce irreversible deficits in binocularity[85,86] in esotropic monkeys. We believe it has major implications for the rapidity with which referrals must be made and surgery carried out for children with IET if high grades of binocularity are to be achieved.

The best functional outcome for most infants with IET is the monofixation syndrome:[87] a child with a misalignment less than 10 PD who has fusional ability but only gross stereopsis. However, Wright reported excellent motor alignment and high grade stereopsis in two of seven patients operated on between 13 and 19 weeks of age.[88] Ing reported on 16 patients aligned before 6 months of age;[89] only one achieved high grade stereopsis. Helveston et al. cautioned that children operated on before 6 months of age had an average of one additional subsequent procedure in order to retain satisfactory alignment.[90]

There are several studies reporting delayed development in children with IET prior to surgery with improvement within months after surgery.[91-93] Drover et al. tested fine and gross motor development in infants with IET.[91] The presurgery group showed delayed sensorimotor and gross motor milestones (Fig. 74.11). After surgery, the delays disappeared

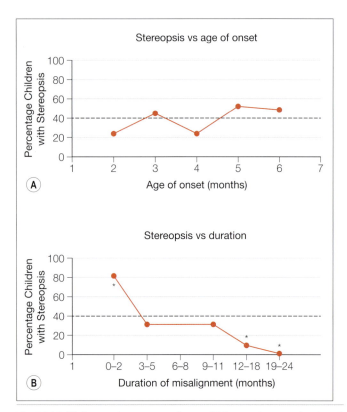

Fig. 74.10 (A) Stereopsis versus age of onset. (B) Stereopsis versus duration of misalignment. There is an inverse relationship between duration of misalignment and development of stereopsis. (From Birch EE, et al. J AAPOS 2000; 4: 10–14. Reprinted by permission of Elsevier.)

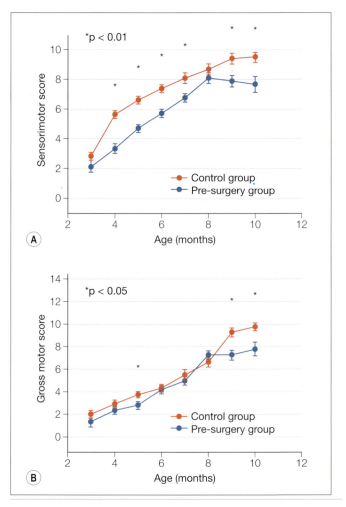

Fig. 74.11 Comparison of fine motor (A) and gross motor (B) score of presurgery and control groups. Bars represent one standard error. Asterisks represent significant differences. Planned comparisons indicated that the delay of sensorimotor milestones was significant at 4, 5, 6, 7, 9, and 10 months of age (p < 0.01). Delay of gross motor milestones was significant at 5, 9, and 10 months of age (p < 0.05). (From Drover JR, et al. Improvement in motor development following surgery for infantile esotropia. J AAPOS 2008; 12: 136–40. Reprinted by permission of Elsevier.)

suggesting that surgery is beneficial to infant development (Fig. 74.12).

Using a decision analysis approach, Trikalinos et al. concluded it is probably warranted to attempt surgery for IET "as early as possible."[94] In one series, parental satisfaction with their child's surgical outcome was reported as 85% and this correlated with a postoperative alignment in the microsquint range.[95] After surgery, parents noted improved eye contact and appearance of their children. The psychosocial benefits of surgery should not be underappreciated.

Why delay primary surgery?

The reasons advanced for delaying surgery include:

1. Difficulties measuring the angle of misalignment.
2. The lack of stability of deviation.
3. The possibility of spontaneous resolution.
4. Anesthetic risk.
5. Technical difficulties of surgery on infant eyes.

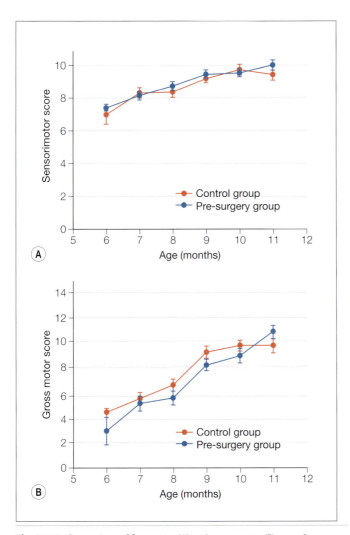

A

B

Fig. 74.12 Comparison of fine motor (A) and gross motor (B) score for postsurgery and control groups. Bars represent one standard error. (From Drover JR, et al. Improvement in motor development following surgery for infantile esotropia. J AAPOS 2008; 12: 136–40. Reprinted by permission of Elsevier.)

6. The difficulty of diagnosing amblyopia in infants with microtropia after successful surgery.

Spontaneous resolution has been reported in a small percentage of patients.[32] The CEOS reported that spontaneous resolution usually occurs when the deviation is <40 PD and is intermittent or variable in infants <20 weeks of age.[32] In infants with a constant deviation >40 PD only 2.4% of cases spontaneously resolved. In a series of infants less than 1 year of age with intermittent, small angle, and variable ET, Fu et al.[96] reported that patients with intermittent ET had a 46% chance of spontaneous resolution or were controlled with spectacle correction alone. However, patients with a constant small or variable angle ET progressed to a constant large angle ET requiring surgery.

Calcutt and Murray reported a series of adult patients with unoperated IET. The prevalence of amblyopia was 14% in whom two-thirds were anisometropic.[97] Later, they reported an improvement in sensory status in 88% of IETs operated on after 8 years of age and a widening of the visual field in 76% of patients.[98]

Posterior segment eye growth is rapid in the first few months of life[99] producing alterations in the insertion sites of the muscles relative to the equator so the determination of surgical dosage under the age of 6 months might be difficult. However, Helveston reported that this was not an issue when surgery was carried out at 4 months of age or later.[100]

Surgical management

The majority of patients with IET require surgical correction. Orthotropia or microesotropia gives better long-term results than microexotropia.[101] Surgery for IET can be technically demanding in children less than 2 years of age. Surgical approaches include BMRc, unilateral recess/resection, and for larger angles adding unilateral or bilateral lateral rectus resection(s) muscle surgery.[102-104] We no longer perform four horizontal muscle surgery due to an unacceptable rate of over-corrections. Our surgical table (BMRc- based on Helveston) provides surgical amounts up to 80 PD of ET (Table 74.1).[105]

We perform BMRc rather than a unilateral recess/resect procedure because it is technically easier, quicker, and does not

Table 74.1 – Horizontal muscle surgery dosage for infantile esotropia

Preoperative deviation (PD)	BMRc (mm) Age <1 year	BMRc (mm) Age >1 year	LLRs (mm)
30	9.5	10.0	–
35	10.0	10.5	–
40–55	10.5	11.0	–
60–65	10	10.5	4
70	10	10.5	5
75	10	10.5	6
80	10.5	11	6
85	10.5	11	8

NB. Amount of recession is measured from the limbus and recession amounts for 3MSR are reduced to lower the risk of consecutive exotropia.

involve a loss of muscle tissue. Nevertheless, a controlled randomized comparison of BMRc and unilateral recession/resection procedures in older children reported no difference in outcome.[106] In children with IET, the position of the medial rectus insertion varies from 3 to 6 mm from the limbus[107] and can also vary according to the degree of traction exerted during surgery.[108] Kushner and Morton proposed that unreliable results may be minimized by measuring recession from the limbus rather than the insertion.[109] They reported success in 84% of cases (mean preoperative deviation 53 PD) after performing 10.5 mm BMRc from the limbus. This was significantly better than graded recession from the insertion. We prefer measuring from the limbus because this is a constant ocular landmark (Fig. 74.13).

Successful alignment with BMRc in children with IET (30–100 PD) has been reported to be between 30% and 90%.[89,90,102,110-113] The prevalence of larger angles (>60 PD) in IET is 18%.[53] Few studies have reported the results of surgery for this group in isolation. Undercorrection rates are still significant and may be due to inadequate surgery amounts and/or the variability of the medial rectus insertion.[102,107] Scott compared BMRc 5–6.5 mm from insertion with three horizontal muscle surgery (graded BMRc measured from the limbus with lateral rectus resection) in angles >50 PD.[102] Success was 37.3% for the two horizontal muscle group with residual ET in 58%. Success in the three muscle group was 64.5%.

We conducted a validation study of a table guiding surgical dosage for three horizontal muscle surgery for larger angle IET. We reported successful alignment to within 10 PD of orthotropia in 91.3% at 1 year, 77.8% at 4 years, and 73.6% at 8 years.[105]

Inferior oblique surgery can be incorporated at the time of initial surgery if the IOOA is significant, especially with significant V pattern (>20 PD). The options for inferior oblique weakening include recession, anterior transposition, and myectomy. Mims et al. reported that successful bilateral anterior

transpositions also reduced the need for DVD surgery.[114] We do not perform inferior oblique myectomy in patients with IET because this prevents its use to treat DVD at some future time. If IOOA exists in isolation, we perform a graded IO recession. If IOOA and DVD coexist, we prefer a graded IO anterior transposition. If DVD is present alone, we perform a large superior rectus resection.[114]

Review of botulinum and the rationale of its use

The role of botulinum toxin A (Botox) injections in children as a primary or secondary treatment for failed surgery is still being debated (see Chapter 84).[115,116]

Motor "success" after 1–2 injections has been reported as greater than 80%.[117,118] Ing reported 50% of patients achieved sensory and motor fusion at 3 years follow-up; however, this was significantly less than those who had surgery.[119]

De Camponmanes et al. demonstrated that botulinum toxin had comparable success rates to surgery for smaller angles (<30 PD). However, for larger angles, surgery was better in achieving orthotropia.[115] Tejedor et al. compared botulinum toxin to reoperation for residual ET after unsuccessful BMRc and found similar sensory and motor results.[120] Botulinum toxin injection was most effective if given in the first 6 months after initial surgery.

Sedation is required for these injections. Injection risks include transient ptosis, secondary vertical misalignment, and the rare complications of globe perforation and retrobulbar hemorrhage.[121] Follow-up of children after botulinum toxin treatment is similar to those undergoing surgery.[118] Despite the reasonable motor and sensory outcomes with multiple botulinum toxin injections, its use as the primary therapy in IET has not become widespread. Surgery remains the standard in most centers.

Postsurgical management

In the immediate postoperative period, the most important considerations are to exclude a lost muscle, conjunctival dehiscence, and postoperative infection. We review patients on day 1, week 1, week 3, and week 6 postoperatively. The 6-week postoperative alignment correlates with the likelihood of long-term success.[122] Postoperatively, we prescribe antibiotic drops four times a day and steroid drops (twice daily only – to reduce steroid induced ocular hypertension)[123] for 2 weeks. At week 1, if the strabismus is undercorrected, cycloplegic refraction should be repeated and the full plus correction given. Miotic drops (e.g. Ecothiopate (phospholine iodide) 0.06% twice daily) can also be used for undercorrections as a temporizing measure but it is not widely available.

If the alignment is ≥15 PD at the 6-week postoperative visit, further surgery needs to be considered. We perform lateral rectus resections rather than medial rectus re-recessions due to a lower rate of consecutive XT (11% vs. 57%).[124,125] A small angle XT with normal ductions in the immediate postoperative period usually resolves spontaneously. An underacting medial rectus in the immediate postoperative period is a predictor for consecutive XT. We review patients 3-monthly for 2 years after surgery, then 6-monthly until age 6, then yearly until 8. After

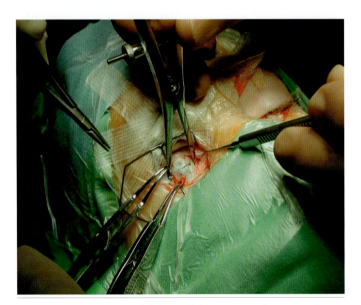

Fig. 74.13 Measurement of right medial rectus recession 11 mm from the limbus. Left arm of caliper at 3 o'clock position on limbus. Note infantile type insertion approximately 3 mm from limbus. (Measurement technique is described in Camuglia JE, et al. Three horizontal muscle surgery for large angle infantile esotropia. Eye; 2011.)

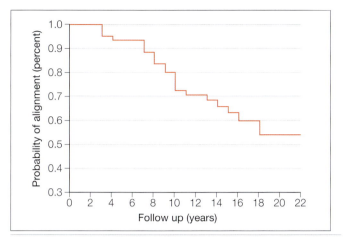

Fig. 74.14 Kaplan-Meier survival curve showing the percentage of patients with long term success after two muscle surgery for IET. (From Prieto-Diaz J, Prieto-Diaz I. Long term outcome of treated congenital/infantile esotropia: does early surgical binocular alignment restoring (subnormal) binocular vision guarantee stability? Binoc Vision Strab Q 1998; 13: 249–54. Reprinted by permission of Binoculus Publishing.)

the age of 8, if the uncorrected alignment is satisfactory and the visual acuity is normal, it may be reasonable to discharge the child but the parents should be warned of the risk of consecutive XT even decades into the future.

Such follow-up of IET is essential for the early detection of amblyopia, refractive errors, accommodative ET, and secondary associations of DVD and IOOA. Postoperative amblyopia rates are between 17% and 39%.[10,80,126-128] Risk factors for its development include preoperative amblyopia and uncorrected refractive errors (particularly anisometropia). DVD occurs in up to 90% of patients and is unrelated to the timing of surgery if carried out in the first 2 years of life.[23]

Despite early postoperative motor success, alignment can fail over time. Prieto-Diaz et al. estimated that 75% patients would have successful alignment at 10 years[129] and 55% at 18 years (Fig. 74.14). Helveston reported failed alignment in 70% after initial BMRc.[90] Over an 8–12 year follow-up period there was a 52% reoperation rate. Louwagie et al. reported that repeat surgery was required in 51% by 10 years and 66% by 20 years.[130] Preoperative moderate amblyopia is a risk factor for loss of alignment.[131]

Approximately 60% of patients with IET develop accommodative ET,[132,133] but it is unclear whether surgery unmasks a pre-existing accommodative ET or whether it develops as a consequence of poor sensory outcomes.[65,132] Birch et al. identified three risk factors for the development of accommodative ET after surgery:

1. Delay from diagnosis to surgery >3 months.
2. A sustained increase in hyperopia.
3. Absent or poor stereopsis.[65]

The usual decrease in hyperopia seen in normal infants in the first 9 months of life does not occur in infantile esotropes.[134]

Conclusion

It is now well established that we should operate early (<2 years) to promote the development of binocular vision and some stereopsis. The onset of IET is around 4 months of age.

This produces profound deficits in binocular vision if not corrected promptly. We are now able to identify which patients are most likely to benefit from surgery at a much earlier age than two years. Much earlier alignment appears to produce better functional results. Much of our clinical practice is based on retrospective case series. The only new treatment for IET in recent decades has been botulinum toxin and we cannot yet resolve the controversies regarding type of surgery, non-surgical options, and age of intervention in patients with IET.[135]

Acknowledgment

GG would like to acknowledge the generosity and patience of his strabismus teachers, especially William E Scott MD, G Frank Judisch MD, and Graham Pittar FRANZCO. They were greatly inspired to me and set a high standard to follow.

References

10. Ing MR. Early surgical alignment for congenital esotropia. Trans Am Ophthalmol Soc 1981; 79: 625–63.
15. von Noorden GK. Bowman lecture. Current concepts of infantile esotropia. Eye (Lond) 1988; 2(Pt 4): 343–57.
17. Helveston EM. 19th annual Frank Costenbader Lecture – the origins of congenital esotropia. J Pediatr Ophthalmol Strabismus 1993; 30: 215–32.
20. MacEwen CJ, Chakrabarti HS. Why is squint surgery in children in decline? Br J Ophthalmol 2004; 88: 509–11.
30. Birch E, Stager D, Wright K, et al. The natural history of infantile esotropia during the first six months of life. Pediatric Eye Disease Investigator Group. J AAPOS 1998; 2: 325–8; discussion 29.
31. The clinical spectrum of early-onset esotropia: experience of the Congenital Esotropia Observational Study. Am J Ophthalmol 2002; 133: 102–8.
33. Wong AM. Timing of surgery for infantile esotropia: sensory and motor outcomes. Can J Ophthalmol 2008; 43: 643–51.
40. Ciancia AO. Infantile esotropia with abduction nystagmus. Int Ophthalmol Clin 1989; 29: 24–9.
47. Tamura EE, Hoyt CS. Oculomotor consequences of intraventricular hemorrhages in premature infants. Arch Ophthalmol 1987; 105: 533–5.
52. Ing MR. Progressive increase in the quantity of deviation in congenital esotropia. Ophthalmic Surg Lasers 1996; 27: 612–17.
53. Birch EE, Felius J, Stager DR, Sr, et al. Pre-operative stability of infantile esotropia and post-operative outcome. Am J Ophthalmol 2004; 138: 1003–9.
58. Choi RY, Kushner BJ. The accuracy of experienced strabismologists using the Hirschberg and Krimsky tests. Ophthalmology 1998; 105: 1301–6.
59. Thompson JT, Guyton DL. Ophthalmic prisms. Measurement errors and how to minimize them. Ophthalmology 1983; 90: 204–10.
60. Interobserver reliability of the prism and alternate cover test in children with esotropia. Arch Ophthalmol 2009; 127: 59–65.
77. Tychsen L. Can ophthalmologists repair the brain in infantile esotropia? Early surgery, stereopsis, monofixation syndrome, and the legacy of Marshall Parks. J AAPOS 2005; 9: 510–21.
80. Birch EE, Stager DR Sr. Long-term motor and sensory outcomes after early surgery for infantile esotropia. J AAPOS 2006; 10: 409–13.
81. Birch EE, Fawcett S, Stager DR. Why does early surgical alignment improve stereoacuity outcomes in infantile esotropia? J AAPOS 2000; 4: 10–14.
86. Tychsen L. Causing and curing infantile esotropia in primates: the role of decorrelated binocular input (an American Ophthalmological Society thesis). Trans Am Ophthalmol Soc 2007; 105: 564–93.

87. Parks MM. The monofixation syndrome. Trans Am Ophthalmol Soc 1969; 67: 609–57.

88. Wright KW, Edelman PM, McVey JH, et al. High-grade stereo acuity after early surgery for congenital esotropia. Arch Ophthalmol 1994; 112: 913–19.

91. Drover JR, Stager DR Sr, Morale SE, et al. Improvement in motor development following surgery for infantile esotropia. J AAPOS 2008; 12: 136–40.

98. Murray AD, Orpen J, Calcutt C. Changes in the functional binocular status of older children and adults with previously untreated infantile esotropia following late surgical realignment. J AAPOS 2007; 11: 125–30.

101. Kushner BJ, Fisher M. Is alignment within 8 prism diopters of orthotropia a successful outcome for infantile esotropia surgery? Arch Ophthalmol 1996; 114: 176–80.

109. Kushner BJ, Morton GV. A randomized comparison of surgical procedures for infantile esotropia. Am J Ophthalmol 1984; 98: 50-61.

115. de Alba Campomanes AG, Binenbaum G, Campomanes Eguiarte G. Comparison of botulinum toxin with surgery as primary treatment for infantile esotropia. J AAPOS 2010; 14: 111–16.

121. Rowe F, Noonan C. Complications of botulinum toxin A and their adverse effects. Strabismus 2009; 17: 139–42.

122. Bateman JB, Parks MM, Wheeler N. Discriminant analysis of congenital esotropia surgery. Predictor variables for short- and long-term outcomes. Ophthalmology 1983; 90: 1146–53.

127. Weakley DR Jr, Parks MM. Results from 7-mm bilateral recessions of the medial rectus muscles for congenital esotropia. Ophthalmic Surg 1990; 21: 827–30.

129. Prieto-Diaz J, Prieto-Diaz I. Long term outcome of treated congenital/infantile esotropia: does early surgical binocular alignment restoring (subnormal) binocular vision guarantee stability? Binocul Vis Strabismus Q 1998; 13: 249–54.

135. Elliott S, Shafiq A. Interventions for infantile esotropia. Cochrane Database Syst Rev 2008; (1): CD004917.

Access the complete reference list online at

http://www.expertconsult.com

Part 2
Esotropias

The accommodative esotropias

David R Weakley • Erika Mota Pereira

Characteristics

Accommodative esotropia describes an esotropia caused in whole, or in part, by the use of accommodation to clear vision in the presence of uncorrected hypermetropia. This association is widely attributed to Donders.[1] Accommodative esotropia is one of the most common forms of childhood strabismus accounting for about a third of all strabismus patients in most studies in Europe and North America.[2]

The typical age of onset ranges from 2 to 5 years old, but may present earlier ("infantile accommodative esotropia") or, less commonly, at a later age. Caregivers typically report crossing that is intermittent initially and most apparent when the child is fixing on a near object or when fatigued. With time, the crossing occurs more frequently and, without treatment, often becomes constant. Accommodative esotropia may manifest suddenly following a minor illness, trauma, or without any obvious precipitating event.

Classification

The most widely accepted classification of accommodative esotropia includes four distinct types:

1. Fully accommodative esotropia (refractive esotropia): those patients in whom the distance and near deviation are equal and the esotropia is caused entirely by uncorrected hypermetropic refractive error. In one study, these patients had a mean age of onset of 3½ years and a

mean refractive error of +4.75 D.[3] They have a normal accommodative convergence to accommodation (AC/A) ratio and respond to correction of the full cycloplegic refractive error (Figs 75.1 & 75.2).

2. High AC/A ratio accommodative esotropia: those patients who have a significant near–distance disparity in the magnitude of the esotropia, with the deviation being at least 10 prism diopters (PD) more at near than at distance. They have a younger age at presentation (mean 2.7 years old),[4] and a lower degree of hypermetropia, than patients with typical fully accommodative or refractive esotropia. They have a normal hyperopic refractive error for age and little or no esotropia in the distance

3. Arguably, the most common form has elements of both of the preceding types. These patients have a significant hypermetropic refractive error and some level of high AC/A ratio that leads to a deviation that is greater at near than distance by at least 10 PD.

4. "Early onset esotropia" or "infantile accommodative esotropia" refers to patients with fully accommodative esotropia presenting at a very early age. They may present

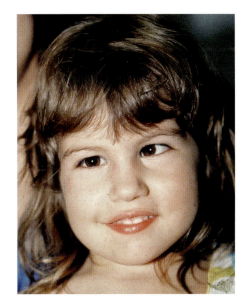

Fig. 75.1 A 3-year-old girl presents with a new onset of left esotropia (with strong fixation preference for the right eye). The deviation is 35 PD at near and distance fixation. The cycloplegic refraction is +4.25 OD and +4.50 OS.

with esotropia as early as 6 months of age and typically have very high hypermetropia and are more likely to have inferior oblique ove.raction.

The accommodative convergence/accommodation ratio

The accommodative convergence/accommodation ratio (AC/A) plays an important role in the development, treatment, and prognosis in accommodative esotropia. Patients with a high AC/A ratio present earlier, are more likely to require surgery, and to have a poorer prognosis for long-term binocular vision.[5] There are different ways to calculate the AC/A ratio although in clinical practice this is not necessary. A clinical comparison of distance to near deviation is most commonly used to determine whether or not the AC/A ratio is high. Patients can be further classified based on the degree of near–distance disparity:

Grade I: 10–19 PD more deviation at near.
Grade II: 20–29 PD more deviation at near.
Grade III: 30 PD or more deviation at near than distance.

To calculate the AC/A ratio, either the gradient or heterophoric method can be used. For the gradient method, measure the deviation at a fixed distance while relaxing accommodation by introducing plus lenses as follows:

$$AC/A = (D1 - D0)/p$$

where p is the power of the lens used, D0 the deviation without lenses, and D1 the deviation with lenses.

In the heterophoric method, near and distance deviations are compared while taking into account the interpupillary distance (IPD) as follows:

$$AC/A = IPD\ (cm) + (Dn - Dd)/D$$

where D is the fixation distance at near, Dn is the deviation at near, and Dd is the deviation in the distance. The gradient method is more easily performed and more accurate. By this method, a normal AC/A ratio is between 3:1 and 5:1.

Risk factors for accommodative esotropia

The most commonly recognized risk factor for the development of accommodative esotropia is excess hypermetropia. Its prevalence increases with increasing levels of hypermetropia. Other factors including family history, subnormal binocularity, and the presence of anisometropia all increase the risk of developing accommodative esotropia.

The prevalence of affected first-degree relatives in patients with accommodative esotropia is 18–23% with as many as 75% of patients having an affected sibling, parent, grandparent, aunt, or uncle. Subnormal stereopsis or fusion, preceding the onset of accommodative esotropia, is a contributing factor in its development. These patients may develop accommodative esotropia with lower levels of hypermetropia.[6] Anisometropia of >1 D and amblyopia, in patients with hypermetropia, increase the likelihood of developing accommodative esotropia, particularly in patients with lower levels of hypermetropia.[7]

Clinical evaluation

Evaluation of patients with presumed or suspected accommodated esotropia requires a systematic approach. First determine if a family history is present and if the child has any developmental issues or recent illness. The caregivers should be questioned about duration, frequency, and constancy of the crossing. Triggering factors such as near viewing or fatigue should be ascertained. Though accommodative esotropia is typically intermittent in the early stages, delay in treatment will often result in deterioration of fusion and development of a constant deviation and amblyopia.

The examination should include age-appropriate acuity testing, extraocular motility evaluation with attention to other causes of acquired esotropia (e.g. decreased abduction in sixth nerve palsy, etc.) as well as measurement of the deviation at near and distance. Evaluation for oblique muscle dysfunction and the presence of A or V patterns should be assessed. Inferior oblique muscle overaction, though less common than in infantile esotropia, may occur, particularly in cases of infantile accommodative esotropia or in the presence of significant amblyopia.[8,9] As noted, the AC/A ratio need not be calculated but can be graded based on the near distance disparity.

A cycloplegic refraction is essential. Though some believe atropine refractions are necessary, the additional hypermetropia detected with atropine compared to cyclopentolate is unlikely to be of clinical significance especially if blue-eyed because they dilate and cycloplege more readily. We feel adequate cycloplegia can be obtained using 0.5% cyclopentolate (Mydrilate, Cyclogyl, Pentolair) under 6 months of age, 1% cyclopentolate from 6 months up to age 2, and 2% cyclopentolate in patients over 2 years of age. We typically use 2.5% neosynephrine (phenylephrine) to facilitate dilation. The drops may be repeated in 5 minutes if needed and 30–40 minutes should be allowed to pass before refracting the patient. Children who do not dilate or become cyclopleged with cyclopentolate should be atropinized.

A fundus examination is critical; attention should be directed to any structural lesions that could result in a sensory deviation as well as assessment of the optic disc to detect swelling that that could indicate increased intracranial pressure.

Non-surgical treatment

Initial treatment of presumed accommodative esotropia is proper spectacle correction. In most cases, the full cycloplegic refraction should be prescribed (Fig. 75.2). In a patient in whom the angle of deviation is small and the hypermetropia significant an undercorrection of 1 to 2 D can be prescribed to facilitate initial compliance with spectacles. However, one should increase to the full cycloplegic refraction if the child is not well aligned at the first follow-up visit. We do not initially prescribe bifocals even if the AC/A is high. It is important to correct any anisometropia as well as astigmatic error even if the full spherical correction is not prescribed.

If significant amblyopia is present, treatment should be instituted initially although in mild to moderate cases it may

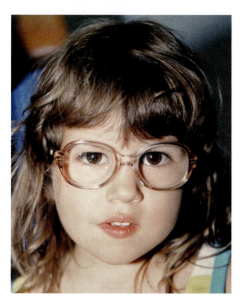

Fig. 75.2 The same girl as in Figure 75.1 4 weeks later wearing her full hyperopic correction. She has a small left esotropia with fixation preference for her right eye. Part-time occlusion therapy of the right eye is begun.

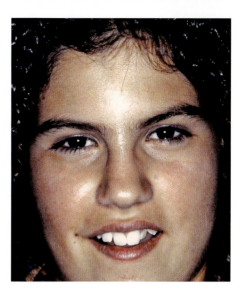

Fig. 75.3 The same girl as in Figure 75.1 and 75.2. She is 15 years old. She has been weaned from glasses. Her cycloplegic, refraction is +1.50 OD, +1.50 OS. Visual acuity is 20/20 in each eye and she is orthotropic at near and distance fixation with high-grade stereoacuity.

be preferable to wait until the child has been in the glasses for a few weeks before beginning amblyopia therapy. Spectacle correction alone improves acuity in amblyopic eyes even in the presence of strabismus.[10] Once the child has adapted to the spectacles, a more accurate baseline acuity can be determined to assess the response to amblyopia therapy. Both atropine penalization or patching are effective (see Chapter 70), though decreasing the spectacle power of the sound eye when using atropine does not significantly improve its effectiveness.[11]

Alignment in spectacles should be assessed after about 6–8 weeks. If the eyes are well aligned at near and distance, the child can be seen in 6 to 12 months unless amblyopia therapy necessitates more frequent follow-up. If alignment is unsatisfactory, longer observation in spectacles is generally acceptable particularly if compliance with glasses is in question. Administration of atropine 1% to both eyes each morning for 1 to 2 weeks often improves compliance. Repeat cycloplegic refraction can be performed if its accuracy is in question.

If distance alignment is good, but significant esotropia persists at near after 3 months of spectacle wear, +3.00 bifocals can be considered. The bifocals should be executive or flat topped and set at the level of lower edge of the pupil. Miotics, such as phospholine iodide, may be considered though their potential side effects and difficulty of administration limit their usefulness.

Surgical treatment

Surgery is indicated when the eyes are not aligned adequately with glasses; the definition of what constitutes "adequate" differs among clinicians. The decision to proceed with surgery involves a number of factors in addition to alignment with glasses including patient age, family or patient desires, presence or absence of amblyopia, and previous experience and compliance with spectacle or contact lens correction.

In the visually formative years, alignment that allows for fusion and prevention of amblyopia is paramount. Surgery should not be delayed if alignment is unsatisfactory. Fusion disruption for as little as 4 months can risk permanent loss of

binocularity.[5] Two common situations in which surgery is indicated are:

1. Partially accommodative esotropia: patients who never achieve good alignment in glasses alone.
2. Deteriorated accommodative esotropia: patients with initially good response to spectacles who later lose it. Deterioration of previously controlled accommodative esotropia has been associated with early onset, high AC/A ratio, and amblyopia.[7,12]
3. Surgery may be indicated in patients with marginal control, those with good distance alignment but residual esotropia at near who do not tolerate or desire bifocals.[13]
4. Older patients whose hypermetropia may have normalized but who cross without correction.

Surgery need not be deferred until amblyopia therapy is complete. Amblyopia therapy may benefit from improved alignment.[14]

In general, bilateral medial rectus recessions are the preferred surgical approach. Undercorrection is common in patients with accommodative esotropia if standard surgical dosages are followed. This is particularly true in the presence of a clinically high AC/A ratio. Various approaches can improve results, including adding additional recession to standard surgical dosages,[15] operating for the near deviation,[16] or combining medial rectus recessions with traditional or "muscle pulley" posterior fixation sutures[17]

Long-term prognosis

One of the most commonly asked questions by parents of children with accommodative esotropia is "Will my child always have to wear glasses?" While it is important to keep patients in their full hyperopic correction through the visually formative years, many clinicians "wean" patients out of their full correction (and bifocals, if worn) to decrease spectacle dependence over time.

Mohney et al. reported 20% of accommodative esotropes will be free of spectacles by 10 years after diagnosis (Fig. 75.3).[18] Patients with high hypermetropia, high AC/A ratio (bifocal dependence), and anisometropia are more likely to need glasses long term. Those with low hypermetropia, normal AC/A ratio, and those that undergo surgery are more likely to be successfully weaned from spectacles.

For those patients that need correction beyond 10 years of age, contact lenses are a viable option and may improve compliance.

References

1. Donders FC. On the Anomalies of Accommodation and Refraction of the Eye. London: New Sydenham Society; 1864.

2. Mohney BG. Common forms of childhood strabismus in an incidence cohort. Am J Ophthalmol 2007; 144: 465–7.

3. Dickey CF, Scott WE. The deterioration of accommodative esotropia: frequency, characteristics, and predictive factors. J Pediatr Ophthalmol Strabismus 1988; 25: 172–5.

4. Parks MM. Abnormal convergence in squint. Arch Ophthalmol 1958; 59: 364–80.

5. Fawcett SL, Birch EE. Risk factors for abnormal binocular vision after successful alignment of accommodative esotropia. J AAPOS 2003; 7: 256–62.

6. Birch EE, Fawcett SL, Morale SE, et al. Risk factors for accommodative esotropia among hypermetropic children. Invest Ophthalmol Vis Sci 2005; 46: 526–9.

7. Weakley DR, Birch EE, Kip K. The role of anisometropia in the development of accommodative esotropia. J AAPOS 2001; 5: 153–7.

8. Wilson ME, Parks MM. Primary inferior oblique overaction congenital esotropia, accommodative esotropia, and intermittent exotropia. Ophthalmology 1989; 96: 950–5.

9. Weakley DR Jr, Urso RG, Dias CL. Asymmetric inferior oblique overaction and its association with amblyopia in esotropia. Ophthalmology 1992; 99: 590–3.

10. Cotter SA, Edwards AR, Arnold RW, et al. Pediatric Eye Disease Investigator Group. Treatment of strabismic amblyopia with refractive correction. Arch Ophthalmol 2007; 125: 655–9.

11. Pediatric Eye Disease Investigator Group. Pharmacologic plus optical penalization treatment for amblyopia: results of a randomized trial. Arch Ophthalmol. 2009; 127: 22–30.

12. Ludwig IH, Imberman SP, Thompson HW, Parks MM. Long-term study of accommodative esotropia. Trans Am Ophthalmol Soc 2003; 101: 155–60.

13. Leuder GT, Norman AA. Strabismus surgery for elimination of bifocals in accommodative esotropia. Am J Ophthalmol 2006; 142: 632–5.

14. Weakley DR, Holland D. The effect of ongoing treatment of amblyopia on surgical outcome in esotropia. J Pediatr Ophthalmol Strabismus 1997; 34: 275–8.

15. Wright KW, Bruce-Lyle L. Augmented surgery for esotropia associated with high hypermetropia. J Pediatr Ophthalmol Strabismus 1993; 30: 167–70.

16. Kushner BJ. Fifteen-year outcome of surgery for the near angle in patients with accommodative esotropia and a high accommodative convergence to accommodation ratio. Arch Ophthalmol 2001; 119: 1150–3.

17. Clark RA, Ariyasu R, Demer JL. Medial rectus pulley posterior fixation is as effective as scleral posterior fixation for acquired esotropia with high AC/A ratio. Am J Ophthalmol 2004; 137: 1026–33.

18. Mohney BD, Lilley CC, Green-Simms AE, Diehl NN. The long-term follow-up of accommodative esotropia in a population-based cohort of children. Ophthalmology 2011, 118: 581–5.

Special esotropias (acute comitant, sensory deprivation, myopia associated and microtropia)

John J Sloper

These esotropias mostly occur later in childhood when binocular fusion is stable. There is considerable overlap between some groups and all patients do not fit neatly into a category. They are best approached by trying to understand the pathophysiology of each individual case and attempting to identify the cause of the breakdown of fusion.

Acute comitant esotropia

In a child presenting with sudden onset comitant esotropia a reason needs to be sought for loss of fusion at an age when binocular function is usually stable. This is commonly a benign condition, but children with intracranial pathology, particularly posterior fossa tumors, can present in this way.[1,2]

Children with acute onset comitant esotropia can be divided into three groups:[3]

1. Acute onset esotropia following artificial interruption of fusion. This can occur with patching for anisometropic amblyopia, but has also been described following patching for a corneal abrasion. Loss of fusion may be associated with uncorrected hypermetropia. It can also occur following visual loss in one eye (see below, Sensory esotropia).
2. Comitant esotropia of the "Franceschetti" type. This is an acute onset comitant esotropia with diplopia and good potential binocular co-operation. It may be intermittent at first. The accommodative element is usually minimal. In most patients no immediate cause can be found: in some an illness or shock may precede the onset.[3]
3. Comitant esotropia of the "Bielschowsky" type. These patients have up to 5 diopters (D) of myopia. There is uncrossed diplopia for distance, with fusion for near. The mechanism of the causal relationship between the myopia and esotropia is debated.

In groups 1 and 3 there is generally a clear cause for loss of fusion and investigation is not indicated in the absence of any other abnormalities. In group 2 there is no clear cause for the breakdown of fusion and there is concern about underlying neurological disease.

The decision on neuroimaging depends on the features of each case.[4] The risk of underlying pathology must be balanced against the risks associated with the X-ray dose for a CT scan and a general anesthetic for CT or MRI imaging if required.

History taking and examination should determine whether there is evidence of a pre-existing cause for the esotropia and whether there is evidence of any associated neurological disease. If there is a cause for the esotropia (significant uncorrected hypermetropia or myopia, a high AC/A ratio or anisometropic amblyopia), without other suspicious features, imaging is not required. Untreated anisometropic amblyopia may result in decompensation. Patching can precipitate a manifest squint in a child with a pre-existing microtropia.

Features suggesting neurological disease include age of onset after the age of 5 years and distance diplopia prior to the onset of the esotropia. Diplopia at presentation indicates the absence of pre-existing suppression and an esotropia of recent onset and so higher risk. Suspicious features of the examination include a distance angle larger than the near angle, an increase in esotropia in lateral gaze, lateral rectus underaction, and nystagmus. Lack of fusion on testing with prisms or the synoptophore is more common where there is a brain lesion. An "A" esotropia may be associated with hydrocephalus secondary to an Arnold-Chiari malformation, a tumor, or aqueduct obstruction. Papilledema or optic nerve dysfunction as shown by reduced acuity or color vision or abnormalities of pupil responses mandate imaging.[4] Visual fields and clinical electrophysiological testing may provide valuable information.

Headache, clumsiness, evidence of developmental regression, or abnormalities of other cranial nerves may indicate neurological disease.

Initial treatment consists of full correction of any refractive error and treatment of amblyopia. If re-alignment is not achieved with refractive correction alone, then early surgery is indicated to realign the eyes before the potential for fusion is lost. As an alternative treatment botulinum toxin may result in the long-term re-establishment of high-grade stereoscopic function.[5]

Early re-alignment carries a good prognosis for re-establishing fusion. The failure to re-establish fusion may be an indicator of an underlying neurological problem.[1] However, fusion following strabismus surgery has been reported in patients with a tumor.[2] Patients with treated intracranial tumors and *incomitant* strabismus have a better chance of re-establishing fusion.[6] In the absence of involvement of brainstem fusion centers, the duration of misalignment is a major prognostic factor for the re-establishment of binocular function. However, the time-frame for loss of fusion potential varies from child to child. Some older children have regained fusion after several years; in some younger children fusion potential is lost in a few months. Early surgery or botulinum toxin to re-establish alignment is likely to be beneficial even in children with (treated) intracranial tumors.

Sensory deprivation esotropia

The visual cortex fuses the images from the two eyes into a single image. If the image from one eye is severely degraded or lost, fusion cannot occur. In adults, divergence is common,[7] but in children an eye with poor vision and absent binocular function will commonly become convergent, perhaps because they are hyperopic. Sensory esotropia may occur with early onset conditions (monocular congenital cataract or optic nerve anomalies; Fig. 76.1), or with later acquired visual loss (trauma; Fig. 76.2). Correction of hypermetropia in the fixing eye has a variable effect on reducing the deviation and should be undertaken before surgery is considered.

Management must address whether vision can be restored in the affected eye and whether fusion can be re-established if vision is recovered. A common cause of reversible monocular visual loss in an older child is a traumatic cataract. In the absence of other ocular damage, the visual prognosis is good. Amblyopia does not develop in older children, but fusion may be lost rapidly and restoration of vision following cataract surgery may result in intractable diplopia even with straight eyes. For this reason cataract surgery should be undertaken as early as possible.

In a child with no prospect of visual improvement strabismus surgery can be undertaken if the appearance of the deviation is unacceptable. All hypermetropia of the fixing eye should be corrected. I prefer medial rectus recession and lateral rectus resection of the deviating eye, with the goal to leave a small convergent deviation with no adduction deficit to minimize consecutive exotropia.

Some children adopt a face turn towards the fixing eye because of manifest latent nystagmus in this eye that can substantially reduce their acuity. Acuity is maximized by adducting the fixing eye and turning the head. The abnormal head posture can be improved by recession of both medial recti or medial rectus recession and lateral rectus resection of the fixing eye provided that parents and patient are comfortable with surgery to the only good eye. Inferior oblique overaction may also develop in both eyes. In the fixing eye this results in downdrift of the non-fixing eye on abduction ("the fallen eye syndrome"). This can be improved by weakening the inferior oblique in the fixing eye.

Myopia-associated esotropia

Different esotropias have been described associated with different degrees of myopia.

Bielschowsky[8] described distance esotropia occurring in patients with myopia of up to −5.00 D. This can be of acute onset, but the time of onset can be difficult to determine because the diplopia is intermittent. This occurs mainly in adults, but also in older children.[3] Inadvertent overcorrection of the myopia stimulates accommodation and convergence and must be avoided. There is typically a small distance esotropia with diplopia, and binocular function for near,

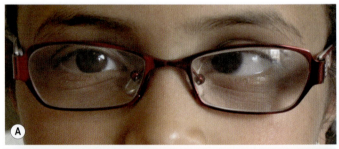
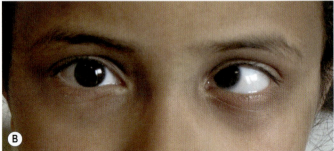

Fig. 76.2 Left sensory esotropia with left inferior oblique overaction in a 9-year-old girl following blunt trauma to her left eye as a baby. The left acuity is logMAR 1.30 (6/120, 20/400, 0.05). The fundus was normal, but electrodiagnostic testing showed left optic neuropathy and maculopathy. Although the deviation is smaller with glasses (A) than without (B), surgery will be needed to improve the appearance.

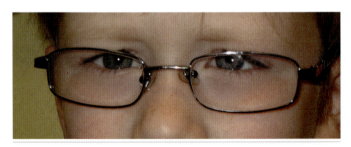

Fig. 76.1 Left sensory esotropia in a 6-year-old boy with left optic nerve hypoplasia. The left acuity was logMAR 1.1 (6/76, 20/250, 0.07). The esotropia is controlled to an acceptable appearance by his hypermetropic spectacle correction.

although this may eventually break down.[9] Slight lateral rectus underactions may occur. Prisms give good symptomatic control. Most patients eventually undergo strabismus surgery, with good results. In any patient with a distance esotropia care needs to be taken to exclude a sixth nerve palsy.

Patients with high myopia develop esotropia by two overlapping mechanisms. With esotropia of high myopia there is good corrected acuity in each eye and a purely convergent deviation with good motility and mild restriction of abduction. Such patients do well with ipsilateral medial rectus recession and lateral rectus resection. Histological examination of the resected lateral rectus may show fibrotic change. This may be an important etiological factor.[10]

Other patients have the eso-hypotropia of high myopia.[11] This is due to stretching and dehiscence of the connective tissue band running between the pulleys[12] of the superior and lateral recti in the super temporal quadrant which leads to downward slippage of the lateral rectus and nasal slippage of the superior rectus muscles.[13,14] There is superolateral dislocation of the posterior pole of the globe out of the muscle cone, with inferonasal displacement of the cornea resulting in an eso-hypotropia. This has been confirmed by high-resolution MRI studies.[13,14] Significant secondary contracture of the medial rectus may occur. Motility may be very restricted and vision in one or both eyes is often poor from myopic macular change or amblyopia. Binocular function is commonly absent.

Horizontal recess–resect procedures are of limited value, but several forms of "muscle-path" surgery have been reported as successful.[15,16] The lateral border of the superior rectus is sutured to the superior border of the lateral rectus at 15 mm behind the muscle insertions using a non-absorbable suture to appose the muscle borders and reposition the posterior pole of the globe into the muscle cone.[17,18] If the medial rectus is contracted, it is recessed. This improves both the deviation and ocular motility[17,18] and is valuable in patients with a wide range of myopia and eso-hypotropia, even those with good vision in both eyes and binocular function who present with intermittent diplopia.[19]

Microtropia

A microesotropia is a small angle convergent squint with anomalous binocular function. Microtropia is best considered as a description of the binocular status of the patient who may have any of a number of different types of squint. It represents the first stage in the breakdown of binocular function caused by abnormal visual experience during visual development. It is often seen with anisometropic amblyopia,[20] but may be a primary abnormality.[21] It may be the result of reduced binocularity from intermittent misalignment of the eyes during visual development, e.g. Duane's syndrome. In patients with accommodative esotropia it may be the end result of treatment rather than bifoveal binocular fusion. A microtropia is often the outcome of early strabismus surgery,[22] particularly in younger children.

Patients with a microtropia demonstrate the monofixation syndrome, with peripheral fusion but a central area of suppression in the deviating eye (PD).[23] However, not all patients with monofixation have a clinically demonstrable microtropia.[23] Anomalous binocular function can be maintained up to an angle of about 8 prism diopters.[23] Stereopsis is present, but

reduced, with a smaller deviation being associated with better stereopsis.[24] Receptive fields of visual cortical neurons in the foveal part of the visual field representation are small and become progressively larger with increasing eccentricity. For a small angle of ocular misalignment the fields no longer overlap centrally, but binocular correspondence can be maintained with the larger, more peripheral fields. Thus, there is central suppression of the deviating eye while peripheral binocular function is maintained.

Patients with a microtropia may demonstrate central monocular fixation with their deviating eye, in which case there is a small flick on cover–uncover testing. However, some children have eccentric monocular fixation with their deviating eye and fixate monocularly using the same eccentric retinal point that corresponds to the fovea of the non-deviating eye under binocular conditions. In this case, there is no movement on cover test.[25] Eccentric fixation can be demonstrated with the visuoscope. A few patients fix monocularly with an eccentric point which differs from that corresponding to the normal fovea and they show a flick on cover test.

The central suppression scotoma can be demonstrated by the 4 D base-out prism test. When a 4 D base-out prism is placed in front of one eye, a patient with bifoveal fixation makes a small conjugate movement of both eyes to re-establish fixation, followed by a small vergence movement to re-establish bifoveal alignment. In monofixation, this latter vergence movement will not occur if the prism is placed in front of the fixing eye, and no movement at all occurs if the prism is placed in front of the eye with the suppression scotoma. Testing with Bagolini glasses shows lateral displacement of the arm of the cross seen by the deviating eye, together with a break in the center of the line corresponding to the central suppression area.

A stable microtropia is not amenable to surgical or prismatic treatment. The microtropia, acuity, and stereopsis may improve with patching for anisometropic amblyopia.[26]

A microtropia occasionally decompensates to a large esotropia in childhood, particularly following patching or in hypermetropic children who do not wear their glasses. If this happens, full hypermetropic correction is required. If this is unsuccessful then early re-alignment by surgery or botulinum toxin will likely lead to recovery of binocularity. Patients with a microtropia have good motor fusion and stable ocular alignment. Arthur et al.[27] studied 80 early onset esotropes surgically aligned to within 8 PD. Those achieving monofixation were aligned at a significantly earlier age than those without monofixation. Seventy-five percent of those with monofixation remained stable, whereas only 45% of non-monofixators maintained stability. Patients who have monofixation and subsequently lose alignment have a good prognosis for recovering monofixation with surgery.[28]

Synthesis

Different esotropias have been described. The distinction between them is not always clear-cut and there is considerable overlap. Patients are best approached by attempting to understand the underlying pathophysiology of each case. The common thread in many cases is the breakdown of binocular fusion relatively late in childhood. The reasons for this can be divided into three main categories:

1. Sensory impairment.
2. Motor imbalance.
3. Impairment of central fusion centers.

In some cases more than one factor may contribute. Some patients show weak fusion easily disrupted by one of the other factors. In a child where there is no sensory or motor reason for the loss of fusion, symptoms or signs of neurological disease must be sought and neuroimaging considered.

In a child with previously normal binocular function, diplopia occurs until suppression develops and binocular potential will be retained for an unpredictable period of misalignment. Binocular function can often be recovered by early re-alignment. In an older child fusion potential is likely to be retained for longer, but if it is lost and suppression does not develop, intractable diplopia results.

References

1. Williams A, Hoyt C. Acute comitant esotropia in children with brain tumors. Arch Ophthalmol 1989; 107: 376–8.
2. Lyons C, Tiffin P, Oystreck D. Acute acquired esotropia: a prospective study. Eye 1999; 13: 617–20.
3. Burian H, Miller J. Comitant convergent strabimsus with acute onset. Am J Ophthalmol 1958; 45: 55–64.
4. Hoyt C, Good W. Acute onset comitant esotropia: when is it a sign of serious neurological disease? Br J Ophthalmol 1996; 79: 498–501.
5. Dawson EL, Marshman WE, Adams GG. The role of botulinum toxin A in acute-onset esotropia. Ophthalmology 1999; 106: 1727–30.
6. Shalev B, Repka M. Restoration of fusion in children with intracranial tumors and incomitant strabismus. Ophthalmology 2000; 107: 1880–3.
7. Havertape SA, Cruz OA, Chu FC. Sensory strabismus – eso or exo? J Pediatr Ophthalmol Strabismus 2001; 38: 327–30.
8. Bielschowsky A. Das Einwartsschielen der Myopen. Ber Dtsch Ophthalmol Ges 1922; 43: 245–8.
9. Webb H, Lee J. Acquired distance esotropia associated with myopia. Strabismus 2004; 12: 149–55.
10. Meyer E, Ludatscher R, Lichtig C, et al. End-stage fibrosis of the lateral rectus muscle in myopia with esotropia: an ultrastructural study. Ophthalmic Res 1990; 22: 259–64.
11. Hugonnier R, Magnard P. Les desequilidres oculo moteurs observes en cas de myopie forte. Ann Ocul (Paris) 1969; 202: 713–24.
12. Demer J. Pivotal role of orbital connective tissues in binocular alignment and strabismus. Invest Ophthalmol Vis Sci 2004; 45: 729–38.
13. Krzizok TH, Kaufmann H, Traupe H. Elucidation of restrictive motility in high myopia by magnetic resonance imaging. Arch Ophthalmol 1997; 115: 1019–27.
14. Yokoyama T, Tabuchi H, Ataka S, et al. The mechanism of development in progressive esotropia with high myopia. Transactions of the 26th Meeting of the European Strabismological Association, 2000, Barcelona, Spain. Swets and Zeitlinger; 2000: 218–21.
15. Hayashi T, Iwashige H, Maruo T. Clinical features and surgery for acquired progressive esotropia associated with severe myopia. Acta Ophthalmol Scand 1999; 77: 66–71.
16. Krzizok TH, Kaufmann H, Traupe H. New approach in strabismus surgery in high myopia. Br J Ophthalmol 1997; 81: 625–30.
17. Yokoyama T, Ataka S, Tabuchi H, et al. Treatment of progressive esotropia caused by high myopia – a new surgical procedure based on its pathogenesis. Transactions of the 27th European Strabismological Association, 2001, Florence, Italy. Swets and Zeitlinger; 2001: 145–8.
18. Yamaguchi M, Yokoyama T, Shiraki K. Surgical procedure for correcting globe dislocation in highly myopic strabismus. Am J Ophthalmol 2010; 149: 341–6.
19. Child C, Khawaja A, Sloper J, et al. A review of the Yokoyama procedure for eso-hypotropia associated with high myopia. Transactions of the 32nd Meeting of the European Strabismological Association, 2008, Munich, Germany. European Strabismological Association; 2008: 141–4.
20. Hardman Lea SJ, Snead MP, Loades J, Rubinstein MP. Microtropia versus bifoveal fixation in anisometropic amblyopia. Eye 1991; 5: 576–84.
21. Matsuo T, Kawaishi Y, Kuroda R, et al. Long-term visual outcome in primary microtropia. Jpn J Ophthalmol 2003; 47: 507–11.
22. von Noorden GK. Bowman Lecture. Current concepts of infantile esotropia. Eye 1988; 2: 343–57.
23. Parks MM. The monofixation syndrome. Trans Am Ophthalmol Soc 1969; 67: 609–57.
24. Hahn E, Cadera W, Orton RB. Factors associated with binocular single vision in microtropia/monofixation syndrome. Can J Ophthalmol 1991; 26: 12–7.
25. Helveston EM, Von Noorden GK. Microtropia: a newly defined entity. Arch Ophthalmol 1967; 78: 272–81.
26. Houston CA, Cleary M, Dutton GN, McFadzean RM. Clinical characteristics of microtropia – is microtropia a fixed phenomenon? Br J Ophthalmol 1998; 82: 219–24.
27. Arthur B, Smith J, Scott W. Long-term stability of alignment in the monofixation syndrome. J Pediatr Ophthalmol Strabismus 1989; 26: 224–31.
28. Hunt MG, Keech RV. Characteristics and course of patients with deteriorated monofixation syndrome. J AAPOS 2005; 9: 533–6.

Part 3
Exotropias

Intermittent exotropia

Alvina Pauline D Santiago • Michael P Clarke

Definition

Intermittent exotropia (X(T)) is a strabismus condition with outward drifting of either eye interspersed with periods of good alignment or orthotropia (Fig. 77.1). Monocular eye closure may occur during exodeviation. Near stereoacuity is often normal during periods of alignment, though it may deteriorate if the condition progresses.

Cause

The causes of intermittent exotropia are not fully understood. Proposals which have been advanced are as follows:

1. An imbalance between active convergence and divergence,[1] although it is not clear that divergence is active.[2]
2. Abnormal orbital anatomy.[3]
3. Abnormalities of extraocular muscle proprioception,[4] although the existence of active proprioceptors in extraocular muscles is disputed.[5]

   It is tempting to speculate that the cause of X(T) relates to the ability to switch between a state of suppression and relatively normal binocular function seen in children with the condition.

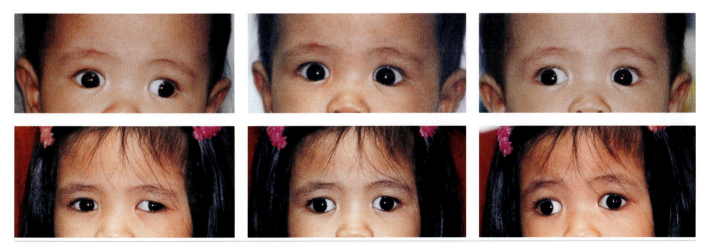

Fig. 77.1 A 7-month-old child with intermittent exotropia that progressed to constant exotropia. (Top center) At age 7 months note orthotropia in primary gaze; (top left) large angle exotropia with right eye fixing; (top right) large angle exotropia with left eye fixing. Patient was initially managed conservatively with patching and convergence exercises with good control of the deviation after only 3 months. Patient failed to follow-up regularly. (Bottom) At the time of last evaluation at age 2 years, she had a large angle constant exotropia with a left eye preference. Photos also show deviation with either eye fixing.

Epidemiology

X(T) is the most common form of divergent strabismus.[6,7] As divergent strabismus is much more common than convergent strabismus in Asia, it is now the most common form of strabismus worldwide.[8] The prevalence of exotropia in children less than 11 years of age was estimated as 1%.[9] X(T) accounted for approximately half of all cases of exotropia.[6] In Singaporean children aged between 6 and 72 months, the prevalence of strabismus was 0.8%, with an exotropia : esotropia ratio of 7 : 1. Sixty-three percent of cases of exotropia were intermittent.[10] In Japanese elementary school children, the incidence of X(T) was estimated as 0.12%[11] with a slight female predominance.[12]

Clinical features

The onset is typically in the second to third year of life,[13,14] when an intermittent outward drift of one eye or monocular eye closure in bright sunlight is noted (Fig. 77.2). Monocular eye closure in X(T) has been attributed to photophobia,[15] although it is difficult to explain why more light should enter exotropic than orthotropic eyes. Monocular eye closure may be due to diplopia or an abnormal visual percept, or reduction in threshold for bright lights, induced by divergence of the eyes.[16,17] It may resolve following surgery.[18]

It is usually not possible to accurately measure stereoacuity at presentation because the children are too young, but older children with X(T) have normal, or near normal (for age), near stereoacuity.[14] One study found reduced visual acuity in one or both eyes of 26% of children at presentation, although this reduction was generally just below age-related normal thresholds and due to anisometropia.[14]

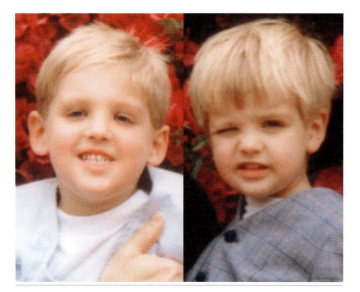

Fig. 77.2 Two brothers standing in Southern California sunshine. Boy on the left has no strabismus. Boy on the right has intermittent exotropia with monocular eye closure, a common sign of intermittent exotropia.

X(T) is traditionally classified into three types:

1. *True divergence excess*: the deviation is more than 10 prism diopters (PD) larger when measured at distance fixation than at near.
2. *Simulated divergence excess*: initially greater at distance fixation, but the misalignment at near fixation increases to within 10 diopters of the angle at distance following disruption of near binocular vision by monocular occlusion.
3. *Basic*: the size of the misalignment is equal, to within 10 PD, whether the misalignment is measured at distance or near fixation.[19,20]

The distinction between the types is important in determining the appropriate surgical treatment,[21] although this has been disputed.[22] The measurements required may be difficult in young children.

One of the most striking neurophysiologic features of X(T) is that children with the condition alternate between a state of apparently normal (or near normal) binocular vision, with normal stereoacuity when the eyes are aligned and a state of suppression, or anomalous retinal correspondence, when the eyes are divergent.[23-25] However, binocular function is not entirely normal during ocular alignment in X(T); children with X(T) have reduced positive fusional vergences (reduced convergence in response to a base-out prism).[26] Furthermore, suppression can be demonstrated even during periods of normal ocular alignment, indicating that it can be triggered by purely retinal information.[27]

A subset of children with X(T) have subnormal binocular function even during periods of ocular "alignment" because the "alignment" is actually a small constant divergent misalignment.[28] This may underlie the lack of normal stereoacuity seen following treatment of X(T) in some cases.[29]

While X(T) is not associated with neurodevelopmental abnormalities, it has been associated with the subsequent development of psychiatric disorders.[30,31] The reason for this is unknown, but it is unlikely to be due to the consequences of an abnormal appearance in childhood, as it is not seen in children with esotropia.[30]

Quality of life in intermittent exotropia

The Pediatric Quality of Life Inventory has been used to investigate quality of life in X(T) without significant effects being observed.[32] Hatt et al.[33] developed a specific quality of life measure based on interviews with children with X(T). They identified concerns about the presence of exotropia, particularly relating to awareness of exotropia by observers, but also awareness on the part of the child of strategies to control exotropia, such as blinking. They also identified parental anxiety about exotropia as the most significant concern.[34]

Clinical evaluation

Possible measures of progression or outcome in X(T) are:

- Angle (size) of misalignment.
- Stereoacuity (for near and/or distance fixation).

- Deterioration of convergence.
- Control of misalignment.
- Deterioration to constant exotropia (+/− development of strabismic amblyopia).

Accurate measurements of stereoacuity and convergence are not consistent in children under the age of 4 years, and control, constancy, and angle (particularly at distance) are also challenging to measure in this group. Any therapy for children under the age of 4 years with X(T) is necessarily based on imperfect clinical measurements, making assessment of the effect of therapy difficult. Thus, many clinicians defer treatment until later, despite the theoretical benefits of early therapy.[14]

The traditional outcome measure for the effect of therapy on X(T) is the size of the angle of the misalignment, with successful outcomes following therapy often taken as angles of between +/− 10 PD of orthophoria.[35-38]

Ocular alignment (usually with a range of +/−10 PD), is, however, an inadequate outcome measure for treatment of X(T). The measurement given usually includes latent and manifest (tropia and phoria) components of the misalignment. Thus small constant misalignments, both esotropic and exotropic, with worse functional correlates than X(T)s, are included as treatment "successes."[38]

Assessing the control of intermittent exotropia

A more relevant measure of treatment of X(T) is the degree of control of the misalignment, as measured by the frequency with which a strabismus is manifest, and the ease with which an induced misalignment can be realigned. Diplopia is not a feature of X(T), and the mechanisms underlying control are obscure, but some children report awareness of their misalignment.[33]

Two scoring systems for the measurement of control of X(T) are in common usage: the Mayo office based scale,[39] and the Newcastle Control Score.[40,41]

The Mayo scoring system is outlined in Table 77.1. The Mayo Scale is based solely on timed observations.

The second scoring system is the Newcastle Control Score for Intermittent Exotropia (NCS).[41] The criteria for assigning an NCS are given in Table 77.2. The NCS is based on the criteria for surgical intervention popularized by Rosenbaum.[42] These criteria consist of a parental report of the frequency with which a divergent misalignment of the eyes is observed (home control) and an objective assessment of the ease with which the eyes can be realigned following the induction of strabismus with a cover test (office control). Rosenbaum suggested that surgery should be considered if the strabismus was present more than 50% of the time and was poorly controlled on examination. The relationship between these two criteria requires further study, but correlations have been shown between home and office control.[43]

One study using the Mayo control score showed that control varied over time, which limits its value as an outcome measure.[44] Variability has not been demonstrated with the Newcastle score, but the office control component is likely to behave in the same way. The home control element is potentially subject to observer bias but does have the merit of being a parent-reported outcome measure.

Measuring the deviation

For measurements to be reproducible any significant refractive error must be corrected. This is usually the maximum tolerated plus or the least minus prescription. An accommodative fixation target slightly above threshold must be used; for example, a patient with 20/20 vision in both eyes needs to be presented with a 20/50 line. In preverbal children, videos or toys presented as targets should have sufficient detail to control accommodation.

Distance measurements should be made at more than 20 ft to eliminate accommodation. In some cases, distance deviation may have to be measured at true infinity, beyond the confines of the standard visual lane. Breaking fusion by prolonged monocular occlusion for 30 to 60 minutes may be required to eliminate all fusional vergence. The patch is removed by the examiner, and fusion, no matter how momentary, is not allowed.

Table 77.1 – The Mayo scale for scoring control in X(T)[39]

5 = Constant exotropia
4 = Exotropia >50% of the exam before dissociation
3 = Exotropia <50% of the exam before dissociation
2 = No exotropia unless dissociated, recovers in >5 seconds
1 = No exotropia unless dissociated, recovers in 1–5 seconds
0 = No exotropia unless dissociated, recovers in <1 second (phoria)

Notes:
The score is measured at distance and near fixation, and so yields an overall control score ranging from 0 to 10.
Levels 5 to 3 are assessed during an initial 30-second period of observation at distance fixation and repeated at near fixation for another 30-second period.
Levels 2 to 0 are then graded as the worst of three rapidly successive trials; an occluder is placed over the right eye for 10 seconds and then removed, measuring the length of time it takes for fusion to be re-established. The left eye is then occluded for 10 seconds and the time to re-establish fusion is similarly measured.
A third trial of 10-second occlusion is performed, covering the eye that required the longest time to re-fuse.
The worst level of control observed following the three 10-second periods of occlusion should be recorded.
If the patient has a microesotropia by simultaneous prism and cover test, but exodeviation by alternate cover test, the scale applies to the exodeviation.

Table 77.2 – The Revised Newcastle Control Score for Intermittent Exotropia[41]

NCS criteria	Score
Home control (XT or monocular eye closure seen)	
Never	0
<50% of time fixing in distance	1
>50% of time fixing in distance	2
>50% of time fixing in distance + seen at near	3
Clinic control (scored for near and distance fixation)	
Immediate realignment after dissociation	0
Realignment with aid of blink or re-fixation	1
Remains manifest after dissociation/prolonged fixation	2
Manifest spontaneously	3
Total score: n/9	

Stereoacuity in intermittent exotropia

In X(T), the eyes usually remain aligned for near fixation, or are capable of realignment in response to the stimulus of presentation of a stereoscopic image. Values of near stereoacuity in X(T) are within age-related norms,[45-47] making near stereoacuity a poor measure of severity. Near stereoacuity may be lost completely if X(T) deteriorates to a constant exotropia, although, in some cases, restoration of near stereoacuity can be achieved with surgery.[48]

The initial abnormality in X(T) is binocular misalignment at distance fixation. Measurement of stereoacuity at distance fixation is, therefore, a potential measure of X(T) severity. The tendency to diverge at larger viewing distances may introduce a "pedestal disparity" between the reference surface and the fixation point, thus lowering stereoacuity.[25]

Measurement of stereoacuity at distance fixation is technically challenging. Previous studies (Binocular Visual Acuity Test)[49] used a liquid crystal system requiring goggles during measurement, limiting its use in young children. It is no longer available. Subsequent studies have utilized the Frisby Davis Distance Stereotest[50] and the Distance Randot Test.[51]

Variable results have been reported of the effect of X(T) on distance stereoacuity, depending on the characteristics of the test used. Distance stereoacuity has been reported as normal or absent.[52] In contrast, other authors have found distance stereoacuity to be degraded in X(T),[53] and to be improved by surgery.[54,55] This may be due to the way in which absent distance stereoacuity was recorded, as in some studies a nominal value was ascribed to absent stereoacuity. It remains uncertain whether improvements in distance stereoacuity following surgery represent regression to the mean of a series of measurements, with surgery being more likely to be performed when poor distance stereoacuity is measured.

Differential diagnosis

X(T) is not associated with neurologic pathology.[6,56] Constant exotropia with a variable angle can mimic X(T), particularly in children who are too small to perform accurate monocular visual acuity and binocular vision testing. It is associated with neurologic and ocular pathology[56] (see Chapter 78). Children with poor vision in one eye due to optic nerve glioma or retinoblastoma may masquerade as cases of X(T).[57-59]

Children with craniofacial anomalies are frequently exotropic (see Chapter 28). Alphabet pattern deviations are common. V patterns mimic inferior oblique overaction; A patterns mimic superior oblique overaction. Dynamic magnetic resonance imaging (MRI) of the rectus muscles may suggest heterotopic rectus muscles (Fig. 77.3). These patients benefit from transposition surgeries correcting the muscle displacements to improve the pattern deviations. Surgical procedure on the oblique muscles is usually unnecessary.

Management of intermittent exotropia

There are uncertainties about the best management of X(T).[60] Most outcome studies of treatment of X(T) consist of highly selected retrospective case series, which use multiple, often conflicting, outcome measures. Assessing the true effects of treatment must await the results of robust, prospective, randomized studies.

There are no studies indicating the long term outcome in an unselected cohort of patients with X(T). Studies of untreated patients are biased by the drop out of patients with more severe X(T) who go on to have treatment. However, a significant proportion of children with X(T) do not progress to constant exotropia. One study of 73 patients, with an average 10 year follow-up, showed a reduction in the angle of exotropia over time; however, 82% of the patients received some form of nonsurgical treatment[61] which the authors suggested might represent regression towards the mean of varying measurements. Many children with X(T) do not have to undergo active management.[14]

Parents should be counseled about the current uncertainties regarding the evidence for the treatment of X(T) prior to any intervention.

Overminus lenses

Minus lenses may have a beneficial effect on angle and control of X(T),[43,62] and be useful as a temporizing measure allowing surgery to be deferred until an age when amblyopia is unlikely to develop in the event of a surgical overcorrection. The amount of overminus used should be assessed with trial frames. It commonly is around 2 diopters. Overminus lenses may have a particular application for children with X(T) and a high accommodative convergence/accommodation (AC/A) ratio. The lack of a randomized controlled trial of their use in X(T) leaves open the possibility that the beneficial effect observed may be due to spontaneous improvement.

Orthoptic/occlusion treatment

Occlusion for early onset unilateral exotropia[63] for 4–6 hours per day for 3–6 weeks has been advocated to modify suppression. Orthoptic/occlusion treatment prior to surgery may improve surgical success rates.[64]

Chemodenervation

There are few reports of the use of botulinum toxin in X(T)[65] and its use in X(T) is not widespread except in the management of surgical overcorrection of X(T).

Surgical management

X(T) is commonly treated with surgery. Some authorities, supported by work on visual physiology,[66] recommend surgery shortly after diagnosis because restoration of normal ocular alignment as soon as possible is the best method of promoting normal visual development. There are practical difficulties, however, with X(T) surgery in young children: obtaining full assessment and inaccuracies in assessment mean that measurements are uncertain and the diagnosis can only be provisional. Furthermore, in the event of a surgical overcorrection, young children may respond by developing constant suppression of diplopia and amblyopia. This represents a worsening of sensory status compared to preoperatively, when normal stereoacuity is usually achievable.

Thus, many surgeons defer surgery until the age of 4 years or older, provided that there is no deterioration in the

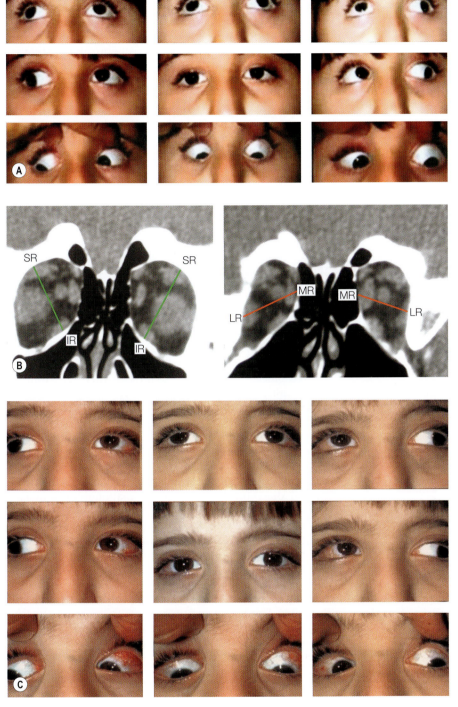

Fig. 77.3 (A) Patient with craniosynostosis showing a V pattern deviation with apparent pseudo-overaction of the inferior oblique. (B) Dynamic MRI shows lateral displacement of the superior rectus muscles (SR) downward displacement of the lateral rectus muscles (LR) and medial displacement of the inferior rectus (IR) muscles. (C) After repositioning of the lateral rectus muscle bellies superiorly, the V pattern deviation is improved.

condition with the threat of a constant exotropia. These views are supported by retrospective case series with some arguing that age at surgery does not influence outcome.

Ekdawi et al.[67] reported 33% of X(T) patients had surgical treatment, with 19.7% undergoing a second procedure. While recovery of stereopsis has been reported in cases of X(T) which have progressed to constant exotropia,[37] Wu et al. reported significantly better stereoacuity results in X(T) compared to constant exotropia and a history of previous X(T),[48] despite similar rates of motor alignment. Initial overcorrection of the

deviation has been associated with improved long term alignment;[38] however, others have challenged this view.[68]

Exotropias tend to recur following initially successful surgery; in one large study, orthotropia or mini-microtropia was achieved in 60.2% of patients 1 month after surgery, but half of these patients developed recurrent X(T) by 4 years after surgery.[22] Ekdawi et al. found the rate of developing greater than 10 diopters of misalignment at distance after the first surgery for X(T) was 54% by 5 years, 76% by 1 year, and 86% by 15 years.[67]

Surgical procedures

Rectus muscle surgery for X(T) consists of a weakening procedure on the lateral rectus muscle and/or a strengthening procedure on the medial rectus muscle. Operating on the lateral rectus muscle is believed to affect the distance deviation more than near; the reverse is believed to be the case for the medial rectus muscle. The choice as to which muscle to perform surgery on is suggested by the clinical pattern of the deviation.

If a patient has true or simulated divergence excess exotropia, bilateral lateral rectus recession (Table 77.3) is appropriate; patients with basic exotropia with equal near and distance deviation are treated with a recess–resect procedure (Table 77.4). A prospective, randomized clinical trial revealed only a 52% success rate in patients with basic exotropia if only lateral rectus recessions are performed. This increased to 82% if a recess–resect procedure was chosen[21]

Desired early postoperative alignment

Within the first 2 weeks, the aim is to achieve a small angle (5–10 PD) esotropia. The eyes are brought beyond

the temporal hemiretinal suppression scotoma to increase diplopia awareness. This may stimulate fusional vergences and stabilize postoperative alignment. Intentional overcorrection has risks in children with an immature visual system. In the immediate postoperative period, base-out prisms to neutralize residual deviation to maintain bifoveal fixation may be useful to prevent development of monofixation esotropia with foveal suppression.

In older children and adults who develop X(T) after the visual system has matured, diplopia and visual confusion occur with little or no suppression. The surgical goal in these cases should be orthotropia even on the first postoperative day aided by adjustable sutures. Base-out prisms are used temporarily if overcorrection occurs. Non-surgical management of postoperative overcorrection should be tried for at least a month before reoperation is contemplated because of the high likelihood of spontaneous resolution.

Other associations

Pattern deviations (see Chapter 80)

In patients without significant oblique muscle dysfunction, vertical transposition of the horizontal recti is our preference.

In A pattern exotropia with superior oblique overaction our preferred procedure is a posterior three-quarters tenectomy of the superior oblique tendon (Fig. 77.5). In V pattern deviations with inferior oblique overaction (Fig. 77.6), we prefer an inferior oblique weakening procedure.

In patients with craniofacial syndromes, dynamic MRI may show that rectus muscles are excyclorotated and that the X(T) in upgaze is due to the lateral displacement of the superior rectus with downward displacement of the lateral rectus. Repositioning the muscle to its normal anatomic position may improve the pattern deviation (see Fig. 77.3).

In patients with long-standing exodeviations, a tight lateral rectus muscle may cause an X pattern deviation (Fig. 77.7). Both the inferior oblique and superior oblique muscles appear to overact. The tight lateral rectus muscles cause a leash effect, creating pseudo-overaction of the oblique muscles. The apparent oblique muscle dysfunction disappears after lateral rectus weakening. The tight lateral rectus syndrome is uncommon and probably found only in a very large poorly controlled decompensated X(T). It is more common with long-standing constant exotropia.

Lateral or horizontal incomitance

Patients whose primary position deviation exceeds right and left lateral gazes by 20% or at least 10 PD have significant horizontal incomitance, which is associated with postoperative overcorrection and reoperation.[69] They may benefit from reducing the intended surgical weakening procedure on the lateral rectus muscle. This modification prevents overcorrection on lateral gazes but risks undercorrection in primary position. When lateral incomitance is due to a tight medial rectus muscle, resection procedures on this muscle worsens the incomitance. Recession of the tight medial rectus with enhanced lateral rectus recession to compensate for the effect of the medial rectus recession is recommended. Adjustable

Table 77.3 – Surgery for exotropia

Exotropia (PD)	LR recession (mm each eye)
20	4.5
25	5.0
30	6.0
35	6.5
40	7.0
45	7.5
50	8.0

Lateral rectus (LR) recession both eyes for intermittent exotropia. Designed for 5–10 PD of esotropia in the early postoperative period. The numbers in this table should be modified based on clinical findings (such as horizontal incomitance), the surgeon's technique, and results of the surgeon's personal series.

Table 77.4 – Surgery for exotropia

Exotropia (PD)	LR recession (mm)	MR resection (mm)
20	4.0	3.0
25	5.0	4.0
30	5.5	4.0
35	6.5	4.5
40	7.0	4.5
50	8.0	4.5

Lateral rectus (LR) recession and medial rectus (MR) resection (recess–resect). The numbers in this table should be modified based on clinical findings (such as horizontal incomitance), the surgeon's technique, and results of the surgeon's personal series.

sutures improve results, but are challenging to perform in young children.

High AC/A ratio

Patients with X(T) and a high AC/A ratio are at risk of postoperative overcorrection,[70] and may be better managed with over-minus lenses. There is significant test/test variability in the measurement of AC/A ratio, particularly in the young.

Concomitant vertical deviations

Small vertical deviations may occur with X(T). Vertical deviations of less than 10 PD can be corrected by vertical transposition of the horizontal rectus muscles. For example, the recessed lateral rectus and the resected medial rectus muscle may be displaced superiorly one-half to a whole tendon width in the hypotropic eye (directions are reversed for a hyperdeviation). This adds an additional upward vector assisting in the control of the vertical deviation. Large vertical deviations should be addressed with the appropriate surgery on the cyclo-vertical muscle at the time of exotropia surgery.

Postoperative undercorrection

Severe early postoperative undercorrection may arise because of a slipped, resected, medial rectus muscle. There is usually restriction of adduction and widening of the palpebral fissure on attempted adduction. Treatment is with early surgical exploration and repair. More commonly, X(T) persists or recurs following surgery (Fig. 77.4). Further treatment including surgery should be considered and discussed with the parents.

Postoperative overcorrection

Overcorrection that persists beyond the immediate postoperative period is less common than undercorrection, even when surgery for the largest recorded angle of exodeviation is the target. Transient esotropia for near targets is common in the first few postoperative weeks. A small angle esotropia that persists at distance, with only exophoria or orthotropia at near, is usually stable and best left untreated, provided diplopia is not problematic. Rarely, a large overcorrection following an over-recessed, slipped, or lost lateral rectus muscle may occur. It is most bothersome in the field of gaze of the weakened lateral rectus (Fig. 77.8).

In the early postoperative period, a rather large esotropia may not necessarily mean a poor response to surgery. Long term stability of alignment after bilateral lateral rectus recession was achieved in patients who demonstrated up to 20 PD of esotropia in the first 10 days after surgery.[36,38]

Esotropia at near that persists beyond 3 weeks is worrisome, especially in children susceptible to suppression and deterioration of fusional status. Children can develop monofixational esotropia even if aligned to within 8 PD of orthotropia. Older children and adults, on the other hand, tolerate overcorrection poorly because of diplopia.

Further treatment with occlusion, prisms, and botulinum toxin injection to the medial rectus and further surgery (usually medial rectus recession) should be considered if the overcorrection does not settle within an acceptable time period.

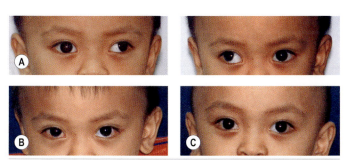

Fig. 77.4 Patient with intermittent exotropia who underwent three muscle surgery consisting of lateral rectus recession OU and a right medial rectus resection. (B) Preoperative photos showing exotropia. (A) Early postoperative photo showing minimal lid fissure narrowing in the right eye following a recess–resect procedure. (C) Two months postoperative photos show improvement in lid fissure height and symmetry but shows small angle exotropia with dissociated vertical deviation. Amblyopia OD persisted despite occlusion therapy.

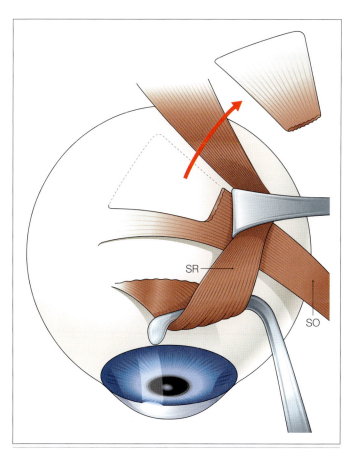

Fig. 77.5 Posterior 3/4 superior oblique tenectomy. A quadrilateral posterior tenectomy is performed on the superior oblique tendon (SO) where it fans out, leaving the anterior 1–2 mm of the tendon intact to preserve intorsion. (From Shin GS, et al. Posterior superior oblique tenectomy at the scleral insertion for collapse of A-pattern strabismus. J Pediatr Ophthalmol Strabismus 1996; 33: 211–8. Reprinted with permission from Slack, Inc.)

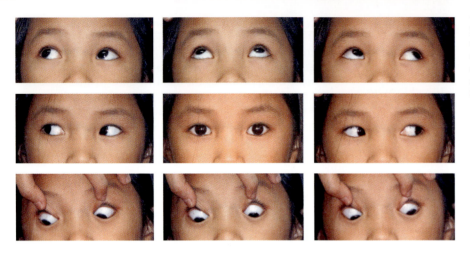

Fig. 77.6 Four-year-old patient with intermittent exotropia with V pattern and inferior oblique overaction. Center photograph shows right exotropia that increased in upgaze and reduced in downgaze. Note also the mild overaction of the right inferior oblique in up and left gaze.

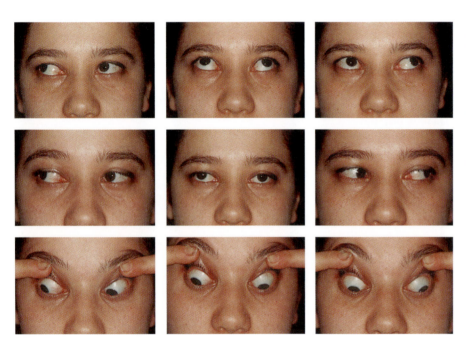

Fig. 77.7 Patient with X pattern deviation because of long-standing exotropia. Tight lateral rectus muscles act as a leash. Forced duction testing will show resistance to full adduction. Only weakening procedures on the lateral rectus are necessary to relieve the X pattern. No surgery is required on the oblique muscles. (From Santiago AP, et al. Intermittent exotropia. In: Rosenbaum AL, Santiago AP, editors. Clinical Strabismus Management: Principles and Surgical Techniques. 1st ed. Philadelphia: Saunders; 1999. With permission of Elsevier.)

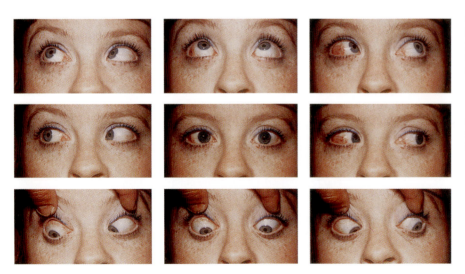

Fig. 77.8 Overcorrection after bilateral rectus recession for intermittent exotropia. Patient developed 25 PD of right esotropia with abduction deficit in right gaze. Differential diagnosis should include slipped or lost lateral rectus muscle. A lost muscle, however, seems less likely because of relatively good right lateral rectus rotation despite the observed deficit. (From Santiago AP, et al. Intermittent exotropia. In: Rosenbaum AL, Santiago AP, editors. Clinical Strabismus Management: Principles and Surgical Techniques, 1st ed. Philadelphia: Saunders; 1999. With permission of Elsevier.)

References

3. Kim SH, Yi ST, Cho YA, Uhm CS. Ultrastructural study of extraocular muscle tendon axonal profiles in infantile and intermittent exotropia. Acta Ophthalmol Scand 2006; 84: 182–7.

4. Tamura O, Mitsui Y. The magician's forceps phenomenon in exotropia under general anaesthesia. Br J Ophthalmol 1986; 70: 549–52.

7. Mohney BG. Common forms of childhood strabismus in an incidence cohort. Am J Ophthalmol 2007; 144: 465–7.

8. Chia A, Roy L, Seenyen L. Comitant horizontal strabismus: an Asian perspective. Br J Ophthalmol 2007; 91: 1337–40.

10. Chia A, Dirani M, Chan YH, et al. Prevalence of amblyopia and strabismus in young Singaporean chinese children. Invest Ophthalmol Vis Sci 2010; 51: 3411–17.

13. Chia A, Seenyen L, Long QB. A retrospective review of 287 consecutive children in Singapore presenting with intermittent exotropia. J AAPOS 2005; 9: 257–63.

14. Buck D, Powell C, Cumberland P, et al. Presenting features and early management of childhood intermittent exotropia in the UK: inception cohort study. Br J Ophthalmol 2009; 93: 1620–4.

19. Kushner BJ, Morton GV. Distance/near differences in intermittent exotropia. Arch Ophthalmol 1998; 116: 478–86.

20. Jung JW, Lee SY. A comparison of the clinical characteristics of intermittent exotropia in children and adults. Korean J Ophthalmol 2010; 24: 96–100.

21. Kushner BJ. Selective surgery for intermittent exotropia based on distance/near differences. Arch Ophthalmol 1998; 116: 324–8.

25. Serrano-Pedraza I, Clarke MP, Read JC. Single vision during ocular deviation in intermittent exotropia. Ophthalmic Physiol Opt 2011; 31: 45–55.

28. Kushner BJ. The occurrence of monofixational exotropia after exotropia surgery. Am J Ophthalmol 2009; 147: 1082–5.

33. Hatt SR, Leske DA, Holmes JM. Awareness of exodeviation in children with intermittent exotropia. Strabismus 2009; 17: 101–6.

34. Yamada T, Hatt SR, Leske DA, Holmes JM. Health-related quality of life in parents of children with intermittent exotropia. J AAPOS 2011; 15: 135–9.

35. Ing MR, Nishimura J, Okino L. Outcome study of bilateral rectus recession for intermittent exotropia in children. Trans Am Ophthalmol Soc 1997; 95: 433–43.

36. Ruttum MS. Initial versus subsequent postoperative motor alignment in intermittent exotropia. J AAPOS 1997; 1: 88–91.

39. Mohney BG, Holmes JM. An office-based scale for assessing control in intermittent exotropia. Strabismus 2006; 14: 147–50.

40. Haggerty H, Richardson S, Hrisos S, et al. The Newcastle Control Score: a new method of grading the severity of intermittent exotropia. Br J Ophthalmol 2004; 88: 233–5.

41. Buck D, Clarke MP, Haggerty H, et al. Grading the severity of intermittent distance exotropia: the revised Newcastle Control Score. Br J Ophthalmol 2008; 92: 577.

54. O'Neal TD, Rosenbaum AL, Stathacopoulos RA. Distance stereo acuity improvement in intermittent exotropic patients following strabismus surgery. J Ped Ophthalmol Strabismus 1995; 32: 353–7.

55. Adams WE, Leske DA, Hatt SR, et al. Improvement in distance stereoacuity following surgery for intermittent exotropia. J AAPOS 2008; 12: 141–4.

56. Eibschitz-Tsimhoni M, Archer SM, Furr BA, Del Monte MA. Current concepts in the management of concomitant exodeviations. Compr Ophthalmol Update 2007; 8: 213–23.

62. Rowe FJ, Noonan CP, Freeman G, DeBell J. Intervention for intermittent distance exotropia with overcorrecting minus lenses. Eye (Lond) 2009; 23: 320–5.

63. Freeman RS, Isenberg SJ. The use of part-time occlusion for early onset unilateral exotropia. J Pediatr Ophthalmol Strabismus 1989; 26: 94.

64. Figueira EC, Hing S. Intermittent exotropia: comparison of treatments. Clin Exp Ophthalmol 2006; 34: 245–51.

65. Spencer RF, Tucker MG, Choi RY, McNeer KW. Botulinum toxin management of childhood intermittent exotropia. Ophthalmology 1997; 104: 1762–7.

68. Leow PL, Ko ST, Wu PK, Chan CW. Exotropic drift and ocular alignment after surgical correction for intermittent exotropia. J Pediatr Ophthalmol Strabismus 2010; 47: 12–6.

69. Pineles SL, Ela-Dalman N, Zvansky AG, et al. Long-term results of the surgical management of intermittent exotropia. J AAPOS 2010; 14: 298–304.

70. Brodsky MC, Fray KJ. Surgical management of intermittent exotropia with high AC/A ratio. J AAPOS 1998; 2: 330–2.

Access the complete reference list online at
http://www.expertconsult.com

Special forms of comitant exotropia

Stephen P Kraft

Chapter contents

Introduction

Exodeviations in children can be comitant or non-comitant. Non-comitant exodeviations result from either innervational causes, i.e. third nerve paresis and Duane's syndrome, or mechanical causes, such as tumors or trauma (see Chapters 82 and 83).

The most common comitant type in children is intermittent exotropia, and there are other comitant exodeviations whose management can be challenging. This chapter deals with infantile exotropia, monofixational exotropia, exotropia associated with hemianopic visual field defects, and sensory exotropia. Although they are considered as comitant deviations, they may develop incomitance from secondary changes in the lateral rectus muscles in long-standing cases, especially in sensory exotropia or infantile exotropia with a large deviation, or where the exodeviation is due to amblyopia or structural abnormalities in the misaligned eye.

Infantile exotropia

Introduction

Infantile exotropia is an exodeviation that develops within the first few months of life and persists. While infantile esotropia is generally defined as having its onset by age 6 months, the term infantile exotropia is used for exodeviations that first manifest up to 1 year of age.[1-6] It can be a primary disorder or secondary to an ocular or systemic problem.

Primary infantile exotropia, unrelated to a systemic or ocular disorder, is rare, roughly 1 per 30 000 births.[7] In primary strabismus in infancy, for every case with exotropia there are between 150 and 300 cases with esotropia.[8] Intermittent exotropia can manifest by age 12 months, and it may represent a large minority of cases of exotropia seen before age 1 year (see Chapter 77).[6] Infantile exotropia is often associated with ocular or systemic disorders. It is seen with ptosis, albinism, ocular motor apraxia (saccadic initiation failure), optic nerve anomalies, and with diseases that lead to vision loss, including retinoblastoma, retinoschisis, iridolenticular abnormalities, and cataracts.[8-10] Exotropia can be a feature of several congenital strabismus syndromes, including third nerve palsies, Duane's syndrome, congenital fibrosis of the extraocular muscles, and strabismus fixus[8,9] (see Chapter 82). It is described in association with many systemic disorders including prematurity, cerebral palsy, seizure disorders, hydrocephalus, craniofacial syndromes, and various chromosomal anomalies.[1,4,5,8,10,11]

Ocular or systemic disorders are more common in infantile exotropias than in esotropias, and infants with constant exotropia have a much stronger chance than those with intermittent exotropia of having a coexisting problem.[5,9] The incidence of systemic anomalies may also be positively correlated with the size of the angle of deviation:[5] it is prudent to consider a neurodevelopmental assessment of a child with infantile exotropia.

Etiology

Vergence abnormalities

Exodeviations appear in over one-third of healthy neonates, while esodeviations are rare.[12,13] Mostly, they are transient and resolve by 6 months as the vergence system matures.[13] Therefore, primary infantile exotropia may be an arrested development of the convergence system.

Abnormal convergence may be a primary or secondary phenomenon. There may be a primary convergence deficit in the convergence system, or it may arise from defective cortical binocular development.[14] Disruption of binocular connections in the immature visual cortex potently disrupts development of vergence, leading to strabismus and to functional deficits, loss of fusion, asymmetric monocular smooth pursuit, and asymmetric monocular motion perception.[14] The asymmetries are characterized by better tracking and detection of targets when they are followed from the temporal to the nasal visual field than when they are tracked in the reverse direction. This directional asymmetry should lead to infantile esotropia, rather than exotropia. Therefore, the severity of a primary or secondary convergence system deficit must override the other abnormal processes such that divergence is predominant. The identical pursuit asymmetry seen in infantile esotropia also occurs in infantile exotropia (L Tychsen, personal communication, 2001).

Anatomic factors

An asymmetry in the structure of the lateral and medial rectus muscles occurs with the length–tension curve of the lateral rectus showing more stiffness than the medial rectus and the diameter of the lateral rectus may be congenitally larger than normal, allowing it to "overpower" the medial rectus.[8] Finally, orbital dysmorphism, as in craniofacial syndromes, can produce a divergent positioning of the eyes.

Genetic factors

Infantile exotropia occurred in three consecutive generations of one family, suggesting autosomal dominant inheritance.[11] It may be more common in Asians and Africans than in Caucasians.[8]

Clinical features

Infantile exotropia occurs by 12 months of age.[1,3,8] It can have a wide range of angles, from 20 to 90 prism diopters (PD), with most cases more than 35 PD[7,9,11,15] (Fig. 78.1). The angle is usually stable initially, increasing slowly.[6] Amblyopia occurs in up to 25%, usually caused by strabismus rather than anisometropia.[8] It responds to the usual treatments (see Chapter 70). There is a normal distribution of refractive errors.[7,8] If the deviation is large, an "X" pattern strabismus is common, as also seen in adults with large angle exotropia who have a tight lateral rectus syndrome. The deviation is larger in upgaze and downgaze than in the primary position with mild limitation of adduction in one or both eyes and upshoots and downshoots in adduction (see Fig. 78.1) which have been ascribed to contracture with overactions of the oblique muscles, to sideslip of the lateral rectus around the globe (a "leash effect"), or to the globe having more room to elevate and depress when it is not fully adducted.[8,16,17] Alternatively, there may be "A" or, more commonly, "V" patterns.[1,4,7,11,15] Latent nystagmus, dissociated vertical deviations, and inferior oblique overactions may occur, as with infantile esotropia, but less frequently.[1,3,4,6]

Examination

Some pertinent points must be noted in the evaluation of infantile exotropia.

1. The general behavior and physical features of the child may suggest a systemic or orbital association.
2. Anterior and posterior segment disorders can be associated with infantile exotropia. A cycloplegic refraction is vital.
3. The examiner must observe the corneal light reflexes to rule out a positive angle kappa that gives a false appearance of exotropia:[8] the cover test will confirm a true exodeviation rather than a pseudo-exotropia (see Chapters 7 and 72).
4. When the angle is large, the examiner needs to use two prisms oriented base-in and split between the two eyes to

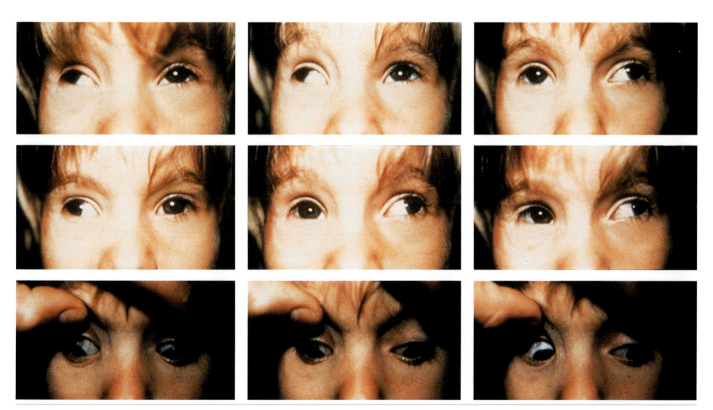

Fig. 78.1 Photos of nine diagnostic gaze positions of a child with infantile exotropia. Note the large angle of exotropia in the primary position (central photo). There is limited adduction of each eye and an "X" pattern. Each eye shows an upshoot and downshoot in the adducted position. (From Kraft SP. Selected exotropia entities and principles of management. In: Rosenbaum AL, Santiago AP, editors. Clinical Strabismus Management. Philadelphia: Saunders; 1999: 176–201. Copyright Elsevier 1999.)

get an approximation of the total angle, whether the angle is measured by the Krimsky or prism and alternating cover methods (see Chapter 72).

5. The examiner should search for features of the infantile strabismus complex including dissociated vertical deviations and oblique muscle overactions. Optokinetic testing may detect monocular nasal–temporal motion asymmetries.

Management

Non-surgical therapy

Infantile exotropia usually requires surgery after any refractive errors and amblyopia have been treated. Although the angle of the deviation is generally stable, the strabismus angle may reduce with occlusion.[1]

Botulinum toxin injections have been used for infantile esotropia, but there are no reports on series of cases of the rarer infantile exotropia and success rates range from 50% to 70%, with bilateral, not unilateral, lateral rectus injections.[18,19] Most had intermittent exotropia: the success rates for exotropia over 35 to 40 PD was much lower, and, since most infantile exotropias are larger than this, botulinum toxin may be less successful than surgery for deviations over 35 PD.

Surgery

Timing

Patients with primary infantile exotropia should be approached in the same manner as those with infantile esotropia where the general consensus among pediatric ophthalmologists for many years was to align the eyes before the age of 24 months to achieve optimal motor and sensory results.[2,3,7,20] In recent years, earlier surgery has been favored in the belief that it is more effective in reversing the binocular vision and vergence deficits. Evidence suggests that the optimal "window" for treating infantile esotropia may be the first 8 to 10 months of life[21] but whether it is applicable to infantile exotropia is not known. The consensus still favors realigning the eyes before 24 months of age. Once the diagnosis of infantile exotropia is confirmed and any refractive error or amblyopia is corrected, the child should be followed for a few weeks to be sure the angle of the strabismus is stable.

Surgical planning

Strabismus surgery techniques for exotropia are described in Chapter 85, but there are some specific recommendations for surgical treatment of infantile exotropia:

1. The aim in primary infantile exotropia is to create an esotropia in the immediate postoperative period, as in most exotropias in older children and adults.[1,7] This principle also applies to children with infantile exotropia and developmental delay or cerebral palsy, as the postoperative drift is usually in the divergent direction whether they originally had esotropia or exotropia immediately after surgery.[8] For either category, the best result in a single operation seems to require an immediate postoperative angle in the range of 10 to 14 PD, which is slightly larger than is usually targeted for later-onset intermittent exotropia.

2. The strategy generally involves weakening (usually recession) of one or both lateral rectus muscles, as they

are often tight. If the near exotropia is larger than that at distance, then a strengthening (usually a resection) of a medial rectus muscle should be included.[8]

3. Strabismus angles under 40 PD can usually be successfully treated with surgery on two horizontal muscles, either bilateral lateral rectus recessions or a unilateral lateral rectus recession with a medial rectus resection.[1] Treatment of angles over 40 PD may require "supramaximal" amounts of recessions or resections if surgery is limited to two muscles. Alternatively, surgery of more "regular" dosages can be planned on three or four horizontal muscles.[1,3,4,7,11,15,20] Another strategy involves large recessions of both lateral rectus muscles combined with simultaneous injections of botulinum toxin into the two muscles.

4. Surgery for any coexisting dissociated vertical deviations or oblique overactions can be planned for the same sitting or for subsequent surgery, as in infantile esotropia.

Results

The success rates for infantile exotropia surgery are not high. Reoperation rates are as high as 50% of patients: undercorrections are more common than overcorrections.[1,3,11,15,20]

Young children who are aligned before age 24 months develop peripheral fusion in up to 50% of cases: some may show gross stereopsis.[1,11,15,20] The best binocular outcomes reported are monofixation syndromes.[6] Realigning patients with infantile exotropia after age 2 years can lead to stable long-term results, but sensory fusion is rarely achieved after this age.[7,8]

Monofixational exotropia

Introduction

The monofixation syndrome is characterized by fixation with the fovea of only one eye under binocular conditions.[8,22] Sensory features include intact peripheral fusion, preserved gross stereopsis and, frequently, amblyopia of the non-foveating eye. The motor features include manifest heterotropia of under 8 PD, a larger heterophoria, and preserved convergence and divergence fusional amplitudes.[22-24] Some cases show no heterotropia on cover test: they are termed monofixational phorias. Some show a heterotropia without a heterophoria: these are sometimes termed microtropias (see Chapter 76).[22]

In most cases of monofixation syndrome, if there is a small angle heterotropia, it is an esotropia, and any associated heterophoria is an esophoria. However, about 20% have an exotropic orientation for the tropia and the phoria.[22,23,25-28] Most cases of monofixational exotropia are secondary, either associated with anisometropia or following surgery for exotropia. However, a monofixation syndrome may underlie some cases of intermittent exotropia and its true nature may only become evident after surgery for the total exodeviation.[23,29]

Most cases of monofixational exotropia, by virtue of intact vergence amplitudes, retain a stable long-term small exotropia under binocular conditions. In a minority, fusion control is disrupted and the exophoria becomes predominant: this is termed a decompensated monofixational exotropia.[22,23,25]

Etiology

The monofixation syndrome can be primary or secondary. The secondary form may be associated with anisometropia, a macular lesion, or previous surgery for infantile or acquired strabismus. Otherwise, it is considered a primary disorder.

Primary monofixation exotropia

Patients with the primary form have a deficit in fovea-to-fovea correspondence: they cannot attain bifoveal fusion.[22] This may be an hereditary error in foveal correspondence that may exceed the capability of Panum's fusional space to compensate for it, leading to suppression of the less dominant fovea.[8] Alternatively, there may be a reversal of the normal dominance of the nasal over the temporal hemifield. As a result, any degree of foveal disparity can lead to a facultative scotoma on the temporal side of the fovea rather than in its usual location on the nasal side.[8,24,30]

A primary monofixational exotropia can decompensate because of an acute illness or chronic fatigue and the "all or none" suppression in exodeviations is less flexible than that in esodeviations.[30,31] If the latent heterophoria begins to manifest, then the strong hemiretinal suppression mechanism may increase the propensity for the exodeviation to decompensate.[8,31]

Secondary monofixational exotropia

The majority of secondary forms in children result from surgery for constant or intermittent exotropia.[26] Monofixation after surgery suggests a pre-existing defect in bifoveal fusion, and this may underlie a minority of cases of seemingly typical intermittent exotropia.[22,25,26,29] Anisometropia is a less common cause but, as an obstacle to bifoveal fusion, it leads to suppression of the less dominant fovea. Finally, a unilateral macular lesion can lead to a progressive manifest exotropia; small lesions can result in a small scotoma with the attributes of a monofixation syndrome.[8]

Secondary monofixation exotropia has the same propensity for deterioration as the primary form. There is an abnormal binocular state, and any loss of the "peripheral fusion lock" allows the heterophoria to manifest. If the control deteriorates then the hemiretinal suppression adaptation may take over and increase the likelihood that the exotropia becomes constant.[31]

Clinical features

Motor features

Most patients with a monofixation syndrome show a heterotropia of 2 to 8 PD under binocular conditions. Up to one-third of cases will show no shift on cover test: most commonly in the form secondary to anisometropia.[8,22]

The exophoria uncovered on alternating prism and cover test tends to be larger than that seen in bifoveal patients who have exophoria, although it rarely exceeds 25 PD[23,25] and the fusional amplitudes are nearly normal.[22] When exotropia and exophoria coexist, the simultaneous prism and cover test should be performed initially to measure the static heterotropia. Then the prism and alternating cover test measures the superimposed heterophoria[8] (see Chapter 72).

Cases of decompensated monofixational exotropia can appear as intermittent exotropia: chronic cases may show a constant exotropia. Children whose monofixation exotropias decompensate may complain of asthenopia as their deviations stress their fusional amplitudes, or give them diplopia if the separation of the perceived images exceeds their suppression scotoma. These symptoms are more common with decompensating monofixation exotropia than for esotropia, but asthenopia in monofixation exotropia is less frequent than in bifoveal patients with exophoria.[23]

Sensory features

Binocular sensory testing in monofixation confirms a foveal scotoma in the non-dominant eye with preservation of peripheral fusion. In monofixation exotropia there may be a suppression scotoma extending temporally from the fovea. Depending on the test, the size of targets, the patient's age, and the size of the heterotropia, they can indicate either normal retinal correspondence or anomalous correspondence, even in the same patient.[8,22,27,31] Eccentric fixation may also be demonstrated in the non-dominant eye, especially if amblyopia is severe.[27]

Stereopsis is subnormal in this syndrome but often detectable in monofixational exotropia.[25,26] Stereoacuity is higher in the primary than in the secondary form, in both monofixational esotropia and exotropia.[26]

Where the exodeviation has decompensated and manifests almost constantly as an exotropia, sensory testing with the angle offset with prisms may show subnormal binocular vision, suggesting an underlying monofixation syndrome.[8,29]

Amblyopia (see Chapter 70)

The incidence of amblyopia in monofixation exotropia ranges from 30% to 65%, slightly less than in monofixational esotropia.[8,22,25-28] It occurs most commonly with anisometropia and least often with the postsurgical form.[22,27] Up to 50% of patients with monofixation and moderate to severe amblyopia may also show eccentric fixation on monocular testing.[27]

Treatment

Once a primary or secondary monofixation syndrome develops, it is difficult to gain bifoveal fixation.[22,24] Aggressive attempts to break down the facultative macular scotoma to achieve this may risk diplopia.[22-24] There are anecdotal cases of conversion of monofixation to bifoveal situations with aggressive therapy in children.[24]

In children there are two clear indications for treatment in monofixation exotropia: the reversal of amblyopia and the restoration of alignment in a decompensated exotropia.

Amblyopia

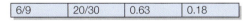

| 6/9 | 20/30 | 0.63 | 0.18 |

Amblyopia of worse than logMAR 0.40 (6/15, 20/50, 0.40) should be treated, even in a monofixation syndrome, including spectacles for refractive errors and anisometropia, and patching or penalization.[24] In decompensated monofixational exotropia, treatment of the amblyopia can improve control of the exotropia and reduce symptoms such as asthenopia. Success includes improving vision to logMAR 0.18 (6/9, 20/30, 0.63) or better and a stable monofixation – a small angle exotropia with peripheral fusion.[8,24]

Alignment

No treatment is indicated for asymptomatic patients with small, infrequently manifest exodeviations, but those with

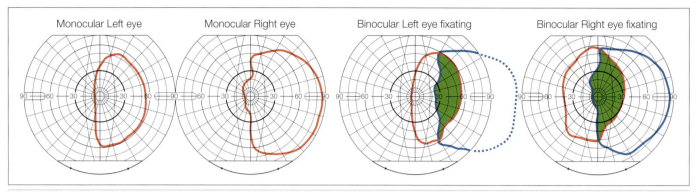

Fig. 78.2 Monocular and binocular visual fields in a patient with congenital complete left homonymous hemianopia and exotropia. The first two plots show the monocular visual fields of the left and right eyes. The third plot shows the binocular field with the left eye fixating, and the fourth plot shows the binocular field with the right eye fixating. The shaded area is the overlap of the monocular fields. Note that the panorama of the binocular field is greater when the right eye is used for fixation than when the left eye takes up fixation. (From Kraft SP. Selected exotropia entities and principles of management. In: Rosenbaum AL, Santiago AP, editors. Clinical Strabismus Management. Philadelphia: Saunders; 1999: 176–201. Copyright Elsevier 1999; after Gote H, Gregersen E, Rindziunski E. Exotropia and panoramic vision compensating for an occult congenital homonymous hemianopia: a case report. Binocul Vis Eye Muscle Surg Q 1993; 8: 129–32, with permission of Binoculus Publishing.)

frequent exotropia who complain of asthenopia or diplopia warrant intervention. The goal is comfortable single vision, usually by achieving monofixation exotropia rather than bifoveal fixation.[22,25,29,31]

Non-surgical options include part-time occlusion, prisms, and minus lens overcorrection (see Chapter 84). Orthoptic exercises are not usually indicated for decompensated monofixation exotropia as the fusional amplitudes are good. Anti-suppression therapy is contraindicated, as in decompensated monofixational esotropia, to avoid breaking down suppression.[22]

Botulinum toxin and surgery are used to treat children whose exodeviations have decompensated or are not corrected by amblyopia treatment or non-surgical interventions. Botulinum toxin has a good success rate for small angles in children[18,19] as the exotropia is rarely more than 20 to 25 PD. Surgery has about the same rate of success as for the common forms of intermittent exotropia. However, the result is a monofixation syndrome, rather than bifoveal fixation.[8,25,29]

Exotropia with hemianopic visual field defects

Introduction

Exotropia occurs with both homonymous and bitemporal hemianopias; binasal hemianopias are very rare. The field loss is usually extensive when an exotropia develops in association with one of these disorders.

Homonymous hemianopias

Etiology

Exotropia can occur with homonymous hemianopias caused by congenital or acquired intracranial disorders. It is mostly acquired before the age of 2 years, but it can be an adaptation with hemianopia onset as late as 7 years.[32-34] The normal binocular visual field is compromised by the bilateral loss of the field on one side. The divergent strabismus is likely an adaptive

compensation to enlarge the binocular field[32-35] (Fig. 78.2). This is challenged by those who feel that the exodeviation is an epiphenomenon, not adaptive.[36,37]

Clinical features

In contrast to patients who develop homonymous hemianopias later, children with congenital or early-acquired brain lesions adapt well. They are often unaware of their field loss[36-38] and develop eye movement strategies that include large saccadic movements into the blind field followed by smooth pursuit into the intact field to fixate a target.[37] They may develop a face turn to the side of the hemianopia in order to better center their remaining hemifield.[8,34,36,37]

Children who later develop a homonymous hemianopia do not adapt as well: they often bump into objects on the side of the hemianopia, and reading is difficult.

Motor features

An exotropia occurring as an adaptation to field loss may be limited to cases that are congenital or early acquired. The compensatory exotropia can be seen either in childhood or later.[32-35] In early acquired cases the onset can be as soon as 8 weeks after the cause of the hemianopia. They usually show a constant deviation, which contrasts with the intermittent exodeviations reported with later-acquired hemianopias. The angle in early-onset cases ranges from 20 to 70 PD and it is often larger for distance fixation than for near.[32-35] It may be associated with a vertical heterotropia or a pattern strabismus.[8,33]

Children with later-acquired hemianopia and exotropia usually have deviations less than 20 PD.[38] They can be an exophoria or an intermittent or constant exotropia. Exotropias in such cases may not be adaptive.[8,27,32,38]

Sensory features

Young children adapt better to homonymous defects than do older children; those who develop exotropia have complete and congruous defects.[32,33,35,36] With the exotropia, the expansion of the visual field to the side of the missing field ranges from 20° to 45°. This strategy is only relevant if the exotropia develops in the eye ipsilateral to the field loss, while the child fixates with the eye on the side of the intact field (see Fig. 78.2). The amount of expansion is proportional to the size of the exotropia.[32,33,35,36]

Children with exotropia with congenital or early-onset hemianopia rarely complain of diplopia or asthenopia because they may develop anomalous retinal correspondence (ARC).[32,33,35] They suppress within the overlapping portions of the monocular fields, and elsewhere they show ARC.[32,33] This can be tested by the synoptophore or with sensory tests performed while the angle of exotropia is offset with base-in prisms.[8,32,33,35]

Patients with later-acquired hemianopias generally complain of diplopia since they retain normal correspondence, cannot develop ARC,[8,32,38] and cannot develop suppression.

Treatment

Surgery for exotropia with congenital or early-onset homonymous hemianopia is undertaken with caution. First, the realignment of the eyes reduces the total binocular visual field. Second, patients who develop ARC in response to the exodeviation may experience paradoxical diplopia if the eye is realigned once the adaptation is complete.[32,33,35] Patients should be tested before surgery with a monocular patch to see whether they can adapt to the smaller binocular field and then with a prism to see whether they develop diplopia.

Patients with later-onset hemianopia who develop diplopia or asthenopia because of an exodeviation may be treated initially with a prism or a patch, or they may require surgery or botulinum toxin.

Bitemporal visual field defects

Etiology

Bitemporal hemianopia results from lesions of the optic chiasm. Extensive bitemporal field loss disrupts peripheral fusion and compromises the vergence system, which, in turn, increases the risk that an existing exophoria decompensates.[38,39]

Clinical features

The disruption of the vergence reflex may lead to exodeviation which can cause several sensory phenomena especially if the field loss in each eye is extensive enough to involve the two maculae.

Motor features

The exodeviation measures a few PDs,[8] often variable because of poor fusional vergences and the endpoints can be difficult to measure.[38,39] The extraocular movements are usually normal.

Sensory features

Patients with bitemporal hemianopia may have two unusual and often missed symptoms. First, the loss of overlapping visual fields can lead to "hemiretinal slide" as the intact nasal visual fields of the two eyes cannot be synchronized.[38-40] The exotropia then leads to reduction of the binocular field and overlap of the partial images seen by the intact nasal fields. Any target appears elongated, and there is duplication of features within the target[8,40] (Fig. 78.3). This leads to reading difficulties.

Second, complete bitemporal hemianopia produces "postfixation blindness" from stimulation of non-seeing nasal retina by objects that lie within that area of space beyond the fixation target[8,38] (Fig. 78.4). An exotropia places the area of postfixation blindness further from the eyes and any proximal object including the fixation target may be double, as most patients have normal retinal correspondence (NRC)[8,39,40] (Fig. 78.4). This leads to difficulty with daily chores such as reaching accurately, pouring fluids, and picking things up off a flat surface.

Very young children with bitemporal hemianopia and exotropia may not have symptoms. They may be able to develop suppression as an adaptation to diplopia.[38,40] Others may adapt to their abnormal binocular vision in the same way that children can learn strategies to overcome symptoms of bilateral homonymous hemianopia.[8]

Treatment

There is no adequate therapy for exotropia with total or almost complete bitemporal hemianopia, whether it appears in young or older children. Prisms can be tried to alleviate diplopia, but they are not always helpful due to the variability of the exodeviation.[40] Patching one eye reduces the visual field. Surgery to eliminate diplopia and exotropia can help if the misalignment is eliminated. However, the result is rarely stable due to lack of adequate fusional vergences.[8,40]

Sensory exotropia

Sensory exotropia – a unilateral exodeviation – develops as a result of loss of vision or chronic poor vision in one eye.[2,8,24] Children under age 5 or 6 years who develop strabismus due to vision loss in one eye have an equal chance of developing esotropia or exotropia; after 6 years, exotropia develops more often.[24]

Etiology

Sensory exotropia occurs in children as a result of congenital and acquired ocular disorders. Congenital disorders compromise vision development; normal binocular vergence reflexes cannot develop and strabismus is a frequent result. Acquired causes include traumatic and non-traumatic diseases, such as cataracts, that disrupt the fusion reflex[8,24] (Fig. 78.5). One specific cause is anisometropic amblyopia, especially anisohyperopia. Older children whose vision remains reduced are at particular risk of developing exotropia.[41-43]

The mechanisms for the development of exotropia when vision is lost in one eye are the following.

1. *Binocular rivalry.* When the retinal image of one eye is degraded, it sets up a rivalry between that and the fellow eye. Normal visual signals becomes inhibitory to the disadvantaged eye: this is even more powerful with partial than with total loss.[41] Also, there is a superiority of the nasal retina over the temporal retina in response to bright and formed stimuli, and this becomes exaggerated when an eye loses vision. These factors lead to disruption of the vergence system, and an active retinomotor divergence takes hold with a progressive exodeviation, especially in older children.[42]

2. *Decompensation of exophoria.* A well-controlled exophoria can decompensate from loss of fusion if one eye loses vision. This appears to be a settling of the poorer eye into its "elastic" rest position, not an active divergence reflex.

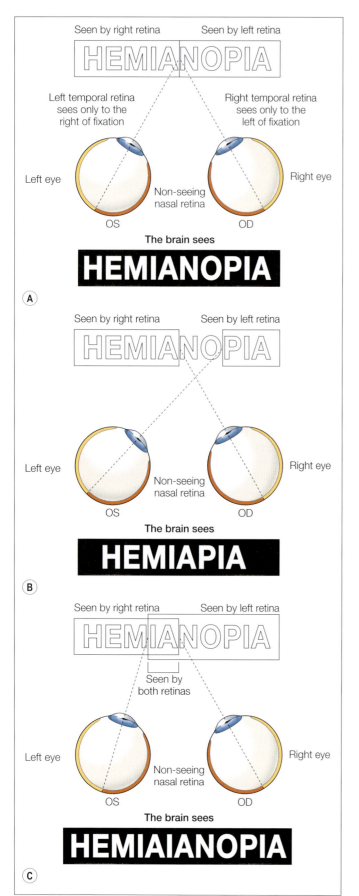

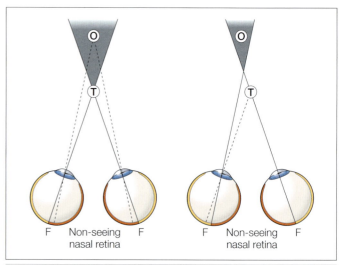

Fig. 78.3 Hemifield sliding and abnormal binocular phenomena in a patient with complete bitemporal hemianopia. (A) Straight eyes: the two separate monocular visual fields juxtapose to form a complete image of the target. (B) Left esotropia: central portions of the target are missing. (C) Left exotropia: central portions of the target are duplicated as a result of redundant reception by the functioning temporal retinas of both eyes. (From Kraft SP. Selected exotropia entities and principles of management. In: Rosenbaum AL, Santiago AP, editors. Clinical Strabismus Management. Philadelphia: Saunders; 1999: 176–201. Copyright Elsevier 1999; after Fritz KJ, Brodsky MC. Elusive neuro-ophthalmic reading impairment. Am Orthoptic J 1992; 42: 159–64, with permission of University of Wisconsin Press.)

Fig. 78.4 Postfixation blind area in a patient with complete bitemporal hemianopia. (Left) The diagram shows the situation when the eyes are straight. When both foveae (F) fixate on a target (T), the retinal image of any second object (O) located within the shaded area would fall on the non-functioning nasal retinas of both eyes and not be seen. (Right) The diagram shows the situation in the presence of a left exotropia with the right eye fixating. The target (T) may be seen as diplopic because the image falls on the fovea of the right eye and on the functioning temporal retina in the left eye. A second object (O) is not visualized as it is located in the postfixation blind area, which is more remote from the patient compared to the orthotropic state. (From Kraft SP. Selected exotropia entities and principles of management. In: Rosenbaum AL, Santiago AP, editors. Clinical Strabismus Management. Philadelphia: Saunders; 1999: 176–201. Copyright Elsevier 1999; after Roper-Hall G. Effect of visual field defects on binocular single vision. Am Orthoptic J 1976; 26: 74–82, with permission of University of Wisconsin Press.)

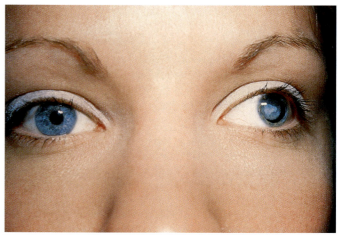

Fig. 78.5 Child with sensory left exotropia due to traumatic cataract. Note the large angle of the deviation. (From Kraft SP. Selected exotropia entities and principles of management. In: Rosenbaum AL, Santiago AP, editors. Clinical Strabismus Management. Philadelphia: Saunders; 1999: 176–201. Copyright Elsevier 1999.)

The divergent position results from an imbalance of muscle tone between the lateral and medial recti.[42]

3. *Mechanical factors.* Orbital dysmorphism or muscle anomalies predisposes to an exotropia if one eye suffers a loss of vision. Strabismus in which there is congenital tightness or stricture of the lateral rectus, such as in Duane's syndrome, can show progressive exotropia if vision deteriorates in the affected eye.

Clinical features

Motor features

Sensory exotropia is usually over 30 PD.[2,8] If the cause of the vision deficit persists, then the angle can increase progressively. A long-standing large exotropia leads to secondary muscle changes. The lateral rectus contracts and the overlying soft tissues shorten, creating a tight lateral rectus syndrome (see the Clinical features subsection of Infantile exotropia, above): an updrift and downdrift in the adducted position, and possibly an "X"[14] (see Fig. 78.1), "A", or less commonly, a "V" pattern.[8,29] The exotropic eye may exhibit a small hypertropia.

Measuring the angle of the exotropia can be tricky when the vision is poor in one eye. The prism and alternating cover test may not be accurate since the poor fixation in the eye does not allow the examiner to see a stable endpoint during the measurement; thus, the angle is better measured with the modified prism and light reflex (Krimsky) test: after the angle kappa is noted for the fixating eye, progressive base-in prism power is placed over that eye until the exotropic eye is drawn over sufficiently in the nasal direction to create a matching angle kappa in that eye[8] (see Chapter 72).

Sensory features

Several adaptations can occur in sensory exotropias. If the vision is very poor, there may be deep suppression and no binocular responses. Children whose vision is not severely reduced and who have exotropia not exceeding 40 PD may develop ARC.[43] Children with anisometropic amblyopia and exotropia may retain NRC.[41] Young children can avoid diplopia by suppressing the displaced image. Older children with sensory exotropia may experience diplopia because they cannot develop ARC.

Sensory tests in a patient can vary, ARC or NRC, depending on the depth of suppression and the dissociating ability of the tests,[8,43] the brightness of ambient lighting, the distance of the testing apparatus from the patient, and the size of the exotropia.[8,43]

Management

Treating the underlying cause of the vision loss is paramount: cataracts, corneal opacities, anisometropic amblyopia, ptosis, eyelid hemangioma, retinoblastoma, and retinal detachments are potentially reversible examples. If the problem is present early, then the exotropia can be prevented if vision can be restored by treatment, especially of amblyopia. If exotropia has already developed, it may still reduce if vision can be recovered.[8]

If exotropia persists despite correction of the underlying disorder, or if the vision loss is chronic and irreversible, it can be treated with either non-surgical or surgical options.

Non-surgical therapy and safety precautions

Prescription of safety lenses for patients with unilateral vision loss is important: those who already wear glasses should be sure that their lens and frame designs meet safety specifications.

Patients with diplopia or asthenopia can be helped with prisms if the angle of the exotropia is not over 30 PD. Children who are aware of the second image but are not helped by base-in prisms may be helped by base-out prisms to further separate the two images. Patients with intractable diplopia may be helped by Bangerter or MIN occlusion foils to reduce the clarity, and therefore awareness, of the displaced image in the exotropic eye.

Botulinum toxin injections are successful in realigning angles of exotropia under 35 PD.[18,19] However, the angles in sensory exotropia tend to be larger, with a lower long-term success rate. Patients with a large exotropia angle who choose botulinum injections rather than surgery must accept the likelihood that periodic re-injections will be needed.[8]

Surgery

Surgical planning

Children with sensory exotropia should undergo preoperative prism testing to see whether they can be realigned without inducing intractable diplopia. If a prism, placed base-in and matching the strabismus angle, is introduced before the misaligned eye and the child does not complain of diplopia, then the surgeon can plan to align the eyes close to orthotropia. If the child complains of diplopia with exact prism offset, then a reduced amount of prism for determining whether a partial correction is possible can be tried. However, a diplopia response to an offset of the angle does not necessarily mean diplopia postoperatively. In such a case, a prolonged prism trial for determining whether the child can adapt sensorially to a complete correction of the angle can be done.[8]

A complete eye examination is mandatory prior to surgery. The surgeon must be sure that the eye is healthy enough to undergo strabismus surgery. Problems such as phthisis, corneal compromise, and orbit factors may make it risky to perform muscle surgery. Older children may allow a forced duction test to be done on their eye to detect a contracture of the lateral rectus and any other restrictive phenomena that will help in the planning of surgery.

Most cases of sensory exotropia require surgery on two muscles due to the large angles typically seen in these patients. Weakening of the lateral rectus is almost always a component of the surgery plan, and, if the overlying conjunctiva is also tight, it should be recessed as well.[16,44] The medial rectus can be lax and may be strengthened. The surgeon should perform several forced ductions at surgery as each layer is dealt with, to be sure that restrictions are released. The addition of ipsilateral inferior oblique and superior oblique weakening to the horizontal rectus surgery can increase the success of surgery for angles over 50 PD.[44]

If the surgical goal is orthotropia, then the immediate postoperative alignment should be a small angle esotropia, as there is typically a drift toward exotropia of several PD in the first few weeks.[8,45] In general, the postoperative target angle should be slightly larger than that recommended for routine cases of intermittent exotropia, of the order of 10 to 14 PD, similar to that recommended above for infantile exotropia. To achieve this and to improve the long-term stability, the forced duction at the conclusion of surgery should be mild to moderately limited to abduction and the spring-back balance test should be biased in the esotropic direction.[16] Some authors caution against aligning to orthotropia any older patient with sensory exotropia caused by anisometropia, and they recommend leaving such patients undercorrected.[41]

Results

Patients with preoperative exotropia angles under 40 PD have a 75% chance of a stable small angle heterotropia. Over 45 PD, the results decrease dramatically to 40% to 50% long-term success.[44] Once the eye is realigned, the secondary muscle phenomena such as upshoots and downshoots and "X" patterns often resolve within weeks.[8]

References

1. Biglan AW, Davis JS, Cheng KP, et al. Infantile exotropia. J Pediatr Ophthalmol Strabismus 1996; 33: 79–84.
3. Rubin SE, Nelson LB, Wagner RS, et al. Infantile exotropia in healthy children. Ophthalmic Surg 1988; 19: 792–4.
5. Baeteman C, Denis D, Loudot C, et al.Interet de l'IRM cerebrale dans les exotropies precoces. J Fr Ophtalmol 2008; 31: 287–94.
6. Hunter DG, Kelly JB, Buffenn AN, Ellis FJ. Long-term outcome of uncomplicated infantile exotropia. J AAPOS 2001; 5: 352–6.
8. Kraft SP. Selected exotropia entities and principles of management. In: Rosenbaum AL, Santiago AP, editors. Clinical Strabismus Management. Philadelphia: Saunders; 1999: 176–201.
9. Hunter DG, Ellis FJ. Prevalence of systemic and ocular disease in infantile exotropia: a comparison with infantile esotropia. Ophthalmology 1999; 106: 1951–6.
12. Nixon RB, Helveston EM, Miller K, et al. Incidence of strabismus in neonates. Am J Ophthalmol 1985; 100: 798–801.
14. Tychsen L. Neural mechanisms in infantile esotropia: what goes wrong? Am Orthoptic J 1996; 46: 18–28.
15. Williams F, Beneish R, Polomeno RC, et al. Congenital exotropia. Am Orthop J 1984; 34: 92–4.
19. Spencer RF, Tucker MG, Choi RY, et al. Botulinum toxin management of childhood intermittent exotropia. Ophthalmology 1997; 104: 1762–7.
20. Hiles DA, Biglan AW. Early surgery of infantile exotropia. Trans Pa Acad Ophthalmol Otolaryngol 1983; 36: 161–8.
21. Wong AMF. Timing of surgery for infantile esotropia: sensory and motor outcomes. Can J Ophthalmol 2008; 43: 643–51.
23. Boyd TAS, Budd GE. Monofixation exotropia and asthenopia. In: Moore S, Mein J, Stockbridge L, editors. Orthoptics: Past, Present, Future. Miami: Symposia Specialists; 1976: 173–7.
24. von Noorden GK. Binocular Vision and Ocular Motility, 6th ed. St Louis: Mosby; 2002: 340–5, 370–1.
25. Baker JD, Davies GT. Monofixational intermittent exotropia. Arch Ophthalmol 1979; 97: 93–5.
26. Galloway-Smith K, Kaban T, Cadera W, et al. Monofixation exotropia. Am Orthoptic J 1992; 42: 125–8.
27. Lang J. Lessons learned from microtropia. In: Moore S, Mein J, Stockbridge L, editors. Orthoptics: Past, Present, Future. Miami: Symposia Specialists; 1976: 183–90.
28. Johnson F, Cunha LAP, Harcourt BR. The clinical characteristics of micro-exotropia. Br Orthoptic J 1981; 38: 54–9.
29. Kushner BJ. The occurrence of monofixational exotropia after exotropia surgery. Am J Ophthalmol 2009; 147: 1082–5.
32. Herzau V, Bleher I, Joos-Kratsch E. Infantile exotropia with homonymous hemianopia: a rare contraindication for strabismus surgery. Graefes Arch Clin Exp Ophthalmol 1988; 226: 148–9.
34. Donahue SP, Haun AK. Exotropia and face turn in children with homonymous hemianopia. J Neuro-ophthalmol 2007; 27: 304–7.
35. Levy Y, Turetz J, Krakowski D, et al. Development of compensating exotropia with anomalous retinal correspondence after early infancy in congenital homonymous hemianopia. J Pediatr Ophthalmol Strabismus 1995; 32: 236–8.
37. Hoyt CS, Good WV. Ocular motor adaptations to congenital hemianopia. Binocul Vis Eye Muscle Surg Q 1993; 8: 125–6.
38. Roper-Hall G. Effect of visual field defects on binocular single vision. Am Orthoptic J 1976; 26: 74–82.
39. Fritz KJ, Brodsky MC. Elusive neuro-ophthalmic reading impairment. Am Orthoptic J 1992; 42: 159–64.
40. Shainberg MJ, Roper-Hall G, Chung SM. Binocular problems in bitemporal hemianopia. Am Orthoptic J 1995; 45: 132–40.
41. Jampolsky A. Unequal visual inputs and strabismus management: A comparison of human and animal strabismus. In: Symposium on Strabismus: Transactions of the New Orleans Academy of Ophthalmology. St Louis: Mosby; 1978: 358–492.
42. Jampolsky A. Ocular divergence mechanisms. Trans Am Ophthalmol Soc 1970; 68: 730–822.
44. Velez G. Surgical treatment of exotropia with poor vision. In: Reinecke RD, editor. Strabismus II: Proceedings of the Fourth Meeting of the International Strabismological Association. Orlando: Grune and Stratton; 1984: 263–7.

 Access the complete reference list online at
http://www.expertconsult.com

CHAPTER **79**

Vertical strabismus

Burton J Kushner

Chapter contents

Overview and definitions

For a patient with vertical strabismus, one should first determine whether the deviation is comitant or incomitant. If the latter, one next determines if the problem is paretic, restrictive, or a manifestation of primary oblique muscle dysfunction. Finally, one determines if the deviation is dissociated (e.g. does not appear to follow Hering's Law with respect to the vertical component).

It is best to describe the deviation as it is actually manifested. Thus, if a patient fixes with the left eye and has a restrictive right hypotropia, you should call it a right hypotropia rather than using the old convention of describing it in terms of a hypertropia – in this example a left hypertropia. If the patient freely alternates fixation, you should then use the old convention. There has also been confusion about the terminology for describing dissociated vertical divergence (DVD). Terminology should be descriptive by addressing three issues; indicate if the deviation is:

1. Constant or intermittent.
2. Latent of manifest (e.g. a phoria or tropia).
3. Dissociated or not dissociated.

The most common presentation for DVD is for one eye to have a hypertropia that is intermittently manifest and for the other to have a hypertropia that is latent (only present in the dissociated state, e.g. under cover). Appropriate terminology for describing such a patient would be intermittent manifest DVD in one eye and latent DVD in the other. An alternative would be an intermittent dissociated hypertropia in one eye and a dissociated hyperphoria in the other.

Physiology

The cyclovertical muscles have a triple function that includes a vertical, torsional, and, to a lesser degree, horizontal action. With head tilt right or left, there is a small partial compensatory torsional rotation of each eye, which corrects for about 5–10% of the head tilt.[1] This comes from stimulation of the intorters (superior oblique and superior rectus) in the eye on the side to which the head is tilted, and the extorters (inferior oblique and inferior rectus) in the fellow eye, and forms the basis for the Bielschowsky Head Tilt Test and the Parks' 3-Step Test.[2] Although the vertical rectus muscles have their main vertical action in adduction, they are still the primary elevators and depressors across the horizontal gaze fields. Oblique muscles have a relatively weak vertical action. If the superior rectus is detached from the globe, the inferior oblique alone cannot elevate the eye above the midline. The superior oblique, however, has a stronger vertical action than the inferior oblique.

Patient evaluation

History

Before measuring the deviation, observe whether the patient has a spontaneous compensatory head posture (CHP) with visual effort. Although there are many causes for CHPs, I find they mostly serve to place the eyes in a gaze field in which the deviation is less, or to damp nystagmus (see Chapters 87, 88, and 89). The presence of facial asymmetry typically identifies the CHP as dating back to early childhood. There is a shortening of the midface between the horizontal canthus laterally and the corner of the child's mouth on the side to which the head is habitually tilted[3] (Fig. 79.1). Measure the deviation with the head posture using the prism and alternative cover test, and then in the head erect position. Although a diagnosis can often be made by just measuring a patient in seven fields of gaze (primary, up, down, right and left) and on head tilt right and left, an optimum treatment plan often requires additional measurements in the four oblique fields. Ductions and versions should be assessed with particular attention to the presence of overelevation or overdepression in the oblique fields. If there is overelevation of the adducting eye on side

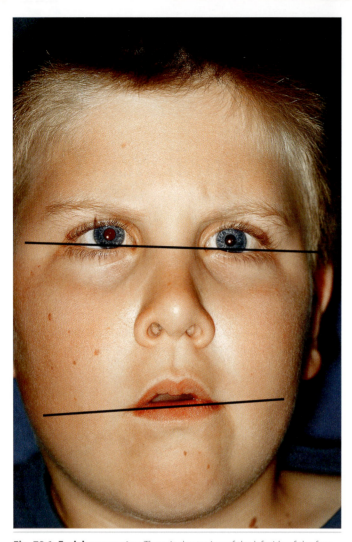

Fig. 79.1 Facial asymmetry. There is shortening of the left side of the face in this boy with a long-standing head tilt to the left for control of a right superior oblique palsy.

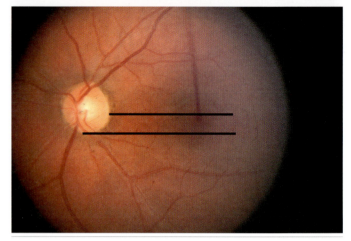

Fig. 79.2 Normal relationship of fovea to disk with respect to torsion. The fovea is normally positioned level with the lower third of the optic disk. The borders of normal lie between the two black lines in the figure. This photograph indicates an absence of objective torsion but is near the border for intorsion.

Box 79.1
Situations in which the Parks' 3-step test may be misleading[4]
DVD
Multiple muscle involvement
Bilateral fourth nerve palsy
Multiple other muscle weakness
Pulley heterotopia
Superior rectus overaction/contracture
Inferior rectus restriction
Superior rectus palsy
Inferior rectus palsy
Skew deviation
Prior extraocular muscle surgery

gaze, do a cover test in that gaze field to ascertain if the vertical deviation is a manifestation of DVD or true inferior oblique overaction.

Determine if the deviation is dissociated or not. With a non-dissociated deviation, a hypotropia is present in the contralateral eye when fixation is with the higher eye. Unless a secondary deviation is present due to paresis or restriction, the hypotropia in one eye will be of equal size to the hypertropia of the other eye. With DVD, the hypotropia of the fellow eye is either smaller or absent when fixation is with the eye with the DVD (see section on Dissociated vertical divergence).

The Parks' 3-Step Test will tell, in theory, which of the eight cyclovertical muscles is paretic; however, in practice it works best for confirming the diagnosis of unilateral superior oblique palsy.[2,4] Even in cases of isolated superior or inferior rectus palsy, it may be misleading. Most importantly, it does not tell whether a vertical strabismus is due to a palsy of one of the cyclovertical muscle, but is based on the assumption that it is. Box 79.1 lists some of the common situations in which the 3-Step Test leads to an incorrect diagnosis (see Video 79.1). The man in this video developed vertical diplopia immediately after closed head trauma from a motor vehicle accident. He

had a left hypertropia which increased in right gaze and on left head tilt, thus meeting the 3-Step Test criteria for a left superior oblique palsy. In fact, he had an orbital floor fracture in his right eye. He consistently fixed with his right eye due to mild amblyopia in his left eye. His diplopia resolved when the fracture was repaired

You should test for the presence of torsion both objectively and subjectively. The latter is accomplished with the double Maddox rod test using two red lenses, because the use of one red and one white lens frequently leads to a localization artifact; if the eye behind the white lens is the one that is torted, the patient will frequently perceive the torsion as being in the eye behind the red lens.[5] However, even when I use two red lenses, I sometimes find that the double Maddox rod test just tells me the total amount of torsion between the two eyes, and may be misleading with respect to localizing to the specific eye affected. Objective torsion is determined with the indirect ophthalmoscope and may be more useful in determining which eye actually is torted.[6] Normally the position of the fovea should be level with the lower one-third of the optic disk (Fig. 79.2). The absence of subjective torsion in the presence of objective fundus torsion usually means the deviation is long-standing and sensory adaptations have occurred. If a patient describes torsion, determine if the patient can fuse when the vertical and horizontal deviations are offset with prisms. If the patient can fuse comfortably despite the presence of torsion, it may be possible to ignore the torsion when designing a surgical strategy. If they cannot fuse, there may be a central disruption of fusion. Testing on the synoptophore, which can offset the torsion and may determine whether you can expect fusion if the strabismus is successfully treated.

General diagnostic pointers

1. Are history and symptoms helpful in determining etiology? Is there diplopia, childhood strabismus (if the patient is an adult), and is there DVD?
2. Is incomitance greater vertically or horizontally? If it is greater vertically, consider a restriction or palsy of a vertical rectus. If the largest difference is horizontal, consider an oblique problem.
3. Is there a limitation of rotation? Differentiate restriction from paresis with forced duction and active force generation testing.
4. Is there substantial torsion? If so, consider oblique problems or a vertical restriction.
5. Might the patient be fixing with the involved eye? Always consider this if there is asymmetric corrected visual acuity. Check for a secondary deviation.

General treatment principles

You should choose a treatment plan that will give the maximum correction in the field of gaze in which the deviation is greatest. Thus, you need to pay attention to the pattern of incomitance and the presence of torsion. Keep in mind that the primary position and downgaze (for reading) are the two most important fields of gaze and should not be sacrificed for the benefit of eccentric gazes. Oblique muscle surgery will give much more correction in adduction than abduction, but with vertical rectus surgery the difference in correction between abduction and adduction is less dramatic. Also, oblique muscle surgery causes more torsional change than rectus muscle surgery. An exception is with vertical rectus restrictions in which releasing the restriction may correct substantial torsion.

In general, surgery on the inferior rectus or superior oblique is least "forgiving." Inferior rectus recessions of 5 mm or more may cause a lag of that eye in downgaze unless there was a hypotropia that increased in downgaze prior to surgery. Also, large recessions of the inferior rectus may cause lower eyelid retraction postoperatively, minimized by advancement of the capsulopalpebral head at surgery.[7] Large resections of the inferior rectus muscle may cause narrowing of the palpebral fissure, and large recessions of the inferior rectus using a suspension technique (hangback adjustable suture) have a higher incidence of muscle slippage or non-adherance. This is probably caused by the shorter arc of contact of that muscle, which can cause the muscle to lose apposition with the globe in downgaze after surgery if the muscle is not fixed to the sclera.[8] Slippage can be prevented by using the semi-adjustable suture technique,[9] or a non-absorbable suture.

Specific clinical entities

Pseudohypertropia

Some patients may appear to have a hypertropia when in fact they do not. These include cases of orbital dystopia, anterior segment anomalies, or vertical angle kappa (Fig. 79.3). This latter may be due to a displaced fovea secondary to retinopathy

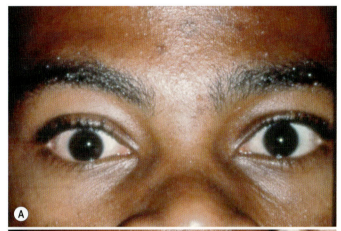
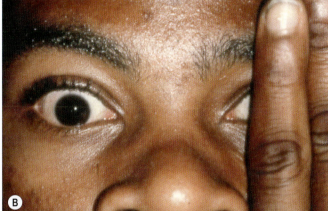
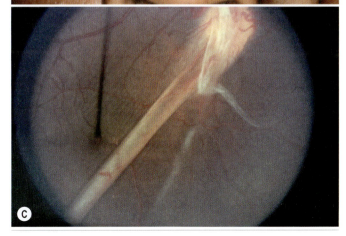

Fig. 79.3 Pseudohypotropia. (A) Patient with what appears to be a right hypotropia. (B) Cover test shows he is actually fixating with the eye when it appears to be infraducted. (C) His right fovea is dragged inferiorly due to traction secondary to retinopathy of prematurity, resulting in a large vertical angle kappa.

of prematurity (see Chapter 43) or other causes of retinal dragging.

Comitant deviations

Small comitant hypertropias, unrelated to prior strabismus surgery, are common. If they are more than several prism diopters, they may cause symptoms of asthenopia or diplopia, often managed with prisms. Large comitant vertical deviations not associated with horizontal strabismus are relatively uncommon. When present they most likely represent a spread of comitance in a patient that initially had paralytic strabismus. If the deviation is large but comitant, vertical rectus muscle surgery is usually appropriate.

Incomitant deviations: non-restrictive non-paretic

Primary oblique dysfunction

Primary overaction of the inferior oblique muscles, and to a lesser degree the superior oblique muscles, is a common accompaniment of primary horizontal strabismus. Oblique muscle overaction is not usually present at birth but after 1 year of age. Inferior oblique overaction is characterized by an overelevation in adduction and is associated with a "V" pattern. Superior oblique overaction is associated with overdepression in adduction and is associated with an "A" pattern (see Chapter 80). Typically objective extorsion is present with inferior oblique overaction and intorsion with superior oblique overaction. Subjective torsion may not be present as the patient develops sensory adaptations. The main differential diagnosis between primary oblique overaction and palsy of the antagonist oblique muscle is settled with the head tilt test. With bilateral superior oblique palsy, the Bielschowsky Head Tilt Test should reveal alternating hypertropias (right hypertropia on right head tilt and left hypertropia on left head tilt) for the reasons above. With primary oblique dysfunction, the difference in the vertical deviation with head tilting is minimal[10] (Video 79.2). The boy in this video has marked inferior oblique overaction, superior oblique underaction, and a large V pattern. On head tilt right and left there is a negligible hypertropia, thus distinguishing primary inferior oblique overaction from bilateral superior oblique palsy. He had a history of previously undergoing medial rectus recessions for infantile esotropia. Subsequently, a CT scan for unrelated reasons showed the superior obliques were of normal size. I believe primary inferior oblique overaction is primarily due to inferior oblique muscle contracture,[10] possibly due to a chronic excyclorotation of the eye. It can be treated with inferior oblique muscle weakening.

It is rare for bilateral superior oblique overaction to be secondary to inferior oblique palsy. If superior oblique overaction is bilateral and symmetric, there will be no hypertropia in the primary position, but an "A" pattern is typically present. If the superior oblique overaction is unilateral, there may be a small hypertropia in the primary position. For mild superior oblique overaction, I prefer a posterior 7/8 tenectomy performed at the insertion of the superior oblique. For greater amounts of superior oblique overaction, the split tendon lengthening procedure[11] allows titration of the effect, is potentially reversible, and unlike the silicone expander, does not place a foreign body in the orbit.

Paralytic strabismus (see Chapter 83)

Fourth cranial nerve palsy

Fourth nerve palsy is the most common form of paralytic vertical strabismus. The diagnostic criteria include a hypertropia of the affected eye that increases on adduction and ipsilateral head tilt (Fig. 79.4). A useful test for differentiating fourth cranial nerve palsy from skew deviation is to measure the deviation in the head erect and supine position. A decrease in the hypertropia by 50% or more is strongly suggestive of skew deviation.[12]

When treating fourth nerve palsy, slightly undercorrect the deviation or the patient may have bothersome diplopia. The primary position measurement determines how many muscles need surgery, and the pattern determines which muscles. Although Knapp's classification of superior oblique palsy is sound, it does not take into account the use of adjustable sutures and some newer observations about superior oblique anatomy and function.[13] I follow this approach:

1. If the deviation is 15 prism diopters (PD) or less, I do one muscle. That threshold may be lowered to 10 PD if adjustable sutures are used.

2. If the deviation is greater in the inferior oblique field, I recess the ipsilateral inferior oblique. If it is greater in the superior oblique field, I tuck the superior oblique. An alternative to tucking the superior oblique in this setting is to recess the contralateral inferior rectus muscle for the vertical deviation, and transpose the ipsilateral inferior rectus nasally for the torsion.[14] This is useful for surgeons who are not comfortable tucking the superior oblique; however, it should not be done if there is anything more than a few prism diopters of eso-deviation in downgaze, as it may exacerbate a downgaze eso-deviation.

3. If the deviation in primary mandates more than a one muscle procedure, I recess the ipsilateral inferior oblique and the contralateral inferior rectus. I find the semi-adjustable suture technique useful in this setting.

4. If there is 10 PD or more of hypertropia in the horizontal abducted field, there is most likely some degree of superior rectus overaction/contracture. Often this is more a manifestation of overaction than contracture, and may not be detectable by forced ductions.[10] I then recess the ipsilateral superior rectus a small amount along with the ipsilateral inferior oblique. Small superior rectus recessions are indicated to avoid decreasing upgaze.

Many patients with congenital superior oblique palsy have lax superior oblique tendons.[15] The dogma is that, if a lax tendon is found, it is tucked and, if it is not lax, a tuck is avoided. This is based on the belief that the primary problem is a tendon anomaly. I feel this philosophy has never been validated clinically and may not be sound. Lax tendons are associated with atrophy of the superior oblique muscle,[16] so trying to strengthen a paralyzed superior oblique would be comparable to resecting a paralyzed and flaccid lateral rectus muscle, for which a transposition of the vertical rectus muscles would be a better choice. Tucking a non-lax superior oblique would be akin to resecting a mildly paretic lateral rectus, which is often successful. Perhaps the wisest approach is to tuck tendons that are not lax if the incomitance pattern justifies it, but do a small tuck.

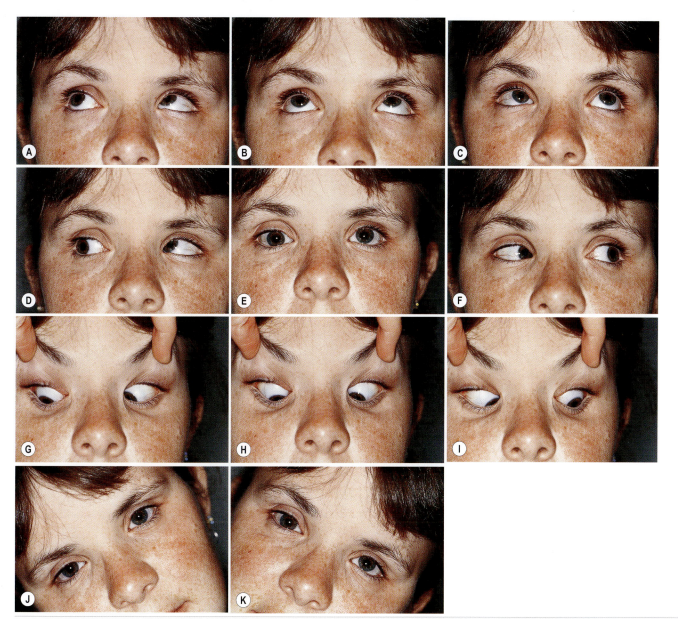

Fig. 79.4 Three-step test for left superior oblique palsy. This girl has a left hypertropia that increases on right gaze and left head tilt, meeting the 3-step test criteria for a left superior oblique palsy. There is overaction of the left inferior oblique muscle and mild underaction of the left superior oblique muscle.

Fourth nerve palsy, particularly if acquired, is often bilateral. If the degree of paresis is very asymmetric, the palsy in the lesser affected eye may not be evident on routine testing, and only becomes apparent after surgery is performed on the more paretic eye. This is called a bilateral masked superior oblique palsy. Diagnostic signs of a bilateral problem include a large V pattern, more than 10 degrees of excyclotropia, bilateral objective fundus torsion, a relatively small Bielschowsky head tilt difference, and reversal of the hypertropia in any field of gaze (particularly the contralateral superior or inferior oblique field) or on forced head tilt.[17] This is one of the reasons that proper surgical planning necessitates measuring in all nine diagnostic fields of gaze plus on head tilt right and left. If there are findings which suggest a bilateral masked palsy, I do bilateral surgery even without reversal of the hypertropia in the routinely measured gaze fields. Surgery depends on the specific

pattern of incomitance, but usually involves bilateral oblique muscle surgery. This may be bilateral but asymmetric inferior oblique recessions, a Harada-Ito procedure in one eye, and a superior oblique tuck in the other, or symmetric oblique surgery to treat torsion and a vertical rectus recession to treat primary position hypertropia.

Inferior oblique palsy

Inferior oblique palsy is relatively rare and can be treated with ipsilateral superior oblique weakening. It must be differentiated from Brown's syndrome, which has a similar appearance on versions in the inferior oblique field. A diagnostic criterion is an "A" pattern, which is typically present with inferior oblique palsy whereas a "V" pattern is typical of Brown's syndrome (see Fig. 79.4).

Vertical rectus palsy

Vertical rectus palsy is usually treated with recession of the antagonist vertical rectus if mild, the same combined with a resection of the paretic muscle if moderate, or a transposition procedure of the horizontal rectus muscles if severe. In mild cases, recession of the same vertical rectus muscle in the other eye to match the deficit can give good results. The head tilt test is inconsistent with vertical rectus palsy.[4]

Dissociated vertical divergence

DVD is a marker for early-onset strabismus, but it is unusual at birth. Most commonly it appears after 1 year of age, and may not be evident until after surgery for infantile esotropia. It may present as a subtle deviation, which may be small and only present on cover testing. Or it may be associated with a large and frequently manifest vertical deviation that can be as cosmetically disfiguring as the initial horizontal strabismus. Although DVD is a bilateral disease, it may appear to be unilateral because only the preferred eye has a latent deviation. This is particularly the case with amblyopia: fixation always occurs with the non-amblyopic eye. However, this can also occur in patients with equal vision.

DVD is characterized by a slow upward drifting of the eye; the eye extorts when it elevates, simultaneously, intorsion occurs in the fixing eye. It is typically associated with latent or manifest latent nystagmus. The hallmark is that, when the fixing eye is covered and the patient regains fixation with the deviating eye, the previously fixing eye does not have a commensurate hypotropia. If the DVD is significant in both eyes, the formerly fixing eye will elevate under cover. Thus, it appears that DVD is characterized by an uncoupling of Hering's Law. Often DVD appears worse in adduction simulating inferior oblique overaction. Differentiating the two conditions includes performing a cover test on side gaze to see whether there is hypotropia of the abducting eye when it is occluded. With DVD the abducting eye will not show a hypotropia and may be hypertropic if the DVD is bilateral (Fig. 79.5). Because of the nature of DVD, and that there is not an equal hypotropia of the contralateral eye, one cannot neutralize this deviation with the alternate prism and cover test. To accurately measure DVD, one must use the prism under cover test. This test is carried out by first estimating the size of the DVD. Then a prism equal to the estimated size of the deviation is placed base down in front of the affected eye, while the eye is dissociated behind a cover. The cover should then be rapidly switched to the other eye. If the estimated amount of prism was correct, no movement of the eye being tested should occur. If there is still a downward movement, the test should be repeated with a larger prism; if an upward movement occurs, it should be repeated with a smaller prism. However, many patients with DVD have a marked redress movement and an accurate endpoint cannot be obtained, even with the prism under cover test. In that case, the deviation must be estimated by determining whether the upward and downward components of the redress movement were of equal magnitude, or by using a light reflex test.[18]

Approximately one-third of patients with DVD have a spontaneous abnormal head posture (see Chapter 81).[18] Most patients with DVD show an increase in the size of the DVD on contralateral head tilt (e.g. right DVD increases with left head tilt); however, some show the converse (Fig. 79.6).

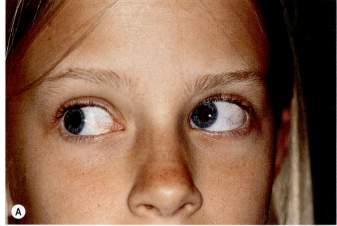
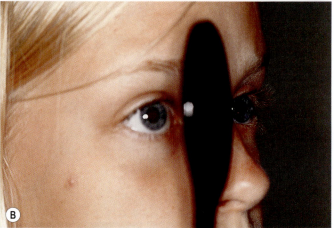

Fig. 79.5 DVD mimicking inferior oblique overaction. (A) This girl shows overelevation of the left eye in adduction, which is consistent with left inferior oblique overaction. (B) Under cover, however, a hypertropia is seen in the right eye, confirming that this child in fact has DVD.

Recent theories have shed light on the etiology and pathophysiology of DVD. They suggest that DVD is a result of damping of nystagmus by complex interactions of the cyclovertical muscles, possibly via a vestigial remnant of the dorsal light reflex of lower animals.[19,20]

Surgical management of DVD depends on whether inferior oblique overaction is present, the size of the deviation, and if it is bilateral or unilateral. If it is unilaterally manifest, the possibility that the patient may shift fixation after surgery should be taken into account. If amblyopia is present, a shift in fixation is unlikely. If inferior oblique overaction is present concurrently with DVD, I prefer to anteriorly transpose the inferior oblique muscle to a point level with the inferior rectus insertion.[21] Weakening the inferior oblique without anterior transposition may not adequately treat DVD. If anterior transposition of the inferior oblique is planned, it should be done bilaterally or there will be a resultant hypotropia of the operated eye in upgaze. It should not be performed if the inferior obliques are not overacting, or if there is substantial superior oblique overaction.

If DVD is significant and there is no overaction of the inferior obliques, recession of the superior rectus muscles is the treatment of choice. Even if DVD is unilaterally manifest, bilateral surgery is advisable if the dominant eye shows latent DVD

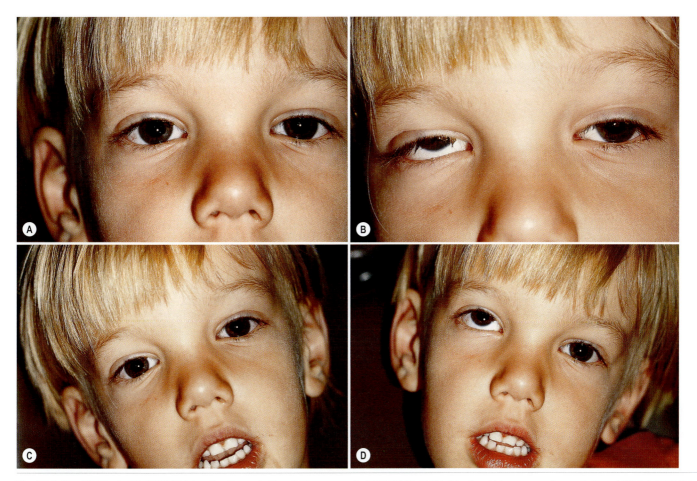

Fig. 79.6 Head tilt test with DVD. This boy has the typical head tilt response for DVD. (A) His DVD is latent and his eyes are often well aligned. (B) A right DVD is intermittently manifest. (C) The deviation is absent on head tilt to the right. (D) The deviation increases on head tilt to the left, which is common for a right DVD.

under cover and if equal vision is present. Then, if unilateral surgery is performed, it is likely that the patient will shift fixation postoperatively and manifest a DVD in the previously preferred eye. For guidelines for the magnitude of superior rectus recession for DVD see Table 79.1. As is depicted in the table, with unilateral surgery (which is desirable if amblyopia is present) the amount of superior rectus recession for a given amount of DVD should be less.

Symmetric inferior rectus resections in the range of 4–7 mm can be used to treat DVD. This procedure is generally reserved for use as a secondary procedure after other treatments have failed. This magnitude of inferior rectus resection will often cause narrowing of the palpebral fissure by raising the height of the lower eyelid.

Special forms of vertical strabismus

Brown's syndrome

Brown's syndrome is caused by a mechanical restriction of the superior oblique tendon moving through the trochlea, which results in a restriction of elevation in adduction. On version testing it mimics an inferior oblique palsy, except that a "V" pattern is present; an "A" pattern is expected with inferior oblique palsy. Most cases of Brown's syndrome are congenital,

Table 79.1 – Amount of superior rectus recession for DVD

Deviation (PD)	Bilateral superior rectus recession (mm)	Unilateral superior rectus recession (mm)
<10	7	5
10	8	6
15	9	7
20	10	8
25 and up	10	9

but can be acquired due to either trauma or inflammation. If an inflammatory etiology is suspected, a systemic work-up for autoimmune disease is appropriate. Inflammatory Brown's syndrome may resolve spontaneously. If not it can be treated with steroid injection in the region of the trochlea. Systemic anti-inflammatory medications may play a role, but I have found the results disappointing.

Some cases of congenital Brown's syndrome resolve spontaneously. Treatment may be indicated if a child needs to assume an unacceptable head posture for fusion. At surgery, forced ductions with attention to elevation in adduction should be performed. They will be positive if Brown's syndrome is present and negative if there is an inferior oblique palsy. The surgical treatment of Brown's syndrome consists of one of many procedures to weaken or lengthen the superior oblique tendon.

Duane's syndrome (see Chapter 82)

Patients with Duane's syndrome frequently have an upshoot or downshoot of the affected eye on adduction (Fig. 79.7). Although this appears to be caused by overaction of an oblique muscle, it is in fact caused by co-contraction of the lateral rectus muscle. This causes the lateral rectus to slip above or below the midline on adduction, creating the vertical deviation. Treatment in the form of oblique muscle weakening is usually not helpful. Successful treatment involves releasing the lateral rectus muscle in the form of either recession or Y splitting with recession. In severe cases it should be disabled by suturing it to the lateral orbital periosteum.

Restrictive strabismus

Common forms of restrictions that cause vertical strabismus include orbital floor fracture, primary ocular muscle fibrosis, Graves' orbitopathy, myotoxicity from local anesthetic, and scarring after prior strabismus surgery. In these cases there will be a limitation of rotation of the eye in the field opposite the affected muscle. Treatment involves recession of the affected muscle and freeing of any scar tissue (Fig. 79.8).

Oblique muscle incarceration

Surgery on one of the vertical rectus muscles and/or the adjacent oblique muscle may result in the oblique muscle becoming incarcerated in the insertion of the rectus muscle. When this occurs with the superior oblique tendon, a restrictive hypertropia and incyclotropia results[22] (Fig. 79.9). With the inferior oblique muscle a restrictive hypotropia is found.[23] Treatment can be difficult and consists of freeing the incarcerated oblique muscle or tendon, and often recessing the adjacent vertical rectus muscle.

Altered rectus muscle path

Alteration of the normal path of the rectus muscles due to pulley heterotopia or pulley laxity may result in a vertical strabismus that may mimic other more common forms of vertical strabismus.[24] Inferior slippage of the lateral rectus muscle can mimic Brown's syndrome and high-quality imaging is needed to make the diagnosis. It can be treated by using posterior fixation sutures to reposition the muscle in the proper position

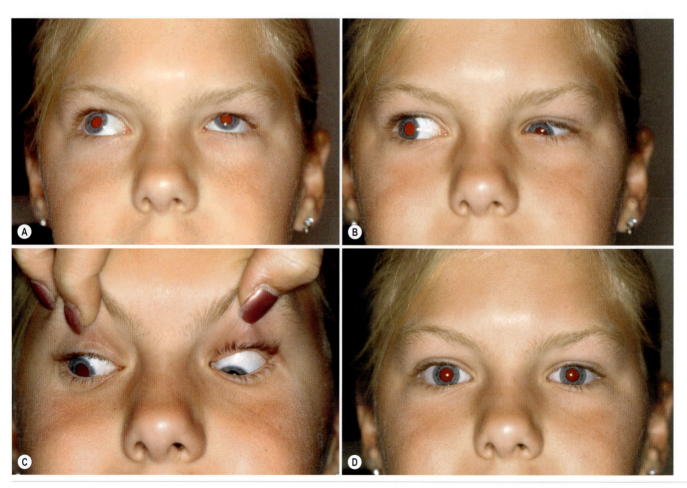

Fig. 79.7 Exotropic Duane's syndrome with upshoot. This girl has a small left exotropia associated with limited adduction in her left eye secondary to Duane's syndrome. There is a marked downshoot of the left eye with adduction and a large upshoot of the left eye with adduction above the midline. Although this resembles oblique muscle overaction, weakening of the apparent overacting oblique muscle is ineffective but weakening the lateral rectus may be effective (see Chapter 82).

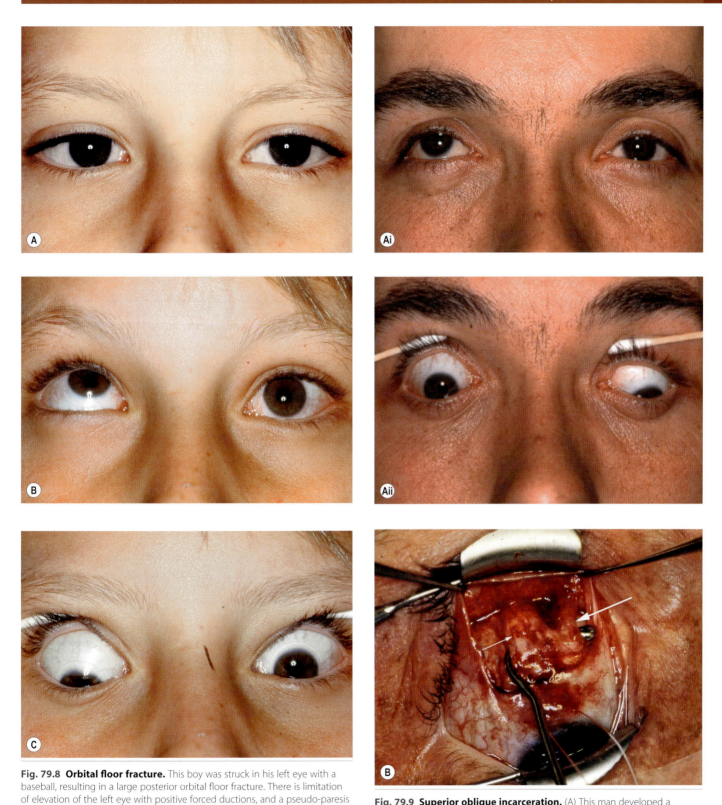

Fig. 79.8 Orbital floor fracture. This boy was struck in his left eye with a baseball, resulting in a large posterior orbital floor fracture. There is limitation of elevation of the left eye with positive forced ductions, and a pseudo-paresis of the left inferior rectus resulting in a limitation of depression.

Fig. 79.9 Superior oblique incarceration. (A) This man developed a restrictive right hypertropia and large right incylotropia after undergoing a small right superior rectus muscle resection. (B) At subsequent surgery the right superior oblique tendon (large arrow) was found scarred into the right superior rectus insertion (small arrow) causing the restriction.

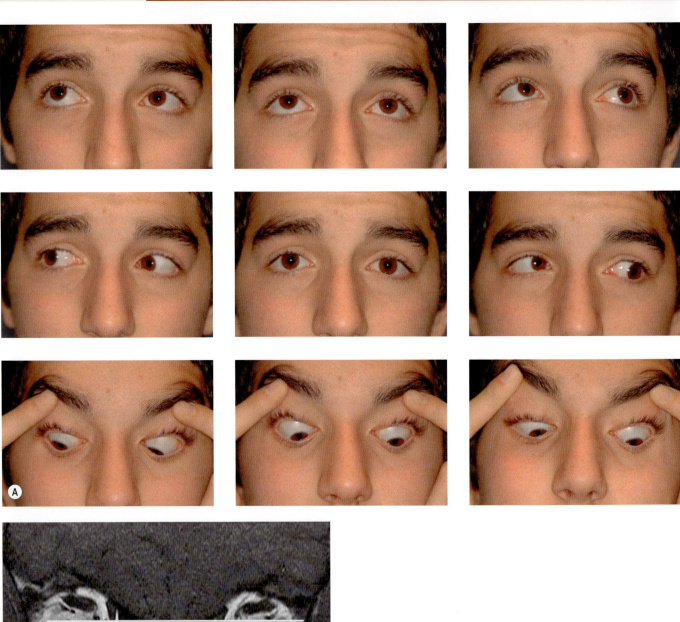

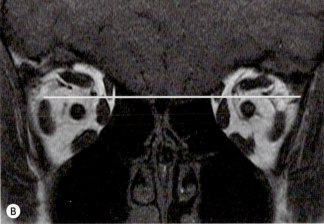

Fig. 79.10 Pulley heterotopia. (A) This 14-year-old boy has a left hypotropia with diplopia to the right and left of the primary position. There is a downshoot of the left eye on adduction and a mild limitation of elevation in adduction. (B) Orbital imaging shows inferior displacement of the left lateral rectus muscle.

(Fig. 79.10 and Video 79.3). The 14-year-old boy in this video has diplopia to the left and right of the primary position. His left eye has a downshoot on abduction and is mildly limited in adduction. Orbital imaging shows the left lateral rectus is to be slipped inferiorly.

References

1. Kushner BJ. Ocular torsion: rotations around the "WHY" axis. J AAPOS 2004; 8: 1–12.

2. Parks MM. Isolated cyclovertical muscle palsy. Arch Ophthalmol 1958; 60: 1027–35.

3. Wilson M, Hoxie J. Facial asymmetry in superior oblique muscle palsy. J Pediatr Ophthalmol Strabismus 1993; 30: 315–8.

4. Kushner BJ. Errors in the three-step test in the diagnosis of vertical strabismus. Ophthalmology 1989; 96: 127–32.

5. Simons K, Arnoldi K, Brown MH. Color dissociation artifacts in double Maddox rod cyclodeviation testing. Ophthalmology 1994; 101: 1897–901.

6. Kushner BJ, Haraharan L. Observations about objective and subjective ocular torsion. Ophthalmology 2009; 116: 2001–10.

7. Kushner BJ. A surgical procedure to minimize lower eyelid retraction with inferior rectus recession. Arch Ophthalmol 1992; 110: 1011–4.

8. Chatzistefanou KI, Kushner BJ, Gentry LR. Magnetic resonance imaging of the arc of contact of extraocular muscles: implications regarding the incidence of slipped muscles. J AAPOS 2000; 4: 84–93.

9. Kushner BJ. An evaluation of the semiadjustable suture strabismus surgical procedure. J AAPOS 2004; 8: 481–7.

10. Kushner BJ. Multiple mechanisms of extraocular muscle "overaction". Arch Ophthalmol 2006; 124: 680–8.

11. Bardorf CM, Baker JD. The efficacy of superior oblique split Z-tendon lengthening for superior oblique overaction. J AAPOS 2003; 7: 96–102.

12. Wong AM. Understanding skew deviation and a new clinical test to differentiate it from trochlear nerve palsy. J AAPOS 2010; 14: 61–7.

13. Knapp P. First Annual Richard G. Scobee Memorial Lecture. Diagnosis and surgical treatment of hypertropia. Am Orthopt J 1971; 21: 29–37.

14. Kushner BJ. Vertical rectus surgery for Knapp class II superior oblique muscle paresis. Arch Ophthalmol 2010; 128: 585–8.

15. Helveston EM, Krach D, Plager DA, Ellis FD. A new classification of superior oblique palsy based on congenital variations in the tendon. Ophthalmology 1992; 99: 1609–15.

16. Sato M. Magnetic resonance imaging and tendon anomaly associated with congenital superior oblique palsy. Am J Ophthalmol 1999; 127: 379–87.

17. Kushner BJ. The diagnosis and treatment of bilateral masked superior oblique palsy. Am J Ophthalmol 1988; 105: 186–94.

18. Bechtel RT, Kushner BJ, Morton GV. The relationship between dissociated vertical divergence (DVD) and head tilts. J Pediatr Ophthalmol Strabismus 1996; 33: 303–6.

19. Brodsky MC. Dissociated vertical divergence: a righting reflex gone wrong. Arch Ophthalmol 1999; 117: 1216–22.

20. Guyton DL. Dissociated vertical deviation: etiology, mechanisms, and associated phenomena. Costenbader Lecture. J AAPOS 2000; 4: 131–44.

21. Elliott RL, Nankin SJ. Anterior transposition of the inferior oblique. J Pediatr Ophthalmol Strabismus 1981; 18: 35–8.

22. Kushner BJ. Superior oblique tendon incarceration syndrome. Arch Ophthalmol 2007; 125: 1070–6.

23. Kushner BJ. The inferior oblique muscle adherence syndrome. Arch Ophthalmol 2007; 125: 1510–4.

24. Rutar T, Demer JL. "Heavy eye" syndrome in the absence of high myopia: a connective tissue degeneration in elderly strabismic patients. J AAPOS 2009; 13: 36–44.

Part 4
Vertical, "pattern" strabismus and abnormal head postures

"A", "V" and other strabismus patterns

Burton J Kushner

Overview and definitions

The terms "A" and "V" pattern describe horizontal strabismus that is vertically incomitant. It is characterized by a substantial difference in the horizontal deviation between the midline upgaze and downgaze positions. A patient with a "V" pattern is more esotropic or less exotropic in downgaze than upgaze (Fig. 80.1); an "A" pattern is characterized by the converse (Fig. 80.2). By convention, the difference between upgaze and downgaze must be 15 PD (prism diopters) or greater to diagnose a clinically significant "V" pattern and 10 PD to diagnose an "A" pattern. Less commonly, there are variations of pattern strabismus in which there is minimal change from downgaze to the primary position, but the eyes diverge in upgaze resulting in a "Y" pattern. The girl shown in Figure 80.3 and Video 80.1 was first diagnosed to have this motility pattern at 3 years of age. I have continued to care for her over the subsequent 33 years and her motility is unchanged. She is symptom free without treatment.

Converse to a "Y" pattern, the main exo shift may be between the primary position and downgaze to form a "λ" (lambda) pattern.

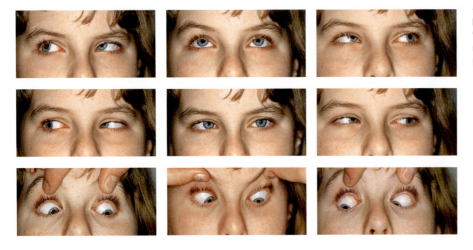

Fig. 80.1 "V" pattern esotropia. This girl has a "V" pattern esotropia with associated inferior oblique muscle overaction and superior oblique muscle underaction.

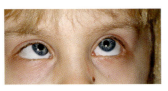
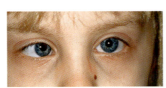
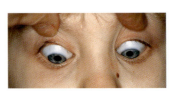

Fig. 80.2 "A" pattern esotropia. This girl has an "A" pattern esotropia showing an increase in the deviation in upgaze and orthophoria in downgaze.

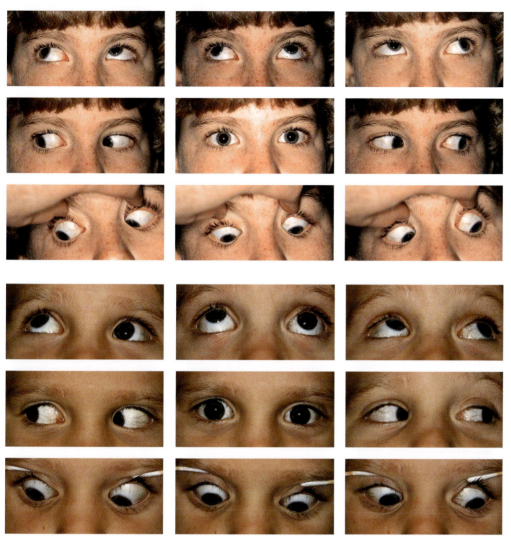

Fig. 80.3 "Y" pattern exotropia. This girl has a "Y" pattern exotropia with pseudo inferior oblique overaction. She is orthophoric in the primary position, horizontal sidegaze, and all downgaze fields. In all upgaze fields she has a large exotropia.

Fig. 80.4 Brown's syndrome (see Chapter 79). This girl has limitation of elevation of her left eye in adduction as is characteristic for Brown's syndrome. Note that a "V" pattern is present.

History

Duane first described a "V" pattern in 1897 in a patient with bilateral superior oblique palsy.[1] Subsequently little attention was given to the importance of measuring the angle of strabismus in upgaze and downgaze until Urrets-Zavalia in 1948.[2,3] Urist brought the "A" and "V" patterns into the English literature in 1951.[4]

Occurrence

Estimates of patients with strabismus having an "A" or "V" pattern range from 12% to 50%.[5-8] This wide range is because ethnic and systemic factors influence the incidence of pattern strabismus and the make-up of each series. In one series of 421 patients with "A" or "V" patterns, 58% had an onset of strabismus prior to 12 months of age.[6] "A" or "V" pattern strabismus occurs much more frequently in congenital or paralytic strabismus than in non-paralytic acquired strabismus. Brown's syndrome (see Chapter 79) characteristically has a "V" pattern, differentiating it from inferior oblique palsy, in which an "A" pattern is found (Fig. 80.4). Duane's syndrome (see Chapter 82) often presents with a "V" or "Y" pattern, and less commonly an "A" or "λ" pattern (see Chapter 79, Fig. 79.7). "A" patterns with overdepression in adduction are frequently seen in patients with spina bifida and/or hydrocephalus with a 31% incidence having been reported.[9,10] Although frontal bossing in children with hydrocephalus (see Chapter 55) may result in anterior displacement of the trochlea, mechanically enhancing the vertical vector of the superior oblique tendon with strengthening of the depressing action of the superior oblique. However, the exact mechanism is unclear.

Etiology

There are differing theories as to the etiology of "A" and "V" patterns, in part because different mechanisms may be responsible in different patients.

Oblique muscle dysfunction

The most popular theory, suggested by Knapp in 1959,[11] attributes most cases of "A" and "V" pattern to oblique muscle dysfunction. Abduction is a tertiary action of the oblique muscles. Thus, if the inferior obliques are overacting and the antagonist superior obliques are underacting, one would expect a relative convergence in downgaze and divergence in upgaze, resulting in a "V" pattern. The converse occurs if the superior obliques are overacting and the inferior obliques are underacting, resulting in an "A" pattern. One typically finds the oblique muscles to be dysfunctional in this manner in most patients with pattern strabismus. This clinical observation, combined with the theoretical construct, has led to the justified implication of oblique muscle dysfunction as a cause of "A" and "V" patterns.

Torsion as a cause of "A" and "V" patterns

The torsion that accompanies oblique muscle dysfunction should theoretically cause or contribute to "A" and "V" patterns.[12] Patients with a "V" pattern typically have an excyclotropia, which is most likely secondary to the accompanying inferior oblique overaction. This excyclotropia results in rotation of the rectus muscles (Fig. 80.5). The superior rectus muscles would become partial abductors and the inferior rectus muscles partial adductors, which will contribute to a "V" pattern. The medial rectus muscles will also have elevating force vectors and the lateral rectus muscles depressing force vectors, contributing to the elevation seen in adduction with overacting inferior obliques. I believe, however, that torsion is only a minor contributing cause of pattern strabismus rather than the main cause. Several observations support this belief.[13] First, the rise or fall of an eye with oblique muscle overaction, as it moves into adduction is curvilinear. If the rise or fall were primarily caused by the change in force vectors of the rectus muscles as seen in Figure 80.5, one would expect a linear trajectory. Secondly, surgery like the Harada-Ito procedure that mainly corrects torsion has a negligible effect on the overelevation in adduction in patients with fourth cranial nerve palsy, even when it eliminates the excyclotropia. In addition, it has been shown that objective extorsion may precede the development of overelevation in adduction and a "V" pattern in patients with infantile esotropia (see Chapter 74), by as much as several years. If the torsion caused the overelevation in adduction and the pattern, they should occur concurrently. Finally, surgery in the form of vertical transposition of the horizontal rectus muscles that successfully eliminates an "A" or "V" pattern will predictably worsen the underlying torsion (see section Horizontal transposition of vertical rectus muscles below).

Orbital structural anomalies

Orbital anomalies are often associated with "A" and "V" patterns. There is a frequent occurrence of "A" pattern esotropia accompanied by inferior oblique underaction in patients with upslanting palpebral fissures and an association of "V" pattern exotropia with inferior oblique muscle overaction.[14] In patients with downslanting palpebral fissures the opposite occurs. There is also a very high incidence of "A" and "V" patterns in patients with craniofacial syndromes[15,16] (Fig. 80.6). Recently Clark et al. and Demer have attributed some cases of "A" and "V" patterns to orbital pulley heterotopia or laxity.[17,18] This is an evolving concept with no good data as to the frequency that pulley issues are at fault.

Iatrogenic

An "A" or "V" pattern may develop as a result of prior strabismus surgery. This can result from an overcorrection from prior treatment of "A" or "V pattern strabismus. On occasion, a marked "Y" pattern can occur in the form of the anti-elevation syndrome after anterior transposition of the inferior oblique muscles[19] (Fig. 80.7). Also, an "A" pattern frequently occurs following large bilateral recessions of the inferior rectus muscles, commonly in thyroid eye disease. This occurs from a loss of the adducting effect of the inferior rectus muscles in downgaze secondary to surgical weakening, and by an increase in innervation to the yoke superior oblique muscles.[20]

Horizontal rectus muscles

Urist felt overaction or underaction of the horizontal rectus muscles were responsible for "A" and "V" patterns[4,5] and that the medial rectus muscles were more active in downgaze and the lateral rectus muscles were more active in upgaze. His surgical recommendations involved weakening the offending muscles. Although this theory is less compelling than others, it may explain the occurrence of some cases of "A" or "V" pattern where there is no other apparent cause. It can also explain the small decrease in "V" pattern observed after bilateral medial rectus recessions.

Other less popular theories

Brown felt that "A" and "V" patterns were caused by a weakness of the inferior and superior oblique muscles respectively, resulting in apparent overaction of the yoke oblique muscles due to fixation "duress."[21] This theory is not widely accepted.

Gobin suggested that the primary event that causes a "V" pattern is an abnormal sagittalization of the inferior oblique muscles which decreases its vector for torsion resulting in an incyclotropia. Subsequently, to correct this abnormal incyclotropia, there is increased innervation to the excyclorotary muscles, resulting in inferior oblique overaction.[22] In my opinion, this theory is inconsistent with the clinical findings of torsion in patients with pattern strabismus. According to the sagittalization theory, a patient with a "V" pattern should have no fundus torsion as the inferior oblique overaction served the purpose of eliminating an abnormal intorsion. In fact, these patients typically have objective extorsion.

Presentation

The manner of presentation of a patient with an "A" or "V" pattern depends on the underlying strabismus and the size of the deviation. If there is a sufficiently large deviation in the primary position such that, despite the presence of an "A" or "V" pattern, there is no head position in which fusion is possible, the pattern may not affect the presentation. If the deviation is small enough that fusion is possible in upgaze or downgaze, the patient may assume a chin-down or chin-up head posture in order to fuse. Some adults with an "A" or "V" pattern may not become symptomatic until they become presbyopic. Their symptoms may not become manifest until they need to get their eyes into downgaze to read through a bifocal segment. Prior to becoming presbyopic they may have unconsciously held reading material closer to the primary position. Similarly, some presbyopic patients with strabismus that is only significant in downgaze may become symptomatic if they switch from a flat-top to a progressive bifocal which have a wide transition zone that requires the eyes to move further into downgaze in order to permit vision through the prescribed add.

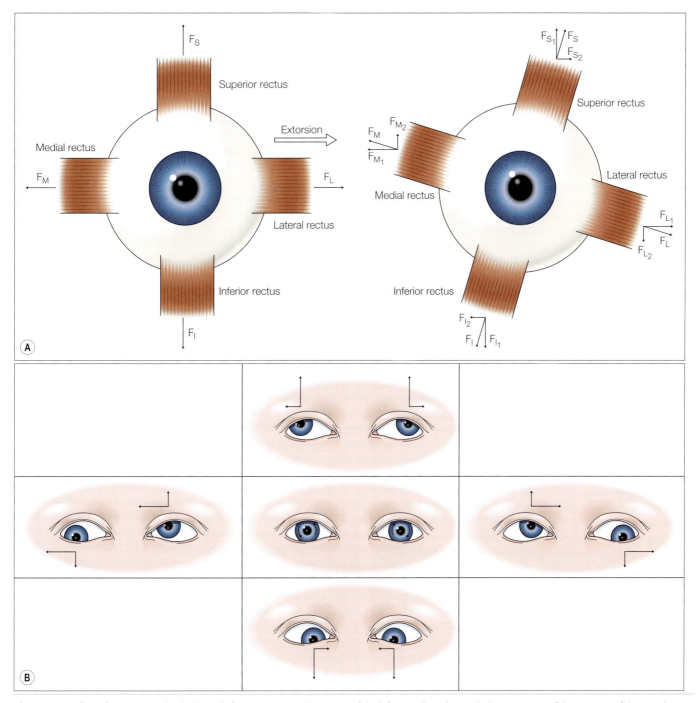

Fig. 80.5 (A) Effect of torsion on individual muscle function. An excyclorotation of the left eye will result in a clockwise rotation of the insertion of the muscles. This will create a vector for elevation for the medial rectus muscle, abduction for the superior rectus, depression for the lateral rectus, and adduction for the inferior rectus. (B) Effect of torsion on motility pattern. If the torsional changes that are depicted in (A) occurred in both eyes, the new force vectors would cause divergence in upgaze and convergence in downgaze. In addition there would be an elevation of the adducting eye and depression of the abducting eye. Thus, these torsional changes that occurred as a result of extorsion contribute to both the "V" pattern and the elevation seen in adduction.

Examination

Motor exam

The diagnosis of an "A" or "V" pattern must be made by measuring with the prism and alternate cover test 25–30 degrees above and below the midline. Testing should be done at 6 m to eliminate the near reflex. You can be misled by assessing the size of the deviation on version testing using a light reflex, as this will not bring out the latent deviation. Particularly in patients with intermittent exotropia, the deviation may be controlled in the primary position; however, fusion may break down when the eyes are rotated into extreme fields of gaze giving the false appearance of a "Y", "λ", or "X" pattern. Testing should be done with full optical

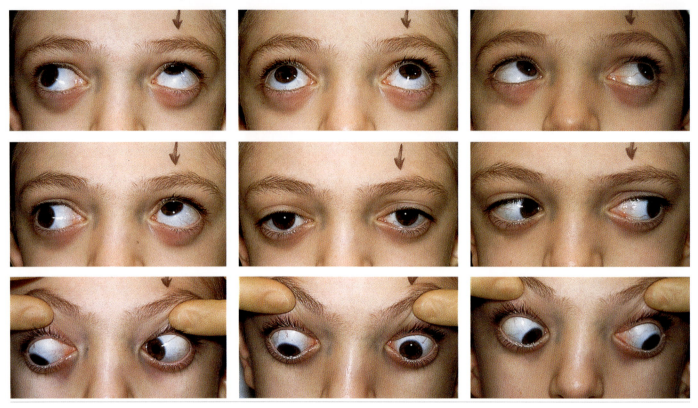

Fig. 80.6 Craniofacial anomaly with associated pattern: Crouzon's syndrome. This boy shows the classic "V" pattern seen in Crouzon's syndrome (see Chapter 28). There is overelevation and underdepression of each eye in adduction. (Photo courtesy of Ken K. Nischal FRCOphth.)

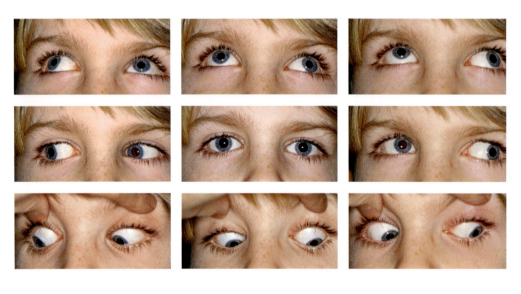

Fig. 80.7 The antielevation syndrome. This boy has a large "V" pattern after previously undergoing inferior oblique anterior transposition bilaterally to treat dissociated vertical divergence. What looks like residual inferior oblique overaction is actually a result of fixation duress to the abducting eye on attempted elevation, due to the anti-elevating property of the transposed inferior oblique muscle. This drives the adducting eye superiorly and mimics contralateral inferior oblique overaction.

correction in place *and* while fixation is maintained on an accommodative target: if not, a pseudo "A" or "V" pattern may be observed.

Special care should be taken to assess any relative overelevation or overdepression in adduction, and the presence or absence of fundus torsion should be assessed with indirect ophthalmoscopy.

Sensory findings

Sensory findings depend on whether the patient is orthotropic in any field of gaze. Patients who are well aligned in the primary position may have surprisingly good fusion. If the patient is tropic in all fields of gaze, suppression and varying depths of anomalous retinal correspondence (ARC) may be found. In many patients with ARC and pattern strabismus, the angle of anomaly varies with the angle of deviation, thus resulting in ARC that is harmonious in all fields of gaze. This speaks to the fluidity of ARC.

Surgical treatment of "A" and "V" patterns

If a pattern needs to be eliminated, the treatment is surgery. However, first you need to determine whether the pattern itself needs to be addressed. If the patient has a significant chin-up or chin-down head posture in order to fuse, surgery is appropriate. A continuous change in the size of the deviation that varies with change in gaze direction is destabilizing for binocular fusion. Thus if an "A" or "V" pattern is clinically significant, it should be addressed in any child undergoing horizontal strabismus surgery, in whom there is any likelihood of some degree of binocularity being gained. This is probably the case in all children unless there is dense amblyopia. You should also pay attention to the location of the pattern. The primary position and downgaze are the two most important fields of gaze. You might ignore the pattern completely in an asymptomatic patient with a "Y" pattern who only manifests a deviation in upgaze. This is particularly true if treating a pattern might be at the expense of the good alignment in the primary position and downgaze. If the strabismus is cosmetically unacceptable because of an "A" or "V" pattern, surgery for the pattern is appropriate. For most adults undergoing surgery for other reasons, a pattern should be treated if also present. Exceptions include patients in whom treating the pattern might adversely affect the outcome in the primary position or downgaze, or if dense amblyopia is present.

Oblique muscle surgery

If you decide to treat a pattern in a patient in whom there is substantial oblique muscle overaction, the overacting oblique muscles should be weakened because:

1. It decreases the excessive abducting force in the gaze direction in which the eyes diverge (upgaze for a "V" pattern, downgaze for an "A" pattern).
2. It decreases the torsion which contributes to the pattern and may be an obstacle to fusion.
3. It corrects any cosmetically unacceptable upshoot or downshoot occurring in adduction.

Oblique muscle surgery should be combined with any necessary horizontal surgery, the latter based on the angle of misalignment in the primary position. No allowance is necessary for the loss of abducting force of the oblique muscles, because it is negligible in the primary position. Weakening both inferior oblique muscles will result in 15–25 PD of esotropic shift in upgaze, depending on the degree of overaction of the inferior oblique muscles; the greater the degree of overaction, the more effect is obtained. There will be little or no effect on the horizontal deviation in the primary position. Initially, there will also be no horizontal effect in downgaze from weakening the inferior oblique muscles. Later, however, there may be some increased divergence in downgaze because the previously underacting superior obliques may recover function after the antagonist inferior obliques have been weakened.

The effect of weakening the superior obliques depends on the technique. Weakening the superior obliques nasally, by any technique, has a large effect and can correct up to 40 PD of exotropia in downgaze. Weakening the superior obliques temporally is a less powerful operation, but is also less likely to cause complications. A posterior 7/8 tenectomy will cause a reduction of approximately 15–20 PD of exotropia in downgaze.[23,24] A somewhat more powerful operation than a posterior tenectomy is a complete disinsertion of the superior oblique tendon. A still greater effect can be obtained with a tenectomy of the superior oblique tendon at the insertion or a graded recession. Weakening the superior oblique has no effect on the horizontal deviation in upgaze. In the primary position it will only correct between 0 to 3 PD of exotropia.[25,26] You need little or no adjustment in your horizontal surgery if you do bilateral superior oblique weakening.

When treating a pattern by weakening oblique muscles, it is important to perform the surgery symmetrically unless you are also trying to correct a vertical deviation in the primary position. Otherwise you will create an unwanted vertical strabismus. Complete weakening procedures of the superior obliques, such as nasal tenectomy or tendon expansion, have a powerful effect on torsion. They may lead to a disruption of fusion in a patient with bifoveal fusion and can create postoperative torsional diplopia in a fusing patient. Exercise extreme caution when weakening the superior obliques in such patients! A posterior tenectomy procedure may be adequate for addressing the pattern and is safer than doing a complete superior oblique tenectomy or tendon expansion. Alternatively, it might be prudent to address the pattern with vertical transpositions of the horizontal rectus muscles, and just decrease, rather than eliminate the pattern, if it is large.

If oblique muscles are not overacting, they should not be weakened when treating an "A" or "V" pattern. Finally, "V" patterns with superior oblique underaction can be treated with superior oblique tucks.

Vertical transpositions of the horizontal rectus muscles

Many patients with "A" or "V" patterns can be treated effectively with transpositions of the horizontal rectus muscles combined with the usual recession or resection you would perform based on the primary position deviation. You should not make any adjustment in your standard surgical formula because of the transposition.

Horizontal rectus transpositions are based on the principal that, when a rectus muscle is transposed, its primary action is decreased when the eye rotates into the field of gaze toward which the muscle was moved, and its action increases when the eye moves in the opposite direction (Fig. 80.8). For example, if a medial rectus muscle is transposed inferiorly, it becomes a weaker adductor when the eye is in downgaze and a greater adductor when the eye is in upgaze. This occurs because the insertion of the transposed muscle has a new relationship to the center of rotation of the globe as seen in Figure 80.8. Thus, for treating a "V" pattern esotropia, you can recess and infraplace the medial rectus muscles, because downgaze is the field in which you want them to have less adducting action. However, when transposing rectus muscles, it is important to consider that two additional changes in their function occur simultaneously (Fig. 80.9). One effect is the creation of

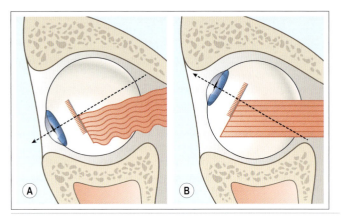

Fig. 80.8 Effect of vertical transposition of rectus muscle on its primary action. If a muscle is infraplaced, there will be more slack in the muscle when the eye is in downgaze (A) than in upgaze (B). This weakens the primary action of the muscle more in downgaze than in upgaze.

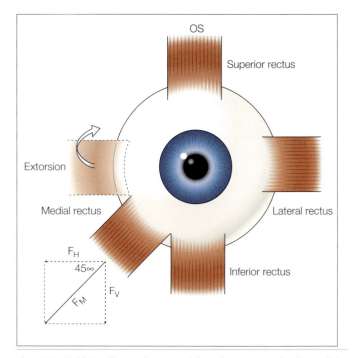

Fig. 80.9 Multiple effects of transposition of rectus muscle. If a medial rectus muscle is infraplaced, a new force vector for depression will be created. In addition, a torsional force vector will be created in the direction toward the original insertion. With infraplacement of the medial rectus, a vector for extorsion is created.

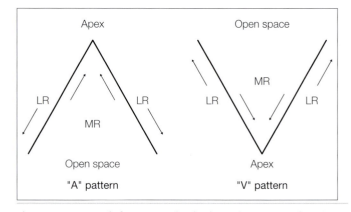

Fig. 80.10 Mnemonic for transposing horizontal rectus muscles. This diagram depicts the directions to move the horizontal rectus muscles for the treatment of an "A" pattern (left) and a "V" pattern (right). The lateral rectus muscles (LR) are always moved toward the open space and the medial rectus muscles (MR) always move toward the apex of the pattern.

a force vector in the direction in which the muscle is moved. Thus, if a medial rectus muscle is infraplaced, an additional force vector for depression is established. For this reason, it is important to always use this treatment symmetrically; otherwise an unwanted vertical deviation in the primary position will be induced. The exception might be those circumstances in which you want to treat a pre-existing primary position vertical deviation, in which case you might perform a unilateral transposition or a bilateral transposition that is asymmetric.

The other effect of transposition of rectus muscles relates to torsion. When a muscle is transposed, a torsional vector is created in the direction from which the muscle is moved. For example, moving a medial rectus inferiorly creates a force vector that results in extorsion as shown in Figure 80.9. Importantly, this torsional rotation is in the opposite direction to the torsional correction one desires when treating most "A" or "V" patterns. A "V" pattern esotropia is typically associated with inferior oblique overaction and excyclotropia. Transposing the medial rectus muscles inferiorly successfully treats a "V" pattern but makes excyclotropia worse.[13] This rarely results in adverse symptoms, probably because most patients with "A" and "V" patterns do not have bifoveal fusion, and also because the amount of torsional change is small.

A simple mnemonic for remembering the direction in which to transpose the horizontal muscles for treating pattern strabismus is presented in Figure 80.10. The medial rectus muscles are always transposed toward the apex of the pattern (down for a "V" pattern and up for an "A" pattern) and the lateral rectus muscles are always transposed toward the open space of the pattern (up for a V pattern and down for an "A" pattern). This holds true whether the muscles are recessed or resected, and if the patient is esotropic or exotropic. Vertical transposition of the horizontal rectus muscles is generally effective for treating pattern strabismus if there is no significant oblique dysfunction, but is less effective if the obliques are significantly overacting. This is understandable in light of the fact that transpositions worsen the torsion that is already present if there is oblique dysfunction and because torsion contributes to the pattern.

I find that, in most cases of "A" or "V" pattern without oblique muscle dysfunction, a symmetric vertical transposition

of the appropriate horizontal rectus muscles by one-half tendon width (0.5 mm) is effective in reducing an average of 15–20 PD of pattern. In most cases in which the pattern is more than 20 PD, there is usually significant oblique muscle dysfunction, and I usually address the pattern with oblique muscle surgery. If oblique muscle surgery is not indicated in a patient with a large pattern (perhaps it has already been performed but a pattern persists), transposition of the appropriate horizontal rectus muscles three-quarters or a full tendon width can be effective for patterns that are greater than 20 PD. Also, transpositions of the horizontal rectus muscles can be combined with oblique muscle surgery. For example, a patient with a very large "V" pattern (perhaps 40 PD or more), and inferior oblique overaction plus superior oblique underaction, might benefit from bilateral medial rectus recessions with infraplacement and bilateral inferior oblique weakening.

You can also apply the principles of transposition when doing unilateral surgery in the form of a recess-resect procedure. One muscle can be raised and the other lowered. Keep in mind, however, that doing so does not create an equal balance of forces. If you raise a weakened (recessed) muscle the same amount as you lower a tightened (resected) muscle, you are creating an increased force vector in the direction the resected muscle was moved. I have seen unwanted vertical deviations created from this surgical approach. Although unilateral transposition is often successful, I prefer symmetric surgery when performing transpositions.

Horizontal transposition of vertical rectus muscles

Horizontal transposition of the vertical rectus muscles can treat "A" and "V" patterns.[27,28] The theoretical efficacy of this approach is based on a different principle than that of vertical transposition of the horizontal rectus muscles. It is predicated on one of the effects depicted in Figure 80.9 – specifically that a force vector is created in the direction a muscle is moved. This same principle is the basis for transposition procedures to treat paralytic strabismus. Thus a "V" pattern esotropia can be treated by temporal transposition of the inferior rectus muscles along with appropriate recessions of the medial rectus muscles; typically the vertical rectus transpositions are 7 mm. A summary of the directions to transpose the vertical rectus muscles for treating "A" and "V" patterns is presented in Table 80.1.

Notably, horizontal transposition of the vertical rectus muscles may create a torsional shift that exacerbates a pre-existing cyclotropia for the reasons depicted in Figure 80.9. This is particularly relevant in treating patients with Graves' orbitopathy with large bilateral inferior rectus recessions, which often results in a postoperative "A" pattern with intorsion. I have seen such patients in whom the inferior rectus muscles were transposed nasally at the time of recession in hopes of preventing the occurrence of an "A" pattern, and an unexpectedly large and symptomatic incyclotropia was created. I prefer to combine large inferior rectus recessions with posterior tenectomy of the superior oblique tendon to prevent an "A" pattern in this setting.

Horizontal transposition of the vertical rectus muscles never gained popularity for treating routine cases of "A" or "V" pattern strabismus. I feel this is largely because it involves operating on an additional rectus muscle in each eye, which is not necessary when oblique muscle surgery or vertical transposition of the horizontal rectus muscles can be performed.

Surgery to correct pulley abnormalities

If pulley heterotopia or laxity is the cause of an "A" pattern, surgery could be performed to stabilize or reposition the orbital pulleys. Diagnosis of pulley abnormalities requires orbital imaging.[17,18]

Insertion slanting surgical procedures

Mathematical modeling of extraocular muscle mechanics indicates that one can theoretically consider an extraocular muscle as inserting at a point in the middle of its insertion[29] (Fig. 80.11A). If there is unequal tension along the edges of the muscle, one can still consider the muscle as inserting at a point which is then shifted toward the edge with greater tension (Fig. 80.11B). In theory, this principle can be used to treat pattern strabismus by selectively slanting the superior or inferior pole of the recessed muscles to simulate transposition. For example, for a "V" pattern esotropia the superior poles of the medial rectus muscles are recessed more than the inferior poles which simulates the effect of an infraplacement. This approach has been used successfully to treat pattern strabismus.[30] Paradoxically, good results have been reported with slanting the muscles in an opposite manner by numerous authors.[29,31] For a "V" pattern esotropia these authors would recess the inferior pole of the medial rectus muscles more than

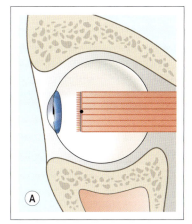
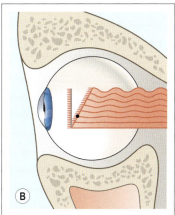

Fig. 80.11 (A) Mathematically one can consider a rectus muscle to insert at a point (black dot) at the middle of its insertion. (B) If there is unequal tension along the edges of a muscle as occurs with a slanting procedure, the muscle still can be thought of as inserting at a point (black dot). However, the point shifts toward the edge under greater tension. If the superior pole of a horizontal rectus muscle is slanted back, the point shifts toward the inferior edge, which is akin to infraplacing the muscle.

Table 80.1 – Summary of directions in which to transpose vertical rectus muscles

Strabismus	Transposition
"V" esotropia	IR OU temporally
"V" exotropia	SR OU nasally
"A" esotropia	SR OU temporally
"A" exotropia	IR OU nasally
OU = both eyes, IR = inferior rectus, SR = superior rectus.	

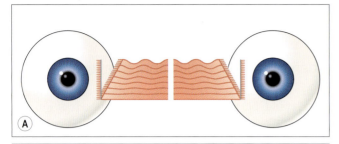

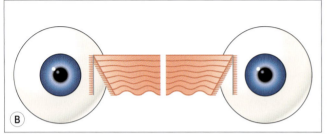

Fig. 80.12 (A) The treatment of a "V" pattern esotropia with insertion slanting according to the principles shown in (B). The superior poles of the medial rectus insertions are slanted back which simulates infraplacement. (B) The treatment of a "V" pattern esotropia according to the concept that the inferior fibers are more taut in downgaze.

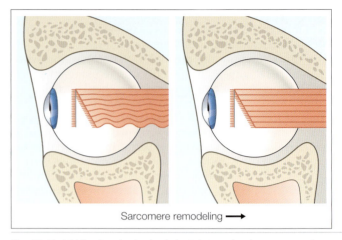

Sarcomere remodeling ⟶

Fig. 80.13 Initially after slanting back the inferior pole of a rectus muscle, there is substantial slack induced in the inferior muscle fibers (A). After a period of several weeks, sarcomere remodeling should even out the differential edge tension and largely negate the effect of the slanting procedure (B).

the superior poles. The rationale for this approach is based on the thought that the inferior edge of a horizontal rectus muscle is more taut in downgaze and the superior edge more taut in upgaze. The authors arrived at this conclusion through a misinterpretation of known facts about extraocular muscle mechanics. In fact, the opposite is true. This leads to a conundrum: How can opposite methods of slanting both produce good results (Fig. 80.12)? For the same "V" pattern esotropia some investigators would slant in the manner depicted in Figure 80.12A and others would use the configuration shown in Figure 80.12B. I believe that, despite their popularity, insertion slanting procedures in either manner should have a negligible effect on pattern strabismus. Sarcomere remodeling should rapidly occur and even out the edge tension after an insertion slanting procedure (Fig. 80.13). Probably the good outcomes reported with these procedures were the result of the recession or resection performed.

Summary of surgical planning

In all cases, I do the standard horizontal surgery based on the primary position measurement except perhaps allowing for up to 3 PD of eso shift in the primary position with superior oblique weakening. Table 80.2 summarizes my recommendations for the surgical management of "A" and "V" patterns.

Optical management

Some patients with "A" or "V" patterns may have good alignment in the primary position but have an esotropia or exotropia in downgaze. As stated earlier, such patients may first become symptomatic as they become presbyopic. Some patients of this type can be managed by either using single vision reading glasses, or having a separate bifocal for prolonged reading with a segment that is higher than is typically prescribed.[32]

Table 80.2 – Summary of surgical recommendations

If oblique dysfunction is present[a]	
"V" eso with IO OA	Recess MR or resect LR & weaken IO OU
"V" exo with IO OA	Recess LR or resect MR & weaken IO OU
"A" eso with SO OA	Recess MR or resect LR & weaken SO OU[b]
"A" exo with SO OA	Recess LR or resect MR & weaken SO OU[b]
Without oblique dysfunction[a]	
"V" eso	Recess MR and infraplace or resect LR and supraplace OU
"V" exo	Recess LR and supraplace or resect MR and infraplace OU
"A" eso	Recess MR and supraplace or resect LR and infraplace OU
"A" exo	Recess LR and infraplace or resect MR and supraplace OU

[a]Perform the usual amount of recession or resection of the horizontal rectus muscles based on the deviation in the primary position.
[b]Avoid a powerful superior oblique weakening procedure in patients with bifoveal fusion.
IO = , OA = , OU = , SO = , LR = , MR = .

References

1. Duane A. Isolated paralysis of the extraocular muscles. Arch Ophthalmol 1897; 26: 317–34.
2. Urrets-Zavalia A. Abducción en la elevación. Arch Oftalmol 1948; 23: 124–34.
3. Urrets-Zavalia A. Paralisis bilateral congenita del musculo oblicuo inferior. Arch Oftalmol 1948; 23: 172–82.
4. Urist MJ. Horizontal squint with secondary vertical deviations. AMA Arch Ophthalmol 1951; 46: 245–67.
5. Urist M. The etiology of the so-called "A" & "V" syndromes. Am J Ophthalmol 1958; 46: 835–44.
6. Costenbader F. The "A" and "V" patterns in strabismus. Trans Am Acad Ophthalmol Otolaryngol 1964; 58: 354–86.
7. Harley RD. Bilateral superior oblique tenectomy in A-pattern exotropia. Trans Am Ophthalmol Soc 1969; 67: 324–38.

8. Knapp P. "A" and "V" patterns. In: Symposium on Strabismus Transactions of the New Orleans Academy of Ophthalmology. St Louis: Mosby; 1971.

9. France TD. Strabismus in hydrocephalus. Am Orthopt J 1975; 25: 101–5.

10. Biglan AW, Walden PG. Ophthalmic complications of meningomyelocoele: a longitudianal study. Trans Am Ophthalmol Soc 1990; 88: 389–461.

11. Knapp P. Vertically incomitant horizontal strabismus: the so-called "A" & "V" syndromes. Trans Am Ophthmol Soc 1959; 57: 666–9.

12. Kushner B. The role of ocular torsion on the etiology of A and V patterns. J Pediatr Ophthalmol Strabismus 1985; 22: 171–9.

13. Kushner BJ. Effect of ocular torsion on A and V patterns and apparent oblique muscle overaction. Arch Ophthalmol 2010; 128: 712–8.

14. Urrets-Zavalia A, Solares-Zamora J, Olmos HR. Anthropological studies on the nature of cyclovertical squint. Br J Ophthalmol 1961; 45: 578–96.

15. Miller M, Folk E. Strabismus associated with craniofacial anomalies. Am Orthopt J 1975; 25: 27–37.

16. Robb RM, Boger WP, 3rd. Vertical strabismus associated with plagiocephaly. J Pediatr Ophthalmol Strabismus 1983; 20: 58–62.

17. Clark RA, Miller JM, Rosenbaum AL, Demer JL. Heterotopic muscle pulleys or oblique muscle dysfunction? J AAPOS 1998; 2: 17–25.

18. Demer JL. The orbital pulley system: a revolution in concepts of orbital anatomy. Ann N Y Acad Sci 2002; 956: 17–32.

19. Kushner BJ. Restriction of elevation in abduction after inferior oblique anteriorization. J AAPOS 1997; 1: 55–62.

20. Kushner BJ. Thyroid eye disease. In: Dortzbach R, editor. Ophthalmic Plastic Surgery: Prevention and Management of Complications. New York: Raven Press; 1994: 381–94.

21. Brown H. Vertical deviations. Trans Am Acad Ophthalmol Otolaryngol 1953; 57: 157–62.

22. Gobin M. Sagittalization of the oblique muscles as a possible cause for the "A" and "V" phenomena. Br J Ophthalmol 1968; 52: 13–8.

23. Prieto-Diaz J. Posterior partial tenectomy of the SO. J Pediatr Ophthalmol Strabismus 1979; 16: 321–3.

24. Shin GS, Elliott RL, Rosenbaum AL. Posterior superior oblique tenectomy at the scleral insertion for collapse of A-pattern strabismus. J Pediatr Ophthalmol Strabismus 1996; 33: 211–8.

25. Parks MM. Doyne Memorial Lecture, 1977. The superior oblique tendon. Trans Ophthalmol Soc UK 1977; 97: 288–304.

26. Diamond GR, Parks MM. The effect of superior oblique weakening procedures on primary position horizontal alignment. J Pediatr Ophthalmol Strabismus 1981; 18: 35–8.

27. Fink WH. "A" and "V" syndromes. Am Orthopt J 1959; 9: 105–10.

28. Miller JE. Vertical recti transplantation in the "A" and"V" syndromes. Arch Ophthalmol 1960; 61: 689–700.

29. Kushner B. Insertion slanting strabismus surgical prodedures. Arch Ophthalmol 2011; 129: 1620–5.

30. van der Meulen-Schot HM, van der Meulen SB, Simonsz HJ. Caudal or cranial partial tenotomy of the horizontal rectus muscles in A and V pattern strabismus. Br J Ophthalmol 2008; 92: 245–51.

31. Bietti GB. Su un accorgimento tecnico (recessione e reinserzione oblique a ventaglio dei muscoli orizzontali) per la correzione di atteggiamenti a V o A di grado modesto negli strabismi concomitanti. Boll Ocul 1970; 49: 581–8.

32. Kushner B. Management of diplopia limited to down gaze. Arch Ophthalmol 1995; 113: 1426–30.

Abnormal head postures: causes and management

Stephen P Kraft

Chapter contents

General considerations

Abnormal head postures (AHPs) are frequent in pediatric ophthalmology. The medical term is torticollis from the Latin prefix "tortus" (twisted) and "collum" (neck).[1,2] The term is applied to muscular or neurologic disorders that cause unnatural positions of the head.[1,3] The eye-related conditions that lead to AHPs are termed ocular torticollis.[4-6]

Physiological basis of head postures

Normal head position is maintained by inputs from the otolith apparatus, the semicircular canals within the labyrinth, the proprioceptors in the neck and the retina. The labyrinth is the sense organ for static and dynamic head movement. The otolithic apparatus responds to static head position. It is activated during maneuvers such as head tilting to one shoulder. The semicircular canals respond to dynamic head movements in any of the three dimensions.[1,3,7]

Input from these sources travels to the vestibular brainstem nuclei and from there to the vestibular cortex and to the cervical cord and neck muscles. There are also direct pathways from the labyrinth to the extraocular muscles in response to changes in the semicircular canals. Cerebellar projections and cervical proprioceptive input are integrated into the system.[2,4,7] Integration of input from the retinas leads to fine adjustments in head position.[2]

The muscles of the neck that maintain the vertical column which in turn supports the head are the sternocleidomastoid, thoracic, and semispinalis muscles. Torticollis manifests when the forces in these muscles are unbalanced due to a congenital or acquired problem within the spinal column, the muscles themselves, or as a result of abnormal neural inputs from a variety of sources including the vestibular apparatus.[3] It is also a rare presenting sign of a psychiatric disorder.[2,3]

Ocular torticollis arises from disturbances in the input from the afferent visual pathway, ocular motor nerves, or the vestibular apparatus. Any of these disorders leads to alterations in the inputs to the neck muscles. In ocular torticollis, the abnormal posture is adopted for the following reasons:[2,5-9]

1. To optimize visual acuit.
2. To maintain single binocular vision.
3. To center a narrowed visual field with respect to the body.

Torticollis due to an ocular problem that persists long-term can lead to a secondary musculoskeletal torticollis and even scoliosis.[3-5,9-13] Torticollis is not a diagnosis, but a sign of an underlying disorder:[3] a cause must be sought. The assessment in a child is often multidisciplinary, involving pediatricians, orthopedic surgeons, neurologists, and physiotherapists.[3,14] It is common for an ophthalmologist to be consulted to rule out ocular causes for torticollis.

General categories of head postures

By orientation (Fig. 81.1)

Torticollis can involve rotation of the head around any of the three main axes. These include:

1. The vertical axis: the head is rotated to one side or the other away from the primary gaze.
2. The horizontal axis: the chin is elevated or depressed relative to the primary position.
3. The anteroposterior axis: the head is tilted to one or the other shoulder.
4. A combination of any of these three orientations.

By onset

Most cases of childhood torticollis are not seen at birth but within a few months. There are cases of true congenital torticollis due to muscular or skeletal anomalies.[1,3,14] Ocular

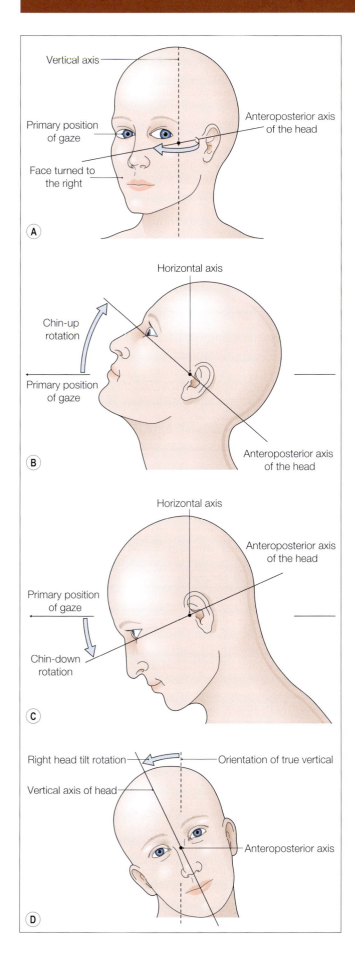

Primary position of gaze

Face turned to the right

A

Chin-up rotation

Primary position of gaze

Anteroposterior axis of the head

B

Horizontal axis

Anteroposterior axis of the head

Primary position of gaze

Chin-down rotation

C

Right head tilt rotation — Orientation of true vertical

Vertical axis of head

Anteroposterior axis

D

Fig. 81.1 Orientations of abnormal head postures. (a) Face turn to the right. The anteroposterior axis of the head is rotated from primary gaze direction to the right about the vertical axis. (b) Chin-up posture: the anteroposterior axis of the head is rotated upward from the primary gaze direction about the horizontal axis. (c) Chin-down posture: the anteroposterior axis of the head is rotated downward from the primary gaze direction about the horizontal axis. (d) Head tilt to the right shoulder: the vertical axis of the head is rotated away from the vertical axis about the anteroposterior axis.

torticollis almost never presents within the first few weeks of life. Trauma must be ruled out as a cause of any acquired AHP, whether as a result of damage to the neck or due to disruption of eye muscle balance.[3]

By timing

An AHP can be paroxysmal or persistent. It can be temporary in transient diseases, such as otitis media or benign paroxysmal torticollis of infancy. It can be constant, as with congenital nystagmus with an eccentric null zone or with restrictive strabismus. The head posture can be consistent in its orientation, as occurs in cases of superior oblique muscle paresis (see Chapter 83) and congenital nystagmus (see Chapter 89) or it may constantly change, as PAN.

Non-ocular causes of head postures (Box 81.1)

There are many non-ocular causes of torticollis, both congenital and acquired. This discussion will be limited to the most common and serious conditions.

Congenital disorders

Muscular causes

Congenital muscular torticollis

Congenital muscular torticollis (CMT) is the most common type of congenital torticollis: it occurs in 0.4% of newborns. It manifests within 2 to 6 weeks of age, and in many cases there is a painless, discrete "fibroma" on one side of the neck adjacent to the sternocleidomastoid muscle.[1,3,5,14-16] The infant develops a head tilt to the side of the involved muscle, with a forward flexion. The mass resolves with time over several months.

As the neck and facial bones enlarge, the fibrotic sternocleidomastoid muscle may fail to elongate properly. As a result, CMT can lead to various deformities including hemifacial hypoplasia, plagiocephaly, and compensatory thoracic scoliosis: these changes can be arrested by early intervention with passive physiotherapy.[1,2,15] In a minority, surgery is needed.[1,15]

Postural torticollis

The head posture is evident shortly after birth but it is not associated with any mass in the sternocleidomastoid muscle. It may result from an abnormal fetal position. It is usually transient, although some cases require physiotherapy early in childhood to release muscle stiffness.[1,16]

Skeletal or osseous causes

Abnormalities in the cranial junction or cervical spine, including atlantoaxial rotatory displacement and odontoid hypoplasia, can lead to chronic torticollis.[1,3]

Box 81.1

Non-ocular causes of torticollis

I. Congenital
  A. Muscular
    1. Congenital muscular torticollis
    2. Postural torticollis
    3. Absent cervical muscles
  B. Skeletal/osseous
    1. Atlantoaxial bony deformity
    2. Klippel-Feil syndrome
    3. Sprengel's deformity
    4. Miscellaneous anomalies
II. Acquired
  A. Traumatic
    1. Skeletal/osseous
      a) Atlantoaxial displacement
      b) Subluxation of C2–C3 joint
      c) Fractures
    2. Ligament
    3. Muscle or soft tissue
  B. Non-traumatic
    1. Skeletal/osseous
      a) Inflammation
      b) Tumors
      c) Ligamentous laxity
    2. Postural
    3. Neurologic
      a) Spinal and posterior fossa pathology
      b) Dystonia
      c) Infections
    4. Otolaryngologic
      a) Nasopharyngeal infections
      b) Benign paroxysmal torticollis of infancy
      c) Deafness
      d) Ocular tilt reaction
    5. Miscellaneous
      a) Gastroenterologic
      b) Metabolic
      c) Pharmacologic
      d) Psychogenic/functional

The Klippel-Feil syndrome can lead to torticollis as a result of the associated cervical vertebral anomalies, including congenital vertebral fusion and hemivertebrae, which can lead to reduced neck motion. Sprengel's deformity is seen in 30% of Klippel-Feil cases. It is characterized by an elevated scapula with limited shoulder movement, and is associated with scoliosis, renal anomalies, and an omovertebral bone.[1,3]

There are several clinical syndromes that place the child at high risk of cervical spine instability as a result of congenital laxity of ligaments or abnormalities of their vertebral bodies. These include Down's syndrome, mucopolysaccharidoses (see Chapter 62), and osteogenesis imperfecta.[1]

Acquired disorders

The acquired causes are divided into traumatic and non-traumatic. Trauma must be considered in any child with torticollis.[1,16,17]

Traumatic causes

Trauma can damage bones, ligaments, or muscle or soft tissue. The most common trauma affecting the neck involves rotatory subluxation of the atlantoaxial joint or subluxation of C2 and C3.[1,3,16,17] Fractures of the scapula or clavicle can lead to AHPs.[3] There is pain and limitation of movement, although there may be little or no neurologic deficit.[3] Ligament injuries are less common, but they can be associated with severe neurologic complications, especially if the transverse ligament is ruptured.[16] Direct trauma to the neck can lead to hematomas or tearing of muscle fibers, especially the sternocleidomastoid or the posterior capitis.[3,16]

Non-traumatic causes

Skeletal or osseous torticollis

Bone erosion in the cranial junction or cervical spine can lead to chronic torticollis. Erosion can arise from inflammation due to osteomyelitis, rheumatoid arthritis, or tuberculosis or from tumors. It leads to rotatory subluxation or anterior dislocation.[1,3,16]

Atlantoaxial rotatory displacement can arise from excessive transverse ligament laxity following a local infection, especially cervical adenitis or a retropharyngeal abscess.[1,16] It can also arise from intrinsic changes in the ligament, e.g. in patients on prolonged systemic steroids.[3] Most cases resolve spontaneously or once an underlying cause is reversed. A minority require immobilization or cervical traction.[1,3]

Postural torticollis

Rarely, torticollis can be produced by prolonged maintenance of the head in an awkward position that causes undue neck strain. Usually seen in older children, it develops gradually with permanent changes in the neck muscles.[3]

Neurologic

Posterior fossa and spinal pathology Torticollis may be the only sign of a spinal cord or central nervous system anomaly or neoplasm.[18] Acquired torticollis may be the presenting sign of syringomyelia leading to scoliosis and hyperhidrosis. Torticollis has also been described with colloid cysts of the third ventricle and with tumors of the posterior fossa, including ependymomas and hemangioblastomas.[3] Astrocytomas of the cervicomedullary junction can stretch the meninges and cause neck muscle spasms on attempted passive flexion of the head, especially in young children.[1] Tumors in the lower brain stem and cervical spine can cause anomalous head postures in young children, usually head tilts or chin-up postures. Torticollis accompanied by hyperactive tendon reflexes or extensor plantar responses may indicate a cervical cord disturbance, indicating the need for radiologic examination.[2]

The Arnold-Chiari malformation, in which there is a downward displacement of the cerebellar tonsils in the cervical canal, can lead to symptoms and signs including scoliosis, headache, and neck pain with torticollis.[1] There is a triad of photophobia, epiphora, and torticollis associated with posterior fossa lesions. The postulated mechanism for the torticollis is irritation of the vestibular nuclear complex, herniation of the tonsils, oblique muscle paresis, or a combination of these.[19,20]

Dystonia Spasmodic torticollis is a form of dystonia of the facial and cervical muscles that results from neurologic diseases or as an effect of medications that affect the basal ganglia. Loss of interneuron inhibition is a factor.[1,2,5] Affected patients show sustained muscle contractions with repetitive movements and AHPs.

Spasmodic torticollis in children can be a reaction to psychiatric medications such as phenothiazine. It may be accompanied by other dystonic reactions such as trismus and oculogyric crises.[2] Idiopathic spasmodic torticollis in children is rare; it often progresses from a focal dystonia to a more generalized disorder.[1] Two other conditions that can present in the first two years of life are benign paroxysmal dystonia of infancy and paroxysmal choreoathetosis.[2,3]

Infections AHPs, usually head tilts, have been reported with acute bacterial meningitis; the mechanism may be involvement of the cranial nerves, especially the fourth cranial nerve.[2,5] Torticollis can also follow encephalitis with damage to the basal ganglia.[3] It can occur after systemic infections including scarlet fever, measles, influenza, poliomyelitis, and diphtheria, or from postinfectious neuritis or as a result of osteomyelitis from a cervical abscess.[3]

Otolaryngologic

Nasopharyngeal torticollis Non-traumatic acute torticollis in children commonly results from inflammations and infections of the the pharynx, tonsils, sinuses, mastoids, and the ears.[16] The deep cervical lymph nodes are frequently enlarged and the sternocleidomastoid muscle becomes painful due to spasm,[1,3,16] a condition termed Grisel's syndrome.[16]

The head postures seen with otitis media may be due to labyrinthine disturbances.[3] Retrotonsillar and retropharyngeal abscesses can lead to torticollis. A presumed cause is fluid accumulation between the ring of C1 and the odontoid bone.[3,16]

Benign paroxysmal torticollis of infancy This consists of recurrent attacks of head tilting often accompanied by vomiting, pallor, and agitation[21] in female infants. When the child begins to walk there is ataxia and older children may have headaches or vertigo.[1,2,16,21] It is considered a migraine variant that affects the vestibular system. There is often a strong family history of migraine. This tends to subside over several months or years.[2,16,21]

Deafness In infants an intermittent, unilateral, recurring face turn may be the presenting sign of a unilateral hearing deficit.[2,3]

Ocular tilt reaction This triad of vertical divergence of the eyes, bilateral ocular torsion, and head tilt is a postural reflex originating in the otolithic apparatus. It can be caused by lesions of the vestibular nucleus or its central connections.[2,7] See the section on head tilt postures, below.

Miscellaneous causes

Gastroenterologic

Hiatus hernia and gastroesophageal reflux can be seen in children, usually those with cerebral palsy. This combination can lead to intermittent neck extensions or head tilts to decrease the amount of reflux, known as Sandifer's syndrome.[1,2,4,5,13,16] Such infants with this rarely present with vomiting.[1,2,16] Antireflux treatment can help. Abnormal neck postures have also been described in infants with pyloric stenosis.[3]

Metabolic disorders

Torticollis with dystonia and dyskinesia occurs in glutaric aciduria. Affected children may also have severe motor and language deficits and global developmental delays.[1,3]

Pharmacologic

There are a number of drugs that cause torticollis including the phenothiazines and metoclopramide.[1,3]

Psychiatric and functional disorders

Unexplained head deviations may occasionally be functional in nature. The most common psychological disorder that leads to torticollis is a conversion reaction:[17] these patients require close follow-up for signs that require further investigation.[1]

Ocular causes of head postures

General considerations

Children adopt head postures with several ocular conditions. When the child derives a demonstrable advantage by adopting the head position it is more correctly termed a compensatory head posture[22,23] and the ophthalmologist's goal is to determine an ocular cause. If there is an underlying ocular cause, treatment can eliminate or reduce the problem and restore a normal head posture.

If a non-ophthalmologist has a patient with an AHP, referral for an eye examination should be made early because:

1. An untreated ocular cause can lead to changes in the neck muscles and produce a secondary torticollis,[4,9,10,14] which may persist even if the underlying ocular situation is rectified.

2. A child with incomitant strabismus may adopt a compensatory posture to maintain fusion. If the posture is difficult to sustain, the child may assume a more normal position which creates a heterotropia with loss of fusion, suppression, and amblyopia.[2]

3. Some ocular head tilts early in childhood can be associated with changes in the facial bones and even plagiocephaly. The facial bony changes may be secondary to, or coincident with, the head position. The bony alterations can be prevented by early treatment of the eye disorder.[9,10-12]

4. The binocular visual acuity of a child with a compensatory posture may not be optimal in the adopted position, especially if nystagmus is the cause (see Chapter 89). Eye muscle surgery for the head posture may improve the binocular acuity.[13,23-26]

Compensatory head postures have four advantages.[4,22] They serve to:

1. Optimize visual acuity.
2. Maintain binocularity.
3. Center the field of binocular vision.
4. Generate miscellaneous benefits.

Optimize visual acuity

Children adopt a compensatory posture either to optimize their binocular visual acuity or, if unable to maintain that, to maximize vision in the fixing eye.[2,6,22]

825

Examples in the first category include infantile nystagmus (see Chapter 89) and ptosis (see Chapter 19). In the case of infantile nystagmus, the vision is best because the nystagmus intensity (amplitude × frequency) is least or else the fovation times within the waveforms are maximized in the AHP.[23,24,26] The AHPs of spasmus nutans and ocular motor apraxia (saccadic initiation failure) fall into this category.[4,6,23,26]

The second category includes significant refractive errors (especially astigmatism), manifest latent nystagmus in a monocular patient, severe restrictive strabismus, and infantile esotropia with cross fixation. It also includes cases of eccentric fixation associated with macular heterotopia and head tilts adopted in order to reorient the retinal meridians in the presence of cyclotropia.[6,27]

Maintain binocularity

Many forms of incomitant strabismus have a gaze position featuring zero, or minimal, heterotropia and where fusion is maintained. Usually the posture is adopted to gain the benefit of bifoveal fusion, but it can also achieve anomalous retinal correspondence.[9] The causes can be subdivided into horizontal incomitance (such as sixth nerve paresis; see Chapter 83), Duane's syndrome with esotropia (see Chapter 82), and oblique muscle paresis (see Chapter 83) and vertical incomitance (such as monocular elevation deficits and "A" and "V" pattern strabismus; see Chapter 80).

The causes in each plane can also be grouped under innervational and mechanical causes.[28] Innervational problems include both underaction of muscles (e.g. muscle paresis and myasthenia; see Chapter 83) and excessive innervation of muscles (e.g. overaction of oblique muscles; see Chapter 80). Mechanical problems can affect any of the structures within the orbit such as bony abnormalities (e.g. orbit fractures), muscle disorders (e.g. thyroid orbitopathy, Brown's syndrome and congenital cranial dysinnervation disorders), soft tissue diseases (e.g. pseudotumors), and neoplasms in the orbit.

Center the field of binocular vision

A child with congenital homonymous hemianopia may turn their faces to the hemianopic field when they fixate to centralize the intact visual field with the body.[2,9,29,30] Altitudinal field defects may also include chin-up or chin-down head postures.[2] Finally, monocular patients may turn slightly to the blind side to maximize their panorama of vision.[9]

Miscellaneous causes

Children with unilateral horizontal gaze palsies may adopt a face turn toward the side of the gaze deficit to allow the eyes to move in a range that is centered with respect to the body.[2]

Occasionally a patient with diplopia due to an incomitant strabismus will adopt a head posture to maximize the separation of images. This is occasionally seen in acquired unilateral superior oblique paresis whereby the child tilts to the shoulder ipsilateral to the involved eye so that the vertical tropia is maximized.[6,9,22,31]

A head posture may not directly improve vision or binocular functioning. A classic example is the ocular tilt reaction.[2,7,9] Children may also adopt an abnormal posture for cosmetic reasons to hide a physical deformity in the eyes, such as a postsurgical conjunctival scar.[6]

Box 81.2

Ocular causes of a right face turn

I. Nystagmus
   A. Infantile
      1. Conjugate form (infantile nystagmus syndrome)
      2. Disconjugate forms (including fusion maldevelopment syndrome)
   B. Acquired
      1. Periodic alternating nystagmus
      2. Spasmus nutans
II. Incomitant strabismus
   A. Horizontal muscle abnormalities
      1. Right eye/left eye
         a) Innervational causes
         b) Mechanical causes
      2. Both eyes: gaze palsy
   B. Vertical muscle abnormalities
      1. Left superior oblique dysfunction
      2. Left inferior oblique dysfunction
   C. Paradoxical face turn
III. Uncorrected refractive errors
IV. Eccentric fixation
V. Right homonymous hemianopia
VI. Miscellaneous etiologies
   A. Ocular motor apraxia
   B. Monocular blindness
   C. Very high myopia with esotropia

Face turn: differential diagnosis (Box 81.2)

Nystagmus

Infantile nystagmus

Infantile nystagmus causes face turns for two reasons:

1. Presence of conjugate null zones: the eyes are normally aligned but the nystagmus null zone lies to the same side for both eyes. This is the typical pattern of infantile nystagmus syndrome (see Chapter 89).[26] The child adopts a face turn to the side contralateral to the null zone in order to fixate in the null zone and optimize binocular visual acuity. If the null zone is located to the right of fixation, the child will adopt a left face turn. Although CN can create any orientation of compensatory posture, at least 80% of patients with a posture have a face turn as the chief component.[22,32] Rarely, there is more than one null zone, sometimes different for distance and near.

2. Presence of disconjugate null zones: this is usually seen with infantile esotropia (see Chapter 74). The patient has a large-angle esotropia with either eye fixing in adduction; they develop nystagmus on attempting to abduct either eye. This was previously referred to as manifest latent nystagmus or Ciancia's syndrome, but is now termed fusion maldevelopment nystagmus syndrome.[23,26,33] These children have a null zone in the adducted position in either eye and adopt a left face turn to fixate with the left eye, and a right face turn to fixate with the right eye (see Chapters 74 and 89).

A similar mechanism accounts for the face turn in patients with early-onset vision disorders of one eye. They are forced to fixate with the better eye and may develop a manifest latent nystagmus with an eccentric null zone. The null zone is usually in the adducted position with an adoption of an ipsilateral face turn to allow the eye to fixate steadily.[2,5,6]

Patients with nystagmus blockage syndrome may converge the eyes to dampen the intensity of nystagmus and improve their vision. However, the improved vision is gained at the expense of the alignment of the eyes because a large esotropia develops. This forces the child to adopt a face turn to fixate with one or the other eye.[4,9]

Acquired nystagmus

Two forms of (usually) acquired nystagmus that can cause face turns are periodic alternating nystagmus (PAN) and spasmus nutans. PAN is a rhythmic shifting of a conjugate null zone from right to left with periods of between 90 seconds and 10 minutes. It causes a periodic oscillation of the face turn from right to left and back again. Many cases are benign, but some are caused by posterior fossa pathology (see Chapter 90).[4,26]

Spasmus nutans is a triad of fine rapid frequency nystagmus, head nodding, and torticollis. Although the most common head posture is a head tilt, some have a face turn.[2,23,26] It usually resolves by age 2 to 3 years. It is usually benign, but chiasmal tumors can cause a similar picture (see Chapter 90).[2,4,26]

Incomitant strabismus

Incomitant horizontal strabismus can force a child to adopt a face turn to maintain fusion to avoid both diplopia and the need to suppress one image. There are two categories of horizontal plane incomitance, one involving the horizontal rectus muscles and the other involving the oblique muscles. *For purposes of this discussion the child has a right face turn; the differential diagnosis for a left face turn is the mirror image.*

Horizontal rectus muscle abnormalities (Fig. 81.2)

The child may adopt a right face turn to maintain fusion. This implies that there is a horizontal heterotropia whose magnitude is least in the left gaze position. The angle of deviation increases progressively as the eyes move from left gaze into the primary position and then into the contralateral gaze field. In some cases fusion may not be a factor, but the preferred eye for fixation may not be able to fixate in the primary position. Therefore, the differential diagnosis of a right face turn may be problems of abduction of the right eye or adduction of the left eye. Then, for each eye, in turn, one must consider both innervational and mechanical disorders.[28]

For the right eye Innervational causes include such entities as a sixth nerve paresis, Duane's syndrome with esotropia, or a slipped lateral rectus muscle after strabismus surgery. Mechanical restrictions on the medial side of the orbit include orbital wall fractures, fibrosis syndromes, and thyroid orbitopathy.

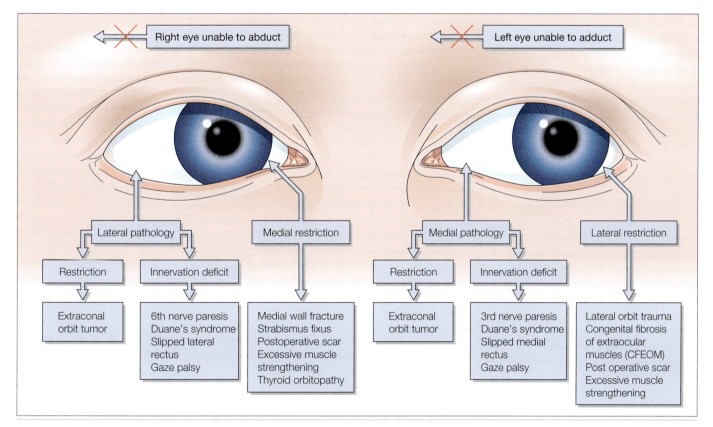

Fig. 81.2 Horizontal strabismus causes of compensatory right face turn. A useful approach is to address the reasons for a deficit of abduction of the right eye and/or of adduction of the left eye. The causes are classified into innervational and restrictive etiologies, and these are assigned to the lateral or medial sides of the two eyes, as illustrated.

Restriction of abduction can be due to a large extraconal tumor. Patients with bilateral strabismus fixus have to adopt a face turn to keep the fixing eye in adduction.

For the left eye Innervational causes include a partial third nerve (medial rectus) paresis (see Chapter 83) or palsy, Duane's syndrome with exotropia and limited adduction (see Chapter 82), or a slipped medial rectus muscle after surgery. An internuclear ophthalmoplegia causing limited adduction of the left eye may also force the patient to adopt a right face turn (see Chapter 90).

Mechanical causes include restrictions from lateral orbit scarring from trauma, congenital cranial dysinnervation disorders, thyroid orbitopathy, prior surgery, or medial orbital tumors which limit adduction.

For both eyes A complete gaze palsy to the right side may force the patient to adopt a right face turn to allow easier fixation in the remaining intact field.[2]

Vertical alignment abnormalities (Fig. 81.3)
Strabismus disorders that cause incomitant vertical heterotropias can create face turns. These include oblique muscle anomalies and disorders that create up- or downdrifts in the adducted position of one eye. The vertical actions of the inferior and superior oblique muscles are strongest when the eye is adducted and are least when abducted. If an oblique muscle in one eye is overacting or underacting, there is a vertical heterotropia, most marked in the lateral gaze position where the oblique muscle has its strongest vertical action, and least in the opposite gaze field.

Although head tilts are usually the main component of the head posture in oblique muscle disorders, torticollis with mainly a face turn may occur.[14,22] For a right face turn, the oblique muscles with abnormal actions are those of the left eye, with a paresis or overaction of either muscle. A right face turn is adopted to avoid the right field where the vertical deviation is most noticeable.

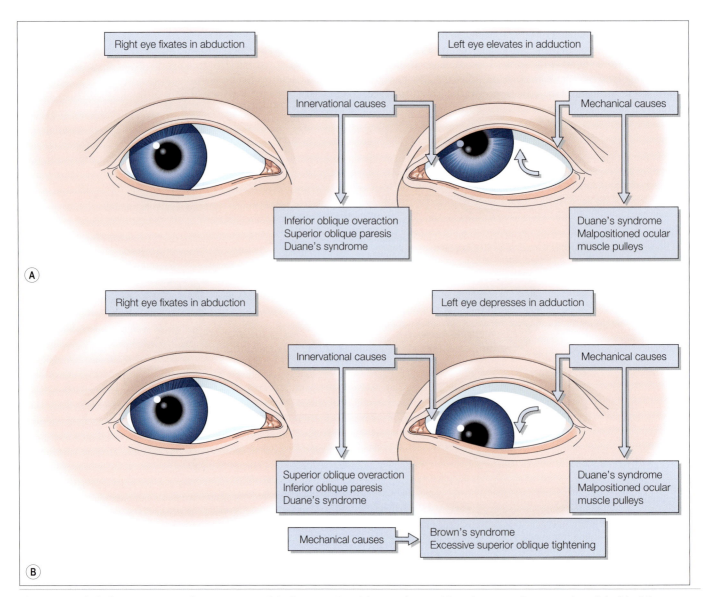

Fig. 81.3 Vertical alignment causes of compensatory right face turn. A useful approach is to address the causes of an up- or downdrift of the left eye on attempted adduction. (A) An updrift of the left eye causes an incomitant left hypertropia that is worse on right gaze. (B) A downdrift of the left eye causes an incomitant left hypotropia that is worse on right gaze. In both situations, the causes are divided into innervational and mechanical etiologies.

Alternatively, an up- or downdrift of the left eye can result from various mechanical and innervational disorders such as left Brown's syndrome (see Chapter 79), Duane's syndrome (see Chapter 82), or abnormal positioning of the extraocular muscle pulleys in the orbit (see Chapter 79).

Paradoxical face turn

Rarely, diplopia due to an acquired incomitant strabismus causes a head posture that brings the eyes into their maximum deviation. For example, a patient with a left sixth nerve paresis may not have fusion even when a left face turn is adopted so they may adopt a right face turn to spread the diplopic images as much as possible to allow the false image to be ignored.[2,9,22]

Uncorrected refractive errors

The most common uncorrected refractive errors that cause face turns are myopia and against-the-rule astigmatism.[2,4] Correction of the refractive error usually eliminates the face turn, but if a prescription is too weak, a face turn to fixate through the peripheral parts of the lenses generates added power by astigmatism of oblique incidence.

Eccentric fixation

Children who are forced to fixate with an eye that cannot foveate may adopt a face turn to position the new eccentric retinal fixation point in the primary position. This is seen in patients with macular heterotopia due to retinopathy of prematurity (see Chapter 43) and in macular dystrophies (see Chapter 46).[2,6]

Congenital homonymous hemianopia

Patients with a right complete homonymous hemianopia may adopt a right face turn to better center the remaining field with the body.[30] They may also develop an exotropia to expand the field of vision (see Chapter 78).[29,30]

Miscellaneous causes

Ocular motor apraxia (saccadic initiation failure) usually presents with horizontal head thrusting in order to overcome the lack of saccadic drive to fixate on a target (see Chapter 90). However, rarely the child may adopt a face turn while fixating a stationary target.[6] Monocularly blind patients may turn the head to maximize the panorama of vision in the remaining eye.[9]

Patients with enlarged eyes (e.g. high myopia) may have restricted abduction due to a combination of medial rectus contracture, inferior displacement of the lateral rectus muscle, nasal displacement of the vertical rectus muscles, and herniation of the posterior wall of the globe through defects in the lateral intermuscular septum.[34] This causes a face turn due to the fixed adducted position of the eye. Although this is usually seen in adults, its onset can be earlier.[34]

Chin-up: differential diagnosis (Box 81.3)

Nystagmus

Infantile nystagmus syndrome (see Chapter 89)

Infantile nystagmus can lead to any orientation of head posture. If the null zone is located in the downgaze position, the child may adopt a chin-up posture to maximize the binocular visual acuity[23,26] when both eyes have conjugate null zones in downgaze.

Box 81.3

Ocular causes of a chin-up posture
I. Nystagmus
   A. Infantile
   B. Acquired
II. Strabismus
   A. Elevation deficits
      1. Right eye/left eye
         a) Innervational causes
         b) Mechanical causes
      2. Both eyes
   B. Pattern strabismus
      1. "A" pattern esotropia
      2. "V" pattern exotropia
III. Ptosis
IV. Uncorrected refractive errors
V. Supranuclear gaze disorders
VI. Superior visual field defects

Acquired nystagmus (see Chapter 90)

Acquired disorders that cause nystagmus which is exaggerated in upgaze may lead to a chin-up posture to maintain optimal visual acuity.[2] In the dorsal midbrain syndrome there is limitation of upward movements along with a retraction nystagmus elicited by attempted upgaze. Thus the child maintains fixation below primary position.

Strabismus

There are two categories of eye muscle problems that can lead to a chin-up posture.

1. A limitation of eye movements in the vertical plane: a chin-up position will manifest if the child can maintain fusion in downgaze. There can be a limitation of upward movement of one or both eyes, and if the process involves both eyes it may be symmetric or asymmetric (see Chapter 79).
2. "A" and "V" patterns (see Chapter 80).

Elevation deficits (Fig. 81.4)

The differential diagnosis is formed from innervational and mechanical causes for each eye, similar to face turns.

For the right or the left eye Innervational causes include weakness of one or both elevators of the eye, the inferior oblique and superior rectus. Limited upgaze can occur from an infranuclear disturbance (such as an isolated inferior oblique paresis or as part of a third cranial nerve paresis) or from a supranuclear disorder (see below). Isolated paresis of either muscle can lead to hypotropia in primary position that may be smaller or absent in downgaze. Combined paresis of both muscles, while not a common entity, is termed a "double elevator paresis."

Mechanical causes include restrictions arising in the inferior part of the orbit: orbit floor fractures, fibrosis syndromes, and thyroid orbitopathy. There can also be a restriction to elevation due to processes superiorly in the orbit such as primary or secondary Brown's syndrome and extraconal masses superior to the globe. A large glaucoma-filtering device or sclera buckle can displace the eye downward and force a chin-up posture. The syndrome of high myopia with esotropia frequently has

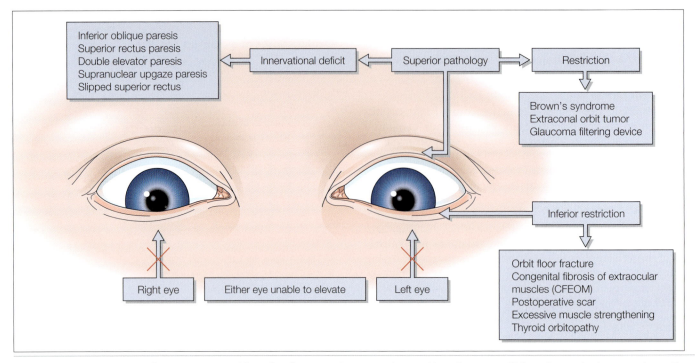

Fig. 81.4 Strabismus causes of a compensatory chin-up head posture. One approach is to address the causes of failure of one or both eyes to elevate. The causes are classified into innervational and restrictive etiologies, and these are assigned to the superior or inferior aspects of one or both of the eyes, as illustrated.

an associated hypotropia, leading to a chin-up component to the posture.[34]

Most cases of double elevator palsy or weakness are restrictive, due to inferior rectus contracture or fibrosis.[35] It is best to label an upgaze deficiency as a "monocular elevation deficit" until the cause is determined to be innervational or mechanical.

For both eyes The processes listed for either eye can occur bilaterally; some are prone to affect the two eyes, especially the fibrosis syndromes, thyroid orbitopathy, acquired Brown's syndrome, and supranuclear gaze disorders. The involvement can be asymmetric, but a head posture may arise if the vertical and horizontal heterotropias in downgaze are small enough to allow fusion.

"A" and "V" patterns
Two causes of chin-up postures are an "A" pattern esotropia and a "V" pattern exotropia. In both, the horizontal heterotropia is minimal in the downgaze field, while it increases progressively as the eyes move upward.[4,9]

Ptosis (see Chapter 19)

Ptosis, congenital or acquired, of one or both eyelids can lead to a chin-up posture if the lid margins obstruct the pupil.[4,6,9]

Uncorrected refractive errors (see Chapter 5)

Children with refractive errors may adopt a chin-up posture to take advantage of the stenopeic slit effect of the narrowed palpebral apertures most commonly used in myopia or astigmatism.

Supranuclear gaze disorders (see Chapter 90)

Damage to the vertical gaze centers in the brain stem can lead to upgaze paresis. Most common in children are hydrocephalus and the dorsal midbrain syndrome:[2] the latter

includes convergence-and-retraction nystagmus, eyelid retraction, and light–near dissociation of the pupils. Most cases of supranuclear gaze deficits are bilateral, but unilateral monocular elevation deficit can also have a supranuclear cause.[7,36]

Visual field defects

Patients who have lost a significant portion of their superior visual fields may adopt a chin-up posture to centralize the range of residual field relative to the body.[2] The most common causes are retina and optic nerve diseases that lead to altitudinal field deficits.

Chin-down: differential diagnosis (Box 81.4)

Nystagmus

Infantile nystagmus syndrome (see Chapter 89)
Infantile nystagmus can lead to any head posture. If the null zone is located in upgaze, the child adopts a chin-down posture to maximize the binocular visual acuity when both eyes have conjugate null zones in the upgaze field.[23,26]

Acquired nystagmus (see Chapter 90)
Acquired disorders (e.g. lower brainstem trauma or disease) that cause nystagmus whose intensity is greatest in downgaze may induce a chin-down posture for best visual acuity.

Strabismus

Eye muscle causes of a chin-down posture include:

1. A limitation of eye movements in the vertical plane: a chin-down position occurs if the child can fuse in upgaze. There can be a limitation of downward movement of one or both eyes; if bilateral, it may be symmetric or asymmetric.
2. "A" and "V" patterns.

Depression deficits (Fig. 81.5)

As for chin-up postures, the differential diagnosis is also formed from innervational and mechanical causes for each eye.

For the right or the left eye Innervational causes include weakness of one or both depressors of the eye, the superior oblique and inferior rectus. This can result from an infranuclear disturbance (third nerve paresis or fourth nerve paresis) or from a supranuclear disorder. Isolated paresis of either muscle can lead to a hypertropia in primary position that may be smaller or absent in upgaze. Combined paresis of both muscles is often termed a "double depressor paresis;" it is most commonly seen after orbital trauma.

Box 81.4

Ocular causes of a chin-down posture

I. Nystagmus
   A. Infantile
   B. Acquired
II. Strabismus
   A. Depression deficits
     1. Right eye/left eye
       a) Innervational causes
       b) Mechanical causes
     2. Both eyes
   B. Pattern strabismus
     1. "A" pattern exotropia
     2. "V" pattern esotropia
III. Uncorrected refractive errors
IV. Supranuclear gaze disorders
V. Inferior visual field defects

Mechanical causes include restrictions arising in the superior part of the orbit, such as orbit roof fractures, postoperative or post-traumatic scarring, and, rarely, thyroid orbitopathy. There can also be a restriction of depression due to mass lesions in the inferior orbit.

For both eyes Although the processes for either eye can occur bilaterally, some are particularly prone to affect the two eyes, especially bilateral superior oblique paresis after closed head trauma. It can be asymmetric, but a head posture may arise if the vertical and horizontal heterotropias in upgaze are both small enough to allow fusion.

"A" and "V" patterns (see Chapter 80)

The two causes of chin-down postures are an "A" pattern exotropia and a "V" pattern esotropia. In both, the horizontal heterotropia is minimal in upgaze, whereas it increases progressively as the eyes move down to primary position and downgaze.[4,9]

Bilateral superior oblique paresis that is fairly symmetric is a common cause of a chin-down posture that compensates for the "V" pattern esotropia and excyclodiplopia.[13,22,31]

Uncorrected refractive errors

Children who have uncorrected or undercorrected refractive errors may adopt a chin-down posture. Children with moderate hyperopia may be more apt to adopt a chin-down posture rather than a chin-up orientation. Children who have incorrect prescriptions in their glasses may peek over the frames in order to improve their vision.

Supranuclear gaze disorders

Damage to the vertical gaze centers can lead to paresis of downgaze, especially if it involves the rostral interstitial nucleus of the medial longitudinal fasciculus.[7] Bilateral downgaze paresis may also be a feature of neuropathic Gaucher's disease,

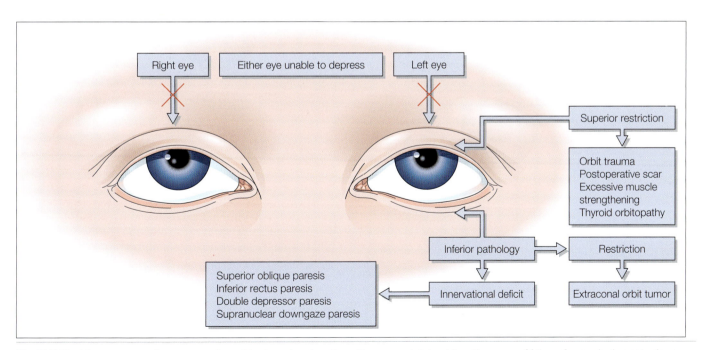

Fig. 81.5 Strabismus causes of a compensatory chin-down head posture. One approach is to address the causes of failure of one or both eyes to depress. The causes are classified into innervational and restrictive etiologies, and these are assigned to the superior or inferior aspects of one or both eyes, as illustrated.

Niemann-Pick disease type C, and it can be induced by several drugs and infectious causes.[2,7]

Visual field defects

Patients who have significant inferior visual field loss, as a result of retina or optic nerve diseases, may adopt a chin-down posture to centralize the range of residual field relative to the body.[2]

Head tilt: differential diagnosis (Box 81.5)

Nystagmus

Infantile nystagmus syndrome (see Chapter 89)
Infantile nystagmus can cause any head posture. A head tilt is usual, but there is often a face turn.[22,23] The nystagmus intensity decreases when the head is tilted toward one shoulder, whereas it increases as the head is positioned into primary gaze position and further increases on tilting to the opposite shoulder.

Acquired nystagmus (see Chapter 90)
The most common orientation of the torticollis in spasmus nutans is a head tilt, although a face turn may occur.

Strabismus (Fig. 81.6)

Causes of a head tilt include vertical muscle problems, cyclotropia, and horizontal deviations. For the purposes of

discussion, the child has a right head tilt. The differential diagnosis for a left tilt is the mirror image of that presented.

Vertical muscle problems (see Chapter 79)
The vertical muscle abnormalities that can lead to a head tilt can be divided into innervational and mechanical entities. In each case, the vertical deviation differs on tilting to one

---

Box 81.5

Ocular causes of a right head tilt

I. Nystagmus
   A. Infantile
   B. Acquired
II. Strabismus
   A. Vertical muscle problems
      1. Right eye/left eye
         a) Innervational causes
         b) Mechanical causes
   B. Cyclotropia
   C. Horizontal muscle problems
   D. Paradoxical head tilt
   E. Ocular tilt reaction
III. Refractive errors

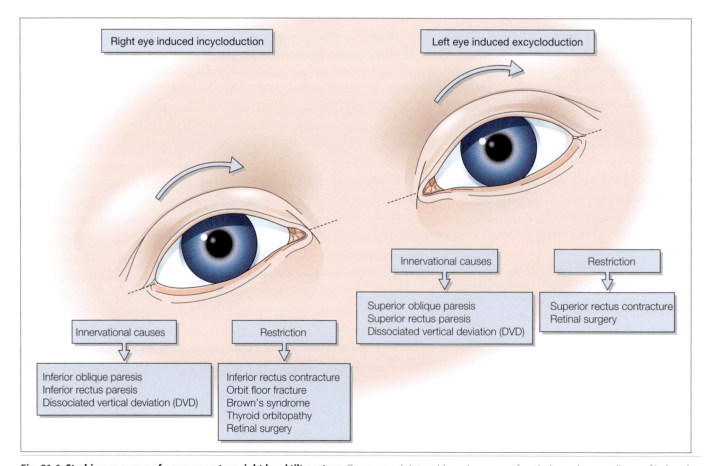

Fig. 81.6 Strabismus causes of a compensatory right head tilt posture. One approach is to address the causes of vertical muscle anomalies or of induced or compensatory cycloduction of one or both eyes. The etiologies are classified into innervational and restrictive etiologies, as illustrated.

shoulder compared to that on tilting to the other shoulder. In most cases the vertical heterotropia is minimal or absent when the compensatory posture is adopted.

For the right eye Innervational causes include inferior oblique paresis, inferior rectus paresis, and dissociated vertical deviation (DVD). Inferior oblique paresis creates an incomitant hypotropia, minimized on tilting to the ipsilateral side.[6,37-39] Most cases are congenital and benign. Acquired cases are usually caused by facial trauma, dog bites, and myasthenia gravis. The head tilt may be accompanied by a face turn or chin-up position.[38] Inferior rectus paresis can also lead to a head tilt to the ipsilateral shoulder.[39]

DVD is frequent in the infantile strabismus complex. The spontaneous upward and excyclotropic drift of one eye can be large and cosmetically displeasing (see Chapter 88). It may be associated with a head tilt posture to the side of the eye with the hyperdeviation or to the contralateral side.[11,40,41]

Mechanical causes include a contracture of the inferior rectus muscle causing a hypotropia smaller and better controlled on tilt to the ipsilateral shoulder. This can arise after chronic fixation by the fellow eye affected by a depressor weakness, such as a superior oblique paresis.[2] A blow-out fracture or thyroid orbitopathy can create a head tilt posture by the same mechanism, but also cyclodiplopia may be a cause.[6,40] Unilateral Brown's syndrome may rarely cause an ipsilateral head tilt.[6,39]

For the left eye The most common innervational disorder that leads to a head tilt is a superior oblique paresis.[6,14,39,40] A head tilt is usually the dominant posture even if a patient has other components including a face turn or chin-down posture.[4,14,22,27,31,39] The patient typically has a hypertropia of the paretic eye that increases on gaze to the contralateral side and on ipsilateral head tilt (the Bielschowsky head tilt test). The child compensates by tilting the head to the opposite shoulder to minimize the hyperdeviation and maintain fusion.[31,37,39] A right head tilt posture would compensate for a left superior oblique paresis.

DVD may show a head tilt to the side contralateral to the eye manifesting the hypertropia,[2,9,40,41] but it may also be seen as a head tilt to the hyper side. A compensatory head tilt can also arise with the rare isolated paresis of a superior rectus muscle.[6,40] If the left superior rectus were weak, the resulting left hypotropia would be expected to worsen on tilting to the ipsilateral shoulder, and lessen on tilting to the right shoulder. This finding is the final step of the three-step test to differentiate a left superior rectus paresis from a right superior oblique paresis.[37] However, there are also cases of superior rectus paresis that lead to compensatory tilts to the ipsilateral side.[39]

A mechanical disorder causing a head tilt is a contracture or fibrosis of a superior rectus muscle. This can be idiopathic or secondary to thyroid orbitopathy or a chronic superior oblique paresis. Contracture of the left superior rectus muscle creates a large hyperdeviation on tilt to the left shoulder which lessens on tilt to the right shoulder.[42]

Cyclotropia

Cyclotropia of one eye causes a head tilt that may be a sensory compensation for disinclination of the retinal meridians of the fixating eye:[4,6,22,27,43] if a patient fixates with an excyclotropic left eye, it may promote a tilt of the head to the right

shoulder.[22,43] It can also occur after a scleral buckle or macular translocation surgery.[6,31]

Horizontal muscle problems

There are rare cases of horizontal tropias, usually esotropias that are larger on tilt to one side than the other. Some cases may be due to congenital nystagmus that is worse on head tilt to one side and where convergence is used as a dampening strategy. The patient tends to tilt to the opposite shoulder where the nystagmus intensity is less and little or no convergence dampening is required. However, there are other cases where nystagmus dampening may not be the only factor. The esotropia differs on right versus left tilt.[6] This has been described in Down's syndrome.[44]

Paradoxical head tilt

Occasionally a patient will adopt a paradoxical head tilt to maximize the separation of images to facilitate suppression or ignoring of one image.[6,9,22,31] This occurs in 2% to 3% of cases of superior oblique paresis presenting with head posture.[22]

Ocular tilt reaction

This is a triad of vertical divergence of the eyes, bilateral ocular torsion, and tilting of the head resulting from a lesion of either the vestibular nucleus or its connections to the contralateral interstitial nucleus of Cajal.[2,7,9,45] The ocular torsion characteristically is ipsiversive (if the head is tilted to the right shoulder, the right eye is excyclotorted while the left eye is incyclotorted). The ipsilateral eye, in this case the right eye, is hypotropic.[7,46]

Refractive errors

High astigmatism in the fixating eye can induce a head tilt, especially if the cylinder is oblique.[4,6,9] Correction of the astigmatic error alleviates the posture.

Bilaterally dislocated lenses may cause a head tilt to place the eyes in a position that optimizes the refractive correction.[47]

Diagnostic considerations

The approach to torticollis can be summarized in Figure 81.7. The main focus is to differentiate ocular from non-ocular causes. In the examination of a child with torticollis, the ocular causes must be ruled out before a non-ocular basis can be considered.

There are several clinical tests that are helpful in the assessment (see Chapters 7, 72, and 89).

Observation

Physical features

The presence of facial asymmetry or dysmorphism, neck deformities, or anomalies of the trunk or the extremities suggest either a musculoskeletal cause or a chronic ocular muscle palsy. Nystagmus or a manifest strabismus can help the examiner focus on specific ocular conditions.

Observing the child

Watching the child for an extended period determines whether the torticollis is consistent. Does it manifest only under certain conditions, such as with fixation on fine visual targets, or with reading.

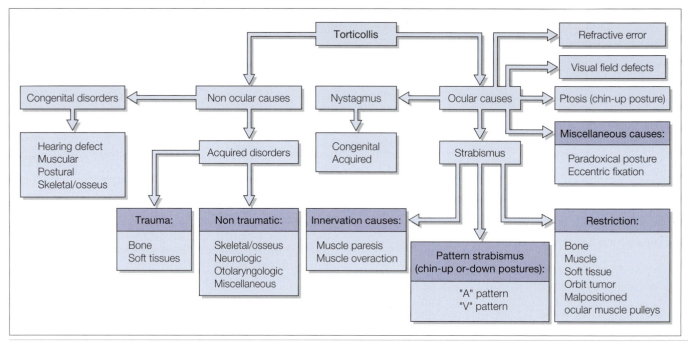

Fig. 81.7 Differential diagnosis of torticollis in children. The causes are divided into non-ocular and ocular causes (ocular torticollis). The non-ocular disorders include congenital and acquired conditions. Nystagmus, strabismus, and refractive errors must be ruled out as possible etiologies for any head posture orientation, whereas other etiologies apply to selected orientations.

Observe a patient with nystagmus for several minutes. A periodic alternation of a head posture suggests PAN, whereas a thrusting of the head with changes in fixation is characteristic of ocular motor apraxia (saccadic initiation failure). The orientation of the posture in all three planes must be noted, especially if it changes with different tasks.

Review of old photographs or videotapes

Documentation from the early life can confirm the chronic nature of a head posture especially when the time of onset is unclear. Serial photographs provided by the family can be useful.

Occlusion of one eye

If a child has ocular torticollis to maintain binocularity, then occluding one eye abolishes or reduces the magnitude of the posture. However, this test can be falsely negative if a chronic problem has led to a "habit" posture in addition to the original compensatory head position.

Eye movements

By asking the child to move the eyes into the nine diagnostic positions of gaze the examiner can detect an incomitant strabismus or a nystagmus null zone. An alternative is to move the head from its abnormal orientation into a position opposite to that adopted. This may reveal a zone of increased nystagmus intensity or a larger heterotropia.

Measuring the head posture

In addition to documenting the orientation of the posture, measuring it with an orthopedic goniometer or torticollometer may assist in documenting change in the head posture.[48,49]

Visual fields

In cases where strabismus or nystagmus does not seem to be causative, it is helpful to identify a hemifield or altitudinal field defect.

Refraction

One cause of vision-driven head postures is an uncorrected or partially corrected refractive error, or an incorrect prescription. A refraction is essential and a trial of spectacles may eliminate the head posture.

Fundus examination

The detection of any anomalies such as retinal traction or fundus pathology can account for some forms of head postures, and the evaluation of the fundus for cyclotropia can help confirm some cases of oblique muscle paresis or overaction. Indirect or direct ophthalmoscopy may also detect low-amplitude nystagmus that may not be seen on direct examination.

Eye movement recordings

In cases where the ocular diagnosis is not clearly evident after a thorough examination, sensitive eye movement recordings may reveal subclinical nystagmus. The waveform may determine the etiology and guide further management.

Palpation of the neck muscles

In musculoskeletal torticollis, the neck muscles are tight. Passive straightening of the head is difficult. In CMT the pseudotumor in the neck can be located.[1,3,5] In contrast, it is rare for cases of ocular torticollis to develop the extreme neck muscle contracture seen with congenital or early-onset musculoskeletal anomalies.[14,22]

Consultations with other specialists

Orthopedic surgeons, otolaryngologists, neurologists, neurosurgeons, physiotherapists, and occupational therapists may be part of the treatment team.[14] Imaging may be indicated.

References

1. Boutros GS, Al-Mateen M. Non-ophthalmological causes of torticollis. Am Orthoptic J 1995; 45: 68–74.
4. Rubin SE, Wagner RS. Ocular torticollis. Surv Ophthalmol 1986; 30: 366–76.
5. Nucci P, Curiel B. Abnormal head posture due to ocular problems: a review. Curr Pediatr Rev 2009; 5: 105–11.
6. Kushner BJ. Ocular causes of abnormal head postures. Ophthalmology 1979; 86: 2115–25.
7. Wong AMF. Eye Movement Disorders. New York: Oxford University Press; 2008: 24–45, 137–46.
9. Caldeira JA. Abnormal head posture: an ophthalmological approach. Binocul Vis Strabismus Q 2000; 15: 237–9.
12. Greenberg MF, Pollard ZF. Ocular plagiocephaly: ocular torticollis with skull and facial asymmetry. Ophthalmology 2000; 107: 173–9.
14. Nucci P, Kushner BJ, Serafino M, Orzalesi N. A multidisciplinary study of the ocular, orthopedic, and neurologic causes of abnormal head postures in children. Am J Ophthalmol 2005; 140: 65–8.
17. Webb M. Acute torticollis: identifying and treating the underlying cause. Postgrad Med 1987; 82: 121–8.
18. Kumandas S, Per H, Gumus H, et al. Torticollis secondary to posterior fossa and cervical spinal tumors: report of five cases and literature review. Neurosurg Rev 2006; 29: 333–8.
20. DeBenedictis CN, Allen JC, Kodsi SR. Brainstem tumor presenting with tearing, photophobia, and torticollis. J AAPOS 2010; 14: 369–70.
21. Snyder CH. Paroxysmal torticollis in infancy: a possible form of labyrinthitis. Am J Dis Child 1969; 117: 458–60.
22. Kraft SP, O'Donoghue EP, Roarty JD. Improvement of compensatory head postures after strabismus surgery. Ophthalmology 1992; 99: 1301–8.
23. Hertle RW, Zhu X. Oculographic and clinical characterization of thirty-seven children with anomalous head postures, nystagmus, and strabismus: the basis of a clinical algorithm. J AAPOS 2000; 4: 25–32.
24. Dell'Osso LF, Flynn JF. Congenital nystagmus surgery: a quantitative evaluation of the effects. Arch Ophthalmol 1979; 97: 462–9.
25. Scott WE, Kraft SP. Surgical treatment of compensatory head position in congenital nystagmus. J Pediatr Ophthalmol Strabismus 1984; 21: 85–95.
26. Hertle RW. Nystagmus in infancy and childhood. In: Wilson ME, Saunders RA, Trivedi RH, editors. Pediatric Ophthalmology: Current Thought and A Practical Guide. Berlin: Springer-Verlag; 2009: 243–54.
27. von Noorden GK, Ruttum M. Torticollis in paralysis of the trochlear nerve. Am Orthoptic J 1983; 33: 16–20.
29. Hoyt CS, Good WV. Ocular motor adaptations to congenital hemianopia. Binocul Vis Eye Muscle Surg Q 1993; 8: 125–6.
30. Donahue SP, Haun AK. Exotropia and face turn in children with homonymous hemianopia. J Neuro-ophthalmology 2007; 27: 304–7.
31. von Noorden GK, Murray E, Wong SY. Superior oblique paralysis: a review of 270 cases. Arch Ophthalmol 1986; 104: 1771–6.
34. Krzizok TH, Kaufmann H, Traupe H. Elucidation of restrictive motility in high myopia by magnetic resonance imaging. Arch Ophthalmol 1997; 115: 1019–27.
36. Ziffer AJ, Rosenbaum AL, Demer JL, et al. Congenital double elevator palsy: vertical saccadic velocity utilizing the scleral search coil technique. J Pediatr Ophthalmol Strabismus 1992; 29: 142–9.
37. Parks MM. Isolated cyclovertical muscle palsy. Arch Ophthalmol 1958; 60: 1027–35.
38. Pollard ZF. Diagnosis and treatment of inferior oblique palsy. J Pediatr Ophthalmol Strabismus 1993; 30: 15–8.
41. Santiago AP, Rosenbaum AL. Dissociated vertical deviation and head tilts. J AAPOS 1998; 2: 5–11.
43. von Noorden GK. Clinical observations in cyclodeviations. Ophthalmology 1979; 86: 1451–61.
44. Lueder GT, Arthur B, Garibaldi D, et al. Head tilt-dependent esotropia associated with trisomy 21. Ophthalmology 2004; 111: 596–9.
46. Donahue SP, Lavin PJM, Hamed LM. Tonic ocular tilt reaction simulating a superior oblique palsy: diagnostic confusion with the three-step test. Arch Ophthalmol 1999; 117: 347–52.
49. Hald ES, Hertle RW, Yang D. Application of a digital head-posture measuring system in children. Am J Ophthalmol 2011; 151: 66–70.

 Access the complete reference list online at
http://www.expertconsult.com

Congenital cranial dysinnervation disorders

Neil R Miller • Thomas M Bosley

Chapter contents

The congenital cranial dysinnervation disorders (CCDDs) result from abnormal development of individual or multiple cranial nerve nuclei or their axonal connections. Most are either proven or suspected to have a genetic basis.[1,2] Although many of these conditions are characterized only by abnormal extraocular muscle innervation, facial innervation, or both, others have associated systemic and/or neurologic abnormalities, such as cerebrovascular, cardiovascular, and skeletal malformations that also are attributable to the underlying genetic defect.[2] At present, a total of seven disease genes and ten phenotypes have been identified.[2] In this chapter, only those CCDDs characterized wholly or in part by abnormalities of eye movement will be discussed. These include the three main types of congenital fibrosis of the extraocular muscles (CFEOM), Duane's retraction syndromes (DRS), homeobox A1 (*HOXA1*) spectrum, horizontal gaze palsy with progressive scoliosis (HGPPS), and Möbius' syndrome.

Congenital fibrosis of extraocular muscles

This group of disorders is characterized by congenital ocular motility abnormalities, congenital ptosis, and fibrotic extraocular muscles. To date, three primary CFEOM main phenotypes have been described – CFEOM1, CFEOM2, and CFEOM3 – with CFEOM3 having three phenotypic variants: CFEOM3A, CFEOM3B, and CFEOM3C.[2,3]

Congenital fibrosis of the extraocular muscles type 1 (MIM #135700)

CFEOM1 is the most common of the CFEOM phenotypes. It is autosomal dominant with full penetrance and has been reported worldwide.[4] It is characterized by congenital bilateral ptosis and a bilateral ocular motility disorder with the globes infraducted in primary position, restricted upgaze, and variably restricted horizontal gaze. These abnormalities result in many affected individuals adopting a chin-up head posture (Fig. 82.1). These patients have positive forced ductions and misdirected eye movements such as a marked synergistic convergence on attempted upgaze. They are rarely noted to have retraction. Neuropathologic studies reveal significant atrophy and fibrosis of the superior rectus and levator palpebrae muscles, with variable reduction in the size of the other extraocular muscles. The ocular motor nerves are absent or hypoplastic, and the diameter of the optic nerves is reduced by 30–40%.[5] CFEOM1 is caused by a heterozygous missense mutation in *KIF21A*, a gene located on chromosome 12 (12q12).[3] This gene encodes a kinesin microtubule-associated protein associated with anterograde organelle transport in neurons.[6]

Congenital fibrosis of the exraocular muscles type 2 (MIM #602078)

CFEOM2 is an autosomal recessive disorder characterized by bilateral ptosis associated with bilaterally absent adduction, upgaze, and downgaze (Fig. 82.2).[7] Although abduction is present, it is limited and the pupils are often irregularly shaped and sized and non-reactive to both light and near stimulation. The appearance is that of bilateral oculomotor (third) nerve palsies and neuroimaging has shown what appears to be bilateral absence of the third nerves.[8] This condition is caused by homozygous mutations in the *PHOX2A* gene located on chromosome 11 (11q13.3–q13.4)[7] that codes for a homeodomain transcription factor expressed predominantly in developing oculomotor and trochlear neurons and that is essential for their survival. Mutations alter the factor sufficiently that the oculomotor (and probably trochlear) nerves never develop.

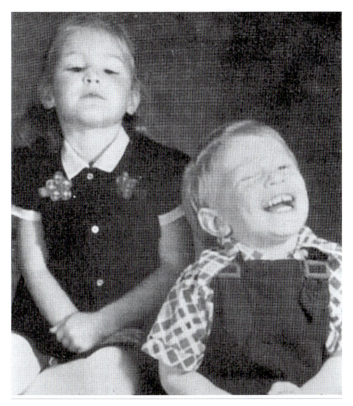

Fig. 82.1 Congenital fibrosis syndrome type I (CFEOM1) in a brother and sister. Because of their bilateral ptosis and deficient upgaze, both children have adopted a head posture with the chin elevated. (Image courtesy of Dr Stewart M Wolff.)

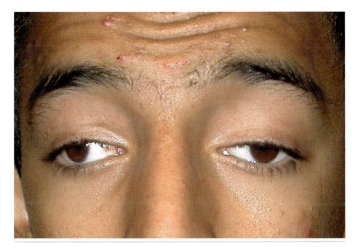

Fig. 82.2 Congenital fibrosis syndrome type 2 (CFEOM2). This patient with homozygous mutations in *PHOX2A* demonstrates the typical congenital exotropia and bilateral ptosis (note furrowed brow to elevate lids) associated with CFEOM2. He had no upgaze or downgaze of either eye, no adduction of either eye, and mild limitation of abduction of both eyes. His pupils were both mid-position, irregular in outline, and unreactive to light.

Congenital fibrosis of the extraocular muscles type 3

CFEOM3 is an autosomal dominantly inherited disorder that has clinical features similar to those of CFEOM1 except that they are more variable and sometimes associated with the ability to elevate the eyes above the midline.[9] The phenotypic

variability results, at least in part, because the condition may be caused by heterozygous mutations in at least two genes: *TUBB3* (CFEOM3A; MIM #600638) and, rarely, *KIF21A* (CFEOM3B).[10,11]

Several different missense mutations may occur in the *TUBB3* gene which codes for a component of microtubules. Thus, some patients with CFEOM3A have isolated ocular motor deficits (some even have isolated absence of upgaze), whereas others have bilateral facial weakness, peripheral sensory or sensorimotor neuropathies, wrist and finger contractures, cognitive dysfunction, or a combination of these features. Magnetic resonance imaging has shown dysgenesis of the corpus callosum and anterior commissure in some cases.[11] Patients have been described who have a phenotype similar to CFEOM1 except for the presence of some upgaze and who have a mutation in *KIF21A*. They are said to have CFEOM3B.[2] A single family has been described in which three generations have what appears to be CFEOM3 but who carry a reciprocal translocation involving chromosomes 2q and 13q,[12] termed CFEOM3C (MIM #609384).

Practical management of CFEOM patients

Once the diagnosis of CFEOM is made, it is crucial to help the patients and their parents live with their complex and unremitting problems, particularly when they have not only ocular motor deficits and ptosis, but also systemic and/or neurologic deficits. The outlook is guarded, and, as the condition is rare, even the most experienced pediatric ophthalmologist can offer little in the way of a confident individual prognosis. Nevertheless, all children with CFEOM should undergo a refraction, be treated for amblyopia with part-time occlusion therapy or atropinization when appropriate (see Chapter 70), and be evaluated periodically throughout their period of visual development. In patients whose ptosis requires surgical treatment, one must be careful not to overcorrect, as this may result in exposure keratopathy because of the restricted eye movements and lack of a Bell's phenomenon in most of these individuals. We find that a sling procedure is usually more effective than a levator resection and, in addition, allows overcorrection to be more easily managed. If a decision is made to perform a levator resection, the eyelids should be raised only so that they are above the pupillary axis.

Unfortunately, the strabismus associated with CFEOM is not particularly amenable to surgery. Results are poor because of the marked lack of ocular motility even when the eyes are able to be aligned in primary position by performing very large recessions and occasionally resections.[13] Thus, the patient's parents should be counseled accordingly so that they have realistic expectations regarding the goals of the surgery.

Duane's retraction syndrome

Duane's retraction syndrome (DRS) is the most common CCDD affecting ocular motility.[2] There are several variants; however, the most common presentation is characterized by marked limitation or absence of abduction, variable limitation of adduction, and palpebral fissure narrowing with globe retraction on attempted adduction (Figs 82.3–82.5). Vertical ocular movements are often noted on adduction, most frequently in an upward direction (see Fig. 82.5).

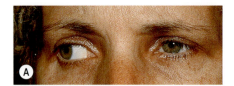 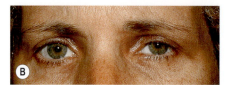 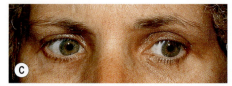

Fig. 82.3 Unilateral (left) Duane's retraction syndrome type 1 in a 42-year-old woman. Note limitation of abduction of left eye and widening of left palpebral fissure on attempted left gaze. On attempted right gaze, there is mild limitation of adduction of the left eye and narrowing of the left palpebral fissure.

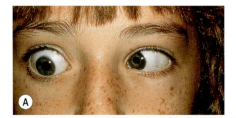 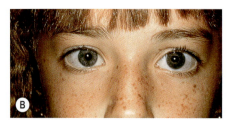 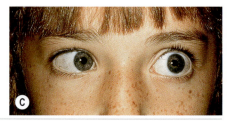

Fig. 82.4 Bilateral Duane's retraction syndrome type 1 in a 4-year-old girl. Note bilateral moderate limitation of abduction, bilateral mild limitation of adduction, and widening of the ipsilateral palpebral fissure on attempted right and left gaze. (Images courtesy of Dr Michael X Repka.)

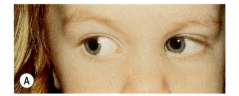 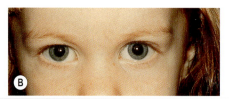 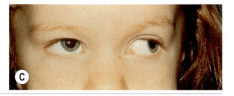

Fig. 82.5 Unilateral (right) Duane's retraction syndrome type 2 in a 3-year-old girl. Note full abduction of right eye on right gaze and moderate limitation of adduction with upshoot of right eye on attempted left gaze.

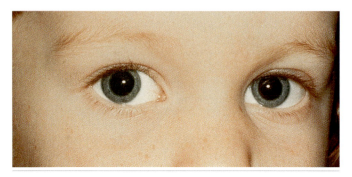

Fig. 82.6 Unilateral (right) Duane's retraction syndrome type 2. Same patient as that in Fig. 82.5 showing patient's typical head position consisting of a face turn to the left to maintain binocularity.

In most cases, DRS is unilateral (see Figs 82.3 and 82.5), but bilateral DRS occurs in 15–20% of affected patients (see Fig. 82.4). The syndrome occurs more commonly in females than males, and the left eye is more frequently affected than the right. Gaze is usually directed toward the side of the unaffected eye and, in some instances, the face is turned toward the affected side to allow binocular single vision. Visual symptoms are conspicuous by their absence. Vision is almost always normal unless there is associated anisometropia and amblyopia. Thus, in the majority of cases, no treatment is necessary unless the patient has a marked head turn (Fig. 82.6).

Early histologic studies demonstrated abnormalities of the lateral or medial rectus muscles and led investigators to conclude that DRS was a local, myogenic phenomenon. It was generally believed that the cause of the abduction deficiency was fibrosis of the lateral rectus muscle and that limitation of adduction was caused by a posterior insertion of the medial rectus muscle. Adhesions between the medial rectus muscle and the medial orbital wall were also reported. Subsequently, electromyographical studies, magnetic resonance imaging, and histological studies established that the disorder is caused by absence or hypoplasia of the abducens nerve with innervation of the ipsilateral lateral rectus muscle by a branch of the oculomotor nerve.[14-16]

A modest number of patients with DRS have associated congenital neurologic deficits that localize to the brainstem, such as crocodile tears and sensorineural hearing loss or structural defects involving ocular, skeletal, and neural structures.[2]

Most cases of DRS are sporadic, but familial unilateral and bilateral cases occur.[17] Familial DRS usually is transmitted in an autosomal dominant pattern. Affected individuals in such families show substantial clinical diversity.

Duane's retraction syndrome 1 (MIM #126800)

In the DURS1 phenotype, the syndrome may be unilateral (see Fig. 82.3) or bilateral (see Fig. 82.4) and, depending on the size of the deletion, may occur in association with other features including mental retardation, branchio-oto-renal syndrome, genital tract anomalies, and other somatic mutations. The gene disrupted by overlapping cytogenic abnormalities at the DURS1 locus located on chromosome 8(8q13) may be CPAH, a carboxypeptidase gene with eight exons.[18,19]

Duane's retraction syndrome 2 (MIM #604356)

In the DURS2 phenotype, the condition is almost always bilateral (Fig. 82.5). Associated findings can include a variety of vertical deviations such as apparent underaction of the superior oblique and dissociated vertical deviation. Patients have been noted to have decreased abduction with or without decreased adduction. No patients have had adduction defects without abduction defects. Amblyopia is common. No associated somatic abnormalities have been found. Inheritance is autosomal dominant. The responsible gene, CHN1, is located on chromosome 2 (2q31).[20-22] It is involved with ocular motor path finding during the development of the abducens nerve and, to a lesser extent, the oculomotor nerve.[23,24]

Duane's radial ray syndrome (Okihiro syndrome, MIM #607323)

This condition is characterized by a unilateral or bilateral Duane syndrome associated with radial dysplasia that also may be unilateral or bilateral. Thumb hypoplasia is most common, but the defect ranges from hypoplasia of the thenar eminence to phocomelic limbs. The syndrome often includes deafness and somatic malformations. Inheritance is autosomal dominant and is caused by truncating SALL4 mutations on chromosome 20 (20q13).[25,26] SALL genes encode putative zinc finger transcription factors.

Wildervanck's cervico-oculo-acoustic syndrome (MIM #314600)

This syndrome of congenital deafness, Klippel-Feil anomaly (fusion of cervical vertebrae giving a short neck), and bilateral abduction palsy with retraction on adduction (Duane's phenomenon) is almost completely limited to females, suggesting X-linked dominance with lethality in the hemizygous male.

Practical management of Duane's retraction syndrome

The majority of patients with DRS have few problems other than a head turn and do not require surgery. Indeed, the head turn allows these patients to develop and maintain binocular single vision; however, surgery is appropriate for patients with significantly abnormal head posture associated with strabismus. When the abnormal head posture is associated with an esotropia, the optimum procedure is an ipsilateral medial rectus recession or, in some cases, bilateral medial rectus recessions. Horizontal transposition of the vertical rectus muscles and posterior fixation sutures may be appropriate in some cases, but the results of straightforward medial rectus recessions are sufficiently good in nearly all cases to make these procedures unnecessary.

Recession of the ipsilateral lateral rectus is appropriate for the rare cases of abnormal head position associated with exotropia, with the amount of the recession varying with the angle in the primary position.

Eye retraction and the consequent narrowing of the palpebral fissure is a cardinal feature of DRS and is caused by co-contraction of the medial and lateral recti. Only very rarely are these phenomena alone cosmetically bothersome enough

to warrant surgery. Nevertheless, weakening of the medial or lateral rectus for other reasons, such as an anomalous head position, is invariably accompanied by a reduction in retraction.

It is unusual for young children to have sufficient retraction to need surgery, but some have increasing retraction caused by one of the horizontal rectus muscles, usually the lateral rectus, being "tight," with an abnormal forced duction test. If this becomes cosmetically significant, a large lateral rectus recession may be helpful, although it usually must be combined with a recession of the ipsilateral medial rectus to prevent further strabismus. This is an effective procedure but the results are somewhat unpredictable; thus, appropriate preoperative counseling is mandatory.

As noted above, many patients with DRS have upward or downward movements of the affected eye on attempted horizontal gaze. Although some of these movements may be related to the branch of the oculomotor nerve that is innervating the lateral rectus muscle, most appear to result from progressive stiffness of the lateral rectus, which on attempted adduction slips under (to give an upshoot) or over (downshoot) the globe. Accordingly, these movements usually can be treated effectively by a large recession of the affected lateral rectus, balanced by a medial rectus recession on the same side. The amounts recessed depend on the amount of the shoot, the magnitude of any strabismus, and the presence of marked retraction. Some have suggested posterior fixation sutures on the lateral rectus, combined with recession. Another option is to split the lateral rectus longitudinally and then recess the two split portions of the muscle, elevating the superior portion and infraplacing the inferior portion thus cradling the eye in between the "Y-split" portions.

Human homeobox A1 spectrum (MIM #601536)

The HOXA1 spectrum is autosomal recessive and characterized by bilateral DRS with absent abduction and reduced adduction (Fig. 82.7) associated with deafness, cerebrovascular and cardiovascular malformations, and, in some cases, autism that may be profound.[27-29] Some affected persons, particularly those with the Native American variant, have associated facial weakness, cognitive dysfunction, central hypoventilation, or a combination of these features.[30] Magnetic resonance imaging has demonstrated absence of both abducens nerves and almost completely absent development of the acoustic and vestibular structures in the petrous bone of many patients.[27-29]

The HOXA1 spectrum is caused by homozygous mutations in the HOXA1 gene on chromosome 7 (7p15.3), a gene that has been shown in animal models to be critical for hindbrain development.[3]

Practical management of the HOXA1 spectrum

Patients with this condition may be quite impaired by their non-ophthalmologic disease. Nevertheless, it is appropriate to insure that they have an adequate refraction on a regular basis and that any significant refractive error is corrected with spectacles. Most do not have strabismus and, thus, do not require extraocular muscle surgery; however, it is appropriate to consider surgery if the parents request it and if there is no contraindication to general anesthesia.

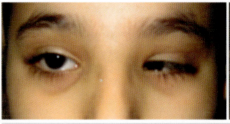
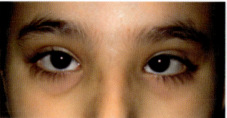
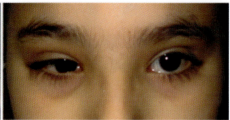

Fig. 82.7 Human homeobox A1 (*HOXA1*) spectrum. This patient with homozygous mutations in *HOXA1* has the classic triad of congenital bilateral type 3 Duane's retraction syndrome, deafness due to almost complete absence of inner ear development bilaterally, and cerebrovascular malformations. She has a moderate esotropia in primary gaze, no abduction of either eye, and limited adduction of both eyes associated with obvious globe retraction and narrowing of the palpebral fissure; however, she has full upgaze and downgaze bilaterally.

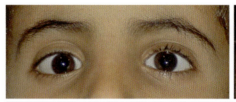
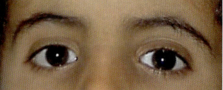
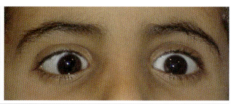

Fig. 82.8 Horizontal gaze palsy with progressive scoliosis. This young man with homozygous mutations in *ROBO3* has a horizontal gaze palsy and a severe progressive scoliosis. His eyes are orthophoric in primary gaze, and he has excellent visual acuity in both eyes, binocular fusion, and no diplopia. He has essentially no conjugate gaze to the right, and can only move both eyes minimally to the left; however, he has full upgaze and downgaze. He also has small-amplitude horizontal pendular nystagmus. The disturbance of ocular motility was present at birth.

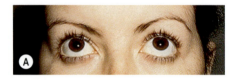
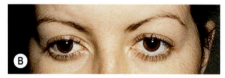
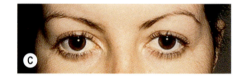
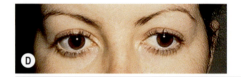
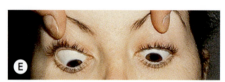

Fig. 82.9 Horizontal gaze palsy with progressive scoliosis. Note intact vertical movements. (A) Patient looking up. (B) Patient in primary gaze. (C) Patient attempting to look right. (D) Patient attempting to look left. (E) Patient looking down.

Horizontal gaze palsy and progressive scoliosis (MIM #607313)

HGPPS is an autosomal recessive syndrome characterized by complete or near complete bilateral horizontal gaze limitation (Figs 82.8 and 82.9), normal vertical gaze, variable convergence, variable congenital nystagmus, and asynchronous blinking.[31] Scoliosis begins in early childhood and may be both rapidly progressive and severe. Magnetic resonance imaging shows intact abducens nerves but deep anterior and posterior clefts in the medulla and lower pons, a large fourth ventricle, and no decussation of the axons of the corticospinal tract, medial lemniscus, or superior cerebellar peduncle.[32,33]

The mutations responsible for this disorder are in the gene *ROBO3* located on chromosome 11 (11q23–q25), a gene responsible for producing a transmembrane cell adhesion molecule that is a receptor for axon guidance during development of the hindbrain.[3,34]

The explanation for absence of horizontal gaze in patients with HGPPS is unclear; however, it may be due to aberrant supranuclear input onto the abducens motorneurons by axons from the paramedian pontine reticular formation that cannot cross the midline and/or to inability of developing axons in the medial longitudinal fasciculus to cross the midline.[35]

Practical management of horizontal gaze palsy and progressive scoliosis

Because the horizontal gaze deficit in patients with HGPPS is always bilateral and symmetric, such patients almost never have diplopia and, thus, do not require treatment for their ocular motility disturbance; however, they often benefit from surgery to correct their scoliosis.

Möbius' syndrome (MIM #157900) and its variants

Congenital facial weakness can be accompanied by an ocular motility disorder that usually includes abduction weakness (Video 82.1). The eponym "Möbius' syndrome" is reserved for the congenital combination of non-progressive facial weakness and at least an abduction deficit in one or both eyes. Möbius' syndrome usually is a sporadic disorder frequently accompanied by lingual or pharyngeal dysfunction, craniofacial dysmorphisms, and limb malformations. Several cytogenetic abnormalities have been reported in association with Möbius' syndrome.

Characteristically, the defect in Möbius' syndrome involves the face and horizontal gaze mechanisms bilaterally. Affected patients have a mask-like facies, with the mouth constantly held open (Figs 82.10 and 82.11). In some infants, this defect prevents adequate nursing and the appearance may interfere with normal bonding and attachment. The eyelids often cannot be completely closed, and, in some patients, they cannot be closed at all. There may be excess lacrimation and epiphora. Some patients have only an esotropia (see Fig. 82.10) associated with unilateral or bilateral limitation of abduction, and some may even be able to converge. In most cases, however, the eyes are straight but do not move horizontally (see Fig. 82.11). Henderson reviewed 61 cases of Möbius' syndrome in the literature.[36] He found that bilateral abducens palsy was present in 43 cases, unilateral abducens palsy in two cases, and horizontal gaze palsy in the rest. In rare cases, vertical eye movements are also abnormal.

Other congenital defects found in patients with Möbius' syndrome include deafness, webbed fingers or toes, congenital "amputations," supernumerary digits, defects of the muscles of the chest, neck, and tongue, and even absence of the hands, feet, fingers, or toes (Fig. 82.12). Abnormalities of lower cranial nerves, with speech and swallowing difficulties, are extremely common. Occurring less frequently are low-set ears, a small mouth opening, micrognathia, epicanthal folds, congenital heart defects, or a combination of these abnormalities. Tachypnea and other respiratory difficulties occur in some patients with Möbius' syndrome, whereas others have a combination of anosmia and hypogonadotrophic hypogonadism (Kallmann's syndrome). Many patients with Möbius' syndrome have some degree of mental retardation, and some degree of autism also is common.

Patients with Möbius' syndrome who undergo neuroimaging have the same heterogeneity of findings as their variable clinical presentation would suggest. Some show no abnormalities, whereas others have intracranial calcifications, brainstem hypoplasia, or changes consistent with ischemia.

Most cases of Möbius' syndrome are sporadic, although some patients with Mobius-like phenotypes have mutations in TUBB3 or HOXA1.[2] Baraitser concluded that the risk of another affected sibling is no greater than 2% in pedigrees in which the syndrome includes limb abnormalities.[37]

Pathologic findings in patients with Möbius' syndrome were separated by Towfighi et al. into four groups according to the neuropathologic findings in the brainstem nuclei.[38] Group I consisted of four cases with hypoplasia or atrophy of cranial nerve nuclei. Group II consisted of two cases in which, in addition to neuronal loss, there was evidence of active neuronal degeneration in the affected facial nerve nuclei. It was postulated that these neuronal changes were caused by physical injury to the facial nerve, arising from a malformed temporal bone or from application of forceps during delivery. Group III consisted of six cases in which, in addition to a decrease in the number of neurons and reactive changes in the affected cranial nerve nuclei, there was frank necrosis of the tegmentum of the lower pons. These lesions are probably acquired later during fetal life rather than during early embryonic development, and both hypoxia and viral infections are implicated in their etiology. The final group, Group IV, consisted of three cases in which no lesions were found in the brainstem or cranial nerves. A primary myopathy may have been responsible for these cases.

The diversity of pathologic findings in patients with Möbius' syndrome suggests that the syndrome is a heterogeneous group of congenital disorders caused by genetic and/or developmental defects related to a variety of insults, such as ischemia or toxic effects of prenatal prescribed drugs including misoprostol, a synthetic prostaglandin, or one of the benzodiazepines.

Practical management of Möbius' syndrome

Most patients with Möbius' syndrome do not require strabismus surgery because they have bilateral and symmetric horizontal gaze paresis; however, some children have strabismus

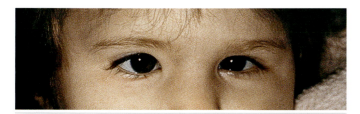

Fig. 82.10 Möbius' syndrome in a 3-year-old girl. Note esotropia and bilateral facial weakness. (Image courtesy of Dr Michael X Repka.)

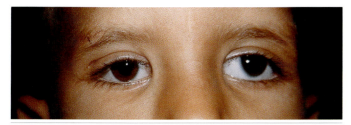

Fig. 82.11 Möbius' syndrome in a 6-year-old boy. Note bilateral facial weakness associated with mild bilateral ptosis. The patient's eyes are fairly straight. (Image courtesy of Dr Michael X Repka.)

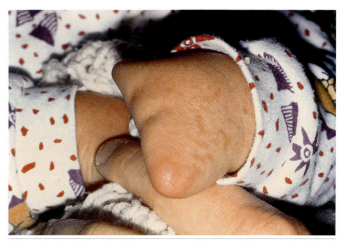

Fig. 82.12 Absent fingers in same patient as that seen in Figure 82.11. (Image courtesy of Dr Michael X Repka.)

characterized by an esotropia. Treatment in such cases includes bilateral medial rectus recessions, medial rectus recession combined with lateral rectus resection, and, in severe cases, muscle transposition. A reasonable cosmetic appearance can be achieved in most cases, although more than one operation may be required.

Patients with Möbius' syndrome who have associated corneal anesthesia are at risk of developing exposure keratopathy, particularly when there also is an abnormality of blinking. This complication is of particular concern in infants and young children, who may require a temporary or even permanent tarsorrhaphy when simple corneal lubrication is not sufficient to provide adequate corneal lubrication.

Summary

Based on both neuropathologic and genetic evidence, it is clear that there exists a group of disorders for which absent or anomalous innervation of the extraocular and/or facial muscles is the most likely pathophysiology. These disorders are appropriately referred to as "congenital cranial dysinnervation disorders" and include CFEOM types 1, 2, and 3, Duane's retraction syndromes 1 and 2, the Duane's radial ray syndrome, the *HOXA1* spectrum, congenital horizontal gaze palsy with progressive scoliosis, and Möbius' syndrome. The above list of clinical phenotypes and genetic loci is almost certainly incomplete and will undoubtedly increase with time.

References

1. Gutkowski NJ, Bosley TM, Engle EC. 110th ENMC International Workship: the congenital cranial dysinnervation disorders (CCCDs). Naarden, The Netherlands, 25–27 October, 2002. Neuromusc Disod 2003; 13: 573–8.

2. Oystreck DT, Engle EC, Bosley TM. Recent progress in understanding congenital cranial dysinnervation disorders. J Neuro-ophthalmol 2011; 31: 69–77.

3. Engle EC. Oculomotility disorders arising from disruptions in brainstem motor neuron development. Arch Neurol 2007; 64: 633–7.

4. Traboulsi EI, Engle EC. Mutations in KIF21A are responsible for CFEOM1 worldwide. Ophthalmic Genet 2004; 25: 237–9.

6. Yamada K, Andrews C, Chan WM, et al. Heterozygous mutations of the inesin KIF21A in congenital fibrosis of the extraocular muscles type 1 (CFEOM1). Nat Genet 2003; 35: 318–21.

7. Nakano M, Yamada K, Fain J, et al. Homozygous mutations in ARIX(PHOX2A) result in congenital fibrosis of the extraocular muscles type 2. Nat Genet 2001; 29: 315–20.

8. Bosley TM, Oystreck DT, Robertson RL, et al. Neurological features of congenital fibrosis of the extraocular muscles type 2 with mutations in PHOX2A. Brain 2006; 129: 2363–74.

9. Doherty EJ, Macy ME, Wang SM, et al. CFEOM3: a new extraocular congenital fibrosis syndrome that maps to 16q24.2-q24.3. Invest Ophthalmol Vis Sci 1999; 40: 1687–94.

11. Tischfield MA, Baris HN, Wu C, et al. Human TUBB3 mutations perturb microtubule dynamics, kinesin interactions, and axon guidance. Cell 2010; 140: 74–87.

12. Aubourg P, Krahn M, Bernard R, et al. Assignment of a new congenital fibrosis of extraocular muscles type 3 (CFEOM3) locus,

FEOM4, based on a balanced translocation t(2;13) (q37.3;q12.11) and identification of candidate genes. J Med Genet 2005; 42: 253–9.

13. Yazdani A, Traboulsi EI. Classification and surgical management of patients with familial and sporadic forms of congenital fibrosis of the extraocular muscles. Ophthalmology 2004; 111: 1035–42.

15. Miller NR, Kiel SM, Green WR, et al. Unilateral Duane's retraction syndrome (type 1). Arch Ophthalmol 1982; 100: 1468–72.

16. Parsa CF, Grant E, Dillon WP Jr, et al. Absence of the abducens nerve in Duane syndrome verified by magnetic resonance imaging. Am J Ophthalmol 1998; 125: 399–401.

18. Pizzuti A, Calabrese G, Bozzali M, et al. A peptidase gene in chromosome 8q is disrupted by a balanced translocation in a Duane syndrome patient. Invest Ophthalmol Vis Sci 2002; 43: 3609–12.

19. Lehman AM, Friedman AM, Chai D, et al. A characteristic syndrome associated with microduplication of 8q12, inclusive of CHD7. Eur J Med Genet 2009; 52: 436–9.

20. Appukuttan B, Gillanders E, Juo SH, et al. Localization of a gene for Duane retraction syndrome to chromosome 2q31. Am J Hum Genet 1999; 65: 1639–46.

21. Evans JC, Frayling TM, Ellard S, et al. Confirmation of linkage of Duane's syndrome and refinement of the disease locus to an 8.8 cM interval on chromosome 2q31. Hum Genet 2000; 106: 636–8.

22. Chan W-M, Miyake N, Zhu-Tam L, et al. Two novel CHN1 mutations in 2 families with Duane retraction syndrome. Arch Ophthalmol 2011; 129: 649–52.

23. Demer JL, Clark RA, Lim KH, et al. Magnetic resonance imaging evidence for widespread orbital dysinnervation in dominant Duane's retraction syndrome linked to the DURS2 locus. Invest Ophthalmol Vis Sci 2007; 48: 194–202.

24. Miyake N, Chilton J, Psatha M, et al. Human CHN1 mutations hyperactivate alpha2-chimaerin and cause Duane's retraction syndrome. Science 2008; 321: 839–43.

25. Al-Baradie R, Yamada K, St. Hilaire C, et al. Duane radial ray syndrome (Okihiro syndrome) maps to 20q13 and results from mutations in SALL4, a new member of the SAL family. Am J Hum Genet 2002; 71: 1195–9.

26. Kohlhase J, Heinrich M, Schubert L, et al. Okihiro syndrome is caused by SALL4 mutations. Hum Mol Genet 2002; 11: 2979–87.

28. Bosley TM, Salih MA, Alorainy IA, et al. Clinical characterization of the HOXA1 syndrome BSAS variant. Neurology 2007; 69: 1245–3.

29. Bosley TM, Alorainy IA, Salih MA, et al. The clinical spectrum of homozygous HOXA1 mutations. Am J Med Genet A 2008; 146: 1235–40.

31. Bosley TM, Salih MA, Jen JC, et al. Neurologic features of horizontal gaze palsy and progressive scoliosis with mutations in ROBO3. Neurology 2005; 64: 1196–203.

32. Pieh C, Lengyel D, Neff A, et al. Brainstem hypoplasia in familial horizontal gaze palsy and scoliosis. Neurology 2002; 59: 462–3.

33. Sicotte NL, Salamon G, Shattuck DW, et al. Diffusion tensor MRI shows abnormal brainstem crossing fibers associated with ROBO3 mutations. Neurology 2006; 67: 519–21.

34. Jen JC, Chan WM, Bosley TM, et al. Mutations in a human ROBO gene disrupt hindbrain axon pathway crossing and morphogenesis. Science 2004; 304: 1509–13.

35. Marillat V, Sabatier C, Failli V, et al. The slit receptor Rig-1/Robo3 controls midline crossing by hindbrain precerebellar neurons and axons. Neuron 2004; 43: 69–79.

38. Towfighi J, Marks K, Palmer E, et al. Möbius syndrome. Neuropathologic observations. Acta Neuropathol 1979; 48: 11–7.

Access the complete reference list online at
http://www.expertconsult.com

Cranial nerve and eye muscle palsies

John S Elston

Introduction

Apart from congenital IVth nerve palsy, childhood congenital and acquired infranuclear ocular motor palsies are uncommon. Because of this and concerns about the potential serious underlying pathology, these cases are usually referred to specialist centers. However, the principles of history taking, examination, diagnosis, and documentation are the same as those applied to more routine ocular motility cases. All ophthalmologists whose practices include child referrals should be familiar with the investigation and management of these cases and establish a network of contacts with pediatric neurology and neuroimaging colleagues to optimize outcomes.

Congenital IIIrd nerve palsy: classification

Bilateral

A. Congenital cranial dysinnervation disorder (CCDD) (see Chapter 82). This is the commonest cause of bilateral congenital IIIrd nerve palsy. Inherited genetic mutations lead to primary maldevelopment of either the IIIrd (CFEOM1) or the IIIrd and IVth cranial nerve nuclei

(CFEOM2). Clinical features include bilateral ptosis and symmetrically reduced elevation and adduction. High resolution MRI shows cranial nerve hypoplasia.[1]

B. Rarely, sporadic bilateral infranuclear congenital IIIrd nerve palsy has been described usually in association with extensive neurodevelopmental anomalies.

Unilateral congenital IIIrd nerve palsy

A. Clinical features suggesting pre- or perinatal peripheral IIIrd nerve damage, viz. variable IIIrd nerve innervated muscle involvement and signs of misdirection regeneration. The palsy may be isolated or associated with additional perinatal neurologic damage (Fig. 83.1).[2]

B. With features suggesting a primary nuclear maldevelopment, viz. bilateral partial ptosis and contralateral superior rectus palsy. A hypoplastic peripheral IIIrd nerve may be seen on MR imaging and specific genetic mutations known to be associated with CCDD identified.

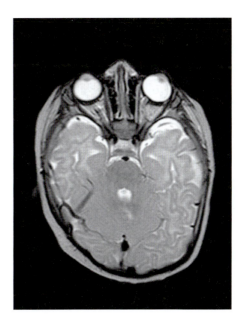

Fig. 83.1 Congenital left IIIrd nerve palsy. Axial T2-weighted scan shows superior vermis lesion (other presumed perinatal hypoxic ischemic lesions seen elsewhere).

C. Unilateral congenital IIIrd nerve palsy has also been reported in:

- Neurofibromatosis 2 (NF2) – this can be the presenting feature.
- PHACE syndrome. The posterior fossa malformations described include unilateral IIIrd nerve palsy (Fig. 83.2).
- Septo-optic dysplasia. Both unilateral and bilateral congenital IIIrd have been described.
- Rarities, e.g. congenital neurenteric cyst.

D. Variants:

- Cyclic ocular motor palsy. This occurs following congenital or early onset acquired IIIrd nerve palsy. The child has a complete IIIrd nerve palsy but with superimposed episodic activity in IIIrd nerve innervated muscles. The muscles involved are usually the levator, which may elevate to a normal position or even retract, plus the superior and medial recti. A dilated pupil may constrict. These "spasms" of IIIrd nerve function are short-lived lasting 30 seconds to a minute and may be induced by contralateral eye movement or attempted fixation with the paretic eye, but may also occur spontaneously and in sleep. It is presumed that variable prenuclear activation of intact motor neurons is responsible for this phenomenon.
- Double elevator palsy. A hypotropia and deficit of elevation of an eye is due to an isolated palsy of the superior rectus and inferior oblique muscles. Differentiation from primary isolated ocular muscle fibrosis may require a forced duction test.
- Congenital medial rectus palsy with synergistic divergence. Isolated congenital medial rectus palsy is associated with divergence of both eyes on attempted adduction of the affected eye. This is probably a CCDD variant.
- Brown's syndrome variant. Congenital failure of elevation in adduction may be associated with

elevation of the ipsilateral lid on adduction which elevates further on gaze down and in. The lid movements are those of "misdirection regeneration" of the IIIrd nerve and this Brown's syndrome variant may be due to IIIrd nerve pathology.

Management

Important steps in the management of congenital IIIrd nerve palsy are:

- Establishing the etiology if possible. This may be clear from the history or require investigation and neuroimaging.[1]
- Advising the parents about the possible outcomes.

Vision

Amblyopia of the affected eye in unilateral cases is invariable. Patching of the uninvolved eye is essential but the visual outcome is usually poor. No binocular single vision (BSV) will develop.

Eye position and movement

Whether or not it will be possible to successfully align the affected eye with strabismus surgery will depend on the extent of the palsy. The outcome in a complete IIIrd nerve palsy is likely to be disappointing. The eye position should be corrected first before considering ptosis surgery. Ptosis surgery should not be undertaken unless corneal protection can be guaranteed.

Acquired IIIrd nerve palsy

Most cases are unilateral and likely to occur in a clinical context that helps establish the etiology.[2]

Trauma

The commonest cause is accidental closed head injury, e.g. in a road traffic accident. Isolated IIIrd nerve palsy is due to avulsion of the nerve rootlets from the brain stem. With basal skull fracture there are likely to be multiple cranial neuropathies.

IIIrd nerve palsy occurring after minor head trauma may indicate an underlying predisposing factor. IIIrd nerve palsy has been described after non-accidental injury in infants and following surgical trauma. Some spontaneous recovery for up to a year can be expected, often with misdirection–regeneration.

Infection

A. Bacterial meningitis. In neonates, due to group B streptococcal infection (also *Escherichia coli*/listeria with brain stem encephalitis), it may be complicated by unilateral or bilateral IIIrd; recovery is likely to be poor. Cerebral visual impairment is also common (see Chapter 56). IIIrd nerve palsy can also occur in infantile or childhood meningitis.

B. TB meningitis. This can present with or be complicated by unilateral or bilateral progressive IIIrd nerve palsy.

C. Para-infectious palsy. A presumed immune-mediated pathology is responsible for cases described after, for

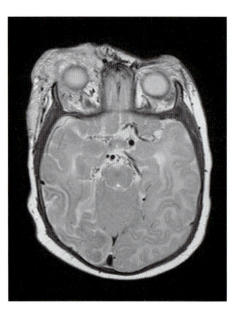

Fig. 83.2 PHACES. Axial T2-weighted scan shows facial hemangiomata plus absent right internal carotid artery and dilated perforators in Sylvian fissures. Patient had congenital left IIIrd nerve palsy.

example, influenza vaccination or MMR (measles, mumps, rubella) vaccination. The condition can be recurrent.

D. Viral meningitis. Causal viruses include herpes simplex, Epstein-Barr virus, cytomegalovirus, and herpes zoster virus.

Tumor

Intracranial and intraorbital tumors can present with signs including a IIIrd nerve palsy, usually progressively worsening (Fig. 83.3). External compression, direct involvement of the nerve (e.g. by schwannoma), infiltration, or malignant meningitis may be responsible. Compression can be anywhere along the course of the nerve (e.g. brainstem glioma or parasellar tumor). Raised intracranial pressure may be a contributory or primary cause.

Additional neuro-ophthalmic signs should be sought to help localize the pathology: neuro-imaging is mandatory.[1]

Rare causes

Vascular

A. Aneurysmal compression. This may occur in the first or second decade due to posterior communicating artery aneurysm: also (usually with a VIth nerve palsy) due to intracavernous internal carotid artery aneurysm in, for example, Loewys-Dietz syndrome (Fig. 83.4).

B. Vasculitis. Cases have been described secondary to Kawasaki's disease with or without aseptic meningitis and raised intracranial pressure, also polyarteritis nodosa.

C. Vascular malformation. A hemorrhage in a brain stem cavernoma or other vascular malformation can present with a partial IIIrd nerve palsy.

Ophthalmoplegic migraine

This is a diagnosis of exclusion after full investigation.[3] It cannot be made on clinical grounds alone. The syndrome is not certainly due to migraine. The diagnostic criteria are:

- Childhood onset IIIrd nerve palsy associated with headache, photophobia/photopsia, and nausea.
- Pupillary involvement and usually a complete palsy.
- Neuroimaging normal except for enlargement and gadolinium enhancement of the cisternal portion of the IIIrd nerve on MRI (not invariable).[4] The cerebrospinal fluid (CSF) is normal.
- Steroid responsive (but self-limiting without treatment).
- Family history of migraine.

The differential diagnosis includes schwannoma, hemangioma, and lymphoma. The condition may be recurrent (Fig. 83.5).

It characteristically affects the IIIrd nerve but can affect the IVth or VIth.

Neuroma

IIIrd nerve neuroma producing a slowly progressive palsy can complicate NF2 or as an isolated tumor. The signs may fluctuate initially.

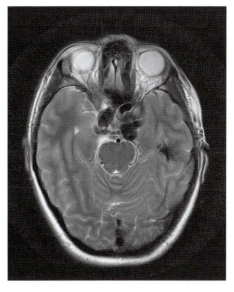

Fig. 83.4 Loeys-Dietz syndrome. Axial T2-weighted scan showing large flow voids in bilateral internal carotid artery aneurysms. Patient has bilateral VIth nerve palsies.

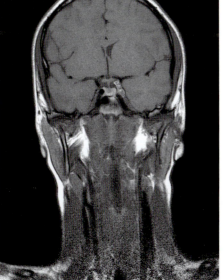

Fig. 83.3 Left intracavernous dermoid. Coronal T1-weighted scan; presented with progressive left IIIrd nerve palsy in an 8-year-old.

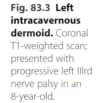

Fig. 83.5 Recurrent right IIIrd nerve palsy × 3 from ages 5 to 9. Axial T1-weighted FS post gadolinium shows enhancing nodule on right IIIrd nerve. The scan also shows bilateral vestibular schwannomas indicating NF2.

Inflammatory

Fascicular IIIrd nerve palsy may occur in ADEM (acute disseminated encephalomyelitis) and in childhood onset multiple sclerosis (MS).[5]

Idiopathic/cryptogenic

Despite full investigation, a small proportion of childhood onset IIIrd nerve palsies remain unexplained. It is important to be prepared to reinvestigate if new signs develop; ocular myasthenia, for example, can present as a unilateral pupil sparing IIIrd nerve palsy with negative antibodies and normal electromyography.[6]

Management

Establishing the etiology is the first priority. Treatable underlying pathology must be identified and managed appropriately.

In visually immature children, amblyopia is inevitable in the affected eye and should be managed in the conventional way.

At least 1 year from onset (e.g. of a traumatic palsy) should be allowed for spontaneous recovery before considering surgical treatment. Attempts to correct a neurogenic hypotropia by inferior rectus recession always lead to an abnormal recessed lower lid position: a better option is to move both horizontal muscles upwards with augmenting sutures if necessary.

IVth nerve palsy

Congenital palsy

This is the commonest congenital cranial nerve palsy and the commonest cause of hypertropia in children.[7] It is usually unilateral.

The clinical signs are:

- An abnormal head posture (AHP) – possibly detectable from early infancy onwards. This consists of a tilt and turn of the head away from the side of the lesion (for differential diagnosis, see Box 83.1).[8]
- Without the AHP, a hypertropia of the affected eye which increases in adduction and reduces in abduction. This is associated with ipsilateral inferior oblique overaction/superior oblique underaction and contralateral superior rectus underaction/inferior rectus overaction.
- The Parks' three step test is a useful way of identifying the primary underacting muscle (see Chapter 80).

Box 83.1

Differential diagnosis of a head tilt/turn in childhood

A. Ocular
  - Unilateral IVth nerve palsy
  - Duane's syndrome
  - VIth nerve palsy
  - Homonymous hemianopia
  - Nystagmus with a null-zone
B. Non-ocular
  - Sternomastoid torticollis
  - Cervical spine torticollis

Etiology

Central pathology

Primary hypoplasia or aplasia of the IVth nerve nucleus and nerve may be demonstrable on MRI. This is probably a variant of CCDD. It may occur as a component of CFEOM2 (see Chapter 82) or be isolated. Polymorphisms of the ARIX and PHOX2B genes may be pathogenic or genetic risk factors for this condition. These genetic factors probably account for the condition of autosomal dominant congenital IVth nerve palsy.

Peripheral pathology

The following factors may be relevant alone or in combination.

- Primary muscle hypoplasia. This may be demonstrated on orbital imaging but may be due to a primary muscle deficit or secondary to reduced innervation.
- Superior oblique tendon laxity. Laxity of the tendon and/or abnormalities of insertion on the eye have been noted peroperatively.
- Orbital maldevelopment. Primary orbital maldevelopment may affect the position of the trochlear causing an effective weakening of superior oblique function. Extensive facial hypoplasia may explain superior oblique palsy and changes in facial morphometry in cases previously described as "superior oblique palsy plus" – i.e. in addition to the IVth nerve palsy, a horizontal misalignment of the eyes and amblyopia of the hypertropic eye. Alternatively, an infant with a superior oblique palsy and an abnormal head posture may always adopt the same resting position in sleep leading to positional plagiocephaly.
- Heterotopic muscle pulleys. Theoretically this could unbalance the cyclovertical muscles and produce partial IVth nerve palsy signs. There is evidence from targeted orbital MRI to support this hypothesis.[9]

Most infants and children with congenital IVth nerve palsy of whatever etiology do not have amblyopia and develop good BSV. There is, however, a sub-group who adopt a head posture reducing the vertical deviation, but always have a manifest vertical tropia and do not have BSV. In spite of this, ipsilateral inferior oblique recession (see below) may reduce the AHP.

Rarities

A number of brain stem developmental anomalies may be associated with a congenital IVth nerve palsy. PHACE syndrome is another association (see Chapter 20).

Management

The first priority is to be certain that the physical signs are due to a congenital IVth nerve palsy (see Box 83.1). Orthoptic investigation of binocular status is important. Most cases should be followed in the Orthoptic Department to make sure that BSV is developing satisfactorily. Surgery is required if binocular function is deteriorating or if the child has a marked AHP.

Acquired IVth nerve palsy

The signs of acquired IVth nerve palsy are those noted above in congenital cases. Symptoms are diplopia with a combined vertical/horizontal separation plus (subjective incyclo) torsion maximal in downgaze, particularly symptomatic in bilateral cases.

The differential diagnosis is skew deviation, i.e. a supranuclear vertical dissociation of the eyes (see Chapter 90). Skew deviation may be isolated or associated with additional signs which may help in localizing the lesion, e.g. lateral medullary syndrome or ocular tilt reaction, the triad of:

1. Skew deviation (vertical squint).
2. Paradoxical head tilt (toward the hypotropic eye).
3. Bilateral conjugate ocular rotation (toward the hypotropic eye).

Causes

Trauma

Closed head injury is the commonest cause of acquired unilateral or bilateral IVth nerve palsy in childhood. It is attributed to IVth nerve root avulsion by traumatic distraction. There may be scan evidence of focal dorsal mid brain hemorrhage attributable to concussive impact against the tentorium cerebelli.

Traumatic IVth nerve palsy has been described after shaking injury in infancy.

Other causes

IVth nerve palsy may be a presenting feature of posterior fossa tumors, e.g. childhood astrocytoma. There are rare cases of trochlear nerve schwannoma demonstrated on MRI and presenting under the age of 16 as progressive IVth nerve palsy.[9]

ADEM, childhood onset MS, arteritis (e.g. polyarteritis nodosa), and rarely idiopathic intracranial hypertension are other rare causes. Also Lemierre's syndrome (see below, VIth nerve palsy) and after halo traction for cervical spine trauma (also with VIth nerve palsy).

Management

Traumatic IVth nerve palsy has a strong propensity for spontaneous improvement which, combined with binocular fusional adaptations, leads to a satisfactory outcome in many cases. At least a year should be allowed for spontaneous recovery before considering surgery.

In unrecovered or partly recovered bilateral IVth nerve palsy with torsional double vision and an esotropia on downgaze, anterior half superior oblique tendon advancement is a useful intervention.

VIth nerve palsy

Congenital VIth nerve palsy

A. A small percentage of normal neonates have an isolated unilateral VIth nerve palsy presumed to be traumatic in origin and related to delivery. It seems likely that many of these cases go undetected as full spontaneous recovery within 6 weeks is common. The differential diagnosis of congenital VIth nerve palsy includes infantile esotropia with cross fixation[10] (see Chapter 74). This condition is often not diagnosed until the child is a few months old.

B. Primary abducens nuclear aplasia/hypoplasia. The child presents during the first year of life with a parental observation of a misalignment of the eyes. This is a variant of CCDD and recognized as Duane's syndrome. In its most characteristic form this consists of a failure of abduction of one or both eyes with a normal primary position alignment of the eyes or a normal alignment with a head posture toward the involved side. Most cases of unilateral Duane's syndrome develop normal sensory binocularity and good motor fusion.

Duane's syndrome may be unilateral or bilateral and sporadic or inherited. Some cases are secondary to teratogens such as thalidomide. Duane's syndrome may be isolated or a component of a more extensive cranial nerve dysinnervation syndrome such as Möbius' syndrome or in Poland's and Goldenhar's syndromes (see Chapter 82).

Acquired VIth nerve palsy

Young children rarely complain of double vision. The presentation of VIth nerve palsy in the first decade is often with the observation by the parents that the child's eye is squinting or that he or she is shutting one eye when concentrating visually. Alternatively, the child may adopt a head posture to align the eyes. An older child is more likely to complain of double vision, particularly (with a partial VIth nerve palsy) distance diplopia.

The history should concentrate on possible explanatory events (e.g. trauma, recent infections, etc.) and additional symptoms of potential localizing or diagnostic value. In many cases, the context of the onset of the symptoms and signs will provide the explanation for the palsy.[10]

Examination

Cover and alternate cover testing at distance and far distance may be necessary to reveal a subtle eso-deviation. A Hess chart in an older child is useful for both documentation and assessing progress. Potential localizing signs such as facial weakness or asymmetry, nystagmus, sensory trigeminal neuropathy, and Horner's syndrome should be sought. Myasthenia can mimic any infranuclear (or inter-/supra-nuclear) ocular motor disturbance; check orbicularis oculi forceful eye closure.[11] Exclude spasm of the near reflex (convergence spasm) – checking the pupils and dynamic retinoscopy may be helpful. Optic disk examination is important.

The differential diagnosis includes:

1. Divergence paralysis: viz. a normal near alignment, esotropia for distance but full abduction. This has been attributed to diverse brain stem lesions.
2. Supranuclear paresis of abduction: a uni- or bilateral abduction paresis with slow abducting saccades +/– nystagmus of the adducting eye; the VOR is intact. This is a "posterior internuclear ophthalmoplegia of abduction" and due to a rostral pontine/mesencephalic lesion.

Important causes

Tumor

Isolated, usually progressive, VIth nerve palsy may be the presenting sign of an intracranial tumor, usually an intrinsic neoplasm, either pontine glioma (Figs 83.6 and 83.7) or other posterior fossa tumor such as ependymoma or medulloblastoma. Clivus chordoma can also present this way. Parasellar tumors such as craniopharyngioma or pituitary tumor may invade the cavernous sinus and present with VIth (or other) ocular motor palsies.

Trauma

Closed head injury – sometimes apparently quite minor – without skull fracture is a recognized cause of VIth nerve palsy. In basal skull fracture, it may be accompanied by an ipsilateral facial nerve palsy. Bilateral traumatic VIth nerve palsies result in a huge esotropia and cross fixation using an abnormal head posture and can be seen in bitemporal crush head injury which mostly occurs in childhood with VIIth nerve palsies and hearing loss.

Benign/post viral/idiopathic/inflammatory

This condition is well recognized, but it is a diagnosis of exclusion by normal neuroimaging and CSF and blood studies. The VIth nerve palsy is usually unilateral, sudden in onset, and complete. Any presumed triggering illness such as a viral upper respiratory tract infection is usually fairly trivial. However, VIth nerve palsies can occur with more serious neurotropic virus infections such as varicella. Prognosis for full recovery is good beginning approximately 6 weeks after onset and complete within 3 to 4 weeks.

Benign VIth nerve palsy of childhood may be recurrent either on the same side or contalateral eye. The location and nature of the pathology is uncertain.

Focal demyelination affecting the VIth nerve fascicles in the pons can occur in ADEM (Fig. 83.8) and childhood onset MS.[5] Neurosarcoid can present with a cranial mononeuritis, most often involving the VIIth but also the VIth nerve (or cranial polyneuritis.)

Raised intracranial pressure

VIth nerve palsy may be a consequence of raised intracranial pressure (Fig. 83.9). It may occur as the presenting feature of tumor obstructing the CSF flow or in idiopathic intracranial hypertension. Children with the latter condition do not necessarily have the body habitus and BMI (body mass index) characteristic of adults with this condition.

Infection

VIth nerve palsy is a recognized complication of meningitis, both neonatal and infantile/childhood, also TB meningitis. It can occur following middle ear infection complicated by petrous apicitis, i.e. Gradenigo's syndrome (Fig. 83.10). This consists of ipsilateral VIth nerve palsy and Vth nerve distribution pain and earache/otorrhea. Middle ear infection can lead to cerebral venous sinus thrombosis and secondary raised intracranial pressure with VIth nerve palsy.

Lemierre's syndrome is when *Fusobacterium necrophorum* (or other anaerobic infection) develops in a peritonsillar abscess

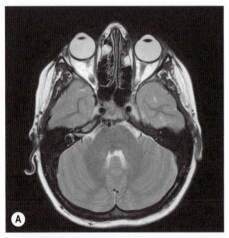

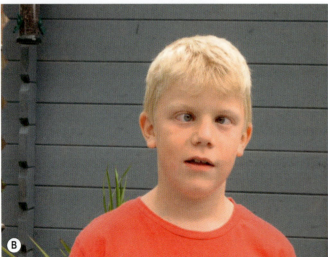

Fig. 83.6 Pontine glioma. (A) The axial T2-weighted scan shows enlargement of the right facial colliculus; the child has bilateral VIth and right partial VIIth nerve palsies. (B) Clinical photo.

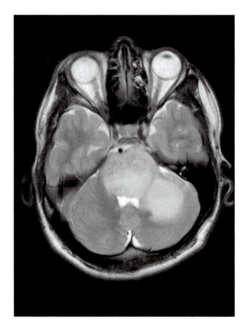

Fig. 83.7 Bilateral progressive VIth nerve palsies in a 12-year-old. Axial T2-weighted scan shows large intrinsic mass in brainstem and left cerebellar hemisphere; aggressive pontine glioma.

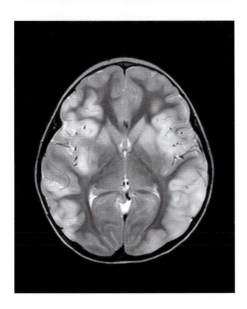

Fig. 83.8 ADEM. Axial T2-weighted scan shows multifocal cortical swelling and signal change plus deep gray matter involvement. Patient had bilateral VIth nerve palsies.

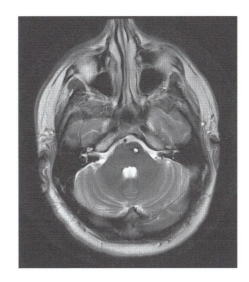

Fig. 83.11 A 16-year-old presented with sudden onset left VIth nerve palsy. Axial T2-weighted scan shows pontine cavernoma with signal rim from hemosiderin.

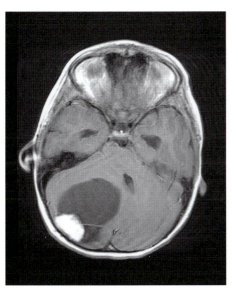

Fig. 83.9 NF1. A 6-year-old girl presented with raised intracranial pressure, bilateral VIth nerve palsies and papilledema. Axial T1-weighted post gadolinium scan shows large right cerebellar cyst and enhancing nodule plus obstructive hydrocephalus.

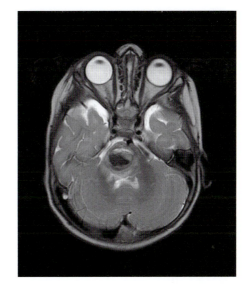

Fig. 83.12 Right VIth and VIIth nerve palsies in an 18-month-old due to pontine cavernoma shown on axial T2-weighted scan.

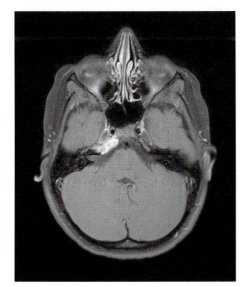

Fig. 83.10 Petrous apicitis presenting with painful right VIth nerve palsy in a 6-year-old. Axial T1-weighted (FS) post gadolinium scan showing enhancement of the petrous apex.

and is complicated by internal jugular vein thrombosis and septic thrombophlebitis. Ipsilateral VIth nerve palsy or rarely IVth nerve palsy may occur. Successful treatment of the infection may not lead to resolution of the palsy.

Vascular

Pontine vascular malformations, such as cavernoma, may be complicated by or present with ipsilateral VIth nerve palsy (Figs 83.11 to 83.13).

Other causes

VIth nerve palsy can develop after a lumbar puncture due to intracranial hypotension. The palsy is sudden in onset, complete and accompanied by low pressure headache. Most cases resolve spontaneously. Idiopathic intracranial hypotension can rarely occur in childhood causing recurrent headache, sometimes with double vision due to VIth nerve palsy. The MRI findings are characteristic.[1]

Management

In acquired VIth nerve palsy, treatment of the underlying cause is the priority. Once the condition has been stabilized, time

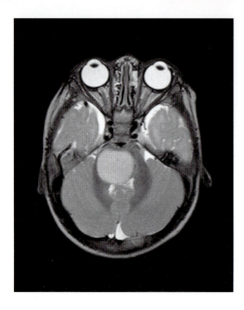

Fig. 83.13 A 10-year-old presenting with right VIth then right gaze palsy. Pontine cavernoma shown on axial T2-weighted scan.

Table 83.1 – The following conditions are known to cause multiple ocular motor palsies in childhood; most will be identifiable from the history and associated findings, including localizing neuro-ophthalmic signs

Trauma	Basal skull fracture, e.g. road traffic accident Closed head injury without fracture
Tumor	Pontine glioma Parasellar tumors including pituitary apoplexy Craniopharyngioma Suprasellar germinoma
Infection	Meningitis Botulism Post infectious cavernous sinus thrombosis
Vascular	Intracavernous carotid aneurysm Aneurysm (traumatic/associated with collagen disorder, e.g. Ehlers-Danlos syndrome)
Inflammatory	ADEM MS Tolosa-Hunt syndrome
Autoimmune	Ocular myasthenia gravis Miller-Fisher syndrome

for spontaneous improvement of up to a year should be allowed before surgical treatment is considered. In visually immature children, patching to prevent the development of amblyopia is essential.

Unrecovered VIth nerve palsy with esotropia does not respond to standard strabismus surgical techniques. Temporary weakening of the medial rectus muscle with an injection of botulinum toxin (see Chapter 84) should be followed by temporal transfer of the whole superior and inferior rectus muscles to the insertion of the lateral rectus muscle, usually with augmentation sutures. A subsequent medial rectus muscle recession may be required.

Multiple ocular motor palsies/complex ophthalmoparesis (Table 83.1)

Tolosa-Hunt syndrome

The defining characteristics of this condition, a few cases of which have been described in childhood, are the following:

1. One or more episodes of unilateral orbital pain persisting for weeks if untreated.
2. Unilateral IIIrd, IVth, and VIth nerve palsy, alone or in combination, coincident with the pain or within 2 weeks of it.
3. Pain and palsies steroid responsive within 72 hours.
4. Enhancing soft tissue visible on MRI in the cavernous sinus/orbital apex (or granuloma on biopsy).
5. Exclusion of other causes. The differential diagnosis includes ophthalmoplegic migraine, orbital pseudotumor, and pituitary tumor with apoplexy.

Infant botulism

This is very rare but a few cases occur annually in the USA and Europe. The child is usually previously breast fed and late weaned at the age of about 12 to 15 months. *Clostridium botulinum* spores are ingested and because of the lack of the normal protective bowel bacterial flora, colonization and absorption of endogenously produced toxin occurs.

The child presents with muscle weakness including feeding and respiratory difficulties plus ptosis and internal and external ophthalmoplegia with other evidence of parasympathetic blockade. The treatment is supportive and includes yogurts and other foods to alter bowel flora. Prolonged bilateral ptosis may occur but visual development is normal.

Cavernous sinus thrombosis

Cavernous sinus thrombosis in children is associated with a high incidence of serious morbidity and mortality. Presenting symptoms include headache, vomiting, and visual disturbance and signs include papilledema, fever, and VIth nerve palsy. The commonest underlying conditions are middle ear infection and paranasal sinus infection with or without associated orbital cellulitis. Despite vigorous antibiotic and thrombolytic therapy, many patients die or have residual serious neurologic deficits. Early diagnosis is the key to successful treatment.

Autoimmune ocular motor disturbances in childhood

Neuromuscular junction disorders

Congenital myasthenia

This is a heterogeneous group of genetic disorders of neuromuscular transmission, the differential diagnosis of which includes congenital muscular dystrophies and myopathies.[12] Most cases present in infancy but they can present in childhood or adolescence. The clinical characteristics are similar in all the identified disorders with modest phenotype/genotype correlation. Severe cases may be fatal in infancy.

The ophthalmologic features include ptosis, lower lid retraction, weak eye closure, and ophthalmoplegia usually with divergence of the visual axis and reduced upgaze. Amblyopia is unusual.

These disorders are genetic with autosomal recessive inheritance but a male preponderance.[12] The defect in neuromuscular transmission may be:

- Presynaptic (8%): reduced synthesis or release of acetylcholine.
- Synaptic basal laminar (16%): acetylcholinesterase dysfunction.
- Postsynaptic (76%): mutations in acetylcholine receptor subunits including rapsyn, the protein needed for acetylcholine receptor concentration and organization.

Treatment with pyridostigmine or 3,4-diaminopyridine may be helpful. Immunosuppression is not. Do not attempt squint or ptosis surgery.

Neonatal myasthenia

A pregnant woman with autoimmune myasthenia gravis may have antifetal acetylcholine antibodies which cross the placenta. In untreated cases, neonatal myasthenia results and in severe cases, arthrogryposis multiplex congenita, i.e. congenital muscle contractures.

Juvenile autoimmune myasthenia gravis

Fifty percent of cases present to ophthalmologists in the first decade with ptosis and double vision; an exodeviation is typical. The features are variability and fatiguability of extraocular muscle and levator function with normal pupils (Video 83.1). Orbicularis oculi weakness may be marked. Thirty percent have detectable anti-acetylcholine receptor antibodies and an even smaller number have anti-MusK (muscle specific kinase) antibodies.

The diagnosis is clinical supported by antibody studies and electromyography. Treatment is with immunosuppression and anticholinesterase drugs. Up to 50% of cases will develop amblyopia and require patching treatment. There is an approximately 25% risk of the development of generalized myasthenia gravis but up to a third go into remission.[6,11]

Miller-Fisher syndrome

MFS consists of external (and sometimes internal) ophthalmoplegia, ataxia, and loss of tendon reflexes. It is a variant of Guillain-Barre syndrome and can present in childhood. Facial palsy may be associated; the CSF protein is elevated. There is frequently a mixed infranuclear/internuclear/supranuclear picture. Detection of serum anti-GQ1b antibodies is diagnostic; the anti-GQ1b epitope is particularly concentrated in the paranodal region of the extramedullary IIIrd nerve. The condition may develop after viral or other infections, notably *Campylobacter* jejuni enteritis. Full spontaneous recovery is usual.

MFS associated IIIrd nerve palsy may recover with misdirection regeneration (10% of reported cases) indicating the peripheral nature of the palsy.

There is a wide spectrum of disorder and isolated ptosis, rectus muscle involvement, or internal ophthalmoplegia alone ranging up to acute bilateral ophthalmoparesis may be due to anti-GQ1b antibodies. There may be MRI and electrophysiologic evidence of brain stem involvement and an overlap with Bickerstaff's brain stem encephalitis.

Ocular muscle disease

Ocular myopathies

Chronic progressive external ophthalmoplegia

CPEO is a heterogeneous group of disorders associated with large scale mitochondrial DNA deletions or mutations and characterized by slow progressive symmetric ophthalmoparesis with ptosis and orbicularis oculi weakness.[13] The pupils are normal. The muscle weakness is invariable and does not fatigue. Muscle biopsy shows ragged red fibers on Gomori staining.

Children with CPEO may present to the ophthalmologist in the first decade with an exodeviation with or without mild bilateral ptosis. Other systemic features such as growth retardation may not be present at this stage.

CPEO is classified as:

1. Congenital.
2. Isolated.
3. Oculofacial.
4. Occurring with pigmentary retinopathy.
5. Occurring with pigmentary retinopathy, heart block, cerebral dysfunction, and raised CSF protein (Kearns-Sayre syndrome).
6. Occurring with systemic features such as growth retardation.

Definitive diagnosis is by muscle biopsy and genotyping. The child should be referred to a pediatric neurologist. The ptosis and ophthalmoparesis are slowly progressive. Surgery for the ptosis is usually contraindicated because of the risk of corneal exposure, and muscle surgery for the exotropia is ineffective.

Muscular dystrophies

Myotonic dystrophy

This usually presents in the first decade with muscle weakness and wasting involving the face, neck, and limbs with myotonia.[14] There is symmetric bilateral ptosis with lower lid retraction and a slowly progressive external ophthalmoplegia, rarely symptomatic.

The condition is autosomal dominant and systemic features include cataracts ("Christmas tree" cataract) (see Chapter 36) and learning difficulties.

The condition is due to an unstable trinucleotide repeat (CTG) on the long arm of chromosome 19. The number of abnormal repeats determines the severity of the condition. Management is supportive, but cataract surgery may be required.

Oculopharyngeal muscular dystrophy

This is inherited (AD) and can present in the first or second decade with ptosis and exotropia. The diagnosis is made on muscle biopsy and the genetic defect is GCG repeat expansions on the *PABP2* gene.[15]

Congenital myopathy

This group of disorders presents in infancy with delayed motor development and reduced muscle tone and bulk.

Ophthalmologic features include ptosis and ophthalmoparesis, e.g. in myotubular myopathy.

Neurodegenerative disorders

Ophthalmoplegia and/or ptosis may be a feature of childhood onset neurodegenerative disorders. Examples include:

1. Juvenile spinal muscular atrophy.
2. Infantile progressive spinal muscular atrophy (Werdnig-Hoffman disease type 1).
3. Childhood lactic acidosis where ptosis is occasionally seen but optic atrophy much more commonly.
4. Abetalipoproteinemia (ocular motor nerve palsies may occur).
5. Spinocerebellar degeneration.

Ocular myositis

Ocular myositis presents with eye pain, redness, conjunctival edema, and watering, sometimes with proptosis and reduced eye movements. It may affect single or multiple muscles and be uni- or bilateral. Painful globe retraction on attempted movement of the eye against the inflamed muscle may be evident.

The differential diagnosis is wide. The following specific disease entities can present in childhood as described above:

- Granuloma/inflammatory: Wegener granulomatosis/sarcoid/Tolosa-Hunt syndrome.
- Immune mediated: Graves' ophthalmopathy.
- Infections: Lyme borreliosis/herpes zoster ophthalmicus/trichinosis/orbital cellulitis.
- Malignancy: rhabdomyosarcoma/lymphoma/(paraneoplastic).

Ocular myositis more frequently occurs as an isolated idiopathic condition characteristically affecting one or two muscles in one orbit. Idiopathic cases can be recurrent.

Investigation

All cases should have imaging. Blood tests for specific conditions may be required. A pediatric opinion should be sought.

If there is any doubt about the diagnosis, an extraocular muscle biopsy is needed.

Treatment is with systemic and topical immunosuppression (steroids). Idiopathic cases usually respond promptly and fully. Exceptionally after resolution of the acute inflammatory condition, the eye muscle becomes fibrotic and squint surgery may be needed.

References

1. La Rocca V, Gorelick G, Kaufman LM. Medical imaging in pediatric neuro-ophthalmology. Neuroimag Clin North Am 2005; 15: 85–105.
2. Scummacher-Feero LA, Yoo KW, Solari FM, Biglan AW. Third cranial nerve palsy in children. Am J Ophthalmol 1999; 128: 216–21.
3. Lyerly MJ, Petersch BW, Lara AK, McGrath TM. Ophthalmoplegic migraine. Headache 2011; 1526–9.
4. Ferreira T, Verbist B, van Buchem M, et al. Imaging the ocular motor nerves. Eur J Radiol 2010: 74: 314–22.
5. Benwell B, Ghezzi A, Bar-Or A, et al. Multiple sclerosis in children: clinical diagnosis, therapeutic strategies and future directions. Lancet Neurol 2007; 6: 887–902.
6. Pinelis SC, Avery RA, Moss, et al. Visual and systemic outcomes in pediatric ocular myasthenia gravis. Am J Ophthalmol 2010; 150: 453–59.
7. Tarczy-Hornoch K, Repka MX. Superior oblique palsy or paresis in pediatric patients. J AAPOS 2004; 8: 133–40.
8. Nucci P, Kushner BJ, Serafino M, Orzalesi N. A multi-disciplinary study of the ocular, orthopedic and neurological causes of abnormal head postures in children. Am J Ophthalmol 2005; 140: 65–8.
9. Choi BS, Kim JH, Jung C, Hwang JM. High resolution 3-D MR imaging of the trochlear nerve. AJNR 2010; 31: 1076–9.
10. Merino P, Gomez de Liano P, Villalobo JM, et al. Etiology and treatment of pediatric sixth nerve palsy. J AAPOS 2010; 14: 502–5.
11. Ortiz S, Borchet M. Long term outcomes of pediatric ocular myasthenia gravis. Ophthalmology 2008; 115: 1245–8.
12. Barisic N, Chaoch A, Muller JS, Lochmuller H. Genetic heterogeneity and pathophysiological mechanisms in congenital myasthenic syndromes. Eur J Paediatr Neurol 2011; 15: 189–96.
13. Gronlund MA, Honarvar AK, Holme E, et al. Ophthalmological findings in children and young adults with genetically verified mitochondrial disease. Br J Ophthalmol 2010; 94: 121–7.
14. Ekstrom AB, Tulinius M, Sjostrom A, Aring E. Visual function in congenital and childhood myotonic dystrophy type I. Ophthalmology 2010; 117: 976–82.
15. Emery AEH. The muscular dystrophies. Lancet 2002; 359: 687–95.

SECTION 6
Amblyopia, strabismus and
eye movements

CHAPTER **84**

Part 6
Strabismus treatment

Strabismus: non-surgical treatment

Alejandra de Alba Campomanes

Many treatments used to manage children and adults with strabismus are non-surgical. Even in patients who require surgery to restore normal alignment and/or binocular function, our surgical approaches are usually complemented by many non-surgical treatments ranging from altering the refractive correction to using pharmacological chemodenervation with botulinum toxin. The treatment of some forms of strabismus is entirely non-surgical. For example, the treatment of convergence insufficiency includes vergence-accommodative exercises, or passive treatment with base-in prisms: surgery is rarely required.

Optical correction

It is important to recognize that refractive errors, whether corrected or uncorrected, have a major impact on strabismus and its management. Correcting a refractive error may result in better control of a misalignment solely by gaining optimal visual acuity. Conversely, previously uncorrected strabismus patients can be made symptomatic by correcting their refractive error by encouraging spontaneous alternation or switch of fixation to their non-dominant eye.[1]

All children with strabismus or suspected strabismus require a cycloplegic refraction to determine the basic refractive state without the influence of accommodation. This can be done with 0.5% to 2% cyclopentolate (Mydrilate, Cyclogyl), 1% tropicamide (Mydriacyl), or 1% atropine. Cyclopentolate is commonly preferred over atropine due to its shorter onset and duration of action. The mean residual accommodation of these agents is less than 0.1 D for a 3-day administration of 1% atropine, and between 0.4 and 0.6 D for 1% cyclopentolate or 1% tropicamide in children with dark irides.[2] The difference between atropine and cyclopentolate cycloplegia has consistently been measured to be between 0.4 and 0.7 D,[2-5] but it is important to recognize that 15–20% of children who have a cycloplegic refraction with 1% cyclopentolate alone will have a hyperopic undercorrection of 1 D or more.[2-3] Therefore, in accommodative esotropia with a residual deviation, an atropine refraction is still essential to uncover the maximal amount of hyperopia that needs to be corrected. Atropine eye drops do not sting: cyclopentolate drops do. The pupillary dilation achieved with any of these agents allows the funduscopic exam which is mandatory during the initial evaluation of a strabismus patient to exclude visual axis opacification or abnormalities of the posterior segments.

Considering the optimal optical correction for each patient is essential in the management of their strabismus. In acquired esotropia, particularly accommodative esotropia, all degrees of hypermetropia may be significant, and should be fully corrected with spectacles. The full hyperopic correction should be prescribed in order to remove all accommodative convergence. In most forms of esotropia (including essential infantile esotropia) following surgical alignment, spectacle correction may be of considerable value in improving a small residual deviation. In patients with surgical overcorrections of partially accommodative esotropia, reduction of the hypermetropic correction of more than +2.50 D may be associated with long-term instability of the alignment: such overcorrections should be avoided.[6,7]

In intermittent exotropia (X(T)), it may seem logical not to correct moderate to high hypermetropia since the convergence induced by the hypermetropia has a beneficial effect on the control of the exodeviation. A small study of children with moderate to high hyperopia (3–7 D) and X(T) showed that full hyperopic prescription corrected the manifest deviation and improved the binocular status in all the patients.[8] A larger study demonstrated that with partial spectacle correction the mean exodeviation increased on average 10 PD (prism diopters) in one-third of patients with X(T) and moderate hyperopia compared to patients with fully corrected hyperopia, emmetropia, or myopia.[9] Nevertheless, high hyperopia, anisometropia, significant astigmatism, and myopia should always be corrected in patients with X(T). High hyperopic patients may not be accommodating fully and experiencing blur, resulting in poor control of the X(T). It is unclear if moderate hyperopia needs to be corrected unless the patient has decreased vision, or if surgical planning should be done wearing moderate hyperopic corrections to improve long-term surgical outcomes.[9]

For the treatment of X(T), over-minus lens therapy has been proposed (1.5–4 D additional minus) to stimulate accommodative convergence and improve control of the deviation. In three prospective studies of children treated with over-minus glasses, some form of improvement (depending on the outcome measure used) was seen in 45–70% of patients.[10-12] This improvement was seen irrespective of the initial angle of deviation and in some patients was maintained after discontinuation of therapy. Since the reports on the natural history and spontaneous improvement of X(T) are contradictory, and there is a lack of control groups for these interventions, it is difficult to ascertain their real efficacy. Over-minus therapy does not appear to increase myopia.[12,13]

Other non-surgical interventions prescribed for the treatment of X(T) include part-time occlusion, fusional vergence exercises, and atropine. The rationale behind these interventions is that they may improve the control of the intermittent deviation, preserve stereoacuity and eliminate, or at least delay, surgical treatment. Most of these interventions have not been rigorously studied and their efficacy remains unclear.[14,15] (see section on Occlusion therapy).

Bifocals are indicated in children with a high AC/A (accommodative convergence to accommodation ratio) accommodative esotropia (convergence excess esotropia), where the full hypermetropic spectacle correction aligns the eyes for distance fixation, but a residual esotropia is seen at near. It is important to make sure that when the child looks down, as when reading, the line of sight will be through the bifocal segment (executive style or large flat-top segment bisecting the pupil is often prescribed). Some physicians order an add of +3.00 D, on the grounds that the average fixation distance at near is 3 cm. Others prescribe the minimum near addition which controls the near esotropia. The recommended strategy is then to gradually and incrementally reduce the bifocal correction.

Occlusion therapy

Some authorities recommend treating amblyopia fully before strabismus surgery even though in some cases this means delaying surgery for many months. Two prospective studies evaluated the need for completion of amblyopia therapy versus early operation with continuation of occlusion postoperatively. Neither study detected a significant difference in motor or sensory outcome whether amblyopia was fully or only partially treated before surgery.[16,17]

A recent study reported that, with partially accommodative esotropia, the mean angle of deviation decreased significantly after occlusion treatment for amblyopia and noticed that occlusion may resolve the non-accommodative component of the deviation obviating the need for surgery. Surgery would have been performed in 81% of patients if planned before the termination of amblyopia treatment, compared to 38% of patients that ultimately required surgery.[18] Another study showed that 61% of 46 small-angle strabismic children 1.5 to 9 years of age, undergoing part-time treatment with Bangerter foils for amblyopia, developed motor fusion with no additional interventions.[19]

Occlusion therapy, even in the absence of amblyopia, may be effective in improving the control of some forms of strabismus. Part-time (3–4 hours a day) unilateral or alternating occlusion is commonly prescribed for the treatment of X(T).[20,21] Occlusion may improve the control of the deviation by eliminating suppression. Commonly, the angle of the deviation decreases, and the relationship between distance and near deviation may change, altering the X(T) pattern.[21] Unfortunately, most data supporting this and other non-surgical treatments for X(T) come from small retrospective and/or non-controlled studies. It remains unclear what is the most effective treatment for this condition.[14]

Prisms

Prisms have very limited value in the management of childhood strabismus. Where a child has a temporary deviation that might confidently be expected to improve, as in consecutive esotropia after surgery for exotropia, or in a post-viral sixth nerve palsy, temporary Fresnel membrane prisms may be used to maintain binocularity while the deviation resolves. Occasionally, prisms can be used to move unwanted images into an area of the retina that is suppressed in patients with diplopia. However, in anything other than the lowest powers, prisms significantly degrade the visual acuity, in addition to attracting dirt, fingerprints, etc.

Prism adaptation

In the prism adaptation test for esotropia, the patient has base-out prisms applied to the glasses to correct the angle of deviation. In cases where the esodeviation increases, the power of the prisms is increased until the angle stabilizes. Subsequent surgery is then based on the maximum prism-adapted angle. Results are claimed to be superior to those based on the manifest angle without prism adaptation. The Prism Adaptation Study was a prospective randomized controlled clinical trial of prism adaptation in acquired esotropia in which 60% of patients underwent prism adaptation and 40% did not. Of the group that responded to prism adaptation with a stable motor angle and sensory fusion, half had strabismus surgery based on the prism-adapted angle and half had a conventional amount of surgery. The best rates of alignment were obtained in prism responders who underwent surgery (89%), and the lowest were in patients who were not prism adapted (72%).

Prisms in nystagmus

In children with congenital nystagmus and a compensatory head posture, when Kestenbaum surgery is being contemplated, it may be helpful to conduct a short trial of prismatic glasses to allow the parents to confirm that the face turn is abolished. The Fresnel prisms should not be stronger than 15–20 PD, and should be applied with the bases to the side to which the head is habitually turned. In some patients with nystagmus the amplitude is decreased on convergence and an attempt to induce this artificially can be made with base-out prisms.

Orthoptic exercises/vision therapy

Orthoptic exercises are sometimes used to teach patients how to use their fusion ability more efficiently. Orthoptic exercises may help in establishing control of strabismus in a very small group of patients with good fusion potential. The effectiveness of orthoptic exercises (and the broader practice of vision therapy) in treating most forms of strabismus is debated. A comprehensive review of the evidence supporting orthoptic exercises/vision therapy from the UK concluded that there was little evidence-based research to support these practices.[22] A notable exception is the management of convergence insufficiency.[23]

The Convergence Insufficiency Treatment Trial, a placebo-controlled randomized clinical trial, demonstrated that a 12-week office-based program of vergence and accommodative exercises (such as string-convergence and barrel-convergence) with home reinforcement was more effective than home-based "pencil push-ups," home-based computer therapy plus "pencil push-ups," or office-based placebo therapy in treating convergence insufficiency in children.[24] A similar conclusion was reached by the same researchers investigating convergence insufficiency treatment in young adults.[25]

Drugs

Irreversible cholinesterase inhibitors, such as Ecothiopate (phospholine iodide 0.125%, 0.0625% and 0.0325%) drops, can be used to control accommodation and, thereby, accommodative convergence. Pilocarpine, a muscarinic receptor agonist, can be used to decrease the synkinetic convergence response. Contraction of the ciliary body produces increased convexity and forward-shifting of the lens, resulting in a myopic shift and reduction in the active accommodation effort made. The most common indications for these medications include persistent consecutive esotropia after surgical overcorrection of exotropia, small residual post-operative esotropia, and as a supplement to glasses in patients with high AC/A accommodative esotropia with residual esodeviation at near.

Phospholine iodide is rarely used now due to its limited commercial availability and side effects (supraorbital pain, poor vision especially at night, and iris cysts and lens opacities with long-term use). Systemic absorption of the drops causes a depletion of plasma cholinesterase making the patient susceptible to depolarizing muscle relaxants. If a child treated with cholinesterase inhibitors requires general anesthesia, a depolarizing relaxing agent such as succinylcholine should be avoided as prolonged respiratory paralysis may result. The depletion may last up to 6 weeks and parents should be advised appropriately. To reduce the risk of iris cyst formation, phenylephrine (5%) eye drops can be prescribed concurrently.

In hypermetropic esotropic children who do not tolerate their newly prescribed spectacles, atropine 1% once daily for 5 days can be used to blur the vision and give the child an incentive to wear glasses.

Botulinum toxin

The pharmacologic treatment of strabismus was pioneered by Scott, who experimented with the direct injection of various substances into the extraocular muscles. In 1990, botulinum toxin type A was granted FDA approval. Botulinum toxin type A (BTX-A) is a large protein molecule of 150 000 daltons. After intramuscular injection, the toxin enters and remains at the nerve terminal for several days to weeks inhibiting the release of acetylcholine by cleaving SNAP-25, a protein integral to the successful docking and release of the neurotransmitter in vesicles within the nerve endings resulting in muscle weakness or paralysis maximal within 3 to 5 days after the injection. Although an irreversible binding occurs, extrajunctional acetylcholine receptors may develop. The nerve reinnervates the muscle with a reversal of the paralysis and eventual recovery. Extraocular muscle paralysis usually lasts from 2 to 8 weeks.

The mechanism by which permanent alignment can occur after the paralyzing effect of botulinum toxin is gone is not completely understood. One theory is that if the antagonist muscle remains contracted for a certain time because of reduced force in treated muscle, it will develop structural alterations that shorten it[26,27] and decrease its elasticity (contracture). Conversely, the chemodenervated muscle will undergo lengthening as its antagonist contracts. This length adaptation is believed to occur through the addition and deletion of sarcomeres.[27] The alterations induced in extraocular muscles by botulinum treatment have been shown to be specific to the orbital singly innervated muscle fibers.[26,28] This fiber-type specificity is thought to explain the permanent effect on static alignment but sparing the saccade kinematics after BTX-A injection.[28,29] Sensory mechanisms must also play a role in the permanent realignment after treatment with BTX-A in selected types of strabismus.[30] The structural theory (selective fiber-type atrophy) is clearly an insufficient explanation, as permanent double vision is rarely seen in patients who have diplopia immediately after periorbital BTX-A injections.[28]

The lyophilized drug is supplied in 100-IU vials and is reconstituted with non-preserved saline solution (0.9% sodium chloride injection), resulting in doses from 1 IU/0.1 mL to 12 IU/0.1 mL. One unit is equivalent to one-fiftieth of a lethal dose in a rat or 4 ng. The estimated systemic toxic dose is 40 U/kg body weight.

Injection technique

Transconjunctival injection of botulinum toxin can be done with or without electromyography (EMG) guidance (Fig. 84.1). Adult patients can have the procedure with topical anesthesia; in younger patients, injections should be administered under sedation using very low doses of ketamine if EMG is used. When the injection is done without EMG assistance, sevofluorane, propofol, ketamine, or nitrous oxide can be used.[31] The efficacy and complication rates with and without EMG control appear comparable.[32-34]

We perform most of the injections using a closed conjunctival technique without EMG (Fig. 84.2; Video 84.1). Others prefer to inject under direct visualization using an "open sky" technique,[30] but this negates some of the advantages of BTX-A treatment over surgery (shorter anesthesia time, reduced scarring, etc.) We reserve the open sky technique for patients with previous large muscle recessions (Fig. 84.3; Video 84.2). After placing a lid speculum, the eye is rotated into the opposite direction of the muscle being injected using conjunctival forceps. The insertion is identified and firmly grasped using toothed forceps[34] (Fig. 84.4) and a 25- to 27-gauge needle with the bevel toward the sclera, on an insulin syringe is passed through the grasped tendon. The eye is then rotated to the straight position and the needle is introduced to the hub. The desired dose of the drug is injected and the needle is retrieved.

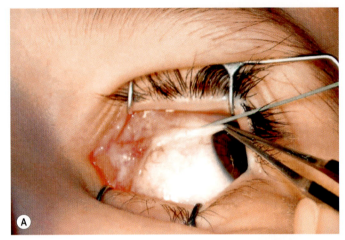

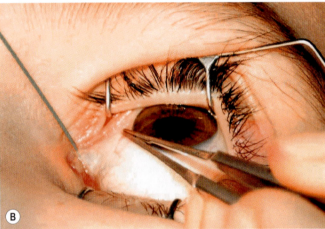

Fig. 84.1 BTX-A injection with EMG. (Courtesy of Pilar Gómez de Liaño, Madrid, Spain.)

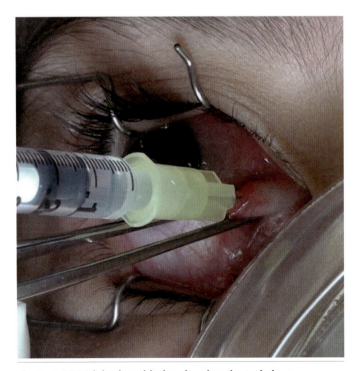

Fig.84. 2 BTX-A injection with closed conjunctiva technique.

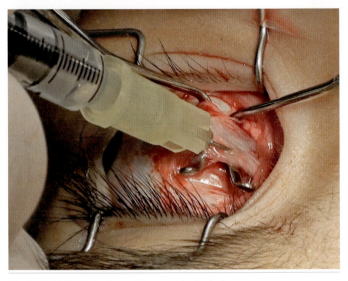

Fig. 84.3 BTX-A injection with open sky technique.

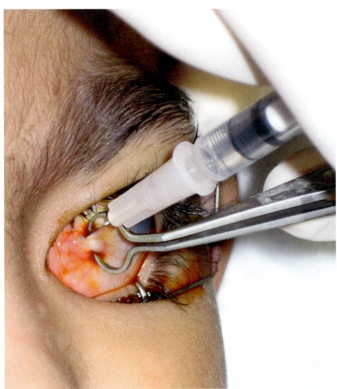

Fig. 84.4 BTX-A injection using Mendonça forceps.

Under EMG guidance a special needle acts also as an EMG electrode connected to an amplifier that converts the electrical signal from the muscle to sound. The needle is introduced through the conjunctiva and conducted to the muscle until a characteristic cracking sound is heard, confirming that the tip is in the muscle body. The needle must penetrate the muscle posteriorly, close to the nerve insertion.

The doses used vary, most authors recommending 1.25 to 7.5 IU per muscle[35-37] in a volume of 0.05 to 0.15 mL per muscle (Table 84.1).

Table 84.1 – Examples of BTX-A doses

Horizontal/vertical strabismus <20 PD	1.25–2.5 IU
Horizontal/vertical strabismus 20–50 PD	2.5–5.0 IU
Reinjection	1.5–2× original dose
Childhood esotropia	
Initial	2.5–5 IU
Reinjection	5–7.5 IU
Sixth nerve palsy	
Initial LR weakness	1.5–2.5 IU
Recovered LR function, persistent small ET	2.5 IU
Large ET, paretic LR	5 IU
With transposition	2.5–5 IU

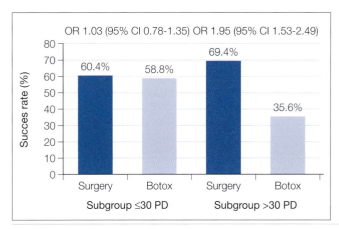

Fig. 84.5 Effectiveness of surgery vs. Botox (BTX-A) by angle of deviation. The pretreatment angle of deviation was statistically associated with a successful outcome in the BTX-A group only (the mean angle in the success group was 35.2 PD compared to 41.6 PD in the group with an unsuccessful outcome, p < 0.0001).The magnitude of deviation did not predict a successful outcome in the surgical group (p = 0.17). A post hoc subgroup analysis of those deviations classified as "small-angle esotropias" (<30 PD) was performed. Stratification by this angle of deviation revealed that among subjects with deviations ≤30 PD, there was no statistical difference between groups (surgery 60%, botulinum toxin 59%; OR 1.03, 95% CI 0.78–1.35). At deviation >30 PD, surgery achieved 69% success vs. 36% with botulinum toxin (OR 1.95, 95% CI 1.53–2.49).

Box 84.1

Common current indications of BTX-A

- Infantile ET without vertical deviations, little or no contraction and moderate to small angle in patients less than 2–3 years old
- Acquired ET of less than 30 PD
- Residual ET of <30 PD (after surgery)
- ET in patients with developmental delay (especially with angle variability)
- Consecutive exotropia if no duction deficit
- Acute sixth nerve palsy
- Diagnostically for the investigation of sensory or motor status in complex strabismus cases
- Treatment of oscillopsia in acquired nystagmus (retrobulbar or 4 muscle injection)

Indications

Infantile esotropia with a small or moderate deviation, acquired nerve palsies in the acute phase, post-surgical residual deviations, and restrictive conditions such as thyroid-related strabismus and Duane's syndrome currently are the most common indications. Box 84.1 summarizes the most common applications of BTX-A for strabismus currently used. Unfortunately most studies supporting or rejecting the efficacy of BTX-A as an alternative to surgery have lacked the methodological rigor of evidence-based medicine.[38,39]

In two randomized controlled trials BTX-A injection was as effective as reoperation in the treatment of residual esotropia after surgery for acquired[40] or infantile[41] esotropia, in terms of both motor and sensory outcomes. For acquired esotropia in children, the same authors reported that 1–3 injections of BTX-A as primary treatment was effective in 88% of patients.[37]

The success rate of BTX-A for the treatment of infantile esotropia (alignment within 10 PD of orthotropia) varies between 33% and 89%.[30,35,36,42-45] McNeer reported a high success rate of alignment (89%) in selected patients with infantile esotropia and a small to moderate angle of deviation.[44] Campos reported similar findings with a single injection in patients younger than 8 months old and small to moderate deviations.[30] Other studies have found an unacceptable rate of treatment failure, concluding that the prolonged period of misalignment and the need for multiple injections could interfere with early alignment and establishment of binocular vision.[46,47] The validity of these studies is limited due to no randomization and masking, small sample sizes, short follow-up, or ill-defined patient populations.

We conducted a prospective, single center, non-randomized comparison between BTX-A and surgery as primary treatment in infantile esotropia presenting by the age of 36 months. The primary outcome was alignment within 10 PD of orthotropia after one surgery or 1–3 bilateral botulinum injections.[36] BTX-A was injected in 322 patients and 120 patients underwent surgery. The odds of achieving a successful outcome at the average angle of deviation pretreatment (38.60 PD) was 2.3 times higher in the surgical group than in the patients receiving BTX-A. However, there was a significant interaction between treatment group and pretreatment angle of deviation (p < 0.001). A post hoc subgroup analysis was conducted using stratification by angle of deviation. This revealed that in subjects with deviations ≤30 PD, there was no statistical difference between groups (surgery 60%, botulinum toxin 59%; RR 1.03, 95% CI 0.78–1.35). At deviation >30 PD, surgery achieved 69% success vs. 36% with botulinum toxin (RR 1.95, 95% CI 1.53–2.49) (Fig. 84.5).

The relationship between the size of the strabismus angle and BTX-A effectiveness is well documented.[36,37,45] Studies that do not include appropriate stratification and effect modification analysis will fail to demonstrate BTX-A true efficacy. Other possible interactions and confounders such as sensory status,[48] age,[30,44] and duration of misalignment may also play an important role in predicting which patients will have a favorable response to this treatment. The paucity of randomized clinical trials and well-conducted prospective studies have limited our understanding of which patients will obtain the greatest benefit from BTX-A.[38]

BTX-A is less frequently used for exotropia and vertical deviations. Some use it in residual XT <15 PD or in young children (less than 3) with poorly controlled X(T) with the objective of delaying surgery until the age of 5 to 6 years. It has also been used successfully in patients with overcorrected exotropia and fusion potential.[49]

For cranial nerve palsies the most common application of BTX-A is in the acute phase of a sixth nerve palsy to prevent contracture of the unopposed ipsilateral medial rectus muscle. Such contracture may lead to persistent esotropia even when there is recovery of the lateral rectus function. Reports of cases successfully treated with BTX-A injection even after years of the onset of the esotropia supports this concept, but whether this secondary contracture can be prevented is controversial. If truly effective, botulinum toxin injection into the medial rectus soon after the onset of the esotropia would improve the spontaneous recovery rate of sixth nerve palsies and decrease the rates of surgery.

Lee et al. reported their experience with non-traumatic acute sixth nerve palsy randomized to observation versus BTX-A injection to the ipsilateral medial rectus muscle.[50] At 6 months, no statistically significant difference was observed. Control of the deviation (within 10 PD of ortho) and single vision was achieved in 86% of the patients treated with BTX-A, and in 80% of the control patients. Despite randomizations, the two groups were different with respect to their initial angle of deviation (10 PD larger on average in the BTX-A group) and duration. Multivariate analysis adjusting for these differences (re-analyzed from published data) suggests that there may be an advantage to using BTX-A (odds ratio 5.9, 95% CI 0.6 to 57.8) although the power was insufficient to reach statistical significance. A non-randomized study conducted by the Pediatric Eye Disease Investigator Group reported that in 84 patients, age 2–79 years, with acute traumatic sixth nerve palsy, the adjusted relative risk of recovery in patients that received BTX-A within 3 month of injury was only 14% higher than in patients managed with observation alone (RR 1.14, 95% CI 0.70–1.35).[51]

The same investigators prospectively studied 56 patients with sixth nerve palsies of more than 6 months duration nonrandomly allocated to observation, BTX-A alone, surgery alone, or a combination of surgery plus BTX-A. The success rates (absence of diplopia and ET <10 PD in primary gaze) were 10% (95% CI 0–45%) in the BTX-A and 39% (95% CI 17–64%) in the surgical groups. However, the authors warned that the different success rates might be due to selection bias and confounding by indication. For example, patients that received BTX-A were on average 27 years older than those who received surgery; 40% of patients that received BTX-A had complete paresis of the sixth nerve compared to 27% in the surgical group and most of the cases with a neoplastic etiology were treated with BTX-A alone. This study is also limited by its small sample size; the 95% confidence interval for the success rates in these two groups overlap significantly. Additional care should be taken when interpreting these results since these patients had a chronic longstanding deviation (median 270 days from onset to injection) and prevention of secondary contracture would not be expected.[52]

Medial rectus muscle injection of BTX-A prior to or during vertical muscle transposition can be used as an alternative to medial rectus recession, especially when anterior segment ischemia is of concern.

Complications

The complications of BTX-A treatment include subconjunctival hemorrhage, transient ptosis (Fig. 84.6) and hyperdeviations

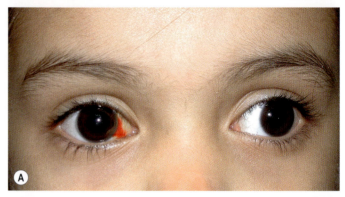
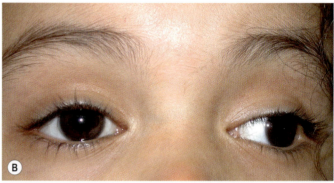

Fig. 84.6 Exotropia, ptosis and subconjunctival hemorrhage are commonly seen after BTX-A injection.

that usually resolve within 6 months (most resolving within several weeks of the injection). Transient vertical deviations occur in 5–30% of patients and ptosis in 15–35%. It is usually unilateral, and the risk increases with higher volume or concentration. The amblyogenic potential of ptosis must be considered in young children, but most authors report only partial reversible ptosis with no amblyogenic effects observed. Rare, but severe complications include globe perforation and retrobulbar hemorrhage. No systemic paralytic effect has been observed or suspected in any patient treated with the small doses of BTX-A used for strabismus. Antibodies to the toxin have not been detected in patients given small doses for ocular use. Therefore, repeat injections can be given when necessary.

In infantile esotropia, a temporary exotropia is not considered a complication of treatment; it is not only expected, but considered a sign of good prognosis.[30] It usually resolves by 6 weeks (4 to 10 weeks). Reinjection is recommended after 4 months if the angle of deviation is more than 10 PD ET although, in many cases, we would consider earlier reinjection, especially in those cases in which an initial exodeviation was not obtained. Permanent exotropias are rare.[30,36,37,53]

References

2. Ebri A, Kuper H, Wedner S. Cost-effectiveness of cycloplegic agents: results of a randomized controlled trial in Nigerian children. Invest Ophthalmol Vis Sci 2007; 48: 1025–31.

3. Rosenbaum AL, Bateman JB, Bremer DL, Liu PY. Cycloplegic refraction in esotropic children: cyclopentolate versus atropine. Ophthalmology 1981; 88: 1031–4.

8. Iacobucci IL, Archer SM, Giles CL. Children with exotropia responsive to spectacle correction of hyperopia. Am J Ophthalmol 1993; 15; 116:79–83.

9. Chung SA, Kim IS, Kim WK, Lee JB. Changes in exodeviation following hyperopic correction in patients with intermittent exotropia. J Pediatr Ophthalmol Strabismus 2011; 48: 278–84.

10. Caltrider N, Jampolsky A. Overcorrecting minus lens therapy for treatment of intermittent exotropia. Ophthalmology 1983; 90: 1160–5.

11. Watts P, Tippings E, Al-Madfai H. Intermittent exotropia, overcorrecting minus lenses, and the Newcastle scoring system. J AAPOS 2005; 9: 460–4.

12. Rowe FJ, Noonan CP, Freeman G, DeBell J. Intervention for intermittent distance exotropia with overcorrecting minus lenses. Eye (Lond) 2009; 23: 320–5.

14. Hatt S, Gnanaraj L. Interventions for intermittent exotropia. Cochrane Database Syst Rev 2006; 3: CD003737.

18. Koc F, Ozal H, Yasar H, Firat E. Resolution in partially accommodative esotropia during occlusion treatment for amblyopia. Eye (Lond) 2006; 20: 325–8.

19. Abrams MS, Duncan CL, McMurtrey R. Development of motor fusion in patients with a history of strabismic amblyopia who are treated part-time with Bangerter foils. J AAPOS 2011; 15: 127–30.

20. Freeman RS, Isenberg SJ. The use of part-time occlusion for early onset unilateral exotropia. J Pediatr Ophthalmol Strabismus 1989; 26: 94–6.

22. Barrett BT. A critical evaluation of the evidence supporting the practice of behavioural vision therapy. Ophthal Physiol Opt 2009; 29: 4–25.

23. Scheiman M, Gwiazda J, Li T. Non-surgical interventions for convergence insufficiency. Cochrane Database Syst Rev 2011; 3: CD006768.

24. Convergence Insufficiency Treatment Trial Study Group. Randomized clinical trial of treatments for symptomatic convergence insufficiency in children. Arch Ophthalmol 2008; 126: 1336–49.

25. Scheiman M, Mitchell GL, Cotter S, et al. A randomized clinical trial of vision therapy/orthoptics versus pencil pushups for the treatment of convergence insufficiency in young adults. Optom Vis Sci 2005; 82: 583–95.

30. Campos EC, Schiavi C, Bellusci C. Critical age of botulinum toxin treatment in essential infantile esotropia. J Pediatr Ophthalmol Strabismus 2000; 37: 328–32; quiz 54–5.

35. Scott AB, Magoon EH, McNeer KW, Stager DR. Botulinum treatment of childhood strabismus. Ophthalmology 1990; 97: 1434–8.

36. de Alba Campomanes AG, Binenbaum G, Campomanes Eguiarte G. Comparison of botulinum toxin with surgery as primary treatment for infantile esotropia. J AAPOS 2010; 1: 111–6.

37. Tejedor J, Rodriguez JM. Long-term outcome and predictor variables in the treatment of acquired esotropia with botulinum toxin. Invest Ophthalmol Vis Sci 2001; 42: 2542–6.

39. Rowe FJ, Noonan CP. Botulinum toxin for the treatment of strabismus. Cochrane Database Syst Rev 2009; 2: CD006499.

40. Tejedor J, Rodriguez JM. Retreatment of children after surgery for acquired esotropia: reoperation versus botulinum injection. Br J Ophthalmol 1998; 82: 110–4.

41. Tejedor J, Rodriguez JM. Early retreatment of infantile esotropia: comparison of reoperation and botulinum toxin. Br J Ophthalmol 1999; 83: 783–7.

43. McNeer KW, Tucker MG, Spencer RF. Botulinum toxin therapy for essential infantile esotropia in children. Arch Ophthalmol 1998; 116: 701–3.

44. McNeer KW, Tucker MG, Spencer RF. Botulinum toxin management of essential infantile esotropia in children. Arch Ophthalmol 1997; 115: 1411–8.

45. Gomez de Liano R, Monplan B, Gomez de Liano P, Rodriguez JM. Tratamiento del estrabismo infantil mediante toxina botulinica. Acta Estrabologica 1993: 37–42.

49. Dawson EL, Marshman WE, Lee JP. Role of botulinum toxin A in surgically overcorrected exotropia. J AAPOS 1999; 3. 269–71.

50. Lee J, Harris S, Cohen J, et al. Results of a prospective randomized trial of botulinum toxin therapy in acute unilateral sixth nerve palsy. J Pediatr Ophthalmol Strabismus 1994; 31: 283–6.

51. Holmes JM, Beck RW, Kip KE, et al. Botulinum toxin treatment versus conservative management in acute traumatic sixth nerve palsy or paresis. J AAPOS 2000; 4: 145–9.

52. Holmes JM, Leske DA, Christiansen SP. Initial treatment outcomes in chronic sixth nerve palsy. J AAPOS 2001; 5: 370–6.

53. Tejedor J, Rodriguez JM. Management of nonresolving consecutive exotropia following botulinum toxin treatment of childhood esotropia. Arch Ophthalmol 2007; 125: 1210–3.

 Access the complete reference list online at
http://www.expertconsult.com

Part 6
Strabismus treatment

Strabismus surgery

Craig A McKeown • Kara Cavuoto • Robert Morris

Introduction

The management of strabismus involves careful assessment of patients, and various forms of treatment, including correction of refractive error, orthoptics, amblyopia therapy, and surgery. Amblyopia should generally be treated prior to performing strabismus surgery.

The goals and risks of surgery should be clearly delineated to the parents, the child, and in the case of adults with strabismus, the patient. Parents should understand the importance of ongoing follow-up, particularly during the period of visual development, which extends through roughly the first decade of life.

The evaluation of surgical patients should include historical information, such as age of onset, direction of the strabismus, changes in the strabismus magnitude or direction over time, prior non-surgical or surgical treatment, and family history. A comprehensive ophthalmologic evaluation is essential, including cycloplegic refraction. Visual acuity should be documented at near and distance with appropriate correction. Refractive error should be fully corrected prior to determining the angle of deviation. The current prescription needs to be measured and, if a prism is present, this should be noted.

An appropriate sensory and motor examination is important. Sensory examination should include tests of fusion and stereopsis in patients old enough to perform them. In older children as well as adults with incomitant strabismus and diplopia, a diagram of the field of single binocular vision may be included. Motor examination is tailored to the unique features and age of the patient. Complex, multiplanar non-concomitant strabismus with limited range of movement requires special attention. A diagram of ocular range of motion for both ductions and versions is helpful.

In patients with prior ocular surgery, anterior segment and retinal findings may influence the choice and technique for surgery. Examination should identify conjunctival surgical scars and, the status of anterior ciliary vessels over the rectus tendons and insertions. Chorioretinal scars from prior surgery should be identified before additional strabismus surgery is performed.

Anatomy is important to strabismus surgery

Conjunctiva

The conjunctiva is a thin mucous membrane comprising the external surface of the eye posterior to the limbus. The conjunctiva fuses with Tenon's capsule and intermuscular septum 1 mm posterior to the limbus. This zone of fusion is useful during traction testing and when positioning the eye with forceps during surgery. Posterior to the zone of fusion, the conjunctiva can be separated from the underlying Tenon's capsule.

The conjunctiva is nearly transparent and well vascularized (Fig. 85.1). Adjacent to the limbus, it contributes to the rich anastamotic vascular network providing collateral flow to the anterior segment.[1] After topical 2.5% phenylephrine, normal conjunctival vessels constrict; the underlying anterior ciliary vessels do not. The anterior ciliary vessels, their scleral penetration sites and anastamotic branches to neighboring rectus muscles can be seen. The insertion sites of the four rectus muscles can be visualized. The anterior termination of the extraconal fat pad is seen through the conjunctiva roughly 10 mm posterior to the limbus. These features help determine if there has been prior surgery and guide placement of the surgical incision.

The conjunctiva permits full movement of the globe. With scarring the conjunctiva can limit globe movement.

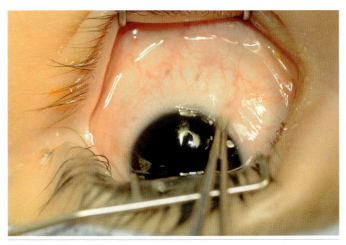

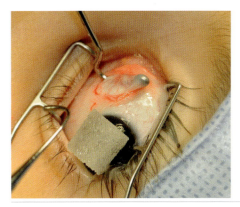

Fig. 85.2 Left medial rectus with Jameson hook behind insertion (surgeon's view). The conjunctiva and Tenon's capsule have been retracted over the tip of the hook, exposing the intermuscular septum, which remains intact on the superior pole of the medial rectus insertion. The anterior ciliary vessels are on the surface of the medial rectus tendon and the surface of the sclera.

Fig. 85.1 Forceps grasp the left globe at the limbus in the inferior nasal quadrant (surgeon's view). Small conjunctival vessels run anteriorly from the fornix, mostly meridional. Larger caliber anterior ciliary vessels are traveling on the scleral surface anterior to the insertion of the inferior rectus. The anterior edge of the extraconal fat is seen inferonasally and inferotemporally.

Tenon's capsule

Tenon's capsule is a dense, translucent and nearly avascular fascial layer extending from the limbus to the optic nerve. Anteriorly, it is located just beneath the conjunctiva. The conjunctiva can easily be separated from the underlying Tenon's capsule, beginning 1 mm posterior to the limbus. Three millimeters posterior to the limbus, Tenon's capsule fuses with the underlying intermuscular septum, forming a single fascial layer.[2] Posterior to this zone, Tenon's capsule envelops the globe, forming a potential cavity (sub-Tenon's space).

In young people, Tenon's capsule is thick, white and glistening, becoming thinner in adulthood. The bulbar surface of Tenon's capsule is smooth, providing movement of one fascial plane over another.

Tenon's capsule is penetrated by the four rectus muscles, just posterior to the equator of the globe. The penetration sites are approximately 10 mm posterior to the insertion of the rectus muscles. The inferior oblique muscle and superior oblique tendon penetrate Tenon's capsule just anterior to the equator. The penetration sites of the extraocular muscles resemble a cuff on the sleeve of a sweater and represent a point of attachment between Tenon's capsule and the capsule of the four rectus muscles, the inferior oblique muscle, and the superior oblique tendon. This point of attachment is an important landmark during strabismus surgery and in the recovery of lost muscles.

The penetration sites of the rectus muscles form a division between anterior and posterior Tenon's capsule. Anterior Tenon's capsule extends from the penetration sites to the limbus, while posterior Tenon's capsule extends from the penetration sites to the optic nerve.

Tenon's capsule separates the orbital fat from the globe. Anterior Tenon's separates extraconal fat from the eye; posterior Tenon's separates intraconal fat from the globe. Fibrous septae extend from the outer surface of Tenon's capsule to the orbital periosteum.[3] It is important to avoid violating Tenon's capsule during surgery. Failure to do so permits fat to prolapse into sub-Tenon's space. Scarring may result in fat adherence with restricted eye movement.

Muscle capsule and intermuscular septum

The rectus and oblique muscles and tendons are enveloped in connective tissue capsules. The capsules on the rectus muscles are well developed anterior to the site of the muscles' penetration of Tenon's capsule. With age, the capsules thin. Postoperative scarring is reduced if the muscle capsule is left intact in areas not involved with the procedure. Posterior to the penetration site in Tenon's capsule, the muscle capsules become quite thin.[4]

The intermuscular septum is a thin, avascular layer of connective tissue that is continuous with the muscle capsules, extending from the border of each rectus muscle to the adjacent rectus muscles (Fig. 85.2). Anterior to the rectus muscles' penetration of Tenon's capsule, the intermuscular septum forms a thin, separate layer just beneath Tenon's capsule, adjacent to the sclera. Posterior to the rectus muscles' penetration, the intermuscular septum has been thought to separate intraconal from extraconal fat. However, the existence of this portion of the intermuscular septum has recently been questioned: it may be the anterior aspect of the connective tissue pulleys.[5] The intermuscular septum is associated with the inferior oblique and forms a roughly 2 mm wide band, extending off the posterolateral margin of the muscle.

Blood supply

The ophthalmic artery supplies the extraocular muscles. The lateral muscular branch of the ophthalmic artery supplies the lateral rectus, superior rectus, superior oblique, and levator palpebrae superioris. The lateral rectus is also supplied by the lacrimal artery. The medial muscular branch of the ophthalmic artery supplies the inferior rectus, medial rectus, and inferior oblique muscles. The inferior rectus and inferior oblique muscles are also supplied by the infraorbital artery.

Each of the four rectus muscles carries anterior ciliary vessels that contribute to the blood supply of the anterior segment; the two oblique muscles do not. In the classic description, each rectus muscle has two anterior ciliary arteries, except the lateral, which has one.[6] This diagram of the ocular circulation is reproduced repeatedly in ophthalmic literature[6,7] and shows the anterior ciliary vessels traveling within the muscle and

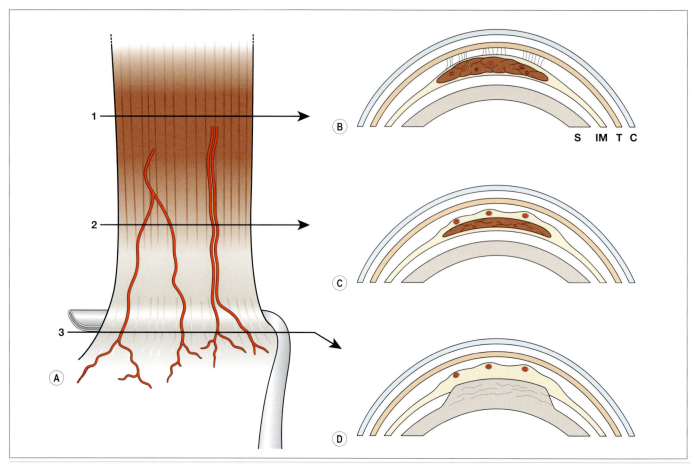

Fig. 85.3 Diagram of typical rectus muscle showing position of anterior ciliary vessels (ACVs). (A) Surgeon's view of inferior rectus. The ACVs emerge from the substance of the muscle posterior to the transition from muscle to tendon. Anterior to this point, the ACVs travel on the surface of the muscle and tendon, following somewhat serpentine course in a plane that is continuous with the muscle capsule, continuing onto the surface of the sclera. (B) Transverse section of rectus muscle at position a-1, posterior to the point of emergence of the ACVs. The vessels are deep in the muscle, not visible to the surgeon. S = sclera; IM = intermuscular septum (continuous with the muscle capsule); T = Tenon's capsule; C = conjunctiva. (C) Transverse section at position a-2 showing three ACV "groups" on the surface of the tendon, in a plane that is continuous with the capsule of the muscle and tendon. Each anterior ciliary vessel group can contain more than one anterior ciliary vessel. (D) Transverse section at position a-3: the tendon insertion site. The ACVs remain on the surface and continue onto the sclera, anterior to the tendon insertion.

tendon. However, the vessels emerge from the substance of the muscle, posterior to the transition from muscle to tendon, and travel on the surface of the tendon[8] (Figs 85.3 and 85.4). The number of anterior ciliary vessels is variable.[9,10]

The contribution of the anterior ciliary vessels to anterior segment blood flow has been studied by iris fluorescein angiography.[11] Tenotomy of either of the vertical rectus muscles produces a significant delay in vascular filling in the corresponding segment of the iris.[12] Surgery on the vertical rectus muscles impacts more on anterior segment blood flow than surgery on the horizontal rectus muscles and may influence the risk of anterior segment ischemia.

Innervation

The extraocular muscles receive innervation from the oculomotor (III), the trochlear (IV), and the abducens (VI) nerves. The abducens nerve innervates the lateral rectus. The trochlear nerve innervates the superior oblique. The oculomotor nerve divides into a superior and an inferior division. The superior division innervates the levator palpebrae muscle and the superior rectus muscle while the inferior division innervates the

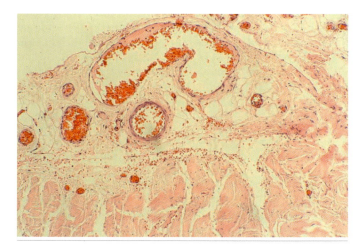

Fig. 85.4 Transverse section of resected lateral rectus. A single ACV group is shown, which contains three vessels of significant size, surrounded by loose connective tissue, which is continuous with the capsule and separates the vessels from the underlying tendon. A potential surgical dissection plane exists between the vessels and the tendon (hematoxylin-eosin; original magnification, ×200).

medial rectus, inferior rectus, and inferior oblique muscles. The nerves supplying the rectus muscles penetrate the bellies of the muscles at roughly the junction of the posterior and middle thirds of the muscles. The inferior oblique muscle receives its innervation lateral to the inferior rectus muscle. The superior oblique muscle receives its innervation from the inferior surface in the middle third of the muscle.

Sclera

The sclera is composed of highly organized collagen fibers. It ranges from 1 mm thick just posterior to the limbus to 0.33 mm thick just posterior to the rectus muscle insertions, where it is most at risk of perforation during strabismus surgery.

Pulleys of the orbit

Highly complex pulleys in the anterior orbit have been described. Each rectus muscle passes through an encircling ring of connective tissue near the equator of the globe, which attaches to the orbital wall. The pulleys are composed of collagen, bands of smooth muscle, and elastin.[13,14] They have an intimate and active relationship with the extraocular muscles, which can include acting as the functional origin and limiting side-slipping.[15,16,17] Orbital malformations, disease, trauma, and surgical procedures that affect the integrity of the orbital pulleys may be significant in ocular motility disorders.

Rectus muscles

There are four striated rectus muscles arising from the annulus of Zinn in the apex of the orbit. Each is 40 mm in length and inserts on the sclera anterior to the equator of the globe. Following the "spiral of Tillaux," the medial rectus inserts 5.5 mm from the limbus, the inferior rectus 6.5 mm, the lateral rectus 6.9 mm, and the superior rectus inserts 7.7 mm from the limbus (Table 85.1). The location of the insertions is actually somewhat variable.[18] The insertions of the rectus muscles are curvilinear, particularly the vertical rectus muscles, in which the temporal border is further from the limbus than the nasal border.

The medial rectus is responsible for adduction, the lateral rectus for abduction. The superior rectus supraducts and the inferior rectus infraducts; they have additional actions – adduction and torsion.

Table 85.1 – Rectus muscle dimensions

	Distance from limbus (mm)	Width at insertion (mm)	Length of muscle (mm)	Length of tendon (mm)
Medial rectus	5.5	10.3	40	3.7
Inferior rectus	6.5	9.8	40	5.5
Lateral rectus	6.9	9.2	40	8.8
Superior rectus	7.7	10.8	40	5.8

The medial rectus muscle courses anteriorly along the medial wall of the orbit inserting on the sclera with a 6 mm arc of contact with the globe. It is at risk for inadvertent damage during ethmoid sinus procedures and nasal pterygium excision. Without fascial attachments to an oblique muscle and its innate tension and relatively short arc of contact, the medial rectus is at the greatest risk of inadvertent loss during surgery.

The lateral rectus courses anteriorly along the lateral orbit inserting on the sclera with a 10 mm arc of contact with the globe. The insertion of the inferior oblique is in close proximity to the lower border of the lateral rectus, 8–10 mm posterior to the lower pole of the lateral rectus insertion. Due to fascial attachments between the lateral rectus and the inferior oblique, the surgeon can often locate the lateral rectus muscle if it becomes detached during surgery or trauma.

The inferior rectus muscle courses anteriorly, laterally, and inferiorly to insert on the sclera. The inferior rectus forms a 23° angle with the visual axis when the globe in the primary gaze position. It has fascial attachments to the inferior oblique muscle and the lower eyelid retractors (Fig. 85.5). If these attachments are not severed during recession or resection of the inferior rectus, eyelid fissure changes may occur. Connective tissue attachments between the superior rectus and the superior oblique may assist the surgeon in locating a 'lost' superior rectus muscle.

The superior rectus muscle courses anteriorly, laterally, and superiorly to insert on the sclera. It forms a 23° angle with the visual axis when the globe is in the primary gaze position. The superior rectus has fascial attachments to the superior oblique tendon and the levator palpebrae muscle. If the attachments to the levator palpebrae are not severed during recession or resection of the superior rectus, eyelid fissure changes may occur. Connective tissue attachments between the inferior rectus and the inferior oblique may assist the surgeon in locating a "lost" inferior rectus muscle.

Superior oblique muscle

The actions of the superior oblique are incyclotorsion, depression, and abduction. The superior oblique is an antagonist of the inferior oblique, with respect to torsion. The other actions are not strictly antagonistic with the inferior oblique.

The superior oblique muscle arises from periosteum in the orbital apex above the annulus of Zinn and travels anteriorly along the superomedial orbital wall. It becomes a cord-like tendon, passing through the trochlea to run in a posterolateral direction at an angle of approximately 51° to 54° with the sagittal plane. The tendon passes under the superior rectus and fans out, inserting on the sclera in the superotemporal quadrant (Fig. 85.6). The anterior pole of its insertion is located close to the lateral border of the superior rectus, beginning 4 to 6 mm posterior to the superior rectus insertion. Its tendon is thin and broad, extending posteriorly for about 11 mm, but with considerable variability. The posterior end of the insertion lies 6–7 mm from the optic nerve. The superior temporal vortex vein can exit the sclera temporal to the superior oblique insertion, under the insertion or sometimes split the fibers of the insertion and pass through them.

The superior oblique tendon can be abnormal.[19] It may be redundant, lax, or misdirected. It can have an anomalous insertion nasal to the superior rectus or may insert into Tenon's capsule and the trochlea, or be absent.[20] Intraoperative

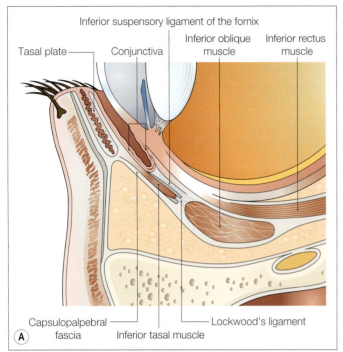

Inferior suspensory ligament of the fornix

Tasal plate — Conjunctiva — Inferior oblique muscle — Inferior rectus muscle

Capsulopalpebral fascia — Inferior tasal muscle — Lockwood's ligament

(A)

Fig. 85.5 Relationship of inferior rectus to lower lid: surgeon's view from above. (A) Diagrammatic illustration. (B) Lower lid retractors on surface of inferior rectus muscle being held with forceps. (C) Thickened Tenon's fascia beneath inferior rectus muscle seen as a glistening membrane with ridges between the muscle and the globe. (D) Inferior rectus muscle seen within Tenon's capsule. The original muscle insertion is seen under the left muscle hook. (Patient of Dr R. Morris.)

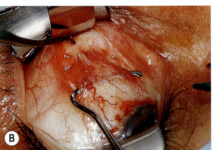
(B)

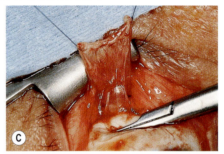
(C)

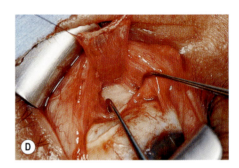
(D)

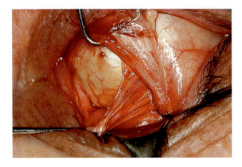

Fig. 85.6 Superior oblique tendon (held in lower hook) inserting beneath the superior rectus: surgeon's view from above. (Patient of Dr R. Morris.)

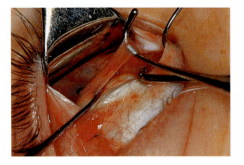

Fig. 85.7 Strabismus hooks beneath superior oblique tendon demonstrating tendon laxity. (Patient of Dr R. Morris.)

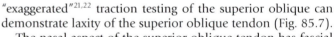

"exaggerated"[21,22] traction testing of the superior oblique can demonstrate laxity of the superior oblique tendon (Fig. 85.7).

The nasal aspect of the superior oblique tendon has fascial relationships with the intermuscular septum, which envelops it to form a capsule. If the nasal intermuscular septum is thin, atrophic, or is damaged while performing a nasal tenotomy, the cut ends of the tendon may separate excessively, creating a superior oblique palsy. The ends of the tendon may be difficult to recover. There is a frenulum between the capsule on the underside of the superior rectus and superior surface of the superior oblique tendon. The frenulum must be lysed for significant procedures on either muscle (Fig. 85.8).

Inferior oblique muscle

The actions of the inferior oblique are excyclotorsion, elevation, and abduction. The inferior oblique forms an antagonist pair with the superior oblique with respect to torsion. The additional actions of the inferior oblique are not strictly antagonistic with the superior oblique.

The inferior oblique muscle originates from the maxillary bone adjacent to the lacrimal fossa. It passes posteriorly and laterally, forming approximately a 51° angle with a sagittal plane passing through the origin of the muscle. After passing beneath the inferior rectus, the inferior oblique travels upward

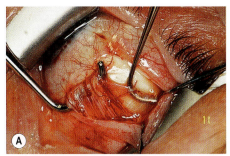

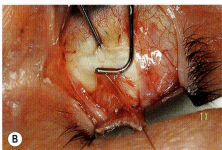

Fig. 85.8 Relationship between superior oblique and superior rectus: surgeon's view from above. (A) Chavasse muscle spreading hook (left) beneath superior rectus and Stevens hook beneath the superior oblique tendon showing the fascial attachment between them. It passes obliquely between the crook of the Stevens hook to just by the insertion of the superior rectus. (B) Undersurface of disinserted superior rectus (below, held on sutures) showing fascial attachment between it and the superior oblique tendon. (Patient of Dr R. Morris.)

inserting on the sclera, close to the macula.[23] The tendon of the inferior oblique is 1–2 mm long, the shortest of the extraocular muscle tendons. The inferior oblique insertion is 8 to 12 mm posterior to the lateral rectus insertion, adjacent to its lower border. There is considerable variability in the location and configuration of the inferior oblique insertion.

The inferior temporal vortex vein lies close to the inferior oblique. It can be damaged when the surgeon isolates the inferior oblique muscle or when placing an inferior oblique muscle to be recessed at its new insertion site, which may be close where the vortex vein exits the sclera. The scleral exit of the inferior temporal vortex vein is variable, but is often close to the lateral border of the inferior rectus, 8–10 mm posterior to the lateral pole of the inferior rectus insertion.

The neurovascular bundle enters the inferior oblique muscle as it passes beneath the inferior rectus muscle. The neurovascular bundle may serve as the effective origin of the inferior oblique, particularly after anterior transposition of the muscle.[24]

Overaction of the inferior oblique is common, particularly in congenital esotropia, intermittent exotropia, and superior oblique palsy. Overaction of the inferior oblique is clinically graded on a scale of 1–4.[25] Overaction of the inferior oblique must be distinguished from other causes of elevation of the globe in adduction. Overaction of the inferior oblique commonly coexists with dissociated vertical deviation.[26]

General principles of surgery

Preoperative examination

The preoperative examination should include a comprehensive eye examination with history, sensory, and motor

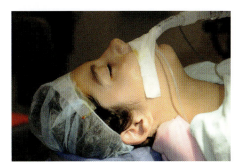

Fig. 85.9 Patient correctly positioned for surgery with neck slightly extended.

evaluation and refraction. Of particular importance are issues of prior surgery and which extraocular muscles were involved. It is not uncommon for adults to not recall childhood surgery. The examination should identify prior surgical scars as well as alterations in the course of the anterior ciliary vessels. Certain systemic and orbital disorders are associated with anatomic abnormalities affecting the extraocular muscles.

Preoperative counseling

The patient and/or the patient's guardians must be informed regarding the indications, potential benefits, risks, and alternatives to the procedure. Realistic expectations are essential. The discussion includes the potential effects on binocular vision, the possibility of overcorrection, undercorrection, and future sequential deviations that may require additional treatment.

Anesthesia

For young strabismus patients, surgery is usually performed under general anesthesia. Because strabismus procedures are relatively quick, short acting inhalational anesthetic agents are typically utilized. Sevoflurane is the most commonly used inhalational agent and a laryngeal mask airway or endotracheal tube is employed for its administration. Using a right angle endotracheal tube or a flexible tube laryngeal mask airway avoids the airway interfering with the drapes and reducing exposure.

Postoperative nausea and vomiting in strabismus patients receiving general anesthesia is common. Short acting inhalational anesthetics reduce, but do not eliminate, this problem.[27,28,29] Dexamethasone and ondansetron decrease postoperative nausea and vomiting.[30,31]

Patient preparation

Patient preparation is essential for efficient and safe surgery. Patient identification, diagnosis and laterality for surgery should be verified before operating. One drop of 2.5% phenylephrine is instilled in the operated eye(s) prior to the surgical preparation to provide vasoconstriction and dilate the pupil should postoperative fundoscopy be needed.

The patient should be positioned with the head level and the neck slightly extended (Fig. 85.9). The exposed skin is cleaned with aqueous povidone-iodine. One drop of 5% aqueous povidone-iodine is placed in the conjunctival cul-de-sac prior to surgery. The eyebrows are covered with drapes or an adhesive plastic strip (Fig. 85.10) and one is placed over the upper eyelid eyelashes. A separate speculum is used on each eye, when the procedure is bilateral.

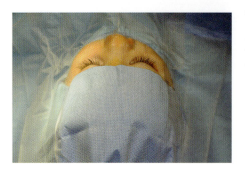

Fig. 85.10 **Surgical drape covering face while exposing both eyes for bilateral surgery.**

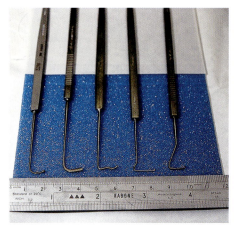

Fig. 85.11 **Strabismus hooks.** From left to right: a Stevens tenotomy hook, a von Graefe hook, a Chavasse hook, a Helveston hook, and a Green muscle hook.

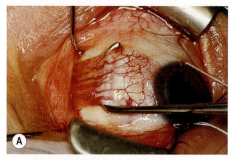

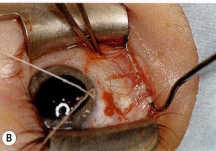

Fig. 85.12 **Surgical use of muscle hooks.** (A) Chavasse muscle hook under medial rectus. Note even spreading of the tendon on the hook and the anterior ciliary arteries. (B) Muscle spread evenly on Helveston hook. (Patient of Dr R. Morris.)

Surgical instruments

A selection of strabismus hooks is essential (Fig. 85.11). Hooks with tips slightly longer than the width of the rectus muscle insertion allow the tendon to be spread evenly on the hook, which facilitates dissection and suture placement (Fig. 85.12).

Traction testing

Traction testing is performed at the beginning of every procedure. If abnormal, the test may be repeated several times intraoperatively as the muscles are released. The position of the surgeon should be consistent for each traction testing. Traction testing consists of two components: force generation and passive range of motion.

Force generation testing is performed with the patient awake and able to follow commands, with no anesthetic induced akinesia or hypokinesia of the extraocular muscles. It qualitatively assesses the strength of the extraocular muscles by stabilizing the globe in one position and asking the patient to voluntarily move the eye in specific directions.

Passive range of motion testing can be performed in the office or the operating room. It qualitatively assesses the resistance imparted by the extraocular muscles as well as orbital tissues during manual rotation of the globe. It can be performed with the patient awake or under general or local anesthesia. The "volume effects" of any anesthetic agent injected in the orbit may alter the passive range of the traction test.

Intraoperative traction testing can be performed using different techniques. Most commonly, it is performed with two toothed forceps placed 180° apart adjacent to the limbus. The rectus muscles are evaluated by rotating the globe medially, temporally, superiorly, and inferiorly, while placing gentle

anterior traction on the globe, to place tension the rectus muscles.

To test the oblique muscles, the globe is rotated into extorsion and intorsion with gentle posterior pressure on the eye (retropulsion). This places the oblique muscles, with their anterior functional origins, under tension.

The exaggerated traction test of the superior oblique determines whether superior oblique laxity is present and may be helpful in Brown's syndrome.[32] It is performed by grasping the eye with two toothed forceps adjacent to the limbus. The eye is adducted while placing the eye in retropulsion, external rotation, and elevation. While maintaining this position, the eye is moved into abduction. A palpable "thump" is perceived with a normal superior oblique. An absent or reduced "thump" is evidence of superior oblique laxity. This test requires a considerable experience.

Incisions for strabismus surgery

Limbal incision

The limbal incision is a common approach for access to extraocular muscles (Fig. 85.13). The fusion of conjunctiva, Tenon's capsule, and intermuscular septum a few millimeters from the limbus permits the three layers to be retracted together, providing direct access to the sclera. It provides an excellent view of the extraocular muscles.

This incision is ideal for the inexperienced surgeon. Compared to the fornix incision, the limbal incision does not require as much anatomic knowledge on the part of the surgical assistant.

Fornix or cul-de-sac incision

The fornix or cul-de-sac incision is also commonly employed. It reduces postoperative discomfort and places the surgical scar is beneath the eyelid (Fig. 85.14). It requires a skilled assistant, familiar with ocular anatomy.

The fornix incision does not gain direct access to the sclera by penetrating the conjunctiva, Tenon's capsule, and intermuscular septum together in a single incision. Proper placement

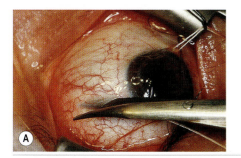
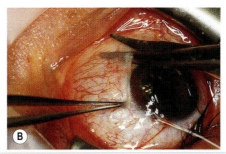
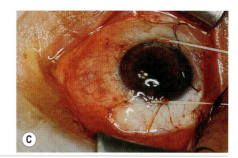

Fig. 85.13 Limbal conjunctival incision: surgeon's view from above. (A) Inferior conjunctival "relaxing" incision. (B) Superior conjunctival relaxing incision parallel to inferior conjunctival incision following completion of peritomy. (C) Accurate apposition of conjunctiva following rectus muscle surgery using four 7–0 Vicryl sutures. (Patient of Dr R. Morris.)

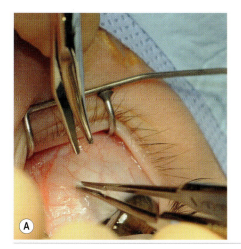
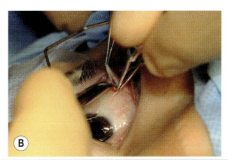
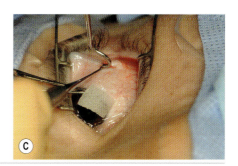

Fig. 85.14 (A) Cul-de-sac conjunctival incision is made 8 mm from the limbus parallel to the fornix in the inferonasal quadrant. (B) Tenon's capsule is held up with two Castroviejo forceps and incised at a right angle to the conjunctival incision. (C) A tenotomy hook engages the edge of the medial rectus behind the insertion. It is replaced with a Jameson or other long tipped hook to hold the entire width of the tendon just posterior to its insertion.

is important, particularly to avoid bleeding, inadvertent entry into the orbital fat, and, potentially, surgery on the wrong muscle.

The conjunctiva is opened as an isolated layer. Depending on the location of the anterior termination of the extraconal fat, the incision is placed 1–2 mm anterior to the fornix extending for 8 mm parallel to the fornix. A second incision is made through Tenon's capsule and the underlying intermuscular septum at a right angle to the conjunctival incision. It is important to avoid extending the incision in Tenon's capsule more than 10 mm posterior to the limbus, due to the anterior border of the extraconal fat. When the sclera is exposed, a muscle hook is used to engage the extraocular muscle to be operated.

Fornix incisions may be performed in any of the four oblique quadrants. By employing only an inferior temporal and superior nasal incision, the surgeon can gain access to all six extraocular muscles. Avoid incising the plica semilunaris when performing an inferonasal quadrant fornix incision.

Swan incision

The Swan incision is made directly over the rectus muscle insertion.[33] It is less popular due to the interpalpebral location of the wound with scar formation and potential bleeding from the underlying anterior ciliary vessels. A modified Swan incision may be useful in reoperations.

Minimal incision

Minimally invasive incisions are performed via small openings away from the limbus placed over the location on the muscle in which sutures are required. This may reduce discomfort and scarring.[34-36]

Extraocular muscle surgery

Principles

Attention to detail makes extraocular muscle surgery proceed smoothly. Confirmation of the proposed procedure should be re-verified immediately prior to starting surgery.

A history of prior muscle surgery warrants special consideration. Surgical scarring may alter the location of the extraocular muscles and other structures.

Careful dissection and hemostasis provide better exposure, reduce adhesions, and minimize muscle and vessel trauma. This diminishes the potential for inadvertent penetration of Tenon's capsule and fat prolapse. Light bipolar cautery under saline irrigation reduces tissue damage, in comparison to thermal cautery: its judicious use prevents tissue shrinkage and excessive scarring.

A moistened flat cellulose sponge placed on the corneal surface throughout the procedure helps reduce drying of the cornea and postoperative discomfort.

Sutures

Spatulated, side cutting needles are a major advance in strabismus surgery. They provide for easier and safer scleral passes and reduce the risk of scleral perforation.

Most strabismus surgery is performed using absorbable sutures, such as 6-0 coated polyglactin 910. A number of needle choices are available. Double armed 6-0 coated polyglactin 910 needle choices for strabismus surgery include S-14, S-24, S-28, S-29, and TG-100 needles.

Non-absorbable suture is sometimes desirable: 5-0 and 6-0 polyester white braided suture is available with S-14 and S-24 spatulated needles.

Conjunctival closure can be accomplished with a wide variety of techniques including no suture, cautery, 6-0 gut, and 8-0 polyglactin. The choice of needle for conjunctival closure is less critical than for suture placement in the sclera.

Tissue adhesives

Tissue adhesives have been used in conjunctival closure during strabismus surgery[37,38] but have not gained popularity in securing the muscles to the sclera.[39-41]

Magnification

Some surgeons routinely use the operating microscope; most use magnifying loupes of 2× to 3.5× power. Wide field 3.5× loupes provide excellent magnification, a comfortable depth of field, and a field wide enough to include the entire orbit. However, higher magnification and a wide field create a larger ring scotoma than the more commonly used 2× non-wide field loupes.

Rectus muscle surgery

Proper exposure of the extraocular muscles is essential for successful strabismus surgery. Dissection of excess connective tissue at the suture line provides better exposure for precise suture placement and decreases the risk of slipped or lost muscles (Fig. 85.15). This requires excision of redundant muscle capsule and intermuscular septum. The muscle capsule and intermuscular septum can be lifted off the rectus muscle adjacent to the insertion and excised without disrupting the anterior ciliary vessels. Cauterizing anterior ciliary vessels prior to passing sutures or making incisions in the tendon or muscle reduces bleeding and decreases scarring.

Weakening procedures on the rectus muscles

Recessions

Recessions are the most common weakening procedure on the rectus muscles. The maximal effect is in the field of action of the recessed muscle. However, recessions also have a significant effect on primary gaze alignment. Recessions are generally more comfortable postoperatively than resections; causing less swelling, dellen formation, inflammation, and scarring.

Recession results in a small resection of tendon. The method and point of measurement for recessions varies. Because of this and other factors, a 5 mm recession performed by one surgeon is not identical to one performed by another. Suture placement 1 mm posterior to the insertion minimizes the concurrent resection and allows disinsertion to be performed without inadvertent suture transection. Techniques to place the suture securely in the tendon include placement of a central tie in the tendon and double locking sutures at each border of the tendon.

The preferred site for measuring a recession varies. Measurement from the limbus avoids the potential variability in the position of the muscle insertion.[42] Those who measure from the insertion of the tendon feel the amount of recession is dependent upon the change in position relative to the original scleral attachment point, rather than the limbus. Measurement from the insertion should be determined prior to disinsertion; the elastic properties of the sclera allow the insertion to shift anteriorly following detachment of the muscle,[43] especially with tight extraocular muscles.

Recessions can be performed by attaching the muscle to the sclera at the desired position or by employing "hang-back," "hemi hang-back," or various modifications.

Direct fixation of the recessed muscle to the sclera is widely used (Fig. 85.16A,B). The scleral entry position of the needles is at the location of the desired recession and should be directly posterior to the original insertion site. Each pole should be spaced to maintain the width of the recessed muscle to avoid "central sag." If sagging occurs, the center of the muscle can be sutured to the sclera (Fig. 85.17). Because the muscle is sutured directly to the sclera, it allows accurate supra- and infraplacement and "slanting" the recession, if desired, in "A" and "V" patterns.

Hang-back and hemi hang-back techniques are commonly employed in recessions (Fig. 85.16C,D).The hang-back technique suspends the muscle on a suture attached at or near the terminal poles of the original insertion or can be located near

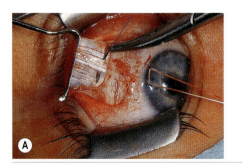
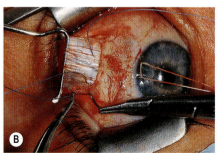
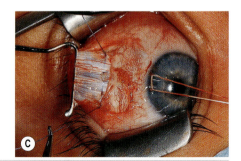

Fig. 85.15 Muscle suture placement: double-armed suture through lateral rectus: surgeon's view from above. (A) Central suture placement. (B) Superior locking bite. (C) Completed suture placement prior to muscle disinsertion. (Patient of Dr R. Morris.)

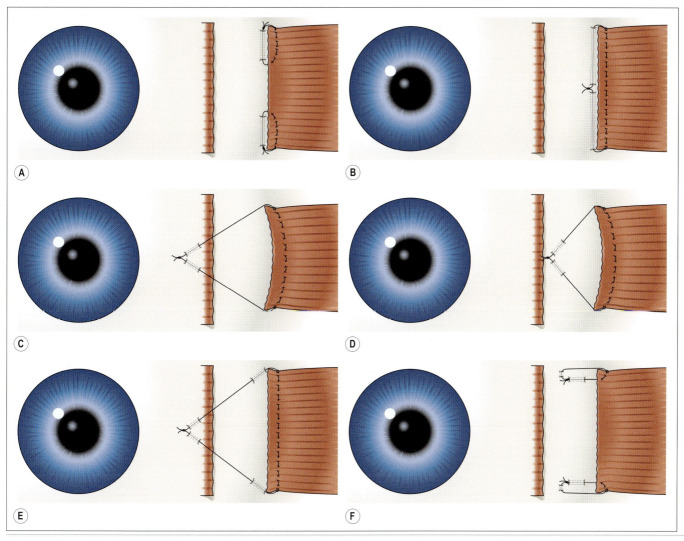

Fig. 85.16 Rectus muscle recession. (A) Fixed recession (two single sutures). (B) Fixed recession double armed suture. (C) Hang-back recession (note central bowing). (D) Hemi hang-back recession. (E) Anchored hang-back suture. (F) Gobin's loop recession.

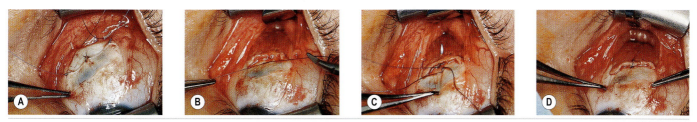

Fig. 85.17 Inferior rectus fixed muscle recession, double-suture technique: surgeon's view from above. (A) Needle placement through two scleral tunnels. (B) Muscle tied in recessed position. (C) Needle placed back through center of muscle. (D) Sutures tied down: note absence of central sag. (Patient of Dr R. Morris.)

the mid-portion of the original insertion (see Fig 85.20). Hang-back recessions may reduce scleral perforations by placing the sutures in thicker sclera at the original insertion. However, with large recessions, the muscle may side-slip or creep anteriorly during or after surgery; this is reduced by placing shallow scleral "belt-loops" close to the recessed muscle or using an anchored hang-back suture (Figs 85.16E and 85.18).

In the hemi hang-back technique, the suture engages the sclera posterior to the original insertion site but anterior to the recessed muscle (Fig. 85.16D). Indications include: surgical exposure, thin sclera, scarring, the presence of an oblique muscle (particularly the superior oblique tendon), or a scleral buckle, glaucoma implant or other device on the sclera. Hemi hang-back sutures with large recessions may reduce the potential for side-slipping or muscle creep.

In a loop recession, a non-absorbable suture is placed through each pole of the muscle and sutured to the sclera behind the insertion (Fig. 85.16F).

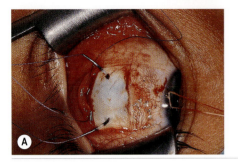
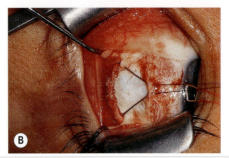
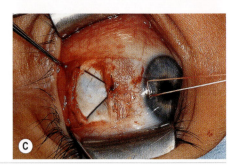

Fig. 85.18 Medial rectus. Anchored hang-back suture. (A) The needles of the double armed sutures (already attached to the muscle, as in Figure 88.13, and the muscle detached) are passed through the sclera. (B) Sutures passed through muscle insertion. (C) Sutures tied down: note minimal central sag. (Patient of Dr R. Morris.)

Table 85.2 – Esotropia[a]

Angle of esotropia (prism diopters)	Recess MR OU (mm)	Resect LR OU (mm)	Recess MR/ Resect LR
15	3.0	4.0	3.0 /4.0
20	3.5	5.0	3.5 /5.0
25	4.0	6.0	4.0 /6.0
30	4.5	7.0	4.5 /7.0
35	5.0	8.0	5.0 /8.0
40	5.5	9.0	5.5 /9.0
50	6.0	9.0	6.0 /9.0

[a]Quantity of surgery to consider for uncomplicated esotropia according to angle. Recess MR OU = recession of medial rectus in both eyes; Resect LR OU = resection of lateral rectus in both eyes; Recess MR/Resect LR = recession of medial rectus and resection of lateral rectus in one eye.

Table 85.3 – Exotropia[a]

Angle of exotropia (prism diopters)	Recess LR OU (mm)	Resect MR OU (mm)	Recess LR/ Resect MR
15[b]	4.0	3.0	4.0/3.0
20	5.0	4.0	5.0/4.0
25	6.0	5.0	6.0/5.0
30	7.0	6.0	7.0/6.0
40	8.0	6.0	8.0/6.0
50[c]			9.0/7.0
60			10.0/8.0
70			10.0/9.0
80			10.0/10.0

[a]Quantity of surgery to consider for uncomplicated exotropia according to angle.
[b]Up to 40 prism diopters for exotropia without profound amblyopia.
[c]For up to 80 prism diopters with profound amblyopia, use a unilateral recession and resection.
Recess LR OU = recession of lateral rectus in both eyes; Resect MR OU = resection of medial rectus in both eyes; Recess LR/Resect MR = recession of medial rectus and resection of lateral rectus in one eye.

Horizontal muscle recession

Dose-response tables for horizontal rectus recessions and resections are available. As a general rule, the medial rectus can be recessed a maximum of 7 mm without reducing adduction and the lateral rectus recessed up to 10 mm. Exceptions to these limits are common, particularly with restrictive and paretic strabismus, when much larger recessions are commonly employed. However, 7 mm bilateral medial rectus recessions may increase the risk of consecutive exotropia in children with congenital esotropia.[44-46] The dose-response with large recessions is non-linear and less predictable. The guideline values listed in the dose-response tables are most useful in uncomplicated strabismus (Tables 85.2 and 85.3).

The quantity of surgery required to correct horizontal deviations is dependent upon a number of factors, especially the magnitude of the preoperative deviation. Axial length and refractive error are not usually significant.[47] Recession of unoperated rectus muscles is more predictable than recession of previously operated muscles. Restrictive disorders, particularly thyroid orbitopathy, and recession of antagonist to a paretic muscle are associated with a reduced effect per millimeter of recession. Very large recessions combined with resections may result in limitation of movement.

Recessions can be measured using a curved ruler or calipers. Curved rulers follow the circumference of the sclera, measuring the length of the arc (Fig. 85.19). Calipers measure the length

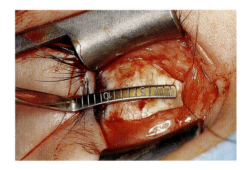

Fig. 85.19 Curved ruler measuring 11 mm from medial limbus. (Patient of Dr R. Morris.)

of the chord: this disadvantage can be reduced by measuring the total recession as two small chord lengths, whose sum is equal to a large recession.

Inferior rectus muscle recession

Inferior rectus recessions are employed in complex nonconcomitant vertical strabismus. Indications for inferior rectus recession include thyroid orbitopathy, blowout fracture, congenital fibrosis of the extraocular muscles, "double elevator" palsy, superior rectus palsy, superior oblique palsy in the contralateral eye, and anesthetic block induced vertical strabismus.

Recession of the superior rectus in the contralateral hypertropic eye is often preferred over recession of the inferior rectus in the hypotropic eye in non-restrictive strabismus. In patients with over 15 prism diopters (PD) of deviation, recession of the ipsilateral inferior rectus and contralateral superior rectus can be considered.

Although inferior rectus recessions employ basic techniques similar to horizontal recessions, there are several differences. The inferior rectus is closely associated with the inferior oblique muscle and the retractors of the lower eyelid.

There are no dose-response tables for vertical rectus recessions or resections. On average, 1 mm of inferior rectus recession will result in correction of 3 PD of vertical deviation in primary gaze and 5 PD in downgaze.[48]

Recessions of the inferior rectus for non-paretic, non-restrictive disorders should generally be limited to 5 mm or less; larger recessions commonly cause lower eyelid retraction. However, inferior rectus recessions of less than 5 mm may cause lower eyelid retraction in restrictive strabismus, particularly thyroid orbitopathy. Severe restrictive disorders often require large recessions resulting in significant retraction of the lower eyelid. The patient should be warned of this preoperatively.

Techniques to reduce lower eyelid retraction include:

1. Dissection and lysis of fascial attachments to the inferior rectus as far posteriorly as possible, including: intermuscular septum, check ligaments, and Lockwood's ligament connections.
2. Suture the lower eyelid retractors to the inferior rectus.[49] An adjustable suture can be placed on the capsulopalpebral head and passed through the inferior rectus insertion. Adjustment of the capsulopalpebral head is performed after the inferior rectus adjustment.[50]
3. Disinsertion of the lower eyelid retractors from the tarsal plate.[51]

Delayed overcorrection is a significant problem following inferior rectus recession. This is usually accompanied by limited depression in the operated eye with diplopia, particularly in downgaze. Delayed overcorrection is more likely to occur with thyroid orbitopathy treated with adjustable sutures. It occurs in 10–21% of cases.[52,53,54]

A number of mechanisms may contribute to "late slippage" of the inferior rectus.[55,56,58] These include:

1. Thickened Tenon's capsule under the inferior rectus muscle allowing the muscle to slip posteriorly after absorption of the sutures, forming a pseudo-tendon anterior to the insertion.
2. Inferior rectus attachments to Lockwood's ligament and the lower eyelid retractors.
3. Hang-back adjustable sutures hold the recessed inferior rectus in place centrally. When the eye makes horizontal movements, the inferior rectus does not move fully with the eye; repeat side-slipping prevents firm reattachment of the muscle to the sclera.
4. Laterally directed traction of the inferior oblique may prevent adherence of the inferior rectus to the sclera.

5. Scarring around Lockwood's ligament pulls the inferior rectus muscle anteriorly, creating slack in the anterior aspect of the muscle, weakening its depressor function.[57]
6. Following a large recession, the inferior rectus is not in apposition to the globe when the muscle is contracting and the eye is in downgaze.[58] MRI studies demonstrate that an inferior rectus recession of 6.0 mm and a medial rectus recession of 7.5 mm in a normal eye leads to loss of inferior rectus apposition, with lower values in thyroid associated patients.[59]
7. Ipsilateral contraction of the superior rectus in thyroid orbitopathy leads to late overcorrection.

Undercorrections after inferior rectus recessions are associated particularly with restrictive processes and reduced contractility of the opposing superior rectus. In severe thyroid orbitopathy, even recessions of 15 or more millimeters from the insertion may fail to correct the hypotropia. Significant restriction in elevation may persist, even while the inferior rectus is disconnected from the globe during surgery. Postoperative undercorrection in primary gaze with hypertropia in downgaze indicates a tight superior rectus. Restriction following orbital blowout fractures frequently is associated with alterations in the elastic properties of the surrounding orbital tissues.

Poor or absent superior rectus function is a cause for undercorrection. "Double elevator" palsy and superior rectus palsy are likely to be undercorrected with inferior rectus recessions alone. Failure of superior rectus development in congenital fibrosis of the extraocular muscles causes disappointing results following inferior rectus recession.[60,61] Retrobulbar and peribulbar block induced vertical strabismus can be complex and is often associated with paretic and restrictive components.[62-67]

Bilateral recessions of the inferior rectus muscles can create exotropia in downgaze, forming an "A" or "λ" pattern, especially in thyroid orbitopathy where large inferior rectus recessions have been performed. Nasal displacement of the inferior rectus muscles reduces the tendency for exotropia in downgaze. However, this may be associated with intorsion.[63]

Superior rectus muscle recession

There are also no dose response tables for superior rectus recessions or resections. Each millimeter of superior rectus recession generally corrects 3 to 4 PD of vertical deviation up to 6 mm of recession. Recessions of greater than 6 mm are avoided, except in dissociated vertical deviation (DVD), when hang-back recessions of up to 10 mm may be performed (Fig. 85.20).[64,65] Superior rectus recessions beyond 4 mm require lysis of the fascial attachments between the underside of the superior rectus and the superior oblique

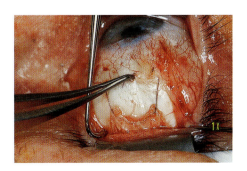

Fig. 85.20 Superior rectus hang-back recession: surgeon's view from above.
(Patient of Dr R. Morris.)

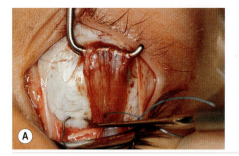
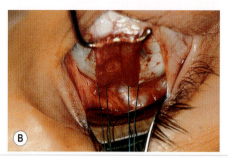
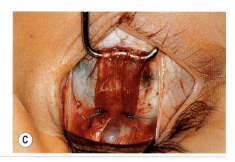

Fig. 85.21 Right superior rectus posterior fixation suture: surgeon's view from above. (A) Scleral placement of suture on a half-curved needle at medial border of superior rectus; it will next be passed through the muscle. The lateral suture is already placed through sclera and muscle. (B) Sutures prior to tying. (C) Completed procedure. (Patient of Dr R. Morris.)

tendon (see Fig. 85.8B). For very large recessions, it is important to dissect and cut fascial attachments and check ligaments on the superior rectus as far posteriorly as possible and identify the superior oblique tendon, both nasal and temporal to the superior rectus. The superior oblique insertion is in close proximity to the temporal border of the superior rectus. The thin fibers of the superior oblique near its insertion can be mistaken for intermuscular septum and inadvertently transected (Fig. 85.6).

Superior rectus recessions do not commonly cause upper eyelid retraction.[66] Because of the potential problems associated with inferior rectus recessions, surgery for concomitant vertical deviations of up to 15 PD is often performed by superior rectus recession in the hypertropic eye.

Non-concomitant hypertropia that increases on downgaze is usually treated by recession of the ipsilateral superior rectus. In the absence of oblique dysfunction, hyperdeviations that increase in abduction are treated by superior rectus recession in the hypertropic eye. However, hyperdeviations that increase in adduction (without oblique dysfunction) are commonly treated by recession of the inferior rectus of the hypotropic eye. Deviations larger than 15 PD in primary gaze are often treated with recession of the superior rectus in the hypertropic eye and recession of the inferior rectus in the hypotropic eye.

Faden operation or posterior fixation suture

The faden operation, or posterior fixation suture, reduces the effect of a rectus muscle in its field of action. Two separate non-absorbable sutures are placed through each edge of a rectus muscle in a location behind the equator (Fig. 85.21). The sutures alter the arc of contact of the muscle by changing the point of tangency on the globe. There is little effect on the primary gaze position, but as the globe rotates into the field of action of the muscle the lever-arm length is reduced.[67] Posterior fixation sutures with recessions create a weakening effect in primary gaze and increase the weakening effect overall, requiring a smaller recession.

Posterior fixation sutures are most effective on the medial rectus; the arc of contact can be increased from 6 mm to 12–16 mm. Similar effects can be achieved on the superior and inferior rectus muscles. With its already long arc of contact, posterior fixation sutures on the lateral rectus muscle have limited effect, although this has been challenged.[68]

Posterior fixation sutures are useful in non-concomitant strabismus, particularly when the deviation is small in primary gaze and increases as the eye moves into the field of action of the muscle. The procedure is particularly useful in non-concomitant vertical deviations with limited infraduction:

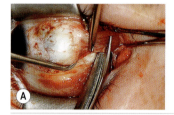
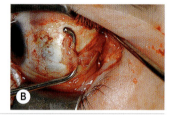

Fig. 85.22 Marginal myotomy. (A) With a strabismus hook under a previously recessed medial rectus, two pairs of scissors are positioned so as to make overlapping myotomy cuts through the muscle. (B) Appearance of muscle postmyotomy: the overlapping cuts allow the muscle to stretch. (Patient of Dr R. Morris.)

blowout fractures, scleral buckle, or previously recessed inferior rectus muscles in thyroid orbitopathy.[69] Another indication is accommodative esotropia with a high AC/A ratio.[70] Posterior fixation of the medial rectus to the medial pulley has been proposed.[71]

Two separate non-absorbable braided 5-0 or 6-0 polyester sutures with spatulated needles are used. A 1/2 circle spatulated needle makes suture placement in the sclera easier. The two separate sutures are placed 12–16 mm posterior to the insertion (as far posterior as possible) in the sclera adjacent to the border of the muscle. The sutures are then passed through 30% of each border of the muscle. If a recession is to be included, the sutures are passed through the muscle in the appropriate position. Extensive posterior dissection is important for good exposure. The vortex veins are typically in close proximity to the site of suture placement. It is usually easier to pass the scleral sutures before they are passed through the muscle.

Marginal myotomy

Marginal myotomy is rarely employed today. The effects are variable and unpredictable. It is occasionally used when a muscle has been maximally recessed or if recession is contraindicated. Marginal myotomy is performed by cutting the opposing margins of the rectus muscle for a distance occupying 75% of the width of the muscle, with the cuts 5 mm apart (Fig. 85.22).

Strengthening procedures on the rectus muscles

Resections

Resection of a muscle tightens it by removing all or part of the tendon with large resections, some muscle may also be removed. The shortened muscle is reattached to the original insertion. Resections are usually combined with recession of the antagonist muscle.

Resections generally produce more postoperative discomfort, redness, and swelling. The edematous conjunctiva is more likely to produce postoperative dellen than following recession.

Resections require careful dissection of the intermuscular septum and check ligaments, to a position approximately 4–5 mm posterior to the proposed site of the resection. Care should be taken to avoid disruption of Tenon's capsule and the muscle capsule during the dissection. Two hooks are placed under the muscle: one at the insertion and one posterior to the site of suture placement that can be marked with light bipolar cautery. Caution should be exercised while placing the suture, since traction on the muscle capsule can move the capsule and cautery marks up to several millimeters, leading to suture misplacement. Most resections are performed with 6-0 absorbable sutures, such as coated polyglactin 910. Occasionally, non-absorbable polyester sutures are preferred, particularly on the inferior rectus. A double armed spatulated needle is introduced in the muscle at the proposed resection site. When using a single suture for a resection, a single tie is placed in the mid-portion of the muscle with double locking bites at each border (Fig. 85.23). A narrow straight clamp is temporarily placed just anterior to the suture line. The tendon is severed at its insertion on the sclera, leaving as little stump as possible. The muscle/tendon anterior to the clamp is excised and the stump cauterized. Each arm of the suture is then passed in the sclera at the original insertion. Supra- or infra-placement can be combined with resection. The eye is rotated in the direction of the resected muscle to relieve tension on the muscle; the sutures are advanced, tightened, and tied. The two arms of the suture can be passed back through the mid-portion of the resected muscle, creating a horizontal mattress suture and avoiding central sagging.

When a resected muscle is tight or a muscle is advanced from a previously recessed position, it may be appropriate to use two double armed sutures. Each suture passes through half the width of the muscle[72] (Fig. 85.24).

Horizontal rectus muscle resections do not usually affect lid position. Significant tightening can cause globe retraction and narrowing of the palpebral fissure. Vertical rectus resections of less than 5 mm do not typically affect lid position.

Resections are more likely to be associated with lost muscles than recessions. This is related to tightness of the muscle following a resection and the need for placement of the anchoring sutures in muscle rather than tendon with large or repeat resections. A resected medial rectus is the most common muscle to be lost.

A temporary overcorrection is commonly seen after resections. Advancement of previously recessed muscles has more effect than an identical quantity of resection. The predictability of advancement is less than with unoperated muscles.

Tucking and plication procedures

A rectus muscle can be tucked or plicated as an alternative to a resection. One of the early plication procedures was the O'Connor cinch.[73,74] Tucking or plication may also be used in an attempt to preserve anterior ciliary vessels during tightening procedures on the rectus muscles.[75,76]

Inferior oblique surgery

Indications

Weakening the inferior oblique by recession or anteriorly transposing the muscle is commonly done. Tightening procedures, such as resection or advancement, are rarely performed in isolation. Resection in combination with anterior transposition has been described.[77,78]

The main reason for a weakening procedure on the inferior oblique is overaction of the muscle. Inferior oblique overaction is associated with "V" or "Y" pattern horizontal

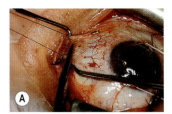 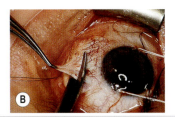 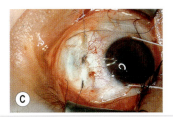 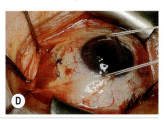

Fig. 85.23 Single-suture, double armed needle rectus muscle resection. (A) With a suture placed 4 mm from muscle insertion, the muscle is being cut anterior to the suture. (B) Removal of redundant muscle tissue. (C) Scleral placement of sutures anterior to insertion. (D) Final position of muscle following suture tying after a pass through the center of the muscle. Note absence of central sagging of resected muscle. (Patient of Dr R. Morris.)

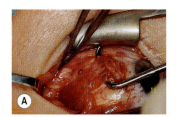 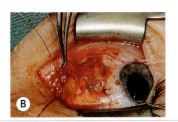 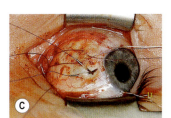 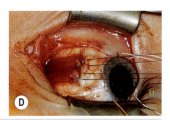

Fig. 85.24 Two-suture, double armed needle rectus muscle resection. (A) Hook under medial rectus muscle. Note the pseudotendon attached to the muscle, which can be seen on the left. (B) Redundant pseudotendon about to be excised. (C) Sutures placed just anterior to original muscle insertion. (D) Muscle advanced to insertion: the four ends of the two sutures are about to be tied to its corresponding end. This configuration gives minimal central sag. (Patient of Dr R. Morris.)

strabismus. Reducing the overaction reduces the horizontal deviation in upgaze by up to 20 PD, with little or no effect on the horizontal deviation in primary gaze or downgaze.[79]

Superior oblique palsy with overaction of the ipsilateral inferior oblique is another common indication for inferior oblique surgery. Weakening the ipsilateral inferior oblique is effective when there is significant overaction of the muscle, extorsion measures less than 5° and there is less than 15 PD of hyperdeviation in primary gaze. Large vertical and torsional fusion amplitudes can make the procedure effective, even when these numbers are exceeded. We avoid anterior transpositions on unilateral superior oblique palsy, although some have advocated it.[80,81]

Patients with combined overaction of the inferior oblique and DVD are frequently treated with anterior transposition of the inferior oblique.[82] An uncommon indication for inferior oblique weakening is "inverted Brown pattern" deviation, in which a tight inferior oblique masquerades as superior oblique underaction.[83]

Surgical procedures

Surgical procedures performed on the inferior oblique include: disinsertion (tenotomy), myectomy, graded recession,[84] denervation and extirpation,[85,86] extirpation of the nasal portion of the inferior oblique, anterior transposition of the inferior oblique[87] (standard temporal anterior transposition), nasal

transposition of the inferior oblique,[88-90] fixation of the inferior oblique muscle to the orbital wall,[91] and others.

Tenotomy of the inferior oblique is rarely performed. This involves isolating the muscle, exposing its insertion, and severing the tendon at its insertion. The tendon of the inferior oblique is 1 millimeter in length and there is no bleeding as long as the tenotomy occurs in the tendon. Reattachment of the inferior oblique to the sclera after this procedure is unpredictable.

Myectomy of the inferior oblique is commonly performed (Fig. 85.25). Exposure of the muscle is the same as with a recession or anterior transposition. A clamp is placed across the muscle. The muscle is severed on the insertion side of the clamp and the tendon is severed at its attachment to the sclera. Objections to this procedure include the random site of reattachment, its irreversibility, and the remote potential for unplanned myectomy of the inferior rectus or lateral rectus.

Recession is the most common weakening procedure performed on the inferior oblique (Fig. 85.26). Direct measurement on the scleral surface from the original inferior oblique insertion to the proposed position of the recession is not practical. Anatomic landmarks on the globe are used to guide placement of the inferior oblique muscle in recessions.

We perform inferior oblique recessions of 10, 12, or 14 mm. All recessions should place the new insertion at or posterior to the equator of the globe. Inferior oblique recessions are

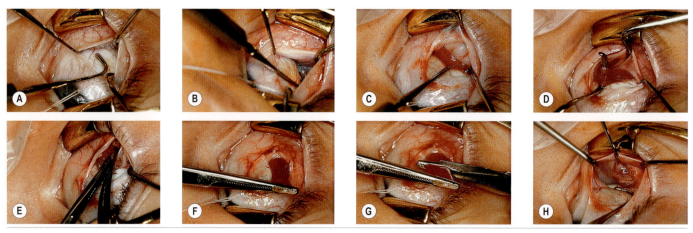

Fig. 85.25 Inferior oblique myectomy: surgeon's view from above. (A) Inferolateral conjunctival fornix incision. (B) Visualization of posterior border of inferior oblique, seen at the tip of the hook. (C) Stevens tenotomy hook under both inferior oblique muscle and orbital fat. (D) Hook under inferior oblique, the orbital fat having been freed, showing the intermuscular septum between inferior oblique and Tenon's capsule. (E) The inferior oblique is held in a straight artery clamp and is being disinserted from the globe. (F) Inferior oblique muscle having been disinserted. (G) A segment of muscle being removed with scissors. (H) Cut border of inferior oblique visible, retracting into Tenon's capsule. (Patient of Dr R. Morris.)

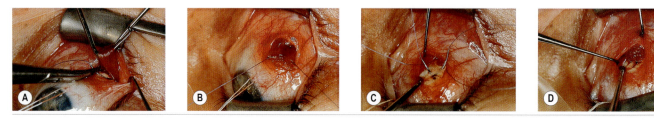

Fig. 85.26 Right inferior oblique recession: surgeon's view from above. (A) Suture being placed at insertion of inferior oblique muscle having been disinserted with double armed Vicryl suture. (B) Double armed Vicryl suture through inferior oblique muscle. (C) Needles placed lateral and posterior to the lateral border of the inferior rectus (the strabismus hook in the bottom left of the picture is under the insertion of the inferior rectus). (D) Muscle in recessed position. (Patient of Dr R. Morris).

performed with a muscle hook behind the insertion of the inferior rectus, elevating the globe. Care should be taken not to rotate the globe inward or outward; as this will alter the position of the lateral border of the inferior rectus.

A classic 10 mm inferior oblique recession[92] places the anterior border of the recessed inferior oblique 3 mm posterior and 2 mm temporal to the lateral border of the inferior rectus insertion. We modify this by placing the inferior oblique further posteriorly and more temporally, with the anterior border of the inferior oblique in a position 6 to 8 mm posterior to the temporal pole of the inferior rectus insertion and 4 mm temporal to the lateral border of the inferior rectus. This is anterior to the scleral exit of the inferior temporal vortex vein.

A 12 mm inferior oblique recession places the anterior border of the new insertion 2 mm temporal to the lateral border of the inferior rectus and 6 to 8 mm posterior to the temporal pole of the inferior rectus insertion.

A 14 mm inferior oblique recession places the anterior border of the new insertion adjacent to the lateral border of the inferior rectus and 8 to 10 mm posterior to the temporal pole of the inferior rectus insertion. The 14 mm inferior oblique recession[93] often places the sutures in a position to "straddle" the exit site of the inferior temporal vortex vein, when it is located adjacent to the lateral border of the inferior rectus.

Anterior transposition of the inferior oblique places the new insertion anterior to the equator of the globe, adjacent to and parallel with the lateral border of the inferior rectus insertion.[94] The more anterior the muscle is transposed, particularly the posterior fibers, the greater the effect. The effect can be further enhanced by combining it with a small myectomy of the inferior oblique.

Anterior transposition converts the muscle from an elevator to a depressor of the globe, which can limit elevation. With anterior transposition, the neurovascular bundle creates a J-shaped deformity in the muscle, becoming the effective origin of the inferior oblique.[95,96] Spreading the transposed inferior oblique fibers excessively is associated with limited elevation, particularly in abduction. This is the "anti-elevation syndrome;" overaction of the contralateral inferior oblique may result.[97,98] The transposed inferior oblique insertion should be kept compact, avoiding lateral placement of the posterior (lateral) corner of the inferior oblique muscle. When the anti-elevation syndrome is significant, it can be improved by converting the inferior oblique transposition to a recession.[99] Bilateral inferior oblique nasal myectomy is an alternative.[100]

Anterior transposition of the inferior oblique is indicated when there is marked overaction of the inferior oblique or when overaction coexists with DVD.[108] It is unwise to combine anterior transposition of the inferior oblique with significant recessions of the superior rectus; elevation may become markedly limited.

Anterior and nasal transposition of the inferior oblique involves disinserting the muscle and reattaching it to the sclera 2 mm nasal and 2 mm posterior to the insertion of the inferior rectus. This may be used to treat carefully selected patients with superior oblique palsy, inferior oblique overaction, anti-elevation syndrome, and Duane's syndrome.[101]

General approach to expose and isolate the inferior oblique

Inferior oblique surgery is most commonly performed using an inferior temporal fornix incision. The conjunctival incision is 8–10 mm from the limbus, depending upon anterior border of the extraconal fat and the anterior border of the inferior oblique. The incision in Tenon's capsule and the intermuscular septum is at a right angle to the conjunctival incision. A muscle hook is placed behind the insertion of the lateral rectus. A temporary traction suture (typically 4-0 polyester or silk on a taper needle) is placed beneath the lateral rectus and attached to the drapes to adduct and elevate the globe. A fiberoptic head lamp may be helpful. A Stevens tenotomy hook is placed along the inferior border of the lateral rectus; the conjunctiva and Tenon's capsule are retracted posteriorly. A von Graefe hook is used to retract the same tissues in an inferior temporal direction. Gentle "hand-over-hand" traction may be required to gain exposure to three important structures: the scleral surface, the inferior temporal vortex vein, and the posterior border of the inferior oblique. This is the so-called "golden triangle" of inferior oblique surgical exposure (Fig. 85.27). Under direct visualization, a Stevens' tenotomy hook engages the posterior border of the inferior oblique; the muscle is retracted anteriorly. Splitting the inferior oblique may cause bleeding and obscure the anatomy. Alternatively, the inferior oblique is located at its insertion, adjacent to the lower border of the lateral rectus 10 to 12 mm posterior to the lateral rectus insertion. The inferior oblique is retracted anteriorly, residual orbital fat is lifted and allowed to retract posterior to the hook. Two millimeters of intermuscular septum separates the posterior border of the inferior oblique from Tenon's capsule. A small opening is made in the intermuscular septum posterior to the inferior oblique and a muscle hook introduced under the muscle. Intermuscular septum attachments to the inferior oblique fan out near the insertion of the muscle and require lysis, exposing the insertion. A 6-0 absorbable suture is preplaced before disinsertion or after the inferior oblique is separated from the sclera. A 6-0 coated polyglactin 910 double armed with $\frac{1}{2}$ circle S-28 spatulated needles works well. Because the inferior oblique is thick and compact, it is not necessary to place the suture in the mid-portion of the muscle and extend the pass to each border. A single pass from one border to the other with a single locking bite at each border is sufficient. Following disinsertion, the inferior oblique does not retract significantly; a "lost" inferior oblique is not a concern. Following disinsertion and suture placement, the traction suture is released. A muscle hook is placed behind the insertion of the inferior rectus, elevating the globe. It is important to keep the inferior rectus well centered; medial or lateral rotation of the globe will displace the inferior rectus and may result in erroneous placement of the inferior oblique on the sclera.

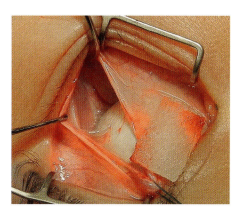

Fig. 85.27 Surgeon's view of left inferior temporal quadrant showing the "golden triangle". The scleral surface, the inferior temporal vortex vein, and the posterior border of the inferior oblique.

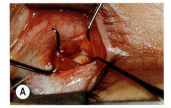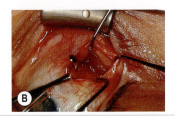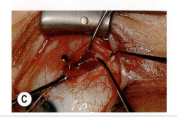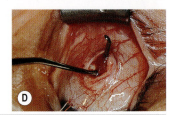

Fig. 85.28 Inadvertently split right inferior oblique muscle: surgeon's view from above. (A) A Green hook placed through apparently intact inferior oblique muscle. (B) The posterior part of the muscle seen in the V formed by the hooked muscle. (C) The Stevens tenotomy hook lifts the split posterior portion of the muscle onto the Green hook to join the two halves together for suturing. (D) No further muscle tissue seen in the V formed by the inferior oblique, which is now complete and held on the Green hook. (Patient of Dr R. Morris.)

Problems with inferior oblique surgery

1. Persisting overaction of the inferior oblique can be caused by inadvertently splitting the inferior oblique, creating a "dual head" or bifid appearance, making the weakening procedure incomplete[102,103] (Fig. 85.28).

2. DVD can be responsible for elevation in adduction, creating pseudo-overaction of the inferior oblique. This commonly occurs with infantile onset strabismus.[104]

3. Consecutive overaction of the opposite inferior oblique can occur when a unilateral procedure is performed.

4. Masked bilateral superior oblique palsy can result in overaction of the opposite inferior oblique after a unilateral weakening procedure.

5. Esotropia can occur following a weakening procedure on the inferior oblique, converting an esophoria to an esotropia, in spite of improved vertical misalignment.

6. Pupil dilation and paresis of the ciliary muscle.[105,106] This is rare; it may improve spontaneously or persist. When it occurs, care must be taken with respect to the amblyogenic potential of accompanying ciliary muscle paresis.

7. Hemorrhage from the inferior oblique muscle or disruption of the inferior temporal vortex vein.

8. Inferior oblique fat adherence syndrome causing hypotropia and restriction of elevation in adduction, postoperatively. This can be caused by rupture of Tenon's capsule, prolapse of orbital fat, and hemorrhage, leading to scarring.

9. Inadvertent disinsertion or myectomy of the inferior rectus or lateral rectus muscle. This can occur when an inferior oblique myectomy was the intended procedure.

10. The "anti-elevation syndrome"[107] can occur after anterior transposition of the inferior oblique. What appears to be overaction of the inferior oblique in the contralateral eye, with a "Y" or "V" pattern and exotropia in upgaze, occurs. This pseudo-overaction of the inferior oblique may be the consequence of limitation of elevation in abduction in the operated eye(s). This can be avoided if inferior oblique fibers are sutured close to the inferior rectus and not spread laterally more than a few millimeters.[108]

Superior oblique surgery

Both weakening and strengthening procedures are performed on the superior oblique. The surgery can be technically challenging and improper technique or patient selection may cause loss of fusion or intractable diplopia. Overcorrections and other undesirable effects cannot be as predictably reversed as surgery on the rectus or inferior oblique muscles.

Superior oblique weakening procedures

Weakening procedures of the superior oblique include tenotomy, tenectomy, posterior tenectomy, recession, disinsertion, Z-tenotomy, and superior oblique tendon spacer.

Indications

Weakening procedures on the superior oblique may be performed for Brown's syndrome and significant overaction of the superior oblique(s) causing a vertical deviation and/or "A" or "λ" pattern horizontal deviations. Rarely, superior oblique tenotomy is performed for superior oblique myokymia.[109]

Most Brown's syndrome patients, do not have a significant vertical a deviation in primary gaze and therefore do not require surgical intervention. Spontaneous improvement and resolution can occasionally occur.[110] When Brown's syndrome interferes with binocular vision or causes significant torticollis with a vertical deviation in primary gaze, surgery should be considered.

Individuals without fusional capabilities and no diplopia potential can be relatively safely operated; patients with diplopia potential should be approached with caution.

Superior oblique tenotomy

The superior oblique tendon is usually transected just nasal to superior rectus, where the tendon is well formed and cord-like. It is more difficult to cut the entire tendon at its insertion; the frenulum-like connections between the superior rectus muscle capsule and the superior oblique tendon are difficult to transect without first disinserting the superior rectus. For these reasons, a nasal tenotomy is preferred.[119]

The superior oblique tendon is usually approached through a superior fornix incision (Fig. 85.29). A temporal incision is more challenging, but leaves the intermuscular septum intact nasal to the superior rectus. A muscle hook is placed behind the insertion of the superior rectus and the globe infraducted. Exposure may be improved by removing the eyelid speculum. Two Stevens tenotomy hooks retract Tenon's capsule, exposing the broad, sheet-like check ligament attached to the superior rectus muscle capsule. The nasal half of the check ligament is incised; the muscle hooks are shifted nasally. Better exposure may be obtained by replacing the Stevens hooks with a small Desmarres lid retractor. Slight temporal traction on the muscle hook beneath the superior rectus places the superior oblique tendon under tension and elevates it, making it more apparent. A Stevens hook is introduced posterior to the superior oblique tendon and passed forward, between the tendon and sclera. This places the tendon on the hook, but includes intact intermuscular septum enveloping the tendon. Proper visualization of the superior oblique tendon is important to reduce the risk of "blind hooking" with its potential complications.

A small incision is made in the external aspect of the intermuscular septum overlying the superior oblique tendon, while attempting to keep the deeper layer of the intermuscular septum intact. Two Stevens hooks are introduced under the tendon, avoiding damage to the intact deeper layer of the intermuscular septum. In a tenotomy, the superior oblique tendon is transected between the two Stevens hooks and the ends retract. The distance the tendon retracts is controlled by the surrounding intermuscular septum, which should be left intact, except for the small incision in the intermuscular septum overlying the tendon. This also reduces the potential for adhesions between the cut ends of the tendon and the scleral surface while at the same time controlling the separation of the cut ends of the tendon. The use of a "chicken suture" makes recovery of the tendon ends possible and increases the potential reversibility of the procedure.[111]

Superior oblique tendon spacer

The superior oblique tendon spacer has several potential advantages: providing graded weakening of the superior oblique and avoiding potential problems with the ends of the tendon fusing together following surgery. It may also reduce the risk of secondary superior oblique underaction.[112]

Following nasal tenotomy, a segment of a silicone band is inserted between the cut ends of the nasal portion of the tendon and secured with a non-absorbable suture (Fig. 85.30). A #240 band (cross section 2.5 × 0.6 mm) is used, although a #40 band (2.0 × 0.75 mm) can be utilized. The length of the silicone spacer is 4 to 7 mm. The silicone spacer is secured with a 5-0 or 6-0 preplaced non-absorbable polyester suture at the nasal and temporal cut ends of the tendon. A 7-0 monofilament polypropylene suture with double armed vascular needles also works well. Adjustable techniques have been described.[113-115]

Superior oblique tendon spacers are contraindicated in superior oblique myokymia; the contractions of the superior oblique are transmitted to the globe through the tendon spacer.

Other weakening procedures

Bilateral posterior tenectomies may treat mild "A" pattern esotropia associated with overaction of the superior oblique muscles. The procedure consists of wedge excision of posterior and medial fibers. This weakens the abduction and depression effects of superior oblique, while preserving the anterior fibers responsible for intorsion. Bilateral posterior tenectomies can correct up to 15 PD of "A" pattern.

Tenotomy, disinsertion, and recession of the superior oblique tendon at its insertion is less predictable than nasal tenotomy. The procedures are challenging due to the long and thin insertion, the proximity of the superior temporal vortex vein, and the presence of fibrous connections between the underside of the superior rectus and the superior oblique tendon.[114]

For large "A" pattern deviations associated with superior oblique overaction, superior oblique tenotomies or superior oblique tendon spacers can be combined with horizontal muscle surgery, with vertical displacement. This may correct up to 45 PD of "A" pattern.[115]. The correction in the primary position is greater in exodeviations than esodeviations.

Superior oblique myectomy with trochlear resection has been proposed to treat superior oblique myokymia.[116]

Problems after superior oblique weakening procedures:

1. Inadvertent transection of the superior rectus.[117]
2. Consecutive underaction of the superior oblique.[118,119]
3. The cut ends of the tendon may separate excessively, especially in elderly patients with a very thin and friable intermuscular septum.
4. Production of superior oblique palsy.
5. Diplopia from consecutive hypertropia, excyclotropia, and/or esotropia.
6. Consecutive development of inferior oblique overaction.

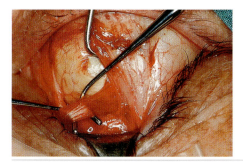

Fig. 85.29 Right superior oblique tenotomy: surgeon's view from above. The superior rectus is held with a Chavasse hook (above). The superior oblique tendon can be identified via nasal approach and is held with two Stevens tenotomy hooks beneath it. The muscle is divided between the hooks for a superior oblique tenotomy. (Patient of Dr R. Morris.)

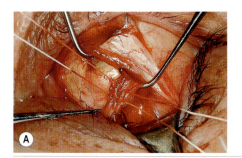 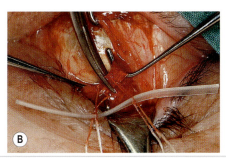 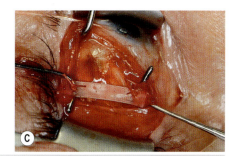

Fig. 85.30 Superior oblique tendon expander: surgeon's view from above. (A) Two non-absorbable double armed sutures are passed through the superior oblique tendon. (B) A segment of silicone band is inserted and transfixed by each end of the double armed sutures. The tendon is being divided with scissors. (C) Tendon following division and insertion of the silicone band, which is held by the double armed sutures. (Patient of Dr R. Morris.)

7. The cut ends of the tendon grow back together.

8. Adhesion between the cut ends of the tendon and the sclera.

9. Downgaze restriction following insertion of a superior oblique tendon spacer.[120]

10. Bleeding from superior temporal or superior nasal vortex vein.

11. Inability to recover the cut ends of the superior oblique tendon when overcorrection has occurred.

Strengthening procedures

Indications

Strengthening procedures of the superior oblique are used to treat superior oblique palsy with superior oblique underaction, hypertropia, and significant extorsion and "V" pattern esodeviations, in which there is significant underaction of the superior oblique and esotropia occurs predominantly in downgaze.

Superior oblique tuck

The superior oblique tendon can be resected, plicated, or tucked, nasal or temporal to the superior rectus. We prefer a superior oblique tuck along the temporal border of the superior rectus.

Superior oblique tucks can be performed with specifically designed instruments; our preference is to use a "free hand" technique (Fig. 85.31).[121]

The superior oblique tendon is approached using a superior nasal fornix incision. The nasal intermuscular septum is incised and a muscle hook is placed behind the insertion of the superior rectus. The globe is maximally infraducted. A Stevens hook is placed under the superior oblique tendon. The intermuscular septum along the posterior border of the tendon is incised. Intermuscular septal attachments to the superior oblique tendon are lysed, both nasally and temporally.

A non-absorbable suture is placed 6–9 mm from the insertion of the superior oblique with double locking bites at each border. The sutures are passed in the sclera starting at the anterior and posterior terminations of the original superior oblique insertion. The sutures are passed back through the mid-portion of the tendon and through the preplaced suture at the plication site. The sutures are tightened and tied.

Modified Harada-Ito procedure

The modified Harada-Ito procedure is useful for superior oblique weakness causing excyclotorsion without significant vertical misalignment.

Advancement of the anterior one-third to one-half of the superior oblique tendon increases its intorsion, while having little effect on vertical deviation. The original procedure[122] has been modified.[123-125]

It is utilized for torsional diplopia of 7° to 20°. The effect is variable but averages 6° to 9°.[138] Some regression of the torsional effects 2 and 12 months postoperatively is common.[124]

A superior temporal fornix incision is utilized (Fig. 85.32). A muscle hook is placed behind the superior rectus insertion. A Stevens hook engages the anterior aspect of the thin superior oblique tendon near its insertion. After engaging the superior oblique tendon, the Stevens hook is replaced with a larger hook. Dissection of the intermuscular septum from the superior rectus is completed. The tendon of the superior oblique is exposed by placing a retractor that nasally displaces the superior rectus. The anterior 1/3 to 1/2 of the superior oblique tendon is longitudinally divided using two Stevens hooks, beginning at the insertion and extending for 10 to 15 mm nasal to the insertion.[125]

A 6-0 coated polyglactin 910 with S-28 or S-29 needles is preplaced in the anterior portion of the split superior oblique tendon, with locking bites placed at each border. A non-absorbable suture can be utilized instead of an absorbable suture. The anterior portion of the tendon is disinserted.

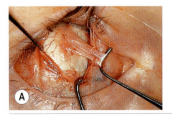 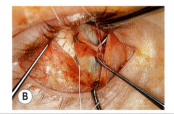 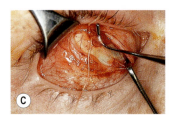 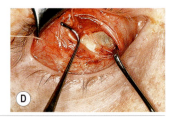

Fig. 85.31 An 8-mm superior oblique free tuck. Right eye, viewed from the front. (A) Superior oblique identified and double armed non-absorbable suture placed 8 mm from insertion. The lateral rectus is held to one side by the hook on the left. (B) Needles placed in sclera at insertion of tendon. (C) Muscle tied with a Stevens tenotomy hook through redundant loop of muscle. (D) Final position of muscle after tuck. Note Stevens tenotomy hook through redundant loop of muscle. (Patient of Dr R. Morris.)

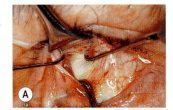 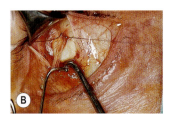 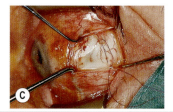 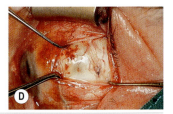

Fig. 85.32 Modified Harada-Ito procedure. Left eye, frontal view. (A) After a superior temporal fornix conjunctival and Tenon's incision, the superior rectus is held with a Chavasse hook and the insertion of the superior oblique identified and the tendon held between two Stevens hooks. (B) The anterior third of the tendon is split and a double armed 6-0 Vicryl suture placed through it at the insertion of the split anterior third. The posterior two-thirds can be seen under the retractor. (C) The anterior third of the tendon is divided from the globe and the double armed suture placed above the superior border of the lateral rectus 8 mm from insertion. (D) Final position of tendon. (Patient of Dr R. Morris.)

A muscle hook is placed behind the insertion of the lateral rectus and its upper border exposed. Each arm of the double armed suture attached to the anterior portion of the superior oblique tendon is passed into the sclera, adjacent to the superior border of the lateral rectus, beginning 8 mm posterior to the lateral rectus insertion. The ends of the suture are tightened to advance the anterior portion of the superior oblique tendon. The transposed anterior portion of the superior oblique tendon remains on the equator of the globe, imparting torsional, rather than vertical, forces.

A greater abducting effect in downgaze is achieved if the anterior tendon fibers are placed more posteriorly.[126] Adjustable techniques may be utilized.[127]

Transposition procedures

Muscle transposition procedures are performed to alter the direction of the vectors of force of extraocular muscles. Transpositions are used when there is a reduction in force generated by one or more of the extraocular muscles. Examples include sixth nerve palsy, "double elevator" palsy (monocular elevation deficiency) and selected patients with third nerve palsy, Duane's syndrome, and other congenital cranial dysinnervation disorders. Transpositions can be employed when trauma or surgical complications result in loss of function of extraocular muscles.

Treatment of "A" and "V" patterns

Vertical displacement of the horizontal rectus muscles is used to treat "A" and "V" patterns. Vertical displacement of the horizontal muscles can be used alone or in combination with oblique muscle surgery.

"V" patterns exist when there is a difference of 15 PD or more between 25° upgaze and 25° downgaze. "A" pattern strabismus occurs when the difference is 10 PD or more. Surgical treatment can be considered for a chin-up or chin-down head position, when the pattern precludes fusion or is otherwise symptomatic. The appropriate horizontal rectus muscles are displaced in the direction in which the greatest weakening effect is desired.[128]

In "V" patterns, the medial recti are moved inferiorly, toward the apex of the "V" (Fig. 85.33). If the lateral rectus muscles are operated, they are displaced superiorly. The direction of displacement of the respective muscles is the same for "V" esotropia and "V" exotropia.

In "A" patterns, the medial recti are moved superiorly, toward the apex of the "A" (Fig. 85.33). If the lateral rectus muscles are operated, they are moved inferiorly. The direction of displacement of the respective muscles is the same for "A" esotropia and "A" exotropia.

A half tendon width displacement of the horizontal rectus muscles can alter the pattern deviation by 10–20 PD; a full tendon width displacement by 25–30 PD. Full tendon width displacements are not as predictable. The displaced muscles should follow the spiral of Tillaux (Fig. 85.34). The quantity of horizontal surgery performed is governed by the deviation in primary gaze. Unilateral surgery can be effective for "A" and "V" patterns, which can be accomplished by moving the medial and lateral recti vertically in opposite directions.[129]

Transposition of the rectus muscles

The many transposition procedures of the rectus muscles can be divided into muscle splitting and full tendon techniques.[146]

Muscle splitting techniques include the Hummelsheim[130] and Jensen procedures.[131] They are generally used to treat sixth nerve palsy.

Hummelsheim procedure

When the Hummelsheim procedure is used for a sixth nerve palsy, superotemporal and inferotemporal incisions are utilized. A muscle hook is placed behind the insertion of the superior rectus. After lysing the intermuscular septum and

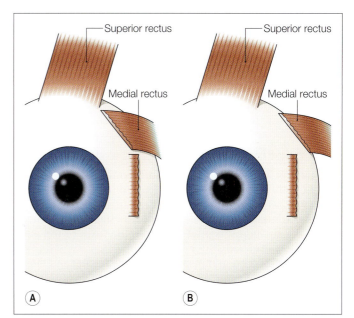

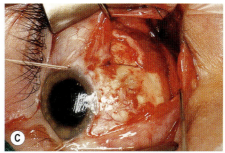

Fig. 85.34 (A) Medial rectus supraplaced. (B) The medial rectus is recessed and supraplaced (anchored hang-back technique). (Patient of Dr R. Morris.)

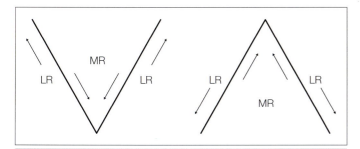

Fig. 85.33 Direction in which medial (MR) and lateral recti (LR) are moved in "V" and "A" patterns.

check ligaments, the muscle is split longitudinally for a distance of 15 mm posterior to the center of the insertion. Before splitting the muscle, the anterior ciliary vessels can be "combed" to the nasal side to preserve them. A double armed 6-0 coated polyglactin 910 suture is preplaced in the temporal half of the rectus muscle, 1 mm posterior to its insertion. Double locking bites are placed at the nasal and temporal borders of the split temporal half of the tendon. The temporal half is severed from its attachment to the sclera. A muscle hook is placed behind the insertion of the lateral rectus and the globe adducted. Each arm of the suture attached to the temporal half of the muscle is passed through the sclera, adjacent to the superior border of the lateral rectus. An identical procedure is performed on the inferior rectus.

Jensen procedure

The Jensen procedure is performed without disinsertion of the rectus muscles in an effort to preserve the anterior ciliary vessels. For sixth nerve palsy, the Jensen procedure is performed using superotemporal and inferotemporal incisions. A muscle hook is placed behind the insertion of the superior rectus. After lysing the intermuscular septum and check ligaments, the superior rectus is split longitudinally for a distance of 15 mm posterior to the insertion. Care is taken to avoid damage to the anterior ciliary vessels. A muscle hook is placed behind the insertion of the lateral rectus. After lysing the intermuscular septum and check ligaments, the lateral rectus is split longitudinally for a distance extending 15 mm posterior to the insertion. The temporal half of the superior rectus and superior half of the lateral rectus are joined together using a 4-0 or 5-0 non-absorbable suture placed 10 mm posterior to the insertions of the two muscles. The suture is tied relatively loosely to avoid strangulation of the anterior ciliary vessels. The suture can also include a scleral bite to reduce the tendency for post-operative migration of the transposed muscles. An identical procedure is performed on the inferior rectus.

Full tendon transposition

Full tendon transpositions are more commonly used than muscle splitting techniques for rectus muscle paresis. They work best when only one muscle is affected and there is minimal contracture of the antagonist. If significant contracture of the antagonist is present, botulinum toxin or recession should be considered.

Superior full tendon transposition of the medial and lateral rectus muscles (Knapp procedure) is used to treat "double elevator" palsy (monocular elevation deficiency). In one study, the procedure corrected an average of 38 PD of hypotropia.[132] The operation is used in patients with hypotropia in primary gaze and significant chin-up head posture. The insertions of the medial and lateral rectus muscles are transposed to a position adjacent to the respective border of the superior rectus insertion (Fig. 85.35). The procedure is most effective when there is no restriction to upgaze on traction testing. If traction testing reveals significant restriction, recession of the inferior rectus should be considered. The amount of hypotropia corrected may increase over time; it does not correlate with the size of the preoperative deviation and is less predictable if there has been prior inferior rectus surgery.[133] The procedure can be modified by performing recession and resection of the transposed muscles to concurrently treat a horizontal

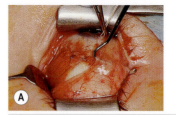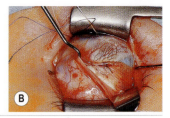

Fig. 85.35 Knapp procedure: surgeon's view of right eye. Vertical transposition of (A) medial and (B) lateral recti on the spiral of Tillaux. The superior rectus is held in a Helveston hook. (Patient of Dr R. Morris.)

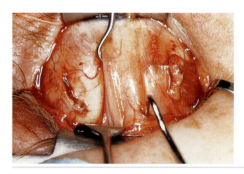

Fig. 85.36 Knapp procedure: surgeon's view of left eye. Vertical transposition of medial and lateral recti parallel to the medial and lateral borders of the superior rectus. The medial rectus has also been resected and the lateral recessed. (Patient of Dr. R. Morris.)

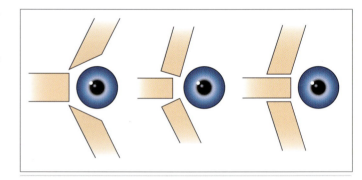

Fig. 85.37 Three different positions at which full tendon transpositions have been anchored to the sclera by different strabismus surgeons.

deviation (Fig. 85.36). Inferior transposition of the horizontal rectus muscles can be used to treat depressor palsies (Dunlap procedure).[134]

Full tendon transposition of the vertical rectus muscles is performed in the treatment of rectus muscle palsies. Full tendon transposition of the vertical rectus muscles has also been used to treat Duane's syndrome in an attempt to expand the field of single binocular vision.[135,136] There is some concern regarding the potential for the induction of vertical deviation and the loss of binocular vision and/or diplopia, which occurred in 8.5%[154] of a series of these patients. Altering or reversing transpositions can be difficult and somewhat unpredictable.

Placement of the insertion of transposed muscles varies by surgeon (Fig. 85.37), from a position that splits the pole of the insertion of the paretic muscle to placing them adjacent to the inferior and superior borders of the paretic lateral rectus running parallel for 8 mm. Most surgeons place the transposed muscles in a position that follows the spiral of Tillaux.

The effectiveness of transpositions can be augmented by placing a fixation suture in the transposed muscle posterior to its new insertion and securing it to the sclera (Foster modification)[137] (Fig. 85.38). Transposition of the vertical rectus muscles can be applied to hypofunction of any horizontal rectus muscle as well as treatment for Duane's syndrome.[138]

Technique for augmented full tendon transposition

Full tendon transposition for lateral rectus dysfunction is performed using superotemporal and inferotemporal fornix incisions. A muscle hook is placed behind the insertion of the superior rectus. Intermuscular septum and check ligaments are lysed from the insertion to the point at which the muscle penetrates Tenon's capsule. Tenon's capsule and the muscle capsule should remain intact and the underlying superior oblique tendon undisturbed. If not selected for preservation, anterior ciliary vessels receive light bipolar cautery. A 6-0 coated polyglactin 910 suture is passed in the tendon of the superior rectus, 1 mm posterior to the insertion. A single tie is placed in the central portion of the tendon and double locking bites are placed at the nasal and temporal borders. The total width of the superior rectus insertion is measured with calipers. The superior rectus is severed from its attachment to the sclera. The frenulum-like attachments from the underside of the superior rectus to the superior oblique tendon are lysed. A muscle hook is placed behind the insertion of the lateral rectus muscle and the globe adducted. The suture attached to the temporal pole of the superior rectus is passed in the sclera, adjacent to the upper pole of the lateral rectus, following the spiral of Tillaux in a superonasal direction for a distance of 5 mm. The suture attached to the nasal pole of the superior rectus is passed in the sclera, one tendon width away from the scleral entry site of the other suture. This is roughly 10 mm

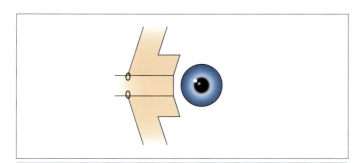

Fig. 85.38 Augmented full tendon transposition. The superior and inferior recti are transposed to the new insertion site, following the spiral of Tillaux. Non-absorbable sutures are placed in the sclera 8 mm posterior to the insertion of the lateral rectus and incorporate 25% of the adjacent transposed muscle, which is anchored to the sclera, creating the augmentation.

superior and nasal to the upper pole of the lateral rectus insertion. The needle exits the sclera adjacent to the previously placed needle in "crossed-swords" fashion. The sutures are tied. A 5-0 white braided non-absorbable suture (polyester) with spatulated needles is placed in the sclera, adjacent to the upper border of the lateral rectus, 8 mm posterior to the insertion of the lateral rectus. This is 16 mm posterior to the limbus. The 5-0 non-absorbable suture is passed through 25% of the lower portion of the transposed superior rectus, 8 mm posterior to the new insertion site. The 5-0 suture is tied and the gap between the lateral rectus and the transposed superior rectus is closed. An identical procedure is performed on the inferior rectus. Traction testing should be repeated to check for surgically induced restriction.

Superior oblique transposition

Transposition of the superior oblique tendon is useful in the treatment of complete third nerve palsy, when palsy of the superior rectus and inferior rectus make transposition of these two muscles ineffective. Transposition of the superior oblique tendon is usually combined with a "supramaximal" recession of the lateral rectus recession and sometimes a large resection of the denervated medial rectus. Repeat resections of denervated muscles eventually leave a relatively inelastic cord-like structure that serves as a "tether" holding the eye close to primary gaze.

Superior oblique transposition is accomplished by cutting the superior oblique tendon at the nasal border of the superior rectus. The superior oblique tendon is resected and attached to the sclera adjacent to the upper border of the medial rectus insertion (Fig. 85.39). This provides a medially directed vector force on the globe. Concurrent dislocation of the trochlea may make the sub-Tenon's course of the superior oblique follow closer to the path of the medial rectus. This procedure is controversial; bleeding and scarring may result. Postoperative traction sutures may temporarily hold the eye in adduction.[139]

Adjustable suture techniques

Reasonably standardized dose-response surgical tables are commonly used to determine the quantity of surgery to be employed in conventional strabismus surgery. However, there are many shortcomings to this approach. Over- and undercorrection are common.

Adjustable sutures serve to reposition extraocular muscles after surgery, potentially reducing the failure rate of conventional surgery. The first adjustable suture was probably the

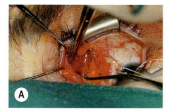
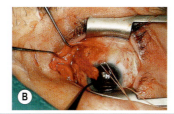
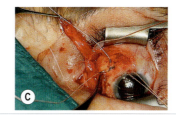
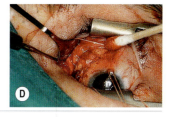

Fig. 85.39 Superior oblique tendon transposition. (A) The tendon is over a Green hook, and an artery forceps is being used to fracture the trochlear. (B) The tendon is disinserted and moved nasally. (C) Suture placed through tendon and sutured above the insertion of the medial rectus. (D) The tendon is sutured to sclera, the redundant tendon tissue having been excised. Note the medial rectus has been resected. (Patient of Dr R. Morris.)

O'Connor cinch.[140,141] Jampolsky re-introduced the concept of practical and clinically useful adjustable suture techniques.[142]

Adjustable suture techniques are of greatest benefit for patients where the effect of surgery is unpredictable and the risk of postoperative over- or undercorrection is increased. This includes patients with complex, non-concomitant, multi-planar strabismus, particularly those with scarring, orbital abnormalities affecting the elasticity of the orbital tissues, and paretic, myopathic and restrictive disorders affecting the contractility and elasticity of the extraocular muscles.

Strabismus with variation in the angle of deviation is not as amenable to adjustable suture techniques. This includes variable angle strabismus with central nervous system disorders and dissociated deviations.

Adjustable sutures are generally restricted to use in adults. However, adjustable sutures can be used in selected children less than 10 years of age and infants and young children with postoperative intravenous sedation.[143]

Surgical technique for adjustable sutures

Anesthesia for the primary procedure with placement of adjustable sutures can be performed using topical, peribulbar, retrobulbar, sub-Tenon's, or general anesthesia.

Most adjustable sutures are performed on rectus recessions; adjustable suture techniques can be used in resections, transpositions,[144] and superior oblique surgery.[145,146] The inferior oblique is rarely adjusted. With complex strabismus, adjustable sutures may be placed on more than one muscle.

The most common adjustable suture techniques are:

1. The "bow tie" technique. The sutures are placed just anterior to the insertion through scleral tunnels emerging 1.5 mm apart (Figs. 85.40A,B and 85.41). At adjustment, the bow is undone and the muscle advanced or recessed. When the muscle is in the desired position, the knot is tied. Two scleral passes for each suture can be made to form a "Z"[147] (Fig. 85.40B).

2. The sliding noose (sliding knot or cinch) technique. A second suture is tied tightly around the two arms of the suture attached to the muscle (Fig. 85.40C). The sliding noose can be slid up or down the muscle sutures to enable adjustment. It produces a larger knot and more tissue reaction but it is easier to estimate the amount of adjustment.

3. Other techniques in which the sutures are cut flush with the sclera and require no manipulation of the globe, if adjustment is not required, have been described.[148]

Technique for adjustable suture using sliding noose technique

Fornix or limbal incisions can be employed. If a fornix incision is used, inferior incisions are preferred; exposure is better and discomfort less during adjustment. However, superior rectus surgery, superior oblique surgery and superior transpositions of the horizontal rectus muscles require superior incisions.

After the sclera is exposed through the fornix incision, a muscle hook is placed behind the tendon insertion. Check ligaments and intermuscular septum are lysed for the distance appropriate to the procedure. After exposing the rectus muscle, the anterior ciliary vessels receive light bipolar cautery. This reduces bleeding during the procedure and suture adjustment.

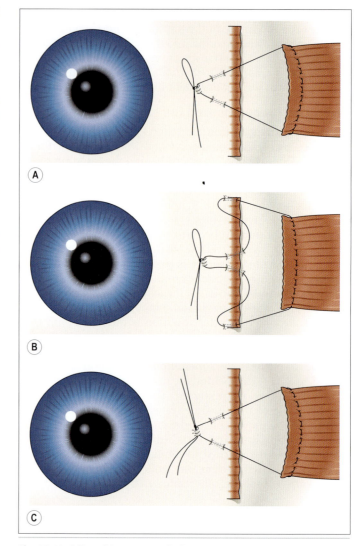

Fig. 85.40 Adjustable suture techniques. (A) Bow-tie technique. (B) Fells' technique. (C) Cinch technique.

A double armed 6-0 coated polyglactin 910 suture is placed in the tendon of the rectus muscle, 1 mm posterior to the insertion. Double locking bites are utilized at each of the two borders of the tendon. The tendon is severed at the insertion and allowed to retract. Each arm of the double armed suture attached to the rectus muscle is passed in the sclera at the original insertion site. The scleral exit points should be close to each other. This reduces movement of the knot securing the hang-back adjustable suture and an inadvertent tilted muscle. The muscle is temporarily advanced to the original insertion site and the sutures tied approximately 4 cm anterior to the cut end of the tendon. This allows room for the sutures to be tied after adjustment.

A sliding noose is fabricated from 6-0 coated polyglactin 910 and placed in a position to recess the muscle the planned distance. A removable sliding noose with 6-0 coated polyglactin 910 has been described.[149] For long hang-back adjustable sutures, a belt-loop of 6-0 polyglactin can be placed to reduce the risk of the muscle side-slipping.

When a fornix incision is used, a temporary 5-0 or 6-0 polyester traction suture is placed in the sclera, adjacent to the border of the original insertion. The traction suture controls

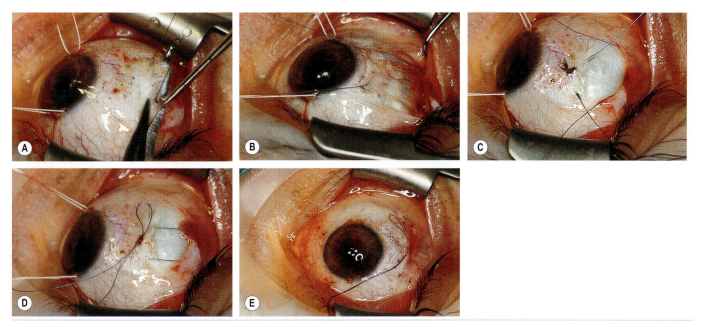

Fig. 85.41 Bow-tie adjustable suture technique using limbal conjunctival approach: left lateral rectus. (A) Double armed Vicryl suture placed through the muscle, which is then disinserted. (B) The disinserted muscle. (C) Suture needles are placed in "crossed-swords" position anterior to the muscle insertion. (D) A bow-tie knot is placed. (E) The conjunctiva is recessed to the level of the knot to facilitate adjustment of the suture. (Patient of Dr R. Morris.)

eye position during adjustment and retracts the conjunctiva and Tenon's capsule, exposing the adjustable suture.[150]

The conjunctiva is approximated with 6-0 plain gut suture. In some instances, the suture is left loose, to be tied after suture adjustment.

After completion of the surgical procedure, the adjustable sutures are tucked in the fornix and antibiotic/steroid ointment is applied. The longer exposed adjustable sutures are taped to the orbital rim.

Suture adjustment after using the "sliding noose" technique

Suture adjustment is performed when the effects of the anesthetic and other pharmacologic agent(s) have worn off.

Most suture adjustments are performed on the day of surgery. Suture adjustment can be performed immediately upon the completion of surgery, while the patient is on the operating room table[151] or delayed up to 14 days postoperatively.[152] Some employ viscoelastics[153,154] to facilitate delayed adjustment.

The patient should wear their usual spectacles (without prism) when postoperative measurements are obtained for suture adjustment. An accommodative fixation target is used.

The end-point for suture adjustment depends upon a number of factors. In many patients, the goal of surgery is fusion and the elimination of diplopia. Blurred vision immediately after surgery often degrades fusional ability at the time of adjustment, making objective prism and cover measurements important.

Suture adjustment is performed using topical anesthesia. The patient is supine, an eyelid speculum is inserted and the sutures identified.

The patient is asked to look in a direction that facilitates exposure of the adjustable suture. A small tenotomy hook placed on the polyester traction suture exposes the sliding noose and adjustable suture.

If it is necessary to advance the muscle forceps grasp the two adjustable sutures anterior to the sliding noose and pull the muscle anteriorly, while counter-traction is applied by holding the polyester traction suture. Use another forceps to grasp the sliding noose sutures and move the noose toward the insertion, securing the muscle in the new advanced position.

If it is necessary to recess the muscle, forceps grasp the two adjustable sutures anterior to the sliding noose and pull the muscle anteriorly, creating a space behind the sliding noose. Forceps or non-locking needle holders grasp the adjustable sutures posterior to the noose. The sliding noose is pulled anteriorly, increasing the recession. The noose and the adjustable suture are released. The globe is moved in a direction opposite to the adjustable suture by placing tension on the polyester traction suture. The patient is asked to look in the direction that places tension on the adjustable sutures and pulls the sliding noose back to the insertion. If the suture fails to move, the conjunctiva is retracted to expose the hang-back adjustable sutures. Non-toothed forceps pull each hang-back adjustable sutures posteriorly, moving the noose to the insertion site and allowing the muscle to be recessed.

The usual magnitude of each adjustment is 1 or 2 mm. After each adjustment, ocular alignment is re-evaluated.

When the desired end-point is reached, the adjustable sutures are tied after cutting one of the sutures. After tying the adjustable sutures, the ends are cut, preferably not shorter than 1.5 mm. The sutures attached to the sliding noose are cut, flush with the sliding noose. The conjunctiva is slid over the adjustable suture, covering the knot.

Problems with adjustable sutures

Careful patient selection is critically important with respect to success in adjustable sutures. Only a small number of children with strabismus are candidates for adjustable sutures with the patients awake.

Reoperations

A significant number of strabismus patients require more than one operation. In some forms of childhood strabismus, particularly infantile strabismus, this may approach 50%.

Adults may not know or remember that they received strabismus surgery during childhood. The presence of latent nystagmus and dissociated deviations imply that strabismus was present very early in childhood. The surgeon should look for evidence of previous surgery, particularly conjunctival scarring and disruption of the anterior ciliary vessels.

Reoperations require careful surgical planning. Special surgical equipment may be required including fiberoptic head lamps, special (e.g. Frazier) suction cannulas, malleable ribbon neurosurgical retractors, and other instruments.

Scarring and its many manifestations present the greatest challenge in reoperations. Scar tissue may cause alterations in the resting position of the globe, including torsion. This may alter the position of the extraocular muscles and orbital tissues, increasing the likelihood of bleeding, fat prolapse, muscle or tendon injury, and wrong muscle surgery.

Conjunctival scarring to the sclera, Tenon's capsule, orbital fat, and the muscle capsules can make exposure difficult. Sometimes, a limbal incision provides better exposure and a safer dissection. If there are significant adhesions between the conjunctiva and the sclera surface near the limbus, a more posterior incision may be preferred. Previous large limbal dissections create significant scarring adjacent to the limbus. In these circumstances, a perilimbal incision or modified Swann incision may be useful.

Prior rectus surgery may create anomalies in the position of the nearby extraocular muscles, particularly the oblique muscles. Prior superior rectus surgery frequently alters the position of the superior oblique tendon, which may be adherent to the nasal aspect of the superior rectus insertion, and can easily be cut or damaged. Previous lateral rectus surgery is often associated with anomalies affecting the course of the inferior oblique.[155] The inferior oblique may be anteriorly displaced and adherent to the inferior aspect of the lateral rectus. It can be inadvertently included in a hook intended to be placed behind the insertion of the lateral rectus.

Particular challenges occur in patients who have received scleral buckling procedures, glaucoma implant surgery, and the insertion and removal of radioactive plaques. Muscles and tendons, particularly the superior oblique, may be adherent to the capsule surrounding the implants or may be disrupted. It is common to encounter adhesions between the muscle capsule and the scleral surface, posterior to the capsule surrounding the scleral buckle or glaucoma implant. These create a mechanical effect similar to a posterior fixation suture. It is important to lyse these adhesions at the time of surgery.

Emerging techniques

Anterior ciliary vessel preservation during strabismus surgery

Strabismus surgery on the rectus muscles usually utilizes a full-width tenotomy which disrupts all of the anterior ciliary vessels (ACVs) on the operated rectus muscles. Anterior

segment ischemia is rare in children but a potentially serious complication.[156]

Most strabismus operations involve surgery on one or two rectus muscles in an eye, imparting little risk of anterior segment ischemia. However, cranial nerve palsies, restrictive disorders, and reoperations may require surgery on multiple rectus muscles in one eye. The mechanically ideal procedure may create a risk of anterior segment ischemia.

Avoidance of this complication includes staging surgery, limiting the total number of rectus muscles tenotomized and using techniques that spare the anterior ciliary circulation.[157] ACVs do not generally recanalize after strabismus surgery.[158,159]

Muscle splitting procedures, such as the Hummelsheim and Jensen transposition procedures and marginal myectomy and myotomy techniques may spare some anterior ciliary circulation. A modified rectus tuck that preserves anterior ciliary blood flow without dissection of the anterior ciliary vessels has been described.[160,161] Dissection and preservation of some ACVs during full tendon width strabismus surgery has been described.[160,162]

Surgical technique for dissection and preservation of the anterior ciliary vessels during strabismus surgery

The operating microscope is recommended and supplemental microvascular equipment[162] is necessary. This is a technique which has specific indications and is usually performed by a highly specialized surgeon. An outline of the surgery is shown in Figs 85.42 to 85.45.

Anterior segment ischemia has occurred after attempted dissection and preservation of the anterior ciliary vessels.[163] Although loupe techniques have been used,[164-166] we recommend the use of the operating microscope.

Titanium T-plates in the management of refractory strabismus

Several forms of complex strabismus do not respond well to conventional strabismus surgery. These include restrictive and paralytic (particularly multiple) disorders or when muscles have been surgically transected,[165-169] traumatically avulsed or lost.

Techniques to replace the force of an absent or dysfunctional muscle move the eye closer to the primary gaze position and counteract the antagonist. They tether the globe near primary gaze with permanent sutures,[166,167] alloplastic materials,[168,169] non-vascularized[170,171] and vascularized[172] autogenous tissues, or tendon.[173,174] The posterior fixation point is outside the muscle cone and usually adjacent to the affected muscle. The most common fixation structures have been the periosteum[175-177] and bone.[176] The effectiveness of these techniques depends on durability, tensile strength, and direction of resistance imparted by the connecting element and the position of the anchoring material or tissues. A titanium T-plate fixation platform allows for a more physiologic pull vector and better simulates the direction of a rectus muscle.[177] A patient who could potentially benefit from this procedure might have absence of medial rectus function from paresis, trauma or surgical transection of the muscle, when vertical rectus muscle transposition is not an option or has failed. The titanium T-plate is attached to the orbital wall with a non-absorbable

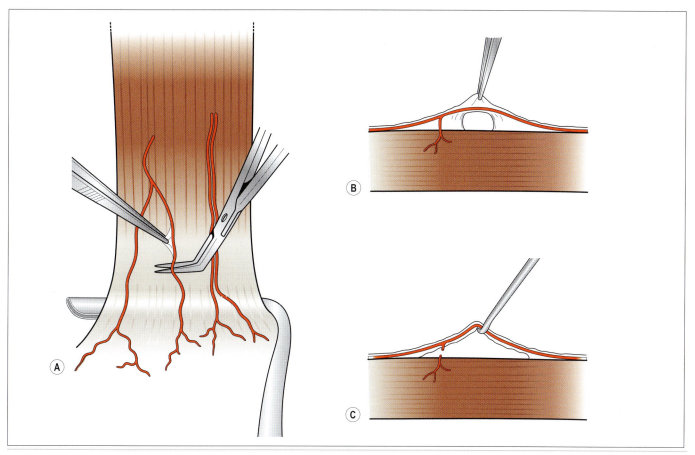

Fig. 85.42 Preservation of anterior ciliary vessels. (A) Initiation of dissection by creation of surgical plane beneath anterior ciliary vessels using microscissors. (B) Microvascular forceps grasp connective tissue and lift vessel to expose plane of dissection between vessel and tendon. (C) Right angle blunt micro hook lifts partially dissected vessel. A branch vessel has been cut after light bipolar cauterization away from the main anterior ciliary vessel.

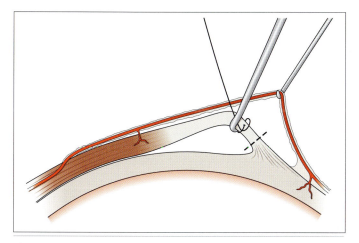

Fig. 85.43 Diagram of sagittal section of a rectus muscle with completed dissection of an anterior ciliary vessel. The vessel emerges from the muscle on the left and is suspended on the small hook on the right. The inherent "slack" in the vessel and the continuation of the dissection onto the sclera anterior to the tendon insertion provides space for suture passage adjacent to the insertion. The proposed tenotomy site is marked with a dashed line.

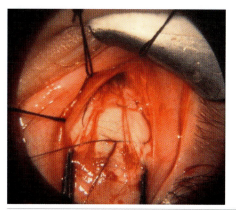

Fig. 85.44 Retracted right inferior rectus following tenotomy. Four anterior ciliary vessel groups have been dissected and preserved, which are silhouetted against the sclera. The scleral sutures have been passed 4 mm posterior to the original insertion. (Same muscle as shown in Figure 85.42.)

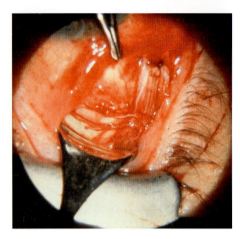

Fig. 85.45 Right superior rectus transposed temporally to the upper pole of the lateral rectus. Three dissected and preserved anterior ciliary vessel groups span the region between the transposed muscle and its original insertion site.

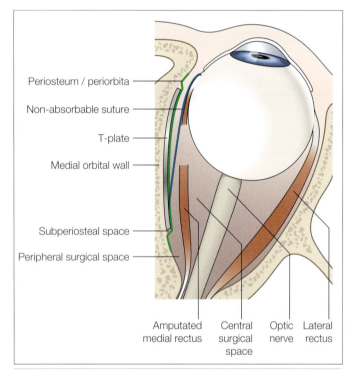

Periosteum / periorbita

Non-absorbable suture

T-plate

Medial orbital wall

Subperiosteal space

Peripheral surgical space

Amputated medial rectus   Central surgical space   Optic nerve   Lateral rectus

Fig. 85.46 Diagram of axial view of right orbit with transected (partially amputated) medial rectus (in red). The titanium T-plate (in blue) is in the subperiosteal space along the medial orbital wall. The equatorially oriented short arm of the T-plate is located anteriorly and extends superiorly and inferiorly out of the plane of this axial view and is secured to bone with titanium screws. A non-absorbable polyester suture (white) is tied to the posterior hole in the titanium T-plate; it passes through a surgical fenestration in the periorbita and travels anteriorly into sub-Tenon's space where it is secured to the sclera adjacent to the insertion of the medial rectus.

suture secured to the apex of the long arm of the T-plate, which is located in the posterior aspect of the orbit. The suture is passed in an anterior direction through an opening made in the periorbita and Tenon's capsule. The suture is then attached to the sclera, adjacent to the insertion of the dysfunctional muscle (Fig. 85.46).

References

1. Sedwick LA, Fishman PH, Repka MX, et al. A primate model of anterior segment ischemia after strabismus surgery. The role of the conjunctival circulation. J Neuro-ophthalmol 1990; 10: 295–300.

5. Demer JL. Mechanics of the orbita. Dev Ophthalmol 2007; 40: 132–57.

8. McKeown CA, Lambert HM, Shore JW. Preservation of the anterior vessels during extraocular muscle surgery. Ophthalmology 1989; 96: 498–506.

11. Hayreh SS, Scott WE. Fluorescein iris angiography. I. Normal pattern. Arch Ophthalmol 1978; 96: 1383–9.

12. Hayreh SS, Scott WE. Fluorescein iris angiography. II. Disturbances in iris circulation following strabismus operation on the various recti. Arch Ophthalmol 1978; 96: 1390–400.

19. Helveston EM, Krach P, Plager DA, et al. A new classification for superior oblique palsy based on congenital variations in the tendon. Ophthalmology 1992; 99: 1609–15.

25. Vivian AJ, Morris RJ. Diagrammatic representation of strabismus. Eye 1993; 7: 565–71.

26. Scott WE, Morris RJ. Dissociated vertical deviation and inferior oblique overaction in infantile esotropia. Arch Ophthalmol 1990; 108: 1081–4.

29. Oh AY, Kim JH, Hwang JW, et al. Incidence of postoperative nausea and vomiting after paediatric strabismus surgery with sevoflurane or remifentanil–sevoflurane. Br J Anaesth 2010; 104: 756–60.

32. Guyton DL. Exaggerated traction test for the oblique muscles. Ophthalmology 1981; 88: 1035–40.

39. de Alba Campomanes AG, Lim AK, Fredrick DR. Cyanoacrylate adhesive use in primary operation and reoperation in rabbit eye muscle surgery. J AAPOS 2009; 13: 357–63.

43. Kushner BJ, Preslan MW, Vrabec M. Artifacts of measurement during strabismus surgery. J Pediatr Ophthalmol Strabismus 1987; 24: 159–64.

44. Stager DR, Weakley DR, Everett M, et al. Delayed consecutive exotropia following 7-millimeter bilateral medial rectus recession for congenital esotropia. J Pediatr Ophthalmol Strabismus 1994; 31: 147–52.

49. Kushner BJ. A surgical procedure to minimize lower lid retraction with inferior rectus recession. Arch Ophthalmol 1992; 110: 1011–4.

59. Chatzistefanou KI, Kushner BJ, Gentry LR. Magnetic resonance imaging of the arc of contact of extraocular muscles: implications regarding the incidence of slipped muscles. J AAPOS 2000; 4: 84–93.

62. Hamed LM. Strabismus presenting after cataract surgery. Ophthalmology 1991; 98: 247–52.

68. Holmes JM, Hatt SR, Leske DA. Lateral rectus posterior fixation suture. J AAPOS 2010; 14: 132–6.

79. Stager DR, Parks MM. Inferior oblique weakening procedures: effect on primary position horizontal alignment. Arch Ophthalmol 1973; 90: 15–6.

81. Keskinbora KH. Anterior transposition of the inferior oblique muscle in the treatment of unilateral superior oblique palsy. J Pediatr Ophthalmol Strabismus 2010; 47: 301–7.

97. Kushner BJ. Restriction of elevation in abduction after inferior oblique anteriorization. J AAPOS 1997; 1: 55–62.

111. Knapp P, Moore S. Diagnosis and surgical options in superior oblique surgery. Int Ophthalmol Clin 1976; 16: 137–49.

113. Suh DW, Guyton DL, Hunter DG. An adjustable superior oblique tendon spacer with the use of nonabsorbable suture. J AAPOS 2001; 5: 164–71.

120. Wilson ME, Sinatra RB, Saunders RA. Downgaze restriction after placement of superior oblique tendon spacer for Brown syndrome. J Pediatr Ophthalmol Strabismus 1995; 32: 29–34; discussion 35–6.

124. Nishimura JK, Rosenbaum AL. The long-term torsion effect of the adjustable Harada-Ito procedure. J AAPOS 2002; 6: 141–4.

132. Knapp P. The surgical treatment of double elevator paralysis. Trans Am Ophthalmol Soc 1969; 67: 304–23.

136. Rosenbaum AL. Costenbader Lecture. The efficacy of rectus muscle transposition surgery in esotropic Duane syndrome and VI nerve palsy. J AAPOS 2004; 8: 409–19.

142. Jampolsky A. Strabismus re-operation technique. Trans Am Acad Ophthalmol Otolaryngol 1975; 79: 704–17.

148. Saunders RA, O'Neil JW. Tying the knot. Is it always necessary? Arch Ophthalmol 1992; 110: 1318–21.

152. Robbins SL, Granet DB, Burns C, et al. Delayed adjustable sutures: a multicentred clinical review. Br J Ophthalmol 2010; 94: 1169–73.

162. McKeown CA, Lambert HM, Shore JW. Preservation of the anterior vessels during extraocular muscle surgery. Ophthalmology 1989; 9: 498–506.

168. Bicas HE. A surgically implanted elastic band to restore paralyzed ocular rotations. J Pediatr Ophthalmol Strabismus 1991; 28: 10–3.

169. Scott AB, Miller JM, Collins CC. Eye muscle prosthesis. J Pediatr Ophthalmol Strabismus 1992; 29: 216–8.

177. Tse DT, Shriver EM, Krantz KB, et al. The use of titanium T-plate as platform for globe alignment in severe paralytic and restrictive strabismus. Am J Ophthalmol 2010; 150: 404–11.

 Access the complete reference list online at

http://www.expertconsult.com

Part 6
Strabismus treatment

Strabismus surgery complications and how to avoid them

John A Bradbury • Rachel F Pilling

Chapter contents

INCIDENCE

MILD COMPLICATIONS

SEVERE COMPLICATIONS

CONSENT IN STRABISMUS SURGERY

REFERENCES

Severe complications of strabismus surgery are rare but they can be devastating. This chapter will discuss the frequency and management of problems our patients may encounter after surgery and how we might approach consenting patients to ensure their expectations are well informed.

Incidence

The incidence and outcomes described are from a 2-year prospective survey of severe complications of strabismus surgery carried out by the author through the British Ophthalmic Surveillance Unit (BOSU) and the available literature. The incidence of severe complications of strabismus surgery was 2.5–3 per 1000. Globe perforation is the most common complication with almost an incidence of 1:1000. Retinal detachment and endophthalmitis are the least common reported (Fig. 86.1, Box 86.1 and Table 86.1). Anterior segment ischemia was not part of the BOSU study, but may be 1:13 000 operations.[1] Eighteen percent of patients with a complication had a poor or very poor outcome: about 0.05% or 1:2000 of patients operated on.

Mild complications (Box 86.2)

We devised a 5 point scale depending on the severity of outcome of the complication. This is outlined in Figure 4. The number of complications in the 5 categories split into adults and children is shown in Figure 5 with the p values. Although there were more infections and globe perforations in children and more SINS and lost muscle in adults only SINS reached statistical significance.

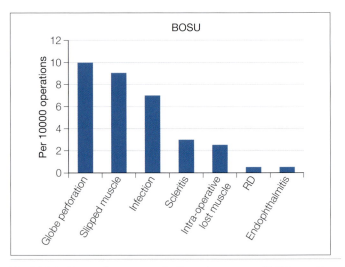

Fig. 86.1 Incidence of severe complications of surgery, per 10 000 operations. RD = retinal detachment.

Box 86.1

Classification of outcome

Grade 1: Good outcome

Grade 2: Surgical or medical intervention but good outcome

Grade 3: Surgical or medical intervention asymptomatic but compromised outcome

Grade 4: Surgical or medical intervention but poor outcome, e.g. double vision or up to 2 lines of loss of vision on a Snellen chart

Grade 5: Very poor outcome, greater than 2 lines of visual loss on a Snellen chart

Box 86.2

Mild complications of strabismus surgery

Dellen

Chronic red eye

Pyogenic granuloma

Tenon's fascia prolapse

Epithelial inclusion cyst

Chemosis

Table 86.1 – Number of complications reported in BOSU study. The p value compares adult and child rates for each complication

	Infection	SINS	Perforation	Lost muscle	Slipped muscle	Retinal detachment	Endophthalmitis	Total
Adults								
1			1					
2	2	3	2	1	7			
3			4	3		1		
4	1	2		1				
5		1						
								29
Children								
1			1					
2	8		10		4			
3	1				4			
4	2				3			
5			1				1	
								35
P values	0.0573	0.0312	0.3591	0.0625	0.4805	1.00		1.00

SINS = surgically induced necrotizing scleritis.

When we look at outcome, 18% of patients with a complication had a poor or very poor outcome. This means about 0.05% or 1:2000 of patients operated on had a poor or very poor outcome.

Dellen

Dellen tend to occur in the peripheral cornea, specifically nasal and temporal quadrants in the first 1–2 weeks following strabismus surgery. Dellen are thinning of the cornea due to the drying out of the collagen in the stroma related to poor corneal wetting. They are related to tear film disruption and altered anterior segment contour due to swollen conjunctiva which prevents the smooth travel of the eyelids. They are more common in adults, but may occur in children (who are rarely examined on the slit-lamp). The reported the incidence is between 0.3% and 22.45%.[2] It is usually self-limiting or responds to topical lubricants; rarely a contact lens is required.

Chronic red eye

Redness is common, especially after repeated strabismus surgery, but some patients have a persistent red eye for many weeks or months. These patients are unhappy, feeling their appearance is harmed. Some of this may be related to more long term problem with corneal wetting and responds to topical lubricants. Prolonged postoperative inflammation or violation of the orbital fat may contribute to a chronic red eye, most often of the medial rectus and surrounding tissue. Prevention includes meticulous surgery, hemostasis, avoidance of orbital fat, and thinning and reduction of thickened and redundant medial conjunctiva. This often occurs in adults with long standing (especially consecutive) exotropias. We give such patients intensive topical steroid drops for a month following strabismus surgery; occasionally, long term lubricants and topical steroids are required. If the eye is still red after 3 months, we may give subconjunctival depot steroids to whiten the eye, and reduce the conjunctival bulk.

Pyogenic granuloma

This fleshy mass appears a few weeks after surgery and is composed of inflammatory cells and capillary proliferation. It may be confused with a suture granuloma. They respond to topical steroids but occasionally require surgery.

Prolapsed Tenon's capsule

This occurs in children and young adults with a prominent Tenon's layer. It is caused by poor conjunctival closure. If the prolapse is large, it may need to be trimmed, but it usually resolves spontaneously.

Epithelial inclusion cyst (Fig. 86.2)

This rare complication is caused by deposition of conjunctival epithelial cells into deeper tissues. Most are small, some can be large, especially those at muscle insertions. They enlarge and need surgical removal.

Chemosis

Chemosis occurs after most strabismus surgery. It is rarely severe, but it can be so severe that the conjunctiva is exposed and the chemosis is exacerbated by drying: intensive topical lubricants and steroids usually resolve it. Rarely, it may be necessary to tape the lid shut or perform a temporary "superglue" tarsorrhaphy (with caution in children because of distress and amblyopia risk). An option is to suture the conjunctiva into the fornices.

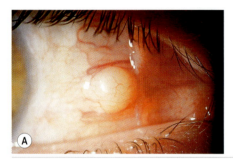
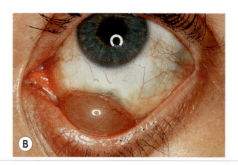
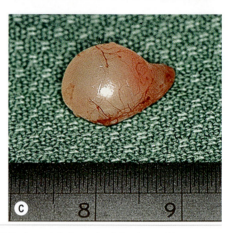

Fig. 86.2 **Conjunctival epithelial inclusion cysts.** (A) Cyst over medial rectus. (B) Cyst over inferior rectus. (C) Cyst over inferior rectus following excision. (Courtesy of Mr Robert Morris.)

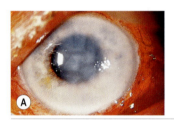
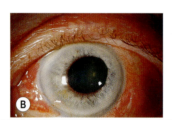
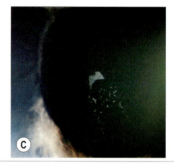
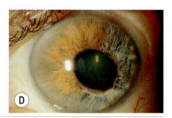

Fig. 86.3 **Anterior segment ischemia.** (A) Severe ischemia causing corneal edema. (B) Same eye 6 months later; note mid-dilated pupil. (C) Anterior lens opacities following anterior segment ischemia. (D) Iris atrophy following anterior segment ischemia. (Courtesy of Mr Robert Morris.)

Box 86.3

Severe complications of strabismus surgery

Globe perforation
Orbital infection
Endophthalmitis
Surgically induced necrotizing scleritis
Slipped muscle
Lost muscle
Retinal detachment
Adherence syndrome
Anterior segment ischemia

Table 86.2 – Grading of anterior segment ischemia

Grade 1	Grade 2	Grade 3	Grade 4
Reduced iris perfusion	Pupillary abnormalities	Postoperative uveitis	Keratopathy

Severe complications (Box 86.3)

Anterior segment ischemia (Fig. 86.3)

Two anterior ciliary arteries (branches of the ophthalmic artery) supply each rectus muscle apart from the lateral rectus which has only one: the obliques have no anterior ciliary arteries.

The incidence of significant anterior segment ischemia (ASI) may be 1 : 13 000 cases.[1] It was not surveyed in the BOSU study because ASI would be grossly underreported, especially in children where postoperative slit-lamp examination is not normally performed. Severe outcomes are rare although there is a report of phthisis bulbi.[1] Risks factors for ASI include

increasing age, previous rectus surgery, operations on multiple muscles (especially recti) in the same eye, circulation problems (i.e. hypertension or diabetes), similar surgery on adjacent rectus muscles, surgery on vertical rectus muscles, and a limbal incision.

In children, it may be safe to operate on more than two recti muscles at once: most surgeons avoid operating on all four recti muscles simultaneously. If it is necessary to operate on more than two recti muscles in an adult or if the patient has a very high risk of developing ASI, anterior ciliary artery sparing surgery can be performed by dissecting out the anterior ciliary arteries from the muscle or performing a partial tendon transposition, sparing at least one of the anterior ciliary arteries.

Symptoms and signs of ASI can vary from mild uveitis and reduced iris perfusion to a keratopathy[1,3] (Table 86.2).

Grade 1 ASI can only be detected by iris angiography.
Grade 2 ASI is caused by areas of iris hypoperfusion, sometimes an abnormally shaped pupil. It rarely requires treatment.
Grades 3 and 4 ASI usually require treatment with topical or systemic corticosteroids. Unusual treatments include

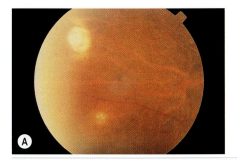
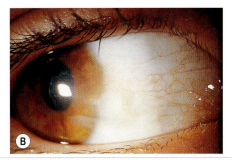
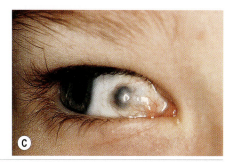

Fig. 86.4 Globe perforation complications. (A) Localized chorioretinal scar following scleral perforation at strabismus surgery. (B) Bleb formation following unrecognized scleral perforation from limbal traction suture 3 years previously. (C) Scleromalacia 4 years after strabismus surgery at site of original muscle insertion. (Courtesy of Mr Robert Morris.)

hyperbaric oxygen. The vast majority recover with only minor sequelae including iris atrophy, corectopia, or a poorly reacting pupil.

Globe perforation (Fig. 86.4)

Globe perforation is the commonest severe complication of strabismus surgery, reported in 0.13% to 1% of cases.[4,5] In the BOSU study, the incidence was 1 : 1000. The incidence was more common in children, this has been noted previously but did not reach statistical significance, This may be due to surgical access. In one case the outcome was very poor. The patient developed endophthalmitis and had to have an evisceration. Although globe perforation is common, a poor or very poor outcome is extremely rare. Complex surgery, i.e. faden procedures, may have a higher incidence of globe perforation.

In the BOSU study, globe perforation sometimes occurred when placing a traction suture. This resulted in some cases of penetration into the anterior chamber and a soft eye making strabismus surgery difficult. Most cases of posterior segment perforation had peroperative treatment, usually cryotherapy or laser. There was one case of retinal detachment in a high myope who had bilateral globe perforation from bilateral Harada-Ito procedures.

Management of globe perforation is not evidence based. Ninety percent of cases are treated with cryotherapy and/or laser.[6] In children, where globe perforation is more likely, retinal detachment is unlikely as they have formed vitreous. We perform a fundus examination to confirm the diagnosis with the pupil dilated peroperatively by injection of 1 or 2 mL of local anesthetic sub-Tenon's. We do not perform peroperative treatment ourselves but seek a vitreo-retinal opinion, if available. In adults, we do a fundus examination and, in patients with a high risk of retinal detachment (i.e. high myopes), we perform peroperative treatment of the hole and then seek vitreo-retinal opinion. We do not treat those at low risk, but would seek a later vitreo-retinal opinion. All patients have systemic antibiotics to reduce the risk of endophthalmitis. The BOSU study reported one case of endophthalmitis leading to evisceration in a 3-year-old. Rathod[6] reported two cases of endophthalmitis, two retinal detachments, one suprachoroidal hemorrhage, and one choroidal scar.

Strategies to prevent globe perforation include:

1. Avoiding suturing in areas with scleral thinning.
2. Techniques (i.e. hang-back procedures) that do not involve direct scleral suturing in thinner areas or where access is difficult.

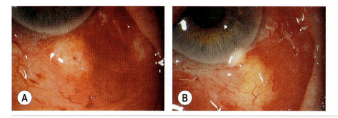

Fig. 86.5 Localized abscess. (A) Localized subconjunctival abscess. (B) Pus released by pressure on abscess. (Courtesy of Mr Robert Morris.)

Orbital infection (Fig. 86.5)

Orbital infection following strabismus surgery tends to be equally either diffuse orbital cellulitis or an abscess at the muscle insertion. In the BOSU study there were 13 cases, only two in adults. Three muscle insertion abscesses developed a slipped muscle requiring surgical exploration. Kothari[7] reported a similar bilateral case. Management depends on whether it is a diffuse orbital infection: systemic antibiotics are usually curative. A muscle insertion abscess, if associated with a slipped muscle, requires surgical exploration and drainage and systemic antibiotics.

Histology of endophthalmitis has shown that infection gained access to the eye from a postoperative muscle insertion infection suggesting a more aggressive approach to postoperative muscle insertion infections. No such cases occurred in the BOSU study.

Surgically induced necrotizing scleritis

Surgically induced necrotizing scleritis (SINS) is a rare but serious complication of strabismus surgery. There is only one pediatric case in the literature[8] but the BOSU study had six adult cases which presented 1–6 weeks postoperatively, usually with ocular pain. They were treated usually with topical and systemic non-steroidal anti-inflammatory drugs (NSAIDs) or steroids. One severe case required treatment with cyclophosphamide and developed posterior synechiae and a cataract reducing the vision to logMAR 0.60 (6/24, 20/80, 0.25). Fifty percent of cases had a poor or very poor outcome. Most patients were elderly; two were in their 20s. Figure 86.6 shows a case of surgically induced necrotizing scleritis. This responded to oral and topical non-steroidal agents with no significant sequelae. Patients with SINS may best be seen by an inflammatory diseases specialist, bearing in mind the poor prognosis in the BOSU study.

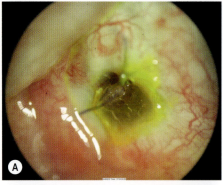

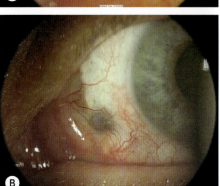

Fig. 86.6 (A) This 16-year-old male developed surgically induced necrotizing scleritis having had medial rectus recession on adjustable sutures for a blow out fracture. There is a suture holding the conjunctiva covering the area of scleritis. (B) The appearance after treatment with topical steroids and oral non-steroidal agents.

Mild scleritis may be common following strabismus surgery, presenting with pain, more severe and deep-seated than normal with diffuse scleral inflammation requiring oral NSAIDs. Risk factors include advancing age, poor circulation, scleral diathermy, and ischemia.

 ## Lost muscle

In the BOSU study, lost muscle was defined as a muscle lost peroperatively. There were six lost muscles, five in adults. Most were in elderly patients, four of whom had had previous strabismus surgery. Four were medial recti, two were lateral recti. Medial recti are the most common muscles lost at surgery.[9] This may relate to how frequently the muscle is operated on, or to its anatomy. The other recti have attachments to the oblique which prevent the muscle retracting into the orbit. All patients in the BOSU study had the muscles found peroperatively: only one had a poor or very poor outcome.

Should a muscle be lost peroperatively it is best to find the muscle immediately. A common mistake is to look for the muscle around the globe when in fact the recti muscles lie slightly away from the globe. Get help from an experienced surgeon, use suitable retractors for exposure, and control hemostasis. Careful exploration usually finds the muscle sheath and the muscle within. Some authors have suggested using the oculo-cardiac reflex as a way of finding the muscle as pulling on the muscle would slow the heart rate, this is only partially useful. If the muscle cannot be found, suture the check ligaments and Tenon's surrounding the muscle to the original muscle insertion:[9] some muscle action may be transferred though these tissues to the eye. A muscle transposition could be performed; however, beware of anterior segment ischemia in adults. A more experienced strabismus surgeon may be able to find the muscle at a subsequent exploration. Postoperative investigations may include MRI and CT scans

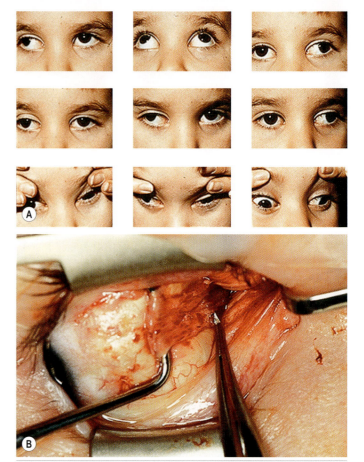

Fig. 86.7 Patient with slipped right medial rectus muscle. (A) Note large exodeviation and underaction of medial rectus. (B) Findings at surgery: strabismus hook under pseudotendon of medial rectus 11 mm from limbus. Forceps indicating proximal end of medial rectus muscle. Note the change in color between muscle tissue and pseudotendon. (Courtesy of Mr Robert Morris.)

especially with lost muscles due to trauma or with congenital or acquired abnormal orbits. An orbital approach may help with a posteriorly situated muscle.[10]

Slipped muscle (Fig. 86.7)

In the BOSU study slipped muscle was defined as the patient presenting with an overcorrection and 50% or more reduction in movement in the action of a previously operated muscle. There were 18 cases, and it was slightly more common in children. In three of these, the slipped muscle resulted from a muscle insertion infection. Three had a poor or very poor outcome; all were children.

Slipped muscles take two main forms. A true slipped muscle is similar to a lost muscle: a problem with the sutures or insertion soon after the operation. The suture fails and the muscle slips. One deals with this like with a lost muscle. The more common presentation occurs many weeks to even years later, with a gross limitation of action of the muscle that has slipped. Exploration often finds the muscle on a large pseudotendon, not attached directly to the sclera but indirectly via stretchy scar tissue. This may occur due to stretching of a poorly inserted muscle over time. The pseudotendon is removed and the muscle re-attached to the globe. Shortening of the antagonist may require recession of it and the conjunctiva.

Adherence syndrome

This is a restrictive condition, often progressive, caused by orbital fat coming through a surgical disruption of posterior Tenon's, as a result of strabismus surgery commonly to the inferior oblique. Occasionally it is caused by trauma or lid surgery. To prevent this, care must be made to visual the posterior edge of the inferior oblique so only the muscle is hooked, sometimes excessive bleeding leads to poor visualisation and contributes to the scarring process. If orbital fat prolapses at surgery the fat can be excised and the posterior tenons repaired. Often the problem is found postoperatively as the patient develops progressive hypertropia and limitation of elevation (Fig. 86.8). Surgical options are to explore the inferior fornix, excise any orbital fat, repair the posterior Tenon's capsule defect, and then recess the inferior rectus, Tenon's, and conjunctiva followed by an amniotic membrane graft.

Endophthalmitis

There was one case of endophthalmitis in the 2 years of the BOSU giving an incidence of 1 : 24 000 cases. For diagnosis and treatment of endophthalmitis, see Chapter 14.

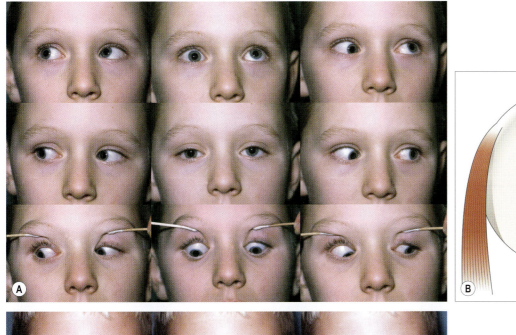
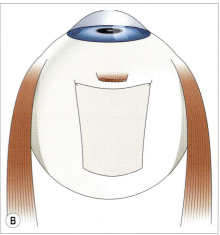
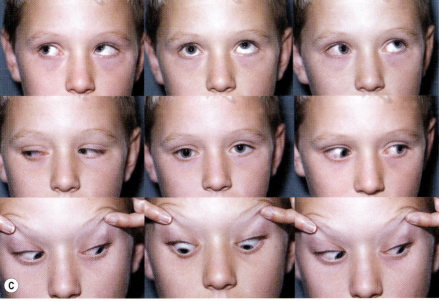

Fig. 86.8 A 14-year-old boy underwent routine right inferior oblique myectomy for a right fourth nerve palsy. (A) Two weeks postoperatively he developed restriction in elevation in the right eye as a result of right inferior fornix adherence syndrome. (B) He underwent recession of inferior rectus recession of the conjunctiva and Tenon's capsule together with an amniotic membrane graft placed between the sclera and the inferior rectus (C). His postoperative ocular motility showed improvement in elevation of his right eye.

Consent in strabismus surgery
(see also Chapter 58)

The act of placing a signature on a consent form should be the terminal event in a patient's journey from first appointment to eye theater.[11] The principle of taking consent prior to treatment is directed towards protecting a patient's autonomy. To be valid, it must be given voluntarily by an informed patient with capacity to consent.[12,13] According to the Mental Capacity Act 2005[13] (UK Law) capacity is defined by a person's ability to fulfill the following four conditions below. The patient is able to:

1. Retain information.
2. Understand the information.
3. Use the information to weigh up risk and benefit.
4. Communicate the decision.

Consent is a process, not an event

During consent, the patient should develop a clear understanding of options, rationale, and outcomes, then weigh risks and benefits to make an informed decision and develop reasonable expectations for surgical results.

It is considered best practice to document the discussions you have with your patient at each stage of the consent journey and record what written information is given. Adequate time for discussion in clinic and gaining consent before the day of surgery allows the patient to reflect upon their decision and any additional queries can be answered during confirmation of consent on the day of surgery.[14] Some authorities recommend that consent should be performed by the physician providing treatment;[15] whilst others countries allow delegation of consent to another team member so long as they have sufficient knowledge to describe risks and benefits and to answer questions.[16]

Contrary to popular belief, there is no specific "risk threshold" which mandates which complications you should or should not discuss with your patients. The legal standard describing what risks should be disclosed to the patient varies within and between countries. The standard of ethical care expected of health care professionals by their regulatory bodies may exceed the legal requirements. It is advisable to inform your patient (Box 86.4) of all significant possible adverse outcomes or unavoidable risks of surgery and make a record of the information given.[12]

Encourage a dialogue between you and your patient

A careful balance needs to be struck between listening to what your patient wants and ensuring they have sufficient information (Box 86.5) to make an informed decision.[18]

It is the duty of the surgeon to ascertain the patient's needs and wishes and discuss everything relevant to the individual,[16] to present information in a balanced way, and check that the patient has understood the information. In many countries, the surgeon also explains the risks of anesthesia, including morbidity and death; in others this is done by the anesthetic team.

Decision making in children should be centred around shared responsibility between surgeon and parents

For minors, informed consent is required from a parent or legal guardian prior to medical treatment.

In most cases, a decision will be made which represents the best interests of the child. Although only one parent signature is required, it may be appropriate to involve both parents in decision making.

Consider an adolescent's developing capability for involvement in decision making[20,21]

A young person's ability to consent depends more on their understanding of the nature of the proposed treatment and its possible consequences than on their age.[18,22] There is no simple criterion or measure of competence; your skill lies in assessing the young patient's competence in a particular context for a specific decision.[23] The legal at which a minor may give consent varies widely from country to country and should be considered on a case by case basis. The law on consent is constantly evolving and varies internationally. Legal advice should always be sought if there is doubt as to the legal validity of a proposed intervention.

Box 86.4

Informed consent should cover these areas[16,17]

Diagnosis

Treatment options, including no treatment

Other possible procedures which may be necessary during surgery

Common side-effects/complications

Rare, significant complications

Anesthetic options and risks

Box 86.5

Ophthalmic Mutual Insurance Company Informed Consent for Strabismus Surgery

Major risks of strabismus surgery:

1. Need for additional surgeries
2. Persistent misalignment, altered eyelid position, limitation of eye movements, persistent visual problems
3. Double vision
4. Scar tissue formation
5. Infection
6. Hemorrhage or bleeding
7. Severe infection or bleeding leading to damage to the eye or rarely visual loss
8. Allergic reaction
9. Temporary side-effects, such as corneal abrasion, conjunctivitis, eye ache

Ophthalmic Mutual Insurance Company (OMIC). Strabismus Surgery Consent Form. Version 4/16/09 ed, 2009.[19]

References

1. France T, Simon J. Anterior segment ischemia syndrome following muscle surgery: The AAPOS Experience. J Pediatr Ophthalmol Strabismus 1986; 23: 87–91.

2. Maig Jang S. Relationship in corneal dellen tear break up time. Yan Ke Xue Bao 1991; 7: 43–6.

3. Lee JP, Olver JM. Anterior segment ischaemia. Eye 1990; 4: 1–6.

4. Noel LP, Bloom JN, Clarke WN, Bawazeer A. Retinal perforation in strabismus surgery. J Pediatr Ophthalmol Strabismus 1997; 34: 115–17.

5. Simon JW. Scleral perforation during eye muscle surgery, incidence and sequelae. J Pediatr Ophthalmol Strabismus 1992; 29: 273–5.

6. Rathod D, Goyal R, Watts P. The management of globe perforation during strabismus surgery. J AAPOS, 2010; 14: 25.

7. Kothari M, Sukri N. Bilateral *Staphylococcus aureus* sub-Tenon's abscess following strabismus surgery in a child. J AAPOS 2010; 14: 193–5.

8. Kearney FM, Blaikie AJ, Gole GA. Anterior necrotising scleritis and strabismus surgery in a child. J AAPOS 2007; 11: 197–8.

9. MacEwan C, Lee J, Fells P. Aetiology and management of the detached rectus muscle. Br J Ophthalmol 1992; 76: 131–6.

10. Lenart T, Reichman O, MacMahon S. Retrieval of lost medial rectus muscle with a combined ophthalmological and otolaryngologic surgical approach. Am J Ophthalmol 2000; 130: 645–52.

11. Jackson E. Consent I: Capacity and Voluntariness – Medical Law: Text Cases and Materials. Oxford: OUP; 2006.

12. Department of Health. Reference Guide to Consent for Examination or Treatment, 2nd ed; 2009. http://www.dh.gov.uk/en/PublicationsandstatisticsPublications/PublicationsPolicyAndGuidance/DH_103643. Accessed 11 April 2011.

13. Crown Copyright. Mental Capacity Act; 2005.

14. American Academy of Ophthalmology. Practice Guidelines for Informed Consent. December 2011. http://one.aao.org/ce/practiceguidelines/patient_content.aspx?cid=500f9f05-9ebf-43fa-a02e-426c8f4fb860. Accessed 11 April 2011.

15. American Medical Association. Informed Consent. March 2005. http://www.ama-assn.org/ama/pub/physician-resources/legal-topics/patient-physician-relationship-topics/informed-consent.page. Accessed 11 April 2011.

16. General Medical Council. Consent: Patients and Doctors Making Decisions Together, 2008. http://www.gmc-uk.org/static/documents/content/Consent_0510.pdf.

17. American Academy of Ophthalmology. Advisory Committee on the Code of Ethics: Informed Consent; 2008. http://www.aao.org/about/ethics/code_ethics.cfm#informed. Accessed 14 April 2011.

18. British Medical Association. Consent Toolkit, 5th ed. http://www.bma.org.uk/images/consenttoolkitdec2009_tcm41-193139.pdf.

19. Ophthalmic Mutual Insurance Company (OMIC). Strabismus Surgery Consent Form. Version 4/16/09 ed; 2009.

20. Committee on Bioethics. Informed consent, parental permission, and assent in pediatric practice. Pediatrics 1995; 95: 314–17.

21. American Academy of Pediatrics. AAP publications retired or reaffirmed. Pediatrics 2007; 119: 405.

22. General Medical Council. 0–18 Years Guidance; 2007. http://www.gmc-uk.org/static/documents/content/0-18_0510.pdf. Accessed 25 April 2011.

23. Shaw M. Competence and consent to treatment in children and adolescents. Adv Psychiatr Treat 2001; 7: 150–9.

Part 6
Strabismus treatment

Bupivacaine injection of eye muscles to treat strabismus

Alan B Scott • Joel M Miller • Kenneth K Danh

Introduction

Correcting misalignment of deviating eyes is essential to developing and maintaining binocular vision and achieving a normal cosmetic appearance. Surgery on the extraocular muscles (EOM) and optical correction of refractive errors are the classic methods; injection of drugs into the eye muscles to change their action is a third method of altering eye alignment. I will describe the use of bupivacaine (BUP) injection of EOM, the first pharmacologic technique to strengthen the EOMs. It is safe, reliable, and long lasting for small to moderate comitant deviations, about equal in these regards to surgery, with which it will be compared in a pending trial.

Drugs injected into human eye muscles

Alcohol

Behrens, inspired by alignment changes after injection of alcohol into the orbit to reduce eye pain in absolute glaucoma, injected alcohol into the muscles of a few patients with strabismus. The effect was nerve paralysis in one or two and no effect in most. It is reasonable to credit him for this pioneering effort to treat strabismus by direct injection of the extraocular muscles.

Botulinum toxin A

This drug weakens EOM. It was first used for strabismus in 1978; a large experience of its use has been reported since. Chapter 84 addresses this topic.

Collagenase

In 1992, we found that purified bacterial collagenase easily dissolved scleral fibers and intramuscular fibrous tissue in rabbits. We injected the EOM of eight patients in increasing doses, trying to remove fibrous tissue in the EOM in thyroid eye disease and restricting scar formation after orbit fracture. Positive effects were beginning to become evident as the dose was increased, but hemorrhaging from dissolution of collagen in vascular tissues also occurred. It is likely that we terminated these experiments prematurely. Collagenase is now approved by the FDA for use in Dupytren's contracture; injections with good results are usually accompanied by mild bleeding. Application of this drug to restrictive strabismus should be re-visited.

Bupivacaine

BUP enlarges, shortens, and strengthens EOM. We first injected it into EOM as treatment for strabismus in 2006. We have experience with 52 cases of various types, using a range of BUP concentrations and volumes.

Bupivacaine

Mechanism of action

Small lipophilic local anesthetic molecules penetrate cell walls and attach to voltage gated sodium channels of nerves and muscles, blocking propagation of nerve and muscle action potentials. It is reversible and leaves no damage. BUP is especially lipophilic and strongly penetrates the sarcoplasmic reticulum of muscle fibers where it causes myotoxic damage by releasing the stored calcium into the cytosol and blocking calcium re-uptake by the sarcoplasmic reticulum. The high calcium concentration in the cytosol damages the mitochondria of the muscle fiber and activates an enzyme that dissolves the Z-band fibers of the muscle, resulting in separation of the sarcomeres.[1-3] The damaged fibers are not repaired, but are removed over the next few days by macrophages leaving the cell membranes, nerves, and blood vessels intact.[1-8] Within a few hours of exposure to BUP, autocrine growth factor molecules such as insulin growth factors IGF-I and IGF-IEc or mechano growth factor (MGF) are released from the damaged area. These molecules activate the satellite cells that are scattered around each muscle fiber. The satellite cells proliferate and coalesce to form new muscle fibers and myocytes to replace the damaged muscle, a process taking 3 weeks.[1,4,7,9,10,11] In EOM, regeneration builds a muscle that has larger muscle fibers and is increased in size 5–10%, especially in its posterior third. The regenerated muscle is stiffer than before, probably due to added non-contractile fibrous tissue within the muscle.[9,11,12] These biomechanical alterations change eye alignment.

An EOM treated with BUP appears to regenerate to the length at which it is held during the process of regeneration. Physically restraining the eye to do this is impractical. A small dose of Botox® to the antagonist to weaken it for 3–4 weeks prevents stretching of the BUP injected muscle during the phase of regeneration. This allows the BUP injected muscle to regenerate to a shorter length, doubling the correction effect as compared to use of BUP alone.[13]

Injection volume

The BUP molecule is small and rapidly taken into the blood stream after injection into the highly vascular EOM. Therefore, one cannot deposit a bolus and count on diffusion to carry it through the muscle as occurs with Botox®. A sufficient volume must be injected throughout the muscle to expose the fibers to the BUP. The injection should extend to include the important posterior one-third of the muscle that contributes strongly to contraction and power of the EOM.

The lower volume limit is 2.0 mL, sufficient for the smaller vertical rectus muscles and for small horizontal deviations of 10–15 prism diopters (PD); 3.0 mL is our standard volume. Magnetic resonance imaging (MRI) taken a few minutes after injection shows that the horizontal rectus muscles are fully expanded and are starting to leak after injection of 3.0 mL. The upper useful limit appears to be 4.0 mL. At this volume, BUP breaks out of the EOM and surrounds it, penetrating into the muscle and having a positive effect. Some muscles that were shown by MRI to have been inaccurately injected still achieved a good effect from this outside-in penetration of BUP.

Concentration

Our data show that the effect of BUP on correcting strabismus is dose-related. The usual anesthetic preparations of 0.50% and 0.75% BUP are adequate for strabismus of 10–15 PD. We use 1.50% to 2.50% BUP for larger deviations, reserving 3.00% for the largest angles. Compounding pharmacies can provide 3.00% BUP, which then can be diluted with saline to effect lower concentrations.

Toxicity and safety

Orbital tissues

BUP has been injected into innumerable orbits for cataract anesthesia. Except for rare physical damage from the needle and occasional myotoxic damage when inadvertently injected into EOM, the drug appears harmless. Bathing the anterior EOM and surrounding tissues with 2–3 mL of 0.75% BUP for postoperative pain relief after strabismus surgery is innocuous and without myotoxic effect. In our patients, injection of BUP into the orbit in concentrations up to 3.00% does not damage any tissue except muscle. Even when complete block of the optic nerve and motor nerves has occurred it has reversed fully.

Increased fibrosis around muscles treated with BUP injection might be a mechanism of action. However, we did not encounter this in the muscles of two patients we operated after injection, nor is it remarked in the many reports of surgery for

myotoxic strabismus after cataract surgery. Nevertheless, the muscle damage caused by BUP does cause inflammation; this must be considered an open issue.

Muscles

BUP damage to muscle causes inflammation with removal of the necrotic fibers and myocytes by macrophages. With small BUP doses, this is usually subclinical inflammation. However, necrosis of most of the EOM from a large dose such as 3.0 mL of 3.00% BUP creates redness, swelling, and discomfort for 2–3 days before the EOM tissue is absorbed. Preventive use of oral prednisone, starting with 50 mg on the day of BUP injection for an average adult and declining by 10 mg steps for three subsequent daily doses, will markedly reduce such inflammation.

Systemic toxicity

BUP in healthy patients is considered safe in intravenouis doses below 1.5 mg/kg body weight. We have used up to 2.0 mg/kg to inject multiple EOMs without adverse reaction. Large vessels exist in the posterior part of the EOM and orbit where the BUP is injected; needle aspiration should be routine before orbital BUP injections.

Injection technique (Video 87.1)

We use topical proparacaine 0.5%, then a vasoconstrictor such as brimonodine, then proparacaine each minute for 4 minutes. For previously unoperated muscles, insert the electrode needle 12 mm posterior to the limbus. If there was earlier recession surgery, insert the needle further posterior. The posterior extent of the EOM is at least 10–15 mm further back than usual Botox® injection sites. With electromyography (EMG) guidance showing that the needle is in the EOM, the necessary posterior location of the injection can be done with assurance. Aspirate to ensure the needle is not intravascular. Inject 0.25 mL of BUP and wait for the EMG sound to become quiet as the muscle and nerves are anesthetized. Then continue to inject, slowly so as not to blow up the muscle suddenly. Plan to put about two-thirds into the posterior third of the EOM; the remainder is injected into the middle third of the EOM. If resistance to injection develops, retract forward a few millimeters until injection can proceed easily.

Results of BUP injection

In 23 patients with comitant strabismus, the average correction of the deviation was 70% at 6 months after injection. Except for technical errors of injection and some early trials with doses too small, all BUP injections have had an effect; BUP injection into EOM is reliable in changing alignment.

In an earlier report, six patients with comitant esotropia treated with BUP alone were corrected an average 8.2 PD after an average of 343 days.[14] Revisiting these patients at an average postinjection interval of 736 days, we find the average deviation to be 7.4 PD.

In an earlier report, seven patients with comitant strabismus injected with both BUP and Botox® were corrected an average of 19.7 PD at 193 days after injection.[13] Revisiting these patients at an average postinjection interval of 602 days, we find the average deviation to be 19.3 PD.

Wutthiphan and Srisuwanporn injected one horizontal rectus muscle in 20 patients with horizontal strabismus, using

4.50 mL of 0.50% BUP. Thirteen of 15 comitant patients were improved. The average improvement was 8–9 PD, and was the same at 1, 3, 6, and 12 months after injection.[15] They found improvement in 13 of 15 comitant patients, but only two of five incomitant cases. This is similar to our experience (see below); paralyzed, restricted, or damaged muscles do not respond as well to BUP injection as do the muscles in comitant strabismus.

Clinical course after injection

BUP alone gives a day of anesthesia of the injected EOM (and often of other tissues) followed by a week of mild weakness from the myotoxicity, then 2–3 weeks of progressive improvement. The outcome of the injection procedure will be evident at 1 month.

BUP and Botox® given together weaken agonist and antagonist about equally, reducing ductions in both directions. This typically leaves the treated eye with little alignment change until regeneration gives improved muscle function at 3 to 4 weeks after injection (Fig. 87.1).

Increased muscle action

In mild incomitant deviations without muscle paralysis, it is often desirable to increase action of an EOM. BUP makes this possible. The ambylopic 32 mm diameter left eye in Figure 87.2 (upper panel) could be only partially corrected to 20 PD left exotropia by multiple Botox® injections to the left lateral rectus (LLR). BUP injection of the left medial rectus (LMR) both aligned and retracted the left eye with a result that was stable for over 2 years (Fig. 87.2, lower panel).

Josephson and Mathias treated patients with symptomatic convergence insufficiency unresponsive to orthoptic training or prismatic glasses by injection of one or both medial rectus muscles with BUP. They corrected the average deviation of 11 patients from 12.6 PD to 5.3 PD, measured at 1 year after injection. Nine patients were without symptoms, one patient required prism glasses, and one patient required surgical correction.[16]

Special cases

Muscle atrophy

BUP did not work in five patients with atrophic lateral rectus muscles after sixth nerve paralysis. Some of these EOMs were injected several times, attempting to "grow" a bigger and stronger muscle. All patients remained without substantial change. We suggest that the absence of satellite cells around these atrophic muscles is the reason for this lack of response. Direct injection of stimulating molecules such as MGF may yet be useful in these muscles, as may be transplantation of muscle cells with BUP or transplantation of stem cells. The great need

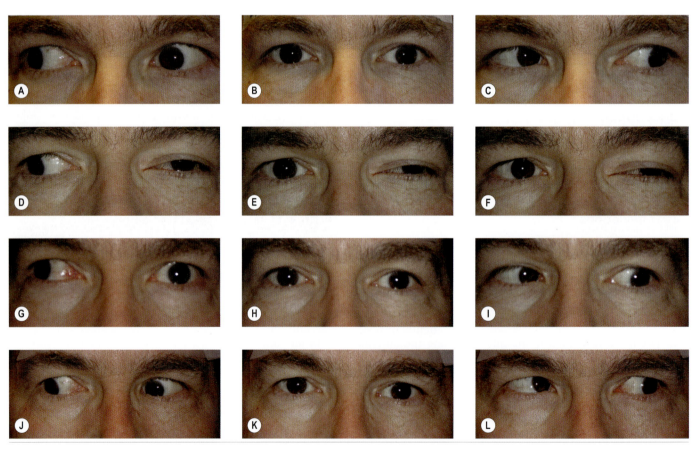

Fig. 87.1 Sequence of events after injection of BUP to LMR and Botox® to LLR. (Top row) Pre-injection, 16 PD exotropia following two operations for esotropia and three Botox® injections of the LLR for exotropia. (Second row) 30 minutes after injections with paralysis of the LMR. (Third row) 13 days after injections, 16 PD exotropia, with weakness of both the LMR and LLR. (Bottom row) 355 days after injection, 6 PD exotropic. (Modified from Scott AB, et al. Treating strabismus by injecting the agonist muscle with bupivacaine and the antagonist with botulinum toxin. Trans Am Ophthalmol Soc 2009; 107: 104–109. Republished with permission of the American Ophthalmological Society.)

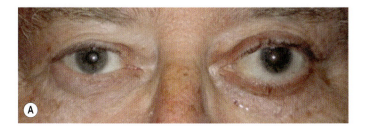

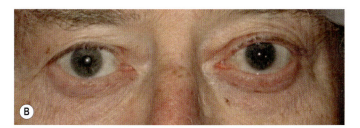

Fig. 87.2 (A) 20 PD exotropia of amblyopia 32.0 mm long myopic left eye after three injections of left lateral rectus with Botox®. (B) Left eye straight and also retracted 2.0 mm at 722 days after BUP injection of LMR and Botox® injection of LLR.

for a technique to strengthen weak EOM will attract several solutions beyond BUP.

Denervation without atrophy

BUP worked well in one partially paralyzed lateral rectus muscle without atrophy and in the muscles in one case of cranial third nerve paresis with anomalous regeneration. It appears that the extent of muscle atrophy, not the extent of innervation, determines BUP effectiveness.

Injection of BUP and Botox® into the same muscle

In three patients we injected both BUP and Botox® into the same muscle, testing the idea that the treated muscle would be stretched by the antagonist during regeneration and thereby result in a longer muscle. This did not elongate the muscle; two of the three cases experienced slight worsening of the strabismus as the muscle shortened.

Larger deviations

The limit of effect of BUP and Botox® injected together seems to be about 30 PD. However, repeated injections are additive. Figures 87.3 and 87.4 show the change in alignment and in EOM sizes in one such case.

High myopia with acquired esotropia from muscle displacement

One case has a correction of 30 PD of esotropia from combined BUP and Botox® and remains stable at 1 year. A second case has reduction of 40 ET to 18 ET. We suggest that the enlarged and stiffened lateral rectus muscle remains effective as an abductor and does not slide inferiorly as it did in its stretched pre-injection condition. Both cases required two injection treatments to effect these changes.

Ptosis correction

Four of six adults with acquired ptosis and apraxia of eyelid opening associated with blepharospasm have shown 1–3 mm of upper eyelid elevation after treatment of the levator

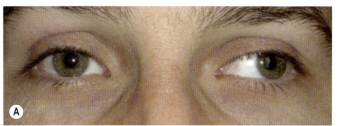

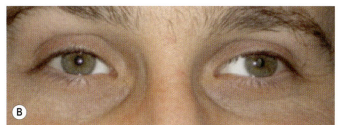

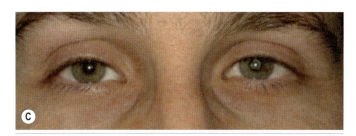

Fig. 87.3 (A) Congenital cataract with amblyopia, 50 PD exotropia. (B) 55 days after injection of left medial rectus with BUP, and left lateral rectus with Botox®. (C) Left eye re-injected at 55 days after first injection; this image 2.5 years after second injection.

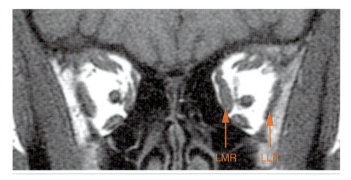

Fig. 87.4 MRI of patient from Figure 87.3 at 224 days after second injection of left medial rectus (LMR) with BUP and left lateral rectus (LLR) with Botox®. Notice that the LMR is larger, and LLR is smaller than the corresponding muscles in the right eye.

palpebrae with 3.0 mL of 3.0% BUP. These are presumed to be normal muscles that have been stretched. The utility of BUP injection in patients with ptosis due to abnormally developed levator muscles remains to be defined.

Children with strabismus

We have no data on the effect of BUP in children. Patients aged 18 to 89 have shown little variation in response to BUP, and our experience in the laboratory with animals of various ages shows no discernible effect of age on the action of BUP. We suppose that BUP action in children will be about the same as that in adults (Table 87.1).

Table 87.1 – Usage of BUP in adults

Condition	Treatment
Comitant strabismus of 6–12 PD	2.0–3.0 mL of 1.5% BUP
Comitant strabismus of 12–30 PD	3.0 mL of 1.5% to 2.5% BUP and 1.0 to 2.0 units Botox®
Comitant strabismus of >30 PD	3.0 mL of 3.0% to 2.5% BUP and 2.0 to 5.0 units Botox®
Non-paralytic ptosis	3.0 mL of 3.0% BUP injected through the upper lid

Summary

BUP injection of EOM, initially an accidental event causing unwanted strabismus following retrobulbar anesthesia, has emerged as a controllable and useful treatment modality. BUP alone, or together with Botox® is safe and effective in the treatment of moderate deviations of up to 30 PD in adults. Its place in the treatment of other forms of strabismus remains to be defined.

Acknowledgments

This work was supported by NIH Grant NEI RO1 EY018633 to Alan B Scott and Joel M Miller at the Smith-Kettlewell Institute of Visual Sciences, San Francisco, and by Pacific Vision Foundation, San Francisco. Patent 11/867,532 covers the use of local anesthetics to treat muscle disorders. Federal law does not allow this patent to restrict BUP use for medical treatment by physicians.

References

1. Hall-Craggs EC. Early ultrastructural changes in skeletal muscle exposed to local anesthetic bupivacaine (marcaine). Br J Exp Pathol 1980; 60: 139–49.

2. Bradley WG. Muscle fiber splitting. In: Mauro A, editor. Muscle Regeneration. New York: Raven Press; 1979: 215–32.

3. Nonaka I, Takagi A, Ishiura S, et al. Pathophysiology of muscle fiber necrosis induced by bupivacaine hydrochloride (Marcaine) Acta Neuropathol 1983; 60: 167–74.

4. Hall-Craggs EC. Survival of satellite cells following exposure to the local anesthetic bupivacaine (Marcaine). Cell Tissue Res 1980; 209: 131–5.

5. Rosenblatt JD, Woods RI. Hypertrophy of rat extensor digitorum longus muscle injected with bupivacaine: a sequential histochemical, immunohistochemical, histological and morphometric study. J Anat 1992; 181: 11–27.

6. Benoit PW, Belt DW. Destruction and regeneration of skeletal muscle after treatment with a local anaesthetic, bupivacaine (Marcaine(r)). J. Anat 1970; 107: 547–56.

7. Park CM, Park SE, Oh SY. Acute effects of bupivacine and ricin mAb 35 on extraocular muscle in the rabbit. Curr Eye Res 2004; 29: 293–301.

8. Komorowski TE, Shepard B, Okland S, et al. An electron microscopic study of local anesthetic-induced skeletal muscle fiber degeneration and regeneration in the monkey. J Orthop Res 1990; 8: 495–503.

9. Plant DR, Beitzel F, Lynch GS. Length-tension relationships are altered in regenerating muscles of the rat after bupivacaine injection. J Appl Physiol 2005; 98: 1998–2003.

10. Hill M, Wernig A, Goldspink G. Muscle satellite cell activation dur ing local tissue injury and repair. J Anat 2003; 203: 89–99.

11. Anderson BC, Christiansen SP, Grandt S, et al. Increased extraocular muscle strength with direct injection of insulin-like growth factor-I. Invest Ophthalmol Vis Sci 2006; 47: 2461–7.

12. Rosenblatt JD. A time course study of the isometric contractile properties of rat extensor digitorum longus muscle injected with bupivacaine. Comp Biochem Physiol Comp Physiol 1992; 101: 361–7.

13. Scott AB, Miller JM, Shieh BS. Treating strabismus by injecting the agonist muscle with bupivacaine and the antagonist with botulinum toxin. Trans Am Ophthamol Soc 2009; 107: 104–9.

14. Scott AB, Miller JM, Shieh KR. Bupivacaine injection of the lateral rectus muscle to treat esotropia. J AAPOS 2009; 13: 119–22.

15. Wutthiphan S, Srisuwanporn S. Bupivacaine injection to treat exotropia and esotropia. Strabismus 2010; 18: 137–41.

16. Josephson ME, Mathias SA. Bupivacaine treatment of intermittent exotropia of the convergence insufficiency type. J AAPOS 2011; 15: e4.

SECTION 6
Amblyopia, strabismus and
eye movements

Part 7
Nystagmus and eye movements

CHAPTER 88

Latent nystagmus and dissociated vertical–horizontal deviation

Lawrence Tychsen

Overview

Latent nystagmus (LN) is the byproduct of fusion maldevelopment in infancy originating as an afferent visual pathway disorder. Because fusion maldevelopment – in the form of strabismus and amblyopia – is common, LN is a prevalent form of pathologic nystagmus. We have studied patients and non-human primates (NHP) with maldeveloped fusion. We have demonstrated that loss of binocular connections within area V1 (striate cortex) in the first months of life is the necessary and sufficient cause of LN. The severity of LN increases with longer durations of binocular decorrelation and greater losses of V1 connections. Decorrelation durations that exceed the equivalent of 2–3 months in human development result in a 100% LN prevalence. The binocular maldevelopment originating in area V1 is passed on to downstream, extrastriate regions of cerebral cortex that drive conjugate gaze (notably medial superior temporal-dorsal, MSTd, neurons). Conjugate gaze is stable when MSTd neurons of the right vs.

left cerebral hemisphere have balanced, binocular activity. Fusion maldevelopment in infancy causes unbalanced, monocular activity. If input from one eye dominates and the other is suppressed, MSTd in one hemisphere becomes more active. Acting through downstream projections to the ipsilateral nucleus of the optic tract (NOT), the eyes are driven conjugately to that side. The unbalanced MSTd drive is evident as the nasalward gaze-holding bias of LN.

LN is the cause of dissociated vertical deviation (DVD) and dissociated horizontal deviation (DHD). Vertical vergence damping of LN evokes DVD. Relaxation of convergence damping of LN releases a latent exodeviation, or DHD. Abnormal head postures (turns and tilts) are also used to damp LN.

Latent nystagmus distinguishing characteristics and associations

Latent nystagmus (LN) is a common subtype of pathologic nystagmus observed in humans and NHPs.[1] It is linked strongly to binocular maldevelopment in infancy, either from strabismus or amblyopia.

LN is characterized by a conjugate, horizontal slow-phase drift of eye position that is directed nasalward with respect to the viewing eye.[2,3] When viewing switches from eye to eye, the direction of the slow-phases reverse instantaneously: leftward when the right eye is fixating and rightward when the left eye is fixating (Fig. 88.1). The severity of the nystagmus (and its visibility during clinical examination) increases when one eye is covered, hence the term "latent." When the nystagmus is evident with both eyes open, it is called manifest LN (MLN).

LN is distinguished from congenital ("idiopathic infantile") nystagmus (CN, or the infantile nystagmus syndrome – INS) by the feature of instantaneous reversal-of-direction with alternating fixation. By eye movement recording, it is distinguished also in waveform which is always that of decreasing velocity and linear trajectory, whereas that of CN/INS is of increasing velocity and pendular trajectory.[2] Eye movement recordings, or high magnification clinical inspection with a slit-lamp or ophthalmoscope, frequently reveals a superimposed small torsional movement.

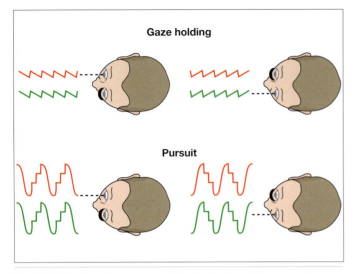

Fig. 88.1 Nasalward gaze asymmetries in strabismic human and monkey. Gaze-holding latent nystagmus: viewing with the right eye, both eyes have a nasalward slow-phase drift, followed by temporalward refoveating fast-phase microsaccades. The direction of the nystagmus reverses instantaneously when the left eye is fixating, so that the slow-phase is nasalward with respect to the fixating eye. Tracking pursuit/ OKN (optokinetic nystagmus): horizontal smooth pursuit is asymmetric during monocular viewing. Pursuit is smooth (normal) when target motion is nasalward in the visual field. Pursuit is cogwheel (low gain–abnormal) when the target moves temporalward. The movements of the two eyes are conjugate, and the direction of the asymmetry reverses instantaneously with a change of fixating eye, so that the direction of robust pursuit is always for nasalward motion in the visual field.

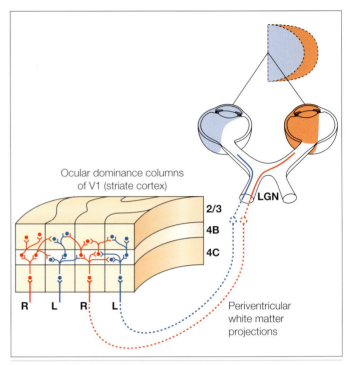

Fig. 88.2 Neuroanatomic basis for binocular vision. Monocular retinogeniculate projections from left eye (temporal retina-nasal visual hemifield) and right eye (nasal retina-temporal hemifield) remain segregated up to and within the input layer of ocular dominance columns (ODCs) in V1, layer 4C (striate visual cortex). Binocular vision is made possible by horizontal connections between ODCs of opposite ocularity in upper layers 4B and 2/3 (as well as lower layers 5/6, not shown). RE inputs = red; LE inputs = blue.

Our understanding of the clinical features of LN have been clarified by Dell'Osso et al.,[2,4] who have described the historical origins of LN's various terms. In 1872, Faucon[5] first described manifest LN (MLN). In 1912, Fromaget and Fromaget[6] introduced the term "nystagmus latent." These early reports of LN were reviewed by Sorsby[7] in 1931. The oxymoron "manifested latent" nystagmus was introduced by Kestenbaum[8] in 1947, who emphasized that LN is often observed in patients with strabismus when they view with both eyes open.

Although infantile esotropia is the leading association with LN, any disorder that perturbs development of binocular fusion in infancy, such as monocular or severe binocular deprivation, will produce LN and MLN.[9,10] The NIH Committee on Eye Movement and Strabismus (CEMAS) classification[11] recommended that the terms LN/MLN be replaced by the etiologic descriptor fusion–maldevelopment nystagmus.

Development of fusion eliminates nasalward visual cortex biases

The postnatal development of binocular sensory and motor functions in normal infant monkeys parallels that of normal infant humans, but on a compressed time scale; 1 week of monkey development approximates 1 month of human.[12-15] Binocular disparity sensitivity and binocular fusion are absent in human and monkey neonates. Stereopsis emerges abruptly in humans during the first 3–5 months of postnatal life,[16-20] and in monkeys during the first 3–5 weeks,[14] achieving adult-like levels of sensitivity.

V1 horizontal axonal connections are key components of fusion development and maldevelopment (Fig. 88.2). Binocularity in primates begins with horizontal connections between V1 ocular dominance columns (ODCs) of opposite ocularity.[21-23] These connections are immature in the first weeks of life, conveying crude, weak binocular responses.[24-26] Maturation of binocular connections requires correlated (synchronous) activity between right eye and left eye geniculostriate inputs.[27,28] Decorrelation of inputs (Fig. 88.3), produced by binocular non-correspondence, causes loss of horizontal connections over a period of days in V1 of kittens.[27,29] Similar losses occur over a period of weeks in V1 of monkeys, and over a period of months in V1 of children. Binocular decorrelation also promotes interocular suppression (Fig. 88.4) as a further hindrance to fusion.[1]

In the first months of life in humans and weeks of life in monkeys, monocular motion VEPs (visually evoked potentials) reveal a nasotemporal asymmetry.[30-33] Monocular preferential-looking testing reveals greater perceptual sensitivity to nasalward motion.[34] Monocular pursuit and optokinetic tracking both reveal biases favoring nasalward target motion.[12,35-38] These nasalward motion biases are pronounced before onset of sensorial fusion and stereopsis, but systematically diminish thereafter. They are retained in subtle form in normal adult humans, and can be unmasked using contrived, monocular stimuli.[39,40] If normal maturation of binocularity is

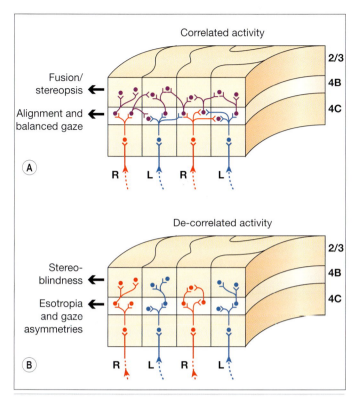

Fig. 88.3 Horizontal connections for binocular vision in V1 of normal (correlated activity) vs. strabismic (decorrelated) primate, layer 2–4B. V1 of normal primates is characterized by equal numbers of monocular and binocular connections. In strabismic primates, the connections are predominantly monocular (i.e. a paucity of binocular connections). RE inputs = red; LE = blue; binocular = violet.

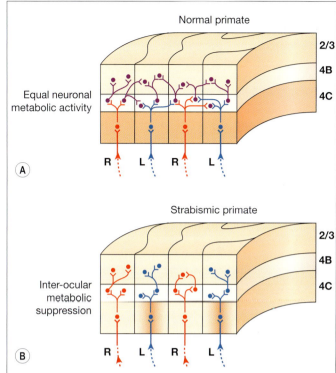

Fig. 88.4 Metabolic activity in neighboring ocular dominance columns (ODCs) within V1 of normal vs. strabismic primate. In normal primates, layer 4C stains uniformly for the metabolic enzyme cytochrome oxidase (shown as brown), indicating equal activity in right eye vs. left eye columns. In strabismic primates, a narrow monocular zone within the dominant ODCs (shown here as left eye) shows normal metabolic activity (brown), but ODCs belonging to the suppressed eye (shown as right eye) and binocular border zones between ODCs are pale, connoting abnormally low – i.e. suppressed – activity.

impeded by eye misalignment or monocular deprivation, the nasalward biases persist and become pronounced.[34,41-47] The nasalward gaze bias is the key feature of the fusion maldevelopment syndrome. Other common findings are loss of stereopsis, interocular suppression, strabismus, and smaller amplitude torsional/vertical oscillations of the eyes.

Binocular decorrelation from various causes begins the LN cascade

Clinical studies of children[43] and adults[2,4,44,48] with LN have inspired a series of behavioral, physiologic, and neuroanatomic studies in NHPs who had LN associated with naturally occurring[22,23,49-55] or experimentally induced[1,10,56-65] infantile strabismus. The common finding is that the prevalence and severity of LN correlates with the age of onset and duration of binocular decorrelation in infancy.

The most common clinical cause of binocular decorrelation is strabismus, which in human infants is overwhelmingly esotropic (convergent).[66] Early-onset esotropia exceeds exotropia by a ratio of 9:1. Esotropia is also the most common form of naturally occurring strabismus in NHPs.[67,68] However, any prolonged deprivation of normal binocular experience in early infancy (monocular congenital cataract, uniocular high hyperopia, myopia or astigmatism, uniocular neonatal vitreous

hemorrhage, uniocular corneal clouding, dense bilateral cataracts, NHP models) can cause binocular decorrelation, including monocular deprivation (uniocular amblyopia) or severe binocular deprivation (bilateral amblyopia),[10,57,63] eyelid suturing (the thin, translucent eyelid of NHPs mimics a congenital cataract, allowing diffuse luminance to the retina but blocking spatial vision). Loss of spatial vision is not required; the majority of human and NHP infants with strabismus alternate fixation initially and have no amblyopia.[69] The necessary and sufficient factor is binocular decorrelation, not lack of sharp visual acuity.

Decorrelation durations that exceed the equivalent of 3 months in human infant development result in an LN prevalence of 100%.[1,65,70] Perturbing these inputs from week 1 of life causes LN, but delaying the perturbation to the time of onset of normal fusion and stereopsis (the equivalent of age 2–4 months in humans) is equally effective.[71] The severity of the resultant LN corresponds to the severity of loss of binocular connections between ODCs of opposite ocularity in visual area V1, and the severity of interocular suppression.[1,72] Area V1 feeds forward to extrastriate areas (areas MT/MST) important for gaze-holding and gaze-tracking, such as smooth pursuit, OKN, and the short-latency ocular following response.[73-76]

Maldevelopment in V1 is passed on to areas MT/MST

Visual areas V1, V2 (prestriate cortex), MT (medial temporal), and MST (medial superior temporal) of the cerebral cortex are major components of the conjugate gaze pathway.[77] Each of these areas in normal primates contains directionally selective, binocular neurons.[78-81] MST in each cerebral hemisphere encodes ipsiversive gaze.[74,82-84] MST projects downstream to the brainstem visuomotor nuclei that generate eye movements: the NOT, medial vestibular nucleus, and interconnected abducens and ocular motor nuclei.[77,85] In primates, subcortical inputs to NOT may play a minor role.[9,10,86] The dominant pathway is cerebral – from MST to brainstem. The dominant role of the cortical pathway, and the minimal role of a subcortical pathway, is reinforced by studies of children. Neuroimaging of visual cortex, combined with eye movement recordings, have shown absence of visually driven pursuit or OKN in cerebrally blind infants.[87,88]

One mechanism for the gaze-holding asymmetry would be over-representation of nasalward neurons within visual areas V1 through MT in the immature/strabismic cortex. However, directional and binocular responses of neurons in V1, V2, and MT have been investigated in infant monkeys, as well as in monkeys with early-onset strabismus, and no over-representation of neurons selective for nasalward motion has been found.[26,61,89,90] In strabismic animals, binocular (excitatory) responses are reduced and interocular suppression is increased.[89-91] These physiologic abnormalities have neuroanatomic correlates. In V1 of strabismic monkeys, binocular connections are deficient[22,23] and interocular metabolic activity is suppressed.[53,92,93]

Binocular decorrelation unmasks an innate nasalward monocular bias

LN is always linked to abnormal binocular development in infancy. This important clinical observation motivated the studies of NHPs reviewed above, which have in turn provided the functional-structural correlations needed to explain the pathophysiology of LN. The NHP studies have motivated pediatric ophthalmologists to repair fusion earlier in infancy,[94] thereby preventing LN or reducing its severity.

Latent nystagmus is caused by an afferent binocular visual pathway defect. The binocular defect unmasks a directional bias encoded in the cerebral gaze pathways. Normal binocular development (fusion) – in the first months of life – eliminates the directional bias; abnormal development (maldeveloped fusion) exaggerates the bias. If fusion goes unrepaired in infancy, the directional bias persists throughout adult life.[1,95]

The visual cortex in each cerebral hemisphere is wired innately for nasalward motion. The innate wiring is monocular. To generate temporalward gaze-holding, signals must traverse binocular connections, unimpeded by interocular suppression. If normal binocularity fails to develop, the system remains predominantly monocular and asymmetric, incapable of driving temporalward gaze-holding or robust, temporalward pursuit/OKN.[10,43,44,61,66,90] LN is an abnormal monocular bias added on to a normal, ipsiversive hemispheric gaze bias.

Hypothetical signal flow for LN

Figure 88.5 illustrates the mechanism for LN, showing the circuit mediating gaze-holding in primates and the role of binocular connections. Shaded structures indicate less active visual and motor neurons caused by occlusion of one eye and/or interocular suppression. The circuit on the left depicts the pathways and visuomotor component structures in a primate with LN.

The flow is from top to bottom, starting from the monocular visual field of the fixating (or viewing) right eye. The nasal and temporal visual fields (VF) in primates are unequal in area, with a bias favoring the larger, temporal hemifield. Retinal ganglion cell fibers (RGC) from the nasal and temporal hemiretinas decussate at the optic chiasm (chi), synapse at the lateral geniculate nucleus (LGN), and project to alternating, monocular right eye (RE) and left eye (LE) ODCs in V1. During development, RGCs from the nasal retina outnumber and establish connections earlier than those from the temporal retina (not shown). The LGN lamina corresponding to the nasal retina – lamina 1, 3 and 5 (also not shown) – contain more neurons and develop earlier than those from the temporal hemi-retina, 2, 4, and 6. Within the LGN, the neurons remain monocular, with no binocular interlaminar interaction.

The monocular bias, favoring nasal hemi-retina inputs, is passed on to the ODCs of area V1. In each V1, ODCs representing the nasal hemi-retina (temporal visual hemifield) occupy slightly more cortical territory (in the diagram are larger) than those representing the temporal hemi-retinas (nasal hemifield), but each ODC contains neurons sensitive to nasalward (in this case rightward) versus temporalward (leftward) visual motion. Receptive field neurons in V1 and MT are simplified here as half circles to match their corresponding hemi-fields. The arrows indicate the directional preference of the neurons. Visual area neurons (including those beyond V1 in area MT) are sensitive to both nasalward and temporalward motion,[26,61,89] but only those encoding nasalward motion are wired innately, through monocular connections, to gaze (eye motion) neurons in area MST (congregated in the dorsal-medial portion, or MSTd). MSTd in each cerebral hemisphere encodes ipsiversive gaze,[74,82-84] which is nasalward gaze in relation to the contralateral eye (leftward for MST in the left cerebral hemisphere and rightward for MST in the right hemisphere).[90]

The only difference between the LN primate's visual cortex and the normal primate's visual cortex is a paucity of binocular horizontal connections[23,72] (compounded by interocular suppression).[53,92,93] The paucity is depicted as a lack of diagonal right eye ODC to left eye ODC connections, absent in the LN cortex (left side of figure) and present in the normal cortex (right side of figure). In the cortex of normal primates, access to MSTd for temporalward gaze requires binocular connections to homoversive neurons within neighboring ODCs that have opposite ocularity (LE ODC neurons when viewing with the RE). The pathway from V1/MT to MSTd requires efferent projections through the splenium of the corpus callosum (labeled as "call").[96,97]

MSTd efferents project to the ipsilateral brain stem NOT,[85,98] and to ipsiversive-related brainstem structures (medial vestibular nucleus, dorsolateral pontine nucleus, and ocular motor nuclei of the third and sixth cranial nerves).

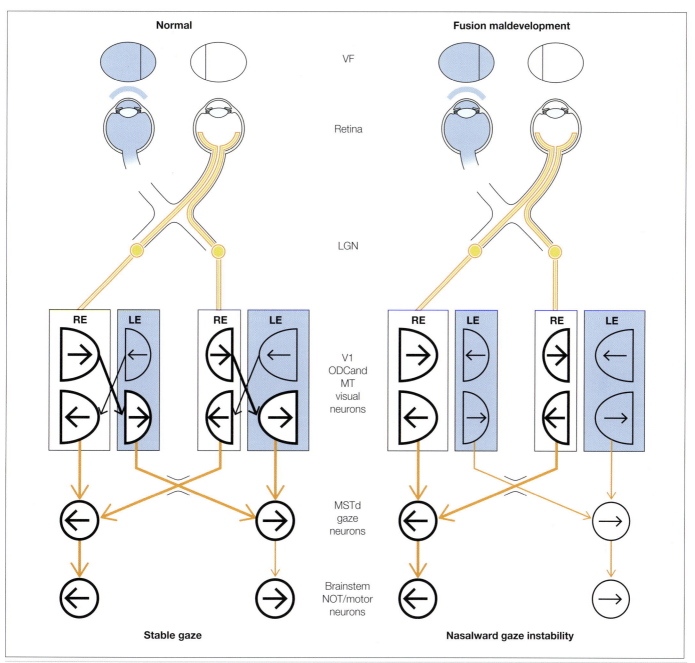

Fig. 88.5 Neural network diagrams showing visual signal flow for pursuit and gaze-holding in strabismic vs. normal primates. Paucity of mature binocular connections explains behavioral asymmetries evident as asymmetric pursuit/OKN and latent fixation nystagmus. In all primates, pursuit area neurons in each hemisphere encode ipsilaterally directed pursuit. Signal flow is initiated by a moving stimulus in the monocular visual field, which evokes a response in visual area neurons (i.e. V1/MT). Each eye at birth has access – through innate, monocular connections – to the pursuit area neurons (e.g. MSTd) of the contralateral hemisphere. Access to pursuit neurons of the ipsilateral hemisphere requires mature, binocular connections. Strabismic/nasalward gaze instability: Moving from top to bottom, starting with target motion in monocular visual field of right eye. Retinal ganglion cell fibers from the nasal and temporal hemiretinae (eye) decussate at the optic chiasm (chi), synapse at the lateral geniculate nucleus (LGN), and project to alternating rows of ODCs in V1 (visual area rectangles). In each V1, ODCs representing the nasal hemiretinae (temporal visual hemifield) occupy slightly more cortical territory than those representing the temporal hemiretinae (nasal hemifield), but each ODC contains neurons sensitive to nasally directed vs. temporally directed motion (half circles shaped like the matching hemifield, arrows indicate directional preference). Visual area neurons (including those beyond V1 in area MT) are sensitive to both nasally directed and temporally directed motion, but only those encoding nasally directed motion are wired innately – through monocular connections – to the pursuit area. Normal/stable gaze: binocular connections are present, linking neurons with similar orientation/directional preferences within ODCs of opposite ocularity (diagonal lines between columns). Viewing with the right eye, visual neurons preferring nasally directed motion project to the left hemisphere pursuit area; visual neurons preferring temporally directed motion project to the right hemisphere pursuit area. Temporally directed visual area neurons gain access to pursuit area neurons only through binocular connections. Call = corpus callosum, through which visual area neurons in each hemisphere project to opposite pursuit area. Bold lines = active neurons and neuronal projections.

Mechanism of dissociated vertical deviation: damping vertical and cyclotorsional components of LN/MLN

DVD is upward deviation of an eye without a corresponding hypotropia of the fellow eye. DVD occurs spontaneously or may be evoked by reducing the vision in that eye (e.g. by cover test, a dark filter, an obscuring lens, or foil). The upwardly deviating eye also excyclotorts.

LN/MLN has cyclotorsional and vertical components. DVD occurs when vertical vergence is activated to damp the cyclotorsional and vertical components of LN/MLN. To understand DVD is to understand normal vertical vergence.

Vergence eye movements are disconjugate. In the case of horizontal vergence, one eye moves leftward and the other rightward. In the case of vertical vergence, one eye moves up and the other down. With normal vertical vergence, the eyes also execute a conjugate cyclotorsional movement.[99] One eye intorts while the other extorts. The combined disconjugate vertical and conjugate torsional eye movements that typify vertical vergence in normal humans and monkeys are shown in Figure 88.6. In the trial shown, a base-down prism is introduced in front of the right eye to cause vertical binocular disparity and evoke vertical fusion. To eliminate the disparity and restore fusion, the right eye moves upward and the left eye downward. The upward-downward vergence is accompanied by counter-clockwise conjugate torsional movements of both eyes. The left eye depresses and intorts, the right eye elevates and extorts. Normal vertical vergence tends to be nystagmoid, with the slow-phases intorsional in the depressing eye and extorsional in the elevating eye.[100]

The fixating (or dominant) eye in LN/MLN displays downward and intorsional slow-phases; the non-dominant eye downward and extorsional slow-phases (Fig. 88.7).[101] The oscillations of LN cause retinal image slip, which degrades visual acuity. To improve acuity, nystagmus is damped by moving the fixating eye further in the direction of its slow-phase ("Alexander's Law"). The patient moves the fixating eye

further in the direction of the slow-phases by activating vertical vergence. Vertical vergence depresses and intorts the fixating eye, stabilizing it. Vertical vergence also elevates and extorts the non-fixating eye, precipitating DVD.[102]

Why does activating vertical vergence cause a DVD in patients with LN/MLN, but not in normal persons? Because normal persons have robust vertical fusion, which acts as a brake to prevent a runaway hyperphoria in the elevating eye. The threshold for manifesting a DVD and the amplitude of DVD will vary depending upon the intensity of LN in each eye, and the amount of vertical vergence invoked to damp the nystagmus and improve acuity. That threshold is multifactorial, encompassing fatigue, attention, anxiety, and the acuity demanded (head position also contributes, see below).

Mechanism of dissociated horizontal deviation: exodeviation when convergence damping of LN/MLN relaxes

Dissociated horizontal deviation (DHD) is an intermittent exodeviation of the non-fixating eye in a patient with LN/MLN. Patients with DHD also have DVD in one or both eyes. If the magnitude of the exodeviation is greater than that of the DVD, DHD will tend to be the major complaint. DHD, like DVD, may occur in patients with LN/MLN due to primary infantile microtropias, but the typical patient has a secondary microtropia (usually eso but sometimes exo) after surgical correction of larger angle infantile strabismus. Superimposed on the baseline microtropia is an intermittent exodeviation controlled by convergence damping of horizontal LN/MLN. When convergence damping relaxes, the DHD is manifest (Fig. 88.8). That is why DHD is expressed when fixating with the dominant eye – the eye with less intense LN/MLN and better acuity – but controlled when fixation switches to the eye with more intense LN/MLN and poorer acuity. The eye with less intense nystagmus requires less convergence damping to

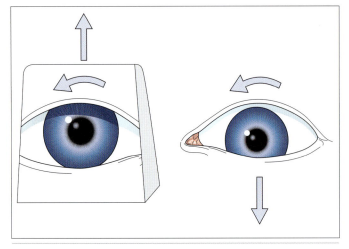

Fig. 88.6 Normal vertical vergence by base-down (e.g. 2Δ) prism. Right eye elevates and left eye depresses to eliminate binocular disparity (diplopia) and restore fusion. The depressing eye incyclotorts and the elevating eye excyclotorts.

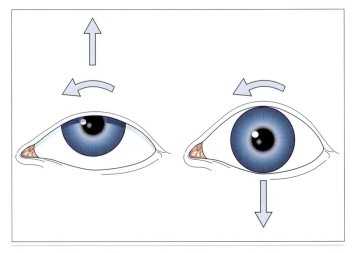

Fig. 88.7 DVD resembles normal vertical vergence, but is exaggerated. Vertical vergence is activated to damp the vertical and cyclotorsional slow-phase of LN/MLN in the fixating (dominant or preferred) eye.

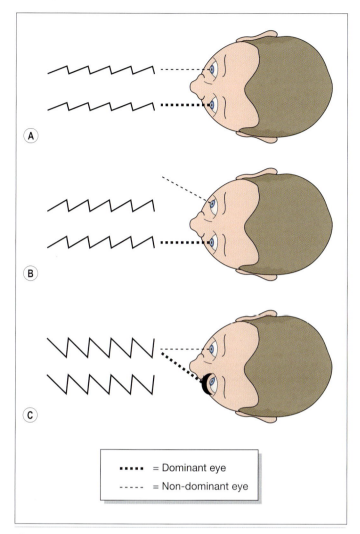

Fig. 88.8 **Right DHD triggered by relaxation of convergence damping.**
(A) Fixation with preferred left eye; mild convergence damps MLN. (B) Fixation left eye, convergence relaxed, right eye DHD (exodeviation). (C) Forced fixation with non-preferred right eye (left eye covered), LN more intense right eye promoting intense convergence to damp, triggering left esodeviation.

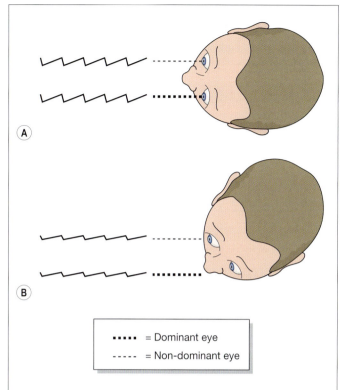

Fig. 88.9 **Damping of MLN achieved by head turn – evoked-gaze position.** Dominant left eye is moved nasalward toward slow-phase MLN.

see clearly, releasing the intermittent exodeviation. When fixating with the eye with more intense nystagmus, more convergence damping is required. More convergence damping not only controls the exodeviation, but also begets a larger esodeviation on cover testing.[103] DHD is variable because its expression, like that of DVD, is dependent on the acuity task at that moment. The amount of relaxation of convergence damping defines the threshold for expression of the DHD in an individual patient.

How head postures affect LM/MLN and DVD

Vergence damping will vary with the visual resolution required, the viewing distance, the choice of fixating eye, the interocular acuity difference (e.g. refractive error or amblyopia), and the difference in nystagmus intensity in the two eyes. To reduce the need for vergence damping the patient may use a head posture and eccentric gaze (versional) damping (Fig. 88.9). The head turn moves the fixating eye to a more nasalward position in the orbit – the direction of the slow-phases of the nystagmus ("Alexander's Law," e.g. a leftward face turn when fixating with the left eye, and vice versa).[104] If the acuity task is easy, little head turn and gaze eccentricity may be needed. If the acuity task is taxing and the patient fatigued, a larger head turn will be employed. A patient with LN/MLN may use a head-turn-driven gaze position for different reasons. The gaze position can be employed to reduce convergence and control a residual esodeviation, preserving a degree of binocular fusion. Or alternatively, a head-turn-driven gaze position and convergence damping can be used in additive fashion, to further stabilize the fixating eye and boost acuity.

Head tilts may be used as well. Head tilting evokes cyclotorsional counter-rolling, driven by the normal vestibular ocular reflex. A patient with LN/MLN who prefers to fixate with the left eye, can reduce the demand for vertical vergence damping by tilting the head to the left. The left head tilt evokes counter-rolling intorsion of the left eye, adding to vertical vergence evoked left eye intorsion. These "spontaneous" or adaptive head tilts in patients with LN/MLN and DVD are, however, multifactorial and highly idiosyncratic. The head tilt will depend upon the robustness of vertical fusion, the need to control a baseline micro-hypertropia, the intensity of the vertical cyclotorsional components of LN/MLN, and the acuity task.

References

1. Tychsen L. Causing and curing infantile eostropia in primates: the role of decorrelated binocular input. Trans Am Ophthalmol Soc 2007; 105: 564–93.

2. Dell'Osso LF, Schmidt D, Daroff RB. Latent, manifest latent, and congenital nystagmus. Arch Ophthalmol 1979; 97: 1877–85.

13. Boothe RG, Dobson V, Teller DY. Postnatal development of vision in human and nonhuman primates. Annu Rev Neurosci 1985; 8: 495–546.

15. Brown RJ, Wilson JR, Norcia AM, et al. Development of directional motion symmetry in the monocular visually evoked potential of infant monkeys. Vision Res 1998; 38: 1253–63.

17. Birch EE, Gwiazda J, Held R. Stereoacuity development for crossed and uncrossed disparities in human infants. Vision Res 1982; 22: 507–13.

18. Birch EE, Gwiazda J, Held R. The development of vergence does not account for the onset of stereopsis. Perception 1983; 12: 331–6.

21. Hubel DH, Wiesel TN. Ferrier Lecture: Functional architecture of macaque monkey visual cortex. Proc R Soc Lond [Biol] 1977; 198: 1–59.

26. Hatta S, Kumagami T, Qian J, et al. Nasotemporal directional bias of V1 neurons in young infant monkeys. Invest Ophthalmol Vis Sci 1998; 39: 2259–67.

30. Norcia AM, Garcia H, Humphry R, et al. Anomalous motion VEPs in infants and in infantile esotropia. Invest Ophthalmol Vis Sci 1991; 32: 436–9.

31. Norcia AM. Abnormal motion processing and binocularity: infantile esotropia as a model system for effects of early interruptions of binocularity. Eye 1996; 10: 259–65.

35. Naegele JR, Held R. The postnatal development of monocular optokinetic nystagmus in infants. Vision Res 1982; 22: 341–6.

37. Jacobs M, Harris C, Taylor D. The development of eye movements in infancy. In: Lennerstrand G, editor. Update on Strabismus and Pediatric Ophthalmology Proceedings of the Joint ISA and AAPO&S Meeting, Vancouver, Canada, June 19–23, 1994. Boca Raton: CRC Press; 1994: 140–3.

44. Tychsen L, Lisberger SG. Maldevelopment of visual motion processing in humans who had strabismus with onset in infancy. J Neurosci 1986; 6: 2495–508.

54. Tychsen L, Yildirim C, Anteby I, et al. Macaque monkey as an ocular motor and neuroanatomic model of human infantile strabismus. In: Lennerstrand G, Ygge J, editors. Advances in Strabismus Research: Basic and Clinical Aspects. London, UK: Wenner-Gren International Series, Portland Press Ltd.; 2000: 103–19.

50. Tychsen L, Leibole M, Drake D. Comparison of latent nystagmus and nasotemporal asymmetries of optokinetic nystagmus in adult humans and macaque monkeys who have infantile strabismus. Strabismus 1996; 4: 171–7.

62. Tychsen L, Yildirim C, Foeller P. Effect of infantile strabismus on visuomotor development in squirrel monkey (Saimiri sciureus): optokinetic nystagmus, motion VEP and spatial sweep VEP. Invest Ophthalmol Vis Sci 1999; 40: S405.

65. Richards M, Wong A, Foeller P, et al. Duration of binocular decorrelation predicts the severity of latent (fusion maldevelopment) nystagmus in strabismic macaque monkeys. Invest Ophthalmol Vis Sci 2008; 49: 1872–8.

67. Kiorpes L, Boothe RG. Naturally occurring strabismus in monkeys (Macaca nemestrina). Invest Ophthalmol Vis Sci 1981; 20: 257–63.

72. Tychsen L, Richards M, Wong A, et al. Spectrum of infantile esotropia in primates: behavior, brains and orbits. J AAPOS 2008; 12: 375–80.

79. Albright TD, Desimone R, Gross CG. Columnar organization of directionally selective cells in visual area MT of the macaque. J Neurophysiol 1984; 51: 16–31.

80. Orban GA, Kennedy H, Buillier J. Velocity sensitivity and direction selectivity of neurons in area V1 and V2 of the monkey: influence of eccentricity. J Neurophysiol 1986; 56: 462–80.

85. Mustari MJ, Fuchs AF, Kaneko CRS, et al. Anatomical connections of the primate pretectal nucleus of the optic tract. J Comp Neurol 1994; 349: 111–28.

88. Werth R. Residual visual functions after loss of both cerebral hemispheres in infancy. Invest Ophthalmol Vis Sci 2007; 48: 3098–106.

90. Mustari MJ, Ono S, Vitorello KC. How disturbed visual processing early in life leads to disorders of gaze-holding and smooth pursuit. Prog Brain Res 2008; 171: 487–95.

92. Horton JC, Hocking DR, Adams DL. Metabolic mapping of suppression scotomas in striate cortex of macaques with experimental strabismus. J Neurosci 1999; 19: 7111–29.

94. Tychsen L. Can ophthalmologists repair the brain in infantile esotropia? Early surgery, stereopsis, monofixation syndrome, and the legacy of Marshall Parks. J AAPOS 2005; 9: 510–21.

101. van Rijn LJ, Simonsz HJ, ten Tusscher MPM. Dissociated vertical deviation and eye torsion: relation to disparity-induced vertical vergence. Strabismus 1997; 5: 13–20.

103. Zubcov AA, Reinecke RD, Calhoun JH. Asymmetric horizontal tropias, DVD, and manifest latent nystagmus: An explanation of dissociated horizontal deviation. J Pediatr Ophthlamol Strabismus 1990; 27: 59–65.

Access the complete referece list online at

http://www.expertconsult.com

Part 7
Nystagmus and eye movements

Nystagmus in childhood

Frank A Proudlock • Irene Gottlob

Introduction

Nystagmus consists of rhythmic ocular oscillations of the eyes. Pathologic nystagmus is involuntary although it may be modulated when performing certain tasks such as reading. Infantile nystagmus develops in the first 3–6 months of life. Nystagmus can be acquired later in life, usually due to neurologic diseases. Patients with acquired nystagmus have oscillopsia, the illusion that the environment is moving. Patients with infantile nystagmus usually have a stable view of the environment probably due to neuronal plasticity and adaptation during visual development.

Nystagmus in childhood can be idiopathic or associated with retinal diseases, low vision in infancy, and a variety of syndromes and neurologic diseases. Nystagmus associated with neurologic disorders may be similar in appearance and pathophysiology to acquired nystagmus. Onset may also be after 6 months of age. The estimated prevalence of nystagmus (including both infantile and acquired nystagmus) is 24 in 10 000. The prevalence of infantile nystagmus is 14 per 10 000.[1] Among the infantile forms of nystagmus, idiopathic nystagmus is the most common, followed by nystagmus associated with ocular disease. The diagnoses associated with infantile nystagmus are shown in Figure 89.1.

Causes of infantile nystagmus

The causes of most forms of infantile nystagmus are unknown. Infantile nystagmus is considered to be a disorder

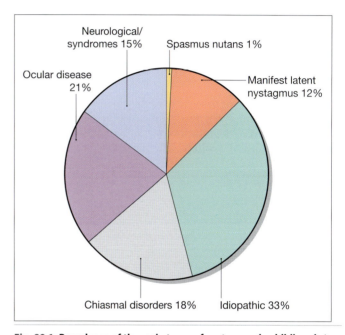

Fig. 89.1 Prevalence of the main types of nystagmus in childhood. A breakdown of the various disorders in individuals 18 years and under with infantile nystagmus from the Leicestershire Nystagmus Survey. The majority of patients with chiasmal disorders had albinism. (From Sarvananthan N, Surendran M, Roberts EO, et al. The prevalence of nystagmus: the Leicestershire Nystagmus Survey. Invest Ophthalmol Vis Sci 2009; 50: 5201–6.)

of gaze-holding and slow eye movement systems,[2] leading to sinusoidal oscillations and/or drifts of the eye away from fixation. These involuntary slow eye movements constitute nystagmus slow phases. The slow phases are interrupted and shaped by the interposition of nystagmus quick phases which serve to realign the eyes.

Many types of infantile nystagmus are associated with sensory abnormalities during early visual development.[3] With "afferent" diseases such as achromatopsia and congenital cataract, the nystagmus is the result of changes in the otherwise healthy ocular motor systems in response to afferent deficits present during visual development. For other conditions, such as albinism and various syndromes, it is uncertain whether the nystagmus is also due to afferent deficits or abnormalities in ocular motor neural circuitry.

Quality of life and infantile nystagmus

Quality of life studies of adults and children with infantile nystagmus show that the effects on visual function are considerable and are comparable to diseases such as age-related macular degeneration.[4] Infantile nystagmus has a much wider impact than simply reducing vision. It affects social interaction, due to lack of confidence caused by the cosmetic appearance of nystagmus, and causes restriction in mobility of many patients, as they are not able to drive.[5] Treatment of nystagmus should not only aim at improving visual acuity (VA) but also at improving cosmesis. This might include, for example, the correction of abnormal head postures and the reduction of nystagmus intensity in patients with poor visual potential. Patients may also benefit from counseling services and support groups such as:

- Nystagmus Network, UK (http://www.nystagmusnet.org).
- American Nystagmus Network (http://www.nystagmus.org).

Classification of infantile nystagmus

There is significant controversy over the classification and terminology used in nystagmus. Some researchers have been mainly interested in the morphology of nystagmus waveforms and others in clinical etiology.

The advantages of using a classification of infantile nystagmus based on the associated diseases are that the clinical implications such as prognosis, possible genetic counseling, or treatment options are highlighted.[6] Figure 89.2 lists examples of disorders using this type of classification. Idiopathic nystagmus is a diagnosis of exclusion where all other eye examinations are normal. VA is logMAR 0.3 (6/12, 20/40, 0.5) or better in most patients.[7,8] Mutations in the *FRMD7* gene have been identified as a major cause of X-linked idiopathic nystagmus.[9,10] Several genetic mutations are known for other disorders such as albinism[11,12] and achromatopsia.[13] It is likely that the nystagmus genotype will be the principal method of classification in the future.

The Committee for the Classification of Eye Movement Abnormalities and Strabismus Workshop (CEMAS, http://www.nei.nih.gov/news/statements/cemas/pdf) have grouped idiopathic nystagmus, nystagmus associated with ocular diseases, and nystagmus associated with chiasmal misrouting into one category, "infantile nystagmus syndrome." This classification makes unconfirmed assumptions about a common mechanism leading to nystagmus in all of the underlying pathologies.

Terminology used in nystagmus

Nystagmus can be characterized by clinical examination of the patient. Eye movement recordings can provide greater

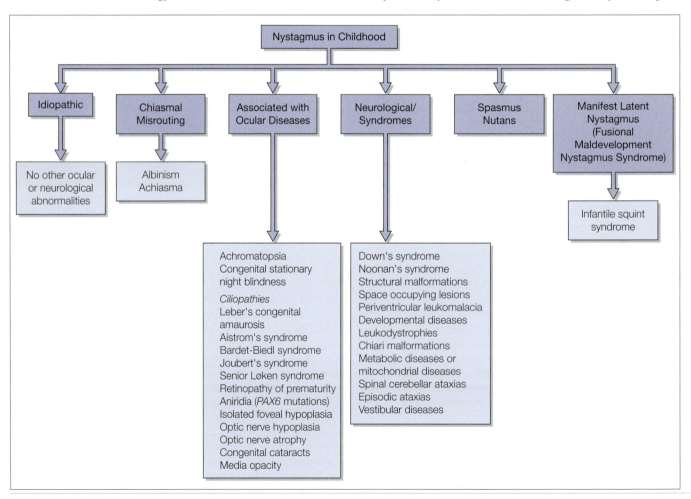

Fig. 89.2 Classification of nystagmus based on associated diseases.

precision in detecting and describing nystagmus waveforms which can assist in the diagnosis (Figs 89.3 and 89.4). The following parameters can be used to describe nystagmus:

Plane The plane of oscillation can be horizontal, vertical, torsional, or a combination of more than one plane (e.g. Fig. 89.3C,2).

Intensity The intensity of the nystagmus is a measure of the speed of the eye movements and is obtained by multiplying the nystagmus amplitude (in degrees) and frequency (oscillations per second in Hertz).

Waveform Nystagmus can be classified into jerk and pendular waveforms. Jerk nystagmus consists of alternating slow and quick phase eye movements. The nystagmus direction is defined using the quick phase. Slow phases can have increasing velocity profiles where the eyes start slowly and accumulate speed (e.g. Fig. 89.4A in right gaze). Alternatively, slow phases may have decreasing velocity (e.g. Fig. 89.4C) or linear velocity profiles. In contrast, pendular nystagmus consists of sinusoidal oscillations with small or no quick phases (e.g. Fig. 89.4A at null region). Dual jerk nystagmus is a combination of large jerk nystagmus waveforms with small pendular nystagmus waveforms superimposed along the same plane.

Conjugacy If both eyes move together, i.e. with the same amplitude, frequency and plane, the nystagmus is conjugate. Disconjugacy (dissociated nystagmus) occurs if the eyes move with different amplitude (e.g. torsional eye movements in Figure 89.3A,3), frequency, phase (e.g. vertical eye movements in Figure 89.3C,2), or along different planes.

Foveation Most types of infantile nystagmus show periods when the eyes move at a slower velocity. These slow periods are used to align the fovea to improve VA, and hence are called foveation periods.

Null region Many patients with infantile nystagmus prefer to use a particular gaze direction where the nystagmus is reduced in intensity and the VA is optimal. This is called the null region. If the null region is not in the primary position, patients may adopt an abnormal head posture (AHP) using the null region to improve vision when looking straight ahead (see Chapter 81). An example is shown in Figure 89.4A,2 where the null region is in right gaze.

Infantile nystagmus can change depending on several factors:

Change with gaze Patients with albinism and idiopathic nystagmus usually have a null region. The nystagmus becomes more jerk-like (Fig. 89.4A,1) and intense (Fig. 89.4A,2) away from the null region.

Change with time Most patients have a consistent oscillation when attempting to maintain a fixed gaze position. However, certain types of nystagmus vary with time. In periodic alternating nystagmus (PAN) the fast phase beats periodically to the right and to the left with quiet periods at the change-over periods (Fig. 89.4B).

Change upon covering one eye In manifest latent nystagmus (MLN) the fast phase of nystagmus changes direction beating toward the fixing eye (Fig. 89.4C).

Clinical assessment

History

It is important to establish the time of onset for the nystagmus. Infantile nystagmus occurs usually in the first 3, or sometimes 6, months of life.

As several forms of infantile nystagmus are hereditary, establishing whether other family members have nystagmus or associated ocular diseases can help with the diagnosis. If there is a positive family history, determining the mode of inheritance is important. Idiopathic nystagmus often occurs in an X-linked pattern in which heterozygous females are fully affected in approximately 50% of cases (i.e. 50% penetrance).[9,10] In contrast, only males are fully affected in X-linked congenital stationary night-blindness,[15] blue cone monochromatism,[13] or ocular albinism.[12] Oculocutaneous albinism[11] and achromatopsia[13] are usually autosomal recessive. The most common form of autosomal dominant nystagmus is caused by mutations in *PAX6* genes.[16]

Where neurologic deficits are present, they are likely to play a key role in the etiology of the nystagmus.

Establish whether the parents think the child has poor vision. Nystagmus can be of very large amplitude at onset and parents can have the impression that the child is visually unresponsive. Usually the amplitude is considerably smaller by 6 to 9 months of age[17] Video 89.1). Explaining to parents that nystagmus changes and becomes less evident with age is important. Caution should be taken about predicting poor vision later in life.

Often children with nystagmus have head nodding or bobbing. This is an independent abnormal head movement which can decrease or disappear with age (Video 89.2). Only in spasmus nutans has head nodding been shown to be compensatory (minimizing the nystagmus) (Fig. 89.3D, Video 89.3).

A history of photophobia should be specifically asked for. This indicates retinal disease, particularly achromatopsia (Video 89.4) or blue cone monochromatism. A history of night-blindness should be specifically asked for. This suggests a rod disorder and is common in congenital stationary night-blindness.

Oscillopsia seldom occurs in infantile nystagmus. Some children, however, perceive oscillopsia if they look away from the null region[18] or if the nystagmus changes, for example in MLN which can change with the degree of strabismus (Video 89.18). Oscillopsia in acquired nystagmus is usually sudden in onset and severe. When it occurs in infantile nystagmus, the time of onset is generally not well defined and the symptoms are milder.

Clinical examination

Visual acuity

VA needs to be examined with the best optical correction and tested with both eyes open and either eye covered with a free head position. MLN, alone or superimposed on infantile nystagmus, can increase the nystagmus and decrease VA when one eye is covered. VA should be measured at distance and near. In infants, VA tests can be performed using preferential looking cards. In patients with horizontal nystagmus, measurement of

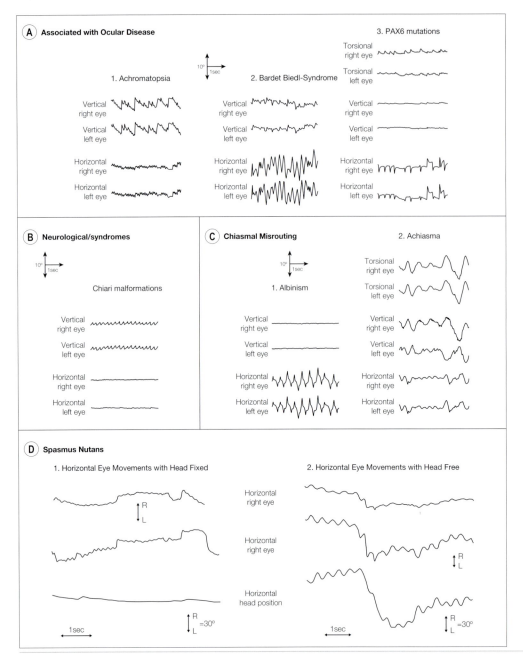

Fig. 89.3 The use of eye movement recordings in the diagnosis of nystagmus. Examples of eye movement recordings from patients with infantile nystagmus associated with (A) ocular diseases, (B) neurologic disorders and syndromes, (C) chiasmal misrouting disorders, and (D) spasmus nutans. (A) Ocular diseases. In achromatopsia a fine pendular nystagmus with a vertical component is often present. In the achromat shown (A,1) a fine mainly horizontal pendular nystagmus of 1–2° amplitude and 8 Hz frequency coexists with a vertical upbeat jerk nystagmus of approximately 5° amplitude and 1.5 Hz frequency. A patient with Bardet-Biedl syndrome (A,2) has horizontal pendular oscillations that are much larger than in the achromat (8–10° amplitude and 3 Hz frequency in the example shown) but the vertical component to the nystagmus is smaller. *PAX6* mutations (A,3) lead to a variety of waveforms with the two eyes sometimes showing disconjugate eye movements. The example here shows unusual horizontal waveforms with both increasing and decreasing velocity components. A significant torsional component is apparent which is larger in the right eye. (B) Neurologic disorders and syndromes. These can be associated with vertical eye movements. The example shown is from a patient with a Chiari malformation leading to a downbeat jerk nystagmus of 2–3° amplitude and 3–4 Hz frequency with little horizontal nystagmus. (C) Chiasmal routing disorders. Similar to idiopathic infantile nystagmus (Fig. 89.4A), nystagmus associated with albinism (C,1) can have pendular or jerk waveforms but always along the horizontal plane and usually with a null region. Jerk waveforms can be left beating, right beating, or bidirectional as shown. Achiasmic disorders (C,2) lead to see-saw nystagmus: the eyes give the appearance of rotating around an invisible pivot positioned somewhere between the two eyes. As one eye moves up the other eye moves down leading to a disconjugate vertical waveform. The eye moving up intorts and the eye moving down extorts leading to a large amplitude torsional nystagmus. There is also a horizontal component to see-saw nystagmus. (D) Spasmus nutans. Nystagmus in spasmus nutans is altered by head movements. When the head is fixed, a rapid pendular oscillation develops which is disconjugate between the two eyes. When the head is free, head bobbing occurs with the eyes moving in the opposite direction due to the vestibulo-ocular reflex. This leads to suppression of the rapid oscillation. (Reproduced from Gottlob I, Zubcov AA, Wizov SS, Reinecke RD. Head nodding is compensatory in spasmus nutans. Ophthalmology 1992; 99: 1024–31.)

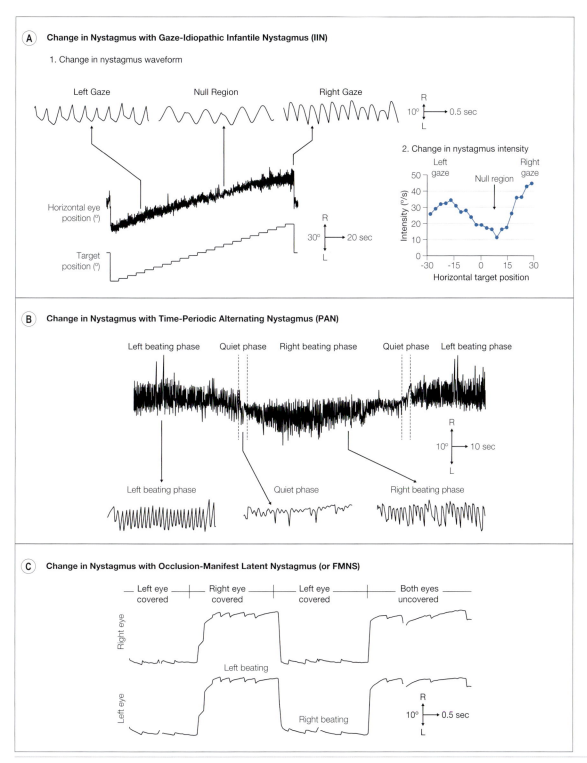

Fig. 89.4 Change in nystagmus with (A) gaze, (B) time, and (C) occlusion. (A) An example of the null region in a patient with idiopathic infantile nystagmus. The patient follows a target moving from the left to right in steps of 3° every 8 seconds (lower traces). The horizontal nystagmus changes both in waveform (A,1) and intensity (A,2) as the direction of gaze changes. The changing waveforms can be seen from the expanded views in the upper traces. At the null region, which is 9° to the right of central fixation, the nystagmus waveform is predominantly pendular with occasional foveating saccades. Jerk waveforms are present to the left and right of the null region with the nystagmus beating to the left in left gaze and right in right gaze. A plot of the nystagmus intensity in relation to the horizontal gaze angle is shown in A,2. (B) A patient with idiopathic infantile nystagmus and periodic alternating nystagmus. The nystagmus completes a full cycle of left beating and right beating nystagmus every 200 seconds with short quiet phases of several seconds between each change in beating direction. Expanded views are shown in the lower traces. (C) A patient with manifest latent nystagmus illustrates the change in beating direction on covering either eye. The eyes always beat toward the open or fixing eye. The waveforms all show decreasing velocity slow phases. Note the step change in eye position on covering either eye which is due to a large esotropia. The left eye is the dominant eye. The nystagmus is less intense when both eyes are open.

VA can be assisted by vertically aligning the cards[19] making it easier to identify changes in fixation when the child looks up or down. This can be masked by the horizontal nystagmus if the card is aligned horizontally. The presence of vertical (optokinetic nystagmus) OKN suggests the likelihood of better VA in horizontal nystagmus.

Abnormal head posture (torticollis)

AHP occurs commonly in nystagmus because patients can reduce their nystagmus by looking in a certain direction of gaze. In most patients, the full extent of torticollis is only observed during visual effort. To identify the full amount of AHP, ask the patient to read or look at pictures (Fig. 89.5A, Video 89.5). Glasses can prevent the patient adopting the full head turn due to the spectacle frame and optical decentration. VA measurements should be repeated, therefore, without spectacles. Figure 89.5B and Video 89.6 show a child with idiopathic infantile nystagmus (IIN) and a right head turn increasing as he reads smaller letters. With a greater visual demand, a large head turn is adopted and he looks over his glasses or prefers to read without glasses since the full head turn is prevented by the glasses.

MLN dampens on adduction. As a result, the patient adopts a head turn to keep the fixing eye adducted (Fig. 89.5C, Video 89.7). In MLN the head position needs to be examined with each eye covered, as the head position can change depending on the fixing eye (Fig. 89.5D, Video 89.8). Patients with "A" or "V" pattern strabismus may adopt a chin up or down position to maintain binocular function and thus reduce the amplitude of the nystagmus (Fig. 89.5E, Video 89.9). Eye movement recordings are helpful in understanding AHPs for example in establishing whether the head posture is due to idiopathic nystagmus (Fig. 89.4A) or manifest latent waveforms (Fig. 89.4C) and whether the adopted head posture leads to a reduction in the nystagmus.

Orthoptic examination

This should include an assessment of strabismus at distance and near, the range of motility of each eye, binocularity, stereopsis, and fusion ranges if binocular vision is present.

Color vision testing

This is important to detect achromatopsia and other retinal or optic nerve diseases.

Examination of light sensitivity and nyctalopia

Photophobia is easily noted on slit-lamp or fundus examination and points to achromatopsia (Video 89.4) or other retinal dystrophies. Nyctalopia can be objectively measured using dark adaptometry and indicates congenital stationary night-blindness or other retinal dystrophies.

Structural examination

The most common abnormal sign of the anterior segment is iris transillumination which is strongly associated with albinism. The amount of iris transillumination varies and can be easily missed if it is mild, especially in patients with dark irides or in small children. Slit lamp examination should be performed in a completely dark room with retro-illumination. Examine the parents as carriers commonly have mild iris transillumination. It is important to examine for corneal changes, aniridia or abnormal iris structure and the presence of cataracts. The retina can appear normal in the early stages of retinal dystrophy. Foveal hypoplasia often manifests as a missing foveal reflex and abnormal vessels in the foveal area. This can be difficult to establish in a child with nystagmus. In retinal diseases such as achromatopsia and congenital stationary night-blindness, the retina can appear normal. Optic nerve hypoplasia or atrophy can cause nystagmus, particularly if it is bilateral. Large refractive errors are also commonly a sign of retinal dystrophies, albinism, *PAX6* mutations, or other diseases associated with low vision. Paradoxical pupillary response (initial pupillary constriction when room light is turned off) can be a sign of retinal diseases.

Electrophysiology

Every patient with infantile nystagmus should have an electrophysiologic examination. Hemispheric visual evoked potentials (VEPs) are the gold standard for determining increased crossing of the optic nerves in albinism and reduced crossing in achiasma (see Chapters 40 and 54).

Electroretinography (ERG) is essential to investigate possible retinal dystrophies (Fig. 89.6).

Eye movement recordings

Eye movement recordings are useful in clarifying the pathophysiology of the nystagmus, in differential diagnosis, and in planning surgery. Figures 89.3 and 89.4 show examples of eye movement recordings in each of the main classes of infantile nystagmus.

Nystagmus associated with albinism (Fig. 89.3C,1) or idiopathic nystagmus (Fig. 89.4A) is conjugate, almost always horizontal, with a combination of pendular and jerk waveforms that vary with gaze.[7] Away from the null region the slow phases typically increase in velocity and drift toward the null region (Fig. 89.4A). In contrast, nystagmus associated with MLN usually has decreasing velocity slow phases (Fig. 89.4C). Nystagmus waveforms associated with retinal diseases are variable and can be dissociated, vertical, and can have increasing or decreasing slow phase velocities (Fig. 89.3A). Vertical nystagmus may be associated with neurologic disorders (Fig. 89.3B).

Optical coherence tomography

Optical coherence tomography (OCT) is a useful tool for the differential diagnosis of nystagmus.[20-22] It is particularly helpful in identifying foveal hypoplasia. Figure 89.7 shows OCT images of a control subject and patients with albinism, *PAX6* mutations, isolated foveal hypoplasia and achromatopsia. If foveal hypoplasia is detected on OCT, the most likely diagnosis is albinism.[20] However, mutations in the *PAX6* gene or idiopathic foveal hypoplasia cannot be ruled out.[22] These diseases have similar morphologic changes in the fovea. In contrast, foveal hypoplasia in achromatopsia is atypical.[21,22] In many patients with achromatopsia there is a pathologic continuation of inner and outer plexiform layers. Typically, there is disruption of the inner segment/outer segment junction and cone outer segment tip and thinning of the outer nuclear layer. The most striking sign is a "punched out" hyporeflexive zone, which often only appears in older patients. Morphologic changes in achromatopsia increase with age on OCT.[21]

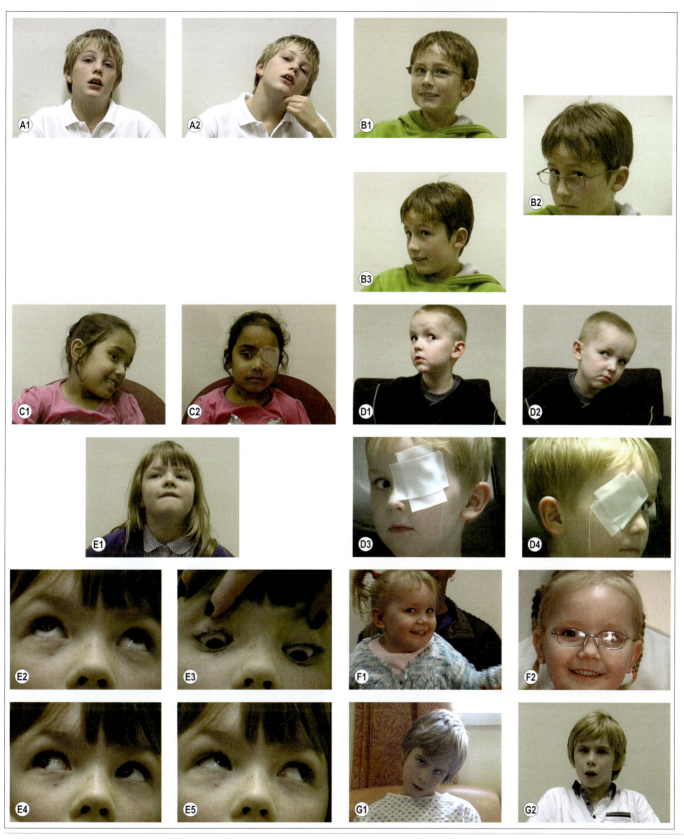

Fig. 89.5 Abnormal head postures. (A) Patient with idiopathic infantile nystagmus (IIN) and a mild head tilt to the left when reading large letters on a VA chart (A1), which significantly increases (A2) when reading smaller letters. (B) Moderate head turn to the right due to IIN when reading large letters (B1). As the patient reads smaller letters the head increasingly turns to the right and the patient looks over his glasses as the frames do not allow a larger head turn to the right (B2). He prefers to read without glasses in order to adopt a large head turn (B3). (C) Child with a blind right eye due to optic nerve hypoplasia adopting an extreme head turn and tilt to the left to dampen manifest latent nystagmus (C1). When the left eye is covered and there is no vision the head turn is absent (C2), which shows that there is no muscular torticollis. (D) Manifest latent nystagmus and alternating exotropia. The patient turns the head alternately to the right to fix in adduction with the right eye (D1), or the left to fix in adduction with the left eye (D2) to dampen the manifest latent nystagmus. When one eye is patched, he turns the head continuously to the right when the right eye is open (D3) and to the left when the left eye is open (D4). (E) Girl with manifest latent nystagmus adopting chin elevation while reading (E1). She has "V" pattern exotropia with bilateral inferior oblique overaction (E2-E5). On down-gaze she has some binocularity (Bagolini positive) which causes the nystagmus to dampen. Hence, she adopts a chin up position when reading. (F) Head turn to the left due to IIN (nystagmus null region to the right) which does not allow the patient to wear glasses as the frame is obstructing her vision (F1). After Kestenbaum surgery (F2) her head is straight and she is able to wear her 4 diopters of astigmatic correction, significantly improving her vision. (G) A patient with albinism and pronounced head tilt to the left before surgery when reading the visual acuity chart (G1). After surgery he reads the same line on the acuity chart without a head tilt (G2).

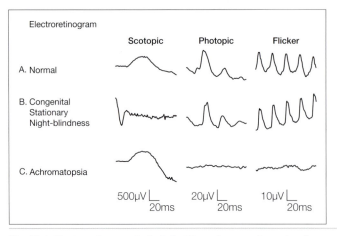

Fig. 89.6 **Electroretinography in infantile nystagmus.** Examples of scotopic, photopic, and flicker electroretinograms (ERGs) of (a) a normal subject, (b) a patient with congenital stationary night-blindness (CSNB) with a negative scotopic ERG, and (c) a patient with achromatopsia with extinguished photopic ERG and flicker ERG.

Structural grading of foveal hypoplasia based on retinal imaging using OCT may be used to estimate VA (Fig. 89.7B).[20,22]

Magnetic resonance imaging of the brain

MRI is necessary if the nystagmus is not typical of idiopathic nystagmus (i.e. disconjugate, vertical, or oblique) and cannot be explained by ocular or systemic disease. MRI is generally not indicated when the associated disease (e.g. albinism, achromatopsia or MLN/infantile squint syndrome) has been determined and when no other neurologic/developmental problem is present. Any suspicion of neurologic disease, optic atrophy, optic nerve hypoplasia or developmental delay should prompt neuroimaging. In the presence of optic nerve hypoplasia, investigation for septo-optic dysplasia (de Morsier's syndrome) and hormone deficiency is important (see Chapter 51).

Clinical characteristics of infantile nystagmus types

Idiopathic infantile nystagmus

Idiopathic infantile nystagmus (IIN) is diagnosed by excluding other ocular or neurologic pathology (Video 89.10). Anterior segment, fundus examination, VEPs, and ERGs are normal. If the IIN is familial, the most frequent inheritance mode is X-linked where approximately 50% of female carriers are clinically affected.[9,10] Autosomal dominant inheritance has also been described. The first gene (*FRMD7*) in which mutations cause X-linked IIN has been found.[9,10] Knockdown of *FRMD7* during neuronal differentiation results in altered neurite function.[23]

Patients with IIN have a median VA of logMAR 0.18 (6/9, 20/30, 0.63), strabismus is uncommon (less than 10%), and good stereoacuity is often present.[8] Patients with mutations in the *FRMD7* gene often have fewer AHPs compared to patients with IIN without mutations in this gene.[8] Nystagmus is conjugate and usually horizontal especially when associated with *FRMD7* mutations (Fig. 89.4A).[8] Nystagmus waveforms in IIN often have increasing velocity slow phases. However, the nystagmus can be more complex, consisting of underlying pendular oscillations regularly interrupted by quick phases (Fig. 89.4A). Increasing velocity slow phases are more apparent away from the null region.

Nystagmus waveforms are often of very large amplitude in the first few months of life but become smaller as children become older. Changes in waveform characteristics also occur with more jerk waveforms becoming apparent with age (Video 89.1).[17] Possibly these are adaptive mechanisms to allow better vision through the development of foveation periods, where the eyes move at a relatively slower velocity. Typically, the nystagmus has a null region where nystagmus intensity is reduced causing an AHP if the null region is not in the primary position (Fig. 89.4A, Videos 89.5, 89.6, 89.10). Over 20% of patients with idiopathic nystagmus due to mutations in *FRMD7* have periodic alternating nystagmus. This is usually not detected clinically but only on eye movement recordings (Fig. 89.4B, Video 89.11).[24] IIN can be vertical, albeit rare (Video 89.12).

Chiasmal misrouting

Albinism has very similar nystagmus characteristics as IIN (Fig. 89.3C,1, Video 89.2). Albinism can be easily missed and signs such as iris transillumination, hypopigmentation of the retina, optic nerve hypoplasia, and abnormal crossing on VEP need to be assessed carefully. OCT is very helpful in detecting foveal hypoplasia (see Fig. 89.7A(a,b,c); see also Chapter 40).

Patients with achiasmia have congenital see-saw nystagmus (Video 89.22). The diagnosis is confirmed using MRI and VEP (see Chapters 8 and 54).

Nystagmus associated with ocular disease

Nystagmus can occur in most types of retinal dystrophy. The 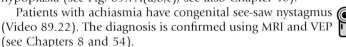 diagnosis of achromatopsia (Fig. 89.6, Video 89.4) or blue cone monochromatism is likely in a patient with marked light sensitivity, poor vision, poor color discrimination with a small amplitude, and high frequency nystagmus. Inheritance in achromatopsia is autosomal recessive, and mutations in four genes have been described for which molecular genetic testing is available.[13] Patients with mutations in the same gene can have widely varying phenotypes.[13] This can range from profound visual impairment with no color vision, to incomplete achromatopsia with some color perception and, less commonly, to "oligocone trichromacy" with almost normal color vision and VA as good as logMAR 0.1(6/7.5, 20/25, 0.8).[25] Patients with achromatopsia often have fast pendular nystagmus superimposed on jerk nystagmus and also vertical nystagmus (Fig. 89.3A,1).[26] Typical findings on OCT examination have been described in achromatopsia (Fig. 89.7A(h,i)).[21] The diagnosis can be confirmed by extinguished or severely reduced photopic electroretinography (see Fig. 89.6C). In blue cone monochromatism the VA is usually better and the inheritance is X-linked.[13]

Congenital stationary night-blindness (CSNB) is often associated with nystagmus with waveforms corresponding to infantile or MLN (Video 89.8). Patients have variable VA,

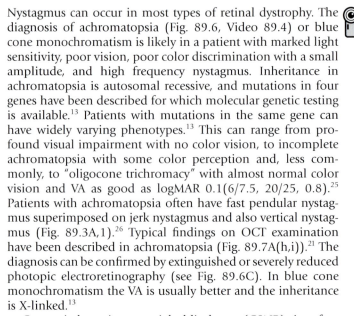

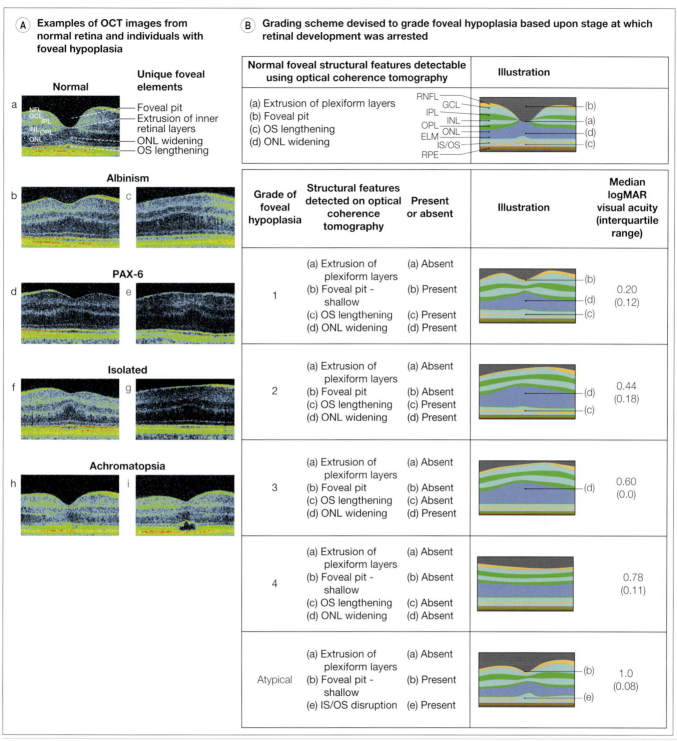

Fig. 89.7 Optical coherence tomography in infantile nystagmus. (A) Optical coherence tomograms for (a) a normal fovea, (b, c) albinism, (d, e) associated with *PAX6* mutations, (f, g) isolated cases, and (h, i) an atypical form of foveal hypoplasia seen in achromatopsia. In (i) hyporeflective zone (cavitation) is also seen indicating cone photoreceptor degeneration. Foveal hypoplasia of varying degrees is seen in all disorders. In achromatopsia, there is an atypical form of foveal hypoplasia with a shallower pit, incursion of the plexiform layers, and disruption of the inner segment (IS)/outer segment (OS) junction. INL = inner nuclear layer; NFL = nerve fiber layer; ONL = outer nuclear layer. (B) The unique features of a normal fovea detectable on optical coherence tomography are shown with the typical and atypical grades of foveal hypoplasia through a series of schematics. All grades of foveal hypoplasia had incursion of inner retinal layers. Atypical foveal hypoplasia also had incursion of the inner retinal layers. Grade 1 foveal hypoplasia is associated with a shallow foveal pit, outer nuclear layer (ONL) widening, and outer segment (OS) lengthening relative to the parafoveal ONL and OS length, respectively. In Grade 2 foveal hypoplasia, all features of grade 1 are present except the presence of a foveal pit. Grade 3 foveal hypoplasia consists of all features of grade 2 foveal hypoplasia except the widening of the cone outer segment. Grade 4 foveal hypoplasia represents all the features seen in grade 3 except there is no widening of the ONL at the fovea. The final image shows an atypical form of foveal hypoplasia in which there is a shallower pit with disruption of the inner segment/outer segment (IS/OS) junction, possibly a sign of photoreceptor degeneration. The atypical form of foveal hypoplasia is seen with achromatopsia, whereas grades 1 through 4 are seen with albinism, *PAX6* mutations, and isolated cases. ELM = external limiting membrane; GCL = ganglion cell layer; INL = inner nuclear layer; IPL = inner plexiform layer; OPL = outer plexiform layer; RNFL = retinal nerve fiber layer; RPE = retinal pigment epithelium. (Reproduced from Thomas MG, Kumar A, Mohammad S, et al. Structural grading of foveal hypoplasia using spectral-domain optical coherence tomography: a predictor of visual acuity? Ophthalmology 2011.)

reduced night vision, often high myopia, and the ERG is negative (see Fig. 89.6B). Pendular, oblique, and mostly disconjugate nystagmus of high frequency and low amplitude have been described often with and dual jerk nystagmus waveforms present. Inheritance is commonly X-linked and mutations of two causative genes have been identified.[15] Nystagmus in retinal dystrophies can occur in ciliopathies, which consists of dysfunction of the primary cilium, an organelle involved in intracellular and intercellular sensing and signaling (e.g. Alström's syndrome, Bardet-Biedl syndrome (Video 89.13), Joubert's syndrome, Senior-Løken syndrome, and Leber's congenital amaurosis) (see Chapter 44). In retinal dystrophies, nystagmus can occasionally appear later in life as the vision deteriorates.

Nystagmus can be associated with retinopathy of prematurity, congenital cataracts, corneal opacity, and optic nerve hypoplasia. In these patients nystagmus can have the same characteristics as in achromatopsia or CSNB, or have characteristics of MLN (Videos 89.7, 89.8). Early treatment of cataract or other media opacities can prevent the development of nystagmus. Mutations in the *PAX6* gene, inherited in an autosomal dominant pattern, are associated with nystagmus which can be horizontal, vertical, or torsional (Fig. 89.3A,3, Video 89.14).[16] OCT shows foveal hypoplasia (Fig. 89.7A,D,E), but the VEP does not show misrouting of the optic nerve that is characteristic of albinism. Aniridia is common.

Nystagmus in neurologic diseases or syndromes

Childhood nystagmus is a common feature of a range of syndromes, developmental and neurologic disorders, for example Down's syndrome, Noonan's syndrome (Video 89.15), structural malformations, space occupying lesions, periventricular leukomalacia, cerebral palsy, leukodystrophy, Chiari malformation, metabolic disease, or mitochondrial disease.[27] Vertical, torsional, see-saw, or disconjugate nystagmus waveforms are common in neurologic disorders (see Fig. 89.3B showing vertical nystagmus in Chiari malformation). MRI is essential if there are other neurologic symptoms, developmental delay, optic atrophy or any suspicion of atypical nystagmus.

Spasmus nutans

Spasmus nutans consists of a triad of nystagmus, head nodding, and AHP (Video 89.3). The onset is later than in infantile nystagmus, usually developing after 6 months of age. The nystagmus is of high frequency and pendular. The nystagmus may be intermittent and disconjugate. Sometimes it is clinically apparent in only one eye (Fig. 89.3D).[14] The nystagmus usually disappears spontaneously 1 to 2 years after onset although subclinical nystagmus persists on eye movement recordings. Head nodding suppresses the nystagmus since the vestibulo-ocular reflex stabilizes the eyes, which can permit development of binocular vision (Fig. 89.3D).[14] The etiology of spasmus nutans remains unclear. It has been associated with a lower socioeconomic status.[28] The same nystagmus characteristics, head nodding and torticollis, can occur in suprasellar tumors such as chiasmal glioma.[29] If there is an afferent pupillary defect or optic nerve pallor, suspicion of a tumor is high. Some

retinal diseases, achromatopsia and CSNB, can mimic spasmus nutans.[30] We recommend that ERG and/or MRI be performed in all children presenting with spasmus nutans.

Manifest latent nystagmus

MLN, or "fusional maldevelopment nystagmus syndrome" (FMNS), is part of the congenital strabismus syndrome. The nystagmus is typically larger upon covering one eye, the fast phase beats to the fixing eye and the slow phase has decreasing velocity (Fig. 89.4C, Video 89.16) (see Chapter 88).

Treatment

Spectacles and contact lenses

The incidence of refractive error in nystagmus is high.[31] Children with nystagmus under 6 years of age need frequent refraction to prevent amblyopia. Contact lenses can be helpful because they may give better optical correction. Contact lenses allow patients to adopt large AHPs with better optical correction as contact lenses do not have the problems of decentration and obstruction of the visual axis by spectacle frames (Fig. 89.5B, Video 89.6). Some studies suggest that contact lenses may reduce nystagmus by providing sensory feedback through the eyelids although this is unconfirmed.

Surgical treatment and treatment with prisms

Patients often use compensatory strategies to reduce nystagmus. These strategies are different in individual patients. Compensatory mechanisms can often be assisted using surgery or prisms. Surgery for AHPs usually yields excellent and sustained improvement.

Kestenbaum-Anderson type procedures

Patients with infantile nystagmus, especially idiopathic nystagmus and nystagmus associated with albinism, commonly have a null region. If the null region is not in primary position, patients often adopt an AHP using the eccentrically positioned null region for better vision (Fig. 89.4A, null region on eye movement recordings, Fig. 89.5A,B,F,G, Videos 89.5, 89.6, 89.10, 89.19, 89.20). Usually the null region is either in the primary position of gaze or along the horizontal plane. Some patients with horizontal nystagmus have vertical head postures or head tilts (Videos 89.5 and 89.20), or a combination of AHPs in different planes. Patients with infantile vertical nystagmus can also show horizontal head postures (Video 89.12). These mechanisms are not well understood.

If patients have vertical head postures, recess or resect procedures can be performed on vertical and/or oblique muscles. For head tilt, rotatory Kestenbaum procedures can be performed either by recession and resection of oblique muscles or by inducing torsion by moving the insertion of the rectus muscles.[32] If the two horizontal or vertical rectus muscles are operated on in either eye, they can be shifted up and down or left and right to induce a rotator effect. If the patient has manifest strabismus, surgery for the AHP needs to be performed on the fixing eye. The amount of strabismus resulting from preoperative strabismus and possibly surgery for the AHP can be corrected in the non-fixing eye (Case study 2). Significant

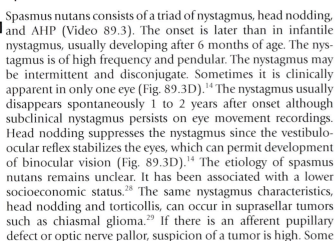

amounts of horizontal muscle recession and resection are necessary for large head turns.[33]

Surgery for AHPs is usually successful. Surgery can be performed at any age, but it is best to wait until the cause of the head turn is established. If amblyopia is caused by the child not being able to wear glasses due to a large AHP, surgery should be performed early. Otherwise a convenient age for surgery is around 6 to 8 years of age when the child is cooperative and can be easily examined. Head turns do not often fully develop until school age when the head posture may become more frequent and pronounced with increasing school work. Kestenbaum-Anderson type procedures are effective even in adults.

Case study 1

A 4-year-old girl with IIN needed spectacle correction of 4 diopters astigmatism in each eye. Since she had a large head turn to the left, she could not wear her glasses because the frame obstructed the view. She had a 12 mm recession of the right lateral rectus muscles and left medial rectus muscle and 12 mm resection of the right medial rectus muscle and left lateral rectus muscle. After surgery her head was straight. Because she could now wear her glasses, her binocular VA increased from 0.6 to 0.2 logMAR (Fig. 89.5F, Video 89.19). The head position remained straight 8 years later.

Case study 2

A 9-year-old boy had nystagmus and a pronounced head tilt increasing on visual effort. He had "V" pattern esotropia and bilateral inferior oblique overaction. Surgery consisted of moving the right lateral rectus and left medial rectus muscle one tendon width down and the right medial rectus and left lateral rectus muscle one tendon width up. In addition, recession of the left medial rectus for esotropia and bilateral inferior oblique recession to correct overaction and a "V" pattern was performed. After surgery, the head tilt was significantly reduced (Fig. 89.5G, Video 89.20).

Artificial divergence

Convergence may reduce the intensity of infantile nystagmus. Artificial divergence can be induced to increase convergence and to trigger a convergence impulse even at distance. Good binocular vision is essential for the effectiveness of artificial divergence. Without binocular vision, surgery or prisms would simply change the angle of squint without inducing convergence. Fusion range and the optimal strength of base out prisms to reduce the nystagmus should be tested. It is often best to wear Fresnel prisms for at least 1 or 2 weeks during normal activities and to adjust the amount of prisms. If prisms are small, they can be incorporated into glasses.

Nystagmus blockage syndrome

Some patients with MLN or infantile nystagmus can dampen nystagmus by over-convergence. Bilateral medial rectus recession can help to permanently dampen the nystagmus. This forces the patient to maintain convergence in order to keep the eyes straight.

Case study 3

A patient with congenital nystagmus complained about constant "unquiet eyes" and needing to turn in one eye in order

to have better vision. He had nystagmus and intermittent large angle esotropia. Eye movement recordings showed jerk nystagmus with waveforms showing IIN and MLN reducing on convergence. Bimedial rectus recessions of 5 mm reduced the nystagmus and esotropia. VA with both eyes open improved from 6/12 to 6/9 (Fig. 89.8, Video 89.17).[34]

Adduction

Adduction dampens MLN. If the left eye is dominant, the patient will fix in adduction with the left eye and turn the head to the left (Fig. 89.5C, Video 89.7). If strabismus surgery is performed, the dominant fixing eye should be operated on to correct the abnormal head turn. If a patient with MLN has an alternating strabismus, the head turn can change in the direction of the fixing eye and this can give the false appearance of periodic alternating nystagmus where more than one head posture can be adopted (Fig. 89.5D, Video 89.8). If a patient with MLN fixes with one eye at near and the other at distance, the head turn may change accordingly.

Case study 4

A 5-year-old boy complained of an alternating head turn and exotropia. He had MLN on eye movement recordings, bilateral inferior oblique overaction, and a large exotropia. To correct the head turn unusually large bimedial rectus recessions of 10 mm were performed to limit adduction. However, since medial rectus recession would increase the exotropia, simultaneously bilateral lateral rectus recessions of 16 mm were performed. The head turn disappeared but a moderate exotropia remained. Seven years after surgery, however, the exotropia and the nystagmus were reduced (Fig. 89.5D, Video 89.8).

Reduction of strabismus

Reduction of strabismus and improvement of binocular vision in MLN can reduce nystagmus intensity.[35] Patients with "A" and "V" pattern strabismus may adopt a chin up or chin down head position in order to reduce the angle of strabismus and improve the nystagmus (Fig. 89.5E, Video 89.9). In patients with MLN, strabismus surgery can substantially improve nystagmus.

Case study 5

A patient reported having nystagmus since birth, but his vision had deteriorated over the last year. He had MLN and exotropia without any binocular function. Pictures from several years ago showed that the patient had a small esotropia. Base in prisms were fitted to restore the esotropic microstrabismus. The patient had subnormal binocular vision (Titmus fly positive) and reduced nystagmus. Binocular VA increased by 2 logMAR lines (Video 89.18).

Periodic alternating nystagmus

If the quiet phase of periodic alternating nystagmus (PAN) is not static, the head posture can slowly oscillate from left to right. It is important to recognize a patient has PAN before surgery is performed. Kestenbaum-Anderson procedures may increase the head turn to one side in PAN. Twenty-three percent of patients with IIN and mutations in *FRMD7* and 29% of patients with albinism have PAN.[7,24] Ideally, patients should have eye movement recordings over a period of at least 8 minutes as the cycle of PAN in infantile nystagmus has been

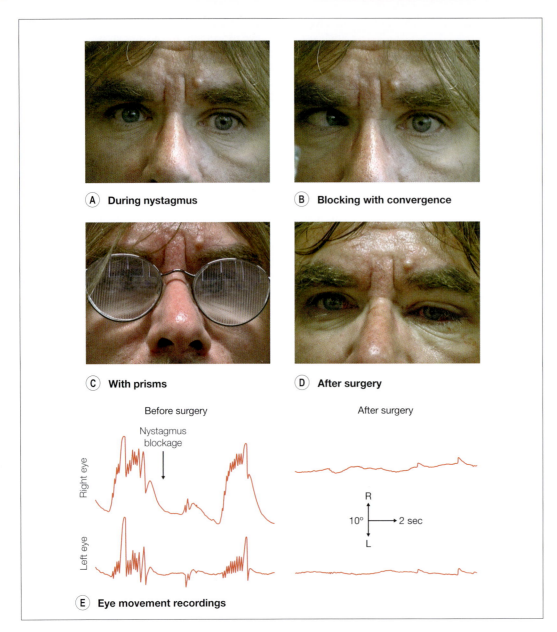

Fig. 89.8 Nystagmus blockage syndrome (see Case study 3).

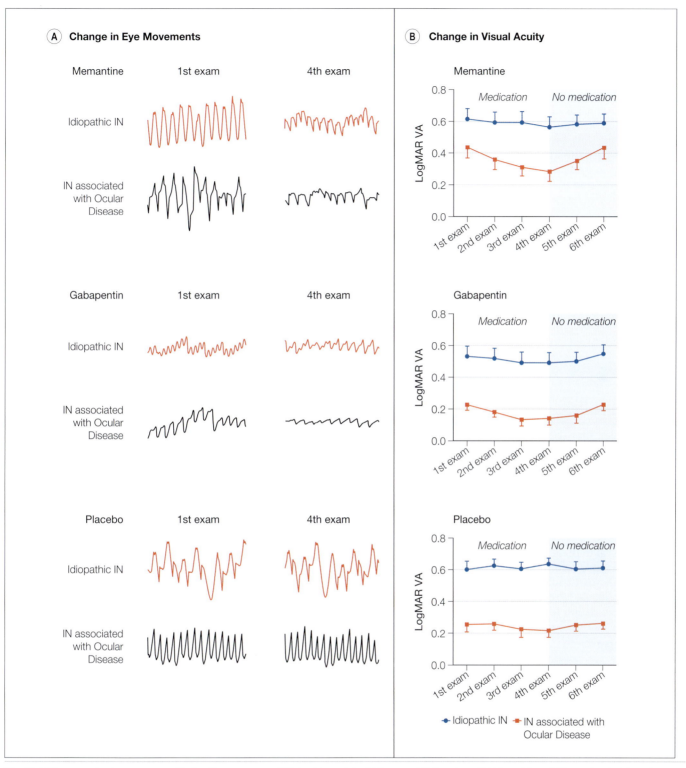

Fig. 89.9 Pharmacologic treatment of infantile nystagmus (IN). In this study by McLean et al.[40] 48 patients (21 idiopathic and 27 associated with ocular disease) were randomized into three treatment arms receiving either memantine, gabapentin, or placebo (between visits 1 and 4). (A) The change in eye movements before and after treatment. (B) The change in logMAR visual acuity during treatment and in the washout period of 2–3 months following (shaded area between visits 4 and 6) during which no medication was received. (Reproduced from McLean R, Proudlock F, Thomas S, et al. Congenital nystagmus: randomized, controlled, double-masked trial of memantine/gabapentin. Ann Neurol 2007; 61: 130–8.)

found to be between 90 and 280 seconds (Fig. 89.4B).[24] Many patients with PAN do not have alternating head position probably because their null region is not moving (Video 89.11). In PAN, one can recess all four horizontal muscles to improve head position.

Tenotomy of four rectus muscles

This procedure consists of detaching and reattaching the rectus muscles at their insertion. Tenotomy may reduce nystagmus and broaden the null region possibly due to changes in proprioceptive feedback from the eye muscles.[36] The procedure can be performed on horizontal or vertical muscles and be combined with correction of strabismus. The value of tenotomy of four rectus muscles has yet to be determined.

Pharmacologic treatment

Baclofen, gabapentin, cannabis, memantine, aminopyridines, and several other drugs have been used in acquired nystagmus.[37,38] Baclofen is effective in infantile PAN.[39] Gabapentin and memantine have been found to be effective in patients with infantile nystagmus.[40] Gabapentin (up to 2400 mg) and memantine (up to 40 mg) were used in slowly increasing dosages. Although the medications are effective in IIN, it is not clear which patients respond best to which type of treatment. Larger trials are underway (Videos 89.21 and 89.22, Fig. 89.9).

Other treatments

Botulinum toxin may reduce infantile nystagmus.[41] However, injections need to be repeated and can induce strabismus and ptosis. Auditory feedback is ineffective or impractical in infantile nystagmus.

Acknowledgment

The authors wish to thank Rebecca McLean for help with preparation of the video recordings and figures in the chapter. We would also like to thank Geoffrey Woodruff for his careful and critical feedback in reading the manuscript. We thank the Ulverscroft Foundation for their continuous support.

References

1. Sarvananthan N, Surendran M, Roberts EO, et al. The prevalence of nystagmus: the Leicestershire Nystagmus Survey. Invest Ophthalmol Vis Sci 2009; 50: 5201–6.

2. Thurtell MJ, Leigh RJ. Nystagmus and saccadic intrusions. Handb Clin Neurol 2011; 102: 333–78.

3. Harris C, Berry D. A developmental model of infantile nystagmus. Semin Ophthalmol 2006; 21: 63–9.

4. Pilling RF, Thompson JR, Gottlob I. Social and visual function in nystagmus. Br J Ophthalmol 2005; 89: 1278–81.

5. McLean RJ, Windridge KC, Gottlob I. Living with nystagmus: a qualitative study. Br J Ophthalmol 2012; 96: 981–6.

6. Casteels I, Harris CM, Shawkat F, Taylor D. Nystagmus in infancy. Br J Ophthalmol 1992; 76: 434–7.

7. Kumar A, Gottlob I, McLean RJ, et al. Clinical and oculomotor characteristics of albinism compared to FRMD7 associated infantile nystagmus. Invest Ophthalmol Vis Sci 2011; 52: 2306–13.

8. Thomas S, Proudlock FA, Sarvananthan N, et al. Phenotypical characteristics of idiopathic infantile nystagmus with and without mutations in FRMD7. Brain 2008; 131: 1259–67.

9. Tarpey P, Thomas S, Sarvananthan N, et al. Mutations in FRMD7, a newly identified member of the FERM family, cause X-linked idiopathic congenital nystagmus. Nat Genet 2006; 38: 1242–4.

10. Thomas MG, Thomas S, Kumar A, et al. FRMD7-related infantile nystagmus. In: Pagon RA, Bird TD, Dolan CR, Stephens K, Adam MP, editors. GeneReviews Feb 12, 2009 ed. Seattle: University of Washington; 2009.

11. Gronskov K, Ek J, Brondum-Nielsen K. Oculocutaneous albinism. Orphanet J Rare Dis 2007; 2: 43.

12. Lewis RA. Ocular albinism, X-linked. In: Pagon RA, Bird TD, Dolan CR, Stephens K, Adam MP, editors. GeneReviews Mar 12, 2004 ed. Seattle: University of Washington; 2004.

13. Kohl S, Jagle H, Sharpe LT, Wissinger B. Achromatopsia. In: Pagon RA, Bird TD, Dolan CR, Stephens K, Adam MP, editors. GeneReviews 17 Feb, 2004 ed. Seattle: University of Washington; 2004.

14. Gottlob I, Zubcov AA, Wizov SS, Reinecke RD. Head nodding is compensatory in spasmus nutans. Ophthalmology 1992; 99: 1024–31.

15. Boycott KM, Bech-Hansen NT, Sauve Y, MacDonald IM. X-linked congenital stationary night blindness. In: Pagon RA, Bird TD, Dolan CR, Stephens K, Adam MP, editors. GeneReviews Jan 16, 2008 ed. Seattle: University of Washington; 1993.

16. Hingorani M, Williamson KA, Moore AT, van Heyningen V. Detailed ophthalmologic evaluation of 43 individuals with PAX6 mutations. Invest Ophthalmol Vis Sci 2009; 50: 2581–90.

17. Reinecke RD, Guo S, Goldstein HP. Waveform evolution in infantile nystagmus: an electro-oculo-graphic study of 35 cases. Binocul Vis 1988; 3: 191–202.

18. Cham KM, Anderson AJ, Abel LA. Factors influencing the experience of oscillopsia in infantile nystagmus syndrome. Invest Ophthalmol Vis Sci 2008; 49: 3424–31.

19. Weiss AH, Kelly JP. Acuity development in infantile nystagmus. Invest Ophthalmol Vis Sci 2007; 48: 4093–99.

20. Mohammad S, Gottlob I, Kumar A, et al. The functional significance of foveal abnormalities in albinism measured using spectral-domain optical coherence tomography. Ophthalmology 2011 Aug; 118(8): 1645–52.

21. Thomas MG, Kumar A, Kohl S, et al. High-resolution in vivo imaging in achromatopsia. Ophthalmology 2011; 118: 882–7.

22. Thomas MG, Kumar A, Mohammad S, et al. Structural grading of foveal hypoplasia using spectral-domain optical coherence tomography a predictor of visual acuity? Ophthalmology 2007; 118: 1653–60.

23. Betts-Henderson J, Bartesaghi S, Crosier M, et al. The nystagmus-associated FRMD7 gene regulates neuronal outgrowth and development. Hum Mol Genet 2011; 19: 342–51.

24. Thomas MG, Crosier M, Lindsay S, et al. The clinical and molecular genetic features of idiopathic infantile periodic alternating nystagmus. Brain 2011; 134: 892–902.

25. Andersen MK, Christoffersen NL, Sander B, et al. Oligocone trichromacy: clinical and molecular genetic investigations. Invest Ophthalmol Vis Sci 2010; 51: 89–95.

26. Gottlob I, Reinecke RD. Eye and head movements in patients with achromatopsia. Graefes Arch Clin Exp Ophthalmol 1994; 232: 392–401.

27. Leigh RJ, Zee DS. The Neurology of Eye Movements, 4th ed. Oxford: Oxford University Press; 2006.

28. Wizov SS, Reinecke RD, Bocarnea M, Gottlob I. A comparative demographic and socioeconomic study of spasmus nutans and infantile nystagmus. Am J Ophthalmol 2002; 133: 256–62.

29. Arnoldi KA, Tychsen L. Prevalence of intracranial lesions in children initially diagnosed with disconjugate nystagmus (spasmus nutans). J Pediatr Ophthalmol Strabismus 1995; 32: 296–301.

30. Gottlob I, Wizov SS, Reinecke RD. Quantitative eye and head movement recordings of retinal disease mimicking spasmus nutans. Am J Ophthalmol 1995; 119: 374–6.

31. Hertle RW. Examination and refractive management of patients with nystagmus. Surv Ophthalmol 2000; 4: 215–22.

32. de Decker W. Kestenbaum transposition in nystagmus therapy: transposition in horizontal and torsional plane. Bull Soc Belge Ophthalmol 1987; 221–222: 107–20.

33. Graf M, Droutsas K, Kaufmann H. Surgery for nystagmus related head turn: Kestenbaum procedure and artificial divergence. Graefes Arch Clin Exp Ophthalmol 2001; 239: 334–41.

34. Lorenz B, Brodsky MC. Pediatric ophthalmology, neuro-ophthalmology, genetics. Strabismus – New Concepts in Pathophysiology, Diagnosis, and Treatment. Berlin, London: Springer; 2010.

35. Zubcov AA, Reinecke RD, Gottlob I, et al. Treatment of manifest latent nystagmus. Am J Ophthalmol 1990; 110: 160–7.

36. Hertle RW, Dell'Osso LF, FitzGibbon EJ, et al. Horizontal rectus tenotomy in patients with congenital nystagmus: results in 10 adults. Ophthalmology 2003; 110: 2097–105.

37. McLean RJ, Gottlob I. The pharmacological treatment of nystagmus: a review. Expert Opin Pharmacother 2009; 10: 1805–16.

38. McLean RJ, Gottlob I, Proudlock FA. What We Know about the Generation of Nystagmus and Other Ocular Oscillations: Are We Closer to Identifying Therapeutic Targets? Curr Neurol Neurosurg 2012; 12: 325–33.

39. Solomon D, Shepard N, Mishra A. Congenital periodic alternating nystagmus: response to baclofen. Ann N Y Acad Sci 2002; 956: 611–5.

40. McLean R, Proudlock F, Thomas S, et al. Congenital nystagmus: randomized, controlled, double-masked trial of memantine/gabapentin. Ann Neurol 2007; 61: 130–8.

41. Carruthers J. The treatment of congenital nystagmus with Botox. J Pediatr Ophthalmol Strabismus 1995; 32: 306–8.

Supranuclear eye movement disorders, acquired and neurologic nystagmus

Richard W Hertle • Nancy N Hanna

Chapter contents

Introduction

Abnormal eye movements in the infant or young child can be congenital or acquired, associated with abnormal early visual development, or a sign of underlying neurologic or neuromuscular disease or orbital disease. Abnormal eye movements in an apparently well child should never be labeled as congenital or benign without careful investigation, including medical history, clinical examination, neuroimaging, laboratory testing, and electrophysiologic investigation of the visual sensory system. Ocular motility analysis can indicate the type of eye movement disturbance and whether this is associated with an underlying ocular or neurologic condition.

Anatomy and physiology (Table 90.1)

Neural integrator

The neural integrator is an engineering term applied to an ocular motor "function" carried out by groups of cells in the cerebellum (flocculus and paraflocculus) and the prepositus hypoglossus and medial vestibular nucleus.[1] The neural integrator is needed for all conjugate eye movements. To move the eyes at a constant speed or hold them in an eccentric gaze position, two neural signals must overcome the elastic tendency of the eyes to go back to their "resting" position. These signals are the desired speed (phasic component) and a tonic component that counterbalances the elastic restoring forces. A

changing tonic component can be precisely generated by a premotor neural signal that mathematically computes the "integration" of the velocity signal, thus the term neural integrator. The role of the neural integrator in generation of saccades and maintenance of eccentric gaze positions occurs after inhibitory burst neurons (IBN) are inhibited and excitatory burst neurons (EBN) fire rapidly, yielding an intense phasic signal that is transmitted to the appropriate yoked pair of extraocular muscles via the appropriate cranial nerves. The "burst" signal is also transmitted to the neural integrator, which "integrates" that burst signal (counts the number of discharge spikes) and generates a neural signal (again transmitted via the cranial nerves) appropriate to hold the eye steady at the new position (tonic discharge).

The neural integrator is not perfect and the "tonic" signal slowly decays or "leaks" over time. This decay is normally not seen in lighted conditions because visual feedback, with the use of the smooth-pursuit/fixation system, aids in holding the eye steady.[2] At birth the neural integrator is leaky but by about 1 month of age it functions well.[3]

Saccadic system

A saccade is a rapid eye movement, which may occur volitionally (voluntary saccade), reflexively, or as part of the fast phases of nystagmus, which serves to purposefully redirect the fovea to a specific target. Voluntary saccades may be predictive command-generated (i.e. look right), memory-guided, and antisaccades. Involuntary saccades include the fast phase of nystagmus, spontaneous saccades, and reflexive saccades. The pathway of saccades proceeds through the anterior limb of the internal capsule and then through the diencephalon. It then divides into dorsal and ventral pathways, the dorsal limb going to the superior colliculi and the ventral limb (which contains the ocular motor pathways for horizontal and vertical eye movements) to the pons and midbrain. The superior colliculus acts as an important relay for some of these projections.[4] In the brainstem, the rostral interstitial nucleus of the medial longitudinal fasciculus (riMLF) and pontine paramedian reticular formation (PPRF) provide the saccadic velocity commands, by generating the "pulse of innervation" immediately

Table 90.1 – Types of eye movements

Type of eye movement	Function	Stimulus	Clinical tests
Vestibular	Maintain steady fixation during head rotation	Head rotation	Fixate on object while moving head; calorics
Saccades	Rapid refixation to eccentric stimuli	Eccentric retinal image	Voluntary movement between two objects; fast phases of OKN or of vestibular nystagmus
Smooth pursuit	Keep moving object on fovea	Retinal image slip	Voluntarily follow a moving target; OKN slow phases
Vergence	Disconjugate, slow movement to maintain binocular vision	Binasal or bitemporal disparity; retinal blur motion	Fusional amplitudes; near point of convergence

OKN = optokinetic nystagmus.

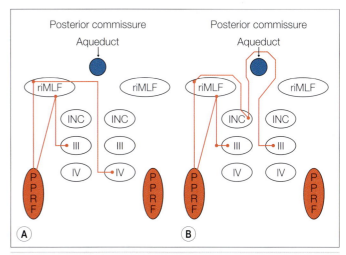

Fig. 90.2 Schematics of brainstem pathways coordinating downward (A) and upward (B) saccades. (A) The PPRF activates neurons in the riMLF that send fibers caudally to synapse upon the inferior rectus subnucleus of the ipsilateral third nerve and the contralateral superior oblique nucleus. Not shown in this diagram, fibers from the contralateral PPRF carry corresponding signals simultaneously. (B) The PPRF activates neurons in the riMLF that send fibers through the posterior commissure to the superior rectus subnucleus of the contralateral third nerve and fibers to the inferior oblique subnucleus of the ipsilateral third nerve. Not shown in this diagram, fibers from the contralateral PPRF carry corresponding signals simultaneously. riMLF = rostral interstitial nucleus of the medial longitudinal fasiculus, INC = interstitial nucleus of Cajal, III = third cranial nerve nucleus, IV = fourth cranial nerve nucleus, PPRF = paramedian pontine reticular formation.

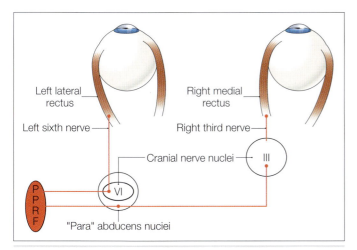

Fig. 90.1 Schematic of brainstem pathways coordinating horizontal saccades. The PPRF, after receiving input from the ipsilateral cortical centers and superior colliculus, stimulates two sets of neurons in the abducens nucleus: (1) those that send axons to innervate the ipsilateral lateral rectus and (2) those whose axons join the MLF and subsequently activate the medial rectus subnuclei of the contralateral third nerve. PPRF = paramedian pontine reticular formation, VI = sixth cranial nerve nuclei, III = third cranial nerve nuclei.

before the eye movement, to cranial nerves III, IV, and VI. Horizontal saccades are generated by EBNs in the PPRF, which are found just ventral and lateral to the MLF in the pons, and by IBN in the nucleus paragigantocellularis dorsalis, caudal to the abducens nucleus in the dorsomedial portion of the rostral medulla (Fig. 90.1). Vertical and torsional components of saccades are generated by EBN and IBN in the riMLF, located in the midbrain[4] (Fig. 90.2).

Following a saccade, a "step of innervation" occurs during which a higher level of tonic innervation to ocular motor neurons keeps the eye in its new position against orbital elastic forces that would restore the eye to an anatomically "neutral"

position in the orbit. For horizontal saccades, the step of innervation comes from the NI, most importantly from the nucleus prepositus-medial vestibular nucleus complex. The eye is held steady at the end of vertical and torsional saccades by the step of innervation provided from the interstitial nucleus of Cajal in the midbrain.[4,5] Other burst neurons termed long-lead burst neurons (LLBNs) discharge 40 ms prior to saccades, whereas EBNs discharge 12 ms prior to saccades. Some LLBNs lie in the midbrain, receiving projections from the superior colliculus and projecting to the pontine EBN, medullary IBN, and OPNs. Other LLBNs lie in the nucleus reticularis tegmenti pontis, projecting mainly to the cerebellum but also to the PPRF. It appears that LLBNs receiving input from the superior colliculus may play a crucial role in transforming spatially coded to temporally coded commands, whereas other LLBNs may synchronize the onset and end of saccades.[4,5]

The saccadic system is not fully developed until about 1 year of age; infants make multiple hypometric saccades to reach the target.[6] If the head is held still, this hypometria can be seen clinically in infants less than 3 months of age, especially for large saccades. There is a progression toward "normometria" during the first 7 months of life.[7] In healthy adults and children older than 1 year, saccades are typically hypometric, reaching about 90% to 100% of the target distance, followed by secondary saccades–normometria. In optokinetic nystagmus (OKN) and vertical nystagmus, quick phases occur less frequently in children than in adults.

Smooth-pursuit system

The function of smooth pursuit (SP) is to hold fixation on a moving target, and both eye and head movements are required.

This requires a prediction to overcome the time delays of the visuomotor system and the ability to suppress the vestibulo-ocular reflex (VOR).[8] VOR suppression is required because, when the head moves, there is a reflexive VOR that moves the eyes equally in the opposite direction. SP and VOR suppression are probably the same ocular motor functions. The frontal and extrastriate visual cortexes transmit information about the motion of both the target and the eyes to the dorsolateral pontine nuclei, thence to the paraflocculus, flocculus, and dorsal vermis, and then via the vestibular and fastigial nuclei to the ocular motor nerve nuclei III, IV, and VI. Unilateral lesions in the cortex and cerebellum affect ipsilateral SP. Brainstem lesions are less well defined clinically.[1]

SP is present in the first week of life but is immature in the young infant. Horizontal gaze probably develops before vertical gaze.[9] SP gain increases with age, and at 5 months the SP is more apparent. It is not known at what point in time pursuit matures to the adult form. It does not appear to happen before 6 months of age, and may not be until late adolescence.[10]

Vestibulo-ocular response system

The vestibular apparatus drives reflex eye movements to keep images steady on the retinas as we move our heads. The eyes move in the opposite direction to the head so that they remain in a steady position in space. The three-neuron arc – vestibular ganglion, vestibular nuclei, and ocular motor nuclei – are the principal connections. The direct neuronal pathways include both excitatory and inhibitory contributions. Each semicircular canal influences a pair of extraocular muscles that move the eyes in the plane of that canal (Table 90.2). The anatomy of the vestibular nuclei has been well characterized;[11] they receive projections from the 14 000 to 18 000 axons of the vestibular nerve.[11]

There are four major vestibular nuclei and accessory subgroups, including the interstitial nucleus, with its cells distributed among the vestibular rootlets as they enter the brainstem, and the y-group, near the superior cerebellar peduncle. The MVN has the greatest volume and is the longest vestibular nucleus. The LVN also has projections to the spinal cord, mainly via the ipsilateral lateral vestibulospinal tract but also through the contralateral medial vestibulospinal tract. In its most rostral aspect the DVN also projects to the ocular motor nuclei.

The primary vestibular afferents enter the medulla at the level of the lateral vestibular nucleus. Almost all bifurcate, giving a descending branch to terminate in the MVN and DVN and an ascending branch to the SVN, with a final destination in the cerebellum, especially the anterior vermis and the nodulus and uvula. All canals and otoliths project to the borders of ventromedial LVN, medial MVN, and dorsomedial DVN. All canals also converge on a small patch in the ventromedial SVN. Utricular afferents project to the rostral MVN and saccular afferents project to the y-group. For both the horizontal and vertical VOR, many neurons in the vestibular nuclei that receive inputs from primary vestibular afferents encode head velocity, eye position, and varying amounts of SP and saccadic signals. Vestibular nuclei neurons do not project just to motor neurons; they also send collaterals to the nucleus prepositus hypoglossi, the nucleus of Roller, and the cell groups of the paramedian tracts.[11]

When testing the VOR in the infant it is not unusual to find a slightly high VOR gain, which gradually decreases during preschool years, and a short VOR time constant.[12] In the premature infant and in some healthy full-term infants, rotation induces a tonic deviation or "locking up." The eyes deviate in the direction opposite to rotation when the doll's head maneuver or the Barany chair rotation test is used. They deviate in the same direction as the rotation when the infant is rotated at arm's length. A "corrective" fast phase develops at approximately 45 weeks postconceptual age.[6] This lock up may be prolonged in the infant with delayed visual maturation. Usually there is no more than a couple of beats of postrotational nystagmus when the child stops spinning; if there are more than a few beats of nystagmus, a severe visual deficit, or abnormality of the SP pathway, should be suspected.[13] This test can be influenced by behavioral state and wakefulness.

Vergence system

Vergences are eye movements that turn the eyes in opposite directions so that images of objects will fall on corresponding retinal points. In other words, it is the ability to change the angle between the two visual axes to permit near

Table 90.2 – Effect of stimulating a single semicircular canal

Canal	Head movement	Eye movement in		Agonist		Antagonist	
		R gaze	L gaze	R	L	R	L
R Post	R and up	L Tors	Down	SO	IR	IO	SR
R Ant	R and down	Up	L Tors	SR	IO	IR	SO
R Lat	R	L	L	MR	LR	LR	MR
L Post	L and up	Down	R Tors	IR	SO	SR	IO
L Ant	L and down	L Tors	Up	IO	SR	SO	IR
L Lat	L	R	R	LR	MR	MR	LR

Based on R. John Leigh and David S Zee, The Neurology of Eye Movements, 2006, Oxford University Press.
R = right, L = left, Post = posterior, Ant = anterior, Lat = lateral (horizontal canal), Tors = torsional (cyclotorsion with upper poles of eyes moving to subject's right/left), SO = superior oblique, IO = inferior oblique, IR = inferior rectus, SR = superior rectus, MR = medial rectus, LR = lateral rectus.

(convergence), far (divergence), and torsional (cyclovergence) foveation, for binocular vision. Three major stimuli are known to elicit vergences: (1) retinal disparity that leads to fusional vergences; (2) retinal blur that evokes accommodative vergences; and (3) motion induces both disparity and accommodative vergence. The neural substrate for vergence lies in the mesencephalic reticular formation, dorsolateral to the oculomotor nucleus where neurons discharge in relation to vergence angle (vergence tonic cells), velocity (vergence burst cells), or both angle and velocity (vergence burst-tonic cells). Although most of these neurons also discharge with accommodation, some remain predominantly related to vergence.[2,14] Like versional movements, a velocity-to-position integration of vergence signals is necessary: the nucleus reticularis tegmenti pontis (NRTP) is important in this integration. The cells in NRTP that mediate the near response are separate from cells that mediate the far response. Lesions of NRTP cause inability to hold a steady vergence angle. NRTP has reciprocal connection with the cerebellum (nucleus interpositus) and receives descending projections from several cortical and subcortical structures.[2,14]

The eyes of neonates, particularly if premature, often appear divergent, and there is little voluntary convergence until 2–3 months. By 3 to 6 months of age, 75% of premature and 97% of full-term infants have no deviation.[9] Fusion is not completely established until 6 months. Accommodation-driven vergence can be detected at 2 months of age and disparity-driven vergence at about 4 months, which is when stereopsis and fusion develop.

Optokinetic system

The optokinetic system is responsible for conjugate slow following of the eyes to movement of large areas of the visual field. Optokinetic nystagmus (OKN) is a reflex conjugate physiologic nystagmus in which a slow-phase pursuit response to movement of the visual surround (optokinesis) is followed by a corrective saccade or quick phase. OKN is elicited naturally during head and eye movements, or unnaturally by looking out of the window of a moving vehicle. Together with the vestibular system, the optokinetic system holds images steadily on the retina during sustained motion of the head or world or both. The neural substrate for optokinesis includes the nucleus of the optic tract and accessory optic pathways. Optokinesis can be elicited by either full-field (natural head or eye movements) or small field (foveal) motion (a moving drum or tape). Both SP and optokinetic systems contribute to the stabilization of images of stationary objects during head rotations. In primates, OKN has two components, each of which has a separate but parallel neural pathway[11] Delayed (indirect, slow) OKN (OKNd) has a slow buildup (tens of seconds) and gives rise to optokinetic after-nystagmus (OKAN), which is a gradual decay of the nystagmus after the lights have been extinguished. OKNd is closely related to VOR and is driven by visual motion signals in the visual cortex via the nucleus of the optic tract in the pretectum and the vestibular nuclei.[15] Early (direct, fast) OKN (OKNe) has a rapid buildup (<1 s) and does not give rise to OKAN; it ceases promptly in the dark. The OKNe pathway is similar to the SP pathway, which is mediated by a corticopontocerebellar route, and it is doubtful that the pretectum has a direct role in OKNe/SP, although it may be involved in its adaptive control.[15]

Finally, the cerebellum plays an important role in eye movements. Together with several brainstem structures, including the nucleus prepositus and the medial vestibular nucleus, it appears to convert velocity signals to position signals for all conjugate eye movements through mathematical integration.

Clinical assessment

General patient investigations

The workup of supranuclear eye movement disorders and nystagmus is directed toward identifying associated ophthalmic and neurologic features with which, if found, the etiology is usually apparent by history, examination, or neuroimaging.

General examination

The history and physical examination determines whether the nystagmus has been present from early or acquired later. A family history of neonatal eye disease, the pregnancy, labor, delivery, and growth and development since birth should be sought. Neonatal forms are generally benign, while acquired forms require further investigation. Since anxiety can affect nystagmus, the eye movements should be observed at a comfortable distance, in a non-threatening manner, while talking to the child or the parent. The most important features of nystagmus can usually be ascertained while "playing" with the child. Head turns or tilts while the child is viewing distant or near objects should be noted. An adequate fundus examination is a necessary part of the evaluation of eye movement disorders and involuntary ocular oscillations in infants and children (Figs 90.4 and 90.5).

Vision testing

Subjective accuracy of vision testing depends on the patient's age and their neurologic status. The "binocular acuity" should be tested first. The patient must be allowed to assume any anomalous head posture (AHP). During the examination of visual acuity in nystagmus patients with an AHP the direction of the posture must be observed over a 5- to 7-minute period. Up to 17% of patients with infantile nystagmus and some forms of acquired nystagmus have a periodicity to the direction of their fast phase with a changing head posture.

Binocular acuity is the "person's" acuity and monocular acuity is the "eye's" acuity; they are often very different in patients with nystagmus. In a non-verbal child or adult, various tests can be used to help determine both binocular and monocular acuity. These include fixation behavior, the 10-prism-diopter base-down test, Teller acuity cards, and matching of single, surrounded, HOTV optotypes or Lea symbols. Simple testing of binocular function is always attempted as the results are important if convergence is to be stimulated or fusion is to be aided by refractive therapy, e.g. Worth 4-dot and near stereopsis.

Refraction

In older children a subjective refraction is the foundation for any type of refractive therapy. All refractionists develop their own idiosyncrasies that assist them with rapid and accurate refraction. Try to ignore the oscillation and start with the distance retinoscopy in a phoropter in those patients without an AHP or trial frame (in those with a significant AHP). The next step is to do binocular refraction: this is the most important step in these patients because some patients have significant changes in their nystagmus under monocular conditions. The best way to do this is to fog the eye not being refracted with enough extra plus to decrease the vision 1–3 lines.

It is important in infants and young children to perform an objective refraction procedure; a cycloplegic refraction provides additional and important data for treatment decisions. In those patients in whom there is a different refraction under cycloplegia, record both subjective and objective refraction for decision making regarding spectacle prescription.

Ocular motility evaluation

Clinical evaluation of the ocular oscillation includes fast phase direction, movement intensity, conjugacy, gaze effects, convergence effects, and effect of monocular cover. The amplitude, frequency, and direction of the nystagmus in all directions of gaze can be documented with a simple diagram (Fig. 90.5). The clinician can also observe the nystagmus while moving the patient's head. Associated motility systems (e.g. strabismus, pursuit, saccades, and VOR) can be clinically evaluated and recorded. Changes in the nystagmus with convergence or monocular viewing should be noted. If the nystagmus increases beneath closed eyelids, vestibular or brainstem pathology should be suspected since visual fixation may suppress nystagmus from lesions in these regions. Conjugacy of eye movements should be observed.

Ocular motility recordings

Eye movement recordings provide a basis for eye movement abnormality classification, etiology, and treatment and have impacted on eye movement systems research (Figs 90.6 and 90.7). There are four commonly used methods:

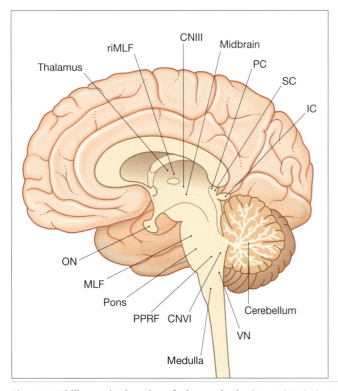

Fig. 90.3 Midline sagittal section of a human brain. Sites within the brain responsible for the "localizing" forms of acquired nystagmus.

- Electro-oculography.
- Infrared reflectance oculography.
- Scleral contact lens/magnetic search coils. This is the most sensitive technique and is minimally invasive, but its use in children between 6 months and about 10 years is unpredictable (Figs 90.6 and 90.7).
- Video oculography.

Practical applications of eye movement recording technology in clinical medicine include diagnosis/differentiation of eye movement disorders and utility as an "outcome measure" in clinical research.[16,17] Eye movement recordings display the data during continuous periods of time. Position and velocity traces are clearly marked with up being rightward or upward eye movements and down being leftward or downward eye movements. The basic types of nystagmus patterns observed after eye movement recordings are shown in Figure 90.8.

Specific system evaluation

Neural integrator

To test the neural integrator clinically, observe primary position fixation, fixation in eccentric gaze, saccades, pursuit, and OKN and also test for rebound nystagmus and VOR cancellation. To examine for rebound nystagmus, first ask the patient to fixate on a target from the primary position, then to refixate on an eccentric target for 30 s, and then return to the primary position target. A patient with rebound nystagmus shows transient nystagmus with the slow phases toward the previous gaze position. To evaluate a child's VOR cancellation, it is easiest to place your hand on top of the patient's head to control both the head and a fixation target that will extend in front of the child's visual axis. If the child is unable to cancel the VOR, you will observe nystagmus instead of the steady fixation expected in normal subjects.

"Gaze-evoked" nystagmus is a sign of a leaky neural integrator and occurs with attempts to maintain eccentric gaze. These "beats" of nystagmus toward the eccentric position persist as long as the child attempts to view a peripherally placed target. This is different to physiologic endpoint nystagmus where only a few beats of nystagmus, gradually decreasing in amplitude, are present while viewing eccentrically placed targets.

Saccades

If an abnormality of saccadic eye movements is suspected, the quick phases of vestibular and OKN can be easily evaluated in infants and young children. To produce and observe vestibular nystagmus, hold the infant at arm's length, maintain eye contact, and spin first in one direction and then in the other (Fig. 90.9A,B). An OKN response can be elicited in the usual manner by passing a repetitive stimulus, such as stripes or an OKN drum, in front of the baby first in one direction and then in another (Fig. 90.9C). In addition, reflex saccades will be induced in many young patients when toys or other interesting stimuli are introduced into the visual field. Older children are asked to fixate alternately upon two targets so that the examiner can closely observe the saccades for promptness of initiation, speed, and accuracy (Fig. 90.10). However, do not confuse a saccade toward sound as a visually guided saccade in a child with poor vision; it should first be established that the child can see. In children with strabismus it is necessary to test saccades monocularly. The OKN drum/tape or the VOR

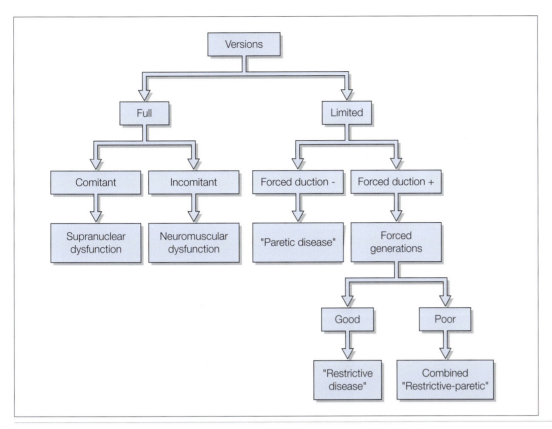

Fig. 90.4 Clinical evaluation of range of eye movements. Versions and cover test measurements allow the examiner to decide whether the eye movements are normal (no limitation) or limited. Forced duction testing is used to differentiate a restriction (positive resistance to movement of the globe) from a "paresis" (no resistance to movement of the globe).

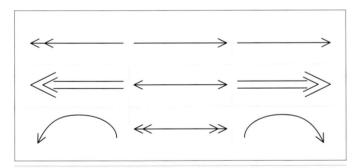

Fig. 90.5 Diagram of nystagmus in nine positions of gaze. Arrowheads indicate direction of jerk fast phase if on one end, pendular nystagmus if on both ends, and increasing frequency with more arrowheads. Additional lines indicate increased nystagmus amplitude. The curved lines indicate torsional nystagmus.

response can also be used to assess saccadic function. It is sometimes easier to observe the eyelashes moving vertically while testing vertical saccades using a vertically rotating OKN drum (Fig. 90.9C).

Smooth pursuit and vestibulo-ocular response systems

SP is tested by having the child follow a slow-moving easily seen target (e.g. a brightly colored toy or mirror), both horizontally and vertically. The child's head should initially be kept still. If the child is uncooperative or is thought to have hysterical blindness, a mirror should be slowly rotated before his/her eyes, or an OKN drum or tape can be used. When examining the pursuit system, one should always include an assessment of VOR suppression, which is an essential component of the SP task during motion. In the older child, VOR suppression can be examined by asking the child to hold his/her finger about 6–8 cms in front of their face. The child is then asked to slowly rotate his/her head with their finger from left to right while maintaining fixation on their finger. If the VOR response is suppressed there is no movement of the eyes relative to the head. Failure of VOR suppression results in a jerk nystagmus beating in the direction of the rotation. In an infant or young child you can test VOR suppression by holding the child in outstretched arms and spinning in both clockwise and counterclockwise directions, while encouraging the child to fix on your face.

Vergence system

Vergence is usually tested by objective tests such as cover/uncover testing, alternate cover testing, prisms in front of the eye, and manual tests of near point of accommodation and vergence. Subjective aspects of vergence are tested by measuring the child's ability to perceive stereopsis. Many of these tests are dependent on the child's ability to cooperate but alternate cover testing can be performed as soon as the child is able to fix on a near object.

Optokinetic system

Both slow and fast phases of OKN can be elicited by using OKN drum, tape, or full-field OKN stimuli (Fig. 90.9C). OKN responses are observed with both eyes open in the full-term

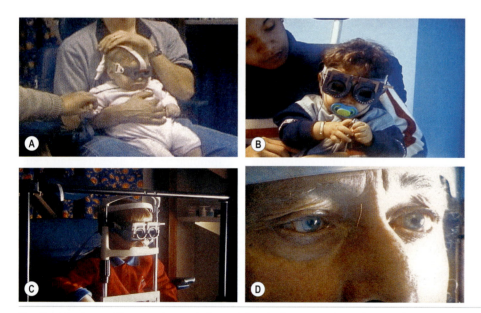

Fig. 90.6 Ocular motility recording equipment. Ocular motor laboratory showing infrared reflectance goggles (front (A), back (B)), silicone contact lens (C), flexible exam chair, chin rest, and stimulus screen (D).

Fig. 90.7 Ocular motility recording techniques. Infrared reflectance performed on an infant (A), toddler (B) and a young child (C), and scleral search coil recordings performed on an adult (D).

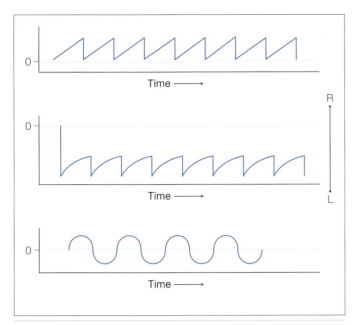

Fig. 90.8 Ocular oscillations. Artist's representation of major types of nystagmus waveforms. Continuous periods of time are depicted in each tracing. Rightward eye movements are up and leftward eye movements are down.

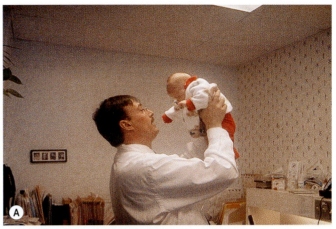
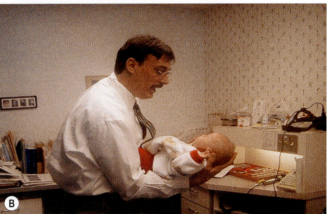
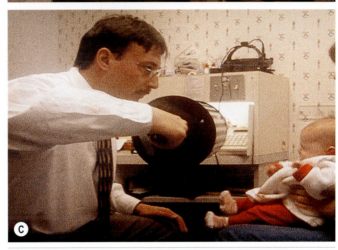

Fig. 90.9 Clinical evaluation of infant eye movements. The child is rotated in the examiner's arms in the vertical (A) and horizontal (B) planes to test the vestibulo-ocular, optokinetic, and saccadic systems. (C) An optokinetic drum is rotated close to the child in the vertical direction to assess visual fixation and saccadic and optokinetic functions.

infant on the first day of life.[18] In healthy neonates, a monocular OKN response can be obtained when the stimulus is moved in the temporal-to-nasal direction, but not in the nasal-to-temporal direction (physiologic/developmental, monocular OKN asymmetry). After 3 months, this monocular OKN asymmetry declines for moderate stimulus speeds, but persists beyond 6 months of age at high stimulus speeds.

Disorders of supranuclear eye movements

Neural integrator

Neural integrator dysfunction

Neural integrator dysfunction manifests clinically as gaze-evoked nystagmus and is often associated with low pursuit gain (gaze-holding deficiency nystagmus, eccentric gaze nystagmus) and rebound nystagmus. Quick phases are away from the central position (Fig. 90.8). Neurologic signs and symptoms include vertigo, nausea, dizziness, and oscillopsia. Gaze-evoked nystagmus is induced by moving the eye into lateral or vertical gaze, with sustained attempts to look eccentrically (Fig. 90.11). After the eyes are then returned to the central position, a short-lived nystagmus with quick phases opposite to the direction of the prior eccentric gaze occurs (rebound nystagmus). Abnormal suppression of the VOR and low-gain OKN responses are also associated clinical findings and, again, probably reflect cerebellar disease[19,20] (Fig. 90.11).

Most types of pathologic nystagmus increase their intensity as the eyes move in the direction of the fast phase (Alexander's law); this is believed to be due to a physiologically adapted "leaky" neural integrator responding to the pathologic vestibular imbalance that is part of the nystagmus.[19,20]

Most frequently, gaze-holding deficiency nystagmus is seen in conjunction with use of anticonvulsants and sedatives, cerebellar and brainstem disease, or other drug intoxication. MRI/CT scan of brain reflects underlying disease and ocular motility recordings show slow phases that have decelerating velocity characteristics.[19,20] Acquired eye movement abnormalities suggesting defective neural integration, whether isolated or associated with other neurologic deficits, alert the examiner to

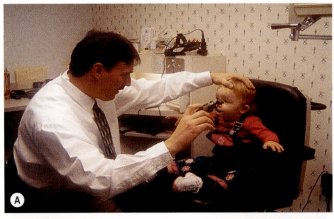

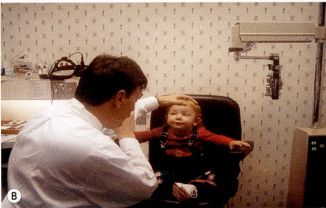

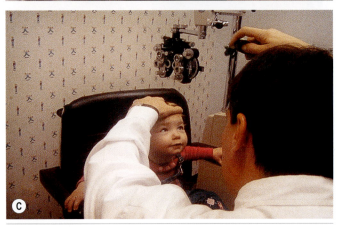

Fig. 90.10 Clinical evaluation of child voluntary saccadic eye movements. The child is seated while the head is held steady and targets are placed in the peripheral visual field horizontally (A,B) and vertically (C).

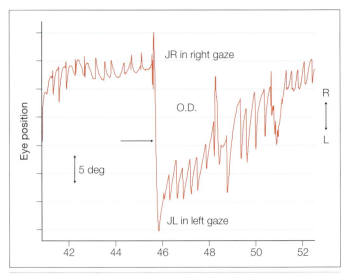

Fig. 90.11 Ocular motility recording of gaze-evoked nystagmus. This is a typical 10 s position trace of ocular motor recordings from a patient with gaze-evoked nystagmus. Right gaze shows jerk right with linear/decreasing velocity slow phases while left gaze shows jerk left with linear and decreasing velocity slow phases. The horizontal arrow points to where the patient's gaze shifted from right 15° to left 15°. O.D. = right eye, R = rightward eye movements and right gaze, L = leftward eye movements and left gaze, deg = degree, JR = jerk right nystagmus, JL = jerk left nystagmus.

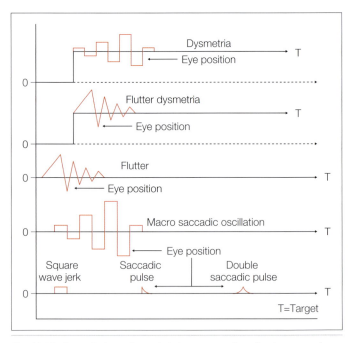

Fig. 90.12 Saccadic intrusions. Artist's representation of major types of saccadic instabilities and their ocular motor characteristics. Continuous periods of time are depicted in each tracing. Rightward eye movements are up and leftward eye movements are down. 0 = primary position fixation, T = target.

investigate for a serious central nervous system (CNS) abnormality. Structural anomalies affecting the brainstem and cerebellum, e.g. the Arnold-Chiari malformation, as well as metabolic, vascular, and neurodegenerative disorders may also produce abnormalities of the neural integrator.

Disorders of saccades

Saccadic accuracy

Normal and abnormal saccades are often dysmetric (inaccurate). Saccadic inaccuracy can be a result of gain dysmetria or pulse-step dysmetria. In saccadic dysmetria, the saccade misses the target and corrective saccades are needed for foveation (Fig. 90.12). If the saccades fall short of the target, they are known as hypometric; if they overshoot the target, they are hypermetric. In both cases, one or more secondary saccades are needed to eventually fixate the target. Hypometria is often seen in cerebellar disease, including autosomal dominant spinocerebellar ataxia type 3, and ocular motor apraxia (OMA). It is far more common than hypermetria. Consistent marked hypometria below 90% that persists beyond 7 months of age suggests neurologic disease. Hypometric saccades can be secondary to changes in visual magnification; for example, the removal of aphakic spectacles may lead to a temporary hypometria until adaptation takes place.[21]

Hypermetria is much less common and appears flutter-like (but should not be mistaken for ocular flutter). With the exclusion of centripetal saccades, hypermetria is abnormal at any age, and, when conjugate, it is almost always associated with cerebellar disease, including spinocerebellar ataxia type 1. If hypermetria is severe, the corrective saccade may be as large as the primary saccade, thus causing the eyes to oscillate back and forth with saccades. This phenomenon has been termed macrosaccadic oscillations. After recovery of opsoclonus, there may be persistent hypermetric saccades (Fig. 90.12).[22,23]

Saccadic velocity

Slow saccades may not be obvious clinically, especially in children. They may result from an abnormality involving the paramedian pontine reticular formation and have been thought to be pathognomonic of burst cell dysfunction. Slow saccades may be seen in mitochondrial disorders, progressive external ophthalmoplegia, myasthenia gravis, basal ganglia disease, Duane syndrome, and families with spinocerebellar ataxia type 2. Slow horizontal and sometimes vertical saccades may occur in patients with Gaucher type 3 disease.[24]

Saccadic latency

The time between the onset of a stimulus and the beginning of a saccade in healthy infants is up to about 1 s (about 200 ms in adults). In childhood, prolonged saccade latencies usually occur in association with saccade initiation failure.

Saccade initiation failure/ocular motor apraxia

The term saccade initiation failure (SIF) or ocular motor apraxia (OMA) is used to specify impaired voluntary saccades and variable deficit of fast phase saccades during vestibular or OKN.[24] Congenital OMA is characterized by defective horizontal saccades, but it does not represent a true apraxia since reflex saccades may also be impaired.[25]

Patients with congenital SIF show abnormal initiation and decreased amplitude of voluntary saccades; saccadic velocities in these patients are normal and fast phases of nystagmus of large amplitude can occasionally be generated. This suggests that the brainstem burst neurons that generate saccades are intact.[24,26] Acquired SIF may be due to conditions as listed in Table 90.3. Some of these patients with the acquired type, such as those with Gaucher's disease (types 1 and some type 3 patients), have abnormal saccadic velocities.[41] Although the exact cause or localization of the defect in congenital SIF has not been determined, there is strong evidence that most can be localized subtentorially, particularly to the cerebellar vermis.[24,26]

Affected infants and children with poor head control are commonly thought to be blind since the expected refixations are not observed. In such an infant demonstration of vertical saccades, vertical pursuit, OKN response in any direction, and normal acuity on visual-evoked response testing suggests the diagnosis of SIF. Another clinical sign in young infants is an intermittent tonic deviation of the eyes in the direction of

Table 90.3 – Congenital and acquired saccade initiation failure

Classification by cause	Specific etiologies
Idiopathic	
Perinatal problems	Cerebral palsy; hypoxia; hydrocephalus; seizures
Congenital malformations	Agenesis of corpus callosum; fourth ventricle dilation, and vermis hypoplasia; Joubert's syndrome; macrocerebellum; dysgenesis of cerebellar vermis and midbrain; Dandy-Walker malformation; immature development of putamen; heterotropia of gray matter; porencephalic cyst; hamartoma near foramen of Munro; macrocephaly; microcephaly; posterior fossa cysts; chondrodystrophic dwarfism and hydrocephalus; encephalocele; occipital meningocele; COACH syndrome (cerebellar vermis hypoplasia, oligophrenia, congenital ataxia, coloboma, hepatic fibrocirrhosis)
Neurodegenerative conditions with infantile onset of SIF	Infantile Gaucher's disease (types 2 and 3); Gaucher's disease type 2; Pelizaeus-Merbacher disease; Krabbe's leukodystrophy; propionic acidemia; GM1 gangliosidosis; infantile Refsum's disease; 4-hydroxybutyric aciduria
Neurodegenerative conditions with later onset of SIF	Ataxia telangiectasia; spinocerebellar degenerations; juvenile Gaucher's disease (type 3); Huntington's disease; Hallervorden-Spatz disease; Wilson's disease
Acquired disease	Postimmunization encephalopathy; herpes encephalitis; posterior fossa tumors
Other associations	Alagille syndrome; Bardet-Biedl syndrome; carotid fibromuscular hypoplasia; Cockayne's syndrome; Cornelia de Lange syndrome; juvenile nephronophthisis; Lowe's syndrome; neurofibromatosis type I; orofacial digital syndrome; X-linked muscle atrophy with congenital contractures

Adapted from Cassidy L, Taylor D, Harris C. Abnormal supranuclear eye movements in the child: a practical guide to examination and interpretation. Surv Ophthalmol 2000; 44: 479–506.

slow-phase vestibular or OKN; in these infants fast phase saccades may be impaired.

By 4 to 8 months of age, the child develops a striking "head thrusting" behavior in order to refixate. First, the eyelids blink ("synkinetic blink") and the head begins to rotate toward the object of interest (Figs 90.13 and 90.14). Next, the head continues to rotate past the intended target allowing the tonically deviated eyes, which are now in an extreme contraversive position, to come into alignment with the target. Finally, as the eyes maintain fixation, the head rotates slowly back so that the eyes are in primary position. This apparent use of the VOR to refixate continues for several years, but with increasing age, patients demonstrate less prominent head thrusting and may even be able to generate some saccades though they are abnormal. The blink-saccade synkinesis adaptation may persist.

In some infants, generalized hypotonia may be associated.[27]

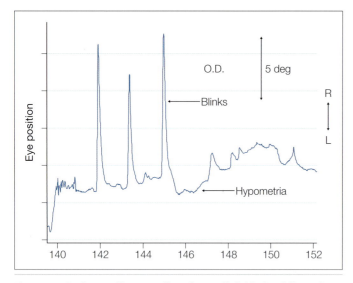

Fig. 90.13 Ocular motility recording of saccadic initiation failure. This is a 12 s position trace of ocular motor recordings from a patient with saccadic initiation failure. "Synkinetic" blinks are followed by hypometric saccades. O.D. = right eye, R = rightward eye movements and right gaze, L = leftward eye movements and left gaze, deg = degree.

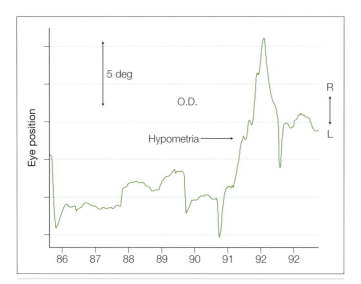

Fig. 90.14 Ocular motility recording of saccadic initiation failure. This is an 8 s position trace of ocular motor recordings from a patient with saccadic initiation failure. Multiple hypometric ("staircase") saccades are illustrated. O.D. = right eye, R = rightward eye movements and right gaze, L = leftward eye movements and left gaze, deg = degree.

A brain MRI is necessary for suspected neurologic disorders, to look for midline malformations, particularly around the fourth ventricle and cerebellar vermis.

Gaucher's disease, ataxia telangiectasia and its variants, and Niemann-Pick variants may also present with the inability to generate saccades as well as blinking and head thrusting prior to refixation. Unlike SIF, these disorders generally involve vertical as well as horizontal saccades and eventually manifest systemic signs.

The prognosis of the congenital type is good. Many adapt to allow gaze shifts with less head thrusting and can generate some saccades, albeit abnormal. There is no treatment for SIF,

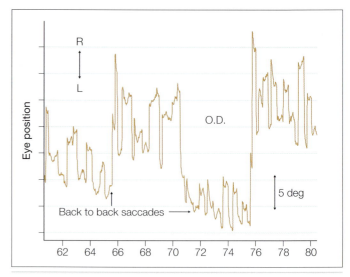

Fig. 90.15 Ocular motility recording of flutter and saccadic oscillations. This is a typical 18 s position trace of ocular motor recordings from a patient with ocular flutter. Back to back saccades with (macro-sacccadic oscillations) and without (flutter) an intersaccadic interval, both interrupting fixation and occurring on refixation are demonstrated (arrows). O.D. = right eye, R = rightward eye movements and right gaze, L = leftward eye movements and left gaze, deg = degree.

but children who have this condition should be investigated appropriately and recognized as having learning and living difficulties, and they should receive extra help and other educational benefits at school. Whether the condition improves with age is not known; any apparent improvement may be a result of the improvement of the adaptive strategies these children use to enable rapid shifts of gaze.

Opsoclonus/ocular flutter

Opsoclonus, also referred to as "saccadomania" or dancing eyes, is a rare, but striking saccade disorder, characterized by intermittent involuntary bursts of wild conjugate multidirectional back to back saccades.[23] When the eye movement is purely horizontal, it is known as ocular flutter (Fig. 90.15). During resolution, opsoclonus may revert to ocular flutter, and finally saccadic dysmetria, before eventually reverting to normal eye movements. Opsoclonus is often triggered by attempted fixation, SP, convergence, up-gaze, eyelid closure, or OKN or vestibular nystagmus. The frequency is high, usually ranging between 5 and 13 Hz, and the amplitude can be tens of degrees, although it may be so small that the oscillations cannot be seen without a slit-lamp, ophthalmoscope, or eye movement recordings (Figs 90.16 and 90.17). Opsoclonus usually persists during sleep, although it may be diminished or even absent.[23] Acquired opsoclonus is often associated with limb myoclonus. In such cases, it is described as opsoclonus–myoclonus, dancing eye–dancing feet syndrome, myoclonic encephalopathy of infants, or infantile polymyoclonia.[23] The opsoclonus–myoclonus syndrome is more common in children.[23]

Onset may be acute or subacute and is often accompanied by ataxia, vomiting, and irritability. It may be a manifestation of occult malignancies, in particular neural crest tumors (neuroblastoma, ganglioneuroblastoma, ganglioneuroma), hepatoblastoma, infection (Coxsackie B, HIV, mumps, parainfluenza

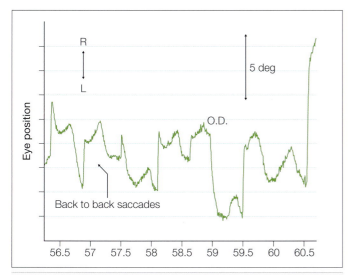

Fig. 90.16 Ocular motility recording of opsoclonus. This is a typical 4 s position trace of ocular motor recordings from a patient with opsoclonus. High-frequency back to back saccades without (flutter) an intersaccadic interval are demonstrated (arrows). O.D. = right eye, R = rightward eye movements and right gaze, L = leftward eye movements and left gaze, deg = degree.

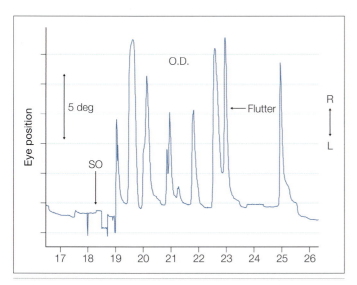

Fig. 90.17 Ocular motility recording of opsoclonus + saccadic intrusions. This is a 10 s position trace of ocular motor recordings from a patient with opsoclonus and saccadic oscillations. Small amplitude back to back saccades with an intersaccadic interval are followed by large amplitude back to back saccades without an intersaccadic interval (flutter). SO = saccadic oscillation, O.D. = right eye, R = rightward eye movements and right gaze, L = leftward eye movements and left gaze, deg = degree.

virus, psittacosis, salmonella, syphilis, St. Louis encephalitis, rickettsia, enterovirus, Epstein-Barr virus infection), toxic (amitriptyline, cocaine, diazepam, lithium, and phenytoin), or metabolic disorders (biotin-responsive multiple carboxylase deficiency, hyperosmolar non-ketotic coma).[6]

In children with neural crest tumors or brainstem encephalitis, opsoclonus is commonly accompanied by diffuse or focal myoclonus. Although opsoclonus–myoclonus is rarely a presenting feature of neuroblastoma, it is seen in about 50% of children with an occult neuroblastoma, and the presence of

opsoclonus confers a favorable survival rate.[28] Paraneoplastic opsoclonus is associated with a single copy of the N-*myc* oncogene, and those children with amplification of this oncogene who do not develop opsoclonus and carry a worse prognosis.[29] It is hypothesized that in paraneoplastic opsoclonus, the tumor and some CNS structures share an epitope, and that this common epitope triggers an immune response against the tumor and the CNS, resulting in the neurologic symptoms.[29]

Opsoclonus may be mistaken for nystagmus and vice versa. Formal eye movement recordings will differentiate the two, demonstrating that opsoclonus is a burst of back to back saccades with no intersaccadic interval, without the slow phases of nystagmus (Figs 90.15–90.17). However, on rare occasions there may be a constant high-frequency acquired pendular nystagmus. Once opsoclonus has been confirmed, children should be screened for urinary vanillylmandelic acid (VMA) and homovanillic acid (HVA) and have an oncologic workup. This may include chest and abdominal CT and/or MRI. Elevated levels of urinary VMA and HVA are diagnostic; however, normal levels occur in 26% of children with paraneoplastic opsoclonus.[29] Blood and cerebrospinal fluid (CSF) samples should also be taken and sent for virology and bacteriology. CSF pleocytosis has been reported in children with paraneoplastic opsoclonus and there are occasional oligoclonal bands. There have been occasional reports of autoantibodies, including anti-Hu and antibodies against neurofilaments, in the sera of children with paraneoplastic opsoclonus.

Acquired opsoclonus is probably immune-mediated. Its neural substrate remains a mystery, and there may be no single site involved in the causation of opsoclonus.

Opsoclonus–myoclonus, especially when it occurs with brainstem encephalitis, may be a benign self-limiting condition. Although children with paraneoplastic opsoclonus tend to have a better oncologic prognosis, the neurologic outcome is unpredictable. Children who have become cancer free may have significant neurologic sequelae. Adrenocorticotrophic hormone or systemic steroid treatment has a dramatic short-term effect on symptoms in 50% to 90% of children with opsoclonus.[30] However, not all children have such a good response, and the opsoclonus and ataxia may become steroid-dependent, re-emerging when treatment is tapered or during intercurrent illnesses. Other drugs used to treat opsoclonus–myoclonus include intravenous IgG, azathioprine, propranolol, and divalproex sodium. A combination of systemic steroids and high-dose immunoglobulin can be used for the treatment of opsoclonus–myoclonus in patients who do not respond to first-line therapy with steroids.

Regardless of the short-term response, these children often have long-term developmental problems, including speech, motor, and cognitive disabilities.[43] Abnormal eye movements may persist. Parents, teachers, and carers should be informed of such problems. Occupational therapists, psychologists, and social services should be involved at an early stage.

Antisaccades

An antisaccade requires the subject to suppress a reflexive saccade to an abruptly appearing peripheral target, and generate a voluntary saccade in the equidistant but opposite direction. The ability to suppress reflexive responses in favor of voluntary motor actions is necessary in everyday life, and both of these abilities can be assessed with use of the antisaccade task. The correct execution of an antisaccade requires at least two functioning subprocesses: an intact fixation system and the ability to generate a voluntary saccade in the opposite direction. Infants as young as 4 months have a fixation system adequate to allow inhibition of reflex saccades, but the ability to generate a voluntary antisaccade develops much later, usually over 10 years old, with a steep decrease in the mean error rate from 10 to 15 years, then a more gradual decrease toward 20 years.[31] Difficulty in making antisaccades has also been described in people with schizophrenia, children with attention deficit hyperactivity disorder, autosomal dominant cerebellar ataxia type 2, male dyslexics, and Tourette syndrome.[32]

Saccadic intrusions and oscillations

There are saccadic eye movements that may intrude on steady primary position fixation or interrupt refixation and, hence, mimic nystagmus (Figs 90.12, 90.17, and 90.18). Saccadic intrusions (SIs) must be differentiated from nystagmus, in which a drift of the eyes from the desired position of gaze is the primary abnormality, and from saccadic dysmetria, in which the eye over- or under-shoots a target, sometimes several times, before achieving stable fixation. Only eye movement recordings can definitively distinguish SIs and saccadic oscillations (SOs) from nystagmus.

Square wave jerks consist of a conjugate displacement of the eyes up to 5° from fixation, followed by a refixational saccade after a normal intersaccadic interval of 200 ms. They are seen in normal healthy subjects of any age. However, if they are more frequent (more than nine square wave jerks per minute in a young person should be considered abnormal), they are referred to as square wave oscillations, and are seen in cerebellar disease, progressive supranuclear palsy, and multiple sclerosis.[33] Square wave jerks and oscillations are rarely seen in childhood (Fig. 90.18).

Macro-square wave jerks are also rare in childhood. They consist of conjugate displacement of the eyes away from fixation by more than 5°, and, after a shorter than normal latency of 80 ms, there is a refixation saccade. They occur in bursts and may be mistaken for flutter. The amplitude is variable, and they are present in the dark. They occur in diseases that disrupt cerebellar outflow, i.e. multiple sclerosis or olivopontocerebellar degenerations, including Huntington's disease.[33]

Macrosaccadic oscillations represent a severe form of saccadic hypermetria. They are characterized by conjugate oscillations of the eyes around fixation, with a normal intersaccadic interval of 200 ms. The oscillations increase and then decrease in amplitude during each episode. They are a result of lesions affecting the midline cerebellum and underlying nuclei. They are not present in darkness.

Disorders of smooth pursuit

Smooth-pursuit asymmetry–initiation failure

Monocular SP asymmetries may persist in patients with early-onset, but not with late-onset, strabismus. Impaired SP to the side of the lesion has been most frequently reported in patients with lesions restricted to the posterior cortical areas and underlying white matter, but it also occurs with frontal lobe lesions and in hemidecortication. Ipsilateral pursuit deficit may also be seen in unilateral lesions of the lower portions of the pursuit pathway, including the thalamus, midbrain tegmentum, dorsolateral pontine nucleus, and cerebellum. Nuclear vestibular lesions may affect either ipsilateral or contralateral SP.[34]

Abnormal smooth pursuit gain

Low pursuit gain, which may be seen clinically as saccadic or jerky pursuits, occurs in the elderly and in patients with basal ganglia disease, and cerebellar disease, large cerebral lesions, or posterior cortical lesions. Low pursuit gain has been described in spinocerebellar ataxia types 1 and 3. If gaze-holding deficiency nystagmus is associated with saccadic pursuit, the lesion is most likely to be cerebellar, whereas saccadic pursuit in the absence of gaze-holding deficiency nystagmus is more likely to indicate a cerebral lesion.

Abnormal visual fixation

Steady fixation may be disrupted by slow drifts, nystagmus, or involuntary saccades. The frequency of square wave jerks increases in certain neurologic conditions, i.e. progressive supranuclear palsy, Friedreich's ataxia, and focal cerebral lesions. Detection of nystagmus during attempted steady fixation is abnormal. If the slow-phase velocity or intensity of nystagmus is similar both during fixation and when fixation is prevented (e.g. by Frenzel goggles or in darkness), then a disorder of the fixation system is inferred.

Disorders of the visual system lead to instability of gaze, the extreme example being blindness. Monocular loss of vision may lead to unstable gaze in the affected eye, which is predominantly due to slow, low-frequency vertical drifts. Binocular loss of vision causes loss of gaze stability and a continuous horizontal and vertical nystagmus.[35] This nystagmus characteristically changes direction over the course of seconds and minutes, a feature also encountered following experimental cerebellectomy. Thus, the nystagmus that follows bilateral visual loss reflects a gaze-holding mechanism that has never been calibrated by visual inputs. Acquired lesions of the

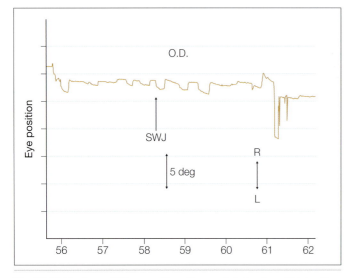

Fig. 90.18 Ocular motility recording of saccadic intrusions. This is a 7 s position trace of ocular motor recordings from a patient with saccadic intrusions. Small to moderated amplitude back to back saccades with an intersaccadic interval are present throughout the recording at about 1 Hz. SI = saccadic intrusions, SWJ = square wave jerks, O.D. = right eye, R = rightward eye movements and right gaze, L = leftward eye movements and left gaze, deg = degree.

cerebellum without specific involvement of the visual pathways may disrupt fixation with SIs and with slow drifts, especially in the vertical plane, that lead to nystagmus. The pathogenesis of pendular oscillations occurring in association with visual loss is unknown.[36]

Disorders of vergence

Strabismus

See Section 6.

Spasm of the near reflex (convergence spasm)

Spasm of the near reflex, also referred to as convergence spasm, is characterized by intermittent spasm of convergence, of miosis, and of accommodation. Symptoms include headache, photophobia, eye strain, blurred vision, and diplopia. Patients may appear to have bilateral sixth nerve palsies, but careful observation will reveal miosis and high myopia (8–10 D) on dry retinoscopy, accompanying the failure of abduction. This key clinical clue will prevent misdiagnosis and misdirected testing. Most commonly, spasm of the near reflex is psychogenic, and treatment may include simple reassurance, psychiatric counseling, or cycloplegia with bifocals.

Spasm of the near reflex associated with organic disease has been reported with encephalitis, tabes, labyrinthine fistulas, pituitary adenoma, Arnold-Chiari malformation, posterior fossa lesions, trauma, myasthenia gravis, anticonvulsant toxicities, midbrain lesions, metabolic problems, and cyclic oculomotor palsy. Disturbances that are clearly functional do not exclude coexisting organic disease!

Divergence insufficiency/paralysis

Divergence insufficiency is characterized by an esotropia for distance and orthophoria for near and normal convergence; the esotropia may be constant or intermittent. The fusional divergence may be reduced or completely absent. Divergence paralysis is characterized by complete loss of divergence amplitude. It appears as a constant esotropia for distance, with normal convergence, and it usually indicates an underlying neurologic problem, such as a tumor or head trauma resulting in elevated intracranial pressure, or the onset of Miller Fisher syndrome. Bilateral sixth nerve paresis should be excluded in these cases.

Convergence insufficiency/paralysis

Convergence insufficiency is characterized by reduced fusional convergence at near and a variable exophoria (occasionally intermittent exotropia) at near. It usually appears in adolescence and gives rise to vague symptoms of eye strain, headache, diplopia, and blurring associated with close work. Eye movements and reading acuity are normal, and there should be no neurologic abnormalities.

Convergence insufficiency usually has no underlying cause, but it can be associated with stress, fatigue, and anxiety, and it may follow infection or trauma.[37] Underlying intracranial lesions are rare. The child and parents should be reassured that there is no disease, and orthoptic near point exercises can be tried. If orthoptic exercises fail, prisms may be required.

Complete convergence paralysis is highly suggestive of an intracranial lesion, such as encephalitis, demyelination, neurosyphilis, or a condition resulting from trauma or toxins. The patient is usually completely unable to converge.

Disorders of the vestibulo-ocular response system

Abnormal VOR gain

VOR gain is the peak slow-phase velocity divided by rotation speed and is higher in infants than in adults. Abnormalities of VOR gain in the small child are not easily detected clinically but require eye movement recordings. If VOR gain is abnormal, a child's visual acuity will deteriorate by several lines while moving the head compared to the acuity taken with the head stationary. Abnormally high gain has been described in lesions of the cerebellar flocculus and the inferior olive. Mildly high gains have also been reported in familial vestibulocerebellar disorders.[38]

Abnormal VOR time constant

The time constant is measured as the time taken for the eye velocity of per-rotational or postrotational nystagmus measured in the dark to fall to 37% of its initial value. As a rule of thumb, the nystagmus will persist for a total time of about three times the time constant. Measurements on animals have shown that the time constant of the decay of per-rotatory or postrotatory nystagmus as measured at the vestibular ganglion is about 5 or 6 s. However, the nystagmus takes much longer to decay, with a time constant of approximately 12 s in humans. This augmentation of the cupula time constant is known as the velocity storage mechanism (VSM). It is also under adaptive control by the nodulus and uvula in the cerebellar vermis, and experimental lesions result in a prolonged VSM time constant. Abnormally short time VSM constants can be caused by disease of the end organ, the vestibular nerve, or central disease. Very short time constants have been reported in Chiari type I malformation, olivopontocerebellar degeneration, demyelinating disease, congenital and acquired blindness, and bilateral vestibulopathy secondary to ototoxic drugs. Abnormally long time VSM constant is rarely seen.

Absent VOR quick phases

Absent quick phases are seen in children with SIF. Most of these children will show a similar failure during OKN, but occasionally only vestibular nystagmus demonstrates the failure. This may indicate a very subtle form of saccade failure, and as an isolated phenomenon it is probably of little clinical significance. Absent quick phases may also be seen in neonates up to 2 to 3 weeks, or in older infants with delayed visual maturation.[13]

Absent VOR

The VOR appears clinically absent or very erratic in children with infantile nystagmus, whether elicited by calorics, constant rotation, or sinusoidal oscillation.[39] The VOR may be absent in children with the CHARGE association and in children with Usher syndrome type 1.

Disorders of the optokinetic system

Absence of OKN

No OKN can be elicited in a completely blind child, as it is a visually induced reflex. However, the absence of OKN alone must not be used as an indicator of visual acuity as the sighted infant who may appear visually unresponsive may have absence of OKN for another reason. The response to a full-field OKN stimulus is difficult to suppress, so the very presence of OKN demonstrates some vision. Bilateral lesions of the optokinetic pathway in the cortex, cerebellum, or brainstem may completely obliterate all OKN and SP. Infants with cortical dysplasia may have absent OKN, they may be cortically blind, or they can have a normal VEP and no OKN. If the optokinetic response is assessed with a hand-held device in the clinic, quick phase failure in children with SIF can be mistaken for absent OKN if the eyes are not driven to the limit of gaze. If there is any doubt, the child should have full-field OKN assessment, which will readily demonstrate the typical "locking up" of SIF.

Binocular asymmetry of OKN

Any unilateral lesion in the optokinetic pathway, as it passes through the brainstem, cerebellum, or parietal lobe, can result in asymmetric abnormalities of binocular OKN and SP. With brainstem and cerebellar lesions, there may be accompanying localizing neurologic signs, whereas isolated binocular OKN asymmetry is suggestive of a parietal lesion and has been reported in children as young as 4 to 5 months.

Monocular asymmetry of OKN

With early disturbances of binocular vision caused by strabismus, anisometropia, or unilateral congenital cataract, the normal early monocular OKN asymmetry persists in both eyes;[40] after 1 to 2 years, the monocular asymmetry persists.[40] The persistence of monocular OKN asymmetry and poor binocular vision together with the fact that OKN becomes symmetric in normal infants around the time that binocular function is detectable has led to the hypothesis linking binocularity and OKN asymmetry but they may be separate processes.[19]

Miscellaneous disorders

Induced convergence retraction (dorsal midbrain syndrome)

Lesions of the posterior commissure in the dorsal rostral midbrain may result from many disease processes and can affect a variety of supranuclear mechanisms, including those that control vertical gaze, eyelids, vergence, fixation, and pupils. Other terms such as pretectal syndrome, Koerber Salus-Elschnig syndrome, Sylvian aqueduct syndrome, posterior commissural syndrome, and collicular plate syndrome all refer to this condition.

Among the many underlying causes of this condition are hydrocephalus, stroke, and pinealomas. Table 90.4 lists other reported etiologies and systemic associations.

Limitation of upward saccades is the most reliable sign of the convergence retraction. Upward pursuit, Bell's phenomenon, and the fast phases of vestibular and OKN may also be affected either at presentation or with progression of the underlying process. It is rare for up-gaze to be unaffected. Pathologic lid retraction and lid lag are also common (Collier's sign).

Unlike the pathways from upward saccades, the pathways for downward saccades do not appear to pass through the posterior commissure (Fig. 90.2). Perhaps because of this, disturbances of down-gaze are not as predictable or uniform. Usually down-going saccades and pursuit are present, but they may be slow. Sometimes, especially in infants and children,

Table 90.4 – Causes of childhood dorsal midbrain syndrome

Classification by cause	Specific etiologies
Tumor	Pineal germinoma, teratoma and glioma; pineoblastoma; others
Hydrocephalus	Aqueductal stenosis with secondary dilation of third ventricle and aqueduct, or with secondary suprapineal recess compressing posterior commissure, commonly caused by cysticercosis in endemic areas
Metabolic disease	Gaucher's; Tay-Sach; Niemann-Pick; kernicterus; Wilson's disease; others
Midbrain/thalamic damage	Hemorrhage; infarction
Drugs	Barbiturates; carbamazepine; neuroleptics
Miscellaneous	Benign transient vertical eye disturbance in infancy; trauma; neurosurgery; hypoxia; encephalitis; tuberculoma; aneurysm; multiple sclerosis

there is a tonic downward deviation of the eyes that has been designated the "setting sun" sign, and downbeating nystagmus may also be observed. The setting sun sign may also be seen in children with hydrocephalus.

Convergence spasm may occur during horizontal saccades and produce a "pseudoabducens palsy" since the abducting eye moves more slowly than the adducting eye. All children with convergence retraction deserve thorough, prompt neurologic and neuroradiologic evaluation, since timely intervention may be decisive. The natural history of this disorder is dependent on the underlying etiology.

Transient vertical gaze disturbances in infancy

Vertical gaze abnormalities may be benign and transient in infants. Infants with episodic conjugate up-gaze that became less frequent over time have been described. During these episodes, normal horizontal and vertical vestibulo-ocular responses could be observed.[41]

Tonic down-gaze has been observed in 5 of 242 consecutively examined healthy newborn infants as well as in other infants. Again, the eyes can easily be driven above the primary position with the VOR. Premature infants with intraventricular hemorrhage may also develop tonic down-gaze, usually in association with a large-angle esotropia. These infants do not elevate the eyes with vestibular stimulation. Up-gaze often returns during the first 2 years of life, but the esotropia does not resolve when up-gaze returns.

Internuclear ophthalmoplegia

In the absence of peripheral lesions such as myasthenia gravis, failure of adduction combined with nystagmus of the contralateral abducting eye is termed internuclear ophthalmoplegia (INO) and localizes the lesion to the medial longitudinal fasciculus (MLF) unequivocally.

The abducens nucleus consists of two populations of neurons that coordinate horizontal eye movements (Fig. 90.1). Fibers from one group form the sixth nerve itself and innervate the ipsilateral lateral rectus muscle; fibers from the second group join the contralateral MLF and project to the subnucleus of the third nerve, which supplies the contralateral medial rectus muscle. In this way, the neurons of the sixth nerve nucleus yoke the lateral rectus with the contralateral medial rectus.

Clearly, lesions of the abducens nucleus will cause ipsilateral conjugate gaze palsy. Lesions of the MLF between the midpons and oculomotor nucleus will, in turn, disconnect the ipsilateral medial rectus subnucleus from the contralateral sixth nerve nucleus and cause diminished adduction of the ipsilateral eye on attempted versions. The signs of INO may be accompanied by an ipsilateral hypertropia or skew deviation.

A host of structural, metabolic, immunologic, inflammatory, degenerative, and other processes can interfere with the function of the MLF and nearby structures. In young adults, multiple sclerosis is by far the most common cause of INO.[71] Additional causes of INO include Arnold-Chiari malformation, hydrocephalus, meningoencephalitis, brainstem or fourth ventricular tumors, head trauma, metabolic disorders, drug intoxications, paraneoplastic effect, carcinomatous meningitis, and others. Peripheral processes, particularly myasthenia gravis and Miller Fisher syndrome, may closely mimic INO and should be considered in any patient with INO-like eye movements.[42]

Variable diplopia and/or ptosis most often prompt an ophthalmologic evaluation. Since there is no stereotypical myasthenic eye movement, this diagnosis should be considered in any child with an unexplained, acquired ocular motility disturbance and clinically normal pupils – particularly when the deviation is variable – whether or not ptosis is present. Any pattern of abnormal motility is suspect including an apparent gaze palsy, INO, isolated cranial nerve palsy, one and one-half syndrome, incomitant strabismus, accommodative and vergence insufficiency, and gaze-evoked nystagmus. Prolonged OKN may demonstrate slowing of the quick phases; large saccades may be hypometric; small saccades may be hypermetric; and characteristic "quiver movements," which consist of an initial small saccadic movement followed by a rapid drift backward, may be seen.[42]

Acquired and neurologic nystagmus

Eye care practitioners may be among the first to evaluate infants and children with involuntary ocular movements, producing anxiety in the medical care provider as well as the family. The eye care professional choosing to specialize in infants and children may, in fact, see more patients with nystagmus than any other specialist. This is due to the frequent association of nystagmus with strabismus.[17] It may be that nystagmus gets "less press" (e.g. literature, teaching, research, education) because there is less we understand or can do about it than strabismus or other childhood eye diseases.

Historical perspective

Nystagmus comes from the Greek word "nystagmos," to nod, drowsiness and from "nystazein" to doze, probably akin to Lithuanian "snusti," also to doze. It is a rhythmic, involuntary oscillation of one or both eyes. Using the information obtained from a complete history, physical examination, and radiographic and oculographic evaluations over 40 types of

nystagmus can be distinguished. Some forms of nystagmus are physiologic, whereas others are pathologic. Although the nystagmus is typically described by its more easily observable fast (jerk) phase, the salient clinical and pathologic feature is the presence of a slow phase in one or both directions. Thus, clinical descriptions of nystagmus are usually based on the direction of the fast phase and are termed horizontal, vertical, or rotary, or any combination of these. The nystagmus may be conjugate or disconjugate. The nystagmus may be predominantly pendular or jerky, the former referring to equal velocity to-and-fro movement of the eyes, and the latter referring to the eyes moving faster in one direction and slower in the other. Involuntary ocular oscillations containing only fast phases are "saccadic oscillations and intrusions" and not nystagmus. It is well documented that these differences may be difficult, if not impossible, to differentiate clinically. Recent advances in eye movement recording technology have increased its application in infants and children who have clinical disturbances of the ocular motor system (Figs 90.8 and 90.12).

Incidence

In 1991 Stang retrospectively reviewed the records of Group Health Inc. (White Bear Lake, MN) and in their pediatric population of 70 000 found a prevalence of clinical "nystagmus" of 1 in 2850.[43] Other estimates of its incidence range from 1 in 350 to 1 in 6550.[44,45] It is difficult if not impossible to give accurate prevalence/incidence on all types of nystagmus combined, but it is known that up to 50% of the infantile strabismic population will have some associated nystagmus. This could increase the prevalence of nystagmus to up to 0.5% of the population.

Etiology

All the theoretical neuronal mechanisms of nystagmus are constantly evolving and are beyond the scope of this chapter. Particularly controversial is the role of cortical motion processing in the development of some forms of infantile nystagmus. However, major supranuclear inputs to the oculomotor system are reasonably well accepted for their role in stabilization of eye movements. These include the pursuit system, vestibular system, and the neural integrator. The vestibular system maintains a constant resting firing rate that tends to drive the eyes contralaterally. This tendency is counterbalanced by the vestibular system on the opposite side unless the balance is changed by head rotation. The counterbalance is lost with unilateral vestibular damage, and the eyes tend to drift toward the affected side. A corrective saccade is then made toward the unaffected side. The slow phase of the nystagmus toward the affected side is of constant velocity as recorded by ocular motility recordings. This is a distinguishing feature of vestibular nystagmus. Most forms of acquired nystagmus are due to disease of the vestibular system (centrally or peripherally). Ocular motility recordings show various combinations of uniplanar or multiplanar, simple pendular, linear, or decelerating velocity slow phases[46] (Fig. 90.19).

Neurologic and acquired nystagmus types

Spasmus nutans

Spasmus nutans is an ocular oscillation beginning in infancy and consisting of the association of high-frequency, small

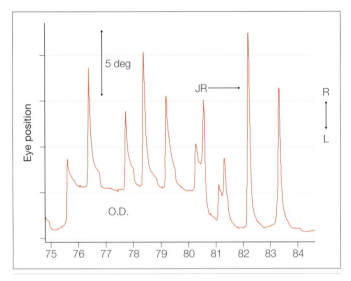

Fig. 90.19 Ocular motility recording of acquired jerk nystagmus. This is a typical 10 s position trace of ocular motor recordings from a patient with acquired jerk nystagmus. The jerk right nystagmus has decreasing velocity slow phases. O.D. = right eye, R = rightward eye movements and right gaze, L = leftward eye movements and left gaze, deg = degree.

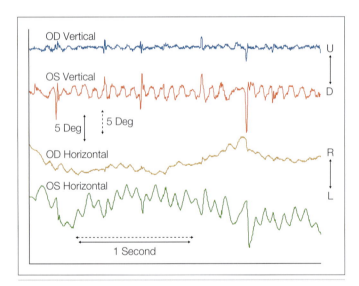

Fig. 90.20 Ocular motility recordings of spasmus nutans. OU open high-frequency (12–14 Hz), asymmetric, disconjugate, multiplanar (torsional), pendular nystagmus typical of spasmus nutans. Continuous periods of time are depicted in each tracing. Rightward eye movements (R) are up and leftward eye movements (L) are down. OD = right eye, OS = left eye.

amplitude, disconjugate oscillations, a head nodding oscillation, and a head tilt (Fig. 90.20). The head nodding associated with SNS is a combination of vertical head nodding together with a lateral shaking of the head in an unpredictable pattern. The head nodding is of lower frequency than the nystagmus and becomes prominent when the child attempts to inspect something of interest. It disappears during sleep but may persist when the child is lying down. The head tilt in SNS is a variable finding that is present in less than half of cases. Although the reason for the associated head tilt is unclear, Gottlob et al. have suggested that it may serve to directionalize the head nodding to its optimal trajectory.

The characteristic feature of spasmus nutans is the very fine, rapid pendular nature of the nystagmus. The eyes appear to have a shimmering movement. It may be horizontal, vertical, or torsional. It is usually asymmetric to the point that it may appear unilateral. Pure unilateral forms are not uncommon. It may appear to switch eyes with changes in direction of gaze, and frequently appears worse in the abducting eye. Tremendous asymmetry is associated with amblyopia of the more involved eye.[17,47] A key clinical eye movement recording observation is the variable phase difference between the two eyes, which is reflected clinically as an asymmetry in the oscillations between the two eyes.

Spasmus nutans may be a completely benign condition with onset in infancy and resolution within 2 years. However, tumors of the diencephalon can cause a condition indistinguishable from spasmus nutans. Consequently, neuroimaging or careful monitoring for visual, neurologic, or endocrinologic decline is essential. An intracranial tumor should be strongly suspected in any child who develops spasmus nutans after 3 years of age. Neurodegenerative disorders such as Pelizaeus–Merzbacher disease and Leigh disease may produce nystagmus and head nodding that are indistinguishable from spasmus nutans. These disorders should be suspected in children with clinical signs of ataxia or developmental delay or with MRI evidence of white matter signal abnormalities. Achromatopsia, congenital stationary night blindness, and Bardet-Biedl syndrome can also masquerade as spasmus nutans.

Drugs/toxins

Many drugs (some in therapeutic dosages) or toxins can cause nystagmus. The most common of these include anticonvulsants (i.e. phenobarbital, phenytoin, and carbamazepine), sedatives, hypnotics, and alcohol. Aspirin and quinine drugs causing nystagmus include chloroquine, quinidine, and quinine. Loop diuretics causing nystagmus include bumetanide, ethacrynic acid, furosemide, and torsemide. Aminoglycoside antibiotics causing nystagmus include amikacin, dihydrostreptomycin, gentamicin, neomycin, netilmicin, ribostamycin, streptomycin, and tobramycin. Antineoplastic drugs causing nystagmus include carboplatin and cisplatin. Environmental chemicals/toxins causing nystagmus include butyl nitrite, carbon disulfide, carbon monoxide, hexane, lead, manganese, mercury, styrene, tin, toluene, trichloroethylene, and xylene.[48,49]

Intracranial disease

Developmental, traumatic, and inflammatory brain diseases commonly cause acquired nystagmus. Consequently, nystagmus associated with other systemic, historical and physical findings nearly always requires further neurologic and radiologic evaluation. (See "Localizing" forms of nystagmus below for further discussion.)

Voluntary flutter

Voluntary flutter ("nystagmus") (present in 7% to 15% of the population) is a misnomer referring to a series of volitional, rapid alternating saccades with little to no intersaccadic interval[25] (Figs 90.12 and 90.15). They are usually horizontal, but may be vertical or torsional, and can only be sustained for a few seconds. Voluntary nystagmus is a popular "party trick," and is often seen in patients with functional visual complaints. It is frequently associated with convergence of the eyes or facial grimacing. Voluntary nystagmus warrants no laboratory or radiographic investigation.

"Localizing" forms of nystagmus due to neurologic disease (Box 90.1)

(A)periodic alternating nystagmus

(A)periodic alternating nystagmus may resemble infantile nystagmus or be "acquired." Patients with acquired form usually have vertigo, nausea, dizziness, and oscillopsia. The key clinical

---

Box 90.1

Neurological nystagmus types

See-saw nystagmus

Rostral midbrain lesions

Parasellar lesions (e.g. pituitary tumors)

Visual loss secondary to retinitis pigmentosa

Downbeat nystagmus

Lesions of the vestibulocerebellum and underlying medulla (e.g. Arnold-Chiari malformation, microvascular disease with vertebrobasilar insufficiency, multiple sclerosis, Wernicke's encephalopathy, encephalitis, lithium intoxication)

Heat stroke

Approximately 50% have no identifiable cause

Upbeat nystagmus

Medullary lesions, including perihypoglossal nuclei, the adjacent medial vestibular nucleus, and the nucleus intercalatus (structures important in gaze holding)

Lesions of the anterior vermis of the cerebellum

Benign paroxysmal positional vertigo

Periodic alternating nystagmus

Arnold-Chiari malformation

Demyelinating disease

Spinocerebellar degeneration

Lesions of the vestibular nuclei

Head trauma

Encephalitis

Syphilis

Posterior fossa tumors

Binocular visual deprivation (e.g. ocular media opacities)

Pendular nystagmus

Demyelinating disease

Monocular or binocular visual deprivation

Oculopalatal myoclonus

Internuclear ophthalmoplegia

Brainstem or cerebellar dysfunction

Spasmus nutans

Usually occurs in otherwise healthy children

May be caused by chiasmal, suprachiasmal, or third ventricle gliomas

Torsional

Lateral medullary syndrome (Wallenberg's syndrome)

Abducting nystagmus of internuclear ophthalmoplegia

Demyelinating disease

Brain stem stroke

Gaze-evoked

Drugs: anticonvulsants (e.g. phenobarbital, phenytoin, carbamazepine) at therapeutic dosages

---

component is that the null point shifts position in a cyclic pattern. This results in changes in the amplitude and direction of the nystagmus every few minutes. Adequate observation of the patient for several minutes should exclude this diagnosis. However, it should be considered any time a patient's head turn is different from one examination to the next. This is more common in patients with oculocutaneous albinism.[50,51]

Periodic alternating nystagmus is usually congenital and benign. However, it may be associated with vestibulocerebellar lesions, neurodegenerative conditions such as Friedreich's ataxia, or even visual loss. Neuroimaging is warranted in all cases unless the nystagmus has been stable for a prolonged period of time. Periodic alternating nystagmus may respond to treatment with low doses of baclofen in acquired forms of periodic alternating nystagmus.[52]

Gaze-evoked nystagmus

Gaze-evoked nystagmus is a jerk nystagmus that occurs in the direction of eccentric gaze. In contradistinction to infantile nystagmus most forms of gaze-evoked nystagmus can be stabilized by visual fixation and are accentuated by darkness or image blur (Fig. 90.11). Gaze-evoked nystagmus is called gaze-paretic nystagmus if it occurs in the direction of limited eye movement, as it may be associated with a cranial nerve palsy or myasthenia gravis. Gaze-paretic nystagmus may appear dissociated if the limitation of eye movement is asymmetric between the two eyes. One form of gaze-evoked nystagmus that is completely benign is endpoint nystagmus. This occurs in extreme positions of lateral or upward gaze. It can be distinguished from pathologic forms of gaze-evoked nystagmus by its low amplitude, symmetry on right and left gaze, poor sustainability, and absence of associated neurologic abnormalities. With endpoint nystagmus, the eyes attempt a saccade out to an extreme gaze position and have an initial difficulty finding this position. After a short amount of jerk nystagmus, the position is found, and the eyes maintain the eccentric gaze. Endpoint nystagmus is a normal finding and differs from gaze-evoked nystagmus by the fact that gaze-evoked nystagmus is a constant nystagmus with larger amplitude (defined as 4 degrees or more) and is often asymmetric. Gaze-evoked nystagmus is caused by a deficiency, usually a structural lesion, in the neural integrator network. Gaze cannot be held at an extreme position, and the eyes drift back toward the null point of the integrator, which often is straight-ahead gaze. A corrective saccade is attempted to move the gaze back to the eccentric position, and the process repeats.

Disease in the posterior fossa or drugs, particularly anticonvulsants and sedatives, are the most common causes of pathologic gaze-evoked nystagmus. Disease of the cerebellum or vestibular system usually results in asymmetry of gaze-evoked nystagmus between directions of gaze. For example, tumors of the cerebellopontine angle may result in high-amplitude, low-frequency nystagmus (caused by cerebellar damage) when looking to the side of the lesion, and low-amplitude, high-frequency nystagmus (caused by vestibular imbalance) when looking to the contralateral side, a condition known as Brun's nystagmus. Associated neurologic abnormalities such as ataxia, hearing loss, tremor, or hemiparesis should always be sought.

Vestibular nystagmus

Certain characteristics of vestibular nystagmus can localize the etiology to the peripheral or central neuronal pathways of the vestibular systems. Central vestibular nystagmus is frequently uniplanar in contrast to peripheral vestibular nystagmus, which is usually torsional or multiplanar. Visual fixation easily inhibits peripheral vestibular nystagmus, but not central vestibular nystagmus. Vertigo and tinnitus are common in peripheral vestibular nystagmus, and uncommon in central vestibular nystagmus.

Acquired pendular nystagmus

Acquired pendular nystagmus may be due to tumors, infarction, inflammation, or degeneration of the brainstem or cerebellum. The nystagmus may be horizontal, vertical, or both. A single lesion in the brain will result in horizontal and vertical components that oscillate at the same frequency of 2 to 7 cycles per second. If the horizontal and vertical components are in phase, the nystagmus will appear oblique. If they are out of phase, it will appear circular or elliptical. Circular or elliptical nystagmus that is constantly changing character is due to horizontal and vertical components oscillating on different frequencies. (90.21).

See-saw nystagmus

See-saw nystagmus is a pendular, upward incyclotorsion of one eye with a simultaneous downward excyclotoresion of the other eye. The pendular-waveform see-saw nystagmus is commonly due to a midline mesodiencephalic, bilaterally compressing mass[53] (Fig. 90.21). See-saw nystagmus can also be associated with traumatic or congenital chiasmal abnormalities,[53] and is mostly due to a unilateral lesion in the mesodiencephalic junction. Congenital see-saw nystagmus is a rare form of neonatal nystagmus with upward excyclotorsion of one eye and concomitant downward incyclotorsion of the other eye.

Downbeat nystagmus

Downbeat nystagmus is usually produced by lesions in the cerebellum that also damage pathways that control horizontal tracking and visual–vestibulo-ocular interactions.[52,54] The most frequent causes are infarction, cerebellar and spinocerebellar degeneration syndromes, and multiple sclerosis and developmental anomalies affecting the pons and cerebellum.[52,54] It is also commonly due to drugs (particularly lithium or sedatives) or lesions at the cervicomedullary junction.[52,54] In children, it is usually due to Arnold-Chiari malformation or syringomyelia. Without a drug history, downbeat nystagmus should be evaluated in all patients with a sagittal MRI scan of the brainstem and cervical spinal cord. All patients have jerk-down nystagmus in some positions of gaze and a few patients have jerk-down nystagmus only with convergence, in the dark, or with positioning of the head and body. Horizontal gaze increases the nystagmus. The nystagmus slow components usually have constant velocity or increasing-velocity waveforms. Associated patterns of abnormal horizontal eye movements are characteristic of damage to the midline structures of the cerebellum (impaired pursuit, impaired OKN, and inability to suppress VOR).

Upbeat nystagmus

Upbeat nystagmus with its fast upward movement usually increases on extreme up gaze and generally follows Alexander's Law. The oscillations may be enhanced by a head tilt, and with convergence the nystagmus can increase or change to downbeat nystagmus. Upbeat nystagmus is probably caused by midbrain dysfunction or cerebellar disease. It is very similar to downbeat nystagmus but is generally less common.

Treatment and prognosis

There are a number of signs and symptoms due to nystagmus that are amenable to treatment. The first and most obvious is decreased vision ("central visual acuity," "gaze-angle" acuity, near acuity). Correction of significant refractive errors in children with nystagmus is the single most powerful therapeutic intervention for improving vision and visual function in these patients. Refractive etiologies of decreased "vision" include either one or a combination of conditions, e.g. myopia, hyperopia, astigmatism, and anisometropia. These refractive conditions can contribute significantly to already impaired vision in patients with other "organic" etiologies of decreased vision, e.g. amblyopia, optic nerve and/or retinal disease, oscillopsia, and the oscillation itself. The use of telescopes, magnification, and other low vision aids are valuable refractive adjuncts that can be used situationally in nystagmus patients with and without associated sensory system deficits. The second is AHP. The etiology of the AHP includes a "gaze null" due to INS or acquired nystagmus (e.g. chin-down in downbeat nystagmus), an "adduction null" due to infantile nystagmus or latent/manifest latent nystagmus (manifest strabismus with the preferred eye fixing in adduction), convergence damping ("nystagmus blockage"), and a periodically changing head posture due to (a) periodic alternating nystagmus. The third is oscillopsia, which is usually due to either acquired nystagmus or a change in the sensory/motor status of the patient with infantile nystagmus (e.g. "decompensated" strabismus, a change in the gaze null angle, or decreasing acuity).[55] Other less common associated signs and symptoms include hypoaccommodation and photophobia (i.e. congenital cone dystrophy and albinism).

The prognosis of all these ocular oscillations depends on the type of underlying ocular and systemic disease. In general, infantile forms improve with time unless they are associated

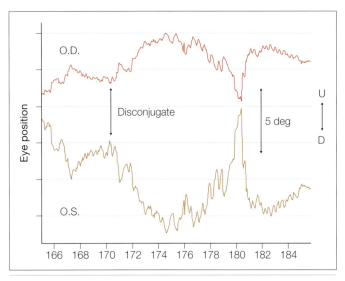

Fig. 90.21 Ocular motility recording of see-saw + pendular nystagmus. This is a 20 s vertical position trace of ocular motor recordings from a patient with see-saw and pendular nystagmus. On a background of a continuous, 2–4 Hz, pendular, small amplitude, conjugate, ocular oscillation there is a slower, vertically, out of phase disconjugate oscillation representing the see-saw component. O.D. = right eye, O.S. = left eye, U = upward eye movements and up-gaze, D = downward eye movements and down-gaze, deg = degree, JL = jerk left nystagmus.

with a degenerative ocular or systemic disease. Acquired forms are more visually disturbing and follow the course of the underlying neurologic disease.

References

1. Cannon SC, Robinson DA, Shamma S. A proposed neural network for the integrator of the oculomotor system. Biol Cybern 1983; 49: 127–36.
2. Büttner-Ennever JA, Horn AK, Graf W, et al. Modern concepts of brainstem anatomy: from extraocular motoneurons to proprioceptive pathways. Ann NY Acad Sci 2002; 956: 75–84.
4. Quaia C, Lefevre P, Optican LM. Model of the control of saccades by superior colliculus and cerebellum. J Neurophysiol 1999; 82: 999–1018.
5. Pierrot-Deseilligny C, Rivaud S, Gaynard B, et al. Cortical control of saccades. Ann Neurol 1995; 37: 557–67.
6. Cassidy L, Taylor D, Harris C. Abnormal supranuclear eye movements in the child: a practical guide to examination and interpretation. Surv Ophthalmol 2000; 44: 479–506.
7. Harris CM, Walker J, Shawkat F. Eye movements in a familial vestibulocerebellar disorder. Neuropediatrics 1993; 24: 117–22.
9. Nixon RB, Helveston EM, Miller K, et al. Incidence of strabismus in neonates. Am J Ophthalmol 1985; 100: 798–801.
10. Jacobs M, Harris CM, Shawkat F, et al. Smooth pursuit development in infants. Aust NZ J Ophthalmol 1997; 25: 199–206.
11. Cohen B, Reisine H, Yokota JI, et al. The nucleus of the optic tract: its function in gaze stabilization and control of visual-vestibular interaction. Ann NY Acad Sci 1992; 656: 277–96.
14. Büttner-Ennever JA, Horn AK. Anatomical substrates of oculomotor control. Curr Opin Neurobiol 1997; 7: 872–9.
16. Hertle RW, Dell'Osso LF. Clinical and ocular motor analysis of congenital nystagmus in infancy. J AAPOS 1999; 3: 70–9.
17. Hertle RW, Zhu X. Oculographic and clinical characterization of thirty-seven children with anomalous head postures, nystagmus, and strabismus: the basis of a clinical algorithm. J AAPOS 2000; 4: 25–32.
20. Büttner U, Büttner-Ennever JA. Present concepts of oculomotor organization. Rev Oculomot Res 1988; 2: 3–32.
22. Bronstein AM, Rudge P, Gresty MA, et al. Abnormalities of horizontal gaze. Clinical, oculographic and magnetic resonance imaging findings. II. Gaze palsy and internuclear ophthalmoplegia. J Neurol Neurosurg Psychiatry 1990; 53: 200–7.
23. Shawkat FS, Harris CM, Wilson J, et al. Eye movements in children with opsoclonus-polymyoclonus. Neuropediatrics 1993; 24: 218–23.
24. Harris CM, Shawkat F, Russell-Eggitt IM, et al. Intermittent horizontal saccade failure ("ocular motor apraxia") in children. Br J Ophthalmol 1996; 80: 151–8.
28. Cooper R, Khakoo Y, Matthay KK. Opsoclonus-myoclonus-ataxia syndrome in neuroblastoma: histopathologic features – a report from the Children's Cancer Group. Med Pediatr Oncol 2001; 36: 623–9.
30. Moretti R, Torre P, Antonello RN, et al. Opsoclonus-myoclonus syndrome: gabapentin as a new therapeutic proposal. Eur J Neurol 2000; 7: 455–6.
34. Pierrot-Deseilligny C. Saccade and smooth-pursuit impairment after cerebral hemispheric lesions. Eur Neurol 1994; 34: 121–34.
35. Huo R, Burden SK, Hoyt CS, et al. Chronic cortical visual impairment in children: aetiology, prognosis, and associated neurological deficits. Br J Ophthalmol 1999; 83: 670–5.
36. Good WV, Jan JE, Hoyt CS, et al. Monocular vision loss can cause bilateral nystagmus in young children. Dev Med Child Neurol 1997; 39: 421–4.
39. Abadi RV, Bjerre A. Motor and sensory characteristics of infantile nystagmus. Br J Ophthalmol 2002; 86: 1152–60.
40. Aiello A, Wright KW, Borchert M. Independence of optokinetic nystagmus asymmetry and binocularity in infantile esotropia. Arch Ophthalmol 1994; 112: 580–3.
43. Stang HJ. Developmental disabilities associated with congenital nystagmus. J Dev Behav Pediatr 1991; 12: 322–3.
46. Stahl JS, Averbuch-Heller L, Leigh RJ. Acquired nystagmus. Arch Ophthalmol 2000; 118: 544–9.
48. Leigh RJ, Ramat S. Neuropharmacologic aspects of the ocular motor system and the treatment of abnormal eye movements. Curr Opin Neurol 1999; 12: 21–7.
49. Jaanus SD. Ocular side effects of selected systemic drugs. Optom Clin 1992; 2: 73–96.
51. Leigh RJ, Robinson DA, Zee DS. A hypothetical explanation for periodic alternating nystagmus: instability in the optokinetic-vestibular system. Ann NY Acad Sci 1981; 374: 619–35.
52. Leigh RJ, Das VE, Seidman SH. A neurobiological approach to acquired nystagmus. Ann NY Acad Sci 2002; 956: 380–90.
54. Baloh RW, Spooner JW. Downbeat nystagmus: a type of central vestibular nystagmus. Neurology 1981; 31: 304–10.
55. Hertle RW, Fitzgibbon EJ, Avallone JM, et al. Onset of oscillopsia after visual maturation in patients with congenital nystagmus. Ophthalmology 2001; 108: 2301–7; discussion 2307–8.

 Access the complete referece list online at
http://www.expertconsult.com

I think my baby can't see!

Ingele Casteels

Normally, a full-term baby shows visual fixation at birth or shortly afterward. Absent, poor, or delayed visual contact is a common reason parents bring their baby to their ophthalmologist. They are anxious to understand why the baby seems not to see, and want to know the cause and prognosis. Although this is not usually a medical emergency, parents need to have their baby diagnosed soon. This is a challenge. In some babies the underlying cause is evident on clinical examination; in others, additional investigation will be necessary. The diagnosis depends on a thorough birth, family and clinical history and a systematic clinical examination (Fig. 91.1). The clinician should verify the cause and degree of visual impairment, give a prognosis, and make a plan of management and counseling for the family.

History

It is important to take a detailed history from the parents, grandparents, and caretakers. While talking to the parents, you can observe the infant's visual behavior. The history of the pregnancy, delivery, and postnatal development is important.

Was the baby premature? Visual development depends on the postmenstrual age at birth. Premature infants with intraventricular hemorrhage are at risk of optic atrophy (see Chapter 53), hydrocephalus, and cerebral visual impairment (CVI) (see Chapters 56 and 57). Visual development in premature babies can also be delayed due to associated retinal or neurological problems. The presence of seizures, developmental delay, and dysmorphic features may suggest a brain problem. Maternal infections, medication during pregnancy, trauma, and hypoxia can have significant visual consequences.

It is important to find out if there is a significant problem or is the baby just different from others? Some normal babies can just be less responsive.

Has there been a change in visual behavior since birth? Vision can deteriorate after the onset of seizures or progressive neurological or ocular diseases.

A positive family history, or a history of consanguinity, makes certain diseases more likely. For instance, a baby born to first cousin parents with searching eye movements and hypermetropia is very likely to have a congenital retinal dystrophy (see Chapter 44). The pediatric ophthalmologist should inquire about other family members, examine them and the first-degree relatives. Specific questions to parents or caregivers

on the visual behavior in dark or bright light can give a clue to the diagnosis. Some congenital retinal disorders, especially achromatopsia, cone–rod dystrophy, and Leber's congenital amaurosis, may present with photophobia or day-blindness (see Chapter 44). Babies with CVI can show reluctance to look at a light, or, in contrast, will develop lightgazing[1] (see Chapter 56). Lens (see Chapter 36) and corneal opacities (see Chapters 33 and 34), i.e. congenital glaucoma (see Chapter 37), albinism (see Chapter 40), and aniridia (see Chapter 38), can cause photophobia.

Did the parents notice wobbling eyes? Nystagmus and searching eye movements can be the presenting symptoms in many babies with poor vision from birth, but usually appear at 2 to 3 months of age. Roving or drifting eye movements are often seen in babies with very poor vision.

Are there any specific hand movements? Blind babies tend to press or poke their eyes (Fig. 91.2). Babies with limited vision due to retinal disorders may wave their hands between their eyes and a light source (Fig. 91.3).

Examination

It is often difficult to quantify visual acuity in babies, especially in those with poor visual contact. Parental estimations of vision and changes in vision can be helpful, but it is relevant to obtain a measure of overall visual function. Despite advances in research, behavioral observations remain of primary importance in assessing visual function in infancy. In a term baby, a visual following response should be present by 2 months, and the baby should smile responsively to a parent. At 4 months, a child should reach for an object. Complex stimuli with contrast should interest a happy and wakeful baby.

The presence of optokinetic nystagmus (OKN) in a baby excludes a very severe visual problem. In congenital ocular motor apraxia (saccadic initiation failure) the eyes will deviate on being spun around without developing the fast phases of nystagmus ("locking up"). OKN examination in most cases shows normal vertical OKN. A measure of vision can also be achieved with the dynamic vestibulo-ocular reflex (VOR) by evaluating the "after" nystagmus, which is much longer in a blind baby. In addition to the normal immaturity of pursuit and saccadic movements in the newborn, congenital ocular motor apraxia, Möbius' syndrome, and bilateral Duane's

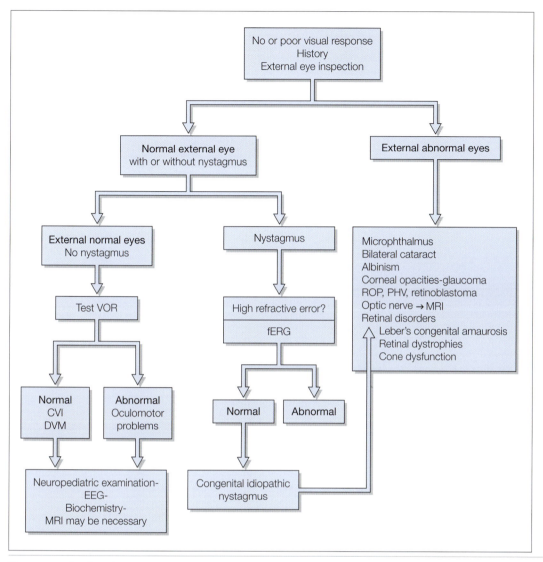

Fig. 91.1 Evaluation of an apparently blind infant. ROP: Retinopathy of prematurity; PFV: Persistent fetal vascular.

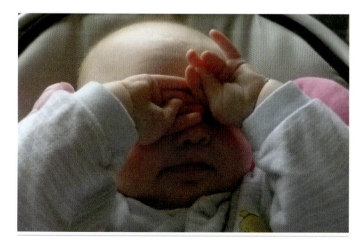

Fig. 91.2 Eye poking in a baby with Leber's amaurosis.

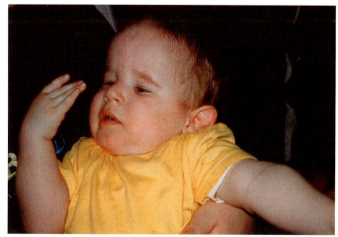

Fig. 91.3 Babies with limited vision due to retinal disorders tend to wave their hands between their eyes and a light source.

Table 91.1 – Common causes of poor vision in infants with apparently normal eyes on clinical examination

Diagnosis	Clinical signs apart from poor vision	Pupils	Slit-lamp	Ophthalmoscopy	Refraction	Flash ERG	Flash VEP	Pattern VEP	MRI	Neuropediatric examination/ EEG	Visual outcome
DVM	Pour visual contact	Normal	Normal	Normal	Normal	Normal	Normal	Normal	Normal	Normal	Normal
Cerebral visual Impairment	Eccentric viewing/light gazing	Normal	Normal	Usually normal	Normal	Normal	Usually abnormal	Usually abnormal	Usually abnormal	Usually abnormal	Usually poor perceptual defects
Idiopathic nystagmus syndrome	Nystagmus Head tilt	Normal	Normal	Normal	Normal/ abnormal	Normal	Normal	Abnormal	Normal	Normal	Good
Leber's congenital amaurosis	Roving eyes Photophobia Eye poking	Paradoxical Sluggish or normal	Normal	Usually normal	High hypermetropia	Absent	Abnormal	Absent	Usually normal	Normal	Poor
Retinal dystrophy	Nystagmus Night-blindness	Usually normal	Normal	Usually abnormal	Usually normal	Abnormal	Usually normal	Abnormal	Normal or abnormal	Normal or abnormal	Poor
Achromatopsia/ cone dystrophy	Photophobia Day-blindness Color-blindness Nystagmus	Paradoxical or normal	Normal	Normal	Normal or high hypermetropia Blue cone dystrophy, myopic	Absent cone response	Normal	Abnormal	Not indicated	Normal	Poor, photophobia Stationary
Bilateral optic nerve hypoplasia or atrophy	Poor vision Roving eye movements	Afferent defect	Normal	Abnormal, direct ophthalmoscopy necessary	Normal	Normal	Abnormal	Abnormal	Normal or abnormal	Normal or abnormal + endocrine exam	Variable
Albinism	Nystagmus Photophobia	Normal	Abnormal	Abnormal	Myopia or astigmatism	Normal or enhanced	Crossed asymmetry	Crossed asymmetry	Usually not indicated	Normal	Variable

syndrome may be the cause of apparently poor visual contact because the baby cannot move the eyes. Rotation to induce VOR should exclude an eye movement defect.[2]

Examination of the external eyes and eye movements may reveal nystagmus and strabismus. It is difficult to distinguish between nystagmus waveforms clinically. Eye movement recordings have shown some useful clinical information. A high-frequency, low-amplitude pendular nystagmus in otherwise normal eyes is often seen in cone dystrophies[3] (see Chapter 44). Searching eye movements with very poor vision are seen in Leber's congenital amaurosis (see Chapter 44). Early-onset nystagmus can be divided into three groups: sensory defect nystagmus, in which there is a proven sensory defect; congenital idiopathic nystagmus (sometimes called motor nystagmus), in which no visual or neurological impairment can be found; and neurological nystagmus, which is associated with neurological disease.[4]

Pupil reactions can be useful and should be examined carefully (see Chapter 63). In most babies the cause of poor vision from birth is obvious to a pediatric ophthalmologist after clinical examination. A structural abnormality (e.g. microphthalmos) may be obvious at a glance. The use of the red reflex to identify media opacities is a useful quick and non-threatening screening technique. I find it easy to evaluate with the retinoscope. Hand-held slit-lamp examination may reveal anterior segment problems: cataracts (see Chapter 36), colobomas, aniridia (see Chapter 38), albinism (see Chapter 40), etc. Slit-lamp examination is particularly important in infants with nystagmus. In cases of albinism, iris transillumination is evident. Especially in ocular albinism the diagnosis is less straightforward without a good look at the anterior segment. Slit-lamp examination should be repeated after dilatation of the pupils in order to better visualize lens opacities or lens subluxation.

Bilateral pupillary dilatation with cyclopentolate 0.5% is necessary in order to perform indirect and direct funduscopy and retinoscopy. On funduscopy, attention is paid to both the vitreous and the retina. Vitreous haze and hemorrhages, seen in bleeding disorders, uveitis (see Chapter 39), retinal vasculitis, non-accidental injury (see Chapter 66), retinopathy of prematurity (see Chapter 43), retinal dysplasia (see Chapter 44), hyaloid abnormalities, and retinoblastoma (see Chapter 42), may be found. Indirect ophthalmoscopy will reveal retinal problems such as chorioretinal colobomas, macular toxoplasmosis (see Chapter 39), retinal detachment (see Chapter 50), retinal folds, chorioretinal dysplasia, and sometimes retinal dystrophy. However, many cases of congenital retinal dystrophies will present with a normal appearing retina on ophthalmoscopy.

Direct ophthalmoscopy is best for subtle optic disc anomalies such as colobomas and optic disc hypoplasia or dysplasia (see Chapter 51). An examination under sedation or anesthesia may occasionally be necessary to see the optic nerve in detail.

Refraction is vital. High refractive errors – hypermetropia in particular – can give rise to poor visual contact from birth. Correction of moderate and high myopia in babies with apparent delayed visual maturation may improve poor visual behavior.[5] Refractive errors can provide a clue to the underlying diagnosis.

When the eyes of a baby with poor visual contact appear to be normal, with or without nystagmus, further investigation is necessary (Table 91.1). The flash electroretinogram (fERG) may diagnose retinal diseases. The fERG and flash VEP (visually evoked potential) have conspicuous immature features during the early months and may not aid in establishing the diagnosis. The fERG may be more useful at a later age.[6,7]

A pediatric neurological consultation and further investigations, such as biochemistry and brain magnetic resonance imaging (MRI), are carried out where indicated. Babies affected with CVI usually have a normal eye examination, no nystagmus or strabismus; some have associated optic nerve atrophy (see Chapter 56).

An electroencephalogram (EEG) should also be included in the initial investigation of every infant with apparent delayed visual maturation (DVM) in order to detect a treatable underlying epileptogenic abnormality.[8] "Delayed visual maturation" is a term used to describe a normal baby with a transient visual deficit (see Chapter 4). There are no data to establish that any primary visual system is delayed in its development (see Chapter 3). DVM is a retrospective diagnosis, which can only be made after a long enough follow-up to exclude neurological problems. DVM is not a single diagnostic condition but rather a sign common to neurological abnormalities affecting several areas of the brain (see Chapter 3).

An incorrect or unclear diagnosis of visual impairment in an infant can be devastating to the family. In most infants presenting with poor visual contact, clinical signs are diagnostic, but additional studies may be necessary to establish the correct diagnosis. A long enough follow-up by the ophthalmologist in collaboration with the pediatrician should be planned and it is essential to be encouraging whenever you can but not to be dogmatic about either the diagnosis or the prognosis as both can change!

References

1. Jan JE, Groenveld M, Anderson DP. Photophobia and cortical visual impairment. Dev Med Child Neurol 1993; 35: 473–7.
2. Hoyt C. Costenbader Lecture. Delayed visual maturation: the apparently blind infant. J AAPOS 2004; 8: 215–9.
3. Yee RD, Baloh RW, Honrubia V. Eye movement abnormalities in rod monochromacy. Ophthalmology 1981; 88: 1010–8.
4. Casteels I, Harris CM, Shawkat F, Taylor D. Nystagmus in infancy. Br J Ophthalmol 1992; 76: 434–7.
5. Winges KM, Zarpellon U, Hou C, Good W. Delayed visual attention caused by high myopic refractive error. Strabismus 2005; 13: 75–7.
6. Lambert SR, Kriss A, Taylor D. Delayed visual maturation: a longitudinal study: clinical and electrophysiological assessment. Ophthalmology 1989; 96: 524–8.
7. Kriss A, Russell-Eggitt IM. Electrophysiological assessment of visual pathway function in infants. Eye 1992; 6: 145–53.
8. Shahar E, Hwang PA. Prolonged epileptic blindness in an infant associated with cortical dysplasia. Dev Med Child Neurol 2001; 43: 127–9.

My baby's got a red eye, doctor!

James Elder

The eye appears red when blood is visible. This is usually the result of vessel dilatation or hemorrhage as a consequence of infection, inflammation, trauma, or abnormality of blood vessels. Frequently, this is associated with other symptoms or signs such as pain, blurring of vision, photophobia, purulent discharge, tearing or blepharospasm. With babies, symptoms can only be inferred.

Assessment with simple magnification or a portable slit-lamp augmented with fluorescein dye staining affords a clinical diagnosis in most babies. Measurement of intraocular pressure and fundal examination will be required in some instances to make a diagnosis. Infectious causes are common and microbiology is the most frequent additional investigation.

The baby with a red and discharging eye

Neonatal conjunctivitis presents with a red and discharging eye and is the most common cause of a red eye in a baby (see Chapters 12 and 93). Frequently, discharge is more prominent than red eye.

Ligneous conjunctivitis will rarely present in a baby as a recurrently red eye that discharges. Eversion of the lid will reveal granulomatous lesions with a fibrinous mass forming an approximate cast of the conjunctival fornix. The parents may describe pieces of this fibrinous mass breaking free. Serum plasminogen will be near zero in such infants.[1]

The baby with a painless red eye

Birth trauma may result in conjunctival hemorrhage and, rarely, hyphema. There may be direct injury following forceps delivery. Corneal edema secondary to Descemet's membrane splits may be present. Conjunctival hemorrhage may be the result of non-accidental injury.

Juvenile xanthogranuloma can cause a spontaneous hyphema and may present as a painless[2] or painful red eye. This can be mistaken for a non-accidental injury if the typical skin changes (yellow to reddish brown "waxy" papules) are not detected.

A corneal dermoid presents as a red fleshy lump on the surface of the eye. It may be associated with systemic conditions such as Goldenhar's syndrome.

Occasionally, a newborn with albinism and iris transillumination will present with the parents describing red eyes prior to recognition of the other features of albinism.

Infrequently, infantile hemangiomas or orbital venous anomalies may present primarily in the conjunctiva and appear as a painless red eye.

The baby with a watery red eye

Corneal abnormalities frequently cause a red and watery eye (see Chapter 33). Portable slit-lamp examination with fluorescein staining is useful to establish a diagnosis.

Corneal ulceration due to any cause presents with a red and watery eye. Most commonly, this will be simple trauma (either direct or due to subtarsal foreign body). Less commonly, primary corneal infection presents in infancy with a red eye. Herpes simplex viral infection is the most common, but bacterial infection following corneal trauma needs to be considered. Corneal epithelial abnormalities such as epidermolysis bullosa dystrophica can present early with a red watery and painful eye.[3]

Corneal hypoesthesia may present with a recurrently red and watery eye with varying degrees of epithelial loss from punctate erosions to frank ulceration.

KID syndrome[4] (keratitis, ichthyosis, and deafness) and Cogan's syndrome (keratitis, deafness, aortitis, systemic inflammatory disease) can present with a red eye from limbal stem cell failure, recurrent ulceration, and corneal neovascularization.

Rarely, other causes of a dry eye or meibomian gland disease may present with a red eye in infancy.

The baby with photophobia or blepharospasm and a red eye

Acute glaucoma in an infant may present with photophobia and a red eye (see Chapter 37) from pupil block due to an ectopic or anteriorly displaced lens, as seen in Marfan's syndrome, homocystinuria, or retrolental membranes. Corneal enlargement and clouding, with photophobia and watering, are prominent in infants with glaucoma.

A masquerade syndrome caused by advanced retinoblastoma presents with a red eye, photophobia, and blepharospasm. Endogenous endophthalmitis can present similarly and is usually seen in an otherwise extremely unwell and septic child.

Anterior uveitis is seldom seen in infancy and less commonly causes a red eye. Kawasaki's disease in an infant may be associated with conjunctivitis and mild anterior uveitis.[5]

The author has seen a single case of non-accidental injury caused by deliberate installation of an unidentified caustic agent in both eyes of a baby (see Chapter 67). This baby presented with red eyes, photophobia, blepharospasm, and total corneal epithelial loss. This form of child abuse is unusual and can be blinding.[6]

References

1. Mehta R, Shapiro AD. Plasminogen deficiency. Haemophilia 2008; 14: 1261–8.

2. Liang S, Liu YH, Fang K. Juvenile xanthogranuloma with ocular involvement. Pediatr Dermatol 2009; 26: 232–4.

3. Pfendner EG, Lucky AW. Dystrophic epidermolysis bullosa. In: Pagon RA, Bird TD, Dolan CR, Stephens K, editors. GeneReviews [Internet] (updated 2010 Nov 04). http://www.ncbi.nlm.nih.gov/books/NBK1304/

4. Djalilian AR, Kim JY, Saeed HN, et al. Histopathology and treatment of corneal disease in keratitis, ichthyosis, and deafness (KID) syndrome. Eye 2010; 24: 738–40.

5. Che Mahiran CD, Alagaratnam J, Liza-Sharmini AT. Leucocoria in a boy with Kawasaki disease: a diagnostic challenge. Singapore Med J 2009; 50: 232–4.

6. Ong T, Hodgkins P, Marsh C, Taylor D. Blinding keratoconjunctivitis and child abuse. Am J Ophthalmol 2005; 139: 190–1.

SECTION 7
Common practical problems in
a pediatric ophthalmology
and strabismus practice

CHAPTER **93**

The sticky eye in infancy

David Laws

Ophthalmia neonatorum

Purulent discharge within 48 hours of birth should alert the physician to *Neisseria* whereas chlamydial infection presents at around 10 days (see Chapter 12). Conjunctival culture is useful to identify the organism but, increasingly, microarray techniques are being used for more rapid diagnosis.[1] The parents should undergo contact tracing in a genitourinary clinic. Systemic therapy is required for chlamydial disease to treat other complications such as pneumonitis. Neonatal prophylaxis of ophthalmia neonatorum has been abandoned in the UK and Sweden. Povidone iodine 1.25–2.5%, topical tetracycline, or fusidic acid can be used particularly where antenatal care has not been well documented, but iodine may cause irritation.[2]

Bacterial conjunctivitis

Bacteria cause the majority of cases of acute conjunctivitis in infants.[3] Although most clear without treatment, antibiotic therapy results in earlier clinical and microbiological resolution. Most comparative studies of treatment of acute conjunctivitis show little difference between the broad-spectrum antibiotics.[4] Antibiotic resistance is increasingly recognized, particularly with Gram-positive isolates.[5]

Viral and allergic conjunctivitis

Viral conjunctivitis causes most of the other acute cases, with epidemics of adenovirus in winter months. Viral hemorrhagic conjunctivitis epidemics caused by coxsackievirus and enterovirus are increasingly reported.[6] Primary herpes simplex or chickenpox may also affect the conjunctiva. A small molluscum lesion on the lid margin may be easily missed and result in chronic conjunctivitis. Allergic conjunctivitis is unusual in infancy, but should be considered in the presence of other atopic disease.

Nasolacrimal duct obstruction

The commonest association of the recurrently sticky eye is congenital nasolacrimal obstruction (see Chapter 21) and superinfection by opportunistic bacteria. The majority are associated with epiphora. Clinically, 20% of young infants have evidence of obstruction but 95% of these resolve by a year.[7] The presence of a lacrimal sac mucocele should be excluded and the child examined for abnormalities of or for supernumerary lacrimal puncta. Initial care is by massage to the lacrimal sac and cleaning the lids from nasal to temporal using clean cotton wool and water; persistent epiphora (past 1 year of age) or severe recurrent infection is treated with probing of the nasolacrimal duct. Cases that have persistent watering after one or more probings may undergo silicone rod intubation. Several studies suggest that monocanalicular is as successful as bicanalicular intubation.[8] Balloon dilation may be used but there are conflicting results in the literature.

Lashes and lids

The soft lashes of small children are normally well tolerated in epiblepharon. Persistent corneal staining, however, may be an indication that intervention is required.[9] Multiple rows of lashes or congenital lid anomalies such as lid notch associated with trichiasis may be found. Blepharokeratitis is associated with recurrent corneal ulceration leading to vascularization and scarring of the cornea. Systemic therapy with erythromycin is useful in reducing the severity of lid disease. Systemic tetracyclines should be avoided in children.

Malnutrition and other causes

In developing countries malnutrition, including vitamin A deficiency, may contribute to recurrent infection.

Rarely, recurrent conjunctivitis may be associated with systemic disease in infants. Lymphadenopathy, a high fever, and conjunctivitis should alert the physician to the possibility of Kawasaki's disease, which is associated with coronary aneurysms. Stevens-Johnson syndrome may result in a severe cicatrizing conjunctival inflammation. Dry eyes with a mucous discharge and corneal anesthesia may be associated with familial dysautonomia. Ligneous conjunctivitis also rarely affects infants. All infective disease should be treated with great caution in the immunosuppressed.

Epiphora and photophobia raise the possibility of congenital glaucoma (see Chapter 37), corneal dystrophy (see Chapter 34), or corneal ulceration (see Chapter 33) (Fig. 93.1).

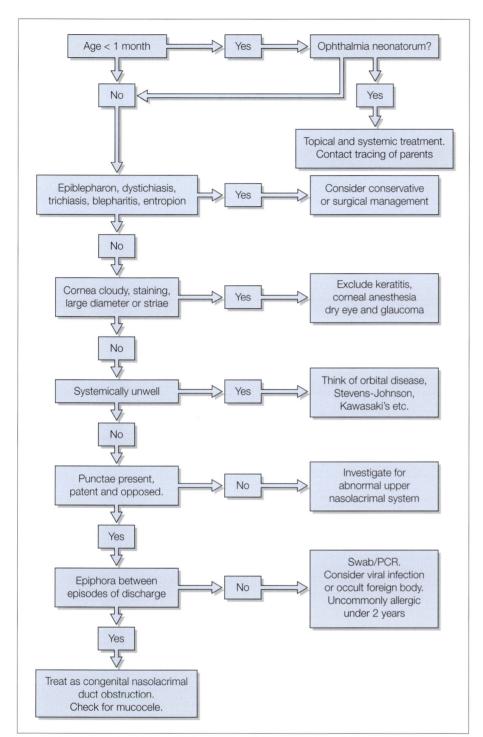

Fig. 93.1 Assessment of recurrent sticky eyes in infancy.

References

1. Yip PP, Chan WH, Yip KT, et al. The use of polymerase chain reaction assay versus conventional methods in detecting neonatal chlamydial conjunctivitis. J Pediatr Ophthalmol Strabismus [Comparative Study]. 2008; 45: 234–9.

2. Zuppa AA, D'Andrea V, Catenazzi P, et al. Ophthalmia neonatorum: what kind of prophylaxis? J Matern Fetal Neonatal Med 2011; 24:69–73.

3. Wong VW, Lai TY, Chi SC, Lam DS. Pediatric ocular surface infections: a 5-year review of demographics, clinical features, risk factors, microbiological results, and treatment. Cornea 2011; 30: 955–1002.

4. Sheikh A, Hurwitz B. Antibiotics versus placebo for acute bacterial conjunctivitis. Cochrane Database Syst Rev 2006: CD001211.

5. Adebayo A, Parikh JG, McCormick SA, et al. Shifting trends in in vitro antibiotic susceptibilities for common bacterial conjunctival isolates in the last decade at the New York Eye and Ear Infirmary. Graefes Arch Clin Exp Ophthalmol 2011; 249: 111–9.

6. Kono R. Apollo 11 disease or acute hemorrhagic conjunctivitis: a pandemic of a new enterovirus infection of the eyes. Am J Epidemiol 1975; 101: 383–90.

7. Maini R, MacEwen CJ, Young JD. The natural history of epiphora in childhood. Eye 1998; 12 (Pt 4): 669–71.

8. Andalib D, Gharabaghi D, Nabai R, Abbaszadeh M. Monocanalicular versus bicanalicular silicone intubation for congenital nasolacrimal duct obstruction. J AAPOS 2010; 14: 421–4.

9. Sundar G, Young SM, Tara S, et al. Epiblepharon in East Asian patients: the Singapore experience. Ophthalmology 2010; 117: 184–9.

Doctor, my baby's eye looks strange

John A Bradbury

Parents find it easier to describe the behavior of their child than an anatomical abnormality of the eye. For example, parents can usually tell you that their child can't see or has night-blindness rather than describe accurately leukocoria or aniridia. Usually they say that the eye looks "funny" or "unusual." However, a careful history from the parent can often clarify how long the abnormality has been present, whether this has coincided with any deterioration in visual function, and if the physical abnormality is static or progressive. Closer questioning may reveal exactly what the abnormality is, but in general this is found by your own careful examination (Fig. 94.1).

If no clue is available from the parent or child's history, the best way to approach the problem is anatomically – looking at each tissue systematically. If an abnormality is found, examining other systems may help in the diagnosis, e.g. umbilical hernia + dental abnormality + corectopia = Rieger syndrome. If the abnormality is not easily explained, examination of parents and siblings is always worthwhile to try and exclude an inherited condition. Also, one must always bear in mind trauma as a cause of an ocular abnormality.

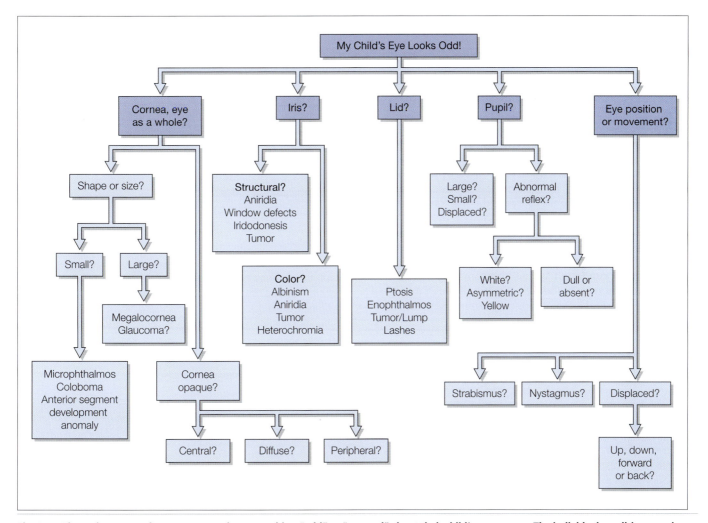

Fig. 94.1 The main causes when a parent notices something "odd" or "unusual" about their child's eye or eyes. The individual conditions can be found via the index.

My baby has a lump in the lid

Gerd Holmström

A lump in the lid is common in children either as an isolated finding or as a manifestation of a systemic disease (Table 95.1). The causes are mostly benign, although malignancies need to be considered (Box 95.1).

Rhabdomyosarcoma (see Chapter 24)

Rhabdomyosarcoma is a rapidly progressing malignant tumor, which must be considered in the differential diagnosis of a lid lump in children. Although proptosis is the most common feature of ophthalmic rhabdomyosarcoma, manifestation in the lid can be the presenting finding. The history is typically short: days or weeks, and the tumor often presents before 10 years of age.[1,2] The tumor may simulate an inflammatory process or vascular lesions such as capillary hemangioma or lymphangioma.

If rhabdomyosarcoma is suspected, the child should promptly be investigated with MRI, and a biopsy should be taken for diagnosis and histopathological classification. Molecular diagnostics may sometimes be helpful in the classification. Modern treatment with multiagent chemotherapy, sometimes supported by radiotherapy, has resulted in increased survival rates to more than 90%, although tumors of an alveolar type and presentations in infancy show a worse prognosis.[1,2]

Dermoid (see Chapter 29)

Dermoids are common in children. They are developmental, cystic, lesions usually at the supratemporal margin of the orbit. Histologically they are lined by keratinizing, stratified squamous epithelium and may contain fat, hair follicles, sebaceous glands, and sweat glands. Inflammation occurs if the cyst ruptures. A dermoid usually appears as a smooth mass and is variably movable due to attachment to underlying structures.[3] Superficial lesions are most common: some are deep.

Dermoids in the lid usually do not affect vision, although amblyopia may occur due to pressure on the eye resulting in

Box 95.1
Causes of lumps in the lid
Benign
Nevus
Acquired melanocytic nevus
Congenital melanocytic nevus
Inflammatory
Chalazion
Stye/abscess
Molluscum contagiosum
Warts
Sarcoidosis
Wegener's granulomatosis
Pseudorheumatoid nodules
Neural
Neurofibroma – NF1
Schwannoma
Vascular
Capillary hemangioma
Nevus flammeus/Sturge-Weber
Lymphangioma
Pyogenic granuloma
Miscellaneous
Dermoid
Juvenile xanthogranuloma
Histiocytosis
Angiofibroma (in tuberous sclerosis)
Pilomatrixoma (calcifying epithelioma of Malherbe)
Malign
Rhabdomyosarcoma
Lymphoma
Leukemia
Metastatic tumor
Melanoma

Table 95.1 – Presentation and Pathology of Lumps in Lid

Lesion	Elevated or flat	Focal	Color	Location	Pathology
Nevus	Flat	Focal	Brown/black	Lid or margin	Benign melanocytic cells
Nevus sebaceous	Plaque	Geographic	Tan/brown	Lid	Epidermal hyperplasia, absence of hair follicles
Chalazion	Nodule	Focal	Pink/red	Lid margin	Lipogranulomatous inflammation
Stye	Nodule	Focal	Red	Lid Margin	Inflammation sebaceous gland
Molluscum contagiosum	Papules	Multiple	Pink/flesh	Lid or margin	Intracytoplasmic inclusion bodies in epidermis
Warts	Papules	Multiple	Flesh/white	Lid or margin	Benign proliferation of skin/mucosa
Sarcoidosis	Nodules	Multiple	Flesh	Lid/orbit	Non-caseating granulomas/Langerhans' giant cells
Wegener's granulomatosis	Ulcer	Focal	Red	Lid/orbit	Necrotizing granulomatosis vasculitis
Pseudorheumatoid nodule	Nodule	Focal	Normal	Lid	Palisading granuloma/central necrosis
Neurofibroma	Thickened	Diffuse	Non-pigmented	Lid/orbit	Proliferation of all elements of peripheral nerve
Schwannoma	Mass	Focal	Non-pigmented	Lid	True capsule/fascicles of Schwann cells
Capillary hemangioma	Variable	Focal	Pink/bluish-red	Lid/orbit	Proliferation of vascular channels/mostly veins
Nevus flammeus	Flat	Geographic	Red/pink	Lid	Abnormal aggregation of capillaries
Lymphangioma	Fullness	Diffuse	Bluish	Lid/orbit	Irregular sized/shaped vascular channels, fibrous
Pyogenic granuloma	Pedicle	Focal	Pink/red	Lid	Lobulated proliferation of capillaries/stroma edema
Dermoid	Mass	Focal	Non-pigmented	Eyebrow	Thick wall, hair follicles, fat, sebaceous glands
Juvenile xanthogranuloma	Papules	Multiple	Red, yellow, brown	Lid	Histiocytic proliferation, non-Langerhans' giant cells
Histiocytosis	Swelling	Diffuse	Non-pigmented	Lid/orbit	Histocytic proliferation, Langerhans' giant cells
Angiofibroma	Papules	Multiple	Reddish-brown	Lid	Spindle cells, collagen, thick-walled vessels
Pilomatrixoma	Hard nodule	Focal	Flesh/purple	Lid	Small basaloid cells, foreign body reaction, calcification
Rhabdomyosarcoma	Mass	Focal	Non-pigmented	Lid/orbit	Rhabdomyoblasts, variable muscle morphogenesis
Lymphoma	Mass	Diffuse	Salmon patch	Lid/orbit	Atypical lymphocytes, no follicles, minimal vascularity
Leukemia	Mass	Diffuse	Non-pigmented	Lid/orbit	Increased white blood cells, proliferation of blasts
Primary mucinous carcinoma	Mass	Focal	Non-pigmented	Lid/orbit	Epithelial nests, mucin, fibrovascular septa
Metastatic carcinoma	Mass	Focal	Non-pigmented	Lid/orbit	Depends on primary site
Melanoma	Flat	Focal	Brown, black	Lid	Proliferation melanocytes/mitotic figures
Kaposi's sarcoma	Variable	Multiple	Red, purple, brown	Lid	Intracellular hyaline, spindle cells, high vascularity

anisometropia. Treatment may be conservative, observation only, or surgical removal. Usually they are removed for cosmetic problems, inflammation, or growth. Dermoids may extend into the orbit. Unless the tumor is fully movable, a CT scan should therefore be performed prior to surgery. The aim should be to excise the dermoid as a whole cyst and avoid rupture, which may cause chronic inflammation.

Capillary hemangioma
(see Chapter 20)

Capillary hemangiomas are common, benign, tumors, most often affecting the upper lid and the orbit of the child. Superficial hemangiomas have a red, lobulated appearance and are often referred to as "strawberry lesions." Subcutaneous hemangiomas have a more bluish color. They present during the first months of life and grow rapidly during the following months. Rarely, they are very extensive and markedly affect the appearance of the child. After a period of stabilization they slowly regress. Most involution occurs before 7 years. Capillary hemangiomas are often isolated, but may be associated with ocular and systemic abnormalities.

Amblyopia may occur due to occlusion of the visual axis or distortion of the globe, leading to astigmatism and anisometropia.

Chalazion (see Chapter 15)

Chalazia are lipogranulomatous inflammations that result from an obstruction of a meibomian gland duct. They usually present as a localized and painless nodule in the lid or lid margin with a swollen, red lid. Small chalazia usually resolve spontaneously. Warm compresses, lid hygiene, and topical antibiotics can be useful if the lesion is inflamed. Larger chalazia may need incision and curettage under general anesthesia in young children. Chronic chalazia warrant a suspicion of malignancy, such as rhabdomyosarcoma.

As in all young children with a lump in the lid of any cause, the risk of amblyopia by distortion of the globe or partial occlusion of the visual axis must not be overlooked.

Molluscum contagiosum and warts (see Chapter 19)

Molluscum contagiosum and warts are common viral infections of the lid in children. The lesions are small (a few millimeters) and often multiple, with an umbilicated center and may be associated with a symptomatic follicular conjunctivitis. They sometimes require treatment with incision, curettage, or diathermy.

Stye/abscess

A stye is a painful abscess of the sebaceous glands of Zeiss in the lid often associated with *Staphylococcus aureus*. The stye may resolve spontaneously, but antibiotic ointment may be helpful and relieve some of the discomfort. Larger abscesses may require systemic antibiotics, incision, and drainage.

Other less common causes of lumps in the lid

Malignancies

Lymphoma, leukemic infiltrates, melanoma, and metastases of other tumors are all rare (Box 95.1).

Nevi (see Chapter 18)

Both acquired and congenital melanocytic nevi of the lid occur. The acquired nevi usually present between 5 and 10 years of age; they are flat or slightly elevated, and they darken with age. Malignant transformation is rare.

Inflammatory lesions

Sarcoidosis, Wegener's granulomatosis, and pseudorheumatoid nodules are granulomatous inflammations that may involve the lids.

Neural (see Chapter 65)

A neurofibroma of the lid usually occurs with neurofibromatosis, often giving the lid an "S-shaped" appearance. Gradual growth of the tumor may cause ptosis, distortion of the globe, and amblyopia. Surgical debulking is often needed but the mass frequently recurs. Ipsilateral glaucoma is frequent.

Schwannomas are tumors arising from the Schwann cells of the peripheral nerve sheath. They may also occur in association with neurofibromatosis.

Other vascular lesions (see Chapter 20)

A lymphangioma usually presents in infancy and gradually grows over many years. Due to hemorrhage, the presentation is often sudden. Lymphangiomas are difficult to manage, and, unlike capillary hemangiomas, they do not regress spontaneously.

Nevus flammeus may be isolated or associated with the Sturge-Weber syndrome. Congenital or juvenile glaucoma is a common complication (see Chapter 65).

Pyogenic granuloma appears as a fleshy red mass and is a proliferative fibrovascular response to previous trauma, inflammation, or surgery.

Miscellaneous

Juvenile xanthogranuloma (see Chapter 27) is a benign, yellow/orange-colored, granulomatous inflammatory disorder of the skin, which may also affect the lids. It predominantly occurs in infancy and early childhood. The lesions usually regress spontaneously.

Histiocytosis (Langerhans' cell histiocytosis, histiocytosis-X) is an uncommon disorder that may affect the lid.

Angiofibromas of the skin and lid often occur in the first decade of life as early manifestations of tuberous sclerosis.

Pilomatrixoma (calcifying epithelioma of Malherbe) is a benign tumor originating from the hair matrix cells. It is usually solitary and appears in the lid or eyebrow as a subcutaneous red to blue, *hard* mass. The lesion should be surgically excised.

References

1. Kodet R, Newton WA, Hamoudi AB, et al. Orbital rhabdomyosarcomas and related tumors in childhood: relationship of morphology to prognosis – an intergroup rhabdomyosarcoma study. Med Pediatr Oncol 1997; 29: 51–60.
2. Shields JA, Shields CL. Rhabdomyosarcoma: review for the ophthalmologist. Surv Ophthalmol 2003; 48: 39–57.
3. Shields JA, Kaden IH, Eagle RC Jr, et al. Orbital dermoid cysts: clinicopathologic correlations, classifications, and management. The 1997 Josephine E. Schueler Lecture. Ophthal Plast Reconstr Surg 1997; 13: 265–76.

My child keeps blinking and closing his eye

John S Elston

Introduction

This is a relatively common referral to the pediatric ophthalmologist. In the vast majority of cases the diagnosis will be evident from a targeted history and a standard ophthalmological examination. Tic disorder and ocular surface disease are the two common causes.

History

1. Enquire about associated symptoms and signs. Redness, tearing, discharge, mucus, and clouding of the cornea indicate an ocular surface disorder. There may be a history of atopy, or recent eye lid vesicles suggesting primary herpes simplex virus infection. Potentially significant ocular trauma or foreign body exposure is often unreported by children unless specifically asked about.
2. Ask about the circumstances in which the blinking or unilateral eye closure is most evident. There are characteristic factors that exacerbate or ameliorate tics (see below). Previous episodes of self-limiting unilateral or bilateral increased blinking at the appropriate age also suggest tic disorder.
3. Ask if there is a family history of refractive error, amblyopia, or squint (see below).

Examination

1. Whilst questioning the parents, observe the child surreptitiously for the characteristics of an eye winking or blinking tic or other simple motor or phonic tics.
2. The ophthalmological examination should include elimination of uncorrected refractive error as a potential cause and an orthoptic assessment for heterophoria.
3. Slit-lamp examination should include exclusion of lid margin malposition, lash abnormalities, and a foreign body (including subtarsal). Superior limbal vernal keratoconjunctivitis may be missed unless specifically looked for; look also for signs suggesting corneal anesthesia such as opacity and superficial vascularization.

Tic disorder

Simple motor tics are sudden brief repetitive stereotyped motor movements involving discrete muscle groups. Eye winking (one eye) or eye blinking (both eyes) tics are the commonest and affect boys more than girls (3 to 10 times more frequent) at an average age of 6 years. In 12% the onset is before the age of 4 years and development after the end of the first decade is very unusual. 10% to 15% of boys between school starting age and 10 years will have a simple motor tic at some stage. Tics may be triggered by minor focal trauma, e.g. in the case of eye winking a lash in the eye.

There may be a family history of simple motor tic in first degree relatives. Also, childhood onset obsessive compulsive disorder (OCD), which may be familial and often has tic co-morbidity and there is a genetic susceptibility to the spectrum of tic disorder, OCD, and attention deficit hyperactivity disorder (ADHD).

Eye winking and blinking tics characteristically increase with stress, fatigue, boredom, and anxiety. They reduce with absorption in activities including books, games, and sport. Tics are voluntarily suppressible for a short period only – the underlying sensory premonitory urge is irresistible and "released" by the motor tic. The child will be able to stop the tic for a while but then "have to do it" – like an itch that has to be scratched. Some boys with eye winking or blinking tics also have, or have had, other simple motor tics such as head shaking or vocal or phonic tics, particularly throat clearing.

Simple motor tics characteristically wax and wane over a period of months before spontaneously remitting within about a year; occasionally they recur a few months later.

There is a spectrum of disorder determined by the duration, severity, and characteristics of the tics from simple tic disorder to Tourette's syndrome. It is likely that this spectrum of disorder is determined by genetic susceptibility. It is important to note that most cases of Tourette's syndrome are not severe and the highly publicized, socially embarrassing features are rare.

Eye movement tics – characteristically large concomitant diagonal saccades – may occur in both simple tic disorder and Tourette's syndrome.

Management

The vast majority of children with eye winking or blinking tics do not require any form of investigation or referral. When the typical features are present, parents can be reassured that this common condition invariably resolves spontaneously. The parents may want to notify the school authorities to ensure the child is not punished or teased about the tic. There is no role for parental admonishment of the child or need for routine referral to a pediatrician.

Tourette's syndrome should be suspected if in addition to motor tics there is a history of vocal tics (including swear words, etc.), motor hyperactivity, impulsivity, and disruptive behavior. These children should be referred to a pediatric neurologist or psychiatrist for definitive diagnosis and management.

Ocular surface disorders

Mostly, these are common acquired conditions such as meibomian gland dysfunction/blepharitis and allergic eye disease. Occasionally, rarities such as childhood onset corneal dystrophy or deposits may present with eye blinking or closure. A specific diagnosis can usually be made on clinical examination which should include eversion of the superior tarsal plate. If this is not possible in a young child, an examination under anesthetic is essential. A subtarsal foreign body can be retained for months in a young child or an unsuspected self-sealing traumatic ocular perforation may have occurred.

Ocular alignment/movement/refraction

Intermittent exotropia and uncorrected refractive error have been designated the underlying cause of excessive blinking in childhood in up to 25% of cases. Forceful blinks may help to control an exophoria. Unilateral eye closure in bright sunlight is a feature of intermittent exodeviations, but the explanation is uncertain as diplopia is unusual even when the deviation is manifest.

Children with an ocular misalignment of any cause may not complain of double vision but shut one eye to avoid it, presenting with unilateral eye closure. Cover testing in all positions of gaze is required as the deviation may be small and not evident in the primary position.

Photoreceptor dystrophy

Photophobia, increased tearing, and excessive blinking are features of photoreceptor dystrophies particularly congenital achromatopsia, also cone–rod dystrophies. Other potential ocular causes, such as opacities in the media and intraocular inflammation, must be excluded.

Other possibilities

Ocular myasthenia can present as an isolated unilateral ptosis; there may also be flickering lid movements – lid twitches on vertical eye movement and lid hops on horizontal movement – which can be a prominent feature.

Orbicularis oculi myokymia can cause persistent irritating rippling contractions unilaterally. This is usually a benign self limiting disorder; if persistent or spreading, it can also be due to dorsal pontine pathology and has been reported in demyelinating disease and pontine glioma.

Hemifacial spasm causes bursts of flickering rapid unilateral eye closure, often involving the ipsilateral mid to lower face and synchronous eyebrow elevation. In adults it is almost invariably due to microvascular compression of the ipsilateral facial nerve in the root exit zone.

Infantile or childhood onset hemifacial spasm is very rare and although vascular pathology may be responsible a number of cases have been reported due to intrinsic pontine tumours; all cases must be fully investigated with neuroimaging.

Familial hemifacial spasm is a rare phenomenon probably due to genetically determined vascular malformation which can present in the second decade.

Blink-saccade synkinesis is the descriptive term for the use of eye blinks to break fixation and initiate saccadic eye movements. It is seen most obviously in saccade initiation failure syndromes (ocular motor apraxia), but also in some apparently normal children.

Tardive dyskinesia is involuntary dystonic muscle hyperactivity that may develop and sometimes persist after usually long-term exposure to neuroleptic drugs used in the treatment of childhood onset schizophrenia and sometimes ADHD. Metoclopramide used to treat gastro-esophageal reflux can also be responsible. Increased forceful eye blinking, brow elevation, and facial grimacing may be seen. Drug withdrawal may not lead to resolution of the signs.

My baby keeps closing one eye

Manoj V Parulekar

Introduction

The child who closes one eye can cause considerable anxiety to the parents, and pose a diagnostic conundrum. The presentation could be in the acute clinical setting or as a chronic symptom, and the symptoms may be intermittent.

The approach to a case

The parents often describe the child as "screwing up the eye" or "squinting one eye," or covering the eye with the hand.

The history includes which eye is involved, duration and frequency of symptoms, aggravating factors such as bright lights,[1] cold windy weather, stressful situations, and relieving factors, if any. Associated symptoms such as redness and watering are relevant. A history of trauma must be sought.

A full eye examination is mandatory until the cause is found, although the approach depends on the mode of presentation.

With the direct ophthalmoscope on +4 D magnification it is useful to assess corneal and media clarity followed by slit lamp examination. A drop of short-acting topical anesthetic such as proxymetacaine 0.5%, with or without fluorescein, may facilitate the examination. If no cause is evident, dilated fundus examination is warranted. Tonometry (see Chapters 7 and 37) can be difficult in the acute setting, but the advent of the I-care tonometer has made this easier. Other useful maneuvers include examining the younger child when feeding or asleep.

If an adequate examination is impossible, and it is important to exclude a foreign body, uveitis or glaucoma in the presence of an unexplained red eye, examination under anesthetic or sedation may be needed.

Acute presentation

The common causes in the acute setting are given in Box 97.1. The child is often distressed, usually seen in the emergency department, and examination might be difficult. The commonest cause is a *corneal abrasion* or *foreign body*, less common is *infective keratitis* (see Chapter 15). Fluorescein staining is very useful in these situations. It is important to evert the lids and look for subtarsal foreign bodies if multiple linear abrasions are seen.

Diffuse punctate staining could result from *chemical injury*[2] (see Chapters 15 and 33).

Although *acute meibomitis* or *preseptal cellulitis* (see Chapter 13) is evident on external examination, anterior segment pathology can similarly present with lid swelling and must be excluded.

Rarely, *acute hydrops* in *keratoconus* (see Chapter 33) or corneal edema from raised intraocular pressure (see Chapter 37) can present with unilateral eye closure.

An acute rise in intraocular pressure from traumatic or spontaneous *hyphema* (see Chapters 37 and 66) can be excluded with a hand-held slit-lamp examination.

Sub-acute or chronic presentation

The approach is quite different when the child presents with long-standing symptoms. A detailed history taking is essential.

Box 97.1

Causes of unilateral eye closure

Acute causes of unilateral eye closure

Lid – angioneurotic edema, blepharochalasis syndrome, inflamed meibomian cyst, preseptal cellulitis

Ocular surface
corneal abrasion, conjunctivitis – infective, allergic, or chemical keratitis – bacterial, viral, or fungal

Trauma – corneal or subtarsal foreign body, hyphema

Anterior segment – acute glaucoma, acute uveitis

Neurological – acute ptosis from myasthenia, oculomotor palsy, migraine

Sub-acute and chronic causes of unilateral eye closure

Media opacities – cataract, colobomas (cause glare)

Diplopia – from acute onset strabismus, intermittent exotropia

Ocular surface – allergic eye disease

Lid problems – fatiguable ptosis

Neurological – cyclic oculomotor palsy, myasthenia, Marcus Gunn jaw wink, epilepsy, ophthalmoplegic migraine

Functional – tic, conversion disorder

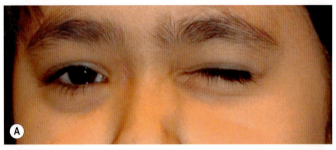

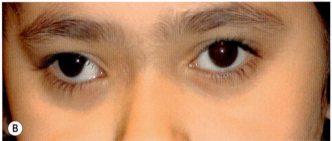

Fig. 97.1 Unilateral eye closure. (A) From acute onset exotropia;
(B) following orbital trauma.

Photographs and videos demonstrating the eye closure, often recorded by parents on mobile phone cameras, are invaluable where the symptoms are infrequent and do not manifest during the consultation (see Chapter 7).

Photophobia is an important sign, and usually points to an ocular surface problem. The assessment in such cases is similar to that described above. It is important to look for *cataract* or other *media opacities* (see Chapter 36), and *colobomas* (see Chapter 38) that can result in light scatter and glare.

Episodic unilateral ptosis (see Chapter 19) could be mistaken for eye closure, and can occur in *cyclical third nerve paralysis*,[3] and *ophthalmoplegic migraine* (see Chapter 83). It is important to look for signs of *hemifacial spasm*, which is usually due to brainstem pathology in children and needs neuroimaging. Eyelid *myoclonia with absences (Jeavons' syndrome)*[4] and *Marcus*

Gunn jaw winking ptosis (see Chapter 19) could both be reported as intermittent eye closure.

A history of diplopia must be sought, and cover testing and ocular motility examination are useful in detecting *intermittent exotropia*[5] (see Chapter 77), not uncommonly a cause of unilateral eye closure. Similarly, *new onset strabismus* might produce diplopia and unilateral eye closure (Fig. 97.1). Associated features such as abnormal head posture might provide useful clues to the underlying diagnosis.

Finally, one must consider the possibility of a *tic*, or *functional causes* (including conversion disorder) for the eye closure (see Chapter 60). Tics are more common in boys and are, rarely, the first manifestation of *Tourette's syndrome*.

Unilateral or bilateral asymmetric eye closure

Some cases of apparently unilateral lid closure can be bilateral or asymmetric (see Chapter 96).

References

1. Wiggins RE, von Noorden GK. Monocular eye closure in sunlight. J Pediatr Ophthalmol Strabismus 1990; 27: 16–20; discussion 21–2.
2. Macdonald EC, Cauchi PA, Azuara-Blanco A, Foot B. Surveillance of severe chemical corneal injuries in the UK. Br J Ophthalmol 2009; 93: 1177–80.
3. Bateman DE, Saunders M. Cyclic oculomotor palsy: description of a case and hypothesis of the mechanism. J Neurol Neurosurg Psychiatry 1983; 46: 451–3.
4. Striano S, Capovilla G, Sofia V et al. Eyelid myoclonia with absences (Jeavons syndrome): a well-defined idiopathic generalized epilepsy syndrome or a spectrum of photosensitive conditions? Epilepsia 2009; 50 (Suppl 5): 15–9.
5. Serrano-Pedraza I, Manjunath V, Osunkunle O, et al. Visual suppression in intermittent exotropia during binocular alignment. Invest Ophthalmol Vis Sci 2011; 52: 2352–64.

My child's eyes are dry and sore

Gillian G W Adams

Introduction

The eye is protected against damage and infection by the lids and by a lubricating tear film. The tear film consists of three layers: mucous (produced by conjunctival goblet cells), aqueous (secreted by the lacrimal glands), and lipid (secreted by the meibomian glands). Dysfunction in any layer of the tear film can result in ocular surface drying and damage. Dry eye disease may be categorized as either aqueous deficient (caused by disorders affecting the lacrimal gland) or evaporative (due to meibomian gland dysfunction or abnormalities of the lid, lid closure and globe leading to exposure).[1] Ocular dryness results in increased osmolarity of the tear film and inflammation of the ocular surface. The presence of corneal anesthesia exacerbates the effects of drying and exposure and puts the eye at risk of defective epithelial healing, corneal ulceration, and perforation.

Dry eye in childhood is underdiagnosed and whilst a severely dry and ulcerated eye is easily recognized, milder forms may go unrecognized. Many cases of dry eye have a simple and easily identified explanation, e.g. a lid notch or, most commonly, secondary to allergic eye disease. However, a dry eye in childhood may be the sign of a rare, but serious systemic disorder, and the ophthalmologist should be alert to this possibility.[2] Tables 98.1 and 98.2 give details of ocular and systemic diseases/conditions associated with dry eye in children.

Presentation and symptoms

Children rarely complain of a dry eye, but usually complain of a gritty, itchy, or scratchy eye, a foreign body or burning sensation, or blurred vision and light sensitivity. The child may blink excessively or be photophobic.

History

A dry eye may be associated with a local ophthalmic disorder, systemic disease, environmental factors, or effect of medication. The history should clarify birth history, medical problems, and medications. For example, if the child was premature

Table 98.1 – Ocular disease causing dry eye

Allergic eye disease	Papillae, giant papillae, corneal erosions
Anesthetic cornea from corneal disease	Damage to trigeminal nerve, e.g. herpes simplex, herpes zoster
Aniridia	Abnormal tear film stability and meibomian gland dysfunction
Chemical burns	Conjunctival scarring
Congenital alacrima	Primary form limited to lacrimal gland (also occurs as part of syndromes)
Contact lens wear	Reduced tear film volume
Dacryoadenitis	Secondary to infection, e.g. Epstein-Barr virus
Incomplete lid closure, proptosis, facial palsy	Intensive care patients, VII palsy, shallow orbits, orbital tumors
Lid margin disease	Telangiectatic lid margin vessels, scaly debris in lashes, blocked meibomian glands
Lid notch	Allows evaporation of tear film
Ocular surface abnormalities	Conjunctival scarring (including strabismus surgery), dermolipomas, corneal dellen
Post-ptosis surgery	Incomplete lid closure, aggravated by reduced Bell's or reduced upgaze
Reduced blink rate	May be associated with prolonged computer or electronic games use
Topical drug therapy	Preservatives can cause conjunctival irritation and dryness

and underwent gastrointestinal surgery for necrotizing enterocolitis, this could place the child at risk of short bowel syndrome and vitamin A deficiency. Some medications such as antihistamines, antispasmodics or retinoids, and topical drugs containing preservatives may cause a dry eye. Checking if the child attends other physicians will identify concurrent disease such as diabetes or cancer.

The parents should be asked if the child produces reflex or emotional tears. It has been said that babies do not produce tears until 6 weeks of age, but tears are produced from the first

Table 98.2 – Systemic disease causing dry eye

Allgrove's syndrome	Triple A syndrome: adrenocorticoid deficiency, achalasia of the cardia, alacrima
Autoimmune polyendocrinopathy syndrome type 1	Reduced tear production, hypoparathyroidism, mucocutaneous candidiasis, adrenocortical insufficiency
Blepharophimosis syndrome	Absent lacrimal glands giving alacrima
Chronic renal failure	Reduced tear secretion and tear film stability
CIPA: congenital insensitivity to pain with anhidrosis	Dry eye, reduced corneal sensivity and ulceration, recurrent fever, anhidrosis, delayed healing
Complete androgen insensitivity syndrome	Sex hormone related dry eye may occur before sexual maturation
Craniofacial syndromes	Proptosis with exposure
Cystic fibrosis	May be vitamin A deficiency or a direct manifestation of cystic fibrosis
Diabetes	May relate to autonomic dysfunction
Down's syndrome	Incomplete lid closure is common leading to dry eye
Ectodermal dysplasia	Anomalies include ectrodactyly, defects of hair, teeth and sweat glands, cleft lip and palate
Environmental factors	Heating, low humidity, air-conditioning, extensive computer use
Epidermolysis bullosa	Skin and mucous membrane disease with conjunctival scarring
Goldenhar's syndrome	Dermolipomas, epibulbar dermoids
Graft-versus-host disease	Common after pediatric bone marrow transplantation
HIV	Lacrimal gland infiltration
Juvenile dermatomyositis	Dry eye reported in dermatomyositis and secondary Sjögren's syndrome
Juvenile idiopathic arthritis	Reduced basal tear secretion
Juvenile localized scleroderma	Particularly form involving face (en coup de sabre)
KID syndrome: keratitis-ichthyosis-deafness	Hyperkeratotic skin lesions, sensorineural hearing loss and vascularizing keratitis
LOC: laryngo-onycho-cutaneous syndrome	Ocular granulation tissue with progressive scarring of conjunctiva and cornea
Medication	Antihistamines, antispasmodics, retinoids, topical drugs containing preservatives
Möbius' syndrome	Reduced blinking with facial weakness
Multiple endocrine neoplasia type IIB	Marfanoid appearance, thick lips and eyelid neuromas, may have prominent corneal nerves
Neuroparalytic keratitis	Trigeminal nerve damage: acoustic neuroma, pontine tumors, Goldenhar syndrome, leprosy, after trauma
Pierre Robin sequence	May be associated with congenital alacrima
Post-orbital radiotherapy	Lacrimal gland damage
Riley-Day syndrome	Affects autonomic and sensory nervous system with dry, anesthetic eye
Sjögren's syndrome	Lacrimal gland infiltration producing aqueous deficiency
Stevens-Johnson syndrome	Blisters or pseudomembrane in the early stages, later scarring and symblepharon
Trachoma	Common in developing world, mucopurulent conjunctivitis then cicatrization and corneal scarring
Turner's syndrome	May relate to hormonal effect on meibomian gland function
Vitamin A deficiency	After bowel surgery, restricted diet, cystic fibrosis, dry conjunctiva, Bitot's spots, keratomalacia, night blindness
Xeroderma pigmentosum	Dry pigmented skin, photophobia, reduced tearing, ocular surface squamous neoplasia

day of life.[3] Congenital alacrima is rare but the eye surface is often moist despite the absence of reflex or emotional tears.[4] Ask if the child sleeps with their eyes open. This may occur in normal children, in those with craniofacial disorders, proptosis, and lid abnormalities, or after ptosis surgery.

Examination

Some tests will only be possible in the older child. If the child has severe dry eyes it is likely to be photophobic and difficult to examine unless it has corneal anesthesia. Be alert to the possibility of loss of sensation as the combination of dry eye and corneal anesthesia can result in severe keratitis.

Assessment

1. Best corrected visual acuity.
2. External inspection: face, lid closure and blink rate, external eye, and tear strip.
3. Ocular surface examination.
4. Staining patterns.
5. Other tests: Schirmer's test, impression cytology, and corneal sensation.

Visual acuity

The visual acuity is usually normal unless the cornea is severely dry or ulcerated.

External inspection

Look at the child, its face, eye, and eyelids. Check the facies for a syndromic disorder that may be associated with dry eyes such as ectodermal dysplasia. Normally, an eye should be "white" with a bright, moist surface. If the eye is mildly injected with a dull surface and little moisture visible in the tear film the child has a dry eye.

Assess the blink rate and lid closure. Check for an abnormality that causes ocular surface exposure and drying such as proptosis or a craniofacial syndrome (see Chapter 28). Look for lid abnormalities such as scarring, notches, or colobomas (see Chapter 18), and for blepharitis and meibomianitis, which may destabilize the tear film and cause surface drying (see Chapter 15). Assess lid closure: if inadequate the tear film cannot maintain corneal wetting and the ocular surface will desiccate. After ptosis surgery a poor Bell's phenomenon or reduced upgaze will result in ocular drying. If there is evidence of facial weakness or poor lid closure, the presence or absence of Bell's phenomenon and corneal sensation should be noted.

Ocular surface examination and staining patterns

If possible, this should by undertaken by slit-lamp examination, which is achievable in most children from about the age of 3 years, but if not possible a 20 D lens and hand-held flashlight can be substituted. The examination should inspect the conjunctiva, the cornea, the tear film, the tear break-up time, and the surface staining patterns. In children with significant dry eye the inferior tear meniscus is reduced and contains mucus strands and debris. The tear meniscus is easier to see after the instillation of fluorescein. The tear break-up time, which assesses tear film stability, should be estimated after the instillation of fluorescein drops without anesthetic as fluorescein strips or topical anesthetic will reduce the break-up time. The time is the interval between the end of a blink and the first appearance of dry spots in the fluorescein-stained corneal tear film; less than 10 seconds is abnormal.

Ocular surface damage is assessed with fluorescein or Rose Bengal staining. Rose Bengal staining of devitalized epithelial cells is a very sensitive test of dryness but is irritating to the eye so as little solution as possible should be used. The degree of ocular surface dryness can be graded from no staining to staining of the whole cornea and corneal ulceration.

The conjunctiva should be examined for scarring or other abnormality. Inspect the bulbar conjunctiva, the tarsal conjunctiva, and if possible evert the upper lids and examine the conjunctiva of the tarsal plate. The finding of redundant conjunctival folds parallel to the eyelid in the lower temporal quadrant is a marker of a dry eye. Severe conjunctival chemosis may cause incomplete lid closure with drying of the eye. The conjunctiva may be hyperemic with blisters or pseudomembrane in the early stages of Stevens-Johnson syndrome, followed later by scarring and symblepharon. A mucopurulent conjunctivitis is followed by cicatrization, dry eyes, and corneal scarring in trachoma (see Chapter 15). The initial signs of hypovitaminosis A occur in the conjunctiva, which is dry and wrinkled with Bitot's spots in the exposed areas followed by keratomalacia as the cornea becomes involved. Surface drying may occur with dermolipomas and epibulbar dermoids or conjunctival scarring after strabismus surgery.

The corneal surface should be inspected for dellen, scarring, ulceration, the presence or absence of corneal nerves, and mucus filaments or plaques. Prominent corneal nerves may be present in patients with MEN (multiple endocrine neoplasia) 2B.

Other tests

Schirmer's test

The Schirmer's test assesses tear secretion. It can assess basal (unstimulated) secretion if done with anesthetic, or reflex (stimulated) secretion if performed without the use of local anesthetic. The test may be difficult to perform in children, and may be possible only after the instillation of local anesthetic. To perform the test, a filter paper of standard size and width is hung over the lower lid into the conjunctival fornix usually at the junction of the middle and outer one-third without touching the cornea. The child then shuts their eyes gently for 5 minutes, after which the filter paper is removed and the wetted portion of the paper is measured. An abnormal result is a wetting of 5 mm or less.

Tear osmolarity

The chemical properties of the tear film can be measured by testing osmolarity, which is increased in dry eye. This test is not in general clinical practice.

Impression cytology

Conjunctival impression cytology, performed by gently rubbing Millipore filter paper against the conjunctival surface, obtains a sheet of cells, which can be stained for epithelial cell morphology and goblet cell density[5] (Fig. 98.1). Epithelial cell cytology is abnormal in damaged eyes and the density of goblet cells, which produce mucus, decreases with an alteration in the normal staining patterns in various diseases including chronic cicatricial change and inflammation (Fig. 98.2). In

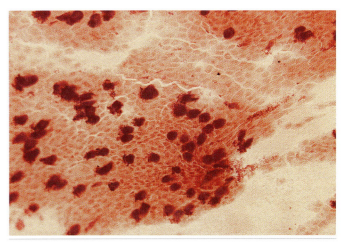

Fig. 98.1 Normal impression cytology showing a confluent sheet of epithelial cells and goblet cells with deep pink-staining intracellular mucus.

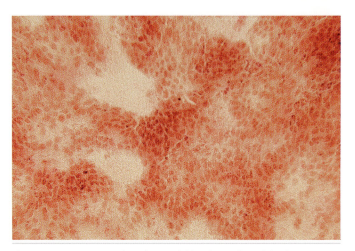

Fig. 98.2 Impression cytology from a child with ectodermal dysplasia showing an almost complete absence of goblet cells.

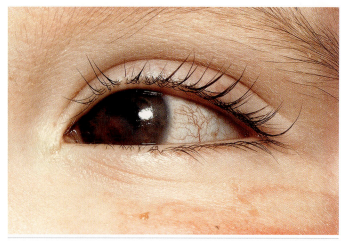

Fig. 98.3 Corneal drying, ulceration, scarring, and vascularization in Riley-Day syndrome. The combination of anesthesia and dryness makes keratitis a significant problem for many of these children.

dry eyes the bulbar ocular surface has been shown to have abnormal epithelium with reduced goblet cell density. This test is only usually possible in the older more cooperative child or in the younger child during an examination under anesthesia.

Corneal sensation

Reduced sensation from the ocular surface results in reduced tear secretion and a reduced blink rate producing a dry anesthetic eye, with a high risk of ulceration.

Corneal sensation can be tested using a fine wisp of cotton wool, for example from the tip of a cotton bud, to gently touch the corneal surface. A child with normal sensation will either tell you they can feel it, or blink and draw away. Observation of the child's reaction to the instillation of drops will also give an indication of sensation. Corneal sensation is reduced in dry eye and should be unequivocal to be of clinical importance.

Congenital loss of corneal sensation can occur in Goldenhar's syndrome and in rare autosomal recessive diseases such as congenital insensitivity to pain with anhidrosis (CIPA) and Riley-Day syndrome.

Riley-Day syndrome (familial dysautonomia) is a recessively inherited disorder that affects the development and function of the sympathetic, parasympathetic, and sensory nervous system with neurologic, systemic, and ophthalmologic manifestations.[6] It is almost exclusively found in Ashkenazi Jews (those of European origin). It is caused by a mutation of the IKBKAP gene on chromosome 9. Dysfunction of the autonomic nervous system produces labile blood pressure, skin blotching, unstable temperature, and excessive sweating. Sensory disturbance produces insensitivity to pain and reduced taste perception. Other signs are hyporeflexia, motor incoordination, poor swallowing, drooling, anxiety, and emotional lability. Ophthalmologically, the two most significant findings are dry eyes due to absence of tears and either absent or significantly reduced corneal sensation. This combination of deficits produces corneal ulceration (Fig. 98.3). There is evidence of denervation hypersensitivity with pupillary constriction after instillation of dilute (0.1%) pilocarpine (Fig. 98.4A,B). Other reported findings are exodeviations, myopia, anisocoria, retinal tortuosity, anisometropia, and

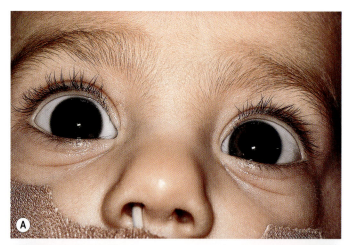

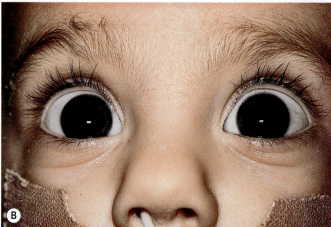

Fig. 98.4 (A) Riley-Day syndrome at the time of instillation of pilocarpine 0.1%. (There is no change in pupil size in normal children.) (B) Same patient, same lighting conditions, 20 minutes later. The denervation hypersensitivity is indicated by the pupil constriction.

ptosis. Non-ophthalmic diagnostic features are a wheal without the normal erythematous response to an intradermal injection of histamine and the absence of the fungiform papillae of the tongue.

In neuroparalytic keratitis (NPK) there is sensory denervation of the cornea and conjunctiva due to damage to the trigeminal nerve. This can be seen with acoustic neuroma or pontine tumors, after trauma or herpes zoster, and in leprosy.

Causes of dry eye

Tables 98.1 and 98.2 give details of ocular and systemic disease/conditions associated with dry eye in children.

Management

When managing patients with dry eye it should be remembered that symptoms do not always correlate with clinical signs; if the child has an anesthetic cornea, they may be untroubled by a dry ocular surface and even by corneal ulceration.

General advice

The aim of treatment is to improve surface wetting and reduce the child's symptoms. If there is an obvious treatable cause of drying such as a lid that cannot close fully after ptosis surgery or a lid defect causing ocular surface desiccation, the child should be referred to an oculoplastic specialist. A child with significant ocular exposure due to proptosis from facial deformity or orbital tumor may need to be considered for craniofacial surgery. Drugs contributing to ocular surface drying should be stopped if possible. Vitamin A deficiency should be treated with supplementation. Acute dacryoadenitis is treated with antiviral and anti-inflammatory therapy where indicated. If the ocular surface dryness is related to reduced blinking associated with prolonged computer or games use, then appropriate advice about taking regular breaks should be given. General advice about avoiding low humidity, drafts and high-temperature environments, or taking precautions if exposed to them is helpful. The management becomes more complex if there is also reduced corneal sensation.

When considering topical medication it should be noted that many drugs are not licensed for pediatric use or only for use in the older child, but are still frequently used by pediatric ophthalmologists.

Protection

Children at significant risk of ocular surface exposure; for example, in intensive care situations or with lack or significant loss of lid closure, eyes require protection, in addition to lubrication (Fig. 98.5A). The lids may be taped shut, but care should be taken to apply tape safely and effectively to provide adequate corneal cover. A protective bubble shield can be taped to the face or a polyacrylamide gel (Geliperm) placed over the eyes (Fig. 98.5B).

Lubrication

The mainstay of treatment is ocular lubrication using topical preparations, either drops or ointment. There are many

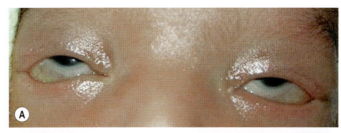
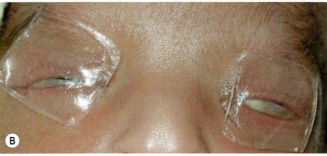

Fig. 98.5 Infant with Wolf-Hirschorn syndrome. (A) He had ocular exposure with dryness due to incomplete lid closure. (B) Same patient with the eyes protected with Geliperm and demonstrating a good Bell's phenomenon.

preparations available.[7] Drops are more useful as ointment will blur the vision, but an ointment preparation, preferably preservative-free, may be helpful at night. If drops are needed more than four times a day, or long-term, consider the use of preservative-free drops as preservatives may cause corneal drying and exacerbate the problem. Lubricant drops are now available in a variety of single-dose, preservative-free preparations.

Artificial tears containing hyaluronic acid may give greater relief than other artificial tear substitutes.

Autologous serum tears produced from the patient's serum can be used to treat severe dry eye; they are unpreserved but can be frozen and require a blood donation 2–4 times a year to produce them.

Allergic eye disease

Allergic eye disease causes dry eye and is probably the commonest reason for a dry eye in childhood. Topical medications for allergic eye disease include antihistamines, mast cell stabilizers and dual-acting agents. It is probably helpful to use medication such as olopatadine that need to be instilled only twice a day rather than drops that require more frequent instillation.[8] Oral antihistamines may be required, remembering that they may also worsen a dry eye. Anti-inflammatory treatment with topical steroids or the non-steroidal anti-inflammatory ketorolac may be required. The topical immunomodulator cyclosporine A has also been advocated for the control of difficult disease.

Cyclosporine A

Topical ciclosporin increases tear production and also has an anti-inflammatory effect. It is commercially available in 0.05% concentration (higher concentrations up to 2% can be obtained from specialist pharmaceutical suppliers) and is used twice daily.

Acetyl cysteine drops

If the presence of corneal filaments and mucus is significant and contributing to discomfort, topical acetyl cysteine (10% or 20%) may be helpful.

Lid margin disease

The mainstay of treatment is lid hygiene using eyelid scrubs with either cotton-tipped swab sticks or a clean face flannel, and warm compresses with lid massage to open the meibomian glands.[7] Topical antibiotic ointment massaged into the lid margin after cleaning will help control any infectious component. Topical steroids may be intermittently required for flare ups. Long-term low-dose systemic antibiotics can be helpful. Oral erythromycin (not tetracycline because of the risk of yellowing the secondary teeth in young children) in dosages of 25–50% of normal treatment levels (e.g. 62.5–125 mg bd) is recommended; this will need to be continued for approximately 3 months, and courses may need to be repeated. Oral flaxseed oil (2.5–5 mL) may be helpful in some children.

Punctal occlusion: temporary or permanent

The use of drops more than four times a day is difficult unless the child is old enough to instill them. In this situation ointment can be used, but this does produce blurring, which may not be acceptable. If considerable lubrication is required, punctal occlusion should be considered. This can be achieved temporarily with collagen implants, or more permanently with intracanalicular or external lacrimal plugs. External punctal plugs have the advantage that they can be removed if occlusion is overeffective with epiphora. In small children plugs need to be inserted under general anesthesia, but in older cooperative children this can be performed at the slit-lamp. Permanent punctal occlusion using cautery is occasionally required in chronic conditions, such as Riley-Day syndrome.

Glasses and moisture-retaining goggles

Glasses with side shields (or goggles for more effect) to reduce evaporative tear loss and to increase local humidity may be helpful. These are not always aesthetically popular, particularly with the older child.

Contact lenses

Soft contact lenses have been tried, but most patients do not have sufficient tear film to support their use, and there is a significant risk of infection. Scleral contact lenses have been used in severe ocular surface disease.[9] They provide a precorneal reservoir giving better hydration, but they require expert fitting and training of the caretaker in insertion and removal of the lens. Parents should be asked to bring the child back for immediate review if the eyes become sore and cannot be opened, or if a discharge is noted.

Tarsorrhaphy: temporary, permanent

A child with an anesthetic eye, especially if associated with a facial palsy, has a significant chance of developing corneal ulceration, which is difficult to treat. In this situation a tarsorrhaphy is often required to produce healing and prevent future

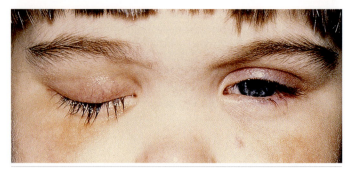

Fig. 98.6 Botulinum induced ptosis of the right eye. Performed for corneal protection in a 2½-year-old child with Stevens-Johnson syndrome.

damage. The most effective type of tarsorrhaphy for this condition is a central one, which is rarely a popular option with either the child or parents.

With long-term facial palsy and intact corneal sensation, protection can be provided by a combination of small lateral and medial tarsorrhaphies, which are both more effective and cosmetically better than a large lateral closure. If there is temporary facial weakness, with ocular surface exposure, which is expected to improve, as in a Bell's palsy, then a botulinum toxin protective ptosis should be considered. It will provide short-acting protection without damage to the lid margins (Fig. 98.6). It is easily achieved by injecting a low dose of botulinum toxin A (from 2.5 to 20 units of Dysport in 0.1 mL of saline), passing a 25 G, 25-mm needle just beneath the supraorbital margin along the roof of the orbit to its full length prior to injecting the toxin, or by an anterior transcutaneous approach using 10–15 units of Botox.[10,11] Complications include an induced vertical deviation due to underaction of the ipsilateral superior rectus muscle and preseptal hemorrhage. The risk of these is reduced by using a small volume. Full closure may not be achieved in the presence of a facial palsy, but the eye will be closed sufficiently to protect the ocular surface. Maximum ptosis will last about 2 weeks. Levator function will return to pretreatment levels in 2 to 3 months. It can be repeated as required. Although it can easily be undertaken in awake adults and older children after application of anesthetic cream to the skin of the lid, in the younger child the procedure should be undertaken under general anesthesia or sedation.

Temporary lid closure has been attempted with cyanoacrylate glue but in the main is not very effective as it lasts only a few days to about a week, may be uncomfortable, and prevents examination of the ocular surface.

Salivary gland transplant

Submandibular gland autografts have been performed in adults for severe dry eyes. It improves ocular comfort and wetting, but does not improve vision.[12] It is probably not appropriate for use in very small children but may have a place in the older child with significant problems. Following this procedure the eye is bathed in salivary tears not lacrimal tears, which have a different enzyme and electrolyte composition. Corneal edema occurs in some cases. This is not an option for anything other than severe dry eye.

References

1. The definition and classification of dry eye disease: Report of the Definition and Classification Subcommittee of the International Dry Eye WorkShop. Ocul Surf 2007; 5: 75–92.

2. Mac Cord MF, Silvestre de CR, Leite SC, et al. Management of dry eye related to systemic diseases in childhood and longterm follow-up. Acta Ophthalmol Scand 2007; 85: 739–44.

3. Patrick RK. Lacrimal secretion in full-term and premature babies. Trans Ophthal Soc UK 1974; 94: 283–90.

4. Sjogren H, Eriksen A. Alacrimia congenita. Br J Ophthalmol 1950; 34: 691–4.

5. Nelson JD, Havener VR, Cameron JD. Cellulose acetate impressions of the ocular surface: dry eye states. Arch Ophthalmol 1983; 101: 1869–72.

6. Liebman SD. Riley-Day syndrome: long-term ophthalmologic observations. Trans Am Ophthalmol Soc 1968; 66: 95–116.

7. Wong IB, Nischal KK. Managing a child with an external ocular disease. J AAPOS 2010; 14: 68–77.

8. Kari O, Saari KM. Updates in the treatment of ocular allergies. J Asthma Allergy 2010; 3: 149–58.

9. Gungor I, Schor K, Rosenthal P, Jacobs DS. The Boston scleral lens in the treatment of pediatric patients. J AAPOS 2008; 12: 263–7.

10. Adams GG, Kirkness CM, Lee JP. Botulinum toxin A induced protective ptosis. Eye 1987; 1 (Pt 5): 603–8.

11. Naik MN, Gangopadhyay N, Fernandes M, et al. Anterior chemodenervation of levator palpebrae superioris with botulinum toxin type-A (Botox) to induce temporary ptosis for corneal protection. Eye (Lond) 2008; 22: 1132–6.

12. Geerling G, Sieg P, Bastian GO, Laqua H. Transplantation of the autologous submandibular gland for most severe cases of keratoconjunctivitis sicca. Ophthalmology 1998; 105: 327–35.

My child seems to hate the bright light

Charlotte L Funnell

Although mild photophobia is fairly common in normal young children, photophobia must be taken seriously as there are a wide variety of conditions including serious disorders such as infantile glaucoma and anterior visual pathway tumors which may present with photophobia.

Presentation

A variety of behavioral patterns suggest a child is sensitive to light. Babies and young children may get upset and close their eyes when outside, in the car, or under fluorescent lighting, but play happily under natural light indoors. Photophobic children are often thought of as shy or sad as they have a tendency to look down, furrow their brows, and screw up their eyes. Frequent blinking, watering, and rubbing of the eyes are common. Children may complain of pain in their eyes, blurred vision, and headaches, especially when it is bright.

The approach to a photophobic child

It is critical that a good rapport is built with the child and as much information as possible gathered before formal examination is attempted. The lighting in the examination room should be lowered to aid the child's comfort. The differential diagnosis for photophobia is considerable. Taking into consideration the age of the child (see Table 99.1) and getting a good history (see Table 99.2) help to focus the examination toward finding the diagnosis.

During the examination it is best if tests that can be done remotely, with lower illumination levels, are attempted first. Visual acuity assessment, a cover test to examine for latent strabismus and observation for nystagmus should be undertaken. A hand-held slit-lamp, topical anesthesia, and fluorescein staining all assist with anterior segment examinations. In young children corneal diameters should be assessed and intraocular pressure measurements undertaken if possible. Corneal haze may not be obvious when a child initially presents with glaucoma. Examining for iris transillumination using a slit-lamp aids in the diagnosis of albinism. Dilated fundal examination is important. Electrophysiology studies (electroretinograms and visual evoked potentials) and neuroradiological imaging may be required to confirm or rule out certain diagnoses.

Occasionally, treatment may need to be started for the suspected condition without a detailed examination being possible. In this situation the child should be followed up very closely. If the child is not responding to treatment, or in cases where a diagnosis or examination has not been possible, prompt examination under sedation or general anesthesia should be undertaken.

The pathophysiology of photophobia

Research has provided us with a better understanding of the mechanisms behind photophobia. Ocular photophobia is most commonly caused by corneal epithelial surface disturbance with or without stromal involvement and anterior uveitis. This occurs due to activation of the ocular

Table 99.1 – Important causes of photophobia in each age group

Infants	Infantile glaucoma
	Inherited corneal dystrophies, especially congenital hereditary endothelial dystrophy (CHED)
	Keratitis
	Descemet's break due to forceps delivery
	Stationary cone disorders, e.g. achromatopsia
Young children	Glaucoma
	Corneal abrasions and foreign bodies
	Blepharokeratoconjunctivitis
	Vernal keratoconjunctivitis
	Herpes simplex or bacterial keratitis
	Inherited corneal dystrophies
	Cataract
	Albinism
	Aniridia
	Stationary cone disorders, e.g. achromatopsia
	Acquired central nervous system (CNS) pathology
School-age children	Progressive cone dystrophies
	Partial aniridia
	Cataract or ectopia lentis
	Intermittent exotropia
	Migraine
	Acquired CNS pathology

Table 99.2 – Questions and considerations in photophobia

Severity?	If severe photophobia, consider infantile glaucoma, corneal surface disease, acute CNS pathology (e.g. meningitis or migraine), achromatopsia, oculocutaneous albinism, or aniridia
Recent onset or present since very young?	Acquired corneal pathology is common in children New onset photophobia with a normal ocular examination may be due to acquired CNS pathology Long-standing problem more likely to be due to an inherited corneal or retinal disease
Associated watering?	Infantile glaucoma, keratoconjunctivitis, keratitis, and epithelial dystrophies have associated epiphora In retinal and CNS disorders epiphora tends to be less prominent
Associated redness of eyes?	Suggests corneal pathology
One or both eyes?	Acquired corneal disease is often asymmetric
Constant or intermittent?	Consider migraine or fluctuating corneal pathology
Reduced vision?	Most corneal and retinal pathologies causing photophobia also reduce visual acuity
Squint?	Monocular eye closure and photophobia are common in intermittent exotropia
Family history or history of consanguinity?	Meesman's corneal dystrophy, aniridia, and many congenital cataracts are dominantly inherited Cystinosis, tyrosinemia type II, and achromatopsia are recessive Albinism has multiple modes of inheritance Congenital hereditary endothelial dystrophy (CHED) can be autosomal dominant or recessive
Past medical history?	Especially history of CNS disease such as birth asphyxia, meningitis, encephalitis, cerebral bleed, or brain injury

nociceptors which stimulate the trigeminal nucleus via the trigeminal nerve.[1]

It is proposed that light causes release of parasympathetic neuropeptides, via a pathway involving the pretectal nucleus, and these cause intraocular vasodilation and neurogenic inflammation, activating the ocular nociceptors.[1]

Potentially, retina-damaging shorter wavelengths of visible light induce more photophobia than longer wavelengths, suggesting photophobia protects the retina.[2] Macula pigment also has a retinal protective function and the increased photophobia in people with poorly pigmented maculae is consistent with this finding.[2] A lack of functioning cones, as in achromatopsia, also is associated with photophobia.

Photophobia occurs at lower light intensities when the pupil is abnormally large or there is a lack of iris pigmentation to prevent light from passing through the iris. Scattering of incipient light, via corneal or lens opacities, also appears to cause photophobia, although the exact mechanism remains unclear.

Migraine headaches appear to be exacerbated by light via the recently discovered retino-thalamo-cortical pathway that carries signals from the retina to the thalamic trigeminovascular neurons and to cortical areas involved in somatosensory and visual perception.[1,3] The photophobia that may accompany migraine headaches has been attributed to several mechanisms: neurovascular, cortical spreading depression, vasoactive substances, neurotransmitters, or brainstem activation.

The photophobia found associated with expanding central nervous system (CNS) pathology appears to result from stretching of pain-sensitive structures in the meninges or blood vessels at the base of the brain, resulting in transmission via trigeminal afferents or by direct damage to the thalamus.[4-6]

Diseases causing photophobia

Conjunctivitis

Conjunctivitis causes photophobia when there is associated corneal surface disease such as in acute follicular keratoconjunctivitis or Stevens-Johnson syndrome.

Corneal disorders

Corneal disorders are the most common cause of photophobia.

The following are associated with epiphora, conjunctival hyperemia, and eyelid involvement including edema and hyperemia:

(a) Acquired epithelial injury such as corneal abrasions and foreign bodies.
(b) Blepharokeratoconjunctivitis and vernal keratoconjunctivitis (see Chapter 15).
(c) Herpes simplex keratitis or bacterial keratitis, which usually occurs in the setting of compromised corneal epithelium (see Chapter 15).

The following cause photophobia and epiphora but usually with less conjunctival or lid hyperemia:

- Inherited conditions affecting the integrity of the epithelium such as tyrosinemia type II, xeroderma pigmentosa, and Meesman's corneal dystrophy (see Chapters 33 and 34).
- Inherited conditions affecting the clarity of the cornea such as the deposition of corneal crystalline deposits in cystinosis (Fig. 99.1), the mucopolysaccharidoses, and the corneal edema secondary to congenital hereditary endothelial dystrophy (CHED) (see Chapters 33 and 34).

Glaucoma

Infantile glaucoma classically presents with photophobia, epiphora, and blepharospasm. This should always be considered when a young child presents with photophobia (see Chapter 37).

Uvea

(a) Aniridia results in photophobia secondary to a lack of pupil function, the poor ocular surface, and cataract (see Chapter 32).

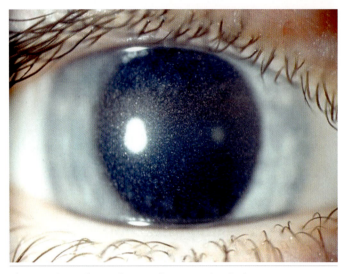

Fig. 99.1 Corneal crystals secondary to cystinosis. (Patient of Manchester Royal Eye Hospital, UK.)

(b) Iris transillumination, foveal hypoplasia, and nystagmus are classically found in ocular and oculocutaneous albinism (see Chapter 40).

(c) Anterior uveitis commonly presents with photophobia and a red eye in older children, usually associated with HLA-B27 or blunt trauma. The anterior uveitis associated with juvenile idiopathic arthritis does not usually cause photophobia (see Chapter 39).

Lens

Partial cataracts, particularly posterior subcapsular, lamellar, or zonular cataracts, and ectopia lentis may cause photophobia (see Chapters 35 and 36).

Retina

Stationary cone disorders including achromatopsia usually present in young children with marked photophobia, reduced vision, and nystagmus. Visual function is often markedly worse in bright light conditions (see Chapter 44). Progressive cone dystrophies usually present in later childhood or early adult life with photophobia and gradual reduction in visual acuity and color vision (see Chapter 44).

Central nervous system

Photophobia can be severe in encephalitis, meningitis, subarachnoid hemorrhage, trigeminal neuralgia, and migraine. Persistent, usually mild, photophobia has been reported to occur in about a third of children with cortical visual impairment.[7] When congenital, the photophobia is present from birth and when acquired it appears immediately after the brain insult, with intensity tending to diminish over time.

Worsening photophobia may be the presenting complaint in a variety of compressive lesions of the optic chiasm including pituitary adenomas, craniopharyngiomas, clivus chordomas, and anterior communicating artery aneurysms, with only subtle visual acuity and visual field abnormalities.[4,6] Young children may present with photophobia, epiphora,

torticollis, and good visual function due to posterior fossa tumors. In most of these cases, the diagnosis was significantly delayed.[8] Acute onset photophobia occurs secondary to optic neuritis and to demyelination in the retrochiasmal visual pathway.[9]

CNS pathology should be considered in children with persistent and especially progressive photophobia unexplained by ocular abnormalities.

Strabismus

Mild to moderate photophobia is common in patients with latent and dissociated deviations; however, even patients with manifest strabismus may display these behaviors, including monocular closure in bright light. This is classically seen in intermittent exotropia (see Chapters 77 and 96).

Physiological and functional

Some children with fair complexions and physiologically low levels of ocular pigmentation complain about photophobia. This tends to improve with age. Children tend to have larger pupils than adults which may contribute. Other diseases should be ruled out if this symptom persists.

Management

Management should be aimed at identification and treatment of the underlying disease. Supportive measures are important in helping improve the quality of life of children with significant photophobia. They should be advised on the importance of sunhats and provided with tinted or photochromic glasses. Letters should be sent to school explaining the problem, ensuring children are sat out of the direct sunlight in class and allowed to use sunhats and glasses during the school day. Involving the teachers for the visually impaired is invaluable.

References

1. Noseda R, Burstein R. Advances in understanding the mechanisms of migraine-type photophobia. Curr Opin Neurol 2011; 24: 197–202.
2. Stringham JM, Fuld K, Wenzel AJ. Spatial properties of photophobia. Invest Ophthalmol Vis Sci 2004; 45: 3838–48.
3. Noseda R, Kainz V, Jakubowski M, et al. A neural mechanism for exacerbation of headache by light. Nat Neurosci 2010; 13: 239–45.
4. Kawasaki A, Purvin VA. Photophobia as the presenting visual symptom of chiasmal compression. J Neuro-ophthalmol 2002; 22: 3–8.
5. Lee AG, Miller NR. Photophobia in anterior visual pathway lesions. J Neuro-ophthalmol 2003; 23: 106.
6. Hagihara N, Abe T, Yoshioka F, et al. Photophobia as the visual manifestation of chiasmal compression by unruptured anterior communicating artery aneurysm: case report. Neurol Med Chir (Tokyo) 2009; 49: 159–61.
7. Jan JE, Groenveld M, Anderson DP. Photophobia and cortical visual impairment. Dev Med Child Neurol 1993; 35: 473–7.
8. Marmor MA, Beauchamp GR, Maddox SF. Photophobia, epiphora, and torticollis: a masquerade syndrome. J Pediatr Ophthalmol Strabismus 1990; 27: 202–4.
9. Kawasaki A, Borruat FX. Photophobia associated with a demyelinating lesion of the retrochiasmal visual pathway. Am J Ophthalmol 2006; 142: 854–6.

My child's eyes keep watering!

Anthony G Quinn

Up to 20% of infants have a watery eye in the first month of life.[1] The vast majority have congenital nasolacrimal duct obstruction; the rest may have potentially serious problems. Acquired watering eyes present another range of diagnoses.

Congenital nasolacrimal duct obstruction and its management are discussed elsewhere in this book (see Chapter 21).

Signs and symptoms

History

A child with excessive tearing can cause parents and primary care doctors concern. Build-up of mucus in the tear film causes "stickiness" and constant spillage of tears causes redness and irritation of the lower lid skin. The lids may be stuck together on waking and require frequent cleaning. Parents may complain that the appearance "ruins" childhood photographs and they may feel the child's appearance reflects poorly on them as a parent. The primary care physician may feel compelled to prescribe repeated courses of topical antibiotics, to no lasting effect.

Try and establish whether the watering had its onset soon after birth, or if it is recent. Photophobia must specifically be asked about, as it is common in congenital glaucoma. The typical presentation is a child who avoids opening their eyes in normal daylight, often burying the eyes behind an arm or hand. Photophobia is also a symptom of corneal disease (such as cystinosis; see Chapter 33), uveitis, and a foreign body in the conjunctival sac. The possibility of trauma needs to be kept in mind, as children cannot always give a detailed history. The child with excessive lacrimation, rather than blocked tear drainage, may have a watery nose on the same side as the watery eye. A history of eye rubbing or poking and concerns about whether the child can see suggests a retinal dystrophy, such as Leber's congenital amaurosis (see Chapter 44).

Examination

External inspection

Tearing, red macerated skin, and stickiness may be seen. In nasolacrimal duct obstruction, the tear lake is thickened, brimming the lower lid margin. Normally, the tear film is virtually invisible, and, with fluorescein staining of the tear film, measures less than 1 mm. With obstruction, it typically measures 2 mm or more. Secondary bacterial conjunctivitis can occur, causing generalized conjunctival redness, whereas perilimbal injection may be more specific for keratitis or uveitis. Generalized corneal haze with secondary corneal epithelial edema may be a sign of glaucoma. An estimate should be made of horizontal corneal diameters using a ruler held close to the lid. A congenital swelling over the nasolacrimal sac is probably a dacryocystocele.

Slit-lamp examination

This is often best done with a portable model in young children. Look for presence or absence of puncti, punctual ectopia, or epiblepharon with inturned eyelashes. Inspect the inferior conjunctival fornix looking for diffuse redness and swelling of the conjunctiva, suggesting chlamydia conjunctivitis. Everting the upper lid is very unlikely to be possible in a young, awake child, but it is possible to retract the upper lid digitally and inspect the tarsal conjunctiva and fornix with the portable slit-lamp, looking from below. Corneal crystals, abrasions, scars, ulcers, and foreign bodies can be excluded, as can signs of uveitis, e.g. keratitic precipitates, hypopyon, posterior synechiae, or cataract (also check red reflex). Haab's striae and corneal edema should be excluded.

Fluorescein testing

This is a very sensitive test for detecting any defect in the corneal epithelium, and fluorescein will diffusely stain the cornea with epithelial edema. The fluorescein dye disappearance test is excellent for confirming nasolacrimal duct obstruction (see Chapter 21). It may also appear in the nose, confirming drainage.

Intraocular pressure

It is possible to check this in the majority of awake infants or young children with a "Tonopen,"® Icare® tonometer, or an "air puff" tonometer (see Chapter 37). If congenital glaucoma is likely, an examination under anesthesia or with ketamine sedation may be necessary. Tactile measurement is inaccurate and may mislead.

Cycloplegic refraction, fundus examination

Refraction and fundus examination will highlight unilateral myopia in a child with unilateral glaucoma, posterior synechiae, disc cupping, and any posterior segment pathology such as retinoblastoma, which can present as a red, watery eye with a "pseudo-hypopyon."

Causes and treatment

Non-patent nasolacrimal drainage system (see Chapter 21)

Spontaneous resolution occurs in about 70% of affected children free of symptoms by 3 months of age and over 90% having resolved by their first birthday. Spontaneous resolution may also occur later than 12 months of age and those children whose epiphora does not resolve spontaneously after age 2 years are likely to have more complex lacrimal drainage problems. Children with white eyes (no evidence of secondary conjunctivitis) should not be treated with antibiotic drops. Antibiotics should only be given when there is clinical evidence of infection. Many physicians advocate massage of the lacrimal sac, but its efficacy is not known. Lid cleaning may help prevent secondary infection and skin excoriation.

Treatment

There are a number of treatments (see Chapter 21); the commonest, probing, is safe,[2] but even in the best circumstances can have complications; it is sometimes traumatic and may, rarely, cause canalicular stenosis.

Foreign body/corneal abrasion

A history of sudden onset of pain, epiphora, conjunctival redness, and a foreign body sensation suggest either a corneal/conjunctival abrasion or a foreign body in the conjunctival sac or cornea. A careful history from the child and/or caregivers is essential in understanding the likely injury and predicting its severity. Fluorescein stains a corneal or conjunctival abrasion, and staining vertical scratches suggest a superior subtarsal foreign body caused by the foreign body being dragged over the corneal surface with blinks. If there is a full thickness corneal laceration, the Seidel (fluorescein leak) test will sometimes be positive. A corneal foreign body is often visible with a check of the red reflex using the direct ophthalmoscope, but the portable or table-mounted slit-lamp is the ideal way to examine the cornea. If a portable slit-lamp is not available, loupes or a +20 diopter lens, with a good light, may be useful.

Corneal abrasions usually settle quickly with antibiotic ointment and no patching is required. Removal of an embedded corneal foreign body in a child may require general anesthesia. Loosely adherent foreign bodies in the conjunctival sac or on the cornea may be removable with a sterile cotton bud.

Keratitis and conjunctivitis (see Chapter 15)

A watery eye is a common symptom in keratitis (Fig. 100.1). There is frequently associated photophobia, conjunctival injection, increased mucus production, and a foreign body sensation. Visual acuity is often reduced in keratitis. Conjunctivitis

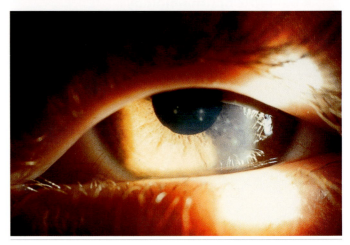

Fig. 100.1 Thygeson's superficial punctate keratitis (TSPK). This 8-year-old child had a variably watering eye for 9 months that did not respond to a variety of treatments. TSPK follows a relapsing and remitting course over several months.

is not associated with photophobia, unless there is an accompanying keratitis. Conjunctivitis is commonly infective (viral, bacterial) or allergic or traumatic. Allergic conjunctivitis typically presents as itchy, watery eyes, and is usually a bilateral problem. There may be a family history of allergic disease, and a clinical history of exacerbations in spring/summer, or of other allergic diseases such as eczema, hay fever, or asthma. "Shield" ulcers associated with giant subtarsal conjunctival papillae produce a characteristic loss of corneal epithelium and are easily seen with fluorescein and slit-lamp microscope.

Contact lens-related epiphora

In the older child, or the aphakic infant with contact lenses, epiphora may result from numerous causes. Poorly fitting, change in corneal curvature, build-up of deposits on the contact lens, and chips or tears at the edge of the contact lens can all cause watery eyes from epithelial trauma or drying. The superior tarsal conjunctiva must be assessed for giant papillary conjunctivitis (GPC) in the long-term contact lens wearer. Treatment may include revising contact lens hygiene, replacing lenses, refitting lenses, replacing lenses with a different material or edge design, and treatment of GPC with appropriate pharmacologic agents (see Chapter 15). Infectious keratitis or corneal abrasion should be actively excluded and parents warned to be sure to remove the lens and seek ophthalmological advice within a few hours if the child's eye becomes red, sticky, watery, or photophobic.

Congenital glaucoma

Epiphora with photophobia may indicate a diagnosis of congenital glaucoma. Buphthalmos, corneal clouding, Haab's striae, increased intraocular pressure (compared to normal for infants), and enlarged optic disc cup are also usually present. Anisometropia and strabismus may occur (see Chapter 37). Prompt treatment, usually surgical, is needed to prevent further optic nerve damage.

Crocodile tears

One peculiar from of tearing occurs only when the patient salivates, most typically when eating, but it is also possible when the patient is thinking of a good meal. This usually occurs as a congenital problem, and is an example of a range of disorders known as "congenital cranial dysinnervation disorders" (see Chapter 21). Crocodile tears can also occur after trauma or surgery on the ear, or as a sequel to Bell's palsy, representing aberrant nerve regeneration.

References

1. MacEwan CJ. Congenital nasolacrimal duct obstruction. Compr Ophthalmol Update 2006; 7: 79–87.
2. Repka MX, Chandler DL, Beck RW, et al. Pediatric Eye Disease Investigator Group. Primary treatment of nasolacrimal duct obstruction with probing in children younger than 4 years. Ophthalmology 2008; 115: 577–84.

Proptosis at different ages

Christopher J Lyons • Jack Rootman

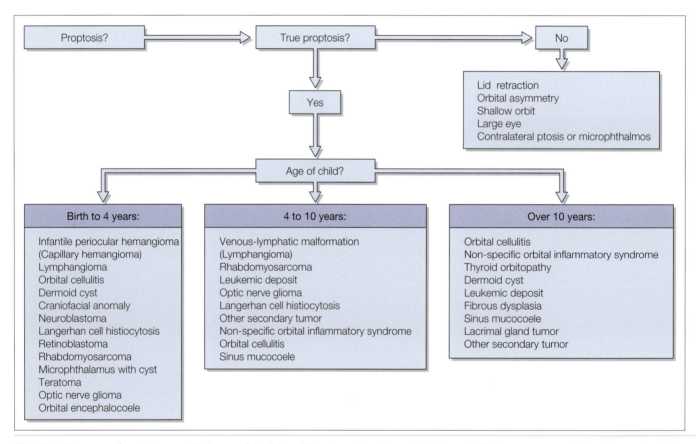

Fig. 101.1 The causes of proptosis vary with the age of the child and there is considerable overlap between both the age groups and the various centers. This figure lists causes in approximate order of frequency. Details of each condition should be sought in the text. In making a clinical diagnosis, the history and progression of the condition as well as the clinical findings are of vital importance. See Chapter 22 for a more detailed and different approach.

My child seems to have a pain in the eye

Peter Hodgkins

In a young child, pain may manifest as eye rubbing, light sensitivity, excessive blinking, and irritability. The older child is able to complain of eye pain when the underlying cause may be anything from a foreign body to an attention-seeking device.

Pain systems

Two fiber systems, myelinated and unmyelinated, transmit pain. The former transmits sharp transient pain, and the latter dull aching pain. Pain fibers innervating the eye and periorbital structures arise from the trigeminal or fifth cranial nerve. Although pain is most commonly generated at the site of the insult, referred pain may occur if the sensory pathway is stimulated in other regions: dural stimulation may result in retrobulbar pain.

The cornea has one of the areas of greatest density of pain nerve endings with the greatest concentration in the central cornea. The retina and optic nerves do not contain pain fibers. Eyelids, caruncle, and conjunctiva show less sensitivity than the cornea. Other ocular structures that can be associated with pain include the uvea, sclera, and optic nerve sheaths. Eye pain may occur with childhood optic neuritis. The pain is initiated by looking from side to side; this causes the inflamed nerve sheath to stretch, eliciting pain. Chronic distension of the nerve sheath such as with optic nerve glioma does not cause pain. Orbital pain may result from local irritation of pain fibers. Such pain usually implies an acute event, such as rapidly expanding mass or infection.

Some patients are left with no pathology to explain their eye pain and one is left with a diagnosis of eye strain, atypical facial pain, or attention seeking. Careful review and working with the parents and child is necessary to achieve a satisfactory outcome.

Classification of eye pains[1]

1. Obvious eye problems.
2. Non-obvious eye problems: refractive; accommodative.
3. Quiet eyes but localizing neuro-ophthalmic findings.
4. No ocular and neuro-ophthalmic findings: functional.

5. Others:
   a. Specific short- or long-lasting headaches or eye pain syndromes.
   b. Pains referred to the eye from other pathology (secondary eye pain).
   c. Pain from orbit, superior orbital fissure, cavernous sinus, intracranial infiltrative, neoplastic, or inflammatory disease process.

History

Where is the pain? When did it start? How long has it been there/occurring? How often is it occurring? What type of pain is it? Are there any other symptoms – e.g. photophobia, visual disturbance, head pain, family history of pains, general health, and recent problems or infections? What does it stop you doing? Have any other family members had problems?

Examination

1. Work systematically through the child and the eye.
2. The whole child: how do they look?
3. Height, weight, and head circumference (if less than 2 years).
4. Temperature, if appropriate.
5. Vision, color vision, and ocular movements: comitant or incomitant squint?
6. The face: any swellings or changes; eyelids especially (may be subtle) and lashes, conjunctiva, cornea, subtarsal (evert lid if possible), pupil, color of iris and comparison of pupil sizes, shape, symmetry, reactions; proptosis or globe displacement. Any localized swellings?
7. Does the redness/swelling stay within the septum's attachment to the periorbital rim (orbital disease) or extend beyond (periorbital)?
8. Dilate and red reflex, refract, fundal examination and optic disc.
9. Intraocular pressure if possible (Icare, air puff)
10. Examine other family members (parents and siblings), especially corneas for dystrophies, systemic problems.

Other investigations

1. Visual fields: confrontation or Goldman/Humphrey.
2. Examination under anesthesia or sedation: may be needed if you can't get a thorough examination of the child especially if there is a red eye and an acute onset where it may be a subtarsal foreign body.
3. MRI, CT scans to look for orbital and neurologic disease.
4. Bloods: full blood count, erythrocyte sedimentation rate/C-reactive protein as an inflammatory marker, antibodies for Epstein-Barr virus, serum glucose.
5. Referral to a pediatrician/pediatric neurologist if there are any systemic concerns.

There is a need to work systematically through the history and examination to ensure all information is gathered (Fig. 102.1). The child who has a foreign body may not have seen the obstacle because of poor vision due to a large refractive error or a visually compromised eye. Recurrent tearing and photophobia could represent a corneal dystrophy that is more obvious on examination of a parent. Poor growth or weight could reflect a systemic problem or abuse. Iritis could represent leukemia or a retinoblastoma. It is not always possible to make a diagnosis at first but careful review and repeat examination will often lead to the cause.

Headache

A child may occasionally talk about eye pain when in fact the complaint is a more generalized headache. The interpretation as "eye pain" may be an important localizing symptom for a further discussion of childhood headache (see Chapter 108). History is the key to diagnosis and it is more common than realized. Its incidence is approximately 50/1000 in school-age children. It increases in frequency with age, but is rare under 2 years. In the prepubertal period, boys outnumber girls by 2 : 1. At puberty this lessens in boys, resulting in the female excess seen in adults. A new classification for headache and overview is best seen in the Third International Headache Classification.[2] There is also a suggestion migraine may be more common in those with child abuse.[3]

The frontal sinus is underdeveloped at birth and appears during the second year. The sphenoid is present at birth but only rudimentary. The ethmoids are properly developed at birth but very small. Sinusitis can develop as a consequence of an upper respiratory infection and show orbital signs with red swollen eyes and restricted movement. Sinus pain is commonly attributed as the cause of pain in young adults yet the IHS (International Headache Society) insists that chronic sinusitis is not a cause of headache and facial pain unless relapsing into an acute phase. The vast majority of children presenting with frontal or temporal headache have tension-type headache.[4]

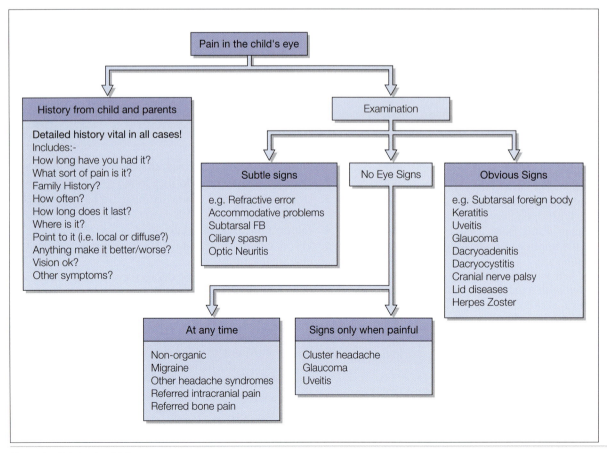

Fig. 102.1 Pain in the child's eye.

Refraction

When refractive errors are large the presenting symptom is reduced vision. When the error is smaller, however, it can present in a variety of ways. These other symptoms arise as a result of the effort to see clearly. Sustained excessive accommodation may be seen in hypermetropia, or discrepancies in the accommodation–convergence association can give rise to strain in the effort to maintain binocular single vision. Myopia may cause peering and periocular pain. These symptoms tend to be grouped together as "eyestrain." These symptoms, however, may be diverse and do not appear in proportion to the causal defect.

Visual symptoms

These are characteristically intermittent, and the symptoms may be most marked in those with good vision who try hard to keep the vision up. There are periods of particular strain, however, when the vision may fall, especially with excessive reading or detailed tasks when there may be sudden confusion, temporary blurring, or the letters running together. The eyes become more tired and the lids heavy with a progressive weariness.

Ocular symptoms

These symptoms are collectively spoken of as asthenopia. The symptoms of "eyestrain" are due to the increased muscular work involved and the direct muscular fatigue that ensues. After long periods of close work the eyes feel hot, tired, and uncomfortable. If work is continued, severe pain may develop in the eyes. These eyes lead to a watery red look when it may be associated with chronic blepharitis or recurrent conjunctivitis. These low-grade infections are exacerbated by rubbing with unclean hands.

Referred symptoms

1. Headaches are the most common symptom, and may take almost any form.
2. Accommodative spasm: the patient presents with diplopia, blurred vision, macropsia, or headaches and eye pain. There will be a variable esotropia, pupil constriction, and pseudomyopia. Refraction is important for the uncorrected hypermetropia; it can also be seen with intermittent exotropia where the patient is using convergence and accommodation to control the exotropia. It can also be functional where no cause can be found.
3. Convergence insufficiency/paresis: typical symptoms are frontal headaches and "eyestrain" associated with close work and blurred vision. Exophorias can also give rise to these symptoms.

References

1. Brazis PW, Lee AG, Stewart M, et al. Clinical review: the differential diagnosis of pain in the quiet eye. Neurologist 2002; 8: 82–100.
2. Olesen J. The Third International Headache Classification Committee of the International Headache Society. Cephalalgia 2011; 31: 4–5.
3. Tietjen GE, Peterlin BL. Childhood abuse and migraine: epidemiology, sex differences, and potential mechanisms. Headache 2011; 51: 869–9.
4. Jones NS. Perspective. Sinus headache: avoiding over- and mis-diagnosis. Expert Rev Neurotherapeut 2009; 9: 439–44.

My child's teacher says she can't see properly!

Hanne Jensen

Mode of presentation

If parents bring their child to the ophthalmologist because of the teacher's suspicion of reduced vision, this indicates that the parents have not been aware of any vision or eye problems. This may be because the child's visual disability has been constant and non-progressive, or that the parents do not expect the child to see any better. The child who never had normal vision will not complain, but as education makes increasing visual demands, problems may become apparent.

The teacher may observe problems with reading (near work), when looking at the blackboard (distance vision), problems with color plates in the book or strange color combinations, or strange behavior in class. The child may miss what is going on or appear uninvolved. The child may need extra time to keep up with the class. There may be recreation problems: the child doesn't want to play, often falls, is photophobic, or has an abnormal head posture. Other symptoms might be squeezing the eyes or complaining of headaches.

In Table 103.1, the signs and symptoms are presented in combination with what may be found at the examination.

Diagnosis

History

Specific questions are necessary because parents may not associate visual problems with change in behavior. Is there a history of trauma? Has the child's situation been long-standing, or has a change occurred with higher demands? Does the child like to play where it is dark, does the child like to walk on her own, or does she always want to hold someone's hand? Has the child suddenly changed her behavior: aggression or passivity can be symptoms of progressive visual loss. Any other systemic symptom must be noted. It is sometimes necessary to talk with the child without the parents. A distinction between blurred and weak vision can only be made by older children who may be able to distinguish the defocused image from subnormal vision.

Blurred vision implies an optical problem. A complaint of decreased vision after strenuous exercise or after warm baths suggests Uhthoff's sign of demyelinating disease.

Examination

Observe the child entering the clinic: are there difficulties, is the child afraid or curious, and can the child hear? Children who have been attending several clinics throughout childhood are often afraid and shy with professionals: it is important to make the child feel safe and cooperative.

Ocular examination

First one measures the visual acuity to establish how reduced the visual function is.

Refraction is a vital and often forgotten part of the examination. The media should be examined before and after the pupils are dilated, either by a slit-lamp, ophthalmoscope, or retinoscope. Direct ophthalmoscopy is used for fundus details, e.g. changes in the retinal nerve fiber layer and in the fovea; indirect ophthalmoscopy gives a panoramic view.

The optic nerve is evaluated by testing pupillary responses, contrast sensitivity, color vision, and visual fields. Electrophysiology may be useful.

Color vision and pupillary responses are often normal in retinal diseases with markedly reduced visual acuity while they can be abnormal even in mild optic nerve disease.

Neurological examination

Neurological examination is necessary in children with reduced vision as many eye symptoms can be part of a systemic disease. It is important to enquire about other symptoms, including hearing problems, in every child with visual loss. Children with concentration deficits must be examined by a neurologist to exclude a seizure disorder, autism, or attention disorders. An MRI scan may be necessary if there are any indications of intracranial pathology. Make certain that no medicine has been given that might influence the vision or the visual field, e.g. vigabatrin.

Table 103.1 – Symptoms and signs giving clues to examination and diagnosis

The teacher described	Examination	Results
Reading difficulties Problems with the blackboard Un-concentrated Squeezing the eyes Headache/asthenopia Abnormal head posture	Refraction	Refractive error: Hypermetropia/ myopia/ Astigmatism
Reading difficulties Un-concentration/asthenopia Problems with the blackboard	Accommodation/ convergence nearpoint	Reduced ANP/CNP Accommodative spasm
Reading difficulties Un-concentration Need extra time to keep up Abnormal head posture Behavioral problems Photophobic	Motor functions/ nystagmus Motility/paresis Pupillary reflex Pursuit/saccade/ ataxia	Retinal dystrophies Neurologic disease Metabolic disease
Problems with the blackboard Problems in the dark Overlooks/falls Behavioral problems	Visual field	Retinal dystrophies Neurological disease Optic nerve disease
Problems with color plates Strange match with color	Color vision tests	Retinal dystrophies Optic nerve disease Congenital color vision defect
Problems in the dark Overlooks/falls	Contrast sensitivity	Media opacities Optic nerve disease
Reading difficulties Problems with the blackboard Photophobic Squeezing the eyes Un-concentrated	Slit-lamp examination	Media opacities: Corneal dystrophies Keratoconus Anterior chamber (uveitis/ glaucoma) Lens anomalies (cataract/ectopia) Corpus vitreum (degeneration/ heme/infection)
Reading difficulties Problems with the blackboard Photophobic Problems in the dark Overlooks/falls	Ophthalmoscopy	Retinal dystrophies Macular dystrophies Optic nerve disease

Causes and treatment

Amblyopia

(see Chapter 70)

Refractive errors

Uncorrected refractive errors are the most important reason for a child not seeing properly. Children must be examined after cycloplegia in order to detect hypermetropic errors

Accommodative anomalies

Older school children often have problems when looking at the blackboard, but not when reading a book. This may be due to a high accommodative tonus that makes them appear

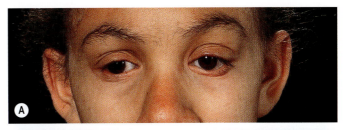
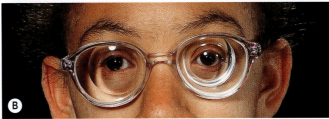

Fig. 103.1 (A) This patient with the diagnosis of hypomelanosis (of Ito which does not often cause defective vision) had acuities of 2/60 in each eye. Despite several examinations (she was difficult to examine), no cause was found. (B) When eventually refracted she was found to be a −25 myope. Corrected, her binocular acuity was 6/12.

myopic, and it is important to measure the refraction with cycloplegia (Fig. 103.1) or the diagnosis will be missed and glasses prescribed in error. Occasionally, treatment with cycloplegic drops and reading glasses is the only way to help the child relax accommodation. In low hypermetropia, they may accommodate to compensate, but some children cannot (e.g. Down's syndrome), and they develop asthenopia: reading glasses may help. Children with convergence insufficiency may have blurred vision while reading; they seldom describe the problem as double vision. Orthoptic treatment may help these cases, but surgery is sometimes necessary.

Orbital disease (see Chapter 22)

Orbital inflammation or a tumor may present with proptosis, but the presenting symptom may be reduced vision accompanied by restriction of eye movement and eventually pain and redness. Distortion of the globe results in astigmatism and hyperopia which, left untreated, may reduce visual acuity.

Media opacities

Corneal diseases (see Chapter 33)

Corneal clouding due to keratitis from any cause may reduce acuity with irritation and watery discharge. Symptoms due to keratoconus usually present during the second decade as slowly progressive visual loss, often leading to multiple attempts at correction with glasses or contact lenses. Dystrophies presenting within the early years of life can result in recurrent epithelial defects or reduced vision (see Chapter 34).

Anterior chamber anomalies

Blurred vision due to anterior segment inflammation is usually associated with pain, redness, and photophobia. In uveitis, vision may be reduced without symptoms (see Chapter 39).

Lens anomalies (see Chapter 35)

Dislocation of the lens is an important cause of reduced vision, as a consequence of the dislocated lens or high myopia. Glaucoma and retinal detachment can arise. Congenital cataract, if present from birth, is usually asymptomatic. Its presence is detected by the parents or by professionals. In older children, blurred vision or photophobia may suggest a cataract, particularly if the child has a predisposing condition such as diabetes mellitus or systemic steroid treatment (see Chapter 36).

Vitreous disorders

Vitreoretinal degenerations such as Stickler's syndrome or juvenile X-linked retinoschisis may be diagnosed at, or before, school age because of reduced visual acuity from myopia or retinal detachment (see Chapter 50).

Vitreous opacities including hemorrhage, vitritis, and retinoblastoma seedlings are uncommon causes of blurred vision. When the vitreous is too opaque to allow visualization, other diagnostic tests may be indicated, e.g. ultrasound, computed tomography (CT), or magnetic resonance imaging (MRI).

Retinal disorders

Congenital vascular disorders (see Chapter 47)

von Hippel-Lindau disease and Coats' disease can present with blurred vision.

Retinal dystrophies (see Chapter 44)

Visual disturbances with retinal dystrophies are variable. A family history of bilateral visual loss may be present, and there may be systemic findings. Blurred vision is rarely a complaint in retinitis pigmentosa in the early stages; night blindness and loss of peripheral visual field are more usual. These children often have high ametropia (hypermetropia or myopia). Macular dystrophies make reading difficult.

Systemic disease

Consider the connection between systemic disease and the retina because the ocular findings may lead directly to the systemic diagnosis. Blurred vision may occur as a consequence of side effects of treatment.

Diabetes mellitus may present early, but retinopathy is uncommon during the first decade of the disease. Blurred vision may result from myopia caused by rapid shifts in blood glucose levels, cataract, or from optic atrophy associated with DIDMOAD (Diabetes Insipidus, Diabetes Mellitus, Optic Atrophy, and Deafness – Wolfram's syndrome).

Many neurometabolic disorders, including Batten's disease, mucopolysaccharidoses, and mucolipidoses, can create blurred vision on a retinal basis, but they will often present with seizures and abnormal behavior before reduced visual acuity is measured. Electroretinography is often needed to diagnose the disease.

In leukemia, vision may be affected by retinal, choroidal, or iris infiltration or hemorrhage.

Optic nerve diseases

When poor acuity, color vision defect, a central scotoma or constricted field, poor pupil response (an afferent defect), and a variably swollen or atrophic optic disc are found in a child, it indicates an optic neuropathy (see Chapters 52 and 53). Optic atrophy without ocular, post-inflammatory, or hereditary causes suggests a central nervous system abnormality. It is usually bilateral, but can initially be unilateral. Congenital optic nerve anomalies (coloboma, hypoplasia) can be associated with poor vision and can be discovered late at school testing (see Chapter 51).

Central nervous system diseases

Blurred or reduced vision can result from involvement of the visual pathways; a lesion proximal to the chiasm results in optic atrophy. Increased intracranial pressure may cause papilledema, usually without visual symptoms, but, if it is severe, there may be episodic or permanent loss of vision. A severely atrophic optic nerve cannot appear swollen despite increased intracranial pressure because there is no retinal fiber layer to become swollen. A child with a central nervous system tumor (especially in the posterior fossa) is often ill, vomiting, and complaining of headache. They may also have varying double vision from a cranial nerve palsy.

The parachiasmal syndrome of visual defect, growth, and other hypothalamic disturbances in children is often caused by optic gliomas or craniopharyngiomas. Various combinations of optic atrophy and papilledema occur, depending on the duration of the process and how rapidly the intracranial disease has developed (see Chapter 55).

Cerebral visual impairment is a particularly frustrating disorder since there are so few ophthalmologic findings. The child may have reduced visual acuity which changes depending on the state of the child (see Chapters 56 and 57).

Non-organic visual disorders

These are often seen in teenage girls with problems either in the family, among their friends, or related to schoolwork. They can be very difficult to diagnose, and some children may undergo several tests in order to be sure that no organic disability is present (see Chapter 60).

Varying degrees of acuity and visual field loss are found, often becoming worse with time, but rarely to an extent that the child becomes blind. It is remarkable how well the child behaves despite marked visual loss.

My child could see perfectly but now the vision is weak

Luis Carlos Ferreira de Sá

Visual loss in an otherwise healthy child is an alarming finding for both the family and clinician. Children often do not complain of decreased vision, and it is common for them to present with severe visual loss. Visual loss may result from congenital problems, only noticed later in life when visual requirements increase at school or when the child had normal vision followed by chronic or acute visual loss (Fig. 104.1).

When investigating acquired visual loss, a comprehensive medical history is essential. Ask about the pregnancy, delivery, gestational age, birth weight, perinatal problems, developmental milestones, ocular and medical anomalies, medications, and family history of systemic and/or visual problems (Fig. 104.2). Seek details regarding trauma, timing, duration, and severity of visual loss.

Irrespective of whether the onset of visual loss is acute or chronic, ophthalmic examination may in most cases reveal abnormalities in the anterior and/or posterior segment, although the site of visual loss may be intracranial (see Chapters 54 and 56). Details about photophobia and eye movement disorders, including strabismus and nystagmus, may be especially helpful in reaching a diagnosis.

Examination

First, observe the child's visual behavior. There may be different degrees of visual loss, including visual inattention. The child may not respond to visual stimuli such as lights, faces, or toys. The examiner should not use animated and noisy objects; the child may be attracted to the sound rather than the visual stimulus. Whenever possible, visual acuity should be measured with different methods appropriate for the age.

Pupillary responses (grade of reactions, presence of an afferent pupillary defect, or paradoxical reaction) and assessment of alignment and eye movement disorders provide the clinician with important diagnostic clues.

Anterior segment

Cornea

Various diseases may affect the cornea. Developmental glaucoma may present with increased corneal diameter because of the elasticity of the collagen fibers in young children. Corneal

transparency may be reduced by several conditions, including developmental glaucoma (see Chapter 37), infectious keratitis (see Chapter 33), and metabolic diseases (mucolipidoses, mucopolysaccharidoses and cystinosis (see Chapter 33). Corneal shape is altered in keratoconus (see Chapter 33), which may be present in childhood and progress at puberty.

Iris

Iris abnormalities are usually not associated with acquired visual loss, although colobomas (see Chapter 38) and iris transillumination (albinism; see Chapter 40) may be related to congenital visual loss.

Lens

The lens should be carefully evaluated. Developmental cataracts can be secondary to trauma, radiation, metabolic/storage diseases, medications, or associated with genetic syndromes that may develop later in childhood (see Chapter 36). Ectopia/subluxated lens may also be observed and can be related to trauma, genetic/syndromes, and metabolic diseases (see Chapter 35).

Posterior segment

Vitreous

Signs of inflammation or hemorrhage related to uveitis, trauma, or tumors may be seen in the vitreous. Vitreous changes are part of a vitreoretinopathy (see Chapter 41). Past medical history of prematurity, high refractive errors, familial history of retinal detachment, joint pains, or cataracts may suggest retinopathy of prematurity, Stickler's syndrome, familial exudative vitreoretinopathy, or congenital stationary night blindness. Electroretinography (ERG) may be useful. Ultrasound, magnetic resonance imaging (MRI), or computed tomography (CT) scans may be indicated when vitreous opacities impede observation of the retina, or when calcification is suspected (retinoblastoma).

Retina/choroid

The retina/choroid should be evaluated. Subtle, but important, anomalies are not always readily observed. Retinal dystrophy and metabolic/storage diseases (see Chapter 44) commonly

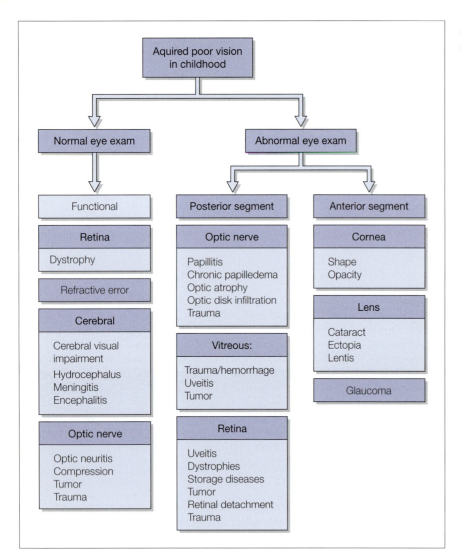

Fig. 104.1 Guidelines for diagnosis of acquired poor vision in childhood.

start without pigmentary changes. They develop later as the disease progresses. When the condition is bilateral and present since birth, nystagmus develops as in cases of Leber's congenital amaurosis, toxoplasmosis, and albinism. Color vision abnormalities and presence of paradoxical pupil reaction may suggest cone dysfunction. Retinal dystrophies will require electroretinography (ERG) for specific diagnosis. Severely reduced electro-oculogram (EOG) is an important diagnostic feature of vitelliform dystrophy (Best's disease). Fluorescein angiography, although difficult in children, is particularly useful in Stargardt's disease ("dark choroid" sign), when visual loss and macular changes may be minimal (see Chapter 45). A work-up for uveitis (see Chapter 39) and retinal detachment (see Chapter 50) may be necessary. Both conditions develop at any age and are important causes of acquired visual loss.

Optic nerve, chiasm, and optic tract

The size, color, and contour of the optic disc merit attention since optic disc abnormalities may be related to congenital and acquired visual loss. In evaluating optic atrophy the color of the optic disc is an important assessment. However, the optic discs may appear pale in infants compared to older children and adults. Moreover, inherited optic atrophy including Leber's hereditary and autosomal dominant forms rarely manifests in

the first year of life. Optic atrophy may be due to panretinal degeneration and ERG may occasionally be necessary. Optic atrophy may occur secondary to long-standing papilledema or compressive lesions of the anterior visual pathway; neuroimaging studies may be indicated. The chiasm and optic tract may be involved in a variety of conditions, including tumors (glioma, craniopharyngioma, neuroblastoma, and retinoblastoma "trilateral"), trauma, infection, inflammation (post-viral, post-immunization, and demyelinating diseases such as multiple sclerosis), vascular anomalies, and radiation.

Central nervous system and cortical visual impairment

Visual loss is frequently associated with disturbances of the visual cortex as the result of trauma, infection, hydrocephaly, hypoxemia, and vascular or metabolic insults (see Chapters 55 and 56).

What if the eye exam is normal?

In a child with acquired visual loss and no ocular explanation for it, it is important to rule out functional visual loss (see

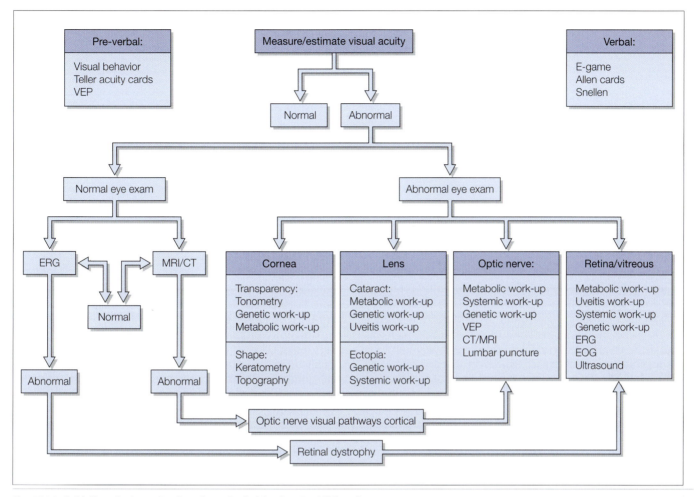

Fig. 104.2 Guidelines for investigation of acquired vision loss in childhood.

Chapter 60) and refractive errors. Electrophysiological tests and neuroimaging studies may be necessary to rule out organic disease. In some patients, acquired visual loss is part of a multisystem disorder.

Electrophysiological tests (see Chapter 8)

ERG is invaluable in diagnosing poor vision in children. It may be performed in a child with poor vision and normal ocular examination because many retinal disorders are not associated with any visible pigmentary changes early in the course of disease. EOG is rarely indicated for small children; conditions in which EOG is indicated (Best's and Stargardt's disease) rarely manifest in the first decade. Visual evoked potential (VEP) can be helpful for estimating visual acuity and in providing information about the neural visual pathway, as in optic neuritis where there may be a prolonged latency.

Neuroimaging studies

MRI and/or CT scan are indicated when the clinical examination and electrophysiological tests fail to explain the poor vision. Resolution of MRI is superior to that of a CT scan, providing better images of the central nervous system (CNS) and it does not expose the child to radiation. However, MRI acquisition time is longer, it does not visualize the bone as well as a CT scan, and may require anesthesia in small children. Neuroimaging studies are important in cases of compressive lesions of the visual pathways, cortical abnormalities, and demyelinating process.

The decision to perform electrophysiological tests before neuroimaging studies should be based on the individual child, availability of an electrophysiological test laboratory, and the possibility of associated CNS pathology.

The deaf-blind child

David Laws

Background

A Danish study estimated the prevalence of deaf-blind children at $1:15\,000$ and congenital deaf-blindness at $1:19\,000$.[1] Visual problems of all severities are found in 40–60% of deaf children.[2] Although profound deaf-blindness is uncommon, it was found in 21.4% of intellectually disabled residents in an Austrian institute and is under-recognized in this setting.[3] Conversely, deaf-blind people may be misdiagnosed as having learning difficulty particularly as behavioral and psychiatric problems are more common.[4] Using a functional definition of deaf-blindness, the US National Deaf-Blind Child Count identified 66% also had cognitive disability, 57% physical disability, and 9% behavioral challenges.[5]

Communication with dual sensory impaired

Communication is often idiosyncratic and depends on several factors:

1. The onset of the disability relative to speech and reading development.
2. Associated neurodevelopmental problems.
3. The absolute and relative severity of each form of impairment.

When communicating with hearing impaired it is best to speak clearly, not too fast, and reduce background noise. Face the child and have good lighting so she/he can lip-read. Follow the child's lead and make use of gestures where appropriate. Dark clothes can help the child to see hand movement when signing. Various methods including fingerspelling (Print on palm) and tactile lip-reading (Tadoma)* are used. Makaton** uses printed symbols that are helpful with learning difficulties. Tablet computers or Braille displays are available.

Faced with a bewildering array of means of communication the carer will often indicate the best method or acts as translator. A mixture of techniques may be most effective.

*Tadoma – the deaf-blind person places their thumb on the speaker's lips and their fingers on the jawline. They feel the lip movement, vibrations of the vocal cords and air produced by nasal sounds.

**Makaton is a program to communicate with people who cannot communicate well with speech. It uses a combination of speech, signs, and graphic symbols.

Neuroadaptation

Like vision, hearing has a sensitive period of cortical development. Cochlear implantation in the congenitally deaf after the period of auditory plasticity has a worse outcome. Early implantation promotes cortical maturation and speech development.[6]

Functional neuroimaging and behavioral studies show that deaf-blindness allows recruitment of the sensory cortex by, for example, tactile stimuli and language processing.[7] Braille alexia in a congenitally blind person following a visual cortex stroke illustrates this cross modal mechanism.[8] Cross adaptation allows behavioral gains, but may prevent rehabilitation of the primary sensory function.

Causes of deaf-blindness

The etiology of deaf-blindness varies with age and geographic distribution. In developing countries infective mechanisms are more common: in developed countries deaf-blindness due to neurological damage is more common (see Chapters 55 and 56).

See Table 105.1.

Management

All children with hearing impairment must be refracted. With neurosensory hearing loss screening for ophthalmic conditions is useful.

If hearing problems have not been addressed, otorhinolaryngology and audiology should be involved. Sleep disorders are common in the deaf-blind and may be helped with melatonin[9] (see Chapter 121). Genetic counseling may be appropriate.

Dual sensory impairment often leads to social isolation for the child and affects all aspects of family life. A seamless link between the hospital and resources in the community is best practice. Many countries have registration procedures for the sensory impaired to promote access to specialist education and welfare support. Education should include mobility and communication training. Referral to specialist educational services is mandatory, even for a newborn. Severe disability causes

Table 105.1 – Expected onset and frequency of deaf-blindness reported to the US National Deaf-Blind Child Count 2009[10]

Diagnosis or syndrome	Usual sequence of sensory loss				Cases (%)
	Congenital/infantile visual and hearing loss	Congenital/infantile visual loss, later hearing loss	Congenital/infantile hearing loss, later visual loss	Later visual and hearing loss	
Unknown					1646 (17.8)
Other: Hereditary					1233 (13.4)
Prematurity	X		X		1171 (12.7)
CHARGE	X		X		746 (8.1)
Other: Prenatal					469 (5.1)
Other: Postnatal					364 (4.0)
Cytomegalovirus	X				332 (3.6)
Microcephaly	X				287 (3.1)
Asphyxia	X			X	241 (2.6)
Hydrocephaly				X	230 (2.5)
Down's syndrome			X		217 (2.4)
Meningitis				X	208 (2.3)
Trauma				X	197 (2.1)
Usher's I			X		194 (2.1)
Stickler's			X		106 (1.2)
Maternal drug use	X				104 (1.1)
Goldenhar's			X		91 (1.0)
Dandy-Walker				X	90 (1.0)
Congenital rubella	X		X		87 (0.9)
Tumor				X	86 (0.9)
Cornelia de Lange				X	80 (0.9)
Encephalitis				X	74 (0.8)
Usher's II			X	X	65 (0.7)
Stroke				X	64 (0.7)
Trisomy 13	X				57 (0.6)
Trisomy 4p	X			X	57 (0.6)
Leber's amaurosis	X	X			46 (0.5)
Infections	X	X	X	X	37 (0.4)
Fetal alcohol	X				36 (0.4)
Pierre Robin				X	36 (0.4)
Norrie's		X			34 (0.4)
Möbius'			X		31 (0.3)
Aicardi's	X				30 (0.3)
Alstrom's		X			29 (0.3)
Refsum's				X	27 (0.3)
Ring chromosome 18	X				25 (0.3)
Chemically induced				X	21 (0.2)
Treacher-Collins			X		20 (0.2)
Waardenburg's	X				20 (0.2)
Marshall's				X	19 (0.2)
Cri du chat	X				17 (0.2)

Continued

Table 105.1 – *Continued*

Diagnosis or syndrome	Usual sequence of sensory loss				Cases (%)
	Congenital/infantile visual and hearing loss	Congenital/infantile visual loss, later hearing loss	Congenital/infantile hearing loss, later visual loss	Later visual and hearing loss	
Batten's disease				X	15 (0.2)
Cockayne's syndrome				X	15 (0.2)
Pfieffer's				X	15 (0.2)
Crouzon's				X	14 (0.2)
Turner's				X	14 (0.2)
Apert's				X	12 (0.1)
Neurofibromatosis 1				X	12 (0.1)
Hurler's				X	10 (0.1)
Sturge-Weber				X	9 (0.1)
Neonatal HSV	X				8 (0.1)
Neurofibromatosis 2				X	8 (0.1)
Smith-Lemli-Opitz	X				8 (0.1)
Usher's III				X	8 (0.1)
Alport's				X	6 (0.1)
Kneist's				X	6 (0.1)
Prader-Willi				X	6 (0.1)
Bardet-Biedel				X	5 (0.1)
Hunter's				X	5 (0.1)
Congental syphilis	X				4 (0.0)
Kearns Sayer				X	4 (0.0)
Klippel-Feil				X	4 (0.0)
Leigh's disease				X	4 (0.0)
Marfan's				X	4 (0.0)
Maroteaux Lamy				X	4 (0.0)
Cogan's syndrome				X	3 (0.0)

financial burden for families and direction to welfare support, if available, is required. Charitable organizations can provide advice regarding communication, sleep, feeding, technical issues, and even family holidays. Technology such as optical character recognition, Braille display, and global positioning systems can improve quality of life.

Resources

Deafblind UK

National Centre for Deafblindness, John and Lucille van Geest Place, Cygnet Road, Hampton, Peterborough, Cambridgeshire PE7 8FD, UK

Tel/text: 01733 358 100; 24-hour helpline: 0800 132 320; Fax: 01733 358 356

Website: http://www.deafblind.org.uk

Sense

101 Pentonville Road, London, N1 9LG, UK

Tel: 0845 127 0060; Fax: 0845 127 0061; Textphone: 0845 127 0062

Website: http://www.sense.org.uk

National Consortium on Deaf-Blindness

The Teaching Research Institute, 345 N. Monmouth Ave, Monmouth, OR 97361, USA

Telephone – Voice: 800-438-9376; Fax: 503-838-8150

Website: http://www.nationaldb.org/

American Association of the Deaf-Blind

8630 Fenton Street, Suite 121, Silver Spring, MD 20910-3803, USA

Tel: 301-495-4403 (voice)

Website: http://www.aadb.org/

Organizations for Deafblind People Throughout the World

http://www.deafblind.com/org.html

References

1. Dammeyer J. Prevalence and aetiology of congenitally deafblind people in Denmark. Int J Audiol 2010; 49: 76–82.
2. Nikolopoulos TP, Lioumi D, Stamataki S, O'Donoghue GM. Evidence-based overview of ophthalmic disorders in deaf children: a literature update. Otol Neurotol [Review] 2006; 27(2 Suppl 1): S1–24; discussion S0.
3. Fellinger J, Holzinger D, Dirmhirn A, et al. Failure to detect deaf-blindness in a population of people with intellectual disability. J Intellect Disabil Res 2009; 53: 874–81.
4. Dammeyer J. Mental and behavioral disorders among people with congenital deafblindness. Res Dev Disabil 2011; 32: 571–5.
5. Killoran J. The National Deaf–Blind Child Count: 1998–2005 in Review. Monmouth, Oregon: National Consortium on Deaf-Blindness; 2007; Available from: http://www.nationaldb.org/NCDBProducts.php?prodID=57.
6. Kral A, O'Donoghue GM. Profound deafness in childhood. N Engl J Med [Review] 2010; 363: 1438–50.
7. Merabet LB, Pascual-Leone A. Neural reorganization following sensory loss: the opportunity of change. Nat Rev Neurosci 2010; 11: 44–52.
8. Hamilton R, Keenan JP, Catala M, Pascual-Leone A. Alexia for Braille following bilateral occipital stroke in an early blind woman. Neuroreport 2000 7;11: 237–40.
9. Bjorvatn B, Pallesen S. A practical approach to circadian rhythm sleep disorders. Sleep Med Rev 2009; 13: 47–60.
10. Deaf-Blindness NCo. Primary etiologies of deaf-blindness – frequency; 2009. Available from: http://www.nationaldb.org/ISSelectedTopics.php?topicID=990&topicCatID=24.

Optic atrophy in infancy and childhood

Yoshiko Sugiyama • Yoshikazu Hatsukawa

Presentation

In childhood, optic nerve disorders occur in three main periods:

1. Prenatal: the result is usually a developmental disorder such as coloboma or optic nerve hypoplasia but an element of optic atrophy may occur when the cause occurs late in gestation.
2. Perinatal: the developmental condition merges with optic atrophy[1] and some cases have both a developmental optic disk anomaly and optic atrophy, as in Figures 106.1 and 106.2, due to loss of neurons at different times.
3. Postnatal: the result is optic atrophy.

Therefore, optic atrophy may occur after damage in the later prenatal, perinatal, or postnatal periods in children. Small children with optic atrophy do not have a pathognomonic mode of presentation connected with the optic atrophy itself. They present with either general behavioral characteristics of visual loss with or without nystagmus or because of other associated symptoms such as pain, headache, or neurologic symptoms.

Causes (Fig. 106.3)

It is not possible to establish a cause in every case; the cause varies enormously between centers. A tertiary referral center sees cases referred to their neurology, neurosurgery, or metabolic departments[2] while developmental centers see mainly cases associated with cerebral palsy. Prevalence is difficult to establish.

If there is a history of pre- or perinatal problems, they may well be the cause, especially if there is a history of significant hypoxia. One should be cautious about attributing optic atrophy to a mild perinatal insult. It is rare for optic atrophy caused by perinatal problems to be unassociated with other, significant central nervous system damage.

In postnatal life, optic atrophy is an indication that the damage is anterior to the lateral geniculate body; before then, trans-synaptic degeneration can occur but is unusual. When optic atrophy is definitely unilateral, the cause is anterior to the chiasm (Table 106.1); when it is definitely bilateral, it is either due to bilateral disease or disease involving pathways posterior to the chiasm.

Postnatal causes of optic atrophy include the hereditary optic neuropathies and metabolic causes. Most underlying metabolic defects are from before birth but many do not present until later in life – in the case of Leber's hereditary optic neuropathy (see Chapter 52), many years later. Babies with lactic acidosis[3] (i.e. Leigh's disease, mitochondrial cytopathy, pyruvate decarboxylase, cytochrome oxidase deficiency, etc.) have a high incidence of optic atrophy, sometimes profound occurring at a variable time after birth.

Postnatal causes include tumors invading or compressing the visual pathways. Hydrocephalus may also occur in optic atrophy but it is an unusual isolated presenting symptom.

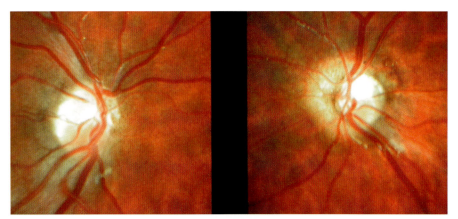

Fig. 106.1 This child has septo-optic dysplasia and presented because of nystagmus at 7 months old. He suffered a near-fatal episode when he was 2½ years old when his parents felt his vision became significantly worse. The optic disks are clearly hypoplastic but the temporal segments, which is where any surviving axons would be, are very pale. The inferior parts contain residual nerve fibers which can be best seen about ½ disk diameter away from the optic disk.

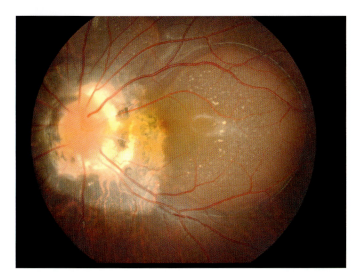

Fig. 106.2 This unilateral optic disk anomaly, a "morning glory disk anomaly," was associated with functionally good vision in infancy. The child has subretinal fluid under the macula which has reduced the acuity. The substance of the optic disk is more pale than one would expect and the peripapillary nerve fiber layer is thin, given the previously good acuity, suggesting an event which has resulted in loss of nerve fibers.

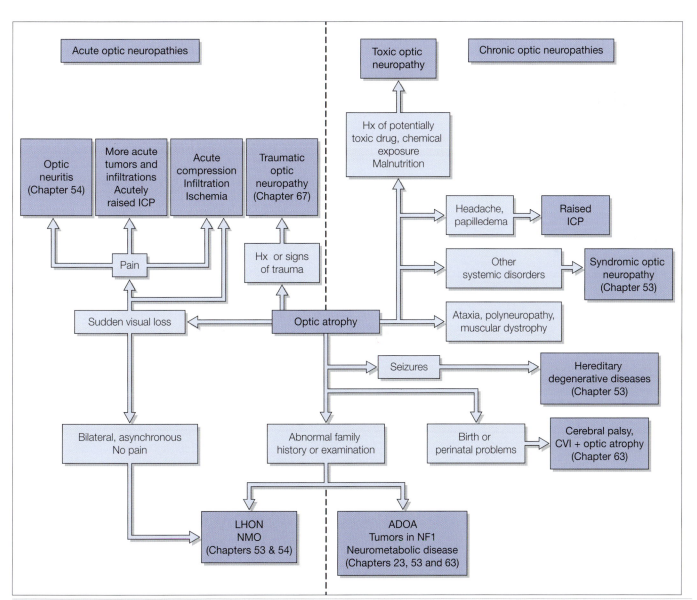

Fig. 106.3 Construct of the more frequent causes, symptoms, and signs of optic atrophy in acute and chronic categories. ADOA, autosomal dominant optic atrophy; CVI, cerebral visual impairment; Hx, history; ICP, intracranial pressure; LHON, Leber's hereditary optic neuropathy; NF1, neurofibromatosis type 1; NMO, neuromyelitis optica.

History and examination

Taking a family history and examining parents and siblings is vital and may suggest the diagnosis. The history of the pregnancy, birth, and how the presenting problem arose or was noticed is elicited (see Chapter 7). Many observant parents make relevant observations about the vision and even the state of the pupils, presence of nystagmus, strabismus, or structural abnormalities of the eye.

Babies are best examined while being fed or sleeping so ask the parents to bring the baby to the clinic hungry and to bring a bottle or be prepared to breast feed them at the most vital part of the examination. Visual behavior can be observed first and any formal assessments such as forced-choice preferential looking studies carried out; after feeding they are likely to be better disposed to more intrusive examinations, using a speculum, etc. Throughout the visit, it is helpful to keep an eye open for the baby's general development and the possibility of developmental anomalies. A more formal examination of the whole baby is made where necessary. Even in children with apparently isolated optic atrophy, for instance that in association with *OPA1* mutations, dominant optic atrophy, may have significant systemic disease.[4] Some cases that need a more detailed clinical examination or further studies are examined under general anesthesia. Examine the fundus with both direct and indirect ophthalmoscopy. The disk appears pale with fewer than normal vessels on the surface; it is helpful to examine the affected optic disk and put equal scrutiny on examining the disk and peripapillary nerve fiber layer of the other eye. The apparently unaffected eye can reveal diagnostic signs (Fig. 106.4), which cannot be found in an already affected eye.

Pupil reactions, if sluggish to light or showing a relatively afferent pupillary defect (Video 106.1), may suggest anterior visual pathway disease, lateralize it, and suggest where the lesion is (see Chapter 63). Color vision, especially if asymmetric or if there is evidence of it changing or if it is specific (as in the blue/yellow tritanopia of dominant optic atrophy), can give vital diagnostic evidence.

Visual field studies, even when using confrontation techniques, but preferably by formal perimetry in older children, provide valuable information for diagnosis and in helping carers and educators understand the child's individual problems.[5]

Further investigations

An electroretinogram (ERG) may be indicated to exclude retinal disease. Careful communication between ophthalmologist and electrophysiologist helps the latter to do the best testing protocol. For instance, if a differential diagnosis includes Stargardt's disease, a pattern ERG could be the only abnormality to suggest the diagnosis. The electrophysiologist needs to be aware of the possible diagnosis in order to do the appropriate test. Fundus imaging can help with optic nerve diseases

Table 106.1 – Laterality, features and causes of optic atrophy in childhood

Laterality and features of optic atrophy	Causes
Purely unilateral causes Other eye clinically normal and ERG/VEPs normal	Glaucoma Compression anterior to chiasm Trauma Leber's hereditary optic neuropathy before other eye (20% of which are normal) affected
Bilateral symmetric +/– nystagmus	Severe hypoxia, tumor, neurometabolic, increased ICP, hereditary optic neuropathy (see Chapters 53 & 54)
Bilateral asymmetric with nystagmus (especially rotary or vertical or asymmetric)	Chiasmal tumor

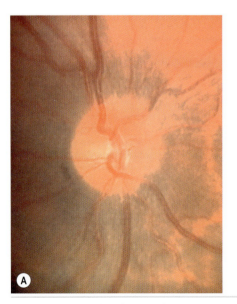
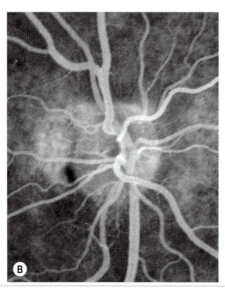
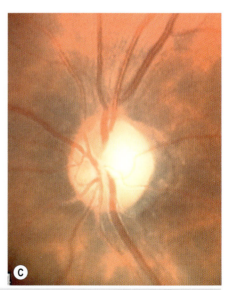

Fig. 106.4 Leber's hereditary optic neuropathy. The optic disk of the first affected left eye (C) shows non-specific optic atrophy. The currently asymptomatic right eye (A) shows the diagnostic peripapillary telangiectasia and nerve fiber layer swelling without fluorescein leakage (B) (see Chapter 52). (Case by courtesy of Dr. Makoto Nakamura, Division of Ophthalmology, Kobe University Graduate School of Medicine.)

(see Chapter 9). CT and, particularly, MRI are indicated for the investigation of most, but not all, patients with optic atrophy. Patients that fit the diagnosis of dominant optic atrophy and have an affected relative, or molecularly diagnosed Leber's hereditary optic neuropathy, normally do not benefit from scanning. If an anesthetic is needed, even an MRI has a risk.

Prognosis

The prognosis depends on the diagnosis and the natural history of the condition. Caution should be used in giving a prognosis to parents whose child has recently suffered optic atrophy from an acute cause such as tumor or hydrocephalus; very dramatic recovery can take place up to 2 or occasionally more years after the onset of the visual loss. As a general rule, it is better to be optimistic rather than pessimistic. This should especially be so if there is still some response to a flash stimulus on the visual evoked responses. Every pediatric ophthalmologist has seen examples of remarkable late recovery in vision with optic atrophy with or without cerebral visual disorders in young children. The uncertainty about prognosis, however, should not inhibit the ophthalmologist from registering the visual handicap with the appropriate authority; periodic re-assessment should be scheduled.

References

1. Hoyt CS, Good WV. Do we understand the difference between optic nerve hypoplasia and atrophy? Eye 1992; 6: 201–4.
2. Repka M, Miller NR. Optic atrophy in children. Am J Ophthalmol 1988; 191: 181–4.
3. Hayasaka S, Yamaguschio K, Misuro K, et al. Ocular findings in childhood lactic acidosis. Arch Ophthalmol 1986; 104: 1956–8.
4. Yu-Wai-Man P, Griffiths PG, Gorman GS, et al. Multi-system neurological disease is common in patients with OPA1 mutations. Brain 2010; 1–16.
5. Rudolph D, Sterker I, Graefe G, et al. Visual field constriction in children with shunt-treated hydrocephalus. J Neurosurg Pediatr 2010; 6: 481–5.

The swollen optic disc

David Taylor

The diagnosis of the cause of a swollen optic disc is made by history and the accompanying visual and other ocular signs and symptoms, not just by ophthalmoscopy of the disc, even though that plays an important role (Figs 107.1–107.23). Figure 107.1 shows the importance of this and how one presentation can progress to another. For instance, papilledema (disc swelling due to raised intracranial pressure) starts with normal acuity and color vision and slightly enlarged blind spots but can progress to severe visual loss.

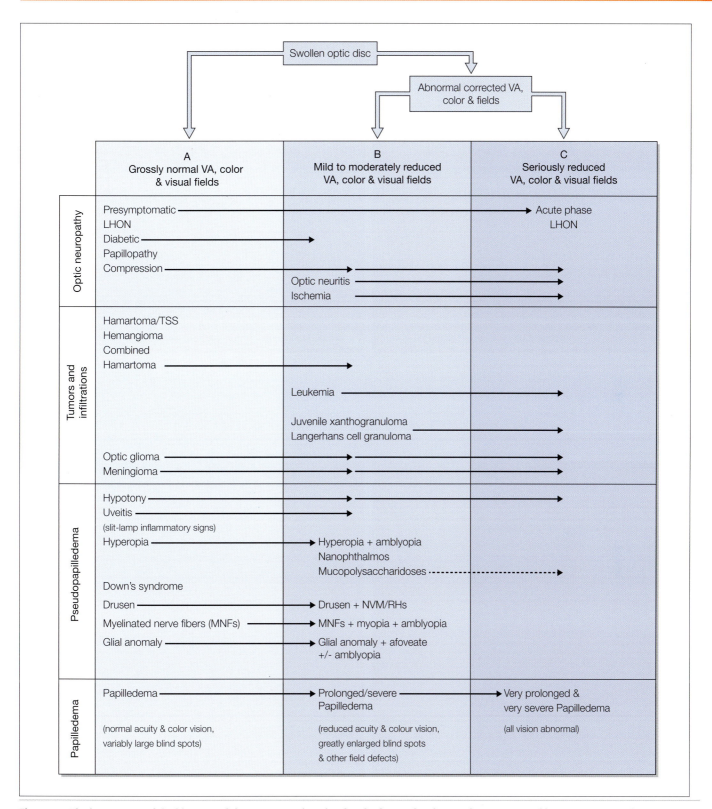

Fig. 107.1 The importance of the history and the accompanying visual and other ocular signs and symptoms and how one presentation can progress to another. For instance, papilledema (disc swelling due to raised intracranial pressure) starts with normal acuity and color vision and slightly enlarged blind spots but can progress to severe visual loss. NVM/RH = Neovascular membrane/Retinal Hemorrhage. MNFs = Myelinated Nerve Fibres.

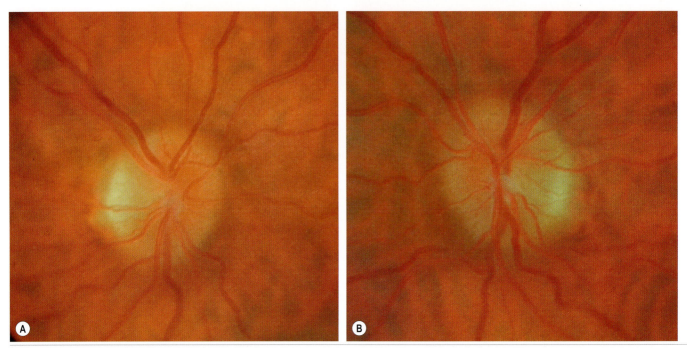

Fig. 107.2 This 10-year-old girl with idiopathic intracranial hypertension (pseudotumor cerebri) had a recurrence of symptoms of headache following cessation of treatment. Both optic discs show slight elevation and indistinct margins due to thickening of the nerve fiber layer around the disc. The lumbar puncture opening pressure was 35 cm of CSF. Visual acuity and color vision were normal. The visual fields showed marginally enlarged blind spots.

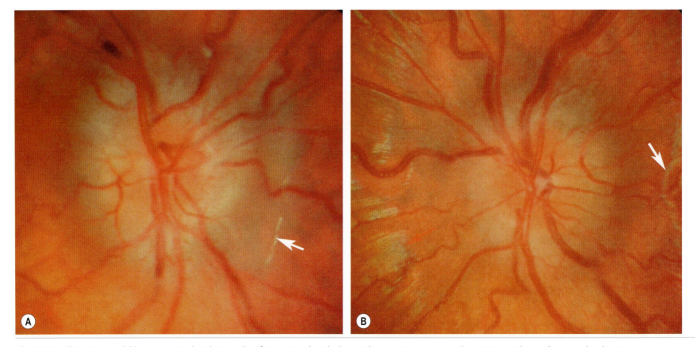

Fig. 107.3 This 10-year-old boy presented with 3 weeks of increasing headaches with morning nausea and vomiting and was diagnosed as having an ependymoma of the fourth ventricle. The optic discs are elevated, the veins dilated and tortuous. The disc capillaries are dilated and the nerve fibers around the optic discs are thickened with the result that the reflexes from the internal limiting membrane (ILM, red arrows) are displaced away from their normal position near the disc margin. Visual acuities were 0.0 logMAR (6/6, 20/20, 1.0) and the visual fields showed larger than normal blind spots on Goldmann fields: papilledema due to raised intracranial pressure.

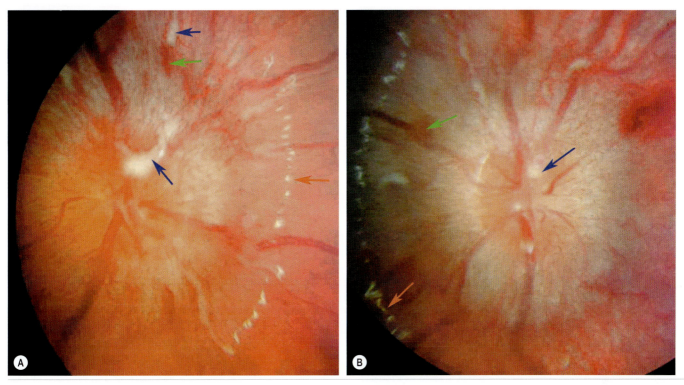

Fig. 107.4 Optic discs of a 6-year-old child with a medulloblastoma who had for a month behaved oddly, lost weight, with illness and vomiting. The optic discs are markedly elevated with dilated capillaries and veins, displaced ILM light reflexes (red arrows), cotton wool spots (blue arrows) which suggest ganglion cell axonal death, and hemorrhages (green arrows). The visual acuity and color vision were normal, but the visual fields showed prominently large blind spots on confrontation testing. The intracranial pressure was markedly raised.

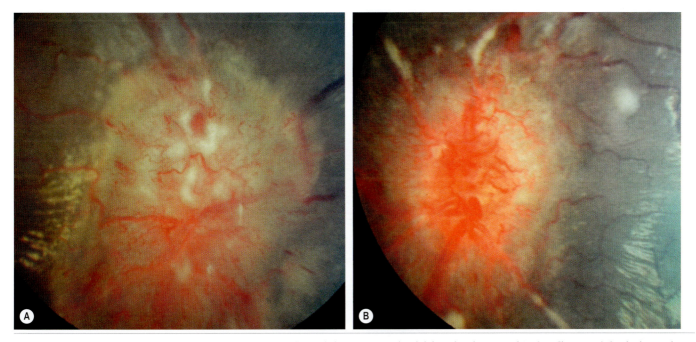

Fig. 107.5 This 7-year-old boy with a brain stem glioma presented with diplopia associated with bilateral sixth nerve palsies (see Chapter 83) that had started gradually about 2 months before and more recent symptoms of raised intracranial pressure. The optic discs are grossly elevated with markedly dilated capillaries and veins, numerous cotton wool spots, and the right eye has a macular star, as a result of protein/lipid accumulation from transudation from disc capillaries. Although the blind spots were very large on Goldmann fields, the visual acuity was 0.1 (6/7.5, 20/25, 0.8) right and 0.0 left.

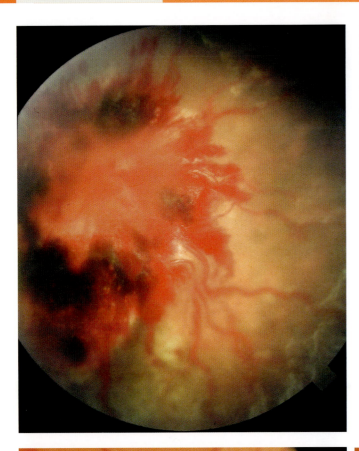

Fig. 107.6 This girl was born with spina bifida and hydrocephalus (see Chapter 56). She was shunted successfully at the age of 2 months and the shunt was revised twice. She was substantially developmentally delayed. At the age of 10 years the shunt blocked leading to a very severe rise in intracranial pressure without many symptoms. The optic discs are grossly swollen and covered in hemorrhage with some cotton wool spots and other ischemic signs are visible. Vision testing was not possible but behaviorally her vision was reduced.

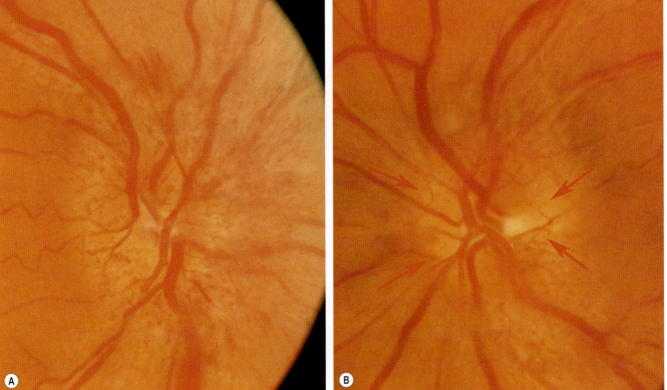

Fig. 107.7 This 18-year-old female with a right optic tract and hypothalamic glioma (see Chapters 23, 54 and 64) has bilateral papilledema as a result of enlargement of the tumor and hydrocephalus. The visual acuities are 0.0 logMAR in each eye, the color vision is normal and there is a total left homonymous hemianopia. The right optic disc is swollen diffusely, but the left disc is swollen mostly in the upper and lower quadrants (above and below the pairs of red arrows). This is where the retinal ganglion cell axons which subserve the intact right visual field that arise temporal to the fovea and arch over the macula are inserted into the optic disc. The axons that subserve the defunct left visual field would be inserted all around the optic disc, but they have atrophied because of pressure from the tumor, leaving a horizontal wedge of pallor and lack of swelling because there are no residual fibers to swell. This is "twin peaks papilledema."

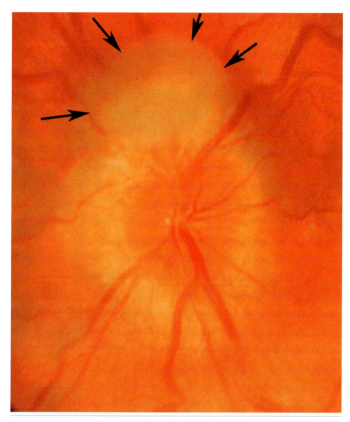

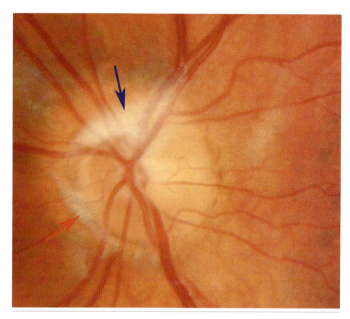

Fig. 107.10 This 6-year-old boy was examined as routine by an optometrist who thought that the right optic disc appeared swollen. All visual functions were perfect and there were no inflammatory signs. There is a pre-papillary white area at the upper pole (blue arrow) and inferiorly (red arrow) which are a congenital developmental anomaly of no functional significance.

Fig. 107.8 This child has hydrocephalus caused by intraventricular tumors associated with tuberous sclerosis (see Chapter 65). The optic disc is chronically papilledematous, but at the upper pole there is an astrocytic hamartoma (black arrows) which makes the disc swelling appear more marked.

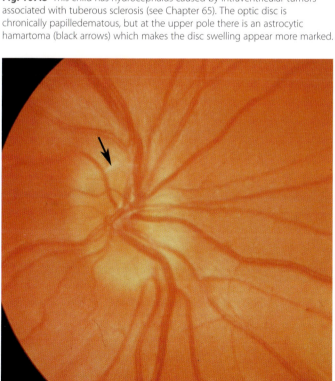

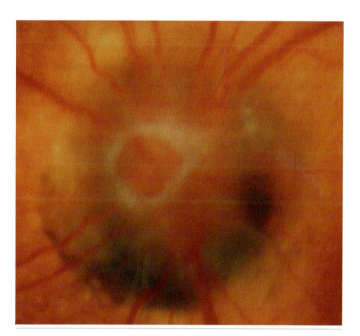

Fig. 107.11 This child presented with left esotropia secondary to very poor vision. The optic disc is anomalous with radial vessels and a pre-papillary "glial" elevation with an optic disc configuration similar to a "morning glory" disc anomaly (see Chapter 51).

Fig. 107.9 The optic disc appears small and "crowded" (the appearance of many vessels given by the small disc size). The retinal nerve fiber layer right up to the disc is normal. The fibers are not swollen. The appearance of swelling is a false one associated with high hyperopia (cycloplegic retinoscopy +6.0). The ultrasound study did not show drusen. There is a small prepapillary glial anomaly near the upper pole (arrow).

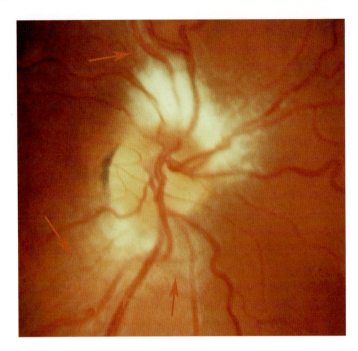

Fig. 107.12 This hydrocephalic child was known to have myelinated nerve fibers. A shunt blockage caused her to develop papilledema which can be seen as thickening of the retinal nerve fibers well away from the optic disc (red arrows).

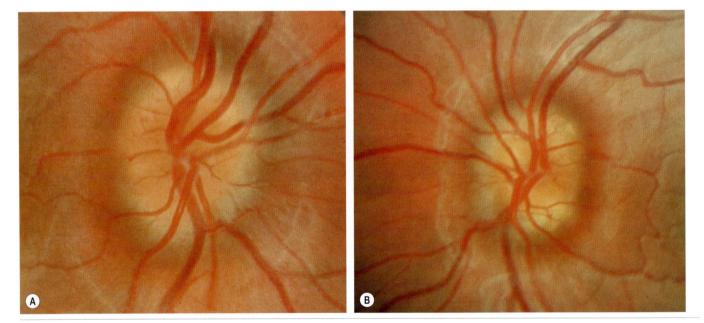

Fig. 107.13 This 12-year-old boy complained of headaches after school and was referred by his optometrist and GP to a neurologist because of the appearance of the optic discs. Both discs are elevated, but the nerve fiber layer around the disc is normal. His visual functions were perfect. The left optic disc shows some drusen bodies (see Chapter 51) which were confirmed in both eyes on ultrasound studies. His intracranial pressure had been found to be normal by the neurologists. The diagnosis of drusen is often difficult and it is said that no neuro-ophthalmologist has ever been correct in every case! Drusen may occur in discs with chronic papilledema.

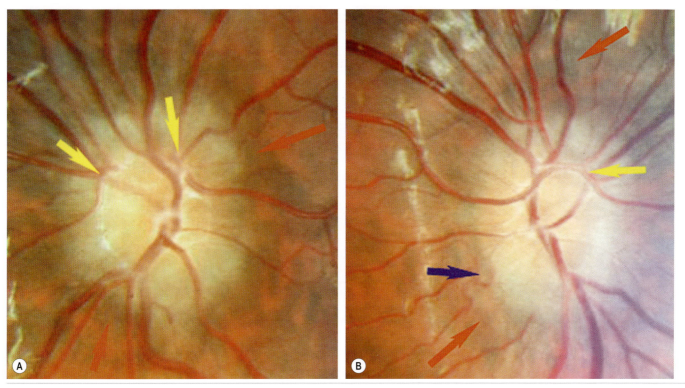

Fig. 107.14 This child with elevated optic discs presented with headaches. A CT scan showed the drusen (see Chapter 51) visible as lumps in the discs. There are anomalous vessels, cilioretinal (blue arrow), and anomalously branching (yellow arrows). The ILM reflexes are well away from the disc because of the elevation, but the nerve fiber layer is normal adjacent to the optic disc.

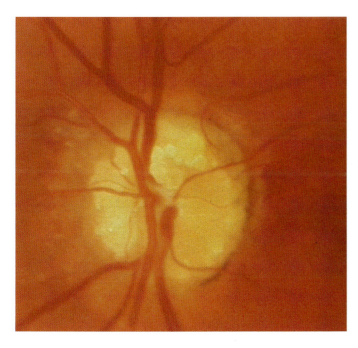

Fig. 107.15 An adult has marked exposed drusen (see Chapter 51). Drusen is a chronic optic neuropathy that is progressive throughout life. The visual loss is insidious and usually mild though occasionally the vision may be compromised by hemorrhages adjacent to the disc or by neovascular membranes.

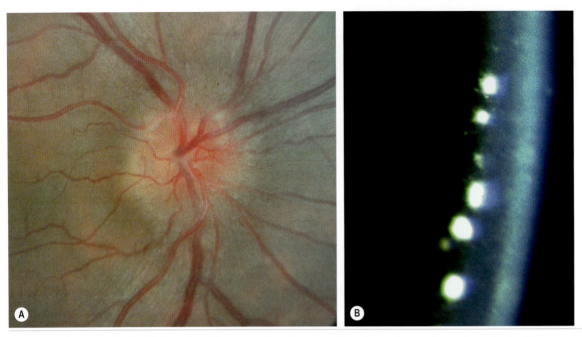

Fig. 107.16 A 16-year-old girl with bilateral uveitis has sarcoidosis. There was bilateral optic disc swelling and vascular sheathing seen near the upper pole of the right disc. Slit-lamp examination showed "mutton fat" keratic precipitates. She had no signs or symptoms of neurosarcoid.

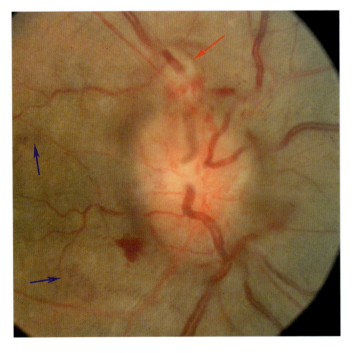

Fig. 107.17 This 6-year-old child of Asian origin had TB meningitis. The right eye developed an esotropia and the visual acuity was less than 1.0 logMAR (6/60, 20/200, 01.). There was a right afferent pupil defect, poor color vision, and a posterior uveitis. The disc was elevated and infiltrated (red arrow). There were superficial and deep (blue arrows) retinal hemorrhages.

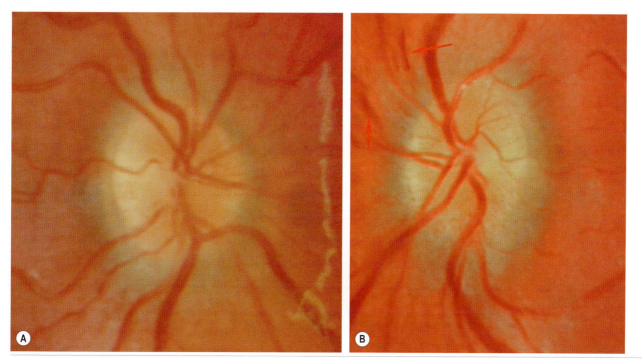

Fig. 107.18 This 8-year-old girl presented with poor vision in both eyes about a week after a non-specific illness. The vision was perception of hand movements in the left eye and counting fingers in the right. She could not accurately discern the color of a bright light. The optic discs are moderately swollen with few hemorrhages (red arrows). She had optic neuritis (see Chapter 53) and regained her vision over a period of 1 month, with some residual optic atrophy.

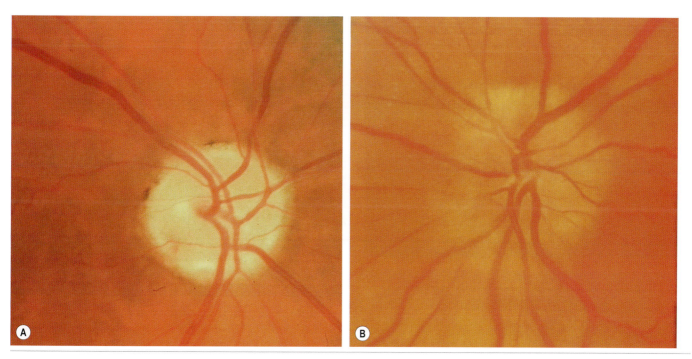

Fig. 107.19 The right eye was blinded by a myeloid leukemia deposit in the sphenoid bone. The child developed raised intracranial pressure and left papilledema in relation to steroid treatment some months later. The right eye did not develop papilledema because, due to the optic atrophy, there are no nerve fibers to swell.

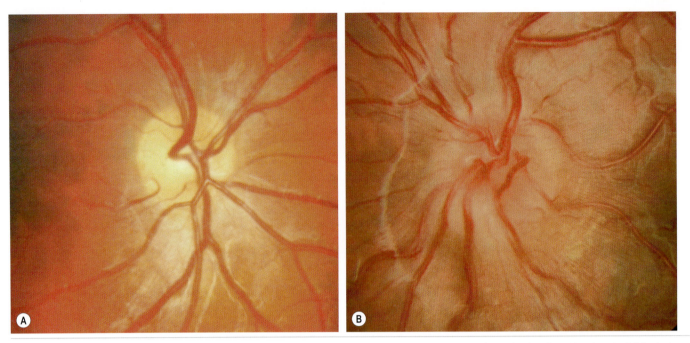

Fig. 107.20 This 7-year-old healthy boy developed left proptosis due to an optic glioma (see Chapter 23). The right eye had perfect vision, but the left had a large central scotoma, an afferent pupil defect, and "count fingers" vision. The left optic disc is swollen presumably due to pressure from the tumor on the intraorbital optic nerve axons.

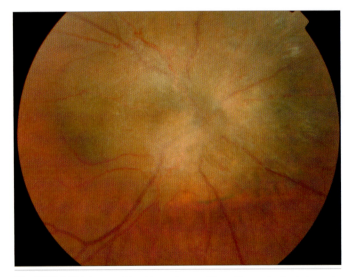

Fig. 107.21 This is a combined hamartoma of the retina and retinal pigment epithelium affecting the optic disc with vision reduced to "count fingers" (see Chapter 47). The pigmentation and telangiectatic capillaries are significant features.

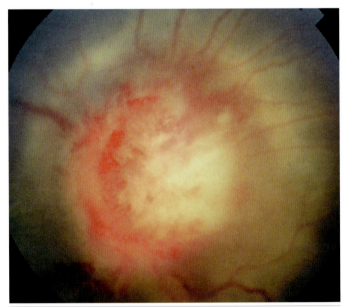

Fig. 107.22 An optic disc is infiltrated with tumor cells in acute myeloid leukemia in a 6-year-old child in relapse with acute myeloid leukemia. The eye is blind.

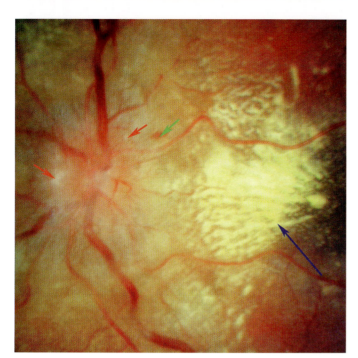

Fig. 107.23 This 12-year-old girl with reflux uropathy has severe arterial hypertension. Both optic discs are swollen with a thickened nerve fiber layer visible up to a disc diameter away from the disc edge, cotton wool spots (red arrows), and a few hemorrhages (green arrow). The vision was reduced (no details available). There is a marked macular "star" (blue arrow). The optic discs are already losing nerve fibers and may infarct if the blood pressure is brought down too rapidly to below the high level that disc blood flow autoregulation has become reset to.

Headache in children

Ian Simmons

Introduction

In a busy pediatric clinic, an ophthalmologist rarely gets the chance to fully explore underlying causes for headaches in one visit, particularly if these are non-organic. Which symptoms should be taken seriously as belying significant pathology and which reflect less severe disease are important to recognize. A simple algorithm which helps make the decision whether to neuroimage is of significant benefit.

Childhood migraine is under-recognized as ophthalmologists tend to use their own diagnostic criteria for adult migraine. Understanding the differences in symptoms and treatment between the pediatric and adult form of migraine is essential.

Classification and etiology

Headaches in children can be classified as primary and secondary. The two most common types of primary headaches are migraine and chronic daily headaches (CDH). Other primary headaches are listed in Box 108.1.

The International Classification of Headache Disorders (ICHD-I) was created to improve the understanding of the

---

Box 108.1

Causes of primary headaches in children

Migraine without aura
Migraine with aura
    Basilar-type migraine
    Hemiplegic migraine
    "Alice in Wonderland" syndrome
Tension-type headaches
Cluster headaches
Paroxysmal hemicrania
Short-lasting unilateral neuralgiform headache with conjunctival injection and tearing
Primary stabbing headache
Primary cough headache
Primary exertional headache
Occipital neuralgia
Neck–tongue syndrome
Cold-stimulus headache ("brain-freeze")

---

range of conditions. It was criticized for a lack of specificity and sensitivity for children's headaches, which prompted some amendments concerning childhood migraine being made in the second edition (ICHD-II).[1] Hershey has proposed further modifications to this classification to aid the diagnosis of pediatric migraine without aura (see below).[2]

Between a third and a half of children have a significant headache by the age of 7 years. Over three-quarters will have one by the age of 15.[3] In a study of Turkish adolescents between 12 and 17, the prevalence of recurrent headaches increased from 42% at the younger end of the spectrum to 61% at the older end; 26% of children had tension headaches and 14.5% had migraine.[4] Other studies have found the prevalence of migraines to be between 2.6% and 6.9% with 50% more girls than boys suffering from this condition.[5-8]

When is a headache worrying?

Young children are poor historians. A new pain for a 4- or 5-year-old can be very difficult to describe. Parents may offer explanations for perceived discomfort, which their child then adopts. Any odd sensations that a child has never experienced before can "become" a "headache" or "pain." A child may copy their parent who may be holding their head regularly out of worry rather than pain, which may then lead to an unsafe diagnosis of headache in a child.

Young children (2 to 4 years old) find describing pain difficult, but they are usually honest and do not suffer from "functional" headache ("medically unexplained symptoms"). A child in this age group who is holding their head in obvious discomfort must be taken seriously. For instance, monocytic acute myeloid leukemia can present with central nervous system disease, which can be associated with severe head pain.

Children under the age of 6 years usually require sedation or general anesthesia for MRI or CT scanning. This organizational hurdle unfortunately can dissuade a physician from neuroimaging even the worrying child. A Korean study looked at 1562 new patients presenting with recurrent headaches to nine pediatric neurology clinics in tertiary hospitals. Seventy-seven percent of these children had brain imaging, but only 9.3% had abnormal findings on the scans. If there were abnormal neurologic exam findings, 50% of the scans identified an organic condition.[9] Lewis et al. developed a practice parameter for evaluating children and adolescents with recurrent headaches,[3] which has been adapted and expanded in Box 108.2.

Box 108.2

Worrying presentations of pediatric headache (after Lewis 2002[3])

Reduced vision

Seizures (focal or generalized)

Focal neurological signs, e.g. cranial nerve palsy

Alteration of consciousness

Papilledema

Systemic evidence of raised intracranial pressure

Change or deterioration of personality/behavior

Reduced growth rate

Diabetes insipidus

Age under 4 (especially with increasing head circumference)

Headaches that are always unilateral (rare in pediatric migraine)

Headaches that last several days and/or do not improve with treatment

Headaches that wake from sleep, are early morning, and associated with, or relieved by, vomiting

Headaches associated with coughing, straining, or changing position (ask about number of pillows used)

Box 108.3

Proposed criteria for pediatric migraine without aura[1,2]

Diagnostic criteria:

A. At least 5 attacks fulfilling criteria B through D

B. Headache attacks lasting 1 to 72 hours (untreated or unsuccessfully treated)

   Sleep is also considered part of the headache duration

C. Headache has at least two of the following characteristics:

   Bifrontal/bitemporal or unilateral location

   Pulsating/throbbing quality (which may need inferring from their behavior)

   Moderate or severe pain intensity (or a numerical or "faces" scale)

   Aggravation by or causing avoidance of routine physical activity

D. During headache at least one of the following:

   Nausea and/or vomiting

   Two of five symptoms (photophobia, phonophobia, difficulty thinking, light-headedness, or fatigue)

E. Not attributed to another disorder

Chronic daily headaches

These children typically suffer continuous diurnal headaches for more than 15 days per month. This may well be on the migraine spectrum as children have often previously had episodic migraine headaches. CDH can develop from episodic tension-type headaches. There can be a precipitating illness or associated stress (changing schools, parental break-up, etc.). Idiopathic intracranial hypertension (IIH) can rarely present without papilledema and can present in a similar way to CDH.[10] CDH appears to have migraine features although they do not reach the diagnostic criteria in ICHD-II.[11]

The progression to daily headaches can be related to medication overuse or concurrent psychologic problems. Primary school children often have regular drinks provided during the day, whereas secondary school adolescents rarely drink sufficient water. Mild dehydration can exacerbate headaches.

Over time, the frequency of headaches improves resulting in a return to episodic migraines or tension-related headaches.[12] Treatment requires a multi-disciplinary approach involving careful use of medication (avoiding overuse) and preventative and bio-behavioral therapies.[11]

Tension-type headaches

These can last from 30 minutes up to 7 days. They are not associated with nausea or vomiting and may be associated with photophobia or phonophobia, but not both. They may be infrequent (less than one per month), frequent (more than one, but less than 15 per month), or chronic (more than 15 per month). Children describe these headaches as pressing rather than pulsating. 50% of children with tension headache manifested teeth-grinding (bruxism) compared to 2.4% of children with non-tension headache.[13] Bio-behavioral strategies using relaxation techniques and coping skills are a better treatment than medical management with amitriptyline.

Cluster headache and paroxysmal hemicrania

Cluster headaches (CHs) are rare in children but significant as they can cause unilateral supra-orbital or retro-orbital pain lasting from 15 minutes to a couple of hours. They can be associated with eyelid edema, conjunctival injection, excess lacrimation, miosis, and ptosis. Paroxysmal hemicrania (PH) has many of the same autonomic symptoms as CH, but has more frequent attacks and a shorter duration of headache. PH differs from CH in that it is exquisitely sensitive to indomethacin.

Migraine

An adult with classic migraine has a visual aura followed by unilateral headache associated with often-severe systemic symptoms. Childhood migraine often presents differently. Headaches are usually bilateral although they may start unilaterally. In one study,[14] 20% had a unilateral onset with 27% complaining of eye pain, 66% frontal pain, and 12% temporal pain. Younger children find the descriptors used in adult migraine ("pounding", "pressing," "vice-like") difficult to relate to and will often agree with the questioner rather than understanding what is being asked. A surrogate marker of migraine severity is how much school is missed. It has been reported that 10% of children with migraines miss 1 day of school in every 2 week period with 1% missing four times that.[14] Using the PEDs QL 4.0, a pediatric quality of life questionnaire, migraines had the same impact on quality of life (in terms of emotional and school development) as rheumatologic, oncologic, and cardiac diseases.[15]

For an adult headache to be classified as a migraine it should last more than 4 hours. Migraine headaches in children often last less than 4 hours, in some cases only 30 minutes. This is one of the principal reasons that there have been proposals made to alter the ICHD-II (see Box 108.3).

A predromal aura of a scintillating scotomata or other sensory or motor symptoms occurs in only a third of pediatric migraine sufferers.[16] These usually occur 20–40 minutes before the headache starts. The typical expanding "C" fortification spectrum of adulthood is rarely reported by children. Facial pallor is, however, commonly described before or during the headache.

Children may not describe classic autonomic symptoms (nausea or vomiting). Migraine is, however, a common cause of syncope in children. Non-specific symptoms may precede the headache. These include light-headedness, irritability, malaise, and hyperactivity.

Precipitating factors include stress, poor sleep, poor or irregular diet, hot weather, menstruation, and significant exercise. Children who are obese, unfit, or cigarette smokers have a higher prevalence of headaches.[17] Obese migraine sufferers who reduce their BMI can reduce their headache frequency. Migraines are more common in children or adolescents taking adrenergic agonists (for ADHD or asthma) or oral contraceptives.

Whilst headaches are the main feature of childhood migraine, there are a number of periodic syndromes that are precursors. These include cyclical vomiting syndrome, abdominal migraine, and benign paroxysmal vertigo (BPV) of childhood. Seventy percent of children with recurrent abdominal pain and cyclical vomiting will have migraine headaches. Only 10% of BPV will be associated with this.[18] Children with migraine often have a history of travel sickness.

To make the diagnosis of migraine, the ICHD-II classification dictates that there should be at least five attacks. However, waiting for all five to occur may delay treatment.

Childhood migraine can be subdivided into migraine with and without aura. The diagnostic criteria for migraine without aura are in Table 108.1. If there are more than 15 migrainous days per month, the diagnosis of chronic migraine is used.

Migraine with an aura requires one or more fully reversible aura symptom(s) indicating focal cerebral or brainstem dysfunction. Auras do not last more than 60 minutes. This may include visual, aural, or speech symptoms followed by headache. Whilst aura without headaches is common in adults, this is very rare in children and should raise concerns of an organic lesion. Rarely, the aura may cause transient (and occasionally permanent) neurologic loss. This is called complicated migraine. Table 108.1 compares migraines in adults and children.

Basilar-type and hemiplegic migraine and "Alice in Wonderland" syndrome are variants of migraine with an aura.

Basilar-type migraine is the most common variant causing symptoms including vertigo (73%), nausea or vomiting (30–50%), ataxia (43–50%), visual field defects (43%), and diplopia caused by cranial nerve palsies (30%).[19] It is most common in adolescent girls, but can present in children as young as 12 to 18 months with episodic pallor, clumsiness, and vomiting.

Hemiplegic migraine occurs both sporadically and as an inherited autosomal dominant trait. Familial patients may develop serious complications such as disproportionate cerebral dysfunction following minor head trauma.[20]

Children with "Alice in Wonderland" syndrome describe bizarre visual illusions and spatial distortions preceding an otherwise nondescript headache. They rarely seem frightened and describe what they have seen enthusiastically rather than fearfully.

"Ophthalmoplegic migraine" is a demyelinating-remyelinating phenomenon and should not be considered a migraine variant.

Etiology and genetics of migraine

Patients with migraine with aura have a higher prevalence of patent foramen ovale. This abnormality may contribute to pathogenesis.[21] The prevalence of mitral valve prolapse is significantly higher in migraine with aura compared to idiopathic headaches.[22] Disrupted sleep with reduced rapid eye movements and slow-wave sleep is associated with severe and chronic migraines.[13]

Current knowledge about the pathophysiology and genetics of migraine comes from studies of a monogenic subgroup of migraine with aura called familial hemiplegic migraine (FHM). Three FHM genes have been identified that code for ion transporters suggesting that disturbances in ion and neurotransmitter balance could be the cause of not only FHM but other more common migraine variants.[23] It is well-accepted that the migraine aura is not caused by reactive vasoconstriction but is neurally driven. It is the equivalent of cortical spreading depression (CSD). CSD is a short-lasting, slowly spreading wave of neuronal and glial cell depolarization which involves massive fluxes of key ions – Ca^{2+}, Na^+, and K^+. This wave of depolarization is followed by a long-lasting (around 20 minutes) inhibition of spontaneous and evoked neuronal

Table 108.1 – Differences between adult and childhood migraine

Feature	Childhood	Adult
Laterality	Bilateral (but may start unilaterally)	Unilateral
Expanding "C" fortification spectrum	Rare	Common
Duration of headache	Often 30 minutes to 2 hours	Usually >4 hours
Systemic symptoms	Variable but often few	Common
Positive family history	Common	Common
Non-visual aura	Common	Infrequent
Visual aura without headache	Very rare	Common
Triggered by certain foods	Very rare	Infrequent

activity (the "depression"). Mutations in FHM genes have not yet been identified. It is likely that migraineurs have a hyper-excitable cerebral cortex, which may have a genetic basis and leads to a lower threshold for internal or external triggers to cause episodes of initial excitation followed by neuronal inhibition. The pain of migraine may have its origin in inflammation of meningeal vessels and "sensitization" of peripheral and central trigeminal afferents.

Management of pediatric migraine

The treatment of migraine can be considered under the following three headings: bio-behavioral strategies, acute therapies, and preventative therapies.

Bio-behavioral strategies

Children suffer less from migraines if they sleep well and eat healthy food regularly. Regular exercise also helps, as does losing weight. Dietary triggers are less common in children but, once identified, should be avoided. Caffeine may cause migraines and may increase their effects by disrupting sleep and aggravating mood. Children who are given over-the-counter medications too frequently may benefit from a gradual reduction in their use. Stress therapy and relaxation techniques are as effective as propranolol in reducing the frequency of migraines.

Acute therapies

Acute treatments (taken within 30 minutes of the onset of the migraine) remain the mainstay of treatment. There are data for the safety and efficaciousness of ibuprofen 10 mg/kg/dose and acetaminophen (paracetamol) 10–15 mg/kg/dose in reducing headache severity. Nasal sumatriptan (20 mg) reduces the severity of the headache, photophobia, and phonophobia. Bad taste is the most common problem with this medication. The use of pretreatment confectionary and aiming the spray upwards into the nose can improve compliance. Oral almotriptan maleate (25 mg) is the first triptan approved for use in adolescents 12–17 years old (Table 108.2).[24] Triptans should not be used for hemiplegic migraine or where there is hypertension or cardiac disease.

Preventative therapies

If a child or adolescent suffers more than three migraines per month, or if acute measures are ineffective, preventative

measures should be considered. A minimum of 6 to 12 weeks is necessary to assess efficacy. Propranolol is consistently effective. It is contraindicated where there is a history of asthma or diabetes. Sleep disturbances related to its use can worsen the life of a migraineur. Antidepressants are the mainstay of migraine prevention in children and adolescents (see Table 108.2). Amitriptyline has a positive effect in up to 89% of subjects. It is best started as a bedtime dose of 5–10 mg increasing slowly over a 6-week period to between 25 and 50 mg (1 mg/kg/day).[19] Divalproex sodium, topiramate, sodium valproate, gabapentin, and levetiracetam (antiepileptic agents) show promise in preventing migraines in children. The calcium channel blocker Flunarizine has been described as "probably effective" for preventative therapy by the American Academy of Neurology, but is not available in the United States.

Secondary headaches

Children with headaches around or behind the eyes are often referred to pediatric ophthalmologists to "rule out anything serious." Headaches in children are infrequently due to ophthalmic problems, even those centered around the orbits. Headaches can be caused by refractive errors and convergence insufficiency. Glaucoma, dry eyes, and optic neuritis can present as "headaches."

Dental malocclusion, tooth problems, temporomandibular joint disease, and bruxism can present as headaches as can referred pain from previous neck trauma.

There are also important secondary intracranial causes for headaches (Box 108.4).

Epilepsy

Preictal headaches

Up to 20% of adolescents with epilepsy have moderately severe, throbbing headaches in the 24 hours before a secondary generalized tonic–clonic seizure. These can last around 8 hours. Treatment of the seizure usually treats the headache.[25]

Table 108.2 – Medical treatment for migraine in children

Under 10	10 and over
Acute treatment	
Ibuprofen 7.5–10 mg/kg po	Ibuprofen 400 mg po
Acetaminophen 15 mg/kg po	Acetaminophen 375–1000 mg po
	Sumatriptan nasal spray 20 mg
	Almotriptan 25 mg po
Preventative treatment	
Amitriptyline 5–10 mg nocte	Amitriptyline 5–10 mg nocte (up to 1 mg/kg)
Topiramate (1–10 mg/kg po nocte)	Topiramate (1–10 mg/kg po bid)
	Valproate 250–500 mg po nocte

Box 108.4

Secondary intracranial causes for headache in children

Epilepsy (pre-, per- and postictal)
Raised intracranial pressure and idiopathic intracranial hypertension
Brain tumors
Infections
    Acute viral illness
    Meningitis
    Encephalitis
Structural brain abnormalities
    Arachnoid cyst
    Arnold-Chiari malformation
Vascular abnormalities
    Intracranial hemorrhage and arteriovenous malformations
    Cerebral venous sinus thrombosis
    Vasculitis
Acute disseminated encephalomyelitis and multiple sclerosis
Trauma

Postictal headaches

Up to 70% of children with complex partial seizures will complain of postseizure headache. These headaches can mimic migraine and respond well to triptan therapy.[25]

Raised intracranial pressure and idiopathic intracranial hypertension

Raised intracranial pressure (ICP) can cause progressive headaches that may wake a child from sleep and are made worse by Valsalva's maneuver or exertion. Associated findings are nausea and vomiting, lethargy, and personality defects.

Intracranial hypertension (IIH) (see Chapter 56) is elevated ICP without an underlying organic cause such as a space-occupying lesion or hydrocephalus. Headaches are usually daily and associated with nausea and vomiting. Children may complain of transient visual obscurations, tinnitus, paresthesia, ataxia, and arthralgia. Young children are often irritable or apathetic and sleepy. They complain of neck stiffness and dizziness and often demonstrate a change of personality. IIH can be associated with inflammatory conditions such as sarcoidosis and Behçet's disease and metabolic disorders such as cystinosis. IIH is more common in adolescents than in younger children. Girls are more likely to be affected than boys.

Brain tumor

This is the diagnosis parents (and children to a lesser extent) worry about. It is important to reassure them that headaches in children are common and brain tumors are rare (around 5 per 100 000 person years).

Headaches that awake the child from sleep, cause confusion and vomiting, are of recent onset, and exist in patients with no family or personal history of migraine-like symptoms are worrisome. Migraines and other benign headaches uncommonly cause occipital headaches or ones made worse by straining, so these should also be warning symptoms. A significant number of pediatric brain tumors affect midline structures (pinealomas, craniopharyngiomas, cerebellar tumors, and ependymomas) and the examination may not reveal any neurologic disorders. Intrasellar tumors, such as craniopharyngiomas, commonly present with headache due to stretching the dural plate.

Infections

An acute viral illness is the most common reason that a child will present with a headache to an emergency department. True "sinus" headache in children is rare. The dull periorbital, pressure-like pain, associated with nasal congestion, that adults complain of, rarely gets better when "sinusitis" is treated in children. It is usually an atypical form of one of the primary headaches discussed above. Meningitis and encephalitis account for 5% of children with an acute headache.

Structural abnormalities

Arachnoid cysts are usually diagnosed incidentally on an imaging study. They are collections of cerebrospinal fluid (CSF) contained in a sac of arachnoid membranes that can be congenital or secondary to trauma (Fig. 108.1). Cysts become symptomatic with mild to moderate headaches in around 40%. Other features include seizures, weakness, vision loss,

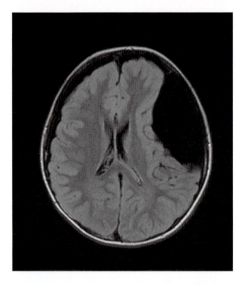

Fig. 108.1 Arachnoid cyst. (Photo courtesy: Dr Atul Tyagi.)

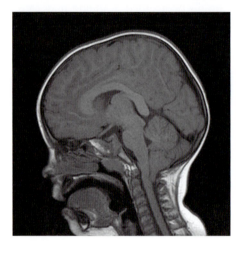

Fig. 108.2 Chiari 1 malformation. (Photo courtesy: Dr Atul Tyagi.)

hydrocephalus, and scoliosis. Surgical treatment can include fenestration or shunt insertion.[25]

A Chiari 1 malformation is the herniation of cerebellar tonsils more than 5 mm below the foramen magnum (Fig. 108.2). Symptoms include headaches (sometimes occipital which worsen with straining or coughing), sensory disturbance, neck pain, vertigo, and ataxia. Only 70% of patients will be symptomatic.[26] Surgical enlargement of the posterior fossa is often successful but needs careful consideration.

Vascular abnormalities

Pediatric hemorrhagic strokes are rare (around 1 per 100 000 per year).[26] Three-quarters of sufferers will complain of headaches and around 50% will have a pre-existing arteriovenous malformation. Around 20% will have an aneurysm.

Cerebral venous sinus thrombosis occurs at the same frequency as hemorrhagic strokes in children. Headache is less common (around 20%). Patients present with seizures, coma, and motor weakness.

Summary

A careful history and thorough ophthalmic and systemic neurologic examination can usually prevent unnecessary investigations in children with headaches. There are symptoms and signs that can identify the patient with serious pathology. An understanding of the presentation, management, and treatment of primary headaches will help the pediatric ophthalmologist.[27-30]

References

1. Headache Classification Subcommittee of the International Headache Society. The International Classification of Headache Disorders. Cephalalgia 2004; 24(Suppl 1): 1–160.

2. Hershey AD, Winner P, Kabbouche MA, et al. Use of the ICHD-II criteria in the diagnosis of pediatric migraine. Headache 2005; 45: 1288–97.

3. Lewis DW, Ashwal S, Dahl G, et al. Practice parameter: evaluation of children and adolescents with recurrent headaches: Report of the Quality Standards Subcommittee of the American Academy of Neurology and the Practice Committee of the Child Neurology Society. Neurology 2002; 59: 490–8.

4. Karli N, Akis N, Zarifoglu M, et al. Headache prevalence in adolescents aged 12 to 17: a student-based epidemiological study in Bursa. Headache 2006; 46: 649–55.

5. Fendrich K, Vennemann M, Pfaffenrath V, et al. Headache prevalence among adolescents: the German DMKG headache survey. Cephalalgia 2007; 27: 347–54.

6. Winner P, Diamond S, Reed ML, et al. Migraine prevalence, disability and prevention need in a community sample of adolescents: results from the American Migraine and Prevalence and Prevention (AMPP) study. Presented at the 48th Annual Scientific Meeting of the American Headache Society, Los Angeles, CA, June 22–25, 2006.

7. Diamond S, Bigal ME, Silberstein S, et al. Patterns of diagnosis and acute and preventive treatment for migraine in the United States: results from the AMPP study. Headache 2007; 47: 355–63.

8. Silberstein S, Loder E, Diamond S, et al. Probable migraine in the United States: results of the AMPP study. Cephalalgia 2007; 27: 220–34.

9. Rho Y-I, Chung HJ, Suh E-S, et al. The role of neuroimaging in children and adolescents with recurrent headaches: multicenter study. Headache 2011; 51: 403–8.

10. Beri S, Gosalakkal JA, Hussain N, et al. Idiopathic intracranial hypertension without papilledema. Pediatr Neurol 2010; 42: 56–8.

11. Hershey AD, Kabbouche MA, Powers SW. Chronic daily headaches in children. Curr Pain Headache Rep 2006; 10: 370–6.

12. Wang SJ, Fuh JL, Lu SR. Chronic daily headaches in adolescents: an 8-year follow-up study. Neurology 2009; 73: 416–22.

13. Vendrame M, Kaleyias J, Valencia I, et al. Polysomnographic findings in children with headaches. Pediatr Neurol 2008; 39: 6–11.

14. Stang PE, Osterhaus JT. Impact of migraine in the United States: data from the National Health Interview Survey. Headache 1993; 33: 29–35.

15. Powers SW, Patton SR, Hommel KA, et al. Quality of life in pediatric migraine: characterization of age-related effects using PedsQL 4.0. Cephalalgia 2004; 24: 120–7.

16. Mortimer MJ, Kay J, Jaron A. Epidemiology of headache and childhood migraine in an urban practice using Ad Hoc, Vahlquist and HIS criteria. Dev Med Child Neurol 1992; 34: 1095–101.

17. Robberstad L, Dyb G, Hagen K, et al. An unfavourable lifestyle and recurrent headaches among adolescents: the HUNT study. Neurology 2010; 75: 712–17.

18. Al-Twaijri WA, Shevell MI. Pediatric migraine equivalents: occurrence and clinical features in practice. Pediatr Neurol 2002; 26: 365–8.

19. Lewis DW. Headaches in children and adolescents. Curr Probl Pediatr Adolesc Health Care 2007; 37: 207–46.

20. Curtain RP, Smith RL, Ovcaric M, et al. Minor head trauma-induced sporadic hemiplegic migraine coma. Pediatr Neurol 2006; 34: 329–32.

21. McCandless RT, Arrington CB, Nielsen DC, et al. Patent foramen ovale in children with migraine headaches. J Pediatr 2011; doi:10.1016/j.peds 2011.01.062.

22. Termine C, Trotti R, Ondei P, et al. Mitral valve prolapse and abnormalities of haemostasis in children and adolescents with migraine with aura and other idiopathic headaches: a pilot study. Acta Neurol Scand 2010; 122: 91–6.

23. de Vries B, Frants RR, Ferrari MD, et al. Molecular genetics of migraine. Hum Genet 2009; 126: 115–32.

24. Linder SL, Mathew NT, Cady RK, et al. Efficacy and tolerability of almotriptan in adolescents: a randomised, double-blind, placebo-controlled trial. Headache 2008; 48: 1326–36.

25. Ahad R, Kossoff EH. Secondary intracranial causes for headaches in children. Curr Pain Headache Rep 2008; 12: 373–8.

26. Blume HK, Szperka CL. Secondary causes of headache in children: when it isn't a migraine. Pediatr Ann 2010; 39: 431–9.

27. Lewis DW, Gozzo YF, Avner MT. The "other" primary headaches in children and adolescents. Pediatr Neurol 2005; 33: 301–13.

28. Fenstermacher N, Levin M, Ward T. Pharmacological prevention of migraine. BMJ 2011; 342: 540–3.

29. Kandt RS, Johnston M. Childhood migraine. On-line summary article last updated Jan 2011. http://www.medlink.com/cip.asp?UID=mlt0007c&src=Search&ref=31157496.

30. Winner PW, Silberstein SD. Headache in children: overview and treatment approaches. On-line summary article March 2010. http://www.medlink.com/cip.asp?UID=mlt002pb&src=Search&ref=31157496.

SECTION 7
Common practical problems in
a pediatric ophthalmology
and strabismus practice

CHAPTER **109**

My little girl tells me she sees strange things

Göran D Hildebrand

Introduction

Unusual visual experiences are not rare in children, but are often difficult to interpret due to the difficulty for the child to express the peculiar sensation. Most complaints will be of a benign and usually transient nature requiring only reassurance. However, a visual complaint may have a more significant meaning, signifying a serious underlying disorder. It is important to take the child's and parents' complaint at face value and to approach its evaluation systematically.

I have made a short mnemonic which I find helpful when dealing with such cases. "OSCE" stands for:

1. **O**-ptical (refractive, optic media).
2. **S**-ensory (visual pathway).
3. **C**-erebral (neurologic, psychologic/functional, psychiatric.
4. **E**-fferent (motor, e.g. nystagmus, superior oblique neuromyokymia, or accommodation spasm) causes.

This should ensure the approach to the evaluation of the problem is complete (Table 109.1). This can usually be achieved by appropriate history taking followed by a clinical examination, but may require ancillary investigations and referral to other specialists (Box 109.1). It has to be remembered that not all cases have a definitive diagnosis made (Fig. 109.1) and that even apparently bizarre symptoms can arise from organic disease (Fig. 109.2).

Typical peculiar visual complaints are broken up into individual visual symptoms and presented from common to rare. There are excellent reviews of this subject.[1-8]

Table 109.1 – Systematic approach to children who complain of seeing peculiar things

Systematic approach (mnemonic "OSCE")	
O-ptical	Refractive Optic media (red reflex)
S-ensory (visual pathway)	Anterior segment Posterior segment Optic nerve, chiasma, optic tract, visual cortex
C-erebral	Neurologic Psychologic/functional psychiatric
E-fferent (motor)	Extraocular movement exam (nystagmus, superior oblique myokymia) Lid movements (myokymia) Accommodation (loss/spasm)

Box 109.1

Overview of diagnostic management

History

Sensory assessment
  Visual acuity
  Color vision
  RAPD
  Amsler grid
  Visual field test (confrontation if young)

Optical media and refraction
  Red reflex/Brückner test
  Refraction

Ocular exam
  Examination of anterior segment
  Examination of posterior segment

Motor
  Hirschberg corneal reflex
  Cover and alternating cover test
  Extraocular movements (pursuit, saccades, convergence)
  Accommodation

Investigations
  Corneal topography (in keratoconus)
  Ocular imaging (OCT, AF, FFA, ultrasound)
  Neuroimaging (MRI, CT)
  Electrodiagnostic, electroencephalogram testing
  Referral (pediatrician, neurologist, psychologist)

RAPD, relative afferent pupillary defect; OCT, optical coherence tomography; AF, autofluorescence; FFA, fluorescein angiography; MRI, magnetic resonance imaging; CT, computed tomography.
See also Chapters 7, 8 and 9.

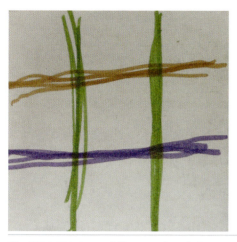

Fig. 109.1 This 9-year-old boy complained of constantly seeing a color grid in front of both eyes. Five months later, the color grid in one eye persisted, but changed to constant black and white vision in the other eye. He has no history of seizures or systemic illness or trauma. He is a well adjusted boy who likes school. All his investigations, including his ocular and pediatric examination, objective pupillary testing, his MRI brain, and electrodiagnostic testing (ERG, VEP, and EEG), have remained normal.

Entoptic phenomena

Entoptic phenomena are visual perceptions from sources within the eye rather than the outside world. Most are harmless curiosities which are usually not perceived or ignored, but may be noticed by a bright young child. They are noticed under special viewing or light conditions. Most people will have experienced some of them at some point in their life. Clinicians use them to assess the presence of gross retinal and optic nerve visual function when no direct fundal view is possible due to dense medial opacities. On the other hand, children with very poor sight will often rub and poke their eyes to stimulate entoptic phenomena (oculodigital sign; see Chapter 59).

Scheerer's (or blue field entoptic) phenomenon consists of seeing tiny bright spots that rapidly move in squiggly lines, especially when looking into the bright clear blue sky or an open field of snow. They are due to the movements of white cells in the capillaries near the macula. Blue field entoptoscopy has been used to measure retinal capillary flow.

Most children with normal vision will notice *Purkinje's trees* which are images of the own retinal circulation. This is best seen when a bright light is shone through the closed eye lids, resulting in the retinal vessels casting a shadow on the unadapted, underlying photoreceptors.

Other harmless entoptic phenomena include *Purkinje's blue arcs, Haidinger's brushes, light diffraction through eye lashes,* as well as *floaters, photopsia,* and *phosphenes.*

Photopsia and phosphenes

Phosphenes and photopsia are brief entoptic phenomena. Phosphenes can be induced by mechanical (eye rubbing, sneezing), electrical, and magnetic stimulation of the retina and visual cortex as well as by the spontaneous firing of retinal cells. *Pressure phosphenes* consist of seeing colors and lights with eye rubbing. *Flick phosphenes* are flashes of light that are seen

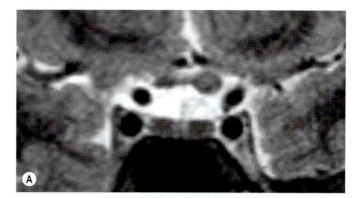

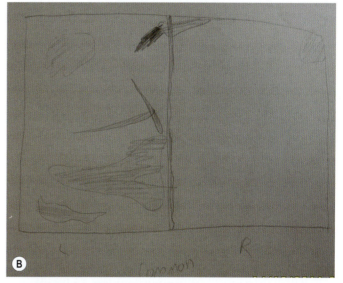

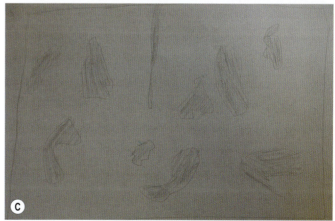

Fig. 109.2 A 14-year-old boy with known neurofibromatosis type 1 and a known glioma of the left optic nerve and chiasm (A) was complaining of seeing intermittently patches in his left and sometimes also in both eyes (B,C).

during eye movements, especially when the retina is dark-adapted and the lids are closed. *Accommodative phosphenes of Czermak* occur with sustained accommodative effort and may be due to ciliary muscle traction on the peripheral retina.

Photopsia and phosphenes may also be pathologic and associated with a number of important pathologies of the retina (retinal traction, tear, detachments, retinal inflammation, outer retinal disease), the optic nerve (optic neuritis, papilledema), or the brain (typically migraine). In the anterior segment, irritating reflections, glare, and dysphopsia may be caused by corneal pathology, cataracts, the edge effect of a dislocated or scratched intraocular lens, or posterior capsular opacification. Only a thorough ocular examination, especially of the peripheral retina, can exclude potentially sight-threatening pathology.

Floaters (myodesopsia, mouches volantes)

At birth, the tertiary vitreous is perfectly transparent. *Myodesopsia* is the perception of a floater and is caused by the development of imperfections or deposits within the vitreous body that cast a moving shadow on the retina. Floaters have been likened to "flying flies" (synonyms *mouches volantes* in French or *muscae volitantes* in Latin). The floater is most noticeable against a uniform, bright background and when it comes closest to the retina. Unlike a scotoma which is fixed in space, a floater comes and goes and moves position from second to second.

Most floaters are entirely harmless, albeit annoying, and require reassurance only. These are due to normal degenerative changes in the vitreous (vitreous syneresis, uncomplicated posterior vitreous detachment, Weiss ring) and are a ubiquitous visual complaint with growing age, affecting myopes earlier than emmetropes. Occasionally, asteroid hyalosis, synchysis scintillans, or a persistent primary vitreous remnant of the hyaloid artery in Cloquet's canal is causative and is of no further consequence.

However, new floaters may point to a more concerning condition, especially if associated with photopsia, a sudden shower of black spots, a shadow, or reduced vision. This always warrants an ophthalmologic examination to exclude a retinal tear, retinal detachment, vitreous hemorrhage, or uveitis.

A visual sensation similar to a vitreal floater may be seen with precorneal tear film abnormalities (dry eye, meibomian gland dysfunction, foreign body), but can easily be differentiated from these by the clearing effect of blinking, the associated external symptoms of ocular irritation, and by ocular examination.

Benign blurred ("fuzzy") vision

Children will frequently complain of their vision being "fuzzy" or "blurry." The most common cause will be an unrecognized refractive error. Other frequent causes include intermittent or constant strabismus, amblyopia, afterimages following looking at bright light, entoptic phenomena and tear film, and conjunctival or corneal abnormalities (e.g. dry eye, unstable tear film with meibomian gland dysfunction).

Transient loss of vision

Important *non-ischemic* causes of transient visual loss include *migraine* (associated with nausea and headaches and photopsia/teichopsia), *ictal/postictal visual loss* in epilepsy (may be associated with motor, sensory, autonomic signs, or automatisms), *visual obscurations* in papilledema (associated with symptoms of raised intracranial pressure that are worse with postural change and Valsalva maneuvers), *optic neuritis* (associated with discomfort with eye movements and recent infections/

immunizations in children), *Uhthoff's phenomenon* in optic neuropathy (loss of vision associated with rising body temperature, e.g. in a hot shower), *post-traumatic transient cerebral blindness* (associated with occipital lobe injury), *gaze-evoked amaurosis* due to transient compression of the intraorbital optic nerve or ophthalmic artery (associated with eye movements), transient *intraocular pressure* rise, poor diabetic control, *intraocular inflammation*, and *hemorrhages*.

Ischemic causes include hypertensive/hypotensive, cardiac (arrhythmia, septal defects), arterial (dissection, aneurysmal, vasculitis, moyamoya disease, vasospasm), and prothrombotic and rheologic/hematologic (polycythemia, leukemia) disorders and require an urgent pediatric referral.

Movement illusions (oscillopsia and Pulfrich phenomenon)

Visual perception of movements may be motor, sensory, or cerebral in origin. Motor causes are *oscillopsia* due to either *nystagmus*, in which case it tends to be acquired, or *superior oblique myokymia*. In superior oblique myokymia, the oscillopsia is monocular and vertical and/or torsional. The diagnosis is made by making the patient look into the field of action of the superior oblique and looking for brief saccadic movements on ophthalmoscopy. *Eye lid myokymia* are involuntary and usually harmless lid contractions that are differentiated from true oscillopsia by history and examination.

A sensory cause is the *Pulfrich phenomenon*, caused by delayed conduction in optic neuropathy. The stereoscopic effect is a result of the retinal disparity cue caused by the latency disparity between the two optic nerves. This can be tested by swinging a ball in a line perpendicular to the subject from side to side. Instead of seeing the object swing from side to side, an elliptical movement towards and away from the patient is perceived.

Epileptic kinetopsia is an ictal illusory perception of motion seen in temporal lobe epilepsy.

Color (dyschromatopsia)

Loss of color vision is physiologic under scotopic light conditions due to the relative insensitivity of cones compared to rods ("all cats are gray in the dark").[9] Children may describe colorful afterimages after looking at a bright object, which persists for a while, even when closing both eyes. A clear history and a simple explanation will reassure the child and parents.

True *dyschromatopsia* is a disturbance in color vision. Congenital color blindness is the most common cause for dyschromatopsia, deuteranomaly affecting approximately 5–8% of boys, but only 0.4% of girls. Commonly, this is noticed by others rather than the child, for example when observing the child naming or drawing objects' colors incorrectly or during vision screening at school. Acquired dyschromatopsia is common with media changes (e.g. cataract, vitreous hemorrhage), optic nerve disease (e.g. optic neuritis), and, less often, with retinal and macular disease (e.g. retinal and macular dystrophies). *Köllner's rule* pertains to the causes of acquired color vision loss and states that diseases of the outer retina (e.g. in macular disease) typically result in blue–yellow color defects, while disorders of the inner retina, the optic nerve, and beyond tend to cause red–green color loss. Relative bitemporal red desaturation on confrontation is an early clinical indicator of compression of the optic chiasm. Cerebral causes of color loss are rare (cerebral achromatopsia).

Seeing multiples (monocular diplopia, triplopia, and polyopia)

A child may use "seeing double" to simply express visual blur or shadowing around an object rather than true diplopia. A bright child noticing physiologic diplopia in front of or behind a fixation point is not an uncommon cause of referral. Most pathologic diplopia is binocular due to ocular misalignment. In patients with chiasmal disease and strabismus, complete bitemporal field loss can result in the slide phenomenon, diplopia, or central visual field loss. The hallmark of binocular diplopia is that the double vision disappears under monocular cover. True monocular diplopia and polyopia, however, persist under monocular conditions. Most monocular diplopia is due to an abnormality of refraction, the precorneal tear film, corneal pathology, cataract formation, lens dislocation, polycoria, or rarely a retinal cause. Cerebral causes of diplopia and polyopia are very rare and often associated with other defects (e.g. visual field) and are discussed in the section on Visual perseveration.

Size (micropsia, macropsia, teleopsia, lilliputianism)

Objects may appear abnormally large (*macropsia*), far away (*teleopsia*), or small (*micropsia*) (Fig. 109.3). In *lilliputianism*, people appear to be very small. Simple benign global micropsia is an isolated complaint, affecting children mostly at school age. It may be associated with prior reading at night and resolve spontaneously after some months. Micropsia of macular origin is associated with reduced or distorted vision. Cerebral causes include migraine and less frequently epilepsy and infections.

If the micropsia is isolated and present in an otherwise healthy child with no distortion of reality or hallucinations, full visual fields, and normal orthoptic and ocular findings, clinical observation is reasonable. In all other cases or where symptoms do not resolve, investigations (pediatric assessment, infective screen, neuroimaging) are indicated.

Distortion (dysmetropsia, metamorphopsia and "Alice in Wonderland syndrome")

Dysmetropsia and metamorphopsia are related visual illusions where object shapes appear distorted and straight lines bent. Metamorphopsia is best assessed with an Amsler grid. Even relatively young children will be able to say whether the lines are straight or not and report "funny lines." Visual distortions are either optical (common), macular (occasional), or cerebral (rare) in origin: optical causes include high corneal, lenticular or retinal (staphylomatous) astigmatism, high ametropia,

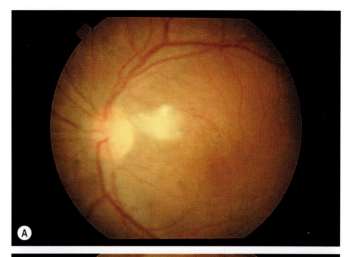

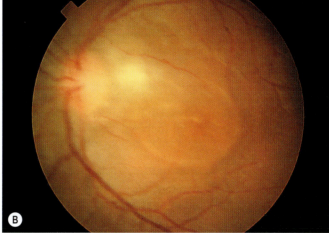

Fig. 109.3 Neuroretinitis with micropsia. This 9-year-old girl complained of dullness of vision in both eyes and smallness of objects with distortion on the left. (A) The white area temporal to the optic disk represents retinal nerve fiber swelling and vascular leakage, extending to the fovea. (B) As the retinal edema increased and extended across the macula, the acuity dropped to 6/36 and the micropsia disappeared.

anisometropia, and new glasses. Macular causes include macular edema and choroidal neovascularization (e.g. associated with myopic Fuchs' maculopathy, inflammatory ocular disease, and macular dystrophies). Rarely visual distortion is of cerebral origin, as in the "Alice in Wonderland syndrome." With a cerebral cause, other associated neurologic symptoms and signs will likely be found.

If the Amsler grid confirms the presence of distortions, management includes refraction, corneal topography (if keratoconus is suspected) and detailed slit-lamp examination of the anterior and posterior segments. Investigations may include optical coherence tomography or fundus fluorescein angiography with macular disease and neuroimaging (MRI) if a cerebral cause is suspected.

Metamorphopsia, micropsia, macropsia, and the Alice in Wonderland syndrome are more common in children than in adults with migraine. Alice in Wonderland syndrome is frequently associated with migraine, but may also be due to epilepsy, drugs/medication (topiramate), varicella infection, or infectious mononucleosis (see Chapter 9).

Bradyopsia

Rarely, children may take excessive time to adapt to changing levels of bright- and darkness and finding it difficult to track moving objects due to a defect in the photoreceptor deactivation mechanism in the phototransduction cascade. In addition to markedly delayed dark and light adaptation, they may also display moderately reduced visual acuity and mild photophobia with normal color vision and normal fundi (see Chapters 44 and 45).

Visual perseveration and other rare cerebral visual disturbances

Palinopsia is the visual perseveration of an image in time (Fig. 109.4). In the immediate type, the image persists for minutes after the true object has disappeared. In the delayed type, the image of a previously seen object reappears, sometimes for days or weeks. The picture is formed and different from afterimages created by retinal overstimulation by prolonged looking at a light, for example. In *cerebral diplopia* or *polyopia*, the visual image persists in space and two or more copies of the same image are seen simultaneously. Unlike binocular diplopia, cerebral diplopia and polyopia is monocular and is differentiated from ocular causes of monocular diplopia and polyopia by refraction followed by examination of the eye to exclude corneal pathology, lens displacement, iris defects (polycoria), or a cataract. In cerebral diplopia/polyopia, each perceived image is equally clear, pinhole viewing has no beneficial effect, and no difference is seen with binocular versus monocular viewing. In *illusory visual spread*, the image expands beyond the real object size. Palinopsia, polyopia, and illusory visual spread will often be seen in the context of other cerebral

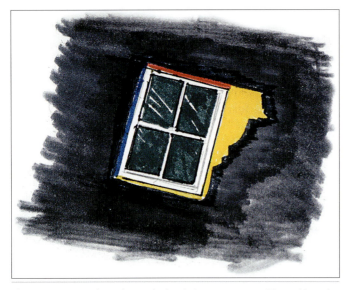

Fig. 109.4 Picture drawn by a right-handed young person with an ultimately fatal metastatic carcinoma in the right parietal lobe. The presenting symptom was the recurrence of an image of the kitchen window that impinged itself involuntarily on the visual environment in different circumstances for several hours after the original stimulus.

disturbances, such as homonymous visual field defects. In *cerebral akinetopsia*, any perception of motion is completely lost due to bilateral cerebral lesions. "*Visual disorientation*" and "*simultanagnosia*" is the ability to interpret individual parts of a picture, but not the totality of the image seen and is part of *Balint's syndrome*.

Visual disturbances associated with migraine

Children with migraine can have a large spectrum of visual disturbances, classically visual hallucinations with enlarging scintillating scotomas and fortification patterns (*teichopsia*) or simple unformed light flashes (*cerebral photopsia*). Visual field loss (e.g. hemianopia) is a well recognized complication. Visual illusions of micropsia, macropsia, metamorphopsia, and Alice in Wonderland syndrome are associated with migraine. Other reported visual disturbances in migraine include palinopsia and polyopsia. Rarely, complex visual hallucinations containing people or animals (*zoopsia*) and out of body experiences may be experienced in which the migraineur views his own body (*autoscopy*). Other rare disturbances are complete achromatopsia (cerebral color loss), prosopagnosia (no recognition of faces), and visual agnosia (no recognition of objects).

Hallucinations

Hallucinations are sensory perceptions generated by the mind *sui generis* in the absence of true external stimulation (Fig 109.5). Illusions are misinterpretations or distortions of existing external stimuli.

Hallucinations in darkness and with social deprivation

Non-formed random noise of tiny lights and dark points are seen with eye closure or in complete darkness (*closed-eye hallucinations and visualizations*). *Eigengrau* (German for "intrinsic gray") or *Eigenlicht* (German for "intrinsic light") is the gray or light seen in perfect darkness as a result of baseline intrinsic retinal electrical activity. The **Ganzfeld effect** describes visual hallucinations caused by prolonged staring into a featureless field of vision or field of color. Prolonged **sensory deprivation** in darkness (e.g. at night or in a dark room) may give rise to hallucinations of formed light of different colors or even human figures.

Charles Bonnet syndrome (visual release phenomenon)

Visual hallucinations may be release phenomena.[10] Visual hallucinations associated with visual loss in a lucid person who realizes that the hallucinations are not real are called Charles Bonnet syndrome. They can occur after simultaneous or sequential, not necessarily complete, bilateral visual loss (Fig 109.6) due to any cause in the visual pathway (e.g. dense

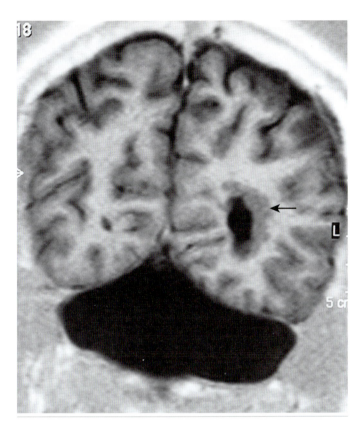

Fig. 109.5 This boy with a Möbius-like syndrome started, at the age of 18, to get unformed hallucinations in the right half of his visual field accompanied by nausea followed by sleepiness, without seizures. The MRI shows an area of dysplastic ectopic gray matter in the left posterior parieto-occipital region (arrow).

cataracts, macular, optic nerve, or cortical disease, after enucleation). The hallucinations are typically vivid, formed, and complex (often people or scenes), filling in the blind scotoma. The hallucinations are strictly visual (e.g. people do not speak in the hallucinations). They represent release visual phenomena caused by the loss of cortical stimulation after visual loss and are potentially reversible (e.g. after successful cataract surgery). Many patients may be understandably very reluctant to admit to these hallucinations. The individual is typically relieved, once reassured of their true nature.

Hypnagogic and hypnopompic hallucinations

Visual hallucinations at sleep onset (hypnagogic) and on awakening (hypnopompic) are normal, but a child with daytime somnolence should be investigated for narcolepsy, if hypnagogic hallucinations are associated with sleep attacks, cataplexy, or sleep paralysis.

Occipital and temporal lobe epilepsy

Another important cause of hallucinations is occipital and temporal lobe epilepsy (rarely parietal lobe). Visual hallucinations tend to be simple (photopsia, white phosphenes, steady colored lights) with occipital and more often complex (e.g. faces, people) with temporal lobe epilepsy. Visual seizures will often be accompanied by other ictal signs, such as focal motor seizures, automatisms (e.g. lip pursing, chewing), and sensory (e.g. olfactory hallucinations) and autonomic changes (e.g. pupillary changes, salivation, urinary incontinence). Occipital lobe epilepsy with visual hallucinations only may be difficult to differentiate from acephalic migraine with visual aura.

Benign childhood epilepsy with occipital epilepsy is an idiopathic epilepsy syndrome in children of school age that ceases spontaneously when they become teenagers. The seizures are associated with simple or complex visual hallucinations (or transient visual loss), may progress to motor or partial complex seizures, and be followed by postictal headaches similar to migraine. EEG is diagnostic and pharmacologic treatment is available.

Peduncular hallucinosis

In this rare syndrome, vivid, colorful, kaleidoscopic images, geometric patterns or elaborate pictures of landscapes, flowers, animals or even human beings are seen. The pathology typically involves the midbrain and may be associated with other signs of midbrain disease as well as sleep and cognitive disturbances.

Drug-induced hallucinations

Visual hallucinations and illusions may be caused by medication (e.g. steroids, lamotrigine, ciclosporin, digoxin, sildenafil (for pulmonary arterial hypertension), ganciclovir, vincristine, lidocaine, itraconazole, lithium, levodopa), its withdrawal (e.g. barbiturates in epileptic children, baclofen), anesthetics (ketamine), eye drops (idiosyncratic response to atropine and cyclopentolate), alcohol as well as hallucinogens (e.g. LSD, phencyclidine (PCP), cocaine, marijuana).

Psychogenic ("functional") visual loss

Psychogenic, or "functional", visual loss is not uncommon in children (estimated incidence of 1.4/1000 per year, girls more common, clustered in immediate prepuberty and puberty teenage years) and should be suspected when an unexplained discrepancy exists between purported subjective visual loss and objective findings (see Chapter 60). It is a diagnosis of exclusion. Some children with an element of psychogenic visual loss will also be found to have an underlying organic disease with time. The manifestations can be diverse and range from purported total loss of vision to relatively unusual visual experiences. Some children clearly are pretending, but most affected teenagers appear genuinely affected. Brodsky has classified these into four groups:

Group 1: the visually preoccupied child.
Group 2: conversion disorder.
Group 3: possible factitious disorder.
Group 4: psychogenic visual loss superimposed on true organic disease.

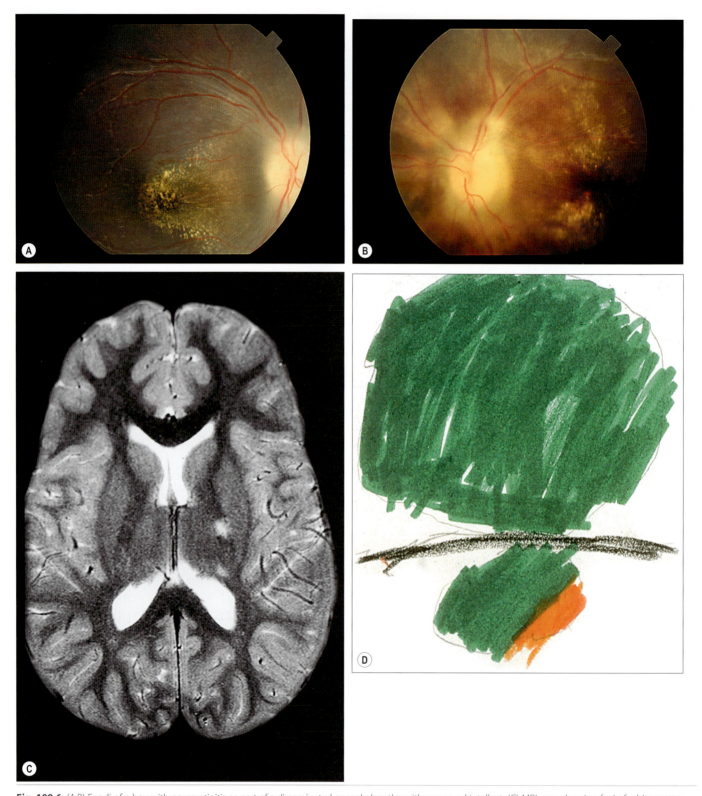

Fig. 109.6 (A,B) Fundi of a boy with neuroretinitis as part of a disseminated encephalopathy with preserved intellect. (C) MRI scan showing foci of white matter inflammation. (D) His vision at this stage, 4 weeks after the onset, was "counting fingers." He later (when his vision had partially recovered) drew the figures that he had seen.

Medical conditions

Visual hallucinations and illusions may be seen in a number of medical conditions, including febrile delirium, encephalitis, and encephalopathy from metabolic disease. Urgent medical referral is required in the management of these cases.

Psychiatric dis ease

Hallucinations, in which all insight in the false nature of the perception is lost, are part of psychosis, a profound thought disorder in which the individual loses the control over his sense of reality. Unreal voices and visions become real. Often frightening visual and acoustic (hearing voices) hallucinations are associated with delusional beliefs, bizarre behavior, and a general decline in self-care as part of this grave thought disorder. Recognizing a teenager with frank psychosis (not infrequently following the consumption of illicit drugs) is usually not challenging. Urgent referral to a psychiatric team is indicated due to the substantial risks of harm to the affected individual and others.

Psychiatric patients can have genuine visual problems as well. One should therefore give the psychiatric patient the benefit of the doubt when complaining of a visual problem, if his complaint is persistent and consistent after his mental state has stabilized. The author recalls being asked to see a young psychiatric inpatient who said that he could neither read well at near nor see people in the distance. His psychiatrist was doubtful of any organic basis to this, but referred him: he had marked keratoconus!

References

1. Zeki S. Vision of the Brain. Oxford: Blackwell Scientific Publications; 1993.
2. Brodsky M. Transient, unexplained, and psychogenic visual loss in children. In: Pediatric Neuro-Ophthalmology, 2nd ed. Heidelberg: Springer; 2010: 213–252.
3. Liu GT, Volpe NJ, Galetta SL. Disorders of higher cortical visual function. In: Neuro-Ophthalmology: Diagnosis and Management, 2nd ed. Philadelphia: Saunders Elsevier; 2010: 339–362.
4. Liu GT, Volpe NJ, Galetta SL. Transient visual loss. In: Neuro-Ophthalmology: Diagnosis and Management, 2nd ed. Philadelphia: Saunders Elsevier; 2010: 363–375.
5. Liu GT, Volpe NJ, Galetta SL. Functional visual loss. In: Neuro-Ophthalmology: Diagnosis and Management, 2nd ed. Philadelphia: Saunders Elsevier; 2010: 377–392.
6. Liu GT, Volpe NJ, Galetta SL. Visual hallucinations and illusions. In: Neuro-Ophthalmology: Diagnosis and Management, 2nd ed. Philadelphia: Saunders Elsevier; 2010: 393–412.
7. Rizzo M, Barton JJS. Retrochiasmal visual pathways and higher cortical function. In: Glaser JS, editor. Neuro-Ophthalmology, 3rd ed. Philadelphia: Lippincott, Williams & Wilkins; 1999: 239–91.
8. Miller NR, Newman NJ, editors. Central disorders of visual function. In: Walsh & Hoyt's Clinical Neuro-Ophthalmology: The Essentials, 5th ed. Philadelphia: Williams & Wilkins; 1999: 369–408.
9. Hildebrand GD, Fielder AR. Anatomy and physiology of the retina. In: Reynolds JD, Olitsky SE, editors. Pediatric Retina. Heidelberg: Springer; 2011: 39–65.
10. Cogan DG. Visual hallucinations as release phenomena. Graefes Arch Klin Exp Ophthalmol 1973; 188: 139–150.

My little boy isn't doing as well as he should at school

Alison Salt

Many children present to the eye clinic because of school difficulties. Parents and teachers quite reasonably ask if a problem with vision could be the explanation for poor school progress. This chapter outlines the problems that may present with school failure and suggests appropriate referral routes.

It is usually children with less severe problems who you are likely to be asked to see. Those with severe learning difficulty are usually identified before they start school, although visual difficulties affecting learning should be detected by routine vision assessment as part of their care. The increased demands of a school curriculum will often bring to light less severe problems.

Schools may take several routes in seeking advice when a child is not reaching expected targets; an educational psychologist may be asked to undertake an assessment of a child's abilities, a pediatrician may be asked to exclude a medical diagnosis, and the child may be referred to an eye clinic or an audiologist to exclude a visual or hearing impairment.

Possible reasons for poor school progress

Global learning difficulty

Learning difficulties affecting all areas of development occur in between 3% and 10% of children. The most common causes are chromosomal anomalies; Down's syndrome and fragile X syndrome are the most common, although they are most likely to present before school age. Mild or moderate learning difficulties may not present until the child starts school; in a majority no cause can be identified. Nevertheless, referral to a pediatrician to consider the possible etiology and appropriate intervention is appropriate.

Specific learning difficulty

Some children whose general cognitive abilities are average have specific problems with learning. However, these specific problems may also present in combination, i.e. more than one difficulty may coexist.

Dyslexia or specific difficulties with reading are described in detail in Chapter 61. These problems frequently lead to referral to the eye clinic so that vision problems can be excluded. The diagnosis will be confirmed by a detailed assessment by an educational psychologist or neuropsychologist and specific educational support will be required.

Developmental coordination disorder (DCD) (or dyspraxia) is a specific problem of motor coordination affecting the coordination of large and fine movements and may lead to difficulty with physical activities, writing, and speech clarity. These children may have difficulty with visual and spatial perception, general organization, and self-help skills, e.g. dressing. They may experience additional emotional and social difficulties. A physiotherapist or an occupational therapist (OT) can provide assessment, advice, and treatment. A psychologist can help in assessing any associated specific cognitive difficulty which may coexist.

Speech and language disorders usually present prior to starting school, but more subtle difficulties of comprehension may not be recognized without detailed assessment. Assessment and support from a speech and language therapist will be necessary and may include a language program delivered as part of the school curriculum. Specific difficulties with literacy are associated with particular speech and language disorders.

Other developmental disorders

Problems with attention and concentration may lead to underachievement and may present with behavior difficulties. The possibility of attention deficit hyperactivity disorder (ADHD) should be considered in these children. The diagnosis is based on early onset and pervasive (occurring in all environments) problems with overactivity, impulsivity, and problems with attention and concentration. The diagnosis requires collection of information about behavior from parents and teachers using standardized questionnaires. Treatment may include medication with methylphenidate or similar psychostimulants, but will also require modification of the environment with reduction in distraction and additional adult support to assist with concentration. Referral to a pediatrician for diagnosis is appropriate.

Problems with concentration may indicate a hearing difficulty. Most severe hearing difficulties will present early with concern about hearing behavior in the young child or speech delay. However, conductive hearing loss is very common in childhood and some of the progressive sensorineural hearing impairments present after the age of routine screening. Hearing assessment should always be considered if a child appears to have problems of attention or concentration in the classroom.

Children may also present with difficulties with peer relationships and social interaction. When these children have problems with the use of language for communication and limited or obsessional interests a diagnosis of autistic spectrum disorder may be considered. If this type of problem is suspected a referral to a pediatrician will be necessary.

Other problems with peers may be secondary to external factors. School failure or reluctance to attend school may result from emotional and social difficulties in school through difficult relationships with peers, e.g. bullying, or a difficult interaction with the teacher. Difficulties at home may also lead to school failure.

Beware of the child who appears to be losing skills. This suggests a degenerative neurological condition. Vision loss may occur in these conditions. Urgent referral to a pediatrician or pediatric neurologist is essential.

Assessment and intervention

Assessment by a pediatrician, psychologist, and other therapists can provide a description of a child's strengths and weaknesses in verbal and non-verbal abilities. A child's learning needs can be identified and appropriate suggestions made for intervention. This may include additional support in the classroom, specific educational interventions, e.g. for reading difficulty, or intervention and advice from other therapists, e.g. a speech and language therapist, occupational therapist or physiotherapist (Fig. 110.1).

The role of the ophthalmologist

The ophthalmologist will need to exclude significant eye disease, refractive error, or ocular motor dysfunction. Subtle visual problems are a rare cause of educational difficulties, but mild refractive errors or problems such as convergence insufficiency play a role.

School difficulty in a child with visual impairment

Children with visual impairment may present with school failure. These children may have additional learning difficulty or they may be experiencing difficulty because educational material is not being sufficiently adapted to meet their visual needs (Box 110.1).

Distance access

For those children with mild visual impairment simply ensuring that they are sitting at the front of the class with

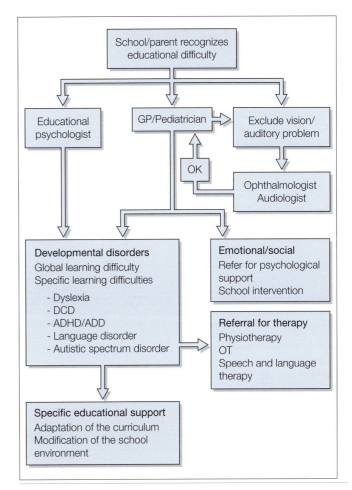

Fig. 110.1 Referral pathways and possible reasons for educational difficulties.

appropriate lighting conditions may be all that is required. In children with moderate to severe visual impairment (worse than 6/18), education material that is usually accessed visually should be provided in a readily accessible format (appropriately enlarged and with suitable contrast).

Children may also experience difficulties in the playground. They may not be able to identify their friends at a distance so that support systems to assist them at playtime need to be put in place. They may have difficulty identifying facial expression and body language at a distance and therefore do not pick up on social cues. School staff should be advised to give additional auditory cues.

Near access

Print size used should be that which is read easily at standard reading distance (approx. 30 cm), not the minimum size seen at very close range. In the early stages of reading it is essential that text is enlarged even beyond that level (as it is for all early readers who have full sight) and that good contrast is ensured. Avoid print overlying pictures thus reducing contrast.

Low vision aids including magnifiers are only useful for accessing small amounts of text and rarely useful for prolonged spells of reading especially in younger children. A sloping desk will help children to come closer to text without adversely affecting the child's posture and the lighting of the text. A

Box 110.1

The child with visual impairment failing in school

1. Exclude additional learning difficulty (see Fig. 110.1)
2. Ensure visual material appropriately adapted
   Distance
      Mild impairment
        – sit close to front of class
      Moderate/severe
        – provide all visual material at near reading distance
        – adapt font size as for near
   Near
      Appropriate enlargement (font size read at approx. 30 cm)
      Sloping desk
      Good contrast of print and background
3. Provide low vision aids
   CCTV
   Hand-held magnifiers
   Other low vision aids
4. Consider alternatives for written work
   Laptop
   Audiotape
   Scribe
5. Lighting
   – sufficient
   – not too bright (in some eye conditions)
6. Social
   Playground assistance
   Use auditory as visual cues may not be seen

CCTV can be useful where small amounts of text are too difficult to enlarge or for maps or pictures.

Lighting conditions in the classroom need to be considered. Some children, e.g. those with albinism and cone dystrophies, will find bright lighting conditions uncomfortable or will actually have reduced vision in these conditions.

The effort involved in reading for children with visual impairment should not be underestimated. Children will often tire towards the end of a school day. If possible, therefore, tasks with high visual demand should be confined to the early part of the school day. Alternative means for producing written work will also be necessary, e.g. access to a laptop or audiotape. A specialist advisory teacher for children with visual impairment should be available to give advice to the class teacher and to monitor progress.

My child's pupils look odd!

Susan M Carden

Neonates may be suspected of having abnormalities of their pupils by parents, nurses, and neonatologists. The possiblity of an associated anomaly or syndrome is often raised. Referrals may be vague because the palpebral fissures of premature infants are small, the infants spent most of their days asleep, and, in some instances, the eyelids are edematous due to prolonged respiratory intubation or treatment with steroids.

Any vagueness of a pupillary description by referring doctors, nurses, or parents should not be dismissed or criticized because it is rarely a finding without foundation. A full eye examination usually reveals the cause and often a portable slit-lamp can be helpful (Fig. 111.1). After careful examination, the pupils should be dilated and fundoscopy performed because associated retinal problems are not infrequent.

The size of the pupils is smallest during infancy, which adds to the difficulty for pediatricians in their assessments, particularly in infants with dark irides. An increase in size begins to occur sometime during the first 6 months of age.[1] It is not until adolescence that the pupils attain their fullest size (see Chapter 6).

Some patients have an intermittent abnormality in the pupil size. Alternating anisocoria has been described.[2] It is not unusual for the pupil abnormality to be absent on the day of examination and hence it is very important to listen carefully to the history given by parents and to encourage them to describe what they have seen.

Box 111.1 gives guidelines on the causes of abnormal pupils in infancy.

Box 111.1

Guidelines on the causes of abnormal pupils in infancy

Abnormal shape

Coloboma (inferonasal)

Atypical coloboma

Polycoria/corectopia

Partial aniridia

Persistent pupillary membrane

Abnormal size

1. Relatively too small

Horner syndrome

Microcornea

Uveitis with posterior synechiae

Drugs (e.g. narcotics)

Severe retinopathy of prematurity (failure of pupils to dilate)

2. Relatively large

Third nerve palsy

Tonic pupil (Adie's)

Drugs

Aniridia/partial aniridia

Coloboma

Trauma – sphincter rupture

Surgical mydriasis for a congenital problem

Abnormal position

Corectopia

Polycoria

Coloboma

Abnormal iris color

Congenital heterochromia

Waardenburg's syndrome[3]

Hirschsprung-associated heterochromia[4]

Postuveitis or severe intraocular congenital defects

Congenital horner's syndrome

Incontinentia pigmenti

Heterochromic cyclitis

Neovascularization/rubeosis

Trauma

Rubella

Other pupil abnormalities observed by parents

Unusual reflection from the pupil (see leukocoria in Table 42.1 in Chapter 42)

Persistent pupillary membrane

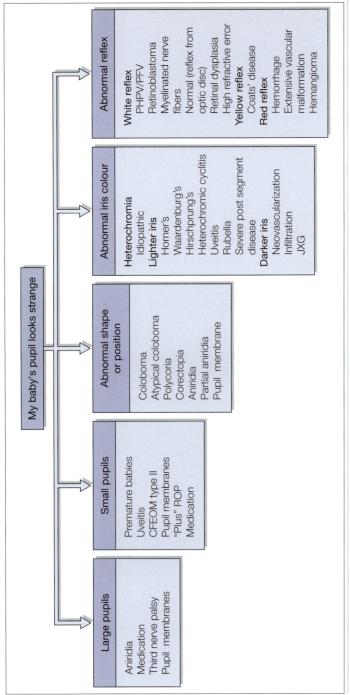

Fig. 111.1

References

1. MacLachlan C, Howland HC. Normal values and standard deviations for pupil diameter and interpupillary distance in subjects aged 1 month to 19 years. Ophthalmic Physiol Opt 2002; 22: 175–82.

2. Brodsky MC, Sharp GB, Fritz KJ, et al. Idiopathic alternating anisocoria. Am J Ophthalmol 1992; 114: 509–10.

3. Mullaney PB, Parsons MA, Weatherhead RG, et al. Clinical and morphological features of Waardenburg syndrome type II. Eye 1998; 12: 353–357.

4. Lai JS, Lan DS, Yeung CK, et al. Bilateral iris sector heterochromia with or without Hirschsprung's disease. Eye 1998; 12: 1024–7.

Unequal pupils

Susan M Carden

When anisocoria is found in a child, a simple step-by-step routine can be followed as outlined in Fig. 112.1. Anisocoria can be thought of as being due to one of four problems:

1. An abnormality of the sympathetic nervous supply to the dilator muscle.
2. An abnormality of the parasympathetic nervous supply to the sphincter.
3. A structural abnormality of the iris (congenital or acquired).
4. Benign or physiologic.

Horner's syndrome

In most cases, concern about possible Horner's syndrome should be foremost. The pupils are unequal with the difference being greatest in the dark: 1–2 mm of upper lid ptosis is expected; the lower lid may also be affected. Heterochromia is variable, but, if present, usually a congenital lesion is causative. The possibility of an associated neuroblastoma or ganglioneuroma should be considered.

Oculomotor palsy

Anisocoria caused by congenital oculomotor palsy is rare and will virtually always be accompanied by some degree of ocular motility disturbance[1,2] (see Chapters 82 and 83). The pupil may be spared or paradoxically miotic in congenital oculomotor palsies and congenital dysinnervation disorders. Adie's pupil is extremely uncommon in the first decade of life except in association with chicken pox infection.

Structural anomalies

Structural anomalies of the iris (see Chapters 32 and 38), especially persistent pupillary membranes, may produce smaller or larger pupils than normal. Congenital idiopoathic microcoria is usually unilateral, often eccentric with a pupil 2 mm or less. The cause is unknown. Congenital pupillary-iris-lens membranes are usually unilateral and cause pupillary distortion, iris adhesions to the lens with rigidity of the pupil, and progressive occlusion of the pupil. This is thought to be due to iridogoniodysgenesis. Acute angle closure glaucoma may occur.

Physiological anisocoria

Physiological anisocoria is common, occurring in at least 20% of normal infants. The asymmetry is rarely more than 1 mm but may vary from time to time. The pupillary asymmetry persists in bright light or the dark.

Pharmacological testing

Pharmacological testing may be helpful, but most cases of anisocoria can be diagnosed clinically by the pupil size variation under different lighting conditions, examination of the iris and anterior chamber, and by neurological accompaniments. In some clinics, it is convenient to use topical apraclonidine 0.5% instead of topical cocaine 4%, 5%, or 10% to diagnose whether there is a sympathetic defect. We do not use apraclonidine in infants due to the occasional prolonged and severe soporific effect.[3]

Slit-lamp examination

Slit-lamp examination is important to detect developmental abnormalities of the pupil and sinuous (uneven) pupillary reactions. Eccentricity of the pupil suggests an underlying structural cause of pupil asymmetry. Hippus (physiologic pupillary unrest of the entire pupil) is present in normal pupils.

Light and near reactions

The pupil reactions to a bright light and to a near stimulus should be noted. A bright light is essential in examining the pupil. Light–near dissociation (better reaction to a near target than a bright light) occurs in Argyll Robertson pupils, the Sylvian aqueduct syndrome, and Adie's pupils. The pupil sizes in the dark and in bright light are recorded and photographed where possible. Examination of family photos is useful.

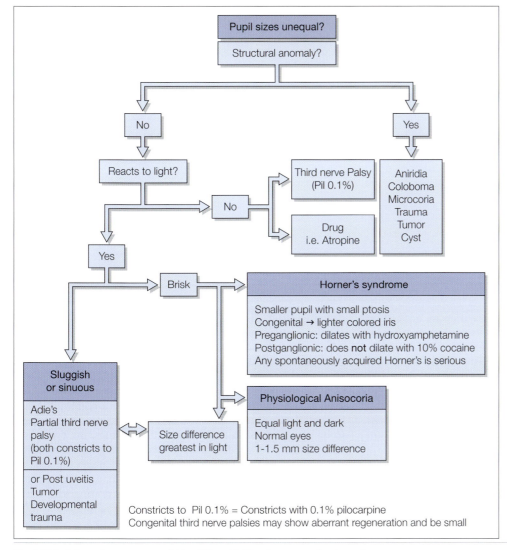

Fig. 112.1 A flow diagram as an aid to differentiating the cause of anisocoria.

Physiological anisocoria is common in minor degrees and is the most common cause of pupillary asymmetry at any age.[4]

Refraction

It may be useful to perform retinoscopy while eliciting a visual response to a near target. A dynamic change in retinoscopy reveals important information about pupillary reaction to accommodation and about visual response per se (accommodation is induced by a sense of a near visual target). Although poor accommodation is common in cerebral palsy and Down's syndrome the pupillary light response to near is unaffected.

When to investigate Horner's syndrome

The overwheming concern when evaluating a child with unequal pupils is whether it is a sign of serious systemic or neurologic disease. This is especially true in the evaluation of pediatric Horner's syndrome where there is concern about the possibility of an associated neuroblastoma.[5] The question arises as to how far such a child should be investigated. Experts are divided, with some arguing in favor of investigations, others preferring repeated testing. We believe that the child should be investigated only if there is any question about its congenital onset, if the child is unwell in any way, or if there are signs of involvement of the superior cervical ganglion such as in anhidrosis.[6]

References

1. Balkan R, Hoyt CS. Associated neurologic abnormalities in congenital third nerve palsies. Am J Ophthalmol 1984; 97: 315–9.
2. Good WV, Barkovich AJ, Nickel BL, Hoyt CS. Bilateral congenital oculomotor nerve palsy in a child with brain anomalies. Am J Ophthalmol 1991; 111: 555–8.
3. Watts P, Satterfield D, Lim MK. Adverse effects of apraclonidine used in the diagnosis of Horner syndrome in infants. J AAPOS 2007; 11: 282–3.
4. Roarty JD, Keltner JL. Normal pupil size and anisocoria in newborn infants. Arch Ophthalmol 1990; 108: 94–5.
5. Musarella MA, Chan HS, DeBoer G, Gallie BL. Ocular involvement in neuroblastoma: prognostic implications. Ophthalmology 1984; 91: 936–40.
6. George ND, Gonzalez G, Hoyt CS. Does Horner's syndrome in infancy require investigation? Br J Ophthalmol 1998; 82: 51–4.

Wobbly eyes in infancy

J Raymond Buncic

Jiggly or wobbly eyes in infant are often first spotted by a family friend or relative, sometimes before they are noticed by the parents. Sometimes what is more noticeable is the associated strabismus, ocular structural abnormalities, e.g. microphthalmos, or poor visual responsiveness. The parents ask: What is the problem, can it be repaired, and can or will the child see? The two main issues are the spontaneous abnormal eye movements and any accompanying impairment of vision.

The two main categories of spontaneous eye movement abnormalities in infants in general are:

1. The less common abnormal saccadic (rapid movement) disorders, and often related to fixational changes.
2. Those which are repetitive oscillations (nystagmus), more constant though variable and not as closely related to fixational changes.

The most important saccadic disorder is the bursts of spontaneous saccades, multidirectional, often part of a startle response, seen as an early manifestation of the generalized clonic movements that sometimes accompany a neuroblastoma. This "opsoclonus" should prompt the physician to investigate for this treatable tumor although opsoclonus may be part of the benign "dancing eyes and dancing feet" syndrome of childhood.

Spontaneous jiggling of the infant's eyes is more commonly due to nystagmus, which can be regarded as either ocular or neurologic in origin. The ocular types, more often seen in infants, can be due to some form of visual impairment (sensory infantile nystagmus) or idiopathic (formerly referred to as a motor congenital nystagmus).

Clinical "wave forms"

Nystagmus can take many forms in its movement (usually variations of pendular and jerk type of oscillations), as well as in direction and speed. Some movements form a pattern that is helpful in diagnosis, but, many times, other clues in the history or examination lead to the definition of the problem. Some patterns of nystagmus are highly characteristic and suggestive of an ocular problem while, less commonly, others suggest a topographically localizing neurological problem.

The history of prenatal/natal difficulties (maternal diabetes, drug ingestion, difficult delivery) and a neonatal and developmental course need to be considered as well as the child's visual responsiveness, ocular symptoms (poor vision, photophobia, head nodding, strabismus), and the family history of any visual impairment and nystagmus.

Most infantile nystagmus disorders show horizontal oscillations, but sometimes vertical, rotatory, or a combination of several planes of movement occurs. Visual fixation may appear to be good, or vision may be poor. Sometimes, the eye movements are typical of idiopathic infantile nystagmus, sometimes called "congenital nystagmus" or "motor congenital nystagmus" (horizontal, variable in intensity, changing with gaze movements, dampening by convergence, increasing with visual effort, and no conversion to vertical nystagmus on vertical gaze, i.e. remaining horizontal on vertical gaze). A null point with compensatory head turn may be present. Nystagmus on the basis of sensory defects (sensory congenital nystagmus) may appear similar. It is not always possible to detect milder degrees of associated visual loss. Vertical nystagmus in infants is more often ocular in origin than neurological. Severe visual impairment commonly produces more irregular, slow, wandering horizontal movements with intermittent vertical jerking and little response to the usual visual stimuli and optokinetic testing. Very valuable is the history of the time of onset of the nystagmus, because visual system gliomas may masquerade as forms of infantile nystagmus with good vision, even the so-called "congenital nystagmus" and spasmus nutans. In most cases, infantile wobbly eyes are recognized early in life, but sometime the "time of onset" may be unclear. A useful rule is that in cases with onset not recognized until after approximately 3 months of age, neuroimaging of the head and visual system, preferably with MRI, should be carried out to rule out structural brain abnormalities.

Latent, or occlusion nystagmus, often accompanies infantile esotropia, with or without congenital nystagmus. This is a binocular horizontal jerk form of oscillation, precipitated by occlusion of one eye, resulting in conjugate nystagmus jerking toward the fixating eye. Sometimes, the same form of nystagmus exists without being initiated by occlusion, usually in the presence of strabismus, but is further exaggerated by occlusion, i.e. a spontaneous binocular deficiency nystagmus syndrome (sometimes called by the oxymoron "manifest" latent nystagmus). Latent nystagmus is a motor sign of strabismus-related developmental loss of binocular vision and, for isolated cases, usually requires no electrophysiologic or neurological investigation.

Monocular nystagmus in infancy is unusual and usually is associated with amblyopia requiring occlusion therapy. Occasionally, it is the harbinger of a brain tumor such as a hypothalamic glioma. For this reason, an MRI of the head is recommended.

Symptoms related to the visual system (poor vision, head nodding, anomalous head positions, photophobia, strabismus) in the absence of CNS problems point the way to ocular causes of the infant's nystagmus.

The ocular examination may reveal the cause of the nystagmus (e.g. bilateral macular toxoplasmosis, bilateral optic nerve hypoplasia, or bilateral cataracts), but sometimes the eye exam seems normal, specifically the retina. In these cases, an electroretinograom (ERG) will help define nystagmogenic conditions such as congenital stationary night-blindness and rod monochromatism (achromatopsia). If both the ocular structures and ERG are normal, an MRI is recommended. If no causal condition is uncovered after these investigations, then one labels the nystagmus as "idiopathic congenital nystagmus."

Photophobia occurs in a number of nystagmus-associated conditions such as retinal dystrophies, Leber's amaurosis, aniridia, and albinism, but is perhaps most dramatic with rod monochromatism (achromatopsia), in which it is especially exaggerated out of doors. Multichannel visual-evoked potentials (VEPs) usually show evidence of chiasmal misrouting in albinism.

It is unusual for infantile nystagmus forms to take the characteristic CNS pattterns that are neuroanatomically localizing ones and more often seen in later years, but these do occur in brain disorders and are helpful in directing investigation and suggesting etiologies. It is essential to work with a neurological specialist or pediatrician to complete the patient's management since a great many CNS diseases have nystagmus as part of their clinical picture, e.g. Joubert's, Pelizaeus-Merzbacher, Leigh's disease, and cerebral palsy. Very often

---

Box 113.1

Abnormal eye movements in infants: nystagmus vs. saccadic intrusions

Infantile nystagmus

I. Identified shortly after birth (<3 months) or at birth
  A. Monocular
    Amblyopia
    Brain tumor
    Highly asymmetric binocular nystagmus
  B. Binocular
    1. With visual loss
      a. Severe visual loss
        Wandering searching movements of the blind infant
        Eye exam and erG most important, e.g. Leber's amaurosis
      b. Some/little visual loss and recognizable structural abnormality
        Aniridia
        Albinism (ocular/oculocutaneous)
        Coloboma involving maculae
        Macular scars
        Optic nerve hypoplasia
        Optic atrophy
        Foveal hypoplasia
        Retinopathy of prematurity (macular drag)
        ERG may be helpful in doubtful cases
      c. Some/little visual loss and normal ocular exam (erG is essential)
        Rod monochromatism
        Retinal dystrophies
        Leber's amaurosis
        Congenital stationary night blindness
    2. Without visual loss
      a. Motor or idiopathic
        "Congenital" motor nystagmus (MrI and erG normal)

3. With strabismus
  a. Binocular deficiency nystagmus syndrome
    Spontaneous
    Occlusion elicited (occlusion or latent nystagmus)
  b. Nystagmus blockage syndrome/Ciancia's syndrome

II. acquired nystagmus (onset >3 months)
  A. Spasmus nutans
    Glioma masquerade
    True spasmus nutans (transient childhood nystagmus)
  B. "Congenital"-like nystagmus
    Glioma masquerade
  C. Non-ocular (CNS) nystagmus
    1. Vestibular
      a. Peripheral, i.e. vestibular nerve/end organ complex
      b. Central vestibular
        Periodic alternating nystagmus
        Upbeat, downbeat, see-saw, rotary
    2. Gaze-evoked jerk nystagmus
      Internuclear ophthalmoplegia, $1\frac{1}{2}$ syndrome, gaze-paretic nystagmus,
      Brun's nystagmus, cerebellopontine angle tumor, dorsal midbrain syndrome (convergence retraction syndrome)
    3. Pendular
      Oculopalatal myoclonus, multiple sclerosis
    4. Monocular
      Brain tumor
    5. Others

Saccadic intrusions and other oscillations

May mimic nystagmus but have a different clinical significance

Square wave jerks

Opsoclonus

Macro-oscillations

Voluntary nystagmus

Ocular flutter

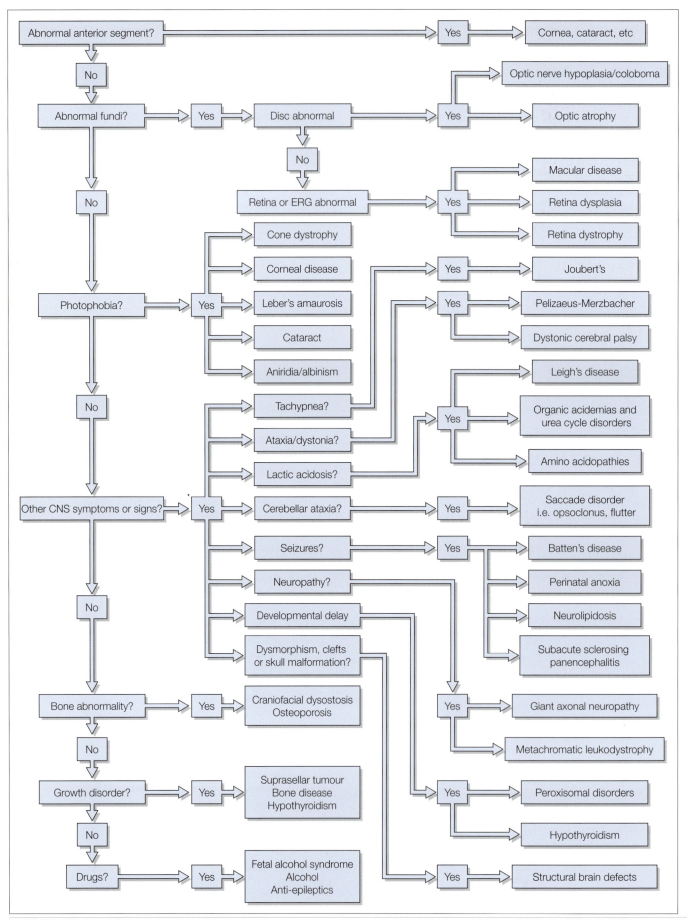

Fig. 113.1 Systemic diagnosis of wobbly eyes in infancy.

these children are ill systemically in addition to having nystagmus; this differentiates them from the majority of those with purely ocular forms of eye movement disturbances. Although oscillopsia accompanies most neurologically related nystagmus, and not ocular forms, this symptom is clearly not one of infancy.

Vision

The simplest way to assess vision in an infant with wobbly eyes is by history and observation of the child's visual behavior. What can the child do and not do visually, especially when compared to the behavior of normal siblings? Use of pattern VEPs is helpful, but the oculomotor instability degrades the response in some. In the presence of a significantly reduced VEP result, it is helpful to repeat the study and base one's comments more heavily on the visual behavior of the child.

Some congenital structural abnormalities are untreatable. Early removal of congenital cataracts does eradicate the development of sensory deprivation nystagmus. Sensory forms require full optical treatment but the nystagmus remains, although its intensity may decrease with age. In idiopathic varieties, the use of induced convergence to diminish the spontaneous movements in older children with concave lenses and base-out prisms may enhance visual acuity. Surgical methods to diminish the intensity of nystagmus have been attempted with unconvincing success. Bilateral extraocular muscle surgery to center the null point to eliminate a compensatory head position may be useful.

Box 113.1 illustrates a working schema of spontaneous eye movement disorder in infancy, with neuroimaging suggested if the time of onset is unclear or late (e.g. after 3 months of age), or in the presence of other clinical clues suggestive of neurologic etiology.

Figure 113.1 is an algorithm outlining a systematic approach to the diagnosis of wobbly eyes in infancy regardless of their movement characteristics.

Further reading

Hertle RW. Congenital nystagmus: characteristics and evidence for treatment. Am Orthopt J 2010; 60: 48–58.

Thurtell MS, Leight J.Therapy for nystagmus. J Neuro-ophthalmology 2010; 30: 361–71.

Tychsen L, Richards M, Wong A, et al. The neural mechanism for latent (fusion maldevelopment) nystagmus. J Neuro-ophthalmol 2010; 30: 276–83.

Wong A. Eye Movement Disorders. Oxford: Oxford University Press; 2008.

SECTION 7
Common practical problems in
a pediatric ophthalmology
and strabismus practice

CHAPTER 114

Practical problems: abnormal head postures

Ankoor S Shah • David G Hunter

Introduction

We describe a practical approach to the patient presenting with an abnormal head posture (AHP).[1,2,3] Chapter 81 details the causes, types, and physiologic basis of abnormal head postures.

Nomenclature

The three axes of rotation are "yaw" (about the vertical axis), "pitch" (about the anteroposterior axis), and "roll" (about the left-to-right axis) (Fig. 114.1). An AHP is described by these axes: *yaw* corresponds to *head turn* or *face turn*, *pitch* to *head tilt*, and *roll* to *chin up* or *chin down*."Torticollis" refers to any abnormal head posture; sometimes, it is reserved for head tilt. "*Compensatory head posture*" is an AHP adopted to improve vision.

Patient history

The age of onset of a head posture is infrequently available. The patient and family do not recognize an AHP unless extreme. Old photographs provide reliable historical information about the onset and severity.

Characterization of the head position

Clinicians estimate the angle of head positions in degrees. Orthopedic goniometers (Fig. 114.2A), arthrodial protractors (Fig. 114.2B),[4] and other devices including cervical range of motion devices (Fig. 114.2C)[5] have been used to improve precision. Placing a prism (or yoked prisms) of increasing power in the line of sight until the head appears straight also may be used to measure the head position. Clinical photographs are a convenient, accurate, and reproducible way to document a head position (unpublished data). To obtain an accurate photograph, provide a target requiring fine visual resolution to ensure that the patient is fixating on the camera as the photograph is taken. Eliminate confounding background objects. Have a child sit up straight, off of the parent's lap, to minimize

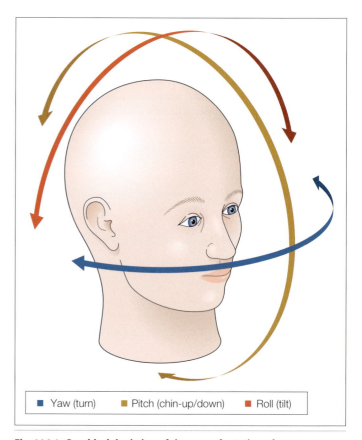

Fig. 114.1 **Graphical depiction of the axes of rotation of a three dimensional object.**

| ■ Yaw (turn) | ■ Pitch (chin-up/down) | ■ Roll (tilt) |

leaning. Obtain similar photographs with each eye covered if head position changes with monocular viewing.

Force the head in the opposite direction and observe the response: the drive to maintain the AHP against resistance may also be characterized while the patient is watching a movie or reading an eye chart. Strong resistance to movement may represent a strong drive for binocularity with strabismus or a non-ocular, musculoskeletal anomaly. Lower resistance followed by a prompt return to the preferred position when the patient requires best visual acuity suggests a desire to improve vision related to nystagmus or dissociated vertical deviation (DVD). Minimal resistance, with prolonged maintenance of

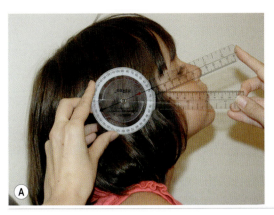
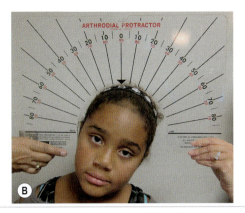
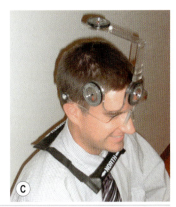

Fig. 114.2 Instruments used for quantifying head position. (A) Orthopedic goniometer (HiRes™, Baseline® Diagnostic and Measuring Instruments, Fabrication Enterprises, Inc., White Plains, NY, USA). (B) Arthrodial protractor (Reedco Research, Geneva, NY.) (Image courtesy Donny Suh, MD.) (C) Modified cervical range of motion device. (Image courtesy of Burton Kushner, MD.)

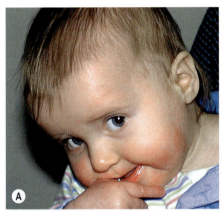
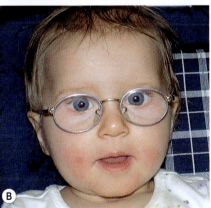

Fig. 114.3 (A) This 6-month-old girl presented with a 3-month history of a head turn and tilt. The magnitude of the head turn was variable, and the patient did not resist forced head repositioning. Motility was full. Cycloplegic refraction was +8.50 +0.50 × 90 OU. Note use of brow for "pinhole" effect on right eye. (B) 3 months later the patient returned wearing partial hyperopic correction of +6.50 +0.50 × 90 OU. The head posture had completely resolved.

the newly forced head position, suggests habitual head turn or possibly periodic alternating nystagmus with variable head posture, but may also be acuity-based positioning. Forced head position testing should be repeated with one eye occluded to determine whether the head posture is used to preserve binocular function.

Examination

Visual acuity/refraction

Uncorrected refractive error may cause a compensatory head posture (Fig. 114.3) by using the brow or eyelid margins to achieve a pinhole effect. If there is no refractive error but visual acuity is subnormal, the examiner should seek other ocular causes of a head posture, such as nystagmus. When the head posture persists after monocular occlusion, measure visual acuity with the head held straight; re-measure visual acuity after allowing the patient to adopt the preferred head posture, or observe for a change in head position as the patient reads progressively smaller letters.

External examination

Palpate the neck muscles; tightness suggests a non-ocular etiology. Ptosis is obvious when severe enough to produce a head posture. Assess for facial asymmetry by imagining two horizontal lines, one connecting the lateral canthi and the second connecting the corners of the mouth. If these lines are not parallel, there is facial asymmetry. In congenital superior oblique palsy, the side where the lines diverge is usually the side of the paresis (see Fig. 79.1).[6]

Ocular motility

When nystagmus causes an abnormal head position, it is frequently obvious but subtle cases can easily be missed. To identify subtle nystagmus, hold the head in the position opposite to the preferred position and assess the stability of the eye. Magnification (using, for example, a 20-diopter fundus lens) may help.

Assess ductions and versions, and perform prism-and-cover testing in the diagnostic positions of gaze: incomitant strabismus in a fusing patient often leads to a compensatory head posture (Fig. 114.4). Comitant intermittent exotropia may lead to a head turn as control decompensates. Perform sensory testing with and without the AHP. Dissimilar target projection tests (Hess screen, Lancaster red-green) map the gaze position in the nine diagnostic gaze positions.

Other aspects of the examination

Slit-lamp evaluation and indirect ophthalmoscopy may reveal micro-nystagmus. Visual field evaluation can reveal a hemifield defect, which could cause an AHP. Detection of fundus torsion by indirect ophthalmoscopy may reveal unrecognized malfunction of a cyclovertical muscle.[7]

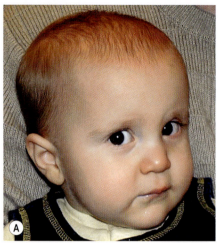

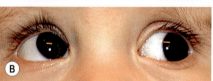

Fig. 114.4 (A) This 11-month-old boy presented with a constant left head turn and a slight chin-down position. He strongly resisted left gaze. (B) On forced gaze left, a left hypotropia was noted, with limited elevation in abduction. Imaging revealed no orbital or extraocular muscle abnormality. He underwent a left inferior rectus recession, followed years later by horizontal strabismus surgery.

Treatment[4,8,9,10]

While treatment of an underlying condition (e.g. refractive error, ptosis, or strabismus) normally eliminates an AHP, there are exceptions. Head positions may become habitual, though this may be overdiagnosed when the examiner cannot locate a cause. Other causes of persistent (most commonly, undercorrected) AHP after surgery must be ruled out before concluding that it is habitual. Marked facial asymmetry may create the false appearance of a head tilt. DVD is difficult to treat: surgery that eliminates the vertical drift may not alter the head tilt. DVD may coincide with other conditions causing AHP and treatment does not eliminate the DVD or the head posture. Nystagmus surgery may reposition the null point, but the nystagmus may persist and the null point may drift.

Correction of an abnormal head posture secondary to nystagmus may be a challenge (see Chapter 81). Head turns may respond to bilateral recess/resect procedures, but the surgical dosage must be selected to avoid inducing heterotropias and adjusted to compensate for pre-existing horizontal strabismus. Chin-up or chin-down head postures may respond to symmetric vertical recess/resect procedures, or to weakening

matched vertically acting muscles in both eyes. For head tilts, horizontal transposition of the vertical rectus muscles to induce torsion may be effective.

Summary

An AHP is a diagnostic clue. When a patient presents with an anomalous head position, the comprehensive eye examination and sensorimotor evaluation may need to be supplemented by:

1. Assessing resistance to head repositioning.
2. Measuring visual function in primary position, preferred position, and the position opposite the preferred position.
3. Determining the response to monocular occlusion.

Non-ocular causes should be considered only after no ocular cause can be identified.

References

1. Kushner BJ. Ocular causes of abnormal head postures. Ophthalmology 1979; 86: 2115–25.
2. Caldeira JAF. Abnormal head posture: an ophthalmological approach. Binocular Vis Strabismus 2000; 15: 237–9.
3. Hertle RW, Zhu X. Oculographic and clinical characterization of thirty-seven children with anomalous head postures, nystagmus, and strabismus: the basis of a clinical algorithm. J AAPOS 2000; 4: 25–32.
4. Suh DW, Oystreck DT, Hunter DG. Long-term results of an intraoperative adjustable superior oblique tendon suture space using nonabsorbable suture for Brown syndrome. Ophthalmology 2008; 115: 1800–4.
5. Kushner BJ. The usefulness of the cervical range of motion device in the ocular motility examination. Arch Ophthalmol 2000; 118: 946–50.
6. Goodman CR, Chabner E, Guyton DL. Should early strabismus surgery be performed for ocular torticollis to prevent facial asymmetry? J Pediatr Ophthalmol Strabismus 1995; 32: 162–6.
7. Guyton DL. Clinical Assessment of Ocular Torsion. Am Orthopt J 1983; 33: 7–15.
8. Kraft SP, O'Donoghue EP, Roarty JD. Improvement of compensatory head postures after strabismus surgery. Ophthalmology 1992; 99: 1301–8.
9. Repka MX. Surgery to correct nystagmus. In: Tasman W, Jaeger EA, editors. Duane's Ophthalmology. Philadelphia: Lippincott Williams & Wilkins; 2011.
10. Guyton DL. Dissociated vertical deviation: etiology, mechanism, and associated phenomena. Costenbader Lecture. J AAPOS 2000; 4: 131–44.

Vital communication issues: the parents

Louise E Allen

Good communication is essential to establishing a positive and trusting relationship with parents: it improves compliance, optimizes clinical outcomes, and reduces complaints and litigation (Box 115.1).[1]

We have all had difficult relationships with parents, but a few techniques maximize the chances of a good relationship with the majority. *Put yourself in their shoes; what would your expectations of your child's care be?*

Before the consultation

Minimize the disruption of the consultation by ensuring that any investigative tests or an interpreter are available on the day and, where possible, coordinate your consultation with other planned hospital visits. All tertiary referrals should all be seen mainly by the consultant: the parents and referring specialist are expecting a knowledgeable discussion and management plan.

It is most effective to arrange the service provided according to guidelines to ease the patient pathway through the clinic. (In the UK it is *The National Service Framework for Paediatric Services*: several other countries have similar.)

1. Waiting rooms should be child-friendly.
2. There should be ready access to clinics for urgent cases.
3. Timely appointment scheduling.[2]
4. In practice, waiting is often unavoidable, resulting in frayed tempers and bored, fractious children. If the clinic is running late, your explanation of the circumstances may diffuse the frustration of the waiting families. The information may enable parents to rebook and the front desk staff will be eternally grateful.

During the consultation

Patients complain that sometimes we interrupt them or appear rushed or distracted; we may miss hearing their concerns and fail to build a rapport with them. The consulting room layout should facilitate good communication: sit at the same eye level as the parents and outside their personal space. Sitting at an angle avoids any awkwardness in breaking eye contact. There should be no barrier (e.g. desk or slit-lamp) between you and the parent and child; try not to turn your back on the child and parents to write notes.

Express empathy and support regularly, and acknowledge the hard work and time that the parent has put into their child's treatment.

Parents of children with a rare condition may be more knowledgeable about it than you are and will want to be fully involved in decision making. Some parents may appear to have a disproportionate level of anxiety: they may have unspoken fears or doubt about the management plan due to information from other sources, such as the internet. Occasionally, parents may not want to follow your management advice and prefer alternative options. It may be necessary to make some compromises to maintain the parents' trust and satisfaction whilst ensuring the child has good care.

In rare instances, parents opt for inappropriate management, for instance treatment of retinoblastoma by faith healing.

Box 115.1

Strategies for establishing a good relationship with parents

- Triage referrals effectively and sensitively
- Appointment letters should inform parents about the potential duration of visit, need for preliminary orthoptic assessment, and dilating drops
- Minimize waiting times and provide a child-friendly waiting area
- Have a consulting room layout which facilitates good communication and privacy
- Give a warm greeting and have an approachable manner, try to avoid medical jargon
- Listen to the parents and let them contribute to the management plan
- Give regular verbal and non-verbal expressions of empathy and support
- Provide written information for the parents to take home
- Provide contact numbers to allow parents access to urgent advice and ensure that there is always someone available to take the call
- Copy clinic letters to the parent – particularly when management decisions are made
- Facilitate a second opinion whenever appropriate: it will enhance the parent's confidence in you

Where this puts the child's sight or life at threat, initial patience for a few days allowing the parents to understand the serious results of such treatment should be followed by consultations with colleagues and the help of the support team and social services workers to gently persuade the parents of the best form of treatment for the child. Legally, in most countries, the life and health of the child is paramount over the desires of the parents. Action appropriate to the country where the child is being treated may need to be taken to protect the child (see Chapter 58). This needs to be handled very sympathetically and carefully so that the relationship with the parents and the treating team is supported.

Once you have discussed the management options with the parents, ensure that they have the information at hand regarding the diagnosis and the potential risks and benefits of treatment options. Information leaflets, details of support organizations and procedure-specific consent forms should be available for them.

After the consultation

Parents will remember only some of the information given during the consultation – so keep them informed; ensure that they get a copy of the letter to the primary care physician written in simple terms outlining the diagnosis, treatment, and/or patching regimen and management plans. Keep any other involved medical teams and visual impairment teachers up to date. It is very reassuring for parents to have contact numbers to ring in case glasses are lost, more patches are required, or urgent problems crop up. Parents often find email communication useful, but it is not a confidential medium – do not write anything that could not be put on the back of a postcard or be sure to send it by a secure system which can be password protected. Do not use your personal email account for professional email communication and ensure that you have the correct email details for the parents. Your hospital may require parents to give signed consent for email communication.

Breaking bad news is hard but, if done well, can make a big difference to the parents' reaction to the problem and their ability to support their child (Box 115.2).[3] Talking to the parents of primary school age children alone about the diagnosis first allows them to think about the diagnosis, ask questions, and compose themselves so that they can offer support to the child. Ask the parents if they would prefer you to talk to the child about the problem or whether they would prefer to discuss it with him/her at home first.

It is helpful to find out what the parents already know. For example, the parents themselves might have raised the concern that their baby is blind and you may be confirming what they already suspect. Try to prepare them that there is bad news coming, break the news gradually, sensing if they are ready for a full explanation or not. Avoid being overcome with emotion yourself, since this can give the impression that things are hopeless. It is helpful to have some positives; for example, that visual function can improve in babies with cerebral visual impairment and that there are visual aids/support processes/research that may help the child in the future. Give the parents a clear plan of follow-up and written information about the condition and contact points for support. Involve the primary care physician to ensure there is community support for the family.

Box 115.2

Breaking bad news

- Prepare yourself by thinking through the conversation and management plan
- Find a private area in which to talk, prevent interruptions
- Talk to parents of children less than (say) 10 years old alone first
- Find out what the parents already know
- Give an open explanation with some positive news as well
- Empathize but do not become overly emotional yourself
- Discuss the problem with the child in a manner appropriate to their age and maturity
- Listen and answer questions honestly and openly
- Give written information and support group contacts
- Inform the primary care team and any involved teachers of the visually impaired
- Give a clear plan of follow-up, arrange an early review
- Offer a second opinion if helpful

Box 115.3

Dealing with the angry parent

- If you are in a public environment, move to a private area with help nearby
- Try and get the aggressive parent to sit down, allow them to vent their anger without interruption
- Calm the parent with soft and slow responses, acknowledge his/her distress
- Apologize to them – even if the cause for the anger is not your fault
- Listen to the issues raised; empathize with them verbally and non-verbally
- Assure them that you will look into what happened and try to put it right
- Do not get defensive or sarcastic, do not tell them to "calm down" (which will have the opposite effect!)
- Avoid showing the parent that you are upset or angry yourself
- Facilitate a second opinion if appropriate
- If the parents want to make a formal complaint, you should inform them how to do this
- Document in detail the conversation in the child's notes

When parents hear bad news about their child, a common reaction is "maybe the doctor is wrong" or "maybe there is a treatment that the doctor doesn't know about." I am sure we would feel the same way in similar circumstances. The parents may not ask because they do not want to upset you, but you should anticipate this and offer to arrange a second opinion if they (or you) feel that this will help them. The parents will usually be relieved and thankful for the offer, even if they decide not to take it up. Second opinions enhance, not diminish, the reputation of the referring doctor in the parents' eyes.

Occasionally, you will be faced with angry relatives even when there has been no issue with the nursing and/or medical care (Box 115.3). They may feel frustrated by the wait or feel helpless about their child's condition. Anger may be part of grieving and may also result from a feeling of guilt. Try and pick up on early non-verbal clues – lack of eye contact, invasion of your personal space and agitated speech – to sense that anger is building so that you can diffuse it before it boils over. Talk slowly and softly, trying to get to the cause of the parents' anger. Emphasize what is being done for the child, offer to facilitate a second opinion, reinforce the message that everybody wants the best care for their child, and try to suggest ways that you can work together to make that happen. If you find yourself getting angry, leave the situation and calm yourself down. The hospital may have a patients' ombudsman or similar person who can act for and advise the parents and can arrange a time to meet with the parents in a non-clinical setting with an independent facilitator.[4]

Complaints and litigation

Our natural response to a complaint is to stop communicating about it in case we increase the risk of litigation. This usually makes things worse, building resentment and giving the impression that there is a conspiracy of silence. If a clinical mistake has been made and a patient has suffered harm, the situation must be honestly and fully explained to the parents. The advice of litigation authorities is that sympathizing and expressing regret does not constitute an admission of liability.[4]

Poor attendance

A significant number of initial and follow-up appointments in pediatric clinics are missed. This may be because the parent has not received the appointment, has forgotten it, or does not feel that it is important.[5] Explaining the importance of the appointment in writing to the referring doctor and parents can often prompt a response to rearrange the appointment. If the condition is sight threatening, a phone call to the parent is necessary. Repeated non-attendance, which could risk the child's sight, is a form of neglect and you should discuss your concerns with the hospital's child protection team.

Summary

One of the best things about pediatric ophthalmology is that we can build a trusting and rewarding relationship with the child and their family. Good communication not only helps improve our ability to diagnose and manage our patients better but makes our job much more enjoyable.

References

1. Myerscough PR, Ford M. Talking with Patients: Keys to Good Communication, 3rd ed. Oxford: Oxford Medical Publications, Oxford University Press; 1996.
2. Department of Health TSO. National service framework for children, young people and maternity services: core standards. National Service Framework, London, 2004. http://www.dh.gov.uk/en/ Publicationsandstatistics/Publications/ PublicationsPolicyAndGuidance/DH_4089102
3. Washer P. Clinical Communication Skills – Oxford Core Texts. Oxford: Oxford University Press; 2009.
4. National Patient Safety Agency. Being Open: Communicating Patient Safety Incidents with Patients and their Carers. London: The National Patient Safety Agency; 2005.
5. Andrews, R. Morgan, JD. Addy, DP et al. Understanding non-attendance in outpatient paediatric clinics. Arch Dis Child 1990; 65: 192–5.

Vital communication issues: the child

Louise E Allen

Good rapport and a trusting relationship with children are vital in order to encourage their cooperation and aid compliance. Your style of communication should be tailored to the age and maturity of the child; they are the center of the consultation.[1]

Infants

To ensure a good examination, babies should be rested and fed. If the baby comes into the consultation sleeping, take the opportunity to perform the ocular examination – visual assessment and eye movement testing can wait until the child is awake. If the baby is crying and the ocular examination is difficult, bottle- or breastfeeding will settle the infant and enable a good examination. Generally, it is unnecessary to use a speculum in term infants unless there is concern about peripheral retinal pathology. If a speculum is necessary, topical anesthetic, swaddling, and oral sugar solution can be helpful.

Toddlers are the most difficult age group to examine (Box 116.1). They don't understand why you are examining them and can rarely be reasoned with. The combination of a tired, hungry toddler and stressed parent can make a full examination impossible. Call the family into the consulting room yourself so that the child can appraise you; give the child lots of smiling, playful banter, and compliments. If the history is complicated, let the child explore and play until you are ready to examine them. If you sense your examination may be limited, do the essential things first and complete other aspects of the examination on a return visit. I very rarely restrain children to examine them – I try all other inducements – drinks,

raisins, cookies, etc. first. If I feel that a fundus check is vital to exclude serious pathology, I will ask the child's parents to briefly hold them in their arms while I take a quick look. If I can't get a good look, I explain this to the parents (who are usually understanding) and arrange another visit. Often an earlier appointment time or having the pupils predilated at home can make a big difference. Many hospitals have play therapists who can help those children who find the examination or procedures like contact lens insertion very frightening.

School-age children

Even children who appear very sophisticated may find understanding visual and eye problems and their treatment difficult (Box 116.2). Video analysis of doctor–parent–child consultations have shown that school-aged children are left out of the conversation in 90% of consultations.[2] Depending on the maturity of the child, you should direct most of the conversation to them, with clarification from the parent when necessary. Don't turn your back on the child to talk to the parent; maintain intermittent eye contact. Break the ice by starting an easy conversation with the child about their age, school, hobbies, friends, etc. They find these questions easy to answer and will be more likely to answer subsequent "medical"

Box 116.1

Tips for communicating with toddlers pre-school children

- Call the child into the consultation room yourself
- Call the child by their usual name/nickname
- Crouch down to their level – SMILE!
- Use simple language and familiar words
- Talk at their pace, use short sentences
- Examine the child on the parent's lap
- Explain to the parent and child what you are going to do
- Demonstrate the examination on their parent, sibling or doll

---

Box 116.2

Tips for communicating with school-age children

- Introduce yourself and start an easy conversation with the child – SMILE!
- Explain why they are seeing you
- Have the examination chair between you and the parent so you can divide your attention between them
- Ask them to describe the problem
- Use simple words and short sentences but avoid speaking down to them
- Tell them truthfully about what to expect in the examination
- Do not continue with the examination if they are crying
- Do not make promises that you cannot keep
- Explain to the child why they need glasses/patching/surgery and try to get their agreement
- Ask if the child has any questions

questions. Always be truthful about any discomfort predicted during the examination and explain the reason why you need to do it. Putting a drop of the topical anesthetic/cycloplegic on their finger or demonstrating the rebound/air-puff tonometer before using it on the eye can show the child that there is nothing to fear.

Children in this age group sometimes develop functional visual symptoms due to problems at school or with their home life. If possible, try and spend some time talking to the child and parents separately to work out what the problem is; sometimes children will not tell their parents about bullying because of feared reprisals at school. It is important to enlist the help of the parents in understanding and ameliorating the causes of the problem.

Although we sometimes feel ineffectual about how little we can do for children with severe visual impairment, a regular consultation allows the child to talk openly about the problem with someone who understands the visual, educational, and social problems they face. As the child matures over the years, further explanation about the condition, treatment, and the future can be given. Most children do not want to feel "different" from their classmates and may avoid talking about it with their peers; this may be one of the few times they can be open about it.

Adolescence is a dynamic time in development, with many physical and psychological changes. Conflicts around these changes can produce challenging behavior, particularly with regard to risk-taking and rebellion through non-compliance (Box 116.3). It is useful to understand what the social and educational expectations are at that age. Young people can be impatient but in general are non-complaining; most silence and sullenness is defensive. It is important to show that you are concerned for them, rather than being interested in superiority and control.[3]

If all else fails

If you are unable to adequately examine a child for whom you have significant concerns, my view is that it is better to arrange examination under sedation or general anesthetic than to attempt a suboptimal examination. Their will never trust you or probably any other doctor again.

If the child is scheduled to have another procedure under sedation or general anesthesia (e.g. tooth extraction, grommets, scans), do not miss the opportunity of a complete ocular examination. Oral sedation for eye examination requires pediatric support. The child should be fasted in the same way as if they were having a general anesthetic and informed written consent taken. Cycloplegic drops should be given prior to the oral sedation. Remember to take topical anesthetic to the ward along with the relevant instruments: conscious sedation does not reduce corneal sensitivity. Buccal midazolam (500 µg/kg, maximum 15 mg) provides excellent sedation; it is effective within 30 minutes and lasts for about the same time. In some countries oral or rectal chloral hydrate (50 mg/kg for infants <4 kg, 100 mg/kg for infants >4 kg up to maximum 2 g dose) is used for infants and toddlers. It takes effect in about an hour and can last several hours. Generally, sedation works well in infants and toddlers but is less effective for school-aged children. Sedation carries about the same level of risk as a general anesthetic and, although the risks are different, children having sedation must have the same safety precautions and level of consent. Sedation should only be carried out in a setting that can cope with anesthetic emergencies.

Summary

A trusting and cooperative relationship between the child and clinician is vital to optimize compliance with the eye examination and ophthalmic procedures. In my view, it is self-defeating to perform an examination or procedure on a child who is crying and heavily restrained, although there may be exceptional circumstances when this is necessary for the child's well-being. Play therapy can be very useful for supporting children who require regular procedures. Conscious sedation is a useful technique when a good examination is essential but impossible to achieve in clinic.

A good pediatric ophthalmologist has the sensitivity and flexibility to adjust their manner of communication to the child's specific needs, and the ability to know which aspects of the examination are essential and which can be left for another day. Perfectionism may not be an ideal personality trait!

References

1. General Medical Council. 0–18 Years: Guidance for Doctors. London: General Medical Council; 2007.
2. Tates K, Elbers E, Meeuwesen L, et al. Doctor–parent–child relationships: a "pas de trios". Patient Educ Couns 2002; 48: 5–14.
3. Myerscough PR, Ford M. Talking with Patients: Keys to Good Communication, 3rd ed. Oxford: Oxford Medical Publications, Oxford University Press; 1996.

My child just will not let me put the eye drops in!

Melanie Hingorani

Introduction

Suboptimal compliance with prescribed medication is widespread in all medical spheres, especially in children. Many parents find it challenging to apply topical medications to a child's eyes.

Causes of poor compliance

1. Child-related factors. Most people do not enjoy putting medication into the eye. It is uncomfortable and intrusive for a sensitive area. The natural instinct when an object nears the eye is to close it, or turn away. Adults are better able to control this instinct than children. Additional factors affecting a child's cooperation may include fear, incomprehension of the disease or need for treatment, unpleasant effects of the drops (e.g. stinging, taste of medication), previous poor experience of eye examinations or drops, and issues that affect behavior and cooperation, in general (e.g. autism, learning difficulties).
2. Parental factors. Parents have a natural urge not to upset or hurt their child. Some are squeamish about dealing with eyes. Parents may not understand the nature of the ocular condition, or why the drops are important. There may be concerns about potential side effects. Parents may be anxious about instilling the drops correctly or accidentally touching the eye. Their anxieties may be unwittingly communicated to the child.
3. Practical factors may be important:
    a. Busy lives with several children to care for.
    b. Other more pressing health concerns.
    c. Scheduling issues – how to deliver frequent drops whilst the child attends school or nursery.
    d. Poor understanding of the technique for instilling the drops.
    e. An element of child neglect.
4. Medication and staff issues. Some medication issues may reduce compliance:
    a. Eyedrops are stingy.
    b. Complicated or time-consuming regimes.
    c. Multiple medications.
    d. Medications that are difficult to administer (ointments are more difficult to administer).
5. Clinician factors may contribute:
    a. Communication difficulties.
    b. Inexperience in pediatric care.
    c. Unsympathetic or poor explanations.
    d. Rushed or rude staff.

Formulating a strategy

Therapeutic strategies need to be tailored to the patient and family. The clinician needs to be sympathetic, professional, and calm. Reassure families that this is a common problem. Acknowledge difficulties identified by the parents as understandable and not their fault. Help to keep the parents calm. Try to explore what factors might be exacerbating the problem. Ask questions about:

1. Understanding of the condition.
2. Practical difficulties.
3. Anxieties.
4. Observe the instillation techniques used. Different personalities and types of staff may offer different approaches which fit better. Ask how much medication they are getting in.

The following may be helpful:

1. Provide a clear and simple explanation of the eye condition and its possible effects, the benefits of treatment, and harm of not treating. Be honest but non-threatening about side effects. Explain the prognosis and how long therapy will be needed. An explanation may be required for the child depending on the age. Explanations need to be comprehensible for the educational level and language of the family. Written information is helpful.
2. Medication changes. Ensure the regime is as simple, infrequent, and pleasant as possible. Reduce frequency of instillation whenever possible. Accept slightly less than recommended frequency if it achieves a reasonable level of therapy. Link drops with other established routines. Use combination preparations whenever possible. If

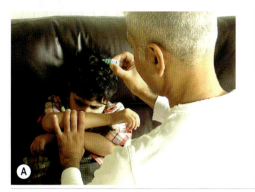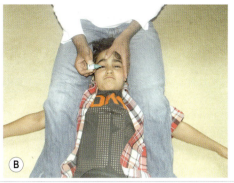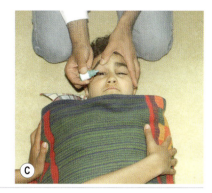

Fig. 117.1 (A) Safely delivering eye drop treatment to the eyes of an uncooperative child can be very difficult but there are ways to deliver the vital medication. (B) One carer alone can gently restrain the child's arms with his or her legs while using both arms to open the lids and put the drop in. Care must be taken not to use excessive force. (C) Firm but gentle restraint by two people is safer and kinder than partial restraint by one person. Here the second person restrains the arms while the first holds the head (which may alternatively be held between the knees) and instills the eye drops. A cuddle and a treat can be given when the procedure is successfully finished.

multiple drops are used, use discretion on how long to wait between the different drops. Change to medications which are easier to instill according to the parents. If drops sting, find a less stingy alternative. If side-effects are a concern, find a safer preparation (e.g. non-steroidals instead of steroids).

3. Technique. Show techniques which may be less "ideal" but still work. If parents use a poor technique which is needlessly painful, or allows contact of fingers or drop bottle with the eye, this needs to be remedied. Watch how the parent attempts drop instillation to observe the child's reaction and the technique and make adjustments if necessary. The ideal is for the child to be still, look up and while the upper or lower lid is pulled, a drop is placed into the fornix. It may be necessary to prize the lids apart. It is possible to put drops on the medial lids and then part the lids, so the drop slips in. Explain that the drops can be instilled in different positions (e.g. sitting, lying back) and places (Fig. 117.1A).

It may be possible to persuade a child by explanation, praise, rewards, play, distraction, or positive reinforcement. If this does not work quickly, it will likely fail. If the child is unable to cooperate, the use of reasonable restraint is acceptable. There are a number of safe methods to restrain children which can be demonstrated and taught (Fig. 117.1B,C). It is important for the parents to see staff, or themselves, use the technique successfully. It is necessary to emphasize that,

even though child and parent might find restraint upsetting, sometimes it is essential for getting the job done quickly rather than having hours of frustrating persuasion and battling.

Discuss who puts the drops in and who helps. The child might be able to put the drops in themselves or at least contribute to, and feel some control over, the process. More than one parent or family member may need to help if restraint is used. Sometimes it is possible to involve the school or nursery staff. Children may cooperate better with such authority figures. The school might find a letter from the clinician useful.

4. Desperate measures. In most cases, success can be achieved. Where the above measures fail, it is necessary to take more extreme actions:
   1. Admission to the ward to begin treatment.
   2. Use of more invasive methods such as depot drugs (e.g. subtarsal long-acting steroids in vernal).
   3. If failure to care for the child is suspected, child protection procedures need to be followed.

Conclusions

Instillation of drops in children is challenging. Explanations, support, simplification of medication regimes, and teaching simple techniques will ensure a reasonable level of compliance with the minimum of upset.

Hand defects and the eye

Luis Carlos Ferreira de Sá

The combination of hand and eye defects is frequent and may be observed in a variety of disorders: Duane's syndrome,[1-3] Möbius' syndrome,[2] CHARGE association,[4] and many others. There may be genetic causes, including specific genes and/or new mutations,[1,5,6] but, due to incomplete penetrance, sporadic events, and association with environmental factors,[2] it is not always possible to determine the underlying mechanism.

Embryology

It is important to consider the embryology of eye and hand development to understand why such defects may occur simultaneously. During the third week of gestation, at about 22 days, the optic primordium becomes identifiable in the human embryo. It is the first morphological evidence of the eyes. At 25 days as the optic cup and embryonic fissure emerge, upper limb buds appear. By 36 days, closure of retinal fissure is almost complete and the retina is incompletely pigmented. At the same time, the hand plate has formed with condensation of mesenchyme. In the hand plate, a central carpal region is surrounded by a crescentic flange, the digital plate, from which originates the five-finger rays. At 45 days, the fingers are partially separated.

Etiology

The etiology of most limb defects (Table 118.1) is unknown. Familial associations indicate a genetic basis for some cases; however, environmental agents such as drugs[2] may be related to the development of limb defects. Developmental abnormalities such as amniotic bands, oligohydramnios, and local vascular disruption are also associated with limb abnormalities.[7] Eye defects and hand/finger anomalies originate usually between the third and the fifth week of gestation. Many loci and gene mutations have been associated with hand and eye anomalies.[1,4-6]

The various hand and eye defects can be grouped according to their similarity in overall features, or according to one major feature among the patterns of malformation, in the same manner as Smith's recognizable patterns of malformation.[8] Many conditions present with occasional hand and eye defects, but only the most important and consistent associations are described in Table 118.2.

Table 118.1 – Common terms used for malformations of limbs and fingers

Anomaly	Definition
Arachnodactyly	Long and thin bones of the fingers
Brachydactyly	Abnormal shortness of the fingers
Camptodactyly	Permanent and irreducible flexion of fingers
Clinodactyly	Deviation or deflection of one or more fingers
Ectrodactyly	Absence of any numbers of fingers
Macrodactyly	Abnormal largeness of the fingers
Meromelia	Absence of part of a limb
Micromelia	Abnormal smallness of a limb
Polydactyly	Extra digits or parts of digits
Syndactyly	Fusion of digits

Table 118.2 – Disease and related eye/ocular region and hand/finger anomalies

Group/disease	Eye/ocular region anomalies	Hand/finger anomalies
Chromosomal syndromes		
Down's syndrome (trisomy 21)	Upslanting palpebral fissures, epicanthal folds, iris Brushfield's spots, keratoconus, strabismus, nystagmus, myopia, cataracts	Short metacarpals and phalanges, fifth finger mid-phalanx hypoplasia, single transverse palmar (Simian) crease
Trisomy 18	Short/slanted palpebral fissure, ptosis, hypertelorism, iris coloboma, cataract, microphthalmos	Clenched hand, overlapping of fingers, absence of distal crease, hypoplasia of nails, hypoplastic or absent thumb, syndactyly, polydactyly, ectrodactyly, short fifth metacarpals

Table 118.2 – *Continued*

Group/disease	Eye/ocular region anomalies	Hand/finger anomalies
Trisomy 13 (Patau's syndrome)	Microphthalmia, iris coloboma, retinal dysplasia, hypotelorism, hypertelorism, anophthalmos, cyclopia, slanting palpebral fissures, shallow orbital ridges, absent eyebrow	Flexion of fingers, overlapping, camptodactyly, polydactyly, syndactyly, retroflexilble thumb
Triploidy syndrome and diploid/triploid mixoploidy syndrome	Hypertelorism, coloboma, microphthalmia, iris heterochromia	Syndactyly, simian crease, clinodactyly, proximally placed thumb
Aniridia-Wilms' tumor association	Aniridia, cataracts, nystagmus, ptosis, glaucoma	Clinodactyly
Very small stature, not skeletal dysplasia		
Cornelia de Lange syndrome[4]	Bushy eyebrow, synophrys, long, curly eye lashes	Micromelia, phocomelia, oligodactyly, simian crease, proximal implantation of thumbs
Rubinstein Taybi syndrome[5]	Heavy/highly arched eyebrows, long eye lashes, epicanthal folds, strabismus, nasolacrimal duct stenosis, ptosis	Broad thumbs with radial angulation, fingers broad, clinodactyly, persistent fetal fingertip pads
Moderate stature, facial, genital		
Smith-Lemli-Opitz syndrome	Ptosis, epicanthal folds, strabismus	Simian crease, occasional flexed fingers, short fingers, polydactyly
Williams' syndrome[6]	Epicanthal folds, stellate iris pattern, occasional strabismus, hypotelorism	Hypoplastic nails, occasional clinodactyly
Noonan's syndrome	Hypertelorism, down-slanting palpebral fissures, prominent corneal nerves, myopia, keratoconus, strabismus, nystagmus	Clinodactyly, brachydactyly, blunt fingertips
Unusual brain and/or neuromuscular findings with associated defects		
Cohen's syndrome	Decreased visual acuity, strabismus, constricted visual fields, chorioretinal dystrophy, optic atrophy	Narrow hands, mild shortening of metacarpals, simian crease
Zellweger's syndrome	Cataracts, optic nerve hypoplasia, retinal pigmentary changes, glaucoma, nystagmus	Variable contractures, camptodactyly
Facial defects as major feature		
Mobius' sequence[7]	Sixth and seventh nerve palsy, strabismus	Syndactyly, limb reduction defects
Fraser's syndrome	Cryptophthalmos, associated with eye defects	Partial cutaneous syndactyly, occasional absent phalanges/thumb
Facial-limb defects as major feature		
Miller's syndrome	Eyelids coloboma, ectropion	Absence of fifth digits, syndactyly
Oculodentodigital syndrome	Microphthalmos, microcornea, short palpebral fissures, epicanthal folds, fine porous iris	Syndactyly, camptodactyly, phalangeal hypoplasia
Stickler's syndrome (hereditary arthro-ophthalmopathy)	Myopia, chorioretinal degeneration, retinal detachment, cataract	Severe arthropathy, occcasional arachnodactyly
Ectrodactyly-ectodermal dysplasia-clefting syndrome (EEC syndrome)	Blue iris, photophobia, blepharophimosis, lacrimal system anomalies, blepharitis	Syndactyly, ectrodactyly, nail dysplasia
Craniosynostosis syndromes		
Apert's syndrome (acrocephalosyndactyly)	Hypertelorism, strabismus, shallow orbits, down-slanting of palpebral fissures	Osseous and/or cutaneous syndactyly, broad distal phalanges of thumb, fingers may be short
Pfeiffer's syndrome	Ocular hypertelorism, shallow orbit, proptosis	Broad distal phalanges, syndactyly
Carpenter's syndrome	Cornea opacity, microcornea, optic atrophy	Brachidactyly, syndactyly, polydactyly, clinodactyly, camptodactyly
Other skeletal dysplasia		
Weill-Marchesani syndrome	Spherophakia, ectopia lentis, myopia, glaucoma	Brachidactyly, broad metacarpals and phalanges, stiff joints (hands)
Connective disorders		
Marfan's syndrome	Lens luxation/subluxation, myopia, retinal detachment, glaucoma	Arachnodactyly
Homocystinuria	Lens subluxation (inferiorly), myopia, cataract, glaucoma, optic atrophy	Arachnodactyly

Continued

Table 118.2 – *Continued*

Group/disease	Eye/ocular region anomalies	Hand/finger anomalies
Ehlers-Danlos syndrome	Blue sclera, myopia, microcornea, glaucoma, ectopia lentis, keratoconus	Hyperextensibility of joints
Osteogenesis imperfecta	Blue sclera (thin and translucent), keratoconus, embryotoxon posterior	Hyperextensibility of joints, fractures, occasional syndactyly
Hamartoses/phakomatosis		
Linear sebaceous nevus sequence	Esotropia, lipodermoid, cloudy cornea, coloboma, optic atrophy, microphthalmia	Polydactyly, syndactyly
Klippel-Trenaunay-Weber syndrome	Glaucoma, cataracts, heterochromia	Asymmetric limb hypertrophy, occasional macrodactyly, syndactyly, polydactyly or oligodactyly
Environmental agents		
Fetal alcohol syndrome	Optic nerve hypoplasia, occasional ptosis, microphthalmos	Small distal phalanges, small fifth finger nail
Miscellaneous syndromes/associations		
Bardet-Biedl syndrome (Laurence-Moon-Biedl)	Retinal dystrophy (retinitis pigmentosa), astigmatism, nystagmus, cataracts	Polydactyly, syndactyly, brachydactyly
Goltz' syndrome	Coloboma, microphthalmia, strabismus	Syndactyly

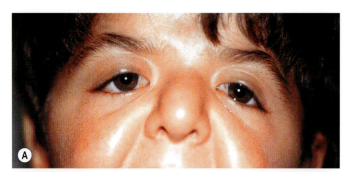
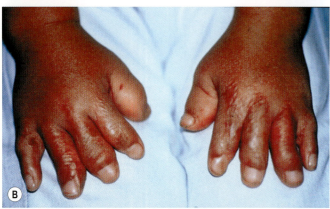
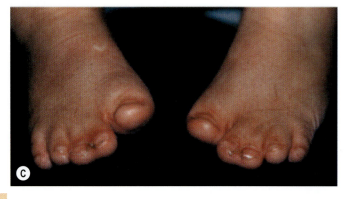

Fig. 118.1 (A) Apert's syndrome. (B) Same patient after surgery for syndactyly. (C) Syndactyly of toes.

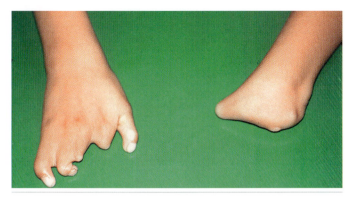

Fig. 118.2 **Möbius' syndrome.** Right hand ectrodactyly and left meromelia.

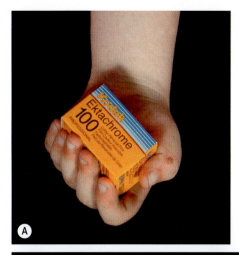

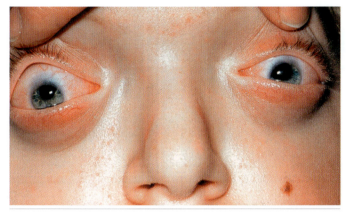

Fig. 118.3 **Atypical iris coloboma in a patient with Pfeiffer's syndrome.**

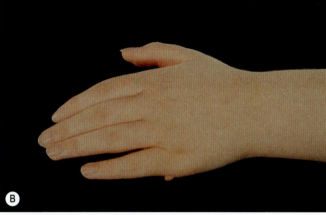

Fig. 118.5 (A) Post-axial polydactyly in a patient with Bardet-Biedl syndrome. (B) Small post-axial polydactyly. By the time of presentation to the ophthalmologist with visual failure, the extra finger has often been removed.

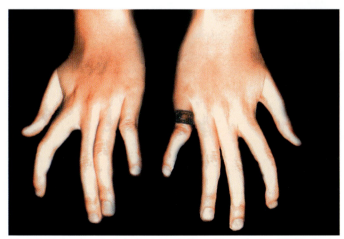

Fig. 118.4 **Arachnodactyly, frequently found in patients with Marfan's syndrome.**

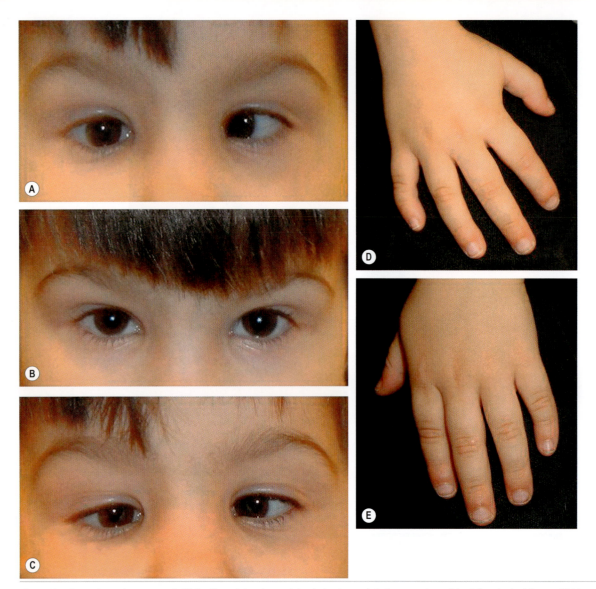

Fig. 118.6 Duane's syndrome type III. (A) Looking right: absent right abduction and slight narrowing of the left palpebral fissure. (B) No strabismus in the straight ahead position but there is bilateral horizontal gaze palsy, abnormal blinking, and tearing. (C) Looking left: absent left abduction and reduced right adduction with narrowing of the right palpebral fissure. (D,E) Bilateral clinodactyly.

References

1. Barry JS, Reddy MA. The association of an epibulbar dermoid and Duane syndrome in a patient with a SALL1 mutation (Townes-Brocks Syndrome). Ophthalmic Genet 2008; 29: 177–80.

2. Miller MT, Ventura L, Strömland K. Thalidomide and misoprostol: ophthalmologic manifestations and associations both expected and unexpected. Birth Defects Res A Clin Mol Teratol 2009; 85: 667–76.

3. Kargi HN, Koç F, Kargi E, et al. Bilateral Duane retraction syndrome associated with an extraordinary hand anomaly. Strabismus 2003; 2: 157–62.

4. Wright EM, O'Connor R, Kerr BA. Radial aplasia in CHARGE syndrome: a new association. Eur J Med Genet 2009; 52:239–41.

5. Alao MJ, Bonneau D, Holder-Espinasse M, et al. Oculo-dento-digital dysplasia: lack of genotype-phenotype correlation for GJA1 mutations and usefulness of neuro-imaging. Eur J Med Genet 2010; 53: 19–22.

6. Chiu YE, Drolet BA, Duffy KJ, Holland KE. A case of ankyloblepharon, ectodermal dysplasia, and cleft lip/palate syndrome with ectrodactyly: are the p63 syndromes distinct after all? Pediatr Dermatol 2011; 28: 15–9.

7. Larsen WJ. Development of the limbs. In: Larsen WJ, editor. Human Embryology, 2nd ed. New York: Churchill Livingstone; 1997: 311–44.

8. Jones, KL. In: Jones KL, editor. Smith's Recognizable Patterns of Human Malformation, 6th ed. Philadelphia: Elsevier Saunders; 2006.

Contact lenses for children

Lynne Speedwell

Parents are the key to successfully fitting children with contact lenses. Explain the reasons why a particular lens type is chosen as well as the risks and advantages of lens wear. With the available range of lenses it is rare to find a case that cannot safely be fitted, but the tolerance of the child or the visual limitations of the parent may make it preferable to avoid or postpone lens wear.

Lens insertion for a child

See Practical tips below.

Types of lenses

Any type of lens can be fitted. The choice of lens depends on the condition being fitted, when the lenses are going to be worn, and the limitations of each material, design, and parameter range (Table 119.1). Rigid lenses have a name for being uncomfortable, but two drops of a local anesthetic can overcome any problems. By the time the anesthetic has worn off, the lens has usually settled.

Hygiene

Stress the need for strict hygiene with a simple, effective, regimen. Solutions that could cause an allergic response should be avoided. Preservative-free solutions may be preferable. The rub and rinse step prior to lens soaking greatly decreases the risk of infection and is recommended by the FDA.[1]

High prescriptions and aphakia

Contact lenses provide a clearer field of vision than spectacles.[2] High myopes have better visual acuity with contact lenses than with spectacles, which reduce the image size. However, high hypermetropes and aphakes have better acuity in spectacles because the image size is larger.[2] This can lead to disappoint-

ment when aphakes with poor acuity are fitted with contact lenses.

High myopia

What lens to fit?

- Any lens type. Disposable lenses may be adequate in powers ≤ –20 D, otherwise tailor-made lenses are required.

Unilateral ametropia

Contact lenses reduce aniseikonia for both unilateral axial and refractive myopia,[3] but amblyopia is usually present and highly myopic eyes (over –9.00 D) do not usually respond well to patching;[4] only 32% of unilateral aphakes achieve vision greater than 0.6 logMAR[5] and, because binocularity is rare, children do not notice much difference when wearing a lens, making compliance poor. However, wearing a contact lens often reduces the angle of any strabismus.

Aphakia

Congenital cataracts

The number of young aphakes requiring contact lenses has decreased in recent years as more infants have intraocular lenses (IOLs) inserted. Many of them are likely to have microphthalmos or other anomalies. Pseudophakes also frequently need to be corrected with contact lenses.

Procedure for lens fitting

Carry out retinoscopy with the trial lens held close to the child's eye. Back vertex powers (BVPs) are usually greater than +20.00 D (the effective power of a +20.00 D trial lens with a back vertex distance (BVD) of 16 mm is +29.41 D at the cornea). Estimate the BVD and calculate the power of the contact lens then add +3.00 D overcorrection to provide a close focus for infants. The final BVP can be more than +40.00 DS.

Determine keratometry (K) and corneal diameter using a printed corneal gauge. Alternatively, fit the lenses empirically using the average radius of a neonate – 7.1 mm.[6]

Table 119.1 – Advantages and disadvantages of available lens types

Lens type	What is it?	Water content	Oxygen permeability (Dk ISO units)	Advantages	Disadvantages
RGP corneal	Rigid gas permeable with lens diameter < corneal diameter	0	Up to 163	Good vision Good for irregular corneas Low risk of infection Low risk of hypoxia	May be uncomfortable Can fall out Time consuming to fit Few tints available
RGP paralimbal	Rigid gas permeable with lens diameter > corneal diameter	0	Up to 163	Good vision Comfortable Stable Low risk of infection Low risk of hypoxia	Time consuming to fit Handling can be difficult Expensive
Soft (hydrogel)	Porous lens that absorbs water	38–75	Up to 32	Comfortable Easy to fit Stable Large range of disposables Can be tinted any color	Poorer vision Low Dk Can dry out Greater risk of infection Greater risk of hypoxia Rubbed out easily in infants
Silicone hydrogel (SiH)	Soft lens polymer includes silicone to increase oxygen permeability	Up to 58	Up to 105	Comfortable Easy to fit Limited tinting available	Poorer vision Greater risk of infection Rubbed out easily
Silicone rubber	Hydrophobic soft lens	0	340	Stable High Dk	Limited parameters Deposit easily Expensive
Hybrid lens	Lens with a rigid center and soft "skirt"	RGP = 0 Skirt = 27	75	Good vision Comfortable Stable	Handling can be difficult Expensive
Piggyback lenses	Rigid corneal lens worn over a soft or SiH lens	Rigid = 0 Soft/SiH various	Varies	Good vision Comfortable	Handling can be difficult Reduced oxygen
Scleral	Large lens covering the whole eye including the sclera	0	83	Good vision Stable Fit very irregular eyes Not rubbed out	Difficult to fit Some resistance to wearing large lens

During the first 2 years, refractive errors reduce, K readings and corneal diameters increase. Contact lens size alters to more adult values and the refraction is changed to distance correction with bifocal spectacles for near. Bifocal or multifocal contact lenses are difficult to fit accurately in high prescriptions.

Beware: excessive eye growth, indicated by a rapid myopic shift or corneal diameter increase, is suggestive of increased intraocular pressure.

What lens to fit?

- Soft or silicone hydrogel (SiH) lens with the back optic zone radius (BOZR) approximately 0.3 mm flatter than average K and total diameter ≥2 mm larger than corneal diameter. With microcornea, larger lenses will help center the lenticular portion over the pupil. These lenses are not available from most multinational companies so order tailor-made lenses from a smaller manufacturer. Infants may rub their lenses out and lenses are prone to dry out and mislocate or fall out.[7]
- Silicone rubber lenses do not dry out and are not easily rubbed out. They are fitted on flattest K and assessed using fluorescein. The high Dk (oxygen permeability) means that they can be worn overnight in emergencies. The steepest lens is 7.50 mm BOZR, too flat for many aphakes.

- Rigid lenses are rubbed out less often. They can be made of hyper Dk materials. Paralimbal lenses with a decreased edge lift will lessen the risk of the lens becoming dislodged.[7] The edge lift may need to be increased when the child is older.

Traumatic aphakia

Intraocular lenses usually give better acuity than contact lenses.[8] After trauma, lens insertion can be difficult; spectacles may be preferable.

What lens to fit?

- Rigid corneal lenses where there is corneal scarring to give the best acuity and least risk of neovascularization.
- Paralimbal or large diameter rigid corneal lenses (Fig. 119.1).
- Soft prosthetic lenses if there is aniridia, poor cosmesis and photophobia, but the low Dk increases the risk of hypoxia. Wearing time should be limited to a few hours a day.

Ectopia lentis or dislocated lens

In Marfan's syndrome, the corneas can be very flat, possibly flatter than 9.00 mm (37.5 D). One eye may be surgically

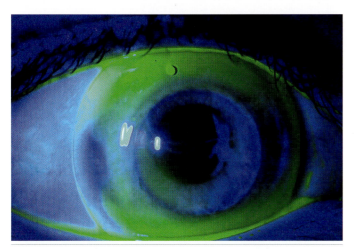

Fig. 119.1 **Paralimbal lens fitted to an aphakic eye with a scarred cornea.**

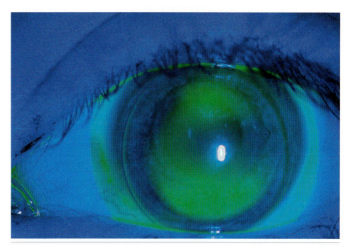

Fig. 119.3 **A piggyback lens system fitted to a scarred cornea resulting from blepharoconjunctivitis.** The eye was originally fitted with a rigid corneal lens but was uncomfortable so a soft lens is worn underneath.

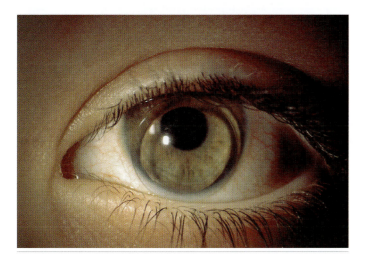

Fig. 119.2 **Aphakic RGP lens riding low on a flat cornea.**

rendered aphakic while the second eye might have a high degree of myopic astigmatism associated with the dislocated lens. Contact lenses provide the best chance of binocularity.

What lens to fit?

- Soft disposable spherical lenses together with spectacles correcting any astigmatism in either eye and a bifocal or multifocal lens for the aphakic eye.
- RGP corneal lenses may give better acuity but aphakic lenses are liable to sit low because the center of gravity of the lens is in front of the cornea. This problem is exacerbated on a flat cornea (Fig. 119.2).

Juvenile idiopathic uveitis

Patients often have band keratopathy and may need ongoing topical medication.

What lens to fit?

- Rigid lenses give the best acuity but are frequently not tolerated.
- Hydrogel or SiH lenses are more comfortable.

The author has found that lens intolerance presages a flare up of uveitis.

Visual development

Irregular corneas

Blepharoconjunctivitis can lead to keratitis and corneal scarring which affects acuity, possibly resulting in amblyopia. Spectacles are unlikely to give the optimum acuity but may be the only option until the acute infection has settled when contact lenses can be fitted.

What lens to fit?

- Paralimbal or large diameter rigid corneal lenses.
- Piggyback system if a rigid lens is not tolerated (Fig. 119.3).
- SiH lens designed for irregular corneas.
- Hybrid lenses.

Keratoconus

This usually presents after puberty, but may emerge earlier especially in those from the Indian subcontinent and Middle East.[9,10] Keratoconus is frequently associated with atopy which is increasing.[11] Many children rub their eyes and a topical mast cell stabilizer and antihistamine, such as olopatadine, should be prescribed to reduce irritation prior to lens fitting.

Once the disease has progressed to a stage where spectacles no longer correct the irregular astigmatism, contact lenses are fitted. Corneal cross-linking is now an option that may be considered (see Chapter 33).

What lens to fit?

- Soft keratoconus lenses, or rigid corneal lenses for early stages.
- Rigid corneal, paralimbal, piggyback, or hybrid lenses for later stages.
- Scleral lenses for very steep cones and keratoglobus.

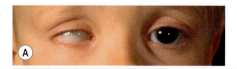
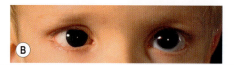
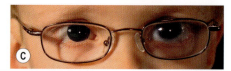

Fig. 119.4 (A) Child with a white eye resulting from failed drainage surgery to a buphthalmic aniridic eye. (B) The same child wearing a soft cosmetic contact lens. (C) The same child also wearing spectacles which enhances the appearance by taking the emphasis away from the eyes.

Keratoplasty

Once the sutures have been removed from a corneal graft, if there is a high residual refractive error, a contact lens should be considered. The optimum fit is often a matter of trial and error.

What lens to fit?

- Large paralimbal corneal lenses avoid pressure on the graft margin.
- Piggyback system.
- SiH tailor-made lenses or hybrid lenses. The latter have a relatively low Dk but the next generation of hybrid lenses with a SiH skirt may prove useful for these eyes.

Colored lenses

Disfigured eyes

Fitting a cosmetic or prosthetic contact lens to a child with a disfiguring eye condition can have a dramatic psychological effect on both the child and the parents. The health of a seeing eye is paramount and if there are any concerns that a lens may adversely affect the eye, it should not be fitted. In an eye with no vision, the priorities are appearance and comfort.

What lens to fit?

- Cosmetic soft lenses with a black pupil or a tinted iris to match the good eye and reduce the initial impact in a young child (Fig. 119.4).
- Prosthetic color matched or hand-painted soft lenses in an older child where good cosmesis is required.
- A cosmetic shell in a pthisical or grossly microphthalmic eye.
- If both eyes are unequally affected, the final result should be a symmetric appearance but if the better eye can safely wear a lens, fitting a pair of prosthetic lenses may provide the best cosmesis.

Photophobia

Each patient needs to find the tint which is most suitable for them so try various tints in spectacles before contact lens fitting. The section below gives a guide of what tint to try first but some patients prefer a neutral density gray tint as this should not alter color discrimination. Manufacturers can match a tint from a spectacle lens (or fragment) if it is sent with the contact lens prescription.

Albinism (see Chapter 40)

Albinos frequently have high degrees of with-the-rule astigmatism. In an older child or adult, spherical lenses may provide the same level of acuity as toric ones.

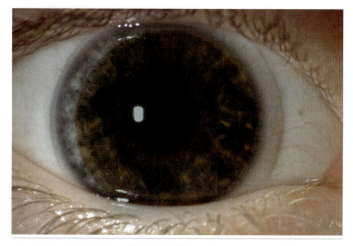

Fig. 119.5 A moderately dark tinted lens worn for achromatopsia or albinism. This lens can be worn the whole time and dark spectacles used outdoors over the top.

What devices or lens to fit?

- A cap or hat with a brim can be adequate if not too photophobic.
- Photochromic spectacles.
- Soft iris tinted lenses of the color and density required indoors (Fig. 119.5) and sunglasses or prescription photochromic glasses can be worn in conjunction when outside. Dark contact lenses will make a striking difference to the patient's appearance so warn them of this in advance.
- Opaque prosthetic iris lenses have a low Dk but may be necessary for some patients.

Achromatopsia (see Chapter 44)

What lens to fit?

- Soft tinted lenses
  - Complete achromatopsia: tinted glasses making patients stand out from their peers. A red tint filters short-wavelengths, allowing better light tolerance.[12]
  - Incomplete achromatopsia: a red–brown tint.
  - Blue cone monochromats: magenta tint.[13]

Aniridia (see Chapter 32)

Tinted lenses do not improve acuity in congenital aniridia but older children are sometimes more comfortable, especially if they have lens opacities. Care is needed when fitting lenses due to the corneal stem cell deficiency, as pannus is common.

In traumatic aniridia, photophobia is reduced and the cosmesis improved by fitting cosmetic contact lenses.

Coloboma

Tinted lenses may help older children. Color matching is easier if a tinted segment is incorporated (Fig. 119.6).

Nystagmus (see Chapter 89)

Contact lenses can reduce the amplitude of nystagmus,[14] perhaps dampened via feedback along the ophthalmic division of the trigeminal nerve leading to an improvement in visual acuity[15,16] and also by improving foveation. Both soft and rigid lenses can be fitted[17,18] but not all nystagmus patients benefit.[18]

Colored lenses

The Chromagen lens system of colored lenses improves color discrimination, in the Ishihara and D-15 color vision tests, in people with red–green color defects.[19] The system is not suitable for young children.

People with dyslexia sometimes wear tinted spectacles (without certain effect)[20] and these can be made up in contact lens form (see Chapter 61).

Occlusive contact lenses

Amblyopes uncompliant with adhesive patches can be fitted with opaque contact lenses, but they often do not work as they rub them out.[21] It is important to consider the risks to the phakic or better eye when an occlusive lens is fitted. Occlusive lenses also improve comfort in intractable diplopia.

Therapeutic or bandage lenses

Children with corneas outside normal dimensions may need a tailor-made therapeutic or bandage lenses (TCL) but most can be fitted with disposable lenses. Measure the less affected eye to decide which lens to fit. A local anesthetic may aid lens insertion.

A TCL can be inserted immediately after surgery for trauma to improve the comfort of the eye (Fig. 119.7).

For conditions such as Stevens-Johnson syndrome or neurotrophic corneal ulcers, scleral lenses may provide the best option.

Conditions more likely to affect children include the following.

Vernal keratoconjunctivitis (see Chapter 31)

Vernal keratoconjunctivitis is uncomfortable: corneal erosions can enlarge and a corneal plaque or shield ulcer can lead to amblyopia. The plaque may be removed surgically and a bandage lens inserted until the epithelium has regenerated.[22] Topical medication is used in conjunction with these lenses.

What lens to fit?

- SiH lenses with a high tensile modulus provide adequate oxygen and are less prone to being rubbed out by the rough tarsal conjunctiva.
- Large diameter hydrogel lenses (22 mm) 74% water content, fitted for extended wear, improve ocular comfort and reduce blepharospasm.[23]

Epidermolysis bullosa

Epidermolysis bullosa may include corneal scarring, symblepharon, conjunctival blistering, and exposure keratitis leading to perforation and corneal transplant.

What lens to fit?

- Medium water content SiH lenses with a low tensile modulus reduce pain and photophobia when the epithelium sloughs.
- Biomimetic hydrogel lens can be used in the short term if SiH does not improve comfort sufficiently.

Lens fitting may be required to visually rehabilitate an eye after a corneal transplant or cataract extraction. In all instances, extreme care is needed. Do not fit rigid lenses even where they are likely to improve acuity, because of the risk of abrasion.

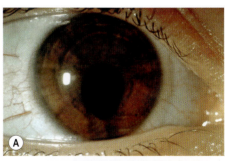
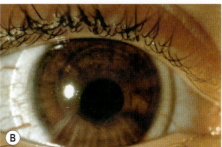

Fig. 119.6 (A) Iris coloboma. (B) The same eye wearing a tinted segment to cover the coloboma. This makes color matching easier.

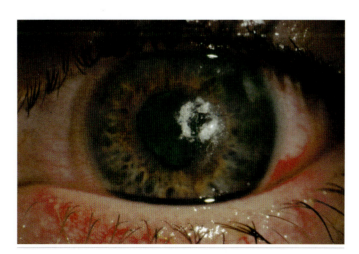

Fig. 119.7 Corneal perforation glued temporarily. A bandage lens is inserted to aid comfort whilst the glue is in situ.

However, scleral lenses may be necessary where there is risk of symblepharon.

Orthokeratology

Fitting lenses overnight to reduce myopia, orthokeratology, is becoming more popular as evidence of success is increasing[24] but overnight lens wear risks microbial keratitis.[25]

Conclusion

Fitting children with lenses can have a dramatic effect on their self-confidence. Many children are subjected to teasing and bullying if they wear high prescription spectacles or if their eyes are abnormal. Aiding the child in their visual and educational development by providing lenses can be extremely rewarding.

Practical tips

- Where possible, involve both parents when inserting or removing lenses. If only one parent is available, a grandparent or friend may help.
- Lens fitting and checking, and also daily insertion and removal can be carried out while the baby or young child is asleep.
- Insist on daily lens removal and cleaning. Warn parents of potential hazards and the importance of good hygiene.
- A child who will not allow fluorescein to be instilled is unlikely to permit lens insertion. Conversely, one who tolerates lid eversion with little fuss is usually unfazed by lenses.
- Vision does not develop better in contact lenses, but that there may be more chance of binocularity developing in cases of anisometropia.
- Do not fit lenses to please the parents except in rare instances (e.g. fitting a cosmetic lens to an unsightly eye). Explain why the child may be better to remain in spectacles.
- For an uncooperative child, make several short appointments, rather than one long one so they become familiar with both practitioner and surroundings.
- If lens insertion is too difficult, prescribe artificial tears to practice with and encourage an older child to touch the conjunctiva with a clean finger.
- Many 2-year-olds start to rebel against having lenses inserted. Prescribe spectacles and return to lenses later. Warn the parents early on that this may happen.
- Contact lenses should not be worn for swimming because of the risk of infection.
- Lenses should be removed or rewetting drops used when flying, as aircraft cabins are very dry.
- *If an eye shows any sign of irritation, the lens must be removed immediately and the eye examined by an eyecare practitioner. Lenses should be left out until the condition has been clear for 3 days.*

References

1. Sweeney D, Holden D, Evans B, et al. Best practice contact lens care: a review of the Asia Pacific Contact Lens Care Summit. Clin Exp Optometry 2009; 92: 78–9.
2. Ford M, Stone J, Rabbetts R. Optics and lens design. In: Phillips AJ, Speedwell L, editors. Contact Lenses, 5th ed. London: Elsevier; 2006: pp 508–13.
3. Winn B, Ackerley RG, Brown CA, et al. The superiority of contact lenses in correction of all anisometropia. Trans Br Contact Lens Assoc Conf 1986; 95–100.
4. Roberts CJ, Adams GG. Contact lenses in the management of high anisometropic amblyopia. Eye 2002; 16: 577–9.
5. Allen RJ, Speedwell L, Russell-Eggitt I. Long-term visual outcome after extraction of unilateral congenital cataracts. Eye 2010; 24, 1263–7.
6. Asbell, P, Chiang, B, Somers M, Morgan K. Keratometry in children. CLAO J 1990; 16 , 99–102.
7. Speedwell L. Paediatric contact lenses. In: Phillips AJ, Speedwell L, editors. Contact Lenses, 5th ed. London: Elsevier; 2006: 508–13.
8. Staffieri S, Ruddle JB, Mackey D. Rock, paper and scissors? Traumatic paediatric cataract in Victoria 1992–2006. Clin Exp Ophthalmol 2010; 38: 237–41.
9. Assiri AA, Yousuf BI, Quantock AJ, Murphy PJ. Incidence and severity of keratoconus in Asir province, Saudi Arabia. Br J Ophthalmol 2005; 89: 1403–6.
10. Georgiou T, Funnell CL, Cassels-Brown A, O'Connor R. Influence of ethnic origin on the incidence of keratoconus and associated atopic disease in Asians and white patients. Eye 2005; 18: 379–83.
11. Downs SH, Marks GB, Sporik R, et al. Continued increase in the prevalence of asthma and atopy. Arch Dis Child 2001; 84: 20–3.
12. Young RSL, Krefman RA, Fishman GA. Visual improvements with red tinted glasses in a patient with cone dystrophy. Arch Ophthalmol 1982; 100: 268–71.
13. Schomack MM, Brown WL, Siemson DW. The use of tinted contact lenses in the management of achromatopsia. Optometry 2007; 78: 17–22.
14. Sédan J. Nystagmus et correction précornéenne de la myopie forte. Bull Soc Ophthalmol Fr 1966; 66: 1053–8.
15. Abadi RV. Visual performances with contact lenses and congenital idiopathic nystagmus. Br J Physiol Optics 1979; 33: 32–7.
16. Dell'Osso LF, Traccis S, Abel LA, Erzurum SI. Contact lenses and congenital nystagmus. Clin Vision Sci 1998; 3:229–32.
17. Allen ED, Davies PD. Role of contact lenses in the management of congenital nystagmus. Br J Ophthalmol 1983; 67: 834–8.
18. Biousse V, Tusa RJ, Russell B, et al. The use of contact lenses to treat visually symptomatic congenital nystagmus. J Neurol Neurosurg Psychiatry 2004; 75: 314–6.
19. Swarbrick HA, Nguyen P, Nguyen T, Pham P. The ChromaGen contact lens system: colour vision test results and subjective responses. Ophthalmol Physiol Opt 2001; 21: 182–96.
20. Huang J, Zong X, Wilkins A, et al. fMRI evidence that precision ophthalmic tints reduce cortical hyperactivation in migraine. Cephalagia 2011; 31: 925–36.
21. Joslin CE, McMahon T, Kaufman LM. The effectiveness of occluder contact lenses in improving occlusion compliance in patients that have failed traditional occlusion therapy. Optometry Vision Sci 2002; 7: 376–80.
22. Solomon A, Zamir E, Levartovsky S, Frucht-Pery J. Surgical management of corneal plaques in vernal keratoconjunctivitis: a clinicopathologic study. Cornea 2004; 23: 608–12.
23. Quah SA, Hemmerdinge C, Nicholson S, Kaye SB. Treatment of refractory vernal ulcers with large-diameter bandage contact lenses. Eye Contact Lens: Sci Clin Pract 2006; 32: 245–7.
24. Walline JJ, Jones LA, Sinnott LT. Corneal reshaping and myopia progression. Br J Ophthalmol 2009; 93: 1181–5.
25. Hsaio CH, Yeung L, Ma DH, et al. Pediatric microbial keratitis in Taiwanese children: a review of hospital cases. Arch Ophthalmol 2007; 125: 603–9.

I just cannot keep the patch on!

Chris Timms

The treatment of amblyopia forms a significant part of the workload of any pediatric eye clinic. Most commonly, it is associated with strabismus and/or anisometropia, but may be the sequelae of congenital glaucoma, ptosis, and congenital cataract. The standard treatment of occlusion of the better eye is a safe and effective treatment for amblyopia. An effective patching regime can improve the visual acuity in the amblyopic eye to within one line of the vision in the better eye in 89% of cases, but as practicing orthoptists and ophthalmologists can attest patching is only successful if the parents or carers of the patient can apply the patch and keep it on for the required period of time each day.

The critical period for development emphasizes the importance of early diagnosis and treatment of amblyopia to produce better results. Treatment of amblyopia after 8 or 9 years of age is unlikely to be successful. The earlier treatment is started the better results will be, and it will be achieved with less patching than when the patient is older. Therefore, we ask parents to patch the better eye in toddlers and small children. We know patching is difficult, even unpleasant, for the child and the parent because it is a new sensation for a young child, being made to wear a sticky patch and forced to use the eye with poor vision. Yet, most children get used to the patch quickly, particularly once the difference between the amblyopic eye and the better eye is lessened and the vision improves. The major improvement in vision occurs within the first 6 weeks of patching – so this very difficult period is short-lived. Improving compliance with patching must involve detailed information to the parent or carer about the need for the patch: the reason why patching must be carried out whilst the child is young and as many tips as possible for helping them to get the child to wear the patch. We also need to admit just how difficult it may be! It is important, when possible, to convey this information to the child and include the child in decisions about the treatment. Patching is easier if everyone, the child, parent and professional, are working together. It is vital that the parents know the reason for patching, i.e. to improve the visual acuity in the amblyopic eye and not to improve the appearance of the squint. Many parents will give up if they cannot see an immediate change in the cosmetic appearance. Regular reviews in the clinic to monitor progress is a great encouragement to both patient and parent. This support from the clinician is vital to successful patching. "Patch clubs" where children who are having difficulty complying with their treatment

are invited to fun, supervised, activities whilst wearing their patches may help. Websites encouraging children to wear a patch whilst playing games are also helpful (e.g. http://www.eyesite.nhs.uk; Fig. 120.1).

Written instructions and information leaflets aimed at children and adults are very effective in improving compliance.[1] Parents may keep a written record of how much patching is achieved each day. Older children can help with this record keeping by making a logbook or star chart. This is to assist the progress of the treatment, rewarding the child and not to be used critically. Parents must know that we understand that patching is difficult as they are the key to success.[2] The professional must be supportive and not judgmental, in much the same way as good compliance with patching should be

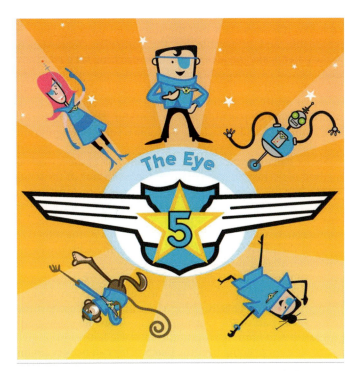

Fig. 120.1 The Eye Five. This is an internet club for children who have to patch. If they are internet-connected, it makes them feel they are not unusual and are connected with others who patch (http://www.eyesite.nhs.uk).

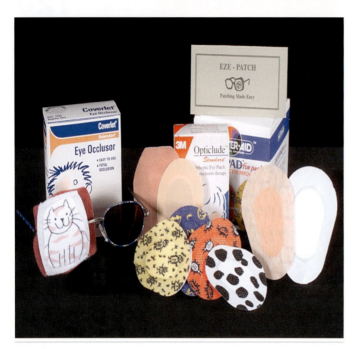

Fig. 120.2 Patches. There are many patches and they are available in most countries. They can be made simply by cutting a wide sheet of sticky tape to an appropriate shape with a non-sticky material attached where the eye, lids, and brow are. Commercially available patches vary in the stickiness of the material used and size. Some include small rewards or encouragements for the child or a chart for the parents or child to enter the amounts patched.

rewarded by the parent with a treat or small gift rather than poor compliance be punished.

There is little evidence of the dose–effect relationship of occlusion, but studies of dose monitored patching[3] show that it is the total amount of patching over a period of time that achieves the result rather than the exact time the patch is on each day. It is important that the amount of patching given is reasonable and achievable for the particular circumstance. Some parents like the idea of full-time patching for a relatively short period of time; others prefer shorter periods each day, knowing it will take longer to reach the required improvement in visual acuity. It is vital to explain that in certain circumstances too much patching may be harmful. The risk of occlusion amblyopia and intractable diplopia is small but significant after the age of 7 or 8 years.

Sticky patches worn on the face (Fig. 120.2) are the ideal method of occlusion, particularly at the beginning of the treatment when the vision in the amblyopic eye is poor. Most bright children will peep over the glasses if the patch is stuck to the lens. There are several commercial companies producing appropriately sticky patches. For most children, the adhesive used on the patch will not cause any difficulty with the facial skin other than a mild temporary redness when the patch is taken off which can be alleviated with face cream. However, if the patch causes significant skin irritation, it is prudent to change the brand of patch. Using a hole punch to remove some of the sticky part of the patch may help. There are some cloth patches that fit entirely around the spectacle lens to minimize the chances of peeping over the patch. They can be very useful if there has been improvement in the vision after wearing a sticky patch: a "reward" for doing well! In the maintenance

phase of treatment a frosted lens or patch on the glasses is enough to ensure that the better eye is disadvantaged.

Most clinicians have a list of their favorite ways of ensuring that recalcitrant patients comply with treatment! Here are a few things we have found that help:

- Choosing the right time to patch is important, not for example when the child is tired. For older children, patching is much more effective when combined with close work. Often the teachers at school or nursery will undertake some of the patching, relieving the parents of the stress of having to continually enforce the occlusion regime. Grandparents may also be very useful in supervising some of the patching.
- The patch sticks better to grease-free skin; clean the skin before the patch is put on.
- If the child pulls the patch off easily, use a stickier patch for a week or so until he gets used to patching.
- Sticky tape over the top of the patch means it takes longer to take the patch off, thus giving the parent time to distract the child before he manages to take the patch off.
- Several devices can be used to prevent the child being able to manipulate his fingers to take the patch off. In a young child a sock pulled up to the elbows over the hands especially if he wears a sweater over the top may be useful. Gloves don't work as well as they are too easy to remove. For a slightly older child, sticky tape on the tips of the thumb and first two fingers of both hands make it very difficult to take the patch off.
- Splints applied to the elbows will allow the child to play with his toys but he will be unable to bend his elbows to get to the patch. These are available commercially or can be made by the physiotherapy department in the hospital. Elbow restraints can be improvised by taping a cardboard tube to the upper and forearm or by using swimming arm bands inflated over the elbows. These restraints do not need to be worn for very long, the child soon realizes that the patch is better than the restraints! They also emphasize to the parents the importance of treating amblyopia. If these mechanical restraints fail, as a last resort some clinics bring children into hospital daily for a few days, where the clinic, nursing, or play staff can supervise the patching.
- If it proves impossible to keep the patch on, it is possible to penalize the better eye with a cycloplegic drop. The PEDIG study showed that in some cases a daily drop of atropine worked as well as patching.[4]

References

1. Newsham D. A randomised controlled trial of written information: the effect on parental non-concordance with occlusion therapy. Br J Ophthalmol 2002; 86: 787–91.
2. Newsham D. Parental non-concordance with occlusion therapy. Br J Ophthalmol 2000; 84: 957–62.
3. Stewart CE, Fielder AR, Stephens DA, Mosely MJ. Design of the Monitored Occlusion Treatment of Amblyopia Study (MOTAS). Br J Ophthalmol 2002; 86: 915–9.
4. Pediatric Eye Disease Investigator Group. A randomized trial of atropine versus patching for treatment of moderate amblyopia in children. Arch Ophthalmol 2002; 120: 268–78.

SECTION 7
Common practical problems in
a pediatric ophthalmology
and strabismus practice

CHAPTER 121

Helping visually impaired children to sleep

James E Jan

Prevalence of sleep difficulties

Sleep disturbances are increasingly common in Western societies due to changing lifestyles. In healthy children, these sleep difficulties tend to be transient and respond well to sleep hygiene techniques (environmental and behavioral promotion of healthy sleep). In contrast, in children with neurodevelopmental disabilities (including visual impairment) they tend to be more frequent, persistent, and severe and may not respond to sleep hygiene interventions.[1] Although, over a hundred different sleep disorders can occur in childhood, circadian rhythm sleep disorders (CRSD) are by far the most common,[2] followed by sleep disordered breathing,[3] parasomnias,[4] and restless legs syndrome.[5] Most of these sleep disorders present differently from those seen in adults.

Adverse consequences of impaired sleep

During the last 20–30 years major advances have been made in understanding sleep physiology. Sleep is a vital restorative neurological function. It is not surprising that severe, persistent sleep deprivation can lead to gradual loss of neurons in various areas of the brain, but more so in the frontal lobes where executive cognitive functions are generated. The behavioral manifestations of inadequate sleep include inattentiveness, aggressiveness, hyperactivity, impulsivity, and mood changes. Cognitive manifestations are impaired comprehension, deficits in reasoning, and memory formation. School failure is common. Health disturbances are also frequent such as impaired immunologic defenses resulting in more frequent infections and even cancer, cardiovascular difficulties, obesity and endocrine disturbances, tendency to accidents, and increased suicide rates among teenagers.[2]

Causes of sleep disturbances

Excessive or inappropriately timed light exposure, leading to CRSD, is the most common cause of sleep difficulties today, which suggests that increasing attention should be paid to environmental light pollution. The retina via a group of ganglion cells has a monosynaptic input into the suprachiasmatic nuclei of the anterior hypothalamus. These paired nuclei, by modulating pineal melatonin production, have a powerful regulatory influence on a large number of circadian rhythms in the body, which include sleep/wake cycles. The final outcome is that light inhibits pineal melatonin production while the absence of light promotes it. Visually impaired children can have a special type of CRSD resulting from their ocular visual loss. Total absence of light input into the hypothalamus results in free-running sleep/wake rhythm. This is rare in children because total blindness is infrequent. In the absence of light, the suprachiasmatic nuclei begin to promote rhythmicity according to their own endogenous neuronal rhythms. These are usually longer than 24 hours. Therefore, the pineal melatonin production is progressively delayed every day and with it the sleep/wake patterns. The only treatment which can stop this persistent shifting is timed melatonin administration given at bedtime.[6] In contrast to ocular visual impairment, children with cortical visual impairments (see Chapter 57) do not exhibit free-running sleep/wake rhythms because the environmental light input via the retina into the hypothalamus is preserved.

Cognitive processes via the cerebral cortex and the thalamus also have strong regulatory inputs into the suprachiasmatic nuclei and pineal melatonin production. The perception of environmental changes and responses to it very much influence human sleep patterns. Thus, when the brain functions are severely disturbed, the prevalence of sleep difficulties may be as high as 80–100%. These sleep disturbances may present as difficulties falling asleep, frequent nocturnal awakenings from minutes to hours, early morning awakenings, day/night reversals, or advanced sleep onset. They are classified under CRSD because the problem is an inability to sleep when dictated by the environment. In response to environmental changes, the brain regulates sleep patterns by modulating pineal melatonin production. Since inadequate or inappropriately timed melatonin production is the underlying cause of CRSD, appropriately timed melatonin replacement therapy can be a very effective treatment.

Management of sleep difficulties

When persistent or recurring sleep difficulties are noted, it is essential to identify the underlying cause because it is only then that appropriate treatments can be chosen. Family physicians and a number of different specialists can deal with the management of many sleep problems, but increasingly multidisciplinary sleep clinics are becoming established for children. A detailed sleep history and a physical examination are necessary. The caregivers are often requested to document their child's sleep in a diary for 7–10 days. Most sleep clinics use wrist actigraphs that record limb movements and, therefore, more objectively identify periods of sleep (inactivity) and wakefulness (activity) than parental logs. Polysomnography, nocturnal video recordings, and neurologic and metabolic tests are occasionally needed for the diagnosis of CRSD and other sleep difficulties.

Sleep disturbances are not an inevitable part of neurodevelopmental disabilities (including visual impairment) and in most instances they can be treated. They must never be ignored. Behavioral, educational, and other types of interventions are ineffective without correcting severe sleep disturbances. Many physicians have received inadequate training in sleep medicine and they tend to overprescribe hypnotics. Persistent use of hypnotics is not recommended for children because of the high frequency of adverse events and because their benefits are usually short lived.

The treatment of CRSD usually starts with the introduction of sleep promotion techniques.[7] For children who do not have significant neurodevelopmental disabilities, modification of sleep environment and sleep habits usually work very well. For the disabled, the sleep hygiene interventions must be individually tailored to their cognitive strengths and weaknesses.

However, with increasing loss of cognition, sleep hygiene is harder to enforce, less effective and may even be ineffective. Melatonin replacement therapy is now recommended by the American Academy of Sleep Medicine for the treatment of CRSD. It is simple and highly effective, lacks adverse effects, and acts quickly. Melatonin is not addictive, does not conflict with other medications, and tolerance does not develop.[2]

References

1. Wasdell MB, Jan JE, Bomben MM, et al. A randomized, placebo-controlled trial of controlled release melatonin treatment of delayed sleep phase syndrome and impaired sleep maintenance in children with developmental disabilities. J Pineal Res 2008; 44: 57–64.
2. Jan JE, Wasdell MB, Reiter RJ, et al. Melatonin therapy of pediatric sleep disorders: recent advances, why it works, who are the candidates and how to treat. Curr Pediatr Rev 2007; 3: 214–224.
3. Gozal D, Kheirandish-Gozal L. New approaches to the diagnosis of sleep-disordered breathing in children. Sleep Med 2010; 11: 708–713.
4. Owens JA, Witmans M. Sleep problems. Curr Probl Pediatr Adolesc Health Care 2004; 34:154–179.
5. Picchietti MA, Picchietti DL. Restless legs syndrome and periodic limb movement disorder in children and adolescents. Semin Pediatr Neurol 2008; 15: 91–99.
6. Lewy AJ, Emens JS, Lefler BJ, et al. Melatonin entrains free-running blind people according to a physiological dose-response curve. Chronobiol Int 2005; 22: 1093–1106.
7. Jan JE, Owens JA, Weiss MD, et al. Sleep hygiene for children with neurodevelopmental disabilities. Pediatrics 2008; 122: 1343–1350.

How should an ophthalmologist tell if a child's development is normal?

Alison Salt

Many eye conditions are associated with developmental disorders. Therefore, the ophthalmologist needs to recognize when to make a referral for an opinion about a child's development.

While a pediatric ophthalmologist is not expected to be as expert in general history taking and examination as a pediatrician, it is essential that he/she understands the rudiments of examining children from a general developmental perspective. It is also important that the ophthalmologist is familiar and confident handling children of all ages. The confidence of parents is greatly enhanced by an ophthalmologist who is confident handling babies and children.

A close collaborative working relationship between the pediatric ophthalmologist and the pediatrician will be essential when there are developmental concerns.

Concerns may arise about children both with normal vision and with severe visual impairment. Children with visual impairment may develop more slowly than their sighted peers. Their progress should be judged against developmental norms appropriate to their level of visual impairment.

The first step is to take a careful history. Remember that parents are usually the best observers of their child's development and their concerns should be taken seriously.

Risk factors

Some common risk factors associated with developmental problems should be enquired about. These include:

- Pregnancy factors: infection (especially cytomegalovirus, toxoplasmosis, and rubella), consumption of drugs or alcohol, smoking, hypertension, and exposure to irradiation.
- Health of the fetus: poor growth, reduced fetal movements, or reduced or excessive amniotic fluid.
- Delivery: the need for resuscitation and signs of significant encephalopathy in the infant, such as significant drowsiness, poor feeding, and seizures soon after birth suggest that damage was sustained around the time of birth. If no such signs are present, the birth is unlikely to have a causal relationship to later developmental problems. A difficult delivery accounts for few subsequent neurological and developmental

problems, although parents often worry about difficulties that they experienced.[1]
- Premature birth (<37 weeks' gestation): gestational age is strongly correlated with the risk of subsequent developmental problems. When considering whether a premature child is reaching developmental milestones it is appropriate to take account of gestational age up to the age of 2 years.
- Serious infection of the central nervous system: meningitis or encephalitis especially in the early weeks or months of life.
- Jaundice in the first days of life: prolonged and severe jaundice (>340 µmol/liter).
- Conditions of the eye that are known to be associated with developmental problems.
- As there are a number of conditions that affect both vision and hearing, always enquire about hearing concerns. Delay in speech development should always lead to referral for assessment of hearing.

Developmental milestones in the fully sighted child

Next, consider whether a child is reaching their expected developmental milestones.

Some key milestones are described in Table 122.1. These are based on normative data from Sheridan,[2] Egan,[3] and the revised Denver developmental screening test.[4] This table shows the average age at which the majority of children achieve particular milestones.

Parents will usually remember the age their child reached major developmental milestones – independent sitting and walking, the development of first words, and when their child was speaking clearly.[5]

Development is generally considered under the following domains:

- Mobility and coordination of movements (gross motor).
- Eye–hand coordination (fine motor).
- Speech and language.
- Personal/social skills.
- Vision.
- Hearing.

Table 122.1 – Key developmental milestones in the fully sighted child

Age	Gross motor	Eye–hand coordination	Speech and language	Personal/social	Vision
4–6 weeks	Pulled to sit – head lags Held sitting – curved back	Hands fisted	Vocalizes not crying	Social smile by 6 weeks	Looks at mother's face Follows dangling ball through 90°
3 months	Prone lifts head and chest Pulled to sit – little head lag Held sitting – lumbar curve only Held standing – sags at knees	Hands open Hands together in midline Holds rattle briefly	Different vowel sounds	Laughs Social response to nearby friendly faces	Follows dangling ball through 180° Horizontal and later vertically Converges on near object
4–5 months	Pulled to sit – no head lag Rolls prone to supine – then supine to prone Bears some weight on legs	Reaches for objects			
6 months	Prone lifts head and chest on extended arms Supine lifts head Sits with support – back straight Held standing – legs are straight and takes weight	Takes toys to mouth Passes toy from hand to hand Uses whole hand in palmer grasp Holds two cubes	Vocalizes tunefully single and double syllables	Socially alert and curious Plays peek-a-boo	Visually attentive for near and far Watches small rolling balls at 5+ feet Full conjugate eye movements
9 months	Sits alone for 10–15 minutes Stands holding on Can get to sitting from lying down Stands momentarily (from 10 months)	Uses index finger approach to objects Immature pincer grasp (between thumb and index finger but not using finger tips) Throws toys to the ground deliberately Looks for fallen toy (even when falls out of sight) Removes object from container	Babbles in long repetitive strings of syllables Situational understanding developing	Feeds self with biscuit Distinguishes strangers from familiars and may be wary	
12 months	Walks holding on to furniture Stands alone well Crawls rapidly Walks hands held	Uses a neat mature pincer grasp Casts repeatedly Retrieves toy hidden in view under cup or cloth Puts object into container	Jargons with conversational cadence Indicates wants (e.g. by pointing) Knows and turns to own name Understands simple commands, e.g. give me and wave "bye bye"	Holds spoon but doesn't use Drinks from cup with help Cooperates in dressing	Sustained visual interest for near and far
18 months	Walks well (75% by 14 months) Stoops without overbalancing	Builds a tower of three cubes Spontaneous scribble Looks at pictures in book and turns pages Tips object out of container	6 to 20 recognizable words and understands many more Shows body parts on request	Uses a spoon Drinks from cup Copies domestic activities Removes some clothing, e.g. simple shoes/socks	

Table 122.1 – *Continued*

Age	Gross motor	Eye–hand coordination	Speech and language	Personal/social	Vision
2 years	Walks up and down stairs two feet per step Runs Jumps on the spot Throws a ball overhand Kicks a ball	Builds tower of 6 cubes Imitates circular scribble (copies a circle by 2.5 years)	Uses 50 or more words Puts two or more words together Much of speech may not be intelligible Asks "what" questions	Uses spoon well Lifts and replaces cup without spilling	Letter matching test possible (BEO) from 2.5 years in 80%
3 years	Stands on one foot momentarily	Builds tower of 9 cubes	Large vocabulary (200+ words) Speech may be unintelligible to strangers	Can undress with fastenings undone	
3.5 years	Hops on one foot	Copies bridge of 3 cubes and copies the drawing of a cross	Uses personal pronouns, regular plurals, and most prepositions Knows some colors Concepts of size and number developing Asks "Who" and "Why" questions	Dresses with some help	
4 years	Balances on one foot for 5 seconds Goes up and down stairs adult fashion	Mature tripod grasp of pencil Draws a man 3 parts	Speech mature and intelligible Knows full name	Dresses without supervision and can manage buttons	Completes letter matching task with each eye
5 years	Can skip on alternate feet	Draws a man 6 parts Copies a square (by 5.5 years a triangle)	Comprehension of abstract meaning and verbal reasoning Asks "Why," "When," and "How" questions	Understands the need for rules and cooperates with other children	

All cells equal averages for age that a milestone is achieved.
Based on Sheridan, Egan, and/or achieved by >50% on Denver Developmental Screening Test.

Remember, however, these areas are fundamentally connected and progress or deficit in one area is likely to have an impact on another.

When should delay in milestones cause concern?

Box 122.1 provides a list of potential developmental warning signs that will help the clinician to recognize when to be concerned about delay in a particular milestone and therefore request further assessment.

Variation in patterns of normal development

Some patterns of normal development are associated with delay in milestones but may not be associated with pathology. A good example is the child who does not crawl but moves around on his/her bottom. This is known as bottom shuffling or scooting and is seen in almost 10% of children. This pattern of prewalking mobility is usually benign and is often familial. Children with this pattern of development on average achieve independent walking at around 18 months but this may be as late as 25 months in a minority.[6] However, this pattern may also be seen in children with neurologic disorders, e.g. cerebral palsy or muscular dystrophy. Therefore, if delay in walking is

beyond 18 months or if there are other concerns, a further opinion should be sought.

The history is key to providing warning signs of developmental problems; Table 122.1 and Box 122.1 are designed to provide guidance on expected developmental stages and to alert the ophthalmologist to the need for further assessment by a pediatrician.

Development in children with visual impairment

Visual impairment has an impact on all areas of development especially when impairment is severe and more so when a child has only light perception or no vision. Parents play a major role in promoting the development of their infants. However, when their child is diagnosed as visually impaired, they need support not only to come to terms with the shock and sadness associated with the knowledge of their child's visual impairment but also to understand how to help their child learn about their world.

The early months are critical in the development of the child's drive to learn. If their natural interest and responsiveness is not stimulated early, it becomes increasingly difficult to

Box 122.1

Developmental warning signs

At any age	Excessive hypotonia (floppiness) or hypertonia (stiffness)
	Marked asymmetry of posture, movements, or muscle tone
	Persistent hand fisting
	Persistent tremor, clonus, jerky movements
	Tendency to push head back and arch body
	Parental concern about hearing or vision
0–3 months	Feeding problems – weak suck
4 weeks	Not fixing on mother's face
	No response to sound
3 months	Not smiling responsively
	Not fixing and following
	Inability to hold toy placed in hand
4 months	Poor head control (head lag when pulled to sit)
	Not lifting head up supine or chest up in prone
	Not engaging hands in midline
	Persistence of infantile reflexes
After 4 months	Grasp reflex
After 5 months	ATNR (asymmetric tonic neck reflex)
	Moro (startle reflex)
	Stepping
6 months	Persistent hand regard
	Not showing interest in surroundings
	Little interest in sounds or does not turn head to sound
7 months	Not reaching, transferring, or taking toys to mouth
9 months	Not sitting steadily unsupported
	Lack of social engagement
10 months	Not using tuneful repetitive babble
12 months	Not mobile on the floor
	No pincer grip
	Showing hand preference before 12 months
	No response to sound
	Has not babbled or has stopped babbling
	Does not participate in vocal interactive play
18 months	Persistence of casting or mouthing
	Does not understand or respond when familiar objects are named
	Showing no interest in communicating his needs through pointing or gesture or attempts at words
24 months	Unsteady walking, not running
	Not pushing or pulling toys
	No constructive or imaginative play
	Poor social interaction
2.5 years	Not using 50+ words
	Not joining 2 words together (e.g. "look bus")
	Does not understand simple commands (e.g. "sit down")
3 years	Unable to throw/kick ball without falling
	Cannot generally be understood by strangers
	Does not use 4 word phrases ("I want a big biscuit")
4 years	Poor vocabulary or sentence construction
	Speech not fully intelligible (except for a few minor articulation difficulties)
4.5 years	Unable to stand on one leg for 3–5 seconds
	Cannot follow stories or a sequence of commands

promote. It is essential that parents receive early support and education about how to help their child.[7] In the UK each Education Authority has an advisory service for children with visual impairment and in most areas a specialist peripatetic teacher will visit the family at home.

The impact of severe visual impairment on development means that children will not always follow the same developmental trajectory as their fully sighted peers. It is important that these children are seen by a pediatrician experienced in assessment of the development of children with visual impairment. Norms for the development of "blind" and "partially sighted" children were produced by Reynell and Zinkin.[8] They recognized that developmental scales for sighted infants were inappropriate for visually impaired infants. While these scales remain the best available there is a need for improved developmental scales that fulfill contemporary rehabilitative and educational aspirations and meet scientific requirements of modern developmental tests.

Below, some of the key developmental milestones for the blind infant are set out and highlight the need for early intervention.

Motor development

Poor vision constrains development of motor skills through a number of complex and interacting mechanisms,[9] including:

1. Reduced drive or motivation to move and explore.
2. Poor realization of the potential functional capacity of hands for reaching and legs for mobility.
3. Reduced opportunity to observe and practice movements.
4. Delay in understanding of concepts such as permanence of people and objects and the floor as a concrete base and continuous surface.
5. Integration of vestibular and proprioceptive sensory inputs to develop postural reactions to changes in position.
6. Fear of moving beyond a secure base.

Blind babies, therefore, show variable delays in motor development with delay in achieving sitting and becoming mobile. Independent walking may not be achieved until 2 years or later.[10]

Exploration of different textures

At 3 to 6 months both the sighted and blind infant begins to actively explore objects in the hands and mouth. The sighted infant will be motivated by sensory feedback and move on by 6 months to active exploration of shape and texture. The blind infant may not explore in this way until 2 to 3 months later. It is important to introduce different shapes and textures early as some children may become alarmed by these different sensations and become oversensitive to certain sensations sometimes referred to as "tactile defensive." They refuse to touch new objects and textures and become distressed if these are introduced. This will severely limit their learning through more complex play and manipulation.

Speech and language/communication

Blind children tend to develop first words later than sighted children. The content of these words tends to emphasize familiar people's names and actions. Social phrases are initially imitated as a whole and then used in context. Expressive language on average lags behind sighted peers by 2 to 3 months and comprehension may lag behind expressive language. The first meaningful word is usually associated with understanding of a simple request ("give me the cup"), but in the blind child there may be a 9-month lag in comprehension of simple phrases. In other blind children first words may not appear until age 2 years.[11]

Sound localization

Understanding where sounds come from requires the integration of hearing, vision, and recognition that sound implies the presence of an object. This is usually integrated with reach at ear level by 5 months, but not above ear level until 8 to 9 months. Blind babies need to be actively taught this skill and without this teaching delay may be even more marked. Parents need to guide their child's arm toward the sound initially in front of them and then in different directions.[7]

Developmental vulnerability

Thirty-one percent of children with profound visual impairment (awareness of light or light-reflecting objects only) were found to be at risk of stasis or regression in cognitive development during the second year of life.[12-14] In this group, disordered social communication was most prominent; this was not specific to any particular visual disorder and was seen in children with a number of different diagnoses. There are likely to be a number of interrelated factors that lead to this vulnerability including underlying structural brain anomalies and genetic factors. In addition, there are the challenges of development in the second year of life including the development of attention control, shared attention, and independence. This highlights the need for intensive support and monitoring of development in these developmentally vulnerable children. The presence of even limited form vision may be protective.

In some visual conditions there is potential for promoting the visual performance and a carefully designed visual promotion program has been shown to be effective in a randomized control trial.[15] This emphasizes that even an improvement from light awareness to limited form vision will have significant benefits.

Severe visual impairment is a developmental crisis that requires experienced developmental and visual management as soon as possible after the diagnosis. It requires close working between the ophthalmologic and developmental teams.

References

1. Stanley F, Blair E, Alberman E. Cerebral Palsies: Epidemiology and Causal Pathways. Clin Dev Med No. 151. MacKeith Press; 2000.
2. Sheridan M. The Developmental Progress of Infants and Young Children, No. 102. London: HMSO; 1975.
3. Egan DF, Illingworth RS, MacKeith RC. Developmental screening 0–5 years. Clin Dev Med 1969; 30.
4. Denver Developmental Screening Test. The Test Agency Ltd, High Wycombe, Bucks, UK.
5. Capute AJ, Shapiro BK, Palmer FB, et al. Normal gross motor development: the influences of race, sex and socioeconomic status. Dev Med Child Neurol 1985; 27: 635–43.
6. Robson P. Prewalking locomotor movements and their use in predicting standing and walking. Child Care Health Dev 1984; 10: 317–30.
7. Dale N, Salt A. Early support developmental journal for children with visual impairment: the case for a new developmental framework for early intervention. Child Care Health Dev 2007; 33(6): 684–90.
8. Reynell J, Zinkin P. New procedures for developmental assessment of young children with severe visual handicaps. Child Care Health Dev 1979; 1: 61–9.
9. Sonksen P, Levitt S, Kitsinger M. Identification of constraints acting on motor development in young visually disabled children and principles of remediation. Child Care Health Dev 1984; 10: 273–86.
10. Fraiberg S. Insights from the Blind. London: Souvenir Press; 1977.
11. McConachie H, Moore V. Early expressive language of severely visually impaired children. Dev Med Child Neurol 1994; 36: 230–40.
12. Cass HD, Sonksen PM, McConachie HR. Developmental setback in severe visual impairment. Arch Dis Child 1994; 70: 192–6.
13. Sonksen P, Dale N. Visual impairment in infancy: impact on neurodevelopment and neurobiological processes. Dev Med Child Neurol 2002; 44: 782–91.
14. Absoud M, Parr JR, Salt SY, Dale NJ. Developing a schedule to identify social communication difficulties and autism spectrum disorder in young children with visual impairment. Dev Med Child Neurol 2011; 53: 285–8.
15. Sonksen PM, Petrie A, Drew KJ. Promotion of visual development of severely visually impaired babies: evaluation of a developmentally based programme. Dev Med Child Neurol 1991; 33: 320–35.

SECTION 7
Common practical problems in
a pediatric ophthalmology
and strabismus practice

CHAPTER **123**

What is a sensible screening program in paediatric ophthalmology?

John R Ainsworth

Why screening is important in pediatric ophthalmology

Young children do not report reliably changes in vision to one or both of their eyes. There are a limited range of professionals who are able to perform an eye examination on children, and this number is possibly reducing. For these reasons many pediatric eye disorders present late. A need for screening is recognized and has led to the detection by screening of over 50% of pediatric eye conditions affecting the child's sight, usually by pediatricians or family doctors.[1]

What is screening?

"Screening is the systematic application of a test or inquiry to identify individuals at sufficient risk of a specific disorder to benefit from further investigation or direct preventive action, among persons who have not sought medical attention on account of symptoms of that disorder".[2] Screening detects individuals within a population who have a disease before they develop signs or symptoms. Alternatively, screening can be used to detect a risk factor for future or asymptomatic disease.

When is screening appropriate?

Criteria for the value and feasibility of screening programs were created by the World Health Organization (Box 123.1)[3,5]. These fall into groups:

Is screening feasible and acceptable to those being screened? (criteria 4,5,6). A test is required that can be performed prior to the development of symptomatic disease that might detect a risk factor for the disease or allow diagnosis at a symptomless stage. The test requires sufficient sensitivity and specificity to be useful, validated, and safe.

Is the disease understood, is treatment possible, is there consensus on who to treat and how, and are facilities in place for investigation and treatment? (2,3,7,8) Understanding of and consensus on the natural history of the disease is necessary to judge the chance of the disease progressing from the asymptomatic screened stage to symptomatic disease. Treatment should be

possible, available, and agreed widely. Screening for untreatable disease, especially in children too young to give consent, carries the risk of significant harm.

Is there a program for widespread and continuing implementation of screening? (1) Screening is complex and it creates expectations of availability. Inequality of access leads to nonparticipation of those most likely to benefit.

What is the cost utility of the whole program, including subsequent investigations and treatments, and how does this relate to resources available for other medical conditions? (1,9) Cost-utility analysis is required. Cost-benefit should exceed that of alternatives – public education via awareness campaigns, medical surveillance to facilitate early detection of symptomatic disease, or increased treatment resources.

Types of screening

Primary screening

A whole population is questioned, examined, or tested. This happens as a single event or can occur at regular intervals. Usually, it is offered at a particular age.

Example: neonatal red reflex examination.

Box 123.1

World Health Organization criteria for screening

1. The condition should be an important health problem.
2. There should be a treatment for the condition.
3. Facilities for diagnosis and treatment should be available.
4. There should be a latent stage of the disease.
5. There should be a test or examination for the condition.
6. The test should be acceptable to the population.
7. The natural history of the disease should be adequately understood.
8. There should be an agreed policy on whom to treat.
9. The total cost of finding a case should be economically balanced in relation to medical expenditure as a whole.
10. Case-finding should be a continuous process, not just a "once and for all" project.

Targeted screening

A test or examination is offered to a population at increased risk of a disease or complication.

Example: diabetic retinopathy screening.

Opportunistic screening

An examination or test is offered when a patient attends a medical appointment for a different reason.

Example: Visual acuity or retinal examination during assessment for congenital nasolacrimal duct obstruction.

Cascade screening

The identification of a person affected by a disease prompts testing of relatives at risk; it is the chief form of screening in clinical genetics. Cascade screening is of heightened value in consanguineous families. In other families, benefit rapidly decreases as testing moves away from the proband, when it detects only a small percentage of the total number of carriers within the wider population.

Example 1: Mutation screening of relatives of a proband with retinoblastoma.

Example 2: Clinical examination of relatives of a person with Marfan's syndrome for major and minor clinical features.

Screening vs. active surveillance

The prevalence of underlying disease in primary screening is low; for example, hundreds of neonatal red reflex examinations will be needed to detect an abnormality and WHO guidelines need to justify screening. When the chance of positive findings within a targeted population is high, then *active surveillance* is used instead of screening (Fig. 123.1).

Genetic screening

The special and changing nature of genetics screening is recognized in program assessment criteria.[4] As costs reduce there is increasing pressure from individuals, families, patient support groups and commercial interests for testing in specific gene disorders or for gene markers of complex traits.[5]

WHO criteria are equally valid for genetic screening, and they have been expanded to address specifics such as the interests of other family members who may inadvertently be found to carry a genetic abnormality during cascade screening, ensuring participants are fully aware of the limitations of the test, that the full effects of the genetic alteration must be understood and the psychological impact taken into account.

Analyzing a screening test[6]

Effective screening needs a test that accurately detects a risk factor or presymptomatic sign that in turn is predictive of later development of disease. The test should be reliable between observers and with time. The optimal threshold between positive and negative test results of a quantitative test (such as visual acuity) varies between conditions; e.g., high sensitivity is required in retinopathy of prematurity screening in view of the severe consequence of each false negative case. Help in making these decisions can be obtained by descriptive statistics, such as ROC plotting to clarify the optimal ratio of sensitivity to specificity.[7] Analysis by prior studies is essential prior to commencement of the program, with subsequent refinement by ongoing quality control.

Setting up a screening service[6]

A governmental public health initiative will secure funding and equality of access. Complex and thorough preparation is key to success.

1. Define objectives. There will be several aims:
   a. Improving disease outcomes.
   b. Limiting harmful consequences of screening.
   c. Maximizing uptake.
   d. Informing participants of a realistic expectation of screening.
   e. Limiting cost.
2. Calculate resources needed. A numerical breakdown is documented, encompassing all aspects of the screening process, including investigation of cases with equivocal results, and treatment of detected cases (Fig. 123.2).
3. Set operational policies. Protocols are created to allow integrated functioning of the program, allocation of responsibilities, and methods of documentation.
4. Create a computerized system for identification and invitation of patients/participants that integrates with the systems used for screening and referral management. The invitation explains what is entailed, and delivers a realistic

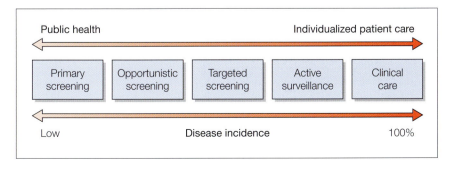

Fig. 123.1 There is a continuous spectrum between primary screening through to clinical care of an individual patient. Clarity is required to define which category of service is being created, as each have different aims.

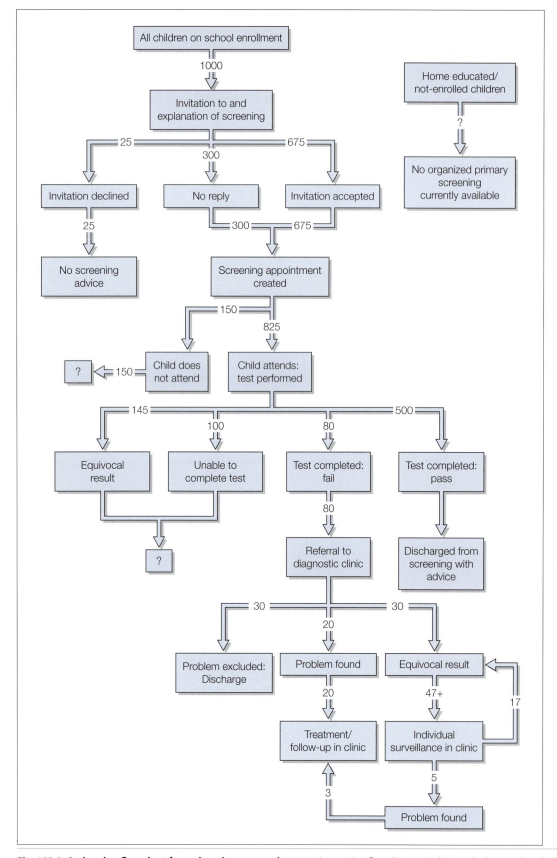

Fig. 123.2 A planning flow chart for an imaginary screening test. A screening flow diagram is the standard means by which resources and protocols are planned for a proposed or active program. All potential care pathways are included, along with estimated or actual numbers of patients following each route.

view of what can and cannot be achieved including the possibility of a false negative screening result.

5. Delivery of screening test. The method and location of the test is defined.

6. Delivery of intervention. Clinical resources need to be in place prior to program commencement to ensure prompt referral and treatment of detected abnormalities.

7. How to deal with uncertain screening outcomes. Patients with an unclear screening result need further management that can absorb considerable resources. Choice of screening test minimizes the number of uncertain outcomes.

8. Service development. The screening program requires management of staff, training, communication, coordination, and quality management, such as audit, research, and development.

Validation of screening

Studies of screening require large numbers of patients and a rigorous protocol. Demonstration of benefit from screening via randomized control trials is essential prior to the setting up of a screening program. Randomization to no screening is difficult once the service is in place.[8]

Benefit from an active screening program is measured by Time Trend Analysis, ideally with data collection extending prior to screening commencement. Alternatively, a comparison can be drawn from a contemporaneous population not subject to screening, for instance a comparison between countries.

Bias

Research studies of screening are prone to bias due to the selection of patients. The major forms of bias create a result that appears to support better outcomes.

Self-selection bias: individuals who accept an invitation to screening are different from those who decline: only random control will fully eliminate the problem.

Lead time bias: earlier detection of cases by screening creates a false impression of prolonged survival or slower progression of disease.

Length bias: screening is more likely to detect slowly progressive or static disease than rapidly progressive cases (Fig. 123.3).

Detection of inconsequential cases: not all cases with pathology will go on to develop clinical disease and remain undetected in the absence of screening. Such cases will create the impression of improved treatment success.

Failure to control these effects is suspected if there is a lack of improvement in population-based rates of treatment success detected by Time Trend Analysis, despite apparent improvement in patient-based outcomes from screening.

Variations in screening practice

Optimal screening practice varies in time and place. The birth age and weight of children developing retinopathy of prematurity varies between countries[9] and over time,[10] so optimal clinical criteria vary for the population targeted for screening (Fig. 123.4). Variations in screening policy also relate to differences in beliefs and values (Fig. 123.5).

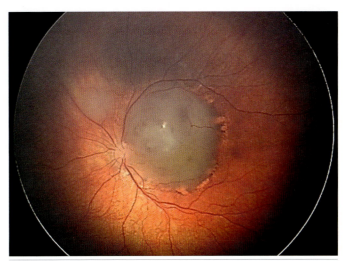

Fig. 123.3 A retinoblastoma detected during vision screening.
Screening will at times detect slowly progressing or inconsequential disease leading to biased outcomes. Surrounding chorioretinal atrophy and intratumoral cystic spaces suggest longstanding static size or early spontaneous regression. The lesion was observed without treatment, and slow regression has continued over the subsequent 24 months.

Screening in developing countries

Health systems in developing countries often lack resources and face overburdening demands, especially in rural areas. Families, particularly mothers, may have limited health and general education and be disempowered. Famine, drought, civil unrest, or war may disrupt services. However, appropriate screening is rewarding if focused on high prevalence diseases with low screening costs and inexpensive treatments (e.g., spectacles, vitamins, basic antibiotics) that can be delivered immediately.

When resources are severely limited, cost utility analysis will facilitate choice between screening and its alternatives, such as education, awareness campaigns, child surveillance services, mass vaccination (e.g. rubella) or disease prevention (e.g. oximetry for premature infants).

Managing expectations

Ideally, screening programs would utilize objective evidence of benefit and prioritization of resources to achieve the greatest benefit (Fig. 123.5A). Other factors influence screening policy (Fig. 123.5B). *Belief* in the benefit of presymptomatic detection of a disease has led to support from the media, public, support groups, and professions for some screening programs that are unsupported by evidence. Societal *values* influence the priority given to support from the media, public, support groups, and professions for some screening policy related to emotive diseases. Commercial interests influence screening at several levels.

Legal implications

Screening can detect only a certain percentage of cases. When a child develops a disease despite previous screening, there is discontent felt by the family and concern by the professionals,

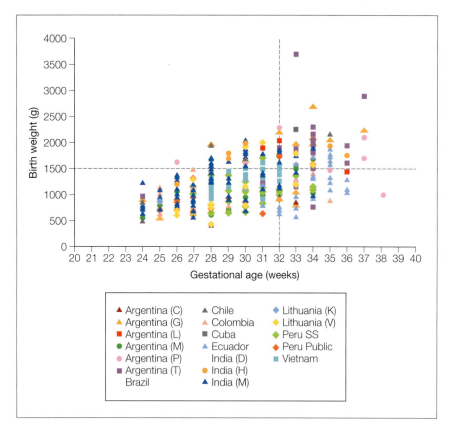

Fig. 123.4 Variation in birthweight and gestational age of children developing severe retinopathy of prematurity among low-, medium-, and high-income countries. The horizontal and vertical lines represent conventional ROP screening criteria. It can be seen that many patients from medium and low income countries fall outside the criteria. (Courtesy of Professor Clare Gilbert and publisher.)

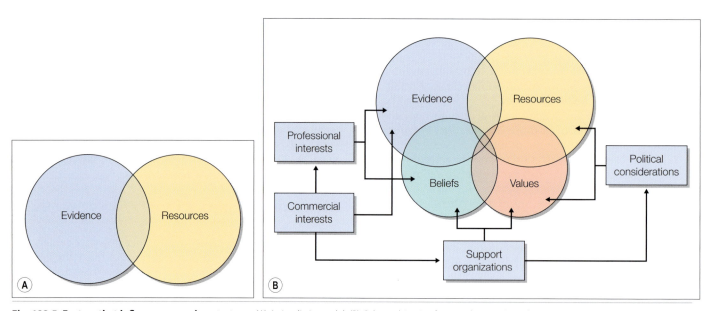

Fig. 123.5 Factors that influence screening strategy. (A) A simplistic model. (B) Other subjective factors play a major role. (From Raffle AE, Muir Gray JA. Screening Evidence and Practice. Oxford: Oxford University Press; 2007.)

even if there was no error. This highlights the difference between screening and individual patient care; all optimal screening tests have less than 100% sensitivity so as to avoid a problematically low specificity which would result in harm from unnecessary investigations and treatment.

Management of such problems commences prior to the screening itself, by ensuring individuals invited for screening are fully informed of the process, including the fact it will only detect a proportion of people who will go on to develop a problem, and why this is necessary. The person is then able to make an informed decision whether they wish to participate in the program. It is necessary to be able to demonstrate retrospectively that informed participation had occurred. The screening service must demonstrate quality controls, with results comparable to set aims and equivalent programs.

Childhood vision screening

The primary aim of most childhood vision screening in developed countries is the detection of amblyopia.

Practice varies widely, incorporating three periods:

Preschool vision screening. The advantage of early detection of amblyopia, or risk factors that may cause amblyopia are balanced against low participation, lack of an ideal test, uncertainties about amblyogenic risk factors, and their natural history.[11] Preschool vision screening is not universally accepted currently, but research continues into criteria, techniques, and instrumentation that may render it practicable.

School entry vision screening has the advantages of enhanced recruitment, and reasonable consensus on tests and treatment. Vision itself is the primary test outcome, rather than examination for risk factors.[11] There is evidence to suggest amblyopia detected at this age of around 5 years remains fully treatable. However, there is an assumption the amblyopia is anisometropic, and that strabismus, media opacities and other causes of amblyopia would have been identified earlier.

School vision screening is most likely to detect uncorrected refractive error and may be justified in developing countries, where it is a major cause of vision impairment. Further screening for amblyopia after the child has entered school is ineffective because new cases of amblyopia will not develop, and the condition becomes irremediable.

Conclusion

Screening is a valuable tool in detecting certain childhood eye diseases at a stage where treatment is possible. However, screening is complex with aspects that are counterintuitive. It is essential to perform high quality research prior to implementing a screening program. It is in the patient's and population's interest to discourage inappropriate screening. National bodies have been set up in several countries to optimize screening public health policy.

References

1. Rahi J, Cumberland PM, Peckham CS, et al. Improving detection of blindness in childhood: The British Childhood Vision Impairment Study. Pediatrics 2010; 126: e895.
2. Wald NJ. Guidance on terminology. J Med Screen 1994; 1: 76.
3. Wilson JMG, Jungner G. Principles and practice of screening for disease. Public Health Paper No. 34, Geneva: WHO; 1968.
4. http://www.screening.nhs.uk/criteria
5. Andermann A, Blancquaert I, Dery V. Genetic screening: a conceptual framework for programmes and policy-making. J Health Serv Res Policy 2010; 15: 90–7.
6. Raffle AE, Muir Gray JA. Screening Evidence and Practice. Oxford: Oxford University Press; 2007.
7. Pepe MS. The Statistical Evaluation of Medical Tests for Classification and Prediction. Oxford: Oxford University Press; 2004.
8. Bhopal R. Concepts of Epidemiology: Integrating the Ideas, Theories, Principles and Methods of Epidemiology. Oxford: Oxford University Press; 2008.
9. Gilbert C, Fielder A, Gordillo L, et al. Characteristics of infants with severe retinopathy of prematurity in countries with low, moderate and high levels of development. Pediatrics 2005; 115: e518–25.
10. Larsson E, Carle-Petreliu B, Cerneurd G, et al. Incidence of ROP in two consecutive Swedish population-based studies. Br J Ophthalmol 2002; 86: 1122–6.
11. Chou R, Dana T, Bougatsos C. Screening for visual impairment in children ages 1–5 years: update for the USPSTF. Pediatrics 2011; 127: e442–79.

My daughter can't be doing this to herself! Self-inflicted injuries

David Taylor

Dermatitis and keratoconjunctivitis

Self-inflicted injury to the surface of the eye and the skin around the eye is rare in childhood and, although not usually sight-threatening, it may be a warning of much more serious problems such as physical or sexual abuse.

In adults there are often a number of associated complex psychological and emotional problems; sometimes these may have more serious underlying psychopathology. When dermatitis or keratoconjunctivitis artefacta affects adults with a long history of psychiatric illness, recovery only occurs with a change in the patient's circumstances. Some adult patients are malingerers, classically trying to escape military service.[1] In factitious disease the patients deny the cause of their injury, are deceptive, and their motivation is to play the sick role; they are much more difficult to treat, requiring skilled psychiatric intervention.[2] When the patient and the parents admit to the self-destructive nature of their problem the outcome is much more benign.

The diagnosis is suggested by the combination of sharply delineated lesions in the inferior and nasal quadrants of the cornea bulbar and lid conjunctiva. Lesions on the skin around the eye are commonly associated with keratoconjunctivitis (Fig. 124.1). This dermatitis is variable in character and it may contain some of the irritant. Keratoconjunctivitis was described in an 11-year-old girl who induced a keratoconjunctivitis with chalk grains.[3] There is often an unconcerned attitude ("belle indifférence") and other psychological features.

In small children, self-inflicted injuries mostly occur in mentally retarded children, especially those with Lesch-Nyhan and Smith-Magennis syndromes.

Management

1. Consider the differential diagnosis and ensure that there is no possible, even rare, natural disease that could cause the symptoms and signs. It is not unusual for an initial diagnosis to be artefacta but end up with the correct one of a significant disease! The diagnosis is not made on the grounds that the ophthalmologist is unable to identify a pathological pattern to the disease but on the finding of POSITIVE evidence of a clearly artefactual cause.
2. Collaborate with a colleague who has appropriate expertise such as an external eye diseases consultant, a dermatologist, or eye trauma expert.
3. Collaborate with a suitably qualified psychiatrist.
4. Rule out congenital anesthesia, which mostly presents in young children.
5. Stop the application of the noxious substance or substances. This is easy if the child and the parents can

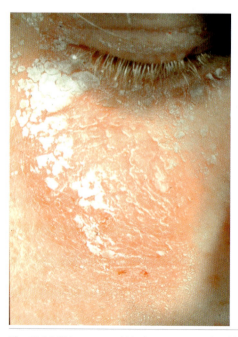

Fig. 124.1 This teenage girl had recurrent attacks of keratoconjunctivitis artefacta which was associated with desquamation of the skin around the affected eye. The agent may have been alum.

be helped to understand the cause and seriousness of the condition but may need admission to an observation unit.

5. Treat the injury in a manner appropriate for the cause. If it is a non-specific irritant or inflammatory agent, then topical steroids are appropriate.

6. The treating ophthalmologist needs to be open and honest with the parents and child, kind to both, and aware that the disease is very serious to the patient and family.

Trichotillomania

Trichotillomania in which the affected person pulls out hair, sometimes the eyelashes and eyebrows, has a prevalence of between 1% and 5%.

Boys, although affected about a half as frequently as girls, have an earlier age at onset (8 years)[4] and they are less likely to pull their eyebrows and eyelashes. Trichotillomanics frequently conceal their habit; the hair pulling can become ritualized, with close inspection of the pulled hair, and the hair may be swallowed.

The lids and brows have healthy skin with multiple broken hair shafts (Fig. 124.2). It is not usually a serious condition and the hair loss is reversible when the pulling stops, but it may become chronic. Some patients are depressed. Stress is implicated as a precipitating factor in many cases.

Management

1. Consider the differential diagnosis. Loss of eyelashes occurs with skin diseases, such as alopecia, ichthyosis, and ectodermal dysplasia, following radiation or chemotherapy, after lid infections, or endocrine disease (see Chapter 19).

2. Most cases respond to reassurance and explanations after a detailed history by the ophthalmologist which must include those details many ophthalmologists are not comfortable with asking. A psychosocial and sexual history is often the key to the underlying cause and it is often best if a pediatrician is invited to collaborate.

3. Behavior therapy, drugs, and other treatment may sometimes help as the condition has some similarities to an obsessive-compulsive disorder.[5]

Ocular self-mutilation: direct eye trauma

Ocular self-mutilation typically occurs in young men with a history of severe psychiatric illness, especially schizophrenia, serious criminality, or drug abuse.[2]

In childhood, self-inflicted injuries occur in the severely mentally retarded. The injury may be by laceration,[6] but is more frequently a result of severe direct blows[7] or headbanging.[8] Self-inflicted injuries occur more frequently in certain syndromes, mostly associated with severe mental retardation. At least 15 syndromes are associated with self-mutilation, of which the Lesch-Nyhan and Smith-Magenis syndromes are the most important to ophthalmologists.

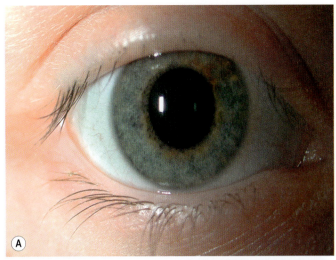
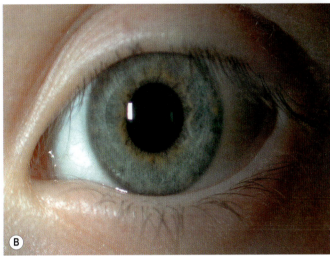

Fig. 124.2 Trichotillomania. The eyelids of both eyes of this 12-year-old girl have broken and missing lashes.

Autoenucleation

This occurs mostly in hallucinating young adult schizophrenics of either sex and is rare in children.[1,9]

References

1. Pokroy R, Marcovich A. Self-inflicted (factitious) conjunctivitis. Ophthalmology 2003; 110: 790–5.
2. Patton N. Self-inflicted eye injuries: a review. Eye 2004; 18: 867–72.
3. Cruciani F, Santino G, Trudu R, et al. Ocular Munchausen syndrome characterised by self-introduction of chalk concretions into the conjunctival fornix. Eye 1999; 13: 598–9.
4. Graber J, Arndt WB. Trichotillomania. Compr Psychiatry 1993; 34: 340–6.
5. Franklin ME, Foa EB. Treatment of obsessive compulsive disorder. Annu Rev Clin Psychol 2011; 7: 229–43.
6. Noel LP, Clarke WN. Self-inflicted ocular injuries in children. Am J Ophthalmol 1982; 94: 630–3.
7. Ashkenazi I, Shahar E, Brand N, et al. Self-inflicted ocular mutilation in the pediatric age group. Acta Paediatr 1992; 81: 649–51.
8. Spalter HF, Bemporad JR, Sours JA. Cataracts following chronic headbanging. Arch Ophthalmol 1970; 83: 182–186.
9. Taylor DSI. Unnatural injuries. Eye 2000; 14: 123–50.

Index

NB: Page numbers in bold indicate major discussions. Page numbers in *italics* indicate boxes, figures and tables.